EDITED BY **ROBERT E. RAKEL, M.D.**

*Professor and Head, Department of Family
Practice, University of Iowa College of
Medicine, Iowa City, Iowa*

HOWARD F. CONN, M.D.

Staff, Uniontown Hospital, Uniontown, Pennsylvania

SPECIAL CONSULTING EDITOR **THOMAS W. JOHNSON, M.D.**

*Medical Director, Blue Cross and Blue Shield of
Kansas City, Missouri*

FAMILY PRACTICE

Second Edition

1978

W. B. SAUNDERS COMPANY
Philadelphia   London   Toronto

W. B. Saunders Company: West Washington Square
                          Philadelphia, PA   19105

                          1 St. Anne's Road
                          Eastbourne, East Sussex BN21 3UN, England

                          1 Goldthorne Avenue
                          Toronto, Ontario M8Z 5T9, Canada

Listed here is the latest translated edition of this book together
with the language of the translation and the publisher.

Spanish (*1st Edition*) — NEISA, Mexico 4 D.F., Mexico

Family Practice   ISBN   0-7216-7447-X

Last digit is the print number: 9   8   7   6   5   4   3   2   1

To the family physician whose dedication to providing quality personalized health care has helped to preserve the dignity of the individual within our modern yet complex health care system.

CONTRIBUTORS

GENE GORDON ABEL, M.D.

Professor of Psychiatry, University of Tennessee Center for the Health Sciences, Staff Psychiatrist, Memphis Mental Health Institute, Memphis, Tennessee.

JOHN E. ALLEN, M.D.

Clinical Professor of Family Medicine, College of Medicine and Dentistry of New Jersey, Rutgers Medical School, Piscataway, New Jersey; Director, Department of Family Medicine, Director, Residency, Family Practice, Monmouth Medical Center, Long Branch, New Jersey; Formerly Professor of Pediatrics, State University of New York, Down-State Medical Center, Brooklyn, New York.

MARTIN H. ANDREWS, M.D.

Clinical Assistant Professor, Department of Family Practice, Oklahoma Health Sciences Center, Oklahoma City, Oklahoma.

JOHN D. BARKER, JR., M.D.

Clinical Assistant Professor of Medicine, University of South Dakota School of Medicine, Gastroenterologist, Central Plains Clinic, Active Staff and Director of Gastroenterology and Laboratories, McKennan Hospital and Sioux Valley Hospital, Sioux Falls, South Dakota.

B. LEWIS BARNETT, Jr., M.D.

Walter M. Seward Professor, and Chairman, Department of Family Practice, University of Virginia Medical School, Charlottesville, Virginia.

FREDERIC BASS, M.D., D.Sc.

Consultant in Preventive Medicine, Vancouver Health Department, Clinical Assistant Professor, University of British Columbia, Vancouver, British Columbia, Canada.

JUDITH V. BECKER, Ph.D.

Assistant Professor of Psychiatry (Psychology), University of Tennessee Center for the Health Sciences, Memphis, Tennessee.

ALEXANDER BERGER, M.D.

Professor, Department of Family Medicine, University of Connecticut School of Medicine, Chairman, Department of Family Medicine, University of Connecticut Health Center, Farmington, Connecticut.

HERBERT R. BRETTELL, M.D.

Professor of Family Medicine, University of Colorado Medical Center, Active Staff, Colorado General Hospital, Rose Medical Center, Denver, Colorado.

PAUL CHARLES BRUCKER, B.S., M.D.

Professor and Chairman, Department of Family Medicine, Jefferson Medical College, Thomas Jefferson University, Chairman, Department of Family Medicine, Thomas Jefferson University Hospital, Philadelphia, Pennsylvania.

THORNTON BRYAN, M.D.

Chairman and Professor of Family Medicine, University of Tennessee Center for the Health Sciences, Memphis, Tennessee.

REMI JERE CADORET, A.B., M.D.

Professor of Psychiatry, University of Iowa College of Medicine, Iowa City, Iowa.

LYNN P. CARMICHAEL, M.D.

Professor of Family Medicine, University of Miami School of Medicine, Chairman, Department of Family Medicine, University of Miami School of Medicine, Miami, Florida.

E. BRUCE CHALLIS, M.D.

Associate Staff, Family Physician, Department of Family and Community Medicine, Toronto General Hospital, University of Toronto, Toronto, Canada.

FREDERICK KEITH CHAPLER, M.D.

Professor, Department of Obstetrics and Gynecology, Director, Division of Reproductive Endocrinology, University of Iowa College of Medicine, Iowa City, Iowa.

EDWARD W. CIRIACY, M.D.

Professor and Head, Department of Family Practice and Community Health, University of Minnesota, Minneapolis, Minnesota.

WILLIAM M. CLEMENTS, B.D., Ph.D.

Assistant Professor of Family Practice, University of Iowa College of Medicine, Iowa City, Iowa, Fellow, American Association of Pastoral Counselors, Clinical Member, American Association of Marriage and Family Counselors.

ROLLO JESSE COBLE, A.B., M.D.

Assistant Professor, University of Iowa College of Medicine, Staff, University of Iowa Hospitals and Clinics, Iowa City, Iowa.

JACK M. COLWILL, M.D.

Professor and Chairman, Department of Family and Community Medicine, University of Missouri–Columbia School of Medicine, Columbia, Missouri.

RICHARD ALLEN CURRIE, M.D.

Associate Professor of Surgery, The Johns Hopkins University School of Medicine, Chief of Surgery, Howard County General Hospital, Surgeon, The Johns Hopkins Hospital, Visiting Surgeon, Baltimore City Hospitals, Baltimore, Maryland.

GORDON H. DECKERT, M.D.

Professor and Head, Department of Psychiatry and Behavioral Sciences, University of Oklahoma Health Sciences Center, Oklahoma City, Oklahoma.

CARMEN A. DELCIOPPO, M.D.

Clinical Assistant Professor, State University of New York, Upstate Medical Center, Full Attending Physician, St.

Joseph's Hospital, Syracuse, New York; Consulting Physician, St. Elizabeth's Hospital, Utica, New York.

JOHN E. DONNELLY, M.D.

Associate Professor, Department of Medicine, University of Connecticut School of Medicine, Director, Family Medicine Residency, University of Connecticut Health Center, Farmington, Connecticut.

ARMANDO R. FAVAZZA, M.D., M.P.H.

Associate Professor of Psychiatry, University of Missouri–Columbia School of Medicine, Chief, Community Psychiatry Service, University of Missouri–Columbia Hospital, Columbia, Missouri.

L. J. FILER, Jr., M.D., Ph.D.

Professor of Pediatrics, University of Iowa College of Medicine, Staff, University Hospitals and Clinics, Iowa City, Iowa.

CARL FLAXER, M.D.

Clinical Instructor of Medicine, University of Colorado Medical Center, Director of Family Practice Residency Program, Mercy Medical Center, Denver, Colorado.

PAUL S. FRAME, M.D.

Clinical Instructor of Family Medicine, University of Rochester School of Medicine, Rochester, New York; Attending Staff, Noyes Memorial Hospital, Dansville, New York.

F. CLARKE FRASER, M.D., C.M., Ph.D., D.Sc. (Acadia), F.R.S.C.

Professor of Medical Genetics, Departments of Paediatrics and Biology, McGill University, Director, Department of Medical Genetics, The Montreal Children's Hospital, Montreal, P.Q., Canada.

SHERVERT H. FRAZIER, M.D.

Professor of Psychiatry, Harvard Medical School, Boston, Massachusetts; Psychiatrist in Chief, McLean Hospital, Belmont, Massachusetts.

EUGENE F. GAURON, Ph.D.

Professor of Psychiatry, University of Iowa College of Medicine, Iowa City, Iowa.

GERALD ROUDOLPHE GEHRINGER, M.D.

Associate Professor of Family Medicine, Louisiana State University School of Medicine in New Orleans, Associate Staff Member, Hotel Dieu Hospital, New Orleans, Louisiana.

ROY J. GERARD, M.D.

Professor and Chairman, Department of Family Practice, College of Human Medicine, Michigan State University, East Lansing, Michigan.

DEREK G. GILL, Ph.D.

Chief, Section of Behavioral Sciences, Associate Professor, Department of Family and Community Medicine and Sociology, University of Missouri–Columbia School of Medicine, Columbia, Missouri.

JOHN GILROY, M.D., F.R.C.P. (C.), F.A.C.P.

Professor and Chairman, Department of Neurology, Wayne State University, Chief of Neurology, Harper–Grace Hospitals and Detroit General Hospital, Detroit, Michigan.

THOMAS JOSEPH GODAR, M.D.

Associate Professor of Medicine, University of Connecticut School of Medicine, Farmington, Connecticut; Associate Clinical Professor of Medicine, Yale University School of Medicine, New Haven, Connecticut; Director, Pulmonary Disease Section, St. Francis Hospital and Medical Center, Hartford, Connecticut.

HARRIS S. GOLDSTEIN, M.D., D.Med.Sc.

Associate Professor of Psychiatry, College of Medicine and Dentistry of New Jersey–Rutgers Medical School, Piscataway, New Jersey.

ROBERT P. GRANTHAM, M.D.

Clinical Instructor, University of British Columbia School of Medicine, Vancouver, Canada; College of Family Practitioners of Canada.

VYMUTT J. GURURAJ, M.D.

Associate Professor of Pediatrics, College of Medicine and Dentistry of New Jersey–Rutgers Medical School, Piscataway, New Jersey; Director, Community Emergency Services, Middlesex General Hospital, New Brunswick, New Jersey.

JACK H. HALL, M.D.

Professor of Medicine and Assistant Dean, Indiana University School of Medicine, Vice-President of Medical Education, Methodist Hospital, Indianapolis, Indiana.

DOUGLAS M. HAYNES, M.D., F.A.C.S., F.A.C.O.G.

Professor of Obstetrics and Gynecology, University of Louisville School of Medicine, Active Staff, Louisville General Hospital, Norton–Children's Hospital, Louisville, Kentucky.

MATTHEW L. HENK, M.S.W.

Medical Social Work Consultant, United States Public Health Service, Regional Office, Kansas City, Missouri.

BRIAN K. E. HENNEN, M.D., M.A., C.C.F.P.

Professor and Director, Division of Family Medicine, Dalhousie University, Consultant Staff, Family Practice, Halifax Infirmary, Associate Staff, Izaak Walton Killam Hospital for Children, Halifax, Nova Scotia, Canada.

JOSEPH W. HESS, M.D.

Professor and Chairman, Department of Family Medicine, Wayne State University, Chief of Family Medicine, Detroit General Hospital, Vice-Chief of Family Practice, Harper–Grace Hospitals, Detroit, Michigan.

DONALD HAMILTON IRVINE, M.D., F.R.C.G.P.

Regional Adviser in General Practice, University of Newcastle upon Tyne, Principal in General Practice, Northumberland, England.

L. PAUL JOHNSON, M.D.

Associate Dean for Ambulatory Care, Professor of Family Medicine, Rockford School of Medicine, University of Illinois College of Medicine, Staff, Swedish-American Hospital, Rockford Memorial Hospital, St. Anthony Hospital, Rockford, Illinois.

SAID A. KARMI, M.D.

Assistant Professor of Urology, University of Maryland, Staff, University of Maryland Hospital, Baltimore, Maryland.

KENNETH F. KESSEL, M.D.

Director, Family Practice Training Program, MacNeal Memorial Hospital, Berwyn, Illinois; Professor, Department of Family Practice, Abraham Lincoln School of Medicine, University of Illinois, Chicago, Illinois; Attending Physician, MacNeal Memorial Hospital, Berwyn, Illinois.

LUCY JANE KING, M.D.

Professor of Psychiatry, Medical College of Virginia, Virginia Commonwealth University, Attending Psychiatrist, Medical College of Virginia Hospitals, Richmond, Virginia.

EDWARD J. KOWALEWSKI, M.D.

Professor and Head, Family Medicine Department, University of Maryland School of Medicine, Head, Family Medicine Department, University of Maryland Hospital, Baltimore, Maryland.

FRANCIS L. LAND, A.B., M.D.

Professor and Director, Division of Family Practice, Georgetown University School of Medicine, Staff, Georgetown University Hospital, Providence Hospital, Washington, D.C.

DONALD G. LANGSLEY, M.D.

Professor and Chairman, Department of Psychiatry, University of Cincinnati College of Medicine, Psychiatrist-in-Chief, Cincinnati General Hospital and Children's Hospital Medical Center, Cincinnati, Ohio.

LARRY LAWHORNE, M.D.

Clinical Assistant Professor of Family Practice and Preventive Medicine, University of Iowa College of Medicine, Active Staff, Mercy Hospital, Clinical Staff, University of Iowa Hospitals and Clinics, Iowa City, Iowa.

IRVING AARON LEVIN, M.D., F.A.C.S.

Clinical Assistant Professor of Surgery, Louisiana State University School of Medicine in New Orleans, Senior Attending Colon and Rectal Surgeon, Touro Infirmary, St. Charles General Hospital, and Charity Hospital, New Orleans, Louisiana.

LOUIS D. LOWRY, M.D.

Assistant Professor, Department of Otorhinolaryngology and Human Communication, University of Pennsylvania, Attending, Children's Hospital of Philadelphia, Graduate Hospital, Pennsylvania Hospital, Senior Attending, Veterans' Hospital of Philadelphia, Philadelphia, Pennsylvania.

IAN R. McWHINNEY, M.D., M.R.C.P., C.C.F.P., F.R.C.G.P.

Professor of Family Medicine, University of Western Ontario, London, Ontario, Canada.

ROBERT J. MASSAD, M.D.

Associate Professor, Department of Family Practice, University of Iowa College of Medicine, Iowa City, Iowa.

L. E. (BRUNO) MASTERS, M.D.

Associate Professor, Department of Family Practice, University of Iowa College of Medicine, Director, Family Practice Residency Program, Iowa Lutheran Hospital, Des Moines, Iowa.

WILLIAM J. MITCHELL, M.D., F.A.C.S., A.A.O.S.

Chief, Uniontown Hospital, Uniontown, Pennsylvania. Orthopedic Consultant, United States Steel Company. Orthopedic Consultant, Fayette County Easter Seal Society for Crippled Children and Adults. Formerly, Consultant in Orthopedics to the Surgeon General, United States Air Forces–Europe.

HAROLD MOESSNER, M.D.

Assistant Professor, Family Practice, University of Iowa College of Medicine, Iowa City, Iowa.

KATHLEEN C. MORTON, M.B;B.S., Sc.M., F.A.A.P.

Dean, Primary Care Education, The Johns Hopkins University School of Medicine, Active Staff, Pediatrics, The Johns Hopkins Hospital, Baltimore, Maryland.

HAROLD A. MULFORD, Ph.D.

Professor of Psychiatry (Sociologist), University of Iowa College of Medicine, Iowa City, Iowa.

KATHARINE A. MUNNING M.S.

Associate in Family Practice, University of Iowa College of Medicine, Iowa City, Iowa.

THOMAS A. NICHOLAS, M.D.

Professor and Chairman, Department of Family Practice, Texas Tech University School of Medicine, Chairman, Department of Family Practice, University Hospital, Active Staff, St. Mary's of the Plains Hospital, Lubbock County District Hospital, Lubbock, Texas.

NICHOLAS J. PISACANO, M.D.

Chairman, Department of Research and Development, College of Allied Health, University of Kentucky, Professor, Biological Sciences, University of Kentucky, Executive Director and Secretary, American Board of Family Practice, Lexington, Kentucky.

JOHN T. QUEENAN, M.D.

Professor, University of Louisville, Chief of Department of Obstetrics and Gynecology, Louisville General Hospital, Chief of Department of Obstetrics and Gynecology, Norton–Children's Hospital, Louisville, Kentucky.

ROBERT E. RAKEL, M.D.

Professor and Head, Department of Family Practice, University of Iowa College of Medicine, Iowa City, Iowa.

DONALD C. RANSOM, Ph.D.

Associate Professor (in Residence) of Ambulatory and Community Medicine, University of California School of Medicine, San Francisco, California; Behavioral Science Coordinator, Family Practice Residency Program, Sonoma Community Hospital, Santa Rosa, California.

WILLIAM REICHEL, M.D.

Chairman, Department of Family Practice, Franklin Square Hospital, Baltimore, Maryland.

SYLVIA O. RICHARDSON, M.A., M.D.

Associate Clinical Professor, Pediatrics, University of Cincinnati College of Medicine, Associate Director, University Affiliated Program for Severe Learning Disorders, Cincinnati Center for Developmental Disorders, Cincinnati, Ohio.

LEWIS C. ROBBINS, M.D., M.P.H.

Consultant, Health Hazard Appraisal, Methodist Hospital of Indiana, Executive Vice President, Health Hazard Appraisal, Inc., Indianapolis, Indiana; Visiting Professor, Jefferson Medical College, Philadelphia, Pennsylvania.

PHILIP L. ROSEBERRY, M.D.

Director and Coordinator, Family Practice Residency Program, York Hospital, York, Pennsylvania.

MELVILLE G. ROSEN, M.D.

Professor and Chairman, Department of Family Medicine, State University of New York at Stony Brook, Stony Brook, New York; Staff, Southside Hospital, Bay Shore, New York; University Hospital, Stony Brook, New York; Good Samaritan Hospital, West Islip, New York; Nassau County Medical Center, East Meadow, New York.

JERRY A. ROYER, M.D.

Associate Professor of Family Medicine, University of Missouri–Columbia School of Medicine, Staff, University of Missouri Medical Center, Columbia, Missouri.

RAYMOND M. RUSSO, M.D.

Associate Professor of Pediatrics, College of Medicine and Dentistry of New Jersey–Rutgers Medical School, Newark, New Jersey; Director, Department of Ambulatory Services, Middlesex General Hospital, New Brunswick, New Jersey.

MARVIN J. SCHWARZ, M.D.

Clinical Director, Riveredge Hospital, Forest Park, Illinois; Clinical Assistant Professor of Psychiatry, Rush Medical College, University of Illinois, Visiting Professor, George Williams College School of Social Work, Chicago, Illinois.

ROBERT H. SELLER, M.D., F.A.C.P., F.A.C.C.

Professor of Medicine and Professor and Chairman, Department of Family Medicine, State University of New York at Buffalo, School of Medicine, Chairman, Department of Family Practice, Deaconess Hospital of Buffalo, Buffalo, New York.

JOYCE G. SMALL, M.D.

Professor of Psychiatry, University of Indiana School of Medicine, Director of Research, Larue D. Carter Memorial Hospital, Indianapolis, Indiana.

GABRIEL SMILKSTEIN, M.D.

Associate Professor, Family Medicine, University of Washington School of Medicine, Attending Physician, University Hospital, Seattle, Washington.

ROBERT SMITH, M.D.

Professor and Director, Department of Family Medicine, University of Cincinnati College of Medicine, Staff, Cincinnati General Hospital, Children's Hospital Medical Center, Veterans Administration Hospital, Holmes Hospital, Cincinnati, Ohio.

FRANK C. SNOPE, M.D.

Associate Professor of Family Medicine, College of Medicine and Dentistry of New Jersey, Rutgers Medical School, Piscataway, New Jersey; Attending Physician, Hunterdon Medical Center, Flemington, New Jersey.

YALE SOLOMON, M.D., F.A.C.S.

Assistant Clinical Professor, Ophthalmology, State University of New York at Stony Brook, School of Medicine, Stony Brook, New York; Attending Ophthalmologist, Southside Hospital, Bay Shore, New York; Attending Ophthalmologist, Good Samaritan Hospital, West Islip, New York; Consultant Ophthalmologist, Smithtown General Hospital, Smithtown, New York; Consultant Ophthalmologist, Brookhaven Memorial Hospital, Patchogue, New York.

G. GAYLE STEPHENS, M.D.

Professor, Family Practice, University of Alabama School of Medicine, Staff, University Hospital, Birmingham, Alabama.

G. LYNN STEPHENS, Ph.D.

Assistant Professor, Department of Philosophy, Notre Dame University, South Bend, Indiana.

THOMAS L. STERN, M.D.

Director, Division of Education, American Academy of Family Physicians, Kansas City, Missouri.

WILLIAM L. STEWART, M.D.

Professor and Chairman, Department of Family Practice, St. John's and Memorial Medical Center, Springfield, Illinois.

HENRY H. STONNINGTON, M.B., B.S., F.R.C.P. (Edin.)

Assistant Professor of Physical Medicine and Rehabilitation, Mayo Medical School, Consultant, Department of Physical Medicine and Rehabilitation, Mayo Clinic and Mayo Foundation, Rochester, Minnesota.

LIBBY A. TANNER, M.S.W., A.C.S.W.

Associate Professor of Family Medicine, University of Miami School of Medicine, Miami, Florida.

GEORGE H. THOMSON, M.D., M.P.H.

Clinical Associate Professor, Department of Family Medicine and Practice, University of Wisconsin, Director, Family Practice Program, St. Mary's Hospital, Milwaukee, Wisconsin.

DONALD F. TREAT, M.D.

Associate Professor of Family Medicine, University of Rochester School of Medicine and Dentistry, Associate Chief, Family Medicine, Highland Hospital, Rochester, New York.

WILLIAM P. VONDERHAAR, M.D.

Professor and Acting Director, Family Practice, University of Louisville School of Medicine, Louisville, Kentucky.

JULIAN A. WALLER, M.D., M.P.H.

Professor and Chairman, Department of Epidemiology and Environmental Health, University of Vermont College of Medicine, Consultant on Injury Control and Emergency Medical Service, Vermont Health Department, Burlington, Vermont.

ALAN A. WANDERER, M.D., F.A.A.A., F.A.A.P.

Clinical Assistant Professor of Pediatrics, University of Colorado Medical Center, Chief of Allergy Section, Mercy Medical Center, Volunteer Staff, National Asthma Center, Volunteer Staff, National Jewish Hospital, Denver, Colorado.

AVERY D. WEISMAN, M.D.

Professor of Psychiatry, Harvard Medical School, Psychiatrist, Massachusetts General Hospital, Principal Investigator, Project Omega, Department of Psychiatry, Massachusetts General Hospital, Boston, Massachusetts.

WILLIAM A. WELTON, M.D.

Professor and Chairman, Department of Dermatology, West Virginia University Medical Center, Morgantown, West Virginia.

JIM L. WILSON, A.B., M.D.

Assistant Professor of Family Practice, University of Iowa College of Medicine, Active Medical Staff, Mercy Hospital, Iowa City, Iowa.

L. THOMAS WOLFF, M.D.

Professor and Chairman, Department of Family Practice, Upstate Medical Center of the State University of New York, Director of Medical Education and Associate Attending Physician, St. Joseph's Hospital Health Center, Syracuse, New York.

CYRIL M. WORBY, M.D.

Professor, Departments of Psychiatry and Family Practice, College of Human Medicine, Michigan State University, Co-Director, Family Life Cycle Studies Program and Clinic, Michigan State University, East Lansing, Michigan.

JOHN D. YOUNG, Jr., M.D.

Professor of Urology, University of Maryland, Head, Division of Urology, University of Maryland Hospital, Baltimore, Maryland.

FOREWORD

In the past decade the concept of the Primary Physician has won substantial acceptance and support among both physicians and laymen. There is, however, some confusion, as is evidenced by the frequent reference to primary *care* physicians. It is important to understand clearly the difference between the two ideas. Family Practice is based upon the concept of the Primary Physician, and there should be no confusion with the idea of a primary care physician.

The Citizens Commission on Graduate Medical Education[1] recommended the education of Primary Physicians as an antidote to the fractionalization of patient care due to the increasing specialization of physicians. The Commission believed that Primary Physicians of several kinds could bring continuity and comprehensiveness to the care of their patients. The word "primary" was used to denote the continuing responsibility of the physician for the care of his patient in sickness and in health, in need of simple or complicated therapy, requiring basic facilities or those of the highest and most complicated technology.

The concept of the "primary *care* physician" is an attempt to define the physician in terms of the severity of the illness of his patient at the moment. The effect of the idea would be to further fractionalize patient care. Physicians would be categorized by the familiar specialties defined by diseases, organ systems, or modalities of treatment and also by the severity of the illness, injury, or disability suffered by the patient at a particular instant of time. Were such a system to develop, there would be less continuity of patient care, and no one would be responsible for any comprehensive and continuing care whatsoever.

There are several dimensions in the concept of continuity. There is the dimension of continuity over time. It involves a continuing relationship of a physician to a patient over a period of years or decades. There is the dimension of continuity through the vicissitudes of life, that is, care in illness and care in health. There is the dimension of continuity in responsibility for the patient through the entire course of an illness and its management; that responsibility lies with the Primary Physician whether he can provide all of the needed services or whether he must have the assistance of colleagues of specialized competence and the resources of the most sophisticated institutions.

The concept of comprehensiveness emphasizes patient *care* in contrast to *cure*. Care includes disease prevention, health maintenance, and health education for those who are in health, as well as therapy to cure those in disease. It deals with the care of the chronically ill, the permanently disabled, and the handicapped.

The development of the field of Family Practice has been based upon the concept of the Primary Physician. It is directed to the whole patient, providing continuing and comprehensive care. The family unit provides one rational base for planning and delivering continuing and comprehensive medical service. It has continuity over periods of health and episodes of illness. It has the continuity of human development. Children are born, reared, and mature. Adults age and their circumstances change.

---

[1]The Graduate Education of Physicians, Report of the Citizens Commission on Graduate Medical Education, Commissioned by the American Medical Association, 1966.

The family presents the opportunity for comprehensiveness of care. The well-being of the group and of each of its members is determined by the same social, cultural, educational, psychological, and emotional circumstances. Diet, life style, risk exposure, and even hereditary factors are common. The well-being of each individual is affected by the health or the illness of his parents and siblings. The care of the family involves attention to all of the factors that affect health — physiological, pathological, neurological, psychological, emotional, and social. Family Practice can and should be that of the Primary Physician.

This textbook begins with the consideration of the social, cultural, psychological, and emotional factors that can and do affect the health of the family and each of its members. It considers the factors of human development and the science of heredity. It covers epidemiology of disease. Finally, it treats the etiology, physiology, and pathology of the commonly encountered diseases and disease processes and their therapy. It should serve as a most useful text for medical students interested in careers as Primary Physicians, for Family Practice residents, and as a reference source for the Family Physician.

JOHN S. MILLIS, Ph.D.

PREFACE

Our purpose in presenting this Second Edition is the same as it was with the first: to provide a text that reflects the comprehensiveness of family practice. It is intended to serve as a reference for the practicing family physician and the family practice resident in training, as well as a text for the student interested in family medicine.

This edition is not merely an updated version of the first, but is a totally new publication. For this text, we have turned to new authors for almost all chapters in order to gain a broader viewpoint of the topic and to approach the subject from a new perspective. Thus, information presented in many chapters, e.g., Family Dynamics and Sexual Counseling, expands upon and complements that provided in the First Edition, allowing this edition to serve as a companion to the first, rather than as a replacement.

The co-author system (pairing an authority in the field with an experienced family physician) that was tested in the First Edition proved to be so successful in maintaining the practical relevance necessary in a clinical reference that it has been used throughout this edition. We have eliminated some chapters that were felt to have limited clinical relevance and thereby created space for new material. In the Clinical Specialties Section, selected areas of Internal Medicine that we consider to be of value to the practicing family physician have been added. The new chapters cover Pulmonary Medicine, Gastroenterology, Cardiology, and Nutrition. A new section on the Problem-Oriented Medical Record has been added as well. The section on Behavioral Problems in Family Practice has been reorganized to permit more specific attention to the dying patient, personality disorders, organic brain syndrome, sexual deviation, psychotherapy, and behavioral modification. Additions to the section on Community Medicine include the Early Diagnosis of Undifferentiated Problems, Use of Consultants, and Geriatrics.

This edition contains over 50 chapters prepared by approximately 100 contributors. We are indebted to these distinguished authors whose talents and co-operation have made this edition possible.

ROBERT E. RAKEL, M.D.
HOWARD F. CONN, M.D.

CONTENTS

Part I THE FAMILY UNIT 1

Chapter 1
THE FAMILY PHYSICIAN 3
Robert E. Rakel

Chapter 2
FAMILY STRUCTURE AND FUNCTION 20
Donald C. Ransom, and Robert J. Massad

Chapter 3
FAMILY DYNAMICS 32
Cyril Worby, and Roy Gerard

Chapter 4
SOCIOCULTURAL INFLUENCES 47
Derek G. Gill, and Jack M. Colwill

Part II PROBLEM-ORIENTED MEDICAL RECORDS 65

Chapter 5
PROBLEM-ORIENTED MEDICAL RECORDS 67
Robert E. Rakel

Part III COMMUNITY MEDICINE 101

Chapter 6
PREVENTIVE MEDICINE 103
Frederic Bass, and Peter Grantham

Chapter 7
PERIODIC HEALTH SCREENING............................. 123
Paul S. Frame, and Brian K. E. Hennen

Chapter 8

EARLY DIAGNOSIS OF UNDIFFERENTIATED
PROBLEMS 138

Ian R. McWhinney

Chapter 9

EPIDEMIOLOGY 147

Julian A. Waller, and George H. Thomson

Chapter 10

PROSPECTIVE MEDICINE 160

Lewis C. Robbins, and Jack H. Hall

Chapter 11

HEALTH CARE DELIVERY 175

Francis L. Land, and Donald Irvine

Chapter 12

UTILIZATION OF COMMUNITY RESOURCES 183

Donald F. Treat, and Matthew L. Henk

Chapter 13

ALLIED HEALTH PROFESSIONALS 188

Edward J. Kowalewski, and Kathleen C. Morton

Chapter 14

USE OF CONSULTANTS 199

Thomas Stern, and Thomas A. Nicholas

Chapter 15

REHABILITATION 210

Henry H. Stonnington, and Edward W. Ciriacy

Chapter 16

CARE OF THE GERIATRIC PATIENT 222

William Reichel, and B. Lewis Barnett, Jr.

Part IV   BEHAVIORAL PROBLEMS 239

Chapter 17

MEDICAL ETHICS 241

G. Gayle Stephens, and G. Lynn Stephens

Chapter 18
THE DYING PATIENT 249
Avery D. Weisman, and Herbert R. Brettell

Chapter 19
INTERVIEWING TECHNIQUES..................................... 258
Gordon H. Deckert, and Martin H. Andrews

Chapter 20
LEARNING DISABILITIES 267
Sylvia O. Richardson, and Robert Smith

Chapter 21
PERSONALITY DISORDERS 276
J. G. Small, and L. P. Johnson

Chapter 22
ANXIETY: ACUTE AND CHRONIC 288
Armando R. Favazza, and Jerry A. Royer

Chapter 23
HYSTERIA AND PHOBIAS.. 297
Shervert H. Frazier, and Nicholas J. Pisacano

Chapter 24
DEPRESSION... 303
Remi Cadoret, and R. J. Coble

Chapter 25
SCHIZOPHRENIA 317
Harris S. Goldstein, and Frank C. Snope

Chapter 26
ALCOHOLISM.. 330
Harold A. Mulford, and Harold Moessner

Chapter 27
DRUG ABUSE.. 341
Kenneth F. Kessel, and Marvin J. Schwarz

Chapter 28
ORGANIC BRAIN SYNDROME 353
Donald G. Langsley, and Gabriel Smilkstein

Chapter 29
SEXUAL ASSAULT, SEXUAL VARIATION, AND
SEXUAL DEVIATION 362
Gene G. Abel, Judith V. Becker, and Thornton Bryan

Chapter 30
PSYCHOPHARMACOLOGIC THERAPY 374
Carmen A. Delcioppo, and L. Thomas Wolff

Chapter 31
PSYCHOTHERAPY AND BEHAVIOR MODIFICATION 390
Lucy Jane King and L. E. Masters

Chapter 32
GROUP PSYCHOTHERAPY 404
Eugene F. Gauron, and Robert E. Rakel

Part V   COUNSELING 413

Chapter 33
MARRIAGE AND FAMILY COUNSELING WITHIN THE
CONTEXT OF FAMILY PRACTICE 415
William M. Clements, and Jim L. Wilson

Chapter 34
SEXUAL COUNSELING 433
Libby A. Tanner, and Lynn P. Carmichael

Chapter 35
CONTRACEPTIVE COUNSELING 450
Paul Brucker, and F. K. Chapler

Chapter 36
GENETIC COUNSELING 465
F. Clarke Fraser, and E. Bruce Challis

Part VI   CLINICAL SPECIALTIES 479

Chapter 37
SURGERY 481
Richard A. Currie

Chapter 38
ORTHOPEDICS **541**
William J. Mitchell

Chapter 39
OTORHINOLARYNGOLOGY **628**
Louis Lowry, and
Philip L. Roseberry (Family Practice Consultant)

Chapter 40
OPHTHALMOLOGY **690**
Yale Solomon, and Melville G. Rosen

Chapter 41
GYNECOLOGY AND OBSTETRICS **731**
John T. Queenan, Douglas M. Haynes, and
William P. Vonderhaar

Chapter 42
UROLOGY **766**
John D. Young, Jr., Said A. Karmi, and William L. Stewart

Chapter 43
PROCTOLOGY **787**
Gerald R. Gehringer, and Irving A. Levin

Chapter 44
PEDIATRICS **830**
John E. Allen, Vymutt J. Gururaj, and Raymond M. Russo

Chapter 45
PULMONARY MEDICINE **883**
Thomas J. Godar, Alexander Berger, and John E. Donnelly

Chapter 46
GASTROENTEROLOGY **941**
John D. Barker, Jr., and Larry Lawhorne

Chapter 47
CARDIOLOGY **986**
Robert H. Seller

Chapter 48
NEUROLOGY **1013**
John Gilroy, and Joseph W. Hess

Chapter 49
NUTRITION 1076
Katharine A. Munning, and L. J. Filer, Jr.

Chapter 50
DERMATOLOGY AND SYPHILOLOGY 1102
William Welton

Chapter 51
ALLERGY AND IMMUNOLOGY 1136
Alan A. Wanderer, and Carl Flaxer

INDEX 1151

PART I

THE FAMILY UNIT

Chapter 1

THE FAMILY PHYSICIAN

by ROBERT E. RAKEL

The practice of medicine is an art, not a trade; a calling, not a business; a calling in which your heart will be exercised equally with your head.

Sir William Osler[20]

The family physician provides continuing and comprehensive care in a personalized manner to patients of all ages and to their families, regardless of the presence or absence of disease or the nature of the presenting complaint. He accepts responsibility for the management of an individual's total health needs, maintaining an intimate, confidential, and personal relationship with the patient. Most of the patient's health needs are taken care of personally by the family physician; for the remainder, he selects appropriate consulting physicians or other health professionals to assist in the care. The efforts of all health professionals are coordinated by the family physician, who has ongoing responsibility for the patient. His training has specifically prepared him to understand and call upon the expertise of those physicians in the more than 40 medical specialties and the personnel in approximately 100 allied health professions — each with specific skills that may be required in the care of any given patient.

Family medicine is the body of knowledge and skills that constitutes the discipline and that — when applied to the care of patients and their families — becomes the specialty of family practice. Family medicine emphasizes attention to responsibility for total health care from the first contact and initial assessment to the ongoing care of chronic problems (from prevention to rehabilitation). Coordination of all necessary health services and integration of these with the least amount of fragmentation are important features of the discipline. Family practice is a horizontal specialty that, like pediatrics and internal medicine, shares large areas of content with other clinical disciplines. It incorporates this shared knowledge and utilizes it in a unique way to deliver primary medical care. This combining of skills is similar to the activities of other specialties that have taken selected components from a variety of other disciplines, creating a new discipline that can function effectively in a unique manner. Thus, ophthalmology selected components of anatomy, surgery, medicine, and physics; and anesthesiology selected from physiology, pharmacology, biochemistry, and clinical medicine. In addition to the content shared with other medical disciplines, family practice emphasizes knowledge in such areas as family psychodynamics, interpersonal relationships, counseling, and supportive psychotherapy. Its basic foundation, however, remains clinical in nature, with the primary focus always on the care of persons who are ill.

The family physician's devotion to continuing, comprehensive, personalized care; the early detection and management of illness; the prevention of disease and the maintenance of health; and the ongoing management of patients in a community setting make him uniquely qualified to deliver primary health care.

BACKGROUND

Francis Peabody, about 1923, commented that the swing of the pendulum toward specialization had already reached its apex, and modern medicine had fragmented the health care delivery system to too great a degree. He called for a rapid return of the generalist physician, who would give comprehensive and personalized care. However, the trend toward specialization increased in momentum rather than decreased, and the deficit of primary physicians became even greater. In 1966, two reports summarized the prevalent attitudes at that time and made correspondingly similar recommendations for correcting the problem. The first of these, published in August, 1966, was the "Report of the Citizens' Commission on Graduate Medical Education of the American Medical Association," with John Millis serving as chairman; it is commonly referred to as the Millis Commission Report. The second, published 1 month later, was the "Report of the Ad Hoc Committee on Education for Family Practice of the Council on Medical Education of the American Medical Association," with William Willard as chairman, commonly referred to as the Willard Committee Report.

Much of the impetus leading to these reviews came from the American Academy of Family Physicians (AAFP), which began in 1947 as the American Academy of General Practice, changing its name in 1971. This name change was intended in part to place increased emphasis upon family-oriented health care and to attempt to gain academic acceptance for the new specialty of family practice. The American Board of Family Practice (ABFP), established in 1969 as the 20th medical specialty board (the first was ophthalmology in 1916), distinguished itself by being the first specialty board to require recertification (every 6 years) to assure the ongoing competence of its diplomates. One basic requirement established for both certification and recertification was continuing education — the foundation upon which the American Academy of General Practice was built 22 years earlier. A diplomate of the ABFP is require to participate 50 hours per year in acceptable continuing education activity to be eligible for recertification. Once eligibility has been attained, he is then examined for competence by cognitive testing and evaluation of performance. The strict emphasis by the ABFP upon quality of education, knowledge, and performance has facilitated the rapid increase in prestige for the family physician in our health care system. The obvious logic of the Board's emphasis upon continuing education to ensure the maintenance of required knowledge and skills has caused this requirement to be adopted by other specialties and state medical societies.

DEFINITIONS

Primary Care. The specialty of family practice is specifically designed to deliver primary care. Primary care has been defined by both the AAFP and the ABFP as:

. . . a form of medical care delivery which emphasizes first contact care and assumes ongoing responsibility for the patient in both health maintenance and therapy of illness. It is personal care involving a unique interaction and communication between the patient and the physician. It is comprehensive in scope, and includes the overall coordination of the care of the patient's health problems, be they biological, behavioral or social. The appropriate use of consultants and community resources is an important part of effective primary care.

Many physicians deliver primary care, in different ways and with varying degrees of preparation. The ABFP added a further clarifying statement:

Primary care is a form of delivery of medical care which encompasses the following functions:

1. It is "first-contact" care serving as point-of-entry for the patient into the health care system;

2. It includes continuity by virtue of caring for patients over a period of time both in sickness and in health;

3. It is comprehensive care, drawing from all the traditional major disciplines for its functional content;

4. It serves a coordinative function for all the health-care needs of the patient;

5. It assumes continuing responsibility for individual patient follow-up and community health problems; and

6. It is a highly personalized type of care.

Primary Physician. The term "primary physician" was defined by the Millis Commission as one who:

. . . should usually be primary in the first contact sense. He will serve as the primary medical resource and counselor to an individual or a family. When a patient needs hospitalization, the service of other medical specialists, or other medical or paramedical assistance, the primary physician will see that the necessary arrangements are made, giving such responsibility to others as is appropriate and retaining his own continuing and comprehensive responsibility.

Few hospitals and few existing specialists consider comprehensive and continuing medical care to be their responsibility and within their range of competence.

Three years after the publication of the Millis Commission Report, the ABFP was established for the purpose of certifying physicians skilled in delivering continuing comprehensive care. Although the nature of this physician was dictated by a myriad of needs and circumstances, it appeared that he specifically satisfied the directive of the Millis Commission.

Family Physician. The family physician was defined as one who:

... serves the public as a physician of first contact and means of entry into the health care system; evaluates his patients' total health care needs; assumes responsibility for his patients' comprehensive and continuing health care and acts as coordinator of his patients' health services; and accepts responsibility for his patients' total health care, including the use of consultants, within the context of their environment, including the community and the family or comparable social unit.[17]

Family Practice. The AAFP and the ABFP have also agreed on a common definition of family practice as:

... comprehensive medical care with particular emphasis on the family unit, in which the physician's continuing responsibility for health care is neither limited by the patient's age or sex nor by a particular organ system or disease entity.

Family practice is the specialty in breadth which builds upon a core of knowledge derived from other disciplines—drawing most heavily on internal medicine, pediatrics, obstetrics and gynecology, surgery and psychiatry—and which establishes a cohesive unit, combining the behavioral sciences with the traditional biological and clinical sciences. The core of knowledge encompassed by the discipline of family practice prepares the family physician for a unique role in patient management, problem solving, counseling and as a personal physician who coordinates total health care delivery.

Any definition of family practice must be built primarily on a base of data that is appropriate to the activities of those practicing this specialty. For this reason, a sincere attempt is being made to design the curriculum for training family physicians so that

it realistically represents those skills and that body of knowledge that they will require in practice. This curriculum definition relies heavily upon an accurate analysis of the problems seen and the skills utilized by family physicians in their practice. The content of residency training programs in the primary care specialties has not always been appropriately directed toward the skills required to solve the problems most commonly encountered by physicians practicing in these areas. The scene is changing rapidly, and training programs should be much more appropriately designed for these needs in the future. The almost randomly educated primary physician of yesterday is being replaced by one specifically prepared to care for the kinds of problems likely to be encountered. It is for this reason that the "model office" is an essential component of all family practice residency programs.

PERSONALIZED CARE

It is much more important to know what sort of patient has a disease than what sort of disease a patient has.

SIR WILLIAM OSLER[20]

Personalized, holistic care is an essential component of family practice. The need for personalized health care is consistently recognized by patients and philosophers alike. Our increasingly fragmented health care system has propelled this issue to major prominence. The steady decline in availability of this type of care—previously taken for granted—has not gone unnoticed by the public sector. This is not a recent phenomenon, however, since even in the 12th century Maimonides cautioned his students to remember that success in treating a patient with asthma depended upon intimate knowledge of the total patient and that the physician should "... not treat the disease, but the patient who is suffering from it."[12] The physician should not think in terms of diseases but in terms of patients who have problems needing attention. The holistic approach to patient care is hampered by focusing primarily upon the disease, since specific diseases require specific treatment and tend to direct the physician's attention away from other needs of the whole patient. Physicians who engage primarily in hospital medicine must make a stronger effort to maintain personalized care because of the added exposure to and the necessary utilization of apparatus and techniques directed toward specific diseases.

The need for physicians to maintain an intimate personal relationship with patients was emphasized by Peabody, who noted, "The treatment of a disease may be entirely impersonal; the care of a patient must be completely personal."[21] If consideration of a patient as an individual remains our prime concern as physicians, then medical care of high quality will persist, regardless of the way it is organized or financed. For this reason, family practice emphasizes consideration of the patient in the full context of his life situation rather than the episodic care of a presenting complaint. To refer once again to the Millis Commission Report, it emphasizes that the family physician "... focuses not upon individual organs and systems but upon the whole man who lives in a complex social setting; and knows that diagnosis or treatment of a part often overlooks major causative factors and therapeutic opportunities." Most of these charges can be answered best by a family physician who knows his patients in their home environment and who assesses the psychosocial factors at play within the family setting in addition to the individual's organic problems. He assesses the illness and complaints presented to him, dealing with the majority himself and arranging special assistance for a few. He serves as the patient's advocate, explaining the causes and implications of illness to the patient and his family, and serves as advisor and confidant for the family—both individually and collectively. The family physician receives many intellectual satisfactions from his practice, but his greatest reward arises from the depth of human understanding and personal satisfaction inherent in family practice.

One of my favorite paintings is by Sir Luke Fildes, entitled "Portrait of a Family Physician." It is a scene at the home of a child with pneumonia, showing worried parents in the background and the physician sitting nearby in a concerned yet helpless pose. The physician's warmth, compassion, and personal dedication are evident, as is the frustration caused by his inability to do more for the child. Although today's antibiotic era would change the nature of this picture, and patients now expect rapid and remarkable cures from our new wonder drugs, they also desire the same degree of personalized concern for their well-being as existed in medical care at the time of the painting. While patients have adjusted somewhat to a more impersonal form of health care delivery and frequently look to institutions rather than to individuals for their health care, their need for personalized concern and compassion remains.

The family physician's relationship with his patients should reflect compassion, understanding, and patience, mixed with a high degree of intellectual honesty. He must be thorough in his approach to problems and must have a keen sense of humor. He must also be capable of creating in his patients attitudes of optimism, courage, insight, and the self-discipline necessary for recovery. If he is unable to cure—as is the physician in Fildes' picture—he must at least comfort.

ATTRIBUTES OF THE FAMILY PHYSICIAN

The following characteristics are certainly desirable for all physicians, but are of greatest importance for the physician in family practice:

1. A strong sense of responsibility for the total, ongoing care of the individual and the family during health, illness, or rehabilitation.

2. Compassion and empathy, with a sincere interest in people.

3. A curious and constantly inquisitive attitude.

4. Enthusiasm for the undifferentiated medical problem and its resolution.

5. An interest in the broad spectrum of clinical medicine.

6. The ability to deal comfortably with multiple problems occurring simultaneously in one patient.

7. A desire for frequent and varied intellectual and technical challenges.

8. The ability to support children during growth and development and during their adjustment to family and society.

9. The ability to assist patients in coping with everyday problems and in main-

taining a homeostatic posture in the family and community.

10. The capacity to act as coordinator of all health resources needed in the care of a patient.

11. An enthusiasm for continued learning and the satisfaction that results from maintaining current medical knowledge through continuing medical education.

12. The ability to maintain composure at times of stress and to respond quickly with logic and effectiveness.

13. A desire to identify problems at the earliest possible stage (or to prevent disease entirely).

14. A strong wish to maintain maximum patient satisfaction, recognizing the need for good continuing patient rapport.

15. The skills necessary to manage chronic illnesses and to ensure maximum rehabilitation following acute illnesses.

16. An appreciation for the complex mixture of physical, emotional, and social elements in holistic and personalized patient care.

17. A feeling of personal satisfaction derived from the intimate relationships with patients naturally developing over long periods of continuous care, as opposed to the short-term pleasures gained from treating episodic illness.

18. A skill for and commitment to educating patients and families about disease processes and the principles of health management.

The ideal family physician is an explorer, driven by a persistent curiosity and the desire to know more. He is part theologian, as was Paracelsus; part politician, as was Benjamin Rush; and part humorist, as was Oliver Wendell Holmes. At all times, however, he holds the care of the patient, the whole patient, somewhat sacred.

Continuing Responsibility

One of the most essential functions of the family physician is the willingness to accept ongoing responsibility for managing a patient's medical care. Once a patient or a family has been accepted into the physician's practice, responsibility for their care is both complete and continuing. The Millis Commission chose the word "primary physician" to emphasize the concept of primary responsibility for the patient's welfare. The family physician is involved in the management of any health problem that arises, whether he manages it completely—as will usually be the case—or whether he utilizes consultants and other allied health professionals. Once a physician accepts responsibility for the initial care of a problem, he likewise assumes the obligation to follow the problem to its conclusion, which means that he has a responsibility to confirm satisfactory results even when the patient has been referred to another physician for a surgical or diagnostic procedure. The commitment to patients does not terminate at the end of an illness but is a continuing responsibility, regardless of the state of health or the disease process. There is no need to identify the beginning or end-point of treatment, since care of a problem can be reopened and dealt with at any time—even though a later visit may be primarily for another problem. This prevents the family physician from focusing too narrowly on one problem and makes it easy to maintain a perspective of the total patient in his environment. Peabody felt that much of the patient's dissatisfaction results from the physician's neglecting to assume personal responsibility for supervision of his care. "For some reason or other, no one physician has seen the case through from beginning to end, and the patient may be suffering from the very multitude of his counselors."[21]

Patient compliance is improved when a single physician provides continuous care and when this care can be given at less cost than when patients with similar problems are treated by a variety of physicians. The physician who knows his patients well can assess the nature of their problems more rapidly and accurately. In addition, because of the intimate ongoing relationship, he is under less pressure to exclude all diagnostic possibilities by the use of expensive laboratory and radiologic procedures than is the physician who is unfamiliar with the patient. The physician who is well acquainted with his patient not only provides more personal and human medical care but does it more economically than the physician involved only in episodic care.

The greater the degree of a physician's continuing involvement with a patient, the more capable he will be of detecting early signs and symptoms of organic disease and functional problems. Patients with problems arising from emotional and social conflicts can also be managed most effectively by a physician who has intimate knowledge of the individual and of his family and community background, resulting from the insight gained by observing the patient's long-term patterns of behavior and his response to changing stressful situations. This longitudinal view is particularly useful in the care of children and allows the physician to be more effective in assisting children to reach their full potential. The closeness that develops between physicians and young patients during their period of growth increases a physician's ability to aid his patient during later periods in life—such as adjustment to puberty, problems with marriage or employment, and changing social pressures. As the family physician maintains this continuing involvement with successive generations within a family, his ability to manage intercurrent problems increases as his knowledge of the total family background grows.

By virtue of this ongoing involvement and intimate association with the family, the family physician develops a perceptive awareness of a family's nature and style of operation. This ability to observe families over time allows him to gain valuable insight that improves the quality of medical care he is able to provide an individual patient. One of the greatest challenges in family medicine is to be alert to the changing stresses, transitions, and expectations of family members over time and to the effect that these and other family interactions have on the health of individuals.

Although the family unit is the family physician's primary concern, his skills are equally applicable to the single individual living alone or to those in other varieties of "family" living. Individuals in each of these alternate forms of "family" living interact with other individuals who have a significant effect on their lives in a manner similar to the nuclear family, and the principles of group dynamics and interpersonal relationships that affect one's health apply to them as well.

The family physician needs to assess an individual's personality so that presenting symptoms can be appropriately evaluated and given the proper degree of attention and emphasis. A complaint of abdominal pain may be treated lightly in one patient with a high functional tendency, but the same complaint would be immediately investigated in depth in another individual who has a more stoic personality. The decision regarding which studies to perform and when they should be done is influenced by knowledge of the patient's life style, personality, and previous response pattern. The greater the degree of knowledge and insight into the patient's background, gained through years of previous contact, the more capable the physician will be in making an appropriate early and rapid assessment of the presenting complaint. The less background information the physician has to rely on, the greater will be his need to depend upon costly laboratory studies and the greater the likelihood of his over-reacting to the presenting symptom. Families receiving continuing comprehensive care have fewer hospitalizations, fewer operations, and fewer physician visits for illnesses compared with those having no regular physician. This is due, at least in part, to the physician's knowing his patients; seeing them earlier for acute problems, and thus preventing complications that would require hospitalization; being available by telephone; and seeing them *more* frequently in the office for health supervision. Care is also cheaper, since there is less need to rely on x-ray and laboratory procedures and visits to emergency rooms.[11]

The increasing complexity of our health care system multiplies expense and wastefulness when a patient self-diagnoses his problems or selects his own specialist rather than developing a firm and ongoing relationship with a family physician. A more efficient and cost-effective system involves a single personal physician, who ensures the most logical and economical management of a problem. Medical care should be made available to patients in the precise degree that it is needed—neither too extensive nor too limited. Only in this manner can one be sure that simple problems will not be magnified out of proportion. The more complex and involved the diagnostic process is, the more costly it becomes, and the greater the potential for error. The need for a primary physician who accepts continuing responsibility for patient care is emphasized by Michael Balint in his concept of "Collusion of Anonymity."[2] In this situation, the patient is seen by a variety of physicians, not one of whom is willing to accept total management of the problem. Important decisions are made—some good, some bad—but without anyone's feeling fully responsible for them.

Francis Peabody emphasized the futility of patients' making the rounds from one specialist to another without finding relief because they

...lacked the guidance of a sound general practitioner who understood his physical condition, his nervous temperament and knew the details of his daily life. Many a patient who on his own initiative had sought out specialists has had minor defects extenuated so that they assume a needless importance and has even undergone operations that might well have been avoided. These are often pathetically tragic figures as they veer from one course of treatment to another—like ships that lack a guiding hand upon the helm, they swing from tack to tack with each new gust of wind but get no nearer to the Port of Health because there is no pilot to set the general direction of their course.[21]

The family physician must also be committed to the management of the common chronic illnesses for which there is no known cure but for which continuing management by a personal physician is all the more necessary to maintain an optimal state of health for the patient. It is a difficult and often trying job to manage these continuing, unresolvable, and progressively-crippling problems, the control of which requires a remolding of the patient's life style and almost always involves a change of life style for the entire family.

Comprehensive Care

Comprehensive medical care refers to a degree of breadth across the entire spectrum of medicine. The effectiveness of a physician's delivery of primary care depends upon the degree of comprehensive involvement attained in his training and practice. The family physician must be comprehensively trained to offer his patient the entire spectrum of medical skills necessary to care for the majority of the patient's problems. The greater the number of disciplines omitted from the family physician's training and practice, the more frequent will be the need to refer minor problems within these disciplines to another physician. The primary physician should be competent in a broad range of medical disciplines in order to minimize the need to delegate his patients' care to other physicians. Only in this manner can maximum cost-effectiveness be realized. A truly comprehensive primary physician will adequately manage acute infections, biopsy skin and other lesions, repair lacerations, treat musculoskeletal sprains and strains, remove foreign bodies, give supportive psychotherapy, and supervise diagnostic procedures. His patients' needs will vary from a routine physical examination, when the patient feels well and wishes to identify potential risk factors, to the need for referral to a narrowly-specialized physician with highly developed technical skills. The family physician must be aware of the variety and complexity of skills and facilities available to his patients and must match these to the individual's specific needs—giving full consideration to the patient's personality and expectations.

Figure 1–1 illustrates the concept of the breadth involved in comprehensive medicine and the varying depths of knowledge utilized in each of the many disciplines that constitute family medicine. A primary physician will require knowledge and skills to varying degrees in each specialty area, depending upon the prevalence of problems encountered in everyday practice or the degree of skills required to become an excellent diagnostician. A physician specializing in only one discipline, however, will have a much more shallow base in comprehensive medicine and a much greater depth in the chosen discipline. The subspecialist is an excellent consultant, but he is not trained and cannot function effectively as a primary generalist. The distribution of his knowledge and skills is not appropriate to that task to any greater degree than the comprehensive physician is competent in the esoteric nuances of a discipline such as neurology.

A patient's personality, fears, and anxieties play a significant role in all illnesses and are factors in all primary care. The family physician has a critical role in the diagnosis and management of psychiatric disorders in the patients under his care. Approximately one-half of them will have a significant emotional problem within any 2-year period. Most frequently, the family physician's role is in the form of providing supportive psychotherapy, but it can involve the management of psychosis as well. This degree of involvement with emotional

Content of a
Consulting Specialty
In this illustration - Neurology

Content of Family Practice

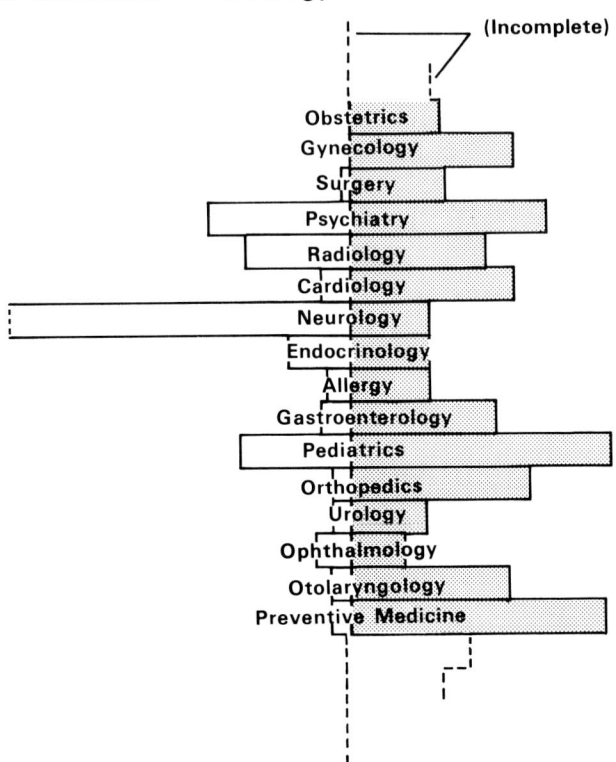

Figure 1–1. *Comparison between content of a consulting specialty and content of family practice. (From Rakel, R. E.: Principles of Family Medicine. Philadelphia, W. B. Saunders Co., 1977.)*

problems requires that skills in dealing with such disorders be taught during the physician's training period.

Some students are more ideally suited to family practice than are others. The student least appropriate for such training is the one who feels insecure with a large volume of material in a breadth of fields. Those receiving greatest satisfaction in family practice enjoy close, personalized relationships with people, like dealing with a broad range of undifferentiated problems, and desire a sense of responsibility for the ongoing management of problems. Management of an illness involves much more than a diagnosis and an outline for treatment. It also requires an awareness of all the factors affecting an individual that may aid or hinder his recovery from the illness. This requires consideration of his religious beliefs; social, economic, or cultural problems; personal expectations; and hereditary background. The outstanding clinician is one who recognizes the effects that spiri-

tual, intellectual, emotional, social, and economic factors have on a patient's illness.

Sickness rarely affects only one person but has ramifications involving other members of the family, friends, or associates at work. A frequent reason for a patient's requesting a complete check-up and electrocardiogram is that one or more acquaintances at work recently had a heart attack; a housewife's anxiety about breast cancer may well stem from a friend's recently having had a radical mastectomy. Thus, influences precipitating a patient's request for care may arise from within the community rather than from within the family.

Interpersonal Skills

One of the essential and foremost skills of the family physician is the ability to utilize effectively the knowledge of interpersonal relations in the management of patients. While sound scientific principles are as important to family practice as they are to the more narrow medical specialties, this powerful element of clinical medicine is perhaps our most useful tool. Modern society considers our medical care system inadequate in those situations in which understanding and compassion are important to the patient's comfort and recovery from illness. Physicians are too often seen as lacking in this personal concern and unskilled in understanding personal anxiety and feelings. The family physician considers this personal concern and understanding among his major strengths.

There is need, however, to nourish the seed of compassion and concern for sick people with which students enter medical school. Family practice emphasizes the integration of compassion, empathy, and personalized concern to a greater degree than is necessary in a more technical or mechanical task-oriented specialty. Some of the earnest solicitude of the old country doctor and his untiring compassion for people must be incorporated as we apply the very effective, yet seemingly cold, modern medical procedures. The patient should be viewed compassionately as a person in distress who needs to be treated with concern, dignity, and personal consideration. He has a right to be given some insight into his problem and a reasonable appraisal of the potential outcome, as well as a realistic picture of the emotional, financial, and occupational expenses involved in his care. Our desire as physicians should be to serve each patient and to learn as much as possible from every patient interaction, much as Sir Francis Bacon, who strove "... to light my torch at every man's candle." To relate well to his patients, a physician must develop the attributes of compassion and courtesy, the ability to establish rapport and to communicate effectively, the ability to gather information rapidly and to organize it logically, the skills required to identify all significant patient problems and to manage these problems appropriately, the ability to be a good listener, the skill necessary to motivate people, and the ability to observe and detect nonverbal clues.

Much of the family physician's effectiveness in interpersonal relationships depends upon his charisma. Charisma is a personal magic of leadership, a magnetic charm or appeal that arouses special loyalty or enthusiasm. The charismatic physician is most likely to engender maximal patient compliance and satisfaction. The physician must be aware of his own feelings, however, and their effect upon the patient. Charisma can be a useful therapeutic tool, but one must learn how and when to use it effectively, since it can also rebound with unfavorable consequences. The physician should be aware of the possibility that he is treating his own ego rather than the patient's needs, since the temptation to take an "ego-trip" is frequent and hazardous. Consider the patient who appeals to the physician's ego by presenting with a functional complaint and asking the physician, in his great wisdom, to cure him. If the physician ignores the opportunity to place part of the burden for treatment and cure on the patient, he may well provide an opening for a continuing series of manipulations by the patient. Just as charisma is therapeutic, so too is the mere *availability* of the physician. The feeling of security that the patient gains by knowing that he can "touch" the physician, either in person or by phone, is psychologically therapeutic and serves as a comforting and calming influence.

Diagnostic Skills — Undifferentiated Problems

The family physician, above all, must be an outstanding diagnostician. Skills in this area must be honed to perfection, since problems are usually seen in their early, undifferentiated state and without the degree of resolution that usually has occurred by the time patients are referred to consulting specialists for further opinion. This is a unique feature of family practice, since symptoms seen at this stage are often vague and nondescript, with signs being either minimal or absent. Unlike the consulting specialist, the family physician does not evaluate the case after it has been preselected by another physician, and the diagnostic procedures used by the family physician must be selected from the entire spectrum of medicine.

At this stage of disease, there are often only very subtle differences between the early symptoms of serious disease and those of self-limited, minor ailments. To the inexperienced person, the clinical picture may appear identical, but to the astute and experienced family physician, one symptom will raise a higher index of suspicion than another because of the greater probability that it is associated with potential serious illness. Diagnoses are frequently made on the basis of probability and the likelihood that a specific disease is present, frequently depending upon the relative incidence of the disease related to the symptoms seen in the physician's community during a given time of the year. Approximately one-fourth of all patients seen will never be assigned a final, definitive diagnosis, since the resolution of a presenting symptom or a complaint will come before a specific diagnosis can be made. Pragmatically, this is an efficient method that is less costly and achieves high patient satisfaction—even though it may be disquieting to the purist physician who feels a thorough work-up and specific diagnosis should always be obtained.

The family physician is an expert in the rapid assessment of a problem presented for the first time. He evaluates its potential significance, often making a diagnosis by exclusion rather than by inclusion, after he first makes certain that the symptoms are not those of a serious problem. Once assured, he allows some time to elapse, using time as one of his most efficient diagnostic aids. Follow-up visits are scheduled at appropriate intervals to watch for subtle changes in the presenting symptoms. The physician usually identifies the symptom that has the greatest discriminatory value and watches it more closely than the others. His most significant clue to the true nature of the illness may depend upon subtle changes in this key symptom. The family physician's effectiveness is often determined by his knack of perceiving the hidden or subtle dimensions of illness and following them closely.

The maxim that an accurate history is the most important factor in arriving at an accurate diagnosis is especially appropriate to family medicine, since symptoms may be the only obvious feature of an illness at the time it is presented to the family physician, with the physical signs still inapparent. Further inquiry into the nature of the symptoms, time of onset, extenuating factors, and other unique subjective features may be the only diagnostic clues available at such an early stage. The family physician must, above all, be a skilled clinician with the ability to evaluate symptoms, verbal and nonverbal communication, and early signs of illness in order to choose those diagnostic tests of greatest value in early diagnosis.

The family physician attempts to minimize the degree of morbidity resulting from illness. For example, he pays close attention to the complete eradication of a urinary tract infection in an effort to prevent permanent damage that could result in renal failure—requiring expensive and incapacitating renal dialysis or kidney transplant. Similar examples would be the early identification of carcinoma in situ of the cervix to prevent the lethal spread of uterine carcinoma, or the early identification of a dysplastic hip that, if undetected, could result in a permanent deformity, similar to an undetected hemolytic streptococcal infection causing rheumatic heart disease.

Arriving at an early diagnosis may be of less importance than determining the real reason that the patient came to the physician. The symptom may be due to a self-limiting or an acute problem, but anxiety or fear may be the true factor that brought the patient to the physician. Although the symptom may be hoarseness resulting from the postnasal drainage accompanying an upper respiratory tract infection, the patient may be afraid that it is caused by a laryngeal carcinoma similar to that recently found in a friend. Clinical evaluation must rule out the possibility of laryngeal carcinoma, but the patient's fears and apprehension regarding this possibility must also be allayed. The patient's expectations are equally as important as the presenting symptom. Every physical problem has an emotional component, and while this is usually minimal, it can be a major precipitating cause. For example, a 42 year old man with influenza and pleuritic chest pain may present himself as anxious and apprehensive because his father died at age 45 of an acute myocardial infarction. Or similarly, a mild thrombophlebitis in a 35 year old woman could bring her to the physician in a more anxious state than is warranted by the problem because her mother died of a pulmonary embolism. The family physician must be a perceptive humanist, alert to the early identification of new problems, and he must apply his comprehensive background and skills with human understanding and compassion.

THE FAMILY PHYSICIAN AS COORDINATOR

Francis Peabody, Professor of Medicine at Harvard Medical School from 1921 to 1927, was a man ahead of his time; his comments are equally appropriate today.

Never was the public in need of wise, broadly-trained advisors so much as it needs them today to guide them through the complicated maze of modern medicine. The extraordinary development of medical science with its consequent diversity of medical specialists and the increasing limitations in the extent of special fields, the very factors indeed which are creating specialists, in themselves create a new demand. Not for men who are experts along narrow lines but for men who are in touch with many lines.[21]

Specialization and the resulting fragmentation of our health care system have resulted in a deficiency of physicians who are broadly trained, competent, and willing to serve as coordinators in this somewhat chaotic system. The family physician, by virtue of his breadth of training in the wide variety of medical disciplines, has unique insights into the nature of skills possessed by physicians who limit their practice to the more narrow specialty areas. He is prepared to select specialists whose skills can be applied most appropriately to a given case, as well as to coordinate the activities of each, so that they are not counterproductive.

The following statement from the Millis Commission Report concerning expectations of the patient is especially appropriate:

The patient wants someone of high competence and good judgment to take charge of the total situation, someone who can serve as coordinator of all the medical resources that can help solve his problem. He wants a company president who will make proper use of his skills and knowledge of more specialized members of the firm. He wants a quarterback who will diagnose the constantly changing situation, coordinate the whole team, and call on each member for the particular contributions that he is best able to make to the team effort.[25]

Such breadth of vision is important for a coordinating physician. He must have a realistic overview of the problem and must be aware of the many alternative routes possible, since he must select that which is most appropriate. Consider, for example, three different patients with peptic ulcer. One may benefit most by medical management, another by psychiatric care, while the third may require surgery. The physician familiar with one form of treatment will tend to rely on it excessively, while the family physician can select the best approach from all possible alternatives.

Bryan refers to medicine today as a social monstrosity, like a pyramid standing on its head, since its management lies at the bottom of the heap and is compressed by the proliferating mass of uncoordinated specialists milling about above.[3] He urges that an attempt be made to right this pyramid and to stand it on its base.

The engineering industry has long ago recognized the value of a project director as the most important member of the team. He knows the special skills of each member or professional involved in the project and is the only person whose breadth of training, knowledge, and perspective ensure that every talent and resource will be used in the most efficient and balanced manner in the completion of the project. Management, which directs the engineer, can be compared with the federal government's interest in delivery of medical care—since both are interested in achieving the most efficient and economical method for producing a quality product.

As we have shown, the complexity of modern medicine frequently involves a variety of health professionals—each with highly developed skills in a particular area—concerned with the care of a seriously ill patient. The family physician, having established rapport with a patient and family and having knowledge of the patient's background, personality, fears, and expectations, is best able to select and coordinate the activities of appropriate individuals from the large variety of other disciplines in planning the patient's care. He can maintain effective communication among those involved, as well as function as the patient's advocate and interpret to the patient and his family the many unfamiliar and complicated procedures to which he is being subjected. This prevents any one consulting physician, unfamiliar with the concepts or actions of all others involved, from ordering a test or medication that would conflict with other treatment. A family physician is also best able to maintain maximum patient and family cooperation during times of stress.

J. E. Dunphy has emphasized the value of the surgeon and the family physician working closely together as a team.

It is impossible to provide high quality surgical care without that knowledge of the whole patient which only a family physician can supply. When their mutual decisions . . . bring hope, comfort and ultimately health to a gravely ill human being, the total experience is the essence and the joy of medicine.[8a]

The ability to orchestrate the knowledge and skills of a variety of diverse professionals is a skill to be learned during residency training and cultivated in practice. It is not an automatic attribute of all physicians or merely the result of exposure to a large number of professionals. These coordinator skills extend beyond the traditional medical disciplines into the many community agencies and allied health professions as well. In order for the family physician to be an effective coordinator, it is essential that all pertinent health information be channeled through him — regardless of what institution, agency, or individual renders the service.

Community medicine is another essential component of family medicine. Because of this close involvement with the community, the family physician is ideally suited to be the integrator of the patient's care, orchestrating the skills of consultants when appropriate and involving community nurses, social agencies, the clergy, or other family members when needed. His knowledge of community health resources and his close personal involvement with the community can be utilized to maximum benefit, not only for diagnostic and therapeutic purposes but also to achieve the best possible level of rehabilitation.

Edmund Pellegrino has emphasized that:

It should be clear, too, that no simple addition of specialties can equal the generalist function. To build a wall one needs more than the aimless piling up of bricks; one needs an architect. Every operation which analyzes some part of the human mechanism requires to be bal-

anced by another which synthesizes and coordinates.[22]

The family physician synthesizes the opinions and skills of a multitude of medical consultants with the individual patient's personal needs and the many community agencies available. These must be matched to the patient's expectations and to his ability to respond to appropriate changes in life style. The recommended changes in life style, however, must be realistic and based on consideration of the patient's ability to comply. Treatment of a newly diagnosed diabetic patient recovering from ketoacidosis who is married to a woman whose main satisfaction in life is cooking for her large family requires a significant amount of tact and skill by the family physician to help them readjust both of their life styles.

PRACTICE CONTENT

The advent of family medicine heralds a renaissance in medical education that involves a reassessment of the traditional medical education environment in a referral hospital. It is now considered more realistic to train a physician in a community atmosphere, providing exposure to the diseases and problems most closely approximating those he will encounter during his future professional life. The ambulatory care skills and knowledge that most medical graduates will need cannot be taught totally within the tertiary medical center. The specialty of family practice emphasizes training in ambulatory care skills in an appropriately realistic environment, utilizing patients representative of a cross section of the community and incorporating those problems more frequently encountered by physicians practicing primary care.

This lack of relevance in the referral medical center applies equally to the hospitalized patient. The majority of hospitalized patients whom our medical graduates will be managing in the future will have acute problems such as appendicitis, gastroenteritis, abscesses, or uncomplicated myocardial infarction. Generally, such cases are not encountered in the referral center. Figure 1–2 is derived from data accumulated in the United States and Great

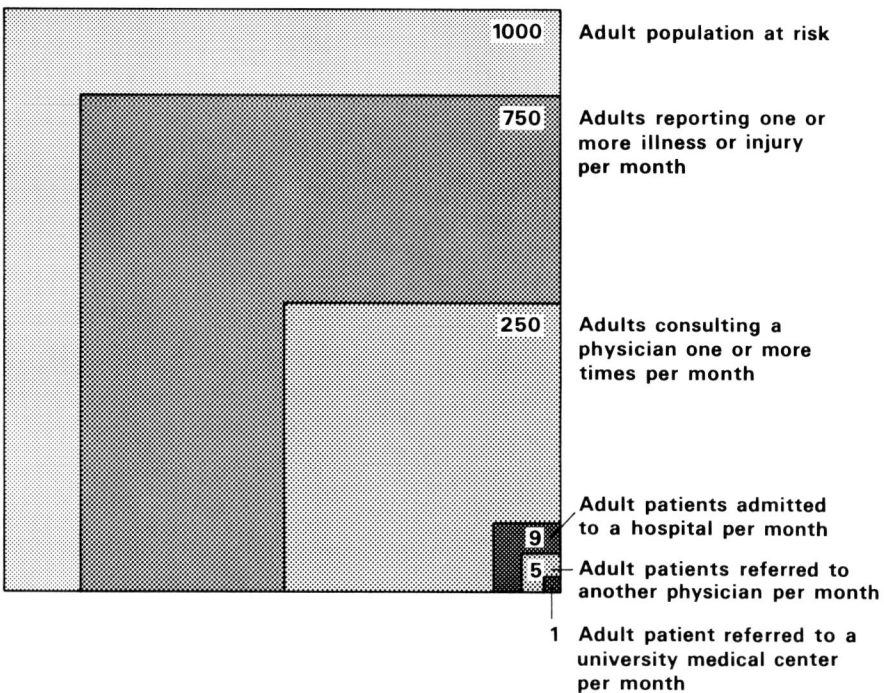

1000 — Adult population at risk

750 — Adults reporting one or more illness or injury per month

250 — Adults consulting a physician one or more times per month

9 — Adult patients admitted to a hospital per month

5 — Adult patients referred to another physician per month

1 — Adult patient referred to a university medical center per month

Figure 1–2. Number of persons experiencing illness or injury during average month, per 1000 adult population. (From White, K. L., Williams, F., and Greenberg, B.: N. Engl. J. Med., 265:885, 1961.)

Britain. In an adult population of 1000 persons aged 16 years or older, 750 will experience one or more illnesses or injuries during an average month. Most of these persons will be managed by self-treatment, but 250 patients will consult a physician. Of these, five patients will be referred for consultation to another physician and nine patients will be hospitalized—eight of them in a community hospital and one in a university medical center. It is obvious that patients seen in the medical center (and frequently the majority of cases used for teaching) represent atypical samples of illness occurring within a normal community. Students exposed in this manner develop an unrealistic concept of the kinds of medical problems prevalent in society. It focuses their training on knowledge and skills of limited usefulness in later practice.

A family physician sees each of his patients an average of four times a year, and in an average practice of 1500 to 3000 individuals, he will see approximately two-thirds of them at least once each year (Fig. 1–3). Many practicing family physicians and most family practice residency programs are currently recording the type and

frequency of problems seen. Undergraduate and graduate curricula are being modified based upon information from these studies regarding the prevalance and nature of problems seen. Until recently, the major classification system was the International Classification of Disease (ICD), which was modified for use in the United States and became the International Classification of Disease Adapted for Use in the United States (ICDA). This was further modified by hospitals into the Hospital International Classification of Disease Adapted for Use in the United States (HICDA), which included perinatal mortality and psychiatric problems and contained a total of more than 4000 items.

This classification system had major deficiencies when applied to the problems most frequently encountered by practicing family physicians, so the Royal College of General Practitioners in England developed a classification system pertinent to their needs in ambulatory practice. This served as the nucleus for an international classification of problems seen by practicing family physicians throughout the world. The sponsoring organization is the

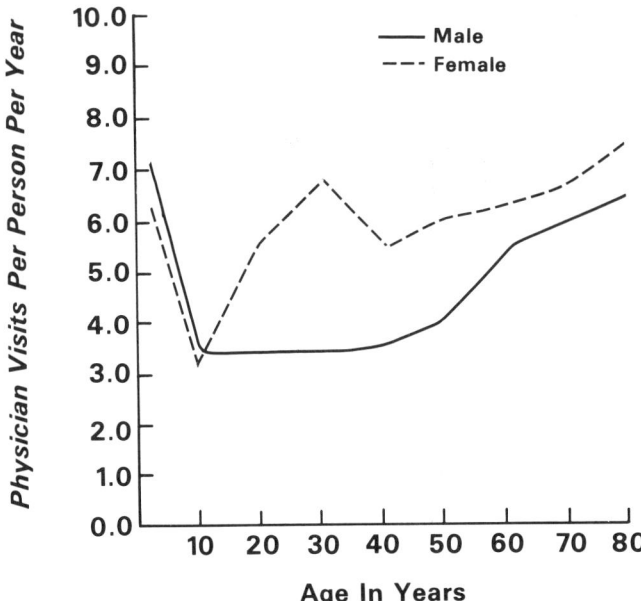

Figure 1–3. Average number of visits to family physician per patient per year. (From Rakel, R. E.: Principles of Family Medicine. Philadelphia, W. B. Saunders Co., 1977.)

World Organization of National Colleges, Academies, and Academic Associations of General Practitioners/Family Physicians (WONCA). The classification was developed by an international working party who gave it the name International Classification of Health Problems in Primary Care (ICHPPC). It is also called Ich-Pic and Pri-Care. This classification system has been developed following a large-scale international trial that isolated the 371 items felt to be most commonly encountered by family physicians. In this manner, a very large number of problems that are included in the ICD but that are infrequently encountered in family practice have been eliminated. The ICHPPC classification is compatible with the larger ICD classification, however, and can be used interchangeably or expanded at will.

The need for such a classification arose when it was realized that as many as 25 per cent of the problems seen by family physicians were not classifiable according to the ICD. Many of these are undifferentiated, indefinite symptoms that resolve either spontaneously or with empiric treatment before progressing to a definitive diagnosis. It is no surprise that respiratory tract infections, emotionally based symptoms and syndromes, skin disorders, gastrointestinal problems, and musculoskeletal and cardiovascular diseases are the most frequently encountered disorders (Table 1–1 and Fig. 1–4).

TABLE 1–1. THE 20 MOST COMMON PATIENT PROBLEMS SEEN IN PHYSICIANS' OFFICES*

Problem	Per Cent of Visits	Cumulative Per Cent
Progress visits	11.7	11.7
Other problems, NEC†	5.8	17.5
Physical examination	4.0	21.5
Pain, etc., in lower extremity	4.1	25.6
Pregnancy examination	4.0	29.6
Sore throat	3.2	32.8
Pain, etc., in upper extremity	2.9	35.7
Pain, etc., in region of back	3.0	38.7
Cough	2.8	41.5
Abdominal pain	2.5	44.0
Cold	2.1	46.1
Gynecologic examination	2.1	48.2
Visit for medication	2.0	50.2
None	2.0	52.2
Headache	1.9	54.1
Fatigue	1.8	56.0
Pain in chest	1.7	57.7
Well-baby examination	1.7	59.4
Fever	1.5	60.9
Allergic skin reaction	1.5	62.4
All other symptoms	37.6	100.0

*From the Department of Health, Education and Welfare, National Ambulatory Medical Care Survey, May, 1973, to April, 1974.
†Not elsewhere classified.

This classification system has permitted family physicians to institute investigative projects that are pertinent to the needs of those supplying primary care and are impossible to conduct utilizing the research methodologies of the tertiary medical

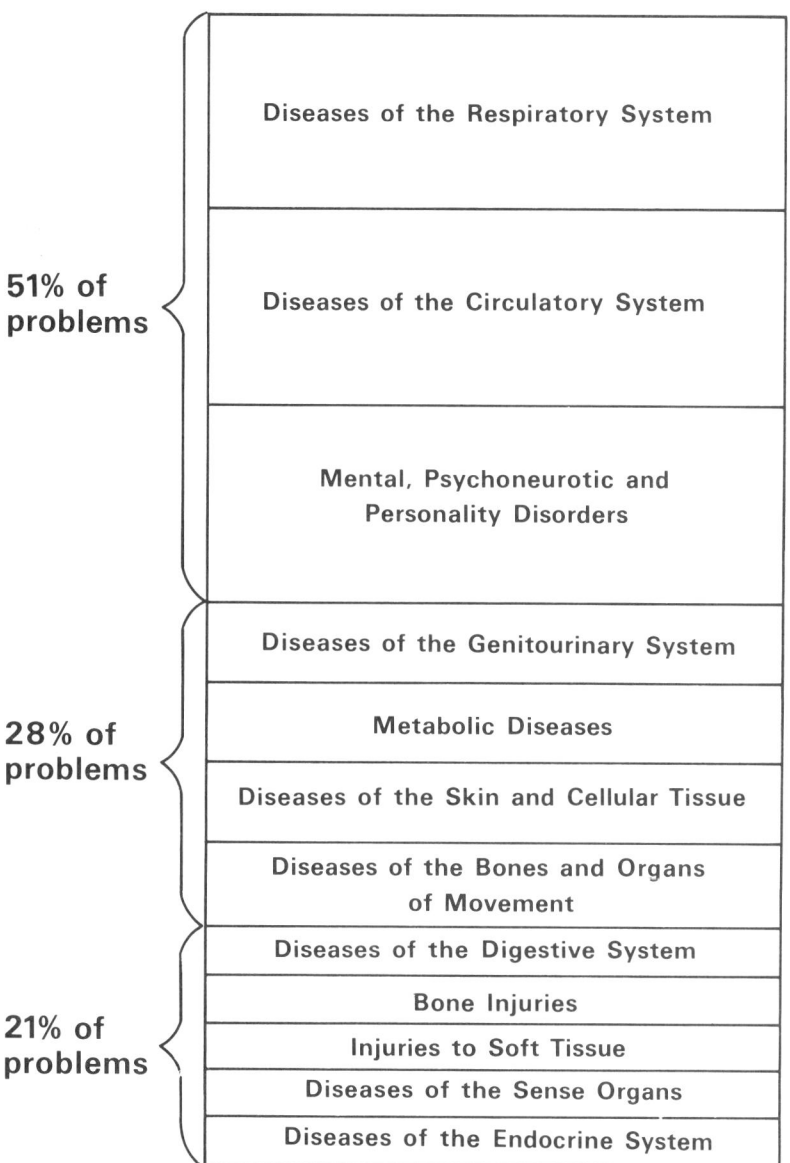

Figure 1–4. *Prevalence of problems in family practice. (From Rakel, R. E.: Principles of Family Medicine. Philadelphia, W. B. Saunders Co., 1977. Modified from McFarlane, A. H., O'Connell, B. P., and Hay, J.)*

center. The National Ambulatory Medical Care Survey being conducted by the United States Department of Health, Education and Welfare measures symptoms or presenting complaints and utilizes its own symptom classification. Table 1–2 compares the nature and the frequency of problems seen by those in the major primary care specialties. The similarity among problems seen by the family physician, general internist, and general pediatrician is readily apparent and emphasizes the fact that physicians in these three specialties will draw increasingly closer together as training programs are redesigned to reflect actual practice content. Family practice, however, remains the most broadly oriented of the primary care specialties, emphasizing involvement in a wide variety of the related disciplines and in the special

skills required to apply these features effectively in everyday practice.

The National Ambulatory Medical Care Survey reverses the previous trend of evaluating the prevalence of disease after the fact (measuring causes of death or diagnosis upon discharge from a hospital) by evaluating the presenting complaints or symptoms at the onset of illness. This change in terminology, from that of standard discharge diagnoses to classifying problems in terms of the presenting complaint, is a formidable and difficult task, but one that should yield a large amount of new and valuable information. During 1972, visits to physicians averaged 4.5 office visits per person per year in the United States, indicating that ambulatory care is the largest component of the nation's health care delivery system.

TABLE 1–2. PER CENT DISTRIBUTION OF PATIENT VISITS TO PRIMARY PHYSICIANS°

Patient's Most Common Problem, Complaint, or Symptom	Totals	Family Physicians	General Internists	General Pediatricians
Progress visits—unspecified condition	7.3	7.4	8.2	5.5
Other problems, NEC†	6.3	6.5	7.8	3.6
Throat soreness	4.6	4.8	1.5	6.5
Cough	4.0	3.8	2.6	1.8
Pain, etc., in lower extremity	3.9	4.3	4.8	1.1
General medical examination	3.2	2.0	2.5	10.6
Pain, etc., in region of back	3.2	3.7	3.6	—
Cold	3.1	3.3	1.8	3.2
Progress visits—specified condition	3.0	2.9	3.5	3.2
Pain, etc., in upper extremity	2.9	3.2	2.7	1.0
Abdominal pain	2.8	2.8	3.9	1.8
Physical examination	2.7	3.1	1.3	1.6
Visit for medication	2.7	2.6	1.7	4.2
Well-baby examination	2.6	0.9	—	14.6
Fatigue	2.4	2.7	3.2	0.1
Fever	2.4	1.5	0.4	9.5
Pregnancy examination	2.3	3.0	0.5	0.2
Pain in chest	2.3	2.2	4.8	0.2
Headache	2.1	2.3	3.0	0.4
Allergic skin reaction	1.7	1.5	1.3	2.9
None	1.6	1.6	2.5	0.5
Pain, etc., of face, neck	1.5	1.7	1.4	0.9
Earache	1.5	1.0	0.9	4.4
Wounds	1.5	1.8	0.7	0.9
Hypertension	1.4	1.6	1.9	—
Vertigo	1.4	1.6	1.7	0.3
Shortness of breath	1.1	1.0	2.8	0.2
Gynecologic examination	0.9	1.2	0.4	0.2
Nasal congestion	0.7	0.5	0.5	1.6
Skin irritations, NEC†	0.7	0.8	0.6	0.5
Eye dysfunction	—	0.1	0.3	—
Weight gain	—	0.2	0.2	—

°Per cent distribution of patient visits to primary physicians classified by the patient's most common problem, complaint, or symptom (United States—from May, 1973, to April, 1974). (From the Department of Health, Education and Welfare, National Ambulatory Medical Care Survey, May, 1973, to April, 1974.)

†Not elsewhere classified.

REFERENCES

1. AAFP Report. Official Definition of Family Practice and Family Physician. AAFP Reporter, 2:10, 1975.
2. Balint, M.: The Doctor, His Patient and the Illness. New York, Pitman Publishing Corp., 1964.
3. Bryan, J. E.: The Role of the Family Physician in America's Developing Medical Care Program. St. Louis, Warren H. Green, Inc., 1968.
4. Byrne, P. S., and Long, B. E.: Learning to Care: Person to Person. Edinburgh and London, Churchill Livingstone, 1973.
5. Canfield, P. R.: Family medicine: an historical perspective. J. Med. Educ., 51:904, 1976.
6. Charney, E., Bynum, R., Eldridge, D., et al.: How well do patients take oral penicillin? Pediatrics, 40:188, 1967.
7. Clute, K. F.: The General Practitioner. Toronto, University of Toronto Press, 1963.
8. Draper, P., and Smits, H. L.: The primary-care practitioner: specialist or jack-of-all-trades. N. Engl. J. Med., 293:903, 1975.
8a. Dunphy, J. E.: Responsibility and authority in American surgery. Bull. Amer. Coll. Surg., 49:9, 1964.
9. Geyman, J. P.: The Modern Family Doctor and Changing Medical Practice. New York, Meredith Corp., 1971.
10. Good, J. M.: Family Practice—An Emerging Specialty. Master's thesis, Program in Hospital and Health Administration, University of Iowa, May, 1971.
11. Heagerty, M. D., Robertson, L. S., Kosa, J., et al.: Some comparative costs in comprehensive versus fragmented pediatric care. Pediatrics, 46:496, 1970.
12. Maimonides, M.: Treatise on Asthma. Vol 1. In The Medical Writings of Moses Maimonides. Philadelphia, J. B. Lippincott Co., 1963.
13. Marinker, J.: The Doctor and His Patient. Leicester, Leicester University Press, 1975.
14. Maultsby, M. C.: Written homework for the patient with an emotional crisis. Am. Fam. Physician, 4:69, 1971.
15. McFarlane, A. H., O'Connell, B. P., and Hay, J.: Demand-for-care model: its use in program planning for primary physician education. J. Med. Educ., 46:436, 1971.
16. McWhinney, I.: The foundations of family medicine. Can. Fam. Physician, April, 1969.
17. Meeting the Challenge of Family Practice. Report of the Ad Hoc Committee on Education for Family Practice of the Council on Medical Education of the American Medical Association (Willard Committee), September, 1966.
18. National Center for Health Statistics: National Ambulatory Care Survey: Background and Methodology, United States. Vital and Health Statistics, Series 2, No. 61. DHEW Pub. No. (HRA) 74–1335. Health Resources Administration. Washington, D.C., U.S. Government Printing Office, March, 1974.
19. National Center for Health Statistics: National Ambulatory Medical Care Survey: Symptom Classification, United States. Vital and Health Statistics, Series 2, No. 63. DHEW Pub. No. (HRA) 74–1337. Health Resources Administration. Washington, D.C., U.S. Government Printing Office, May, 1974.
20. Osler, W.: Aequanimitas with Other Addresses. 3rd Ed. Philadelphia, The Blakiston Co., 1932.
21. Peabody, F. W.: Doctor and Patient. New York, The Macmillan Co., 1930.
22. Pellegrino, E. D.: The generalist function in medicine. J.A.M.A., 198:541, 1966.
23. Robinson, G. C.: The Patient as a Person. New York, The Commonwealth Fund, 1939.
24. Standish, S., Jr., Bennett, B. M., White, K., et al.: Why Patients See Doctors. Seattle, University of Washington Press, 1955.
25. The Graduate Education of Physicians. Report of the Citizens' Commission on Graduate Medical Education, American Medical Association (Millis Commission), August, 1966.
26. Tumulty, P. A.: The Effective Clinician: His Methods and Approach to Diagnosis and Care. Philadelphia, W. B. Saunders Co., 1973.
27. White, K. L., Williams, F., and Greenberg, B.: Ecology of medical care. N. Engl. J. Med., 265:885, 1961.
28. Wolfe, S., and Badgley, R. F.: The family doctor. The Milbank Memorial Fund Quarterly, Vol. I, No. 2, April, 1972.

Chapter 2

FAMILY STRUCTURE AND FUNCTION *

by DONALD C. RANSOM,
and ROBERT J. MASSAD

The special nature of family practice is demonstrated by activity in two related dimensions. The first concerns the uniqueness of the type of practice: the synthesis and application of a wide variety of knowledge and skills in the treatment of a broad range of problems among all age groups over long spans of time. The second dimension concerns the target unit of that practice: persons *plus* the relevant social and physical environments that constitute their immediate ecologic reality. We are concerned in this chapter with the second of these dimensions, specifically with the family both as an environment for those who compose it and as a biosocial unit of health in its own right.

THE MEANING OF "FAMILY" IN FAMILY PRACTICE

Because of the nature of their practice and the types of problems they encounter, family physicians are concerned with the relationship of life in small groups to health, illness, and care. Diagnosis and intervention often occur at the level of interaction among individuals in families and between the family and its surrounding environment. The interactional perspective contained in this approach is the heart of family practice and constitutes a major con-

tribution to health care. It signifies the participation of family practice in the recent medical movement toward continually expanding the focus of attention from the cell to the organ system to the "whole patient," to the patient in his ecologic context. When the problems of specialty and geographic maldistribution have been solved, the enduring contribution of family physicians will be to the understanding and management of health problems that cannot be handled successfully through the narrow focus on the individual, isolated from the pattern of recurrent interpersonal situations that determines and transforms health.

Because of the importance that we place on the interactional view, it is our suggestion that it is not the genetic family or the family as a legal entity or institution that is crucial to family practice but "family" as a type of human relatedness and as a metaphor for primary, self-regulating social systems. This usage purposefully stretches the everyday meaning of the word *family*. In the present context, we feel it is advantageous to do so for both practical and conceptual reasons. On the practical side, the term *family* in the specialty designation *family practice* is too confining in its ordinary application. There is no question that marriage and the family are formal institutions embodying types of affiliations that are different from and, in most cases, more important than other forms of human associations. Yet people are also involved in other intimate relationships, holding memberships in other groups that can rival the literal family in intensity, duration, satisfaction of needs, and the impact of social interaction on the health of the participants. The family physician takes care of all kinds

*We would like to acknowledge the assistance of Elaine Bauserman, Roberta Berg, John Dervin, Patricia Dervin, and Jonathon Rodnick, who read a draft of this chapter and provided valuable comments and corrections that were incorporated into the present version.

of people in all kinds of situations, and this scope should not be hampered by our terminology. Therefore, we shall be using the term *family* to stand for any group of intimates with a history and a future.

On the conceptual side, because of the wide range of interpersonal situations encountered in practice, it follows that the family physician requires a structural model that is not invalidated by variations in family size, composition, or subculture or dependent upon households, bloodlines, or legal ties. Ideally, the model would also provide a basis for conceptualizing change and stability, sources of conflict and disturbance, and strategies of intervention. In short, family practice calls for a framework for thinking about people and contexts that relates productively to its daily activities, yet is abstract enough to bear up under universal application. This is the basis for defining the family in terms of a special type of relationship rather than a particular entity.

To this point, we have been discussing people and families in ecologic terms, i.e., in terms of their relationships. This type of framework suggests a concern with communication, self-regulation, feedback, and purposive change. These, in turn, are characteristics of a general system, and the general systems model is the one we propose as most relevant to family practice as a form of patient care and most heuristic for family medicine as an intellectual discipline.

This chapter, therefore, will undertake the single purpose of describing a systems approach to the general subject of family structure and function. The discussion unfolds in two parts. The first supplies an introduction to family systems theory in formal terms. The aim is to provide an abstract framework capable of being applied to any primary group or social network that may be significant in health, illness, and care. The second part moves from a focus on structure to a discussion of functions and system changes over time. Turning points in system development are illustrated with clinical material. Here we limit our focus to the most frequently acknowledged example of our universal designation of the term *family*—the *nuclear family* made up of a man and a woman, related through marriage, together with their children.

THE FAMILY AS A SYSTEM

While the modern technical language of systems theory may seem strange to many physicians, the basic logic underlying this approach is one that has formed the base of much of medical science for some time. Ruesch[29] traces the developing importance of a working notion of systems in medicine since the late 19th century. He points out that in the extreme mechanistic emphasis of the 18th and early 19th centuries the causal chains for which scientists searched were, almost without exception, lineal, branching, or converging. This meant that a chain of events spaced in time or a set of conditions patterned in space were linked together to build a theory of causality, and what preceded was thought to determine completely what followed.

Profound changes began to occur, however, when what we now call "systems" became perceptible through recognizing that they demonstrated characteristics of self-correction and were capable of predictive and adaptive responses. The behavior of such systems closely resembled the behavior of organisms, and this isomorphism was anticipated by physiologists such as Claude Bernard, who as early as 1860 introduced the term *milieu interne*.[6] The concept of internal environment and its consistency exerted a guiding influence on physiologists through the first quarter of this century, gaining its full and official recognition in medicine with Cannon's formulation of circular, self-corrective homeostatic mechanisms.[11-12]

An example of homeostatic maintenance familiar to all physicians is homeothermy. Von Bertalanffy[7] explains that according to Van't Hoff's rule of physical chemistry, a decrease in temperature leads to slowing of the rate of chemical reactions, as it does in ordinary physicochemical systems and also in poikilothermic animals. In warm-blooded animals, however, it leads to the opposite effect, triggering an increase in metabolic rate, with the result that the temperature of the body in *Homo sapiens*, for example, is maintained constantly at approximately 37° C. This is accomplished through a feedback circuit in which cooling stimulates thermogenic centers in the central nervous system that, in turn, inform heat-producing mechanisms throughout the body to "turn on." Similar feedback patterns are found in a great variety of physiologic processes.

Today, physicians utilize the basic concepts of systems theory as a scientific model to explain many bodily processes. What we are attempting here is simply to make that often implicit model more explicit, to extend it from the level of relations of elements in bodily interaction to the level of relations among elements in social interaction, and to provide a framework for describing how these two levels themselves can be viewed as a larger system connected through subsystemic relations. The logic and structure of the theory are the same in all three applications.

Richardson was the first to apply what was then the beginnings of a general system–communication model to the family and health in *Patients Have Families,* published in 1945.[28] His work anticipated important developments to come. Like other examples in the history of science in which an idea originating in one dimension provides the means for dramatic breakthroughs when applied to another, the application of the system model to the study of the family provided the means for the most important conceptual and therapeutic developments in that field in the past 20 years. The discussion of the family as a general system that follows draws on a wide range of sources, the most important of which are contained in the references at the end of the chapter.

WHAT IS A SYSTEM?

In either the most simple or the most complex form, a system is a special kind of pattern or shape in which attention is focused on the relationships of the component elements and not on the elements alone. This viewpoint stresses the importance of a nonmaterial element, *organization,* per se. In complex systems, the parts become transformed to take on properties that they owe specifically to being components of a larger whole—to being organized in a particular way.

Hall and Fagen define a system as "a set of objects together with relationships between the objects and between their attributes."[16] Applying this definition to a family, the *objects* are the components of the

system and can be organized into a number of shifting, dynamic units: persons, pairs of persons (mother and father as a marital subsystem), generations (the parents or the children), sex subgroupings (males differentiated from females), or any other differentiable parts that, at any given time, may be organized within the whole. The *attributes* of the family system are the properties of the objects, in particular their communicational value and their capacity to make a difference in the behavior of the system. The *relationships* are the patterns of organized behavior that make the family what it is. Kantor and Lehr[18] stress that these patterns of organized behavior are always purposive and move toward system goals. In this sense family relationships are always strategic, although the goals and strategy are not always apparent.

CLOSED AND OPEN SYSTEMS

Systems vary in the degree of complexity of their organization and can be categorized in ascending levels according to their mode of behavior.[8] Most simply they are described as either *closed* or *open,* with open systems being further divided into *closed-loop* and *open-looped* (fully-open) types.

A closed system is defined by Wilden as one "which, in reality or by definition, is not in an essential relation of feedback to an environment."[38] The relation between the momentum of a projectile and the force of gravity or the relations among billiard balls on a table are examples of a closed system. Any modifying influences that may exist between the components are strictly internal and have nothing to do with the surrounding environment. An open system, in contrast, maintains an essential relationship of feedback with its environment that allows for self-regulation through internal processing of information exchanged with that environment. A simple example is the thermostat wired to a furnace. The behavior of a guided missile is another example in which the predetermined goal (the target area) is reached through internal processing of information (speed, direction, and so forth) in order to institute midoperation corrections of its course. Neither the thermostat nor the guided missile, however, is a fully-open system; both are *closed-loop,* mechanical feedback systems that depend entirely on the "environment" to predetermine the behavior of the sytem, i.e., to set the thermostat or to select the missile's target. *Open-looped systems*, in contrast, are capable of using new information to change their internal structure, their relationship with the environment, and, in varying degrees, the environment itself.

To convey the significance of thinking about the family in these terms, it is necessary to describe three widely accepted characteristics of *fully-open systems: wholeness, self-regulation through feedback*, and *equifinality*.

Wholeness

A system does not behave as an aggregate of independent elements but as a unified, irreducible whole that functions as a whole by virtue of the interdependence of its parts. Watzlawick, Beavin, and Jackson[35] emphasize the *emergent quality* that arises when two or more elements form the type of relationship that results in achieving a new whole. When two parts of hydrogen combine (communicate) with one part of oxygen, the result is water, a new whole that has qualities that transcend the properties of its constituents. A family is an emergent whole that results from the relationship of persons who form a system that can never be known from knowledge of only the individuals who compose it.

The aim of viewing the family in this way is not to draw hazy analogies; it is to establish principles and to suggest forms of intervention that derive from the systems perspective. Just as we gain a deeper understanding of how an organism performs an act if we can comprehend how the components of the act are integrated within that organism, we gain a deeper understanding of how a family acts if we look inside it, examining how the behavior of each member combines with the behavior of all the other members to create an emergent reality attributable to the family as a whole.

Self-regulation Through Feedback

Within the constraints imposed by its environment on the one side and by its internal components on the other, a family system, in common with all open systems, is self-regulated through feedback.

Watzlawick, Beavin, and Jackson[35] illustrated the meaning of feedback and the difference between a circular model of causality and a lineal one. If a man out for a walk kicks a pebble, energy is transferred from the foot to the pebble; the latter will be displaced and will eventually come to rest in a position fully determined by such factors as the amount of energy transferred, the shape and mass of the pebble, and the nature of the surface on which it rolls. If, on the other hand, the man kicks a dog, the dog may jump back and bite him. In this case, the relation between the kick and the bite is of a *different order* from the relation between the kick and the rolling pebble. The dog takes the energy for its response not from the kick but from its own metabolism. What makes the difference in this transaction is not the transfer of energy but the transfer of *information*. The kick is a piece of behavior that communicates something to the dog about its relationship to the man, and to this the dog responds with a sequential piece of behavior that, in turn, communicates modifying information. The kick and the bite are *feedback* that become incorporated into the ongoing interaction, influencing its future direction. The system is circular and, for that moment, the dog and the man can be viewed as a fully-open system that is capable of regulating its relationship through the processing of feedback. Families are much more complex systems that exhibit the same characteristic

Systems maintain a range of stability among their internal relations and between themselves and their environment, and the concept of *feedback* refers to the mode of regulation. *Morphostasis* (homeostasis) is supported through "negative feedback" or "constancy feedback loops," whereas *morphogenesis* is achieved through "positive feedback" or "variety feedback loops." There are subvarieties of each type, but it is sufficient for our purposes simply to state here that in morphostasis deviations from the norm are corrected to ensure the conservation of the system in its present form, whereas in morphogenesis deviations are amplified in order to "break the system loose" from one pattern to create another. Both types of feedback are essential for the survival of a family system, whereas too much of either can lead to disordered or distressed behavior in one of the members or to collapse of the family itself.

The observation that open systems be-have as if they are "rule governed" in order to maintain structural and functional stabil-ity led Don Jackson to propose a model of family interaction built around the concept of *family homeostasis*.[17] Jackson repeatedly observed that the families of psychiatric patients often demonstrated significant repercussions when their patient-member improved: marital tensions increased, some-one became depressed or suicidal, psy-chosomatic attacks occurred, and so on. He postulated that "these behaviors and perhaps therefore the patient's illness as well were 'homeostatic mechanisms,' operating to bring the disturbed system back into its delicate balance."[35]

In the time since Jackson's work, we have come to view such a process in a broader context, seeing the role of the pa-tient's symptomatic behavior in both its family-conserving and family-changing functions and as a statement of that per-son's relation to the group. An adolescent's spells of sickness or repeated accidents can serve both as a way to deflect attention from marital discord between his parents onto himself, pulling them together to deal with him, and as a signal that the family is inadequately organized to deal with his needs and must change. In either meaning, the important consideration is that an indi-vidual's behavior, when considered in the context of the family system, can be seen as serving a *function* for the whole. This perspective provides a different view of the problem than if it were examined only as a product of a person or an organism. The *meaning* of the symptom changes as we ad-just the level of organization within which we perceive it.

Having discussed the importance of feedback and the processes of morphostasis and morphogenesis as the means of main-taining and changing the system over time, we are still without an explanation for the specific forms or patterns of organization a system may exhibit. This explanation is best given within a discussion of the last of our universal properties of open systems, *equifinality*.

Equifinality

In open, self-modifying systems, similar states of organization may be reached from different initial states, or by different routes, or both. The corollary concept, *mul-tifinality*, describes the reverse process whereby similar initial conditions, or routes, or both, may lead to dissimilar end states.[9] The immediate practical implica-tion of these properties of open systems for the family physician is that, in attempting to understand the meaning or relevance of family behavior, the historical aspects of a problem are not as central as the ongoing organization of the interaction. This does not mean that the early years of life are not crucial to later development. It simply challenges and offers an alternative to the idea that direct causal relations exist be-tween specific historical events and the later development of illness.

The principle of equifinality can be elu-cidated further by a description of the pat-terns of interaction called *symmetry* and *complementarity*.[1, 2] Remembering that sim-ilar end-states of a system may be reached by different, even opposite, routes, sym-metry and complementarity represent dif-ferent paths that may be followed to main-tain family homeostasis. Symmetrical relationships are those in which a given type of behavior elicits the response of be-havior of the same type, asserting equality. An example of symmetry might be found in the rivalry between an adolescent boy and his father in which escalating attempts by the father to control the son's behavior are met with by more strident demands for in-dependence. Complementary relationships are those in which the responsive behavior is of an opposite type to the initial behav-ior, indicating the acknowledgment of a difference between the system's members, as when a son assumes a dependent role vis-à-vis his father. Each of these opposite patterns of interlocking responses may serve to clarify the relationships among family members and, through repetition, maintain the system's structure.

It was noted previously that the principle of multifinality (the corollary of equifinal-ity) asserts that similar initial conditions or similar routes may lead to dissimilar end-states because the system is open, undergo-ing modification in response to environ-mental feedback. An illustration of multi-finality can be seen in the potential for pathology that exists when the patterns of symmetry and complementarity are ob-served to operate in a system without *re-straint*. In such a system, the repetition of symmetrical or complementary exchanges leads to progressive change that may eventually be destructive.* The potential pathologies—rigidity in complementarity and escalation in symmetry—are examples of *homeostatic impasse,* "the standard pattern of impasse into which the system lapses when it cannot find the means to abort or reverse its self-destroying tendencies."[18]

An example of the symmetrical homeostatic impasse familiar to many clinicians is the marital pattern in which the husband claims his drinking to excess is a response to his wife's nagging, whereas she claims that her increasing nagging is due to his drinking In this situation, it is instructive to note that neither of the participants denies the nature of his or her contribution to the conflict. Their difference arises in the attempt to place blame by labeling their individual behavior as caused by the wrong done by the spouse. Precisely where a participant or observer interrupts ("punctuates") what is, in systems theory, the circle in order to find a "cause" can be seen to be an arbitrary act serving pragmatic or political ends.

FAMILY SYSTEM AND SUBSYSTEM BOUNDARIES

In the discussion of wholeness, it was stated that an open system is not an aggregation of independent elements but a whole that functions through the interdependence of its parts. We can now go further and state that an open system is an *integrated hierarchy* of subsystems that may be composed of still smaller units. The "interdependent parts" of the "organized whole" may themselves be seen as systems, depending only upon the level at which one chooses to focus attention.

The arbitrariness of definition revealed in the choice of focal level indicates the pragmatic nature of deciding both the system composition and where to draw the distinction between system and subsystem. Such decisions are made in response to some felt need, usually in response to a problem at hand. The decision as to which is system and which is subsystem is left to the person dealing with the problem, and, hopefully, the choice will be one that facil-

itates a solution. Minuchin describes family subsystems in the following way:

The family system differentiates and carries out its functions through subsystems. Individuals are subsystems within a family. Dyads such as husband-wife or mother-child can be subsystems. Subsystems can be formed by generation, by sex, by interest, or by function.[23]

Defining subsystems in this way allows attention to be focused on family relations in a way that reveals sources of conflict. For example, symptoms can result from conflict at the *interface* of a subsystem's participation in two or more larger systems simultaneously Efforts to maintain relational integrity in more than one system at a time can lead to confusion, conflict, and potentially disordered behavior when maintaining constancies in relation to one system disrupts or precludes maintaining constancies in relation to the other(s). Thus, an "unresponsive" chronically ill grandparent may not represent a symptom of a disturbed family but rather the lack of integration between the family and the other systems to which the grandparent must perforce relate, such as medical and disability services.

When such sources of structural conflict are recognized, it is possible to map avenues of intervention that can lead to desired change. Any map, in turn, requires the drawing of *boundaries,* and all systems and subsystems can be thought of as bounded in a way that gives shape to the "whole" we have used as a system criterion. Minuchin[23] points out that the boundaries of a subsystem coincide with the explicit and implicit rules defining who participates, how, and around what activities. Again we find the basic units, the subsystems, being defined by relationships rather than by an inherent characteristic.

An example of how boundaries are derived from family rules is the following. A mother may tell an older child, "You aren't your brother's parent. If he's riding his bike in the street, tell me, and I will stop him." She is thus defining a parental subsystem in which children are not invited to participate, maintaining a clear separation of function and responsibility. A different subsystem relationship is defined by the creation of a "parental child" when the mother tells the children, "Until I return, Annie's in charge."[23]

---

*Bateson calls this process *schizmogenesis.*[1]

Perhaps more than anyone else, Minuchin and his colleagues at the Philadelphia Child Guidance Clinic have emphasized the importance of clear boundaries for proper family functioning They argue that the composition of subsystems is not nearly as significant as the *clarity* of subsystem boundaries. A subsystem that has the executive function of parents may include a grandparent, an uncle, or a parental child and may function quite well, for example, as long as the lines of responsibility and authority are clearly drawn. Their work illustrates how a structural concept, the clarity of family boundaries, can be a useful parameter of family functioning. They conceive of a continuum in which one pole is represented by families whose boundaries are diffuse and inconstant. These are labeled *enmeshed* families. At the other extreme are *disengaged* families in which the overly rigid boundaries prevent responsive change to alterations elsewhere in the system.

An illustration of the influence of the family on its members' responses when subsystem boundaries are enmeshed is provided by an experimental demonstration reported by Minuchin.[23] During a structured family interview designed for the purpose of measuring individual physiologic responses to family stress, blood samples were drawn from each member of a family in such a way that obtaining the samples did not interfere with ongoing interactions. The level of plasma-free fatty acids in the samples was later analyzed. (Free fatty acid [FFA] is a biochemical indicator of emotional arousal whose concentration is expected to rise within 5 to 15 minutes following emotional stress.) By comparing the FFA levels at different times during the interview, each family member's response to family stress was physiologically documented.

In the family presented, both children were diabetics. Dede, aged 17, had had diabetes for 3 years; her sister Violet, aged 12, had been diabetic since infancy.

Studies of the children's "physiological lability" showed that there was no obvious difference in their individual responsivity to stress. Yet these two children, with the same metabolic defect, having much of the same genetic endowment, and living in the same household with the same parents, presented very different clinical problems. Dede was a "superlabile diabetic";

that is, her diabetes was affected by psychosomatic problems. She was subject to bouts of ketoacidosis that did not respond to insulin administered at home. In three years, she had been admitted to the hospital for emergency treatment twenty-three times. Violet had some behavioral problems that her parents complained of, but her diabetes was under good medical control.

During the interview designed to measure the children's response to stress, lasting from 9 to 10 A.M., the parents were subjected to two different stress conditions, while the children watched them through a one-way mirror. Although the children could not take part in the conflict situation, their FFA levels rose as they observed their stressed parents. The cumulative impact of current psychological stress was powerful enough to cause marked physiological changes even in children not directly involved. At 10 o'clock the children were brought into the room with their parents. It then became clear that they played very different roles in this family. Dede was trapped between her parents. Each parent tried to get her support in the fight with the other parent, so that Dede could not respond to one parent's demands without seeming to side against the other. Violet's allegiance was not sought. She could therefore react to her parents' conflict without being caught in the middle.

The effects of these two roles can be seen in the FFA results. Both children showed significant increments during the interview, between 9 and 10, and even higher increments between 10 and 10:30, when they were with their parents. After the end of the interview at 10:30, however, Violet's FFA returned to baseline promptly. Dede's remained elevated for the next hour and a half.

In both spouses, the FFA levels increased from 9:30 to 10, indicating stress in the interspouse transactions. But their FFA decreased after the children had come in to the room and the spouses had assumed parental functions. In this family, interspouse conflict was reduced or detoured when the spouses assumed parental functions. The children functioned as conflict-detouring mechanisms. The price they paid is shown by both the increase in their FFA levels and Dede's inability to return to baseline. The interdependence between the individual and his family—the flow between "inside" and "outside"—is poignantly demonstrated in the experimental situation, in which behavioral events among family members can be measured in the bloodstream of other family members.[23] (Fig. 2–1).

FAMILY SYSTEM TRANSFORMATIONS

To this point we have been developing a view of the family as it exists at a given

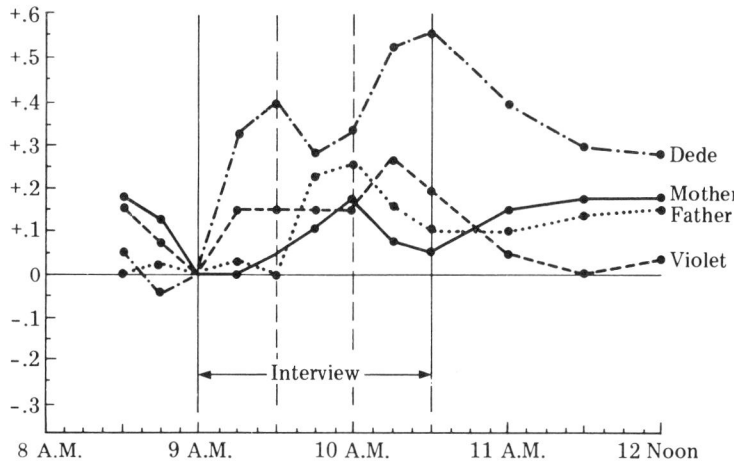

Figure 2–1. *The Collins family—change in free fatty acid. (From Minuchin, S.: Families and Family Therapy. Cambridge, Mass., Harvard University Press, 1974. p. 7.)*

moment in time. Families exist through time, however, and undergo various kinds of changes. For our purposes we can note three sources of family change: historical and societal, catastrophic, and developmental. Historical and societal sources include the effects on the family of external influences such as industrialization, urbanization, changing technology, economic recessions, mass media, and evolving cultural images of what it means to be a person or a family. Catastrophic changes can be historical events such as wars and depressions; natural events such as floods and earthquakes; or personal calamities such as severe illness or unexpected death, financial ruin, or any event that radically disorganizes the normal patterns of a family's life. Developmental sources of change are influenced by external events, but they also occur independently of such events. At pivotal points in its life, the family is confronted with reorganizing itself because of internal changes, such as the addition or loss of members, the growth and maturation of members, the involvement of family and family members with other persons and with outside systems, the changing values or needs of the members and the family as a group, and so on.

Furthermore, it is useful to think of changes within the family as being of two types (Logical Types, actually, in the sense developed by Whitehead and Russell in *Principia Mathematica*[37]): first-order

change and second-order change.[36] First-order change involves alterations that do not affect the organization of the family's basic structure and do not require qualitative change in the members' ways of relating to each other or to the outside world. Second-order change, in contrast, requires the alteration of family patterns, not simply in degree but in kind, leading to qualitative changes in family relationships. Changing from one way of being organized to another entails a break with past forms—a jump from one homeostatic range to another, a discontinuity. In this section, we are concerned with transformative developmental changes within the family.

It has been recognized for some time that families move through a series of phases throughout their life as a group. Several frameworks have been offered to highlight crucial transition points and to categorize the succession of changes into sets of stages.[13, 15, 26, 27, 34] Such frameworks usually describe a *family life cycle.* A discussion of this fruitful concept together with a presentation of the most widely known model of the family life cycle can be found in Chapter 3 of this text.

Haley's account of the work of Milton Erickson provides a discussion of the unfolding stages of family life in terms that are rooted in systems theory and designed for the clinician.[15] The framework presented is based on the view that families and other natural groups undergo developmental processes over time and that human distress appears when this process is disrupted. Such distress can take many forms, including psychiatric symptoms and physical illness. In Haley's formulation, "an anxiety attack in a mother when she gives birth to a child is an expression of the difficulty of that family in achieving the child-rearing stage of development."[15] When the system struggles to create second-order change, distress can result.

Haley discusses the milestones of family change in terms of the important themes arising at each stage, the kinds of tasks that must be accomplished within the group at different times, and the most likely vulnerabilities that arise at different points along the way. He encourages clinicians to be on the alert for problems that may appear as the family goes through the following changes in its structure: marriage and its consequences, childbirth and dealing with the young, middle-stage marriage difficulties, weaning parents from children, and retirement and old age.

To provide an example of the kinds of issues that might be expressed in the family physician's office as problems or symptoms of problems at critical *turning points* in a family's life, we shall focus for a moment on the early phase of the second stage just mentioned, childbirth and dealing with the young. In so doing, we shall limit our previously loose application of the term family to the most widely acknowledged example found in our culture, the nuclear family. The young couple who has successfully married and has learned to live together might find that childbirth raises new issues and unsettles old ones. For some, it becomes a period of distress that takes different forms:

The wife may become extremely upset during pregnancy, she may have mysterious physical problems that prevent carrying a child to term, or she may begin to behave in disturbed and bizarre ways immediately after the birth of the child. Alternatively, the husband or some member of the extended family may develop distress that coincides with the event of childbirth.[15]

Every couple has to cope with the changes brought on by adding a new member to the family system.

It is often not easy to pin down the "cause" of problems during this period because so many established patterns undergo revision with the arrival of a child. If the young couple has considered their marriage a trial, separation is now more complicated and difficult. Others, who thought they were permanently committed to each other, may suddenly feel trapped, recognizing for the first time how fragile the original contract can be. A husband may temporarily be unable to tolerate the felt responsibilities of rearing and supporting a child for the next two decades. A variety of symptoms can result, from accidents and spontaneous physiologic changes to anxiety and depression to abandonment.

Furthermore, the couple who has learned the intimate game of two is automatically entered in a triangle with the birth of a child. Former triangles with friends or members of the families on either side, perhaps successfully resolved, give way to a new kind of triangle embodying new issues. Jealousy of a new kind can develop when one spouse feels the other is more attracted to the child than to him or her. Conflicts in the relationship may now begin to be dealt with through the child. He may become a scapegoat or an excuse for staying together.

The birth of a child is a concrete manifestation of the joining of two families and creates grandparents, aunts, and uncles on both sides. A variety of new relationships must be worked out, a difficult chore that can sometimes result in distressing consequences for some members of the system. In addition, the possibility, or actuality, of a defective child can raise potential doubts about all branches of the family and can be used as ammunition in a family struggle.

Having babies may have been something that both parents looked forward to as a source of self-fulfillment. It is in the phase of caring for young children that a special problem can arise for women in today's world:

Having been educated in preparation for the day when they would be adults and able to make use of their special abilities, they find themselves cut off from adult life and living in a world of children again. In contrast, the husband is usually able to participate with adults in his working world and enjoy the children as an added dimension to his life. The wife who finds herself confined largely to conversation with children can also feel herself denigrated with the label of "only" housewife and mother. A longing for more participation in the adult world for which she was prepared can lead her to feeling discontented and envious of her husband's activities. The marriage can begin to erode as the wife demands more child-rearing help from her husband and more adult activities, while he feels that he is being burdened by wife and children and hampered in his work. Sometimes a mother will attempt to exaggerate the importance of child rearing by encouraging a child to have an emotional problem, to which she can then devote her attention.[15]

The task of the family physician in this case is to join in solving the problems of both members by helping the mother to disengage herself from the child and to find a more fulfilling life of her own.

The complexities and problems involved each time the family transforms itself are far too extensive to present here. The important point is not exactly how many stages should be differentiated and what they should be called, nor is it to develop a laundry list of pitfalls. It is rather to be found in the view contained by this approach, namely, that there are *predictable* developments in the life of natural groups; that these contain elements of change that are novel for the individuals involved, requiring both personal and interpersonal resolution of the issues arising at each turning point; and that both personal distress and illness and interpersonal disorder may be a sign that a family is having difficulty accomplishing the necessary change required for its development. This view adds another dimension to the systems model and provides the family physician with both an expanded framework within which to think about and treat any problem and a rationale for undertaking preventive interventions at critical points in a family's life.

FAMILY SYSTEM FUNCTIONS

In the section on system boundaries, we stated that an open system can be described as an "integrated hierarchy" of subsystems, which themselves may be composed of still smaller units. Koestler states, "The functional units on every level of the hierarchy are double-faced, as it were: they act as wholes when facing downwards, as parts when facing upwards."[19]

The "double-faced" image provides a useful entry into the discussion of family functions. Family functions serve dual sets of purposes, one external and the other internal. External functions are regulated through exchanges with societal units and serve societal and cultural needs. Internal functions relate to the family's members and to the family as a living system itself. Bell and Vogel[4] discuss a variety of external functions by focusing on the family as a subsystem in relation to larger societal systems described as the economy, the polity, the community, and the predominant value system. For example, one functional interchange between the family and the economy is the contribution of labor by the family group in exchange for rewards for services. At the very least, this requires that a family allocate a certain amount of time and performance capacity from at least one member to the economy.

Families carry on internal activities related to these external changes, and they perform internal functions for their own benefit as well. Every group differentiates itself into roles in order to divide labor and distribute power, authority, and leadership. Families also work out patterns of decision-making and norms for regulating their activities. Integration and solidarity must be developed. A family's relation to outsiders must be established, and multiple levels of boundary maintenance must be achieved. Some theorists emphasize the importance of maintaining appropriate generational distinctions and maintaining a marital and parental coalition in relation to the children, whereas others emphasize the importance of adhering to appropriate sex-linked roles. All of these activities—the "work" of family life—require internal differentiation and hierarchic integration among the members and, above all, a capacity to change when change is needed, while still maintaining an identity and structural integrity as a family.

Facing inward, a family performs functions that are vital to its members. These life-maintaining tasks reveal the biologic component in human primary groups more concretely than do the requirements of personality development and the sense of self that are dependent upon family relatedness. From the provision of basic physical needs, such as food, shelter, and clothing, to the subtleties of the ability and the desire to communicate with fellow human beings, the family plays an essential protecting and socializing function.

Pratt[25] has paid special attention to the specific functions families serve in relation to individual health. She documents the centrality of health concerns in family life by demonstrating how health matters are reflected significantly in the family's daily interactions, expenditure of time and energy, and commitment of resources. The family is legally responsible for providing for the needs of all members from the earliest health care and medical treatment to the appropriate disposal of the dead. Families also shape health habits and beliefs, recognize and label health problems, regulate access to professional care, and grant or withhold the sick role. In sum, the family's role in the physical health and psychologic well-being of its members is an ongoing system function that is central to the practice of medicine.

It is apparent from this discussion that family functions serve several "masters"—larger societal systems, its own subsystems, and itself The potential for conflict and disorder at the *interface* of any of these is ever present. This ecologic observation forms the basis for our concluding remarks.

CONCLUSION

As Gregory Bateson tells the story, the evolution of the horse from *Eohippus* was not a one-side adjustment to life on the grassy plain. Changes in the grassy plains were interdependent with the evolution of the teeth and hooves of horses and other ungulates. "Turf was the evolving response of the vegetation to the evolution of the horse."[3] Similarly, in looking at health and illness, it is essential to view any particular development as *part* of the ecologic subsystem here called "family" and not as the result of what remains after we have abstracted the individual from it. Just as in the evolution of the horse, we should not think of a person's state of health or well-being as an adaptation *to* life in society or in the family but as *maintaining a constancy in the relationship* between the person and his various environments.[3]

From this vantage point, the relevant ecosystem becomes the appropriate unit of concern for the health care provider. This

is necessary because the relata—i e., person and family, parents and children—undergo changes not only in relation to each other but also in relation to a number of other relevant ecologies in which they are embedded. Differential participation requires differential adaptation. The important observation is that problems of interest to the family physician often arise because the "logic" of personal, marital, or parental adaptation is a different "logic" from that of the survival of the family or the community. The pathologies of system process "arise precisely because the constancy and survival of some larger system is maintained by changes in the constituent subsystem"[3] and because the constituent subsystems cannot accommodate to all larger system and subsystem compatriots at the same time.

In families each subsystem participates simultaneously in other systems and is continuously involved in efforts to maintain sufficient constancy with them so that the relevant relationships may survive. The "strategies" that result often produce unforeseen and unintended consequences that create conflict or disorder at some nodal point in the total process. Of importance to the family physician is the ecologic law (as expressed by Bateson) that any adaptive change in one part of the family, if uncorrected by some change in the others, will always jeopardize the relationship between them. This conceptual frame proposes a new way to think about the family and medical practice. It provides a basis for the development of what could be the special province of family practice: the relationship of life in families to health, illness, and care.

REFERENCES

1. Bateson, G.: Culture contact and schizmogenesis. Man, 35:178, 1935.
2. Bateson, G.: Naven (1936), 2nd ed. Stanford, Cal., Stanford University Press, 1958.
3. Bateson, G.: Steps to an Ecology of Mind. New York, Ballantine Books, Inc., 1972.
4. Bell, N. W., and Vogel, E. F. (eds.): A Modern Introduction to the Family, rev. ed. New York, The Free Press, 1968.
5. Bernard, C.: An Introduction to the Study of Experimental Medicine. Greene, H. C. (trans.), New York, Collier Books, 1961.
6. Bernard, C.: Lecons sur les Phénomènes de la Vie aux Animaux et aux Vegetaux. Paris, Bailliere, Publisher, 1878.

7. Bertalanffy, L. von: General system theory—a critical review. General Systems, 7:1, 1962.
8. Boulding, K. E.: General systems theory—the skeleton of science. Management Science, 2:197, 1956.
9. Buckley, W.: Sociology and Modern Systems Theory. Englewood Cliffs, N.J. Prentice-Hall, Inc., 1967.
10 Buckley, W. (ed.): Modern Systems Research for the Behavioral Scientist. Chicago, Aldine Publishing Co., 1968.
11. Cannon, W. B.: Bodily Changes in Pain, Hunger, Fear and Rage. New York, Appleton-Century-Crofts, 1929.
12. Cannon, W. B.: The Wisdom of the Body. New York, W. W. Norton & Co., Inc , 1932.
13. Duvall, E.: Family Development, 4th ed. Philadelphia, J. B. Lippincott Co., 1971.
14. Gray, W., Duhl, F., and Rizzo, N. (eds.): General Systems Theory and Psychiatry. Boston, Little, Brown & Co., 1969.
15. Haley, J.: Uncommon Therapy: The Psychiatric Techniques of Milton H. Erickson, M. D. New York, Ballantine Books, Inc., 1973.
16. Hall, A. D., and Fagen, R. E.: Definition of a system. General Systems, 1:18, 1956.
17. Jackson, D. D.: The question of family homeostasis. Psychiatr. Q. (Suppl.), 31(part I):79, 1957.
18. Kantor, D., and Lehr, W.: Inside the Family. San Francisco, Jossey-Bass Inc., Publishers, 1975.
19. Koestler, A.: The Act of Creation. New York, The Macmillan Co., 1964.
20. Lennard, H. L., and Bernstein, A.: Patterns in Human Interaction: An Introduction to Clinical Sociology. San Francisco, Jossey-Bass Inc., Publishers, 1969.
21. Lewis, J. M., Beavers, W. R., Gossett, J. T., et al.: No Single Thread: Psychological Health in Family Systems. New York, Brunner/Mazel Inc., 1976.
22. Miller, J. G.: Living systems: basic concepts; structure and process; cross-level hypotheses. Behav. Sci., 10:193, 337, 380, 1971.
23. Minuchin, S.: Families and Family Therapy. Cambridge, Mass., Harvard University Press, 1974.
24. Minuchin, S., Baker, L., Rosman, B. L., et al.: A conceptual model of psychosomatic illness in children. Arch. Gen. Psychiatry, 32:1031, 1975.
25. Pratt, L.: Family Structure and Effective Health Behavior. Boston, Houghton Mifflin Co., 1976.
26. Rapoport, R.: Normal crises, family structure and mental health. Fam. Proc., 2:68, 1963.
27. Rapoport, R., and Rapoport, R. N.: New light on the honeymoon Hum. Rel., 17:33, 1964.
28. Richardson, H. B.: Patients Have Families. New York, Commonwealth Fund, 1945.
29. Ruesch, J., and Bateson, G.: Communication: The Social Matrix of Psychiatry. New York, W. W. Norton & Co., Inc., 1951.
30 Shands, H. C.: Semiotic Approaches to Psychiatry. The Hague, Mouton, 1970
31. Shands, H. C.: The War With Words: Structure and Transcendence. The Hague, Mouton, 1971.
32. Sluzki, C. E., and Ransom, D. C. (eds.): Double Bind: The Foundation of the Communicational Approach to the Family. New York, Grune & Stratton, 1976.
33. Sluzki, C. E., and Beavin, J.: Symmetry and complementarity: an operational definition and a typology of dyads. In Watzlawick, P., and Weakland, J. H. (eds.): The Interactional View. New York, W. W. Norton & Co., Inc., 1977.
34. Susser, M. W., and Watson, W.: Sociology in Medicine. London, Oxford University Press, 1971.
35. Watzlawick, P., Beavin, J., and Jackson, D. D.: Pragmatics of Human Communication. New York, W. W. Norton & Co., Inc., 1967.
36. Watzlawick, P., Weakland, J., and Tisch, R.: Change: Principles of Problem Formation and Problem Resolution. New York, W. W. Norton & Co., Inc., 1974.
37. Whitehead, A. N., and Russell, B.: Principia Mathematica, Vol. I. 2nd ed. Cambridge, Cambridge University Press, 1910.
38. Wilden, A.: System and Structure: Essays in Communication and Exchange. London, Tavistock Publications, Ltd., 1972.

Chapter 3

FAMILY DYNAMICS

by CYRIL WORBY, and ROY GERARD

Your children are not your children. They are the sons and daughters of Life's longing for itself. They come through you but not from you, and though they are with you, yet they belong not to you. You may give them your love but not your thoughts. For they have their own thoughts. You may house their bodies but not their souls, for their souls dwell in the house of tomorrow, which you cannot visit, not even in your dreams. You may strive to be like them, but seek not to make them like you. For life goes not backward nor tarries with yesterday. You are the bows from which your children as living arrows are sent forth. The archer sees the mark upon the path of the infinite, and He bends you with His might that His arrows may go swift and far. Let your bending in the archer's hand be for gladness; for even as He loves the arrow that flies, so He loves also the bow that is stable.

Kahlil Gibran The Prophet

INTRODUCTION

Whether in solo, group, or team practice, the contemporary family physician is increasingly concerned with the family as the unit of treatment. There are several reasons for this emphasis on the family: (1) illness or dysfunction in one family member strikingly alters relationships among all members of the family, (2) the recovery process from illness is itself affected by the nature of intrafamilial relationships, and (3) the goals of prevention and early detection of illness are more fully realized through a family perspective.

For example, consider the following situation: A 20 year old married woman was a junior at a state university. She presented herself 3 months pregnant to the family practice clinic in town. Neither she nor her husband, also a student, "intended" the pregnancy at this time. They had had some arguments about whose "fault" it was. They considered an abortion for a while and argued about it a great deal, he being more in favor of the procedure than she. Finally, they decided against it. About the sixth

month of pregnancy she experienced considerable nausea and vomiting. Her husband resented her staying in bed so much. He felt neglected, resented his wife's preoccupation with her symptoms, and wondered what would happen to him and his needs when the baby was born. His wife's mother, who lived an hour away, said to her daughter, "Come stay with us. You need us now. We'll take good care of you, just like we did with your sister when she was pregnant." The daughter declined the invitation. However, the fact that it was made led to bitterness between husband and mother-in-law. The baby was born prematurely, and there was concern about his viability. After a month's hospitalization in the neonatal unit, the infant was brought home. The couple told the physician that they feel awkward with the boy. The wife said, "It's funny, but I can't believe he is ours. I'd rather let my mother take care of him."

Let us stop here and consider a number of issues. Who is the patient? Is it the infant, mother, father, or all of them? If the family is the unit of treatment, is the grandmother to be included? And what of the grandfather, who has remained peripheral and quietly sullen? Do we have concepts and skills to bear on this complex yet not uncommon situation?

As we consider the interaction of the complex variables in the example just cited, we become aware that creating a false dichotomy between an individual and a family orientation will not serve us well. The choice is not between these two orientations. Each has something of value to offer in comprehending the total situation. Rather, the task is to evaluate the relative contributions of each perspective to the specific situations at hand.

OBJECTIVES

The aim of this chapter is to provide the family physician with insights into processes underlying key aspects of family functioning so as to enhance the delivery of comprehensive, family-oriented health care. We will not review exhaustively the burgeoning family process literature for pragmatic reasons, believing that the physician's purpose will be served better by a thorough discussion of several major themes rather than by a superficial discussion of many. Likewise, we will place more emphasis on the understanding of family phenomena and less on treatment techniques aimed at altering a family's functioning.

THE SCOPE OF FAMILY DYNAMICS

Families organize themselves in ways that enable them to carry out a number of crucial societal functions. For example, marriage as a social institution provides, among other things, for sanctioned regular access to a sexual partner; and the family, which includes spouses and children, provides a microenvironment for the rearing and socialization of the children. Yet families exist in particular historical periods; and within each historical period they are embedded in larger sociopolitical structures, such as nations, ethnic groups, religious affiliations, and geographic regions. Consequently, the family unit is vulnerable to the ever-shifting environment surrounding it and evolves ways of both adapting to

and altering this changing environment. A contemporary example of such change is the greater prevalence of couples living together outside of marriage and the increasing number of single parent family units. Thus, the family physician must know something of the social, political, and economic forces of his time and have some sense of the impact these forces have on the family unit. In the interests of maintaining our focus, we can do no more than call attention to the importance of the larger social order within which families exist and function.

Our central concern will be with the interior workings of families. How does this group of persons in special relationship with one another go about maximizing individual and family satisfaction of the most basic human needs? In what areas are they likely to experience difficulties, and how might these difficulties manifest themselves in the family practice setting? We will use the term *family dynamics* to denote those regular modes of interactive behavior engaged in by the family group members as a whole to maximize, on the one hand, such interior states of well-being as a sense of safety and predictability, the feeling of pleasure and satisfaction, the sense of meaningfulness and competence, and the clarity of one's uniqueness as a person separate from others; and to minimize, on the other hand, such interior states of distress as panic and anxiety, helplessness and hopelessness, unfulfillment and unworthiness, and sadness and despair.

FAMILY LIFE CYCLE AND EXTENDED FAMILY PERSPECTIVES

Two further concepts will be useful in understanding family dynamics, the family life cycle and the extended family perspective. The family life cycle concept views the family as having a beginning and an end, with a series of sequential stages in between. Each stage is characterized by a number of tasks that must be confronted and worked out in a reasonably satisfactory way. For example, the family cited earlier was in that stage requiring the integration of a third member, a child, into a two-member system of adults.

The other important concept may be

called the extended family perspective. This perspective takes into account a vertical component—the interaction of at least three generations within a family, and a lateral component—the influence of siblings within each generation. Again, consider the example of the couple. Although the daughter had physically separated from her family of origin and, through marriage, formed a new family, old ties were intensified with her parents as a consequence of pregnancy and birth of a son. The family physician in this situation would be more helpful to the couple and infant if he understood something about the three generational relationship, in this case between grandparents, parents, and child. The physician may also need to know something about the lateral component, the sister and her family, in view of the mother's statement, "We'll take good care of you, just like we did with your sister when she was pregnant."

In our discussion thus far we have been guided by a systems view of the family: the family as a system of reciprocal interlocking relationships in which the individual family members continually affect one another by their interactive behaviors. The family system also has subsystems, such as the parental subsystem, the marital subsystem, and the sibling subsystem. In the earlier example, the birth of a son and the grandmother's wish for greater involvement with her daughter led to a problem that affected all of the parties in the relationship.

As we proceed, we will look at the roles the individuals occupy in the family and attend to the "fit" and interchangeability among these roles. We will look at the interior context within which family transactions take place: the tasks inherent in a particular stage of the family life cycle. We will examine important classes of component behaviors that, when taken in their totality, give a family distinctiveness—its "personality." Such behaviors might include the style of communicating within a family; the style of managing feelings; the rules and mechanisms for defining interpersonal closeness and distance between family members; and the style and mechanisms utilized to resolve differences between family members, both intragenerational differences, as might be the case

between parents, and intergenerational differences, as might be the case between parents and children.

The concept of the family life cycle assumes that a new family begins with a man and woman entering into a committed relationship, most usually marriage; that this relationship proceeds for a variable period of time, from months to decades; that children will be a part of most such unions; and that these children will eventually leave the family and lead independent lives, which may include formation of new families, thus repeating the process described.

This trajectory of the family over time may be divided into phases, and within each phase a number of central tasks or issues may be identified that the family unit must address and cope with as best as it can.

How to divide the family life cycle into phases and the selection of tasks most central to a given phase are to some degree arbitrary, since the family is in a continual process of change. Furthermore, certain tasks are addressed throughout the whole of the life cycle, albeit in changing form and intensity. Nevertheless, nodal points of transition do appear, where what is ahead is significantly different either quantitatively or qualitatively from what has gone before.

We will discuss seven sequential phases of family life: (1) early marriage: formation of the family, (2) pregnancy and birth of first child, (3) individuation of first child, (4) emerging sexuality of first child, (5) early and middle school years, (6) adolescence of first child, and (7) parents alone. It will be evident that we rely largely on the child's progressive development as the central stimulus for major reciprocal readjustments within the family. Although this is an oversimplification that excludes childless couples, less conventional arrangements such as same sexed couples, and communal groups not composed of nuclear families, the scheme does address the contemporary modal American family. Following a discussion of the seven sequential phases, we will comment on a number of non–stage-specific crises, such as divorce, serious illness, and death, all of which significantly alter the dynamics of family relationships.

EARLY MARRIAGE: FORMATION OF THE FAMILY

One of the important early tasks in this phase is for each partner to attain sufficient psychologic autonomy from his or her family of origin. This task is not the son's or daughter's alone; it involves a reciprocal letting go and redefinition of the relationship between parent and child. For the young adult, this implies the attainment of a reasonably coherent sense of self, an inner certainty that one can survive as a separate person, and an ability to be by oneself without a feeling of incompleteness and panic. For the parent, the task is to confirm this development despite the sense of loss experienced.

The attainment of a sufficient sense of autonomy as a separate person is an essential prerequisite to the second task for the couple: to enhance the development of genuine mutuality in their relationship with one another. The less one person feels reasonably whole and distinct, the more that person may be driven to merge with the other to complete what is felt as missing in oneself. Rage at oneself and at the other on whom one so desperately depends is a frequent consequence. What follows is an excerpt from a family interview in which a 19 year old man experienced disorganizing panic following a move away from home. He was able to separate from his parents physically; however, he was psychologically unprepared for the task. We have quoted a number of his remarks during the interview, as he tried to articulate how he saw himself in relation to others.

I've gotten a lot of enjoyment out of hearing my father talk. Because, it was like I was living what he was talking about. I used to like it because he's always taking an interest in me. I always had teachers to talk to, and you didn't feel insecure 'cause you thought it was the natural going thing. You had your parents to talk to you. My father talked to me every day at lunch. I had no insecurity about it. But when it came the time that I had to talk to someone else, then I started realizing I don't have anything to say. And I got depressed and insecure. . . .

The paradox described here is not uncommon. A family member, usually a child or adolescent, although sometimes a spouse, appears on the surface to be functioning reasonably well in the familiar context of family and school. However, a precipitating event, such as physical separation from the family; a change in role, such as becoming a parent; or a change in status, such as occurs with graduation or promotion, may evoke in the individual profound doubt about his intactness as a whole, effective, and worthwhile person. Even though the person feels deeply uncertain within himself as to who he is and how he is to be with others, he manages to conceal from himself and others the depth of his dread of being autonomous. Other family members, too, participate in maintaining the fiction that all is well.

The young man continued to explain his view of himself.

I don't think I ever faced very many people as a person. There's always something left out of my character. . . . I wasn't a person. I was more like a pawn and I was playing myself. I wasn't part of anything else. It was like I did this or that; like I was just moving myself around. I had no personal contacts with my work. I just struggled through it alone. And I don't think I enjoyed it too much, but I struggled anyways. . . .

In response to the question "What does it mean to be a person?" he replied,

To be a person is to want to express something—without letting someone else do it for you. Or without saying, "Well, it's not really important." To be a person is to come out and say, "Hey, I want that, or I want to say this or that about something." Well, I think I've gotten to rely on my parents to be my person. Because they were always so talkative and—and you know, I just kinda stood by at the dinner table and listened, and I felt as though I was a person from sitting by. . . . I don't have any personality right now. I'm just a series of problems.

This is an extreme example of a person unable to achieve separateness from his parents and a sufficiently coherent sense of self. As a consequence, his capacity to develop a relationship of shared mutuality with another person, such as a wife, would be seriously impaired. It is important to emphasize that psychologic autonomy from one's parents is never an end-point fully achieved. One is always a child to one's parents, and they are always parents to oneself. What is crucial to achieve is a capacity for reciprocal redefinition of the relationship and to accept this redefinition as an ongoing process across the life cycle.

For example, if the young man just mentioned were to marry and father a child, he would be, in his own eyes, a man, a husband, and a father—all the while remaining a son. The parents' task would be to acknowledge these newer roles acquired by the son, thus confirming his newer, more complex identity. This process is what we intend to call attention to in the phrase "reciprocal redefinition of the relationship."

The following example illustrates this process of mutually working out newer ways of relating to one's family of origin after forming a new nuclear family of one's own. The excerpt is from a family interview with a mother (M), father (F), their 20 year old married daughter (D), and 21 year old son-in-law (SL). At the time of the interview, the marriage was 4 months old, although the couple had lived together for more than a year. The ostensible reason for the meeting was in response to the parents' concern about the son-in-law's smoking pot. A physician (P) and social worker (SW) jointly conducted the session.

The excerpt begins with an exploration of how it felt to the group to have their concerns brought out into the open and talked about.

SW: How has it felt to discuss the issue?

F: Well, I think we should have been talking about it all along. It's good we started.

P: What got in the way of really talking about it?

M: Well, I think I have hang-ups (about drugs). I don't think that talking about it is gonna make us feel that drugs and marihuana are right. And it's better not to talk about some things.

SL: Maybe it's better to keep it hidden.

P: Your assumption has been, "Better not get into it, because if we get into it, it'll be more painful to us (the parents)." Is that right?

SL: Yeah, I think you're right.

M: And we might have harsh words.

P: What do you feel about harsh words occasionally developing?

M: Well, we had harsh words—but not a big break.

P: What's your fear—your big fear?

M: Of having a big break, of saying, "Okay, the heck with you." You know. And I can't do it. And I also was so worried. I couldn't stand to sit at home and worry about it, either. So I figured we better get it out in the open.

P: Have you had experiences with bad breaks?

SW: Big breaks?

Here the social worker and physician want to learn about the characteristic mode utilized by this family in dealing with disagreements. They focus more on the process of dealing with disagreements than on the content of the problem itself. This is so because they sense the parents are expecting a catastrophic rupture in the relationship if they differ with the children. Is this a stylistic pattern in the family? What are the origins of such a pattern, if it exists?

D: (To mother). Sometimes you were threatened by that with your father, from what you've told me.

M: Well, yeah. But not with us (and you).

D: Yeah, but I mean with what happened with you and your father—maybe you had the idea that because you had a break with your parents, you're trying to hold on to us here.

SW: What do you mean by a big break? That's not clear.

F: "Get out of my life," sort of. And meaning it. And sticking to it! "Go away. Don't knock on my door again," or whatever.

P: So you'd lose one another.

M: Yeah.

D: She gets very upset when she discusses her problems with her father when she was my age or younger. He seemed, if you ask me, too strict. It was just always criticism. She feared her father would stop liking her. So she was always trying to please him.

P: So it feels dangerous to you to really disagree because the relationship is liable to get altered. You're liable to really be abandoned, cold turkey. Just cut off.

D: Now my mother has a lot of good points. But I also accept her bad points. When I look at her relationship with *her* mother, I see mother hiding her bad points from her mother. If there is really a close bond between her and her parents, they would be able to accept her bad points. And so I want my parents to accept me as I am with my bad points and my good points. Because then I stand more as a human being. I see that my grandmother has an ideal opinion of them as some sort of epitome of the perfect children. They don't smoke, and they don't drink, according to grandmother.

M: She knows it, honey.

F: She knows it.

D: So she may know that you drink and smoke, but she doesn't accept it.

A number of complex issues have emerged in this segment. The daughter points out the mother's deep vulnerability to the opinions of the mother's parents. The mother has worked out a style of placating her parents and avoiding confrontation for fear of loss of love and abandonment.

The daughter also points up the mother's tendency to equate her (the mother's) situation with her own parents with the daughter's present situation. The mother has projected her own experience with her parents on to her relationship with her daughter, as if to say, "If there is a confrontation between us, we will lose one another."

We see in this excerpt the connectedness between the three generations and how a pattern in one generation may be repeated in the next generation.

The son-in-law, whose family experience has been quite different, offers his view.

SL: Myself, I haven't had this fear of a break, as they call it. It's more like I've always wanted people to accept me the way I am, and if they don't like it, well, that's okay. Goodbye. They can go away, you know. I'm still here. I'll still be doing, you know, whatever I was doing before or after. Other people haven't been that important to me.

D: But you haven't been as close to your parents as I am with mine.

SL: Yeah, I agree. I told you, I haven't.

D: So that a break with your parents wouldn't be as hard for you to accept because you wouldn't see it as that final of a thing. You'd say, "Well, my parents know where I am, and they can find me if they want me." With us, if we had a

break, both parties would be afraid to get back together.

SL: Why wouldn't you just be apart and just go on doing whatever you want to and not worry about it?

D: Because we'd miss each other!

In the remainder of the interview, we learned that the son-in-law was estranged from his family and that he felt he was an outsider in his wife's family. Part of him didn't trust parents, his own or his wife's. Yet he also wanted closeness with his in-laws. Indeed, one of the factors that attracted him to his wife was a sense that she came from a close-knit family. He, too, wanted to belong, but not at the cost of sacrificing his individuality.

PREGNANCY AND BIRTH OF FIRST CHILD

The period of pregnancy, the birth of the child, and the child's first year of life are momentous events in the life of the family. Crowded into a time period of less than 2 years, these three circumstances decisively alter the texture of family life. Husband and wife, as individuals, undergo profound changes in their view of themselves as they prepare to assume a new role, that of mother or father. They also undergo profound changes in their relationship with one another, with their own parents, with siblings, and with peers. The vertical and lateral axes of the extended family take on new dimensions of meaning.

Here are some excerpts from a group of five couples, all in the middle stages of the wife's pregnancy, discussing together the impact pregnancy has had on their lives.

P: How has the fact of becoming pregnant changed the relationship between the two (the couple)?

MR. A: Well, when the wife gets pregnant, you get pregnant. You're both sort of pregnant, in a way. It could draw you closer together because you're aware all of a sudden that something is gonna happen. You're gonna have a child pretty soon, and it's gonna change your life profoundly. You're eagerly or in some cases not so eagerly, perhaps fearfully, anticipating the birth of the child, and you're not sure what it's gonna be like.

MR. B: We've been married 3 years. You become pregnant, you run into responsibility—someone who is gonna be awfully dependent on you. And you have to look at a lot of things you never thought about. Providing for a family now. It kind of jumps on you. It surprises you.

MRS. A: It's going to make a difference, too, whether the pregnancy was planned or not. We've had friends who've had not only unplanned but unwanted pregnancies and, wow, it just makes a big difference in their attitude toward the child, toward each other. I think that a man can resent the woman and the woman can resent the man terribly if the pregnancy's unwanted. "Look what you did to me." You know.

MRS. C: I think it's made us closer in understanding, just the idea that we will soon have something that's a little bit of both of us. For me, 6 years was a long, long time to wait for a baby. And I felt an awful lot of pressure from friends who had them and from family, you know, to have a baby quickly. I kind of got into a defeatist attitude after awhile because I didn't have one. And now that I'm pregnant and everything is going well, it's just great. So maybe it's my feeling of finally accomplishing this thing that I've wanted so much that has changed our relationship for the better.

Turning from a focus on the effect of pregnancy on the couples' relationships, the physician asks how pregnancy altered the relationships with their parents.

MRS. D: When I got pregnant, suddenly we weren't treated as kids anymore. We were adults, and we were treated as adults. It changed the relationship with all of our relatives in that way.

MR. B: We had been overseas for 3 years. As soon as we got back, our parents wanted to know when we were having kids. I have a brother 7 years younger who has three kids already. So this was like, "Get at it kid!"

MRS. C: I only have a mom, and before we got married my mom wanted to break away from me, and I didn't want her to. I knew she had to, but it was very uncomfortable. And then I got married, and I'm pregnant. And now she's coming back, and she's really friendly to me, and nice and helpful, and I love it. I guess she felt that she had to break away for the individual in me to come out. And now that I've got a husband and I'm pregnant, she knows I'm not going to come back, so she doesn't have to be afraid of that.

These excerpts illustrate the interconnectedness of the generations, of the powerful expectations that couples quickly have children. We also learn that whereas for one couple, marriage and pregnancy promoted separateness and confirmation of adulthood, for another woman, marriage and pregnancy permitted an important reunion with her mother, a re-establishment of a relationship for which she had yearned deeply.

In this connection, we wish to emphasize the importance of the physician's not assuming prematurely what a particular patient may feel about an event or process, whether it is pregnancy, diabetes, or impending surgery. Rather, it is the physician's task to discover the meaning each individual patient attaches to the event or process.

Space limitations prevent a detailed consideration of the events surrounding delivery and of the enormous readjustments required during the first year of the child's life. Most central is the fact that the nuclear family now has three members, one of whom is totally dependent on the other two for survival.

The infant commences on a course of extraordinarily rapid development—maturational, social, and psychologic. Rather than being a relatively inert reactor to stimuli around him, as was previously thought, the infant is now known to be an active integrator of internal and external stimuli and to possess a highly individual behavior repertoire from birth onward.

The new father and mother are required to integrate a new role, that of parent, into their previous identities as individuals and as a couple. For them, the first year of life with the infant is a time of considerable complexity. Although at times deeply gratifying and occasionally exhilarating, it is for the most part a demanding, perplexing, and challenging experience. The extreme neediness of the child for intense and continuous care is problematic for many parents, particularly if their own needs for nurturance are insufficiently met. Parents also commonly wonder about their adequacy for the task and experience conflict between themselves as to their proper roles.

In probably no other phase is the family more open to interacting as a unit with the family physician or health care team. For example, there is the opportunity for uncovering parenting problems early, for discovering strain in the "fit" between the child's needs and those of the parents, and for learning of difficulties in the marital relationship. Even if the delivery is to be managed by an obstetrician, the family physician may choose to be centrally involved prior to and after the delivery, thus providing for continuity of care.

INDIVIDUATION OF FIRST CHILD

We begin the next phase with the child's second year of life and carry it through to entry into elementary school. At the time of the child's first birthday the family dynamics have been altered significantly. The original husband–wife dyad has been challenged by another powerful dyad arising from the mother–infant attachment. The mother–infant dyad begins as early as the third month of life, with the infant's capacity to differentiate the mother's face. Toward the end of the first year of life the infant manifests great distress upon separation from the mother and in the presence of strangers.

Thus the stage is set for potential conflict between the parents concerning the infant. The father may feel displaced, the mother insufficiently appreciated and helped. As pointed out earlier, the family physician is in an excellent position to detect these inevitable strains in the relationship, to help the parents express to one another some of their unspoken concerns and conflicts, and to find ways of resolving them.

We chose individuation of the child as a crucial theme of this phase in order to stress its central importance to the child and the parents. At the beginning of this phase the child is starting to walk (a critical development leading to experimentation with being physically separate from the main parenting person) and to explore the environment more independently than before.

The increasing competency with language (the child uses simple sentences by the second birthday) is another important factor fostering the child's capacity to differentiate as a social person. Language, as one of the most powerful tools of the culture, enables the child simultaneously to share in the culture and shape his individuality within it.

Another important development prior to beginning elementary school proper is the increasing play activity with other children. These opportunities are both informal and organized, such as in day care and nursery school settings. There is increasing opportunity to experience interaction with parent surrogates in addition to interaction with peers.

Most parents welcome the child's rapid gains in attaining increasing individuality and autonomy. They facilitate acquisition of competency in locomotion, language development, peer interaction, and the interaction with other adults serving as parent surrogates.

Occasionally, however, the child's movements toward growth and differentiation are experienced by the mother (less usually by the father) as a threat. Rather than supporting the forward maturational thrust of the child, her behavior tends to promote continued attachment. Consequently, there is delayed development by the child of those important skills necessary for interpersonal competence. The normal anxiety experienced by the child in exploring unfamiliar aspects of the physical and "people" environment is heightened, leading to even greater dependency on the parent. The reasons for such dependency are varied and always complex. Sometimes, the relationship between the parents is so ungratifying that the chief sources of the mother's satisfactions come from the intimate bond with the child. The child's movement away from her may lead to feelings of loneliness and even abandonment. The husband may sometimes subtly encourage the wife's overinvestment in the child as a way of diluting his relationship with her. This occasionally occurs with men who find intimacy with their wives threatening. It's as if they are saying, "Your wanting to be close to me is too scary; take the child and give me space."

Another factor leading to excessive fusion between mother and infant may arise out of a mother's uncertainty about herself as a person. The profound dependence of the child on her ministrations may become the chief source of her self-definition as a worthwhile person. Her role as a mother may serve as her central defining characteristic. The child's movement away from her may leave her feeling empty and unfulfilled.

These are some of the intrafamilial factors that may affect the course of early individuation of the child. Clearly, the newer ways of allocating parenting responsibilities between husband and wife, the increasing prominence of day care facilities, the movement of more women into the work force, the longer life span of grandparents, and the changing forms of health care delivery are important developments that will interact to affect the setting within which the young child will develop. These issues are of concern not only to the health planner, the specialist in child development, and assorted other professionals but to the family physician as well. For it is the family physician who often will be in an excellent position to detect early signs of dysfunction in the individuation process and to initiate help for the family.

EMERGING SEXUALITY OF FIRST CHILD

From birth onward, biologic and cultural forces interact to shape human sexual behavior. The biologic characteristics determining sex, e.g., maleness and femaleness, interact with gender identity, e.g., what one learns in a particular culture to feel about being a boy/man or a girl/woman and how one learns to behave in these roles. Each family unit becomes the final common pathway for presenting both attitudes and behaviors concerning gender identity. A central task for the parents is to promote an environment that optimizes the resolution of ambiguities and conflicts in this area.

An extremely complex set of reciprocal interactions ensues within the family as the emerging sexuality of the first child is experienced. The child wants to be like the parent of the same sex, yet is simultaneously in rivalry with that parent as a consequence of a feeling of closeness to the parent of the opposite sex. For the parent of the same sex, there is the problem of controlling annoyance over the competitiveness of the child, while at the same time encouraging the emerging tentative masculine or feminine behavioral roles the 4 to 6 year old child may be experimenting with.

For the parent of the opposite sex, there is the problem of modulating his or her own feelings of attraction to the child, while at the same time being sufficiently responsive to encourage and value the developing sexuality of the child. To complicate things further, the capacity of each parent to value his or her own status as a man or a woman exerts a profound influence on the successful working through of this phase. This is a time of opportunity, a rehearsal, for all the participants in this drama to prepare one another adequately for the more intense drama ushered in by adolescent changes that will emerge in the future.

Consequently, the developing child is enabled to emerge with a reasonably clear view of being a member of one gender in relationship to the other. Aspects of gender identity and of sexual behavior are for the most part products of the culture in which a person develops. Belief systems and values are very powerful forces in defining the range of possibilities permissible to the individual. In general, the culture at large is more permissive in the options offered to the person than is the individual family. This is problematic in our own culture for even the young child in view of the widespread erotization of the mass media.

It should not be forgotten that the parents, usually in their mid-20's at this stage in the family life cycle, are themselves in the middle of two generations. Their own parents are in their late 40's or early 50's and may look with disfavor on the methods of rearing their grandchildren, sometimes criticizing the parents for providing role models discrepant from their own.

EARLY AND MIDDLE SCHOOL YEARS

A useful metaphor in understanding family dynamics is that of the family boundary. Families may be thought of as constructing semipermeable boundaries around themselves and developing rules and mechanisms for controlling crossings into the family by others and out of the family by its own members. The beginning of formal schooling initiates a new and important process for the child and parents: the crossing of the family boundary by the child in a new way. The child now inhabits two worlds simultaneously: the world of the family and the world of the school.

Out of this circumstance, opportunity for growth and for conflict arises. The teacher as a parent surrogate becomes increasingly important. So do classroom peers, who bring different views and mechanisms for dealing with every imaginable interpersonal situation, such as dealing with feelings of anger and love, management of personal property and the property of others, and acceptance of other ethnic, racial, and religious backgrounds. Consequently, parents and child face the task of giving up or modifying their very special way of viewing the world in exchange for new experiences, new relationships, and new and different values.

The child now brings back into the family his own experience of relating to others and of perceiving the world in a way that may challenge the family. This may lead to a conflict between the parents and the school, each asserting their rights and obligations over the child's intellectual, emotional, and social education. The child may become caught in the middle of this struggle, which may then lead to the intervention of yet another social institution, the courts. This has occurred in recent years concerning issues of racial integration, religion, corporal punishment, and the length of a child's hair.

ADOLESCENCE IN THE FAMILY

Adolescence is an intermediate stage between childhood and adulthood. Ushered in by rapid physical growth, its onset is variable and always occurs about 2 years earlier in girls. Throughout the adolescent period biologic (hormonal), psychologic (meanings and feelings), and social (interpersonal) forces interact powerfully. Issues of sexuality (deeply experienced urges), role identity (who am I?), dependence (how much do I need others and in what ways?), and independence (can I stand on my own?) become focal issues for the adolescent and the family group as a whole.

Sexual behavior in the adolescent is an issue often brought to the attention of the family physician. Of the 21 million 15 to 19 year olds in the population, more than half have had sexual intercourse. Venereal disease and teenage pregnancy are the more obvious circumstances in which the physician may be involved. Of the 1 million 15 to 19 year olds pregnant in 1975, 27 per cent had an induced abortion and another 14 per cent had miscarriages. These clearly medical situations bring the physician, adolescent, and family together in a time of crisis. Yet it is important for the physician to see beyond such crises and provide opportunities for the family group to come to terms with an important fact of life, the emerging sexuality of the teenager. The prevention of disease and pregnancy is only part of the goal. Sexuality with pleasure and with respect for one's self and one's partner are equally important attitudes that the physician may help foster. This is an extremely difficult goal to accomplish because of the frequent divergence in views between teenagers and parents concerning the expression of sexuality.

Although the growth spurt and development of secondary sexual characteristics are outward and measurable manifestations of entry into adolescence, the psychologic and interpersonal integration of these changes by the adolescent may follow a more protracted timetable. The integration of these changes by the parents into a different view of their child is a complex process unfolding over time and is characterized by considerable upheaval and readjustment within the family.

The early adolescent is also in a state of flux in his peer world at school. In a given eighth grade class, some children are distinctly pubertal, others are in transition, and yet others are prepubertal. Major shifts in social relationships occur, and as a consequence, the adolescent's intrapersonal world, familial world, and interpersonal world at school become much more complex and problematic than before. It should be noted that the individual's capacity to think more abstractly and to manipulate concepts in a way quite different than was possible before begins with and continues to mature throughout adolescence.

In middle and late adolescence, the "child" and family are disengaging from one another, hopefully without the sense of impending catastrophe as was the case with the 19 year old boy discussed earlier. They are also re-engaging now in a different manner, in an adult-to-adult way, a circumstance unfamiliar and even somewhat strange to all of them. As this process unfolds, the adolescent often seeks physical and psychologic space within the family, such as wanting to shut the door to his room or not reporting the day's events at school. Such behavior is often perceived by the parents as being "self-centered," leading to conflict and feelings of being misunderstood on both sides.

For many adolescents, leaving the parental home will be the next step. For some, this will occur in late adolescence in order to find work in a different geographic location, to go away to school, to marry, to join the Armed Forces, or whatever. For the adolescent and the parents, there is often a mixture of relief and sadness. A watershed in both the individual and the family life cycle has been reached.

This brings us to the last phase of the family life cycle.

PARENTS ALONE

When the last child leaves home, parents frequently are in their mid-40's to mid-50's. A number of important tasks confront them now, as individuals and as a couple. For the woman whose main source of satisfaction derived from the parenting role, there is the task of transcending the "empty nest" syndrome, to find new meanings in her life. A frequent concurrent stress is menopause, experienced by many women as an irretrievable loss of a precious capacity, reproduction.

For the man, his children's entry into the world of work, formation of new relationships, or continued schooling may invite reflection and comparisons with his own life's course, leading to a sense of unfulfilled opportunities and, in extreme cases, despair.

The parents are now thrust into more intimacy with one other. For some couples, this circumstance is welcomed; for others, it is anticipated with dread. This is particularly so for couples who have postponed working out difficulties in their relationship in a continuous manner over the earlier years. The children in such marital

relationships had served to buffer the relational difficulties. With the children gone, the relationship must be attended to if it is to survive and grow.

A third stress for the couple alone is the changing relationship with their own parents, who are likely to be experiencing physical infirmities and economic difficulties requiring the parents to reverse roles and parent their own parents.

This is also a time for confronting their own aging, which is not that far off. The finiteness of life itself as a reality cannot be pushed aside as easily as before.

Some couples emerge from this stage with a sense of rediscovery of themselves as persons with potential for continued growth, both as individuals and as a couple. They approach old age more with serenity than with panic and outrage. Rather than envy their children's vigor and promise of the future, they can take pleasure in it and move on with their own lives. When the time comes for them to rely on their own children more, they can ask of them and receive without shame or guilt.

For other couples, the task is more difficult. Depression is not an uncommon consequence of their attempt to make sense of their lives and find new directions. Divorce, too, may be an outcome.

FAMILY DYNAMICS OF NON–STAGE-SPECIFIC EVENTS

There are events in the family life cycle that are not linked to the family group's development over time. They may occur at any time, and their catastrophic nature immediately alters everyone's lives in the family. Complex readjustments in relationships occur, sometimes temporarily, other times permanently.

Divorce is one such common event. In 1970 there were 2.2 million marriages (10.6 per 1000 of population) and 0.715 million divorces (3.5 per 1000 of population). Approximately 7 million children were members of divorced or separated families in 1970. In 1975 there were 2.1 million marriages (10.0 per 1000 of population) and 1.03 million divorces (4.8 per 1000 of population). The rate of divorce increased, and the rate of marriage decreased.

Family members involved in the process of divorce experience a spectrum of intense and sometimes contradictory feelings. Legally, divorce is a precise event, taking effect at a certain time, in a certain place. Psychologically, divorce is a process with blurred beginnings and an indistinct ending. Divorce means different things to the wife, the husband, and each of the children. Divorce is pain, loss, grief, rage; it is shame, guilt, and failure. Divorce is also freedom, hope, and new beginnings. For the child, divorce is always loss, being in the middle, being used, feeling torn, and being forced to take sides. It can also mean relief: an objectification of the knowledge that something has been terribly wrong for a long time. It is also a "solution."

Remarriage is another such event. One example might be a divorced woman with a son and daughter and a divorced man with a son and daughter. Following remarriage, each child has a sibling and two stepsiblings to relate to, two natural parents and a stepparent, and two grandparents and two stepgrandparents. The increasing incidence and prevalence of divorce and remarriage make it a certainty that the family physician will encounter such families in everyday practice.

Serious illness, such as a coronary, is another event that will alter family dynamics in a decisive way. Here are excerpts from an interview with a group of couples discussing the impact of a heart attack experienced by one partner in each family.

MR. A: I think the hardest part is when you get out of the hospital and go home. Everybody's staring at you, at every move you make, like you're going to do something you're not supposed to. It kind of gripes me. I have to tell them I'm all right. I can do what I want to do.

MRS. A: I was aware every minute that he was home. I was aware he was ill because he was at home and not in the office and I would study him to see if his color was good. And my son's concerned. He comes home from school every day and says, "Dad, did you take your pills?"

MR. B: I certainly appreciated what my wife was doing for me, but I like to do for myself, and when I'm ready to drive the car, I don't want anyone telling me I can't drive the car.

MRS. B: I was just following doctor's orders, and I thought I was there to en-

force those orders and see that they were followed. It's been such a traumatic experience, and I just wonder if I'll ever get over it, really. I feel like things will never be the same. I would hate to be some place and have this thing happen again. And my theory is if it happened once, it can happen again, and this is what I live with over my head. I want to get rid of this feeling, but I can't.

MRS. A: You relive it, don't you?

MRS. B: Yes, I do. I see the spot. I know every minute of it, and I hope I never see that day again.

MR. B: I think this thing has been a real shaker for my Jennie. I think it's been much harder on her than it was on me.

The man experiencing a serious myocardial infarction is forever changed in his view of himself. He has had a brush with death. He now knows he is vulnerable and mortal in a new and profound way. He must sort out his past, present, and future in a highly personal way. He must make new choices for himself. He can attempt to blot out the experience and go on as before, as if nothing has happened and nothing has changed. He can, on the other hand, acknowledge that fundamental changes have occurred in his body. He can make adaptive changes in his life: change his diet, his smoking habits, and his work pace. This work of reorientation is his to do. Yet it is not his alone, for he is part of a family. For his wife, too, a massive change has occurred, which she needs to integrate. She is now vulnerable to being alone, suddenly and unexpectedly. It may happen again, and he may not survive the next time. She feels helpless and tries to control her helplessness by controlling him. Serious stress in the marital relationship can arise.

In the next excerpt, the wife of a man in his mid-30's describes the impact of the coronary on their young children.

MRS. C: I found it difficult to explain something to the kids that I didn't want to believe myself. It happened around Christmas time, and I didn't want to believe it, and by the time I finally did believe it in 3 or 4 days, I had problems with the kids, who are 11 and 12. They were at my folks' house on Sunday, and I picked them up and on the way home my daughter said, "Somebody said Daddy had a heart attack, is that true?" and I said "Yes, he did," and my son looked at me very weirdly and said, "Mommy, is he dead?" And I thought, "I guess I have been ignoring them for 4 days." So we talked then, the three of us, for quite some time about what it meant to have a heart attack and that he wasn't dead.

Here is an instance in which a physician with a family system orientation could have helped the mother earlier by asking if she had thought of ways to help the children make sense of this catastrophic event. The physician can function as a catalyst, enabling the family to mobilize its own resources to deal with a family crisis.

SUMMARY AND SYNTHESIS

We have reviewed a number of dimensions of family process in this chapter. In summary form, these dimensions are:

1. *The Time Dimension:* A family unit has a historical past, a present, and a future. The present family is influenced by its past, and the past and present likewise influence the family's future. A hereditary disease, such as Huntington's chorea, is a concrete and extreme example of how the past, present, and future interact in a lethal way.

2. *The Cultural Dimension:* Nearly all known societies in the past and present have the family as a central structure in their overall organization. Comparative studies of societies indicate wide variability in how families are organized. Within contemporary Western society, there is also wide variability among families, particularly among different ethnic groups and socioeconomic levels.

3. *The Family Boundary Dimension:* Families draw boundaries around themselves, exercising control over which persons are allowed access to the family interior and which ideas and values generated outside the family will be favored. Families also exercise some control over the nature and extent of members' crossing the family boundary to the world outside.

4. *The Social System Dimension:* Family members are connected to one another through a system of reciprocal role relationships that carry both privileges and responsibilities. Thus, roles such as mother, wife, father, husband, daughter, son, brother, or sister carry with them prescriptions for reciprocal behavior vis-a-vis other family members.

5. *The Communication and Feeling Style Dimension:* Families tend to process information arising inside and outside the family in fairly characteristic ways. In some families, communication styles tend to favor direct and open communication. In other families, communication tends to be unclear and indirect. Similarly, there is wide variation in how feelings are handled in a family. These stylistic variables in a given family have important consequences for the capacity of family members to understand one another, meet one another's needs, and act in concert to solve problems effectively.

6. *The Family Life Cycle Dimension:* Families manifest continuous change throughout their life cycle. Dividing the total life course of a family into stages is a useful device for examining the necessary adaptive transitions required of the family over time. The capacity to master the normative tasks of any particular stage is influenced by how well previous tasks had been addressed, i.e., how well a couple work out their relationship with one another before their first child is born will affect the next stage, that of a three-person family and its stage-specific tasks.

7. *The Inter- and Intragenerational Dimension:* As the individual human life span increases, it is not infrequent to encounter families with representatives of four generations in interaction with one another, even though they may not be living under one roof. This interaction may become quite intense, vertically and horizontally, when a member of any generation experiences a health crisis.

We believe that familiarity with these dimensions of family dynamics will enhance the physician's capacity to render the kind of comprehensive, continuous, family-oriented care to which the specialty of family practice aspires.

In addition to having a conceptual framework within which to understand aspects of family functioning, the physician will need skills and resources to apply this framework to the clinical setting. Although medical schools rarely teach skills required to conduct a whole-family interview, they may be learned through reading and continuing education workshops. We have in mind those skills that will enable the physician to assess the strengths and vulnerabilities of a family, particularly as they relate to a health care crisis. Assuming a conceptual foundation and relevant skills for working with whole families, how will the physician find resources to address the family unit and still provide the spectrum of services demanded by the real world of practice?

If in solo practice, the physician may choose to see a whole family together, as time and interest permit. Referral to a psychiatrist, psychologist, or social worker may also be considered. If the physician is part of a health care team, family interviewing, assessment, and counseling may become a shared function, practiced by any member of the team: physician, nurse clinician, or social worker.

There are certain situations, however, in which the family physician may be the most logical and helpful person to conduct the interview. A death of a family member is one such situation in which the physician may want to meet with the remaining family members as a group in order to explore the impact of the death upon them. Another circumstance may be the diagnosis of cystic fibrosis in a child. Here the physician may meet with the parents to explore the far-reaching ramifications of the diagnosis and help them deal with these ramifications.

In bringing a family perspective to the practice setting, the family physician can have an important impact on the quality, depth, and breadth of health care. Preventive efforts may be realized more fully and morbidity lessened. Through such a perspective, the adjective "family" in family physician will take on real meaning.

REFERENCES

1. Ackerman, N. W.: Treating the Troubled Family. New York, Basic Books, Inc., Publishers, 1966.
2. Anthony, E., and Benedek, T. (eds.): Parenthood. Boston, Little, Brown & Co., 1970.
3. Beels, C. C., and Ferber, A.: Family therapy: a view. Family Process, 8:22, 1969.
4. Bodin, A.: Family therapy training literature: a brief guide. Family Process, 8:272, 1969.
5. Boszormenyi-Nagy, I., and Framo, J. L. (eds.): Intensive Family Therapy: Theoretical and Practical Aspects. New York, Harper & Row, Publishers, 1965.
6. Brody, E. H., and Spark, G.: Institutionalization of the aged: a family crisis. Family Process, 5:76, 1966.
7. Duvall, E.: Family Development. 4th ed., Philadelphia, J. B. Lippincott Co., 1971.
8. Erickson, E.: Identity and the Life Cycle. New York, International Universities Press, 1959.
9. Ferber, A., Mendelsohn, M., and Napier, A. (eds.): The Book of Family Therapy. New York, Jason Aronson, Inc., 1972.
10. Ferguson, L.: Personality Development. Belmont, Cal., Brooks/Cole Publishing Co., 1970.
11. Fleck, S.: The family and psychiatry. In Freedman, A., Kaplan, H., and Sadock, B. (eds.): Comprehensive Textbook of Psychiatry/II. Baltimore, The Williams & Wilkins Co., 1975.
12. Glick, I. D., and Haley, J.: Family Therapy and Research: An Annotated Bibliography of Articles and Books Published 1950–1970. New York, Grune & Stratton, 1971.
13. Glick, I., and Kessler, D.: Marital and Family Therapy. New York, Grune & Stratton, 1974.
14. Group for the Advancement of Psychiatry: Treatment of Families in Conflict. New York, Jason Aronson, Inc., 1970.
15. Haley, J., and Hoffman, L.: Techniques of Family Therapy. New York, Basic Books Inc., Publishers, 1967.
16. Haley, J.: Family therapy. In Freedman, A., Kaplan, H., and Sadock, B. (eds.): Comprehensive Textbook of Psychiatry/II. Baltimore, The Williams & Wilkins Co., 1975.
17. Handel, G.: The Psychosocial Interior of the Family. Chicago, Aldine Publishing Co., 1967.
18. Hess, R., and Handel, G.: Family Worlds. Chicago, Univ. of Chicago Press, 1974.
19. Howells, J. G. (ed.): Theory and Practice of Family Psychiatry. New York, Brunner/Mazel, Inc., 1971.
20. Kanter, D., and Lehr, W.: Inside the Family. San Francisco, Jossey-Bass, Inc., Publisher, 1975.
21. King, C.: Family therapy with the deprived family. Soc. Casework, 48:203, 1967.
22. Laing, R. D., and Esterson, A.: Sanity, Madness and the Family. London, Tavistock Publications, Ltd., 1964.
23. Langsley, D., and Kaplan, D.: The Treatment of Families in Crisis. New York, Grune & Stratton, 1968.
24. Lidz, T.: The Person. New York, Basic Books, Inc., Publishers, 1968.
25. McCollum A. T., and Gibson, L. E.: Family adaptation to the child with cystic fibrosis. J. Pediatr., 77:571, 1970.
26. Minuchin, S., Montalvo, B., Guerney, B., et al.: Families of the Slums. New York, Basic Books, Inc., Publisher, 1967.
27. Minuchin, S.: Families and Family Therapy. Cambridge, Harvard Univ. Press, 1974.
28. Morris, P.: Prisoners and Their Families. New York, Hart Publishing Co., 1965.
29. Parkes, C.: Bereavement. New York, International Universities Press, 1972.

30. Prugh, D. G., Staub, E. M., Sand, H. H., et al.: A study of the emotional reactions of children and families to hospitalization and illness. Am. J. Orthopsychiatry, 23:70, 1953.
31. Satir, V.: Conjoint Family Therapy. Palo Alto, Cal., Science & Behavior Books, Inc., 1964.
32. Shapiro, R.: Action and family interaction in adolescence. *In* Marmor, J. (ed.): Modern Psychoanalysis. New York, Basic Books, Inc., Publishers, 1968.
33. Skynner, A. C. R.: Systems of Family and Marital Psychotherapy. New York, Brunner/Mazel, Inc., 1976.
34. Sorensen, R.: Adolescent Sexuality in Contemporary America. New York, World, 1973.
35. Speck, R. V., and Rueveni, U.: Network therapy—a developing concept. Family Process, 8:182, 1969.
36. Steinmetz, S., and Straus, M.: Violence in the Family. New York, Dodd, Mead & Co., 1974.
37. Stierlin, H., Levi, L. D., and Savard, R. J.: Parental perceptions of separating children. Family Process, 10:411, 1971.
38. Stierlin, H.: Separating Parents and Adolescents. New York, Quadrangle, 1974.
39. Stoller, J.: Sex and Gender. New York, Jason Aronson, Inc., 1968.
40. Sze, W.: Human Life Cycle. New York, Jason Aronson, Inc., 1975.
41. Tharp, R.: Marriage roles, child development and family treatment. Am. J. Orthopsychiatry, 35:531, 1965.
42. Weiss, R.: Marital Separation. New York, Basic Books, Inc., Publishers, 1975.
43. Winter, W., and Ferreira, A. (eds.): Research In Family Interaction. Palo Alto, Cal., Science & Behavior Books, Inc., 1969.
44. Worby, C.: Interviewing the Family. *In* Enelow, A., and Swisher, S.: Interviewing and Patient Care. New York, Oxford University Press, 1972.
45. Worby, C., and Babineau, R.: The family interview: helping patient and family cope with metastatic disease. Geriatrics, 29:83, 1974.
46. Worby, C.: The family life cycle. J. Med. Educ., 46:198, 1971.
47. Wynne, L. C., Ryckoff, I. M., Day, J., et al.: Pseudomutuality in the family relations of schizophrenics. Psychiatry, 21:205, 1958.
48. Zuk, G., and Boszormenyi-Nagy, I. (eds.): Family Therapy and Disturbed Families. Palo Alto, Cal., Science & Behavior Books, Inc., 1967.

Chapter 4

SOCIOCULTURAL INFLUENCES

by DEREK G. GILL, and JACK M. COLWILL

The concept that cultural factors impact upon the health status of individuals and families is generally accepted by physicians. Frequently, however, the impact of these influences in specific patient care situations is not recognized or may be ignored. As a consequence, insights, diagnosis, and management suffer. This chapter will attempt to develop a conceptual and organizational framework for incorporating cultural factors, including those of social class, race, ethnicity, and family structure, into family practice. A basic understanding of disease mechanisms and an understanding of the cultural background of the patient and his family assist the physician in interpreting symptoms, predicting stresses, and, consequently, in practicing prospective medicine.

Since cultural influences are pervasive throughout all aspects of our lives, the theme of this chapter will be that biologic, psychosocial, and cultural factors are interwoven in each individual health and illness situation to varying degrees.

We first provide a general overview of the major cultural forces that are characteristic of our society. Many of these factors also influence the health and illness status of the family group; the literature is vast and, consequently, selectivity is inevitable.

The second section deals with cultural determinants of illness episodes. What is perceived as illness may vary among social and cultural groups, and even selection of symptoms has cultural determinants. People seek consultation with a physician in only a small percentage of what they recognize to be illness episodes. Consequently, we examine pre- or protopatient behavior and its effect upon the epidemiology of ambulatory care.

The third section examines the doctor–patient exchange. It develops the thesis that in the ambulatory setting the physician serves not as a provider of health care but as a consultant to the primary providers—the patient and family. Factors leading to success or failure in the relationship are reviewed.

The fourth section focuses upon social class and environmental determinants of disease. Excluded from consideration are diseases transmitted genetically within cultural groups, such as thalassemia among Mediterranean peoples. Thus, this segment will examine the influences of social and cultural factors upon the epidemiology of disease.

The fifth section will attempt to provide a model for utilization of psychosocial and cultural factors in family practice. Much of what has been inappropriately called the "art of medicine" reflects the physican's intuitive recognition of psychosocial and cultural factors in both individual and family care.

THE FAMILY: TRANSMITTER OF CULTURAL HERITAGE

In the study of human behavior, organic, psychologic, social, and cultural factors are often so totally intermixed that the etiologic significance of each component becomes very difficult to separate from the others. Family interaction is the major vehicle for transmitting the social and cultural components of individual behavior. Thus, the impact of the family upon the individual is not only a result of the day-to-day interpersonal relationships but is also the result of the long-term socialization process through which the family's social and cultural heritage has been transmitted to the individual. From this family background and its broader social and cultural environment, the individual develops basic attitudes and habits in such widely varying areas as diet, religious beliefs, definitions of illness, orientation to work and play, sexual mores, and modes of interpersonal communication.

Social Class

In terms of relative impact on contemporary American society, the social class of families may have greater overall influence in determining the attitudes and behaviors of individuals than does cultural background. Social class is a means of describing the educational, economic, and occupational background of the family. These combined factors form the hierarchical divisions that are observable in all sophisticated social systems. People of similar social class tend to have similar means of communication, attitudes about life, and life styles.

In the United States, the social class of families is determined by educational, economic, and occupational characteristics of the head of the household, that is, the socioeconomic status (SES). In Great Britain, a sixfold division of social class is based upon occupation. School teachers in most Western societies are paid relatively little in comparison with other highly skilled occupational categories. Nevertheless, their status and prestige are usually high within their community; consequently, they are in the middle class even though in many cases those in lower classes have higher incomes. In many studies investigators condense the sixfold or greater numerical division of social class into three, upper, middle, and lower. We shall adopt this convention in this chapter.

We tend to assume that the United States is a classless society inasmuch as our Constitution legislated a society in which there was equality of political opportunity. However, in the United States, the disparity between poverty and wealth is perhaps greater than in most other Western countries. Such a wide spectrum between high and low incomes in effect creates differing life opportunities and, as a result, differing life styles.

Social class, therefore, is a means of shorthand expression utilized to summarize different life styles and opportunities available to the upper, middle, and lower sectors of the community. People from the upper social classes tend to enjoy high educational standards and considerable excess of income over expenditure and to enter occupations that are characterized by high autonomy in the work situation. They are able to exercise considerable power in their day-to-day work situation, whether it be power over people or power over resources. They tend to be work-oriented, education-oriented, and achievement-oriented. Failure to achieve expectations has a high likelihood of leading to anxiety, stress, or depression. The life chances of family members in the upper class are greater and more varied than those for the sons and daughters of the poor farmer in Appalachia.

At the very bottom of the social class continuum, the conditions of individuals and their families may create circumstances of absolute or relative deprivation. While in Western countries, this only rarely is of a magnitude to create nutritional deprivation, nevertheless, relative deprivation may be just as stressful and debilitating.[29] Thus, the orientation of the lower social classes is directed more toward day-to-day survival and enjoyment and less toward the abstract. Perspectives are more narrowed and attitudes firmly held. Language itself tends to be more concrete and more preoccupied with the self and indeed very different in terms of syntax, context, and content.

In a society that stresses financial and social success, both achieving and not achieving this success may generate situations in which a variety of pathologic problems emerge. Throughout this chapter, therefore, frequent references will be made to social class divisions and the relevance these have for the behavior of individuals and families in health and illness and in doctor–patient relationships.

Cultural Heritage and the "Melting Pot"

Ethnic origins also have a major impact on individual and family behavior. Our society has arisen from a wide variety of cultural groups. Initially, a series of new groups originating from Anglo-Saxon stock immigrated to this country, each bringing its own cultural traditions. Each cultural group brought its heritage of religious beliefs, social customs, value systems, family structure, and perceptions and orientations toward health and illness.

Viewing the term "culture" broadly, new cultures such as the "hippie culture," the "flower people," and other countercultures have developed within our society in the 1960's. These countercultures embrace a variety of ideologic and value positions. The "hippies," and to some extent the "flower people," generated a separate identity by their objections to the United States involvement in the Vietnamese War. Later, other groups associated with a broader concept of counterculture began to advocate an entirely new set of values directly contrary to their largely middle class origins. Some groups established communes based upon agriculture and handicrafts where the major value orientation seemed to be rejection of middle class culture with its emphasis upon education and social and economic success. The values of cooperation and mutual support rather than competition and individuals striving for success were defined by the countercultures as desirable value orientations.

Our nation has long been termed a "melting pot" of different cultural groups. The "melting pot" thesis suggests that people from different cultural and ethnic backgrounds gradually tend to become "Americanized." With the passage of time and the birth of subsequent generations, cultural traditions and orientations are modified and the values, standards, and practices of the newly emerging culture are incorporated. Thus, for many families in our society, distinct cultural and ethnic traditions have become blurred. A traditional German river town in Missouri becomes "Germanic" only for the period of its annual Maifest celebration. In the "melting pot," intermarriage between individuals of different backgrounds may be one of the major determinants in developing new norms and patterns of behavior that tend to modify the customs derived originally from ethnicity. Thus, intermarriage may also pose the basis for strife based upon different attitudes or orientations within the family. In addition to intermarriage, such forces as the public school system, mass media, slum clearance projects, and others have all had major impact in modifying cultural traditions.

Despite the powerful forces of the "melting pot," groups still persist in our society that maintain a strong emphasis upon and commitment to their ethnic, racial, and cultural backgrounds. Examples are Jewish groups in New York City, Mexican groups in San Antonio, Cubans in Miami, and the black separatist movement. The cultural tradition of each family can be seen in its religious convictions, family structure, orientation toward issues of divorce, abortion, contraception, diet, attitudes about illness, and so forth.

Interrelationships Between Social Class and Culture

In most cases, cultural background and social class influences must be viewed as being interdependent. Irish migration to the United States was typically from the lower class, as was that of Italians. Scandinavian migration was typically rural rather than urban.

The interactions and relationships among social class, ethnicity, and race are well illustrated in the American setting by reference to the black family. In the 1930's, John Dollard[8] suggested that the lower socioeconomic status of the black family owed as much to class distinction as it did to racial background. Staples[31] suggested that research tradition in the investigation of black family structure tended to concentrate upon the "problem families," whereas family sociologists working with white families emphasized research situations involving middle class family life styles. Whenever comparisons are made between black and white family structure, one tends implicitly to think in terms of the black and white cultural differences. In reality, the lower social class status of blacks in general must also be taken into account. For example, in 1972, a significantly larger percentage of black than white households was headed by a female—30 per cent vs. 9 per cent. However, as the level of income rises, so does the number of male-headed families. At family incomes of $15,000 or greater, the percentage of black and white families headed by a woman is comparable.

Family Composition

Family composition is influenced by social class and to a lesser extent by ethnicity. Demographers and family sociologists have long recognized that family size is related to social class. Class differences regarding family size may be related to the ability of upper and middle class families to exercise control over their life situations. Middle class groups, particularly white collar workers, limit family size. Clerical workers and their families with lower class origins struggle to achieve or hang onto newly acquired middle class status. In these circumstances, an extra child disturbs the fine balance between income, life style, and expenditure. In upper class families there are no financial constraints to family size. Among lower social class groups, large family size seems to be a product of a combination of factors—lack of access to and reluctance to utilize contraceptive measures, a lack of knowledge and understanding of the range of available contraceptive techniques, and a traditional preference for large families.

The frequency of three generation families (grandparents, parents, and children) also tends to vary with social class. Thus, Shanas and colleagues,[30] in their study of old age in three industrial societies (the United States, the United Kingdom, and Denmark), found that with lower class groups the most frequent arrangement for taking care of the elderly was to have them live with children and grandchildren when they became incapable of independent existence. On the other hand, middle class groups were more likely to utilize institutional care for the elderly. One factor relating to this observation may be that middle class families tend to have greater geographic mobility than lower class families, who tend toward geographic stability. With the possible exception of Jewish families,[10] it appears that ethnicity is less important than social class in the preservation of three generation family structures.

Our culture is in a constant state of flux, but traditions and values in older generations and in communities isolated from the wider social system persist. Rate and degree of change in our society seem to have increased quite markedly in recent years. Patterns of sexual behavior differ today from those of two decades ago. Improvement in contraception may play a part in generating more liberal attitudes toward sexual behavior, but this process of change is also bound up with the gradual progress of women's liberation.[14] In addition, increasing percentages of the elderly in the population at a time when our society is progressively developing middle class life styles pose a major challenge for the role of the geriatric population in our society. The increasing frequency of divorce and its inherent fragmentation of families pose still another dilemma for a changing society. Changes are also apparent in socialization practices for child rearing. Baby books and child rearing manuals of the 1930's and those of today are different indeed, with the latter focusing much more on permissive schedules of feeding, permissiveness in child behavior, and emphasis on greater freedom for individual growth and development. There is some indication that this trend may well be cyclical, with the future holding a return to a more directive attitude toward socialization of children.

The examples just cited are only a few of the changes occurring within our social system. The evolutionary pattern of our society is also associated with the changing patterns of health and illness.

PERCEPTIONS OF ILLNESS AND PATHWAYS TO THE PHYSICIAN

Perceptions of Illness

Perceptions of illness may vary from individual to individual. Symptoms that may be almost disabling for one person are unimportant for another. A group of physicians at the Peckham Health Center in London from 1939 to 1940 examined a sample of approximately 4000 adults and children. Ninety-one per cent of the population had a defect, but only 50 per cent of those had sought medical care for the defect. There was no relationship between the nature or severity of the disorder and the likelihood of seeking medical care.[27] Apple[1] suggested that interference with day-to-day activities is an important component in the layman's perception and definition of illness. While this is undoubtedly true, it does not explain the fact that those with identical symptoms may or may not seek medical assistance. Multiple social, cultural, psychologic, and economic factors play a role in explaining why some seek medical care and some do not.

Koos[20] and others have documented that

health-seeking behavior shows an inverse relationship to the level of social class. The people from the upper socioeconomic group were more likely to recognize symptoms and seek professional care, whereas those lower on the social class continuum were less likely to perceive even relatively serious conditions, such as blood in the stool, as requiring professional advice and assistance.

Other studies have demonstrated that those of the upper social class are more likely and willing to find psychologic symptoms of anxiety or depression acceptable than those of the lower class. Stress symptoms in the lower class are much more likely to be reflected in vague, poorly defined complaints.

Cultural backgrounds, in addition to social class, may influence patients' perceptions of symptoms. Zola[39] suggested that symptoms that are perceived and acted upon by an individual are defined by his culture, ethnic group, or close associates as those requiring action. He then went on to compare the presenting symptoms of Italian and Irish patients who came to the clinics of the Massachusetts General Hospital. He found that four times as many complaints from the Irish population concerned problems of the ears, nose, or throat, or abdominal disorders as compared with the pattern of complaints from the Italian population. Moreover, only one-third of the Irish patients indicated pain as part of their presenting symptoms, in contrast to over half of the Italian patients.

Pain as a complaint has psychologic as well as organic determinants that may vary from episode to episode for each individual. The individual without feelings of stress might disregard headache, but in a setting of stress from employment or from anxiety about the underlying cause of pain, the same individual might be incapacitated. Pain can be modified by understanding its cause. Vernon[34] and his colleagues demonstrated that patients who are carefully instructed in the type, extent, and nature of pain likely to follow an operation tend to report lower levels of pain and tend to be rehabilitated earlier than those who are given only minimal information. These findings indicate the importance of education in minimizing anxiety and its potentiating effects upon pain.

Acceptability of and reaction to pain as a symptom may vary from group to group, family to family, social class to social class, and cultural group to cultural group. Thus, in our society it is more acceptable for a woman to complain of pain. It is more usual for a Southern European to complain of pain than for a Northern European or an Anglo-Saxon. Zborowski[38] noted that Italians, when complaining of pain, sought relief from the discomfort. On the other hand, Jewish people seemed more concerned about the underlying cause of the pain. Similarly, for the upper classes, anxiety about the underlying cause of pain may be an important trigger in the decision to seek care. Farmers and the Irish and Scandinavians may tend to be stoical and even to deny or downgrade the severity of pain. The woman having marital problems or the man concerned about underlying cancer may tend to exaggerate symptoms. Correct interpretation of the magnitude of the symptoms and their meaning for the patient leads to appropriate diagnoses and approaches to management.

Stress, like pain, tends to be interpreted differently by different social groups. Mechanic and Volkart[24] demonstrated that college students who were under stress were 2.5 times as likely to be frequent users of college health services as those who were not perceived as being under stress. They suggested that students were reporting sick as a means of coping, either consciously or unconsciously, with the stressful situations in which they found themselves. Parsons[26] has suggested that people who are sick are absolved from their normal roles and responsibilities. Students who report sick at examination time may be using the illness episode as an avoidance mechanism consciously, semiconsciously, or unconsciously to escape tests, plead for more time, complete a term paper, or provide an alibi for a substandard performance.

Many groups, particularly those from a lower socioeconomic background in which the cultural tradition inhibits free expression of emotional distress, tend to react to stress situations with physical symptoms. These patients often face serious life difficulties and social stress, but the working class subculture does not permit legitimate expression of their suffering. Such recently was the case of a young woman presenting with a headache and accompanied by her husband, who very clearly asserted to the physician that his wife "cannot have tension headaches because she is under no tension."

David Robinson[28] studied a sample group of English married women with children. Even though they had not seen their physicians in 6 months, he found that they had had a range of illness episodes. Starting from the often expressed opinion that "wives and mothers cannot afford the time to be sick," he suggested that women may use the threat of illness and the disruptions in the family situations that will occur as a bargaining position in family decision-making procedures. This may often be the case in a marital relationship in which the husband has assumed the dominant position.

However, many with major illnesses do not seek the attention of the physician. It may be that the illness is not perceived as unusual. Thus, in many mining communities or among smokers, a hacking cough is so common as to be perceived as "normal." Fry[12] suggests that in the United Kingdom 20 per cent of adults over the age of 45 suffer symptoms of chronic bronchitis, but two-thirds are not seeking medical help and are looking after themselves. Further, "denial" as a defense mechanism causes many to disregard symptoms that intellectually they understand require medical attention. "Denial" may give protection against the anxiety caused by the symptoms.

Clearly, the illness conditions that are presented in the physician's office represent a biased sample of the total illness experience of most families. Take the case of a cold or a sore throat. On one occasion, the individual chooses to consult a physician; on another he does not. The difference between the individual's reaction to the two illness states may be due to the variation in severity of the symptomatology on the two occasions. But it is equally possible that the symptoms were the same on both occasions, and some "trigger" persuaded the sufferer to seek a consultation with a physician.

Behavior regarding preventive health is also influenced by social and cultural factors. The likelihood of participation in vaccination and immunization programs or screening campaigns for conditions as varied as cervical cancer or tuberculosis all tend to be greater in high rather than low social class groups. Individuals from the upper social classes exercise control over

their life situations and seem to be able to orient themselves toward future activities with very little effort. For many working class groups, a future health maintenance orientation may seem to be irrelevant to their life situation.

Pathways to the Physician

Problems presented to physicians by patients represent only the "tip of the iceberg" of the total number of perceived illness episodes. Kerr White,[36] in a 1961 review of British and American literature, estimated that 750 out of every 1000 individuals over age 16 experience some injury or illness episode each month that they perceive to interfere with their activities. He estimated that out of these 750, only 250 seek the advice and counsel of a physician and only 9 ultimately are hospitalized.

The amount of self-medication utilized in Western societies is another measure of the amount of self-care that occurs. In a carefully designed study of a representative sample of the United Kingdom population, Dunnell and Cartwright[9] report:

In a two week period, the ratio of self-prescribed medications taken was roughly 2:1 . . . clearly taking non-prescribed medicines is a popular activity: 2/3 of adults had done so in the two weeks before the interview. Only a small proportion — a 10th — of the non-prescribed medications taken by adults had been first suggested by a doctor; most were the suggestions of parents, friends, neighbors, husbands, wives or other relatives. . . .

In the United States, the Food and Drug Administration estimates that the sale of over-the-counter medications generates 3.5 billion dollars in sales annually.

It would be possible to write an entire book about what Friedson[11] has described as the "lay referral system," a method of health care in which individuals seek advice outside the established medical care system. Within the home, typically the mother assumes the role of healer. She provides the counsel concerning nutrition and the remedies for multiple complaints. In the three generation family, the grandmother is likely to assume this role.

But the referral system also extends beyond the boundaries of the family unit. In some families, especially, but not exclusively working class groups, husbands and wives tend to live in almost separate worlds. Young and Willmott noted that "women have their kin-folk and men have their friends."[37] Husbands tended to be drawn more and more into interaction with friends and acquaintances associated with their work, while wives interacted more frequently with relatives, sisters, cousins, aunts, and especially with their own mothers. The mother's home would be the place where the married sisters would return to meet and gossip and often to discuss health issues. This pattern of findings has been consistent across two cultures, the United States and the United Kingdom, over a 25 year period,[13, 21] although increasingly middle class status with its associated geographic mobility disrupts the separate worlds of husband and wife and encourages development of shared pursuits.

The "two worlds" of husband and wife have a clear significance for an understanding of the family's orientation toward illness. The wife is much more likely to obtain advice on health care issues from her own mother, aunts, sisters, cousins, and neighbors; her husband is more likely to go outside the family setting. Thus, a lay referral system is deeply embedded within our culture, a system that provides the bulk of health care within a framework frequently characterized by a low level of medical knowledge.

It appears that multiple factors trigger the ultimate decision as to whether or not to seek medical care. These factors have social and cultural determinants. They are influenced by immediate family and friends and by the patient's own perception that he is not well and needs assistance in feeling better. We must now examine the nature of the doctor–patient relationship, recognizing that the condition that brings the patient to the physician's office is of sufficient concern to the individual and his family to prevent the primary group, the family, from dealing unaided with the situation.

THE DOCTOR–PATIENT EXCHANGE: A MEETING OF TWO CULTURES

While the patient seeks relief from "dysease" (discomfort, anxieties, and fears), the physician's orientation is to identify "disease." Magraw, in his book *Ferment in Medicine*,[22] suggests that the physician, through the socialization process of his education, tends to have attitudes and perspectives that are disease-oriented. He tends to think in terms of specific diagnoses that are represented by specific pathologic states and by specific symptom complexes. Magraw states.

In the doctor's view, the patient's illness is not defined and in a sense has no reality until it is fitted into a disease frame of reference. Sickness and disease are synonymous. Until the doctor can understand the patient's problem in terms of disease, he does not fully accept the situation as a medical one.

Friedson, in his book *Patients' Views of Medical Practice*,[11] refers to the dilemmas of doctor–patient relationships in another way. He states that,

. . . the separate worlds of experience and reference of the layman and the professional worker are always in potential conflict with each other. This seems to be inherent in the various situations of professional practice. The practitioner, looking from his professional vantage point, preserves his detachment by seeing the patient as a case to which he applies his rules and categories learned during his protracted professional training. The client, being personally involved in what happens, feels obliged to try to judge and control what is happening to him. Since he does not have the same perspective as the practitioner he must judge what is being done to him from other than a professional view. While both professional worker and client are theoretically in accord (with the objectives of their relation to solve the client's problem), the means by which the solution is to be accomplished and the definition of the problem itself are sources of potential difference.

Each brings his own educational and experiential heritage into the doctor–patient exchange. Each has his own expectations. Truly it is a meeting of two cultures.

The Family Physician as a Consultant

Szasz and Hollender[33] have described three basic models of doctor–patient relationships:

1. Activity–passivity (a physician does something to the patient, as in the case of the comatose patient in an acute emergency).

2. Guidance–cooperation (the patient while acutely ill is able to cooperate, and,

thus, the relationship is similar to the relationship of parent and child).

3. Mutual participation (this pattern is common in the management of chronic illness).

During a serious illness, the doctor–patient relationship may pass through two or more of the above models. In the case of an accident victim with a broken leg and concussion, the relationship is likely to pass through all three stages during treatment and rehabilitation.

There is another way of viewing the doctor–patient relationship in the ambulatory setting. The family physician is frequently termed a "primary care physician," implying that he is the *provider* of health care. In reality, as demonstrated in the preceding pages, it is the patient and his family who are the *true* primary care providers. It is their decision as to whether to seek a physician's advice, and it is also their decision as to whether that advice is followed.

Perhaps it is more appropriate to describe the doctor–patient relationship in the ambulatory setting as that of a *consultant* (the physician) to the *primary provider* (the patient and family). The patient seeks assistance from the consultant. Recommendations from the physician consultant may or may not be accepted because the patient may disagree with the recommendations or may have received alternative consultative advice from others. Implicit in the term "consultation" is the expectation of recommendations. Consultants, however, also are sometimes utilized to render a specific service. Physicians frequently "order" an x-ray from their consultant, the radiologist, perceiving which studies they need. So, too, the patient frequently comes to his consultant, the physician, with a perception of what he needs. In such cases, the patient is seeking a specific service rather than recommendations.

The family adds a third dimension to the doctor–patient relationship.

Physician
↗   ↘
Family⟷Patient

Illness of the individual may affect the family, and, conversely, dysfunction of the family may cause illness in the individual.

In the dynamic interaction of the physician, patient, and family, patients may present with symptoms that reflect family problems. Indeed the family may be the patient. Therapy directed at the individual and his stress symptoms may not be successful without involvement of the family in the basic problems. On the reverse side, illness of the patient affects the family. The family may pull itself together to provide sustenance and nurture to the ill patient. Also, the stresses involved may create major problems within the family. The physician must view his patient broadly, considering the family also as the patient. Thus, he may care not only for the pregnant woman but also for the pregnant family. Care for the dying patient becomes care for the entire family.

The family is an important force in determining whether or not the patient follows the physician's recommendations. If the "healer" in the family feels that the recommendations of the physician are inappropriate, it is unlikely that the patient will follow the advice. Conversely, if the physician solicits the assistance of the family by helping them to understand both the problems and the recommendations, to be motivated to implement the recommendations, and to make resources for implementation available, then the likelihood is great that the suggestions will be followed.

The term "compliance" is frequently utilized to indicate whether or not a patient has followed the physician's "orders." These words suggest a highly authoritarian relationship between physician and patient that in reality seldom exists, despite the physician's expectations. While the term "compliance" may be inappropriate in this setting, nevertheless the degree to which patients and families follow the recommendations of a physician may be viewed as a measure of the physician's effectiveness as a consultant.

For the physician to be effective as the family's health care consultant, the following steps must be accomplished: (1) mutual agreement as to the problem, (2) understanding of the recommendations, (3) motivation on the part of the patient and the family to carry out the recommendations, and (4) adequate resources to implement the recommendations.

Effective Communication

Effective communication between physician, patient, and family is a prerequisite for understanding the problem and the basic therapeutic recommendations. When the patient seeks repair of a laceration or care of a respiratory infection, the problem is easily recognized and agreed upon. However, in many settings when the two worlds of physician and patient meet, even a mutual understanding as to the basic problem is difficult to achieve.

The first requirement must be to establish a pattern of communication that allows both participants to understand fully the meaning of the other's remarks. The situation is complicated by the fact that the physician is the possessor of an esoteric body of knowledge acquired over approximately 11 years of training and subsequent experience in the practice of medicine. The patient, on the other hand, frequently has only the haziest ideas of the biologic and physiologic components of illness and disease.[15] Boyle[5] in 1970 administered a series of multiple choice questionnaires listing various medical and anatomic terms and their meanings both to out-patients and to members of the medical staff of a large Glasgow teaching hospital's out-patient clinic. The degree of agreement between the two groups on various terms ranged from 20 per cent to 90 per cent. There was 80 to 90 per cent agreement among physicians and patients on definitions of good appetite, arthritis, heartburn, and bronchitis. Lowest agreement occurred for definitions of flatulence (43 per cent) and diarrhea (37 per cent). While 77 per cent of the patients were able to demonstrate on a chart the location of the intestines and 70 per cent the thyroid gland, only 42 per cent correctly located the heart and only 20 per cent the stomach.

A further complication is the fact that the physician is likely to communicate with his colleagues and within his own social circle in a language code that might be described as elaborated. On the other hand, some groups in the community, particularly those from lower social classes, tend to use a more restricted language code.[3] Distinctions between these two languages may be defined in terms of the kinds of options people utilize when they speak. These linguistic codes seem to be distinguished by the predictability of the syntactic options or alternatives a speaker utilizes. In the case of elaborated language code, the speaker selects from a wide range of syntactic alternatives. It is difficult to predict what the outcome of a verbal exchange will be without paying continuous attention to the content and flow of the communication. However, with a restricted language code, the range of syntactic alternatives is reduced and a much higher degree of prediction is possible.

In doctor–patient exchanges, the situation is exacerbated by the highly technical nature of the medical language. Effective communication requires sensitivity both to the degree of restricted or elaborated language code with which the patient is familiar and also the extent of the patient's understanding of medical vocabularies. The following incident observed in a busy ambulatory clinic in New York City is a clear example of such a communication problem.

Physician: Take this cup over there (nodding vaguely in the direction of the men's room) and void into it.

Patient: (Looks at the cup and hesitates, uncertain of what to do.)

Physician: I need a midstream sample of urine! (Second phrase uttered by the physician with verbal overtones and expressions that indicate frustration.)

Patient: (Still does not understand what is required.)

Physician: Take this cup into the men's room and pee into it and bring me some back.

Patient: Oh! O.K.

The physician initially made a series of assumptions; assuming that the patient was aware of the location of the men's room, that he understood what "void" meant, and that he understood that a sample of urine was required. This is an example of an elaborated language code form of communication. Both the language code and the terminology combined to create a miscommunication. In the second exchange, the physician presented a more precise outline of what he wanted the patient to do and expressed some of his frustration. He also added to the confusion by stating without explanation that he wanted a "midstream sample." Not until the third formulation was the physician's request so defined that the patient did not have to make any interpretation, but the anger exhibited did little to enhance the relationship.

Past experience also has a major impact upon individuals' perceptions of the meanings of various medical terms. Consider the implication of the term "tumor" to a physician, a college graduate, a custodian, a woman whose sister recently died of carcinoma of the breast, and a man who had a sebaceous cyst removed. The meaning of "tumor" to each individual may be very different. The physician in his communications with the patient must be certain that he understands what is being said as well as what is not being said. He must seek the patient's own interpretation of what has been said and also must seek the patient's reaction to the physician's recommendations.

Communications between patient and physician require insights from the physician beyond those of different modes of communication and different technical language. The patient may be unwilling to give the real reason for the visit or occasionally may be unaware of the underlying problem. Consequently, frequently in the ambulatory setting, the physician finds that the patient's underlying problem is quite different from the presenting complaint. Lawrence Henderson[17] has stated:

When you talk with a patient you should listen first to what he wants to tell, secondly for what he does not want to tell, and thirdly for what he cannot tell. He does not want to tell things that are shameful or painful, he cannot tell you his implicit assumptions that are known only to him such as the assumption that all action which is not perfectly good is bad, such as the assumption that everything that is not perfectly successful is a failure, such as the assumption that everything that is not perfectly safe is dangerous.

A recent patient illustrated the importance of listening for what the patient did not want to tell.

A medical student's wife presented for her annual Pap smear. She indicated she was feeling perfectly well other than the fact that her menstrual period was 2 weeks overdue; however, she hastened to state that her periods generally were irregular. Upon questioning, she indicated that she was not utilizing any contraception.

Her examination was totally normal, and she was given a clean bill of health. As an afterthought, the physician suggested that a pregnancy test might be appropriate. When the pregnancy test proved to be positive, the patient was overjoyed.

It was obvious that the patient had really come to ascertain whether she was pregnant. When asked why she hadn't raised the issue, she responded that once before she had seen a physician for possible pregnancy and had been embarrassed when the test proved to be negative. The patient had not told the real reason for coming because as the wife of a medically sophisticated future physician she might "make a fool" of herself by not being pregnant.

Frequently it is only as the physician is about to leave the examining room that the patient obtains the courage to ask about underlying concerns, such as marital or sexual disharmony, fear of cancer, and so forth. Even more frequently the underlying problem will only surface after a number of office visits.

Often, as Henderson has pointed out, the patient may be unaware of the underlying problem.

Recently an elderly woman cared for by one of the authors called to indicate that her husband, a man with a several years' history of an organic brain syndrome, was becoming "impossible." She said, "He is forgetful; he is mean to me! You must do something." Husband and wife were invited to the office. He appeared unchanged, but she was visibly tremulous and agitated. She admitted to having sleeping problems and crying easily. While the wife perceived that the problem was the husband, in reality it was the wife who was in an agitated state of depression. The patient returned to the office following 4 weeks of drug therapy with amitriptyline. Tremulousness was virtually gone. A smile was on her face, and she stated, "Charlie isn't mean to me anymore." When asked what she really meant, she said, "I guess I was the problem."

In the example just cited, there was initially no agreement between the physician and patient as to the problem; in fact, there was no agreement as to who was the appropriate patient. Agreement had to be accomplished through delicate negotiations in which the wife had to accept that her husband would not change and that she, herself, was quite upset and consequently needed assistance.

There are many other situations in which the problem perceived by the physician is vastly different from that recognized by the patient.

A 30 year old vigorously active black man, tremendously proud of his manhood, presented for relief of a respiratory infection. During the physical examination he was found to have a diastolic blood pressure of 110 mm. Hg. The respiratory infection was easily treated, but the patient was unwilling to accept hypertension as a significant problem and refused therapy, even after the physician and the patient's mother exhorted him to return for care.

Without concurrence as to the basic problem and without agreement as to the recommendations, implementation of recommendations was unlikely to occur.

A final component of the communication process is a mutual understanding of expectations. The patient who expects to be "cured" of chronic bronchitis is going to have unmet expectations. These unmet expectations will interfere with his confidence in the therapist and, consequently, with his long-term motivation to continue with the physician's recommendations.

Motivation and Resources to Implement Care

Once effective communication between physician and patient has been established, the decision of the patient to implement the physician's recommendations depends upon the motivation of patient and family and the availability of resources. The very fact that the patient has sought care from a physician suggests he has placed the physician in the role of a "healer" and has expectations of assistance in feeling better. The long-term cultural heritage of respect for the "healer" combined with the patient's psychologic need to be healed provide the physician with strong tools to assist in motivating the patient to implement the recommendations.

Not only may faith in the physician assist in the motivation, it is also an important therapeutic tool and frequently the only therapeutic tool. Placebo responses provide an interesting perspective on the therapeutic effectiveness of the "healer." Numerous studies have demonstrated that approximately 30 per cent of our population are placebo reactors and will have placebo responses to conditions as diverse as emotional difficulties and relief of postoperative pain. The potential placebo component of the response to the physician's ministration must be considered in all aspects of therapeutics.

When the problem perceived by the physician is not felt to be important by the patient or family, then the impact of the "healer" may be less, and the patient may not be motivated to follow recommendations. Our society has long viewed the chubby infant as a healthy infant. It is a major task to convince the young mother not to overfeed the child when all members of the family, as well as their friends, praise the pretty, healthy, obese baby. Smoking for the adolescent may be a means of maintaining social contact with peers, and long-term concern about cancer of the lung seems small in comparison with current social pressures. Drinking for adults may be important, not only for participation in the social group but also as a relief from stress. Motivation to accept procedures designed to maintain health or to continue with long-term therapy for hypertension may be difficult to achieve for those who deny the likelihood of illness. These are all examples of issues perceived as important by the physician but frequently not important by the patient. Typically, the patient has not sought care for these problems, and, consequently, investment on the part of the patient to follow the recommendations is limited.

Bloom[4] described a case history demonstrating social and cultural impacts upon a family's motivation and priorities.

Mrs T. was a 55 year old Italian immigrant who was hospitalized in New York City because of acute congestive heart failure complicating diabetes mellitus. She understood the importance of both dietary management and insulin therapy and while willing to take her insulin seemed not to be able to follow the diet. In fact, she freely admitted that she consumed a large and spicy (and presumably salt-laden) dinner the night before admission. Her continuing care was assumed by a medical student who saw her in the clinic and also made visits to her home. Mr. and Mrs. T. were central figures in a social network of close relatives and friends—the relationship being maintained by frequent banquets at their home. This function symbolized Mr. and Mrs. T.'s role as head of the family. Establishment of a successful dietary program was finally achieved through involvement of the son, daughter, and husband in a program to assist Mrs. T. in maintaining her diet and in fulfilling her duties as the maternal leader in the household.

For Mrs. T., understanding therapeutic recommendations was not enough. Her priority was her role within her family. It required the commitment of the entire family to modify functions while still guaranteeing that Mrs. T's role was maintained.

The problem of unmet expectations has potential to undermine the motivating influence of the physician. The patient who has been socialized to expect an injection of penicillin for a sore throat or an injection of vitamin B_{12} whenever "low" may be distraught when the physician refuses to comply. In the patient's view, these therapies have been effective before, and it is incomprehensible that the physician would not be willing to provide obviously effective therapy. Such situations require careful negotiation, communication, and occasionally some degree of "bending" on the part of the physician in order to best meet the underlying health care needs of the patient and the family. The doctor–patient relationship is established over time and is a negotiated relationship.

The degree to which the physician elaborates upon the rationale of therapy will also influence levels of motivation. Stimpson and Webb[32] provide many illustrations of the ways in which patients, through lack of understanding, often do not comply with physicians' "orders." Comaroff[7] studied 51 general practitioners in a large South Wales town and identified three strategies that physicians utilize in providing information to patients—unelaborated, medium elaborated, and elaborated. Each physician seemed to be consistent in his choice of strategies, with younger physicians seeming to emphasize medium or elaborated communication. Those physicians who placed major emphasis on unelaborated strategies made greater use of placebo therapy.

We suggest that the amount and extent of information conveyed to the patient should reflect the ability of the patient to be comfortable with the uncertainty present in the diagnosis and subsequent treatment. Some patients seek only the therapy and wish to place implicit trust in the physician's ability to cure the illness. On the other hand, others require much additional explanation, wishing to know not only the underlying causes of the problem but the means by which therapy is effective and the possible complications of therapy. The effectiveness of the physician and his ability to motivate the patient will be dependent on his ability to recognize the patient's needs.

Waitzkin and Stoeckle[35] emphasized a potential danger that the physician faces as he attempts to assess an individual patient's needs for elaboration. They suggest that physicians may have a tendency to control information offered the patient as a means of preserving their own power. The physician who provides minimal information will gradually find that the patients seeking his care will be only those who are comfortable in such a setting.

Finally, failure of the patient to implement recommendations may result from relative lack of resources. An expensive prescription may not be filled because of inadequate funds or inability to visit the pharmacy. Strict bedrest as therapy for low back pain may be impossible for the carpenter with a debt to pay or for the mother with small children at home.

A classic example of priorities for utilization of resources is illustrated in Koos' work referred to earlier.[20] One of those studied, a woman, aware that she needed an operation to relieve low back pain, refused the operation on the grounds that she and her family had higher priorities for family resources. The family car was disintegrating, and the family also wished to purchase a radio. She chose not to have surgery but to utilize her resources to accommodate the higher priorities of the family.

While the problems of adequate resources are most marked for the lower social classes, each family must place the cost of health care in its own priority system of needs. As indicated by the previous examples, necessary resources cannot always be purchased with dollars. Thus, even with increasing availability of health insurance, patient and family priorities for health care will still be important determinants of whether the family's resources are utilized.

SOCIAL AND CULTURAL DETERMINANTS IN EPIDEMIOLOGY OF DISEASE

In the preceding sections, we emphasized the social and cultural determinants of specific symptoms, perceptions of illness, decisions to seek health care, and the likelihood of completing care. Social and cultural determinants also may affect the incidence and prevalence of many diseases themselves.

In the Middle Ages the upper classes managed to avoid the plague by moving out of the city. Major infectious diseases have always tended to be more of a problem for the lower social classes. Dramatic drops in the rate of tuberculosis and other infectious diseases can be related to decreasing crowding of lower class populations and to better nutrition in these populations. Indeed the marked drop in incidence of tuberculosis was already occurring before the advent of antituberculosis therapy. Class differences in frequency and prevalence of a wide variety of diseases persist today. The incidence of obstetric complications is far higher among those of the lower social class.[19] The predisposition of lower social class individuals to smoking is a factor resulting in a higher incidence of chronic pulmonary disease and cancer of the lung. The fact that individuals in various occupations tend to come from specific social classes causes some occupational diseases to follow social class lines. The coal miner is more likely to develop chronic pulmonary disease; the farmer, skin cancer; and so forth.

Social class also may be a factor in the incidence of various psychologic illnesses. Depression is a syndrome found almost exclusively in the middle and upper classes. On the other hand, schizophrenia is more common in lower classes. Bagley,[2] in a review of depression, generalized that various classes related to stress in different manners: Class 5 (lower class) "behaves badly," Class 4 "aches physically," Class 3 "defends fearfully," and Classes 2 and 1 "are dissatisfied with themselves." In his review he cites data suggesting multiple explanations for the increased frequency of depression recognized in middle and upper social classes. He suggests that one reason for the differences may be reflected in the fact that lower classes are more likely to present with somatic symptoms, with underlying depression not being recognized. He also provides evidence suggesting both that the stresses of upper and middle class life may predispose individuals to depression and that these individuals may have personalities requiring

that they strive for success, with associated personality factors making them prone to depression. The relationship of social classes and suicide follows patterns parallel to that of depression.

Cultural factors also impinge upon the epidemiology of disease. Suicide rates tend to be low among Catholics and high among Scandinavians, although some of these differences may be related to reporting errors. Suicide rates are higher for upper classes than lower classes. Alcoholism is more prevalent among the Irish than the Jewish populations. Carcinoma of the stomach, so high among the Japanese in Japan, is much lower among Japanese in the United States. On the other hand, coronary heart disease is lower among Japanese in Japan than those in the United States.

Changing cultural patterns may modify patterns of disease. Increasing sexual promiscuity, especially among homosexuals, is associated with increasing prevalence of venereal disease. The advent of the drug culture is associated with an increasing incidence of drug addiction and of liver disease. The recent advent of natural food fads has the potential for creating nutritional deficiencies. Increasing cultural pressure to eliminate obesity is not simply motivated by desires for health maintenance; it represents far broader cultural attitudes about physical attractiveness.

Within each cultural group and within each social class, the social environment creates situations that predispose the individual to illness. A large number of animal and human studies on stress as well as extensive psychosomatic literature all attest to this fact. These psychosocial factors seem to lower the host resistance to a wide variety of diseases. Widowed individuals, especially men, have higher age-matched mortality rates from all causes than married individuals. Holmes and Rahe[18] demonstrated that major illness episodes cluster around life events such as death of a spouse, divorce, marriage, or retirement.

Cassel[6] hypothesizes that individuals faced with stress situations may be cushioned against the possible illness consequences by support from those close to them. Among supporting studies, he cites a study of primigravid women by Nuckolls and colleagues.[25] They studied the relationship of life changes using Holmes and Rahe's rating scale and a measure of the levels of assistance perceived to be available from family and community and related their findings to complications of pregnancy. Those with high life change indices during pregnancy had more complications. High social support levels were associated with much lower frequency of complications, both in those with high life changes and those with low changes. In another study, Marmot[23] demonstrated that coronary artery disease is less frequent among Japanese men living in California who have maintained their cultural ties than among those who have become "Americanized." These findings held true even after effects of diet, blood pressure, serum cholesterol, and smoking were controlled. Cassel felt that while individual studies might be criticized, the weight of evidence supported the thesis that social supports assist in protecting against disease.

Cassel suggests, therefore, that the practice of prospective medicine should include recognition both of psychosocial stress factors and of available social supports. He feels that identification of high risk families and provisions of systems of social support may prove more valuable than systems of screening and early detection of disease.

UTILIZATION OF SOCIAL AND CULTURAL FACTORS IN A PHYSICIAN'S PRACTICE

The outstanding physician integrates his knowledge of disease with the "art of medicine" as he carries out his practice. The "art of medicine" might be defined as the application of the physician's skill in *patient care* as contrasted with *disease care*. Thus, the "art of medicine" is more appropriately termed the "science of patient care." In caring for his patient,* the outstanding physician brings to bear his knowledge of the total environment of the patient—the psychologic, social, cultural, economic, and medical backgrounds. A portion of his knowledge and skill base represents material that has been presented in this chapter.

---

*About half of general practice consultations in the United Kingdom involve more than the doctor–patient dyad, since mothers and young children tend to present together, and elderly persons, whether seen at home or in the physician's office, are often accompanied by their spouse or another relative, usually a son or daughter.[16]

Diagnostic and therapeutic decisions frequently are made on a highly intuitive basis, which the physician himself has difficulty defining. In fact, at all stages of diagnosis, treatment, and prognosis, the physician is consciously or unconsciously utilizing principles of social epidemiology by applying his biomedical knowledge to the social circumstances of each individual patient and family.

When a patient requests consultation from a physician, three processes occur: the diagnostic process, the formulation of therapeutic recommendations, and implementation of therapy. Social and cultural factors outlined in this chapter are operative at each of the three stages.

To demonstrate the method outlined in Figure 4–1, we shall re-examine the case of the elderly woman with agitated depression who perceived that her husband, an elderly man with an organic brain syndrome, was "impossible."

As a result of previous contact with the family, the physician had background knowledge. Mrs. G. had come from basic Anglo-Saxon stock. She had seen the physician for repeated episodes of minor depression, always manifested by vague somatic symptoms. Mr. G., also of similar background, was a retired stoical farmer of few words. The development of dementia by the husband created real anxiety for the wife, not only as a result of day-to-day difficulties but also by generating anxieties about the future. Her foremost concerns were what would happen to each of them, where would they live, who would look after them, and so forth. The husband blandly led an unperturbed existence, sleeping, eating, and maintaining his garden. A concerned daughter living 20 miles from her parents was limited in her ability to assist them as a result of her own familial and occupational responsibilities. Assistance to the couple was available from friendly neighbors living a quarter mile away. This background knowledge provided the physician with a data base with which to begin the diagnostic process.

The presenting complaint was that Mr. G. was "unmanageable." Background knowledge of the family's psychosocial situation was brought to bear. The physician knew not only that the husband had true dementia but also that the wife was more anxious than would usually be expected.

THE MEDICAL CONSULTATION

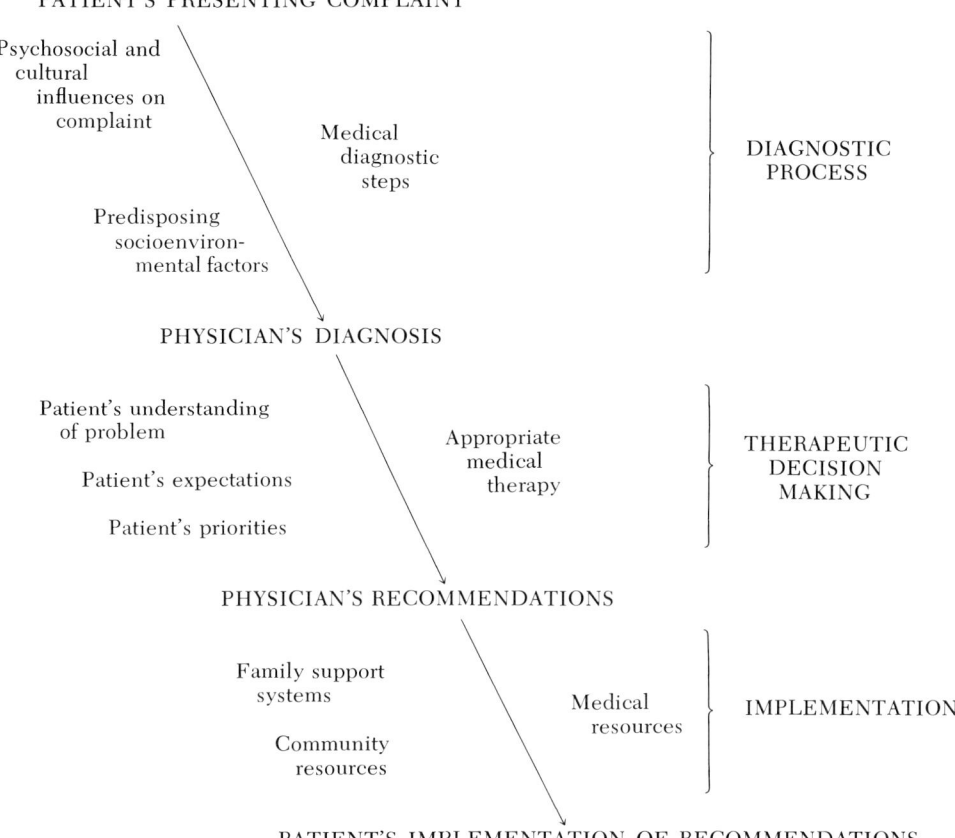

Figure 4–1. Diagram of medical consultation.

Husband and wife were well into the final stage of their life cycle (see chapter 3), and each was at high risk for the social and medical problems of aging. Medical evaluation substantiated that the husband's condition was unchanged but that the wife was in a state of agitated depression with definite sleep disturbance, anorexia, weight loss, constipation, and anxiety. The diagnosis was established.

The next step was to develop realistic therapeutic recommendations. These plans were threefold and had to consider appropriate medical therapy in light of the patients' understanding of their problems, expectations, and priorities. Plans called for (1) drug therapy for depression, (2) long-term support to assist the wife in accepting her husband's reduced biologic and social level of functioning, and (3) development of a long-term plan for care when they were no longer able to care for themselves.

The wife perceived that the husband was the problem and expected that efforts would be made to assist him. Further, notwithstanding a lifelong history of somatic complaints, she basically distrusted medications. The physician had to carry out careful negotiations with Mrs. G. and her daughter to convince each that the husband's situation was chronic and that Mrs. G. herself was upset and needed assistance.

At the implementation stage, the physician encouraged the daughter to monitor her mother's drug therapy. Neighbors checked on the parents' well-being daily. Marked improvement occurred in the wife's depression in approximately 3 weeks. However, 5 weeks later, the patient discontinued medication without telling her daughter and at the end of the 8 weeks was again depressed. The therapeutic program was re-established, and again the patient responded and has remained on medication. More recently, the entire family has been involved with the physician and social worker in a discussion of long-term health and housing needs of Mr. and Mrs. G. The schema outlined in Figure 4–1 assisted in the analysis and treatment of a complex sociomedical problem. While not every illness episode seen by the family physician will be as complex as the example just cited, the application of this schema ensures that the inextricable mix of biologic and social factors in any illness episode is fully considered.

Primary care is broader than simple assistance to the patient in the illness setting. It also includes responsibility for health maintenance. An appropriate attitude would be to view a patient's illness as a sign of failure. Prospective medicine must consider not only diseases for which family members have an increased risk based upon their age, occupation, social class, cultural background, and social habits; it also requires recognition of potential problems facing each family at each stage of its life cycle and the development of support systems to assist the family in these situations. The new widow is at high risk for depression. Other members of the family and the social network can assist in supporting the widow at this time of greatest stress.

At the core of each effective practice is an effective record system that is comprehensive and family oriented. When confronting the problems of individuals, records of the entire family will be of assistance, not only to review the problems of individuals and the family but also to plan health maintenance for each family member. This is particularly relevant to lower social class families whose life styles are not conducive to preventive health care. Comprehensiveness of care may be enhanced through participation of other health professionals, such as social workers and nurse practitioners. Their perspectives and their ability to recognize and treat potential problems complement the physician in his role in patient care.

REFERENCES

1. Apple, D.: How laymen define illness. J. Health Human Behav., *1*:219, 1960.
2. Bagley, C.: Occupational class and symptoms of depression. Soc. Sci. Med., 7:327, 1973.
3. Bernstein, B.: Class, Codes and Control. London, Routledge & Kegan Paul, Ltd., 1971.
4. Bloom, S. W.: The Doctor and His Patient. New York, The Free Press, 1965.
5. Boyle, C. M.: Difference between doctors' and patients' interpretation of some common medical terms. Br. Med. J., 2:585, 1970.
6. Cassel, J.: The contribution of the social environment to host resistance. Am. J. Epidemiol., *104*:107, 1976.
7. Comaroff, J.: Communicating information about non-fatal illness: The strategies of a group of general practitioners. Sociological Rev., *24*:2269, 1976.
8. Dollard, J.: Caste and Class in a Southern Town. Garden City, N.Y., Doubleday Anchor Books, 1957.
9. Dunnell, K., and Cartwright, A.: Medicine Takers, Prescribers and Hoarders. London, Routledge & Kegan Paul, Ltd., 1972.
10. Farber, B., Mindel, C. H., and Lazerwitz, B.: The Jewish American family. *In* Mindel, C. H.., and Habenstein, R. W., (eds.): Ethnic Families in America. New York, Elsevier Scientific Publishing Co., Inc., 1976.
11. Friedson, E.: Patients' Views of Medical Practice. New York, Russell Sage Foundation, 1961.
12. Frey, J.: Common Diseases. Philadelphia, J. B. Lippincott Co., 1974.
13. Gans, H. J.: The Urban Villagers. New York, The Free Press, 1962.
14. Gill, D. G.: Illegitimacy, Sexuality and the Status of Women: Some Sociological Perspectives. Oxford, Blackwells, 1977.
15. Gill, D. G.: Limitations upon choice and constraints over decision-making in doctor–patient exchanges. Washington, D.C., Fogarty International Center, Department of Health, Education and Welfare, 1977 (in press).
16. Gill, D. G., and Horobin, G. W.: Doctors, patients and the state: Relationships and decision-making. Sociological Rev., *20*:505, 1972.
17. Henderson, L. J.: Physician and patient as a social system. N. Engl. J. Med., *212*:819, 1935.
18. Holmes, T. H., and Rahe, R. H.: The social readjustment rating scale. J. Psychosom. Res., *11*:213, 1967.
19. Illsley, R.: The sociological study of reproduction and its outcome. *In* Richardson, A. S., and Guttmacher, A. F. (eds.): Childbearing: Its Social and Psychological Aspects. Baltimore, The Williams & Wilkins Co., 1967.
20. Koos, E. L. The Health of Regionville. New York, Columbia University Press, 1954.
21. LeMasters, E. E.: Blue-Collar Aristocrats: Life-Styles at a Working-Class Tavern. Madison, Wisc., University of Wisconsin Press, 1975.
22. Magraw, R. M.: Ferment in Medicine. Philadelphia, W. B. Saunders Co., 1966.
23. Marmot, M.: Acculturation and coronary heart disease in Japanese Americans. Ph.D. dissertation. Berkeley, Cal., University of California, 1975.
24. Mechanic, D., and Volkart, E. H.: Stress, illness behavior and the sick role. Sociological Rev., 26:51, 1961.
25. Nuckolls, K. B., Cassel, J., and Kaplan, B. H.: Psychosocial assets, life crisis and the prognosis of pregnancy. Am. J. Epidemiol., 95:431, 1972.
26. Parsons, T.: The Social System. Glencoe, Ill., The Free Press, 1951.

27. Pearse, I. H., and Crocker, L. H.: The Peckham Experiment. London, George Allen & Unwin, Publishers, Ltd., 1944.
28. Robinson, D.: The Process of Becoming Ill. London, Routledge & Kegan Paul, Ltd., 1971.
29. Runciman, W. G.: Relative Deprivation and Social Justice. London, Routledge & Kegan Paul, Ltd., 1966.
30. Shanas, E., & Townsend, P., Wedderburn, D. et al. (eds): Older People in Three Industrial Societies. New York, Atherton Press, 1968.
31. Staples, R.: The Black American family. In Mindel, C. H., and Habenstein, R. W. (eds.): Ethnic Families in America. New York, Elsevier Scientific Publishing Co., Inc., 1976.
32. Stimpson, G., and Webb, B.: Going to See the Doctor: The Consultation Process in General Practice. London, Routledge & Kegan Paul, Ltd., 1975.
33. Szasz, T. S., and Hollender, M. H.: A contribution to the philosopy of medicine: The basic models of the doctor-patient relationship. Am. Archiv. Intern. Med., 97:585, 1956.
34. Vernon, T. A., and Bigelow, P. A.: Effect of information about a potentially stressful situation on responses to stress impact. J. Pers. Soc. Psychol., 29:50, 1974.
35. Waitzkin, H., and Stoeckle, J. D.: The communication of information about illness. Adv. Psychosom. Med., 8:180, 1972.
36. White, K. L., Williams, T. F., and Greenberg, G. B.: The ecology of medical care. N. Engl. J. Med., 265:885, 1961.
37. Young, M., and Willmott, P.: Family and Kinship in East London. London, Routledge & Kegan Paul, Ltd., 1957.
38. Zborowski, M : People in Pain. San Francisco, Jossey-Bass, Inc., Publishers, 1969. (See especially Chapter 3.)
39. Zola, I. K.: Culture and symptoms: An analysis of patient presenting complaints. Am. Sociological Rev., 31:615, 1966.

PART II

PROBLEM-ORIENTED
MEDICAL RECORDS

Chapter 5

PROBLEM-ORIENTED MEDICAL RECORDS

by ROBERT E. RAKEL

A well-prepared medical record is among the most useful tools available to a family physician. When functioning effectively, it communicates the relevant facts regarding patient care to all health personnel involved and allows for the easy documentation and retrieval of information vital to the patient's ongoing care. The information should be organized in a systematic, logical, consistent manner and should accurately reflect the patient's state of health. Orderly recording of data is vital to efficient care, and although the information should be simplified as much as possible, it must likewise be both complete and accurate. Information placed in the office record should not be gathered and stored just because it is available and may someday be useful but should be accumulated on the basis that it is presently needed or will at some future time be needed for providing good patient care. We must avoid merely accumulating data and allowing them to be "untouched by human thought."[5] Family medicine involves the care of patients over a prolonged period of time. Acute illnesses cannot be treated as totally isolated events but must be viewed in the total perspective of a person's or a family's long-term care. A pregnant woman, for example, may have a slightly elevated blood pressure, which should be compared with readings prior to and following pregnancy to assess its true importance. Similarly, her smoking habits, weight, and other physiologic and psychologic functions should be noted.

An office record system will maintain its usefulness and efficiency over time only if it is individually designed to match the objectives and the personality of the physi-cian using it. The chart should be developed and organized based upon the individual physician's preferences and needs. Some will enjoy using flow sheets frequently; others will be "turned off" by them. Some will prefer, and will be able to maintain, an adequate medication list; others may find it impossible to keep such a list current. The ideal record for a family physician must also be kept simple and must not handicap or confine the busy physician's productivity by imposing unnecessary paper work. Merely accumulating a large amount of data is not productive: however, a well-organized record may actually require less data and yet be more informative than many present systems. The lengthy, illegible, and poorly organized office record of the past has developed into a logical, well-structured account, which lends itself to quick and easy retrieval of information and ready assessment of the patient's present health care needs and potential health hazards. It also assists the physician in predicting the patient's potential future state of health by identifying significant risk factors.

THE SOMR AND POMR

The traditional office record of the past was structured according to the source of material contained in the record; thus, it is called the source-oriented medical record (SOMR). In such a record, laboratory data, electrocardiographic reports, consultants' reports, physicians' notes, consultants' notes, nurses' notes, and x-ray reports are all filed independently in separate areas.

Material organized in this way becomes primarily a diary of past events and is of relatively limited value in ongoing patient care, although it was probably adequate for the crisis-oriented, episodic care of patients with acute illness, which has too often constituted the bulk of primary medical care.

The stimulus for change in record-keeping came in 1969, when Lawrence L. Weed developed the problem-oriented medical record (POMR). Although this innovative concept was originally applied to the hospital record, its principles have served as the nucleus for major changes in outpatient records as well. The "pure" form proposed by Weed has required some modification to be adapted to family practice, but its basic concepts serve as an excellent foundation for an efficient office medical record. The POMR has also been called the patient-oriented medical record, since it helps to avoid depersonalization and emphasizes individuality of the patient by listing the specific problems unique to that person. Hence, the patient is not just another person with gallbladder disease but an individual with a unique combination of associated problems that identify him as different from other patients with gallbladder disease.

The POMR achieves its maximum potential in the hands of a family physician. It works especially well in the continuing care of patients with chronic illness and in complex cases involving multiple problems. Since these are areas in which the family physician is especially effective, it is no wonder that he is the greatest promoter of the POMR. Now that many patients who suffer from previously fatal illnesses are surviving, the family physician is involved in the continuing care of ever-increasing numbers of the chronically ill. Management of patients with these chronic illnesses requires a dynamic record that accurately reflects at all times the patient's present and past medical problems and assists the physician in remaining aware of other potential problems that can become significant at any time.

Improved Communication

The record is not a static repository of medical observations structured in the meaningless order of source, but a precise instrument of communication.

LAWRENCE L. WEED[8]

In the United States, 73 per cent of the population consults a physician at least once a year, averaging 5.0 visits per person per year. By contrast, only 10.6 per cent of the population is hospitalized each year, for an average of 0.14 hospitalization per individual.

As our society becomes increasingly mobile and medical technology becomes increasingly complex, we need a well-organized medical record system that permits easy communication and transfer of information among health professionals, both within the same office and at separate sites. No longer can the record be a document understood only by the physician who places data in it. It must permit other physicians, as well as an increasing number of other health personnel who also depend on the record, to readily assess the needs of the patient. It must allow the physician, his physician associates, and all health personnel involved to assess the patient's condition, understand the plan of management, and recognize all parameters important to the patient's ongoing care. As long as the record is able to communicate information in this manner, it will serve as an effective tool for all members of the health care team.

The maintenance of a complete and well-organized medical record over a prolonged period of time contributes to high quality care by permitting attention to be focused on preventive measures. The need for a uniform, organized collection of information in the office record will increase as more physicians practice in groups and a larger portion of costs is paid by third parties. Increased emphasis is being placed on the assessment of the quality of care, and outpatient records need to be organized in a manner that permits review, just as hospital records are reviewed. Terminology is also being influenced by third-party payers. The physician and other health professionals, such as the dentist, nurse, and therapist, are now called providers, and the office visit is an encounter. It is hoped that in family practice an encounter will remain a friendly interaction between physician and patient, rather than follow Webster's definition of "a meeting of adversaries or hostile persons to engage in conflict." It is no wonder that many physicians bristle at the use of this term to refer to their caring relationships with patients. An encounter has been officially defined by the Committee on Vital and Health Statistics of the Department of Health, Education and Welfare as "a face to face contact between a patient and a provider (physician, dentist, nurse, or any other health professional) who, at the time of contact, has primary responsibility for assessing and treating or managing the condition of the patient and who exercises independent judgment as to the care of the patient."

Improved patient care must remain the primary objective of any newly structured record system. "Data collection and information systems cannot be justified if they subvert the process of patient care and fail to benefit the patient and provider either directly or indirectly. The growth of public, as opposed to private, responsibility for personal health services means that more and more data requirements will be placed upon the providers of care."[5] Data collection must not be allowed to become threatening to either the patient or the physician but must be an obvious asset to the care and management of all problems related to patients.

Information Retrieval

The medical record is rapidly becoming less the private property and sole responsibility of the physician and more the joint responsibility and common property of the physician, other health providers, and the patient. Information in the medical record should be highly visible, clear, and concise, so that it can be retrieved easily to allow for effective and efficient use of the physician's and other health professionals' time. With such a record, the physician can also easily review data in order to evaluate his effectiveness, just as the research scientist evaluates the results of his experiments.

Medical identification cards are becoming increasingly popular in our mobile society (Fig. 5–1). Such a card contains microfilm of selected portions of an individual's medical record and is carried as a wallet card. This document serves as a "medical passport" and identifies the nature of the patient's medical problems, such as a recent myocardial infarction, diabetes mellitus, drug allergies, anticoagulant medication, and immunization status. These data give an accurate composite picture of the patient's health status to physicians other than the patient's personal physician during an emergency or when the patient is traveling outside the community.

CONVERSION TO A NEW SYSTEM

A well-organized and clearly developed medical record will make the provision of excellent medical care readily apparent. It will also, however, just as readily expose poor or inadequate care. Physicians who have converted their office record systems to the problem-oriented format undergo a humbling experience as numerous weaknesses in their previous care are uncovered. Problems are frequently identified that had been lost in the record, and laboratory abnormalities are uncovered that were not investigated further. One physician discovered that blood pressure readings had been taken on only one-third to one-half of all patients in his practice. Another noted that he had been paying too little attention to preventive measures or to the follow-up of potentially serious problems. The most valuable detection is the uncovering of a considerable amount of buried and almost forgotten clinical data. The conversion of a source-oriented record to any new form of record system, whether it be the POMR or others, will involve a reassessment and reorganization of the record system that will be of value to the physician and his patient by uncovering these problems and placing all facts into a refreshing new perspective.

Transfer of Information

It is important that the family physician incorporate the patient's entire medical background into his record, so that the total comprehensive picture is constantly available to the physician and to other health personnel who have need of it. Valuable medical information is often scattered in a variety of locations, and thus it becomes relatively inaccessible or unavailable when needed. When seeing new patients, a strong effort should be made to acquire all medical information from other physicians, government services, hospitals, and other health agencies previously involved in the patient's care. A great deal of unnecessary effort and expense results when each physician, in turn, must establish full medical data for every patient, since they must needlessly repeat a variety of diagnostic

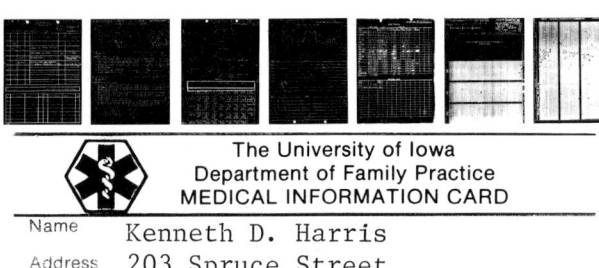

The University of Iowa
Department of Family Practice
MEDICAL INFORMATION CARD

Name	Kenneth D. Harris
Address	203 Spruce Street
	Iowa City, Iowa 52240
Telephone	(319)-356-1990
S.S.#	483-30-9982 Date Prep 10-22-77

Figure 5-1. Medical identification card.

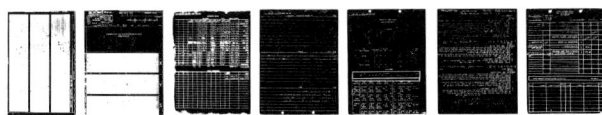

Read film with microscope eye piece,
ophthalmoscope, or microfilm viewer.

Family Physician   R. E. Rakel, M.D.
Family Practice Center - U. of Iowa
Iowa City, Iowa 52242 (319)-356-1787

Special Problems/Allergies   Diabetes Mellitus
                              Penicillin

tests and therapeutic trials. When the transferred record is in the form of the POMR or some similarly concise system, putting it to use is a simple matter for the new physician, and sending it on is a painless experience for the former physician, since he knows that it can be interpreted readily and will be of benefit to his former patient's care. Central computerization of the medical record in the future may obviate much of this problem. In countries with a national health service, such as exists in Great Britain, the medical record is considered state property and is automatically transferred with the patient when he moves to a new community.

A well-organized record system, such as the POMR, also allows the referring family physician to communicate the patient's total health status more effecitvely to consulting physicians, by submitting either the summary sheet or the problem list with the consultation request. This prevents the specialist from merely "treating his own disease" and ensures his awareness of all of the patient's medical, social, and psychiatric problems, as well as the problems for which the consultation is being requested.

When a cardiologist is asked to consult on a seriously ill patient in the coronary care unit, the problem list clearly illustrates other problems to be considered and managed and makes the need for continuing involvement by the family physician readily apparent. Subspecialists are prevented from concentrating on a single part, to the detriment of the whole patient.

Legibility

Legibility is necessary if any data, no matter how systematically organized, are to be retrieved and collated in a rapid, accurate, and useful manner that will permit the quick review of a patient's total health status. The well-known illegibility of physicians' handwriting is an understandable product of conditioning during many years of rapid note-taking. This handicap, the greatest barrier to effective communication and good records, is now being removed, as a rapidly increasing number of physicians turn to dictating their records and utilizing secretarial services for transcription to obtain clearly typed progress notes. This improved legibility is an obvious advantage in group practices, in which more than one physician and several nurses or other health professionals are likely to depend upon the same chart. The POMR, because of its structure, lends itself well to dictation with a minimum of confusion.

Minimum Requirements for the Office Record

A certain minimum amount of basic patient information is necessary for ongoing care. Much of this is demographic information, which is usually obtained at the first office visit and is permanently placed with the chart. It is a ready source of reference for the names and ages of all family members and includes occupational and insurance information as well (Fig. 5–2). A group of national consultants on ambulatory medical records developed a minimum basic set of data that they considered necessary for all records (Table 5–1). This information, although relatively complete, avoids the issue of documenting marital status and race. The American Board of Family Practice has incorporated chart review into its recertification procedure. Table 5–2 lists those items considered by the Board to be essential to a good office record.

UNIVERSITY OF IOWA

FAMILY PRACTICE CENTER

FAMILY REGISTRATION RECORD

FAMILY NAME: JONES FAMILY NUMBER: 50-00-57

NAME (first)	BIRTH DATE (MO/DAY/YR)	EDUC. LEVEL	SOC. SEC. #	SEX	RELIGION	RACE
HUSBAND: JOHN	5/11/40	B.A.	311-46-4700	M	CATHOLIC	C
WIFE: BETTY	8/20/42	COLLEGE-2yrs.	315-45-7646	F	"	"
CHILDREN LIVING AT HOME:						
1. GREG	7/24/65	6th GRADE		M	"	"
2. JUDY	5/7/68	3rd GRADE		F	"	"
3. SUSAN	11/19/72			F	"	"
4. MARK	10/31/74			M	"	"
5.						
6.						
7.						
8.						

OTHER PERSONS LIVING IN THE HOME:	BIRTH DATE (MO/DAY/YR)	EDUC. LEVEL	RELATIONSHIP	SEX	RELIGION	RACE
1.						
2.						

WIFE - PREVIOUS MARRIAGE YES (NO) HUSBAND - PREVIOUS MARRIAGE YES (NO)

MAILING ADDRESS: (Street, city, zip) HOME TELEPHONE:

209 ELMWOOD RD. IOWA CITY, IOWA 52240 338-2375

	OCCUPATION	EMPLOYER	ADDRESS	BUSINESS PHONE:
HUSBAND:	TEACHER	CITY HIGH SCHOOL	IOWA CITY, IOWA	337-2149
WIFE:	HOUSEWIFE			

INSURANCE INFORMATION

COMPANY: BLUE CROSS-BLUE SHIELD POLICY NUMBER: (all numbers)

IN THE NAME OF: JOHN JONES R15358591

COMPANY: POLICY NUMBER: (all numbers)

IN THE NAME OF:

REGISTRATION DATE 11-15-76 COMPLETED BY John Jones

Figure 5–2. *Family registration form, University of Iowa, Family Practice Center. (From Rakel, R. E.: Principles of Family Medicine. Philadelphia, W. B. Saunders Co., 1977.)*

TABLE 5–1. AMBULATORY MEDICAL CARE RECORDS: UNIFORM
MINIMUM BASIC DATA SET*

Items that Characterize the Patient

1. Patient identification
   a. Name—Surname, first name, middle initial
   b. Identification number—A unique number that distinguishes the patient and his ambulatory medical care record from all other patients
2. Residence—Patient's usual residence, to consist of street name and number, apartment number (if any), city, state, and zip code
3. Date of birth—Month, day, and year
4. Sex—Male or female
5. Expected source of payment
   a. Government
      (1) Workmen's Compensation
      (2) Medicare
      (3) Medicaid
      (4) Civilian Health and Medical Program of the Uniformed Services
      (5) Other
   b. Insurance mechanism
      (1) Blue Cross
      (2) Blue Shield
      (3) Insurance company
      (4) Prepaid group practice or health plan
      (5) Medical foundation
   c. Self-pay
   d. No charge (free, charity, special research, teaching)
   e. Other

Items that Characterize the Provider

1. Provider identification
   a. Name—Surname, first name, middle initial
   b. Identification number—A unique number that distinguishes the provider from all other providers
2. Professional address—Street address, office number (if any), city, state, and zip code
3. Profession—The profession in which the provider is currently engaged
   a. Physician—Include specialty, if any, as determined by membership in, or eligibility for, specialty board
   b. Dentist—Include specialty
   c. Nurse
   d. Other (specify)

Items that Characterize the Patient-*Provider Encounter

1. Date of encounter—Month, day, and year
2. Place of encounter
   a. Private office
   b. Clinic or health center (any except hospital outpatient department)
   c. Hospital outpatient department
   d. Hospital emergency room
   e. Home
   f. Other (specify)
3. Reason for encounter—The patient's principal problems, complaints, or symptoms at this encounter, in the patient's own words
4. Findings—All history, physical examination, laboratory, and other findings pertinent to the patient's reasons for visit and/or diagnoses and any other findings the provider deems important
5. Diagnosis and/or problem—The provider's current assessment of the patient's reasons for the encounter and all conditions requiring treatment, with the principal diagnosis and/or problem listed first. Principal diagnosis and/or problem is defined as the health problem that is most significant in terms of the procedures carried out and the care provided at this encounter
6. Services and procedures—All diagnostic, therapeutic, and preventive services and procedures (including history-taking) performed during the encounter and those scheduled to be performed before the next encounter
7. Itemized charges—All charges to be made by the provider for services and procedures performed during the encounter or to be performed by him or his associates before the next encounter
8. Disposition (one or more)—The provider's statement of the next steps in the care of the patient
   a. No follow-up planned
   b. Return, time specified
   c. Return as needed
   d. Telephone follow-up
   e. Referred to other provider
   f. Returned to referring provider
   g. Admit to hospital
   h. Others

*From Consultants on Ambulatory Medical Care Records, U.S. National Committee on Vital and Health Statistics. Dept. of Health, Education and Welfare.

TABLE 5–2. SUGGESTIONS FOR OFFICE CHART CONTENT[*]

A. Basic patient information
 1. Name
 2. Address
 3. Telephone (home and business)
 4. Birth date
 5. Education
 6. Economic status
 7. Pertinent sociologic information
  a. Family structure
  b. Marital status
  c. Occupation
  d. Sex
  e. Race
  f. Religion

B. A summary of the patient's health status (such as a problem list).

C. Historical information, physical findings, laboratory and other test results.

D. A delineation of the plan of treatment (including drugs, diets, treatments, recommendations, etc.) for each element of the patient's health care.

E. A progress record indicating the patient's complaints and observations, health care personnel observations, conclusions, and tests.

In addition

A. Records must be legible.

B. Records should be organized systematically in such a way as to allow efficient and rapid review of the patient's total health picture and any particular health problem by family physicians and associates, consultants, and allied health personnel.

[*]Adapted from the American Board of Family Practice.

FILING FAMILY RECORDS

Family medicine means family care and therefore calls for a family medical record with information about each member occupying a separate area within the family record. Thus, inter-related problems can be identified and followed more easily. Color coding, open filing, and numerical filing systems are now standard features of most practices and work well when filing is done by family, rather than by individual. Even if surnames of children vary within a family because of previous marriages or if maternal parents live with the family, each individual is identified by a one or two digit modifier within the family number. The family folder usually consists of an outer file jacket containing family demographic data (Fig. 5–2) and selected information such as a family problem list, family visit register, or family tree. The outer jacket may be made of plastic or cardboard. Contained within this jacket are the individual charts of each family member, either inside separate manila folders or affixed to rigid dividers (Fig. 5–3). The family chart allows the physician to review shared family problems. During an office visit by one member, a quick review of the problem list of other family members may alert the physician to problems that could be related to the present symptoms or to other disorders that should be considered and evaluated in addition to the presenting problem.

One technique for remaining constantly aware of the presenting problems of other family members is the use of the family member visit register (Fig. 5–4). This is usually placed in a prominent area of the family folder and records the dates, names, and major reasons for visits by all family members. Even though only a single member's chart will be opened during a visit, a glance will show whether other recent problems prominent within the family may have a bearing on the present difficulty. It may also serve as a reminder to the physician to ask about the progress of another family member who was recently ill, in order to assess the degree of recovery or the likelihood of continuing disability. The family physician is thus constantly prepared to deal with family problems, in addition to caring for individual members.

COMPARISON OF THE SOMR AND THE POMR

No medical record can adequately convey the most important element in quality of care, the personal involvement of the physician with his patient. Even though the POMR will improve the physician's ability to retrieve data and analyze the patient's medical status, it does not guarantee that he will utilize the information properly. No medical record can ensure better medical care, and the POMR, like all the rest, can serve only as a tool to assist the physician in rendering better care. Most who have used the POMR, however, feel that it is a better instrument for providing quality health care than is the SOMR.

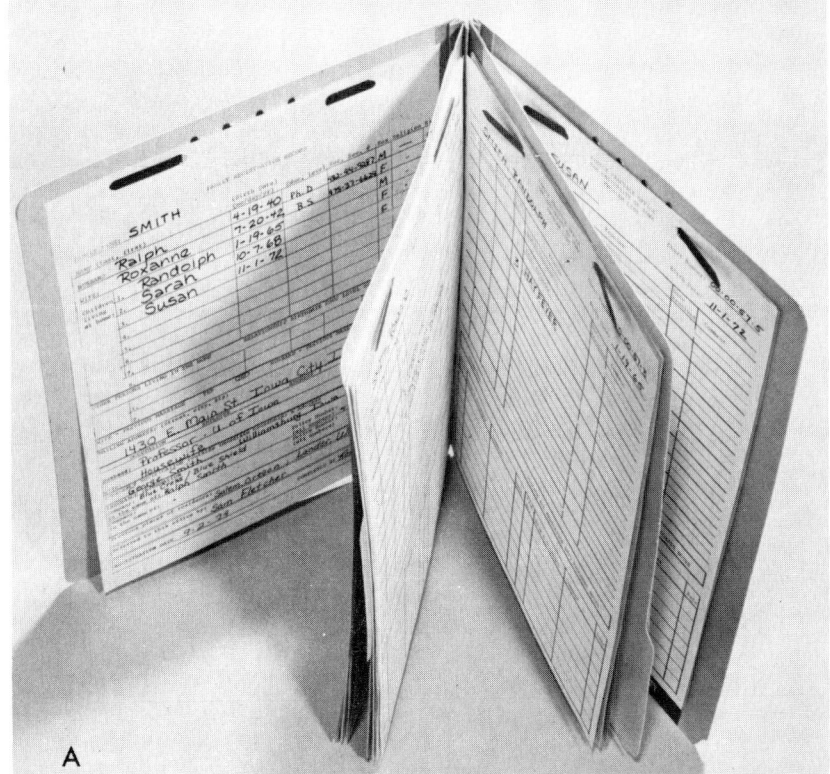

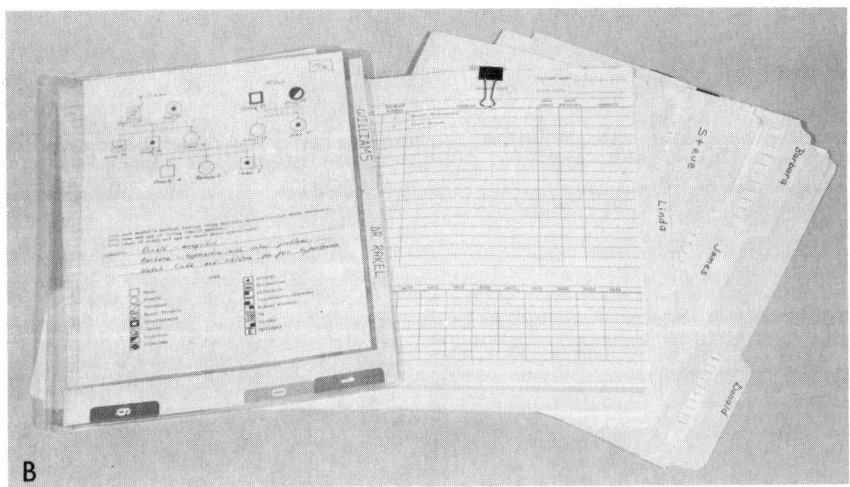

Figure 5–3.   *Two examples of family charts. (From Rakel, R. E.: Principles of Family Medicine. Philadelphia, W. B. Saunders Co., 1977.)*

While the SOMR has material randomly organized in narrative form, the POMR has formally organized material in outline form. The most important difference between the two is the problem list, which serves as the index or table of contents for all significant material within the record. The POMR structures its information in a logical sequence and minimizes word volume by using an outline format, whereas the SOMR resembles a book without a table of contents—the only way to find the information contained is to look through it page by page. Similarly, in the SOMR, unresolved problems are followed with some difficulty, and chronic problems tend to be forgotten or ignored because they are buried within the chart amidst a volume of acute illnesses and relatively unimportant information. The problem list, prominently displayed, serves as a constant reminder of ongoing problems at every patient visit. The POMR presents data in a concise and clearly visible fashion, improving communication and permitting more effective use of physician time while facilitating effective expansion of allied health roles. The SOMR, however, organizes material in a more fragmented manner, has no index,

and makes it difficult to retrace the physician's analytic process and clinical rationale (Table 5–3).

UTILIZING THE POMR

As discussed earlier in this chapter, the POMR was developed by Lawrence L. Weed. Although originally directed toward organization of the hospital record, it was rapidly adapted to the outpatient setting, and its usefulness in family practice was

FAMILY MEMBER VISIT REGISTER

NAME _DALY_

NUMBER _50-00-03_

Given Name	LLOYD	DAWN	PEGGY	KEVIN	MICHELLE	MRS. VAN	
Date of Birth	3/18/39	5/12/41	11/29/60	8/20/64	5/5/71	4/20/02	
DATE	PROBLEM	PROBLEM	PROBLEM	PROBLEM	PROBLEM	PROBLEM	PROBLEM
3/17/75	ulcer						
4/3/75		Headache			well child exam	BP check	
4/7/75				sore throat			
5/12/75			school prob.				
5/30/75	Alcoholism						
7/8/75		Fatigue					
7/23/75		Depression					
8/19/75				Cough			
9/4/75	Ulcer check						
9/22/75						BP check	
10/1/75					Otitis media		
10/10/75					FU-OM		
11/12/75			Drug Prob.				
12/6/75		Depression					
1/17/76				Laceration			
2/10/76		Marital Prob.					

Figure 5–4. *Family member visit register, University of Iowa, Family Practice Center. (From Rakel, R. E.: Principles of Family Medicine. Philadelphia, W. B. Saunders Co., 1977.)*

TABLE 5-3. COMPARISON OF THE SOMR AND THE POMR
AFTER CONVERSION OF AN OFFICE RECORD SYSTEM*

Before Problem-Orienting	After Problem-Orienting
Important problems were frequently forgotten or the chart had to be read completely to find important information, which required much time.	All problems are displayed on one page at the front of the chart.
Office personnel were not aware of all patient problems.	The entire health team not only is aware of the problems but can be active in helping the patient with his problems.
The "insurance girl" frequently had to interrupt me to obtain diagnoses required for insurance forms.	All problems and diagnoses are listed on the page at the front of the chart, which she can read herself.
Since the office girls were frequently not aware of the patient's problems, data such as urinalyses, blood pressures, and weights were not obtained before I saw the patients.	Office girls now see the problem sheet. Protocols have been developed so that data for common problems are collected and entered routinely in the chart before I see the patient. This has increased efficiency and saved considerable time.
Consultants frequently made inappropriate suggestions, repeated studies that had already been performed, or had to read the entire chart to derive needed information.	Consultants are now made aware of *all* the patient's problems. Even though many of the problems are outside a consultant's specialty, they may affect his intervention in one particular problem.
Anesthesiologists had to do a complete evaluation prior to surgery or, more often, were unaware of significant risk factors.	The problem list with *all* problems is at the front of the chart.
When looking for the progress of a particular problem in the record, the entire record had to be read, since the progress notes were not separated by problems.	Only those notes labeled by number and name for a particular problem need be read when evaluating the progress of that particular problem.
Routine systematic audit was impossible because of sketchy, unorganized notes with little assessment information.	Audit is easily obtained because of the structure of the progress notes and the use of flow sheets.
I was unable to assess needs for continuing medical education because there was no way to know the frequency of disease or problem occurrence.	The disease-index file can be used as a guide for further educational efforts. Obviously, if one rarely, if ever, sees a patient with tsutsugamushi disease, there is little reason to attend a conference on it or waste time reading a monograph on that subject. A knowledge of the order of frequency of diseases in my practice has been enlightening and has reordered my priorities for postgraduate education.
There was no way to contact a group of patients with a particular problem for a change in medication, evaluation, etc.	With the disease-index file, *all* patients with a given problem can easily be contacted. This has recently been done in this office to give "flu" immunizations to my patients with chronic obstructive pulmonary disease, diabetes, and coronary artery disease.
There seemed to be little or no continuity of care between the hospital and the office practice.	The problem sheet in the office is duplicated and taken to the hospital when a patient is hospitalized. Therefore, the same problem list is used in exactly the same order in both places. On discharge, the summary is dictated as a problem-oriented progress note, summarizing the hospitalization according to each problem. This is then used in the office record as a continuation of the office progress notes.
There was never a consistent way of planning for future care for a patient. Data were obtained haphazardly. If thought of, information was obtained, but my memory frequently failed.	With a flow sheet, one can "program" future care. This advantage of the Weed system was largely responsible for the conversion of my office to the system.
There never seemed to be a way to evaluate the effectiveness of therapy or evaluation or usefulness of a particular procedure.	An audit on several different levels is possible. From the disease-index file, all charts can be pulled, thereby allowing a comparison of the office practice with the experience of others, as published in the literature. Diagnostic criteria can be established and then performance checked by pulling all the charts with that problem.

TABLE 5–3. COMPARISON OF THE SOMR AND THE POMR AFTER CONVERSION OF AN OFFICE RECORD SYSTEM*—*Continued*

Before Problem-Orienting	After Problem-Orienting
Laboratory, x-ray, electrocardiogram, and consultation data were scattered throughout the chart with no chronologic organization and not organized in relation to specific problems.	All laboratory data are entered on appropriate flow sheets in chronologic order. The lab sheets are then discarded. Results from x-ray and consultation reports are entered in the progress notes under the appropriate problems. The reports are then filed in an envelope in chronologic order at the back of the chart.
Thoroughness and attention to detail were possible but difficult, since there seemed to be little or no organization.	The use of the problem sheet and flow sheets and organization of the progress notes foster thoroughness and highlight detail in patient management. A missing hematocrit here or a blood pressure there stands out like a sore thumb.
Preventive medicine seemed to be an impossible goal and therefore episodic care was given.	Preventive medicine is the name of the game; episodic care is discouraged.

*From Williams, W. L.: Conversion of an established family practice to the problem-oriented system. *In* Walker, H. K., Hurst, J. W., and Woody, M. F.: Applying the Problem Oriented System. New York, Medcom Press, 1973, p. 133.

first demonstrated by Bjorn and Cross.[2] Numerous publications and articles appearing since 1969 have developed the basic concepts further and have suggested many variations, which provide a myriad of choices for the individual physician. Each physician is encouraged to review the literature and then to select those components with which he feels most comfortable and which appear most useful in his particular practice. The design of any component should be varied when necessary to match individual preference. Weed describes four basic elements as the nucleus of the POMR: the data base, problem list, initial plan, and progress notes. While his initial plan applies primarily to the complete work-up of a new office patient or the admission work-up of a hospitalized patient, I prefer to incorporate it into ongoing patient care as a feature of the progress note (Fig. 5–5).

A survey conducted by the author in 1973 showed that 97 per cent of all family practice residency programs at that time were utilizing the POMR in their family practice centers. Although it is obvious that the POMR will play a prominent role in the future design of office medical record systems, it is equally apparent that it will continue to be improved upon as the volume of experience increases.

Chart Organization

The organization of material within the chart will vary with the type of chart se-lected, but in all cases the material should be organized in a consistent and prede-fined manner. If a folder is used, the prob-lem list is usually the top sheet on the left, with the family registration record beneath it. The top sheet on the right contains the most recent progress notes, with previous progress notes beneath it, followed by the data base, electrocardiograms, and corre-spondence. If a flow sheet is used, this is usually placed on top of the most recent progress note. If all of the material is ar-ranged in a single stack, the problem list is always on top, followed by flow sheet, most recent progress note, previous progress notes, data base, electrocardiograms, and correspondence. If possible, each of these sections should be divided by tabs or by some other method to allow easy identifica-tion, for example, by using different colors for each section.

Problem List

Although the problem list is developed largely from information accumulated in the data base, it will be discussed before the data base, since it is the most important single ingredient of the POMR. If there is limited enthusiasm for using all compo-nents of the POMR, development of a problem list alone will be of significant benefit. Addition of a data base will en-hance its usefulness, but full benefits can be realized only when structured progress notes are also incorporated.

A problem is anything that requires

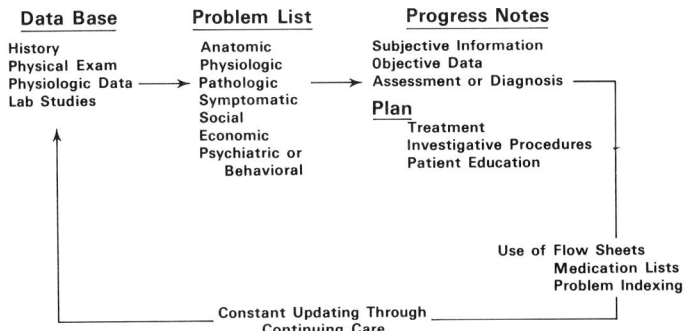

Figure 5-5. *Basic elements and process of the problem-oriented medical record. (From Rakel, R. E.: Principles of Family Medicine. Philadelphia, W. B. Saunders Co., 1977.)*

diagnosis or management or that interferes with quality of life as perceived by the patient. It can be either a firm diagnosis, a physical symptom, or a social or economic problem. It is any physiologic, pathologic, psychologic, or social item of concern to either the patient or the physician. The problem list serves as a comprehensive overview of the patient's present and past state of health. It indicates whether the problems are active or have occurred in the past and are presently inactive. The problems can be:

1. Anatomic (hernia).
2. Physiologic (jaundice of unknown etiology).
3. Symptomatic (dyspnea).
4. Economic (financial difficulty).
5. Social (marital discord, lives alone, husband alcoholic, son in prison).
6. Psychiatric (depression).
7. Physical handicap (paralysis or amputation).
8. Abnormal laboratory test, if it is not part of a more clearly defined item (elevated blood urea nitrogen level).
9. A risk factor (positive family history of diabetes mellitus).

Each problem is numbered, and the progress notes are keyed by number to the appropriate problem on the list, thereby reflecting its present state of resolution. The management of each problem is identified throughout the text by this same number.

The types of illness seen by a family physician are often more appropriately described as symptoms or undifferentiated problems than as diseases. Disease implies a full understanding of the pathology and etiology of the illness, whereas many of the illnesses encountered by the family physi-

cian involve a varying degree of insight into the underlying etiology and a varying severity of the illness, which occasionally resolves while still in the undifferentiated state.

The problem list is a dynamic picture of the patient's health problems and is continually changed by updating, as new problems are added or old problems are carried to a greater degree of resolution. It should contain all of the patient's continuing problems and should have a prominent position in the record, so as to constantly remind the physician to care for the whole patient and not to limit his attention to the problem that may be temporarily outstanding. One value of the problem list is that it continually "stares back at you" and prevents the physician from focusing on too limited an area to the exclusion of the patient's total health picture. With such a format, it is possible to rapidly orient oneself to the most important current problem without forgetting the others.

All problems can be kept in proper perspective. One physician on call for another can rapidly grasp the essential nature of a case by scanning the problem list and thereby can make a more rational decision regarding the acute presenting problem. The POMR also allows for more efficient use of allied health personnel, by permitting the physician to effectively communicate his assessment of the patient's problems and their management.

In the traditional source-oriented record, it is difficult to retrieve and correlate infomation about one particular problem. In the problem-oriented record, this information is arranged according to the problem for which it is intended. The basic concept of the POMR is that the problem is the functional unit. All activities relating to the care of the patient, including progress notes, history, physical findings, and therapy, refer to the specific problem for which they were initiated. The constant surveillance of a patient's state of health by the physician and allied health personnel and their efforts toward establishing effective health maintenance require constant monitoring of health hazards and risk factors. These risk factors should be identified on the problem list and should serve to constantly alert all health personnel to their presence.

Design of the Problem List

The problem list can be structured in a variety of ways. Each physician should select the components he prefers and should arrange them in the manner most comfortable to his style. A survey of 100 family practice residency programs conducted by the author revealed that 85 per cent of them design their own problem list, and 15 per cent purchase commercial systems. One of the most commonly used problem list formats is that employed at the University of Washington (Fig. 5–6). An-

FAMILY MEDICAL CENTER
UNIVERSITY OF WASHINGTON
SCHOOL OF MEDICINE

MASTER PROBLEM LIST

PROBLEM NO.	DATE	PROBLEMS – ACTIVE	DATE	INACTIVE	CODE
1.	5/2/73	Pneumonia- Pneumococcal	5/13/73	X-ray Normal	
2.	9/4/73	Elevated FBS 10/7/73, Diabetes Mellitus			
3.	3/5/74	Overweight			
4.	4/12/74	Marital Problem			
5.	10/5/74	Stasis Dermatitis			
6.	2/3/75	Abdominal Pain GB x-ray → Cholecystitis	6/4/75	Cholecystectomy	

MASTER PROBLEM LIST

Figure 5–6. *Master problem list, University of Washington, Family Medical Center. (From Rakel, R. E.: Principles of Family Medicine. Philadelphia, W. B. Saunders Co., 1977.)*

UNIVERSITY OF IOWA
FAMILY PRACTICE CENTER
PROBLEM LIST

CHART NUMBER: _50-04-42_

NAME: _Williams, Donald_   BIRTH DATE: _9-21-20_

Code No.	Date Recorded	Date Onset	Prob. No.	Problem	Date Resolved	Comment
			1	Health Maintenance		
			2	Acute Episodes		
4010	6/10/68	1962	3.	Hypertension		
5740	6/10/68	1964	4.	Cholelithiasis + Cholecystitis	7/12/68	Cholecystectomy
7130	2/5/70	1970	5.	Pain Rt. Knee —10-7-71→ Osteoarthritis		X-ray Knees
4550	9/8/74	Long Hx	6.	Hemorrhoids		
1084	9/8/74	1974	7.	Marital Problem		
7889	11/14/76	1976	8.	Depression		

ALLERGIES: _Penicillin_   DICTATE ALL MEDICATION INTO PROGRESS NOTES

Prob. No.	Drug & Strength	Comment	Date	Prob. No.	Drug & Strength	Comment	Date
3.	Diuril 500 mg.	ī pd	6/10/68				
5.	ASA gr X	pid	2/5/70				
8.	Elavil 25 mg.	ī AM ii hs.	11/14/76				

Figure 5–7. *Problem List, University of Iowa.*

other is the form used at the University of Iowa (Fig. 5–7), which has a separate column for comments and indicates inactive problems merely by entering the date of resolution.

Twenty-eight per cent of the programs reviewed also use a separate problem list for acute, self-limiting problems, since most feel that only chronic or recurring problems should be placed on the master problem list. Acute-problem lists indicate the frequency of recurrence, so that a chronic minor problem, such as acute bron-

chitis, can be identified as potentially threatening to the patient's future health and can be transferred to the major problem list. Acute problems can be listed on the same sheet as the major problems, as in Figure 5–8, or can be placed on an entirely separate sheet that is kept immediately behind the major problem list.

An alternate method for identifying acute problems is to list them as "problem No. 2" (Fig. 5–7). When using this method, all acute self-limiting problems are labeled problem No. 2 in the progress notes, with the name of the problem also listed next to the heading of No. 2. In a similar manner, the label "problem No. 1" is permanently assigned to health maintenance activities and stresses the emphasis on preventive measures and well-care in family practice. Some prefer to use letters for the acute problems, assigning the next letter in the alphabet to each new acute problem, whether or not a separate acute-problem list is used. Figure 5–9 illustrates a variety of methods for organizing the problem list.

The essential ingredients for any problem list are the patient's name, problem number, problem, date of onset, date of resolution, and code number to permit problem indexing (as described later in this chapter). A variety of methods can be used to illustrate the active or inactive status of each problem. Those problems that have been resolved but may have an impact upon the patient's future health must be retained on the problem list for continued visibility. A resolved problem can be transferred to a separate inactive column, as in Figure 5–6, or can be identified by inserting a date of resolution, as in Figure 5–7, or by drawing a line or arrow through the

Patient folder, page 1

NAME H, B

Prob no.	ICDA no.	*P	PROBLEM — Active	Date entered	PROBLEM — Resolved	Date resolved	CI
1	250.8		Diabetes	4-5-67			
2	277		Overweight ———————		——————>	10-6-71	
3	412.0		HCVD	4-5-67			
4	300		Anxiety Reaction	10-10-67			
5	712.0		Osteoarthritis	9-24-69			
6	308		Callous Lesion	7-8-70	Excised ——>	7-2-71	
7	551.3		~~Occult blood~~ Hiatus Hernia	7-8-70 9-30-70			
8	490		Bronchitis, recurrent	7-8-70			
9							
10							
11							
12							
13							
14							
15							
16							
17							
18							

ACUTE SELF-LIMITED (TEMPORARY) PROBLEMS

Prob no.	ICDA no.	*P	PROBLEM	Dates of Occurrence 1	2	3	4	5	6	CI
A	490		Bronchitis	4-5-67	11-7-68	3-3-69	5-5-69			
B	034.0		Strep pharyngitis	12-2-68						
C	682.9		Cellulitis (face)	3-3-69						
D	796.9		Rash, u.c.	8-19-70						
E	472		Respiratory flu	3-15-71						
F										
G										
H										
I										
J										

MEDICATION TABLE

Medication	Date Begun	1971	1972	1973	1974	1975	1976
Insulin	1961- stopped 1970						
D.B.I. 25 mg	1967	bid ———					
Raudixin 0.1 gm.	1967	bid ———					
Tetracycline 250 mg	1967+5/69						
Penicillin	12/68+3/69						
Erythrocin	3/69						
Librium 10 mg	4/69	tid ———					

KEY: Start —— Continuous —— Stop; Start – – Intermittent / prn – – Stop; * = Short course (7 – 14 days)

Figure 5–8. *Examples of major and acute self-limited problem lists. (From Hurst, J. W., and Walker, H. K.: The Problem Oriented System. New York, Medcom, Inc., 1972.)*

Prob. No.	Code	Active Problem	Onset	Resolved	Inactive Problems
1	4012	Hypertension	1962		
2	5740	Abdominal Pain	7/12/74	7/12/74	Cholecystectomy

Prob. No.	Code	Date of Onset or Entered	Active Problem	Inactive Problems	Comments
1	4012	1962--7/12/74	Hyperten-sion		Diuril
2	5740	7/12/74	Abdominal Pain - - - - - - - -		Cholecystectomy

Prob. No.	Code	Active Problem	Onset	Resolved	Comments
1	4012	Hypertension	1962		Diuril
2	5740	Abdominal Pain	7/12/74	7/12/74	Cholecystectomy

Code	Prob. No.	Problem	Onset	Inactive Problems	Resolved
4012	1	Hypertension	1962		
5740	2	Abdominal Pain	7/12/74 - - - - - - - - - -		7/12/74 Cholecystectomy

Figure 5–9. *Alternate methods for organizing the problem list. (From Rakel, R. E.: Principles of Family Medicine. Philadelphia, W. B. Saunders Co., 1977.)*

problem. When a separate column for inactive problems is used, frequently an arrow is all that is needed to indicate the transfer of the problem from one column to another.

Legibility is an important component of the problem list, and problems should be either typed or printed in large letters to support the major function of the list, that the problems be "visible at a glance." By using the double line format for problem identification, as in Figure 5–7, a problem can be resolved to a higher level, without the need to place it in a new location at the bottom of the list and to assign a new number, by using an arrow to the new problem on the second line. If a comment column is not used, further information can be identified by placing over the arrow the date of the office visit at which information leading to the increased resolution of the problem was obtained, e.g., the glucose tol-

erance test on 10/07/73 in problem No. 2, Figure 5–6.

Once a higher level of understanding or sophistication is reached for any active problem or combination of problems, these should be changed to a single, new problem. For example, the problems of dyspnea on exertion and peripheral edema can be resolved to congestive heart failure, once the presence of renal disease has been ruled out. The physician's analytic ability can be demonstrated by the skill with which related items in the data base and problem list are identified and combined in a meaningful fashion to indicate a specific disease process.

Just as the family visit register focuses attention on the office visit pattern of the entire family, family problem lists depict the problems of each individual member on the same page, along with problems involving the entire family unit (Fig. 5–10). This comprehensive, visible, and concise overview of problems enables the family physician to provide family-oriented care, while keeping the ongoing problems of individual members in proper perspective.

Function of the Problem List

It has been appropriately said that the main value of the POMR is not its structure but its honesty. The POMR demands that all problems be described straightforwardly and at their present stage of development and resolution, no matter how elementary the terms used to describe them may be. It insists that the physician list only what he *knows* is present, not what he *thinks* is present. The principle to be followed is "record what is known, not what

is supposed." The POMR discourages guesswork and insists on an accurate listing of actual problems and observed facts. As Weed has said, "The problem list should not contain diagnostic guesses; it should simply state the problems at a level of refinement consistent with the physician's understanding, running the gamut from the precise diagnosis to the isolated, unexplained finding."[8]

The POMR does not demand excessive compulsiveness but does require that all significant factors be displayed so that they cannot be ignored. All abnormal data should be placed on the problem list and accounted for. The logic behind clinical decisions will be apparent in the POMR, and caution should be taken to avoid drawing conclusions prematurely; for example, a combination of a low hemoglobin level

FAMILY PROBLEM LIST

Simpson   1842 Eastwood   337-2104

NAME   ADDRESS   PHONE

Problem No.	Date	PROBLEM DESCRIPTION	Problem No.	Date	PROBLEM DESCRIPTION
		William DOB 2/6/39			**Margaret** DOB 6/6/41
1	1969	Alcoholism	1	1964	Obesity
2	1969	Chronic underemployment	2	1969	Recurrent tension headaches
3	7/70	Allergic rhinitis	3	1974	Depression
4	2/72	Hypertension, essential	4	1974	Contraception
5			5	1976	Cholecystectomy
6			6		
7			7		
8			8		
9			9		
10			10		
11			11		
12			12		
		Ann DOB 10/29/60			**James** DOB 8/21/64
1	1970	Allergic rhinitis	1	4/70	Asthma
2	11/73	School problem	2	2/75	Behavior problem
3	6/76	Recurrent abdominal pain	3		
4			4		
5			5		
6			6		
		Gary DOB 4/4/71			DOB
1	6/74	Allergic rhinitis	1		
2	10/74	Recurrent otitis media	2		
3	2/75	Penicillin allergy	3		
4			4		
5			5		
6			6		

PROBLEMS OF FAMILY AS A WHOLE

1. Economic problems
2. Marital discord
3. Parent-child conflict
4. Allergies

Figure 5–10. Family problem list. (Used in the private practices of N. T. Grace, M.D.: E. M. Neal, M.D., and C. E. Wellock, M.D., Healdsburg, California.)

and an elevated reticulocyte count does not equal iron deficiency anemia. More information is necessary to reach that conclusion.

Problem-solving techniques are a fundamental component of traditional medical education. Problem recognition, however, is too often modified by a haste to play the academic game of one-upmanship and to establish a diagnosis rapidly and with the least amount of data. The POMR lays bare any attempt to short-cut the establishment of a sound diagnosis based on the logical acquisition of adequate data. This does not mean, however, that a differential diagnosis is to be avoided, since all "rule-outs" and potential causes for the problem should be considered and listed in the progress notes under the heading "plan." Uncertainty of diagnosis is a common and accepted reality in family practice and should be accurately reflected in the record, so that the problem can be pursued to a definite conclusion. This conclusion may be either the complete disappearance of the sign or symptom without a final diagnosis ever being reached or the combining of a variety of symptoms and signs into a definite diagnosis.

Data Base

The data base is the first step toward developing the problem list. It is the platform upon which the structure of the POMR depends for stability. The data base consists of the history, including its components: chief complaint, present illness, past history, systems review, social history, physical examination, physiologic data, and baseline laboratory studies. This information is no different from that traditionally obtained in a new-patient work-up, but it does differ in its method of organization and thoroughness of documentation. A complete patient work-up, however, varies with the age, sex, and race of each patient. Different requirements need to be developed for patients aged 3, 16, 30, and 65 years. Females require a different cancer screening system than males, and blacks require a search for sickle cell disease.

Each physician should define the minimum data that he feels should be collected for all patients in his practice to permit his accurate assessment of their present state of health and potential future needs. He must then establish his own minimum requirements in the age, sex, racial, economic, or cultural categories he considers significant. Every physician has a unique background of training and experience, and each practice is unique in its geographic location and economic and social involvement and in the diseases prevalent within that community. Once the data base has been determined for the assigned categories, data collection should be consistent. The collection of most elements of the data base can be assigned to allied health professionals, who will obtain the information prior to the physician's involvement. Once the content is defined, the physician has a yardstick by which to measure effectiveness. Without an adequate data base, it is difficult for the practice to be oriented toward a preventive and comprehensive standpoint, and care continues to be episodic and crisis-oriented.

The data base serves as the groundwork for each patient's future care and should include those tests that are effective screening procedures for significant disease or are likely to be good reference points for future problems; for example, elevations of blood pressure can have a significant long-term detrimental effect, and a mild elevation may go undetected if an earlier baseline determination is not available for comparison. The data base should concentrate on the problems one cannot afford to miss and should include those tests that are of greatest value in detecting these problems. Active debate will continue regarding the need for various routine tests; the issue of which test is the most reliable indicator of potentially significant disease will be settled only by further research. Tests to be emphasized in the data base are those that detect disease at its earliest, presymptomatic phase, so that the normal course of the disease can be interrupted and its impact minimized. The detection of asymptomatic urinary tract infection by correlation of indicative findings may prevent chronic renal failure and the need for hemodialysis or renal transplantation. The onset of diabetes mellitus may be delayed by the early detection of a diabetic tendency. The use of sigmoidoscopy can prevent carcinoma of the rectum by the early detection and removal of a precancerous polyp.

A complete data base is so essential to

the success of the POMR that many physicians place "incomplete data base" as problem No. 1 on the list, where it remains until all required data have been obtained. A commitment should be made to obtain all of the data within a given period of time. If a complete history and physical examination cannot be obtained at one visit, information can still be collected bit by bit during a series of visits over a period of time. The visibility of an incomplete data base as problem No. 1 serves as a constant reminder to continue accumulating the data, regardless of the nature of the episodic visit.

A variety of new methods for obtaining the medical history have been developed to save the physician time and still allow for an in-depth accumulation of valuable historical information. These health history questionnaires are available as printed forms for the patient to complete, either in the office waiting room or at home prior to the visit. Other forms are manufactured for use with a computer, with the print-out indicating potential problem areas. At least 30 companies market commercial products to assist the physician in obtaining the medical history and other data base information. When the health history questionnaire is completed prior to the office visit, it can be rapidly reviewed and summarized by the physician, and areas requiring further supplementation or amplification are readily identified. An attempt should be made to review symptoms occurring since the last complete examination and to identify genetic, environmental, or other problems that, although they may have been present earlier, are now a problem for the patient. The data base should include a documentation of the patient's usual daily activities to identify those that pose a potential hazard or threat to health and for which education is indicated. Examples include heavy smoking or frequently excessive alcohol use.

One advantage of using the printed history questionnaires and physical examination sheets is the ability to easily identify information that has been obtained in part but has yet to be completed. With the highly structured "check-off" format, as shown in Figure 5–11, it is possible to set a goal for completeness and to know when that goal has been reached or what remains to be done. With a nonstructured, open-ended format, it is difficult to tell how much remains incomplete. The structured method, as developed by the Promis Clinic in Hampton Highlands, Maine, permits the easy identification of items to be obtained by allied health professionals prior to the physician's examination. It also allows for the comparison of data on four successive complete evaluations. When obtaining a complete history, it is important to have available the records from the patient's previous physicians, since the patient may have an unrealistic impression of the pathologic findings present, and accurate assessment of past problems is possible only by reviewing the actual records or a summary from the physicians involved. This information should become a permanent part of the data base and should serve as a reference point for all present and future difficulties in the same areas.

Increasing use is being made of the family tree, or pedigree chart. Some commercial companies place such an outline (Fig. 5–12) in a prominent section of the family record. This chart shows diagramatically the significant medical facts in the family history that may influence the health of present or future generations. The Family Practice Center at the University of Iowa uses an individually drawn pedigree for each family and places it prominently on the front of each chart (Fig. 5–13). Such a "family portrait" allows for visibility and immediate retrieval of this information.

Some practices insist upon a comprehensive data base for all new patients and will not accept patients for treatment beyond the second visit for an episodic illness until the standard comprehensive examination is completed. Following the completion of this examination, the patient is sent a summary of the findings, including a problem list and the plans for following each problem. The patient is asked to review the material for accuracy and to keep it for a permanent record.

A valuable, time-saving practice is to transfer all laboratory report slips to a standard laboratory data sheet (Fig. 5–14). This method avoids the bulk and confusion that a mass of laboratory slips in a variety of colors and sizes contributes to the medical record. The fears expressed that mistakes can be made when transferring the data have been shown to be mostly unfounded, and the significant amount of time saved in

FAMILY PRACTICE OFFICE
UNIVERSITY OF IOWA
PHYSICAL DATA SHEET

Name *TOOKER, LOUIS* Date *11-10-76*

Body Frame	Height/Age	70" / 34	/	/	/
S Ⓜ L	Weight/Pred. W.	206 / 160	/	/	/
Nose	Airway	N			
	Sept./Turb.	N / N	/		
	Sinuses	N			
Mouth	Lips/Tongue	N / N	/	/	/
	Bucc.	N			
	Gums/Teeth	N / N			
	Throat/Larynx	CLEAR / N	/	/	/
Ears	Pinnae/Canals	N / N	/	/	/
	TM's	N / N			
	Audiometry 500	20 / 20			
	1000	15 / 10			
	2000	20 / 20			
	4000	25 / 30			
Eyes	Vision Far	20/30 20/20 20/20			
Glasses	Near	20/30 20/30 20/20			
Yes Ⓝⓞ	ESO EXO	ORTHO			
	R.H. L.H.	ORTHO			
	Fields	INTACT INTACT			
Color	E.O.M. (cover)	FULL FULL			
Ⓝ A	Lips/Pupils	N / N	/	/	/
	Conj/Corn/Schl	N N N			
	Fundi	BENIGN BENIGN			
	Tonometry	14 / 12			
Neck	Carotids(Bruit)	ō / ō			
	Venous Dist.	NONE NONE			
	Thyroid	NOT PALP.			
	Trachea	MIDLINE			
	Mass	ō / ō			
Breasts	Nipple & Areola	N / N			
	Masses	N / N			
	Symmetry	— / —			
Chest & Lungs	Inspection	N / N			
	Palpation	N / N			
	Percussion	N / N			
	Auscultation	N / N			
	FVC/% Pred.	4750 / 103%	/	/	/
	1.0 FEV/% FVC	3500 / 86%	/	/	/
	TB Skin Test	Negative			
Cardiovascular	BP (Sitting)	200/100 196/102			
	BP (Supine)	186/94 190/92			
	BP (Leg)	188/90 186/92			
	Pulse/Irreg.	88 / REG.	/	/	/
	Rhythm	SINUS			
	Murmurs	ō / ō			
	Pulses Radial	++ / ++			
	Femoral	++ / ++			
	Popliteal	++ / ++			
	Post-tibial	++ / ++			
	Dorsalis Pedis	++ / ++			

Figure 5-11. *Physical data sheet, University of Iowa, Family Practice Office. (From Rakel, R. E.: Principles of Family Medicine. Philadelphia, W. B. Saunders Co., 1977. Modified from the Promis Clinic, Hampton Highlands, Maine.)*

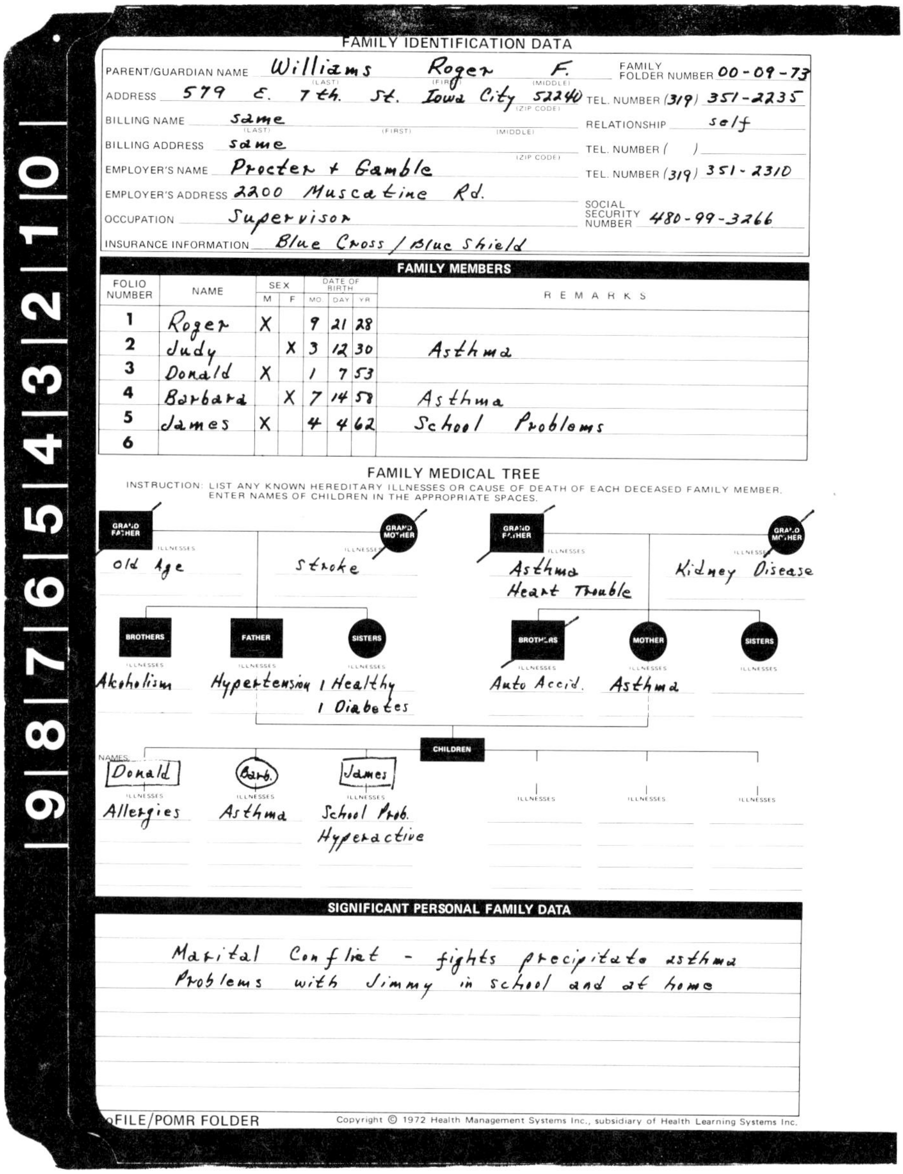

FAMILY IDENTIFICATION DATA

PARENT/GUARDIAN NAME Williams (LAST) Roger (FIRST) F. (MIDDLE) FAMILY FOLDER NUMBER 00-09-73

ADDRESS 579 E. 7th. St. Iowa City 52240 (ZIP CODE) TEL. NUMBER (319) 351-2235

BILLING NAME same (LAST) (FIRST) (MIDDLE) RELATIONSHIP self

BILLING ADDRESS same (ZIP CODE) TEL. NUMBER ( )

EMPLOYER'S NAME Procter + Gamble TEL. NUMBER (319) 351-2310

EMPLOYER'S ADDRESS 2200 Muscatine Rd.

OCCUPATION Supervisor SOCIAL SECURITY NUMBER 480-99-3266

INSURANCE INFORMATION Blue Cross / Blue Shield

FAMILY MEMBERS

FOLIO NUMBER	NAME	SEX M	SEX F	DATE OF BIRTH MO	DAY	YR	REMARKS
1	Roger	X		9	21	28	
2	Judy		X	3	12	30	Asthma
3	Donald	X		1	7	53	
4	Barbara		X	7	14	58	Asthma
5	James	X		4	4	62	School Problems
6							

FAMILY MEDICAL TREE

INSTRUCTION: LIST ANY KNOWN HEREDITARY ILLNESSES OR CAUSE OF DEATH OF EACH DECEASED FAMILY MEMBER. ENTER NAMES OF CHILDREN IN THE APPROPRIATE SPACES.

GRAND FATHER — ILLNESSES: Old Age
GRAND MOTHER — ILLNESSES: Stroke
GRAND FATHER — ILLNESSES: Asthma, Heart Trouble
GRAND MOTHER — ILLNESSES: Kidney Disease

BROTHERS — ILLNESSES: Alcoholism
FATHER — ILLNESSES: Hypertension
SISTERS — ILLNESSES: 1 Healthy, 1 Diabetes
BROTHERS — ILLNESSES: Auto Accid.
MOTHER — ILLNESSES: Asthma
SISTERS — ILLNESSES

CHILDREN

NAMES: Donald — ILLNESSES: Allergies
Barb. — ILLNESSES: Asthma
James — ILLNESSES: School Prob., Hyperactive
ILLNESSES
ILLNESSES
ILLNESSES

SIGNIFICANT PERSONAL FAMILY DATA

Marital Conflict - fights precipitate asthma
Problems with Jimmy in school and at home

FILE/POMR FOLDER

Copyright © 1972 Health Management Systems Inc., subsidiary of Health Learning Systems Inc.

Figure 5–12. *Family identification data and family chart. (From Health Management Systems, Inc., Subsidiary of Health Learning Systems.)*

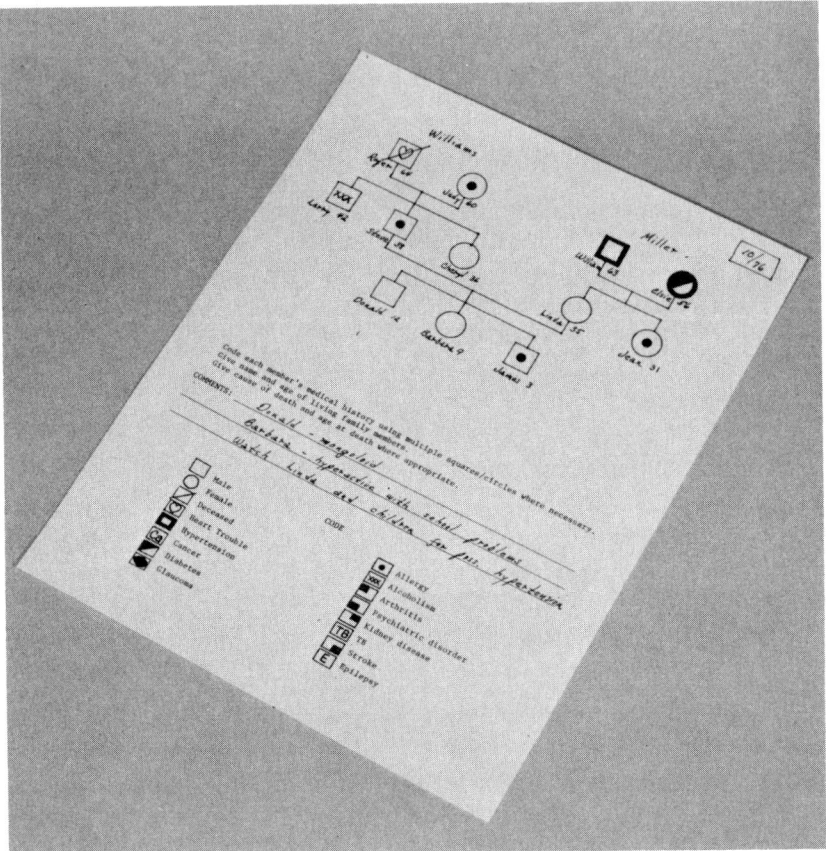

Figure 5-13. *Family pedigree form, University of Iowa, Family Practice Center. (From Rakel, R. E.: Principles of Family Medicine. Philadelphia, W. B. Saunders Co., 1977.)*

retrieving and comparing a sequence of laboratory information arranged side by side chronologically is well worth the time and effort involved. X-ray, electrocardiogram, and Papanicolaou smear test reports are similarly summarized and placed within a specific area of the data base (Fig. 5–15), with the actual report forms (if they contain a more detailed description of an abnormality) being filed to the rear of the chart. Once the information is transferred to the appropriate section of the data base form, the slip is discarded in a manner similar to other laboratory slips. Some laboratories are now reporting the information on adhesive strips, which can be peeled from a backing and reapplied to a data base form (Fig. 5–16). A similar form of perforated record strip can be used when typing progress notes, allowing the typed note to be peeled off and placed in the chart without disassembling the chart for typing.

The data base should also identify all allergies and should include a summary of all immunizations, hospitalizations, and consultations. In this manner, it can be noted at a glance whether a patient has ever been hospitalized, has any allergies, or has ever required consultation by other physicians. Organizing data in this manner may take slightly longer, but the time saved in retrieval more than compensates for this effort. The chronologic order of information in both the progress notes and the laboratory data is particularly useful in family practice because changes over time and frequency of involvement can be visualized and coordinated. When an abnormal laboratory or physiologic finding is identified that cannot be explained by a problem already on the problem list, it is included as a new problem and maintains that visibility until resolved by further diagnosis or treatment.

PATIENT NAME *Jones, Betty*

BLOOD CHEMISTRY

	NORMAL RANGE	PROFILES											
DATE		11-1-74	10-16-75	8-18-76									
TOT PROTEIN	5.9-8.0	7.1	6.8	7.3									
ALBUMIN	3.2-5.0	3.8	4.0	3.7									
Ca	8.8-11.0	9.7	10.0	10.2									
IN. PO$_4$	2.2-4.8	2.9	2.7	3.0									
CHOL	150-220	228	244	215									
GLUCOSE	71-117	85	95	83									
BUN	5-24	10	13	12									
URIC ACID	2.3-6	3.2	3.3	3.7									
ALK PHOS	0.6-2.5	1.1	1.0	1.3									
LDH	280-770	538	544	575									
TOT BIL	0.2-1.0	0.5	0.4	0.5									
SGOT	10-49	20	24	26									
Na	135-150	141	136	142									
K	3.0-5.0	5.4	5.0	4.8									
Cl	94-110	102	98	99									
CO$_2$													
BUN													
CREATININE	0.2-1.7	0.8	1.0	1.2									

INDIVIDUAL TESTS

DATE		11-1-74	10-16-75	8-18-76	9-13-76						
VDRL		Neg									
T3	.80-1.20	.99									
T4	4.0-11.0	9.3									
Free Thyroxine index	3.2-13.2	9.2									
Cholesterol	150-220	228	244	215	220						

Figure 5-14. *Data Base: Laboratory data form, University of Iowa, Family Practice Center. (From Rakel, R. E.: Principles of Family Medicine. Philadelphia, W. B. Saunders Co., 1977.)*

Progress Notes

Well-organized and logically structured progress notes in combination with the problem list are the secret of the POMR's effectiveness in promoting continuing patient care. Progress notes are divided into four main components: subjective information, objective data, assessment, and plan (Fig. 5–17). These components correspond to the history, physical examination, diagnosis, and treatment sections of the traditional record. The acronym SOAP is used to describe the POMR format of a progress note and is a more descriptive and more easily pronounced term than would be the acronym HPEDT. An essential feature of

any useful record is the organization of major components of the progress notes, placing the most important features in consistent and readily identifiable position (Fig. 5–18 *A* and *B*). The historical or subjective data should consistently occupy one specific position and the plan of management or therapeutic data another. The actual location is insignificant, as long as each maintains a separate and readily visible identity.

The *subjective* information includes the following: the history of the problem and all descriptive information perceived as important by the patient, including symptoms and feelings. This is an interpretation of the problem from the patient's point of

Patient Name _Jones, Betty_

DATE	PAP SMEARS (HISTOLOGY & CYTOLOGY)
11-1-74	Pap, negative, Class I
11-16-75	Pap, Class II, atypical cells, probably benign, repeat
8-18-76	Pap, Negative, Class I

DATE TYPE	X-RAYS
11-1-74	Chest, PA + Lateral - normal

DATE	EKGs
11-1-74	EKG - normal

Figure 5–15. *Data Base: Pap smear, X-ray, electrocardiogram results, University of Iowa, Family Practice Center. (From Rakel, R. E.: Principles of Family Medicine. Philadelphia, W. B. Saunders Co., 1977.)*

view. *Objective* data comprise those items noted on examination by the physician or allied health personnel. These data include all measurements and factual information obtained by independent observers, and they represent the facts undistorted by bias. Information within this section should also be arranged consistently in the same order, e.g., data concerning blood pressure, temperature, pulse, and respiration. *Assessment* refers to either the diagnosis or the present stage of resolution of the problem. *Plan* refers to the diagnostic and therapeutic modalities used in the management of the problem. This section should include all present medications, laboratory tests, procedures (such as exercise or inhalation therapy), further diagnostic plans (such as x-ray studies), patient education (such as informative literature and diet instruction), counseling methods, and the use of consultants. The entire plan (or treatment) section is the most important portion of the progress notes and should be prominently located so that it can be easily found, since future evaluation requires the comparison of outcome with previous treatment plans to determine whether the results obtained match previous expectations. In this manner, the success or failure of earlier plans can be measured.

A well-thought-out plan helps to maintain continuity of care and allows the physician to communicate to an associate on

PATIENT NAME: *Jones, Betty*

FAMILY PRACTICE CENTER
UNIVERSITY OF IOWA

Name *Jones, Betty*			URINALYSIS							Rm. *2* #*50-00-03*
Date	Type	Color	Transp.	pH	Sp. Gr.	Alb.	Sugar	Acet.	Blood	Microscopic
9-4-73	Voided ☒ Cath. ☐	*Yellow*	Turbid ☒ Clear ☐	*6*	*1.021*	*trace*	*neg*	*neg*	*neg*	*1-4 WBC/HPF, few bact + yeast, much amorphous mat. + epith. cells*
11-1-74	Voided ☒ Cath. ☐	*Yellow*	Turbid ☒ Clear ☐	*6*	*1.029*	*neg*	*neg*	*neg*	*neg*	Microscopic (Centrifuged) *2-4 WBC/HPF, few bact, mucous threads-amorphous mat, mod epith cells*
6-10-75	Voided ☒ Cath. ☐	*Yellow*	Turbid ☐ Clear ☒	*5.5*	*1.018*	*neg*	*1+*	*neg*	*neg*	Microscopic (Centrifuged) *0-4 WBC/HPF, mod epith cells, mucous threads*
7-22-75	Voided ☒ Cath. ☐	*Straw*	Turbid ☐ Clear ☒	*5*	*1.008*	*neg*	*2+*	*neg*	*neg*	Microscopic *10-20 WBC/HPF 5-10 RBC/HPF no casts, mod bact*
10-11-75	Voided ☒ Cath. ☐	*Yellow*	Turbid ☒ Clear ☐	*6*	*1.025*	*trace*	*neg*	*neg*	*neg*	Microscopic (Centrifuged) *4-6 WBC/HPF, lge # epith cells mod bact (rods), budding yeast present*
11-22-75	Voided ☒ Cath. ☐	*Yellow*	Turbid ☐ Clear ☐	*6*	*1.024*	*trace*	*neg*	*neg*	*neg*	Microscopic (Centrifuged) *18-22 WBC/HPF, large # bacteria (rods)*
12-9-75	Voided ☒ Cath. ☐	*Yellow*	Turbid ☒ Clear ☐	*5.5*	*1.013*	*neg*	*neg*	*neg*	*neg*	Microscopic *3-5 WBC/HPF 0-2 RBC/HPF mod epith cells, few rods*

Name *Jones, Betty*				HEMATOLOGY							Rm. *2* #*50-00-03*
Date	RBC	HB	HT	Sed. R.	WBC	Stab	Seg	Lymph	Mono	Eos	Bas	Other
11-1-74	4.5	13.2	39		5.5	02	47	28	08	13	02	MCV- 8E Platelets--adequate#
10-16-75	4.75	14	42.5		6.0	.3	55	30	6	4	2	Platelets adequate #
8-18-76	4.6	13	39		6.4	0	62	28	5	1	1	Platelets adequate.#

Figure 5-16. *Data base: urinalysis and hematology form, University of Iowa, Family Practice Center. (From Rakel, R. E.: Principles of Family Medicine. Philadelphia, W. B. Saunders Co., 1977.)*

Figure 5-17. *Major components of the POMR progress note. (From Rakel, R. E.: Principles of Family Medicine. Philadelphia, W. B. Saunders Co., 1977.)*

POMR
Progress Note

Date _____ Pt. Name _____ Age _____
Prob. No. _____ Title _____

S Subjective Information
Present Complaint
Symptoms
Family and Social History
Past History

O Objective Information
Physical Findings
Physiological Data
Laboratory Data

A Assessment
Diagnosis
Present Status of Problem

P Plan
Therapy
  Medication
  Procedures
Investigations
  Laboratory Tests
Identify "Rule-outs"
Patient Education

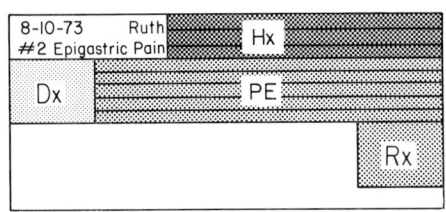

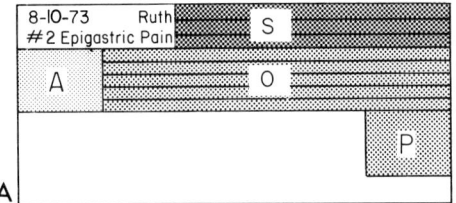

Progress Notes

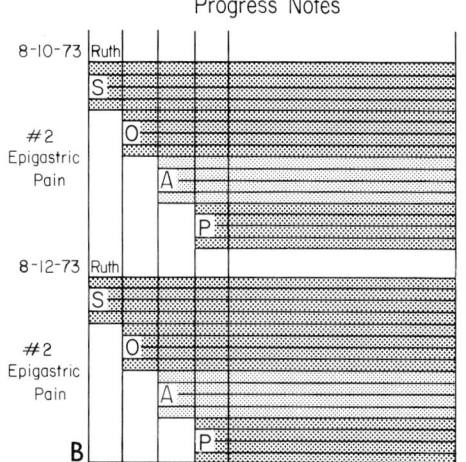

Figure 5–18. *Examples of consistent location of major componentns of progress note.*
A. Equates POMR terminology (SOAP) to the traditional terminology.
B. Illustrates consistent placement of data.
(From Rakel, R. E.: Principles of Family Medicine. Philadelphia, W. B. Saunders Co., 1977.)

call his plans for the patient's management. Three major subdivisions constitute the execution of the plan.

First, *diagnostic studies* should contain the "rule-outs" and the tests to be used in this process of differential diagnosis, e.g., to rule out peptic ulcer, obtain an upper gastrointestinal series, stool guaiac determination, and so forth. Under the heading of diagnostic studies would also be included the laboratory tests to be done at the next visit. The nurse or laboratory technician will then be alerted to obtain these prior to the physician's involvement. The diagnostic studies category really means that more information is needed, and it lists

the tests to be conducted to assist in the further evaluation of a problem.

The second subdivision is *therapeutic measures,* which includes medications and other treatment modalities.

Third is *patient education,* which consists of the factors necessary for patient understanding and compliance. This, too, is often a neglected area and therefore warrants visibility by including it as a regular item in the progress notes. The patient education section is of greatest importance for patients with chronic problems, since treatment of one form or another will be a constant feature throughout their lives. The patient should know what to expect from treatment, what side effects are possible, and how a specific medication might react with other drugs or foods. Unexpected events should be avoided as much as possible, so that maximum compliance will be maintained. The patient also needs adequate insight into the problem to know when to seek help without further delay. When patient instruction is given, whether this be the distribution of an American Heart Association booklet on hypertension or information about the hazards of smoking, it should be documented in the record so that other health personnel who share responsibility for continuing education of the patient will remain informed.

Each progress note is keyed by number to its problem on the problem list, and the problem number and title serve as headings for each progress note. In this manner, all information pertaining to a particular problem and the ongoing plan for managing that problem are easily identified throughout the record. This system allows for rapid assessment of a problem and its stage of resolution by all health personnel. It prevents the POMR from being a disorganized "flight of ideas," as is so frequently the case with the SOMR. Progress notes in the SOMR format are usually long and the information is randomly arranged. Progress notes in the POMR format are in outline form and frequently contain more data, although fewer words (Fig. 5–19).

Every problem need not be described in a progress note at each visit. Comments need only be made regarding those problems that are pertinent to that visit and for which some change of status or new information is noted. Likewise, every item or component of the progress note need not

---

SOMR Progress Note
   Milroy, John
   11/21/75
            Had recurrences of stomach pain 3 days ago similar to that of previous ulcer pain last year.
            Has been drinking again and not sticking to his diet. Has slight tenderness in epigastrium—
            denies tarry stools or change in bowel habits. Stool guaiac was negative. Wife says he won't
            stay on diet when at work or "out with the boys." Reinstructed on diet and need to stay away
            from alcohol and cigarettes. Rx—Maalox
                                          73 words

POMR Progress Note

   Milroy, John
   11/21/75
   Problem #3   Duodenal Ulcer
                   S—Pain recurred 3 days ago—moderately severe—no melena—off diet and drinking
                   O—Mild epigastric tenderness. Stool guaiac negative
                   A—Duodenal Ulcer
                   P—Maalox
                       Instructed regarding diet
                       DC alcohol and smoking
                            31 words

Figure 5–19. *Comparison of volume and organization of SOMR and POMR progress notes. (From Rakel, R. E.: Principles of Family Medicine. Philadelphia, W. B. Saunders Co., 1977.)*

be commented upon at each visit. If there is no change in status or no new information available, then that section, whether it be the subjective, objective, assessment, or plan, should be omitted or a dash inserted to indicate "no need for comment." Certainly, meaningless terms such as "doing well" or "status quo" are of little value and should be avoided. All progress information is documented chronologically, and health professionals other than the physician insert their comments or observations in the same manner as the physician. As new information is accumulated during each visit, the progress notes are used to provide feedback to continually update and modify the problem list.

Hospital discharge summaries should also be organized in the POMR format, with each problem being identified and numbered and the pertinent information "SOAPed." This record (the discharge summary) is then incorporated into the office record at the appropriate chronologic point to assist in the continuing care of the patient during future office visits.

Flow Sheets

Flow sheets are a useful adjunct to any medical record system, particularly when the POMR is used in conjunction with continuing patient care and the management of chronic illnesses. It is sometimes difficult to review the course of a single problem over time using progress notes, since a great deal of page turning is required to pick out that problem on successive visits. Placing the prolonged course of a single problem, or even selected multiple problems, on one flow sheet greatly facilitates comprehension and management. Flow sheets are also useful in any clinical situation requiring the monitoring of multiple laboratory and therapeutic parameters over a long period of time. They present an overview of the illness, compressing events over time onto one page, and allow the physician to identify current values as well as observe trends in the course of a disease. Flow sheets permit speedy retrieval of data and facilitate the ongoing analysis of the stage of chronic illness by indicating changing trends in response to therapy.

Once the parameters to be monitored have been identified, the flow sheet serves as a constant reminder to review these items and acts as an early warning system for potential problems by indicating variations from the previous pattern or baseline. Such sheets allow for a large amount of physiologic and management data to be accumulated in a compact area and observed at a glance.

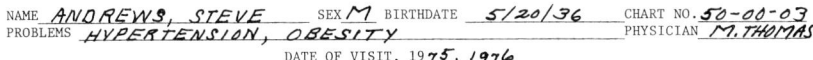
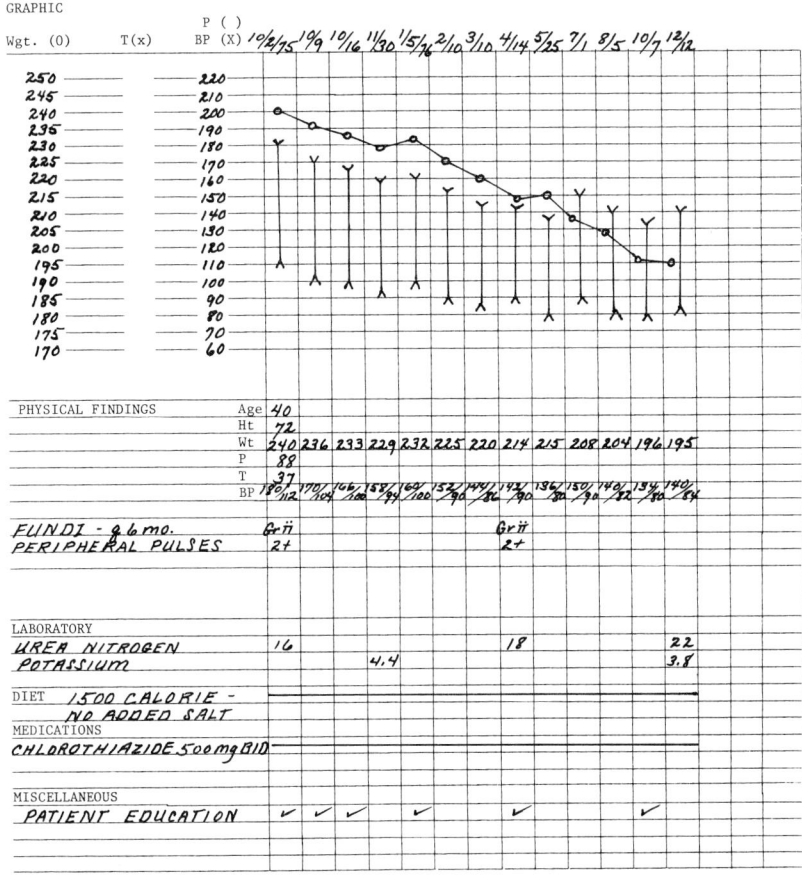

Figure 5-20. *Flow sheet for a patient with hypertension and obesity, University of Iowa, Family Practice Center. (From Rakel, R. E.: Principles of Family Medicine. Philadelphia, W. B. Saunders Co., 1977.)*

When laboratory data have been entered on the flow sheet, they can, but do not need to be, entered on the data base form as well. Just as with the data base form, the laboratory slip is filed elsewhere or discarded and is not retained in the chart. This procedure prevents the chaotic accumulation of a variety of laboratory forms and the frustrating experience of searching for multiple determinations of a particular test when many intervening and irrelevant laboratory slips need to be "leafed through" in order to identify sequential results. The flow sheet permits ready comparison of all determinations of a single test. It also permits physiologic and laboratory data to be monitored on the same time scale as thera-

peutic management. It has been noted, as well, that when material is categorized in this manner, physicians tend to write more concise and clearer notes and to include fewer irrelevant details.

The time required to enter data on a flow sheet is much less than that lost in sorting out disorganized information in the traditional record. A study at the University of Iowa, however, revealed that a partially used flow sheet can be more inefficient than none at all, since the physician is then required to search back and forth among the flow sheet, progress notes, and data base for the complete information. The flow sheet can be a simple piece of graph paper, a self-designed form (Fig. 5-20), or a well-structured, preprinted form (Fig. 5–21). In each instance, the left-hand column should contain the parameters considered essential to the ongoing management of the problems being followed. Just as the data base must be individually designed for each practice, so must the flow sheet be suited to the preferences of the physician and be designed to measure those parameters considered most important in the management of the illnesses for which it is used.

A general purpose flow sheet can be adapted to a variety of chronic problems. Combining more than one problem on a single flow sheet is helpful when one test or variable is used to monitor more than one problem because it avoids duplicating this information in each progress note. For example, a serum potassium determination may be used to follow the management of both hypertension and congestive heart failure, and recording of weight is important in the therapy of both hypertension and diabetes.

Items to be monitored on a flow sheet usually include:

1. Frequency of symptoms.
2. Physiologic data, such as weight, edema, and blood pressure.
3. Laboratory data, such as fasting blood glucose levels, urine cultures, and serum potassium and serum cholesterol levels.
4. Medications.
5. Nondrug therapy, such as diet and physical therapy.
6. Patient compliance.
7. Patient education.

Flow sheets serve as memory aids and guard against the possibility of important aspects of a patient's continuing care being overlooked by the physician. For example, when monitoring the course of a diabetic patient, one may forget to regularly check the fundi or peripheral pulses for potential vascular change. Listing these as param-

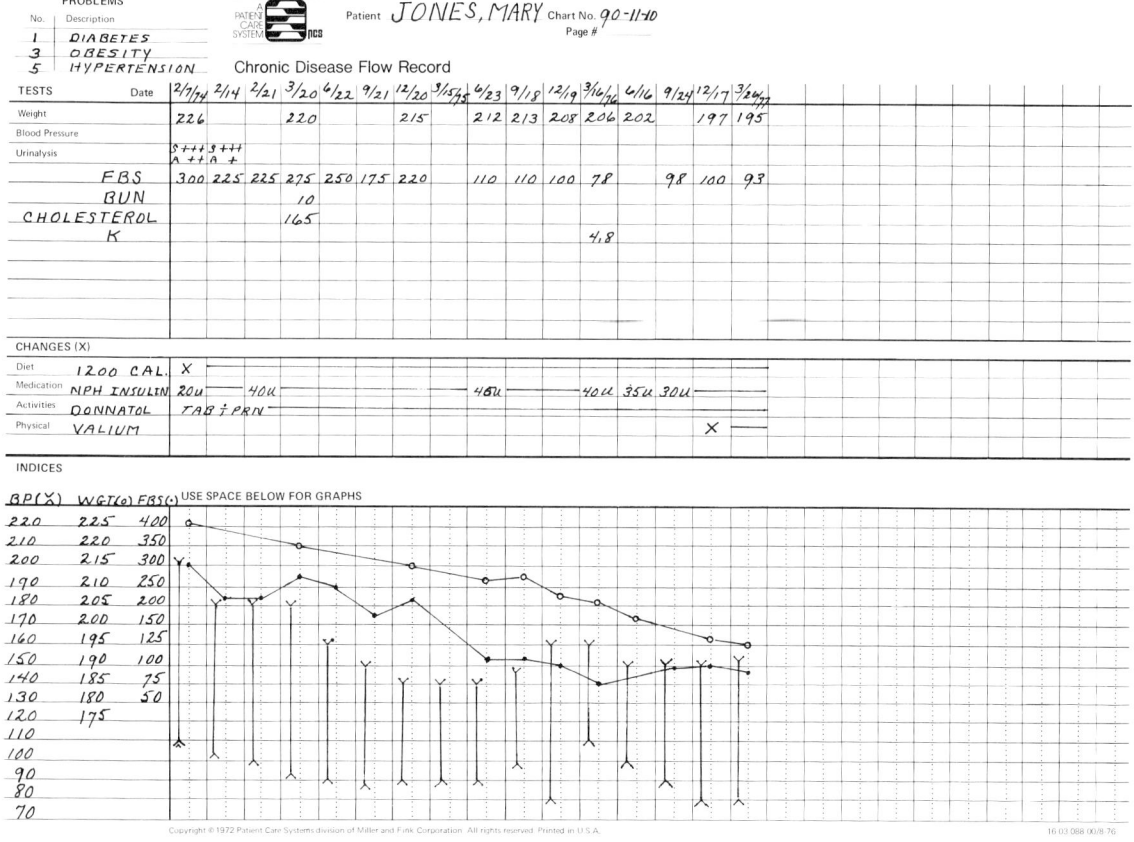

Figure 5–21. *Chronic disease flow record. (Copyright © 1972 Patient Care Systems, Division of Miller and Fink Corporation.)*

eters to be evaluated at prescribed intervals, along with the blood glucose level and other specifics, will serve as a reminder to all office personnel. The data-gathering activities of allied health personnel can easily be incorporated into the structure of the flow sheet by identifying those parameters to be measured at the next visit prior to the physician's examination. The flow sheet should monitor problems at intervals that will reflect the degree of stability of the illness; the more acute and unstable the problem, the more frequently measurements will be required. Items should be monitored often enough to ensure good care without undue expense.

The chart format of a flow sheet also minimizes problems caused by illegible handwriting. Effective use of flow sheets may obviate the need for progress notes when repeated visits relate only to the ongoing management of the chronic illnesses followed on the flow sheet. When progress notes are necessary, "see flow sheet" will frequently suffice in lieu of entries in the objective and plan categories.

This graphic portrayal of the course of disease, when shown to the patient, increases his insight into the problem and thereby improves patient compliance.

EVALUATING QUALITY OF CARE

Many physicians perceive of "audit" as a threatening term, while to others it serves as a source of intellectual stimulation. The challenge is to assess clinical performance and improve professional competence. Bjorn and Cross have designed their practice to include an ongoing audit system, both internal and external, accomplished by review by office staff and visiting consultants.[2] Their enthusiasm for such auditing procedures indicates that such methods can serve as a source of professional stimulation and improved patient care. They feel that if the practicing physician does not develop an efficient audit system, he will "suffer from apathy, bitterness and the general dissatisfaction of conducting a practice devoid of those basic intellectual gratifications integral to continued professional growth."

Family physicians have emphasized continuing education as a requirement for maintaining quality of care and contribut-

ing to professional growth; a willingness to be reviewed by peers can also result in professional stimulation. To be successful, however, audit must be viewed as an experience in learning and as an exciting, intellectually rewarding exercise. Weed emphasizes that to be effective and fair, record audit must relate to defined criteria.[8] Everyone must know what is to be measured and how this is to be done. He equates this process to defining the length and width of a football field and the rules of play before the game has begun, rather than after it is under way. Unfortunately, too many audit procedures utilized in hospitals and clinics today avoid defining specific criteria for audit, or do so after the fact. Both the physician and the reviewer should understand what standards are to be used in the review. This involves developing criteria of excellence that all agree to in advance and against which performance can be measured.

The POMR lends itself well to record audit. Since there is a defined location for all data relating to a particular problem, it is easy to determine the presence or absence of those data. The data base defines the measurements to be obtained for each patient. The plan category relating to each problem clearly indicates the physician's logic and intended course of action. In this manner, the auditor is not required to guess whether the prednisone was intended for the asthma, the arthritis, or some other problem. Such an organized office record system documents the logic of the physician's approach to a problem and preserves it for review by peers, whether the purpose be education, recertification, relicensure, or reimbursement.

In the author's 1973 survey of family practice residency programs (previously mentioned), most were found to have an active outpatient audit program under way. An analysis of the type of audit performed showed that 40 per cent of the auditors were conducting primarily a content review, involving an analysis of whether or not desired components of the record were properly documented and in place. Forty-five per cent were also evaluating the process of care, and 15 per cent were doing a thorough job of establishing criteria of excellence and measuring their performance against those criteria. These 15 per cent were also measuring outcomes and utiliz-

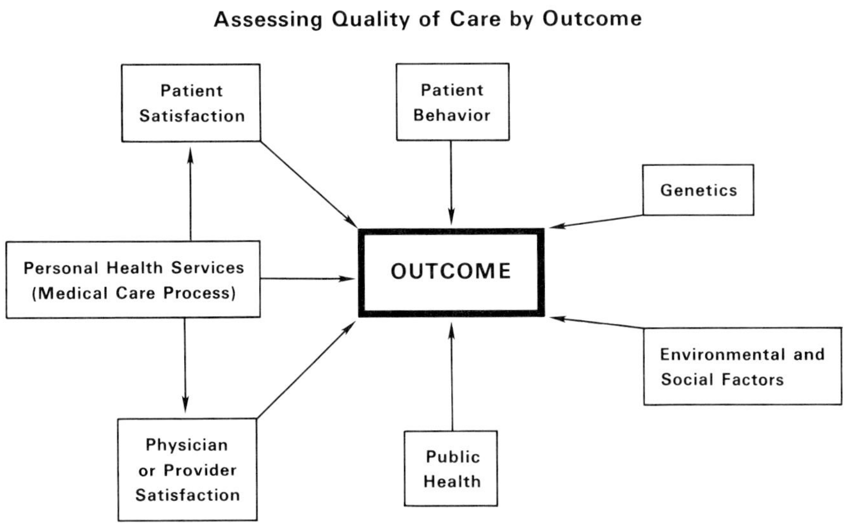

Assessing Quality of Care by Outcome

Figure 5–22. *Assessing quality of care by outcome. (From Rakel, R. E.: Principles of Family Medicine. Philadelphia, W. B. Saunders Co., 1977.)*

ing reviews by visiting consultants. Measurements of outcome of care are the most useful, yet the most difficult, measurements of physician performance. In ambulatory care, outcome is measured not so much by mortality but rather by the degree of disability, discomfort, or interference with functional capacity. Many factors tangential to physician activity can affect the outcome of care (Fig. 5–22). Asking the patient to help review his record results in patient education and in the patient's sharing responsibility for carrying out plans formulated by the physician. This strategy increases patient compliance by improving credibility between physician and patient. The original fears of increasing the patient's anxiety by including him in the record review and thereby destroying the "mystique" of the doctor–patient relationship have been found to be unrealistic. Studies show patient compliance to be increased, rather than decreased, as a result of this involvement. The improved understanding of health risks makes it easier for the patient to effect behavioral changes, such as taking medications or changing diet or smoking habits.

Each physician should design an audit method tailored to the individual needs of his practice, which will allow him to detect errors in management and to identify weaknesses that can be improved by further education of his staff and himself.

PROBLEM-INDEXING

The review or audit of any problem requires that charts of patients with that problem be retrievable. This is made easier by a disease- or problem-indexing system that identifies charts according to the patients' problems. The classification of disease in the past has been keyed to morbid anatomy and to causes of death, neither of which is appropriate to problems encountered by the family physician.

International medical classification was first begun in 1855 by documenting deaths and comparing death rates from selected causes in different countries. In 1948, morbidity was added, resulting in the International Classification of Disease (ICD). This method was further adapted for implementation in the United States as the International Classification of Disease Adapted for Use in the United States (ICDA), and a still further revision by hospitals, which included perinatal mortality and psychiatric problems, resulted in the Hospital International Classification of Disease Adapted for Use in the United States (HICDA). Although the ICD has been the best international system available, it is still heavily disease-oriented and does not allow for adequate documentation of problems at the early, undifferentiated stage frequently seen by the family physician. An international classification designed for family physicians was developed in 1974 at the Sixth World Conference of the World Organization of National Colleges, Academies, and Academic Associations of Family Physicians (WONCA) in Mexico City. This code was specifically designed to document the kinds of problems encountered by family physicians. It is also known as the International Classification of Health Problems in Primary Care (ICHPPC) and as Pri-Care. This classification, while compatible with the ICDA's 4000 items, contains only 371 problems, those defined as most frequently seen by family physicians. This system is more appropriate to family practice because it includes more symptoms and undifferentiated problems than the other classifications. It focuses on the patient's problem rather than the pathology. It also makes possible the classification of abnormal laboratory results, family and psychologic problems, long-term medication usage, and hereditary problems.

The American Board of Family Practice has incorporated a record audit procedure into its recertification process. The diplomate is asked to select and audit four cases from any five of the following 20 categories:

1. Postoperative carcinoma of the breast
2. Pediatric patient
3. Chronic bronchial asthma
4. Hypertension
5. Diabetes mellitus
6. Coronary artery disease
7. Abnormal vaginal bleeding
8. Depression
9. Acute duodenal ulcer
10. Acute cystitis
11. Colitis
12. Appendicitis
13. Lumbar disc disease
14. Rheumatoid arthritis
15. Normal pregnancy through delivery
16. Congestive heart failure
17. Otitis media
18. Obesity
19. Chronic obstructive pulmonary disease
20. Vaginitis

This list of problems will be expanded gradually, increasing the need for family physicians to have some method for easy retrieval of these records. Every family physician should develop some type of disease- or problem-indexing system for his practice. This can be done simply by cataloging only those 20 problems for which charts may need to be retrieved and reviewed for self-audit as part of recertification for the American Board of Family Practice. It would take little additional effort to index the problems encountered in practice more thoroughly by selecting additional, commonly seen problems from among the 371 in the WONCA classification system. A compulsive physician might extend the index beyond the 371 items to incorporate part or all of the 4000 items contained in the ICDA. Practices using computerized billing can usually adapt the computer program to accept such a classification system. The POMR is easily adapted to such indexing, and office personnel merely need to transfer problems from the problem list to the indexing system.

The advantages of problem-indexing include the following:

1. Easy retrieval of records of patients with common problems or of those receiving similar medications.

2. Recall of patients when discoveries indicate new treatments that are likely to be more effective than the one presently being used.

3. Identification of patients for whom medications must be changed when new hazards of therapy are identified, e.g., the need to consider alternate courses of therapy for some women after the discovery of thromboembolic complications of birth control medications.

4. Recall of patients with chronic problems requiring periodic evaluation, e.g., recurrent urinary tract infections or chronic lung disease.

5. Self-audit of physician performance to evaluate effectiveness in selected areas.

6. Audit of the problems encountered in the practice to identify areas of prominence when designing a continuing education program.

7. Analysis of the content of the practice to assist in the design of appropriate curricular objectives for undergraduate and graduate teaching programs.

8. Collection of data for clinical investigation and other research efforts.

9. Retrieval of cases for recertification.

A variety of problem-indexing methods have been developed and are available commercially, such as the E Book, which places the classification into a spiral book

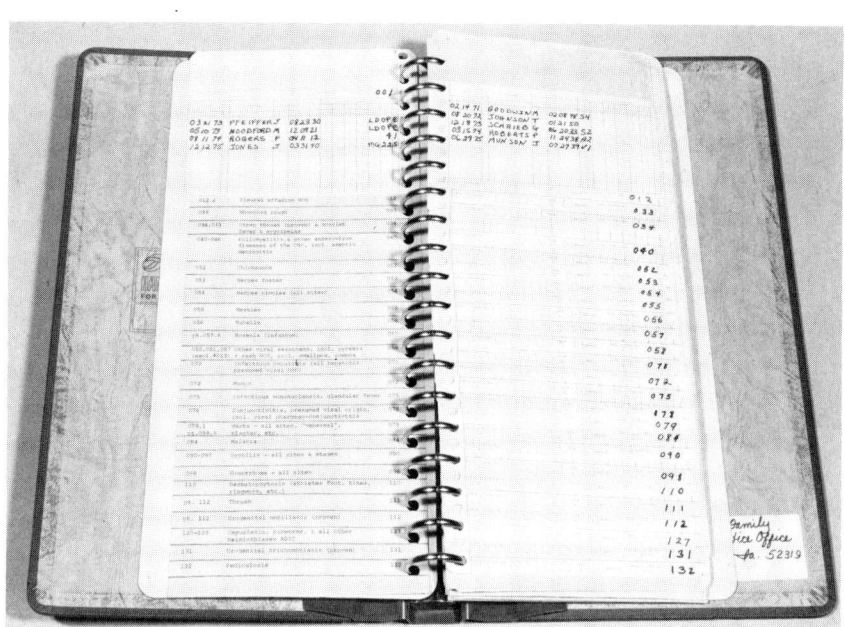

Figure 5-23. *Problem indexing using the E Book. Developed by T. S. Eimerl in Britain. (From Rakel, R. E.: Principles of Family Medicine. Philadelphia, W. B. Saunders Co., 1977.)*

Disease HYPERTENSION Index No. 042 Card No. 17

Patient Name and No.	Birthdate	Date of Dx	Result*	Address and Telephone Number
WILLAMS, J.W. 04131	4-13-30	11-30-68	R	181 CAMBRIDGE, NEW CANAAN 966-8032
BAKER, A.E. 03494	3-4-06	5-30-66	R	14 MERRY LANE, DARIEN 655-4419
VASCO, P.P. 01384	10-1-21	5-2-58	NA	600 WASHINGTON, NORWALK 866-0519
STOWE, J.R. 03641	8-6-25	6-1-62	R	4020 KING, STAMFORD 323-1561
CORNING, P.T. 02210	3-8-18	10-4-54	D	367 SUFFOLK, STAMFORD 348-3062
PELLAM, G.R. 06161	1-11-29	8-8-67	R	32 HOBBY, DARIEN 655-0106

Use this record for followup of chronic disease patients (see Medical Record System instructions).

*Result: R–Recovered D–Died NA–Not Active UT–Under Treatment

A PATIENT CARE SYSTEM pcs

Disease Cross–Index Card

Figure 5-24. *Disease indexing using commercially prepared index cards. (Copyright © 1971, 1977 Patient Care Systems, Division of Miller and Fink Corporation.)*

form or disease index card files (Figs. 5–23 and 5–24). All that is required, however, is a filing system of 3 × 5 cards that contains the names and other selected information of all patients with the designated problem, so that these can be retrieved for review at will. A major advantage of this system is that it promotes an investigative approach to problems seen in a physician's practice and allows him to analyze the effectiveness of his diagnostic and therapeutic skills.

Record review, whether limited to patient care or directed toward recertification, planning, continuing education, research or relicensure, will be a meaningful component of family practice in the future.

REFERENCES

1. Ambulatory Medical Care Records: Uniform Minimum Basic Data Set. A Report of the United States National Committee on Vital and Health Statistics, Lilienfeld, A. M. (chairman). U.S. Department of Health, Education and Welfare, National Center for Health Statistics, Vital and Health Statistics Documents and Committee Reports, Series 4, No. 16, D.H.E.W. Publication No. (HRA) 75–1453.
2. Bjorn, J. C., and Cross, H. D.: Problem Oriented Practice. Chicago, Modern Hospital Press, 1970.
3. Easton, R. E.: Problem-Oriented Medical Record Concepts. New York, Appleton-Century-Crofts, 1974.
4. Hurst, J. W., and Walker, H. K.: The Problem Oriented System. New York, Medcom Press, 1972.
5. Murnaghan, J. H.: Ambulatory medical care data. Review of the conference proceedings. Report of a Conference on Ambulatory Medical Care Records, Chicago, April, 1972. Med. Care, 11:Suppl:13, March-April, 1973.
6. The Problem-Oriented Medical Record and Effective Medical Care. Prepared by Patient Care Projects, Division of Miller and Fink Publishing Corp. for ROCOM, Division of Hoffmann-La Roche, 1973.
7. Walker, H. K., Hurst, J. W., and Woody, M. F.: Applying the Problem Oriented System. New York, Medcom Press, 1973.
8. Weed, L. L.: Medical Records, Medical Education and Patient Care. Chicago, The Press of Case Western Reserve University, distributed by Yearbook Medical Publishers, Inc., 1971.

PART III

COMMUNITY MEDICINE

Chapter 6

PREVENTIVE MEDICINE

by FREDERIC BASS,
and ROBERT P. GRANTHAM

With respect to family practice, we will use the term *preventive medicine* to mean all those activities that offer (1) opportunities on the part of both physician and patient to minimize illness or the consequences of illness, and (2) enhanced abilities on the part of the patient to meet biologic challenges. Whether the patient's problem is chronic illness, the common cold, squabbles with his spouse, or all of these together, the patient and his family physician may have multiple opportunities available to them for bettering the patient's condition, or the patient's abilities to cope, or both. We believe all family physicians should have assembled within their armamentarium a workable set of procedures that the physicians are prepared to apply to a specific, clearly defined set of preventable problems. Since today's causes of disease and death derive principally from unhealthful styles of living, we place particular emphasis on what physicians can do to foster healthful behavioral change among their patients, especially change of habits known to be unhealthy and damaging. Although the family physician is just one of myriad influences upon the patient's behavior, the physician can muster medical skill and influence to support the patient's élan and physical vigor rather than to encourage apathy and resignation.

This chapter begins with some basic definitions used in preventive medicine. Then, for those who wish a specific list of what to do preventively, we present the sets of preventive activities listed for each age group by the 1975 National Conference on Preventive Medicine (Fogarty International Center, the National Institutes of Health). Next, we look at the plagues of this century that have led to many, if not most, of the illnesses found in Western societies—life-style risk factors such as cigarette smoking, overeating, underexercising, abuse of alcohol and other drugs, mismanagement of motor vehicles, and undue psychologic stress. We note what the family physician might do to counter these prevalent conditions and consider the issues family physicians will have to face if they seriously undertake the task of promoting life-style change.

DEFINITIONS

Primary, secondary, and tertiary prevention refer to (1) the points at which, in the natural history of a condition, preventive activities are undertaken, and (2) the objectives of preventive work.

Primary Prevention. Primary prevention averts the development of the condition in the first place by inhibiting or avoiding the early stages of the process in susceptible individuals. For example, the primary prevention of coronary heart disease would inhibit or reverse the early stages of coronary atherosclerosis in at-risk patients, before narrowing of the lumen of the coronary arteries had occurred.

Note that we use the term "condition" in a broad sense. We refer to more than disease, trauma, or problem-causing behavior. Antecedent factors themselves are conditions worthy of systematic attention. These antecedents, or risk factors, may derive from particular bodily reactions, such as a response to tuberculin revealed by skin testing or a pattern of hyperlipidemia revealed by laboratory tests. Or risk factors may be behavioral, such as cigarette smoking and overeating. It makes sense to consider the natural history of risk factors, whether physiologic or behavioral. Thus, the levels of prevention also apply to risk factors themselves. For example, the primary prevention of cigarette smoking would refer to activities that decrease the incidence of persons becoming cigarette smokers.

Secondary Prevention. This term describes activities undertaken during the early stages of a condition that minimize the morbidity or mortality that would otherwise be expected. Secondary prevention of coronary heart disease would ensure that those with myocardial infarction, coronary insufficiency, and angina pectoris were treated so as to minimize their subsequent morbidity or mortality.

Tertiary Prevention. This form of prevention refers to the rehabilitation of those disabled by a condition, so that their disability and discomfort are minimized, allowing them to cope effectively with any residual impairment. Tertiary prevention applied to patients with coronary heart disease would have to do with rehabilitative measures, such as implantation of cardiac pacemakers to correct debilitating arrhythmias and permanent work reassignment and job retraining for those patients whose work had involved high levels of physical stress, mental stress, or both.

Tertiary prevention, at first, does not seem applicable to the risk factors antecedent to a disease; however, there is an analogy. Secondary prevention is directed at risk factors unaccompanied by symptoms or disability, while tertiary prevention attacks the risk factors accompanied by related symptoms and disability. Thus, the secondary prevention of chronic lung disease involves methods to help people stop smoking before they develop the physical signs and symptoms that are complications of smoking. Tertiary prevention involves helping those with the complications resulting from smoking, such as chronic obstructive lung disease, stop their smoking as part of an overall rehabilitative program.

By way of further example, consider the problems for preventive medicine that alcohol abuse presents. The primary prevention of alcohol abuse, when successful, leads to a lower overall consumption of alcohol and fewer people developing drinking problems. Secondary prevention of alcohol abuse involves the treatment of heavy (problem) drinkers so that they maintain or improve internal and social relationships, as well as acceptable functioning in terms of work, automobile driving, family relationships, friends, and self. Tertiary treatment involves rehabilitating those who already have lost major areas of social or physical functioning because of their high alcohol intake. Generally speaking, family physicians find their preventive efforts most successful in secondary prevention (encouraging people with unhealthy habits to change their ways before their ways permanently change them). Success is achieved for two reasons: (1) the patient realizes that there is a problem, and (2) there is an appeal to the physician's traditional interests and training, i.e., the work of healing the sick and of dealing with complaints that are presented.

Natural History of Disease. The concept of the natural history of a disease or condition implies that health problems pattern themselves in time and space. Unless we are acquainted with these patterns, the benefits of our measures, therapeutic or preventive, may be more fancied than real. Unfortunately, the natural histories of few chronic diseases are known (e.g., tuberculosis, coronary heart disease, syphilis), for few have been studied across an entire population and over the necessary decades of time. Thanks to several long-term studies, we have good information about the biologic consequences of several important life-style risk factors, such as cigarette smoking and obesity. Much more of this expensive, time-consuming research is needed.

Prevention implies dealing with risk. Risk implies probability, that is, statistical chance. And probability implies dealing with numbers and with populations. Hence, prevention is bound to *epidemiology*, the study of the distribution and the determinants of health and illness in populations. Traditionally, epidemiology has been the province of "the public health" field, but as this field has become more clinical and as clinicians have become more interested in epidemiology, fields such as community medicine and social medicine have arisen and have gained recognition as specialties within medicine.

TABLE 6–1. MAJOR CATEGORIES OF PROBLEMS IN PREVENTIVE MEDICINE

Accident Prevention Includes motor vehicle, home, industrial, recreational, or school accidents; poisonings.

Environmental Health Air and water pollution, occupational exposures, food sanitation, housing and shelter, and exposure to selected physical factors such as heat, cold, radiant energy, and noise.

Communicable Disease Includes surveillance and reporting of selected diseases, recognition of outbreaks or epidemics of disease, immunization procedures, and counseling of travelers and immigrants.

Reproduction and Promotion of Normal Growth and Development Family planning; genetic counseling; abortion; training for parenting, pregnancy, and delivery; physical and emotional development including height and weight, speech, hearing, vision, motor skills, self-care, and activities of daily living; dental health; intellectual function; and preparing for the successive stages and potential crises of life.

Life-Style Issues Personal health including cigarette smoking, obesity, overconsumption of alcohol, under-exercise, stress management, sexuality, life satisfaction, and fulfillment in work and in play; interpersonal health including family interaction and relationships with friends and workmates.

Coping with Individual and Culturally Induced Stress Particular life events (that represent either positive or negative disruptions of ordinary experience and that are predictive of illness), suicide prevention, and helping handicapped persons and the dying. At a societal level, media violence; health misinformation; and stress associated with crowding, migration, transportation, poverty, racial discrimination, war, and crime.

Chronic Disease Surveillance; screening related to proper diagnostic, therapeutic, and rehabilitative procedures; health counseling; and health education.

Use of Health Care Services Knowledge and practice of first aid, self-care, home care, and chronic and emergency care and defining patients' participation, cooperation, and responsibilities in delivering care.

Iatrogenic Problems Conditions caused by faulty treatment, faulty dispensing, or inadequate instruction and counseling; improper self-administration of drugs; and drug interactions.

The major categories of problems encountered in preventive and community medicine are shown in Table 6–1. These problems reflect many of the interfaces and intersections among medicine, health, and society. Though the family physician may find some of these items unrelated to the usual content of a family practice workload, all physicians still have the responsibility to define their roles in each of these areas of prevention and to decide what the patient should be offered in each, either by the physician directly or by others to whom the patient is referred.

On what basis should preventive procedures be selected? Table 6–2 provides a framework with which to view any problem in preventive medicine. If the objective is to minimize illness and its consequences and to enhance the person's coping abilities, then desirable preventive activities should be measurable in terms that assess illness on the one hand and coping on the other. For measures of illness we can utilize White's "5 D's": death, disease, disability, discomfort, and dissatisfaction.[12] (In countries without comprehensive health insurance, we may add a sixth, debt.) Coping, or functional, capacities have not been conceptualized or organized systematically. However, there are isolated functions that have been studied (more of them biologic than behavioral) such as measurement of the postprandial blood glucose determination, the exercise electro-cardiogram, and the 1 second Forced Expiratory Volume (FEV_1). In each of these biologic examples, there is a standard challenge and a measured response that is judged to be adequate or not. In the realm of behavior, we do not at present have available for clinical use either the means to give a standard challenge or standard measures of the response.

The approach for proving whether a particular preventive procedure produces the desired effect is the same as for any other medical procedure. Cochrane[3] has emphasized the importance of the randomized controlled trial (RCT) in evaluating clinical procedures, and RCT's apply as well to preventive measures, from immunizations to counseling. The actual measurement of the effectiveness of preventive procedures has been confined to the first two D's previously mentioned—death and disease. The assessment of disability, discomfort, or dissatisfaction seldom has been attempted for any therapeutic or preventive procedure, although now more attention is being paid to disability days, work-loss days, and school-loss days as measures of morbidity.

With regard to preventive medicine, changes in the patient's risk factors (especially those mentioned earlier) become an important and tangible outcome of the medical care process when it can be shown that change in life-style risk factors is consequent to the physician's efforts. For example, enough epidemiologic work has

TABLE 6-2. A FRAMEWORK FOR ANALYZING PREVENTIVE PROBLEMS

Definition of the Problem   In terms of the individual, the family, and the community, what precisely is the problem? What illnesses, symptoms, and conditions occur because of the problem? To whom do these occur? When? How? Who is calling for a solution to the problem, whom will the solution affect, and who will provide the resources for the solution?

Significance   What are the medical, social, and economic consequences of this problem:
   in regard to illness:
      deaths caused?
      disability caused?
      discomfort caused?
      dissatisfaction caused?
      other untoward consequences?
   in regard to coping:
      changes in functional capacity
         biologically?
         behaviorally?
      changes in level of emotional and social well-being
         in specific areas?
         in general?
      other coping changes?

Diagnostic Methods   Reliability, sensitivity and specificity, validity, availability, and costs (to patient, physician, public).

Incidence and Reporting   How prevalent is the condition? Do people tend to bring it to the physician's attention? Is the physician required to report the condition? Is information about its occurrence available? What are the actual trends in incidence and prevalence? How does the condition rank with others as a cause of death and morbidity?

Natural History   What etiologic factors pertaining to agent, host, and environment are known? How does the problem start, and what stages can be identified? What is the prognostic significance of these stages? How is the condition transmitted, propagated, and maintained? What are the time relationships, i.e., how soon are people affected following exposure?

Risk Groups   Who is at high risk for the condition and its complications? Are there risk categories into which people can be classified with appropriate preventive services for each category?

Effectiveness of Treatment Measures   Has treatment been proven to make a difference? How uncomfortable, expensive, and difficult is treatment for both patient and physician? What are the current medical practices in the community with regard to treatment, prevention, and counseling related to this condition? Do people cooperate with treatment? Would people prefer to wait for treatment if needed rather than to bother with prevention?

Preventive Measures   Including immunization, health education, chemoprophylaxis, environmental measures, and modification of agent. Several questions must be asked. Do they work? Are they available? What are the current practices in the region? Do people cooperate with these measures?

Potential Costs and Benefits of Prevention   What are the monetary benefits and costs, both direct and indirect? Who benefits and when? Are the estimates of benefit and cost founded on good data?

Social, Cultural, and Political Factors   How do society in general and groups within society view the problem itself, its causal factors, the consequences, and the processes of treatment and prevention? What has been said about the subject by national and local media? What policy statements have been made by governmental agencies? What statements have other agencies and private citizens made? What social conflicts are generated or aggravated by this problem, by its solution, or both?

Ethical and Human Rights Aspects   What ethical, legal, and moral issues are raised by the problem and by the proposed solutions? Is there the danger that coercive methods may be used? Is the legal basis for proposed preventive measures well defined?

Related Organizations and Professions   What other professionals (or laypersons) and organizations are concerned with this problem? Are they providing similar services? How can one work with them most productively?

Related Issues   What priority does this problem have in medical practice and in preventive medicine? Specifically, what procedures and services are more, or less, important than this preventive measure? How can this measure be integrated into other family practice activities? What training, consultation, equipment, supplies, and space are necessary? Which of these are already available? Is financing available to support this preventive work?

Final Plans   What precisely should the family physician do at this point? With which agencies or health workers should the family physician collaborate? What budget is required, and how will financing be arranged?

been done to make good estimates, in terms of mortality, of the value of stopping smoking for a 50 year old man who has smoked 30 cigarettes a day for 30 years. Similarly, estimates can be made for the adverse effects of weight change, heavy drinking of alcohol, and (perhaps) for underexercise. Not enough work has been done to identify the levels of success that physicians should expect their patients to achieve. Nevertheless, a few calculations will show that the effects on life expectancy due to actual change in life style are among the most powerful known to medicine. For example, the 50 year old smoker just mentioned can take no more potent step with respect to his physical health than to stop smoking.

In June, 1975, Task Force III of the United States National Conference on Preventive Medicine drew up a set of recommendations for preventive medicine in the context of the delivery of personal health services.[2] These recommendations constitute a basic set of preventive procedures to be offered to the general population of the United States. The authors noted that for high-risk groups it would be necessary and appropriate to add other procedures. The basic set of procedures is summarized in Table 6–3. In its report, the Task Force noted that there is not conclusive support-

TABLE 6–3. RECOMMENDATIONS FOR PREVENTIVE MEDICINE PROCEDURES

Procedure	Condition	Type Of Prevention (Primary = 1; Secondary = 2)	Intervention
Mother and Fetus			
Urine albumin determination	Toxemia	2	Diagnosis and therapy
Pap smear	Genital tract malignancy	2	Diagnosis and therapy
VDRL determination	Syphilis	2	Diagnosis and therapy, counseling and contact finding
Culture for gonococcus	Gonorrhea	2	Penicillin, counseling and contact finding
Blood grouping and Rh determination	Rh isoimmunization and other blood abnormalities	1	Antibody administration
Blood glucose determination	Abnormal glucose tolerance	2	Diagnosis and therapy
Blood pressure measurement	Hypertension	2	Diagnosis and therapy
Physical examination	Organic heart disease	2	Diagnosis and therapy
Physical examination	Pelvic inadequacy	2	Diagnosis and therapy
Physical examination	Reproductive organ abnormality	2	Diagnosis and therapy
Urine culture	Bacteriuria (after third pregnancy)	2	Diagnosis and therapy
Amniocentesis	Genetic disorders (women over age 40)	2	Diagnosis and therapy
Blood tests	Sickle cell trait (high risk groups only)	2	Diagnosis and therapy
History of menarche	Avoid pregnancy (before unplanned pregnancy occurs)	1	Contraception
Serologic test	Lack of rubella antibody (before pregnancy)	1	Immunization (if not pregnant)
Pregnancy test	Unwanted pregnancy	2	Abortion
History of pregnancy	Unsuccessful prior pregnancy	2	Counseling
History and counseling	Inadequate preparation for pregnancy	1	Counseling
History and counseling	Inadequate preparation for delivery	1	Counseling
History and counseling	Inadequate preparation for parenthood	1	Counseling
History and counseling	Smoking and other risks to developing fetus	1, 2	Counseling
History and counseling	Inadequate recognition of signs and symptoms of abnormalities	1	Counseling

Table continued on following page

TABLE 6-3.   RECOMMENDATIONS FOR PREVENTIVE MEDICINE PROCEDURES—*Continued*

Procedure	Condition	Type of Prevention (Primary=1; Secondary=2)	Intervention
Anthropometric examination and counseling	Nutritional abnormality	2	Counseling and diet
Hemoglobin and hematocrit determinations	Anemia	2	Diagnosis and therapy
Infant†			
History and counseling (parents)	Inadequate preparation for infant (newborn)	1	Parental counseling
Phenylketonuria screening	Metabolic disorders (newborn)	2	Diagnosis and therapy
Silver nitrate administration	Gonorrheal ophthalmia (newborn)	1	Prophylaxis
Observation and measurement	Congenital malformations (newborn)	2	Diagnosis and therapy
Diphtheria and tetanus toxoid combined with pertussis vaccine (DPT)	Diphtheria, tetanus, and pertussis	1	Immunization
Trivalent oral polio-virus vaccine (TOPV)	Poliomyelitis	1	Immunization
Vitamin K administration	Hemorrhagic disease	1	Prophylaxis
Hematocrit determination	Anemia	2	Diagnosis and therapy
Developmental assessment including height and weight	Growth and developmental disorders	2	Diagnosis and therapy
Counseling	Accidents	1	Parental counseling

†Newborn plus four visits after discharge

	Ages 1 to 6 Years†		
Observation and assessment	Growth and developmental disorders	2	Diagnosis and therapy
Observation and assessment	Neurologic disorders	2	Diagnosis and therapy
Anthropometric measurements	Malnutrition and obesity	1, 2	Counseling and diet
Hematocrit determination	Anemia	2	Diagnosis and therapy
Hearing and vision testing	Hearing and visual defects	2	Diagnosis and therapy
Speech testing	Communication disorders	2	Diagnosis and therapy
DPT vaccination	Diphtheria, tetanus, and pertussis	1	Immunization
History and vaccination, if indicated	Measles, mumps, and rubella	1	Immunization
History and TOPV, if indicated	Poliomyelitis	1	Immunization
Dental examination	Dental defects	1, 2	Diagnosis and therapy
Counseling	Accidents	1	Parental counseling
Counseling	Poisoning	1	Parental counseling

†One visit at age 2 to 3 and one at age 5 to 6

	Ages 6 to 16 Years†		
Observation and assessment	Behavioral, intellectual, or communicative maladjustments	2	Counseling, diagnosis, and therapy
History and counseling	Smoking	1, 2	Counseling
Examination and prophylaxis	Dental caries, malocclusions, and peridontal disease	1, 2	Prophylaxis, diagnosis, and therapy
Hearing and vision testing	Hearing and visual defects	2	Diagnosis and therapy
Anthropometric examination	Musculoskeletal disorders	2	Diagnosis and therapy
Anthropometric examination	Malnutrition including underweight or overweight	1, 2	Counseling and diet

TABLE 6–3.   RECOMMENDATIONS FOR PREVENTIVE MEDICINE PROCEDURES—*Continued*

Procedure	Condition	Type of Prevention (Primary=1; Secondary=2)	Intervention
Skin examination	Acne	2	Diagnosis and treatment
History and examination	Sexual immaturity or disorders (2nd visit only)	1, 2	Counseling, diagnosis, and therapy
Counseling	Accidents	1	Counseling
Vaccination	Diphtheria; tetanus (2nd visit only)	1	Immunization boosters
History	Drug abuse and alcohol (2nd visit only)	1, 2	Counseling
Hematocrit determination	Anemia (2nd visit only)	2	Diagnosis and treatment
Blood pressure	Cardiovascular problems (2nd visit only)	2	Diagnosis and treatment
History	Unwanted pregnancy (2nd visit for sexually active patients only)	1	Contraception
VDRL determination	Syphilis (2nd visit for sexually active patients only)	2	Diagnosis and treatment, counseling and contact finding
Culture for gonococcus	Gonorrhea (2nd visit for sexually active patients only)	2	Diagnosis and treatment, counseling and contact finding

†One visit at age 8 to 9 and one at age 13 to 14.

Ages 17 to 34 Years†

Procedure	Condition	Type of Prevention	Intervention
History of completed immunization or booster in past 10 years	Diphtheria, tetanus	1	DT vaccination
Rubella hemagglutination inhibition test	Congenital rubella syndrome (females only)	1	Rubella vaccination
VDRL determination	Syphilis	2	Diagnosis and treatment
Culture for gonococcus in female	Gonorrhea	2	Diagnosis and treatment, contact finding
Height and weight measurements	Malnutrition and obesity	1, 2	Counseling and diet, diagnosis and treatment
Blood pressure	Hypertension and associated conditions and complications	1, 2	Diagnosis and treatment
Cholesterol determination	Coronary artery disease	1	Counseling and diet
Hematocrit determination	Anemia	2	Diagnosis and treatment
Blood glucose determination	Abnormal glucose tolerance and diabetes	1, 2	Diagnosis and treatment
Cervical cytology	Cervical cancer	2	Diagnosis and treatment
Breast self-examination	Breast cancer	2	Diagnosis and treatment
Hearing and vision testing	Hearing and visual defects	2	Diagnosis and treatment
History and life style	Heart and lung diseases	1, 2	Counseling
History and counseling	Alcoholism and drug abuse	1, 2	Counseling
Counseling	Accidents	2	Counseling
History and counseling	Smoking	1, 2	Counseling
PPD tuberculin testing	Tuberculosis (high risk groups only)	2	Diagnosis and treatment

†One visit at ages 17 to 18, 25, and 30

Ages 35 to 64 Years†

Procedure	Condition	Type of Prevention	Intervention
History of completed immunization or booster in past 10 years	Diphtheria, tetanus	1	DT vaccination
VDRL determination	Syphilis	2	Diagnosis and treatment
Height and weight measurements	Malnutrition and obesity	1, 2	Counseling and diet, diagnosis and treatment
Blood pressure	Hypertension and associated conditions and complications	1, 2	Diagnosis and treatment
Cholesterol determination	Coronary artery disease	1	Counseling and diet
Hematocrit determination	Anemia	2	Diagnosis and treatment

Table continued on following page

TABLE 6–3.   RECOMMENDATIONS FOR PREVENTIVE MEDICINE PROCEDURES*—*Continued*

Procedure	Condition	Type of Prevention (Primary=1; Secondary=2)	Intervention
Stool examination for blood	Occult gastrointestinal malignancy	2	Diagnosis and treatment
Blood glucose determination	Diabetes	2	Diagnosis and treatment
Breast examination	Breast cancer	2	Diagnosis and treatment
Mammography or xerography in symptomatic and high risk patients	Breast cancer	2	Diagnosis and treatment
History and life style	Heart and lung disease	1, 2	Counseling
Hearing and vision testing	Hearing and visual defects	2	Diagnosis and treatment
History and counseling	Alcoholism and drug abuse	1, 2	Counseling
History and counseling	Smoking	1, 2	Counseling
Counseling	Accidents	1	Counseling
Pap smear	Cervical cancer	2	Diagnosis and treatment
PPD tuberculin testing	Tuberculosis (high risk groups only)	2	Diagnosis and treatment

†One visit every 5 years from ages 40 to 60

		Age 65 or Greater†	
History of completed immunization or booster in past 10 years	Diphtheria, tetanus	1	DT vaccination
Influenza immunization	Influenza and complications	1	Influenza vaccination
Height and weight measurements	Malnutrition and obesity	1, 2	Counseling and diet, diagnosis and treatment
Blood pressure	Hypertension and associated conditions and complications	1, 2	Diagnosis and treatment
Electrocardiogram	Arrhythmia	2	Diagnosis and treatment
Hearing and vision testing	Hearing and visual defects	2	Diagnosis and treatment
Blood glucose determination	Diabetes	2	Diagnosis and treatment
Hematocrit	Anemia	2	Diagnosis and treatment
Stool examination for blood	Occult gastrointestinal disease	2	Diagnosis and treatment
Breast examination and mammography or xerography	Breast cancer	2	Diagnosis and treatment
History and life style	Heart and lung disease	1, 2	Counseling
History and counseling	Alcoholism and drug abuse	1, 2	Counseling
History and counseling	Depression and suicide	1, 2	Counseling
Counseling	Accidents	1	Counseling

†One visit every 2 years

*From Breslow, L.: Report of Task Force III to the National Conference on Preventive Medicine, Bethesda, Md., Fogarty International Center of the National Institutes of Health and the American College of Preventive Medicine, June, 1975.

ing evidence for many of the recommended procedures; the prudent judgment of Task Force experts served as the ultimate criterion for inclusion. The basis for that judgment centered on three issues: (1) the importance of the problem, (2) the effectiveness of the preventive procedure, and (3) the feasibility of the procedure.

Emphasis was placed upon the need for health care services to develop a long-term programmed approach to preventive medicine rather than to continue with occasional campaigns aimed at particular diseases. These recommendations, because they focus upon prevention as related to personal health services, omit environmental and broad educational measures (which should supplement the measures listed).

LIFE-STYLE RISK FACTORS AND THE FAMILY PHYSICIAN

Upon reading the preventive procedures outlined in Table 6–3 by the Task Force, one is struck by the increasing importance of life-style factors as serious and appropriate concerns for the physician. Most practicing physicians, although informed of the importance of the adverse effects of smoking, obesity, and so forth during their training, were not offered clinical techniques with which to pursue these problems systematically. In the remaining portion of this chapter, we will offer some general comments and some "helpful household hints" on what physicians should do and should avoid doing in helping patients wrestle successfully with life-style problems.

THE EPIDEMIOLOGIC VIEW

Nothing is certain but death and taxes, and when it comes to information about a population's health, or lack of health, the most reliable information available is mortality data. Such data for the white and black populations of the United States are summarized in *Probability Tables of Deaths in the Next Ten Years from Specific Causes,*[4] in which probabilities are listed by five year intervals for each sex. (The tables are obtained from L. C. Robbins, M.D., Health Hazard Appraisal, Methodist Hospital, Indianapolis, Indiana 46202.) See Chapter 10 for a complete discussion of prospective medicine.

When the principal diagnoses listed on United States death certificates are compared, the most frequently noted are arteriosclerotic heart disease, malignant neoplasms of the lungs, motor vehicle accidents, and vascular lesions of the central nervous system. Clearly, life-style and environmental factors are key determinants in these deaths.

In Canada, the Ministry of Health and Welfare has issued a major health policy statement, *A New Perspective on the Health of Canadians,*[5] based upon an anal-

ysis of mortality for those under age 70. In 1971, of the 157,300 deaths in Canada, 75,200 occurred in people below age 70. Of these 75,200 deaths, 10 per cent occurred in children under the age of 5, the majority of these in youngsters with congenital anomalies or in infants who were at high risk postnatally. Twelve per cent occurred in individuals between the ages of 5 and 34, the vast majority of these from accidents and suicide. The remaining 78 per cent occurred in individuals between the ages of 35 and 69; over half of these deaths were due to cardiovascular conditions, respiratory diseases, or lung cancer. When deaths were examined in terms of years lost, before reaching age 70, the same causes of death were listed, but in different order (ranked here in order of total number of person-years lost): motor vehicle accidents, ischemic heart disease, all other accidents, respiratory diseases and lung cancer, and suicide. *A New Perspective on the Health of Canadians* concluded that "self-imposed risks and the environment are the principal or important underlying factors in each of the five major causes of death between age one and age seventy, and . . . unless the environment is changed and the self-imposed risks are reduced, the death rates will not be significantly improved."

One of the important contributions of this study is the formulation of what is termed the *health field concept*, which divides the health field into four components: human biology, environment, life style, and health care organization. *Human biology* refers to those components of health, physical and mental, that spring from the human body directly—man's genetic inheritance, the organ systems of the body, and the occurrence of chronic diseases. The *environment* refers to matters external to the human body over which the individual has little or no direct control—food, water supply, air, and the social environment. *Life style* refers to the sum of decisions and actions by individuals that affects their health and over which they do have direct control. *Health care organization* is the quantity, quality, arrangements, and relationships that constitute health care—medical practice, nursing, hospital care, public health services, pharmacy services, dentistry, and other organized health services. The four components of the health field concept are applied in *A New*

Perspective on the Health of Canadians to potential areas of effort in lowering mortality, in health care financing, and in health care research. These four components bear some semblance to the traditional epidemiologic triad of agent, host, and environment that derived from infectious disease epidemiology. The difference now is that man is his own worst agent and that the organization of health care is a matter of public debate and public policy.

The empirical basis of *A New Perspective on the Health of Canadians* is mortality data; therefore, those aspects of health care not present at death will not be reflected in this type of analysis. Mental health in particular suffers from lack of attention. But without better morbidity data, it is difficult to make definitive statements about remediable disability, discomfort, and dissatisfaction related to either physical or mental illness and assessed across an entire population.

THE POLICY OR POLITICAL VIEW

Pressure is mounting on the health care systems of all nations to improve effectiveness and efficiency. But life expectancy, especially of people beyond the early years of life, seems to bear little relationship to public investment in health care. The general public is repeatedly informed of new developments in health care; yet there is a general disillusionment with physicians and with the complexities and indifference of technical medicine. Furthermore, the cost of medical care has risen dramatically over the past decades to become a leading category of public expenditure. So it is not surprising that the patient has become a "consumer" of medical care and has begun to voice his concerns politically.

Thus, governments have been searching for better ways to contain medical costs and to improve the results of health care. *A New Perspective on the Health of Canadians* makes it clear that the intent of the Canadian government is to spend a greater proportion of funds on life style and on the environment and a lesser proportion on health care organization. But this policy may lead to more than budgetary decisions. *A New Perspective on the Health of Canadians* states:

The following hypotheses...now appear sufficiently valid to warrant taking positive action:
1. It is better to be slim than fat.
2. The excessive use of medication is to be avoided.
3. It is better not to smoke cigarettes.
4. Exercise and fitness are better than sedentary living and lack of fitness.
5. Alcohol is a danger to health, particularly when driving a car.
6. Mood-modifying drugs are a danger to health unless controlled by a physician.
7. Tranquility is better than excess stress.
8. The less polluted the air is, the healthier it is.
9. The less polluted the water is, the healthier it is.
In due course, the validity of the foregoing and similar hypotheses will likely be resolved in a scientific way. . . . Meanwhile, we must move ahead with programs based on precepts such as the foregoing.

The government of Canada has embarked on five strategies based on these conclusions—a *health promotion* strategy to inform and influence the public; a *regulatory* strategy to reduce hazards to health via regulatory governmental powers; a *research* strategy to obtain knowledge relevant to these ends; a *health care efficiency* strategy to balance cost, accessibility, and effectiveness in delivering mental and physical health care; and finally, a *goal-setting* strategy to set specific goals for the physical and mental health of Canadians.

As of this writing, the federal government of the United States seems far less ready to commit its national health policy to an attack on unhealthy aspects of life style and of the environment. *The Forward Plan for Health, Fiscal Years 1978–82* published in 1976 by the United States Department of Health, Education, and Welfare notes:

A characteristic of such conditions as coronary heart disease, cancer, and violent death is that they are often caused by factors in the environment or the life styles of individuals that are not susceptible to direct medical solution. (Most physicians can diagnose and treat patients for chronic disease, but few are trained to prevent further exposure to carcinogenic substances, or to induce their patients to stop smoking or drive safely). . . . While all the options (presented for U.S. Dept. of H.E.W. action) were judged worthy of serious consideration, there was no suggestion that the Department endorsed them, or that they should be undertaken by the federal government rather than some other segment of society.[11]

When presenting the health status of the United States population, this study was careful to distinguish what the health status of the population is from what the health care system does for illness:

Last year's Forward Plan (FY 1977–81) presented a summary of the health status of the population, which is sometimes viewed as an indicator of the effectiveness of the health care system in dealing with illness. However, personal habits and preventive measures also play an important role in the determination of health status.

We find here a recognition, if not a celebration, of the traditional split between what one sector of the health care system does for sick people and what another sector of the system does in the way of prevention. The family physician undoubtedly will be asked to bring together these disparate sectors.

The Forward Plan for Health, Fiscal Years 1978–82, in presenting the nation's health status, devotes considerable space to life-style factors. Cigarette smoking patterns in teenagers and adults are noted, along with the percentage of all smokers who reported having been advised by a physician to stop smoking (only 25.2 per cent of all smokers in 1974 reported being so advised). The number of adults who are obese is noted—one-sixth of the males and more than one-fifth of the females. The percentage of moderate-to-heavy drinkers was 40 per cent among males and 16 per cent among females. The percentages of the population who had various types of preventive care examinations were also noted. Thus, it seems inevitable, regardless of policy, that the preventive services offered by physicians and the preventive behaviors adopted by their patients will receive closer and closer scrutiny in the pursuit of both a healthier population and a more effective health care system.

Other forces will push clinical medicine further into a preventive role. The physician is already engaged in a multitude of preventive services (see Table 6–3) that cannot be divorced from the other educational and behavioral work that needs to be done. The physician is visited more frequently than any other health care provider, except for the pharmacist. It would be most natural and efficient to merge preventive services to this existing pathway that the population now traverses. Many people expect their physicians to play a major role in prescribing important life-style changes. The financing of medical care offers a potential mechanism for the financing of specific counseling procedures directed at life-style changes. If the physician learns even modestly effective ways of helping his patients to change dangerous habits, the payoff for such activity in terms of person-years saved per patient will be high relative to the many other activities in which the physician now engages. Specifically, if the physician is instrumental in helping 10 per cent of patients who smoke to stop smoking, and if the average gain in life expectancy is 3 years per former smoker (a modest expectation), then the average gain per smoker receiving counseling is 0.3 year, a yield far exceeding that of most immunization procedures now available.

Until such preventive activities on the part of physicians are properly funded, the family physician's efforts with respect to life-style change will be a frill rather than a major responsibility. In the meanwhile, voluntary agencies, psychologists, the mass media, some health departments, other health professionals, and various nonprofessional "gurus" will take on the clinical challenges of instituting healthful life-style change.

On the side of the already-overburdened physician is the commentary of J. B. McKinlay, who sees a solely clinical focus on unhealthy behavior as ultimately futile.[7] McKinlay argues that such work is often doing too little, too late. He observes that in Western societies we have "manufacturers of illness—those individuals, interest groups, and organizations, which in addition to producing material goods and services, also produce, as an inevitable byproduct, widespread morbidity and mortality." McKinlay finds that "the promoters of disease-inducing behavior are manifestly more effective in their use of behavioral science knowledge than are those of us who are concerned with the eradication of such behavior." He feels that by ignoring the corporate and political forces that support the manufacture of illness and by devoting preventive attention solely to individuals and groups at risk, we pass up the only weapons with which we can defeat the grand scale of man-made illness we see about us. Those weapons include legislation aimed at advertising, taxation related to generated social costs, closer regulation of lobbying activities, broader public education about manufactured products, and other "upstream" interventions. Not many physicians will have a desire for so political a strategy as McKinlay's, but if the battle is not also fought upstream, the workload may inundate us downstream.

A BEHAVIORAL VIEW

One exciting feature of life-style change over the past decade is the experimental demonstration of effective clinical means of helping individuals gain control over their behavior and enhancing "self-management" or "self-control." In fact, one of the major contributions to the field is the book *Self-Control: Power to the Person* by Mahoney and Thoresen.[8] This progress in behavioral therapy can be ascribed to three factors: (1) the intense empirical and methodologic orientation of psychologists who have been developing the field, (2) a focus on contingency management—that the consequences of behavior (the reinforcers) determine the pattern of subsequent behavior, and (3) a focus on stimulus control—managing differently the environmental stimuli that cue behavior. When these tools have been placed in the hands of persons who wish to change their own behavior, clearcut improvements have been achieved by those with problems such as cigarette smoking, obesity, and excess alcohol intake. No question exists about the findings of clinical, behaviorally-oriented research, but just how these conclusions are to be applied most effectively on a broad scale is not clear. The long-term and large-scale research to determine the degree of behavioral change accomplished by these methods and studies of the ultimate effects on mortality and morbidity have not been done and are not underway; therefore, conclusive results will not be available for decades. In the meantime, it seems wise for us to extrapolate from the many epidemiologic studies that show the perniciousness of certain life-style factors and conclude that life-style change itself is a high priority activity. It seems wise for those with responsibilities for preventive medicine to extend the psychologists' successes in guiding behavioral change by working through medical practice either to refer people to those capable of instituting effective methods of change or to offer direct clinical assistance.

The best documented achievements have come in the control of cigarette smoking and of obesity. McAlister[6] has written an excellent review of efforts to help people quit smoking in which he notes that specific methods have improved one year cessation rates from 15 to 25 per cent a decade ago to over 50 per cent more recently. In their excellent how-to-do-it manual *Slim Chance in a Fat World*, Stuart and Davis[9] review comprehensively the behavioral aspects of obesity and point out that methods are now available that lead to 50 per cent of those in the program losing more than 20 pounds over 1 year, significantly more than the percentage that has been reported with nonbehavioral methods and more than what many physicians expect from their treatment of obesity.

Despite the development of these effective clinical approaches, traditional patterns of physician-patient interaction may impair the broad application of these methods. Two aspects of patient-physician behavior merit comment: (1) the pattern of initiative taken by physician and patient, and (2) the degree to which physicians cue their work to the patient's chief complaint.

Szasz and colleagues[9a] have proposed three models of physician-patient interaction: activity–passivity, guidance–cooperation, and mutual participation. They have pointed out that each model is appropriate for a different medical situation. The first model is applicable in emergency situations, surgical procedures, and other treatments in which technical procedures must be performed for a patient who is essentially helpless. The second model, guidance–cooperation, is suitable in situations that require technical knowledge, professional judgment, and cooperation on the part of the patient. Mutual participation, the third model, is required when the issue is one in which the bulk of the decision-making and expertise rests with the patient, and the physician serves principally as a consultant rather than as an authority.

The latter model is most appropriate for life-style change. However, it is this model of interaction for which most physicians have been least trained, since training tends to occur in settings in which the patient's situation is severe and acute, warranting the activity–passivity model of interaction or the wielding of what Paterson calls Aesculapian authority.*

Another aspect of physician-patient interaction that tends to inhibit the physician's pursuit of life-style change as a legitimate objective of medical care concerns the patient's chief complaint. Magraw[7a] points out that, when successful, the medical contract that develops between physician and patient requires mutual understanding and agreement about what is the nature of the medical problem, what is to be done, and why it is to be done. Thus, the physician who clinically pursues problems such as smoking and overeating when they are not complaints raised by the patient may add to his work the task of showing how these problems are relevant to the patient's health. Furthermore, when the patient initiates a complaint about a problem, the patient is offering an implicit expression of the value and relevance of the problem. When the physician initiates attention to a particular issue, the patient has made no such commitment, nor has he given recognition to the physician's authority, skill, or interest in the matter. Thus, it would seem useful for family physicians who wish to engage their patients in preventive activities to begin by explicitly telling their patients at the outset to expect a preventive emphasis.

In working with any population following an unhealthy life style, partitioning of the population may be useful. We suggest that those with a life-style risk factor of concern be subdivided into four categories:

I. *Changers*—those who are engaged in changing their behavior on their own and who do not need external support to accomplish this change, even though they themselves may seek and obtain external assistance.

II. *Conditional changers*—those who, when given the appropriate treatment methods, whether do-it-yourself, individual counseling, or group approaches, change their behavior. This should be the target group of clinical preventive services.

III. *Doubting nonchangers*—those who do not perceive of themselves as interested in changing their behavior but who wish to learn more about either the associated risks or about the processes of behavioral change.

IV. *Loyal nonchangers*—those who are not interested in changing their life style or not interested in learning more about either its associated risks or its behavioral features.

Instruments have not yet been developed that allow this kind of partitioning of the population, either on a community basis or within a physician's practice. Extrapolating from survey data, we estimate that for cigarette smokers, Category I smokers range from 5 to 10 per cent, Category II about 25 per cent, Category III about 50 per cent, and Category IV about 20 per cent. A completely successful smoking campaign would lead to all of Category I and II smokers becoming nonsmokers and to all of Category III smokers entering Categories I and II. But only when the population is followed systematically over a period of years and when life-style changes are carefully evaluated will a model of this type be validated. We can say unequivocally that clinical methods are now available that help persons change at-risk life-style practices of long-standing. Nevertheless, how these methods are best applied to family practice and what percentage of patients actually responds are not yet known.

WHAT THE FAMILY PHYSICIAN CAN DO

First, we recommend that the physician provide an exemplar role for patients. To smoke, drink alcohol to excess, overeat, or radiate psychologic stress diminishes any encouragement that the physician may give the patient toward changing to a healthful life style. Physicians can be proud of their colleagues in Great Britain who, from 1960 to 1970, dramatically changed their cigarette consumption and also reversed their previously rising mortality rate, the only male occupational group in that nation to do so. If one is to offer good counsel, good

*T. T. Paterson: Management Theory, London, Business Publications Ltd., 1966.

advice, or even good information, it would seem proper to apply these injunctions to oneself, not only for the welfare of patients but also for the promised health and heartiness these offer the physician.

Second, the family physician needs to define explicitly his interest and commitment to this aspect of medicine. Does the physician enjoy maintaining a clinical interest in behavior? Is he willing to read the necessary literature and to obtain the necessary training to do the clinical work? How much does he wish to commit to the area of life-style change, considering the realities of financial compensation and time costs? Will he be duplicating services already available to the patient? Will he have to pioneer to create services that fit the needs of particular patients?

Since no standards are broadly accepted for how the family physician should pursue life-style change, a range of clinical options exists, from doing virtually nothing to offering intensive group therapy. Some physicians choose to say nothing about the patient's smoking, overeating, overconsumption of alcohol, psychologic stress, or automobile safety unless the patient's medical diagnosis demands some action. Other physicians display handouts, cartoons, and posters in the office to communicate their views on particular life-style issues. Some physicians offer their patients an occasional, strategic reminder, hoping to overcome long-standing resistance by attrition rather than by direct confrontation. A few physicians go further than even these measures. Some develop a systematic means of referring patients to available sources of assistance for redirecting life style; some do one-to-one or group counseling; and some, especially those practicing in large, prepaid groups or in occupational medicine, have associated psychologists or behavioral specialists to do the preventive work.

Taking the epidemiologic view, some physicians have worked on more than the host, electing also to work on the environment and on the agent. A good example of this is the group Physicians for Automotive Safety (50 Union Avenue, Irving, New Jersey 07111). Members have lobbied, reviewed automotive safety devices, and studied other factors that relate to automobile injuries. However, in this chapter we will restrict our remaining words to what physicians might do clinically.

THE APPROACH TO LIFE-STYLE CHANGE

To begin, the physician should have a well-thought-out conception of life-style risk factors and of how the patient might proceed to change these. It is useful to regard smoking, overeating, and so forth as overlearned, overpracticed behaviors that have multiple determinants, such as cultural background, family customs, past experiences, the influences of friends and workmates, physical and mental health, previous medical treatment, access to the materials or the opportunities to engage in the behavior, and the person's hopes, preferences, and decisions. Each risk behavior usually serves some function and very legitimate purpose, e.g., a cigarette smoker may use cigarettes to relax in social situations, take a break, structure time, or serve as a reward at the end of a difficult task. Yet, most smokers are unaware of the functional use they make of their "bad" habit. In fact, they usually perceive of a desire only for the cigarette and not for the use to which they will put the cigarette. These uses or functions are best discovered by the patient's monitoring his own behavior by noting down the time, place, circumstances, and feelings during which the problem behavior occurs *and also* when the problem behavior is successfully avoided, the latter because it is important to learn as much about good habits as about bad ones.

It is important to assess the social environment for both sources of stress and sources of support. The person whose spouse has just died is not a good candidate for cessation of smoking, even if the spouse died of lung cancer. On the other hand, positive rewards and encouragement may come from unexpected sources or from casual acquaintances, and these should not be overlooked.

For those who have previously and unsuccessfully attempted a life-style change or who are of a depressive nature, they, rather than the habit, may represent their most formidable opponent. Feeling guilty, celebrating ineptitude, choosing to be overwhelmed, or a combination of these are behaviors that attract attention but that lead to little productive life-style change. When attention is focused on what work has been accomplished and what victories have been won, however minor these may first appear, the odds of successful change increase.

One must not belittle the magnitude of the task for some people. Saying good-by permanently to cigarette smoking or to overeating can be a major and difficult undertaking for many people, perhaps among the most difficult of a lifetime. But when success comes after such a struggle, such individuals will often go on to master other problem areas in their lives, for what had once seemed impossible becomes an accepted daily fact of life.

One last conceptual point concerns the behavioristic view that behavior itself may determine attitudes as much as attitudes determine behavior. This fits with the non-behavioristic "theory of cognitive dissonance," that, given two alternative and competing belief structures, people tend to settle on the one that is most consistent with their experiences. Thus, suppose a smoker, after hearing about the harmful effects of smoking, attempts to stop. If successful, the person will likely believe that stopping smoking was something he always wanted to do and was able to do. If unsuccessful, the person will likely feel that he was not able to stop smoking, that he really did not want to stop, or both. Another way of describing this process is that people rationalize their behavior after the fact. The theory of cognitive dissonance and the behavioral concepts about formation of beliefs help to explain an interesting phenomenon concerning cigarette smoking: smokers who appear to be perfectly happy with their smoking are more likely to succeed in stopping than are those who for some time have been attempting to stop but who have not met with success. The first group tends to be more consistent about life in general. When persuaded that the hazards of smoking apply to them, they stop smoking more quickly and more often than do those who are stuck in "trying hard."

MOTIVATION AND CONTRACTS

Regardless of how expert their interpersonal skills, family physicians cannot supply their patients with motivation. Our view is that each person has his own set of motivations and that these are usually more than enough to generate and maintain his interest in living and in experiencing the good things life has to offer, although many people disguise this interest with self-limiting and self-destructive behavior. But,

at any point in time, only a limited number of those with a risk factor are ready and willing to change their way of life. The physician has one principal and powerful means of motivating the patient—defining, after consultation with the patient, what it is that the patient wants to do about his situation. Then, after the physician identifies what the patient is willing to do and after some bargaining, both can arrive at a mutual understanding, a specific plan, a *contract*. For example, the physician might conclude, "I am willing to spend three visits working with you about your smoking if you are willing to keep the appointments, to keep records of cigarettes smoked, and to talk about both your successful and your unsuccessful attempts to change your smoking patterns."

Contracts must be specific to be meaningful. Rather than stating "to begin exercising regularly," the contract might specify, "to ride a bicycle 2½ miles in 15 minutes on Monday, Wednesday, and Friday afternoons." Contracts should be two-way agreements, i.e., both patient and physician should undertake only that which they are willing to do.

In arriving at the subject matter of the contract, the physician's job is to outline the risk factors that the patient faces and then to offer skill and expertise (the physician's own or another's) to show the patient how the patient can change these risk factors. The patient should choose which risk factors to work on, and the patient should get the credit for success for the work done. The physician's or counselor's job is to show the way but not to do the work. Thus, the contract specifies an active choice on the patient's part and is the first clinical step toward changing risk.

THE SPECIFICS OF BEHAVIORAL CHANGE

Few will question that the major risk factors associated with life style are overpracticed, overlearned behaviors. An approach that many people find acceptable is that of learning theory. Rather than treating smoking, overeating, or underexercising as a manifestation of laziness, of cultural patterning, or of sociologic or economic determinism (although all may be true), it is useful for the individual patient to regard such behaviors as responses he took a long time to learn and therefore as responses that he might take some time and effort to unlearn. Both patient and physician have the option of viewing the patient's venture into changing his behavior as one of problem-solving, rather than one of discovering the inherent worth (or unworth) of the patient, of a particular clinical approach, or of the clinician.

The steps in this problem-solving process, as we view them, are presented as follows.

Monitoring

Monitoring involves systematic notation by the patient of the circumstances of both problem and successful behavior; the time, place, persons, activities, and feelings associated with the response of interest are recorded. The physician or counselor also summarizes both measures of progress and problem situations.

Functional Analysis

The patient decides what uses the undesired behaviors are serving, e.g., cigarette smoking may serve the smoker as a time-out, a reward, a way to structure time, a way to handle angry feelings, or a combination of these. Usually, the functions served are reasonable, necessary matters of everyday life. Thus, a set of daily problems to solve becomes identified, e.g., how else to take time out, to reward oneself, to structure time, or to handle anger other than by lighting a cigarette.

Goal Setting

Setting goals involves particularizing the contract over time so as not to over-reach the patient's interests or capacities and seeing that tangible goals have been specified. These goals ultimately lead to the changes the patient wants. They must each be reasonable and attractive enough so that the patient will not become frustrated and give up. People who tend to be unsuccessful in managing life-style change also tend to set unreasonably high goals for themselves.

A particularly useful approach to goal setting has been developed by Alan Best, a psychologist at the University of British Columbia. He utilizes a behavioral prescription pad much as a physician would use a conventional prescription pad. By writing down the mutually-agreed-upon prescription, with a carbon copy for his own records, the therapist provides the patient with explicit, reasonable goals and simultaneously retains the carbon in the patient's record for follow-up purposes.

Changing the Pattern of and Response to Cues

By acting on the environment and himself, a patient can modify the external and internal cues to the overlearned behavior. For example, by eating before shopping for food, the overweight person can ameliorate the internal impulses that otherwise would cry for cookies and other "goodies."

Or a given cue can be converted to signal other behavior. For example, seeing others light up cigarettes, for the person who used to respond by lighting up his own, might now be met with a loud internal voice that, with practice, has learned to say, "I don't smoke anymore." Such new responses are best derived by the patient's solving his own set of problems rather than by being prescribed by the physician.

Changing the Pattern of Rewards

Rewarding desired behavior and ignoring undesired behavior are potent and necessary steps in behavior change. Many people who have difficulty with life-style change have great difficulty in finding daily, available, modest rewards to offer themselves when they achieve minor, or even major, success. As social primates, most of us treasure the praise and positive murmurings of our fellow creatures. But many people have yet to learn to give and to receive such murmurings with ease and comfort. Instead of welcoming positive recognition, people often respond with disclaimers or by belittling what they have done.

With regard to punishment and other negative reinforcements, we believe it is wiser to ignore undesired behavior rather than to celebrate it with more undesirable consequences or with undue concern.

Feedback (More Monitoring)

Once goals are set and cues and rewards are decided, it is important to check to see that the new behavior takes place. If it doesn't, then the prescription, that is, the self-prescription, ought to be changed. Monitoring must be done at the time of the behavior rather than *ex post facto*. By noting down a piece of food before it is eaten or a cigarette before it is smoked, there remains the opportunity to choose a different behavior. This opportunity disappears when monitoring is done retrospectively. Monitoring disrupts the almost automatic sequence of events that leads to the undesired behavior and inserts a time and place for new learning to occur. If the self-prescription is off the mark, the actual circumstances of the behavior provide an appropriate place and time to rethink another self-prescription.

Internal Dialogue

Most people talk to themselves; some do it more loudly than others. The nature of this talk is very relevant to effective self-management. People who tend to be successful tend to take a positive, problem-solving approach to their conversations with themselves. People with a self-management problem, when conversing with themselves about the problem, tend to be judgmental, negative, and more concerned with establishing blame for the problem than with finding its solution.

When the idea of internal dialogue is presented to patients and when they recognize that they do not have to lock themselves into unproductive behavior, they occasionally change with little further intervention. Psychologists have developed more structured methods for those who require extensive effort to curb their verbal self-harassment.

Dealing with Success

Many people find successful management of a problem to be uncomfortable or even anxiety-provoking. These feelings may appear at the mere thought of success or well after the successful behavior has been achieved. The therapist should check for awareness on the part of the patient of fear of success and, if present, should look further. First, the functional analysis of the problem behavior should have identified some useful and legitimate needs that the behavior had been serving. If the behavior that the patient is changing has served

usefully for many years, the physician should expect the patient to have a sense of loss, even of mourning, for the departed habit. Assurance that the feeling of loss is common is often sufficient.

Does the patient also have anxieties about success in general? Does the patient feel inherently unsuccessful? If the latter is true, then more general or more extensive psychotherapy may be appropriate.

Immunizing for the Future

When attempting to change a life-style behavior, the patient should perceive two major and distinct tasks, the second more important and difficult than the first — initially changing the behavior and then, having changed it successfully, maintaining the new pattern. This requires appropriate responses to the everyday situations that formerly precipitated the undesired behavior and appropriate responses to those infrequent, unpredictable, and disruptive occasions, e.g., an automobile accident or the loss of a job, that also might cue the undesired behavior. The physician should advise patients from the beginning that change and subsequent maintenance of the change are separate and distinct tasks. The physician can help to "immunize" against relapse by asking patients who have successfully changed their habits to describe how they will react to precipitating circumstances without reverting to the old behavioral pattern. The person who wishes to maintain long-term change needs to view his task not so much as never doing this or that again but rather as having available to him a set of skills and behaviors with which to respond to any situation so as to maintain the new behavior. If the exsmoker smokes a cigarette or if the formerly obese person gains 5 pounds, their futures have not been subverted unless they choose to ignore the skills and techniques they have learned and which are still available to them.

An essential ingredient for lifelong change is long-term follow-up of the patient. The patient should be told at the beginning of counseling that the physician will check in the future to see that the new behavior is maintained. Why should the patient and physician go through the bother of counseling and behavioral change if the patient reverts to the original behavior a year and a half later? For those patients and physicians who have a serious interest in maintaining long-term life-style change, a registry or follow-up system may prove to be imperative. From the beginning, we tell our patients that life-style change is forever, or for at least the next century.

IMPLICATIONS FOR FAMILY PRACTICE

The family physician who wishes to counsel and to follow patients in regard to life-style risk factors had better review in detail the practical implications of this kind of clinical activity. First of all, governments and agencies that finance medical care rarely pay for privately delivered preventive services. Physicians who wish to expand the time they invest in life-style change must face squarely a loss of revenue, a loss of leisure time, or the problems of directly billing patients for extra services not covered by health insurance. The physician must remember his role as an exemplar. To work hard without fair compensation is scarcely the role model to offer the overworked patient.

The family physician who is not prepared to make major changes in his style of practice may still offer patients useful services in regard to life style by systematically advising patients to change, by noting whether or not they do, and by inserting a helpful goad or bit of praise when appropriate. When further research is done into the effectiveness of the occasional and well-timed remark offered by the family physician, a potent stimulus may be found that is not now fully recognized.

However, from the point of view of the organizations that finance medical care, there is sense in avoiding a plunge into financing preventive counseling. The potential for abuse is high. The efficacy of widespread counseling by the family physician is not known, and the ultimate effects on health and health care costs are not documented. We expect that ultimately the financing of life-style change will be based upon some reasonable estimate of the amount of time and effort that is shown to be necessary to help patients minimize life-style risk factors.

In family practice, the most precious commodity is time. If physicians choose to reallocate a significant portion of their work to life-style change, which medical activities will they discontinue? Perhaps the most appropriate person to counsel patients is not the physician at all but someone who has been trained to deal with behavioral change. Psychologists, social workers, counselors, nurses, and even preventive technicians may be the most appropriate professionals to do the clinical work. When the methods are sufficiently developed, volunteer workers or even do-it-yourself approaches may work. Nevertheless, we expect a significant minority of family physicians to become involved in providing clinical life-style change services. For these physicians, time would be consumed in training, reading, planning and scheduling, screening patients, and actually providing preventive counseling. Counseling itself requires some decisions about the duration of sessions, their frequency, and their long-term follow-up. Present research suggests that once begun, work to change behavior should be intensive and rapid, with follow-up sessions planned over at least the course of a year, e.g., at 1, 3, 6, and 12 months. Seeing patients in groups is an economical and psychologically-reinforcing approach. Often the group has more collective wisdom than any of its members. If the group leader is willing to act as a convener rather than as a conductor, the success of such groups may be remarkable. But the knowledge and skills of a group leader who successfully encourages group members to solve their own problems are not easy to come by and will not be discussed here.

Record-keeping will be greatly affected by a family physician's involvement in life-style change. With respect to the individual patient, information will be needed over time: basic screening data that note the risk factors and the history of attempts to modify them, specific contracts to monitor and to change behavior, behavioral self-prescriptions as the patient develops them, descriptions of the health professionals' counseling procedures and strategies, actual changes in behavior, the scheduling of follow-up visits, and a system of recall and notification of appointments. With respect to the family physician's patients as a group, there might be some tabulation of the prevalence of the various life-style risk factors, of patients' interests in changing them, of attempts to make changes (with and without the formal help of the family physician), and of successes in achieving change. Follow-up registers similar to infectious disease registers will become useful adjuncts to patients and physicians concerned with long-term behavioral change, if confidentiality is adequately safeguarded. For an approach to the initial appraisal of life style, the reader is referred to the discussion of the process of health hazard appraisal in Chapter 10.

Few practicing family physicians have been trained in helping people to modify their behavior by the techniques that behaviorally-oriented psychologists have developed over the past decade. To explore this area, the reader can review the references listed at the end of this chapter and then consult with the psychiatrists and psychologists locally available who have an interest in life-style change. In terms of orientation, we endorse a major focus on behavior therapy supplemented by selective use of the many other forms of life-style change that have been promoted in recent years, e.g., aerobics, transcendental meditation, transactional analysis, gestalt therapy, assertiveness training, biofeedback, and so forth.

Finally, the family physician who engages seriously in helping patients to change specific life styles may find the need for particular equipment and space, e.g., steps for fitness testing, a soundproof corner for audiovisual presentations, and storage space for printed materials to be given to patients.

As with the patients' attempts to change their life style, family physicians who want to change their style of practice should consider fully the implications, the specifics, the satisfactions, and the problems of long-term maintenance of the new behavior.

ETHICAL AND EDUCATIONAL CONSIDERATIONS

The objective of life-style change services should not be life-style change at any cost but the offer of help to persons so that they can direct themselves to fuller, happier, and more productive lives. If the purpose and financing of such services become myopically focused upon only the behavioral changes themselves, then physicians

and their coworkers may be tempted to use coercive and manipulative methods. It is likely that these would not only fail but would also deprive patients of a rich source of support and assistance in coping with the insults of modern-day living. As with any medical problem, the patient has the ultimate sovereignty of choice among the treatment alternatives available. With the patient as the ultimate judge, the physician's efforts to facilitate life-style change may be both appropriate and effective.

The public should be aware that although community concern and governmental policy may have accurately identified life-style change as a desirable and useful part of family practice, our present physician population, as noted previously, has not been trained entirely appropriately. Our practicing physicians may stimulate, develop, and promote programs of continuing medical education that will teach productive techniques, but there is a more important responsibility on the part of medical schools, i.e., to recognize this need and to properly train graduates as the body of generally acceptable knowledge of this aspect of prevention is developed. Until then, the present blend of amateurism and untested theory, based largely on physician concern and personal experience, will continue to be more prevalent than truly professional expertise.

The necessary data base, the proven techniques, and the corps of properly trained professionals at present are all many years off. These facts must be realized by the public, governments, educational systems, and physicians alike.

SUMMARY

The family physician is in a strategic position to implement preventive medicine. The scope of prevention is broad, and its procedures are only partially defined. Thus, family physicians have the opportunity to stake out their own clinical approach to prevention and to follow their own particular interests.

Life-style factors—cigarette smoking, overconsumption of alcohol, overeating, underexercising, psychologic stress, and behavior predisposing to accidents—are the major risks to which people in technologically advanced nations are exposed.

The family physician can choose from a variety of roles in responding to the risks that patients demonstrate. A physician can warn, goad, refer, educate, or help directly with behavior change, or he can use a combination of these methods. To facilitate such change, the family physician needs a basic approach, and in this chapter we have outlined one. Besides the basic approach, the family physician should recognize the logistic and financial difficulties of dealing clinically with life-style change. But having recognized the obstacles to be surmounted, the incorporation of a balanced set of preventive measures into practice may be as rewarding in terms of professional satisfaction to physicians as it is in terms of health to patients.

REFERENCES

1. Audy, J. R.: The Measurement and Diagnosis of Health. San Francisco, The Hooper Foundation, University of California Medical Center, 1970.
2. Breslow, L. (chairman): Theory and Application of Preventive Medicine in Personal Health Services. Report of Task Force III to the National Conference on Preventive Medicine. Bethesda, Md., Fogarty International Center of the National Institutes of Health and the American College of Preventive Medicine, June, 1975.
3. Cochrane, A. L.: Effectiveness and Efficiency: Random Reflections on Health Services. London, The Nuffield Provincial Hospitals Trust, 1972.
4. Geller, H.: Probability Tables of Deaths in the Next Ten Years From Specific Causes. Indianapolis, Ind., Health Hazard Appraisal, Methodist Hospital of Indiana, 1972.
5. Lalonde, M.: A New Perspective on the Health of Canadians. Ottawa, National Health and Welfare, Government of Canada, April, 1974.
6. McAlister, A.: Helping people quit smoking: current progress. In Enelow, A. J., and Henderson, J. B. (eds.): Applying Behavioral Science to Cardiovascular Risk. Proceedings of a Conference, Seattle, Wash., June 17–19, 1974. New York, American Heart Assoc., 1975.
7. McKinlay, J. B.: A case for refocussing upstream—the political economy of illness. In Enelow, A. J., and Henderson, J. B. (eds.): Applying Behavioral Science to Cardiovascular Risk. Proceedings of a Conference, Seattle, Wash., June 17–19, 1974. New York, American Heart Assoc., 1975.
7a. Magraw, R. M.: Ferment in Medicine. Philadelphia, W. B. Saunders Co., 1966.
8. Mahoney, M. J., and Thoresen, C. E.: Self-Control: Power to the Person. Monterey, Cal., Brooks/Cole Publishing Co., 1974.
9. Stuart, R. B., and Davis, B.: Slim Chance in a Fat World: Behavioral Control of Obesity. Champaign, Ill., Research Press Co., 1972.
9a. Szasz, T., Knoft, W. H., and Hollender, M. H.: The doctor-patient relationship and its historical context. Amer. J. Psychiatry, 115:522, 1958.
10. Thoresen, C. E., and Mahoney, M. J.: Behavioral Self-Control. New York, Holt, Rinehart & Winston Inc., 1974.
11. U.S. Department of Health, Education and Welfare, Public Health Service: Forward Plan for Health, Fiscal Year 1978–1982. Washington, D.C., U.S. Government Printing Office, DHEW Publ. No. (OS) 76-50046, August, 1976.
12. White, K. L.: Primary medical care for families: organization and evaluation. N. Engl. J. Med., 277:847, 1967.

Chapter 7

PERIODIC HEALTH SCREENING

by PAUL S. FRAME,
and BRIAN K. E. HENNEN

They that be whole need not a physician, but they that are sick.
Matthew: 9:12

GENERAL CONSIDERATIONS

Health screening is the presumptive identification of unrecognized or asymptomatic medical problems by history, physical examination, or diagnostic tests. Periodic health screening implies, in addition, that screening tests will be done repeatedly at some stated interval. Screening does not establish definitive diagnoses. All positive findings from screening require further evaluation and work-up before a diagnosis can be made or treatment instituted. Screening should not be confused with finding abnormalities during a work-up initiated specifically to investigate signs or symptoms presented by the patient.

Screening can be carried out on several population levels (Fig. 7–1). *Epidemiologic survey* is the attempt to determine the incidence, prevalence, and natural history of diseases within a general population. Once the general occurrence is known, the disease may then be looked for in specific subpopulations. *Case finding* is the application of tests to selective populations or high risk groups. This can be done effectively within a practice population. *Individualized screening* is the application of screening procedures to a particular patient, taking into consideration his current health status and risk factors.

Periodic health screening is initiated by the formal health care system and is therefore fundamentally different from the usual patient-initiated medical encounter. The patient undergoes screening procedures not because he feels ill or is worried about something but because he has been told by his physician, the news media, the government, organizations such as the Cancer Society or Heart Association that he will benefit from screening procedures and should therefore spend his hard-earned money for them. This creates a unique moral and ethical situation for the physician.

In the normal patient-initiated encounter, the physician's ethical responsibility is to do whatever he can to solve the patient's problem or to give advice and comfort if this is not possible. He is not responsible for current defects of medical knowledge and may pursue investigative hunches or use therapy without conclusive proof of efficacy, provided that he explains the potential uncertainties and risks to the patient.

When a physician suggests screening procedures, the ethical responsibility is different. The physician has a moral responsibility for reasonable proof that screening will beneficially alter the course of disease in a significant number of cases. He should act only when there is evidence that the search will be of value. He should not act when there is a lack of evidence regarding the value or safety of a procedure, although this decision is often called for in clinical situations with symptomatic patients.

The physician must also bear in mind the potential for doing harm to a previously asymptomatic person. This "screening morbidity" includes the direct risk from the procedure itself, the consequences of being

LEVELS OF SCREENING

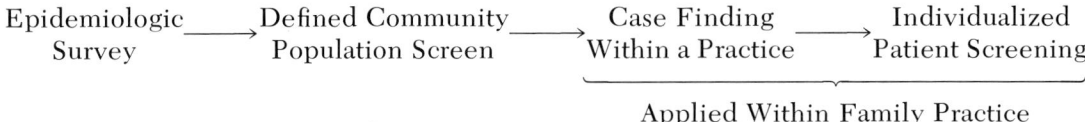

Epidemiologic   ⟶   Defined Community   ⟶   Case Finding   ⟶   Individualized
Survey   Population Screen   Within a Practice   Patient Screening

Applied Within Family Practice

Figure 7–1. Diagram of health screening by different population levels.

identified as "sick" by peers or by oneself, and the likelihood of being discriminated against by employers or insurance companies.

Even a small scale screening program, if applied to the entire practice population, can require a significant investment of time by the family physician and his staff. It should be initiated only after careful consideration of what goals can be realistically achieved, the time and effort required, and the benefits and costs to the patient. Too often, the perpetually busy physician gives his screening efforts low priority and does them haphazardly, not at all, or orders a complete battery of tests, many of which are expensive and useless, for all patients.

A serious problem with most screening tests relates to the inherent limitations of test sensitivity and specificity. *Sensitivity* is the ability of a test to identify persons having the disease being tested for; that is, a high sensitivity means a low number of false negative results. *Specificity* is the ability of a test to distinguish those having a given disease from those not having it; that is, a high specificity means a low number of false positive results. The following example illustrates that even with a highly sensitive and highly specific screening test overidentification of positive results can be a major problem.

Suppose disease X has an incidence of 1 case per 1000 population (slightly higher than the incidence of breast cancer in women). Suppose also that a screening test is 95 per cent sensitive and 95 per cent specific for disease X. This means there will be 5 per cent false positive and 5 per cent false negative results from the test. If a population of 100,000 is screened, the results will be as shown in Table 7–1. 5089 people will have a positive screening test for disease X and will require further work-up, but only 95 people, or 1.9 per cent of those identified as positive, will actually have the disease.

TYPES OF SCREENING PROGRAMS

Health screening is commonly done in many diverse settings and manners. In the United States, screening became popular after World War II. Many of the early programs were financed by large industries, and the populations screened were often executives. Numerous studies reported a high rate of disease detection among these asymptomatic people. However, critical analysis revealed that many of the diseases detected were chronic conditions whose course was not changed by early detection. Many of the abnormalities were not confirmed on follow-up, a large number of patients received no follow-up, and the programs were frequently one-time screening efforts.[4, 26, 27]

Other groups were less quick to advocate mass screening programs. At the 1965 annual meeting of the British Medical Association, the following resolution was pro-

TABLE 7–1. OVERIDENTIFICATION OF POSITIVE RESULTS USING A SCREENING TEST WITH 95 PER CENT SENSITIVITY

	Patients with Disease X	Patients Without Disease X	Total Patients
Positive Test Results	95	4,994	5,089
Negative Test Results	5	94,906	94,911
TOTAL	100	99,900	100,000

posed: "In the opinion of this house, the routine medical check-up in the over-forties does more harm than good."[10]

More recently, organizations such as heart associations and cancer societies have been active in organizing screening clinics. The purpose of these clinics is to reach people who would not normally see a physician for screening and to publicize the importance of detecting and treating certain diseases. Unfortunately, these clinics are often sporadic, are not able to individualize screening to the particular patient, and do not have an assured mechanism for follow-up.

Automated multiphasic testing centers have added a new dimension to screening by being able to offer a large array of tests at a very low unit cost.[9] To be cost efficient, they require a large patient volume and thus are usually only successful in densely populated areas. However, even when a wide variety of tests are coupled with good follow-up provided by a health maintenance organization, it has been difficult to show a significant decrease in morbidity and mortality as a result of multiphasic screening.[8, 23]

The family physician is the logical person to provide periodic screening. He can individualize screening to fit the particular patient, has a longitudinal relationship with that patient, and can provide immediate follow-up for abnormal results. The difficult question is, what screening procedures should be done and how often?

WHAT SCREENING PROCEDURES SHOULD BE DONE AND HOW OFTEN?

The bulk of this chapter will be devoted to this question, which has no single correct answer. Much of the necessary data is unavailable, and many areas are highly controversial.

SCREENING CRITERIA

One immediate problem that arises in any discussion of screening is that the individuals evaluated are not a homogeneous group and are being screened for many different reasons. It is necessary to establish criteria that must be fulfilled before

TABLE 7-2. SCREENING CRITERIA

1. The disease must have a significant effect on the quality or duration of life.

2. Acceptable methods of treatment must be available.

3. The disease must have an asymptomatic period during which detection and treatment significantly reduce morbidity and mortality.

4. Treatment in the asymptomatic phase must yield a therapeutic result superior to that obtained by delaying treatment until symptoms appear.

5. Tests that are safe and acceptable to the patient must be available at reasonable cost to detect the disease in the asymptomatic period.

6. The incidence of the disease must be sufficient to justify the cost of screening.

screening is justified for a given disease. The criteria outlined in Table 7-2 have been used in a recent review of screening, and minor variations in these standards have been proposed by several authors.[11] It is not sufficient for a disease to satisfy one or two of the standards. All criteria must be met if screening is to be justified. For example, ovarian cancer meets criteria 1, 2, 3, 4, and 6. However, there is no adequate diagnostic test that will consistently diagnose cases at a curable stage (criterion 5), so screening for ovarian cancer is not justified.

It is also necessary for purposes of discussion to stipulate that only the hypothetical, asymptomatic person is being considered here. Including people with chronic diseases and those in high risk groups makes the discussion more difficult.

In actual practice there are very few completely asymptomatic persons. The physician must constantly individualize screening for every patient, just as he individualizes management. Indeed, in many cases screening loses its identity as a separate medical function and merges with other procedures for the optimal management of the particular patient. For example, the physician will look for colorectal cancer much more intensively in patients with ulcerative colitis than in the general population. Physicians practicing in low socioeconomic areas may need to screen more actively for such problems as tuberculosis and syphilis. With these qualifications in mind and assuming the patient is asymptomatic, we will proceed to discuss screening for specific diseases according to the criteria in Table 7–2.

To answer the question "what screening tests should be done and how often?" it is necessary to identify which diseases or problems have significant morbidity and then to determine if the disease meets all the screening criteria. To do this, one must obtain information about the incidence and prevalence of the disease; disease progression, both with and without treatment, including morbidity, mortality, and the length of any asymptomatic period; risk factors associated with development of the disease; and the availability of screening tests, their safety, sensitivity, and specificity in the early stages of the disease, their actual or potential risks, and their unit cost.

This information is difficult to obtain, as it is widely scattered in the literature, and much of it is unknown. Many areas are the subject of controversy and ongoing research. Several review articles have attempted to gather this material together and use it to formulate rational longitudinal screening protocols, along with documenting the sources of their information.[3, 11, 22]

PEDIATRIC SCREENING

The periodic well-child examination has a much broader function than periodic health screening. It is difficult to precisely identify the screening component, and in practice it is not essential to do so. Non-screening components of well-child care include child-raising instruction; preventive medicine, including immunization; monitoring of growth and development; and acting as the child's ombudsman to assist parents in providing adequate stimulation, nutrition, and care. In this section we will discuss only screening and will not try to define the content of the well-child examination or suggest how often it should be done.

The most common causes of morbidity and mortality in children are shown in Table 7–3. The conditions with the highest prevalence at the top of this list are relatively minor. They have significant morbidity but very low mortality, even if undetected. Only when one considers congenital heart disease, accidents, phenylketonuria, cancer, and diseases of even

TABLE 7–3. CAUSES OF MORBIDITY AND MORTALITY IN CHILDREN

Cause	Occurrence per 100,000 Population
Dental caries	Over 75,000 (P)
Visual defects	5000 to 20,000 (P)[1]
Anemia	5000 (P)[1]
Positive tuberculin test	1000 to 3000 (P) at school age[1]
Bacteriuria	1200 (P) school-aged girls[1]
Hearing loss	800 (P) at school age[1]
Congenital hip dislocation	400 to 2000 (I)[1]
Hypertension (blood pressure > 140/90)	Rare below age 10 (P)[3] 7000 ages 10 to 13 (P)
Congenital heart disease	500 (P) at school age[1]
Accidents	23 (DR)[2]
Phenylketonuria	10 (I)[1]
Cancer (all forms)	6 (DR)[2]
Congenital malformations	4.1 (DR)[2]
Galactosemia	1 (I)[1]
Homicide	1 (I)[2]

(P) = Prevalence
(I) = Incidence
(DR) = Death Rate

1. Bailey, E. N., Kiehl, P. S., Akram, D. S., et al.: Screening in pediatric practice. *Pediatr. Clin. N. Amer.*, 21:123, 1974.
2. Cancer statistics. CA 25:19, 1975.
3. Lauer, R. M., Connor, W. E., Leaverton, P. E., et al.: Coronary heart disease risk factors in school children: the Muscatine study. J. Pediatr., 86: 697, 1975.

lower incidence is one talking about conditions with significant mortality. The frequency of these lethal conditions is much less than the frequency of many of those screened for in adults (see Table 7–5). Screening for disease in children can be expected to have a much lower yield than in adults. On the other hand, the potential benefit in terms of years of useful life is much greater if disease is detected and corrected in children.

Table 7–4 presents our recommendations for screening asymptomatic children based on the diseases fulfilling the six criteria outlined in Table 7–1. We reiterate that screening must be individualized. These suggestions are useful as a guide, subject to individual modification. Appropriate screening recommendations are certain to change as research and technical advances enlarge medical knowledge.

TABLE 7–4. PEDIATRIC SCREENING FLOW SHEET

Age	Screening Procedures
Newborn	Cardiac auscultation, check for hip dislocation, phenylketonuria, galactosemia, physical examination.
Under 1 year	Cardiac auscultation, check for hip dislocation, gross vision and hearing tests, hematocrit, educate parents about household accidents, use of car seats, and so forth.
1 to 5 years	Cardiac auscultation, cover test for strabismus, tuberculin skin test, review dental care, educate parents regarding accident prevention (especially car seats, poisons, drowning, burns).
School entry	Cardiac auscultation, cover test for strabismus, Snellen chart for visual acuity, hearing test, tuberculin skin test, check for scoliosis, educate parents regarding bicycle accidents.
Age 10	Blood pressure, check for scoliosis.
Age 15	Blood pressure, tuberculin skin test.

Several controversial areas in pediatric screening will be discussed individually. Detailed discussions of each pediatric screening procedure have been presented previously in the literature but exceed the space limitations of this chapter.[3, 22]

CONTROVERSIES IN PEDIATRIC SCREENING

Asymptomatic Bacteriuria

Covert bacteriuria is found in 1 to 2 per cent of school-aged girls. In adult women, the prevalence increases with age to 10 to 15 per cent of women over age 60. Bacteriuria follows a natural course of disappearance and reappearance with the passage of time. There is an association between bacteriuria and urinary tract abnormalities, as demonstrated by radiologic studies. In one study 47 per cent of schoolgirls with bacteriuria had x-ray evidence of abnormal urinary tracts, most commonly showing evidence of pyelonephritis or reflux.[21]

It is unknown whether bacteriuria is a cause, a result, or a coincidental concomitant of the renal abnormalities. It is known that antibiotics can eradicate bacteriuria in most patients. One year after treatment, however, many treated patients again have bacteriuria, and many untreated controls have sterile urines. In some studies there is no statistical difference between the outcomes of the treated and untreated groups 1 year later.[2] This means that continued eradication of bacteriuria will require intensive, continuing, long-term antibiotic treatment for an indefinite period, perhaps even lifetime therapy and surveillance. Furthermore, no study has shown that continued eradication of bacteriuria will prevent or delay the progression of renal abnormalities or even that these abnormalities are progressive.[21]

We do not recommend screening for asymptomatic bacteriuria because although it has a high incidence, there is no conclusive evidence of long-range morbidity, and treatment would be costly, time consuming, and of questionable benefit (fails criteria 1 and 4 of Table 7–1).

Hypertension

The incidence of hypertension in children depends on how it is defined. If a definition of two standard deviations above the mean is used, 2.5 per cent of the population will have hypertension. If the adult definition of hypertension as a blood pressure level greater than 140/90 mm. Hg is used, then hypertension in young children under age 10 is rare.[17] In adolescents, however, hypertension is more common, and blood pressure levels approach adult values.

Londe[18] defined hypertension as a blood pressure level above the 90th percentile for age. Using this definition he studied 74 "hypertensive" children for secondary causes of hypertension. He found abnormalities detected by intravenous pyelograms in three girls, all of whom had had several episodes of symptomatic urinary tract infection. Only three of Londe's patients (ages 9, 11, and 12) had diastolic pressures consistently above 90 mm. Hg. The rest were considered hypertensive even though their pressures were below 140 systolic and 90 diastolic. Thus, most of Londe's hypertensive children were not hypertensive by adult standards, and only three *symptomatic* children had possible secondary hypertension. Interestingly, Londe recommended observation but not treatment of these hypertensive children.

Hypertension in adults is known to increase the risk of cardiovascular disease, especially stroke and myocardial infarction. Antihypertensive treatment has been shown to decrease this risk. It is logical but unproved that hypertension in children causes similar morbidity.

No controlled study has demonstrated morbidity from "hypertension" in children with blood pressure levels below 140/90, and no standards have been established for a "safe" blood pressure at different ages. We are, therefore, left with 140/90 as a clinical borderline level for pathologic hypertension in children as well as adults.

Hypertension as defined by adult standards becomes more common in older children and adolescents.[17] Evidence in adults indicates that treatment of hypertension is beneficial. We therefore recommend screening for hypertension in children at age 10 and in adolescents. In younger children, hypertension by adult standards is rare, and age-specific standards have not been shown to be clinically meaningful. Thus, we do not recommend the routine screening of younger asymptomatic children.

Anemia

Like hypertension, anemia is an entity whose prevalence depends on how it is defined. Except in high risk groups, iron deficiency is by far the most common cause. Other causes either are acute diseases or are too rare to warrant screening. The prevalence of iron deficiency anemia is variously reported as from 5 to 30 per cent or even higher depending on the population surveyed.[3] Decreased iron stores have been noted only when hemoglobin values fall below 10 gm. per 100 ml., and overt cardiovascular morbidity is noted only at hemoglobin levels of 6 to 7 grams per 100 ml. or lower. Thus, much of the high prevalence of anemia is statistical and may not be clinically significant. In infants, the only evidence of morbidity from mild anemia (hemoglobin levels greater than 8 grams per 100 ml.) is a higher incidence of respiratory infection. Growth and develop-

ment of anemic and control infants are not statistically different.[1]

The first year of life is the time of highest risk for anemia. It is also the age when morbidity from increased respiratory infection associated with mild anemia may occur. We recommend screening infants at 9 months of age for anemia by hemoglobin or hematocrit determination. Above 1 year of age there is no evidence that asymptomatic anemia is detrimental or that treatment in the asymptomatic phase is superior to waiting until symptoms occur. Therefore, screening older children for anemia is not recommended (fails criterion 4 of Table 7–1).

ADULT SCREENING

Table 7–5 lists the most common causes of morbidity and mortality in adults and includes recommendations regarding screening for each disease. Most of the problems listed are diseases in the classic sense. The two most prevalent conditions, smoking and obesity, might not be strictly considered diseases. It could also be argued that they are never asymptomatic, since anyone who smokes or is more than 20 per cent overweight is aware of it. However, smoking, obesity, and other behavioral problems are some of society's most serious contributors to disease. Many people either are not aware of the health implications of these problems or deny that they are health problems. It is therefore important that physicians screen for these behavioral factors and educate the patient about the risks they represent.

The incidence, prevalence, and death rate data in Table 7–5 are a guide to occurrence rates of the conditions listed. As such they are useful, but they should not be interpreted too strictly. Comparable data for dissimilar diseases are simply not available in many cases.

Frame and Carlson[11] reviewed each of the conditions listed in Table 7–5 as to their suitability for screening according to the criteria in Table 7–1. They then assembled their conclusions about each disease into a longitudinal screening flow sheet (Fig. 7–2) for adults aged 21 to 70.

In using this flow sheet it is assumed that a complete physical examination and data base will be done on each patient when

TABLE 7-5. CAUSES OF MORBIDITY AND MORTALITY IN ADULTS AND SCREENING RECOMMENDATIONS

Disease	Occurrence per 100,000 Population	Screening Recommendations
Smoking	35,000 (P)	Although not strictly a disease, it leads to serious morbidity. Smoking history should be taken initially and at ages 30 and 40.
Obesity	25,000 (P)	Leads to serious morbidity. Early identified treatment depends on patient motivation. Height and weight should be checked every 4 years.
Hypertension	15,000 (P)	Treatment reduces risk of stroke and heart disease. Slow progression. Screen every 2 years.
Cholelithiasis	11,000 (P)	Screening only indicated if asymptomatic gallstones are to be removed. Not recommended. Fails criterion 4.
Bacteriuria	6,000 (P–W)	No demonstrated long-range benefit from treatment. Fails criteria 1 and 4.
Hyperlipidemia	5,300 (P)	Elevated cholesterol associated with morbidity. Treatment may reduce risk. Screen by serum cholesterol every 4 years.
Anemia	5,000 (P)	No evidence that asymptomatic anemia is harmful. Fails criterion 4.
Alcoholism	4,200 (P)	Long prerecognition phase. Identification can aid patient and family. Ask about drinking habits every 5 to 10 years.
Ischemic heart disease	2,800 (P)	Screen for treatable risk factors, hypertension, smoking, elevated cholesterol. Electrocardiogram not useful.
Diabetes	1,270 (P)	Presymptomatic treatment does not reduce morbidity. Fails criteria 3 and 4.
Open angle glaucoma	360 (P)	No single adequate test. Uncertain whether early treatment prevents morbidity. Fails criteria 4 and 5.
Gonorrhea	285 (I)	Acute symptomatic disease in males, low morbidity in females. Fails criteria 1 and 4.
Rheumatic heart disease	170 (P)	Get initial history of rheumatic heart disease.
Stroke	102 (DR)	Only treatment is reduction of risk factors. Screen for risk factors.
Tuberculosis	80 (P)	Can have morbidity in asymptomatic period. Screen by tuberculin testing every 10 years.
Breast cancer	73 (I–W)	Early detection and treatment shown to improve survival in women over age 50. Self-exam. should be done monthly. Physician exam. biannually to age 50; annually thereafter.
Depression (psychotic)°	70 (P)	No benefit from treating asymptomatic depression. Fails criterion 4.
Colorectal cancer	45 (I)	Rectal exam detects only 10 to 15% of cancers. Sigmoidoscopy has low yield and lower patient acceptance. Screen by stool exam. for occult blood every 2 years in persons aged 40 to 50; every year thereafter.
Lung cancer	26 (I)	Early diagnosis and treatment does not improve survival. Fails criteria 2 and 5.
Cervical cancer	25 (I)	Meets screening criteria but after 2 annual Pap smears, smears every 2 years are adequate.
Prostatic cancer	16.5 (I)	Periodic rectal exam. never shown to increase survival. Fails criteria 2 and 5.
Liver cirrhosis°	14 (DR)	Only specific treatment is cessation of alcohol. Screen for alcoholism only. Fails criteria 2 and 4.
Endometrial cancer	14 (I)	Women should report postmenopausal bleeding. No other adequate test available. Fails criterion 5.
Brain tumors	12 (I)	No adequate screening method. Fails criterion 5.
Syphilis	11.5 (I)	Meets criteria, although incidence low. Screen by serology every 6 years until age 50.
Ovarian cancer	11 (I)	No adequate test for early detection. Fails criterion 5.
Chronic obstructive pulmonary disease°	10.6 (DR)	Only treatment in asymptomatic stage is avoidance of smoking. Fails criteria 3 and 4.

Table continued on following page

TABLE 7–5.   CAUSES OF MORBIDITY AND MORTALITY IN ADULTS AND
SCREENING RECOMMENDATIONS—*Continued*

Disease	Occurrence per 100,000 Population	Screening Recommendations
Pancreatic cancer	9.0 (I)	No suitable test available. Fails criteria 2, 3, 4, and 5.
Stomach cancer	8.5 (I)	Rapid progression. Diagnostic tests all expensive and complex. Fails criterion 5.
Chronic nephritis	7 (DR)	No specific treatment in asymptomatic phase. Fails criterion 4.
Bladder cancer	7 (I)	Low incidence. Early detection not shown to affect ultimate course. Fails criteria 1 and 6.
Lymphoma	6 (I)	Persons should report lymph node swelling. No specific physician screening.
Cancer of the mouth and pharynx	6 (I)	No physician screening. Patients should be taught to report chronic mouth or lip sores.
Chronic leukemia	4 (I)	Early treatment does not affect ultimate course. Fails criteria 4 and 6.
Renal cancer	3 (DR)	No satisfactory screening test. Fails criteria 5 and 6.
Testicular cancer	2.3 (I)	Histologic type affects prognosis more than early detection. Males should be taught to palpate testes.

(I)   = Incidence
(P)   = Prevalence
(DR) = Death Rate
(W)   = Women

*The relative prevalence of these diseases is probably understated in this table because of difficulties in determining true prevalence rates.

first seen. The content of this data base is not specified and is decided by the individual practitioner. After the initial data base has been obtained, no "complete history and physical" is recommended for the asymptomatic patient. Instead, specific examinations and tests are suggested that can rationally be expected to yield significant benefit. For persons under age 50 a screening visit every 2 years is suggested. Persons over age 50 are seen yearly, primarily to screen for breast and colonic cancer.

The omission of the yearly physical examination is perhaps a shock to medical pedagogy but not to medical practice. In fact very few people, asymptomatic or symptomatic, have repeated complete examinations on a regular yearly basis. A physical check-up is the sum of its parts and to justify any part of the examination one must first ask what disease or diseases are being sought? It is then necessary to see if screening for that disease by the examination or test in question fulfills the criteria in Table 7–1. Those procedures that do fulfill the criteria are then included in the screening program.

GERIATRIC SCREENING

Persons over age 65 will soon constitute 10 per cent of a family physician's patient population. Particularly "at risk" are those who live alone, are recently bereaved, or are recently discharged from the hospital. Lowther[19] studied 300 such "at risk" patients in several British physicians' practices by outreach programs (through visiting nurses) and screening procedures (history, physical examination, chest x-ray, urinalysis, hemoglobin level, mean corpuscular hemoglobin concentration, erythrocyte sedimentation rate, and blood urea nitrogen values). He found 16 per cent of the patients studied afflicted with obesity, 14 to 16 per cent with depression or cataracts, 10 to 13 per cent with hypertension, ischemic heart disease, or deafness, and 7 to 9 per cent with chronic bronchitis, osteoarthritis, dyspepsia, or foot defects. The authors, through follow-up, concluded that "to help three patients you must examine twelve, find nothing to do in four, and be unable with certainty to help the remaining five."

For the geriatric population, "asympto-

Figure 1. Screening Flow Sheet

TEST	21	22	23	24	25	26	27	28	29	30	31	32	33	34	35	36	37	38	39	40	41	42	43	44	45	46	47	48	49	50	51	52	53	54	55	56	57	58	59	60	61	62	63	64	65	66	67	68	69	70
Complete History and Physical Examination	●																																																	
History of Rheumatic Fever	●																																																	
Smoking History	●									●										●																														
History of Alcohol Use	●					●		●		●		●		●		●		●		●		●		●		●		●		●		●		●		●		●		●		●		●		●		●		●
Blood Pressure	●	●		●		●				●		●		●		●		●		●		●		●		●		●		●		●		●		●		●		●		●		●		●		●		●
Weight and Height	●	●		●		●		●		●				●						●				●						●				●						●				●				●		●
Pap Smear				●		●		●		●		●		●		●				●		●				●		●		●		●		●		●		●		●		●								
Cholesterol						●		●				●				●				●				●				●								●				●										
VDRL	●																	●																																
PPD	●									●																				●																				
Stool for Occult Blood																				●		●		●		●		●		●										●										●
Teach Self Palpation Breast, Neck, Testes	●									●										●										●										●										
Teach to Report Mouth Sores or Lesions																				●										●										●										
Teach to Report Post Menopausal Bleeding																														●										●										
Tonometry and Funduscopy																●				●				●				●				●				●				●				●				●		
Proctosigmoidoscopy																									●										●															
Physician Breast Check	●	●		●		●		●		●		●		●		●		●		●		●		●		●		●		●		●		●	●	●	●	●	●	●	●	●	●	●	●	●	●	●	●	●

Figure 7-2. Screen flow sheet. (Adapted from Frame, P. S., and Carlson, S. J.: A critical review of periodic health screening using specific screening criteria. J. Fam. Prac.. 2:29, 123, 189, 283, 1975.)

131

matic" may mean "without symptoms" or "reluctance to report presenting symptoms." If we return to our original definition of screening, we can make a case for including "unrecognized" as well as "asymptomatic" diseases. Criteria 3 and 4 of Table 7–1 could be modified to read that "disease must have an *unrecognized* (or ignored) period during which. . ." and "treatment in the unrecognized (or ignored). . .".

If we can indeed help one out of four at-risk geriatric patients by screening, the potential for effective selective screening is probably greater in this age group than in any other.

CONTROVERSIES IN ADULT SCREENING

No chest x-ray or electrocardiogram (ECG) is listed in the flow sheet for adult screening. The chest x-ray might be considered in screening for lung cancer, tuberculosis, chronic obstructive pulmonary disease (COPD), or atherosclerotic cardiovascular disease. In screening for each of these diseases, however, it fails one or more criteria. In lung cancer, because of the rapid progression and inadequate treatment, x-rays even every 6 months do not lead to improved survival.[5] The tuberculin skin test is a cheaper initial screening procedure for tuberculosis. The chest x-ray is a late indicator of COPD, and except for cessation of smoking (which has already been recommended), there is no specific treatment that will arrest the disease. Treatment is aimed only at relieving symptoms. In atherosclerotic cardiovascular disease, chest x-ray abnormalities are inconsistently found prior to the onset of symptoms. Furthermore, in the asymptomatic person, reduction of risk factors (hypertension, smoking, hypercholesterolemia) is the only treatment available. This has already been advocated, and the addition of chest x-ray findings does not lead to any different treatment modality.

The ECG is considered primarily as a test for atherosclerotic cardiovascular disease. It is, however, a poor detector of early ischemic heart disease. The Framingham study showed that only 27 per cent of patients having a first myocardial infarction had previously abnormal ECG's. Seventy-three per cent of patients had a falsely normal ECG within 1 year prior to their first myocardial infarction.[20] In addition, like the chest x-ray, the ECG does not lead to any new treatment modality in the asymptomatic person with ischemic heart disease. Treatment is still the reduction of risk factors, which is advocated regardless of the ECG findings.

Cervical Cancer

Since the development of the Papanicolaou smear test (Pap smear), carcinoma of the cervix has been one of the most frequently screened diseases. It occurs with an overall incidence of from 14 to 36 cases per 100,000 women. It is rare before age 20 but then occurs increasingly until the fifth decade, when an incidence of 85 cases per 100,000 women has been reported. After the fifth decade, the incidence decreases but is still highly significant. Factors that are associated with a higher rate of cervical cancer include low socioeconomic class and frequent sexual contact.[11]

The Pap smear has been established as an inexpensive, reliable test for cervical carcinoma that, when properly done, has a false negative rate of less than 6 per cent.[11] It does, however, have a considerably higher rate of false positive tests that require further evaluation to rule out carcinoma.

In past years there has been considerable debate about the relationship between cervical dysplasia, carcinoma in situ, and invasive carcinoma of the cervix. Recently, there is more agreement that dysplasia, cancer in situ, and invasive cancer are stages in a continuum of malignant cellular changes.

Given this continuum, the key question with respect to screening is "What is the progression time from dysplasia to cancer in situ and from cancer in situ to invasive cancer?" In a prospective study by Richart[25] the average progression time from dysplasia to cancer in situ was 44 months with a range of from 12 months to 86 months. Petersen[24] followed the development of a series of in situ lesions and found 11 per cent became invasive within 3 years, 22 per cent within 5 years, and 39 per cent within 9 years. These studies suggest that cancer of the cervix is a slowly progressive disease requiring between 5 to 10 years to progress from dysplasia to invasive carcinoma.

Gray,[14] discussing the frequency of taking cervical smears, found that the yield of positive smears decreased markedly in women who had had several previous negative smears. He concludes that after two annual negative smears, screening every 3 to 5 years is sufficient. He points out that women who are of low socioeconomic class or who have frequent sexual contact are at much higher risk than the general population and may need more frequent screening.

A Canadian Task Force Report, after a detailed review of the literature on the epidemiology and screening successes for cervical carcinoma, recommended the following as an effective and sufficient frequency of examination for cervical cancer.[7]

1. Initial smears should be obtained from all women over the age of 18 who have had sexual intercourse.

2. If the initial smear is satisfactory and without significant atypia, a second smear should be taken within 1 year.

3. Provided the initial two smears and all subsequent smears are satisfactory and without significant atypia, further smears should be taken at approximately 3 year intervals until the age of 35 and thereafter at 5 year intervals until the age of 60.

4. Women over the age of 60 who have had repeated satisfactory smears without significant atypia may be dropped from a screening program for squamous carcinoma of the cervix.

5. Women who are not at high risk should be discouraged from having smears more frequently than is recommended here.

6. Women at continuing high risk should be screened annually. To facilitate this, provision for taking cytologic smears should be made at family planning clinics, student health clinics, youth clinics, venereal disease clinics, prenatal clinics and medical facilities where women are examined before admission to penal institutions.

In its early stages, cervical cancer is a curable disease. Typical 5 year survival rates are: Stage 0, 99 per cent; Stage I, 90 per cent; Stage II, 60 per cent; Stage III, 30 per cent; and Stage IV, less than 10 per cent.[11] Thus, diagnosis and treatment in the early stages are important to the achievement of a long-term cure.

Cervical cancer meets the criteria for a disease warranting periodic screening. The question is "How often do women need to have a Pap smear?" We recommend that all women over the age of 20 have annual Pap smears for 2 years and if normal have a subsequent smear every other year indefinitely. This is a compromise recommendation between the tradition of annual Pap smears and evidence suggesting a 5 to 10 year progression from dysplasia to invasive carcinoma. Lower socioeconomic populations have a higher incidence of cervical cancer and require more intensive outreach programs.

Breast Cancer

Breast cancer is the leading cause of death due to cancer in women. Its incidence has increased in the past decade to the current level of 73 cases per 100,000 women. It is rare before age 25, but after this age breast cancer becomes increasingly common, reaching an incidence of 150 to 200 cases per 100,000 women in the 45 to 65 age group.[11]

The untreated 5 year survival rate for breast cancer is 15 to 20 per cent. Histologic studies have shown an average tumor doubling time of 28 days, while other studies reported an average tumor growth rate of 1 cm. every 3 months. The rate of growth and progression, however, is exceedingly variable, depending on histologic type and grade, and average figures may be meaningless in the individual case.

Examination by a physician, self-examination, and mammography are three widely used methods of detecting breast cancer.

Ninety per cent of breast malignancies are detected by a patient's self-examination, whether or not the patient has been instructed in systematic, periodic examination of her breasts.[28] In a study of women receiving yearly medical check-up, 38 per cent of all breast malignancies were discovered by patient self-examination at times other than the physician's examination.[29]

There are several problems with self-examination: (1) patient compliance—only 30 to 35 per cent of women with breast tumors, discovered by any method, claimed to be doing routine examinations; (2) there is a lag, averaging 10 months in one study, between the time of self-detection of a lesion and the first physician contact; and (3) small breasts are more easily examined than large, pendulous, or fatty breasts.[11]

The advantages of self-examination are: (1) it is inexpensive, the only cost being the initial educational session and occasional follow-up reminders; (2) it can be done frequently and at any desired interval; and (3) it requires minimal physician or paramedical time.

Examination by a physician and mammography are two other methods of detection. In Shapiro's prospective study of yearly screening for breast cancer, palpation detected 67 per cent of lesions. Forty-five per cent were also detected by mammography, but 22 per cent would have been missed using mammography alone. On the other hand, 33 per cent of all tumors were found only by mammography.[29]

Age and breast size are important variables in the relative yield from mammography and palpation. In women under age 50, 61 per cent of cancers were found by palpation alone, while only 19 per cent were detected by mammography alone. Over age 50, 42 per cent of tumors were detected only by mammography. About the same number, 40 per cent, were found only by palpation. Mammography is most useful for detecting lesions in large, fatty breasts, especially in the lower quadrants.[29] The major problems with mammography are its cost and its unknown potential as an invasive procedure to cause long-term morbidity.

There is little question that treatment improves the survival of patients with Stage I breast cancer. The untreated 5 year survival rate is 15 to 20 per cent. The overall 5 year survival rate for treated breast cancer is 54 per cent with a 10 year survival of 40 per cent. The most improvement occurs in Stage I disease; treatment produces a 5 year survival rate of 74 per cent. By contrast, the 5 year survival rate with treatment of Stage II disease is 28 per cent; that is, not much better than the overall untreated survival rate.[11]

The crucial question is "Does periodic screening improve survival?" No study has shown that screening by a single modality improves survival. Venet and Shapiro, in a prospective study of the effects of annual palpation plus mammography, have shown a significantly decreased 3½ year case fatality rate in women 50 to 60 years old. They were unable to demonstrate an improved survival rate resulting from screening in women under age 50.[29]

Early Stage I breast cancer has a much better prognosis with treatment than do the other stages. There is some evidence that screening improves survival in women over age 50. Self-examination is inexpensive. Mammography is expensive and has a small but unknown potential to cause morbidity. Given these facts, we recommend:

1. At age 20, women should be given detailed instruction in self-examination. This instruction should be repeated every 10 years.

2. Women should be encouraged to do systematic self-examinations at monthly intervals.

3. An examination by a physician should take place every 2 years until age 50, and every year thereafter.

4. Mammography should be used routinely only in women with high risk situations.

Colorectal Cancer

Carcinoma of the colon and rectum has an overall incidence of 45 cases per 100,000 population and a death rate of 21 per 100,000. The disease occurs in all age groups and with equal frequency in both sexes. Ninety-five per cent of cases, however, occur in people 45 years or older and 75 per cent occur in those over age 55. The median age at diagnosis is 60 to 67 years old. Risk factors associated with an increased susceptibility to colonic and rectal cancer include ulcerative colitis, familial polyposis, villous adenomas, and increasing age to the sixth decade.

Adenomatous polyps have, in the past, been thought to be associated with an increased risk of colorectal cancer and the question is still controversial. Their incidence is much higher than the incidence of carcinoma, and they occur in 5 to 10 per cent of people over age 40 undergoing proctosigmoidoscopy. Castleman, in a study of the malignant potential of polyps, concludes "The overwhelming majority of cancers of the colon arise as cancer de novo or in villous adenomas, not in adenomatous polyps. The adenomatous polyp is a lesion of negligible malignant potential."[6]

Seventy per cent of colorectal cancers occur in the distal 25 cm. of bowel. Initial symptoms depend to some extent on the anatomic location of the lesion. Eighty-one per cent of people with cancer of the rectum will complain of bloody stools, while only 22 per cent of those with cancer of the cecum will have this symptom.

The presymptomatic duration of the tumor is not known. As with many other tumors, there is a significant lag of 6 to 7 months between the onset of symptoms and institution of definitive treatment. Even with this considerable delay in reporting symptoms, 42 per cent of tumors are localized when diagnosed.

The 5 year survival rate with surgical treatment for localized disease is 50 to 66 per cent. This decreases to 30 to 35 per cent for disease with regional spread and to 5 per cent if distant metastases have occurred. A 5 year survival rate of 88 per cent was reported in 50 patients who were asymptomatic at the time of diagnosis.[11] Clearly the prognosis is improved if the disease is detected and treated early.

Methods of diagnosing colorectal cancer that must be considered as possible screening studies include barium enema, digital rectal examination, proctosigmoidoscopy, and testing stools for occult blood.

The barium enema is the standard method of diagnosing colonic cancers above the rectosigmoid junction. Excluding the rectum, this procedure is 90 per cent accurate in diagnosing colonic carcinoma. However, it is a poor method of detecting the 40 per cent of cancers occurring in the rectum. A barium enema is expensive and uncomfortable. Furthermore, if periodically repeated, the 1 to 2 rads per test amount to a significant radiation exposure.

Digital rectal examination has long been recommended as a primary diagnostic test for rectal cancer. Close study of the data, however, reveals that its sensitivity has been overrated. No more than 13 per cent of carcinomas of the colon and rectum can be felt on digital examination. In one series of 58 carcinomas, only 9.5 per cent were palpable on rectal examination at the time of diagnosis.[16]

Proctosigmoidoscopy is an important technique in the diagnosis of colorectal cancer. Seventy per cent of carcinomas can be seen on sigmoidoscopic examination. Because of this impressive figure, many have recommended its use as a routine periodic screening procedure. Studies of lesions identified by periodic proctosigmoidoscopy have consistently found a high incidence of adenomatous polyps. The

yield of carcinomas has been much smaller. Hertz found 44 cancers on 47,000 examinations,[16] Greegor found one carcinoma on 2500 examinations,[15] and Gilbertsen found 19 carcinomas on 12,000 initial examinations.[13] Of interest is the fact that there is a much higher rate of carcinoma detection on initial examination than on repeat, periodic proctosigmoidoscopy. Hertz found 70 per cent of his cancers on the initial examination and only 30 per cent on subsequent proctosigmoidoscopies. Gilbertsen did 41,000 repeat examinations and found nine carcinomas at a rate of one per 4400 examinations. This is much less than the one cancer per 630 initial examinations found by Gilbertsen.[12]

Proctosigmoidoscopy costs about $20 and may cause some discomfort for the patient. The incidence of bowel perforations is about one per 1000 examinations. Using Gilbertsen's data, if a family physician were to do repeat yearly proctosigmoidoscopies on 1000 patients (three per day), he would detect one cancer and perforate four bowels in 4 years at a cost of $80,000.

Testing stools for occult blood has been proposed as a screening method for colorectal cancer by Greegor.[15] The procedure involves having patients collect specimens for six slides for occult blood in the stool from three consecutive bowel movements while on a no meat, high residue diet. The special diet is necessary to reduce the number of false positive reactions. Greegor reports detecting nine carcinomas in 900 persons tested over 3½ years by this method. All but one were in early stages. In another uncontrolled report, only one false negative slide was found. These studies have been reported from one source, and further studies to confirm the results are needed. However, the method is cheap, causes no discomfort, and should detect cancer from a wider anatomic area than sigmoidoscopy alone.

Colorectal carcinoma has a high incidence and mortality. It has a significant asymptomatic period of unknown duration. The prognosis is much better if the disease is detected and treated early. The problem with regard to screening is finding an adequate diagnostic test. Barium enema is too expensive and is a poor detector of rectal lesions. Digital rectal examination only detects 10 to 15 per cent of all tumors. Proctosigmoidoscopy is expensive and uncomfortable; its yield decreases markedly with repeated examinations. Testing stools for occult blood is a method that has good potential but has been used on relatively small numbers of patients. All of the methods have advantages and disadvantages.

We recommend that all patients over age 40 have stools tested for occult blood by Greegor's method every 2 years until age 50 and every year thereafter. We do not recommend routine, repeat proctosigmoidoscopies because of the low yield, expense, time, and discomfort involved.

IMPLEMENTING PERIODIC HEALTH SCREENING

There are two levels of implementation of health screening in family practice. First is the periodic screening of those patients who are already coming to the office for some reason. Second is outreach to those people in the physician's practice or the community who do not regularly come to the office. In the first category of patients, screening will probably be blended into their ongoing care. The second group requires direct solicitation to inform them of the need for screening and to obtain their participation.

SCREENING FLOW SHEET

Screening must be efficiently organized so it can be done quickly and with a minimum of paperwork. The person doing the screening should be able to quickly note what screening has been done and what is indicated for a particular patient. One way of doing this is to include a screening flow sheet (see Fig. 7–2) in the patient's chart. The date is placed above the patient's age and a slash is made through the box of each procedure that has been done and is normal. An abnormal result is indicated by an X through the appropriate box. By using this technique, what screening is indicated at a given time is readily apparent.

Patient education and understanding are very important for a successful screening program. Patients who understand the scope and purpose of the program are more likely to be cooperative. Many of the procedures require patient participation at times other than the screening visit. A "screening handout" can serve both to educate pa-

tients about the screening program and to give them specific instructions regarding self-examination procedures. Such a handout may include a copy of a screening flow sheet.

Most, if not all, screening procedures can be done by physicians' assistants or paramedical personnel other than the physician. This is especially true if the patient is coming specifically for a screening visit. It is important that screening be done by the family practice team so that continuity between positive results and follow-up is not lost.

Outreach to inactive patients or to the community at large has not been utilized much in medical practice. In cases where it has been tried, the response is often disappointing, especially if the services offered are not free. Interestingly, outreach in the form of reminders for check-ups is much more common and accepted in dentistry than in medicine.

The simplest form of outreach is the direct mailing of a screening handout or brochure inviting the person's participation. The age, sex register will provide the names and addresses of appropriate people to receive the mailing.

CONCLUSION

Periodic health screening must be considered in the context of what it can and cannot achieve. Screening is not a panacea. It does not guarantee good health and may be potentially harmful. Current screening programs have not been shown to reduce the cost of medical care. Selective screening done by the family physician and blended into the patient's ongoing medical care can be expected (but has not been proved) to decrease the chances of morbidity from certain diseases.

REFERENCES

1. Andelman, M. B., and Sered, B. R.: Utilization of dietary iron by term infants. Am. J. Dis. Child, 111:45, 1966.
2. Asscher, A. W., and Sussman, M.: Asymptomatic significant bacteriuria in the nonpregnant woman—response to treatment and follow-up. Br. Med. J., 1:804, 1969.
3. Bailey, E. N., Kiehl, P. S., Akram, D. S., et al: Screening in Pediatric Practice. Pediatr. Clin. North Am., 21:123–165, 1974.

4. Bates, B., and Yellin J. A.: The yield of multiphasic screening. J.A.M.A., 222:74, 1972.
5. Boucot, K. R., Cooper, D. A., and Weiss, W.: The Philadelphia pulmonary neoplasm research project. Med. Clin. North Am., 54:549, 1970.
6. Castleman, B.: Do adenomatous polyps of the colon become malignant? N. Engl. J. Med., 267:469, 1962.
7. Cervical cancer screening programs. Report of the Canadian Task Force on Screening for Cervical Cancer. Can. Med. Assoc. J., 114:1003, 1976.
8. Collen, M. F., Dales, L. G., Friedman, G. D., et al.: Multiphasic check-up evaluations study for preliminary cost benefit analysis for middle-aged men. Prev. Med., 2:236, 1973.
9. Collen, M. F., Feldman, R., Siegelaub, A. B., et al.: Dollar cost per positive test for automated multiphasic screening. N. Engl. J. Med., 283:459, 1970.
10. Editorial. Can. Med. Assoc. J., 93:613, 1965.
11. Frame, P. S., and Carlson, S. J.: A critical review of periodic health screening using specific screening criteria. J. Fam. Pract., 2:29, 123, 189, 283, 1975.
12. Gilbertsen, V. A.: Adenocarcinoma of the large bowel. J.A.M.A., 174:1789, 1960.
13. Gilbertsen, V. A., Knatterud, G. L., Lober, P. H., et al: Invasive carcinoma of the large intestine — a preventable disease? Surgery, 57:363, 1965.
14. Gray, L. A.: The frequency of taking cervical smears. Obstet. Gynecol. Surv., 24:893, 1969.
15. Greegor, D. H.: Diagnosis of large bowel cancer in the asymptomatic patient. J.A.M.A., 201:943, 1967.
16. Hertz, R. E., Deddish, M. R., and Day, E.: Value of periodic examinations in detecting cancer of the rectum and colon. Postgrad. Med., 27:290, 1960.
17. Lauer, R. M., Connor, W. E., Leaverton, P. E., et al.: Coronary heart disease risk factors in school children: the Muscatine study. J. Pediatr., 85:697, 1975.
18. Londe, S., Bourgoinie, J. J., Robson, A. M., et al.: Hypertension in apparently normal children. J. Pediatr., 78:569, 1971.
19. Lowther, C. P., and MacLead, R. D. M.: Evaluation of early diagnostic services for the elderly. Br. Med. J., 3:275, 1970.
20. Margolis, J. R.: Clinical features of unrecognized myocardial infarction—silent and symptomatic. Am. J. Cardiol., 32:1, 1973.
21. McLachlan, M. S. F., Meller, S. T., Jones, E. R., et al.: Urinary tract in school girls with covert bacteriuria. Arch. Dis. Child., 50:253, 1975.
22. North, F. A.: Screening in child care. Am. Fam. Physician, 13:85, 1976.
23. Olsen, D. M., Kane, R. L., and Proctor, P. H.: A controlled trial of multiphasic screening. N. Engl. J. Med., 294:925, 1976.
24. Petersen, O.: Spontaneous course of cervical precancerous conditions. Am. J. Obstet. Gynecol., 72:1063, 1956.
25. Richart, R. M., and Barron, B. A.: A follow-up study of patients with cervical dysplasia. Am. J. Obstet. Gynecol., 105:386, 1969.
26. Roberts, N. J.: The values and limitations of periodic health examinations. J. Chronic Dis., 9:95, 1959.
27. Sackett, D. L.: The family physician and the periodic health examination. Can., Fam. Phys., August, 1972.
28. Thiessen, E. U.: Breast self-examination in proper perspective. Cancer, 28:1537, 1971.
29. Venet, L., Strax, P., Venet, W., et al.: Adequacies and inadequacies of breast examinations by physicians in mass screening. Cancer, 28:1546, 1971.

Chapter 8

EARLY DIAGNOSIS OF UNDIFFERENTIATED PROBLEMS

by IAN R. McWHINNEY

The problem-solving strategies of family physicians have evolved in response to certain special characteristics of family practice:

1. The pattern of illness in the practice approximates the pattern of illness in the community, i.e., there is a high incidence of transient illness and a high prevalence of chronic illness. There is also a high incidence of minor illness, i.e., illness that is self-limiting and carries no risk to life or health. The early separation of serious and life-threatening illnesses from the much larger category of minor illnesses is one of the most difficult tasks facing the family physician.

2. The illness is undifferentiated, i.e., it usually has not been previously assessed by any other physician.

3. Disease is seen early, often before the full clinical picture has developed.

4. Many of the illnesses (approximately 50 per cent) cannot be diagnosed in the classic sense of the term. By this I mean they are placed in a disease category in which symptoms and signs are linked with a pathologic process. These patients are ill but have no "disease."

5. The relationship with patients is continuous and transcends individual episodes of illness. It follows that the patient is usually personally known to the physician.

PRINCIPLES OF PROBLEM-SOLVING

The basic principles of problem-solving are the same in all branches of medicine and, for that matter, in all branches of science. These are illustrated in Figure 8–1, which is based on the work of Elstein et al.[1] When presented with a problem, the physician identifies certain cues which indicate the category of illness he is dealing with. Cues are of two kinds: certain and probabilistic. A certain cue enables the physician to place the illness into a category immediately and with certainty. In medicine this happens occasionally; for example, if a patient has the typical pain and rash of herpes zoster. More usually, the cue is probabilistic and enables the physician only to form a hypothesis about the illness category.

Physicians usually have between one and four working hypotheses at any one stage of the problem-solving process. These are rank-ordered according to two criteria: probability and pay-off.

Probability

Other things being equal, the more likely diagnoses will be ranked higher than the less likely. Assessments of probability are based on the physician's experience of the incidence of disease in his practice population. They are also influenced by his knowledge of the patient, the patient's constitution, and any special risks he may have been exposed to.

Bayes' theorem, shown here in simplified form, provides a mathematical model for the calculation of probability from a knowledge of the incidence of symptoms and diseases:

$$P(D/S) = \frac{P(S/D) \times P \quad (D)}{P \quad (S)}$$

THE DIAGNOSTIC PROCESS

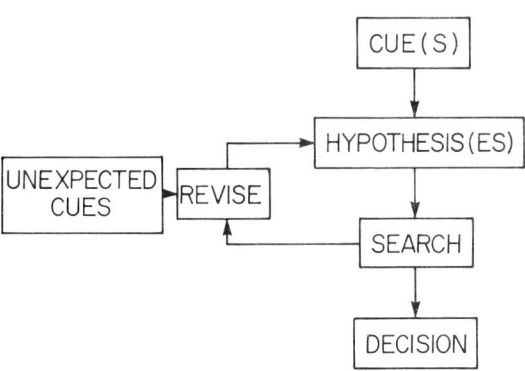

Figure 8–1. Flow chart illustrating the clinical decision-making process.

P(D/S) is known as the conditional probability because it is the probability of disease (D) being present, given a certain symptom (S). To calculate the conditional probability, certain information is needed:

1. The probability of the symptom (S) when the disease (D) is present [P(S/D)].

2. The probability of the disease in the population from which the patient comes (PD).

3. The probability of the symptom in the same population (PS). For example, in a patient with grand mal beginning in adult life, we can calculate the probability of a cerebral tumor [P(D/S)] if we know the incidence of cerebral tumor [P (D)], the incidence of grand mal [P (S)], and the incidence of grand mal in cases of cerebral tumor [P(S/D)].

In clinical practice, of course, we estimate probability intuitively, without being aware of making calculations. Nevertheless, our personal probabilities are based on our experience of the incidence of disease and the significance of symptoms.

Pay-off

This term denotes the consequences of diagnosing or failing to diagnose a disease. If the disease is a serious one in which the outlook depends on early treatment, then the positive pay-off of an early diagnosis is high, and the negative pay-off of failing to make an early diagnosis is also high. Pay-off, in other words, is an expression of a disease's seriousness and treatability. A

disease with a high pay-off may be ranked more highly in the order of hypotheses than one with a greater probability. In a child with abdominal pain, for example, acute appendicitis may be the physician's first hypothesis even though this is very much less probable than gastroenteritis.

Having formulated his hypotheses the physician embarks on a search designed to test them. The search is traditionally divided into three components: the history, the physical examination, and the investigation. In this chapter, all items in these three areas will be referred to as tests. The experienced physician uses tests that have the maximum utility for discriminating between his hypotheses. The concept of utility can be illustrated by the game of 20 questions. If the players are asked to find the name of a city in the United States beginning with *P*, the question "Is it in Pennsylvania?" has a lower utility than "Has it 1,000,000 or more inhabitants?"

In the course of his search, the physician looks for defining attributes of the category to which he has assigned the patient's illness. For example, if he has hypothesized that a patient with fever and cough has red measles, he will look for Koplik's spots and a morbilliform rash. The power of an attribute to define an illness category is a measure of the utility of the test that identifies the attribute. The physician looks for both positive and negative defining attributes. It is obviously important that he should not only seek to support his hypothesis with positive evidence, but also with negative evidence—the exclusion of other disease categories. This is one of the chief purposes of the routine review of systems and the general physical examination. The other important purpose of these procedures is to bring to light new cues to the solution of the patient's problem.

As indicated in Figure 8–1, the process of solving a patient's problem is circular rather than linear. Hypotheses are continually being rejected or revised, either because they have been refuted by the evidence, or because new cues have emerged in the course of the search. It is important to note that in medicine absolute certainty is not usually attainable. Even the final diagnosis is a statement of probability and must remain, like a scientific hypothesis, in Karl Popper's words, "tentative forever."

The end-point of the physician's search

comes when its objectives have been achieved. This is usually a point at which enough evidence has been collected to enable a management decision to be taken. This point is not necessarily equivalent to that at which a diagnosis is made. In a patient with fever of short duration, the search may end at the point at which it can be said that there is no evidence of serious disease. If the fever subsides within 24 hours, then no further search will be necessary. In a patient with acute abdominal pain, a surgeon may end the search when he can say "this is not an acute abdomen."

APPLICATION TO FAMILY PRACTICE[4]

CUES

A cue may be defined as an item of meaningful information. As he deals with a patient's problem, the physician is confronted by a plethora of information: from the patient, from the medical record, from the patient's family and relatives, or from his own store of recollections about the patient.

From this mass of information, the physician must sort the significant from the insignificant. The cues are those pieces of information that he responds to as the most significant and meaningful. His knowledge of the meaning of information comes from his own experience of medicine, from his general knowledge of medicine, and from his own knowledge of what may be significant in a particular patient. The meaning of a piece of information may vary with its context. Facial pallor, for example, will have a different meaning in a new patient and in a patient known to be pale for several years.

One of the physician's first tasks is to establish the patient's meaning. This interpretation takes place at two levels. First the physician determines whether or not the words used to describe the symptoms have the same meaning for him as they do for the patient. Many errors in medicine arise from a failure to understand the patient at this very basic level. The complaint "shortness of breath," for example, can have a number of different meanings. It may mean the deep sighs of an anxious patient who is hyperventilating, or it may mean the exertional dyspnea of a patient

with cardiac failure. Failure to establish the meaning may lead the physician to an erroneous conclusion through a highly inappropriate search strategy.

At the second level, the physician determines whether the patient is communicating his meaning directly or indirectly. Patients frequently do not express their meaning fully or in direct language. This may be because the words are not available, or because the patient is ashamed, or because the problem is a deeply emotional one which cannot be expressed in words. The point may be illustrated by the unspoken meanings that may be conveyed by one symptom, recurrent abdominal pain:

"I have an unpleasant sensation which I would like to have relieved."

"I am concerned about cancer (my mother died from it)."

"I don't like school because I'm afraid of my teacher."

"I'm in despair over my husband's alcoholism, but I can't tell you how I feel."

Cues in the Early Stages of Illness

One of the problems of family practice is the difference between cues in the earlier and later stages of disease. Until recently, clinical training has taken place in hospitals, where the later stages of disease are encountered. Textbooks have usually been written about the later stages of disease. When a textbook describes the symptoms and signs of a disease, it usually does not comment on the discriminatory value of a symptom at different stages of evolution of the disease.

The family physician is concerned about three special aspects of a symptom or cue:

1. Its capacity to bring the patient to see him (i.e., its significance for the patient). Feinstein[2] has called this the "iatrotrophic stimulus." Hemoptysis, for example, is likely to have more meaning for the patient than a cough.

2. Its value as a cue or a defining attribute in the early stages of disease. As an illustration, pyrexia is of little value in the diagnosis of early appendicitis. Pyrexia means that inflammation has spread beyond the appendix and is often not present when the patient presents in the office. The family physician is interested therefore, in the early (presenting) symp-

toms of appendicitis: abdominal pain and anorexia.

3. Cues to more serious or less common conditions. The family physician sees many patients with self-limiting illnesses or with illnesses that do not carry an immediate threat to life or health. In order to distinguish these from the more serious disorders, he must respond effectively to those symptoms (cues) that signify more serious illness. In patients with headache, for example, he responds differently to those with symptoms suggesting an intracranial lesion (progressive, unremitting headaches) or subarachnoid hemorrhage (occipital headaches of very sudden onset). It is the physician's responsiveness to cues which often determines the extent of his search.

HYPOTHESES

Like other physicians, the family physician is influenced in his formulation of hypotheses by the factors of probability and pay-off. Probability is estimated after a consideration of several questions:

1. Given this presenting complaint, what are the most likely reasons for the patient's illness in the population of my practice? Since the incidence of disease in a family practice resembles that in the general population, the probabilities are very different from those in the highly selective populations of a specialty practice or hospital clinic. In patients presenting with fatigue, for example, the most likely diagnosis in family practice is depression; in an endocrinology or hematology clinic dealing with referred patients the conditional probabilities will almost certainly be different.

2. Given this presenting complaint in *this particular patient*, what are the most likely reasons for his illness? Here the family physician uses his personal knowledge of the patient, including such knowledge as the patient's previous illnesses, his previous responses to stress and to illness, his attitudes, his temperament, and his interpersonal relationships. Some of this knowledge is objective and can be documented in the patient's record; some is highly subjective and difficult to express, although no less valuable. Personal knowledge of the patient may prove to be the most important factor in determining the family physician's choice of hypotheses.

THE SEARCH

The purpose of the search is twofold: to test and validate the physician's hypothesis(es), and to bring to light new and unexpected cues. In arriving at a search strategy for a particular problem the family physician has to make three kinds of choice: the choice of tests which he will use, the extent of the search, and the endpoint of the search.

Choice of Tests

This is determined chiefly by three factors:

Utility of the Test. The utility of the test is its capacity to discriminate between the physician's hypotheses. For discriminating between the categories "bronchial carcinoma" and "chest disease other than carcinoma," for example, the presence of cough has a low utility because cough is a very common symptom in both conditions. In a child complaining of aches and pains, however, the erythrocyte sedimentation rate (ESR) is a test of high utility for distinguishing between the categories "acute or subacute rheumatism" and "no active rheumatism." Tests of high utility are obviously far more efficient for solving problems. Because family physicians are often faced with the need to solve problems under the pressure of time, they tend to select and use tests of highest utility.

It is important to note here that tests that have a high utility for discriminating among broad categories may have a low utility for discriminating among narrower categories. By the nature of their work, family physicians often have to begin by placing a patient's illness into one of two broad categories. Examples of these binary categories are given in Figure 8–2. The ESR, previously mentioned, is a useful test for the family physician because of its capacity to discriminate between broad categories. For discriminating between more discrete disease categories it has much less value.

Dividing the complex illnesses encountered by family physicians into binary categories may be an over-simplification. For example, a patient may be suffering from *both* an organic and a psychogenic illness.

Rank Ordering of Hypotheses. The order of the physician's hypotheses determines the initial direction of the search. The most

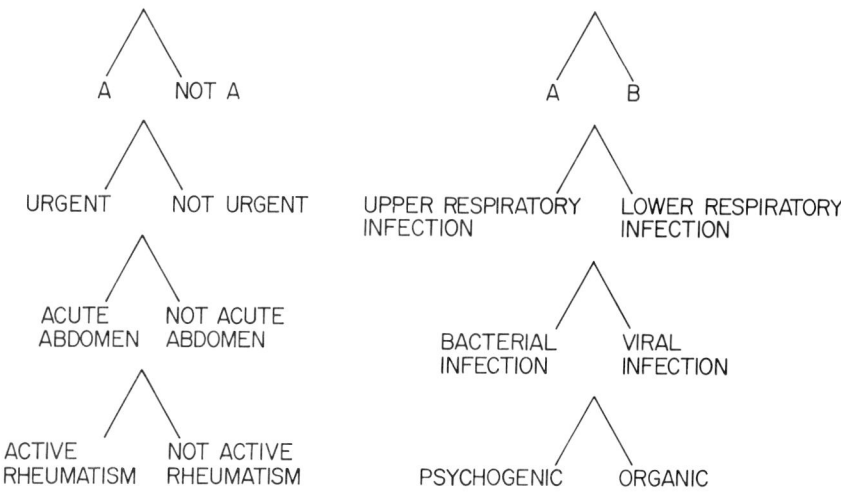

Figure 8–2. *Categorization in primary medical practice. Examples of binary categories.*

logical course is to begin by searching for defining attributes of the first hypothesis. In the example shown in Figure 8–3, the physician has begun by searching for defining attributes of his first hypothesis (depression): patient feels depressed, has insomnia, frequent weeping and loss of interest. Having found defining attributes, he then searches for negative attributes; i.e., he tries to refute his hypothesis by seeking evidence of other disorders which can cause fatigue: thyroid disease, anemia, carcinoma, infection.

Since physicians in different disciplines formulate different hypotheses, their choice of search strategies will be correspondingly different. The physician in an endocrinology clinic, dealing with a patient

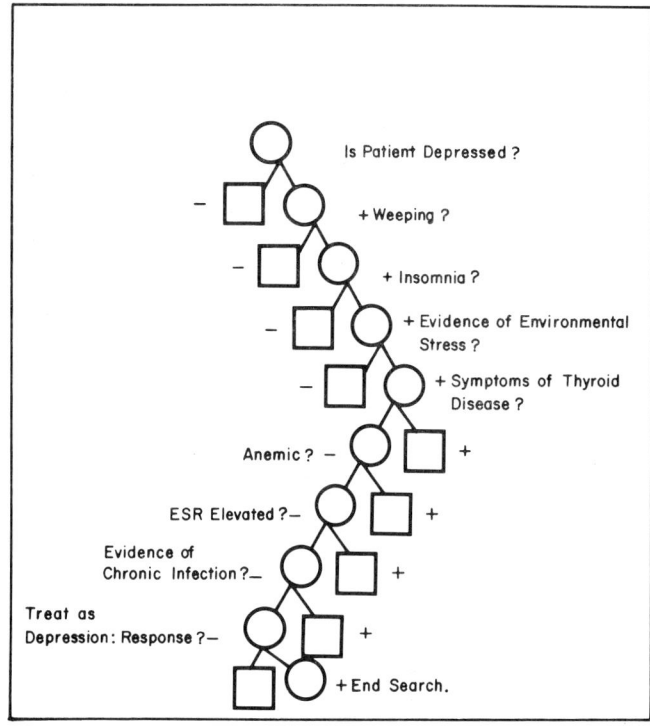

Figure 8–3. *Binary tree illustrating physician's strategy in female patient, aged 30, with fatigue. (After Kleinmuntz, B.: Formal Representation of Human Judgement. New York, John Wiley & Sons, Inc., 1968, Chapt. 6, pp. 149–186.)*

referred with fatigue, might list an endocrine condition as his first hypothesis. He would begin his search, therefore, by seeking different defining attributes. It is important to emphasize that both strategies are correct in their context.

Calculations of Benefit, Risk, and Cost. All tests have some cost. Even a medical history question or an item of physical examination has a cost in the physician's time and patient's time. The physician should know the cost of pathologic and x-ray tests in precise dollar terms.

A large number of tests also have a risk. This may be the risk to the patient of injury or death as a result of the test. Here again, the physician should know precisely the morbidity and mortality risks of any test he is going to use. Other kinds of risks must also be considered. A procedure that has little or no risk to life or health may at the same time be a source of pain and discomfort to the patient. For example, sigmoidoscopy or venipuncture, especially in a child or elderly person, are unpleasant enough to require justification in terms of substantial benefit.

One measure of benefit—utility—has already been discussed. Tests can confer other kinds of benefits. One common example is the test that is necessary to reassure the patient, even though the physician believes it to be redundant.

Tests should be chosen after answering the question, "Do the benefits outweigh the risks and costs?" Unfortunately, much investigation in modern medicine is determined by no rational process whatever. The result is overinvestigation, redundant tests, rising costs, and iatrogenic disease.

Extent of the Search

The extent of the search is a most difficult decision in family practice. The family physician deals with illness of all grades of severity, from upper respiratory infections and furuncles to myocardial infarcts, diabetic comas, and strokes. It is obviously not rational to apply the same search strategy to all problems. Unlike physicians in other branches of medicine, he can make no prior assumptions about the types of problems he will encounter. His search strategies must therefore be extremely flexible.

The extent of the search is determined chiefly by the presenting complaint. A simple complaint of sore throat, for example, will not normally require any examination beyond the head and neck. The presence of a cue to infectious mononucleosis, on the other hand, will indicate a more extensive search. A mild intercostal muscle pain normally will not require more than examination to elicit local tenderness. A man with tight substernal pain of several hours' duration, however, will require an extensive search. Another factor influencing the extent of search is the physician's knowledge of the patient. If, for example, he knows that the patient tends to deny illness, he may carry out a more extensive search than would be warranted by the presenting complaint.

Clinical Routines

As mentioned earlier, the search is designed to reveal unexpected cues as well as to test the physician's hypotheses. This is the reason for routine systematic inquiries and routine physical examinations. It is important to understand that even these routines do not constitute a "complete physical examination." All routines are selections of certain tests from a much larger number of possible tests. Different specialties tend to have different routines, the chief criterion for choice of a test being its value for generating new hypotheses in the patient population with which the specialty is concerned. An internist would probably consider ophthalmoscopy to be routine, but not laryngoscopy. This is because ophthalmoscopy has much greater value for generating hypotheses in patients seen by internists.

Family physicians make less use of standard routines than other physicians. There are several reasons for this. First, the heterogeneity of illnesses encountered in family practice means that no routine can be applied to every case. The family physician may carry out a routine search very similar to that of an internist, but this will be reserved for patients with certain problems. Second, in the situation of continuing personal care, the family physician already has a collection of basic data about the patient and has no need to collect it again.

One additional function of the routine search must be mentioned. A test may be done not because it has any value for solving the patient's problem but for its value in detecting unsuspected disease. This is the screening function of the search. Although it is normal to use tests for problem-solving and for screening in the course of the same search, it is important to be clear about their different purposes. Screening tests are selected according to the usual criteria. A common example is the blood pressure reading taken on a patient who presents with a minor injury or infection.

End-Point of the Search

Traditionally, the end-point of the search has been a diagnosis. In family practice this objective is not always realistic. In the first place, in approximately 50 per cent of the illnesses seen in family practice it is not possible to make a diagnosis in the sense of assigning the illness to a category that links symptoms with pathologic findings. Second, many patients have transient illnesses in which it is more important to know what the patient does not have, than precisely what he does have. In a patient with transient vomiting and abdominal pain, the important label is "not an acute abdomen." Third, illness is seen in its earliest stages, often long before the full clinical picture has developed. Although a diagnosis may emerge in time, this frequently is not possible during the patient's early visits.

In all these patients, however, decisions have to be made, even if no diagnosis is possible. It is more realistic, therefore, to describe the end-point of the search as a decision. The end-point of the search on any particular occasion is the point at which enough information is available to make an informed decision without avoidable risk to the patient.

It is important to understand that end-points are often very different in family practice than in other branches of medicine. A consultant seeing a referred patient will probably feel the need to make a definitive diagnosis before sending the patient back to his own physician. A family physician is not under the same constraint. The continuing relationship with patients means that all problems do not have to be solved immediately. Since the relationship itself has no defined end-point, the search can be discontinued and resumed according to need

The family physician, because of his special role, makes several types of decisions that scarcely arise in other branches of medicine.

The Decision to Wait. In making this decision, the physician is using the evolution of the illness over time as a test of his hypothesis. It is obviously inherent in this decision that no extra risk should be incurred by waiting. The use of time to validate hypotheses in this way can make many investigations redundant. One example of this decision is the *eliminative diagnosis* referred to earlier in which the physician decides that the illness is transient and minor, then waits for his hypothesis to be verified.

The Decision to Refer. The end-point of a search may be the decision to consult with or refer to another physician. This decision may have to be taken before a definitive diagnosis can be made, for example, with a severely ill baby or a patient with an acute abdomen. It is clear that the objective of the family physician in these cases is different from that of the referral specialist. The family physician has fulfilled his obligation if he has decided to refer the patient in time for him to receive effective treatment. He has failed to fulfill his obligation if he has worsened the outcome of the illness by delaying referral in the interests of providing a diagnostic label.

DECISION-MAKING UNDER CONDITIONS OF UNCERTAINTY

All physicians have to make decisions in conditions of uncertainty. Physicians who have to deal with undifferentiated problems work under conditions of maximal uncertainty. For this reason, a capacity for tolerating uncertainty is a necessary attribute in family physicians.

In making such decisions a physician uses the criteria of probability and pay-off referred to earlier. In the normal course of events, the decision-making is intuitive and the calculations that precede it are not formalized. Any clinical decision, however, can be analyzed formally by using the device of the pay-off matrix (Table 8–1). Along the vertical axis are set out the decision alternatives. Along the horizontal axis are set out the expected outcomes. In the interstices of the matrix are the positive

TABLE 8-1. PAY-OFF MATRIX FOR PATIENT WITH ACUTE ABDOMINAL PAIN

Decision Alternatives	Anticipated Event and Outcome Values	
	Appendicitis	*Not Appendicitis*
Diagnose appendicitis and admit	Early appendectomy Quick recovery	Unnecessary admission Quick recovery
Diagnose "not appendicitis" and discharge	Appendix perforates Delayed recovery or death	Quick recovery
Estimated likelihood of events	0.1	0.9

and negative consequences of each decision alternative with one of the expected outcomes. Also expressed is the probability of each outcome. Analysis of clinical decisions by this method is a useful procedure in medical education at all levels. The method can be applied not only to management decisions but also to decisions taken in the course of the search: whether or not to see the patient, whether to see the patient today or tomorrow, whether or not to do a particular test, or whether or not to refer

EXTRANEOUS FACTORS IN CLINICAL DECISION-MAKING

In this chapter, emphasis has been placed on the logic of decision-making. The process has been presented as a rational one, with a logic arising out of the clinical situation itself. It is important to recognize, however, that factors outside the clinical situation may have a powerful influence on the process. Some of these factors are:

Institutional Factors. In deciding on a search strategy a physician may be heavily influenced by what he believes to be the rules of the institution, e.g., "All patients with stroke must have a cerebral angiogram." Institutional rules, applied regardless of individual situations, lie behind some of the overinvestigation that is done in teaching hospitals. The rules are no less powerful for being unwritten.

Patients' Expectations. As a result of reading medical articles in the press, or of hearsay, or of a belief that they are exercising their rights as consumers, patients may demand certain tests when there is no logical justification for them.

Fear of Litigation. The prevalence of mal-

practice suits has been a powerful influence on the search strategies of physicians, the effect being to encourage overinvestigation.

Physician Factors. Another influence on the diagnostic process is the physician's own personality, feelings, and experience. Physicians who feel insecure, or who cannot tolerate uncertainty, tend to carry out more tests than those who feel secure and tolerate uncertainty well. A physician's strategy may be influenced by feelings of anxiety about a particular patient or type of problem. If he feels he has made past errors with a patient, or with a particular problem, for example, he may tend to be overmeticulous in his investigations or especially liable to refer the patient to a specialist.

CUES TO PATIENT BEHAVIOR

As I have implied earlier, the solution of a patient's problem may be more in the understanding of his behavior than in identifying a pathologic process. In many instances, the family physician is carrying out two parallel processes: the process of clinical diagnosis and the process of understanding the patient's behavior. The steps in the second process are essentially the same as those in the first: the physician responds to certain cues, formulates a hypothesis about the patient's behavior, and then conducts a search to verify his hypothesis.

The difference between the two processes is that in clinical diagnosis we have to guide us a precise and universally recognized classification of disease. For patient behavior we have no such universally agreed schema.

It is helpful, however, for the clinician to

formulate hypotheses in answer to certain questions:

1. Why did the patient come at this particular time?

2. What is his own concept of his illness?

3. What does he hope to get from this visit?

4. What is the meaning of the patient's complaints?

It is also possible to formulate simple classification systems which can help us to identify patient behavior just as classifications of disease help us to identify pathology. One schema of this kind describes five categories of patient behavior at the point of contact with the physician:[5]

LIMIT OF TOLERANCE. The patient comes because his pain, discomfort, or disability has become intolerable.

LIMIT OF ANXIETY. The patient comes, not because his symptoms are causing distress, but because he is anxious about their implications. Slight hemoptysis is an example of this category.

PROBLEMS OF LIVING PRESENTING AS SYMPTOMS. The patient's symptoms are a form of communication by which he tries to convey some personal distress that he is unable to convey in words.

ADMINISTRATIVE NEEDS. This category covers doctor–patient contacts whose main purpose is administrative, even though the patient is ill, e.g., the provision of a certificate for a transient illness that would not otherwise lead to a demand for service.

NO ILLNESS. This category includes all attendances for preventive purposes when no symptoms are offered.

REFERENCES

1. Elstein, A. S., Kagan, N., Shulman, L. S., et al.: Methods and theory in the study of medical inquiry. J. Med. Educ., 47:85, 1972.
2. Feinstein, A. R.: Clinical Judgment. Baltimore. The Williams & Wilkins Co., 1976.
3. Kleinmuntz, B.: Formal Representation of Human Judgement. New York, John Wiley & Sons, Inc., 1968.
4. McWhinney, I. R.: Problem solving and decision making in primary medical practice. Albert Wander Lecture. Proc. R. Soc. Med., 65:934, 1972.
5. McWhinney, I. R.: Beyond diagnosis. An approach to the integration of behavioral science and clinical medicine. New Engl. J. Med., 287:384, 1972.

Chapter 9

EPIDEMIOLOGY

by JULIAN A. WALLER,
and GEORGE H. THOMSON

WHAT IS EPIDEMIOLOGY?

In its simplest definition, the etymology of the word *epidemiology* is the study of "what descends upon man." In its broader sense, epidemiology is one of the scientific disciplines that study factors influencing health and disease in living matter.

The objectives of this chapter are to record and review epidemiologic concepts and methods that may be applied to family practice and to assist the physician in developing effective strategies based on valid data for the benefit of the patient, the patient's family, and the community. It is not the intention of this chapter to make family physicians into epidemiologists, but rather to discuss only those aspects of the subject most relevant to everyday practice. The chapter concludes by identifying sources of additional information for those who wish to delve deeper.

As one might infer, historically epidemiology started as an identifiable science by studying epidemics, or disease frequencies that are significantly above the expected norm for a population at a given time. As communicable diseases began to decline somewhat as a major cause of death and disability in the Western world, other uses were found for epidemiologic tools and concepts so that now the techniques are used more often in the study of non-communicable diseases and for the planning and evaluation of health services.

Four applications of epidemiologic techniques are now in common use, and examples of these will be discussed later.

1. The methods are used to define disease entities, their patterns, and their causes.

When several young women appeared at Boston hospitals over a relatively brief time span with an extremely rare form of vaginal carcinoma, studies were initiated to identify what unique exposure they might have had in common. The role of stilbestrol when administered to pregnant women as a latent carcinogenic agent in their daughters was thus identified.

2. Epidemiologic concepts can guide prevention and treatment for individual patients. The selection by the family physician of specific components of a periodic health examination or of specific preventive regimens for a given patient must be based on sound knowledge of relative risks of disease and relative effectiveness of the various preventive options. The individual patient seen in the office may be interacting with others in his family or in the community in the occurrence of the disease that brings him to the physician. While the patient may present as an isolated case, the physician cannot treat him in isolation and hope to achieve a therapeutic triumph.

3. Epidemiology is used to study the availability and utilization of health services. A major diphtheria epidemic occurred in Houston in recent years because immunization practices were not equally distributed within the community. The reasons were identifiable and correctable.

4. Epidemiology is used to evaluate the effectiveness of health programs. Does a new "flu" vaccine really work? Do coronary clubs actually reduce the frequency or severity of subsequent infarctions? The asking and answering of such questions in a methodical and valid fashion are what makes medicine as much a science as it is an art of service to people.

EPIDEMIOLOGIC CONCEPTS

Briefly stated, epidemiology is the study of the *distribution* and *determinants* of disease or health phenomena in a population. Several aspects of this need to be emphasized. First and foremost, epidemiology is population based, getting its data not from theory or laboratory or simulation but directly from observation of the real world, with all the concomitant advantages and disadvantages. Furthermore, such observation is made on groups of people rather than on single individuals or families, as is common in clinical medicine.

Second, the study of distribution implies that the investigator starts with the expectation that the phenomenon to be examined may not be distributed randomly but rather follows specific nonrandom patterns for explainable reasons. This also means that proper study requires examination not only of those periods of time or segments of the population within which the phenomenon exists, but also of the times or segments within which it does not exist, i.e., the control or comparison population.

Here we already begin to get into trouble. A phenomenon may be thought to be absent in a population simply because, although present, it cannot be observed. Unlike clinical medicine, which deals predominantly with correction or prevention of health problems that are obvious, epidemiology deals with what is known as the *biologic gradient* of disease. This term simply means that, if studied carefully enough, virtually all disease will be found to vary not only in frequency but in severity, again for explainable reasons. Thus, a disease may be present but inapparent or subclinical in some; mild, moderate, or severe in others; and fatal in still others. The distribution of this gradient varies with the phenomenon and the circumstances. Rabies is almost always clinically obvious and fatal, while herpes simplex lesions in the mouth are usually subclinical or minor. Thus the epidemiologist is concerned with both frequency and severity.

Third, the study of determinants or causes involves identifying *why* a phenomenon is nonrandomly distributed as opposed to the previous question of *how* the distribution is nonrandom. Here again, some basic tenets should be noted. In studying determinants one commonly examines the host (i.e., person or other living thing affected by the phenomenon), the agent (or factor necessary for the phenomenon to occur), and the environment (the factor that may modify frequency, severity, or both). Also of importance may be the vectors, or vehicles by which the agent is carried to the host. All of these factors contribute to risk, that is, the likelihood that a person with given characteristics will have a given disease and the extent to which he will be incapacitated by it.

Some nonepidemiologists are under the impression that epidemiology seeks out single causes. While it can be and often is used for this purpose, one of the most important basic tenets is that a single cause may have multiple effects and that a single effect may be the result of several causal factors. In some cases, each of these causal factors may be capable of producing the single effect. More commonly, the effect may occur only if two or more factors are present simultaneously or in tandem. In the study of disease, there have been far too few sophisticated studies philosophically oriented toward and capable of examining a multitude of factors simultaneously. This is a fault of the users of epidemiology rather than of the capabilities of the field.

EPIDEMIOLOGIC METHODS

Although there have been many variations, two basic designs exist for testing hypotheses about the association between cause and effect, and a brief discussion of the advantages and disadvantages of each of these designs is warranted. Both designs require examination of two populations over two time frames, the so-called 2×2 model.

Case History Method

The case history, or case-control method, involves comparison of a population that has the disease with a population that does not have the disease. It thus starts with the second time frame, that is, after the disease has occurred. Then, through questioning, studying old records, and so forth, this method attempts to determine how often factors hypothesized to be causal existed during the period antecedent to the disease.

Applied to a study of injury, the researcher would compare persons fatally injured in crashes with those not involved in crashes to determine how often each group had measurable blood levels of alcohol present. The "hooker" is that since the data are from the real world, the populations being compared may differ also in many factors other than alcohol consumption, some of which may be equally or even more relevant to the occurrence of injury events. Thus, the epidemiologist attempts to match the ill and well populations for as many variables as possible, leaving unmatched only those that are subject to hypotheses.

The advantages of the case history method are that it is relatively quick, inexpensive, and can be applied to rare events.

Cohort Method

The cohort method is the exact reverse of the case history approach. The two populations identified are those with and without the variable or variables hypothesized to cause disease or to affect its severity. Both populations are then followed over a specified time, and the resulting proportions with disease or with disease of greater severity are then compared.

Using the case history method, one could say that 42 per cent of fatally injured drivers but only 3 per cent of drivers not in crashes but with similar driving exposure have blood alcohol concentrations (BAC) of 0.10 per cent by weight or greater. Using the cohort method, it would be possible to identify one probability of crashing per 100,000 miles of driving with no alcohol present and a second probability with a BAC of 0.10 per cent. Of course, the cost of following two such populations using the cohort method is prohibitive, and there are very serious and insurmountable ethical issues regarding permitting persons impaired by alcohol to drive and to expose themselves and others to the risk of crashing.

Epidemiologists have agreed upon criteria that are required to establish a *statistical* association between a specified variable and a disease, but establishment of a *causal* relationship remains more subject to judgment. Nonetheless, guidelines can be

offered here also. According to the Surgeon General's report *Smoking and Health:*

"Statistical methods cannot establish proof of a causal relationship in an association. The causal significance of an association is a matter of judgment which goes beyond any statement of statistical probability. To judge or evaluate the causal significance of the association between the attribute or agent and the disease, or effect upon health, a number of criteria must be utilized, no one of which is an all-significant basis for judgment. These criteria include:
(a) The consistency of the association,
(b) The strength of the association,
(c) The specificity of the association,
(d) The temporal relationship of the association,
(e) The coherence of the association."[2]

To clarify these terms, *consistency* refers to the relative comparability of results of several studies using similar methods. *Strength of association* denotes one in which the variable (or variables), when present, is associated with a marked change in the frequency or severity of the disease, while *specificity* means that the disease is rarely, if ever, associated with the presence of other variables in the absence of the variable(s) under question. The *temporal relationship* of the association means that exposure to the variable always precedes the development of the associated disease. *Coherence* refers to the degree to which the causal hypothesis is in agreement with or can be explained by laws of nature.

Commonly, laboratory, clinical, and other studies may supplement epidemiologic data in helping to decide whether a causal or noncausal association exists. Applying these criteria to cigarette smoking and bronchogenic carcinoma: (1) many studies produce similar results; (2) cigarette smoking is associated with a much greater risk of lung cancer than is any other variable yet studied; (3) very few nonsmokers get bronchogenic carcinoma (and most of those who do have other unique exposures, such as miners exposed to uranium); (4) the cancer is virtually always preceded by a history of smoking, mining, or other suspect environmental factors; and (5) the effects of cigarette smoking in man are consistent with bronchial changes observed in laboratory animals and go logically from acute irritation to squamous metaplasia to squamous carcinoma.

CONCEPTS FOR PREVENTIVE AND THERAPEUTIC STRATEGIES

The natural history of disease is a continuum that can be viewed through the following predictable occurrences: No disease risk present; exposure to risk; inapparent disease; clinically evident disease; and resolution with an outcome of being well, disabled, or dead. Prevention is any act that can be done to make the next predictable occurrence either less likely or less serious. Primary, secondary, and tertiary prevention are a series of strategies that can be applied for the benefit of individuals, families, a community, or mankind as a whole.

The goal of primary prevention is to prohibit disease from ever occurring in human hosts. Primary prevention has two major thrusts. The first is the promotion of health through a healthy environment, a healthy population, and a diminution of agents of risk. The second aim of primary prevention is the specific protection of individuals against a specific disease because the risk of that disease persists.

Secondary prevention needs to be applied when the disease has actually occurred. Again there are two aims. In many diseases an advantage may be gained by early diagnosis and treatment. The second aim is management of the disease to limit disability if early treatment fails to eliminate or contain it.

Tertiary prevention is the only strategy left to make less serious the remaining predictable occurrences. When a containable disease has run its course, rehabilitation efforts may regain or vicariously replace lost function. To this may be added another and final dimension—considerate terminal care. This cannot alter the ultimate effect of the disease on the patient but may well decrease suffering and prevent undesirable effects of bereavement in a family.

Therefore, to develop a strategy for health and the treatment of disease for individuals and families requires the identification of risks involved, a manipulation of the balance of host-agent-environment, and application of available measures at appropriate levels in the natural course of diseases.

A word of caution is in order, however, about priorities in choosing strategies. It is commonly but sometimes incorrectly as-sumed that those causal factors most often involved in or most apparently contributing to disease should be attacked first. However, since multiple factors may contribute to disease frequency and severity, more success might be achieved by modifying a contributory factor that is amenable to change than by seeking to affect a primary factor that is often not correctable.

In illustration, a patient may not be convinced to stop smoking, but might be willing to change to low tar and nicotine cigarettes. If he has a myocardial infarction, improved emergency services may then save his life. A problem drinker may not have his drinking arrested, but he need not be injured if he falls asleep while smoking and intoxicated if the fabric of his bed or chair is flame retardant. In both cases secondary prevention may be more feasible—and consequently more effective—than primary prevention and thus should not be scoffed at because it suggests effort "after the fact."

APPLICATION OF PRINCIPLES

A family physician frequently calls upon consultants to perform specialized services. Consequently, a family physician treats acute otitis media but usually seeks the help of consultants for middle ear surgery. The same principle should apply in the approach to problems in the specialty of epidemiology. While there is a vast research and specialty application in the field of epidemiology, there are, however, epidemiologic principles that can be satisfactorily applied in daily practice. Some practical examples of these principles will now be described, starting with applications for the benefit of individual patients and proceeding through the family to a broader community level.

INDIVIDUAL PATIENTS

Developing Appropriate Preventive Strategies

Elsewhere in this book are discussions on preventive medicine, health hazard appraisal, screening methods, and recommended immunization schedules. While each describes an approach to prevention, each is based on common epidemiologic principles. These principles must be kept in mind when developing or applying any preventive measures, as when one needs to make decisions between two or more strategies.

Preventive measures are the application of strategies, and this often requires a weighing of alternative risks of the strategies. The alternatives may relate to the relative severity of the possibilities or to the relative probability of important but less severe consequences. An example of the application of the concept of relative risk is the use of the potentially dangerous passive immunization against rabies after a bite of an apparently healthy dog compared with the low probability of infection from a disease that is almost invariably lethal. An example of strategy-making based on important but less severe consequences is the consideration of the use of sulfonamide preparations to prevent recurrence of beta-hemolytic streptococcal infection in a person known to have rheumatic fever but who is believed to be allergic to pencillin.

To make intelligent decisions among alternatives requires a consideration of probabilities based on epidemiologic information. In the example of the rabies treatment just discussed, one needs to know the condition of the animal, the prevalence of rabies in the community of zoonotic reservoirs, the effect of seasonal variations, the rates of reactions of differing severities to duck embryo vaccine, the probability of compliance to the long regimen, and the availability of newer preparations for passive immunity. In the example of the person with rheumatic fever, one needs to know the extent to which sulfonamides can provide protection, the availability of potentially more effective antibiotics and their possible side effects, the probability of beta-hemolytic streptococcus in the family and community, and the probability of recurrent rheumatic fever if the patient is exposed to the organism.

To make the occurrence of an event less probable requires prediction of the event and an accurate weighing of the probability of its occurrence. For this reason both time and geography are important factors to be considered in choosing strategies to be applied. Programs to control malaria and cholera are appropriate in Africa and India, while those to deal with coronary artery disease or other diseases of an affluent society probably are not. From the temporal and geographic view, cholera has been absent in North America for over 50 years but was epidemic in Pakistan in 1973. With respect to time of life as a variable, mammographic screening is contraindicated in healthy women under age 30, is questionably appropriate for those aged 30 to 59, and may be advisable for women aged 60 or older.

Developing Diagnostic Skills

McWhinney has clearly described the use of hypothesis testing, restating, and retesting as is done by epidemiologists but has applied these methods to problem-solving by clinicians.[3] These principles and the technique of the process are restated in Chapter 8 of this book. While the chapter emphasis is on identification of early and undifferentiated disease, we would like to reiterate here that the epidemiologic principle is applicable in most diagnostic processes in most clinical settings.

Another fundamental epidemiologic concept is that it is usually more than coincidence that a patient has developed a particular disease. For this reason, the clinician must see his patient as a harbinger of epidemiologic characteristics. A patient's description is more than a collection of isolated facts; it is a list of risk factors. In a similar manner, disease processes have epidemiologic characteristics. To fit and refit the patient and disease characteristics until there is an understandable intermeshing is an epidemiologic method that enhances the art of the clinician. Knowing the risk characteristics of a 38 year old balding, hypertensive, sedentary, smoking, overweight, middle-level executive and having knowledge of the epidemiologic characteristics of coronary artery disease makes precordial pain in that patient almost predictable.

To further emphasize the use of epidemiologic reasoning in a clinical setting, we must remind the practicing physician that a most important question to ask a febrile adult patient is, "Where have you been in the past 6 to 12 months?" Failing to ask this single question was a contributing factor in the majority of deaths from malaria in United States in the past few years. In almost every instance specific antimalarial therapy was delayed while the patient was treated for "flu." The same question should be asked of patients with jaundice, persisting diarrheas, subacute chest problems, and even chronic headaches. The question provides a broader data base in identifying the patient's epidemiologic risk characteristics.

Just as knowledge of a patient's travels is important, so it is becoming increasingly important to have very specific information about the nature of work and recreational activities, because exposure of the public to uncommon but toxic chemicals is becoming increasingly frequent.

Aid to Treatment and Management

A fracture including the distal end of the radius and the ulnar styloid process is a clinical entity that cannot be managed successfully with a single method of management for all patients. The risks of unwanted results associated with various treatment options are dependent upon age and sex variables. Hence, it becomes an exercise in prognostic risk calculation to make the correct decision for management. A child may have a successful outcome if the radial fracture is reduced and the arm placed in a midposition in a short-arm cast. A middle-aged person may have a reduction, but the hand should be placed in ulnar deviation, flexed wrist position, with an above-elbow cast for the first 3 weeks. A 72 year old working male may have the same treatment. A 72 year old female should have the wrist placed in a cock-up position and a short-arm cast for only 3 weeks and then should start moderate passive motion. While the advantages and disadvantages of each of these options for specific individuals may be argued, the fact is that each is used by some managers of fractures at some time for some people. The selection of the method for an individual patient should be determined by an evaluation of the relative risks as well as the benefits of each option.

Many careful descriptive and analytic studies have been done by epidemiologists to unravel characteristics and circumstances of conformity or nonconformity and of conformers and nonconformers to management plans made by physicians. Again, one can use the knowledge of the experience reported for groups of people and fit

this to the nature and interests of the individual patient to determine the probability of that particular patient's compliance with a regimen.

Simple but important probability predictions can be made and consequently less promising avenues for treatment may be avoided. Instructions to take one or two doses a day, for example, will be followed better than "q.i.d." or "q.4h." orders. Prescriptions for two medicines will be filled and followed more often than prescriptions for six medicines. Regimens for an illness perceived as being serious will be followed better than if the disease is not perceived as serious. Patients who are meticulously compulsive take medicines more correctly than do those who are erratic and noncompulsive. Compliance by a child relates to behavioral and other characteristics of the significant caretaker The most effective combination of management intent and patient acceptance can be accomplished when the physician applies the knowledge gained from epidemiologic studies on compliance.

Management of Chronic Illness

Epidemiologic variables such as ethnicity, neighborhoods, family size, and social networks exert influences on the physician–patient relationship in the management of chronic illnesses. The fact that these influences are brought by the patient seeking help for his illness must always be recognized and can often be predicted from epidemiologic knowledge. Recognition of such influences prompted the American Diabetes Association to make ethnic-related diabetic exchange diets available for Italian, Jewish, Chinese, Spanish, black, and other patient groups.

Poverty, crowded housing, and isolation are all environmental influences not only on the occurrence of the disease but on the effectiveness of management. An order for bed rest for a rheumatic mother of five small children cannot be accomplished easily. In like manner, suggesting a quiet 15 minutes at toilet rarely can be accomplished by an encopretic boy who lives with five school-aged sisters in a small house.

In developing an integrated plan for long-term care of a chronic illness, a survey of the circumstances of the care program using an epidemiologic model is recommended. Seeing the situation in the light of the disease (agent) is helpful. Is there a need for disposal of contaminated dressings or for provision of ice, heat, filtered air, or special humidity? Seeing the situation in the light of the patient (host) also is helpful. Is there adequate nursing care, communication, entertainment, social stimulation, and reinforcement of personal motivation? Look at the situation of the environment of care. Is there an adequate bed; methods of transportation; management of the environment by the patient; availability, yet control, of visitors; and is the environment adaptable to change with the changes in the disease?

Management of the Terminally Ill

The understanding of the process of dying and its considerate management are discussed in Chapter 18. From an epidemiologic point of view there are three remaining facets that deserve comment. The first is the necessary reporting of death for legal and epidemiologic reasons and the now rare concern for the potential infectivity of the deceased body. The body can in fact become a temporary reservoir for infective matter, but the potential risk has been nearly eradicated in the United States and many other countries by laws governing the handling of the body.

The second facet is an outcome of the concept of biologic gradient. In a lethal disease there is a continuum beyond the obvious early manifestations of the disease. The expected course and its variants are usually predictable enough to permit a skilled physician to establish and stick to a plan for the relief of suffering from the process of dying. Hence, a program for relief of pain can be graduated from aspirin to morphine with fair success.

However, the third facet deserves more emphasis from an epidemiologic view. In the introductory part of this chapter it was noted that multiple causes can precipitate a single effect. Conversely, multiple effects can emanate from a single cause. This epidemiologic principle prompts us to suggest that the practicing physician will increase his skill as a family physician by applying the concept to the care of the family of a terminally ill patient.

Grief at death becomes almost an epidemic in itself, particularly within a family. However, the grief may be from one or several of many causes. Within the family of the deceased there may be some suffering resulting from the loss of the person. Some may be grieving because of a newly increased burden in the care of another survivor, and some may actually grieve because of the release from the burden of care of the deceased. Recognizing these variants of the cause of the common syndrome of grief may aid the physician in understanding the manifestations of other problems in the family.

From this sense of grief caused by the death there are multiple effects that manifest themselves in a variety of ways. Simple helplessness is a common effect in some. Others may exhibit a marked stress–anxiety state, and some a clear depression. But probably the most serious, and potentially the longest lasting, is a fear–anxiety manifestation in children who observe the grieving process in adults without being given an understandable explanation. To recognize this as an epidemiologic threat and to apply preventive measures can be a rewarding effort by a physician which can last for the next 50 years.

MANAGEMENT OF A FAMILY EPIDEMIC PROBLEM

If one wishes to do epidemiologic investigations using the family as the unit at risk and with individuals as subcomponents of the system, there are many technical procedures, methods, and shortcomings to be considered. A guide to this will be reported in a later section. At this point we would like to emphasize the use of the epidemiologic model as a system for integrating a practical plan for managing an epidemic within a family. The problem described was a real one discovered by a family practice resident and is presented in the format of a problem-oriented record. The first part is recorded as it was found on the initial "SOAPing" of the problem (*subjective* findings, *objective* findings, *assessment*, and *plan*). The following commentary is presented as a recommended organization of a management plan based on epidemiologic concepts and a logical expansion of the "plan."

Patient: Job H. . . , white male, aged 6.

Problem: Suppurating cervical lymph node, coagulase-positive staphylococcus.

Subjective: Child has had a sore throat for a week. Had an infected paronychia and a boil on abdomen 2 weeks ago. Now has a swelling in the neck that has started to drain. His mother had some boils about 2 months ago, and a younger sister had some type of skin infection at the same time. An older sibling, aged 8, is said to have a boil on his buttock at present. Father believed to have no boils; works all day, but raises pigeons in cages in the house.

Objective: Throat inflamed and has a foul odor. Left submandibular triangle has a walnut-sized swollen, red, tender area with beginning suppuration from its center. The right triangle is swollen but contains a nonfluctuant, discrete, tender node, 2×3 cm. Patient has temperature of 101° F./os and looks appreciably ill. A culture obtained shows coagulase-positive staphylococci. There is a healing paronychia of the right thumb; remaining fingers are dirty. No epitrochlear or axillary nodes.

Assessment: Staph infection of skin now involving throat and cervical nodes. Mother and two siblings probably have same infection.

Plan:

1. More adequate drainage of node, with culture and sensitivity report.

2. Antibiotic administration after sensitivity report.

3. Public health nurse to visit home.

4. Have mother wash siblings the same way as patient.

5. Get mother to clean house.

6. Wash skin with Betadine or pHiso-Hex.

Commentary on Plan

In reviewing this plan it is apparent that it is only partially complete and was developed without an organization to insure completion. Therefore a new plan was made using a matrix of the essential attributes of a plan and the epidemiologic model. The essential attributes are (A) Investigation, (B) Medical Management, and (C) Patient Education. The attributes of the epidemiologic model are (1) Host, (2) Agent, and (3) Environmental factors. By using this organization it was apparent that many essential unasked questions were posed that required a more complete data base. It was also revealed that essential management factors had been overlooked. The revised plan then developed as follows:

A. Investigation
   1. Host factors
      a. Are there immunologic or cellular deficiencies in the patient or members of his family?
      b. Are there other tissue reservoirs of infection besides the skin and glands?
      c. Are the infected members of the family diabetic?
   2. Agent factors
      a. Is the same organism the infecting agent for all the family?
      b. Has there been culture, sensitivity, and phage typing of samples from all the family?
      c. With the known ability for *Staphylococcus* to vary its antimicrobial resistance, will the antibiotic sensitivity stay constant to eradicate the infection?
      d. Because *Staphylococcus* has a low antigenic nature, what skin barriers can be developed?
   3. Environmental factors
      a. Public health nurse to survey the home and report on habits regarding cleanliness.
      b. Investigate friends, school, and father's employment status (food handler?).
      c. Are adequate washing facilities available?
      d. Is the presence of bird cages in the house a reservoir, an evidence of lack of concern for cleanliness, or a nonrelevant coincidence?
      e. By direct observation, is the family able to or interested in improving their surroundings?
B. Medical Management
   1. Host factors
      a. Scrub hands of all family members frequently with Betadine or pHisoHex, trim nails, careful cuticle care.
      b. Insure adequate nutrition.
      c. Report any new breaks in skin barriers.
      d. Decontaminate or isolate infective exudates.

e. Follow up to insure compliance is continued.
2. Agent factors
  a. Specific antibiotic to be used for tissue spread only. Will not affect skin surface or depths of suppuration. Therefore may need both systemically and locally, or consider no antibiotic.
  b. Coordinate timing of antibiotic in all family members to insure eradication. Follow by surveillance for early identification of recurrence.
  c. Does the organism have growth characteristics that make it especially susceptible to other control measures (heat, cold, acidification, chlorination, etc.)?
3. Environmental factors
  a. Get rid of pigeons and check for other pets.
  b. Clean floor and other surfaces frequently with appropriate antiseptic.
  c. Decontaminate all dressings, clothing, towels, and so forth.
  d. Insure that there is no persisting reservoir for reinfection in the social network.
  e. Insure that there is no spread of the infection to other susceptibles.
  f. Maintain surveillance of the environment until infection is eradicated.
C. Patient Education
1. Host factors
  a. Teach all concerned how to obtain and maintain personal cleanliness.
  b. Instruct parents in the need for compliance in the use of antibiotics.
  c. Instruct family of importance of reporting and caring for any new lesions or new skin injuries, including mosquito bites.
2. Agent factors—probably not applicable.

(It is not uncommon when using a matrical plan that a cell of the matrix may be found empty. However, it is important that the cell be considered and a conscientious effort be made to accept or reject a content. Errors occur most often when there is an omission because the cell was not consid-ered. In this instance, after deliberation, it was felt that no factor needed to be included because it probably would be included elsewhere.)
3. Environmental factors
  a. Instruct family regarding preparation and care of foods and serving of meals.
  b. Encourage family to control presence of vectors.
  c. Encourage family to seek advice on home maintenance.
  d. Instruct family in preparation and use of germicides.

IDENTIFYING AND DEALING WITH COMMUNITY EPIDEMICS

The family physician is literally on the firing line during a suspected or documented epidemic, being bombarded simultaneously by the needs of those patients already ill, the anxieties of others possibly exposed, and the participation in efforts to identify and remove the source of the trouble. Identifying and tracking a possible epidemic is a full-time, frequently frustrating endeavor that requires intensive questioning of both the sick and those not sick and in some cases intensive environmental sampling. Immediate help should be sought from those most skilled in this highly sophisticated speciality. Hence, if an epidemic is suspected, assistance should be sought from staff of the state or local health department, who in turn can decide if further help is needed from the Center for Disease Control (CDC) in Atlanta.

There is much, however, that the practicing clinician can do to limit the ravages in the community.

1. There are two types of epidemics: those emanating from single or point sources either as one time events (such as chemical food poisoning at a picnic) or as continuing events (such as employment of "Typhoid Mary" as a food handler), and those in which there is a secondary attack rate with infected people passing the disease on to contacts. (Note that an epidemic may involve infective organisms, chemical or biologic toxins, or spread of psychologic states of mind, such as hysteria.) In either case, relevant evidence may be extremely evanescent. Therefore, as soon as it is sus-

pected that an epidemic *may* be in progress the family physician should contact other clinicians for their observations and should report his suspicions to the health department.

What constitutes an epidemic? If a disease is quite rare—such as the vaginal carcinoma in young women described earlier—even two or three cases in a year may raise questions. If it is a more common condition, such as influenza, which ordinarily has a highly seasonal incidence, a dozen or more cases within a week may be necessary to alert the physician.

2. As this is being written, epidemiologists from the CDC are attempting to determine precisely how many bona fide cases of "Legionnaires' disease" occurred among persons who attended a convention in Philadelphia in 1976. The problem, so common in epidemics, is that the signs and symptoms may be relatively nonspecific, and it becomes possible to include in the count persons with other diseases who just happened to be ill at this time, as well as to exclude persons with the index disease who have few, mild, or uncommon signs and symptoms.

During a possible epidemic it is especially easy for the overworked family physician to become somewhat lax in making a diagnosis. This can be hazardous because potential sources of spread may be overlooked among people who are inaccurately diagnosed as not having the disease. Furthermore, as the epidemic gains momentum, peaks, and then begins to ebb, there is a tendency to overdiagnose cases without adequate criteria, and the fact that the epidemic is on the wane may be missed for a time, thus obscuring effects of treatment efforts.

During a suspected epidemic, therefore, is *precisely* the time when complete systems review and physical examination, with careful recording of observations, are necessary to get an adequate picture of the nature and variants of the disease and thus to assist in diagnosing new patients. Samples of blood, body tissues, secretions, and excretions, of course, can aid in the diagnosis. The local or state health department can provide guidance concerning these.

3. In addition to good diagnostic criteria, accurate information about the nature and timing of exposures is necessary. It is especially important to get such information

from the earliest persons who come to the attention of the physician. They may be the first to become sick because they have had more intensive exposures (and consequently are able to pass on a larger or more lethal dose of infectious organisms to others), are uniquely sensitive, or were in fact the first to be exposed. The time interval between exposure and disease is shortest for those patients, and memory of recent events thus is likely to be better. It is important when possible and relevant to get a day-by-day listing of activities, people contacted, places visited, and foods eaten. If a patient dies and the family physician has not obtained this information, it may be lost forever to epidemiologists who have not as yet had a chance to question the patient.

4. Obviously, every fatality in suspected or proven epidemics should have a complete autopsy by a pathologist who has first discussed the choice and handling of tissue specimens with the health department.

5. In an epidemic involving an ongoing source of infectious organisms the family physician plays an absolutely crucial role in educating his patients and their families about ways to limit exposure and thus bring an end to the epidemic. These issues have already been considered in the previous discussion of an epidemic in a single family.

STRATEGIES FOR LIMITING THE EFFECTS OF ENVIRONMENTAL HAZARDS

Earlier in this chapter it was noted that the most obvious of several causal factors determining the frequency or severity of disease is not necessarily the most logical factor to be attacked in choosing preventive or therapeutic strategies. William Haddon, a medical epidemiologist concerned with limiting the effects of environmental hazards, has developed an innovative set of ten strategies that consider ways of affecting host, agent, and environment as options not only in primary prevention but often in secondary and tertiary prevention as well.[1] These ten strategies are described with reference to control of physical energy (kinetic, chemical, thermal, radiation, electric) that is the "agent" that causes injury in accidents, suicides, homicides, and most occupational or other environmental-related diseases. But it is clear from the examples that he presents in discussing these strategies that they are applicable to virtually all diseases.

Not all of these strategies are appropriate for the family physician to use in treating all diseases for every patient. But all are appropriate as possible options if both individual practice and community health programs are considered. The strategies are presented here, and the poisoning of young children by aspirin is an illustrative example in most of these.

1. Prevent the initial marshalling of the form of energy. Example—Stop making aspirin (a solution that is not appropriate in the case of aspirin but has been used for various other drugs such as thalidomide).

2. Reduce the amount of energy marshalled. Example—Sell aspirin packaged only in small, sublethal amounts or develop a less hazardous form of the drug.

3. Prevent the release of energy. Example—Educate adults not to leave aspirin around so children can find it, educate children not to eat the aspirin, or provide bottle closures that do not permit children to reach the pills.

4. Modify the rate or spatial distribution of release of energy from its source. Example—Package pills in individual plastic bubbles so the child must take more time to open a lethal quantity and in fact may become bored and stop before reaching that point.

5. Separate in space or time the energy being released from the susceptible structure. Example—This strategy is not appropriate to aspirin but is used in highway safety when a seatbelt slows the transfer of energy to the person, or in cold water treatment of burns when the cold water slows the penetration of heat to subcutaneous tissues.

6. Separate the energy being released from the susceptible structures by interposition of a material barrier. Example—This option also is not appropriate to aspirin but is the basic principle of some suntan or other protective lotions and of motorcycle helmets.

7. Modify the contact surface, subsurface, or basic structure that can be impacted. Example—Nor is this strategy appropriate to aspirin. It is used in safety precautions by providing collapsible steering columns, high penetration resistant

windshields, or by rounding off sharp edges on furniture and toys.

8. Strengthen the living or nonliving structures that might be damaged by the energy transfer. Example—Make tissues less sensitive to the harmful effects of the chemical, an approach not used for aspirin but applied in the use of potassium to reduce sensitivity to toxic effects of digitalis, in immunization programs, and in desensitization regimens for allergies.

9. Move rapidly in detection and evaluation of damage, and counter its continuation and extension. Examples—Provide poison control centers, promote rapid removal of any ingested aspirin not yet absorbed into the bloodstream and, if necessary, remove any chemical already in the blood.

10. Carry out all those measures that fall between the emergency period following damaging energy exchange and the final stabilization of the process (including intermediate and long-term reparative and rehabilitative measures). Example—During and after removal of aspirin in stomach and blood provide effective support of organ systems until reparative processes occur.

PROGRAM PLANNING AND EVALUATION

At this point a still broader example of applied epidemiology will be provided. The family physician who is the sole physician or one of rather few primary physicians serving a community may wonder to what extent his services are affecting the health of the population. It is not our intention in this chapter to state in detail how such studies should be carried out but rather to identify relevant epidemiologic questions to be asked.

First, are all members of the community receiving health services equally, or, as is probably the case, are there some who are seen rarely or never by a physician? Second, what are the characteristics (age, sex, race, marital status, education, socioeconomic status, occupation) of these people as compared with people who do get regular care? Are any identifiable factors associated with nonuse of services amenable to alteration so that a more appropriate utilization pattern might emerge? What are the characteristics of people who overutilize health services, and can any of these be used to change the pattern?

Third, is there any difference in health status overall or in rates of specific types of diseases among those who use services regularly versus those who do not, after taking into consideration such important intervening variables as age, race, occupational exposure, and socioeconomic status? Fourth, if current nonusers cannot be convinced to seek out appropriate services, and if in fact their health is poorer than that of people receiving regular care (a logical assumption but not necessarily a fact), is there any way in which preventive or treatment services for specific health problems can be brought to them through one or more of the ten strategies just described?

Turning now to another area of concern to physicians, let us consider the question of the effectiveness of health education. Commonly, health education activities are not evaluated at all or, if they are evaluated, are examined only inadequately. Three relevant steps need to be considered in applying health education programs, whether for an individual or for a community.

1. An appropriate effort must be made to change skills, knowledge, attitudes, or resources that may be deficient among people who are at greatest risk of disease or of more serious illness. For example, patients with severe obstructive pulmonary disease may lack the skills of pursed lip breathing, knowledge about how to avoid acute infections, appropriate attitudes with respect to regular use of medicines, or a resource such as a Bird apparatus. In order to evaluate the effectiveness of an educational program for such people one would first get information about the baseline level of their relevant skills, knowledge, attitudes, and resources and then determine after this effort if any change occurred.

2. It is generally assumed that if skills, knowledge, and attitudes change, behavioral change will follow. This, however, is not necessarily the case, as evidenced by the number of physicians who still smoke cigarettes despite knowledge of the effects. A second step in evaluation, therefore, would be to determine if, and in what ways, health behaviors have changed in response to an educational effort.

3. It is also generally assumed that appropriate changes in behavior (such as stopping smoking) lead to appropriate changes in disease outcome (such as reduced disability from respiratory disease). Logically then, one should also evaluate a program by examining the effect of the program on outcomes such as death, disability, and discomfort.

Again, the biologic gradient of disease must be considered. Probably the majority of patients treated by physicians get better no matter how inadequate the treatment or stay the same or get worse no matter how expert the care. This happens, of course, because of factors of host, agent, or environment which may be beyond the capabilities of physicians to change. Unless the educational effort happens to be about one of those relatively few conditions for which treatment quite often makes a difference, it may be almost impossible to demonstrate that the effort has had a substantial effect on morbidity or mortality.

SOURCES OF OTHER INFORMATION

The following is a brief review of some additional sources of information for those interested in further readings in the field of epidemiology. A bibliography is provided at the end of this chapter.

Thomas Francis Jr. is an epidemiologist famous for his work on assessment of immunizations for polio and influenza who describes the family as a social group for contracting disease. He points out that the family, not just component individuals, is the unit at risk. This is true not only for genetic disease but for infectious and noninfectious problems.

Frost was a leading epidemiologist who used families extensively as epidemiologic risk groups. His concept of the familial secondary attack rate remains a fundamental method today. In the second Wade Hampton Frost lecture, Fox reviews nearly all the important family-based epidemiologic studies done in the past century. They are carefully reported, analyzed, categorized, and recorded in his bibliography. Fox also records his observations on the advantages and disadvantages of using the family as a risk group.

The position of the family physician in his close relation to the patient and the patient's family makes him an ideal observer of the effect of behavioral factors associated with the etiology of disease. For this reason, epidemiologic investigations by the family physician should include the variables relevant to the sociocultural and behavioral aspects of the population to be studied. In a series of six papers, Bahnson records the effects of social and behavioral pressures on health and disease and describes the role of these pressures as epidemiologic factors.

Section 15 of a book edited by George Thomson contains a listing and short review of the subject "Practice Analysis." Epidemiologic investigations in family practice usually rely on some type of analysis of the practice content. The section reports over 20 such studies, many of them now considered to be classic examples.

Over 250 sources of epidemiologic studies on compliance are recorded and evaluated by Haynes and Sackett. Attribute variables have been classified, and the reader will find references to many articles in each category. Thus, one can find sources on dietary compliance of ulcer patients or the compliance of the elderly in taking digitalis.

Evaluation of the quality of a scientific paper is simultaneously important and difficult. Ashikaga, Waller, and Thomson have listed a number of epidemiologic and statistical principles to help the reader determine if a scientific study has merit and if it is applicable to his practice.

REFERENCES

1. Haddon, W., Jr.: On the escape of tigers: an ecologic note. Am. J. Public Health, *60*:2229, 1970.
2. Smoking and Health. Advisory Committee to the Surgeon General. Public Health Service Publication #1103, 1964, p. 20.
3. McWhinney, I. R.: Problem-solving and decision-making in primary medical practice. Albert Wander Lecture. Proc. R. Soc. Med., 65:934, 1972.

BIBLIOGRAPHY

Ashikaga, T., Waller, J. A., and Thomson, G. H.: On reading medical journals. J. Fam. Pract. *4*:383, 1977.
Bahnson, C. B.: Behavioral factors associated with the etiology of physical disease. Introduction. Am. J. Public Health, *64*(11):1003, 1974.
Fox, J. P.: Family-based epidemiologic studies. (The Second Wade Hampton Frost Lecture.) Am. J. Epidemiol., 99:165, 1974.
Francis, T., Jr.: The family doctor—an epidemiologic concept. J.A.M.A., *141*:308, 1949.
Haynes, R. B., and Sackett, D. L.: An annotated bibliography on the compliance of patients with therapeutic regimens. Available from the Department of Clinical Epidemiology, McMaster University, Hamilton, Ontario, Canada, 1974.
Thomson, G. H. (ed.): Selected References in Family Medicine. 2nd ed., Kansas City, Mo., Soc. Teachers of Family Medicine, 1975.

Chapter 10

PROSPECTIVE MEDICINE

by LEWIS C. ROBBINS,
and JACK H. HALL

INTRODUCTION

Prospective medicine is both the study of the most likely causes of death and disability and the evaluation of what can be done to reduce risk factors associated with these causes. As such, prospective medicine utilizes the principle of *probability,* which is defined as the relative frequency with which events occur. All medicine is practiced by making models of probability based on studies of disease and injury and by placing patients in the appropriate models. Thus, prospective medicine, as does curative medicine, begins with the patient as the unit to be studied. Each patient is evaluated for the specific causes of death and disability that are most threatening to him.

Prospective medicine utilizes results of group studies to apply data regarding the probability of these specific causes to the individual patient. Data derived from studying both high and low risk groups can also give the physician options for providing health maintenance programs for individual patients.

The challenge of prospective medicine is to learn to use the principles of probability to benefit each patient. Utilizing such principles can extend life expectancy for the individual patient and, consequently, for the entire population.

WHAT THE PATIENT WANTS

Health agencies are flooding the media and their own outlets with information about the major causes of death and the factors that place individuals at high risk of death. The patient spends much of his time thinking about his own security and about taking steps to ensure his own preservation. He does not verbalize this well, but the physician is made aware of this concern from his many daily contacts with patients. Health is a personal affair. No one else can enjoy it for the individual. Health has no intrinsic value, for one can neither sell it nor give it away. Health is an enabling function that allows an individual to perform as he chooses. Conversely, disease is a disabling process that may resolve either quickly or slowly or may progress to death. The patient, when he has a chance to choose, asks for an extension of life expectancy, provided he can live in a useful, productive manner.

The medical profession has oriented the majority of its effort toward disease recognition and management. Our concern is whether efforts in the field of prospective medicine are adequate. If we are to make extension of useful, productive life expectancy our goal, changes will have to be made in our practice of medicine.

THE ROLE OF PROBABILITY

Few aspects of our lives elude the effects of chance. An unplanned encounter may decide our choice of a mate or of a job. An inadvertent misstep may land us in a hospital. Our language is replete with adverbs of contingency—"usually," "probably," "perhaps." Every time we contemplate choices, we automatically make estimates of chance before reaching a final decision. The individual looks for as much margin of advantage as possible. He builds his bank account and gauges his chances with life insurance while continually weighing the probabilities of increasing his gains.

Pierre Simon de Laplace, who perfected Newtonian analysis of the solar system in the 18th century, wrote:

Given for one instant an intelligence which could comprehend all the forces by which nature is animated and ... sufficiently vast to submit these data to analysis—it would embrace in the same formula the movements of the greatest bodies of the universe and those of the lightest atom: for it, nothing would be uncertain and the future, as the past, would be present to its eyes.[7]

How can such wishful thinking help us in present day problem-solving? To the patient, this fantasy is an extension of what he now asks for—adequate information with which to make decisions. To the physician, it is a suggestion that he extend his present efforts to acquire the most reasonable data base available as a guide to those regimens that give his patients the best chance for survival. But to those practicing prospective medicine, there is a special significance to the words "... the future, as the past, would be present to its eyes." Why shouldn't the family physician ask about the most likely causes of death and what will reduce those risks for his patient?

An entirely new vista of probability is opened to the physician who knows the natural history of the diseases he treats. Most diseases have a long period of generation. Each precursor of disease (that is, a prognostic characteristic, or risk factor, that appears before an actual disease is diagnosed) has its own natural history (Fig. 10–1). As the patient progresses from the stage

of *no risk* to *vulnerable* to *precursor present* to *signs, symptoms*, and *disability* followed by death, there exists a pattern of probability for each treated and untreated stage. Today, each of the causes of death has been subjected to many studies, and much knowledge about their precursors is available. A prospective study begins with the well person. Certain prognostic characteristics are evaluated to see which individuals will die from which disease and whether these people revealed in their early history telltale omens that predicted the later disease. In medicine, as in the other professions, "Coming events cast their shadows before."*

A new form of prospective medicine is emerging that is best described by the single word "anticipation." Fuller[1] pointed to the evolution of man's desire to go around the world on the surface of the ocean. Many years' experience and many disasters resulted in the development and perfection of sailing ships. Gradually, designs for the tall ships become more "adequately anticipatory of the probable recurrences of yesterday's experiences, both positive and negative."[1] The progressive designs reflected man's anticipation of disaster and his attempt to avoid destruction from storms, shoals, fire, and collisions. Medicine, too, must help man anticipate more adequately the probable recurrence of yesterday's diseases and injuries and must help develop preventive designs for tomorrow. In medicine, as in navigation, one must be able to get a fix on the course

---

*Thomas Campbell—*Lochiel's Warning.*

Natural History of Disease

STAGES IN DEVELOPMENT

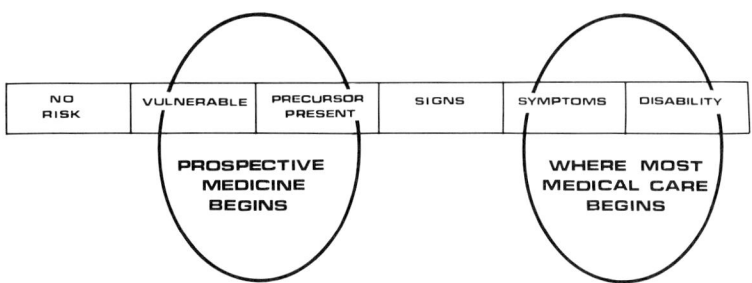

Figure 10–1. Schema showing the natural history of disease.

and make corrections. In prospective medicine, the physician must get a fix on the progression of the antagonist to health and must take every initiative to chart a stronger position for his patient.

HEALTH HAZARD APPRAISAL AS A TOOL

Health hazard appraisal (HHA) is a method or tool used in the practice of prospective medicine that defines the total personal risk of an individual and provides a breakdown of causes plus an outline of possible interventions that will reduce the risk. HHA is a means of combining the science and the art of prospective medicine to benefit the individual patient.

Science has been called the "observation, identification, description, experimental investigation and theoretical explanation of natural phenomena."[11] To the physician, science represents reproducible observations. The science of HHA depends primarily on three sources: the probability tables prepared by the National Center for Health Statistics,[18] the precursors or risk factors derived from prospective studies,[17] and the mortality ratios and prevalence data selected by the epidemiologists.[2]

The art of HHA has a different function. Art has been called "a human effort to imitate, supplement, alter, or counteract the work of nature."[11] While the art of curative medicine attempts to change nature by treating a disease or injury already present in a patient, the art of HHA attempts to change nature by anticipating disease or injury in a well person and by blocking or altering its subsequent course. HHA utilizes three groups or disciplines to perform the art that anticipates and changes nature: the actuary, the primary physician, and the health educator. The actuary's statistical tables are designed to give the physician models that permit him to formulate stages of the disease process and to determine prognosis. The physician applies these models to his patients and draws conclusions that he calls "indications." The health educator determines what the patient actually comprehends about his illness, learns how much he knows about the associated precursors, and estimates how much more he needs to know to make

appropriate decisions about his preventive prescriptions, that is, the treatment interventions planned by his physician.

Prospective medicine seeks, as does curative medicine, the greatest survival advantage for the individual. Some methods of treatment are far better than others, as demonstrated numerically by the treatment of bacterial pneumonia—first treated by serum (85 per cent survival), then by sulfa drugs (90 per cent survival), and finally by antibiotics (95 per cent survival). Utilizing HHA as a tool in patient care has been called a "numbers game," and in the sense that data are collected and used to give the patient the best measurable advantage for survival or freedom from disability, it *is* a numbers game. Without this numerical evidence, the practice of medicine would consist only of individual opinion and personal judgment.

The long-term goal of HHA is to extend useful life expectancy, but the more immediate goal is to "get this patient safely through the next 10 years." The current health status of the well person is defined in terms of his total personal risk for the next 10 years. To what degree that person may increase his survival advantage is determined by his taking certain specific preventive actions.

For the individual, as for the group, there is always a "bunching" of risk, that is, the tendency of only a few specific risk factors to cause a majority of deaths. This is best illustrated by referring to statistical tables evaluating causes of death. Only the leading 12 to 15 causes of death are chosen for appraisal, since these account for two-thirds of all deaths.[13] Below this level, no cause of death contributes to more than 1 per cent of the total deaths. HHA teaches physicians and patients how to reduce this bunching and how to defer many of the less common risk factors. Thus, the physician's practice is directed toward dealing with those risk factors most likely to affect a patient rather than dwelling on those that are unlikely to occur.

CALCULATIONS USED IN HHA

The HHA chart (Fig. 10–2) is designed to give high visibility to risk factors by showing cause, precursor, stage, and intervention, so that the physician can see specific

HEALTH HAZARD APPRAISAL CHART

Quality control. Evaluate performance of a predetermined goal:
(Goal "Get this patient safely through the next ten years.")

40-44 White male

Name John Doe   Patient No. XXXX   Birthdate Dec. 15, 1935
Street Blank Apartments   Race, Sex, Age 41 W M
City Middletown   State ____ Zip ____   Date Dec. 17, 76

AVERAGE TO INDIVIDUAL RISK						RISK REDUCTION FOR INDIVIDUAL					
POPULATION AVERAGE 10 YEAR DEATHS PER 100,000		INDIVIDUAL PROGNOSIS RISK APPRAISAL				PROGNOSIS AFTER INTERVENTION RISK REAPPRAISAL *				SURVIVAL ADVANTAGE	
Disease/Injury	Average Risk	Prognostic Characteristics	Risk Factor	Composite Risk Factor	Present Risk	Prognostic Characteristics	Risk Factor	Composite Risk Factor	New Risk	Amount Reduction	Per Cent Reduction
From Manual	From Manual	Listed in Manual / Physician Select	From Manual	See Instructions	(2) x (5)	After Physician's Prescription	From Manual	See Instructions	(2) x (9)	(6) (10)	**
(1)	(2)	(3)	(4)	(5)	(6)	(7)	(8)	(9)	(10)	(11)	(12)
HEART ATTACK	1629	Blood pres. 180/94	1.3	2.2 / 2.9	4724	Reduce BP to 140/88	1.4 / 1.1	0.8	1303	3421	35
		Cholesterol 220	1.0				1.0				
		Diabetes neg.	1.0				1.0				
		Exercise-walks 1 mi	1.0			Walk 1 mi; stairs 10fl.	0.5				
		Family hist. 60+ 60	0.9								
		Smoking cig. 1 pkg	1.5			Stop smoking	0.7				
		Weight 15% overwt	1.0			Reduce to "optimum"	0.9				
CANCER LUNGS	348	Smoking pack day	1.5	1.5	522	Stop smoking	1.2	1.2	418	104	1
CIRRHOSIS LIVER	343	Alcohol 18 dr/wk	2.0	2.0	686	Reduce to 3-6d./week	1.0	1.0	343	343	4
ACCIDENT: MOT. VEH.	275	Alcohol 18 dr/wk	2.0	2.3	633	Reduce to 3-6 d./week	1.0	1.3	358	275	3
		Mileage 15,000/yr	1.5				1.5				
		Seat belts, 75%+	0.8				0.8				
SUICIDE	260	Depression no	1.0	1.0	260		1.0		260		
		Family hist no	1.0				1.0				
STROKE	178	Blood pres 180/94	1.3	1.3 / 2.7	481	Reduce BP to 140/88	1.4 / 1.1	1.5	267	214	2
		Cholesterol 220	1.0				1.0				
		Diabetes neg	1.0				1.0				
		Smoking 1 pack	1.2				1.0				
HOMICIDE	128	Arrest no	1.0	1.0	128		1.0		128	-	
		Weapon carry no	1.0				1.0				
CANCER COL-REC	86	History polyp no	1.0	3.0	258		1.0	0.3	26	232	2
		Rectal bleedg yes	3.0				1.0				
		Ulcerative col no	1.0				1.0				
		Ann. Proctosig no	1.0			Ann. Procto sigmoidoscopic	0.3				
PNEUMONIA	75	Alcohol 18/wk	3.0	3.2	240		1.0	1.0	75	165	2
		History bact pn no	1.0				1.0				
		Emphysema no	1.0				1.0				
		Smoking 1 pack/day	1.2				1.0				
ACCIDENTS: MACH (non-Mot Veh)	63	Machinery work neg	1.0	1.0	63				63	-	
Other Causes	1750				1750				1750		
Total	5135				9745				4991	4754	49

*Reappraise on assumption that physician's prescription is complied with. Columns (7) through (10) same as columns (3) through (6) except where the physician's prescription changed prognostic characteristics.
**Divide figures in column (11) by total of column (6).

Form CH 969

Health Appraisal Age 46 1/2   Compliance Age 40

Appraiser ____ (SIGNATURE)
Physician Robbins and Hall (SIGNATURE)

Figure 10-2. *Health Hazard Appraisal Chart.*

risks and prescribe possible risk reductions for his patients. The preparation of this chart requires a series of judgments in which the many models of the Geller–Gesner Tables[14] (Fig. 10–3) must be compared to see which models are most applicable to the specific patient. The Geller–Gesner Tables are tables that permit the physician to determine which interventions or which preventive procedures are indicated for the well person. They use the familiar "observed to expected" ratio, which compares the untreated group with the treated group. In clinical trials, this is called the "benefit to risk ratio." These tables are derived from the Geller Tables, which give age-sex-race averages by cause of death (with deviations from the average) and the Gesner Tables, which show how much the group that is treated deviates from average. The Geller–Gesner Tables are designed to perform the HHA that takes the patient from (1) average risk, for his total risk and by cause to (2) risk by precursor to (3) total personal risk without treatment and to (4) total personal risk following the intervention or preventive procedure. The patient must be matched to these tables in order to derive indications. The white male tables were chosen be-cause there is an economic difference between most whites and most blacks that is reflected in the mortality data, which are mostly unfavorable to the blacks.

The HHA chart is largely self-explanatory, with the exception of the composite risk factor and the appraisal age. The composite risk factor is derived by a formula that multiplies the risk factors of 1.0 and under and adds the risk factors greater than 1.0. This treats the precursors as if they were not independent variables and has the effect of dampening the total risk factor, a judgment that has added credibility to the HHA program. The actuary believes that for practical purposes it is better to understate than to overstate the risk.

The health appraisal age is a way of expressing the health of an individual in terms of his total personal risk. Using actuarial tables, one merely matches the individual with averages by age. Thus, the health appraisal age of the individual is the same as the age of that group of people whose average risk approximates his own. For example, if a man has an appraisal age of 46, he carries the total personal risk of people aged 46, even though his chronologic age is 41 years.[14]

Figure 10–2 represents the HHA chart of

WHITE MALE — ENTRY AGE 40–44

POPULATION AVERAGE: 10 YEAR DEATHS PER 100,000   INDIVIDUAL PROGNOSIS: RISK APPRAISAL

RANK	CAUSE OF DEATH: DISEASE/INJURY	NUMBER	PERCENT	PROGNOSTIC CHARACTERISTICS	RISK FACTOR
1.	HEART ATTACK	1629	31.7	BLOOD PRESSURE	
				USE HIGHER FACTOR OF SYST & DIAST	
				EXCEPT BOTH IF BOTH OVER 1.0	
				SYSTOLIC 200	3.2
				180	2.2
				160	1.4
				140	.8
				120	.4
				DIASTOLIC 106	3.7
				100	2.0
				94	1.3
				88	.8
				82	.4
				PRESCRIBED REDUCTION USE AVERAGE	
				OF HIGH & EXPECTED READINGS	
				CHOLESTEROL LEVEL	
				280	1.5
				220	1.0
				180	.5
				DIABETIC	
				YES	3.0
				CONTROLLED	2.5
				NO	1.0
				EXERCISE HABITS	
				SEDENTARY WORK & LEISURE	2.5
				SOME ACTIVITY WORK OR LEISURE	1.0
				MODERATE EXERCISE	.6
				VIGOROUS EXERCISE	.5
				PRESCRIBED EXERCISE FOR SEDENTARY	1.0
				PRESCRIBED EXERCISE FOR OTHERS	.5
				FAMILY HISTORY OF ASHD	
				BOTH PARENTS DIED BEFORE 60	1.4
				ONE PARENT DIED BEFORE 60	1.2
				NEITHER, IF NOW UNDER 60	1.0
				NEITHER, IF NOW OVER 60	.9
				SMOKING HABITS: ONE FACTOR ONLY	
				CIGARETS DAILY AVERAGE	
				1/2 PACK OR MORE	1.5
				UNDER 1/2 PACK	1.1
				CIGARS OR PIPE	1.0
				STOPPED SMOKING WITHIN 10 YEARS	.7
				NONSMOKER OR STOPPED 10 YEARS	.5
				WEIGHT	
				75% OVERWEIGHT	2.5
				50% OVERWEIGHT	1.5
				15% OVERWEIGHT	1.0
				10% UNDERWEIGHT	.8
				REDUCE TO AVERAGE WEIGHT	1.0
2.	LUNG CANCER	348	6.8	SMOKING HABITS: ONE FACTOR ONLY	
				CIGARETS DAILY AVERAGE	
				TWO PACKS	2.0
				ONE PACK	1.5
				1/2 PACK	1.1
				UNDER 1/2 PACK	.8
				CIGARS OR PIPES DAILY AVERAGE	
				OVER 5, OR ANY INHALED	1.0
				UNDER 5, NOT INHALED	.3
				FORMER SMOKER: REDUCE FACTOR	
				20% PLUS 10% PER YEAR STOPPED	
				NOT BELOW NONSMOKER FACTOR	
				NONSMOKER	.2

Figure 10–3. *Page from Risk Factor Manual. Geller–Gesner Tables. (From Robbins, L. C., and Hall, J. H.: How to Practice Prospective Medicine. Methodist Hospital of Indiana. Indianpolis, 1970.)*

WHITE MALE — ENTRY AGE 40-44

POPULATION AVERAGE: 1C YEAR DEATHS PER 100,000   INDIVIDUAL PROGNOSIS: RISK APPRAISAL

RANK	CAUSE OF DEATH: DISEASE/INJURY	NUMBER	PERCENT	PROGNOSTIC CHARACTERISTICS	RISK FACTOR
3.	CIRRHOSIS LIVER	343	6.7	ALCOHOL HABITS	
				ALCOHOLIC	12.5
				HEAVY SOCIAL, DEFINITE EXCESS	5.0
				HEAVY SOCIAL, MILD EXCESS	2.0
				MODERATE & OCCASIONAL SOCIAL	1.0
				INFREQUENT MODERATE SOCIAL	.2
				STOPPED BEFORE SYMPTOMS	.2
				NONDRINKER	.1
4.	MOTOR VEHICLE AC.	275	5.4	ALCOHOL HABITS	
				HEAVY SOCIAL, DEFINITE EXCESS	5.0
				HEAVY SOCIAL, MILD EXCESS	2.0
				MODERATE & OCCASIONAL SOCIAL	1.0
				NONDRINKER	.5
				DRUGS & MEDICATION	
				MILEAGE PER YEAR	
				MILEAGE DIV. BY 10,000 = FACTOR	
				SEAT BELT USE	1.1
				LESS THAN 10% OF TIME	1.0
				10% TO 24%	.9
				25% TO 74%	.8
				75% TO 100%	
5.	SUICIDE	260	5.1	DEPRESSION	
				OFTEN DEPRESSED	2.5
				SELDOM OR NEVER	1.0
				FAMILY HISTORY OF SUICIDE	
				YES	2.5
				NO	1.0
6.	STROKE	178	3.5	BLOOD PRESSURE	
				USE HIGHER FACTOR OF SYST & DIAST	
				EXCEPT BOTH IF BOTH OVER 1.0	
				SYSTOLIC 200	3.2
				180	2.2
				160	1.4
				140	.8
				120	.4
				DIASTOLIC 106	3.7
				100	2.0
				94	1.3
				88	.8
				82	.4
				PRESCRIBED REDUCTION USE AVERAGE	
				OF HIGH & EXPECTED READINGS	
				CHOLESTEROL LEVEL	
				280	1.5
				220	1.0
				180	.5
				DIABETIC	
				YES	3.0
				CONTROLLED	2.5
				NO	1.0
				SMOKING HABITS: ONE FACTOR ONLY	
				CIGARETS	1.2
				CIGARS OR PIPE	1.0
				STOPPED SMOKING	1.0
				NONSMOKER	.8

Figure 10-3. Continued.

WHITE MALE — ENTRY AGE 40–44

POPULATION AVERAGE: 10 YEAR DEATHS PER 100,000   INDIVIDUAL PROGNOSIS: RISK APPRAISAL

RANK	CAUSE OF DEATH: DISEASE/INJURY	NUMBER	PERCENT	PROGNOSTIC CHARACTERISTICS	RISK FACTOR
7.	HOMICIDE	128	2.5	ARREST RECORD	
				BURGLARY, ROBBERY, ASSAULT	10.0
				WITHOUT VIOLENCE OR THREAT	1.0
				NO ARRESTS	1.0
				WEAPONS	
				CARRY ON PERSON	2.0
				DO NOT CARRY	1.0
8.	CANCER COLON-RECTUM	86	1.7	POLYP	
				HAVE HAD	2.5
				HAVE NOT HAD	1.0
				RECTAL BLEEDING, UNDIAGNOSED	
				HAVE HAD	3.0
				HAVE NOT HAD	1.0
				ULCERATIVE COLITIS	
				10 OR MORE YEARS	4.0
				UNDER 10 YEARS	2.0
				HAVE NOT HAD	1.0
				ANNUAL PROCTOSIGMOIDOSCOPY	
				MULTIPLY COMPOSITE OF ABOVE BY	.3
9.	PNEUMONIA	75	1.4	ALCOHOL HABITS	
				HEAVY SOCIAL	3.0
				MODERATE OR NONDRINKER	1.0
				BACTERIAL PNEUMONIA	
				HAVE HAD	2.0
				HAVE NOT HAD	1.0
				EMPHYSEMA	
				HAVE EMPHYSEMA	2.0
				NO SIGNS OR SYMPTOMS	1.0
				SMOKING HABITS	
				CIGARETS, OVER 1/2 PACK	1.2
				OTHERS	1.0
10.	ACCIDENTS DUE TO MACHINES-NON MVA	63	1.2	No risk factors	
11.	OTHER CAUSES	1750	34.0%		
	TOTAL CAUSES	5135	100.0%		

Figure 10–3. Continued.

a 41 year old white male salesman with no history of cancer or heart disease. He had a recent physical examination that was essentially negative, with the following exceptions. His blood pressure was 180 mm. Hg systolic and 94 mm. Hg diastolic, and his cholesterol determination was 220 mg. per 100 ml. He was 15 per cent overweight. There was no evidence of diabetes. He smoked a pack of cigarettes a day, had two drinks each weekday, and had four drinks on both Saturday and Sunday. He drove 15,000 miles per year and used seatbelts more than 75 per cent of the time. He had a history of some rectal bleeding. He got some exercise and had no family history of heart attack. Both parents were over 60 years old and were living and well.

The calculations used in HHA are made by simple arithmetic. The physician, as the patient's advocate, may easily learn to guide the patient on the safest course against the long-term risks. But the patient too must understand the method, for the tool must have high credibility for the patient, who is the one responsible for following the preventive interventions. Hence, the rationale for using the simple arithmetic in HHA.

The following is a sample explanation that could be given to the patient. Most patients are given their calculated HHA, but some are only shown their bar chart (to be explained in the following section). The patient is told:

"While the practice of medicine has been largely directed toward getting you well, HHA is designed to keep you well—to get you safely through the next 10 years. In this, HHA is directed toward extending your life expectancy. The two most important numbers on this chart are your total personal risk and your new risk after all preventive procedures are taken. Your total personal risk is 9680. This means that you have 9680 out of 100,000 chances of dying during the next 10 years. To put this another way, you have 90,320 chances out of 100,000 of survival during the next 10 years. If you would complete all your indicated preventive procedures and take all prescribed preventive measures, you could reduce your total personal risk to a new level of 4992. This big reduction is achieved largely by reducing your risk of death from a heart attack.

While you are actually 41 years old, you have the total personal risk of a man 46.5 years old. This risk can and should be reduced to a level below 5000, which would give you the total personal risk of a man 40 years old. Not bad to go from age 46 to age 40 in a few months! A Canadian health official refers to this as the closest you will get to the fountain of youth.[8]

Let's see what is causing your present risk to be double that of other men of your age.

Heart Attack. The first major risk is that of a coronary, or heart attack. This risk is increased because of your elevated blood pressure and your cigarette smoking. Your blood pressure increases your risk by 150 per cent and your smoking by 50 per cent. By reducing both of these, we can reduce your total personal risk from just a heart attack alone by 36 per cent.

Cancer of the Lung. This is your leading risk of cancer, and you have increased it by 50 per cent by smoking. This gives you a numerical risk of 522. We can begin bringing this down, but it will be more than 10 years before this risk will be as low as it was before you started smoking.

Cirrhosis of the Liver. You are presently consuming 18 drinks per week. This level won't necessarily cause cirrhosis, but it does double your risk in this area. If you reduce your alcohol intake to less than six drinks per week, you can reduce your risk to average for your age groups. Do you have any suggestions?

Motor Vehicle Accidents. We took this, which is your fourth major risk for cause of death, and increased it by 130 per cent. You're 230 per cent of average! A part of this is due to your having 18 drinks per week, and the remainder is due to your large amount of driving, which I assume you cannot change. I've prescribed reducing the number of drinks you take to six per week or less.

Suicide. Your risk is average for suicide.

Stroke. Your risk of stroke is almost tripled because of your high blood pressure and cigarette smoking. The risk of this disease diminishes readily by treating the precursors, such as lowering your elevated blood pressure.

Homicide. There's not much we can do about this, but at least you are not at high risk compared with average.

Cancer of the Colon and Rectum. The rectal bleeding is probably caused by hemor-

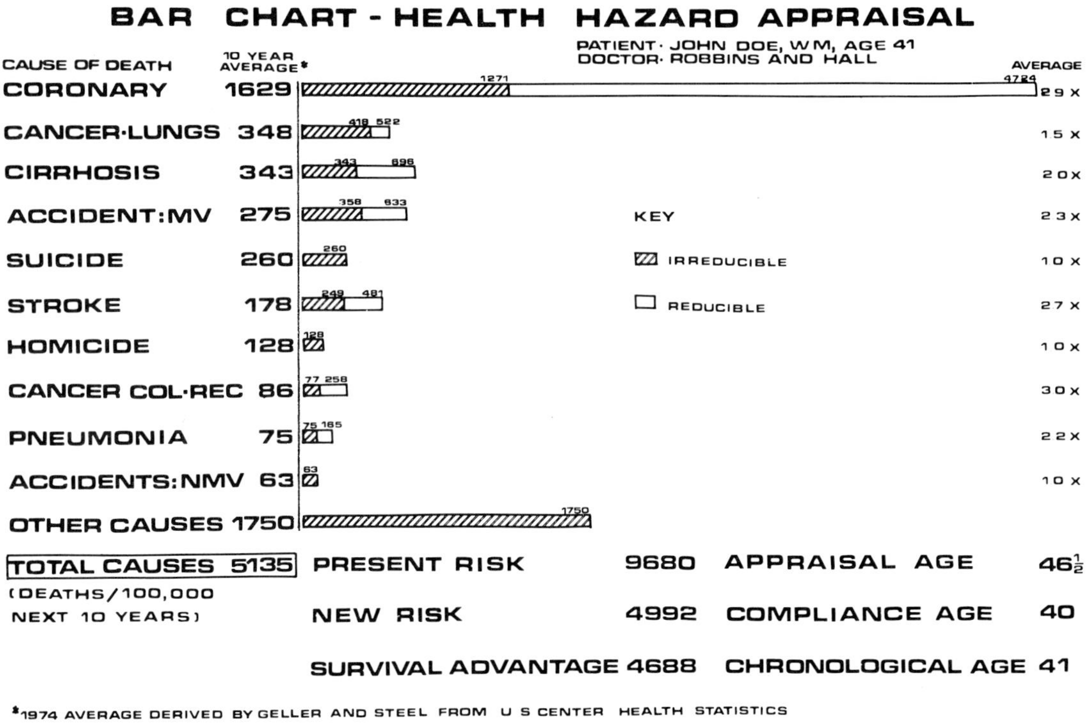

BAR CHART - HEALTH HAZARD APPRAISAL

PATIENT· JOHN DOE, W M, AGE 41
DOCTOR· ROBBINS AND HALL

CAUSE OF DEATH	10 YEAR AVERAGE*		AVERAGE
CORONARY	1629	1271 4724	29 X
CANCER·LUNGS	348	419 522	15 X
CIRRHOSIS	343	343 696	20X
ACCIDENT:MV	275	358 633	23 X
SUICIDE	260	260	10 X
STROKE	178	349 481	27 X
HOMICIDE	128	188	10 X
CANCER COL·REC	86	77 258	30X
PNEUMONIA	75	75 165	22 X
ACCIDENTS:NMV	63	63	10 X
OTHER CAUSES	1750	1750	

KEY

▨ IRREDUCIBLE

☐ REDUCIBLE

TOTAL CAUSES 5135	PRESENT RISK	9680	APPRAISAL AGE	46½
(DEATHS/100,000 NEXT 10 YEARS)	NEW RISK	4992	COMPLIANCE AGE	40
	SURVIVAL ADVANTAGE 4688		CHRONOLOGICAL AGE 41	

*1974 AVERAGE DERIVED BY GELLER AND STEEL FROM U S CENTER HEALTH STATISTICS

Figure 10-4. Bar chart showing patient's personal risks.

rhoids, and we have no choice but to check it out. We can give you a reduced risk if a proctosigmoidoscopy is performed and the results are normal. If you prefer, we can substitute a test of the stool for occult blood, which for most is more comfortable. For the present, I am giving you the same credit for having the test for occult blood in the stool that I would give you if you had the proctosigmoidoscopy, assuming that you follow up on any possible positive tests.

Pneumonia. Your alcohol intake and cigarette smoking more than double this risk.

Accidents—Machinery (Non-Motor Vehicle). We'll put you down for average, since you don't use heavy machinery."

Bar Chart

The bar chart shown in Figure 10-4 is useful in giving the patient a quick picture of his risks and in helping him to visualize the potential risk reduction. This chart was designed as a means of saving physicians' time by explaining numbers that might be confusing to the patient. Each bar refers to a single cause of death. The bar may list several precursors that need to be ex-

plained. The length of the bar shows the patient's chances of dying from that particular cause of death during the next 10 years. The lighter portion of the bar represents that portion of the risk that is reducible. Note the phenomenon of bunching. Following the ten leading causes of death shown in the chart, no other cause contributes even as much as 1 per cent to the total deaths.

DETERMINING RISK FACTORS

The public has been told about risk factors in thousands of releases from health agencies. More and more patients are asking their physicians "What risks really affect people like me?" Physicians are asking "What problems will face my patients during the next 10 years?" The Geller–Gesner Tables and HHA permit 10 year risks to be estimated. What then are the responsibilities of the family physician in applying the findings of prospective medicine to his patient's preventive needs? These obligations including diagnosing those precursors that are most dangerous for the patient, formulating stages, establishing prognoses, and initiating treatment, using HHA as a guide. Utilizing the precision made available by HHA, the physician may take a prospective approach to this patient's long-term risks.

What precursors should be included in the appraisals of people aged 20 and over? While the Geller–Gesner Tables include about 50 precursors, the 25 precursors given in Table 10–1 are especially important and are designed to meet the following criteria:

1. The precursor is associated with one of the leading causes of death included in the Geller Tables.[13] (See Table 10–2.)

2. The presence of the precursor places the individual at an even higher than average risk.

3. The precursor is highly prevalent in the population. The number of people having the precursor should be great enough to justify evaluating each person for its presence. (As a rule of thumb, at least 3 per cent of the population should have the

precursor to justify the expense of searching for it.)

4. Intervention should yield a significant degree of survival advantage. The "payoff" should be high enough to warrant all the effort expended.

5. Prudence dictates its practice. Many prospective procedures adopted in the past lacked the necessary proof required by investigators to establish their efficacy. In HHA, when the evidence supporting the practice is so great that neither the health agencies nor their advisors can accept a default in its practice, that precursor is included in the appraisal.

6. The cost of the procedure should be low. There is always a limited amount of money for risk reduction.

Diagnosis

Precursors should be diagnosed for two reasons. First, early action is necessary. Precursors are usually present for a long time before disease strikes. However, they are subject to the laws of probability, and the chance for prevention may be lost without warning. Second, crisis-oriented care should be avoided. Crisis medicine occurs when a new patient requests treatment for an acute problem. Here, a high quality of medical care is difficult because the data base is incomplete. If an adequate data base, including questions about precursors, has previously been obtained, most crises can be anticipated in part.

Staging

Determine the stage of the disease process. At what point is the patient in the natural history of specific common diseases or injuries? Staging the patient is equivalent to getting a fix in navigation. Appropriate corrections in position must be made. How many cigarettes are smoked, and how much alcohol does the patient consume? What is the blood cholesterol level? How high is the blood pressure?

Prognosis

Some physicians object to telling patients about their risk factors and complain that discussing precursors frightens patients. The issue is whether patients should be advised of their long-term risks if these

---

TABLE 10–1. TWENTY–FIVE PRECURSORS IN HEALTH HAZARD APPRAISAL*

Those that Appear Before the Signs and Symptoms of Disease and Injury

1. Cigarettes to coronary heart disease
2. High blood pressure to coronary heart disease
3. High cholesterol level to coronary heart disease
4. Sedentary life style to coronary heart disease
5. Diabetes to coronary heart disease
6. High blood pressure to stroke
7. Cigarettes to stroke
8. Cigarettes to lung cancer
9. Alcohol to motor vehicle accident
10. Positive cytology to cancer of the cervix
11. Alcohol to cirrhosis
12. Cigarettes to bronchitis–emphysema
13. Obesity to coronary heart disease
14. Not using seatbelts to motor vehicle accident
15. Miles traveled to motor vehicle accident
16. Depression to suicide
17. Carrying weapon to homicide
18. High blood pressure to hypertensive heart disease
19. History of polyp to cancer of colon and rectum
20. Arrest record to homicide
21. Family history (mother, sister) to breast cancer
22. Rheumatic fever to rheumatic heart disease

Those that Appear Before Symptoms but After Signs of Disease and Injury

23. Dominant nodule (lump) to breast cancer
24. Occult blood in stool to cancer of colon and rectum
25. Mammography (cancer image) to breast cancer

*High risk groups selected for their importance as contributors to premature death.

FOUR STEPS TO RISK REDUCTION (HHA)

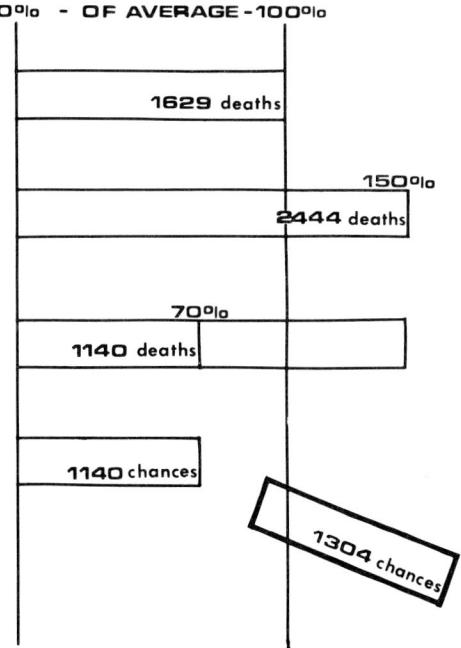

1. AGE AVERAGE RISK. FROM THE GELLER TABLES WE LEARN THAT AMONG WHITE MALES, 40-44, APPROXIMATELY 1629 DEATHS MAY BE EXPECTED IN THE FOLLOWING 10 YEARS PER 100,000 FROM HEART ATTACK.

2. DEVIATION FROM AVERAGE. FROM THE GELLER-GESNER TABLES COME THE DEATHS FROM HEART ATTACK FOR CIGARETTE SMOKERS OF A PACK A DAY. THIS IS 1.5 X AVERAGE, OR 1629. THIS TOTALS 2444 DEATHS AMONG CIGARETTE SMOKERS FOR HEART ATTACK ALONE.

3. CHOOSING THE INTERVENTION. CESSATION FROM SMOKING WILL NOT REDUCE THE RISK TO ZERO. STUDIES SHOW A LESSER REDUCTION: THE RISK FACTOR FOR STOPPED SMOKERS IS 0.7, OR 70% OF AVERAGE. NEW RISK COULD BE 1140 DEATHS.

4. FOR A BETTER PROGNOSIS. COMPLIANCE WITH THE PRESCRIPTION, STOP SMOKING, WILL RESULT IN AN ALMOST IMMEDIATE DROP IN DEATHS FROM HEART ATTACK. THE REDUCTION COULD BE CALLED THE SURVIVAL ADVANTAGE--A DROP IN 1304 DEATHS. THE NEW RISK IS 1140, AS COMPARED TO 2444 CHANCES OF DEATH.

Figure 10–5. *A 41 year old white male who smokes a pack of cigarettes daily is appraised for risk of coronary heart disease.*

risks can be reduced. The dedicated physician tells his patients what they may expect in terms of their illness so that they may share the responsibility for treatment. This is but an extension of the principle on which medicine was founded—prognose so that you may affect prognosis.[5] Those who object to this principle of prospective medicine should be confronted with data and evidence, but their dedication or sincerity should never be questioned. Every block to progress represents an opportunity to discuss the science and the art of prospective medicine.

Treatment

The physician may now prescribe interventions. He does not have a responsibility to see that the patient carries out his preventive prescriptions, but he should make these available. Until the physician has acted, the patient will not know what direction his preventive program should take. Default of the patient is not new to medicine. Some patients will fail to follow the prescribed methods of intervention, and the physician can only make sure that the patient knows his risks and what will reduce them. In this way, the physician shares responsibility with his patient for attempting to prevent those diseases that he someday might otherwise have to treat.

REDUCING RISK FACTORS

The art of prospective medicine must apply the science of this discipline appropriately or else fail to reproduce the research results (that is, a gain in survival advantage). The problem must be broken down into separate segments with known characteristics. Prospective medicine must confront one patient and one precursor of disease in that patient. Prospective medicine, therefore, is an elaboration of this one application. There are four steps in estimating a patient's risk and in evaluating what can be done about it. The process involves moving sequentially from determining (1) *age average risk* to (2) *deviation from*

TABLE 10–2. PROBABILITY TABLES (GELLER TABLES) FOR WHITE MALES, AGE 40

Cause	1974	1968	1960
	1974	*1968*	*1960*
Arteriosclerotic heart disease	1629	1861	1877
Cancer of the lung	348	291	202
Cirrhosis	343	304	222
Motor vehicle accidents	275	339	285
Suicide	260	253	264
Stroke	178	209	222
Homicide	128	87	°
Cancer of the large intestine and rectum	86	88	111
Pneumonia	75	114	111
Accidents caused by machines (non-motor vehicle)	63	70	°
Other causes	1750	1874	2266
TOTAL CAUSES	5135	5490	5560

° Data for this year are not available.

average (or present risk in the high risk group) to (3) *choosing the intervention* (or new risk) to (4) compliance and a *better prognosis.* Figure 10–5 illustrates the four-step process.

Age Average Risk

Let us begin with a 40 year white male and calculate his risk of death from coronary heart disease. Experience has shown that this risk must be expressed in terms of chances of death from specific causes per 100,000 population over the next 10 years. Harvey Geller's tables, modified and updated by Greg Steele (Table 10–2), estimate that 1629 deaths from heart attacks may be expected in this age group.[13] By the time the individual in our example reaches age 51, about 1600 people in his group will have died from a heart attack. This is just under 2 per cent (1.6 per cent) of the total

men in this age group. These data from the National Center for Health Statistics from the year 1974 are the best available and have been corrected by the Reed–Merrell formula. Step 1 of Figure 10–5 shows this graphically. The accuracy of such data is, of course, dependent on each individual physician's judgment at the time that he completes the death certificate and on properly collecting and analyzing information from these death certificates.

Deviation from Average

To the extent that the patient is average, his risk is 1629, but he is not average for he is smoking a pack of cigarettes a day. The actuary now provides us with risk factors, or multipliers, that adjust the average risk (Table 10–3). The actuary must have the appropriate data, however, from the epidemiologist who is asked to judge (1) staging, or degree of severity of the precursor, that is, how much the patient smokes, (2) the mortality ratio, or deaths at each stage, and (3) the prevalence, or per cent, of the population who smoke this amount. The actuary then uses a formula that takes these data and converts them to a relative number, a relative per cent, and, finally, a risk factor.[2] Smoking a pack of cigarettes a day brings this man's risk factor to 1.5 times average (1.5 × 1629 = 2444), which is this man's present risk if his habits don't change.

Choosing the Intervention

How may this high risk be reduced? Present knowledge calls for cessation of cigarette smoking. What if cessation of smoking is prescribed? The epidemiologist is then asked for both the mortality ratio for former smokers and the prevalence data, all

TABLE 10–3. RISK FACTOR FOR WHITE MALES, AGES 40–44*

Cause of Death	Number	Per Cent	Prognostic Characteristics	Risk Factor
Arteriosclerotic heart disease	1629	31.7	Smoking habits: one factor only	
			Cigarette daily average	
			1/2 pack or more	1.5
			Less than 1/2 pack	1.1
			Cigars or pipe	1.0
			Stopped smoking within 10 years	0.7
			Nonsmoker or stopped 10 years or more	0.5

°Example from Risk Factor Manual. Geller–Gesner Tables. (From Robbins, L. C., and Hall, J. H.: How to Practice Prospective Medicine. Indianapolis, Methodist Hospital of Indiana, 1970.)

by stage of cigarette smoking. The actuary applies his formula again and changes his statistics to reflect the risk for a patient who attempts to stop smoking. The patient would now be 0.7 times average (or 70 per cent) for the next 10 years, if he were able to stop (0.7 × 1629 = 1140). Thus, his new prognosis would be 1140 if he could follow the preventive prescription.

A Better Prognosis

The patient has now been given his risk; whether or not he complies depends upon whether he finds an adequate incentive. The last step is his—to stop smoking. He can be offered 1140 chances of death instead of 2444 chances. This reduces his risk from about a 2.5 per cent chance of dying from a heart attack to about a 1 per cent chance. Of course, this is only the "one precursor–one person" estimate, and the total HHA would include all the leading causes of death for that age group. HHA teaches that one must look at the patient's total risk, not just the interests of health agencies, to derive indications from established categories of risk.

CREDIBILITY OF PROSPECTIVE MEDICINE

The philosopher Will Durant once asked during a convocation of college students, "What is your method of faith? How do you choose between the true and the false?" If the family physician is to give his patient meaningful preventive information, what types of health guidance will be most valuable, based on data from prospective medicine? The following eight criteria are utilized by HHA to provide credibility for the principles of prospective medicine.

Age-Oriented

It is well established that survival rates differ for various age groups. The senior author of this chapter is 67 years old and has, to the extent that he is in average health, a 54 per cent chance of a 10 year survival. His coauthor is 47 years old and has a 91 per cent chance of a 10 year survival.[13] Life insurance companies treat these two peo-

ple differently when they apply for insurance.

Averages by Causes of Death

The causes of death are continually changing. Thomas Peery, in a classic address to the American Society of Clinical Pathologists, pointed out that some causes are increasing (the new diseases) and some are decreasing (the old diseases).[12] As mentioned previously, some causes contribute to the great majority of deaths, which is referred to as bunching. Formulations in prospective medicine are made easier because of this tendency of problems to bunch. The Geller Tables of probability for a 40 year old white male, discussed earlier, list the ten leading causes of deaths per 100,000 population, when calculated for deaths that will occur during the next 10 years.[13] (See Table 10–2.) Note that the rates of death from myocardial infarction (ischemic heart disease) and stroke are falling while the rates of death from cancer of the lung, cirrhosis, and homicide are rising rapidly. The Geller Tables omit those causes of death that are so rare that they contribute less than 1 per cent to the total deaths for each age group studied.

High Risk Groups

Even before disease actually occurs, there are some people who fall into high risk groups and who could be said to be in great danger of incurring specific illnesses. Investigators using prospective studies have evaluated well people for their long-term risks and have carefully collected information about those who should be placed in the high risk groups. For the purposes of HHA, which at present is directed primarily toward adults aged 20 and over, there are approximately 25 important high risk groups in the United States. (See Table 10–1.) Those who smoke cigarettes are at very high risk of death from coronary heart disease. The American Heart Association has presented this evidence in the form of a manual for practitioners.[6] Thus, the real public enemies (those that have been demonstrated to cause the most premature deaths in the United States) are the prognostic characteristics that are considered by HHA to be the most crucial for high risk groups of adults aged 20 and over.[14] (See Fig. 10–3.)

Natural History of Disease and Injury

Everyone knows that, as a rule, disease becomes more lethal as it progresses. Figure 10–1, referred to previously, provides a schematic picture of the natural history of precursors of disease and injury. What is not sufficiently appreciated is that there is a long period during which disease can exist before there are any signs or symptoms. The relationship between cigarette smoking and heart disease is one such example.

Staging the natural history of cancer is important to the oncologist, whose treatment changes with the stage of the disease process. In the same manner, the family physician should know at what phase his patient is during the genesis of disease, for there is a growing resistance to intervention at each progressive stage. Most specialists believe that there is a definite relationship between the onset of a disease and the presence of a precursor. The nurse on the lung cancer unit will not believe that a patient's bronchogenic cancer was not caused by cigarette smoking!

Prognosis

In HHA, prognosis is expressed by comparing the individual patient's chances with the average population's risk. The patient can be twice average ($2\times$), or he can have half the average risk ($0.5\times$). The American Heart Association uses this formula in its *Coronary Risk Handbook*.[6] For example, the heavy smoker has a poorer prognosis than the light smoker.

Intervention

Robert Manning, in an address before the predecessor group to the Society of Prospective Medicine, said, "A difference to be a difference must make a difference."[9] There is a great difference between those who smoke and those who have stopped smoking and between those with high blood pressure and those whose blood pressure has been lowered. This is true also of the use or nonuse of alcohol and the consequences of cirrhosis. This difference has been called "survival advantage" by HHA. The family physician cannot promise to prevent or to cure, but he knows that there is a survival advantage for those who can claim to have changed to a low-risk group.

Presence of a Precursor

As mentioned previously, a precursor is a prognostic characteristic that appears before an actual disease is diagnosed in so many cases that its presence is cause for alarm. But can this danger from precursors, derived from group data, be applied to the individual? In the early days of HHA, many epidemiologists said, "You can't apply group data to the individual. He can't be half dead, or twice dead." Their work had been with populations, and, in truth, they couldn't apply group data to specific patients. But two different trillion dollar organizations were applying this data to individuals — life insurance companies and medical practice. The clinician applies group data to his patients in a hundred ways every day. The patient can easily be taught the significance of a precursor and can learn to appreciate the use of probabilities in evaluating his chances for safely surviving the next 10 years.

This Year's Appraisal

One sees changes in the leading causes of death yearly. (See Table 10–2.) Since there is little that is static in the state of health, there must be a continual updating of the tables used by HHA. Nothing is so important to the credibility of the program as the continual review of data to identify changes in prevalence, mortality, and risk reducibility. The work of updating is underway in a program developed by Health Hazard Appraisal, Inc. Health Hazard Appraisal, Inc., is a nonprofit health agency that has assumed the function of updating the risk factors used in HHA. The work is described in the Proceedings of the 12th Annual Meeting on Health Hazard Appraisal and Prospective Medicine.[16] Newsletters of Health Hazard Appraisal, Inc., are available from the Newsletter Office, 3925 North College Avenue, Indianapolis, Ind. 46205. The first ten newsletters are now in print.

SUMMARY

What is HHA? Is it the practice of medicine or the provision of health education? Some of the procedures, such as treatment of high blood pressure and counseling on the use of alcohol, are certainly appropriate for the medical profession, but many kinds of counseling can be performed better by health educators, nutritionists, and others. This is routine in other fields of medicine as well, and the physician who serves patients best will assume the role of captain of the entire health care team. HHA gives the physician a medium by which he can ensure that steps critical to extending useful life expectancy are being taken.

Behavioral scientists profess the ability to provide incentives for better patient compliance. Behavioral modification, normative systems, and many other developments in this field are advancing the day when a person who faces the lonely task of eliminating a habit or changing a life style can get support. But there is an issue here. Should a patient be helped by being provided incentives to prevent disease before knowing his total personal risk? Heart and cancer societies are looking for ways to achieve better patient compliance and have set up demonstrations to study the problem. But to single out heart disease, cancer, lung diseases, or accidents and apply incentives before knowing the patient's real problems is to further fragment medicine. The comprehensive and continuing care program provided by the family physician is a system designed to accomplish just what is needed—ensure that the patient's total health care program is integrated.

One of the most frequently recurring questions directed toward those practicing prospective medicine is, "Do we really know enough about prospective medicine to warrant making all that effort?" The physician must make that decision. The investigator is biased, for he will be looking at each issue to determine those unanswered questions that merit further study. The teacher is biased, for he must prepare the student to make practice decisions and cannot take the time to be an authority concerning all the precursors of disease and injury. This guide to prospective medicine is a practicing physician's guide, and the physician himself must choose what he will do for today's patients. HHA is one such tool that enables the family physician to give comprehensive and continuing care to his patients.

REFERENCES

1. Fuller, R. B.: Intuition. Garden City, N.Y., Doubleday & Co., 1973.
2. Gesner, N. B.: Derivation of Risk Factors from Comparative Data. Proceedings Seventh Annual Meeting, Prospective Medicine and Health Hazard Appraisal. Methodist Hospital of Indiana, Indianapolis, 1970.
3. Gordon, R. D., Bock, W., Egger, R. L., et al.: An Analysis of Patient's Chief Complaints Seen by Indiana Physicians—1974–1975. (In press.)
4. Hall, J. H., Robbins, L. C., and Gesner, N. B.: Whose health problem? Postgrad. Med., 51:114, 1972.
5. Hippocrates: The Book of Prognostics. In Major, R. H. (ed.): Classic Descriptions of Disease. 2nd Ed. Springfield, Ill., Charles C Thomas, Publisher, 1939.
6. Insull, W., Jr.: Estimating risk of coronary heart disease in daily practice. In American Heart Association—Coronary Risk Handbook, Dallas, Am. Heart Assoc., 1973.
7. Laplace, P. S.: Celestial Mechanics (Mecanique Celeste, Tome V, Fr.). Reprint of 1832 ed. New York, Chelsea Publishing Co., 1969.
8. Lauzon, R., Craig, P., and Colburn, H.: Health hazard appraisal: A fountain of youth. Can. Pharm. J., 7:75, 1974.
9. Manning, R. F.: Research into Risk Factors. Proceedings Seventh Annual Meeting, Prospective Medicine and Health Hazard Appraisal. Methodist Hospital of Indiana, Indianapolis, 1970.
10. Marsland, D. W., Wood, M., and Mayo, F.: Rank order of diagnoses by frequency. J. Fam. Pract., 3:38, 1976.
11. Morris, W. (ed.): American Heritage Dictionary of the English Language. Boston, Houghton-Mifflin Co., 1969.
12. Peery, T. M.: The old and new diseases. Am. J. Clin. Pathol., 63:453, 1975.
13. Robbins, L. C.: Geller Tables. Probability Tables of Deaths in the Next Ten Years from Specific Causes. Indianapolis, Methodist Hospital of Indiana, 1972.
14. Robbins, L. C., and Hall, J. H.: How to Practice Prospective Medicine. Indianapolis, Methodist Hospital of Indiana, 1970.
15. Sadusk, J. F., Jr., and Robbins, L. C.: Proposal for health hazard appraisal in comprehensive health care. J.A.M.A., 203:1108, 1968.
16. The Proceedings of the 12th Annual Meeting on Health Hazard Appraisal and Prospective Medicine. Bethesda, Md., Health and Education Resources Publishers, 1976.
17. The Top Twenty-Five Precursors of Disease and Injury. The Health Appraisal Briefing Board. Health Hazard Appraisal Newsletter, Update #9, Health Hazard Appraisal, Inc., 1977.
18. Vital Statistics of the United States, Vol. II, Part A. National Center for Health Statistics, Washington, D.C., Dept. of Health, Education and Welfare, 1974.

Chapter 11

HEALTH CARE DELIVERY

by FRANCIS L. LAND,
and DONALD IRVINE

This chapter will compare the United States system of health care delivery with the delivery system of the United Kingdom. We plan to identify the roles of the participants in health care systems and to provide some historical data.

UNITED STATES

NATIONAL HEALTH PROGRAMS

For many years the United States had several federal health programs that covered members of the military services, Merchant Marine, and Coast Guards, as well as the American Indian population.

In 1965 Congress passed both the "Medicare Act" and the "Medicaid Act," which was the beginning of the implementation of national health insurance. Medicare is targeted for the population of American citizens over the age of 65. It offers complete coverage for physicians' services and hospitalizations, with some deductibles that most recipients defray by supplemental insurance. This coverage has been enlarged to include those citizens who are totally and permanently disabled. Medicare is a *total federal program* funded by employer–employee contributions and general tax revenues.

Medicaid is a *federal–state program* funded by the general tax revenues of both governments. The contribution of the federal government begins at 50 per cent and goes as high as 79 per cent. This contribution is based upon the states' per capita income. Each state determines the monetary level of eligibility and the scope of services offered, although these vary from state to state.

Other federal–state programs have developed that are more disease-oriented, such as programs for end-stage renal disease (dialysis and transplantation), maternal and child health (high-risk pregnancy), and crippled children.

THE REFERRAL SYSTEM

The patient care system in the United States developed in a manner quite dissimilar to that of the United Kingdom. In the late 1800's and the first half of the 1900's, physicians worked in both their offices and the hospitals. Many of the hospitals were owned by the physicians themselves and were called proprietary institutions. Community hospitals were mainly developed by various church groups, but they were usually open to all physicians. After World War II, because of the increasing number of regulations by state health departments and in some instances by specific state laws, physician-owned hospitals began to disappear. Most of the remaining hospitals became truly community-oriented.

A trend began in the mid-50's to move toward a system of specialist-general practice similar to the British system. Hospital staffs began trying to delineate privileges, particularly those concerning the performance of certain surgical procedures by general practitioners. This occurred because more and more physicians were taking residency training before entering practice and were trying to eliminate competition from the general practitioners. However, a vigorous campaign was launched by the American Academy of General Practice and its state chapters that partially thwarted this effort. The Academy did this by insisting that privileges should not be awarded primarily on the basis of training but on the basis of experience and demonstrated competence.

THE EVOLUTION OF FAMILY PRACTICE

The beginning of family practice as a specialty goes back almost 70 years. In 1869 the American Medical Association (AMA) House of Delegates passed a resolution recognizing specialties as a proper and legitimate field of practice, stipulating that specialists should be governed by the same rules of professional ethics as were laid down for general practitioners. The first official specialty was ophthalmology, recognized in 1917, and other specialties followed.

Only 2 years later, in 1919, a resolution was introduced into the House of Delegates of the AMA recommending the designation of "family physicians" as a distinct specialty—the proposal was defeated. A similar resolution was introduced in 1941 and suffered the same consequence. However, a glimmer of hope came immediately after World War II (1946) when a section on general practice was developed by the AMA.

Shortly thereafter, a group of dedicated physicians concerned about the beginning decline in the number of general practitioners organized the American Academy of General Practice (AAGP). This today has grown to a membership of over 38,000, second only to the AMA in size. The Academy's objectives are: (1) to promote and maintain the highest standards of family practice, (2) to preserve the family physicians' rights to practice medicine to the full extent of their abilities, (3) to provide postgraduate training opportunities for the family physician, and (4) to advance the science of medicine and the health and welfare of the nation and to preserve the right of free choice of a physician by the patient.

The AAGP was the first and only national medical organization requiring continuing medical education for membership. The program consists of 50 hours of continuing education every year for a required total of 150 hours every 3 years for a renewal of membership. This is different from the American Board of Family Practice requirements, which will be explained later.

In 1959 an agreement was reached between the Council on Medical Education of the AMA and the AAGP to establish essentials for training in general practice. However, these programs were not well accepted. Few people enrolled and even fewer finished, for they were not able to be certified by any specialty, and medical graduates had become increasingly motivated toward getting the "piece of paper." The AMA recognized this and in 1957 appointed an ad hoc committee on preparation for the specialty of family practice, which made its report in 1959.

Meanwhile, what was happening to the supply of primary physicians in the United States? There was an increase in general internists, general pediatricians, and obstetrics–gynecology practitioners. However, this increase did not make up for the decrease in family physicians, with the result that there were fewer physicians to provide primary care. The medical profession had developed a trend requiring two or three physicians per family rather than one, probably sincerely believing this was the best type of medical care, but also doubling and at times tripling the cost of such care to the family.

It was hoped that the report of 1959 would encourage more graduates to enter the field of general practice, but again the numbers entering these residencies were very few. No medical schools had graduate programs in general practice, and there was no means of affording graduates in general practice academic professional recognition.

At the same time, the supply of primary physicians continued to decline and resulted in the public's asking, "Why can't I find a doctor?" As a result of this aroused public interest, it appeared that more in-depth studies should be made, and in 1964 three separate and completely independent groups began studying the problem. These groups were (1) the National Commission for Community Health Services (Folsom Report),[3] (2) the Report of the Citizens Commission on Graduate Medical Education (Millis Commission),[7] and (3) the Ad Hoc Committee on Education for Family Practice of the Council on Graduate Medical Education (Willard Report).[4] Amazingly, within a 3 month period in 1966, these three committees, using somewhat different semantics, reported many similar findings.

The Folsom Commission stressed the need for every individual to have a *personal physician* for easy access to health care on a coordinated, comprehensive, and continuing basis. This physician should be knowledgeable in preventive medicine and in the use of community resources.[3] The Millis Commission identified a physician somewhat similarly but chose a different name, the *primary physician*. In addition, the Millis Commission Report is having a widespread effect on all medical education.[7] A new term for this physician who would be the new specialist was coined by the Ad Hoc Committee on Education for Family Practice, and this was the *family physician*, the name that has remained viable.[4]

As a result of these very forward-looking reports of 1966, the AAGP placed increased emphasis on the development of a specialty board in family practice. Obviously, this took a great amount of time and discussion. It was not until February 6, 1969, that the American Board of Family Practice became a reality, when it was formally approved as the 20th specialty board in American medicine.

At the time of this writing (1977), almost 11,000 physicians have been certified by the American Board of Family Practice. The eighth examination will be given in October of this year. Twenty-eight per cent of those taking the examination are residency-trained.[5]

In 1970 approximately 250 medical graduates in the United States entered residency training in family practice. In 1971 this increased to more than 500 graduates. It is anticipated that in July 1977 over 2000 students will enter residencies in family practice. This will be approximately 15 per cent of the nation's graduates. There are now 84 departments and 14 divisions of family practice in the United States. There are 304 residency programs and the following number of residents in training: first year—1861, second year—1577, and third year—1237, for a total of 4675 trainees.

In this brief period of 20 years, a revolution in medical education designed to meet the needs of patients rather than medical educators has occurred.

CHANGES IN DELIVERY OF HEALTH CARE

Prior to World War II, most physicians practiced in a solo situation, managing the office as well as taking care of patients. In many instances, the office and home were adjoining. Following World War II, there was a trend away from solo practice and into partnerships or groups. Solo practice, for a variety of reasons, became the least desirable method of practicing. Most observers feel that some of the factors involved in the shift from solo practice to partnerships and groups are:

1. Physicians entering the armed forces in World War II were given ranks based upon the number of years of specialty training, not upon their ability or degree of experience. For example, a physician with 15 years' experience might well enter the service with the same rank as one who had just completed 3 years of residency.

2. Medical knowledge was expanding rapidly, partly due to advances in medicine and surgery made during the war. Physicians began to seek a more limited field, emphasizing depth rather than breadth. The availability of the GI bill after military service certainly aided and abetted the number of physicians taking residency training.

3. Military medicine is, in essence, a partnership or group type of practice. Physicians began to realize the advantages of such an arrangement, such as providing more regular hours, a more organized life, more time with their families, and more time for study and continuing medical education.

4. Some physicians were attracted to partnership or group practice because of the sharing of resources. Expenses were reduced by having a common waiting room, bookkeeping system, and so forth.

Several definitions of group practice have been developed. The one used most commonly is that of the AMA: "The application of medical services by three or more fulltime physicians formally organized to provide medical care, consultation, diagnosis, and/or treatment through the joint use of equipment and personnel and with the income from medical practice distributed in accordance with methods previously determined by members of the group."[2]

These groups were developed in different ways with a variety of fiscal arrangements being represented. In some, all physicians in the group receive the same remuneration; in others, the remuneration is based upon work unit performance; in still others, it is based upon the specialty.

The increase in group practice has been dramatic. In 1946 there were 368 groups in the United States and in 1969 there were 6173. Approximately 50 per cent of the total are single specialty groups.[3] As group practice expanded, there was a concurrent development of prepayment groups in contradistinction to fee-for-service arrangements.

Because of the rapid development of group practice, increased emphasis was placed on disease prevention. Health planners designed a prepayment delivery structure known as the Health Maintenance Organization (HMO). This was designed to provide preventive, diagnostic, and therapeutic services to patients based on a fixed or capitation fee paid by the patient or the employer. These programs were well supported by federal funding but at the time of this writing do not appear to be too successful.

The first medical school faculty group practice was developed at Johns Hopkins University in 1870. In the last 25 years, medical schools have moved toward full-time facilities and have developed what are referred to as practice plans. The arrangements vary from school to school, but in general the faculty physicians' professional fees are pooled, and an agreed-upon distribution is made. Most medical school faculty members see private patients in addition to their teaching, research, and administrative responsibilities.

There has also been an increase in the number of full-time hospital-based physicians. The earliest hospital-based specialists were pathologists and radiologists; however, we are also seeing increasing numbers of other specialists entering full-time activity as chiefs of such services as medicine, pediatrics, cardiology, or physiatry. This is also occurring in many community hospitals (Table 11–1).

FUTURE TRENDS

There are many proponents of national health insurance in the United States, particularly wihin organized labor. President Jimmy Carter has promised in his speeches and in the Democratic platform that there will be such a program. However, it would be expensive and the present high unemployment rate and inflation have led to an unstable economy. Therefore it would appear that national health insurance will be delayed until the economy is stabilized, which may be many years.

TABLE 11–1.   ACTIVE PHYSICIANS IN THE UNITED STATES IN 1966*

In Practice			274,190
Civilian (non-federal)		249,273	
Solo or group practice	190,079		
Full-time hospital practice	16,604		
Interns, residents, and fellows	42,590		
Federal		24,917	
Full-time hospital practice	20,651		
Interns, residents, and fellows	4,266		
Not in Practice			19,882
Civilian (non-federal)		17,247	
Medical faculty	11,166		
Research	3,352		
Administration	2,729		
Federal		2,635	
Research	1,243		
Administration	1,392		
Population per active physician	1 per 700		
Total active physicians			294,072

*(From: The Graduate Education of Physicians: Report of the Citizens Committee on Graduate Medical Education, Chicago, American Medical Association, 1966. Copyright 1966, American Medical Association.)

UNITED KINGDOM

NATIONAL HEALTH SERVICE

To understand the aims, functions, and structure of the National Health Service (NHS) requires an historical perspective because the present Service is the result of an evolutionary process reflecting changes in the patterns of illness, advances in medicine, effects of social legislation, and changes in the function and structure of the medical and other health professions. The NHS provides medical care that is free at the time of use for any person in the country who chooses to use it. A small but important private sector coexists alongside the state Service.

The National Insurance Act of 1911 provided prepaid medical care by general practitioners for a substantial segment of the population but furnished no entitlement to hospital or specialist services. In 1948 the NHS was introduced, with the object of extending health care paid for by a combination of state insurance and direct taxation to the whole population. The main effects of the NHS were (1) to give patients medical care free at the time of use, (2) to increase greatly the number and geographic distribution of consultants (specialists) so that the entire population had reasonable access to specialist services, and (3) to establish in law the right of the entire population to the services of general practitioners who would provide primary, continuing, and terminal care in accordance with Terms and Conditions of Service, which were extremely widely drawn and thus capable of generous interpretation. The NHS did not, however, incorporate those health professions that provided preventive and occupational medicine through local government authorities.

In the early years of the NHS there were thus three main career groups in British medicine. Principals in general practice predominated. They were largely solo practitioners working from their own premises and homes, and they contracted their professional services to the NHS, since they had chosen not to enter salaried employment. Consultants, who now staffed the NHS hospitals, became full- or part-time salaried employees of the NHS. Full-time employees had no right to see private patients; those with part-time contracts retained the right to engage in a limited amount of private work. The smaller number of public health physicians remained salaried employees of local government authorities to provide general preventive services in the community. With one or two minor exceptions, physicians who were not in one of these main career grades were juniors in training.

In 1973 the National Health Services Reorganisation Act was passed. This act was intended administratively to unify the three main elements — general practice, hospital specialist, and local authority preventive services. It has provided an elaborate system of management in which the country is divided into health regions, each region in turn being subdivided into a number of health areas. When the health areas are excessively large, further subdivisions into health districts have been created.

The government health departments in England, Wales, Scotland, and Northern Ireland are at the top of the management pyramid and are responsible for major decisions about the provision of health services. The regional authorities are an intermediate tier of management, intended primarily to supervise major capital building projects, such as the construction of new hospitals, and to coordinate the arrangements for those regionally based specialties such as neurosurgery, radiotherapy, and venereology. The area health authorities are the effective authorities for the provision of local medical services, and at this level there is an elaborate arrangement to ensure collaboration between the medical and social services.

The general management principle is one of accountability upward and delegation of authority downward, with public participation throughout. It is as yet too early to judge the consequences of this reorganization, although it is already evident that there has been a great expansion in the bureaucracy of the NHS, and there is a general feeling among health professionals of all kinds that the Service is now overadministered, with too little time and money being given to the needs of patients, physicians, nurses, and other health professionals and too much to management for management's sake.

TABLE 11–2. MANPOWER SUMMARY (GREAT BRITAIN) FOR YEARS 1966 AND 1974. (From the Annual Reports of the Department of Health and Social Security)

Type of Personnel	Numbers	
	1966	*1974*
Hospital medical staff		
Total	22,802	31,473
Consultants	8,306	11,459
Juniors in training	13,313	18,705
Various types of medical assistants	1,183	1,309
General practitioners		
Total	23,977	25,849
Principals	23,003	24,595
Assistants	820	532
Trainees (residents)	154	722
Hospital nurses	276,858	370,220
Hospital midwives	17,803	21,531
Community nurses°		
Total	24,275	31,591
Home nurses	9,146	12,793
Health visitors	6,427	8,240
Midwives	5,783	4,387
Other general nursing staff	2,919	6,171
Hospital administrative and clerical staff	49,724	80,558
Family practitioner committee staff (NHS administration for general practice)	4,866	5,634 (1973)

° Full-time equivalent

The distribution of health professionals in the Service is shown in Table 11–2.

THE REFERRAL SYSTEM

The health service in the United Kingdom differs distinctly from health care systems in comparable countries in Western Europe and North America in terms of the arrangements made for providing primary and continuing care and the relationship between general practitioners and specialist physicians. Both primary and continuing care are almost entirely in the hands of general practitioners who are each responsible for a defined, registered population of some 2500 people. General practice thus furnishes the normal gateway for patients wanting to use any other part of the NHS.

Specialists work almost exclusively in hospitals. The professional ethic normally forbids them to provide primary medical care; thus, they see patients who are referred by general practitioners rather than accept patients directly. The one general exception to this rule is in the use of hospital accident services in which, for obvious reasons, patients may enter the hospital service immediately. In recent years the division of responsibility between general and specialist practice has become somewhat blurred. An increasing number of general practitioners work part-time in hospitals, and a small number of hospital specialists are beginning to contribute to the work of health centers and group medical practices in the community.

The origin of the "referral" system is interesting. It can be traced to the 17th century, when medical care was provided by a small number of physicians who in the main were recruited from and treated only the upper classes and by apothecaries who were of lower social status and treated the lower classes. In the 18th century, physicians and surgeons, who were nearly all confined to the London area, often gave their services free to charitable hospitals, and they used these appointments to train their successors. Apothecaries, since they were excluded from hospitals, were trained through an apprenticeship with an older apothecary. These divisions between different kinds of practitioners led to much friction and competition for patients. The disputes culminated in the formation of the British Medical Association (BMA), which was designed to counter the established authority of the Royal Colleges of Physicians in London and Edinburgh. By 1858 the new BMA had persuaded government to introduce the Medical Acts, with the object of setting standards for the practice of medicine that would protect the public by distinguishing qualified doctors from charlatans and quacks. The General Medical Council, set up to administer the Medical Acts, acquired effective control of basic medical education provided through the universities, so that shortly afterward there followed a fairly uniform system of training medical students throughout the country. Postgraduate education was excluded from the Medical Acts and thus remained in the hands of the Royal Colleges.

Despite the Medical Acts, the division between those who were specialists and worked mainly in hospitals and those who were generalists and worked mainly in the community persisted for many years. Physicians in hospitals, although they treated some patients privately in their homes, concentrated their work on the institutions and, as they specialized, began to act as "consultants" to other physicians who had a more general interest. In return for this acknowledgment of status, which increased as standards of nursing and general care improved in hospitals, the consultants agreed to accept only work that was referred to them. Thus, in the first half of this century the general practitioners were largely excluded from hospitals but controlled access to patients, and the consultants now enjoyed the prestige and status of specialization through their honorary appointments in the major hospitals but were dependent on the practitioners for their income. This professional division of responsibility was reflected in the structure of the new NHS.

THE EVOLUTION OF GENERAL PRACTICE

The last two decades have seen a radical transformation of general practice. In the 1950's general practitioners were jolted into a painful reappraisal of their effectiveness as providers of primary and continuing medical care by a series of critical reports on the standards of their work, their organization (or rather the lack of it), and their apparently inappropriate education. Thoughtful physicians who recognized that improvements could not be secured by medico-political means alone began to examine and describe their work and to consider how their education could be changed to equip them more adequately for the tasks they were identifying. They coordinated their efforts through the College of General Practitioners, which they founded.

There have been three broadly recognizable stages in the evolution of general practice in the last 20 years. In the 1950's and 1960's group practice (involving only general practitioners) was encouraged, and, as a consequence, the solo practitioner has almost disappeared today. The main emphasis was on finding better ways of organizing general practice, providing a practice administration so that the physician could delegate secretarial tasks, gaining access to NHS diagnostic and treatment facilities, and bringing community nurses, health visitors, and more recently social workers together to form functionally integrated primary health care teams. The movement was given impetus by the "Charter" of 1966, an agreement between general practitioners and government that provided financial incentives to promote group practice, furnished funds to assist the private development of purpose-built premises, initiated a major health center building program for physicians who preferred to work in state-owned premises, and introduced direct subsidies to better enable physicians to provide their own clerical and nursing staff.

Today many of the improvements sought have been secured. All general practitioners have right of access to diagnostic radiology and laboratory services in the NHS, a major rebuilding program is under way, general practice is being reequipped, the framework of local practice administration has been funded and provided, and the development of the primary care health team concept is well advanced.

The second evolutionary stage has been about education and the setting of professional standards. The Royal College of General Practitioners played a prominent role in the initiation of experimental residency programs in the 1960's, and these programs have now been given formal recognition by the passing of the National Health Service (Vocational Training) Act, which will obligate any physician who wishes to work as a principal in general practice in the NHS first to demonstrate that he has completed the required postgraduate training. This is a step forward of immense significance; it should lead to generally improved standards of patient care.

A third stage is now emerging. Since general practice has secured its position as the main provider of primary and continuing care in the NHS, it has moved from a low status to a much higher status career in medicine. This new strength and sense of security are fostering a willingness to look again at the relationship between primary care and the hospital specialties on the one hand and primary care and social services on the other. These new factors also underpin the more questioning approach to continuing education and the thorny question of auditing standards of professional performance. They are also encouraging general practitioners to think more seriously about the contributions they can make to such increasingly relevant but underdeveloped subjects as health education and health care maintenance, in addition to cultivating those areas already revealed as fruitful for research in contemporary practice.

FUTURE TRENDS

The NHS is being looked at critically by many countries which are grappling with the problems of reconciling the potential of technologic medicine with the need for care, the changing expectations that societies have of medicine, and the capacity and willingness of communities to pay for services. The NHS was a remarkable social experiment, and it has brought Britain face to face with these problems at perhaps an earlier stage than in some other countries. The NHS system of care has certainly had its strengths; it has, for example, removed the worry of paying for medical care at a time of illness, and it has achieved a fairly even geographic distribution of physicians, something that is not obtained in every Western country by any means. It has also achieved a reasonably balanced and efficient way of securing primary and continuing medical care, which is local and easily available, and specialist care, which can be used when needed. It is a system that, in certain important respects at any rate, is well geared to meet the main health care problems we are likely to encounter for the remainder of the century.

There are important difficulties that we have to recognize and face. Some in the United Kingdom view the NHS system as fair and equitable and about the best method available. Others argue that the NHS should concentrate on essential services and that certain health needs that do not directly affect survival should be paid for privately by individuals. What is becoming clear is that the piecemeal approach to the provision of health care in the NHS cannot continue, and the decline in our economy has simply brought into sharper focus the problems that would have become inevitable anyway. It is for this compelling reason that there is a new interest in finding ways of evaluating the effectiveness of health services, of devising ways by which the community can make choices and order priorities, of making people more self-reliant than they have become in the welfare state, and of curbing the extensive intrusion of bureaucracy.

REFERENCES

1. Fry, J., and Farndale, W. A. J.: International Medical Care. Baltimore, University Park Press, 1972.
2. Group Practice and Medical Groups in the USA. Report of the Council of Medical Services, Chicago, American Medical Assoc., 1969.
3. Health is a Community Affair. Report of the National Committee on Community Health Services. Cambridge, Mass., Harvard University Press, 1966.
4. Meeting the Challenge of Family Practice, Report of the Ad Hoc Committee on Education for Family Practice of the Council of Medical Education. Chicago, American Medical Assoc., 1966.
5. Personal Communication. Nicholas Pisacano, M.D., Secretary, American Board of Family Practice, Lexington, Ky.
6. Report of the Division of Education. American Academy of Family Physicians, 1976.
7. The Graduate Education of Physicians. Report of the Citizens Committee on Graduate Medical Education. Chicago, American Medical Assoc., 1966.

Chapter 12

UTILIZATION OF COMMUNITY RESOURCES

by DONALD F. TREAT,
and MATTHEW L. HENK

The rising health care expectations of people in today's world are placing increasing demands on those trying to provide the needed care. As a front line provider of primary care for patients and their families, the family physician is often the first professional to whom individuals turn for help when they can no longer cope with their problems. By the time such a step is taken, the problems are often complex and have ramifications in the socioeconomic areas of the patients' lives, as well as psychologic and physical manifestations. One has only to reflect upon the many problems commonly associated with the alcoholic, the pregnant teenager, or the unemployed individual to appreciate the magnitude of the task facing the family physician. Therefore, it is imperative for those physicians dedicated to providing comprehensive and continuing health care to be able to mobilize other resources in an efficient and effective manner.

Except in certain life-threatening crisis situations, the physician must resist the impulse to refer quickly and should, instead, proceed toward the goal of relieving the patient's distress in an orderly, logical manner. The steplike progression toward resolving the patient's problems is analogous to the familiar method of managing straightforward medical problems. The first step is to identify the patient's problems. For this, the time-honored interview between the patient and his physician is still the most effective and versatile diagnostic tool available. In family practice, with the inevitable time constraints, the interview can profitably be regarded as a continuing process occurring over as many visits as are necessary to arrive at an acceptable goal for the patient.

The physician will enhance the possibility of a successful outcome if he brings certain attributes to the interview process. The first attribute is self-awareness. A physician who is aware of his own biases and prejudices is less likely to be judgmental and paternalistic; he is more likely to help the patient deal with his problems rather than to respond on the basis of what he feels would be best for the patient. If strong feelings arise toward the patient (either positive or negative), the physician should recognize that such feelings indicate countertransference, a psychologic reaction that can seriously blur objectivity.

Another facet of self-awareness is knowing and accepting one's own limitations. Often patients will have problems requiring the expertise of others in the helping community—social workers, marriage counselors, attorneys, and clinical psychologists, to name a few. An ability and willingness to work with others is therefore essential. The second attribute is / an appreciation of the many limitations and frustrations workers in other helping professions experience in today's complex, highly regulated society. Having such an understanding can help the physician avoid participating in the frequent blame directed at helpers by disappointed patients.

The interview process for a patient whose complaints suggest an underlying psychologic or social dysfunction, or both, can conveniently and logically be divided into six steps: problems identified, problems clarified, problems defined, plan proposed, plan selected, and plan implemented and follow-up.

SIX STEP PROCESS

Patients usually come to their physician with a complaint that they believe the physician will accept as an appropriate reason for the visit. This "ticket of admission" presents a starting point from which the interviewer can guide and encourage the patient toward a full exposition of the problem. (A description of how this can be accomplished is summarized in Chapter 19.) Step one can be considered completed, at least temporarily, when the patient and the interviewer can agree on what problem, or problems, probably underlie the presenting complaint.

For example, a middle-aged woman presents with the complaint of fatigue. The interview establishes that the patient is also concerned about her "nerves," that her teenaged daughter no longer "respects" her, that she and her husband are "drifting apart," and that she is "worried about the bills." In this example, possible problems in areas of her emotional health, her family relationships, and her economic security are readily identified.

The next step is to clarify the identified problems so that their possible inter-relationships, current status, and relative importance can be understood. This is a time-consuming but necessary step, and one frequently resisted by the patient who will often be pressing the interviewer to "tell me what to do." Clarification includes what the patient has done about the problem in the past, results attained, and who is currently involved in trying to help with the problem. Many patients have been inappropriately moved from one agency, physician, or counselor to another because the primary physician neglected to ask, "Who has been helping you with this problem?" Appropriate and responsible use of a community's health resources requires such knowledge.

To return to our example, clarification of the problem of "nerves" may establish that the patient sought psychiatric help in the past, that her daughter recently moved out of the house after an argument over the daughter's sexual activity, that the patient and her husband are sleeping apart, and that her husband has not received an anticipated pay raise. In addition, appropriate questioning and examinations would have clarified the possibility of organic disease as a contributing factor to the patient's fatigue.

At this point, interviewer and patient work toward definition of the problems in terms acceptable to both. This third step is necessary to focus attention on problems rather than on symptoms and to formulate a priority list of problems. It may be possible to subsume some problems under others. As in the example, the financial and family problems may well be results of a dysfunctional marriage and may be the major factors in the patient's emotional anxiety, depression, or both.

Once the problems have been defined and agreed upon, the fourth step is to examine possible courses of action. It is here that the physician's knowledge about available community resources is important. The more he knows about who can do what for the patient, the more realistic and informed the proposed options can be. Although most patients want to "do something" about their problems, others may not be willing or able to act, at least temporarily. The option of doing nothing should usually be offered. An exception would be a severely depressed patient, particularly if suicidal, or a psychotic patient on whom decisions must sometimes be proposed. In our example, the options might look like this:

1. Do nothing—hope things will not get worse.
2. Bring entire family in for interview with possibility of eventual referral for family therapy.
3. If husband is willing, refer couple to marriage counselor.
4. Invite husband to joint interview for further clarification of marital problems.

At this juncture, the physician may well be pressured again by the patient to "tell me what to do." Again, the physician must recognize that unless the patient has participated in the decision, he will have little invested in the outcome. Also, failure to achieve expected results can easily be shifted to the physician: "He didn't tell me the right thing to do. I guess he can't help me, and I should see another doctor."

Step five involves the joint selection of a plan of action by patient and physician. As each option is considered, the physician should patiently help the patient examine the reasons for or against the option and the feelings it arouses in the patient. The knowledgeable and skillful physician can do much to allay the patient's fear of referral to other agencies, physicians, and so forth. Important in this regard is reassurance of the physician's continuing interest and support. Also, as each option is considered, the physician must clarify what his role might be: therapist, counselor, referring physician, and so forth.

The sixth and final step is the implementation of the agreed-upon plan of action and follow-up. In our example, a decision may have been made to arrange for a family assessment interview by the physician in his office, with the hope that the family would agree to accept referral for therapy. Subsequent referral for therapy may require a repetition of all six steps, because the new individuals were not part of the decision-making process. This is not "wasted" time; a successful outcome depends upon a series of successful steps. Although in some cases the referral process can be shortened, the better course is to offer a full explanation and discussion to all members.

A provision for follow-up is essential for the reassurance of the patient and the education of the physician. The patient knows that there is someone he can return to if things don't work out; the physician learns which community resources seem best suited for specific kinds of problems within his practice.

COMMUNITY RESOURCES

We have presented a description of a process by which a patient's problems can be identified, clarified, and defined and, subsequently, a course of action selected. To adequately present the options for intervention in the patient's problems, the physician must have a good working knowledge of the community resources or work closely with someone who does. Just as the medical resources vary greatly throughout the country, so do the resources available to help meet other human needs vary widely from one community to another. In general, health and welfare resources can be divided into two categories: public, or tax supported, resources and private resources, which may be profit, nonprofit, sectarian, or nonsectarian.

Public (Tax Supported) Agencies
A. Financial—social services
1. Department of Public Welfare
2. State Employment Office
3. Office of Social Security
4. Medicaid and Medicare
5. Child Protective
B. Health services
1. Department of Public Health
a. Disease surveillance and diagnostic laboratories
b. Epidemiology
c. Disease prevention, accident prevention, patient education
d. Screening programs (lead, tuberculosis)
e. Public health nursing
f. Clinics for specific diseases (venereal disease, drug abuse)
g. Mental health services
h. Infant and child health programs
i. Housing inspection
2. Municipal and county hospitals
a. Variety of diagnostic and therapeutic services
C. Employment services
1. Vocational rehabilitation
a. Testing, counseling, placement services
D. Fire and police
E. Courts—legal services
F. Education resources
1. Public school system
a. Testing, counseling, special classes
2. Public libraries
3. Agriculture extension services—rural areas
a. Homemaking, nutrition

Private Agencies
A. Volunteer—self-help, neighborhood, community organizations
1. Examples: *Recovery*—self-help program for former mental patients, *Friends in Service Here* (FISH)—emergency transportation, child care, homemaking services, and so forth, *Drug and Alcohol Council*—volunteer educational programs, *Big Brother Program*—voluntary supportive relationships with the underprivileged

B. Sectarian (religious affiliation)
   1. Extended care facilities, nursing home for aged
   2. Named agencies (e.g., Salvation Army, Catholic Charities)
   3. Churches and synagogues
     a. Counseling, support
C. Nonsectarian (no particular religious affiliation)
   1. Extended care facilities, nursing homes for aged
   2. Named agencies (e.g., Boy Scouts, Senior Citizens, Family Services)
   3. Financial counselors
   4. Hospitals and clinics
   5. Educational agencies (e.g., Childbirth Education Association)
   6. Specific disease services (e.g., American Diabetic Association, American Cancer Society)

Some of these resources are provided at no charge to the patient; others are available for a fee. Some restrict their clientele to a specific age, or religious sect, or certain financial circumstances. Moreover, limitations and requirements that apply to an agency in one community may not apply in another. Therefore, the practicing physician finds it necessary to learn what the resources are in his particular community. As this knowledge is acquired through contact with the various agencies, many find that filing of information about the agencies in a Community Resources File provides a valuable and available reference. We suggest a problem-oriented subject index as most feasible, as shown in Table 12–1.

TABLE 12–1. PROBLEM-ORIENTED SUBJECT INDEX

Abortion – Family Planning	Handicapped Children and Adults
Adoption	Health Education
Alcoholism	Housing
Blind	Information and Referral
Cancer	Library
Child Behavior	Legal
Child Neglect	Mental Health
Consumer Education and Protection	Mental Retardation
Counseling – Family, Geriatric, Marital, Financial, Parenting	Neighborhood Services
	Nursing
Day Care	Public Health
Disability	Recreation
Drug Abuse	Rehabilitation
Education	Shelter and Clothing
Emergency Services	Speech and Hearing
Employment	Transportation
Environmental Health	Unmarried Parents
Family Services	Volunteer Opportunities
Financial Aid	Welfare
Food	Welfare Advocacy

Each indexed subject should contain descriptions of those agencies and organizations that provide services to the community. The entry description of each agency should include:
1. Name of agency
2. Address of agency
3. Telephone number of agency
4. Individual to contact for referral purposes
5. Name of agency administrator
6. Office and service hours per day, days per week
7. Concise list of continuing activities and services
8. Geographic area served
9. Income or age level or other requirements for eligibility
10. Fees
11. Procedure for referring
12. Waiting lists

REFERRAL PROCESS

A child behavior problem is a convenient example of a family practice situation that frequently requires referral to a community resource. The following steps can help the physician obtain the information necessary to make an appropriate referral.

The physician should first determine which agencies accept referral of child behavior problems. He can begin by:
1. Turning to "Social Services Organizations" in the yellow pages of the telephone directory and calling those agencies that appear to work with this type of problem
2. Calling the school principal, nurse, or mental health team
3. Calling the community mental health center
4. Calling the social worker at the hospital
5. Calling the public health nurse
6. Calling an information and referral agency
7. Asking a colleague

Secondly, the physician contacts those agencies that he thinks might respond and asks for an appointment with a staff person. At the same time, the physician can ask for descriptive printed materials that may answer many of the questions. The appointment provides an opportunity to obtain the basic information suggested earlier, such as fees, time involved in obtaining entry, and hours. In the example of a behavior problem, one would inquire about psychologic testing and determine:

1. The qualifications of the workers
2. The types of therapy they provide (individual, drug, group, family)
3. The referral process, i.e., if the patient must call or if the physician can and if a written referral is needed
4. The type of feedback they give and the involvement they allow for the referring source
5. The provisions, if any, for phone consultations

The collected information would then be kept in the Subject Index File. A major objective of this process is not just to obtain information but to develop a professional relationship with the community agency staff. We cannot overemphasize the value of this relationship. The better the physician and the agency staff know each other's abilities and limitations, the more likely it is that appropriate and useful consultations and referrals will result.

Although, ideally, this information would be obtained before the need arose, in practice the physician may need to undertake this process when first encountering the problem. Patients can often wait a few days to obtain a service, particularly if they are reassured that the most appropriate resource will be selected as a result.

For behavior problems in children, the physician will find helpful resources in most communities among the following types of agencies:

1. The community mental health program, usually federally subsidized and operated by the county government
2. The child guidance agencies, such as Family Services, which are funded by the community through private donations
3. Private psychologists, psychiatrists, and social workers on a fee-for-service basis
4. The mental health team at the school

The breadth and depth of available services will vary from community to community, depending upon population characteristics, geographic location, identified needs, special resources, and other factors. In most locations, a combination of private agencies and professionals, along with federal, state, and local government tax-supported agencies, provide for relatively uniform basic health and welfare services. It is the physician's responsibility to call upon these resources wisely and appropriately so that the greatest benefits can be obtained for patients at the least cost to the community.

REFERENCES

1. American Hospital Association Guide to the Health Care Field. Chicago, American Hospital Assoc., 1976.
2. Farley, E. S., and Treat, D. F.: Utilization of community resources. *In* Conn, H. F., Rakel, R. E., and Johnson, T. W. (eds.): Family Practice, 1st ed. Philadelphia, W. B. Saunders Co., 1973.
3. Gross, J. N.: Guide to the Community Control of Alcoholism. New York, American Public Health Association, 1968.
4. Gurevity, H., and Heath, D.: The community and clinical practice. *In* Lamb, H. L. (ed.): Handbook of Community Mental Health Practice. The San Mateo Experience. San Francisco, Jossey-Bass, Inc., Publishers, 1969.
5 Whiting, L., and Hassinger, E. (eds.): Rural Health Services: Organization, Delivery and Use. Ames, Iowa, Iowa State University Press, 1976.

Chapter 13

ALLIED HEALTH PROFESSIONALS

by EDWARD J. KOWALEWSKI,
and KATHLEEN C. MORTON

INTRODUCTION

The authors wish to discuss the topic of the allied health professionals with the reader's full appreciation that we are addressing our thoughts to primary physicians, and specifically to family physicians, based on our own experience. This includes private practice as well as academic involvement and exposure to the development of programs for different categories of allied health professionals. In addition, we have both worked with various levels of personnel in the service arena.

We wish to outline what can be done to assist the physician in providing good quality care in a system that permits him to best utilize his own special skills and training in his medical practice.

We cannot single out or recommend any individual or group of allied health professionals who are the best or who would necessarily be the best for every physician. This must be determined by the specific needs of each physician's practice, his community, and his own personality. We do, however, feel that the family physician should consider the unique responsibilities of family practice that he needs to fulfill in determining the best personnel to work with him. The family physician functions largely, although not exclusively, at the entry point of medical care. His involvement with a patient at any time may be primary, secondary, or tertiary, depending on the complexity of the illness. The family physician must be comprehensive in his approach, offer continuity of care, and be able to work with all ages and sexes. He must be well versed in emergency medi-

cine but holistic in his approach to everyday care. He needs to practice preventive and prospective medicine and to be involved with the individual as well as with the community, although his main concern revolves around the family. He has important managerial responsibilities for patient health care. Therefore, because of the breadth of family practice, the specific requirements for the type of assistance needed, and the variations in the clinical setting, it is impossible to generalize about the recommendations for allied health professionals.

How then does one find reliable assistants, people who can fulfill many needs by being generally trained and who have the flexibility to adjust to an ever-changing situation? Some allied health professionals will be involved with the physician on a full-time basis and will function solely as employees. Others will be part-time, possibly because of family commitments or continuing education requirements. Still others may reside in a community setting and may be called upon only for specific limited purposes. Depending on the level of expertise that the new allied health professional exhibits, there may be a sharing of responsibility with the physician or a total delegation of care with minimal supervision and responsibility by the physician.

Finally, in this introduction, we would like to emphasize the most important factor in the utilization of allied health professionals. This is a generality, but if the physician has neither the personality nor the natural ability to work comfortably with others, he lacks the main prerequisites of potential success in working with someone from the group of allied health professionals.

HISTORICAL BACKGROUND

To appreciate where we are today and how we arrived here, it is important to provide some of the historical background and highlights that occurred in the past 10 years. Our working definition of allied health professionals incorporates many different categories of care. Some demand a specific formal educational requirement, many at the master's level. People in these categories have a clear job description delineated by educational objectives and accepted by proper accrediting bodies. Such people would include:

1. Physician "extenders"—individuals who work closely with a physician, who do not make independent decisions, and who are another arm for the physician so that he may see more patients more quickly and more adequately. The general heading of physician extender includes many designations, such as health assistant, health associate, physician assistant, physician associate, MEDEX, or someone such as an aide trained specifically to help with certain aspects of the office practice.

2. Physician "collaborators"—individuals with previous health care training, whose work and life experiences contribute to the development and subsequent refinement of their techniques, either "on-the-job" or through a didactic program. This group would include graduates from nursing programs and some personnel from the armed services. Titles such as adult, family, or pediatric nurse practitioner, midwife, and clinical specialist are used.

Many titles are therefore used for the same type of role. The common denominator for all the groups is that they have training and experience that enables them to perform certain functions so that they participate in the assessment and care of patients, whether in a dependent, interdependent, or sharing relationship. It can be very confusing to differentiate each category. Indeed, the variation that occurs in the same setting may result in a change of the allied health professional's role from patient to patient, according to the needs as perceived by the allied health professional, the physician, and the patient requiring care.

From the beginning of recorded medical history, physicians have been assisted by individuals with less training than themselves. The term "physician assistant" was first used by Paracelsus in 1524. The arrangement at that time was that the physician's (or academician's) only duty was to read from medical books and the "assistant's" duty was to touch the patient.

In the United States the first actual practical and recognized physician assistant was frequently the wife of the physician. This was feasible both logically and geographically because most physicians had their offices in their homes or very near to where they lived. By and large, before the 1940's the only physicians with offices away from home were limited to a few specialists and to a small number of physicians practicing in the larger cities. Also, the majority of physicians were solo practitioners who did not consider the hospital areas or academic centers appropriate places to deliver ambulatory care.

About the time of World War II, from 1939 to 1945, medical practice began to change. Specialty practice emerged and became the vogue, with group practice gaining in popularity. More physicians chose to settle in the urban and suburban areas, and few new physicians replaced the general practitioners in the community. At the same time, the nurse who graduated from a traditional program spent most of her time within the hospital setting, and third party payment was oriented toward those cared for in this setting. Thus, more patients were admitted to the hospitals, and the nurses attached to these institutions became more specialty-oriented within that setting. Subsequently, a crisis in medical manpower and medical personnel maldistribution developed, resulting in basic health needs being underserved in all geographic areas, with the rural settings suffering most.

Within the office setting, many physicians utilized secretaries to act as their assistants. Many secretaries who were originally hired to type and answer the telephone showed compassion and interest in the patients and quickly expanded their roles to assisting the physician in different areas, which they could quickly learn to handle with minimal supervision. Practical nurses or nurses who for some reason did not wish to work in hospitals were, and still are, employed by physicians in private practice.

These physician-nurse or other personnel associations were really the first "team approaches" that developed. Nurses were utilized the most because of their specific educational background in health care, their recognized role and acceptance by the consumer, and their professional identification as a result of their licensing examinations. Physicians with well-organized offices and large practices recognized the value of this more efficient approach. By demonstrating her adequacy in the role, the nurse could prove a very efficient and effective assistant. By demonstrating her capability, the nurse could, and did, assume many physician functions in the office practice with a high degree of effectiveness and resultant time conservation. By assuming responsibility for performing many of the technical office procedures and by frequently collecting much of the patients' medical history data, the nurse expanded her role to include doing much of the physical assessment as well.

Nurses, therefore, were the first informally trained physician assistants with on-the-job demands guiding their development. They fulfilled a large number of true physician assistant roles and did this without a formal preparatory training program, because most nursing schools concentrated on an educational curriculum based on the needs of hospitalized patients.

Physicians who were very busy utilized whatever office help was available to deliver a large volume of care in the office setting. They were responsible for the first approach to team development. During this period, not just the nurses but also the secretaries, receptionists, technicians, and all office personnel assumed some of the physician's functions. As these highly motivated individuals extended the physician's patient care capabilities, the volume and, in most cases, the quality of care improved. Thus, the individual physician's office was committed to serving more patients more efficiently, utilizing specialized skills as needed in an economical and responsible fashion.

During the early to middle 1960's, the physician manpower maldistribution prob-lem was definitively outlined and became more generally recognized and openly discussed.[2] Pressures were critical, especially in communities where physicians were in short supply. This was true of rural as well as urban settings. Many people found themselves without basic health care services because the number of generalists had fallen rapidly, and there were far too few family physicians emerging from academic programs at that time. Even general internists were emerging in smaller numbers.

Within the academic settings, the strengths of nursing personnel were recognized.[1] In pediatrics the pressure for more personnel was increasing so rapidly that the American Academy of Pediatrics established a subcommittee on pediatric manpower and the delivery of health care to children. This subcommittee decided to pursue the concept of interprofessional care of the ambulatory patient. This concept, of course, involved widespread use of allied health professionals. Although plans and programs to increase the numbers of basic health care physicians were under way, much discussion and action during the late 1960's concerned "physician substitutes." New categories and new titles for these physician extenders emerged almost overnight, and new programs sprang up in many quarters. As so often happens with a new and exciting concept, many programs were educationally well planned and rational endeavors, concerned with and directed toward patient care. However, some of these were not as well structured, without written goals and careful evaluations, so that sound educational training was lacking, and there was no assurance of appropriate placement for the graduates.

A moratorium was declared at this time, and a study was made to determine the status of the entire area of allied health professionals. This was directed particularly toward the role of the physician assistants in the health care setting. The study was directed by the Council of Medical Education of the American Medical Association, under whose authority the allied health professionals, excluding nurses are accredited. Important data from this study revealed that the main concern and need at that time was to provide allied health professional assistance to the primary physician because of the crisis resulting from the shortage of those delivering basic health care.

From this study it was also evident that there was a need for a quality educational process providing academic accreditation. Some clear understanding of the functions and objectives of this new group of allied health professionals was essential. Should an entirely new group provide this service, or should the service be provided by an already existing group, such as "nursing"? Nurses receiving additional training to become nurse practitioners were being utilized by the late 1960's and were meeting many special needs. Leaders in the nursing profession took the position that they wanted to be identified as an independent profession. A practitioner concept was developed, resulting in the title "nurse practitioner" for most of the programs.

Concurrently, aside from nursing, a body of knowledge developed considered essential for the primary care assistant or physician extender training program, which had clearly stated objectives, definitions, and training policies. Strong recommendation was made at this time to have these physician assistants function with and under the supervision of the physician. Programs of this sort had to be reviewed and approved by a specific accrediting body. From their inception, much emphasis was placed on the programs utilizing the large number of people available who had been in the armed services and who had been trained on the job by the military.

One of the important problems faced at that time, and still before us, was whether society would accept such a new category of health manpower and whether physicians would work with this group. The federal government became involved by providing grant support to various physician assistant training programs during this period. In addition, private foundations supported the development of the concept. State governments were also involved, and these developed various controlling mechanisms by establishing guidelines detailing which legal medical care practices would be permitted by the new physician assistants. States rewrote their laws involving medical care, including the laws defining nursing, to embrace the expanded role of nurses that was developing concurrently.

However, as time continued, the primary care manpower situation became worse, and the physician assistant graduates began to become available. Because of necessity, physicians had to incorporate these graduates as their allied health professional help into their health care systems. A variety of evolutionary experiences was gained in many differing health care delivery systems. These ranged from the solo practitioner in a rural setting to sophisticated metropolitan hospital environments.

Today the typical physician assistant training program is quite extensive. It requires a 24 month curriculum including 95 semester credits that approximate to 3 years of college. Most programs require a minimum of 2 years of college for the health associate and at least 1 year of clinical experience for the nurse, after obtaining the R.N. license. The physician assistant graduates must take a board examination now devised by the National Board of Medical Examiners. Again, it is obvious that the physician extender and physician collaborator, called in this chapter the physician assistant and the nurse practitioner, need to recognize their educational and functional similarities and to work together for health care improvement while maintaining their own identities.

An unexpected result of the programs was that educational experiences previously geared exclusively for medical students were incorporated in many of the physician assistant programs. The intimate mingling of the allied health professional students with medical students and residents in training is resulting now in a shared clinical experience. This provides an opportunity to learn each other's capabilities and potentials firsthand and enhances each group's abilities to work together in the future.

It is important to know of this background in order to appreciate the allied health professional concept. As a formal entity, this concept is young and has evolved over a period of less than 10 years. It is a concept that really has a long historical precedent, but its growth and nourishment will require continued patience, guidance, and understanding. All those involved—graduates of the new programs, physicians, governmental bodies, and medical educators, as well as the patients themselves—will need to foster this evolution and to promote a meaningful and honored role for allied health professionals.

THE ALLIED HEALTH PROFESSIONAL'S ROLE

Because of the pluralistic approach in the United States toward meeting the diverse specific health care needs in different areas, the role of the allied health professional is going to vary a great deal. Let us begin with how this relates to the physician who, for the most part, is highly trained in problem-solving and is generally accepted as the leader or advocate of such efforts on the patient's behalf. All of the physician's education has been directed toward developing skills of listening to patients and toward collecting data and sorting out the important from the unimportant. The development of skills in examining the patient and of then directing further diagnostic activities has been practiced repeatedly in the medical school and residency settings. Once a diagnosis is reached, a management plan must be decided upon and transmitted to the patient in terms that can be understood. All these activities call for the physician's fulfilling the role for which he was especially trained and require that a proportionately large part of his time be spent in direct contact with the patient. What has actually happened is that the physician's time with the patient has been rapidly decreasing because he is spending more time performing tasks that could be performed better by others. The unfortunate result is that this "think and direct" time, as well as actual physician-patient contact, has been decreasing in both duration and quality, resulting in a falling off of the overall effectiveness in delivering health care.

Some physicians have difficulty organizing office personnel and sharing or delegating tasks. Other physicians have a long-standing belief that only the physician could and should perform these patient functions. They see the new allied health professional as meddling with time-honored physician rights and fear that there is a planned "take-over" of these rights resulting from the substitution of other health care personnel for the physician. For the most part, it does not appear

that these fears are based on facts, and, indeed, most of the apprehensions arise from a lack of basic knowledge and poor communication. Sufficient data regarding the allied health professionals have now been accumulated, and adequate time for the evaluation of this data has transpired. What has been clearly and unequivocally demonstrated is that properly trained personnel, other than physicians, can and do perform assigned patient tasks at a quality and reliability level at least equal to that of a physician in certain areas.[4]

As programs mature, more physicians and more health care systems are getting involved in the clinical exposure phases of physician assistant education. More graduates are ready for the manpower market. National interest has resulted in an organization of physician assistants, as well as societies for nurse practitioners, and standard certifying examinations have been developed. Many states are formulating new regulations that clearly outline the responsibilities of health care personnel, including physician assistants, as well as delineate the extended health care role. As more experience has been gained and as these groups have demonstrated their credibility and accountability, it is more likely that the individual with these qualifications will be accepted.[3] The key to this increasing acceptance is found in the official definition of the function of the physician assistant delineated in the 1971 "Essentials of an Approved Educational Program for the Assistant to the Primary Care Physician." This outlines what is understood and what is indeed being carried out in practice, as follows:

The Assistant to the Primary Care Physician is a skilled person, qualified by academic and clinical training to provide patient services under the supervision and responsibility of a doctor of medicine or osteopathy who is, in turn, responsible for the performance of that assistant. The assistant may be involved with the patients of the physician in any medical setting for which the physician is responsible.

The function of the assistant to the primary care physician is to perform, under the responsibility and supervision of the physician, diagnostic and therapeutic tasks in order to allow the physician to extend his services through the more effective use of his knowledge, skills and abilities.[5]

Concurrent with these developments in

the physician assistant field and in the nurse practitioner area, more physicians were graduating from family practice programs. Many general practitioners who had been in practice for a number of years sharpened their skills in order to qualify for and pass the American Board of Family Practice certifying examination. Thus, the new physician and the new assistant combinations were already getting into individual practice settings and were able to mutually work out problems created by this new association.

✔ Within different programs across the country, there appears to be a central group of goals in the preparation of allied health personnel. These include the following:

1. To prepare responsible persons to work in collaboration with other health care deliverers in ambulatory health care settings. All curricula that we have reviewed reiterate the requirement of obtaining a pertinent historical data base with careful interviewing of the patient and family. Data collected from reports, charts, or other sources were noted to be needed in order to comprehend the current state of health or deviation from normal of a particular patient.

2. To emphasize the need for looking at social, economic, and environmental implications of health for every patient. Programs highlight consideration of the psychosocial and interpersonal factors that frequently explain the reason for a person's being among the "worried well" or having a continued complaint.

3. To identify the importance of a carefully taken medical history that frequently leads to the diagnosis of the patient's primary problem and may reveal a patient's supportive needs, which are equally important.

4. To teach the ability to perform an accurate physical examination. This is where the greatest change has occurred in the allied health professional's role. Incorporated into the training programs are utilizing the skills of inspection, palpation, percussion, and auscultation (classically those of the physician) and learning the use of the otoscope, ophthalmoscope, and stethoscope, as well as other necessary equipment.

5. To recognize the abnormal. In order to analyze data that have been collected,

allied health professionals need a background in physiology to recognize deviations from normal. This is not to say that diagnosis has been taken from the hands of the physician. On the contrary, this provides another watchful person to call attention to any abnormal finding or abnormal laboratory results that have been uncovered.

Thus, in reviewing the role of the allied health professional, we find both a data collector and an evaluator at work. An important decision that must be made is when to seek consultation and when to feel competent with the assessment of the normal. The policy within the various health care settings will determine whether medical consultation should be obtained for every patient interaction. It has been the policy of the authors to check every patient presented by a new health care provider. In this way, the authors feel comfortable that the new professional is both capable and confident, without any unnecessary imbalance one way or the other. It is also of interest that when the allied health professional rechecks the physician's findings something frequently is found that previously had been missed.

Once the diagnosis and the management plan have been decided upon through consultation, the allied health professional has the opportunity to provide accurate advice and counseling to patients and families in relation to their health care needs. This is particularly important in providing the anticipatory guidance for adult adaptation to illness, as well as for problems of an acute or chronic nature. In addition, providing guidance that aids in child-rearing and in the prevention of common health problems is a vital part of any practice treating growing children.

The allied health professional who is secure and capable is able to share this responsibility with other administrative and professional personnel in order to obtain the highest quality and most efficient patient care services. Many, by virtue of having lived in the community, will have an ability to act as liaisons with other agencies and health workers, since they know many of the people involved.

As with any professional, continuing education in order to grow professionally is an essential part of the allied health personnel's development. It is obvious from this tentative job description that the vital role of the physician will have to determine the function and future of the allied health professional.

THE PRECEPTOR'S ROLE

With hard work, successful relationships will develop between the physician and the allied health professional. The interaction needed for sharing and learning together requires an active, not passive, involvement by both parties. Input from other personnel within the office is also important.

A clearer understanding of the expectations on both sides should precede the hiring of an allied health professional. The allied health professional and the physician will be students of one another, just as each will be teachers of one another. The membership of the office team may be changed by the addition of a newly trained allied health professional or by the assumption of new skills by somebody already on board. There should be a clear understanding of what this new or this redirected person is to do in order to avoid confusion and poor utilization.

During the authors' recent visit to a family physician's practice in a town of 16,000 people, the learning experiences of the health associate affiliated with that practice were discussed. He had completed a 2 year program in a university setting and had been in the practice for 1 year. In order to facilitate communication about hospitalized patients, he made rounds on the day before the physician in charge took his day off. The health associate was then up-to-date on hospital patients and their needs during the physician's absence from the office. The physician covering the practice for the day had more time available to handle his own practice and any emergencies. The health associate saw an average daily census of ten hospital patients, thus giving the covering physician extra time plus freedom from the anxiety of not knowing about the patients for whom he was responsible.

One of the most difficult decisions in the private practice of medicine is the delegation of responsibility. The physician's entire training and orientation are toward the care of patients, and it is difficult to change this habit. Within this system of expanding our own usefulness must be built a worthwhile supervisory function. Supervision is difficult—it is so much easier to do it yourself. Will the quality of the care of the patients suffer? How can one be sure that the care given by someone else is up to one's own standards? When absorbing personnel with different roles into a practice, the physician must be assured that a high standard of quality is maintained. What happens when an allied health professional interacts with a patient can only be found out by direct observation. One of the most difficult tasks is to sit quietly by watching the interaction without intruding. When observing such an exchange, the physician should explain his presence to the patient and write down components of the interaction, particularly the nonverbal behavior, as much as possible.

From these observations of the allied health professional, the physician can determine what aspects of the care do not measure up to his standards. These standards will have been made perfectly clear at the beginning of the allied health professional's joining the office staff. The time allotted to this monitoring can be quite limited, particularly if one picks a single problem and follows it through over a period of months. It is best if the acute care is rendered by the physician and the follow-up care and management by the allied health professional.

Feedback is essential both for approval and for criticism, and this is reciprocal. The allied health professional needs input from the physician, and the physician needs input from the allied health professional. The physician must achieve his goals as a resource person, a supervisor, and a role model. Time for review, particularly during the first few months of the association, must be set aside. It is important to remember that the allied health professional needs encouragement in this new role. Positive comments from patients are a fine reward.

PROBLEM IDENTIFICATION

Within each practice setting, potential problems associated with allied health professionals must be recognized and appropriate preventive actions taken. Many of these have been identified under the following general headings:

1. Medical liability insurance coverage.
2. Delineating specific job descriptions.
3. Financial considerations for the new participant.
4. Patient and community acceptance.
5. Understanding of the functions, limitations, and authority of the new allied health professional by the rest of the staff.
6. Acceptance of the new health professional by the rest of the staff.
7. Developing the team approach with all members, including the physician.

Experience to date has shown that the vast majority of allied health professionals are capable of performing assigned medical tasks and responsibilities very well. A few anecdotes have been heard, but no real problems caused by the allied health professional's usurping the physician's authority seem to have arisen. It is apparent that public opinion and patient demand, together with physician involvement, have helped solve many problems in different areas. This is not to say that difficulties haven't arisen. There are probably many situations in which an allied health professional has left a practice because of such difficulties. However, it is important to realize there have been no real insurance liability problems to date. Medicolegal coverage is available through several companies for most categories of health professionals at reasonable cost.

Composing and discussing a specific job description within an individual practice is a very worthwhile effort. Because of the increased emphasis on a categorical education for the allied health professional, the perception of what the role entails may be confusing to either the new professional or the physician. At present there is still a great deal of confusion in many areas over certain aspects of this problem. When the role of the pediatric nurse practitioner in the outpatient department was introduced to the house officers of a large teaching hospital, the extremes of questions with regard to the nurses' abilities demonstrated the lack of knowledge. One house officer said very firmly, "No nurse is going to take care of my patients." A strikingly different and permissive attitude was shown by another house officer who asked, "Can she do a spinal tap?"

In addition to being ultimately responsible for the care of patients, the family physician, as a preceptor, has a responsibility for the allied health professional as well. As pointed out in the discussion about the preceptor role, a lack of clarity in communication will result in confusion and hurt feelings. This is not the way to take care of patients, and a falling off of quality will result. We feel that to assure the continued success of this category of physician extenders and to have increasing acceptance of this concept, personal discipline and vigilance will be required on the part of all participating groups. Proper utilization and direction by the physician of allied health personnel of all appropriate categories does indeed provide him with the additional time to extend his services through the more effective use of his knowledge, skills, and abilities.

The physician, although usually the team leader, may not always be in that position. In certain cases, patient care (which includes not only the specific drugs ordered by the physician but the counseling and education required to help a patient comply with a treatment program and want to keep well) will frequently be coordinated by the allied health professional. The responsibility for assuring that a two-class health care system does not develop must lie with the physician. We have to assume a major role in the assurance and the maintenance of quality care standards by all the allied health professionals for whom we are responsible. This does not mean that one profession is "policing" another; it does mean applying the standards of quality, integrity, and professionalism as well as high ethical standards that one hopes each physician applies to himself.

The financing of the new participant in the practice must be specifically decided in each individual practice setting. If this financing has been done in a manner made clear to the patient and if the service provided has been of a high quality, generally there has been acceptance of the service charges made. Methods of remuneration seen in different practices range from a salary to profit sharing or incorporation. Income generation by allied health professionals has been shown in many studies to be equal to or in excess of what they are normally paid.[6] As further development occurs and private health insurance companies as well as federal or state programs recognize the quality of the care provided by the allied health professional, financial reimbursement will come more easily. In some programs throughout the country, the office visit, whether to the physician or to the allied health professional, is paid equally by the insurance company or the state program.

Regarding specific remuneration, one must also consider the allied health professional's career mobility. Satisfaction and pride are essential aspects of the delivery of health care. The career ladders that have been adopted in many community college settings, such as nursing training, are examples of the type of mobility that must be considered. After 1 year of training, the student would qualify to be a licensed practical nurse. Another year would provide the qualifications to become a registered nurse with an associate degree. Frequently, 4 or more years are needed for a bachelor's degree, although this in itself is changing, and in some schools this requirement will not take as long. At this time, the physician extender and nurse practitioner programs tend to be on a certificate basis. However, there is a trend toward master's level preparation, particularly in nursing, such as already occurs in the training of midwives. Physician extender groups appear to be tending toward bachelor's degree certification, as they enter practice at a less experienced level.

There will need to be a continued responsibility for the education of health personnel, with the physician's maintaining vigilance in selection, motivation, and training of the students, as well as providing a role model for these candidates. Physicians at the admissions committee level in different schools will have to keep their standards high and be as discerning as possible. This will be particularly true as the number of trainees increases. A further consideration that will have to be faced in the next few years is the possibility of the allied health professional's returning to school and obtaining an M.D. degree.

Indeed, this is a thorny subject. Interestingly enough, in our experience (and we have both served on medical school admissions committees), there have not been a large number of applicants from the nursing group. The nursing profession attracts candidates who wish to support patients and to help them develop coping behaviors. Perhaps the counseling type of personality that predominates in nurses explains the contrast with the authoritarian nature of physicians. However, in our opinion there will be a demand from the health associate group for consideration for medical school admission after suitable work experience.

The acceptance of the allied health professionals has been quite remarkable. The guarded, high standards already set by the physician assistant organization, as well as some guidelines established in nursing, have been fine mechanisms, exemplary in their application. Such self-imposed high standards must be assured, since, to a large degree, it is the maintenance of these high quality levels that will continue to increase public and professional acceptance. Representatives of society who are responsible for setting state or national regulations for medical practice will have to develop more standard regulations that will permit greater utilization of allied health professionals. Progress in this area to date has been properly and understandably cautious and more or less on an individual basis. Because of this and because of the precautions that have already been taken, the assurance of quality as well as of understanding regarding the allied health personnel has been maintained. It seems appropriate to strive for more regulation that will assist in the effective utilization of these people. By repeated and required re-examination of both physicians and allied health personnel, such as now exists in many states and in certifying board regulations, a sound principle can be developed that should be accepted as a regulatory mechanism.

It would appear to us that most of our society is ready to accept the allied health professional as one who functions under the supervision and responsibility of a physician rather than as an independent practitioner. The concept of independent practice has been proposed by some, especially since "The Essentials of an Approved Educational Program for the Assistant to the Primary Care Physician" states, "The assistant may be involved with the patients of the physician in any medical setting for which the physician is responsible."[5]

Lack of guidelines for the physical presence of the physician or for a contact available by telephone as well as for the decision to seek consultation can lead to misunderstanding. Referral to hospital services may be necessary and frequently, in isolated areas, has to be made by the physician extender alone. Here is the core of communication between the physician, the allied health personnel, and the patient, which is so essential for an understanding of the functions and limitations as well as the authority of the allied health professional. Backup, availability, and continuity by the physician make the difference in the type of care that the allied health professional can deliver.

More attention is now being given in the university centers to providing an opportunity for medical students and residents to share classes with allied health personnel during their training period. Intermingling and the resultant opportunity to learn about each other's abilities and capabilities are vitally important for the future. We wish to emphasize that jointly providing quality patient care, even if it is in a "model" setting rather than in real life, is the most practical way for all parties to assess each other's future involvement. We stress and encourage such training for the medical student, with exposure to as many categories of health personnel as possible. The student thus learns the most effective way of giving these new medical manpower categories an opportunity to grow on their own merit.

EDUCATIONAL PREPARATION FOR THE ALLIED HEALTH PROFESSIONAL

Common objectives of most educational programs for allied health professionals, including postgraduate nurses, appear to be as follows:

1. Evaluating the health of the individual through interview techniques, physical assessment, and problem formulation.

2. Planning and maintaining the health of the family through attention to the physical and psychologic problems uncovered, and arranging appropriate consultation for these problems.

3. Managing common acute and chronic illnesses under immediate physician guidance or consultation.

4. Promoting and working as a member of the health care team through cooperation with other members of the team, and participating in individual patient education, family counseling, and community involvement programs.

5. Demonstrating patterns of continued learning in order to ensure personal growth in the allied health professional role.

The experienced nurse who completed a diploma or bachelor's degree program is prepared by didactic presentation, clinical experience, and additional continued education in a service setting. Many programs complete this preparation over a course of 1 year. Those programs incorporating a master's degree include other studies such as epidemiology, biostatistics, and behavioral science.

Physician extender training, originally associated with the armed services, is now incorporated in programs concentrating on the delivery of service under the direct supervision of the physician. The majority of young people entering such training have not had previous health care experience or nursing school training.

In many schools of nursing, the undergraduate nurse preparation approach appears to emphasize the clinical evaluation of patients. These newly graduated nurses, in most cases, are not prepared to take on the practitioner role without further preparation. Therefore, nursing education, although leaning toward a broader exposure to patient evaluation, continues to be directed toward in-hospital care of patients, management skills for ward duties, and carrying out physicians' orders.

Differentiation between the skills of a qualified nurse practitioner and the graduate of a college physician assistant program seems to be mostly dependent on the type of program that the student completed. Of greater importance, the individual response to the needs of the situation, rather than the academic requirements of the preparing program, will determine the quality of the care provided.

SUMMARY

Ample documentation exists that family physicians have successfully utilized allied health professionals for many years. For the most part, people helping in the health care setting received on-the-job training specifically for the needs of the individual setting. Both the physician and the patients understood their roles, and there was little formal standardized training. However, in the last 10 years, with the advent of didactic programs, these trainees come to the physicians better prepared with basic attitudes and skills. Still, it is the joint responsibility of the physician and the new member of the team to develop both initial and continued understanding between them. Thus, they may utilize each other's skills to the best advantage to provide quality patient care. Based on such an understanding, there will be few problems that cannot be handled. Furthermore, a two-class health care system will not arise because both parties are working together in a carefully and clearly delineated system that is openly communicated between them and the patients.

Increasing demands by the public for family physician services and the existing short supply of family physicians require that every family physician must give serious consideration to the increased use of appropriate allied health professionals. This is not an encouragement of physician substitution. On the contrary, it is a voluntary step that positively seeks to improve the quality of care and to provide more of the services that patients need and are searching for. It provides a means for the physician to institute and maintain a practice according to a desired controlled tempo, one that is more apt to bring personal satisfaction and gratification to the physician. A perpetually overexhausted physician makes a very poor medical caretaker, husband, and father. Of equal importance is the effective practice longevity of any physician who must obtain satisfaction, reward and happiness from his chosen career.

We feel that the appropriate use of allied health professionals can provide an important means to ensure that this satisfaction with one's practice will occur. While the use of these new personnel can increase the number of patients seen by a physician and the degree of advice they receive, these expanded services should not be looked upon as the means for paying for the cost of the allied health professional. Admittedly, income will be generated, but better quality health care is generated at the same time. Some of the cost for improved care will, of course, have to be borne by the patient, but, to date, experience has shown that when exceptionally high quality services are provided promptly and are available when requested, the patient is prepared to pay a fair and reasonable price for such services. In general, the system of one fee for the total service provided by the team is the accepted method of reimbursement. When there has been one-class health service and the patient has clearly understood the services of the allied health professional, there have been very few financial reimbursement problems.

Physicians interested in learning more about allied health personnel should visit a training program or practice demonstration in their area. It is useful to observe these processes in university settings and to become acquainted with the educational programs available locally. The authors have, and are, continuing to accumulate gratifying personal experience with regard to the contribution of allied health professionals in the practice setting. Many other physicians have also given testimony as to what contribution a new member on the team of the allied health professional group can make.

REFERENCES

1. Connelly, J. P., Stoeckle, J. D., Lepper, E. S., et al.: The physician and nurse, their interprofessional work in office and ambulatory settings. N. Engl. J. Med., 275:765, 1966.
2. Fein, R.: The Doctor Shortage: An Economic Diagnosis. Washington, D.C., The Brookings Institute, 1967.
3. Garfield, S. R., Collen, M. F., Feldman, R., et al.: Evaluation of an ambulatory medical care delivery system. N. Engl. J. Med., 294:426, 1976.
4. Spitzer, W. O., Sackett, D. L., Sibley, J. C., et al.: The Burlington randomized trial of the nurse practitioner. N. Engl. J. Med., 290:251, 1974.
5. The Essentials of an Approved Educational Program for the Assistant to the Primary Care Physician, AMA Council on Medical Education, Chicago, American Medical Assoc., 1971.
6. Yankauer, A., Tripp, S., Andres, P., et al.: The costs of training and the income generation potential of pediatric nurse practitioners. Pediatrics, 49: 878, 1972.

Chapter 14

USE OF CONSULTANTS

by THOMAS STERN,
and THOMAS A. NICHOLAS

Proper management of the consultation–referral process is of paramount importance in providing quality care for all patients. If a physician recognizes his ethical, legal, and moral duties in referring a patient and if the consultant equally understands what is expected of him and his obligations, the doctor-patient relationship will be enhanced, the incidence of discontent experienced by the patient will decrease, and the amount of litigation resulting from poor communication in medical care delivery will diminish.

The "Principles of Medical Ethics" of the American Medical Association state that "A physician should seek consultation upon request, in doubtful or difficult cases, or whenever it appears that the quality of medical service may be enhanced thereby." This medical ethic is not new; it is a part of our heritage. In earlier times, although the mass of medical knowledge was not great, some people became more expert in certain arts and skills than others. And they were consulted for these skills.

John Halle, in the early 1500's wrote:

When thou arte callde at anye time,
A patient to see:
And doste perceave the cure too grate
And ponderous for thee:

See that thou laye disdeyne aside,
And pride of thyne owne skyll:
And thinke no shame counsell to take,
But rather wyth good wyll.

Gette one or two experte men,
To help thee in that nede:
And make them partakers wyth thee
In that work to procede. [2]

These observations were never more cogent to the practice of medicine than they are today. They apply to all other specialties, as well as to family practice. It is appropriate that all those specifically trained for or skilled in rendering definitive types of care be identified, so as to provide the patient with the best possible service.

Despite the fact that all medicine was general medicine until the early 1920's, there have always been individuals with either special interests or special aptitudes that set them apart from others. Thus, in the 1920's, certain physicians began to limit themselves to that field of general medicine in which they considered themselves especially skilled. The first clearly delineated specialty was ophthalmology. Since then, 22 specialty boards have been created, with family practice being the twentieth board founded. While consultation and referral mechanisms are essential within and among all specialties, family practice has placed special emphasis on the need for such action.

The early health care system in the United States was built on a traditional model of general practitioners serving the large mass of people. In the late 1940's and early 1950's, there was a tremendous explosion in medical knowledge. With this explosion came a need for and an increased emphasis on specialization in certain aspects of health care delivery. Such specialty and subspecialty emphasis upset the balance of the health care delivery system. The prestige of certain specialties created increased desires on the part of physicians to enter these new fields. Indeed, many in highly specialized areas began to look upon the generalist with disdain. But the vast majority of mankind's disease and suffering is of a general nature and does not occur within specialized fields. Maldistribution of physicians by specialty causes health care chaos for most people. Ideally, a health care system is built on a primary physician base that renders most of the care to a large mass of people and then expands, utilizing referrals to or consultations by highly trained organ-system or disease-oriented specialists for special or complicated problems. (See also Chapter 1.)

It is fitting that family practice is a specialty and that within this specialty physicians receive broad training in multiple aspects of health care. This training must include the appropriate and timely use of consultants and referral physicians if quality care is to be ensured for the public. There are no set rules or criteria that can be enumerated that create specific guidelines for obtaining consultations. The competencies and skills of each physician and the situation in which he functions vary widely from one circumstance to another. One of the precepts of the family practice curriculum is to train an individual whose goal is to manage the majority of medical problems that come within the province of his training and knowledge and to be able to request timely and appropriate referral or consultation when indicated. Equally important, the family physician should be skilled in self-assessment, so that at all times he is well acquainted with his own strengths and weaknesses. He must develop neither a false sense of security nor an inordinate sense of insecurity. He must maintain self-esteem and realize that a request for consultation or referral to a physician more skilled in a given area should not be perceived as a failure on his part but rather as indicative of his skillful management of the patient's problem. This tenet should be self-evident to all specialists, as well as to the family physician.

DIFFERENTIATING BETWEEN CONSULTATION AND REFERRAL

Many instances arise in which the family physician needs, desires, or is requested to obtain assistance in the management of a patient. It is well for the family physician to clearly understand the difference between a consultation and a referral. He should communicate these concepts to the consultant so that the consultant clearly understands what is expected of him by the referring physician. Consultants deal with many physicians who have varying expectations. It is well to develop a uniform definition of the consultation that the referring physician, consultant, and patient all understand. Many misunderstandings and, even more importantly, many malpractice suits can thus be avoided.

CONSULTATION

Consultation is a mechanism whereby one physician requests the opinion of a colleague in the management of a patient. This opinion may be from a respected peer and may serve to reinforce the confidence of the one who seeks consultation. It may be the opinion of an esteemed colleague who specializes in a limited discipline of medical or health care or who has expanded skill or knowledge in the management of a specific type of problem. The physician requesting the consultation retains the overall management of the patient during the consultation process. It is the responsibility of the consulting physician to report his assessment of the patient to the referring physician. Information regarding the consultation is transmitted by the family physician to the patient unless a prior agreement between the consultant and the referring physician has altered this sequence of communication.

A suggested outline for requesting consultations is as follows:

A. Request for consultation—a request for consultation is a request for an opinion to be rendered in writing
1. The consultant is not required to write orders on the chart.
2. The consultant is not requested to assume any direct authority for the patient's care.
3. The physician requesting consultation will remain the physician of record for that patient.
4. The physician requesting consultation retains full responsibility, including legal responsibility, for the patient's care.

5. The request for consultation should be a written request; additionally, an oral conversation between the physician requesting consultation and the consultant enhances the effectiveness of such a request.
   a. The request for consultation should not be accomplished through a third party.
6. The report of consultation should be communicated quickly, and in writing, by the consultant and transmitted to the referring physician.

REFERRAL

Referral is the mechanism whereby a physician requests the service of another physician in the management of a patient in order to treat that patient for a specific condition for a specific period of time so that the highest quality of care available is provided to that patient. The consulting physician may be a respected peer or may be a physician trained in depth in another specialty with special qualifications and skills in the management of the specific disease entity. In a referral situation, a specific doctor-patient relationship is established between the consulting physician and the patient. The referring physician delegates his position as primary manager of the case to the consultant and, subsequently, becomes a third party. In some instances, he may become a consultant in other aspects of the patient's management for that specific period of time.

It is incumbent upon the consulting physician to effect a two-part feedback loop to the referring physician. First, the physician who now manages the case should communicate appropriate information regarding his assessment of the patient's condition, and his plan for treatment should ensure that the referring physician is continually aware of the patient's progress and the ultimate plans for disposition. Second, it is the duty of the consultant to return the management of the patient to the referring physician at the conclusion of the disease process or the expiration of the period of time for which the patient was referred. If the consultant feels the need for additional consultations, he should communicate this to the primary physician before initiating further care.

In referral, therefore, the family physician relinquishes the day-to-day continuity of care of the patient to the consulting physician. It is appropriate for, and indeed incumbent upon (whenever possible), the referring physician to communicate with the patient at intervals to signify his continued interest. It is recognized that this is impossible when the referral is made to a geographically remote site. The referring physician should participate in the care of the patient if the condition warrants it or if it is otherwise appropriate. In such cases, economic problems often arise, and the physician should ascertain that the patient does not receive duplicate charges for duplicate services.

A suggested outline for requesting referrals is as follows:

A. Request for referral—a request for referral is a request for transfer of the responsibility of care for a patient from one physician to another physician. The patient must be informed as to the reason and need for the referral and must also be informed that the prime responsibility for management is being transferred to the consultant.
1. The request for referral should be written.
2. The written request, whenever possible, is best preceded by a conversation between the referring physician and the consultant.
   a. This process should not be accomplished through a third party.
3. Clear understanding as to the purpose and duration of the referral should be established between the consultant and the referring physician.
4. The referring physician transfers the responsibility for the patient's care to the consulting physician, as agreed.
5. The consulting physician assumes full responsibility, including legal responsibility, for the patient.
6. Consummation of referral is dependent upon full agreement by the referring physician, consulting physician, and patient.
   a. It is preferable that this agreement be in writing.
7. Upon completion of the referral period, the consulting physician should provide the referring physician with a written resumé of the

treatment process and disposition of the patient and should return the management of the patient to the referring physician.

INDIRECT CONSULTATIVE ACTIONS

Certain consultative actions are less formal but nevertheless should be recognized as consultations. These include instances such as requests by the family physician for certain services by other specialists that assist him in the diagnosis and subsequent management of the patient. Such services include diagnostic radiology, laboratory sciences, nuclear medicine, physical medicine, and other special procedures. These may be provided by physicians or technologists or other medically allied but technically trained individuals.

In these cases, the referring family physician amasses pertinent information without necessarily involving the consultant directly, then makes an assessment, and finally formulates a diagnosis and plan for management of the patient's problem. The consultant provides information, but only in rare circumstances (and then only for short periods) does he assume any responsibility for the patient's management. Other instances of indirect consultation occur when the family physician utilizes the services of an anesthesiologist or a pathologist in the management of the patient. The patient should be made aware that these consultations are being requested, as they often occur without his knowledge, are confusing, and thus may interefere with the smooth management of his care.

MECHANISMS FOR CONSULTATION AND REFERRAL

Solo Practice

The physician in solo practice should develop his own panel of consultants. They should be authorities, recognized and respected by him. If at all possible, they should be personally known to him. The physician should make the decision as to whom the consultant should be and should counsel the patient about the need for the consultation. It is best to choose one consultant and offer this name to the patient

rather than list two or three names and thereby force the patient to make a choice. The patient has engaged the family physician to manage his care and is not in the position, in most instances, to make such decisions. This does not preclude honoring a patient's request if he has a preference and if the family physician is comfortable with the competence of the proposed consultant.

Group Practice

The consultative procedure in a group practice becomes more complex. The first consideration should be maintaining quality of care in the best interest of the patient. Within a family practice group, there may be other physicians having more interest in or expertise about specific problem areas than the referring physician has. It is entirely appropriate to seek consultation from these physicians when indicated. Within multispecialty groups, it is entirely possible that the best consultant is a member of the group, and referral within the group is appropriate. When the best consultant is not in the group, however, it is incumbent upon the referring physician to obtain the best possible expertise, regardless of potential economic loss or loss of prestige to the group itself.

RESPONSIBILITIES OF THE FAMILY PHYSICIAN IN OBTAINING CONSULTATION AND REFERRAL

Medical-Legal Aspects

In addition to the aforementioned moral and ethical responsibilities for a family physician (or any other physician) to seek consultation in certain circumstances, there is also a legal aspect to the consultation process. After a physician has agreed to treat a patient and a doctor-patient relationship has been established, either implicitly or by circumstance, the physician is obligated to conduct the management of the patient's illness or injury with "due care." If he does not do so, he may be negligent in the management of the case. Failure to obtain appropriate consultation from an appropriate consultant at an appropriate time may imply failure to render "due care." The failure to render "due care" constitutes negligence. In most cases, professional liability suits involve allegations that a physician has managed a patient's illness, either by diagnosis or treatment, "negligently." Negligence is the legal term for omission of care in circumstances in which a duty exists to provide such care, with the result that the patient is injured by the physician's failure to fulfill that duty. A physician's legal duty is defined as follows:

By undertaking to render medical services, he (the physician) will ordinarily be understood to hold himself out as having the skill and knowledge possessed by members of the medical profession in good standing under similar circumstances and he will be liable if harm results because he does not possess it.[10]

Thus, in addition to the moral obligation of the family physician to seek consultation in certain instances, there is also clearly a legal obligation to do so.

The Appropriateness of Having the Consultation

The decision to seek consultation for any given patient problem must be made by the family physician with the intent to use the information provided by the consultant. A consultation should be obtained for improving the quality of care to the patient. It is inappropriate to request a consultant's opinion simply to have the record state that a consultation was performed. The referring physician should not seek consultation only to share legal responsibility for the patient. Legally, he cannot do this unless the consultant agrees to accept such responsibility. (This will be discussed later.) Because a contractual relationship is legally established between physician and patient, the physician is obligated to diagnose and treat the patient's illness or injury with due care.[11] He cannot relinquish responsibility unless a satisfactory contract has been made with a consultant for referral and delegation of responsibility. The primary physician may be held liable for abandonment if he does not continue his management duties. Abandonment has been defined as the "unilateral severance by the physician of the professional relationship between himself and a patient without reasonable notice, at a time when there is still necessity of continuing medical attention."[6]

A consultation, therefore, should be sought by a physician not only because of moral purposes involving quality of care but because he is indeed legally required to do so. The principle of negligence applies. While a doctor-patient contract does not include a promise to cure, it does imply a commitment to the treatment of the patient. In law, negligence is not by any means limited to situations that only involve carelessness. A physician who does not have the training to manage a certain condition or who does not ask for the necessary information to make a correct diagnosis may be negligent if he does not refer the patient to another specialist, even though he is extremely careful in dealing with the patient and his care meets the highest possible standards. Thus, the physician must have adequate knowledge and skill and must use these with adequate care in treating a patient, or he must seek a consultant.[1] A physician may be liable for negligence if he does not realize that he is not capable of managing the patient and should therefore refer him to a specialist.[5]

Due care requires the prudent and careful physician to consult with other medical practitioners in many situations.[4] Therefore, the physician should remember that it is his moral and legal duty to seek consultation when in doubt.

When planning a consultation, there are several legal points with which the family physician should become acquainted.

1. In requesting and arranging a consultation, what the consultant is to do and what his ongoing responsibilities are to be should be clarified. The arrangements should include whether the consultant expects to be called in again, whether he will respond to a call directly from the patient, whether he will respond only to another call from the family physician, or whether he will indeed respond at all to a call from anyone. Unless previously agreed upon, he is not legally bound to respond to anyone.[7]

2. A consulting physician who examines a patient at the request of a family physician but who does not intend to continue to treat the patient is not legally required to do so. This should be made clear to the patient by the family physician and should be made clear to the family physician by the consultant.[8]

3. Once an agreement for referral has

been reached, however, a physician who refers a patient to another specialist is generally held to have relieved himself of any further responsibility to the patient in the absence of an understanding that he will be associated with the specialist in caring for the patient.[3] Again, however, this should be agreed upon with the specialist and should be explained clearly to the patient to avoid any possibility of misunderstanding.

4. The family physician should not be threatened by the patient's desire for consultation if that desire stems from the patient's lack of confidence in the management by the family physician. A fearful patient should not be penalized for voicing his fears. The family physician is the advocate of the family in matters of consultation and should be willing and able to make a decision on the appropriateness of any consultation as well as to attest to the ability of the consultant by reputation and observation. The family physician should communicate to his patient that he is always open to suggestion for consultation, so that his patient will always feel free to participate in directing his own destiny. The patient should feel comfortable about asking his family physician to seek consultation. Consultations should be sought when:

    a. The diagnosis is uncertain.
    b. The treatment is proving ineffectual.
    c. A condition is not within the field of training of the family physician and treatment by another specialist is available and would benefit the patient.
    d. It is known by the physician that a problem exists that he is not equipped to solve.
    e. Even though the physician knows the condition and treatment, he knows that another hospital or clinic has better facilities or equipment than that locally available.[4]

TIMING OF A CONSULTATION

In undertaking the care of a patient, a physician represents himself as possessing a reasonable degree of skill in managing the case. Upon consenting to treat a patient, it becomes his duty to use reasonable care and diligence in the exercise of his skill and the application of his learning to accomplish the purpose for which he is employed.[9] When a family physician has even the slightest indication that the progressive management of the patient has exceeded his capabilities, it is prudent to call in a consultant. Timing of a referral is the key to excellent patient management and should be the hallmark of the well-trained family physician.

Family practice involves comprehensive and continuous care, but it also involves personal care. Personal care requires that attention be given to the personal needs of the patient. This should be as true in the area of consultation as it is in the practice of the family physician. The family physician should not confuse personal care with his own personal ego. Too often, the personal relationship between the family physician and his patient prevents the physician from introducing another physician into this relationship, even when such an introduction would benefit the patient.

It is of utmost importance that the family physician not delay seeking consultation until it is too late for the consultant to intervene effectively. The art of obtaining a consultation is such that it should never be demeaning to the family physician requesting this service. The family physician should understand that a properly organized and appropriately utilized consultation is a useful tool in securing patient confidence. The unfamiliar consultant will not usually have the confidence of the patient immediately. It is often unlikely that he will be able to completely gain that patient's confidence during the short period of time available to him in conferring with the patient. While this is not necessarily true in the case of a referral, the consultant is still at a disadvantage, for he has not had the long and continuous relationship with the patient enjoyed by the family physician. Thus, in recognizing this series of relationships, the family physician is well advised to lay a sound foundation for the consultant when discussing this with the patient. The patient will therefore have confidence in the consultant and confidence that the total management of his case is thereby enhanced. The patient always has more trust in a physician who recognizes his limitations and refers appropriately or who seeks a second opinion.

The responsibility for selecting an appropriate consultant lies with the referring physician. The wise family physician will select his consultant carefully. He is the trusted confidant of his patient and he *alone* is able to judge the ability and competency of the consultant in the area for which consultation is needed. He therefore should not expect his patient to do the selecting. The family physician should consider not only the ability and competency of his consultant but also the potential for personal compatibility between the consultant and the patient. Appropriate preparation for the consultation should allow time for the personal attention necessary to provide smooth and orderly care through the consultation period. Patients select a family physician for various reasons, not the least of which are his personality traits. The family physician should realize that the personality traits of the consultant should also mesh with those of the patient if the consultation is to be effective. Proper attention to these details will enhance the quality and effectiveness of the consultation.

TYPES OF CONSULTATIONS

Diagnostic Medical Specialties

By far the most common consultation requested by the family physician will be for radiologic or pathologic testing. This is not often considered a consultation between two physicians, and too often appropriate information is not supplied to the radiologist or pathologist performing these services.

In the area of radiology, pertinent and germane information should be given to the radiologist who is performing the test, whether it be a routine examination or a highly involved technical procedure. The radiologist can perform much more effectively when he is made aware of the possible diagnoses being considered by the family physician and the expected results of the tests.

Examination of tissues by the pathologist is also greatly enhanced by submitting sufficient information with the specimens. This information should include an identification of the region from which the tis-

sue was obtained, the age of the patient, other existing conditions that might have impact on the pathologic diagnosis, the method of preservation of the specimen, and the type of excision or other tissue-removing technique, as well as a tentative diagnosis by the referring physician. The same data should be included in certain aspects of laboratory procedures when special procedures are requested by the referring physician.

The electrocardiographer should also know the expectations of the referring physician when he is asked to consult about an electrocardiogram (ECG). An appropriate consultation request should include the age of the patient; drugs included in the patient's daily management; previous ECG diagnosis, readings, or both; blood pressure; known heart disease; familial heart disease; weight, sex; and even the patient's emotional attitude at the time of the test.

Many studies that outline the scope of the family physician's need for consultation exclude mention of these vital colleagues in the other specialties. Certainly the specialties just described constitute a major factor in the armamentarium of diagnosis and management of many patient problems.

Other Medical Specialties

Physicians in the other traditional specialties also provide a highly utilized and common source of referral and consultation. Consultation requests may occur within one specialty of medicine, and consultation requests between family physicians are not an uncommon occurrence. Some family physicians feel the need of a colleague's expertise. This should not result in a patient's misunderstanding of his physician's particular need to seek advice from other colleagues. Physician-to-physician relationships should be established in which there are both a free exchange of information and appropriate preparation of the consultant by the referring physician. It is often good practice to use the same consultant as frequently as possible in order to reinforce the confidence and understanding between physicians. This gives an opportunity for evaluation of the colleague's results. However, it must be reiterated that the patient's need to be referred to a physician whose personality is compatible with his own should be considered in every consultation. This may result in having available several consultants in a given field in order to select the most appropriate one for a given patient and his current problem. The consultant views with a great deal of pride the fact that other physicians have confidence in his ability, and it is indeed an honor for another physician to be requested to provide consultation.

Referral for Brief Periods to Colleagues

Attention must be given to another area often not considered as a referral or consultation. This referral occurs when one family physician takes calls for a colleague, whether for just one evening or for a prolonged period. To ensure continuity of care, adequate reports need to be submitted by the physician on call to his colleague upon his return. Conversely, critical patient care cases should be reviewed before the referral occurs. Adequate records should be available to the physician covering another physician's practice.

Consultation by Allied Health Workers and Other Professionals

Often physicians consult with public health nurses, psychologists, nutritionists, and others. It is important to remember that this is a necessary part of adequate medical care and that the same tenets apply to such consultations as to those between physician colleagues.

ORGANIZATION OF THE CONSULTATION PROCESS

What to Expect from a Consultation

In requesting a consultation, the referring physician has honored the chosen colleague with trust. The consultant should provide the referring physician with both insight into and added dimension to the patient's problems beyond the scope of the family physician's ability to ascertain these for himself. However, this information must be passed on readily, formally, and completely. The decision as to who will ultimately reveal the results of the consulta-

tion to the patient may be decided upon ahead of time and is often dependent upon the complexity of the consultation. As long as this is decided in advance, there should be no question as to who is to provide the information. Often, as in the case of surgery, the consultant and the family physician report to the patient and the family together.

Information obtained from the consultant should not be used blindly. The referring physician should use this information as he would use the information obtained from a myriad of different tests, and such consultation should not necessarily be the ultimate influence in the decision-making process regarding the patient's future. The patient's future should be decided by a consideration of the conglomerate of information obtained by the family physician's own studies and the use of laboratory, x-ray, and other facilities, as well as the consultant's report.

Training Curriculum and Selection of a Consultant

The family practice resident is trained in the various disciplines of medical care. Although some aspects of medical care will never be delivered entirely by the family physician, the trainee develops knowledge to enhance his ability to select a consultant. The selection of a consultant should embody all of the needs of the patient, including an appraisal by the family physician of the consultant's behavior, competency, and fund of knowledge. In the training program, the consultation is often used as a tool of learning, and the family practice resident is taught to use the consultation freely and without threat of lessening his own stature.

As the trainee becomes a more complete physician, he may use the consultation less frequently, but he must remember that the consultation is a necessary tool in the practice of family medicine. Training programs should teach the consultation mechanisms by including an appropriate consultation model and the appropriate workup required prior to consultation. The goal of the educational program is for the resident to be able to arrange a timely and appropriate consultation and to learn from it.

Proper Utilization of Information from the Consultant

The family physician is expected to provide comprehensive and continuing care for his patient. During the course of delivering comprehensive care, it will be necessary for the family physician to obtain consultation and to sometimes refer the patient to another specialist for care. The proper utilization of the information received from the consultant is of prime importance.

It has been stated before that the referring physician will enhance the entire consultation process if he communicates adequately with the consultant. It is even more important that he communicate properly with the patient. The patient will have unwavering confidence if the physician has carefully explained to him the specific complexities that require consultation. Further explanation should include information about the special expertise of the consultant and how his skill and knowledge will lead to the very best care possible for the particular set of conditions involved.

The family physician and the consultant must have confidence in each other so that the patient does not become confused. Consultations may be delivered in two ways. In the first method, the consultant examines the patient and delivers his findings and recommendations either verbally or in writing to the family physician. It is best to ensure that there is always a written record of the consultation. In the second method, the consultant not only examines the patient but directly advises him as to the diagnosis and the expected course of treatment. He also provides a written report to the family physician. In either case, the family physician must thoroughly familiarize himself in detail with the recommendations of the consultant. He must be certain in the first case that he understands each recommendation and the reason for it. In the second case, he must be equally well informed about the recommendations, since it is possible that the patient will not have understood the explanation by the consultant and will look to the family physician for clarification. In either case, an illness severe enough to warrant consultation will cause anxiety in the patient. A calm, well-informed family physician who can explain in detail the results of the consultation can be most effective in ensuring proper outcome and patient compliance.

The family physician and the consultant who agree upon a reasonable consultation procedure can be confident that the process will not confuse the patient. However, instances occur in which the consultant may communicate information to the patient with which the referring family physician does not agree. When this occurs, the patient's confidence in both the family physician and the consultant is severely disturbed. Careful discussion between the family physician and the consultant will minimize the possibility of this happening. If the family physician intends to continue managing the patient's condition and is simply seeking the consultant's advice to assist him in this management, this information should be clearly explained to the consultant. In such cases, the consultant should communicate his findings and advice to the referring physician rather than directly to the patient. If the family physician does not intend to continue management of the particular condition, this too should be communicated to the consultant. The consultant then may directly inform the patient of his opinion and his plan for further management of the problem for which the patient was referred. If these mechanisms are clearly understood by both the family physician and the consultant, neither will find himself in the position of seeming to criticize the other, the patient will not find himself in the middle of a disagreement, and the integrity of both physicians will be preserved. The patient will thus remain secure in his confidence that he is being treated well.

Elements of the proper utilization of the consultation process therefore include:

1. Special care should be taken by the referring physician to impart all the facts about the patient and his condition to the consultant. It is best to write a review as well as to communicate verbally.

2. Special care should be taken by the referring physician to communicate clearly with both the consultant and the patient.

3. Both the referring physician and the consultant should be certain that the patient and his family fully understand the situation.

4. The patient should be informed of the cost of the consultative service and its justification.

5. Continuity of care should be maintained, if at all possible.

6. Both the consultant and the family physician should take special care in what each says in regard to:

a. Taking credit for specific accomplishments, particularly when not justified.

b. Giving credit for specific accomplishments, particularly when not justified.

c. Adverse criticism of any nature.

Situations will arise that make it necessary to obtain more than one opinion. This creates a special situation in the utilization of information from the consultant. In most cases, careful analysis on the part of the family physician can anticipate that there may be a divergence of opinion or that, because of the particular complications of the problem, more than one opinion will be necessary. The proper analysis of such a situation by the family physician is invaluable. He may then inform the patient prior to consultation that the complexity of the situation requires several consultants and that no final decision will be made until all the evidence is considered and an agreement as to the best course of management is reached.

The most difficult situation is that in which the family physician cannot agree with his consultant and feels the latter's recommendation should not be followed. The patient must be informed that a second consultation is necessary to reach a consensus. If the consultant has already conveyed information to the patient, ethics requires that the family physician communicate to the consultant his concerns and obtain a second consultation. The consultant should then communicate to the patient that a second consultation will take place, and no further direction or information should be given to the patient until a consensus is reached. There is nothing more disconcerting to a patient than to receive divergent opinions from several physicians, especially if they are consultants called in by his own family physician.

Development of Patient Records Utilizing Consultant Information

Proper utilization and preservation of information in the consultation or referral process are ensured by the proper recording of such information. Such data should be recorded in an organized, clear, and concise fashion that will leave no doubt in the mind of the consultant, the family physician, and third party involved or ultimately in the mind of the patient what was intended by the consultant and the family physician in initiating the consultative process and by what means it is to be consummated. It is incumbent upon the family physician to develop a satisfactory record system. The family physician may develop his own system and then ask each of his consultant panel to follow this procedure. Or he may ask each consultant to provide the information in his usual format and then incorporate it into his own system.

The consultation and referral system presents a specific problem in record-keeping. The problem-oriented method (see Chapter 5) has proved to be an effective record-keeping system for family physicians. It is not intended to imply that this is the only system, but simply to point out one good method. The admonition is that a good, clear, concise, and organized record system be established in every instance of consultation or referral.

The family physician should remember that his record is the best mechanism of communication. It is the best tool that exists for precise analysis of the patient's present and future care. The final responsibility for the development, management, and completion of the record should rest with the family physician.

In a problem-oriented system the problem list is the central reference point that will provide the consultant with an overview of all the patient's problems, as well as signal the specific problem for which he is being consulted. While the responsibility for maintaining the list rests with the family physician, the consultant should refer to the problem list so that he may fully understand every aspect of the patient's condition as well as be able to identify the specific problem that he has been asked to assess. After completing his consultation, his report should address the specific problem by number and title and anything else pertinent to the consultation. The consulting physician then assists in refining or redefining a problem and may add to or resolve a problem on the list. The content of the consultant's notes may assume any clear communicative form; however, its organization into subjective and objective findings, assessment of the problem, and suggested plan for management presents a well-organized, easily understandable form consistent with the remainder of the record. In the case of the hospital patient, the problem list and record will be at hand for the consultant to review. In the event of a referral from the outpatient setting, it is important that the family physician include the problem list, resumé of the data base, flow sheet, and progress notes so that the consultant may be fully informed prior to undertaking a consultation. The orderly transmitting of information between the family physician and the consultant can thus be accomplished with a minimum of error or misunderstanding and maximum enhancement of management of the patient.

REFERENCES

1. Armstrong vs. Svoboda. 49 Cal. Report 801, 1966.
2. Burnside, J. W.: Commandments of consultants. Hosp. Physician, 9:53, 1973.
3. Engle vs. Clarke. 346 SW 2d 13, Ky., 1961.
4. Holder, A. R.: Duty to Consult. *J.A.M.A. 226*:111, 1973.
5. Holder, A. R.: Medical Malpractice Law. New York, John Wiley & Sons, Inc., 1975.
6. McIntyre, L. L.: The action of abandonment in medical malpractice litigation. Tulane Law Rev., 36:834, 1962.
7. Nelson vs. Farrisa. 173 NW 715 Minn., 1919.
8. Podvin vs. Honsinger. 128 NW 2d 523, Mich., 1964.
9. Price vs. Honsinger. 49 NE 760, N.Y., 1898.
10. Prosser, W. L.: Torts. 2nd ed., St. Paul, West Publishing Co., 1955.
11. Schneider vs. Little, Co. 151 NW 587–588, Michigan, 1915.

Chapter **15**

REHABILITATION

by HENRY H. STONNINGTON,
and EDWARD W. CIRIACY

As physicians, we are taught to test for weaknesses and deficiencies in a patient. We think about how weak a limb is, how deficient the intellect is, or how much loss there is in the visual fields. These points are indeed important in the diagnostic process. However, as soon as we consider management of the patient as a whole, rather than management of the specific illness, we must reorient our thinking. How much vision *remains*, how *strong* is that limb, and what can we do to *increase* the strength? How can the patient learn to improve his function by compensation, substitution, or other unusual means? That is rehabilitation. No matter how small or how large the disability, there is something that can be done to make life easier, more comfortable, and more worthwhile. To achieve this, we use the body's unending ability to heal and to hypertrophy. We use various modalities of heat and water, orthoses (splints), and prostheses (artificial limbs), along with our knowledge of psychology and physiology, to help remold the patient. Of all the physicians, both the family physician and the physiatrist (specialist in physical medicine and rehabilitation) must most often consider the patient as an individual with individual needs. The rehabilitation process is particularly important for the patient who has a chronic catastrophic disability. It also contributes significantly to the care of most orthopedic, neuromuscular, and arthritic problems. These are all conditions that abound in any family practice, and the family physician must be familiar with the management of many of these problems.

For this management, the physician often needs the help of one or more of the allied health professionals, such as the physical therapist, occupational therapist, speech therapist, social worker, nurse, or workers from community health agencies and agencies that specialize in vocational evaluation and provide a sheltered workshop. The physician should be prepared not only to communicate adequately with these persons but also to help coordinate these programs. The physician must at all times consider the patient's own desires, hopes, and needs and must make sure that the patient and the family take an active part in any decision that will affect their future. This communication may be verbal, but it is often written. It is important that all of the allied health professionals have a clear understanding not only of the patient's disease and disability but also of the goals in his management. These goals are both short-term and long-term. The communication with the physical therapist and occupational therapist needs to be in the form of a written prescription, which includes the history and examination and which sets down the types of modalities and exercises to be used. The physical therapist is concerned with increasing the range of motions, muscle re-education and strengthening, and ambulation and general ability to move. The occupational therapist works particularly on upper extremity function, deals with perceptual deficits, and shows the patient the easiest way to overcome deficits in order to accomplish activities of daily living (ADL). Equally important in this rehabilitation process is the periodic re-evaluation of the patient's progress and the status of the goals. Only by this type of comprehensive approach can the patient's physical and psychologic needs be met. Such a program makes the management of the patient with a long-term disability exciting and rewarding.

A review of the rehabilitation of some long-term disabilities will be presented and will be followed by a discussion of walking aids and gait patterns, postsurgical rehabilitation, and the principles of monitoring progress in rehabilitation.

SPINAL CORD INJURIES

Most patients with spinal cord injuries are young and were healthy people before their accident. They need the help and guidance of a physician, from both a physical and a psychologic point of view. Most of them, with the help of a good rehabilitation program, should ultimately be able to live independently in a home environment. At least 50 per cent of these patients should be able to return to school and work. The likelihood of their returning to such activities increases from categories 1 to 4 as follows: (1) complete quadriplegia, (2) incomplete quadriplegia, (3) complete paraplegia, and (4) incomplete paraplegia.

The level of paralysis is significant. With C5 spared, the patient can only move his shoulders and will be dependent on a helper some of the time. With C7 spared, he will have considerable arm and wrist function that will enable him to make independent transfers and to drive a car. A paraplegic with a level of paralysis lower than T5 has a chance of ambulation with long leg braces. With a conus medullaris lesion, the patient usually can walk with minimal bracing or walking aids. The particular problems that require continued attention are the following:

Neurogenic Bladder

Bladder Training. It is possible to establish bladder control in the majority of these patients. First, one must explain the anatomy and the reason for the abnormality to the patient. Then, together with a urologist, one must establish that there is no current infection or ureteric reflux and that the kidneys function normally. The investigation will include cystoscopy to exclude calculi and other abnormalities. Removal of catheters is usually done under cover of appropriate antibiotics. The patient is taught how to contract the bladder by tapping the suprapubic area and, if appropriate, how to increase abdominal pressure and how to use a Credé type of expression of urine from the bladder. He is asked to do this at regular 2 or 4 hour intervals. At first, intermittent catheterizations are done every 6 hours to find out what the residual urine is. As the residual amounts decrease, catheterizations are decreased and eventually stopped. The aim is to have residual amounts of less than 100 ml. and to have as little spontaneous voiding as possible between tappings. It is important that the intake of liquids stays much the same every day so that the patient will understand his own voiding pattern. Generally, 1800 ml. of liquids spread out over the entire day is an appropriate intake. If spontaneous voidings do occur, an external catheter and a leg bag may help the patient stay dry. If such a pattern cannot be achieved, intermittent self-catheterization can be taught to the patient, and this is preferable to his using an indwelling catheter.

Bladder Infection. Infection of the bladder used to be the greatest cause of morbidity and mortality in these patients. Regular monthly check-ups and cultures, administration of appropriate antibiotics when significant infections occur, and awareness of and management of ureteric reflux are all measures that minimize the problem. Simple measures such as the use of methenamine mandelate (Mandelamine) and the acidification of urine by ascorbic acid ingestion will also help to reduce infection. However, the most important measure for the reduction of infection is the early use of intermittent catheterization and bladder training.

Neurogenic Bowel

Bowel training is a fairly simple matter. The diet should be high in fiber content. Stool softeners such as dioctyl sodium sulfosuccinate (Colace) can be used. Alternate-night use of two glycerin suppositories serves as a mechanical stimulus for emptying the bowel. As with bladder training, regularity is the key to the program.

Skin

The need for care of the skin must be instilled in the patient. This is entirely his responsibility. He must carefully inspect his skin every day, using a mirror for his perineum. He must avoid further pressure on reddened areas and keep his skin clean and dry. At all times he must use a good cushion on his wheelchair, and he must train himself to push himself off the cushion at regular intervals if he sits for a prolonged time. Similarly, he must train himself to change his position in bed every 2 hours. The appearance of a decubitus ulcer requires immediate relief of pressure from the affected area. The best simple treatment is cleaning the ulcer with a watery solution and drying it with a hair blower that has had its heating element removed. This should be done every 4 hours.

Sex

Frank, unembarrassed discussions with the patient and the partner about their sex activities are the best way to approach this subject. These patients can have a full sex life that is satisfying to the patient and the partner alike. Books, courses, and video tapes on this subject are readily available.

Psychologic Needs

Obviously, a catastrophic handicap such as this in a young person will require tremendous adjustments. If the patient has good rapport with his physician, this could be of great help to him. The patient then can come to the physician for advice about his many medical problems and about his psychologic, marital, and vocational problems as well. The physician must use his common sense in deciding when the patient should see an appropriate health professional, such as a psychologist, vocational counselor, social worker, or representatives from various governmental agencies.

Physical Therapy

The rehabilitation center should have trained the patient in strengthening the upper extremities to the fullest, in making transfers, in the use of the wheelchair, and, if appropriate, in the use of braces and crutches.

Occupational Therapy

The occupational therapist should have trained the patient how to be as inde-pendent as possible in activities of daily living and how to use special splints and, for the high quadriplegic, how to use mouth sticks.

The Physician's Role

In addition to his role as coordinator of the rehabilitation process, the physician should be active in community programs to reduce environmental barriers, particularly in apartments, schools, and public places. The physician can be of great assistance in establishing the patient as an independent, useful member of the community and can help him become a taxpayer rather than a social security recipient. These patients need all the help they can get in being accepted in the community and at work, for they are, except for their disability, normal people with normal needs and emotions.

STROKE

The rehabilitation potential (which means the patient's potential to return to independent living as regards activities such as dressing, ambulation, and working) is related to many factors apart from the type of cerebrovascular syndrome that caused the lesion. Factors that generally influence the rehabilitation potential include the site of brain damage, age, sex, and environmental barriers that the patient will return to. Particular factors that influence the rehabilitation potential are listed in Table 15–1.

As soon as the stroke has been completed and has stabilized, an active program can be started as follows:

Physical Therapy

Initially, the main concern is the maintenance of range of motion. This is soon supplemented by procedures that help with the re-education and activation of the paralyzed limbs. For this, the physical therapist uses methods that make use of various spinal, neck, and labyrinthine reflexes that have been released by the cerebral lesion. The procedures are called neuromuscular facilitation techniques. The idea is that after the elicitation of these reflexes, parts of the reflex movements can be inhibited

TABLE 15-1. FACTORS INFLUENCING REHABILITATION POTENTIAL FOLLOWING STROKE

Good Prognostic Signs	Poor Prognostic Signs
Early return of tone	Long delay between onset of disability and start of rehabilitation program
Early return of tendon jerks	Severe degree of flaccidity
Early return of trunk stability	Severe degree of spasticity
Good strength of pelvic and shoulder girdle muscles	Severe degree of contractures
Good strength of hand muscles	Evidence of generalized intellectual impairment
Acceptance of disability by patient and family	Severe sensory and perceptual deficit
Presence of spouse in home	Severe visual deficits
Lack of poor prognostic signs (see opposite)	Sustained bowel and bladder incontinence

by the physical therapist and can be refined and put under volitional control so that the pattern of movement can be re-established.

The therapist also practices trunk control and sitting balance with the patient and teaches him how to transfer from the bed to a chair. Once sitting balance has been established, the therapist begins with standing balance and proceeds to re-establish a gait pattern. Initially this is done with the aid of a stable bar that the patient holds, then with a broad-based cane, and next with a regular cane. Quite often, if there is persistent foot drop, an ankle–foot orthosis (brace) will be used. This could be a metal spring type, a metal double-bar short-leg brace, or the newer molded plastic type of orthosis that fits inside any shoe.

Using this step-by-step approach, with considerable attention to detail and with much repetition, the vast majority of patients who have had a stroke can be taught to walk independently. The more careful the program, the more normal the gait pattern will be.

Occupational Therapy

The occupational therapist is trained to evaluate the patient's perceptual deficits. This is particularly important for the left hemiplegic. The lesion in the nondominant hemisphere often interferes with the patient's orientation and with his spatial and abstract conceptualizations. Superficially, such a patient may seem to have far less deficit than does the right hemiplegic with aphasia. However, it will soon become apparent that he is unreliable, denies his deficits, and has great difficulty in dressing and in finding his way. Having established

what deficits the patient has, the occupational therapist then proceeds to re-educate the patient, helping him to compensate for his deficits. He then teaches him to re-establish his abilities in the "ADL's" (the activities of daily living), that is, dressing, feeding, and personal hygiene. The therapist will help to teach the patient how to cook, write, read, type, calculate, and practice his hobbies. All this, of course, may now have to be done in a one-handed way to a great extent. For this, the occupational therapist will have to devise various gadgets. He will also advise the patient and relatives about how to make the home more barrier-free.

Speech Therapy

The speech therapist is concerned primarily with the following aspects of communication disorders:

1. Dysphasia—resulting from an impairment in the cerebral hemispheres causing a reduction in the patient's ability to formulate or to interpret language.

2. Dysarthria—resulting from a disturbance of muscular control. This may be a weakness, a slowness, or an incoordination of the affected muscles due to damage of the peripheral or central nervous system, causing a disturbance of phonation, articulation, and resonance.

3. Apraxia—resulting from impairment of certain brain circuits needed for programming articulatory movements. Such patients may not be able to put out their tongue or move other articulatory muscles on command or by imitation. However, they can move these muscles for other activities, such as eating and swallowing. Such patients make variable errors, substi-

tutions, and repetitions, particularly with consonants. However, there can also be complete nonspeech (oral apraxia).

The speech therapist works on all of these aspects of speech disability. There comes a point, however, when further therapy is a waste of time, and then the therapist will provide a home program that the patient and his family can continue by themselves.

The Nurse's Role

The nurse helps in the re-establishment of bladder and bowel control, teaches skin care, and helps to prevent contractures by proper positioning of paralyzed parts when the patient is in bed. The nurse also reinforces and practices transfers, dressing, and feeding with the patient and does a great deal of psychologic counseling with the patient and the family.

The Physician's Role

The physician's task, again, is to coordinate all of these aspects of care and to establish the goals to be achieved. Thus, one patient's potential may be so poor that the main goal will be to teach him to help in his transfer from bed to chair, whereas another patient's goal will be complete independence and return to living on his own. The physician will need the help of the social worker, community health services, and vocational rehabilitation services in many instances.

RHEUMATOID ARTHRITIS

Salicylates, rest, and physical therapy are the basic triumvirate in the management of patients with rheumatoid arthritis. The physical therapy should be simple, so that the patient can perform it daily at home without help. The two aspects of this therapy are (1) to increase comfort and decrease stiffness and (2) to prevent deformities and maintain the range of motion of the joints.

Heat

Heat is an important part of the physical therapy. There are two simple methods of providing good, safe heat. One is the heat

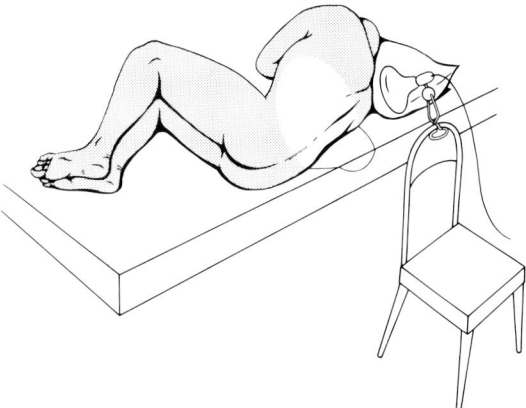

Figure 15–1. Infrared heat lamp used for low back pain.

lamp. This lamp, which has a 250 watt reflector heat bulb and can be clamped to the back of a chair, can be purchased cheaply at a drugstore (Fig. 15–1). It produces the type of infrared rays that cause an increase in local circulation. The lamp is placed at a distance of 18 to 20 inches from the part to be treated and is used for 30 minutes at a time. The intensity of the heat should be comfortable, and this can be varied by moving the lamp. The lamp should be used once or twice a day.

The other method is that of contrast baths for hands and feet. This is far simpler than, and as effective as, the better known paraffin baths. The method of use is as follows:

Fill one large basin or similar container with cold water at 65° F. (use a bath thermometer). Fill another container with hot water at 110° F. Place the hands or feet first in the hot water and then in the cold water, according to the following schedule:

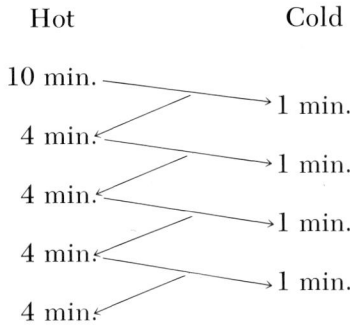

The contrast baths should be used once or twice daily.

For the hands, a basin or sink can be

used for the hot water. For the cold water, a large plastic dishpan about 7 inches deep is satisfactory. A double kitchen sink is useful for contrast baths for the hands.

For the feet, it is sometimes possible to use the bathtub for the hot water. The cold water can be held in a rectangular household bucket or plastic wastebasket measuring about 14 inches deep and about 12 × 12 inches at the bottom. As an alternative, two plastic wastebaskets can be used in the bathtub, one with hot water and one with cold water. Double laundry tubs, placed on the floor, also can be used for the contrast baths for the feet.

Exercise

The most important exercises are those that maintain the range of motion of all the joints. Instructions should be given to perform these once a day. They should not take longer than 20 minutes, otherwise the patient will not keep on doing them. The exercises should become part of the daily routine and should be done whether the joints hurt or not. Often, for example, the shoulder hurts. Instinctively, the patient will protect it. He will avoid reaching for the top shelf. It will not be long before he will be unable to abduct and flex the shoulder fully. If, however, he makes himself put the shoulder through its full range of motion daily, he is less likely to lose the motion. Once the knees are affected, strength of the quadriceps will decrease, and the patient will need instructions for strengthening that muscle. It is important that strengthening be done isometrically (joint does not move) and not isotonically (contraction will move related joint). Isometric strengthening is less likely to injure the joint. Further protection can be given to the weight-bearing joints by the use of walking aids. However, if the upper extremity joints are affected, holding a cane and putting weight on elbows and shoulders might be quite difficult. Therefore, we use aids such as platform canes and crutches.

Patients are often told that if they have arthritis they must keep moving. Nothing is further from the truth. Rest in a good position is far more important than is needless activity. Excessive strain will quickly lead to subluxation of tendons and with it an ulnar drift of the fingers and gross deformities.

Protection from Stress

It is the occupational therapist who can teach the patient to protect his hands. Rest splints that maintain the joints in the functional position are often prescribed to be used at night. The therapist will instruct the patient about how to avoid stresses, such as pulling, pushing, and twisting, by the use of Velcro fasteners and large buttons and by putting a loop of string on a zipper tab. He will show the patient how to avoid carrying heavy objects and how to alter handles. Foam rubber or cloth strips can be wrapped around a handle in such a fashion as to produce a cone-shaped build-up. The cone-shaped built-up portion of a handle should be grasped with the thumb and index finger around its smaller end and with the other digits toward the larger end. Similar handles can be used on toothbrushes, eating utensils, and combs. The therapist will show the patient how to arrange furniture and how to use relatively high seats to minimize strains on hands and knees when getting up. This also applies to raised toilet seats.

BACK PAIN

Back pain is an example of a disability that is often chronic but is not as catastrophic as are the previously described disabilities. Knowledge of some simple physical measures will often help the patient considerably. The first step in the management of back pain is to establish the diagnosis and to exclude any causes that may require surgical or pharmaceutical measures.

The physical therapy program for back pain can often be performed by the patient himself, as long as he is given good instructions. The patient must learn these instructions well, for it is important that he do the exercises daily and continue them as a prophylactic measure even after the pain has subsided.

The physician, therefore, should prescribe a program that a physical therapist can readily transmit to the patient. There is no need for the patient to continue working with the therapist after he has been shown the program three or four times.

Chronic back pain has many causes, but probably the most common cause is a combination of simple trauma causing a strain that is necessary. It does not penetrate more than 3 mm. into the skin, but that is enough to help relax the muscles by reflex mechanisms. Radiant heat can warm a fairly large area with an even intensity and, unlike the heating pad, it does not produce hot spots. Wet packs cool off too rapidly. The heat lamp should be applied as described previously in the section on rheumatoid arthritis and should be directed to the lower part of the back as illustrated in Figure 15–1.

Massage

After the application of heat, massage may help to achieve further relaxation of the muscles so that it is easier for the patient to move about and to perform the prescribed exercises. Massage begins with light stroking of the skin and continues with gentle kneading of the muscles in their affected areas, as shown in Figure 15–2.

Exercise

There are many exercises that can be useful. Generally, the most useful are the spinal flexion exercises that stretch the back and strengthen the abdominal muscles. Once the patient knows how to do these exercises properly, he should slowly start to do them more vigorously and with greater repetition. At no time should he be in a hurry; he must give himself sufficient time to do them correctly. The following are the basic exercises:

1. Spinal flexion exercise 1 (Fig. 15–3). The patient pulls his knees up toward his

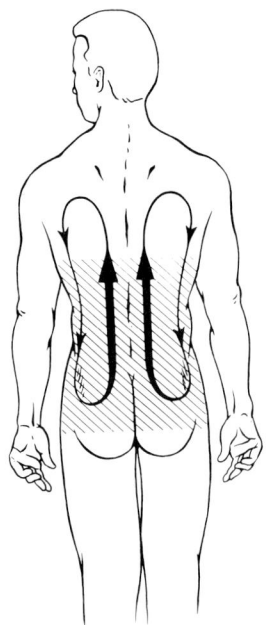

Figure 15–2. *Method of massage for low back pain.*

aggravated by fears, resentments, and other psychologic factors. The physician can alleviate a great deal of the distress by helping the patient in all of these aspects. The patient needs to be treated as a whole person rather than as a backache. This type of approach is often also appropriate when one of the causes of the back pain is chronic degenerative disease or chronic disc disease. The physical therapy prescription would be along the following lines:

Heat

Usually heat will help to relax the muscles. The infrared type of radiant heat is all

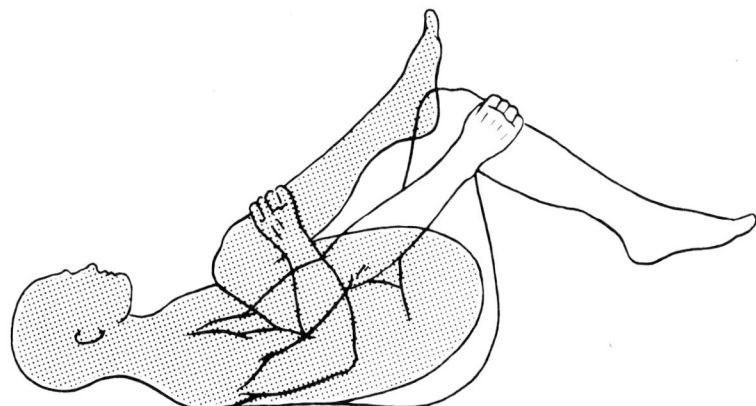

Figure 15–3. *Spinal flexion exercise 1. See text. Shaded figure is final position.*

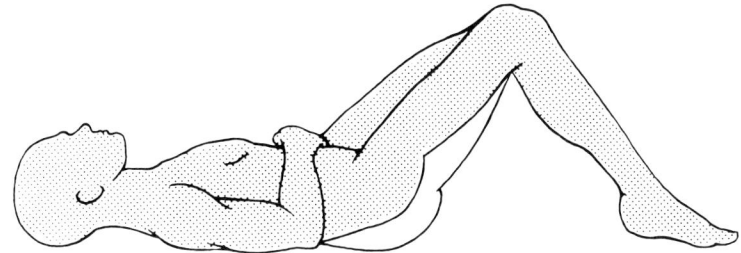

Figure 15–4. *Spinal flexion exercise 2. See text. Shaded figure is final position.*

armpits (the exercise may be done while lying on the side if it is too difficult to do while lying on the back).

2. Spinal flexion exercise 2 (Fig. 15–4). The patient pinches his buttocks together and begins to lift them from the surface. The buttocks should not be lifted too far off the surface because this will increase the swayback (lordosis).

3. Back-stretching exercises. The patient sits on a straight chair with both feet planted firmly on the floor and with his hands on his knees. He then bends forward slowly, as if to put his forehead on his knees. (If he bends so as to put his chest on his knees, he is bending at the hips and will not achieve the desired result.)

4. Isometric abdominal wall-strengthening exercise. The patient lies on his back with his knees and hips bent sufficiently so that the lower part of the back is flattened against the surface. He places his hand behind his head to support its weight. (a) The patient raises his head and shoulders slightly—enough to require a strong contraction of the abdominal muscles but not enough to cause pain in the lower part of the back. (b) While maintaining the position achieved in (a), the patient twists his shoulders slightly to the right—not far enough to cause pain in the back. (c) While maintaining the position in (a), the patient twists his shoulders slightly to the left—not far enough to cause pain in the back. (d) The patient resumes the resting position.

Posture Principles

Since the abdominal muscles are important in helping to support the weight of the trunk, they should be kept contracted when the trunk is upright. The patient should maintain tension in the abdominal wall and should not allow it to protrude. He should

become "belly conscious." A snug nonelastic corset may provide similar support.

Increasing the amount of swayback (lordosis) in the lower part of the back often aggravates low back pain. This may occur because of several circumstances: allowing the abdominal muscles to be too relaxed; reaching above shoulder height with one or both hands; reaching to shoulder height with the elbows straight, with both hands; carrying heavy loads at chest height; lying on the abdomen, particularly on a soft bed; and attempting to lift a window that is stuck.

The wall test (Fig. 15–5) helps to decrease the amount of swayback and to de-

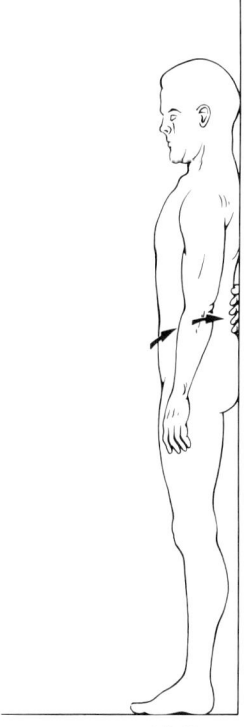

Figure 15–5. *Wall test.*

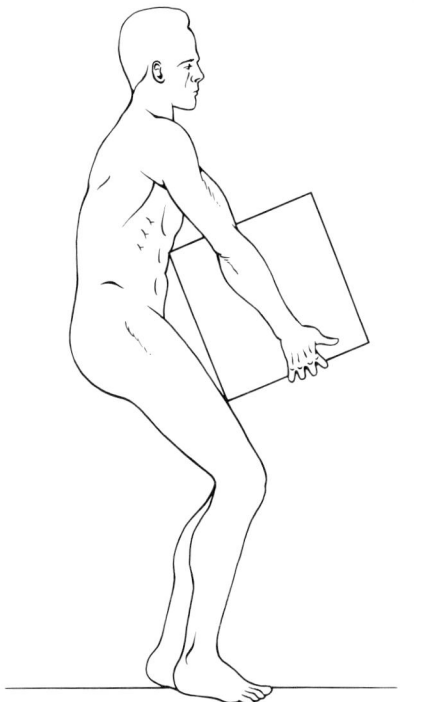

Figure 15–6. *Correct way of carrying heavy object.*

general, one prescribes the simplest aid possible that will provide the maximum compensation and will produce a gait pattern that is the most stable and safe and is the nearest to the normal gait pattern.

Canes

Canes can be used if there is a disability in one leg, the other leg being nearly normal. However, the disabled leg must have at least 50 per cent of its usual weight-carrying capacity. The cane is used on the opposite (the normal) side. For example, if there is osteoarthritis of the right hip, a remarkable amount of relief can be achieved by the use of a cane in the left hand. This is because the weight is redistributed to the left upper extremity. Thus, as one steps on the right leg and lifts one's left leg up to take a step forward, all the weight will be shifted to the arthritic right hip. However, if at that instance the body is balanced by the left-handed cane, nearly 50 per cent of the weight will be taken off the right hip.

velop good posture. The patient stands with his head and back against a flat wall, standing on his heels and 2 inches from the wall. One hand is placed flat behind the small of the back, and the back is flattened by rocking the top of the pelvis backward (Fig. 15–5, *arrows*) and by tightening the abdominal muscles so that the hand is squeezed between the back and the wall. The patient then stands as tall as possible and tries to walk away from the wall while maintaining the posture. He then returns to the wall to check his success.

If it is necessary to carry heavy objects, these should be carried close to the body. Preferably, most of the weight should be supported by the front of the thighs while the trunk is kept bent slightly forward and the abdomen is held in snugly (Fig. 15–6). Objects should be picked up from the floor by squatting rather than by stooping.

WALKING AIDS AND GAIT PATTERNS

The normal gait pattern is very easily compromised. Simple sprains and bruises, fractures, arthritis, and complete paralysis produce different degrees of difficulties. In

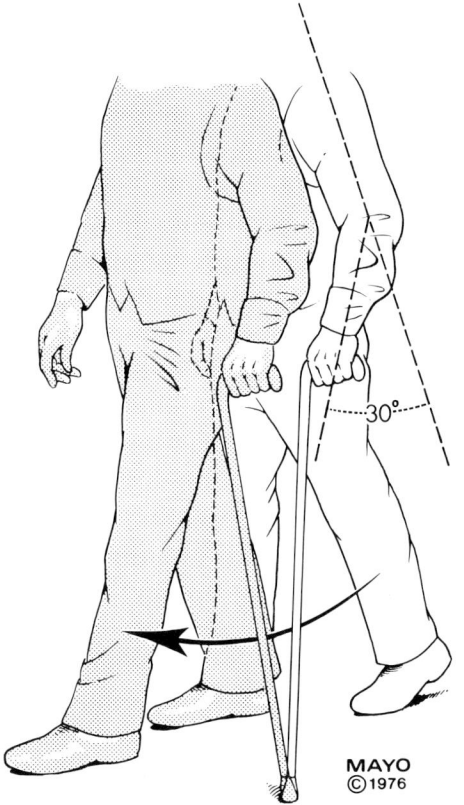

MAYO
©1976

Figure 15–7. *Left-hand cane gait for disability in right leg. See text. Shaded figure is final position.*

Quite often in such an example, the right hip abductors are weak, and this causes drooping of the pelvis; or, because of the pain, a waddling or "antalgic" gait is produced. Either problem can be corrected by the use of a simple cane. Similarly, other conditions, such as pain of the ankle or knee or even some degree of paresis, as with peroneal palsy of one leg, can be helped by a cane.

For conditions in which there is instability as well as weakness, such as after a stroke, a regular cane will be too unstable to begin with and a variety of broad-based canes can be tried. The height of the cane should be such that the elbow is bent 30° in the standing position. This nearly straight elbow allows the patient to put a maximum amount of weight on the cane. As is illustrated in Figure 15–7, the affected leg and the cane in the opposite hand move together at all times. Figure 15–8 illustrates walking up and down a curb. The good leg goes up first, but for stepping down it goes down last.

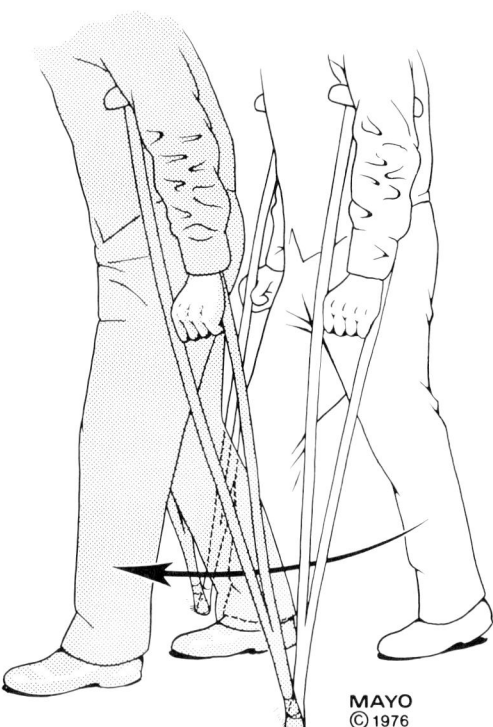

Figure 15–9.   *Three-point crutch gait for disability in right leg. See text. Shaded figure is final position.*

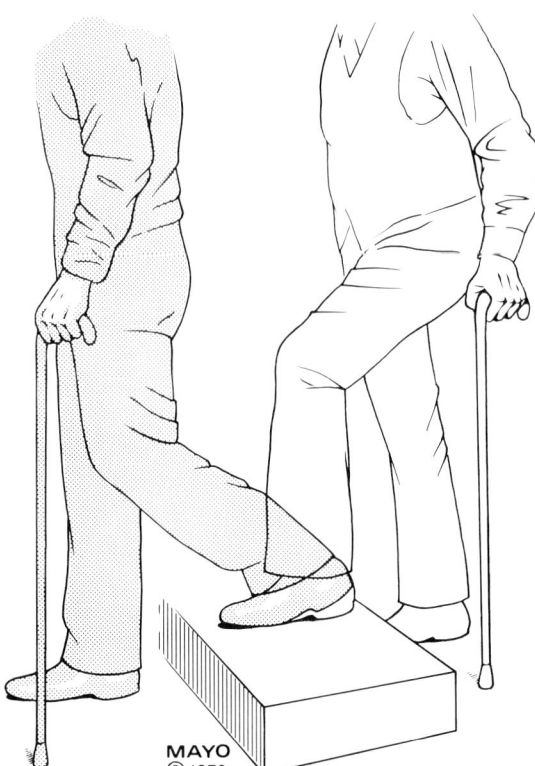

Figure 15–8.   *Going up and down curb with cane. See text.*

Crutches

A number of different crutches are available, but the cheapest and the most stable is the regular wooden variety. Two crutches, of course, give much more stability and weight relief than does one cane. Crutches should always be used if the weakness is so severe as to make walking even with a cane unsafe.

There are various patterns of crutch gait. The most common variety is the three-point gait, which is used for a fracture in one leg. In this pattern (Fig. 15–9) the affected leg and the two crutches go down together. This allows all or part of the weight to be carried by the arms holding the crutches, as the normal leg moves forward. With the normal leg on the ground, the two crutches and the affected leg go forward, leaving all the weight on the unaffected leg. The patient has to have fairly good coordination and stability to use this pattern. If greater stability is needed, another pattern or a walker may have to be used.

The weight of the body should never be carried on the axillae but rather should be borne on the hands. The height of the crutch should be such that the top of the crutch is 3 fingerbreadths below the anterior fold of the axilla, and the hand piece is adjusted to allow 30° of flexion at the elbow. As with use of the cane, for walking up a step or curb with the crutches the good leg goes up first, and the crutches guard the affected leg at all times (Fig. 15–10). Going down, the good leg leaves the step or curb last.

Walkers

Walkers allow much more stability, but they are bulkier and are difficult to use on steps. They are very useful for the old and feeble and the uncoordinated. With walkers, the regular gait pattern is interrupted. A "walk to" pattern is used. One walks up to the walker, moves it ahead, and walks up to it again.

Wheelchairs

Like all walking aids, wheelchairs have to be carefully prescribed. In most cases,

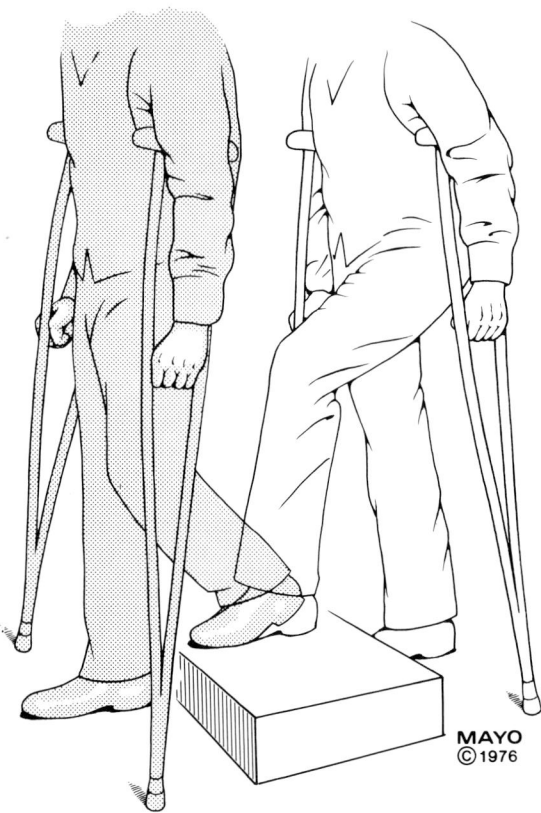

Figure 15–10. *Going up and down curb with crutches. See text.*

these should not be obtained without a carefully thought out prescription. Wheelchairs come in three standard sizes—child's, narrow adult's, and adult's—that differ in width and height. A wheelchair should be snug and should allow only 2 fingerbreadths between the sides of the chair and the patient. Commonly, desk arms are needed. These are armrests that fit beneath a table. They are removable and thereby enable the patient to transfer out of the wheelchair. The leg rests should be removable. One may need heel loops on the footrests. Occasionally, there is need for the elevating type of leg rests. The tires can be pneumatic or solid. Pneumatic tires are useful for carpeted or rough surfaces. Varieties of backrests are also available. Careful selection of a cushion is of particular importance to the patient who has lost sensation.

POSTSURGICAL REHABILITATION PROCEDURES

Knee

The approach is generally similar, whether the knee has been in a cast because of a fracture or has undergone a surgical procedure for an excision of a cartilage or a total knee arthroplasty.

Range of Motion Exercise.   Deliberate, active normal-range exercises are the easiest for the patient to do by himself. He sits on a table, bends the knee as far as possible, and then straightens it; or he can lie on his abdomen and bend and straighten the knee. The therapist can also provide such stretch. The most effective stretch is one that provides a prolonged stretch without pain.

Progressive Resistance Exercise

Before this type of exercise can be done, the physical therapist must show the patient how to contract the muscle (for example, the quadriceps). This is called re-reduction. After nonuse of a muscle for a long time, it is easy to forget how to contract it voluntarily.

The quadriceps muscle is exercised from the sitting position with a 3 inch thick towel roll or pad placed under the knee.

Sandbags are placed over the ankle. The therapist then determines the maximum weight that the patient can lift 10 times without resting. At first, if the muscle is very weak, it may be necessary to use a powdered board to eliminate the effects of gravity. Usually, the amount of weight used can be increased at intervals of 1 to 2 weeks. When no more weight can be added over a 4 week period, maximum strength has probably been achieved.

The weights used are generally based on the maximal number of pounds that can be moved through a full range of motion 10 times (called the 10 repetition maximum, or 10 RM). If the weight is moved through the range, the muscles are exercised isotonically. If the weight is lifted without moving the knee, the exercise is isometric. If the knee is arthritic or has had surgery, it is less damaging to strengthen the knee isometrically.

Gait. While the muscles are weak, the leg needs support. At first a three-point crutch gait is used. As the muscles become stronger, a cane gait is used (cane in the opposite hand). Once the 10 RM is more than 25 pounds, the walking aid can be dispensed with. However, the patient should keep on with the strengthening program if he is very active. Thus, if he is an athlete, the quadriceps 10 RM should be 50 to 60 pounds.

Other Joints

Similar principles of range of motion and strengthening apply to other joints, such as the hip or wrist. Strengthening applies particularly if the weight-bearing joints are involved. With wrist immobilization, the range of motion is the most important. Once the range of motion has been achieved, everyday activities usually will provide the required strength. Everyday activities will also tend to increase the range of motion. However, a deliberate exercise program for improving the full range is also necessary.

PRINCIPLES OF MONITORING PROGRESS IN REHABILITATION

There is no point in having a patient go to a therapist for years if progress is not being made. It is usually more useful for the patient to go daily for a brief period than to go once a week for a prolonged time. The only way progress can be monitored is to take accurate measurements. The range of motion of a joint should be measured (with a goniometer if available, but "eyeballing" can be quite accurate as well). Thus, a knee may lack 15° for full extension and can only flex to 60°. The quadriceps 10 RM may only be 5 pounds. The goal would be to achieve at least full extension, 90° flexion, and a 10 RM of 25 pounds. By keeping a record of these measurements, we have objective data and can give scientific and accurate advice to the patient.

Similarly, with a stroke patient, we record the strength of various muscles and the active and passive ranges of motion. We set down certain goals and with each visit record our measurements. Once a plateau has been reached, we either have to think of a different approach or be content with having a degree of disability remaining. It is then our job to teach the patients to live with that disability and how to substitute for it.

In this chapter, we have tried to illustrate the principles of physical medicine and rehabilitation with a few examples. These principles can be applied to many of the problems that a physician faces in practice. Although the physician needs to be optimistic and give hope, he must also be realistic. He should set realistic goals and be prepared to explain the patient's limitation, not only to the patient but also to the family. Unrealistic hope can be most destructive to the rehabilitation program. A successful rehabilitation program comprises a blend of motivation, acceptance, and faith.

BIBLIOGRAPHY

Guttmann, L.: Spinal Cord Injuries: Comprehensive Management and Research. 2nd ed. Oxford, Blackwell Scientific Publications, 1976.

Krusen, F. H., Kottle, F. J., and Ellwood, P. M., Jr.: Handbook of Physical Medicine and Rehabilitation. 2nd ed. Philadelphia, W. B. Saunders Co., 1971.

Licht, S. H.: Stroke and Its Rehabilitation. Baltimore, The Williams & Wilkins Co., 1975.

Mooney, T. O., Cole, T. M., and Chilgren, R. A.: Sexual Options for Paraplegics and Quadriplegics. Boston, Little, Brown & Co., 1975.

Rusk, H. A.: Rehabilitation Medicine. 3rd ed. St. Louis, The C. V. Mosby Co., 1971.

Chapter 16

CARE OF THE GERIATRIC PATIENT

by WILLIAM REICHEL,
and B. LEWIS BARNETT, JR.

INTRODUCTION

The family physician of the future will be challenged in his practice by a dramatically expanding population of elderly patients. The combined impact of birth control and abortion at one end of the life spectrum, and the increased preservation of life at the other, will generate unprecedented activity in geriatric care. Family physicians and other medical specialists will need to gain increased proficiency in the special problems related to the elderly patient.

At present, there are nearly 32 million Americans over the age of 60, representing 14.7 per cent of the population. From 1970 to 1974, this sector grew 0.6 per cent, more than double the growth rate of the total population. It can only be anticipated that these numbers will increase. Of foremost importance in this expansion of the elderly population is a marked decline in the death rate and a concomitant increase in life expectancy. The average life expectancy has risen steadily from 47.3 years in 1900 to 71.3 years in 1973. For women, life expectancy increased from 48 years in 1900 to 75 years in 1973; for men, the increase was from 46 to 68 years.

Other factors relevant to this remarkable increase in the elderly population include the birth and immigration rates. Since the height of the baby boom in the 1950's, there has been a marked downswing in the birth rate. There has also been a steadily diminishing flow of immigrants. Taking into account mortality rate, birth rate, and immigration rate, one can make reasonably accurate predictions of future population trends. One can assume that the mortality rate will continue to decline slightly. Also, the net rate of immigration to the United States will probably remain at 400,000 immigrants per year. The most labile index is the birth rate or fertility rate. Assuming an intermediate fertility rate—the level of fertility required for the American population to replenish itself indefinitely—one can project the total American population for the year 2000 at 262,484,000. On the basis of these assumptions, one can project that 40,590,000 of the 262,484,000 Americans living in the year 2000 will be 60 years of age or older, that is, 15.5 per cent of the total population. Approximately 30,600,000 individuals, or 11.7 per cent of the populace, will be 65 or older. Among the latter subgroup, approximately two-thirds, or 20 million Americans, will be 75 years of age or older. One can only speculate on the impact of these trends and hope that all of our society's institutions—health care, social security, housing, education, and other areas—will respond to this new human condition.

BIOLOGIC ASPECTS OF AGING

Aging can be described as the progressive decline or loss of physiologic capacity or function in an organism leading to an increased probability of death. There is substantial evidence to suggest that life span, although affected by environmental factors, is influenced principally by genetic control. In animals and plants there appears to be tremendous variation in maximal longevity. The maximal life span attained by each species of animal and plant is one evidence of the genetic control of longevity. Man appears to have a maximal life span of 110 to 115 years. Horses, dogs, cats, rats, and other mammals also show a relatively fixed maximal life expectancy. Similarly, among birds, reptiles, amphibians, fish, and invertebrates, there appears to be a fixed maximal range of longevity for each species. Tortoises seem to be very long-lived. For example, the Galapagos tortoise survives for almost 200 years. What accounts for the giant sequoia living 3000 years or the bristlecone pine living 4600 years according to growth ring information?

There are several other suggestions of genetic control over life span. Another source of evidence is the marked difference in mortality among species. In human studies, important evidence includes twin studies that show that the life spans of identical twins are more similar than the life spans of fraternal twins. Another significant correlate to human longevity is parental longevity. In animals, agricultural and experimental breeding studies also support the concept of genetic regulation of life span. Finally, it is noteworthy that females outlive their male counterparts in virtually all animal species. We have noted earlier the major discrepancy in life expectancy between American women and men — 75 years for women and 68 years for men — in 1973. These changes represent a 56 and 46 per cent increase in longevity for women and men, respectively, since 1900. This major difference between female and male longevity represents an intriguing fact that has not yet been fully explained.

A number of interesting experimental studies of the aging process have been made. In 1935, McKay and associates demonstrated that early deprivation of caloric intake in rodents causes retardation of growth and a prolonged life span. This has been one of the most important experiments in the study of the biology of aging and has been repeated many times. Harman has also prolonged the life of small animals by feeding them antioxidants.

The Hayflick phenomenon is an extremely important model of human aging at the level of the single cell. Over a decade ago, Leonard Hayflick demonstrated the limited capacity of normal human fibroblast cells to multiply in tissue culture. This finite lifetime of cultured cells has become an important model for the study of aging. Also, an inverse relationship seems to exist between the number of in vitro cell divisions and the age of the individual; that is, the older the individual donor, the fewer cell divisions are noted in vitro.

Proponents of the somatic mutation theory of aging have advanced the notion that there is a progressive accumulation of mutations or other chemical damage in DNA, thereby resulting in the incapacitation of individual cells. The autoimmune theory states that mutations or defects in protein specificity could lead to a progressive loss of recognition of "self" by the body's immune system. Burnet long ago proposed the increased incidence of forbidden clones with aging. Considerable evidence has since been assembled supporting this theory.

The theories that attempt to elucidate the mechanisms of aging are plentiful and fascinating. It is conceivable that genetic engineering and environmental modification of life span will be possible in the future, but at present, speculation concerning the retardation of the human aging process remains highly theoretic.

UNIQUE ASPECTS OF THE GERIATRIC PATIENT

There are specific differences between the elderly patient and the patient at other stages in life.[9] We have already indicated that aging is the *progressive deterioration or loss of physiologic capacity*. As life events unfold, the elderly patient witnesses or anticipates the loss of health, income, relations, and friends and must come to terms with this sense of loss.

With aging, not only is there loss but positive attributes as well also may accrue in terms of experience, maturity, and relationships with others in a new dimension with feelings of warmth and love. Geriatric patients may approach death from a different perspective than younger patients. With a different sense of experience, the aging person may have disengaged himself from the ongoing life processes and may be better prepared for the dying process. Attitudes of the aged patient toward dying may be more accepting and less fearful than the attitudes of the younger individual. For example, the elderly patient with impaired health for over 10 years, who has been isolated in an institutional setting with less social interaction, may accept the dying process with greater calm than the middle-aged individual who is caught up in the mainstream of life.

Loss of Physiologic Capacity

Again, the key feature in our understanding of the aging process is the progressive loss of physiologic capacity. A patient suffering myocardial infarction will have a different prognosis if, by virtue of age, he has much diminished lung and kidney function. Certain so-called abnormalities in the geriatric population should be considered normal. What is considered an abnormality in a younger person might be considered normal in an elderly individual. An important example is the decline in glucose tolerance that takes place with age. Hyperglycemia is so common in the older person that to avoid the diagnosis of diabetes mellitus in a high proportion of elderly individuals, Andres has formulated a nomogram that ranks an individual with age-matched peers (Fig. 16–1).[1] The Longitudinal Study on Physiological Aging of the Gerontology Research Center in Baltimore has also shown that the rate of decline in creatinine clearance accelerates with age (Fig. 16–2).[11] It should be noted that this decline in renal function was studied in several hundred normal subjects who were free of specific disease states, and thus might be considered true renal aging.

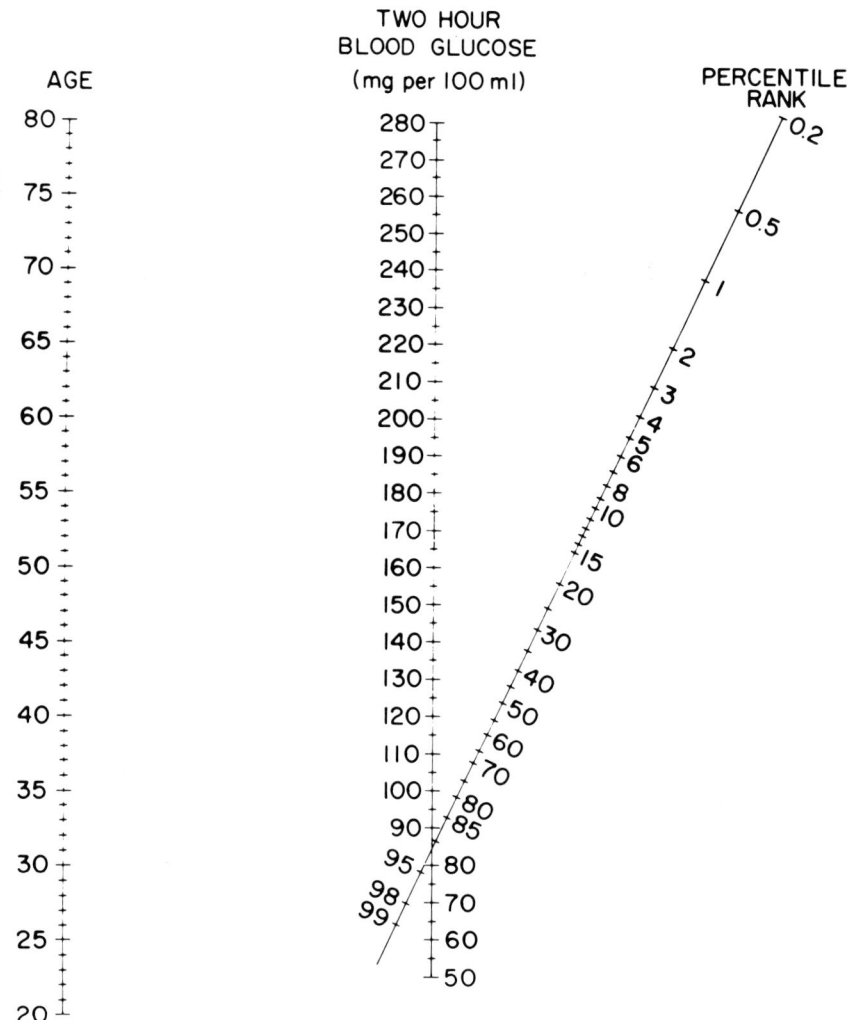

Figure 16–1. Nomogram for judging performance on the oral glucose tolerance test. Dose of glucose was 1.75 gm. per kg. of body weight. Concentration of glucose is measured in venous blood from the ferricyanide reduction method using the AutoAnalyzer. (From Andres, R., Mayo Clin. Proc., 42:674, 1967.)

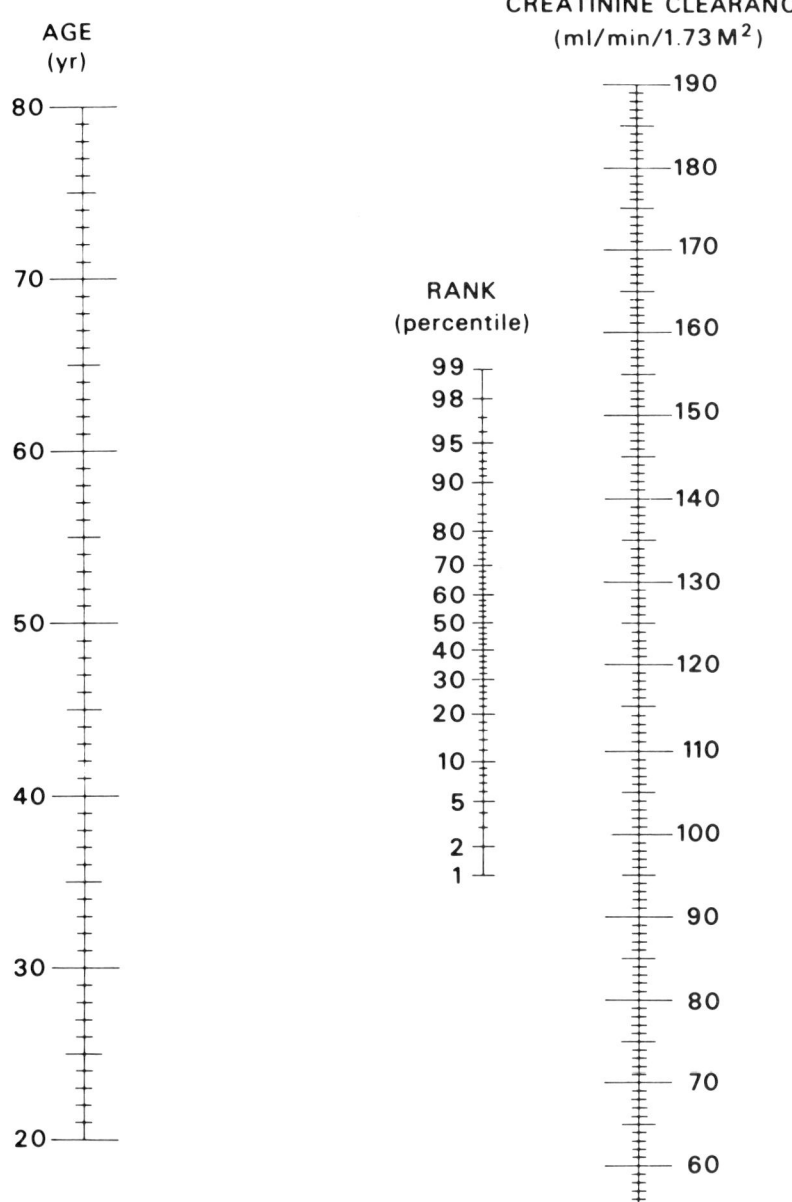

Figure 16–2. Nomogram for determination of age-adjusted percentile rank in true creatinine clearance. (From Rowe, J., J. Gerontol., 31:159, 1976.)

Latency of Disease and Misleading Physical Signs

Another characteristic of the aged population is the latency of disease. Serious disease may be present with few signs. Temperature, white blood cell response, and pain are all diminished in the elderly. The elderly may have pneumonia or pyelonephritis without a temperature elevation or chills. Myocardial infarction, perforated appendix, mesenteric infarction, and ruptured abdominal aorta all may be present without pain in the elderly. Bronchopneumonia can appear as a terminal event with few clinical signs.

In addition to latency of certain signs, there are misleading physical signs. Reluctance of a stuporous patient to breathe voluntarily or poor aeration of the chest may conceal significant pulmonary findings. Local crepitation at the bases of the lungs may simply indicate that the elderly patient has been reclining in bed for a few hours. The patient frequently is not able to cooperate or is too apprehensive to participate in the motor and sensory portions of the neurologic examination. In fact, common problems that face the family physician in the care of the elderly patient include the patient's inability to cooperate, his fearfulness, and the physical conditions of the examination. All of these factors must be considered in the office, hospital, or home. There is often a tendency to avoid various components of the history or physical examination because of such problems. Many elderly patients are not properly evaluated because of their slowness in removing clothing, arthritic pain when getting dressed or changing position, or the dim lighting in the home. In planning the structure and logistics of a busy office practice, these human factors must be taken into account for the proper examination of the elderly patient. Measures that might improve the examination of the geriatric patient include the following: easy access of a wheelchair into an examining room, the presence of an office assistant who can stay with and assist the patient in undressing and dressing, special assistance to the patient in safely getting on and off an examining table, and providing an appointment time when the geriatric patient's visit can be carried out in an unhurried fashion. A physician extender is of extreme value in the examination and care of the elderly, whether in the office, the patient's home, or an institutional setting.

Increased Drug Effect

There is much greater drug effect in the elderly. Older patients tolerate medications poorly. There is an altered response of the central nervous system, and acute confusional states can result not only from barbiturates or tranquilizers but also from antibiotics or digitalis. The rate of elimination of drugs is altered, especially with kidney and hepatic dysfunction. There also is greater variability in response to drugs. In younger persons, the response is well-defined, whereas in the older patient the response is more variable. Drug toxicity is clearly one of the most common problems encountered in geriatric evaluation.

Multiple Disease Processes

The hallmark of the elderly patient is the existence of *multiple disease processes or diagnoses*.[9] Clinical and pathologic studies indicate the long list of problems that each patient over 70 may exhibit. Postmortem examination often reveals as many as 15 or 20 disorders, some of which had been asymptomatic.

In addition to facing the daily challenge of chronic complaints and ailments, the elderly patient remains highly susceptible to disorders easily acquired in a variety of institutional settings.[8] Hospitals and long-term care facilities are replete with potential hazards for the often-frightened, physically compromised older person. In many cases, the elderly patient is oversedated for problems of agitation or confusion. A chain reaction of adverse events is often the result. A patient's acute confusional state or agitation might be the result of drug toxicity or some other type of medical illness. The patient, however, receives further medication and may go on to develop dangerous sequelae, such as pneumonia, or may incur accidents and injuries.

Accidents and injuries can occur with equal ease in the safety and comfort of the patient's own home, complicating pre-existent disorders. Patients with cardiac arrhythmias, cerebrovascular insufficiency, or seizure disorders are all at risk of trauma from falls or automobile accidents. Multiple or even single accidents can diminish self-confidence and lead to serious depressive states. Shoulder dislocations or injuries of the upper extremities can prevent colostomy self-care. Immobilization subsequent to accidents may lead to pulmonary emboli or fat embolization related to fractures of long bones.

Osteoarthritis is another disabling condition often found in association with other ailments among the elderly. It is especially aggravated by superimposed obesity. There are other examples of multiple groups of problems experienced by the aged. The patient's diuretic therapy may precipitate gout. Medications for gout may exacerbate his gastric ulcer problem. The patient with heart failure who requires infusion of fluids or transfusion of blood for gastrointestinal bleeding also poses a management dilemma.

THE PROBLEM-ORIENTED RECORD

The physician dealing with the geriatric patient must cope with multiple problems. Obviously, the problem-oriented record is a valuable tool. Geriatric patients, as a group, are potential beneficiaries of the problem-oriented approach to record-keeping. The voluminous records accumulated by the chronically ill elderly patient include progress notes, hospitalization summaries, and consultations. These data must incorporate not only the medical problems but also an understanding of family, social, and psychologic problems.

The basis of the problem-oriented record is the problem list, which is a table of contents for that individual patient. Symptoms, signs, laboratory findings, and social and psychologic information are included in the problem list. Progress notes are organized in relation to problems. If this system is followed, utilizing flow sheets, an individual problem may be monitored clearly and logically over a period of time (see chapter 5). Using a standard medical record, it is frequently difficult and time-consuming to keep track of the elderly patient's multiple problems. There may be an unwieldy volume of material with important notes hidden away. The simplicity of a comprehensive, concise, and logical approach to record-keeping should add a great deal to the family physician's ability to care for the elderly patient.

The major hazard in evaluating the geriatric patient is the temptation to allow preconceived notions of common patterns of illness to preclude the need for careful individualized evaluation of each elderly patient. Conscientious history-taking and physical examination are essential. Only then can the physician realistically consider every treatment possibility. A judicious analysis of all factors—physical, psychologic, and social—may result in a decision to treat or not to treat certain entities. Attention to less urgent problems may best be postponed rather than complicate an already diverse therapeutic regimen. It may be more important to the patient to remain in the comfortable and familiar environment of his own home despite limited access to therapy than to reside in a long-term care facility. Attention to psychologic problems must sometimes take precedence

over physical illness in the management plan. For example, attempting to treat diabetes, hypertension, or gout may be unsuccessful if the patient is failing to cooperate as a result of depressive preoccupation with a recent loss of spouse.

In some situations, issues raised on the problem list must be left in doubt. Evaluative studies cannot be pursued too aggressively in a frail patient. On occasion, the problem might be identifiable, but good judgment dictates postponement of definitive diagnostic tests or treatment. A resolution of certain other problems, however, may enable the patient to tolerate his total situation better. Relatively minor problems of vision, hearing, dentition, and ambulation may precipitate a crisis with respect to self-sufficiency in the aged patient with multiple disabilities.

The problem-oriented medical record is especially effective in assisting the physician in the organization of complex multidisciplinary therapeutic information. The findings and suggestions of social workers, physical and occupational therapists, nurses, dietitians, psychologists, audiologists, and others can be incorporated into a unified record and treatment plan. A team conference with different types of specialists and health professionals can result in effective care when all of these inputs are well coordinated by the family physician. One should bring members of the family into the multidisciplinary conference in contemplating courses of action, particularly in seeking alternatives to institutionalization.

When possible, it is useful to review the problem and the proposed treatment plans with the individual patient or an interested, alert family member. It is best if the patient is a partner with the physician with a full understanding of the problems that are present. Candor is sometimes not possible, and the physician will receive signals from the patient that he does not want to know the diagnosis or the full implications of the problem. However, others show no reluctance or denial. It is best when the physician and the patient can talk freely and openly about the problems that they face together. In some situations, a family member will ask the physician to shield the patient from frank information about his condition. The physician may need to work with this family member if it is clear that the patient can easily handle the information and it is the family member who needs extra support and guidance.

ORGANIC BRAIN SYNDROMES IN THE ELDERLY

Perhaps the most frequently misinterpreted conditions seen in the elderly are the organic brain syndromes. Neuropsychiatric disturbance in the elderly is often casually accepted as expectable and untreatable, when in reality a treatable cause may be present.

Acute Confusional Reaction (Acute Brain Syndrome)

Acute confusional reaction, or acute brain syndrome, is characterized by recent onset of confusion, disorientation, or delirium—mental changes that are commonly seen in elderly patients in emergency situations. The key word in the description is *recent*. Abrupt change in any patient's customary sensorium, intellectual function, or level of consciousness should be investigated thoroughly as a possible organic disorder. Such mental dysfunction must not be presumed to be dementia, or chronic brain syndrome. For a proper diagnosis of dementia, it is necessary to obtain a history of gradual intellectual decline and memory loss persisting over an appropriate period of time. For example, the elderly patient with an acute confusional reaction who was well until 3 days prior to seeking medical advice, read his newspaper, drove his automobile, and in all respects appeared normal should be evaluated carefully for a hidden medical illness or drug toxicity. Pneumonia or other infectious processes, pulmonary embolism, myocardial infarction, and mild cerebrovascular accidents often do not demonstrate typical findings in the elderly but appear as confusion and disorientation. Other illnesses that produce this situation include cardiac failure, hypokalemia, anemia, and dehydration.

Organic Dementia (Chronic Brain Syndrome)

If the intellectual dysfunction is more long-standing, for example of more than 6 months' duration, chronic brain syndrome, or organic dementia, is the likely diagnosis. Dementia may be described as the gradual deterioration of intellect, memory, or cognitive ability. The physician dealing with the elderly patient must consider testing intellectual function if he suspects dementia. In the presence of a menstrual disorder in a younger patient, the physician must ask the patient about her last menstrual period or about menstrual flow. Similarly, the family physician testing the elderly patient for suspected dementia must ask questions that determine the patient's cognitive ability. The physician should question the patient in regard to immediate recall, memory of recent events, and memory of events of the remote past. Ten questions developed by Kahn and associates[5] are extremely useful: Where are you now? Where is this place located? What is today's date? What is the month now? What year is it? How old are you? What is your birthdate? Where were you born? Who is the President of the United States? Who was the previous President? Other questions can be added about childhood, family, and subjects known to be of interest to the patient. One might ask the name of the patient's first wife or who the President was during World War II. Where was the patient born? When did he move to this state? What are the names of his children? It is important that the patient's responses be verified by family members or other sources. If this substantiation is not possible, a different system of memory testing may be utilized, for example, repetition of a short series of words or numbers, such as "repeat 1, 3, 7" or "repeat house, car, umbrella."

In general, remote memory seems to be preserved to a greater extent than recall of recent events, and impairment of remote memory is associated with a poorer prognosis. It is possible that remote events have been imprinted into the memory system more deeply and recent events are imprinted less deeply. The patient may remember facts pertaining to his childhood or first marriage but will not recall events pertaining to his most recent marriage.

Socioeconomic factors and the accessibility of communications and audiovisual stimuli can also have a considerable bearing on the patient's mental status. In the absence of sufficient stimuli from the environment, the patient may find it difficult to respond properly to common test questions. The patient who has been isolated for a prolonged period without benefit of radio or television may not be able to answer questions related to current events.

The two major forms of organic dementia are primary senile dementia, or Alzheimer's disease, and arteriosclerotic dementia.

Primary Senile Dementia. The chief characteristics of primary senile dementia, or Alzheimer's disease, include memory loss, impaired judgment, and paucity of voluntary movement. There is a gradual loss of ability to perform the normal activities of daily living, and the patient becomes unable to recognize family members and friends. Emotional affect may remain preserved, and social responses may appear intact despite significant intellectual deficit. Neurologic examination may remain normal. Because of intellectual decline, the individual is rendered totally incapable of self-care in the final stages of the disease.

Neuropathologic examination reveals atrophy of the frontal and temporal lobes with loss of cortical cells and symmetrical enlargement of the lateral and third ventricles. Alzheimer's neurofibrillary tangles, amyloid-containing senile plaques, and lipofuscin pigment are noted on microscopic examination. In patients with Alzheimer's disease, little cerebral arteriosclerosis is noted. In fact, Sourander and Sjögren reported that arteriosclerotic changes were noted in only 10 per cent of patients with this disorder.[14] Conversely, they noted few Alzheimer-type changes in patients with cerebral arteriosclerosis. Although the presence of cerebral atrophy can be inferred from clinical signs and symptoms, the diagnosis can be reliably confirmed by pneumoencephalographic demonstration of cortical atrophy and ventricular dilatation. Computerized axial tomography (the EMI scan), however, is preferable for detecting Alzheimer's disease in light of the increased morbidity associated with the pneumoencephalogram.[7]

Alzheimer's disease refers both to the senile form, called primary senile dementia of the Alzheimer type, and to the presenile form, called Alzheimer's presenile dementia. The latter variety tends to occur among individuals in their fourth or fifth decade and is considered at this time to be a more severe variation of the basic Alzheimer's disease. It is characterized by marked memory disturbance, dementia, and loss of spontaneity. The pathologic findings are similar to but much more pronounced than those described in the senile form. Again, computerized axial tomography is valuable in diagnosis.

Arteriosclerotic Dementia. Arteriosclerotic dementia occurs following repeated strokes, or cerebrovascular accidents, which are distinguished by episodic and focal neurologic disease. Other vascular symptoms and signs may be present in the form of headache, dizziness, syncopal attacks, or aphasia. Cerebral softening must be severe and widespread following recurrent vascular insult in order for dementia to occur. Following a series of small strokes, the hypertensive patient may develop pseudobulbar palsy, which is characterized by labile facies, difficulty in speaking and swallowing, and signs of a bilateral upper motor neuron paralysis.

Other Forms of Organic Dementia. Normal pressure hydrocephalus is a syndrome characterized by dementia and gait disturbance and is surgically correctable.[12] There is marked dilatation of the ventricles, but the cortical atrophy present in Alzheimer's disease is not noted. The brain, in a sense, is plastered against the skull. Computerized axial tomography and cisternal scanning are the best tools for diagnosing this condition with less risk than pneumoencephalography.[7] Since 1965, significant improvement has been reported following correction by a shunt operation. It should be pointed out that normal pressure hydrocephalus has been observed following head injury in the elderly. In fact, both chronic subdural hematoma and normal pressure hydrocephalus should be considered in the differential diagnosis of any elderly patient with a history of head injury and deteriorating mental function.

It is clear that certain forms of dementia in the elderly are correctable, and it is up to the physician to decide which cases deserve aggressive investigation. The family physician, knowing the patient and his life situation, may be in the best position to make this judgment. Diagnostic evaluation for normal pressure hydrocephalus is expensive and not without difficulty; the work-up may not be justifiable if the situation offers little hope of improvement. An older individual who has been performing his daily functions until recently and whose physical functions remain reasonably intact would be considered a more appropriate candidate for investigation than another elderly individual with a 5 year history of dementia, other serious illness, and poor physical functioning for the past 10 years. Although the physician must remain alert to the possibility of discovering a correctable disorder, good judgment remains the main factor in determining the extent of diagnostic evaluation.

Other potentially treatable causes of chronic brain syndrome, or dementia, in the elderly include myxedema and pernicious anemia. Other untreatable causes of dementia include general paresis, Wilson's disease, and Huntington's chorea.

Management of Irreversible Dementia

The family physician faces a tremendous challenge in determining what can be offered the patient with irreversible dementia. Not too many years ago, severely demented patients were often committed to state mental institutions. Today, with the prudent support of the physician, these patients can be maintained at home, in a day care facility, or in a nursing home. A warm, familiar, loving environment may be highly therapeutic. The physician, of course, should have a full understanding of the total family picture. Is the health of the patient's spouse stable enough to allow for care of the patient at home? What effect will the patient's illness have on grandchildren or great-grandchildren in the same household? Are there children in the family or neighborhood who might be jeopardized? Does the patient wander away if left unwatched? Does he become agitated or combative? What are the family's financial resources? Are there gas ovens or firearms in the home? How are medications controlled and dispensed? Should the family consider guardianship or other protective legal services at this point?

Whether the patient with dementia is maintained in the community or within an institution, the physician should be careful in the use of psychotropic drugs and restraining devices. Commonly, the mental disturbance may worsen, and chronic oversedation may lead to dehydration, bedsores, pneumonia, and other complications. In dealing with the impaired elderly patient, it is helpful to use his name regularly in conversation. Whenever possible, the patient's orientation to time, place, and person should be reinforced by those attending him.

Differentiation of Neuropsychiatric Disorders

Because of loneliness and losses suffered in old age, many elderly people turn to the increased use of alcohol, making alcoholism a major problem in the geriatric population. In evaluating the patient with acute or chronic brain syndrome, or both, the physician must recognize several types of neuropsychiatric disturbances associated with alcoholism. These include alcoholic intoxication, alcoholic withdrawal, nutritional deficiency (Wernicke-Korsakoff syndrome), hepatic encephalopathy, and miscellaneous degenerative disorders, such as cerebral or cerebellar atrophy.

In addition to acute and chronic brain syndromes, there are also many syndromes with features of both types. The chronically demented elderly patient in a nursing home may develop increased confusion and agitation in response to the development of a major medical illness, such as pulmonary emboli. This is a mixed brain syndrome. The physician must also be able to distinguish a functional disorder from an organic brain syndrome. The elderly patient who has recently suffered the loss of a spouse and is severely depressed may present the appearance of dementia in the form of an immobile posture and unwillingness to communicate. The paranoid patient may also present with the picture of dementia. At some point in the interview, paranoid ideation may become apparent. It is clear that interviewing and observational skills are crucial in making appropriate differentiation of the type of neuropsychiatric disorder. Sensory deprivation is another cause of abnormal behavior that may be mistaken for an organic brain syndrome. The elderly individual living alone in a dimly lit apartment, or alone on a farm without visitors, radio, or television, suffers sensory deprivation. Resocialization, with increased psychologic and audiovisual stimuli, may correct this behavior.

One could provide other illustrations of the need for the most careful evaluation and examination of each impaired elderly patient. Not all mental disturbance in the elderly represents dementia. Not all dementia is arteriosclerotic. One can cite other examples of pitfalls that are common in the daily evaluation and care of the elderly. A cluster of symptoms and signs must be organized into a pattern and then recognized. Are we dealing with acute confusional reaction of recent onset caused by a medical illness or medication? Iatrogenic causes should be ruled out *first.* Are we dealing with a history of intellectual decline over a prolonged period of time? Are we dealing with a picture that is largely functional or emotional, for example, the elderly patient with recent onset of depression following the loss of the patient's spouse? It is rewarding to know that the history, interview, and physical examination will allow us to distinguish these categories—acute confusional reactions, organic dementias, functional disorders, and mixtures of these. Proper diagnosis will allow us to make specific treatment plans, such as the withdrawal of medication in the case of an acute confusional reaction or the treatment of myxedema in the case of a specific dementia.

CARDIAC DISEASE IN THE ELDERLY

Not all cardiac disease in the elderly is arteriosclerotic. Yet an individual past middle age who presents with congestive heart failure is often presumed to have arteriosclerotic heart disease without a proper search for another cause. It is quite possible that the actual cause is long-standing rheumatic heart disease with mitral stenosis. In this situation, the murmur often cannot be heard during the acute episode of cardiac failure. Unless further investigation is pursued after the patient's condition has been stabilized, the patient will not benefit from the correct therapeutic regimen. No cardiac problem should be labeled until all diagnostic possibilities have been considered and the correct diagnosis has been clearly established. In cardiac disease, as in the evaluation of dementia, the physician should avoid the practice of labeling the patient and should continue to reassess a complex diagnostic problem until the etiology is clarified. Congestive heart failure may be caused by rheumatic heart disease, congenital heart disease, recurrent pulmonary emboli, pericardial disease, systemic hypertension, viral myocarditis, alcoholic myocardiopathy, recurrent myocardial infarction, hyperthyroidism, or traumatic heart disease.[4]

Rheumatic Heart Disease. Valvular or rheumatic heart disease, especially mitral stenosis, should be considered in every patient at the onset of congestive heart failure. Although acute childhood rheumatic fever is declining, there are still a significant number of elderly patients who have rheumatic heart disease. In a recent British study, 4 per cent of the patients in a large hospital for the care of the elderly had valvular heart disease.

Consideration of rheumatic heart disease is vital in the individual presenting with symptoms of stroke and thought to have arteriosclerotic heart disease, since he really may be suffering from rheumatic heart disease with systemic embolization. It is crucial that the physician identify the proper diagnosis and initiate long-term anticoagulant therapy, which may significantly prolong the patient's life. Elderly patients may also require cardiac surgery for valvular heart disease and should not be denied this specific form of therapy.

Congenital Heart Disease. A diagnosis of long-standing unrecognized congenital heart disease is probably considered even less frequently than rheumatic heart disease as a potential cause of congestive heart failure in the older patient. Yet, atrial septal defects are being identified more commonly as the cause of congestive heart failure in the older patient. Such individuals may have enjoyed a period of good health for many years prior to the development of cardiac failure. Congenital heart disease should also be considered in the elderly patient with a fever of unknown origin. Subacute bacterial endocarditis can be present in the elderly patient with little evidence of fever, white count elevation, or embolic phenomena. Our minds should be kept open to the possibility of congenital heart disease, even in the aged individual.

Pulmonary Emboli. Therapy for cardiac failure secondary to pulmonary hypertension may prove life-saving. The findings of pulmonary emboli may be extremely subtle in the elderly. Instead of shortness of breath, chest pain, or hemoptysis, the patient may present with recurrent episodes of tachycardia or arrhythmia, worsening of pre-existent heart failure, or some other subtle feature, such as episodes of mental confusion. The bedridden, obese, or crippled elderly patient is especially vulnerable to this problem. Prompt institution of anticoagulant therapy and treatment of venous disease in the lower extremities is essential.

Pericardial Disease. When pericardial effusion is recognized in the elderly patient, tapping this fluid not only will relieve the patient's cardiac failure but also may reveal metastatic carcinoma. Pericardial constriction may also be caused by viral disease or tuberculosis, and again, an erroneous assumption of arteriosclerotic heart disease would preclude proper therapeutic action.

Systemic Hypertension. Systemic hypertension is another cause of congestive heart failure. In this situation, however, therapy may have little to offer. The physician should manage both the hypertension and congestive heart failure, but at this stage the problem is largely irreversible.

Myocardial Disease. Myocardial disease, whether from recurrent myocardial infarction, viral myocarditis, or alcoholic cardiomyopathy, also generally presents a problem with limited therapeutic potential.

Other Causes of Congestive Heart Failure. Other possible causes of unexplained congestive heart failure include traumatic heart disease resulting from an automobile accident, and cardiac failure from hyperthyroidism or Graves' disease. In both cases, careful history and physical examination might prove rewarding.

It is essential to clarify why the patient with congestive heart failure is suddenly becoming increasingly ill. Has he discontinued his medications through forgetfulness? Has he exceeded his dietary limits as far as salt intake, or has he exceeded his physical limits through stressful activity? Is the patient being stressed by pulmonary infection? (In the elderly it is often difficult to tell which problem has developed first—pulmonary infection or congestive heart failure.) Is the patient exhibiting paroxysmal supraventricular tachycardia or another arrhythmia that is resulting in hypotension, cyanosis, and significant heart failure?

Proper diagnosis allows us to determine whether we are dealing with a treatable condition. In the treatment of dementia, we may be able to help the patient with thyroid medication or shunting of normal pressure hydrocephalus. In the case of congestive heart failure, we may be able to help the patient with anticoagulation, cardiac surgery, pericardiocentesis, or antithyroid medication. Evaluation of the elderly patient is made more complex by the diminished physiologic capacities, the latency of disease, increased drug effect, and the multiplicity of physical disease states and psychosocial factors.

DRUG PRESCRIBING FOR THE ELDERLY

In 1974, the aged population spent 2.26 billion dollars on drugs and over-the-counter preparations. This amounted to more than 20 per cent of the national total for these products. Elderly patients averaged more than 13 prescriptions per year, spending approximately $100 per individual for prescriptions and over-the-counter medications. With this phenomenal expense in mind, the family physician should attempt to achieve the greatest degree of effectiveness and the least degree of harm. The admonition "first do no harm" remains a primary consideration in the care of the elderly patient.

Drug Toxicity

Drug toxicity in the elderly patient is an extremely common event and presents with protean manifestations frequently mistaken for the stereotypes associated with old age: confusion, tremor, anxiety, depression, forgetfulness, and weakness. Many of our most valuable drugs are especially hazardous in the aged.[3, 6a, 6b, 8] Digitalis intoxication, as a cause of cardiac arrhythmia, can be triggered by hypokalemia, renal insufficiency, or both. Thiazide and furosemide diuretics are potent potassium depletors and produce elevations of blood glucose and uric acid. In managing hypertensive patients taking these preparations, it is important to check the patients' serum potassium, uric acid, and blood glucose levels periodically. Reserpine often causes serious depression, drowsiness, or peptic ulcer. The physician using methyldopa and other widely prescribed antihypertensive agents should be aware of orthostatic hypotension and a reduction in libido. Phenothiazines are also responsible for significant postural hypotension, which can lead to cerebral infarction. Phenylbutazone toxicity is associated with dangerous blood dyscrasias, gastrointestinal disturbances, and fluid retention. Aspirin, universally used, may be responsible for severe gastrointestinal bleeding. Oral hypoglycemic agents are at this moment the center of continued controversy with regard to the possible correlation between these drugs and increased cardiac morbidity and mortality. Thyroid extract may trigger myocardial ischemia. Anticoagulants may produce episodes of bleeding in susceptible users. Corticosteroids are fraught with many complications. The prescriber should be aware of all the problems associated with corticosteroids and should monitor patients accordingly. Steroid medications should be avoided if a less hazardous drug therapy is available.

Digoxin and the aminoglycosides, such as streptomycin, neomycin, kanamycin, and gentamicin, are eliminated principally through the kidneys and must be used with extreme caution in patients with diminished renal function. The nomogram recently developed at the Gerontology Research Center in Baltimore (see Fig. 16–2) provides guidelines for evaluating creatinine clearance as a function of age. However, nomograms are not yet available for other organ functions. In practice, one should investigate an organ system more thoroughly when there is some reason for suspecting organ dysfunction. Direct measurement of creatinine clearance in the individual patient, for example, provides important information. Drug levels, such as plasma digoxin levels, are often necessary to assure safe use in the presence of renal pathology.

Ninety per cent of all medications are metabolized or detoxified in the liver. Decreased hepatocellular microsomal enzyme activity may lead to excessive drug accumulation and subsequent toxicity. More free drug is available with decreased availability of liver enzymes. Laboratory measurements of liver function, however, are able to detect only major impairment, such as in hepatitis or cirrhosis.

Altered metabolism in the aged may affect drug kinetics. The physician should be aware that fat soluble drugs, such as chloral hydrate, may build up with increased fat deposition, which often occurs with aging. Increased absorption of fat soluble drugs takes place in the obese patient. It should also be noted that with reduced plasma protein, conjugation of drugs proceeds at a slower rate for drugs that are protein-bound. Competition for binding sites is intensified in patients receiving multiple medications. For example, aspirin tends to displace warfarin, resulting in drug-induced bleeding.

Psychosocial Factors

The family physician should be fully aware of the patient's habits and life style that may significantly influence the effects of medications. For instance, there is new evidence that excessive alcohol, coffee, and cigarette consumption may have an adverse effect on the metabolism of various medications.

Loneliness, grief, and various other emotional states may be responsible for reduced food intake. Poor dentition and financial difficulty can also lead to improper diet and nutritional deficiencies. Protein malnutrition, particularly, is an important factor in any consideration of the aged patient's drug therapy.

Patient Compliance

Patient compliance is a vital area of concern in prescribing drugs. The patient may lose or forget to fill a prescription or may stop taking a drug entirely. The patient may fail to record serious side effects, may take the drug along with over-the-counter preparations or previously prescribed medications that were actually discontinued, or may even take medications that were prescribed for other family members. It is essential that the physician determine which medications the patient is currently using. This often involves asking the patient or the family to bring to the office or hospital a shopping basket full of drugs. The physician may have to call several pharmacies in order to determine what each unlabeled bottle contains. Of course, labeling of medications would avoid this latter problem.

Even when regularly prescribed drugs are carefully monitored, the physician may neglect to inquire about over-the-counter products. One of these agents might actually be causing side effects or interfering with the proper function of prescribed medications. For example, belladonna alkaloids can raise intraocular pressure. Aspirin, as mentioned, competes with a variety of drugs for serum protein–binding sites and can cause gastrointestinal bleeding problems.

It is extremely desirable to establish a medication flow sheet on each patient to supplement the progress notes in a patient's file. This flow sheet should give the dates of onset and discontinuation of different medications, as well as any adverse reactions noted. All too often we lose track of which medication is currently being taken. Using the medication flow sheet allows constant surveillance of the patient's drug profile.

In terms of improving patient compliance, there are a number of steps that the physician can take. The family physician should simplify drug schedules, telling the patient to take two pills 3 times per day rather than one pill 6 times per day. If possible, certain medications should be given once per day, such as phenytoin (Dilantin). Medication should be adjusted to meals or other events, such as brushing teeth in the morning and at bedtime. Instructions should be made very specific. Verbal instructions should be reinforced, if necessary, with *written* instructions. The elderly are characterized by decreased speed of learning and immediate recall; hearing and vision are diminished. Written instructions should be stated simply in lay terms. Avoid "Digoxin 0.25 mg. b.i.d."; instead, write "Take one heart pill twice a day." For certain patients, consider using typewritten instructions. Also, consider providing written instructions to family members, particularly in the case of the elderly patient with memory loss. It might be helpful for a family member to lay out the day's medications for the patient, so that it is clear that the patient has four pills to take each day; when the family member returns the next day, he can see how many pills are left.

Advise the patient and the family what side effects to expect, such as orthostatic hypotension from methyldopa. It pays not to order too many pills or capsules initially. For example, prior to ordering 100 analgesic tablets for patients with arthritis, try a smaller number and wait to see whether this medication helps.

Choice of Medication

Prudence is extremely important in prescribing drugs for the elderly. The physi-

cian should determine if the patient's complaint is justification for medication. Is this drug really necessary? The physician should weigh benefits versus risks. This balance is different in the elderly patient compared with the younger patient. Most important, the physician should attempt to keep the total number of drugs down to as few as possible. In general, the physician should try to use only two or three drugs at one time. For example, if a patient is already on three medications, including digoxin, allopurinol, and furosemide, consider holding off using oral hypoglycemic agents if possible. What is a safe total drug load for a particular individual? What medications can be postponed until a later time?

The physician should resist using new untested drugs and should prescribe commonly used drugs of choice for a specific problem. By constantly reinforcing his knowledge of indications, contraindications, and adverse effects, the physician is in a much sounder position than by shifting to unfamiliar drugs based on current promotion of that drug. Most important, the physician should resist the temptation to treat new symptoms that are poorly understood with still more medications. The question must be asked whether the present symptoms, such as confusion or depression, are related to previous drug use.

The elderly patient has a multiplicity of problems, as discussed previously. Clearly, the patient's other problems may interact with the medications prescribed. The older patient with peptic ulcer may not be able to take several types of drugs because of the ulcer problem. *Fewer medications will be required in those situations in which the physician can spend more time with the patient.* In so many instances of anxiety, depression, and sleep disturbance, medications are not necessary. The physician is the chief therapeutic agent for the elderly patient.

ALTERNATIVES TO INSTITUTIONALIZATION

With more than one million elderly Americans confined to institutional care and the over-60 population rapidly expanding, every physician must consider practical alternatives to institutionalization.[10] Nursing homes or other institutions should be prescribed specifically by the physician in the same manner in which digitalis or penicillin is prescribed. Combinations of medical, psychologic, social, and family problems that each patient brings to the family physician must be evaluated, resulting in specific decisions for institutionalization versus other alternatives.

Between 1965 and 1975, a massive push toward institutionalization took place, creating hundreds of thousands of nursing home beds. It is clear that many patients would benefit significantly from careful evaluation and placement at a different level of institutional care or from a noninstitutional alternative. Many, for example, would undoubtedly be more comfortable in the familiar environment of home with the benefit of either visiting supportive services or day care center facilities.

What alternatives are there for the physician who is planning his patient's care? The following is a simple list: homemakers; home health aides; visiting home nurses; friendly visitors; day care centers, domiciliary facilities or churches and other suitable community facilities; foster home care; chore services, home renovation and home repair services; meal programs, both group-feeding and home-delivered, such as Meals-on-Wheels; transportation programs; telephone reassurance; and shopping services. One wonders why during the past decade irrational planning and resistance to change have continued to prevail. At the present time, with evidence of excessive cost and examples of irregular practices in certain nursing homes, there is much interest in creating alternatives and new options to institutionalization.

Home Care Programs

In the United States there are programs that can be studied as models or prototypes of alternatives to institutionalization. A home care program was established at Montefiore Hospital in New York City in 1947. This plan utilized a core group of physician, nurse, and social worker, with additional support provided by physical, occupational, and recreational therapists. In the Montefiore experience, patients suffering from every degree of disability were cared for in the home. Various private and community agencies in different parts of the country have sponsored other home care programs. One program is sponsored by a group of hospitals in Paterson, New Jersey. A private hospital-based program has been developed in Greenwich, Connecticut. In Rochester, New York, a cooperative community plan is supported by a number of organizations. It should be noted that programs supported by hospitals tend to falter when economic conditions worsen. Also, it would seem that home care support is available under Medicare, but in reality only token programming has developed thus far. It would also seem practical to provide reimbursement or tax advantage to relatives who deliver home care to the impaired elderly. This latter approach would offer financial incentives as an alternative to keeping a relative in a long-term care facility under a Medicaid program. In the future, it will also be useful to amplify home care by the use of physician extenders working with the family physician.

Day Care Programs

Geriatric day care alternatives are beginning to appear in greater numbers in the United States. In 1973, the Administration on Aging and the Medical Services Administration funded four demonstration projects utilizing day treatment settings as compared with the more traditional long-term care institutional services. These projects included the Burke Day Hospital of White Plains, New York; the Levindale Day Treatment Center of Baltimore, Maryland; the On Lok Day Care Center of San Francisco, California; and the Montefiore Day Care Center of New York City. These centers and 11 others in the country vary considerably in size, setting, agency, sponsorship, and source of funding. All share similar goals, trying to provide either maintenance, rehabilitation, or both, for the chronically ill and disabled older persons. The Burke program in White Plains is unique as a day hospital that provides direct medical care by physicians connected to the facility as staff members. In contrast, other day care centers do not include the same degree of medical service; they stress social aspects of treatment and other health care supports with various levels of nursing care and ancillary personnel. Advantages of day care include offering the possibility for group interaction with a social worker, providing a mechanism for ventilation of anxieties, forming close interpersonal relationships, and finding relief for the lonely and isolated individual.

The British experience with day treatment alternatives demonstrates the feasibility of both long- and short-term maintenance in the community. In Great Britain, the concept of the day hospital has been implemented within many sections of the country. In the United States, we have seen instead a growth of day care centers rather than day hospitals. Especially with the current attempt to control the proliferation of nursing home beds, we will probably see a significant growth spurt of day care facilities throughout this country.

Specialized Housing

Specialized housing is an important solution for many elderly with a variety of medical and social problems. For example, the Kitay House of New York City offers compact apartments with access to private or common kitchen facilities, cleaning services, and regular medical care. The most imaginative experiments in housing for the elderly exist in Scandinavia. In apartment houses in Oslo, Norway, shops are present on the premises for the elderly to purchase food, tobacco, stamps, and other personal necessities. Bathing facilities are present on each floor; as a preventive safety measure, plastic chairs are available in shower stalls, allowing the aged patient to be safely seated, with access to easily manipulated shower heads. Under Swedish law, compact apartments for the elderly must be incorporated into all new apartment facilities. Thus, the aged are not segregated and, consequently, isolated.

Food Services

Throughout the United States, Meals-on-Wheels services have been established in order to minimize the difficulties encountered by the aged in shopping and food preparation. Ordinarily, a hot meal is delivered every day; a second meal might also be available. Emergency food stores are stocked in case delivery of meals is prevented by inclement weather.

Also throughout the United States, communal or congregate feeding at dining sites is available to the elderly through Title VII of the Older Americans Act. The federal government arranges congregate feeding through State Offices on Aging at senior citizen centers, churches, schools, day care centers, and homes for the aged. Social services, recreational programs, educational lectures, and other types of programs are encouraged at each site.

Homemaking Services

Homemaking service is another valuable alternative in which a homemaker from either a governmental or private agency is available on a variable time basis. As listed previously, there are a host of other programs and alternatives that are helpful, including home health aides, friendly visitors, foster home care, chore services, home renovation and home repair services, transportation programs, telephone reassurance, shopping services, and other community resources that are designed to keep the elderly living independently and outside of long-term care facilities. Certainly, the family physician should be aware of these resources and, in his service to patient and family, should encourage their full usage. In many states and counties, there are information and referral services available through departments of health and offices on aging. These services can assist the physician in identifying a needed resource that could help a specific patient. The family physician can play a key role in his community in the development of these needed resources.

THE ROLE OF THE PHYSICIAN IN LONG-TERM CARE FACILITIES

Although it should be the family physician's goal to prevent unnecessary institutionalization, there will always remain a need for institutionalization of certain impaired elderly patients. Unfortunately, one can cite many factors responsible for the frequently inadequate medical care in our nursing homes.

In our health care system, more attention has always been extended to the treatment of acute disease than to the care of the chronically ill patient whose progress is often slow and frustrating. Many physicians have only a few patients in nursing homes and find it inconvenient to schedule a visit to see them. By and large, our schools of medicine have not paid sufficient attention to long-term care and the special problems that are seen in nursing home facilities. Although hospitals have elaborate systems of peer review and audit, nursing homes are not yet within the mainstream of medical practice. Incomplete medical records, excessive length of the patient's stay, and poor review of drug therapy have all been cited with regard to nursing home care.

An inspiring feature of the new movement of family practice is that many of the ongoing training programs have emphasized the special problems of the geriatric patient and long-term care. Training opportunities have been created in family practice residencies, giving the resident experience in this type of practice. There is a major emphasis on continuity and comprehensiveness of care, a holistic approach, and attention to humanistic factors. More than esoteric knowledge, care of the geriatric patient requires the basic humanism, conscientiousness, and concern for the whole patient that define good medical practice.

Many physicians who are not involved in long-term care may not be aware of the 1973 American Medical Association recommendations that long-term care facilities should have either a medical director, an organized medical staff, or both, to ensure the adequacy and appropriateness of medical care provided the patients in such facilities. The following guidelines were approved concerning the role of the medical director in order to help bring the nursing home into the mainstream of medical practice:

1. Assist in arranging for continuous physician coverage for medical emergencies and in developing procedures for emergency treatment of patients.

2. Participate in the development of a system providing a medical care plan for each patient that covers medications, nursing care, restorative services, diet, and other services, and, if appropriate, a plan for discharge.

3. Be the medical representative of the facility in the community.

4. Develop liaison with attending staff physicians in efforts to ensure effective medical care.

5. In the absence of an organized medical staff, be responsible for the development of written bylaws, rules, and regulations applicable to each physician attending patients in the facility.

6. If there is an organized medical staff, be a member, attend meetings, and help assure adherence to medical staff bylaws, rules, and regulations.

7. Participate in developing written policies governing the medical, nursing, and related health services provided in the facility.

8. Participate in developing patient admission and discharge policies.

9. Participate in an effective program of long-term care review.

10. Be available for consultation in the development and maintenance of an adequate medical records system.

11. Advise the administrator as to the adequacy of the patient care services and medical equipment of the facility.

12. Be available for consultation with the administrator and the director of nursing in evaluating the adequacy of the nursing staff and the facility to meet the psychosocial as well as the medical and physical needs of patients.

13. Be available for consultation and participation in in-service training programs.

14. Advise the administration on employee health policies.

15. Be knowledgeable concerning policies and programs of public health agencies that may affect patient care programs in the facility.

Following these recommendations, new regulations of the Department of Health, Education, and Welfare were published on October 3, 1974 in the *Federal Register*, stating that skilled nursing facilities must employ a part-time or full-time medical director to coordinate care given to patients. The regulations also permit medical directors to be provided through a group of physicians, a local society, or other similar arrangements.

The family physician should be aware of these regulations, although modifications may take place over the next several years.[2, 13] It is not clear whether the current regulations can be carried out in every part of the United States, such as in sparsely populated rural areas. However, the nursing home is a reality in the United States, and the need to bring nursing homes into the mainstream of medical practice and upgrade the quality of medical care within these facilities is also clearly a reality.

These regulations indicate that the part-time or full-time medical director's principal responsibility is for patient care. Patient care policies should be developed by the medical director in cooperation with the attending physician and the nursing home staff and should be designed to monitor the quality of ongoing patient care. The director should be available for consultation with patients, nursing home staff, and attending physicians. The policies should reflect awareness of the total medical and psychosocial needs of patients, and provision should be made for meeting these needs. These policies should cover admission trends and discharge planning in the wide range of patient services.

The medical director must establish and maintain effective liaison with attending physicians. Proper management entails devising medical staff bylaws encompassing such issues as privileges, peer review, and utilization review for all attending staff. The medical director should be informed promptly of the failure of an attending physician to make appropriate patient visits. A delinquent physician should be counseled.

Although the future success of the medical director requirement remains uncertain at this time, the new field of family practice will want to see that all patients receive a high quality of medical care, whether the patient is an infant, an adolescent, or an impaired elderly patient.

It is hoped that family practice, with its clear message of continuity of care and concern for all aspects of the patient and family, will move to find solutions for what is a neglected and troubled area of human concern. While meeting this responsibility, the

family physician will find much gratification in being a caring physician for the elderly population.

REFERENCES

1. Andres, R.: Relation of physiologic changes in aging to medical changes of disease in the aged. Mayo Clin. Proc. 42:674, 1967.
2. Fonrose, H. A.: The medical director in an extended care facility. J. Am. Geriatr. Soc. 24:92, 1976.
3. Hall, M. R. P.: Drug therapy in the elderly. Br. Med. J. 4:582, 1973.
4. Harris, R.: The Management of Geriatric Cardiovascular Disease. Philadelphia, J. B. Lippincott Co., 1970.
5. Kahn, R. L., Goldfarb, A. L., Pollack, M., et al.: Brief objective measures for the determination of mental status in the aged. Am. J. Psychiatry, 117:326, 1960.
6a. Lamy, P. P., and Kitler, M. E.: Drugs and the geriatric patient. J. Am. Geriatr. Soc. 19:23, 1971.
6b. Lamy, P. P., and Kitler, M. E.: The geriatric patient: age-dependent physiologic and pathologic changes. J. Am. Geriatr. Soc. 19:871, 1971.
7. Menzer, L., et al.: Computerized axial tomography—use in the diagnosis of dementia. J.A.M.A. 234:754, 1975.
8. Reichel, W.: Complications in the care of 500 elderly hospitalized patients. J. Am. Geriatr. Soc. 13:973, 1965.
9. Reichel, W. (ed.): Clinical Aspects of Aging. Baltimore, The Williams & Wilkins Co., in press.
10. Rossman, I.: Alternatives to institutional care. Bull. N.Y. Acad. Med. 49:1084, 1973.
11. Rowe, J., et al.: The effect of age on creatinine clearance in men: a cross-sectional and longitudinal study. J. Gerontol. 31:155, 1976.
12. Shenkin, H. A., Greenberg, J., Bouzarth, W. F., et al.: Ventricular shunting for relief of senile symptoms. J.A.M.A. 225:1486, 1973.
13. Solon, J. A., and Greenwalt, L. F.: Physicians' participation in nursing homes. Med. Care 12:486, 1974.
14. Sourander, P., and Sjögren, H.: The concept of Alzheimer's disease and its clinical implications. In Alzheimer's Disease and Related Conditions. A CIBA Foundation Symposium. London, J. & A. Churchill Ltd., 1970, p. 36.

PART IV

BEHAVIORAL PROBLEMS

Chapter 17

MEDICAL ETHICS

by G. GAYLE STEPHENS,
and G. LYNN STEPHENS

PHYSICIANS' DECISIONS

The practice of medicine necessitates the use of power—the power of knowledge, of technologic capability, and of persuasion. Physicians are the custodians of a vast system of biomedical information, and they participate in the governance, management, and even the ownership of almost all institutions of medical care in the United States. They generate and apply a great deal of medical research, and they advise and consult with governmental and private agencies in matters of health and medical care.

Some of the decisions that physicians make are dramatic and more or less public, having to do with abortion, resuscitation, organ transplantation, and heroic surgery. However, these are but the tip of an iceberg of less dramatic but no less important decisions made regularly by every physician in clinical practice. Physicians determine in large part who has access to their care and what risks are to be taken in diagnosis and treatment. They decide when a person is fit for employment or life insurance, as well as when and to what degree a person is disabled. As agents of the law, physicians report contagious diseases and child abuse, assist in the enforcement of public health and sanitation laws, certify causes of death, and make reports to courts about the mental health states of individuals. As counselors to their patients, they influence decisions about occupation, residence, marriage, reproduction, child-rearing, and retirement. It is no exaggeration to say that physicians today regularly make decisions that in former times belonged solely to the gods.

CONTEMPORARY INTEREST IN PHYSICIANS' DECISIONS

For the most part, physicians exercise their power in an amazingly autonomous way. As long as they violate no laws and maintain minimum professional standards, their decisions are subject to little review. This is consistent with the prerogatives that societies have always accorded their highest professions—not only medicine but law, divinity, education, and architecture. The technical aspects of the work of physicians in hospitals are "spot checked" by various committees of the medical staffs, their claims for payment are audited by insurers and other "third parties," and they are subject to litigation by dissatisfied patients—but all these taken together review only a fraction of the work of physicians. Even the courts have recognized and repeatedly affirmed the need for a high degree of autonomy in the practice of medicine by respecting the privacy of physician–patient relationships and by relegating certain decisions to judgments based on the intimacy and responsibility of this relationship.

The winds of change are blowing, however, and there is an increased interest in the decisions of physicians, both within the profession and in the larger society. There is greater public awareness of the capabilities of modern medicine and increased expectations of benefit. This may reflect a number of contemporary social developments, including a new mood of antiauthoritarianism and concerns about consumers' rights and the rising costs of medical care. There is also a rising disenchantment with the impersonality of medical care, expressed poignantly in the women's movement and its attitudes toward obstetrics and gynecology.

Moreover, there is a genre of literature appearing that raises ecologic and economic concerns about the apparently uncritical commitment of modern medicine to more and more technology. Questions are being asked about the appropriateness of prolonging the quantity of life at the expense of quality; about the boundaries of experimentation, especially with humans; and about the total costs of medical care to the nation. Within medicine there is a new level of concern about humanism and ethics, as indicated by a plethora of seminars, conferences, and publications concerning these topics.

What this all adds up to is that the work of physicians in a modern industrial society is of great importance to politicians, economists, social scientists, philosophers, and theologians—as well as to the average citizen. Medicine has always been practiced within the limits of particular social systems and cultural values, and the modern age is surely no exception. Physicians must recognize the legitimate interests of other professionals in medical affairs. They must also be willing to subject their work to critical examination in all respects if they and their patients are not to become merely victims of bias, taboo, prejudice, and unrestrained self-interest.

DECISIONS BEARING SPECIAL ETHICAL AND MORAL SIGNIFICANCE

While it could be argued that all decisions concerning the health and well-being of individuals have ethical and moral significance, some carry a heavier weight of meaning and place special responsibilities on physicians and patients alike.

One characteristic of such decisions is that they generally involve questions of "why" and "whether" more than "what" or "how" and therefore are not resolvable on the basis of scientifically derived data alone. As a matter of fact, the practice of medicine is a great deal more than the application of scientific facts to the treatment of patients who have diseases. Above and beyond the scientific data base and technologic competence of medicine are large areas of human experience that are not explicable by scientific evidence. We are all the bearers of traditions, rules, laws, myths, beliefs, and opinions that exert critical influences on our behavior. This is not to say that such factors are unscientific or antiscientific or that they should not be subject to critical study, but rather it is to recognize the existence of nonscientific categories of great importance.

Ethical and moral dilemmas are encountered primarily at the boundaries between scientific and nonscientific factors in human experience. For the past 300 years particularly, these boundaries have been shifting, as more and more of human life has been subject to scientific inquiry. Many old values and beliefs have been modified or replaced by new, though not necessarily better, ones, but it is safe to say that this "rationalizing" of human experience is far from complete and that the "successes" of science have often created new problems of ethics and morals of greater magnitude than the old ones.

Every age has had its own litany of moral dilemmas, and the present period is no exception. While no claim is made for completeness, the following list, adapted from a *Bibliography of Society, Ethics and the Life Sciences*[1] identifies issues of special concern for physicians and citizens in the United States in the 1970's and beyond.

1. Behavior control
   a. Physical manipulation of the brain
   b. Drugs and drug therapy
   c. Psychotherapy and psychology
   d. Total institutions, incarceration, and the right to treatment
   e. Behavior control through the media
   f. Early education
2. Death and dying
   a. Care of the dying patient
   b. Euthanasia and decisions about life-saving treatment
   c. Suicide
   d. Defining death
3. Experimentation and consent
   a. Clinical investigation: ethical and legal issues
   b. Informed consent
   c. Institutional guidelines for human research
   d. Behavior research
   e. Special questions of consent
      (1). Prisoners and mental patients
      (2). Fetuses
      (3). Children and minors

4. Genetics, fertilization, and birth
   a. Screening for genetic traits and diseases
   b. Genetic counseling
   c. Prenatal diagnosis
   d. Artificial insemination and sperm banking
   e. Gene therapy and genetic engineering
   f. In vitro fertilization and cloning
5. Health care delivery
   a. The right to health and national health insurance
   b. Patients' rights movement
   c. Aging
   d. Women and medicine
   e. The doctor-patient relationship
6. Population and birth control
   a. Contraception
   b. Abortion
   c. Sterilization
7. Scarce medical resources
   a. Transplantation
   b. Hemodialysis

A TAXONOMY OF MEDICOETHICAL ISSUES

From the standpoint of ethics, one may subsume the items in the foregoing list under a three-part taxonomy: (1) problems of distributive justice, (2) duties and conflicts of duty, and (3) problems of the quality of life.

Problems of Distributive Justice

Questions concerning the distribution of medical care occur at every level from national health policy down to the individual physician's decisions about whom to treat and how his time and services should be divided among patients. The goal is to distribute care according to standards that are just. Obviously, the discovery of such standards is itself a moral problem. Further, many of the concepts employed in expressing standards of distribution are moral notions. For example, an appropriate standard will take into account the concepts of *need* and *relative neediness,* that is, one wants to distribute care to those who need it and, in cases in which not all needs can be satisfied, to those who need it most. One's judgments about need and relative neediness depend on assumptions concerning which

ways of living are tolerable, which services people have a right to expect, and which deficiencies are most serious. These matters fall partly or entirely within the province of ethical theory.

Another notion that may figure in standards of distribution is that of deservedness. Some persons may be more deserving of help than others. For example, one whose need arises through no fault of his own may be more deserving, though no more needy, than one who had brought his troubles on himself. In order to make such judgments, one needs principles for assessing moral responsibility, i.e., for deciding whether someone is to blame for his condition.

Duties and Conflict of Duty

Each person has certain moral obligations toward other persons, for example, the obligation to do no harm or to keep one's promises. However, the physician must sometimes choose between conflicting obligations. These cases fall roughly into two classifications: (1) In some instances the physician can meet his obligations to one person only at the expense of his obligations to others. Duties owed to the patient, such as confidentiality, may conflict with duties owed to the patient's family or the general public. (2) One must sometimes choose between different obligations to the same person. Particularly important here are conflicts between one's duty to do what is best for the patient and one's obligation to respect his autonomy. Such conflicts come to the fore in the issue of involuntary treatment or institutionalization. In order to decide these questions, we need standards that inform us of our obligations and that rank these obligations in order of relative importance.

Problems of the Quality of Life

The question of what sort of life is worthwhile for a human being is perhaps the oldest ethical problem. The increasing development of life-sustaining technologies has given special force to the question of whether death is preferable to certain ways of living. Decisions concerning the quality of life also figure prominently in the justification of efforts directed toward population control and genetic engineering.

Further, there is the problem of pain. Pain is an evil; under certain conditions it is a greater evil than death itself. Yet the physician must sometimes inflict pain. One must decide when this is justified and how much suffering may be justifiably inflicted for what ends. Likewise, questions arise concerning whether the patient should be *allowed* to suffer. For example, is some amount of suffering preferable to dependence on narcotics or tranquilizers? Does suffering justify the termination of efforts to sustain life? To cope with such dilemmas, society has developed a system of laws and regulations relative to the education and licensure of physicians. Laws, however, cannot guarantee that physicians will make good and proper decisions on behalf of their patients. Laws can only establish punishment for those who break them and attempt to redress injury and grievance.

Recognizing the limits of the law, physicians historically have developed codes of ethics in an attempt to erect higher standards of conduct among themselves for their patients' benefit and protection. In the famous Hippocratic oath that many medical school graduates still swear ritualistically, they promise to do no harm, to protect their patients' privacy, and to treat all people equally without regard to their social or economic status. Beyond the traditional oaths, however, there are codes of ethics of professional societies such as the American Medical Association that set forth detailed instructions and constraints covering physicians' behavior regarding advertising, fee-splitting, transfer of responsibility for patients, and the like.

However, none of this touches the most difficult decisions in clinical practice. A physician may obey all pertinent laws and abide by all relevant codes of ethics and still experience the uncertainty and anguish of moral decisions.

ETHICS AS AN ACADEMIC DISCIPLINE

Given the nonscientific nature of much of human experience, it is seductively easy to fall into the error of extreme individualism by assuming that no rigorous thinking is necessary and that in all matters of ethics each person's opinion is as valid as any other's. Physicians receive very little formal education in ethics and moral philosophy, and for the most part they depend upon conventional wisdom, armchair philosophy, and their own religious upbringing (or lack of it) to form their decisions.

Although "intuitions" derived from the sources just mentioned play some part in even the most sophisticated moral outlook, there are at least three reasons why they should be subject to systematic examination. First, there are likely to be some cases calling for a moral decision in which one's intuition fails. It is unreasonable to expect that precepts acquired more or less haphazardly will cover all important moral cases. This is true particularly of problems raised by technologic advances and changing social conditions. Second, intuitions sometimes conflict. An individual may accept principles that have mutually contradictory implications in a given case. Likewise, people may honestly disagree about matters of moral principle. Third, in view of the well-known effects of such factors as self-interest and social prejudice on moral judgment, it is not unlikely that some of one's moral beliefs are in error.

The theoretic study of ethics attempts to remedy these defects in our intuitive moral views. It seeks to develop a consistent body of principles covering all moral issues, to set up an ordering among principles that allows us to resolve conflicts of principle, and, finally, to establish standards for evaluating the reasonableness of particular moral judgments and for deciding among competing moral theories.

Three major areas constitute the subject matter of formal study in ethics: (1) normative ethics, (2) metaethics, and (3) metaphysics of morals.

Normative Ethics

Normative ethics encompasses what most people think of as ethics. It is the attempt to formulate comprehensive sets of principles determining which things are *good* or *bad*, which actions are *right* or *wrong*, and which motives and character traits deserve moral *praise* or *blame*. To understand the concerns of normative ethics, let us examine the pairs of notions just emphasized.

Good and Bad. This area of normative theory considers which things are valuable, desirable, or worthwhile in themselves.

Such things are called *intrinsic* goods. Others are good extrinsically, that is, because they serve as a means for the realization of intrinsic goods. In addition, there are intrinsic and extrinsic evils, evils that are either undesirable and degrading in themselves or things that serve as means to such evils.

Philosophers have proposed a number of accounts of the intrinsically good. Some have argued that pleasure alone is good in itself and that only pain is an intrinsic evil. This view, called *hedonism,* has been defended by thinkers who otherwise had very little in common, e.g., Epicurus, Spinoza, and John Stuart Mill. However, owing to the great differences in their understanding of pleasure, such agreement is often more apparent than real. The good has also been identified with the realization of certain human capacities, such as capacities for rational thought or aesthetic appreciation. Such philosophers as Aristotle, Kant, and Nietzsche defended various formulations of this *perfectionist* theory of the good. In the 19th and early 20th centuries, attempts were made to work out a conception of the good based on evolutionary theory. According to such views, only those things conducive to the survival of the species are good. Herbert Spencer is the best known proponent of this theory. Perhaps the most cosmopolitan doctrine is that of Ralph Barton Perry, who held that the good is whatever someone takes as an object of interest or desire. Other theories are possible, but those mentioned provide a fair sample of philosophic opinion on the question of what things are good in themselves.

Right and Wrong.   A theory of the right determines what forms of conduct are permitted, forbidden, or obligatory. An action is *right* if it is morally permitted, *wrong* if it is forbidden, and *obligatory* if it is not permissible to refuse to do it. The theory of justice is that part of the theory of the right concerned with the exercise of political power, the distribution of wealth, and other issues relating to large-scale social organization.

The nature of the relationship between the right and the good provides a point of controversy among moral theorists. Some views, called *teleologic* theories, define the right in terms of the good. An act is right if, and only if, it maximizes the amount of good in the world. Thus, according to John Stuart Mill's *utilitarian* theory, pleasure is the only good, and an act is right if, and only if, it produces a better balance of pleasure over pain than any action one could have performed in its stead. Other thinkers, called *formalists,* hold that the principles of the right are independent of and take precedence over the pursuit of the good. Immanuel Kant, W. D. Ross, and, more recently, John Rawls have defended formalism. Those wishing to follow the debate between teleologic and formalist thinkers are referred to the books by Brandt and MacIntyre mentioned in the bibliography.

Praise and Blame.   While judgments of right and wrong concern actions, judgments of praise and blame refer to the actor, or agent who acts. An action such as giving to charity may be right despite the fact that the giver may have had base motives or contributed under pressure or in ignorance. Similarly, we may praise someone for a wrong act if we think his intentions were good. This brings up the issue of moral responsibility. An agent can be praised or blamed only for those actions for which he is responsible; therefore, any such moral theory must have some account of freedom of the will. Moral philosophers have not been particularly successful in providing such accounts.

Praise also raises the possibility that some actions are above and beyond the call of moral duty. An agent may not reasonably be required to perform a given act, but if he does, he merits special praise. This is referred to as supererogatory action and has been an important element in Roman Catholic theology.

Metaethics

This is a more abstract category about the language of moral discourse—the definition of terms and the logical relations among moral judgments. Professional philosophers are apt to be more concerned with metaethics, since it represents theoretic more than applied aspects. Physicians, unless formally trained, would probably find discussions of metaethics abstruse and not immediately applicable to their clinical work.

Metaphysics of Morals

This term, borrowed from Kant, refers to that area of ethics concerned with the justification of particular moral theories and of the moral life generally. Here, two sorts of questions confront us. First, there are epistemologic questions. How do we know whether a given moral judgment or theory is true? What constitutes evidence for or against a moral opinion? Second, there are questions concerning the rationale of moral conduct and the purpose of moral theorizing. What should one expect a moral theory to do? Supposing that one has an acceptable moral theory at hand, why should one use such a theory to regulate one's actions? Is it reasonable to base one's practical decisions on moral considerations?

Although the metaphysics of morals is the most difficult and the least developed area of ethical philosophy, it is relevant to even the most everyday moral problems. One's decision to accept or reject a particular moral judgment and one's choice between competing normative theories will be based on considerations that belong to the metaphysics of morals.

We have provided only a brief introduction to moral philosophy in this section. More thorough discussions of the issues raised above can be found in the works referred to in the bibliography.

THE PHYSICIAN AS A MORAL AGENT

Where does all this leave us when we consider the decisions physicians must make, as described at the beginning of this chapter? It certainly does not provide us with a formula for action; neither does it remove the burden of responsibility for our actions. No one has written more poignantly about human choices than Jean Paul Sartre.[3] Sartre writes of anguish, forlornness, and despair as characterizing the human condition everywhere. Anguish comes to the individual who understands that in choosing for himself he is also choosing for all mankind. Whatever I allow for myself, I must allow for others, and this deeply felt sense of responsibility for others creates anguish. The individual in reality is a lawmaker when he chooses. Forlornness is a consequence of knowing that I have no authority to tell me what I must do. I act on my own, and the loneliness and isolation of this knowledge produce forlornness. Finally, despair, according to Sartre, is what I feel when I realize what I have actually chosen. He states, "Man is nothing else than his plan; he exists only to the extent that he fulfills himself; he is therefore nothing else than the ensemble of his acts, nothing else than his life."[2] No matter what one may think about Sartre's general philosophy, he has captured accurately the emotions of human decision-making when the stakes are high—as is often the case in medicine. These emotions should not paralyze or deter us, but they should warn us that we should not deny them or become callous and blasé about our responsibilities for others. There is much to be feared from anyone who has become deluded into thinking that moral choice is easy or without cost.

Most of the moral decisions in medicine fall into the category of normative ethics. Most of our debates are between utilitarian and formalist points of view, i.e., between those who think in terms of consequences and those who want to keep the rules. Where one is located between these extremes is largely a matter of upbringing, personality, and religious orientation. Strongly religious persons tend to be formalists, as do persons with obsessive-compulsive personality traits. On the other hand, persons with highly cultivated senses of sympathy and empathy and those who are convinced by the philosophies of pragmatism tend to be utilitarians. Science itself is neutral in this spectrum and may be used in the service of either position. Both positions have been perverted, caricatured, and exploited in history, and it would be hard to estimate which position has done more harm. Societies dominated by formalists are authoritarian and rigid, with medieval Catholicism and New England Puritanism serving as examples. Oddly enough, societies dominated by utilitarians are also subject to authoritarianism, as the various 20th century totalitarian states so aptly demonstrate. When one weds a doctrine of "the most good for the most people" to the political ambitions of a dictator, a holocaust is likely to be the outcome.

Most physicians take an intermediate position between these two extremes, but they tend not to be conscious about how much of each they are appropriating. Such a position of *moral relativism* seems to be a rational compromise, but we need to be more reflective about what we are actually doing. What rules do I accept or reject and why? How thoughtful am I in considering *all* concerned in a decision? How much am I merely the victim of my own feelings when making a medical decision of ethical significance?

Joseph Fletcher has made the clearest modern apology for moral relativism in medicine in his book *Situation Ethics*.[1] He reduces the rules to one, "Love is the only norm," and then tries to apply this to the various contemporary medicoethical situations. Fletcher has become controversial to modern formalists, and his positions are easy to caricature, but he has made a major contribution to modern medicine, particularly in his analysis of the relation of body taboos to organ transplantation.

There is another sense in which the word "moral" has been used in medicine since the time of Pinel. When he became concerned about the inmates of asylums in the early 1800's, Pinel spoke of moral treatment, by which he meant kind treatment. Kindness and consideration for the patient as a person of worth equal to oneself have been hard won achievements in medicine during the past 200 years. Kindness has a long history of effectiveness in human affairs, and it is unthinkable that a physician could be truly moral without it.

There is a third sense of the term "moral" that has meaning for the physician's work in relation to the dominant values of the culture in which he lives. A physician's influence is moral if it supports a value system within the patient. This is a delicate topic that cannot be debated adequately in this chapter. What are the dominant value systems in a pluralistic society? What is the physician's understanding of the value system? It is clear that the family physician in his concern for the family and the community cannot be committed to the destruction of these traditional institutions. Physicians as individuals may be agents of social and political change, perhaps even revolutionaries, but as physicians they stand on the side of moral values, and they cannot cut themselves or their patients

loose from these values. They may help free their patients, and themselves, from ignorant and neurotic misunderstandings of cultural values but that is not the same as destroying the values themselves.

CONCLUSION

In this chapter we have attempted to steer a middle course between those who think that moral questions can be settled by rules alone and those who think that only the consequences count. We have not tried to analyze particular moral questions but have appealed to the study of ethics as an academic discipline and as a rational resource for the physician who wishes to be more reflective and responsible for his decisions. We think that moral decisions are difficult and are surrounded by uncertainty, but they are not impossible. Finally, we hope to have provoked the reader to examine his assumptions, attitudes, and sources of information about these topics.

REFERENCES

1. Bibliography of Society, Ethics and the Life Sciences. Hastings-on-Hudson, N.Y., Institute of Society, Ethics and the Life Sciences, 1975.
2. Fletcher, J.: Situation Ethics. Philadelphia, The Westminster Press, 1966.
3. Sartre, J. P.: Existentialism and Human Emotions. New York, Philosophical Library, Inc., 1957.

BIBLIOGRAPHY OF SUGGESTED READINGS IN MORAL PHILOSOPHY

General Works on Moral Philosophy

Numerous introductions to ethical theory are readily available. William K. Frankena's *Ethics*, second edition, in the Prentice-Hall Foundations of Philosophy Series, Englewood Cliffs, New Jersey, Prentice-Hall, Inc., 1973, provides an excellent short introduction.

R. B. Brandt's *Ethical Theory: The Problems of Normative and Critical Ethics*, also published by Prentice-Hall, Inc., 1959, offers a more detailed account of the major normative and critical theories in ethics.

Alasdair MacIntyre's *A Short History of Ethics*, New York, The Macmillan Co., 1966, surveys the development of ethics from classical Greek philosophy to the present.

Normative Ethical Theories

The following works provide examples of various important normative theories. Most are difficult in at least some respects, and those without philosophic training are well advised to do some preparatory reading before attempting them. In the case of those works available in several editions or translations, we have tried to list the most readily accessible.

Aristotle: The Nicomachean Ethics. Ostwald, M. (trans.), Library of Liberal Arts, New York, Bobbs-Merrill Co., Inc., 1962.

Kant, I.: Foundations of the Metaphysics of Morals. Abbott, T. K. (trans.), Library of Liberal Arts, New York, Bobbs-Merrill Co., Inc., 1949.

Mill, J. S.: Utilitarianism. Acton, H. B. (ed.), London, J. M. Dent & Sons, Ltd., 1972.

Rawls, J.: A Theory of Justice. Cambridge, Mass., Harvard University Press, 1971.

Ross, W. D.: The Right and the Good. Oxford, The Clarendon Press, 1930.

Spinoza, B.: The Ethics. *In* The Chief Works of Benedict de Spinoza. Elwes, R. H. M. (trans.), New York, Dover Publications, Inc., 1955.

Metaethics

W. D. Hudson's *Modern Moral Philosophy*, Garden City, New York, Anchor Books, Doubleday & Co., Inc., 1970, provides a convenient starting point for the investigation of this field. Further bibliography may be obtained from that work.

Metaphysics of Morals

The writings of David Hume available in *Moral and Political Philosophy*, Aiken, H. D. (ed.), New York, Hafner Press, 1972, as well as those of Kant, cited earlier, are excellent examples of traditional philosophic thought in this area.

More recent works by Kurt Baier, *The Moral Point of View*, Ithaca, New York, Cornell University Press, 1958, and G. J. Warnock, *The Object of Morality*, London, Methuen & Company, 1971, provide contemporary introductions to the problems of the metaphysics of morals.

Chapter 18

THE DYING PATIENT

by AVERY D. WEISMAN,
and HERBERT R. BRETTELL

SAFE CONDUCT AND THE FAMILY PHYSICIAN

Sooner or later, everyone dies of something. The aims of medicine are to prevent unnecessary deaths, to help patients live as long and as well as possible, and to circumvent our human obligation to die. The first aim is usually feasible, the second aim is uncertain and difficult, and the third aim is impossible.

Unless a person dies unexpectedly far from home, the family physician is usually the first to evaluate a potentially fatal illness and the last to preside over the actual exitus. Regardless of consultants, specialists, technicians, and care-givers who come and go in the interim, it is the family physician's prerogative and responsibility to provide coherent management by offering treatment, relief, guidance, support, and safe conduct throughout the course of the disease. Although initial symptoms are often ambiguous, telltale signs of fatal illness frequently do show up early. The alert physician will know immediately, even before confirmatory tests are done, that subsequent events are more likely to mean caring for the patient through the vicissitudes of medical and psychosocial problems associated with life-threatening illness than curing that patient.

Every patient has a right to expect (1) accurate diagnosis, (2) prompt treatment, (3) adequate relief, and (4) safe conduct. The first three are self-evident and should occur in approximately that order. The fourth, safe conduct, needs explanation because it is seldom observed scrupulously, especially when dealing with preterminal and terminal patients.

Accurate Diagnosis

A serious illness is not always fatal, nor is a chronic illness necessarily more ominous than an acute disorder. However, for our present purposes, we shall emphasize the chronic illness, because management issues are more apt to be uppermost. Problems occur first when a potentially lethal disease fails to disclose itself promptly. Second, some patients procrastinate, believing that symptoms will go away. Third, physicians may minimize complaints and tacitly encourage further delay.

Delay is less common than ordinarily thought. Using cancer as an example, few patients allow more than 2 months to elapse after their first symptom before consulting a physician, although the length of lagtime may spread out to many months, even years. With the exception of breast or cervical cancer, early diagnosis does not necessarily mean catching the cancer at an early stage of development. However, a long lagtime often tells us more about the patient than it does about the diagnosis.

Highly malignant lesions are sometimes located so that symptoms are late in appearing. Other cancers quickly interfere with ordinary function, and patients are forced to seek diagnosis. When doing so, however, they may be reluctant to reveal their concern, preferring bland explanations that lull physicians into perfunctory examinations and conclusions. Certain patients suspect a serious illness, hope it will go away, and then, when symptoms persist, come to the physician, asking for an allegedly "routine" physical. One woman came to the emergency ward during a holiday, complaining about an upper respiratory infection. Routine chest examination disclosed asymmetry of the breasts that was caused by a sizable tumor.

Prompt Treatment

A family physician may underestimate signs of a life-threatening illness, especially when faced with an indecisive or apprehensive patient. Nevertheless, whether caused by compassion or unfounded optimism, the physician who inordinately delays will always be blamed for not acting sooner. Observation is a form of treatment, but neglect is not observation. "My doctor must have thought I was a neurotic or something. He kept telling me not to worry and to come back in 6 months."

In contrast, few patients accuse their physicians of being alarmists when further consultations, procedures, or tests are ordered *following* a thorough examination and history. "The doctor said that it might be nothing, or something very temporary, but he wanted to be sure." "Just knowing that the doctor took me seriously made me feel better, because I'd been worrying and not letting on about it." Prompt treatment presumes prompt diagnosis. Consequently, no treatment is better than immediate treatment without an accurate diagnosis.

Adequate Relief

Because few illnesses have specific cures, the family physician also offers relief of associated problems. These may be *physical* (pain, local symptoms, or systemic complaints), *psychosocial* (marriage, job, school, religion, and so forth), or *personal* (depression, fears, frustration, hopelessness, and so on). Patients with life-threatening illnesses are likely to have complaints in all three areas. It is the individual who is sick, not simply the individual's organs. Protracted illness usually has a drastic effect upon prevailing psychosocial concerns, more than can be explained by the physical lesions.

Safe Conduct

Safe conduct is uniquely the province of the family physician. Consultants see patients for a few times and under special circumstances. It is only the family physician who follows a patient through thick and thin of diagnosis and disappointment, hope and discouragement, convalescence and then decline. The sick patient fully realizes that the family physician offers much more than physical relief. Specifically, the physician is called upon to sustain patients and families and to guide them through the uncertainties and hazards of an illness destined to end in death.

Safe conduct has two meanings: (1) conducting a patient through peak distress, and (2) the conduct of the physician, which is cautious, courteous, forebearing, and courageous. Safety measures are in general intended to reduce distress and danger, but they cannot eliminate the risk itself. The physician is a guide, not a healer. However, even brief contacts at key moments can be of extraordinary help. Safe conduct is not to be confused with the extremes of extensive psychotherapeutic intervention or with periodic reassurances.

THE TRUTH AND WHAT TO DO ABOUT IT

An informed patient is usually a better and more cooperative patient. From the beginning, regardless of outcome, such a patient participates in decisions and in treatment without sustaining unrealistic expectations or having to maintain a false front. The family physician is also freed from the burden of an unnatural, needless pretense. The objective is *informed collaboration,* which is simply active extension of informed consent. Informed collaboration means sharing concern intelligently; it does not mean that a patient takes over his own treatment.

Whether to Tell

If results of a surgical procedure or a laboratory test are pessimistic, relatives often ask their family physician not to tell the patient. "He'll just give up hope." "He'd commit suicide if he knew he had cancer." As a rule, families are talking about their own despair rather than their knowledge of the patient. Actually, few patients give up hope, and suicide attempts following the diagnosis of a life-threatening disease rarely happen. Patients who do seem to give up are those without effective communication with their physician, not those who face an incurable or threatening illness.

Therefore, the important question is not whether to tell but what to do with the truth at the time we find it. Truth is a way of talking about and perceiving reality, and reality is an evolving idea, not something fixed, certain, and changeless.

Some patients suspect the right diagnosis before it is confirmed by their physician or a pathologist. They may be reticent to talk about it for three reasons. The first is to allow themselves a loophole, as illustrated by a woman who said, "I don't know my diagnosis, and I'm not ready to know it!" The second reason is to protect the physician. The protective idea is shown by a patient who invariably gave an optimistic report, saying, when questioned, "My doctor has tried so hard; I just don't want to disappoint him." A third reason for a patient's reluctance to voice concern or to ask about diagnosis is the physician's own attitude. It is commonplace to hear a physician say, when discussing a serious diagnosis (especially cancer), "No, I haven't mentioned the diagnosis to him, and he hasn't asked. But I think he knows anyway. These people always seem to know without being told." If this is true, why is the physician so timid?

When families adamantly insist that a patient not be informed, it is prudent to agree, but only tentatively. Tell them that you appreciate their shock and determination to protect the patient but that any so-called secret cannot be kept for very long. It might even be harmful. Usually, when the family does get over the shock, they change their minds. In any event, there should not be a conspiracy in which family and physician share something that really belongs to the patient.

To begin the care of a patient with a deception or conspiracy is contrary to principles of safe conduct. While patients may be reticent, diffident, or reluctant to ask about the diagnosis, the physician who has the closest relationship with them should be the one to talk over the situation. The patient may have reasons for withholding information from others. These deserve more adherence than similar prohibitions by families. The family physician cannot forfeit this responsibility or delegate it to others and still hope to maintain a substantial doctor–patient relationship. It is not possible to relinquish care, saying, in effect, "Well, you're Dr. Y.'s patient now. He's an expert." The patient will be puzzled unless he is told either what Dr. Y. is an expert in or why the transfer is being made.

When the task of telling a patient about an onerous diagnosis is too easy, the physician has become callous. When it is too difficult, he needs to examine his own guilt or anxiety. Open confrontation with facts is part of coping with serious illness. The physician can convey pertinent information with compassion and without compromise. He is not imposing a death sentence nor indicating that future treatment is futile.

How to Tell

Learning to listen well is as important as learning how to tell. Glib patter is hypocritical. A fixed speech, rattled off, tends to be confusing. Euphemisms, technicalities, circumlocutions, and half-lies do not clarify or inform, but simply undermine a perplexed patient.

The key phrase is *candor with hope.* This requires compassion, tact, straightforward statements, and common sense. Do not clutter up the situation with platitudes and differential diagnoses. Statistics are useful only for background, not for promises, predictions, or prophecies.

How to tell can be divided into the "hard tell," "soft tell," and "no tell." Hard tell limits itself to bare facts and findings, without tailoring comments to the capacity of the patient to assimilate the information or heeding his personal response. Soft tell is more tactful. It is no less accurate factually, but recognizes that the medical plight of a very sick patient is not relieved by merely learning pathologic findings. No tell occurs when a physician enters a sickroom, hoping that a patient will ask no questions, but if he does, answering with a downright prevarication. "When he's feeling better, then I'll tell him," actually means, "When I'm feeling better, I can tell and not tell at the same time."

The following series of quotes, in descending order, starts with bare facts of hard tell and ends with the more tactful and compassionate candor of soft tell. The family physician is speaking to his patient for the first time after an inoperable cancer of the pancreas has been discovered.

DR.   Mr. A., we found a very bad situation at operation. You have a cancer, and there is no cure for it.

DR.   Mr. B., the cause of your stomach pain turned out to be more serious than we hoped. There is a cancer behind your stomach that can't be removed.

DR.   Mr. C., the operation went all right. I expect you'll be getting over its effects pretty soon. But I'm sorry to say that we found that the stomach pains came from a tumor. We tried to remove as much as we could, but it's the kind of tumor that can't be taken out completely. So some of it is still there. However, while I can't promise you a cure, there are other kinds of treatment, which I'll talk to you about later on.

DR.   Mr. D., we did find a tumor at operation. I wish it could have been all taken out, but it isn't that kind of tumor. There are other kinds of treatment, but that can wait until you're feeling a bit better. I'm sure this news has to be disturbing. Most people would be disturbed; so would I. But you'll have questions, and I'll try to answer them as well as I can.... if not today, then when I see you again.

Note that in the latter examples the physician tells no more than he knows. He mentions tumor, not cancer, because the very term cancer has unfortunate implications. However, if a patient asks, "Do I have cancer?" the physician must answer, "Yes, you have a form of cancer, but cancer means many things. Some cancers can be treated better than others." If a patient continues, "Is my kind of cancer treatable?" the physician is also obliged to answer, "It is not the kind that responds best to treatment, but I do plan to treat you with some medicine we call chemotherapy, or with x-ray treatment, depending on what our consultants say is best."

These comments are not intended as a script. The art of telling and listening is individualized. The physician should allow for an adequate period of time, when he can sit down without looking at his watch. He can talk and give the patient a chance to talk or be silent.

DR.   I'm going to come back again while you're here and before you come to my office

again. We'll talk more about the illness, but I also want to discuss your whole situation with you, because you'll be laid up for some time to come. Meanwhile, don't anticipate too much one way or the other, but let's share worries together.

The rationale of this approach is that of coping through shared concern. The physician offers information that is appropriate, without added gratuitous opinions. He encourages the patient to "share the care." He heeds the person, but without anticipating a fatal result or building up fallacious optimism. This contrasts with the more authoritarian approach.

DR.   Mr. E., I won't bother you with a lot of technical details. It would only be confusing. Everything is okay. Just don't worry. Just get better.

The trouble with this approach is that the physician is not clear about what all the facts are, so he assumes that the patient will get confused. "I know something that you are too uninformed to understand." "Everything is okay" might mean merely that the patient now has a diagnosis. If we think it is helpful to tell any patient not to worry, try it sometime. "Just get better" means, "Don't bother me."

Truth cannot be communicated all at once. Even if it could, no statements are appropriate for every patient under all circumstances. Some patients will become upset, as well they might. But this is never permanent; the degree of distress is more closely connected with *how* a patient is told than with *what* he is told. Safe conduct depends on encouraging hope, trust, and self-regard in the patient, not on promises of recovery or long survival.

EVALUATING THE MORE VULNERABLE PATIENT

Few patients are so stoical when first told about having a potentially life-threatening illness that they show no response. They may, however, be stunned into silence or talk as if they hadn't quite understood. A high level of emotional distress is more common during the first few months than in succeeding months, unless the illness itself is rapidly progressive. In this case, distress usually worsens proportionately.

Psychosocial and emotional factors often aggravate pre-existing conflicts and interfere with efforts to cope. The more prominent factors are likely to be marital problems, indecisiveness, intense worries about living or dying, chronic pessimism, preoccupation with the past, painful recollection of failures and mistakes, suspicion and mistrust, previous psychiatric problems, abandonment by important others, and a generally precarious socioeconomic condition.

The art of listening for these vulnerability factors requires at least rudimentary skills in interviewing and in eliciting information. Interviewing cannot be learned from textbooks, but certain principles are invariable. For example, questions should be open-ended and nonjudgmental, because one seeks individualized, candid answers. For example, a good interviewer does not ask questions that can be answered with a yes or no.

Wrong:

DR.   Have you had any trouble in your marriage?
PT.   No, my husband is a very good man.

Note that the physician is obviously seeking information about marital problems, but he did not ask whether the patient's husband is or is not a "good man." Moreover, his interest in marital problems should be strictly confined to the illness. Mere marital strife is irrelevant unless it interferes with treatment, convalescence, or cooperation.

Right:

DR.   Judging by past experience, how helpful is your husband going to be during your illness, when you're likely to be below par?
PT.   Oh, he'll be all right, I guess. He's a very good man and good father, but not very sympathetic about sickness. He thinks I should be just as I've always been—up and doing.

Most patients like to put themselves in the best possible light and to conceal what they construe as shortcomings.

Wrong:

DR.   Would you call yourself a pessimist?
PT.   No, I always hope for the best.

Right:

DR.   In general, how do things usually turn out for you ... let's say something you really want?
PT.   Sometimes they do, sometimes they don't. I always hope for the best.
DR.   But how do you ordinarily *expect* them to work out?
PT.   Oh, even if they go well, I'm always looking for something to go wrong.

By knowing how to detect certain signs of vulnerability, the physician may be able to correct a patient's perception of events. He can at least realize that this is a patient with a tendency to become distressed, especially if other signs are also found. One must not only know how to ask, but by understanding the impact of questions, know how to appreciate the implications of answers.

VARIETIES OF VULNERABILITY

Patients become distressed in many ways, and their problems are also unique. Consequently, it is most difficult to generalize about individual emotions, such as anger, sadness, anxiety, or joy, except in extreme forms. However, beyond transient moods, there are more enduring forms of distress. These are varieties of vulnerability, such as hopelessness, fear, dread, helplessness, depression, feelings of abandonment and isolation, apathy and exhaustion, bitterness and truculence, shortened or closed time perspective, and so forth.

Emotional responses are not limited to transient depression, anger, or anxiety. The family physician should be able to identify vulnerability and forego the task of differentiating between separate emotions, which overlap, anyway. The following four types of vulnerability may also overlap, but they tell much more about a patient's personality and problems than do very fluid mood changes:

1. *Annihilation.* The patient feels *apprehensive* and convinced that all is lost. He is helpless and hopeless about the future. Having lost self-regard and individuality, he is discouraged and depleted, as if illness itself has taken control of him. He is just a number, a zero, a nothing.

2. *Alienation.* The patient is isolated,

lonely, *depressed*, and feels that those who might have offered support have abandoned him. Such patients also reject offers of help, convinced that they are totally alone and adrift with distressing symptoms and a fatal illness.

3. *Endangerment.* The patient feels frustrated, *angry*, and encroached upon. He is the victim of fate, family, or his physician. Every symptom is construed to be a sign of being killed by illness, in contrast to wasting away.

4. *Denial.* The patient has an *unrealistic optimism*, combined with a tendency to repudiate information and implications about his specific illness. While denial is part of the coping process, this kind of denial is often accompanied both by helplessness and by a paradoxical enthusiasm about a fancied future.

Almost every patient who suffers from a life-threatening illness, especially as that illness draws to a close in death, displays some form of anxiety, depression, or resentment. Others deny their plight and are even somewhat grandiose in their expectations. Fear of extinction is practically universal, but it is more glaring in some patients than in others. For the most part, however, fear of death is disproportionately small to the imminence of death. Patients very close to death have usually left the fear of extinction far behind them.

Utilizing vulnerability, as a concept, is more useful diagnostically than simply assuming that very sick patients are always depressed, anxious, bitter, worn out by futility and frustration, or, in contrast, reconciled. Vulnerability is (1) a state of distress, and (2) a disposition to behavior that confirms or relieves that distress. For example, an angry patient may conceal the resentment he feels, but after complaining about treatment or mistreatment, withdraws and thereafter asks for nothing. The family physician can often find out what bothers a patient by asking *what* and *how* he is feeling and what he would like to *do* about his distress.

It is advisable to anticipate vulnerability early, recognizing that concern about psychosocial problems is probable and that the only question is its variety and degree. Speaking openly means that it is permissible to talk about complaints or discomfort other than symptoms. It does not mean that any topic is thereafter closed. When re-

lapse or recurrence occurs, the physician can again talk about distress in a more knowledgeable way, because he is now familiar with the type of vulnerability his patient customarily exhibits. He can find out what triggered the distress and what, if anything, can be done about it.

A most poignant and painful form of vulnerability is a patient's feeling that it is impossible to convey the depth or extent of his predicament. Desolation and helplessness constitute a condition that means *there is no appeal.* Ironically, this aspect of illness is one that the family physician can do something about, by enlisting the help of significant others and by restoring to the patient a feeling that he is neither completely alone nor insignificant.

HELPING PATIENTS COPE

Competent coping depends upon first identifying the underlying problems correctly. Problems are not always what they seem and seldom what we expect. Psychosocial problems emerging from a fatal illness are often confused with the disease itself. "Anyone would be depressed," is a comment one often hears, but this is not true.

Existential questions about extinction provide the background for problems about religion, work, finances, friends, family, and marriage. The family physician should ask about these issues separately, lest his patient harbor feelings of vulnerability and estrangement from those whom he would naturally turn to. The logic of assuming that fatal disease itself causes everything to go awry runs like this: "Anyone would be depressed about having advanced cancer. No one can do anything about the cancer. Therefore, no one can do anything to help the cancer patient, except, possibly, to give enough medication to keep him comfortable." Such syllogisms may give an incurably ill patient some surcease from physical pain. However, it is not safe conduct, nor does it relieve psychologic suffering.

Since vulnerability is an effort to encompass an infinitude of emotions, it is necessary to propose some general groupings for problems that afflict terminal patients. A detailed catalogue of every kind of psychosocial problem would be even more cumbersome than a list of possible physical symptoms.

Problems may be divided into three groups: (1) *physical* ("I can't walk by myself"), (2) *psychosocial* ("I can't work and support my family"), and (3) *personal* ("I am a burden and worthless").

Patients who dogmatically deny any problems either mistrust the physician or feel so helpless and disappointed that their attitude is "What's the use?" Lest one distort the entire clinical process of coping with terminal illness, however, it should be emphasized that some patients do cope competently. With the support of outside resources or simply out of their own inner strength, they do quite well, needing only physical assistance from time to time. But even these patients have moments of distress. The family physician can also learn from them about coping with physical, psychosocial, and personal problems. For example, the physician can ask, "What's been the most difficult problem you've had to deal with since I saw you last?" Succeeding questions should be a form of "What have you been doing, or have done, about that problem?" Seemingly offhand answers may give a clue as to the coping strategy found most effective or, at least, available:

"I decided to ask my sister's advice."
"I just pushed it out of my mind."
"I got angry and then got drunk."
"I kept very busy, and it went away."
"I took the phone off the hook and went to sleep."
"I left the house, walked around, and took in a movie."
"I did nothing but fret and hope it might let up."
"I yelled at the kids and picked a fight with my husband."

The question that then can be asked is, "How did it work out?" Even better is, "What do you think others might have done in your place?"

In general, preterminal patients have less distress when they confront problems directly and are not constantly preoccupied with illness. Suppression ("I just pushed it out of my mind") is useful for brief periods, but not indefinitely. More effective are distractions consistent with physical status ("I left the house . . . went to a movie . . . read a book . . . watched television"). Blowing off steam relieves tension temporarily, as do drugs and alcohol. However, the physician should be aware of the difference between *showing* distress and *coping* with distress.

Pain relief is mandatory for any form of effective coping. Worry about addiction is almost an absurdity for patients who may soon die. Patients who put regrets behind, without ruminating about the past, are also apt to have higher self-regard and to be somewhat more optimistic, regardless of the outcome. However, putting the past totally behind is not the same as first reflecting on the past, in an endeavor to make sense out of one's life. Optimism does not mean unrestricted cheerfulness or always meeting adversity with a smile or a shrug. Expecting a patient to have equanimity at all times is to expect something even healthy people rarely achieve.

The aims of helping patients cope are to strengthen existing styles of resolving or relieving problems or to suggest other ways of handling an issue. To accomplish these aims, one uses confrontation with distress, clarification of a specific problem, reducing emotional extremes that might distort judgment, and then intervening to implement better control through available resources and options. Total resolution or relief may not be possible, and seldom is. But if the physician can just reduce acute problems to the level of quiet concerns, then distress is lowered and results are surprisingly productive.

Antidepressant drugs are occasionally helpful, but usually disappointing, unless accompanied by a strong dose of human relationship. As a rule, defining a problem helps to suggest a resolution. One woman who had always looked after her husband and children felt she was letting them down by being so ill. Her complaint was that she was so very weak and tearful when they were around. This was clearly a psychosocial problem because she considered her weakness and weeping as visible signs of helplessness and undependability. She was no longer the effective "mother image." Local symptoms of cancer were not important at this point. The physician helped by pointing out (on several occasions) that letting the family see her weep permitted them to help her. It also was another way of her looking after them. This time, however, her behavior was preparing her family for when she would not be around, and they would have to stand on their own. She was still helping them and was not at all helpless or undependable. In other words, her wish to continue controlling the family was fortified in order to bolster self-esteem.

PALLIATION AND PRETERMINALITY

Not every patient with a life-threatening illness is "preterminal," except in a philosophic sense. Preterminality is not synonymous with the diagnosis of an advanced medical illness. Otherwise, physician, family, and patient might wait a very long time for death in many cases. It is, of course, exceedingly difficult to predict when a patient will die. Long-range prophecies are unwise and usually incorrect. For practical purposes, preterminality begins when nothing further can be done to stem definite physical deterioration. In cases of cancer, it might begin in patients with two or more recurrences that are refractory to further treatment. Similar criteria can be promulgated for chronic congestive heart disease, kidney failure, and so forth. While certain patients die unexpectedly or prematurely, preterminality implies that both the physician and patient have some warning that further remissions are unlikely.

In the preterminal phase of illness, patients ask for care, not cure. Those who would seek miracles or untested remedies in far-off places have already done so. Palliation usually poses serious questions for the family physician: What else can be done? Will the price be justified in terms of its value? What is optimum care for this patient? What is consistent with safe conduct?

Everyone needs palliation, i.e., supportive and ameliorative interventions that inflict no further harm and little suffering. Placebos are not palliation. If a patient needs to sleep or to be relieved of pain, then only active drugs should be given. Placebos demoralize both the physician and patient, and preterminal patients are afraid of pain, demoralization, and abandonment. Death cannot be prevented, but demoralization can.

Most patients are aware of preterminality, sometimes before their physicians are.

Many patients prefer to die at home or at least in a familiar hospital environment, rather than be transferred to a nursing facility shortly before death. Commonly, some patients die within 1 or 2 days after an unwelcome transfer. They may suffer from the transfer itself or from overly vigorous rehabilitation efforts in the new and strange place, or they may find unaccustomed neglect. Transfer is not unacceptable, provided that a patient consents and therefore knows that he has not been forsaken. Unfortunately, capitulation by the physician is usually the reason for the transfer. The guiding principle should be whether transfer to a strange place is likely to be confusing or demoralizing.

TERMINALITY AND APPROPRIATE DEATH

When that moment arrives that signifies transition from preterminality to terminality, the patient has usually become obtunded. Goodbyes have been said. Both medication and the inevitable "complications" of disease have taken over. Nevertheless, silent expressions of caring can still be observed. A patient's unresponsiveness does not necessarily mean that he cannot hear or is beyond awareness.

Now is the time for the family physician to look back. How successfully has the patient been guided? What would be done over again, and what might be changed, given another chance? Hectic medical interventions that borrow a little more time are seldom worth the effort, unless the physician feels he must demonstrate something to the family or to himself.

An appropriate death does not mean an ideal or propitious death. It does signify that the patient has been able to live on as high a level of proficiency and esteem as possible, within the limits of physical disability. The patient was not forced to give up or be given up on and therefore arrived at death with a semblance of a satisfactory earlier life. For example, a businessman, accustomed to morning coffee conferences with associates, continued to be visited by one or more partners while he was in the hospital. They had coffee and talked about business prospects and memories of the past. It was good for the patient, and perhaps for his partners.

The physician's aim for his patient's inexorable death is the same as it was at the beginning of illness: survival, as long and as well as possible; symptom relief, as total as possible; and self-regard, as high as possible. If these objectives are reached, so is safe conduct. Death becomes a fact of nature, not a fault of anyone.

REFERENCES

1. Clayton, P. J.: Mortality and morbidity in the first year of widowhood. Arch. Gen. Psychiatry, 30:747, 1974.
2. Coelho, G., Hamburg, D., and Adams, J. (eds.): Coping and Adaptation. New York, Basic Books, Inc., Publishers, 1974.
3. Engle, G. L.: A life setting conducive to illness. The giving-up—given-up complex. Ann. Int. Med., 69:293, 1968.
4. Feifel, H., Freilich, J., and Hermann, L. J.: Death fear in dying heart and cancer patients. J. Psychosom. Res., 17:161, 1973.
5. Fulton, R. (ed.): Death and Identity. Rev. ed. Bowie, Maryland, Charles Press Publishers, Inc., 1976.
6. Glaser, B. G., and Strauss, A. L.: Awareness of Dying. Chicago, Aldine Publ. Co., 1965.
7. Kastenbaum, R., and Aisenberg, R.: The Psychology of Death. New York, Springer Publishing Company, 1972.
8. Leiberman, M. A., and Coplan, A. S.: Distance from death as a variable in the study of aging. Dev. Psychology, 2:71, 1970.
9. Lipowski, Z. J. (ed.): Psychosocial Aspects of Physical Illness, Vol. 8. Advances in Psychosomatic Medicine. Basel, Munchen, Paris, London, New York, Sydney, S. Karger, 1972.
10. Quint, J.: The Nurse and the Dying Patient. New York, The Macmillan Co., 1967.
11. Shneidman, E. S.: Deaths of Man. New York, Quadrangle/New York Times Book Co., 1973.
12. Weisman, A. D.: The patient with a fatal illness—to tell or not to tell. J.A.M.A., 201:646, 1967.
13. Weisman, A. D.: On Dying and Denying: A Psychiatric Study of Terminality. New York, Behavioral Publications, Inc., 1972.
14. Weisman, A. D.: Psychosocial considerations in terminal care. In Schoenberg, B., Carr, A., Peretz, D., and Kutscher, A. (eds.): Psychosocial Aspects of Terminal Care. New York and London, Columbia University Press, 1972.
15. Weisman, A. D., and Worden, J. W.: Psychosocial analysis of cancer deaths. Omega, 6:61, 1975.
16. Worden, J. W., and Weisman, A. D.: Psychosocial components of lagtime in cancer diagnosis. Brit. J. Psychosom. Res., 19:69, 1975.

Chapter 19

INTERVIEWING TECHNIQUES

by *GORDON H. DECKERT,*
and MARTIN H. ANDREWS

"I've never read anything about interviewing that's been worth a damn in my practice!" This statement, made by a family physician during a workshop on psychosomatic medicine, reflects the experience of many of us in our efforts to become efficient and effective interviewers. But how can we expect to become proficient interviewers simply by reading material on this subject? Becoming a skilled interviewer requires more than merely reviewing the literature.[2, 10, 13]

The learning sequence begins with the elaboration of a specific model for interviewing. This model must take into account a particular body of knowledge as well as the nature of a particular interviewer. Yet, at the same time, the model must allow flexibility in dealing with a wide range of patients and their problems.

For most, there must be the opportunity to observe good interviewers in action and to observe role models. Films and video tapes may be helpful if the observer realizes that techniques successful for one interviewer may not be successful for another. Furthermore, techniques that are productive with one patient may be counterproductive with the next. Finally, as with any skill, there must be the opportunity to practice and practice and practice, but to do so with appropriate feedback.

Reviewing audio tapes of one's own interviews with patients can provide useful feedback, especially if done under supervision. However, those who study, research, practice, and teach medical interviewing are increasingly convinced that becoming a truly effective and efficient interviewer requires not only hearing oneself but seeing oneself at work repeatedly, both with self-evaluation and with peer review.[2, 7, 10, 13]

Video tape equipment is becoming more and more available in hospitals and clinics across the United States, especially in those institutions having family practice residency programs.

The experience of physicians with this educational technique follows a typical pattern. They are astonished to discover aspects of themselves that they had not envisioned and are dismayed to note data that simply did not register during the live interview. Although periods of discouragement occur, persistence in using this method will provide pleasure and pride, as physicians modify their particular style to incorporate more efficient and effective techniques. Considerable motivation and effort are required to improve interviewing techniques significantly. Therefore, taking our cue from the family physician already quoted, we would even suggest that further reading of this chapter might be a waste of time if reading is the only step intended toward improving one's interviewing skills.

INTERVIEWING AND PATIENT OUTCOME

What is a good physician? What are the qualities of a good interview and of a good interviewer? Most of us have very strong opinions about this subject. Perhaps it is more useful to attempt to answer these questions by evaluating patient outcome. What are the characteristics of those physicians who have good outcome in terms of patient response, for example, those pediatricians, family physicians, and psychiatrists who have high patient compliance rates compared with those who do not? What qualities differentiate those physicians whose patients lose weight from those whose patients do not?

First, a good physician who is also an effective and efficient interviewer is one who is appropriately nurturing, that is, one who is skillfully supportive of a particular patient at a particular time and in a particular way in response to specific indications. In observing physician–patient interactions in various specialties, it has been found that family physicians tend to be too nurturing and surgeons not nurturing enough.[3]

Second, a good interviewer, as defined by outcome studies, is one who is exceptionally skilled in providing a cognitive model, so that the patient understands both his disease and his "dis-ease." Often, this effort runs counter to a sick role commonly assumed by patients in our society. "I simply need to trust my doctor and do what he tells me, and it is not necessary for me to really understand my disease or my dis-ease." Family physicians are quite effective in providing models of understanding when the patient is suffering from tonsillitis or a urinary tract infection but are less effective in providing such models when the patient's problem is primarily psychosomatic.

Third, good physicians are particularly skilled in involving the patient in the problem-solving process; their interviews are a dialogue.[8] This also runs counter to another sick-role assumption commonly held by many physicians in our culture. "This patient is sick and really not responsible for his illness. I am responsible for telling him what is necessary for him to do to get better, and he is responsible for following my suggestions." Nonetheless, outcome studies show that when patients are involved in the problem-solving process, therapeutic outcomes are more likely.[1]

Note what is not included in this discussion. Those physicians who are good interviewers do not necessarily know more about a given subject than those who are considered less effective, as defined by patient outcome criteria. Nor does one model for understanding human behavior seem more effective than another.

What happens between a physician and a patient during an interview depends considerably on how well the physician accomplishes a series of tasks. This seems to be true whether the encounter takes place in an emergency room, a hospital suite, or a physician's office or whether the encounter logically ends within 10 minutes or the disease/dis-ease process requires multiple interventions over many months. Regardless of these variations, the first several tasks take place even *before* the interview begins.

The Conceptual Task

Anthropologists come to understand the organization and function of a given society by asking and answering a series of critical questions. How does this particular culture view man, how does it view nature, and how does it view the interaction between man and nature? How does this culture view time? An interview can be understood by utilizing a similar exercise. What key concepts does the interviewer bring to the encounter? Does the interviewer become aware of the concepts that the patient brings to the encounter? Are the concepts similar, compatible, complementary, or conflictive? In addition to these key concepts, the medical interview should incorporate the concepts of disease and dis-ease. Does the interviewer, or the patient, or both, hold a reductionistic view? Is disease considered a thing or a process? Are disease and dis-ease regarded as synonymous or antithetical?

Especially useful concepts for the physician to bring to an interview are those of individual and stimulus response specificity. Stimulus response specificity assumes that a particular stimulus results in a particular set of responses. Therefore, given a particular intervention, one should be able to predict fairly accurately what the response will be. Much of our medical school and postgraduate training is based on this assumption, which is frequently useful in an interview situation.

However, family physicians quickly discover, frequently soon after entering practice, that this assumption simply does not work in most instances with most patients. To accurately predict a response to a stimulus or to subsequently deduce which stimulus led to a particular set of responses in a given patient usually requires knowing that patient. Only by knowing the individual can one consistently interrelate stimulus and response.[2] These two concepts will be employed in a complementary fashion by a good interviewer.

Inflexibly maintaining the concept of

stimulus response specificity leads to frustration for the physician and poor outcome for the patient, especially when the problem is primarily psychosomatic or is an adverse psychologic response to a disability. Many physicians continue to ask such questions as "How do you treat muscular tension headaches?" And they even expect an article, or a book, or a consultant to provide a specific answer! On the other hand, a question utilizing individual response specificity, such as "How might I treat this particular patient with muscular tension headaches?", usually allows an answer.

Another factor that influences interview outcome is the set of priorities that the physician brings to the interaction. Certainly, emergency medicine has top priority, and we should first determine whether such a situation exists. But if a medical emergency does not exist, what do we first want to know about a patient? What are our information-gathering priorities?

The usual answer is that we should first elicit the chief or presenting complaint. This, as a top priority, might be an effective and efficient strategy if the situation were usually one of stimulus response specificity. But more often, our strategy should be to observe the patient or to elicit data that will lead us to understand this particular patient at this particular time. This is usually a more efficient and effective focus in medical interviewing and is derived from the concept of individual response specificity. Our initial perceptual task, therefore, is not to elicit the chief complaint (this will come soon enough) but rather to identify the patient's primary emotion.

In summary, the interviewer's first task is to become thoroughly aware of the concepts that he brings to the interview.

The Attitudinal Task

In addition to concepts, the physician and the patient also bring a set of attitudes to the interviewing encounter. The physician can monitor and to some degree modulate his own attitudes. Effective interviewing is partly determined by how honestly and accurately a physician can answer questions such as, "Why did I become a physician in the first place?" "What needs do I have in my role of physician?" Beyond this, effective interviewers monitor their attitudinal

set on a daily basis. Since the interviewer is his own best instrument, he must know that instrument before the interview begins.

One technique to meet this requirement is to conduct a daily psychologic inventory. On a daily basis at a specific time, perhaps before going to work, the interviewer deliberately focuses on such questions as "How do I feel—fatigued, rested, anxious, irritated, excited?" "What task pressures will I experience today?" The physician then turns his attention to his "significant others," asking himself similar questions about how he perceives them, their feelings, and their task pressures. Next, the interviewer reviews his perceptions of the current relationships between himself and his significant others, such as "Today, how do I see my relationship with my son, my mother, my partner?"

Having engaged in this self-inventory, the interviewer then reviews the work anticipated for that day. This should include a review of the anticipated patient schedule. Reflecting on these patients one by one, the physician monitors his feeling and thinking responses concerning each of them and correlates these responses with those already reviewed.

For example, if one interviewer recognizes some difficulty that she is having with her husband or another interviewer recognizes a feeling of sadness in relation to his mother, such perceptions alert them to avoid inappropriate solicitations from particular patients. To cite another example, by being aware of a feeling of annoyance toward his son, a physician avoided an inappropriate behavioral response toward a patient of similar age, demeanor, and behavior. Some physicians who have learned, practiced, and adapted this technique report that their daily psychologic inventory has had dramatic impact on improving their interviewing effectiveness. Their spouses even report that they have become more authentic persons.

Having thus completed the conceptual task and the attitudinal task, the physician is now ready to interview a patient.

The Perceptual Task

The shape and outcome of any interview is mainly a reflection of what the physician sees and hears as well as what the physician does *not* see or hear. The process begins with the first moment of encounter. When making hospital rounds, some physicians behave in a very stereotyped way during their first minute with each patient. This suggests that the physician is structuring his interview from some internal construct, almost as if he were repeating a set speech, as opposed to utilizing his percepts to shape and structure the interaction.

During the interview, there are two main categories of perceptual data.[2] The first category comprises the words used by the patient. Physicians generally are more comfortable with digital than with analog data. Thus, over a period of time, most physicians become fairly skilled in hearing the words used by patients. They hear the patient say, "My belly hurts. It began yesterday." Unless they have had special training, however, they tend to miss what is not being said, nor do they notice what the underlying assumptions seem to be for that patient, given that set of words. The patient said, "My belly hurts," not "*I* have pain in my belly." Furthermore, the patient said, "It began yesterday," and not "*My* pain began yesterday."

A relatively new discipline is bringing considerable understanding to the therapeutic process.[6] Transformational grammarians suggest that when we listen to patients, we listen for complete sentences. In many, perhaps in most, instances, the patient's sentence is not complete. The effective interviewing process encourages patients to finally speak in complete sentences. When a patient says "I am nervous," we note this as a very incomplete sentence. We do not know what the patient means by the word "nervous." Does he mean anxious, afraid, angry, irritated, sad, depressed, or what? The sentence does not include what in the patient's experience has triggered this nervousness. Nor is there any indication that the patient understands his response to this feeling. A more complete sentence might be, "I am feeling scared because I have noticed blood in my urine for the last 2 days, and of course in my imagination I am worrying that I might have cancer and this scares me." Some patients have great difficulty in completing their incomplete sentences. Effective therapeutic intervention assists the patient in doing this and in recognizing and then eliminating distortions. There are specific techniques that the physician can learn to assist the patient in this process. The book by Grinder

and Bandler will be particularly helpful in this regard.[6]

The second category of perceptual data is more analog than digital, more visual than auditory. Such data are particularly helpful in cuing the physician to the patient's character structure, his style of interaction, and, especially, to his primary emotion. With this model of interviewing, one of the higher priorities for the interviewer is the identification of the patient's primary emotion. This priority is based on the assumption that the "royal road" to understanding a given patient at a given time is to conduct an inventory of his primary emotions.

The primary emotions have been fairly well delineated.[2, 4] When communicated by facial expression and in an undisguised fashion, they are universal in form and independent of a particular culture or family. The primary emotions are acceptance, disgust, surprise, joy, fear, anger, and sadness. When interviewers test their ability to accurately identify primary emotions by using standard video tape exercises, they discover that, while they are very expert in identifying some primary emotions, they consistently tend not to see others. This is not surprising, since interviewers are taught certain rules for recognizing emotions by their culture or family long before they enter the medical profession. Each of us has literally been taught not to see certain kinds of data.[2] A training experience corrects this deficiency, once it is recognized.[13] Ekman and Friesen's book is a helpful starting point for those not familiar with this material.[4] Deckert's video tape "Interpreting Body Language in Everyday Practice" allows the observer to come closer to the actual interviewing situation than is possible in book form.[2]

Next, the interviewer should note whether there is congruence between the subjective and the objective messages, that is, whether what the patient says about how he feels (the subjective data) matches how the patient looks to the interviewer (the objective data). One characteristic of psychologically healthy individuals in the interview setting is that they look the way they say they are feeling. The emotion experienced is the emotion communicated. In the disturbed individual the subjective and the objective messages may not agree.

Different patterns of incongruence require different approaches.[5] One example is the patient who communicates anger by the tone of his voice and by his facial expression but, nonetheless, does not use words that suggest that he is feeling angry. In fact, upon direct questioning, he denies experiencing anger. It is quite unlikely that such a patient will be particularly aware of the array of life stresses that precipitate a set of responses leading to severe muscular tension headaches, for example. Others around him, including his physician, may have considerable evidence that such a sequence does occur. However, such a patient usually is very resistant to the idea that there may be a psychosomatic component to his headaches.

Conversely, a woman who uses words that suggest that she is almost overwhelmed by anxiety but, nonetheless, presents these words with a smiling, nonanxious facies presents a different problem. Her communication of emotion lacks facial validity. She tends not to be believed by her significant others, including her physician. And in many areas of her life, she finds herself relatively impotent in resolving her particular problems.

If each of these patients were to have a myocardial infarction, their response to their illness and the subsequent interviewing process would be different. Each would also require a considerably different psychotherapeutic approach. In a specific interview, once congruence has been established between the objective and the subjective evidence, the interviewer usually can elicit the precipitating stress fairly accurately, by simply asking the patient how he accounts for his symptoms or his feelings, or both. Involved dynamic interpretations are not required. However, before this can occur, there must be congruence.

Having seen and having heard the patient, the interviewer is now ready to proceed with the interpersonal task.

The Interpersonal Task

The objectives of the interpersonal task are determined by the accuracy of the perceptual task. That is, success in meeting these objectives depends upon the correctness of the interviewer's perceptions.

Among the initial objectives of the interpersonal task is that of establishing an effective physician–patient doctor relationship as rapidly as possible.[5, 11] An effective technique is to convey explicitly that the message sent by the patient was the message received by the physician.[12] Early in the interview, and repeatedly thereafter, the interviewer reports back or summarizes what he has seen and heard. For example, "I hear you saying that you are anxious because you have noticed blood in your urine for the last 2 days. Indeed you look anxious, you're concerned abut whether this could be cancer, and so your anxiety is understandable." This maneuver gives the patient an opportunity to correct the physician's perceptions and conveys that the physician is attentive and understanding.

Another objective of the interpersonal task is to obtain accurate information. The message sent–message received maneuver facilitates this process. The assistance that the interviewer gives the patient in obtaining congruence between the emotion communicated and the emotion experienced also facilitates this process. To ignore an emotional display is to risk allowing that emotion to interfere with the reporting of accurate data. Anxiety demands attention, anger demands response, and sadness demands recognition. Until these demands are met to some degree, the patient may find that the accurate communication of some data is almost impossible, and the physician may find that the accurate comprehension of some data is equally difficult.

For this reason, the effective interviewer learns how to utilize both the associative interview technique and the interrogative interview technique.[5, 12] The physician using the associative technique follows the patient's thought process and encourages elaboration of his associations by utilizing open-ended questions, by repeating the patient's last few words, by nodding his head, and so forth. The interviewer using the interrogative technique asks a series of questions and expects a series of answers. The patient is asked to follow the interviewer's thought process. This is formalized in an organized fashion and utilizes the review of systems approach learned by all physicians in medical school. For most interviews, the interweaving of these two techniques is indicated. Generally, it is the associative technique that poses particular difficulties for many medical interviewers, especially early in their training.

Finally, another objective of the interpersonal task is to relate to the patient in a way that becomes therapeutic. This is sometimes easier said than done, since neurotic patients tend to solicit neurotic interactions from their physicians. Even so, the interviewer's goal is to utilize interpersonal transactions to accomplish specific therapeutic interventions. This is discussed in greater detail in the section dealing with the therapeutic task.

The Nosologic Task

Very early during the interview, the efficient interviewer begins to compare the pattern of data obtained from the patient with the patterns of data learned from previous training and practice. That is, the interviewer begins to assign a diagnostic label to the patient to facilitate his understanding of both the disease and the disease processes. In the formal sense, the physician first postulates and eventually confirms a diagnosis. Accomplished interviewers do not make a diagnosis by simply following a sequence of "yes or no" logic. When the diagnostic process is studied, physicians who recognize patterns are found to be effective and efficient diagnosticians.

The diagnostic, or naming, process involves several levels of abstraction. Early during the interview, skilled interviewers literally ask themselves such questions as, "What is this patient's diagnosis in terms of his primary emotion?" "What is this patient's personality pattern?" "What is the diagnosis of this patient's disease?" Much of medical training is directed toward the latter question, and this is a critical feature of the nosologic task. But in the practice of medicine, perhaps especially in the practice of family medicine, the answers to the other diagnostic questions are equally critical.

However, simply naming the emotions, the personality pattern, the dis-ease, and the disease is not sufficient.

The Dynamic Task

Having obtained pertinent and accurate data and having made a relatively accurate set of diagnoses, it becomes necessary to put this information into some framework for understanding a patient's physiologic, psychophysiologic, and psychologic make-up. This means utilizing one or more models for understanding behavior at the molecular *and* at the molar level. Physicians have fairly effective physiologic models for understanding their patients' disease processes. However, many physicians, for one reason or another, seem to avoid utilizing available models for understanding human behavior to comprehend patients' dis-ease processes.

Referring once again to the outcome studies mentioned previously, it is important to note that in the field of psychosomatic or psychologic medicine one model is not demonstrably better than another for understanding human behavior. What is significant to outcome is whether an interviewer employs a particular model in a consistent, logical fashion and whether or not the physician is successful in communicating his model for understanding the patient to the patient. This means that a model such as transactional analysis is not necessarily more effective than a psychoanalytic model or a learning model. What is critical is whether the physician and the patient use a given model in an effective manner.

In our view, family physicians should become conversant with more than one model for understanding human behavior. At some point toward the end of the initial interview, an interviewer can begin to utilize the language of a particular model and simply note the patient's response. Some patients respond almost immediately to the language system that flows from the model of transactional analysis, even though they do not necessarily need to become familiar with transactional analysis per se in a formal sense. The same can be said of other language systems from other models for understanding human behavior.

When residents or, for that matter, physicians in practice are observed interviewing a patient, it appears that some do not follow any particular model at all, at least not consistently. It is difficult to move effectively and efficiently through the therapeutic sequence without employing some model for understanding human behavior. While this is not the focus of this particular chapter, the reader is encouraged to become conversant with more than one model. Some suggested materials for further study appear in this chapter's reference list.[3, 9, 10, 11]

The Therapeutic Task

The ultimate task for the health professional is the therapeutic task. Its success, however, is dependent on all those tasks that preceded it. In this chapter, the process is labeled "the therapeutic sequence."

Primary Emotion. As the first step, the interviewer asks himself, "What is this patient's primary emotion?" Even in the first moments of the interaction, this is the interviewer's most important perceptual priority. Is there evidence for the presence of anxiety, anger, sadness, or acceptance? The answer comes by noting the patient's facial expressions, observing his behavior, and listening to his words.[2,4]

Congruence. During the second step, the interviewer seeks to establish congruence between the emotion communicated and the emotion experienced. That is, is the patient aware of what he is communicating, or, conversely, is he communicating what he is feeling?[2] Put simply, does the patient look and feel sad? Does he look and feel puzzled? Does he look and feel irritated? If congruence is not present, the interviewer seeks to establish it by a series of interventions, or, at the very least, he seeks to bring the disparity to the patient's attention. Ideally, congruence is noted or established before proceeding to the next step in the sequence.

Stress. The interviewer next asks himself what class of psychologic or physiologic stress might be precipitating this particular emotion.[2] In psychologically healthy individuals, anxiety or fear is experienced in response to the stress of injury and is then communicated, whether it be fact or fantasy, real or symbolic. The presence of anger usually follows from the frustration of not having particular physiologic or psychologic needs met. Sadness usually relates to the presence of loss. The interviewer begins with the assumption that the category of stress and the usual emotional response to that stress will correspond.

Consensus. During the fourth step, the interviewer obtains consensus. A general agreement is reached between the physician and the patient as to what event or symptom or concern is precipitating the particular emotional response. With psychologically healthy patients, these four steps are usually accomplished fairly rapidly. However, patients with significant areas of neurotic conflict may present considerable difficulty.

Contract. Once congruence and consensus are established, it is possible for the patient and the physician to make a "clean" contract. Too often in the medical setting, the contract is simply assumed by both parties, frequently with each harboring a different set of expectations. What is the patient's goal; what is he requesting? The contracting process may be initiated by the physician's obtaining the patient's chief expectation. For example, "What did you hope would happen by coming to see me?" Now that both the patient and the interviewer have identified the problem and the emotional response to the problem, it is essential that each share his expectations with the other. The contract needs to be explicit, and the terms should include an understanding of suggested diagnostic studies and intervention techniques as well as time and money requirements.

Concurrence. During the sixth step, the physician obtains concurrence. The contract is consummated. Both physician and patient agree to the nature of the intervention process. Both agree, for example, that hospitalization is indicated or that additional interviews will be necessary to delineate the problem, or that specific laboratory tests will be ordered, or that the problem is urinary tract infection, or that the problem is a grief reaction to the loss of a job, and so forth.

Treatment Strategies. The physician, of course, already has been considering various treatment strategies, as he has an expertise that may be helpful to the patient. The patient is often not aware of all the therapeutic options, nor does he possess certain therapeutic intervention techniques, or he simply may not be skilled in problem-solving. On the other hand, the patient may be aware of potential therapeutic options of which the physician is not. For example, the patient may have an employment option that the interviewer does not know about. The skilled interviewer will therefore directly involve the patient in the problem-solving process.

Implementation. The eighth and final step is for both physician and patient to proceed with implementation of a given strategy. If there is difficulty in doing this, the therapeutic sequence will need to be repeated. If there is success, the patient usually says "thank you" and the interviewer hopefully replies "you're welcome," both having been enriched by the encounter.

THE THERAPEUTIC SEQUENCE IN ACTION: AN EXAMPLE

A family physician practicing for 6 years in a town, population 30,000, is about to see a patient already known to him from previous visits. The patient is 45 years old, white, male, married for 23 years, and has three children, ages 16, 18, and 20. He is the manager of a small finance company and has previously been in good health, physiologically and psychologically. The patient walks into the consulting room and takes a seat. The physician shuts the office door.

DR.: "Good morning Jack, you look worried." (The physician has noted the characteristic facies of moderate anxiety and the fidgeting quality of the patient's hand movements as he sits down. He chooses to use a more general term "worried" in his first statement.)

PT.: "Yes sir, to tell you the truth, I'm scared." (The patient acknowledges the physician's perceptual accuracy and specifies more precisely his emotional state.)

DR.: "Scared about what, Jack?" (The physician notes *congruence* between the emotion communicated and the emotion experienced, speculates that this individual has experienced a recent stress of injury or threat of injury, and proceeds to obtain consensus.)

PT.: "Well to be honest, I am scared that I may have heart trouble. You remember my dad had a heart attack several years ago, and it runs in the family. When I walk from my home to my office, you know, up that hill, for the last several weeks I've noticed this discomfort, this pain in my chest, and it kind of goes down my left arm . . . a classic description, I guess. I tried to pass it off at first, but it's happened now 3 or 4 times, especially if I'm hurrying, but I haven't noticed anything else (pause). But I can't help thinking it might be some kind of heart trouble."

DR.: "So you're scared you might have heart trouble. That certainly would be something to be concerned about. It has run in your family, and what you've noticed is this pain in your chest and left arm when you are walking in a hurry up this hill to your office. Is that right?" (The physician already has achieved a degree of *consensus*, is making sure the message sent has been the message

received, is being appropriately nurturing, and accepts the patient's anxiety. In addition, he has introduced a modifying influence by the use of the word "concerned" and is ready to establish an appropriate contract.)

PT.: "Yes, that about says it."

DR.: "So in coming to see me, you want me to check this out?"

PT.: "I sure do."

DR.: "OK. Well, I need to get a little more history, then I will want to examine you, and we may need to run some tests, but we'll talk more about that later. Does that sound reasonable?"

PT.: "Sure does."

Since both the physician and the patient have a clear understanding of what each expects of the other, at this point there is *concurrence*.

The physician proceeds with the history, confirms the absence of other symptoms, confirms the accuracy of the patient's description of the pain, and based on the history seriously considers the diagnosis of coronary artery disease with angina pectoris. He determines that the patient has already discussed these symptoms with his wife and that she is also "very concerned." He then performs the appropriate physical examination, obtains a chest x-ray study and electrocardiogram during this first office visit, orders the appropriate laboratory tests, and tentatively makes the diagnosis of coronary artery disease. He sits down with the patient, reviews the evidence, shares his tentative diagnosis, and outlines a suggested diagnostic plan and a plan for therapeutic intervention. The patient agrees.

DR.: "Are there any questions or concerns?" (The physician is looking for possible difficulties with *implementation.*)

PT.: "No, I guess not." (The patient licks his lips, and an anxious facial expression returns. The therapeutic sequence will be repeated.)

DR.: "Jack, you still seem rather concerned about something. What is it?" (The physician hears the distortion and sees the anxiety and approaches it directly.)

PT.: "Doc, I sure as hell don't want to die."

DR.: "You're worried that somehow this means you're going to die?"

PT.: "Well, I think you can understand that, given my family history."

DR.: "Yes, I certainly can. But you have done several things that make a lot of sense. These symptoms have been present for only a few weeks. You haven't ignored them. You have come to see me. We are going to look at this very carefully before we jump to any conclusions. Even if this turns out to be what we both expect, we have some reason to be optimistic. There are things you can do, things I can do, things we can do. With appropriate treatment, we can anticipate fair success in managing the problem." (The physician continues to set the stage for shared responsibility and joint participation in the development of a therapeutic strategy and its implementation.)

PT.: "Yes, I know. But it is going to take me a while to get used to all of this."

DR.: "I can certainly understand that."

PT.: "And my wife is really worried."

DR.: "What would you think about your wife's coming in with you next time?" (The physician does not say, "I think your wife should come in next time.")

PT.: "I think that's a good idea. Well, I'll go ahead and get those tests and keep track of any other pains like we talked about. I understand about using the medicine, and my wife and I will come to see you in 2 days when we have the results of the tests. OK?"

DR.: "Sounds good."

PT.: "OK, see you then." (Both stand up.) "Thanks, Doc."

DR.: "You're welcome. See the two of you in 2 days."

This is an example of a physician's working with a relatively "easy" patient. The patient is a genital character, that is, someone relatively free from neurotic conflict areas. Even so, the physician's interviewing skill facilitates the therapeutic sequence. As his skill increases, so will his success with "difficult" patients. And as competence increases, physicians consistently find that the interviewing process is one of the more challenging and rewarding aspects of the practice of medicine.

REFERENCES

1. Blackwell, B.: Treatment adherence. Br. J. Psychiatry, 129:513, 1976.
2. Deckert, G.: Interpreting Body Language in Everyday Practice. (Video tape), Los Angeles, Professional Research, Inc., 1974.
3. Deckert, G.: Transactional Analysis for the Practicing Physician. (Video tape), Los Angeles, Professional Research, Inc., 1974.
4. Ekman, P., and Friesen, W.: Unmasking the Face. Englewood Cliffs, N.J., Prentice-Hall, Inc., 1975.
5. Froelich, R. E., and Bishop, M.: Medical Interviewing, A Programmed Manual. 3rd Ed. St. Louis, The C. V. Mosby Co., 1976.
6. Grinder, J., and Bandler, R.: The Structure of Magic. Vol. I and II. Palo Alto, Cal., Science & Behavior Books, Inc., 1976.
7. Helfer, R. E., and Ealy, K. F.: Observations of pediatric interviewing skills. Am. J. Dis. Child., 123:556, 1972.
8. Howe, R.: The Miracle of Dialogue. New York, Seabury Press, Inc., 1963.
9. James, M., and Jongeward, D.: Born to Win; Transactional Analysis with Gestalt Experiments. Menlo Park, Cal., Addison-Wesley Publishing Co., 1971.
10. Kagan, H., Krathwohl, D. R., Goldberg, A. D., et al: Studies in Human Interaction. East Lansing, Mich., Educational Publication Series, Michigan State University, 1967.
11. Magersen, E. W.: Putting the Ill at Ease. New York, Harper & Row, Publishers, 1976.
12. Rogers, C.: Client-Centered Therapy. Boston, Houghton-Mifflin Co., 1951.
13. Werner, A., and Sneider, J. M.: Teaching medical students interactional skills. N. Engl. J. Med., 290:1232, 1974.

Chapter 20

LEARNING DISABILITIES

by SYLVIA O. RICHARDSON,
and ROBERT SMITH

THE PROBLEM

In these modern times, many children are judged not to be normal. They are considered emotionally unstable or mentally retarded or to have low intellectual ability and are often incarcerated in institutions for life.

Approximately 7.5 million such children are estimated to live in the United States.[3] It is now believed that 9 out of 10 of these youngsters are misdiagnosed and that they really suffer from a group of related physiologic problems termed learning disabilities that are primarily neurologic in nature. If early diagnosis and appropriate treatment are provided, enormous suffering can be avoided. A learning disability does not impair intelligence, and this makes failure to diagnose the disorder all the more poignant.

Learning disabilities in children have been called by many names. Among the labels most commonly used are *minimal brain dysfunction* (MBD) and *dyslexia.* MBD is the term most frequently used by physicians and pharmaceutical companies. Dyslexia literally means specific reading disability. Because this term has acquired increasingly broader meanings, the World Federation of Neurology now uses the term *specific developmental dyslexia* to indicate those children, predominantly male, who have a specific language disability in the areas of reading, spelling, and writing, which, in the majority of cases, is familial. Needless to say, the multiplicity of labels and definitions has added to the confusion in the field of learning disabilities. As a result, the United States Congress requested the Bureau of Education of the Handicapped to define children with specific learning disabilites.

The definition that now appears in current federal regulations, recommended by the Office of Education, is as follows:

Children with specific learning disabilities are those children who have a disorder in one or more of the basic psychological processes involved in understanding or in using language, spoken or written, which disorder may manifest itself in imperfect ability to listen, think, speak, read, write, spell, or do mathematical calculations. Such disorders include such conditions as perceptual handicaps, brain injury, minimal brain dysfunction, dyslexia, and developmental aphasia. Such term does not include children who have learning problems which are primarily the result of visual, hearing, or motor handicap, of mental retardation, of emotional disturbance, or environmental, cultural or economic disadvantage.[11]

It is important for physicians to understand the implications of Public Law 94–142,[11] enacted November 29, 1975, which includes provisions designed to assure that all handicapped children have available to them a free, *appropriate* public education. This legislation protects the rights of handicapped children and their parents and says that states and localities must provide for the education of all handicapped children. Its purpose is to guarantee that the effectiveness of efforts to educate such children is assessed and assured.

One of the handicapping conditions listed in Section 602 of the Education of the Handicapped Act, as amended by Public Law 94–142, is the term "specific learning disabilities." The regulations state that evaluation of such children will include a medical examination whenever it is sus-

267

pected that the child has a physical problem relevant to his ability to be educated. The intent of this provision appears to be that an *appropriate* medical examination is required when a child is suspected of having a neurologic impairment that possibly affects his ability to learn. It is therefore important for every physician who treats children to be aware of his responsibilities in this regard. In fact, the regulations state that if questions occur concerning a youngster with a physical problem and associated educational problems, the child shall be referred to an appropriate medical examiner who will determine the type and extent of any medical examination to be performed. When used for support of the determination of the handicap, the relevant medical findings and their relationship to the child's academic functioning shall be stated in writing.

At present, the term *specific learning disability* seems to cover at least four groups of children: (1) Those children with evidence of neurologic impairment, even though the impairment is minor. The history will usually reveal prenatal toxicity or the possibility of birth trauma, anoxia, encephalitis, head injury, and so forth. (2) Those children with exogenous problems such as severe environmental, social, or emotional difficulties that interfere with learning. Children whose learning problems are secondary to such psychosocial problems actually demonstrate learning *inhibition* rather than learning disability. (3) Those children with what may be termed a neurophysiologic developmental or maturational lag, which may be accompanied by other signs of immaturity, by "soft" neurologic signs, and by peculiar configurations of psychologic test findings. Such a lag does not imply that a child will catch up if left to himself and to nature. The lag may continue as a permanent feature of the child's functioning. Such a deviation or "unripeness" will necessitate special help in the early preschool years to assist the child in acquiring preacademic skills and, later, the basic skills of reading, writing, and arithmetic. (Ideally, all children in the primary grades should be allowed adequate instruction time plus flexible teaching using multisensorial educational techniques.) (4) Those children with specific developmental dyslexia, which is most often familial and very specific in nature. The primary disability in these youngsters is the inability to associate sounds with their graphic symbols. MacDonald Critchley refers to this as a type of asymbolia.[5]

That a developmental or maturational lag may have a hereditary anlage or predisposition is quite possible. That minimal insult to the brain during the prenatal or neonatal period might complicate or even create such developmental problems is equally possible. Such questions, however, are still academic. Regardless of why or how a child got where he is (or is not) in the education process, the teacher must work with him at his level and at his pace and must use specific techniques to which the child can respond via the sensory modality through which he learns best. A thorough multidisciplinary evaluation of the child is required to assist the educators in their work.

Because the clues indicating a learning disability must be sought in the complex setting of a child's behavioral reactions, emotional response, and intellectual development, it is necessary to systematize the approach to diagnosis. The clues must be sought in four different areas:

1. Activity level and attention span.
2. Movement and perceptual development.
3. Language and thought development.
4. Emotional and social development.

As these areas are described to him, the family physician will recognize that in most instances a conclusive diagnosis can only be reached after careful consideration of information about the child from the parents, teachers, and other specialists trained to evaluate the learning process. However, by recognizing that such a problem might exist, the family physician can perform the vital function of ensuring that a complete and adequate study of the child takes place.

HOW TO RECOGNIZE THE LEARNING-DISABLED CHILD

No learning-disabled child is exactly like another. There is no specific symptom—rather, these occur in clusters and vary from child to child. One child has a difficult time reading because he cannot perceive the differences between letters, another cannot subtract because the concept of one figure's being less than another cannot be grasped, and yet another child cannot concentrate on the task at hand. The importance of any particular disability can change as the child proceeds through school. Muscular control may improve as a child grows older, so that inability to handle play scissors in kindergarten may not interfere with learning how to write in second grade. On the other hand, a bright preschooler who is unable to discriminate sounds and the rhythm of language may have problems learning to read when he begins school.

Learning disability is not related to level of intelligence. A learning disability may be masked in the especially bright child because he learns to compensate for this. The learning disability, however, will prevent the child from reaching his full potential. The presence of physical problems must be kept in mind. An obviously bright 8 year old who reads poorly may need to have his sight tested. For example, a child was found to have double vision at normal reading distance. When he first tried to read, the youngster believed that everyone saw as he did. Consequently, he said nothing until an astute teacher recognized the difficulty and referred the parents to an ophthalmologist. Exercises corrected the problem, and the child graduated with an "A" average.

ACTIVITY AND ATTENTION SPAN

Many learning-disabled children, but not all, are hyperactive. From birth, they are charged-up, restless, and fidgety. They thrash about, scream, stiffen, and are hard to hold and cannot be comforted by family members, who become discouraged, irritated, and baffled by their behavior. They also may have trouble sleeping. When older, such children will move restlessly about the house, grasping at everything within reach and clumsily upsetting things. Their jagged, spasmodic movements carry over into their thoughts and speech. Such youngsters blurt out embarrassments (for example, exposing personal or family matters before visitors) without inhibition and are apparently unable to learn socially acceptable behavior.

Many learning-disabled children have normal behavior, and some may even be hypoactive. The latter group have little energy and drive, and their slowed movements are matched by their slowed thinking. Such children show little curiosity or eagerness. They appear impassive, stoical, and difficult to rouse. They may also appear even-tempered. These youngsters seem to have little motivation to learn or seem to have a short attention span, not because of distractions but because their attention is difficult to gain in the first place. They tend to be dependent and consequently appear immature. They are rejected by their agemates and subsequently become shy and withdrawn. Although such children may look and act mentally retarded, they are not.

It is important for the physician to remember that the term *hyperactive* refers not to a disease but to a description, with specific inference relative to the person who uses the term. Because of the tremendous amount of literature available to the general public concerning "hyperactivity" in relation to drug management, diet, allergy, and so forth, the term is used indiscriminately in reference to almost any child with highly intense temperamental attributes. The physician must take a very careful history whenever the chief complaint is "hyperactivity" in order to determine whether this is actually the case. Very often, we find that a child may be hyper-*reactive* to stress situations in school or to inappropriate management at home. If the problem is one of hyperreactivity, treatment would necessarily involve modification of the child's environment at home and at school. If, however, the hyperactivity is due to an extremely short attention span, distractibility, and impulsive behavior in a youngster with no inner controls and if this behavior has been noted since infancy, medical management will be indicated.

MOVEMENT AND PERCEPTUAL DEVELOPMENT[4, 6, 7, 9, 17]

The child with a learning disability may be clumsy. This results from inability to coordinate his large muscles, making it difficult for him to maintain balance and causing him to crash about the house or fall easily at play. He may have fine motor incoordination. In particular, poor control of the small muscles of his hands may cause problems with eating, buttoning clothes, and writing.

Poorly controlled movement may be associated with disordered visual perception. Visual acuity may be normal. The perceptual difficulty is caused by inability to interpret what is seen, and this can result in major behavioral and learning problems.

The growing child's organization of his physical environment is based on the vantage point of his own being, whether objects are far from him or near, larger than he or smaller. Inability to sort out these visual impressions can create an environment of confusion and insecurity for the learning-disabled child. He misses objects that he tries to grasp, he cannot make accurate estimates of space and time, and he finds that crossing a road is filled with fear and danger. He does not learn that as objects move and therefore diminish or increase in size, their spatial relationship to him changes. There may be confusion about direction—up and down, right and left, front and back. These children can easily get lost. They also cannot tie objects into a unified whole; their possessions may be scattered in complete disarray. They often demonstrate persistent reversals, erroneous sequencing, or both of letters and words when reading, spelling, or writing.

Some children may have a visual–motor mismatch. In trying to copy letters or shapes, they are unable to guide finger movements accurately, according to what they see, and so writing and drawing are impaired. Such children are said to have eye–hand incoordination or graphomotor problems.

A great deal of learning is dependent upon early sensory–motor integration. The child learns first through his own movements and manipulations, all of which then become associated with the sensory information that he receives and perceives. This sensory–motor coordination occurs primarily in the child's first two or three years of life, but later academic learning is dependent upon the development and integration of these skills. Incoordination, especially fine motor incoordination, and perceptual immaturity can be major obstacles to a 6 year old child trying to learn how to read, write, and cipher. The physician must look for these areas of difficulty during the child's preschool years and must

help the family find appropriate assistance through enrollment in good preschool programs.

LANGUAGE AND THOUGHT DEVELOPMENT[2, 5, 13, 14, 20]

Language and thought processes combine and develop together in the normal child, allowing ideas and concepts to mature and permitting thought-sharing with others to develop through speaking and writing.

Some learning-disabled children cannot organize the sensory impressions on which their language and thought development depends. Such children easily confuse similar-sounding words. They must concentrate intensely if they are to pick up sounds when there is much background noise. These youngsters easily miss the point of what is said, become confused and bewildered, and must strain continuously to understand what is going on about them. Auditory acuity is usually normal, but such children have an auditory perceptual problem. To complicate matters, this impairment may also be combined with a hearing loss.

Speech and language may fail to develop normally when there is an auditory perceptual handicap, since what is said is related to what is heard. In some instances, perception may be normal but speech may be impaired by articulatory dyspraxia (the inability to coordinate the complex movements of lips, tongue, and jaw) or the child cannot remember the precise movements necessary to produce the words he wants.

In some cases, words cannot be thought of as rapidly as the associated ideas normally produce them—the "on the tip of my tongue" syndrome. The more abstract the thought, the greater the difficulty. Such a word-finding problem can prevent development of thought patterns and concepts, thus producing intellectual impoverishment. If a child cannot understand language, he cannot store, categorize, and classify information or draw conclusions that allow him to understand problems and issues. His decision-making ability and judgment are poor.

It is particularly important for the physician to note that delay in acquisition and use of language is often the first indication that a child may later have a learning disability. Any youngster who is not speaking by the age of 3 years or who demonstrates moderate-to-severe articulation problems persistently between the ages of 3 and 6 years should receive a thorough speech, language, and hearing evaluation, and the necessary remediation should be provided as soon as indicated. When these problems are understood and recognized, they can readily be treated by language therapy. Thus, great barriers to human development can be overcome.

Dyslexia[5, 9]

Dyslexia is a specific language disability characterized by disorders in the ability to read, write, and spell. It can occur in isolation or in combination with other learning disabilities.

The child with dyslexia in its "pure" form has no behavior problems, has good attention span, and is physically well-coordinated, even to the extent of becoming an outstanding athlete. He simply cannot associate sounds with graphic symbols and cannot learn the written code for spoken language.

The cause of the condition is unknown. However, it is usually found in boys, is usually hereditary, and may skip generations. Normally, a child learns to translate words heard and words seen rapidly and efficiently. However, the dyslexic youngsters can learn to associate sounds and symbols only with long, intensive tutoring. Such a child can be taught to read adequately but rarely will become a good speller. Yet many bright dyslexic youngsters are superior in mathematics and science, often becoming engineers, surgeons, mathematicians, and so on. Though most benefit from special teaching, it is difficult to predict to what extent a specific child will improve. Much depends on the child's native intelligence and on the provision of family support, early diagnosis, and appropriate teaching.

EMOTIONAL AND SOCIAL DEVELOPMENT[3, 4, 16, 22]

It is not surprising that many learning-disabled children develop emotional disturbances secondary to their handicap. Through preschool and school years, such children are exposed to uncertainties and humiliations, their inadequacies exposed for all to see. They fail to develop self-esteem, a sense of values, or a strengthening of conscience. Things usually go from bad to worse. If they are hyperactive and at the mercy of their impulses, they are soon in conflict with family and school, and their behavior problems may surface sooner than this learning disability. Learning disability in children without a behavior problem may go unnoticed for years, until it is too late to help them.

The unjust pressures and threats of the home and school environment can crush learning-disabled youngsters. Their sense of unfitness mounts as they grow older, and their ego is gradually demolished. Their agemates regard them as "dumb" and socially immature. Learning-disabled youngsters therefore seek out younger children and, feeling safer, may regress to infantile behavior. Such youngsters can become withdrawn or develop a perverse gratification from the upset they cause parents and teachers by their inept behavior and poor achievement.

Normal children learn many things about their environment without being taught. They absorb the signals around them, interpret and understand these signals, and act accordingly. Learning disability prevents the development of "common sense," because in spite of such children's intelligence, their learning depends on clear and explicit messages that may not be apparent in the vast sea of stimuli in their normal environment. As these children recognize easily only the most familiar things, they become confused and even terrified by any change in routine. They may become fixated on one thing, saying the same words over and over or playing interminably with the same object, as if they have at least found gratification in something they clearly understand. If hyperactive, these children cannot delay reacting to impulses and cannot tolerate being denied. Their impatience can destroy relationships with other children and within their family.

Learning-disabled children with emotional disturbances can only be helped through painstaking evaluation by their parents, family physician, teachers, psychologist, and others. First, it must be recognized that a problem does exist, and this is usually initially realized by the child's mother.

THE ROLE OF THE PHYSICIAN

Physicians are approached increasingly by parents and teachers because of child behavior problems at home and at school. The informed family physician is in an ideal position to play a key role. His primary responsibility is to detect any disease or physical handicap that might be present, to refer the child for further evaluation when indicated, and, subsequently, to coordinate and interpret all evaluations for parents and teachers. He should treat the child for any medical conditions present, re-evaluate the youngster on a planned basis, and always be available to counsel the parents or teachers.

PARENT INTERVIEWS AND COUNSELING

Both parents should be interviewed, and their individual attitudes to the child and to each other should be assessed. Since learning disability may be inherited, a history of academic achievement in both parents' families should be obtained. A prenatal and birth history is required to identify possible etiologic factors such as brain damage at birth, maternal bleeding during pregnancy, difficult or prolonged labor, overmedication of the mother, or precipitate delivery. Did the infant breathe and cry normally at birth? Was there jaundice, exchange blood transfusions, prematurity, or infant irritability requiring sedation? Did the baby feed normally? Did he vomit excessively? Maternal reproductive history is important. A birth preceded by prolonged infertility or multiple abortions is more likely to produce a neurologically damaged child. A history of the child's having convulsions, measles with encephalitis, severe dehydration, head injury, or ill-defined chronic illness may be significant in pointing to a neurologic basis for a learning behavior problem.

The mother will give a good assessment of the child's temperament. If the youngster is hyperactive, when was this first noticed? How old was he when he passed the developmental milestones—when did he first sit, creep, walk, ride a tricycle, a bicy-cle? When did he first say words, phrases, and sentences, and was he understandable? A delay in reaching these milestones may be significant, as may be a history of clumsiness (difficulty tying shoelaces and buttoning clothing). How does he behave at nursery school or kindergarten? How is he progressing at school with reading, writing, and arithmetic, and what are his relationships with his agemates?

EXAMINATION OF THE CHILD[3, 4]

Examination of the child begins with general observation, noting the degree of restiveness or, if a school-aged child, the ability to undress and dress. A complete neurologic examination is necessary. Limb reflexes and coordinated large and small muscle movement should be observed, eye reflexes and coordinated movements tested, and auditory acuity and discrimination noted. A 6 year old child should know his own left side from his right and should make few errors in writing letters in proper direction. He should be able to repeat numbers, polysyllabic words, and short sentences. A 6 year old youngster should be able to repeat five numbers in sequence and to remember his own telephone number. Commercially standardized series of paragraphs for oral reading and comprehension are available for each school grade, such as the standardized Oral Reading Paragraphs by Gray.[12]

In addition to physical and neurologic examinations, specific assessment, including paper and pencil tests, should be carried out, especially if the child is younger than 11 years of age. Several functional areas (balance, gross and fine motor coordination, motor speech, extraocular motility, stereognosis, and graphomotor skills) provide clues to potential learning difficulty having a neurologic basis. The Denver Developmental Test is an excellent screening device for the child less than 6 years of age. However, it must be kept in mind that ability to perform certain skills improves by age 7 or 8. Erroneous predictions are possible, unless there is an awareness of the maturational nature of the skills being evaluated. Immature performance persisting beyond age 7 is an excellent indicator of potential difficulty in school.

Following such an examination, testing, and history-taking, the family physician must decide if he should refer the child to an appropriate neurologist, psychologist, special educator, speech and language clinician, or other specialist or diagnostic and treatment unit. The diagnosis may be confirmed and the appropriate special educational process initiated. This process is monitored jointly by the family physician and the specialists concerned for that period of time required to produce maximal effect. An increasing number of special units dealing with the learning-disabled child are being established, and an up-to-date list of addresses and other information can be obtained from the Association of University Affiliated Facilities, Suite 908, 1100 17th Street N.W., Washington, D.C., 20036.

Having helped to initiate the therapeutic process, the physician is responsible for the continuing care of the child. He acts as a liaison between the various specialists involved and maintains and sustains the program, monitoring any medications needed and, above all, caring for the needs of the family as a whole, as periods of hope alternate with periods of doubt and frustration. Throughout this lengthy, complex process, the family physician must especially act as the advocate of the child. Though sensitive to the needs of the parents and others in the family, he must realize that the child with a learning disability has the greatest need for help and the most to lose from failure to obtain this.

THE FAMILY WITH A LEARNING-DISABLED CHILD

Once the child has begun his new educational program, the family physician's most important role is to increase support for the child in the family environment. Failure here can seriously diminish the benefit of the program or even negate it. Time must be taken to discuss problems at home with the mother, perhaps indicating a need for new child-raising techniques. The mother must overcome her self-guilt caused by her apparent failure to achieve the same results as she did with her other children. The affected child will absorb more than his share of time and energy, and the siblings should understand that they may have to do with less parental time.

Fathers sometimes minimize problems in these children and think that their wives are unduly nervous. However, the fathers are not exposed continuously to the child's aberrant behavior, which often improves when they return from work in the evening. Parents must cooperate and jointly accept responsibility for the youngster.

It is essential to emphasize to parents that the child imprisoned by a learning disability is healthy and possesses inherent intelligence. Maturing may be slower, and parents must overcome disappointment because of lack of academic achievement. Ways of dealing with tantrums and sulking must be found, and the child's life must be woven into the total family life. A pessimistic outlook is damaging, and parents often fail to notice the small improvements and advances so important to the child who needs encouragement and approval.

Objectivity and realism are difficult for parents to maintain. Techniques of daily living won't be easily picked up by the child. He must be taught. The extra help given should be gradually withdrawn as dependency diminishes and the child develops self-reliance and initiative. Discovery of areas of unimpaired ability and of latent talent allows parents to give encouragement and even provides new chances for success in life. The real remedial work goes on at home, where variety, repetition, and relevance are found in such mundane activities as cleaning, shopping, cooking, and gardening. These provide an ideal opportunity for the child to develop finger dexterity, visual and auditory perception, a sense of order, principles of logic, and language skills. Such activities also prepare the child to acquire the infinite variety of familiar skills forming the basis of normal daily living. Montessori's "exercises in practical life" give valuable hints about how to use the practical opportunities in the home for such learning.[19]

Parental irritation should be suppressed, as should the temptation to fight all the child's battles. Though kindness and sympathy are essential, firmness, consistency, and clarity will provide the child with boundaries to his life and with a greater sense of security that is essential for his growth. To enable the child to develop an understanding of logical consequences and of achievement and rewards, the handling of problems should be simple, direct, and immediate. Confusion in these matters further handicaps a child having difficulties understanding cause and effect. Physical punishment is rarely useful. When the child's behavior goes out of control and the parents have difficulty handling the situation, physical restraint may be necessary. If this is calmly done and sustained, the behavior may quickly return to normal. Disciplinary techniques should be discussed with the parents and suggestions given on how best to handle such situations. Consistency in discipline is necessary. Inconsistency will lead to inconsistent behavior. Good behavior should be recognized, praised, and at times rewarded with some special treat. This is not bribing but rather helping the child to distinguish between good and bad behavior. Empty threats or promises are quickly recognized by the child, who will continue his bad behavior until the parents' patience is finally exhausted.

Situations causing excessive stimulation should be recognized beforehand, and the child informed so that he can be better prepared and more in control of himself. Parties or visitors should be discussed in advance. Many learning-disabled children thus forewarned make the effort to control their behavior.

If possible, the child should have his own room, where he can relax away from the center of home activity. Mealtime, though a familiar routine, can be formidably complex and overstimulating to such a child and is the scene of many family uproars. Simplification of the routine is important. If behavior gets out of control, the child must be firmly removed from the dining area and taught that return depends on his establishing control. A clear explanation of what is meant by the behavior needed for return is necessary. The child should also be told that such removal is to allow him to regain composure.

He must learn to play with other children and to be prepared for the give and take of games. He must therefore learn to control his temper and to avoid overreacting to losing and winning, so that he can avoid the reputation of bad sportsmanship.

Many marital disagreements originate because of the problems created by a learning-disabled child. Parents must understand this and must develop the insights necessary to handle the situation. Counseling by the family physician can help the parents to relieve tensions and to increase the aid they can give the child.

The greatest gift the parents can give such a child is to provide him with a stable home life and with the feeling that he is a contributing and valued member of the family. In the long run, these lessons are more important than learning how to read, spell, and do sums and can only be acquired within the family. The role of the family physician in such situations is incalculable.

REFERENCES

1. Auckerman, R. C.: Approaches to Beginning Reading. New York, John Wiley & Sons, Inc., 1971.
2. Bangs, T. E.: Language and Learning Disorders of the Pre-Academic Child. New York, Appleton-Century-Crofts, 1968.
3. Brutten, M., Richardson, S. O., and Mangel, C.: Something's Wrong with My Child: A Parent's Book about Children with Learning Disabilities. New York, Harcourt Brace Jovanovich, Inc., 1973.
4. Clements, S. D.: Minimal Brain Dysfunctions in Children—Terminology and Identification. Co-sponsored by the Easter Seal Research Foundation of the National Society for Crippled Children and National Institute of Neurological Disease and Blindness. Washington, D.C., U.S. Dept. of Health, Education and Welfare, 1965.
5. Critchley, M.: Developmental Dyslexia. Springfield, Ill., Charles C Thomas, Publisher, 1964.
6. Crosby, R. M. N., and Liston, R. A.: The Waysiders. New York, Delacorte Press, 1968.
7. DeHirsh, K., DeHirsh, K., and Jansky, J.: Predicting Reading Failure. New York, Harper & Row, Publishers, 1966.
8. Drew, A. L.: Familial reading disability. Univ. Mich. Med. Bull. 21:245, 1955.
9. Duane, D. D., and Rawson, M. B. (eds.): Reading, Perception and Language. Baltimore, York Press, Inc., 1975.
10. Eisenson, J.: Developmental aphasia—a speculative view with therapeutic implications. J. Speech Hearing Dis., 33:3, 1968.
11. Federal Register: Education of Handicapped Children. Washington, D.C., Office of Education, U.S. Dept. of Health, Education and Welfare, Nov. 29, 1976.

12. Gray Oral Reading Paragraphs Test: Indianapolis, Bobbs-Merrill Co., Inc., 1955.
13. Ingram, T. T. S.: Delayed development of speech with special reference to dyslexia. Proc. Roy. Soc. Med., 56:199, 1963.
14. Keenan, J. S.: The nature of receptive and expressive impairments in aphasia. J. Speech Hearing Dis., 33:20, 1968.
15. Kirk, S. A., and McCarthy, J. M. (eds.): Learning Disabilities—Selected ACLD Papers. Boston, Houghton-Mifflin Co., 1975.
16. Lerner, J.: Children with Learning Disabilities. Boston, Houghton-Mifflin Co., 1971.
17. MacKeith, R., and Bax, M.: Minimal brain damage —a concept discarded. *In* Bax, M., and MacKeith, R. (eds.): Little Club Clinics in Developmental Medicine, No. 10, Minimal Cerebral Dysfunction. London, The National Spastics Society and Heinemann Medical Books, Ltd., 1963.
18. McCarthy, J. J., and McCarthy, J. F.: Learning Disabilities. Boston, Allyn & Bacon, Inc., 1970.
19. Montessori, M.: Doctor Montessori's Own Handbook. New York, Schocken Books, Inc., 1964.
20. Orton, S.: Reading, Writing, and Speech Problems in Children. New York, W. W. Norton & Co., Inc., 1937.
21. Richardson, S. O.: Learning disorders and the preschool child. New Jersey Ed. Assoc. Rev., *41*:6, 1968.
22. Solan, H. A. (ed.): The Psychology of Learning and Reading Difficulties. New York, Simon & Shuster, Inc., 1973.

Chapter 21

PERSONALITY DISORDERS

by J. G. SMALL,
and L. P. JOHNSON

INTRODUCTION

The definition of personality disorder in the most recent issue of *A Psychiatric Glossary*[12] provides a convenient point of departure for the discussion of this topic. Personality disorders are described therein as "a group of mental disorders characterized by deeply engrained maladaptive patterns of behavior, generally lifelong in duration and consequently often recognizable by the time of adolescence or earlier." As such, these disorders affect primarily the personality traits of the individual, and thus they are qualitatively different from neurosis and psychosis. The current psychiatric nomenclature in the second edition of the *Diagnostic and Statistical Manual of Mental Disorders*[9] includes descriptions of ten subtypes of personality disorder, each with typical aberrant behavior patterns. Historically, there have been classifications of pathologic personalities since antiquity, but the viewpoint that personality disorders should be regarded as medical and psychiatric problems is of relatively recent origin, beginning about the middle of the 19th century.[21] Since that time, there have been numerous definitions and classifications approaching the topic from various theoretic positions in attempts to distinguish normal variations in personality and social deviance from pathologic states.

NOSOLOGY

Workers in psychiatric research are well aware of the shortcomings of the diagnostic systems in clinical psychiatry, particularly in objective definitions of personality disturbances. As more potent and effective treatments have evolved in psychiatry, primarily in psychopharmacology, the need for precise definitions of clinical syndromes has become more and more important. Several research centers have painstakingly developed their own systems, deriving definitions from attributes in patients that could be observed reliably and that proved on follow-up studies to be stable over time and to appear more often in the first-degree relatives of the patients than in other groups. After more than a decade of painstaking research by the Washington University group, and others, an outline of the conditions that could be so defined was published in 1972 by Feighner and colleagues.[11] In that paper diagnostic criteria for 14 psychiatric illnesses were presented, and two of the personality disorders, hysteria and antisocial personality, were explicitly defined. Further work using this system of classification of psychiatric disorders revealed that most hospitalized psychiatric patients could be classified in terms of 1 of these 14 subgroups. Of those who could not (23 per cent in one series), most were still not classifiable on follow-up nearly 4 years later.[59] Approximately half were still experiencing psychiatric difficulties with manifestations that either did not meet full criteria for any single condition or fit into more than one diagnostic category. The remainder had no definable psychiatric illness on follow-up.

Since that time, more efforts have been exerted to subclassify and refine psychiatric diagnosis to identify homogeneous groups that are predictive of long-term outcome and response to various kinds of therapeutic intervention. Many of the advances in this field are to be incorporated in the third edition of the *Diagnostic and Statis-*

tical Manual of Mental Disorders (DSM-III), which is due to be published in 1978, coinciding with the appearance of the ninth edition of the *International Classification of Diseases.* In addition to the importance of these activities in medical practice, there are other implications in the revised description of mental disease states, including personality disorders, that will have an impact on health insurance claims and hospital admitting practices as well as on treatment planning. As of this writing, the final version of *DSM-III* is not yet available.

A draft version of the new classification contains a separate category for hysterical disorders that includes factitious psychosis and somatization disorder, or Briquet's syndrome (formerly hysteria), with several subcategories relating to various conversion symptoms.[54] The following types are included under personality disorders: paranoid, schizoid, compulsive, histrionic, antisocial, narcissistic, dependent, avoidant, impulsive, borderline, and mixed or other. The specific criteria and descriptions of these categories are not yet available. However, much of *DSM-III* is based upon the latest research on psychiatric diagnosis that is contained in continually updated versions of *Research Diagnostic Criteria (RDC)* issued by Spitzer, Endicott, and Robins and most recently revised in 1975.[53] This document provides definitions of personality disorders that offer potentially useful classifications, albeit tentative at present, since some of them have been recently evolved and have not yet stood the test of time. This system of nomenclature includes categories of cyclothymic, labile, and antisocial personality disorders and Briquet's disorder.

Cyclothymic Personality

Cyclothymic personality disorder is defined in an individual in whom the following characteristics have been present since early adulthood to a greater degree than in most people and have not been limited to discrete affective illnesses. The traits include recurrent periods of depression lasting at least a few days alternating with periods of clearly better-than-normal moods, with or without a normal mood intervening. Such episodes must have been present since early maturity and must be too numerous to count. In addition, the

person is usually not in a normal mood, and changes in mood are often unrelated to external events or circumstances.

Labile Personality

Another *RDC* category is labile personality. This applies to individuals who throughout most of their adult lives have abrupt shifts in mood, ranging from normal to one or more dysphoric states, such as depression, irritability, anger, anxiety, or a combination of these. Such moods usually last several hours to several days. The label should not be applied to anyone still in their 20's unless these traits have been present for at least 6 years. Other criteria required for the diagnosis are that at least three of the following traits have been present since early adulthood, are not limited to discrete episodes of illness, and are present to a noticeably greater degree than in most people: easily disappointed; self-pity, or feelings of being shortchanged; over-reactive to stressful situations; impulsivity, i.e., making quick decisions without reflection; low self-esteem; difficulty maintaining satisfactory intimate relationships, preoccupation with negative aspects of events or situations, or a combination of these. A third requirement for diagnosis is that at least one of the following is present: impairment in social functioning with family, home, school, or at work, taking medication; seeking or being referred for help by someone; or someone else has complained about some manifestations of the condition. An exclusion criterion is also specified in that the affective lability cannot be attributed to any of the other conditions described in the *RDC* classification of more than 25 explicit psychiatric disorders.

Briquet's Disorder

Under this system, hysteria has been renamed Briquet's disorder, thus avoiding some confusing and pejorative associations with the older term. This illness is defined as a chronic or recurrent polysymptomatic disorder beginning early in life with multiple somatic complaints not explained by known medical illnesses. (It is recognized that most people have unexplained aches and pains but most do not mention them—an essential feature of this disorder is that patients *do* mention such symptoms.) The presence of this syndrome does not rule out additional medical or psychiatric diagnoses (with some exceptions for the latter).

In order to be so classified, the patient must have a dramatic, vague, or complicated medical history with onset prior to age 25. For women, a minimum of at least one manifestation in at least five of six groups of symptoms is required for a definite diagnosis and one manifestation in at least four groups for a probable diagnosis. (Since one of the groups applies only to women, one group less is required for diagnosing men.) The examiner does not have to verify that the symptoms were actually present; the patient's report is sufficient if in the judgment of the physician the symptoms are not explained by some physical illness. Physical symptoms that occurred only during periods of other psychiatric or medical illnesses or that developed for the first time after the age of 40 are not to be considered for diagnosis. The specific criteria include the patient's belief of having lifelong illness; neurologic-like manifestations, including conversion reactions such as loss of sensation, aphonia, gait disturbances, or pseudoneurologic symptoms or dissociative phenomena such as amnesia or loss of consciousness; abdominal pain or vomiting spells; gynecologic complaints such as dysmenorrhea, irregular menses, or menorrhagia; and sexual indifference. Another group of symptoms lists pain in the back, joints, or extremities, headaches, or a combination of these.

Antisocial Personality

Antisocial personality is defined much as it was in the paper by Feighner and colleagues.[11] However, the requirements of symptoms in childhood and after age 16 are made more explicit in the *RDC* format. The childhood history should include three or more of the following: truancy, expulsion from school, delinquency, running away from home, persistent lying, unusually early or aggressive sexual behavior, early drinking, theft, vandalism, academic achievement below expected intellectual level, and chronic violations of rules at home or school. After age 16 there must be poor occupational performance over several years, as demonstrated by frequent job changes and significant unemployment and absenteeism. In addition, at least three or more of the following are required for definitive diagnosis: three or more serious arrests, two or more divorces or separations, physical fights, drinking to intoxication weekly or more often, financial irresponsibility, traveling from place to place without a prearranged job, and evidence of impaired capacity to sustain lasting close, warm, and responsible relationships with family, friends, or sexual partners.

Borderline Categories

Other specific categorizations of personality disorder are not included in the *RDC* nomenclature, although there is an applicable section on borderline features. Since there is no consensus in the literature of the definition of the borderline syndrome, the classification is not used as a primary diagnosis.[17] However, it can be added as a secondary diagnosis when a patient can be placed in another diagnostic group.

Borderline features include any one of the following, unless explainable by alcohol or drug abuse or in the context of schizophrenia: at least six different periods of dissociation, depersonalization, or derealization other than during anxiety attacks; odd, bizarre, or eccentric behavior or ideation not commonly seen in other mental disorders such as the neuroses or affective disorders; ideas of reference, extreme suspiciousness, paranoid ideas, or suspected delusions or hallucinations other than during an episode of major psychosis; extreme social isolation for the last 2 years not accounted for by depressed mood; persistent difficulty distinguishing fantasy from reality; recurrent self-damaging, impulsive behavior, e.g., self-mutilation, job quitting, suicidal behavior, or rage reactions not accounted for by the other specific diagnoses; or gross failure to function in any occupational role, including student or housekeeper, for at least a year not clearly due to any other diagnostic conditions. If patients first display diagnostic features of personality disorders and later develop illnesses satisfying criteria for depression, alcoholism, or drug abuse, these subsequent illnesses are listed as additional diagnoses. In the case of depression, the depression is classified as a secondary rather than a primary affective disorder.

Passive-Aggressive Personality

This outline provides a summary of the psychiatric nomenclature as it is evolving in making diagnoses of personality disorders more explicit. There are also other descriptions of personality disorders arising from clinical studies that do not warrant inclusion in the research nomenclature, since the necessary prospective controlled follow-up and family studies have not been done to delineate them from other disorders. Nevertheless, some of this information could be of practical value to the family physician in recognizing additional attributes of persons with disordered personalities. One study attempted to ascertain if passive-aggressive personality disorder could be distinguished from other formally defined psychiatric illnesses. Small and colleagues[49] followed a group of 100 hospitalized patients with this final diagnosis and re-examined them 7 to 15 years later. Independent raters classified the information in the patients' index hospital records in accordance with nosologic systems much like those of Feighner and colleagues.[11] From the initial review of the charts, it was clear that more than half of the patients could be assigned another psychiatric diagnosis, specifically, depression in 30 patients and alcoholism in 18. However, 52 patients did not fit into any other diagnostic category, although all had sufficient numbers of signs and symptoms to be classified as mentally ill. On follow-up, there were few changes in diagnosis or in symptomatology suggesting that the syndrome could be a valid diagnostic entity, although essential studies of prospectively identified patient cohort and control groups remain to be done.

Nevertheless, it seemed that this kind of patient could be described in terms of a disorder recognizable in adolescence and characterized by interpersonal strife, verbal aggressiveness, emotional storms, impulsivity, and manipulative behavior. It was hypothesized that this disorder in some ways occupied an intermediate position between the antisocial personality disorder on the one hand and manic-depressive disease on the other, resembling the antisocial personality in the frequent family history of alcoholism and disrupted social learning, patterns of disturbed interpersonal relationships, and repeated maladaptive behavior. However, these people, unlike the classic antisocial personality, had preservation of some appropriate interpersonal warmth and social interest, as well as episodic variations in mood. The follow-up study established that most patients did not change very much over time, although there were a few (nine in all) who were judged as being without psychiatric illness at the time of follow-up. Good outcome was associated with having received outpatient psychotherapy, although whether this was cause and effect or whether these patients were unusual in some other respect was not known.

Schizoid State

Schizoid state is another category listed among the personality disorders. Heston's studies[19] and Cadoret's review of the literature[4] suggest that the schizoid state is composed of mixed neurotic conditions and character disturbances, the latter of which may be more prominent in males than in females. This condition has variously been described as a temperament or characterologic state characterized by lifelong or chronic aberrant patterns, with shy, retiring, anergic behavior and paranoid and other eccentricities. Whether or not the schizoid state can ultimately be separated from schizophrenia and other disorders and placed into the new nomenclature remains to be determined.

The cyclothymic personality, which has already been discussed, has been shown in some series to predispose to a risk of manic-depressive illness. Whether or not there is also a depressive personality predisposing to episodes of depressive illness is less well established.[6] There have been other discussions of how the syndrome of childhood hyperkinesis may precede development of adult characterologic problems, a subject that will be considered in more detail under etiology and pathogenesis. Nevertheless, there have been several recent reports of adults displaying features similar to those of the hyperactive child, such as irritability, anxiety, emotional lability, impulsivity, and difficulties in concentrating and learning.[45] Whether these clinical features will eventually be thought of as a separate diagnostic entity among the personality disorders remains to be determined.

Episodic Behavior Disorders

Still another area is that of the relationships between personality disorders, epilepsy, and conditions in which there are episodic losses of behavioral control without sensorial clouding, which have been labeled by Monroe and others as episodic behavioral dyscontrol.[28] With regard to epilepsy, there have been conflicting findings. Most controlled studies have shown that there is no specific personality constellation accompanying these diseases, although it is recognized that persons with epilepsy are more prone to psychiatric difficulties than are individuals with other medical problems.[47, 51, 55] The reader is referred to an excellent description and historical perspective on this subject in the monograph by Guerrant and colleagues.[16]

The issue of the episodic dyscontrol syndrome is even more unclear, as the prospective controlled and follow-up studies have yet to be done. However, there are preliminary indications that individuals with this syndrome may benefit from the use of medications with anticonvulsant properties. This will be discussed further in the section on treatment. The use of the electroencephalogram (EEG) in identifying the conditions is also uncertain at the moment, as atypical methods of EEG activation have been employed in most studies. Nevertheless, Monroe's separation of episodic behavior disorders from more or less persistent personality disturbances is interesting and may identify some patients who may benefit from pharmacotherapy.

Thus far, it may appear that biologic psychiatry is becoming preoccupied with minutiae, perhaps in the process leaving the real world and the individual patient and his family far behind. A rebuttal to such a charge is simply that without a system of diagnosis that offers some precision in identifying homogeneous groups, only nonspecific or empirical treatment will be possible in psychiatry. This does not gainsay that there is not another side to the issue, namely the need to integrate behavioral science at its current level of understanding with clinical medicine, which is also important. This has been discussed recently by McWhinney.[27]

LABORATORY AND OTHER DIAGNOSTIC TESTS

Scientific studies in psychiatry must employ structured methods of evaluating mental status and obtaining historical information, insisting upon rigorous definitions of what should or should not be defined as a symptom in psychiatry. Another salient reason for this position is that, unlike almost all other fields of medicine, psychiatry obtains virtually no assistance from laboratory methods or physical examinations for diagnostic guidance. This is not to say that assistance in diagnosis and description from such areas has not been sought and is continuing to be explored. One of the most commonly used laboratory methods in attempting to diagnose personality disorders has been the utilization of psychologic tests. The Minnesota Multiphasic Personality Inventory (MMPI) has probably been most widely used, although differentiation of the syndromes defined by newer, more explicit criteria has yet to be accomplished by either projective or nonprojective methods.[48]

In other situations, neuropsychologic evaluations have been employed,[50] and there has been a recent suggestion that parietal lobe dysfunction, as demonstrated by tests of stereognosis, may underlie abnormal personality development and personality disorder.[20] Other tests have focused on evaluations of so-called neurologic soft signs, i.e., deviations in motor and sensory functions that can be observed reliably but that do not indicate a localized lesion of the central nervous system. Several systems of evaluating such signs have been developed recently, many in connection with studies of hyperactive children. In a recent study by Quitkin and colleagues,[30] such manifestations were found more in patients classified as schizophrenic with premorbid personality disorder and in those with emotionally unstable personalities (similar in many respects to the new classification of labile personality disorder) than in other kinds of psychiatric patients, raising the hypothesis that these illnesses may have an underlying organic basis.

Similar conjectures have been raised about the findings of EEG studies in patients with antisocial personality and other characterologic deficits.[23, 60] Although these findings have not been definitive, there has been a consistent excess of EEG abnormalities reported in these groups, which could relate to underlying central nervous system dysfunction, impairment, or, as some suggest, immaturity. As with psychologic tests, EEG studies have rarely been done in patients classified by *RDC* categories, although this approach seems promising in studies of other diagnostic groups.[52] Other physiologic studies have provided evidence that those with personality disorders share more in common with psychotic patients than with psychoneurotic patients or normals.[43]

Most recently, there has been a suggestion that cytogenetic studies may help to clarify the etiology of some of the personality disorders.[13] There have been reports of an excess of such disorders among individuals with Klinefelter's and Turner's syndromes.[2, 26] Much attention has been given to the association between the male with an XYY chromosomal anomaly and aggressive and criminal behavior.[61] Although this has received too much early publicity, there does appear to be an association between various chromosomal abnormalities and psychiatric problems, including personality disorder and lower intelligence. However, reported associations with aggressiveness are probably not at all characteristic of patients with chromosomal aberrations as a whole, although there are rare exceptions, such as the Lesch-Nyhan syndrome.

An innovative post hoc method of retrospectively identifying new syndromes by evaluating the response to drug treatment has been proposed by Klein and colleagues.[24] This has been a particularly useful approach in undiagnosable patients.[42] One such group of patients was so characterized clinically as hysterodysphoric, a descriptive label applied to individuals with shallow, quickly changing moods and frequent exhibitionistic, seductive, and manipulative behavior. This group was delineated when Klein found that such individuals responded favorably to monoamine oxidase inhibiting drugs, whereas individuals given imipramine often had no response or had worsening of symptoms, with increased somatic distress, racing thoughts, and excitement. It is possible that other subgroups may also be delineated in terms of their response to different pharmacologic agents.

INCIDENCE, ETIOLOGY, AND PATHOGENESIS

The incidence of personality disorders in the population is unknown. Some outpatient figures indicate that 15 per cent of male psychiatric patients and 3 per cent of female psychiatric patients are diagnosed as having antisocial personality disorders.[62] They present for treatment mainly because of associated problems with alcoholism and depression. However, the frequency of antisocial behavior, juvenile delinquency, and crime suggests that such problems are common in the general population, more so in low socioeconomic groups. The prevalence of Briquet's disorder, based on studies of postpartum populations, is between 1 and 2 per cent of the adult female population.[62] No figures are available for the other disorders of personality previously described.

Consideration of the etiology and pathogenesis of personality disorders at this period of our knowledge is at best conjectural. Some indications reviewed in previous paragraphs suggest that both central nervous system dysfunction and heredity may play some role. However, the separation of these factors from the contributions of the environment and family setting is an extremely complicated matter and in some ways detracts from the philosophy of family practice, in which the individual and his environment are viewed together. Nevertheless, such efforts must be made, because advancement of knowledge concerning the origin of personality disorders serves as a prelude to their possible treatment, amelioration, and prevention.

Prior to reviewing the evidence, however, one should be aware of the complex issues involved in the interpretation of social correlates of psychiatric disorders and the demands that an experiment must satisfy in order to separate causes from consequences, as discussed by Robins.[38] There have been many recent studies of patients and prisoners with antisocial personality disorders and Briquet's disorder, all of which agree that these disorders do run in families, with the former syndrome more characteristic of males and the latter of females.[8, 18] In addition, the female relatives of males with antisocial personalities are more apt to be depressed. Male relatives of hysterics tend to have antisocial personality disorders and alcoholism, and the females tend toward Briquet's disorder or depression. However, there is the problem of assortative mating between individuals with the two syndromes and the very frequent occurrence of overlapping clinical features, e.g., conversion symptoms. Such would be anticipated in light of Robins' 30 year follow-up of children with conduct disorders in which the childhood antecedents of both disorders were very similar.[36]

Most recently, there have been adoption studies of the offspring of parents with carefully diagnosed personality disorders that have yielded some interesting findings. Crowe[7] reported an investigation of 46 offspring of female offenders, most of whom were diagnosed as antisocial personalities. The infants were placed in adoptive homes and compared with adoptees known to have biologic mothers without such mental disorders. Enough time was allowed to elapse for all subjects to develop the diagnostic features of antisocial personality. There was a more definite increase in the rate of this disorder among the proband adoptees than among the controls. Nevertheless, important environmental factors were also identified, in that the development of antisocial personality was also related to the length of time spent in foster homes or other temporary placements until final adoption. The antisocial probands had spent an average of 14.2 months in orphanages or other places, whereas the nonantisocial probands had been placed for an average of 4 months. Interestingly, the control group, in which there was a low incidence of antisocial personality and other mental disorders, spent an average of a year in temporary settings before final placement.

Although this study is of great interest, there are alternate explanations of the data, particularly since the paternity of the adoptees was not known with certainty. However, it does suggest that inheritance is important and also that environment may play a role in the development or inhibition of antisocial personality disorder at critical time periods. In this regard, there are many other reports suggesting that there may be another critical time period in late adulthood in which the disorder somehow burns out or becomes less troublesome to the individual, to society, or both. Again, whether this is attributable to social consequences or is the longitudinal course of the illness in some individuals is yet to be determined.

Other recent studies evaluating the contribution of inheritance to the etiologies of personality disorder and alcoholism have focused upon the syndrome of minimal brain dysfunction.[5, 14, 29] There have been several reports of a greater incidence of psychiatric illnesses in the families of such children, especially alcoholism, sociopathy, and Briquet's disorder. The hyperactive child may later develop characteristics of these syndromes, while the hyperactivity and some other typical childhood features disappear. Recently, some individuals have been identified in whom the childhood constellation of symptoms persists into adulthood.[45] Alcoholism is also known to run in families, and adoption studies suggest that alcoholism, although not heavy drinking, may also be explained at least in part by heredity.[15, 41]

Another concept that has developed as an outgrowth of family studies is that the course and outcome of a given psychiatric illness, for example, primary depression, are different in patients with kinships in which there are histories of depression alone versus those with mixed familial pictures of alcoholism, personality disorders, and other conditions considered as "spectrum diseases."[33] Further studies of these issues may clarify some relationships between the major so-called functional psychoses and personality disturbances.

Although more definitive studies of personality disorder and particularly of the recently described syndromes have not been accomplished and will require a great deal of painstaking future effort, the evidence, circa 1976, is that these disorders are familial, are a product of inheritance and environment, have interactions between them, and probably include other factors as well. As such, the family physician should be aware that his management of families with one characterologically disturbed individual will probably lead to the identification of others. Moreover, it is very likely that many such people will come to the attention of the family physician for numerous reasons, for example, the presenting physical complaints in Briquet's disorder; the complications of alcohol and drug abuse, venereal disease, illegitimate pregnancies, and traumatic injuries in antisocial personalities; and the family turmoil, stress, and disruption caused by one, or more than one, socially deviant individual in the family. In addition, persons with aberrant personality structures are as prone as anyone else, if not more so, to develop physical problems and medical illnesses.

TREATMENT

General Issues

There are not many specific approaches known in the treatment of patients with personality disorders. However, there are some general principles. It has already been pointed out that such individuals will frequently come to the attention of the family physician, some for particular presenting complaints related to the type of personality disorder that is present and others for secondary complications or medical problems. Thus, the family physician should be alert to the possibility of an underlying personality disorder and acquainted with the criteria for diagnosis. Thereafter, if physical examination and appropriate laboratory tests fail to confirm the presence of other disorders, the family physician can do a great deal in sparing patients and their families the expense of unnecessary laboratory work and multiple surgical procedures, as in the case of Briquet's disorder. Likewise, the use of habit-forming or addicting drugs or agents that can be used in suicidal gestures are relatively contraindicated. Another general observation is that although such patients frequently seek out physicians, they are not known for maintaining a consistent program of management and treatment. Therefore, short-term, frequent therapeutic endeavors are likely to be more successful than long-range planning. On the other hand, there may be a few individuals with such disorders who can profit from long-term psychotherapy, and this should not be denied to those individuals who appear to be motivated. Faced with a clear diagnostic picture, the physician can offer supportive measures without making the situation worse.

Several recent articles have described various therapeutic approaches to individuals with Briquet's syndrome and other characterologic disorders. Group and psychologic methods of treatment appear to be as helpful as any and are without the complications of potentially toxic chemicals.[40, 42, 58] In general, psychotherapy with these individuals is relatively superficial, although it may vary in depth and intensity depending upon the strengths of the personality, environmental stability, and other factors. Often the focus of therapy is upon the therapist–patient relationship, within which the patient learns to accept limits upon his manipulative, antisocial, or other maladaptive behaviors. If a close therapeutic relationship can be achieved, some personal growth and social learning may occur over time. The family practitioner can manage such treatment if he has the desire, patience, time, and training in psychotherapy. Guidance from a psychiatric consultant will probably be needed in many cases, as such patients are notably resistant to change and frequently reach a therapeutic impasse.

The physician can be relatively secure in the sense that these disorders are fairly stable over time and patients do not tend to develop other psychiatric complications. However, such patients can and do develop significant medical problems, so that the physician must be alert for any changes in the nature or severity of complaints, particularly when these occur in situations that are unlikely to be stressful enough to account for exacerbations.[63] Awareness of the familial nature of these disorders and the possible link with the hyperkinetic child syndrome might also warrant attention to early case finding among the children of such individuals, particularly when both parents are afflicted. Early intervention before repeated disappointments, truancy and failure in school, and social maladjustment have occurred may improve the prognosis of this condition.[37] When adoption is to follow illegitimate pregnancies in such patients, the physician should exert his influence wherever possible to assure early adoptive placement.

Drug Therapy

Many patients with behavioral disorders will present with symptoms of anxiety and depression. In general, it can be said that such patients do not respond as favorably to drug therapy as do patients with other psychiatric illnesses.[42] Poor premorbid adjustment or personality disorder is predictive of poor outcome of drug treatment, with inadequate response, increased incidence of side effects, and drug abuse, including overdosing. Depressed patients with premorbid personality disorders may do as well on placebos as on tricyclic antidepressants or antipsychotic drugs.[31] There is some recent evidence that atypical depression with mixed features of anxiety and personality disturbances may respond better to the monoamine oxidase inhibiting group of drugs than to tricyclic antidepressants.[32, 57] However, choice of such medications must be made in light of the knowledge that they are potentially toxic and may have dangerous interactions with other drugs, food, and alcohol. Also, individuals with a fast acetylator phenotype may metabolize these drugs too rapidly for them to be effective.[22] Because of these complexities, severely depressed patients should probably be referred to a psychiatrist who may elect to avoid drugs and use psychologic methods, electroconvulsive treatment, or both. Similar comments apply to the drug treatment of schizoid personality disorders. Treatment with major tranquilizing drugs is associated with poor response and increased difficulties with side effects, as Klein and others have shown.[25] An exception may be the labile personality, which comprises many of the features described in an earlier nomenclature as emotionally unstable character disorder. Therapeutic studies have shown that such patients respond favorably to chlorpromazine or to lithium carbonate, with considerable amelioration of the rapid shifts in mood.[34, 35]

Lithium is the treatment of choice for the mood swings of the cyclothymic. Lithium has also been proposed for the treatment of aggressiveness in felons and other subjects who would likely be classified as having antisocial personality disorders.[44, 56] However, most of the studies have been conducted over relatively short periods of time. In our experience, lithium does seem to exert favorable short-range effects in the expression of aggressiveness and control of emotionality and impulsiveness in patients with personality disorders, including Briquet's disorder and passive-aggressive subtypes. However, patients in the antisocial personality disorder category rarely comply with long-term drug treatment. An exception to this generalization has been in patients with coexisting epilepsy. Apparently, regular taking of medication is better sustained in these individuals and prolonged improvement has been noted in several cases.

Because of dangers of toxicity, a psychiatrist probably should be involved in the institution of lithium treatment until optimal dosages and plasma levels are established. Thereafter, the family physician may wish to continue the maintenance phase of lithium treatment provided there are facilities for monitoring plasma lithium values as well as for administering renal and thyroid function tests. Another observation is that the minor tranquilizers, with the possible exception of oxazepam, may intensify expression of hostility and aggression.[39]

Partly because of the possible connection with the hyperactive child syndrome, the use of stimulants has been proposed and studied in persons with personality disorders and aggressive behavior. Individuals who continue to have hyperactive symptoms as adults have been reported to respond favorably to stimulant drugs or to imipramine.[45] In other kinds of patients, aggressiveness may be ameliorated by stimulants in some instances and aggravated in others.[1] Interestingly, lithium is known to block the euphoriant effects of amphetamines.[3] In any case, both amphetamines and monoamine oxidase inhibiting drugs should be prescribed with great caution in such individuals because of their known propensities for drug abuse and misuse. Tolerance to either type of drug may also develop.[46]

Other pharmacologic considerations arise in the so-called episodic dyscontrol syndrome, particularly if there are paroxysmal EEG abnormalities. There is some evidence to suggest that a trial of anticonvulsant therapy may be worthwhile. Phenytoin, primidone, and the benzodiazepines have been reported to be of value. In addition, lithium carbonate exerts anticonvulsant effects[10], and might serve a dual purpose in such individuals, with its ameliorating effects upon mood, impulse control, and aggressivity.

Hospitalization

Ordinarily, one does not think of hospitalizing patients who are suffering from a personality disorder. Hospitalization is presumably reserved for the frankly psychotic individual or the dangerously homicidal or suicidal person. Yet, a glance at any inpatient psychiatric service will reveal a large proportion of personality disorders, the more so if the service is in a community hospital rather than a traditional state hospital. Of the personality disorders, those most likely to require hospitalization are the passive-aggressive, antisocial, explosive, and hysterical personalities. It is within these groups that suicidal or homicidal behavior most commonly occurs. Psychotic decompensation may lead to hospitalization of those with paranoid, cyclothymic, or schizoid personality as well as those with hysterical personality. Patients with obsessive-compulsive, asthenic, and inadequate personalities generally do not decompensate or develop behavioral symptoms requiring institutionalization.

Severe depression or agitation, a state of panic, and the threat of, or actual loss of, control over destructive impulses may serve as the symptoms that lead to hospitalization. These may exist in conjunction with progressive deterioration in functioning or a home situation that has become intolerable, serving to aggravate the existing pathology. Occasionally, hospitalization is sought by the patient as a way out of an ego threatening, insoluble conflict. Consciously or unconsciously, he may bring about a crisis that makes hospitalization necessary. The exact nature of the collapse will depend on the particular personality organization and the nature and severity of the stresses. Because of the qualities peculiar to the paranoid defense mechanisms, the paranoid personality is unlikely to decompensate under minor stresses and requires overwhelming sustained pressures to do so. When decompensation does occur, it is likely to move in the direction of a paranoid psychosis, as misinterpretation of reality increases to a frankly delusional point and leads to correspondingly inappropriate behavior.

A similar outcome is apt to affect the schizoid individual subjected to great stress. Withdrawal has become his defense against the world, which he has experienced as cold, ungiving, and frightening. As he digs himself a deeper and deeper hole, a point of isolation is reached that is no longer compatible with living and working in society. Extreme isolation and even catatonic behavior may be the ultimate result.

Depression of varying degrees with the ever-present possibility of suicide is the danger with cyclothymics in particular. It may also occur in hysterical, explosive, and passive-aggressive types. Obviously, depression must reach serious proportions before hospitalization must be considered, but a suicide attempt often occurs before depression attains severe psychotic levels. Such an attempt may be interpreted as the last cry for help made necessary by unresponsive parents and family and, as such, may be an adaptive maneuver, possibly unconsciously determined.

These factors constitute the major developments that may lead to hospitalization of the personality disordered patient. There are many other reasons that may bring a patient with a personality disorder to the admitting office of the psychiatric unit. The following list attempts to outline the more important considerations that make a referral appropriate or not appropriate for admission.

A. Appropriate
  1. Severe depression, with or without suicidal ideation
  2. Suicide attempt (as opposed to gesture)
  3. Decompensation, leading to serious impairment of functioning or actual psychoses
  4. Intoxication with alcohol or drugs leading to a psychotic-like state
  5. Acute situational or gross stress reactions leading to bizarre actions
  6. Episodic dyscontrol ending in rage or destructive behavior
  7. Assaultiveness, particularly if serious or unexplained
  8. Borderline personality with behavior changes indicative of deterioration—the confusing diagnostic problem
B. Inappropriate
  1. Misinterpretation of patient's behavior by others, that is, family or parents over-reacting to a suicidal gesture
  2. Transient alterations of consciousness, such as intoxication, e.g., the

drunken person who is not otherwise in need of hospitalization

3. Malingering, often by patients who want to get off the street or may be seeking to hide from the law

4. Dumping by relatives — some use hospitalization as a form of punishment, others need a respite from a difficult child who really does not require hospitalization

5. Dumping by other institutions or agencies — an age-old practice that usually occurs with difficult disposition problems and may involve misrepresentation of the facts of the case.

SUMMARY

The state of the art at present is such that the family physician needs to be aware of the different constellations of disordered personalities and the criteria by which they are recognized. After diagnostic work-up, including indicated physical and laboratory examinations, management of such individuals should be conservative, with the expectation of long-term, irregular contacts with the patient and most likely with other disturbed family members as well. More than the usual difficulties in treating their physical and emotional problems can be anticipated. Some of these individuals will present with a myriad of symptoms and demand exhaustive medical attention and surgical treatment, but this can ordinarily be avoided if the diagnosis is recognized and supportive treatment is firmly instituted.

Drug therapy has limited application for the relief of symptoms of personality disorders because of inadequate therapeutic response, toxic effects, erratic compliance, and risk of abuse. However, some exceptions to this generalization have recently been recognized. It is possible that early case finding and preventive treatment may be useful in high risk groups, such as the children of these patients. Extrapolating from findings of relationships between stress, life events, and physical and mental diseases indicates that environmental shaping to minimize the impact of stress situations might be protective in these vulnerable individuals. Continued search for clinical and laboratory methods to identify diagnostic subgroups and to provide guidelines for treatment should be pursued. The individual and family distress, social disruption, and financial burden imposed by persons with these disorders and their prevalence in the community should encourage a high priority for conducting these investigations.

REFERENCES

1. Allen, R. P., Safer, D., and Covi, L.: Effects of psychostimulants on aggression. J. Nerv. Ment. Dis., 160:138, 1975.
2. Barker, T. E., and Black, F. W.: Klinefelter syndrome in a military population. Arch. Gen. Psychiatry, 33:607, 1976.
3. Beckmann, H., van Kammen, D. P., Goodwin, F. K., et al.: Urinary excretion of 3-methoxy-4-hydroxyphenylglycol in depressed patients: Modifications of amphetamine and lithium. Biol. Psychiatry, 11:377, 1976.
4. Cadoret, R. J.: Toward a definition of the schizoid state: Evidence from studies of twins and their families. Brit. J. Psychiatry, 122:679, 1973.
5. Cantwell, D. P.: Psychiatric illness in the families of hyperactive children. Arch. Gen. Psychiatry, 27:414, 1972.
6. Chodoff, P.: The depressive personality: A critical review. Int. J. Psychiatry, 11:196, 1973.
7. Crowe, R. R.: An adoption study of antisocial personality. Arch. Gen. Psychiatry, 31:785, 1974.
8. Crowe, R. R.: Adoption studies in psychiatry. Biol. Psychiatry, 10:353, 1975.
9. Diagnostic and Statistical Manual of Mental Disorders, DSM-II. 2nd ed., Washington, D.C., American Psychiatric Assoc., 1968.
10. Erwin, C. W., Gerber, C. J., Morrison, S. D., et al.: Lithium carbonate and convulsive disorders. Arch. Gen. Psychiatry, 28:646, 1973.
11. Feighner, J. P., Robins, E., Guze, S. B., et al.: Diagnostic criteria for use in psychiatric research. Arch. Gen. Psychiatry, 26:57, 1972.
12. Frazier, S. H., Campbell, R. J., Marshall, M. H., et al.: A Psychiatric Glossary. Washington, D.C., American Psychiatric Assoc., 1975.
13. Gerald, P. S.: Current concepts in genetics. N. Engl. J. Med., 294:706, 1976.
14. Goodwin, D. W., Schulsinger, F., Hermansen, L., et al.: Alcoholism and the hyperactive child syndrome. J. Nerv. Ment. Dis., 160:349, 1975.
15. Goodwin, D. W.: Adoption studies of alcoholism. J. Operational Psychiatry, 7:54, 1976.
16. Guerrant, J., Anderson, W. W., Fischer, A., et al.: Personality in Epilepsy. Springfield, Ill., Charles C Thomas, 1962.
17. Guze, S. B.: Differential diagnosis of the borderline personality syndrome. In Mack, J. E. (ed.): Borderline States in Psychiatry. New York, Grune & Stratton, 1975.
18. Guze, S. B.: Criminality and Psychiatric Disorders. New York, Oxford University Press, 1976.
19. Heston, L. L.: The genetics of schizophrenic and schizoid disease. Science, 167:249, 1970.
20. Horton, P. C.: Personality disorder and parietal lobe dysfunction. Am. J. Psychiatry, 133:782, 1976.

21. Jablensky, A.: Personality disorders and their relationship to illness and social deviance. Psychiatr. Ann., 6:375, 1976.
22. Johnstone, E. C.: Relationship between acetylator status and response to phenelzine. *In* Mendlewicz, J. (ed.): Problems of Pharmacopsychiatry. Vol. 10, Brussels, S. Karger, 1975.
23. Kiloh, L. G., McComas, A. J., and Osselton, J. W.: Clinical Electroencephalography. 3rd ed., New York, Appleton-Century-Crofts, 1972.
24. Klein, D. F.: Drug therapy as a means of syndromal identification and nosological revision. *In* Cole, J. O. (ed.): Psychopathology and psychopharmacology. Baltimore, Johns Hopkins University Press, 1973.
25. Klein, D. F., and Rosen, B.: Premorbid asocial adjustment and response to phenothiazine treatment among schizophrenic inpatients. Arch. Gen. Psychiatry, 29:480, 1973.
26. Kolb, J. E., and Heaton, R. K.: Lateralized neurologic deficits and psychopathology in a Turner syndrome patient. Arch. Gen. Psychiatry, 32:1198, 1975.
27. McWhinney, I. R.: Beyond diagnosis—An approach to the integration of behavioral science and clinical medicine. N. Engl. J. Med., 287:384, 1972.
28. Monroe, R. R.: Anticonvulsants in the treatment of aggression. J. Nerv. Ment. Dis., 160:119, 1975.
29. Omenn, G. S.: Genetic issues in the syndrome of minimal brain dysfunction. Semin. Psychiatry, 5:5, 1973.
30. Quitkin, F., Rifkin, A., and Klein, D. F.: Neurologic soft signs in schizophrenia and character disorders. Arch. Gen. Psychiatry, 33:845, 1976.
31. Raskin, A., and Crook, T. H.: The endogenous-neurotic distinction as a predictor of response to antidepressant drugs. Psychol. Med., 6:59, 1976.
32. Ravaris, C. L., Nies, A., Robinson, D. S., et al.: A multiple-dose controlled study of phenelzine in depression-anxiety states. Arch. Gen. Psychiatry, 33:347, 1976.
33. Reich, W.: The spectrum concept of schizophrenia. Arch. Gen. Psychiatry, 32:489, 1975.
34. Rifkin, A., Quitkin, F., Carrillo, C., et al.: Lithium carbonate in emotionally unstable character disorder. Arch. Gen. Psychiatry, 27:519, 1972.
35. Rifkin, A., Levitan, S. J., Galewski, J., et al.: Emotionally unstable character disorder: a follow-up study: I. Description of patients and outcome. Biol. Psychiatry, 4:65, 1972.
36. Robins, L. N.: Deviant Children Grown Up. Baltimore, The Williams & Wilkins Co., 1966.
37. Robins, L. N.: Antecedents of character disorder. *In* Roff, M., and Ricks, D. (eds.): Life History Research in Psychopathology. Minneapolis, University of Minnesota Press, 1970.
38. Robins, L. N.: Social correlates of psychiatric disorders: Can we tell causes from consequences? J. Health Soc. Behav., 10:95, 1969.
39. Salzman, C., Kochansky, G. E., Shader, R. I., et al.: Is oxazepam associated with hostility? Dis. Nerv. Syst., 36:30, 1975.
40. Scallet, A., Cloninger, C. R., and Othmer, E.: The management of chronic hysteria: A review and double-blind trial of electrosleep and other relaxation methods. Dis. Nerv. Syst., 37:347, 1976.
41. Schulsinger, F., Moller, N., Hermansen, L., et al.: Drinking problems in adopted and nonadopted sons of alcoholics. Arch. Gen. Psychiatry, 31:164, 1974.
42. Shader, R. I.: Manual of Psychiatric Therapeutics. Boston, Little, Brown & Co., 1975.
43. Shagass, C., and Schwartz, M.: Observations on somatosensory cortical reactivity in personality disorders. J. Nerv. Ment. Dis., 135:44, 1962.
44. Sheard, M. H.: Lithium in the treatment of aggression. J. Nerv. Ment. Dis., 160:108, 1975.
45. Shelley, E. M., and Reister, A.: Syndrome of minimal brain damage in young adults. Dis. Nerv. Syst., 33:335, 1972.
46. Shopsin, B., and Kline, N. S.: Monoamine oxidase inhibitors: Potential for drug abuse. Biol. Psychiatry, 11:451, 1976.
47. Slater, R., Beard, A. W., and Glithero, E.: The schizophrenia-like psychoses of epilepsy. Brit. J. Psychiatry, 109:95, 1963.
48. Slavney, P. R., and McHugh, P. R.: The hysterical personality. Arch. Gen. Psychiatry, 32:186, 1975.
49. Small, I. F., Small, J. G., Alig, V. B., et al.: Passive-aggressive personality disorder: A search for a syndrome. Amer. J. Psychiatry, 126:973, 1970.
50. Small, I. F., Small, J. G., Milstein, V., et al.: Neuropsychological observations with psychosis and somatic treatment. J. Nerv. Ment. Dis., 155:6, 1972.
51. Small, J. G., and Small, I. F.: A Controlled Study of Mental Disorders in Epilepsy. *In* Wortis, J. (ed.): Recent Advances in Biological Psychiatry. New York, Plenum Press, 1967.
52. Small, J. G., Small, I. F., Milstein, V., et al.: Familial associations with EEG variants in manic depressive disease. Arch. Gen. Psychiatry, 32:43, 1974.
53. Spitzer, R. L., Endicott, J., and Robins, E.: Research Diagnostic Criteria (RDC). Psychopharmacol. Bull., 11:22, 1975.
54. Spitzer, R., and Sheehy, M.: DSM III: A classification system in development. Psychiatr. Ann., 6:102, 1976.
55. Stevens, J. R.: Psychiatric implications of psychomotor epilepsy. Arch. Gen. Psychiatry, 14:461, 1966.
56. Tupin, J. R., Smith, D. B., Clanon, T. L., et al.: The long-term use of lithium in aggressive prisoners. Compr. Psychiatry, 14:311, 1973.
57. Tyrer, P.: Towards rational therapy with monoamine oxidase inhibitors. Br. J. Psychiatry, 128:354, 1976.
58. Volko, R. J.: Group therapy for patients with hysteria (Briquet's disorder). Dis. Nerv. Syst., 37:484, 1976.
59. Welner, A., Liss, J. L., and Robins, E.: Undiagnosed psychiatric patients. Part III: The undiagnosable patient. Brit. J. Psychiatry, 123:91, 1973.
60. Wilson, W. P.: Applications of Electroencephalography in Psychiatry. Durham, Duke University Press, 1965.
61. Witkin, H. A., Mednick, S. A., Schulsinger, F., et al.: Criminality in XYY and XXY men. Science, 193:547, 1976.
62. Woodruff, R. A., Goodwin, D. W., and Guze, S. B.: Psychiatric Diagnosis. New York, Oxford University Press, 1974.
63. Wyler, A. R., Masuda, M., and Holmes, T. H.: Magnitude of life events and seriousness of illness. Psychosom. Med., 33:115, 1971.

Chapter 22

ANXIETY: ACUTE AND CHRONIC

by ARMANDO R. FAVAZZA, and JERRY A. ROYER

To be anxious is to be human. Indeed, a modicum of anxiety is required for survival. Anxiety ensures a vigilance and readiness for action—to cross a busy intersection, to prepare for an examination, or to manage a complicated obstetric delivery. Athletes experience anxiety before a contest; actors experience stage fright before a performance. A hungry infant, unable to verbalize his desires and uncertain about the food supply, vents his anxiety by crying and thrashing; and his parents respond by comforting and feeding him. These are examples of the *adaptive* function of anxiety (Fig. 22–1).

Occasionally, however, anxiety is so intense or so prolonged that it becomes dysfunctional rather than adaptive.* Patients experiencing the taut distress of dysfunctional anxiety frequently consult their physicians. They are frightened but do not know why. Their entire nervous system, especially the autonomic nervous system, becomes overactive. For such patients, anxiety is no longer adaptive. Hence, the focus of this chapter is on *dysfunctional* anxiety.

SYMPTOMS AND SIGNS OF ANXIETY

The anxious patient reports symptoms and shows signs that are varied and diverse. Symptoms and signs are referable to at least five organ systems: nervous, cardiovascular, pulmonary, gastrointestinal, and genitourinary (Table 22–1).

*Our studies of the relationship of anxiety to learning confirm a similar pattern. Anxiety of proper intensity and duration facilitates learning, but overly intense or prolonged anxiety impairs learning.

DIFFERENTIAL DIAGNOSIS

Functional anxiety, in either its acute or chronic form, is the most prevalent type of anxiety seen by the family physician. Nevertheless, it is important to include the following disorders in the differential diagnosis:

Thyroid Dysfunction. Hyperthyroidism does not always appear in its classic form, so thyroid function studies are important. When results are equivocal, the blood chemistries should be repeated. Less frequently, anxiety occurs in hypothyroidism.

Cardiac Pathology. Early congestive heart failure may bring initial symptoms of sleeplessness, nightmares, impaired memory, inability to concentrate, fatigue, and substernal pressure. (In functional anxiety, the electrocardiogram (ECG) is usually normal, except for sinus tachycardia; occasionally there may be S–T segment depression and even depression or inversion of the T-wave.)

Hypoglycemia. It is our impression that hypoglycemia is overdiagnosed in patients

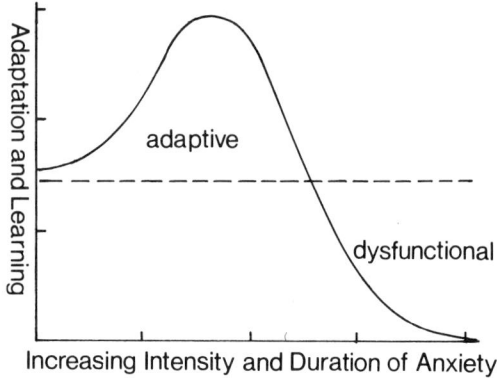

Figure 22–1. *Anxiety and adaptation.*

TABLE 22-1. SYMPTOMS AND SIGNS OF ANXIETY

Symptoms	Signs
Nervous System Tense, unable to relax Difficulty concentrating, difficulty with memory, loss of interest in usual activities Light-headedness, dizziness, syncope "Bad mood," general irritability, unable to tolerate even mild frustration Sleep disturbances: nightmares, difficulty going to sleep Ill-defined fear of the unknown, terrifying sense of dread Fatigue, weakness Headaches, poor coordination Trembling, numbness and tingling of fingers, toes, and face Piloerection ("goosebumps")	*Nervous System* Strained facial expression Stereotypic behavior, e.g., facial tic, nail-biting, chain-smoking Cold, clammy handshake Pacing, restlessness Irritability during physical examination Fine tremor of outstretched hands Occasional exophthalmos
Cardiovascular Palpitations Substernal pressure, precordial pain unrelated to exertion Flushing of face	*Cardiovascular* Sinus tachycardia Transient elevated systolic blood pressure Functional systolic ejection murmur
Pulmonary Difficulty breathing adequately Sense of suffocation	*Pulmonary* Hyperventilation (positive Chvostek's sign, if severe) Increased frequency of sighing respiration
Gastrointestinal Epigastric distress: fullness, belching, heartburn, dyspepsia Diarrhea, constipation Anorexia, compulsive eating	
Genitourinary Increased frequency of micturition Amenorrhea, excessive menstrual cramps and flow Impotence, premature ejaculation	

with functional complaints. The usual glucose tolerance test may be misleading, since blood glucose levels as low as 20 mg. per 100 ml. may be tolerated without producing symptoms in healthy individuals. In diagnosing hypoglycemia, it is important to draw a blood glucose sample *during* an anxiety attack; a blood glucose of less than 50 mg. per 100 ml., followed by the amelioration of symptoms after treatment with 50 per cent glucose given intravenously, suggests the diagnosis of hypoglycemia. Additional procedures such as prolonged fasting or the tolbutamide test may be necessary. The most common causes of spontaneous hypoglycemia in adults are insulin-secreting tumors and retroperitoneal sarcomas.

Drug Reaction. A surprising number of prescribed medications occasionally cause anxiety. Even anxiolytic drugs, e.g., diazepam (Valium), occasionally result in a paradoxical reaction. Physicians also should consider the possibility of amphetamine abuse in all anxious patients; similarly, physicians must inquire about mind-altering drugs such as marijuana and LSD, both of which may cause anxiety. (Anxiety attacks following LSD ingestion may occur months later.) Anxiety also may result from withdrawal from such drugs as alcohol, opiates, and some tranquilizers.

Cushing's Disease. Sudden attacks of anxiety are a common feature of this disorder.

Temporal Lobe Epilepsy. Ictal anxiety attacks, which are brief and sharply defined, may occur as part of this disorder.

Pheochromocytoma. The increased secretion of norepinephrine and epinephrine caused by this tumor may induce attacks in which the patient complains of headaches, sweating, palpitations, anxiety, chest pain, and paresthesias.

Essential Hypertension. Among the many symptoms of this disorder are headache, giddiness, personality changes, chest pain, shortness of breath, cardiac asthma, and increased frequency of micturition.

Postconcussion Syndrome. Following a minor head injury, a patient may complain of anxiety, dizziness, headache, fatigue, and inability to concentrate. This syndrome is extremely difficult to evaluate because objective neurologic signs typically are not present.

Dementias. Included in this group are: Creutzfeldt-Jakob disease, Huntington's chorea, both Alzheimer's and Pick's disease (the presenile dementias), and probably most importantly the senile and arteriosclerotic dementias. In the latter two disorders, prominent early symptoms often include anxiety, memory impairment, irritability, fatigue, and difficulty concentrating.

Other Neurologic Conditions. Although relatively infrequent, anxiety may occur in patients with multiple sclerosis, parkinsonism, brain tumors, and neurosyphilis.

Postinfective Syndrome. Following an infectious disorder, some patients experience anxiety, depression, or both. The psychologic sequelae may persist for months following resolution of the active infectious process. Infectious disorders especially associated with this syndrome include infectious mononucleosis, hepatitis, influenza, Weil's disease, and typhoid fever.

Depression. Among the major disorders that may present with anxiety as a prominent feature are agitated psychotic depression and involutional melancholia.

Schizophrenia. Latent schizophrenia (also known as borderline, incipient, or pseudoneurotic schizophrenia) may be characterized by anxiety, little spontaneity, "clinging" depression, poor interpersonal relationships, and impulsive outbursts of anger. Diagnosis of this controversial entity probably should be left to the experienced psychiatrist.

Transient Situational Disturbance. In response to major environmental stress, an individual may experience considerable anxiety. In the absence of an underlying mental disorder, however, the anxiety will prove transient.

ANXIETY—SYMPTOM OR SYNDROME?

Anxiety occurs both as a *symptom* (associated with various organic and psychiatric disorders) and as a *syndrome* (anxiety neurosis).

The anxiety seen with organic disease is most frequently functional, i.e., a psychologic reaction secondary to the organic disorder. It is not surprising that patients become anxious upon learning of a serious disease process; anticipated surgery is especially anxiety producing. Patients in whom anxiety is part of the primary symptomatology are few in number.

Symptomatic anxiety also occurs frequently in psychiatric disorders such as neurosis, transient situational stress, acute psychotic decompensation, and depressive illness.

The psychoanalytic school maintains that anxiety is central to all neurotic conditions. Anxiety is thought to be so corrosive and so threatening that the mind automatically attempts to defend against it, resulting in defense mechanisms analogous to the physiologic defenses that wall off an abscess. Mental defenses similarly act to contain anxiety, but neurotic symptoms may result in the process. A phobia, for example, is a neurosis in which the mind controls anxiety by focusing it on a feared object, e.g., a spider, or situation, e.g., dread of height. Using this defense tactic, a person feels less anxious as long as he avoids the feared object or situation.

In transient situational disturbances, severe anxiety may result from overwhelming stress, such as personal tragedy or sudden financial failure. In the face of major stress, a usually stable person may behave irrationally, e.g., may have temper tantrums or drink excessively. Once the stress resolves, however, the behavior of a basically healthy person will return to normal.

Anxiety also may occur at the onset of acute psychotic decompensation. Occasionally, a patient reacts to major stress with a brief period of psychosis, a psychosis that typically clears as the stress subsides. An acute schizophrenic reaction, however, is a more serious occurrence, because it may herald a chronic, potentially disabling condition. For example, an acute psychotic decompensation should be considered in the case of a 25 year old patient with a history of marginal or neurotic adaptation to life who presents with sudden marked anxiety and increasingly severe neurotic symptoms such as "out-of-the-body" experiences or feelings of unreality. Such a disorder may progress to hallucinations and paranoia.

Anxiety frequently comingles with depressive illness. Especially noteworthy are those patients with agitated depressive illness. These patients, typically middle-aged or older, experience symptoms both of depression and of anxiety. In addition to feelings of guilt, despair, and unworthiness, they show increased psychomotor activity, such as pacing and handwringing. Such patients are high suicidal risks.

Thus far in this section, we have described anxiety as a symptom of other disorders. Anxiety, however, also exists as a syndrome known as anxiety neurosis. Patients with this syndrome present with any of the signs and symptoms listed in Table 22–1. Anxiety may appear as an acute attack but more often the anxiety is chronic, with acute exacerbations and partial remissions. The anxiety, when extremely intense, may precipitate a panic reaction. The hallmark of an anxiety neurosis is its irrationality; the patient does not know *why* he is so thoroughly distraught or so frightened.

Predisposition to Anxiety

Anxiety is most prevalent during youth and old age. Certain anxieties of childhood, such as nightmares and fears of being left alone, are very common and seldom require therapeutic intervention. Adolescents experience anxiety as they cope with nascent sexuality and new social roles. During adolescence, anxiety frequently finds expression in impulsive behavior, promiscuity, petty crime, shyness or aggressiveness, increased frequency of masturbation, stammering, and inordinate attention to body parts (especially the sexual organs). Middle age, on the other hand, is relatively anxiety free; the middle-aged person usually has developed adequate coping mechanisms, including realistic expectations; has relative financial security; and is in good health. Then in old age, anxiety increases again as physical health declines and the imminence of death becomes more pressing. Anxiety often heightens with the female menopause and the male climacteric.

Physiologic and Character Traits of the Anxious Patient

Body physiology is an important factor affecting a person's threshold for anxiety. For example, the endocrine hormones clearly play a role, as evidenced by the anxiety associated with premenstrual tension, menopause, hyperthyroidism, and Cushing's disease. Anxiety also is associated with any compromise of the cerebral metabolism as seen in hypoglycemia or in hypoxia secondary to arteriosclerotic disease. Anxiety also may be prominent during an epileptic attack.

The anxious patient, usually an offspring of anxious parents, often describes his childhood as having included multiple traumatic events, e.g., the death of a parent, severe medical illness or surgery, abusive or overprotective upbringing, or sexual molestation. The childhood history also may include enuresis, nail-biting, speech pathology, somnambulism, excessive temper tantrums, abuse of animals, and difficulty leaving the mother when first entering school (separation anxiety).

The chronically anxious patient tends to have a dependent, immature premorbid personality and may lack the capacity for mature tenderness and affection. He is frequently insecure and complains of an "inferiority complex" and of feeling unloved. His claim of never achieving anything tends to become a self-fulfilling prophecy. He may be overly concerned about his body image and body functions. He magnifies minor problems and is so self-centered that he may have few friends who are willing to endure his pettiness, his constant self-focus, and his inability to return affection. The inability to offer sexual affection, as manifested by impotence or frigidity, may contribute to serious marital disharmony.

PSYCHOLOGIC CAUSES OF ANXIETY

Probably the most widely held theory about the psychology of anxiety is the psychoanalytic one. The psychoanalytic model traces the origins of adult anxiety to infancy and childhood. Infants experience anxiety in the form of separation anxiety, the earliest separation, of course, resulting from the birth process, when the infant is expelled from the maternal womb, through the constricted birth canal, and into the harsh world. Indeed, some psychiatrists and theologians describe the birth process as the basis for the biblical account of man's expulsion from the Garden of Eden. One developmental task a child faces during the first few years of life is to achieve increasing separation from his mother. Insofar as the process of separation is successful, the child develops a sense of individuality and autonomy. Insofar as this process is arrested, the child experiences heightened anxiety when faced with separation. Frequently, the separation anxiety becomes quite acute when the child must attend school for the first time.

Childhood anxiety also stems from a child's fantasies about mutilation of his body. Some parents actually threaten boys with castration—as punishment for masturbation, for example. More often, however, childhood fears about mutilation stem from fantasies, and these fantasies occasionally have to do with mistaken ideas as to why girls do not possess a phallus. A common fantasy is that a girl is born with a phallus but suffers amputation of this organ as a result of punishment. If not resolved during childhood, such anxiety about mutilation of the body may recur in adulthood. Anxiety about surgery, for example, relates not only to the fear of never awakening from anesthesia but also to the fear that one's body may undergo mutilation in the process.

Heightened anxiety also may arise as the child comes to internalize norms of right and wrong, as he begins to develop a conscience. This process of socialization requires that the growing child develop socially acceptable modes of adaptation and learn to delay the immediate gratification of desires. When a person acts contrary to the dictates of his conscience, he becomes anxious. This anxiety serves as society's lever on its members and forms the basis for societal norms, mores, and even laws. Most people choose to obey the laws, not only because they fear being caught, but also because the very act of law-break-

ing itself leads to increased anxiety. If a child's conscience develops too rigidly, however, or if he encounters exaggerated attention to conflicts between right and wrong, he may experience anxiety from even trivial decisions and actions.

Another major source of anxiety is the fear of losing control over one's own drives, of being consumed by one's animalistic impulses, of literally driving one's self mad. The anxious patient, not able to understand just why he feels so anxious, may fear loss of control and irrational behavior. More frequently, however, the patient's anxiety becomes somatic in focus, and the patient perceives that some part of the body is malfunctioning—hence, hypochondriac symptomatology. For many patients, it is preferable to endure chronic, assorted bodily complaints than to suffer the dread terror of anxiety.

An anxiety state may become increasingly pathologic in the face of mounting stress. A patient's defense mechanisms may not be adequate to cope with increased frustration, threat of personal loss, or imminent danger. The clinical picture may worsen as the increasing anxiety stirs up childhood patterns of coping with stress and anxiety. As an example, consider the extremely anxious woman who consults her family physician, distraught because her husband has announced that he intends to leave her for another woman. The patient has good reason to be anxious. She faces the prospect of raising children as a single parent. Will she have enough money to support herself and her children? Will she have the strength to carry on without the support of a spouse? Over the course of several weeks, the patient's anxiety increases. She calls the physician daily with complaints of palpitations, insomnia, and headaches. She develops frequent episodes of hyperventilation and experiences tingling of her hands and face and faintness. The woman's childhood history proves instructive. As a child, she was enuretic and overly dependent on her mother. Upon entering school, she had acute separation anxiety. When she left for college, she became so homesick that she had to transfer back to a college in her home town. Once married, she frequently experienced anxiety symptoms when her husband was away on business trips. Her physician recognizes that the pathology of her current anxiety state is more deep-rooted than the immediate stress of her husband's leaving; rather, her anxiety has roots in the separation anxiety that originated in childhood and has continued into adulthood whenever she is faced with separation and the threat of the loss of love.

TREATMENT

Acute anxiety requires swift, symptomatic relief. The immediate goal of treatment is to prevent the anxiety from precipitating a psychotic decompensation or a panic reaction. A psychotic or panic-stricken patient may act impulsively, harming himself or others.

The most rapid way to control anxiety is the use of anxiolytic medication in adequate dosage. The most commonly used drugs are the minor tranquilizers, chlordiazepoxide (Librium) and diazepam (Valium). These drugs are preferable to meprobamate or a barbiturate for the following reasons:

1. Suicide is difficult with chlordiazepoxide or diazepam; even massive doses rarely result in fatality (in the absence of taking other drugs).

2. Chlordiazepoxide and diazepam are less likely to lose their clinical effectiveness over time.

3. The anxiolytic effect of chlordiazepoxide and diazepam is more prolonged than that of meprobamate; they need not be taken as frequently.

4. Tolerance and physical dependence occur only when chlordiazepoxide and diazepam are used in high doses over a long period of time.

5. Chlordiazepoxide and diazepam interfere minimally with sleep patterns.

The usual dose of chlordiazepoxide is 5 to 25 mg. t.i.d. and of diazepam, 5 to 10 mg. t.i.d. If a patient does not respond rapidly, the dose should be increased. Although chlordiazepoxide and diazepam are closely related compounds, some patients respond far better to one than to the other. Initially, any prescription written should be limited to a one week supply of the medication. If the patient complains of difficulty sleeping, flurazepam (Dalmane) 30 mg. h.s. may be added to the regimen. But it is important to avoid polypharmacy. Major tranquilizers such as the phenothiazines and the butyro-

phenones (haloperidol [Haldol]) are effective for psychotic conditions but should not be used for an anxiety reaction. A doxepin drug (e.g., Sinequan) is often effective in the treatment of anxiety, especially when mild depression is present.

Before initiating medication, however, it is important to take a careful drug history and to evaluate thoroughly any medication the patient is taking. Inquire specifically about over-the-counter drugs, oral contraceptives, and "nerve" pills. In general, eliminate all medications possible. Medication for organic illness should be given at the lowest therapeutic dosage. Beware of the most common means of self-medication — the use of alcohol to allay anxiety. Assure the patient that the minor tranquilizers are safer and more effective than alcohol.

Clearly, the physician should treat any underlying medical problems. In fact, anxiety often subsides with the resolution of organic disease, although this is not always the case. The anxiety associated with hyperthyroidism may continue long after the patient is again euthyroid.

In addition to immediate drug therapy, the family physician should offer psychologic support to the acutely anxious patient. The patient should be seen briefly on a frequent basis, daily or every few days, until the anxiety attack subsides. By scheduling specific, frequent appointments the number of "crisis" telephone calls can be decreased dramatically. During these visits, assure the patient that the anxiety is psychologic in origin. If the patient's premorbid personality has been stable, and if it is clear that situational stress precipitated the attack, it is safe to predict to the patient that the anxiety will subside as the environmental stress is resolved. Express confidence in his ability to weather the crisis. In working with the patient, practical suggestions may be effective; for example, a patient may be advised to seek legal help or to talk with his minister. Avoid making decisions for the patient, but assist him in considering the alternatives. Decisions that appear to be healthy and adaptive may warrant a supportive statement such as, "That certainly seems like a reasonable thing to do." On the other hand, if the patient seems to be moving toward an unhealthy, maladaptive decision, gently point this out to him. One approach is to share with the patient examples of how other patients have successfully managed similar situations.

Any patient in a state of panic constitutes a medical emergency. In such a case, the physician must be more aggressive in his management. Hospitalization may be indicated; consultation or referral may be advised. The physician must insist that the panicked patient follow explicit instructions.

The management of *chronic* anxiety requires a great deal of patience on the part of the physician. As with any chronic disorder, there will be exacerbations and remissions. Perhaps physicians accept more readily the long-term implications of such chronic disorders as diabetes mellitus and arthritis; because these conditions are primarily organic in nature, we expect exacerbations and remissions. Chronic anxiety is particularly frustrating because of its irrational nature, i.e., the reasons for the anxiety elude both patient and physician. It is important that the physician work through his own frustration so that he is consistent in his management of the patient. The physician who is comforting one week, but irritable the next, only aggravates the anxiety of the patient.

In the management of chronic anxiety it is more important that the physician be a good listener than a good talker. The treatment of chronic anxiety can no more be rushed than the treatment of osteoarthritis. Often, the best therapy is to listen attentively, without interruption; it may be necessary to instruct office staff to hold telephone calls and not to enter your office during the session.

Significant in the treatment is the *trust* a patient develops for his physician. This trust is enhanced if the physician avoids platitudes, poor advice ("Think positively and you'll feel better!"), sarcasm, and forced humor. Also avoid white lies, even though well-intended; avoid telling a patient he is looking much better if, in fact, he is not looking better. Because anxious patients are highly suggestible, words must be chosen carefully. Avoid highly charged, emotional words and metaphors; an anxious man whose wife is mentally abusive will find little solace in the clinical observation, "Your wife certainly is castrating."

The physician should avoid making moral judgments. Rather than saying, "It's shameful the way you are running around on your wife," the physician should gently point out any behavior that is maladaptive. This can be restated in the health context as it pertains to the patient: "Having this affair is important to you now, but is it wise in the long run? It seems to me that your situation would not improve if you were caught. Also, I am concerned that you may feel guilty about this affair in the future." A nonjudgmental approach allows the patient to ventilate his feelings and to examine the consequences of his behavior. Morality is relative; what seems immoral to the physician may not seem immoral to the patient, especially when there is a difference in social class or ethnic background.

What appear to be "common sense" recommendations for alleviating anxiety often fail because of the irrational nature of anxiety. For example, prescribing increased physical exercise to expend one's anxiety provides a momentary respite at best. Similarly, to recommend a vacation may prove futile (unless, of course, environmental stress is a clearcut factor in the anxiety.) Anxious patients commonly do reflect the stresses of some larger social order, but in practical terms, the focus in chronic anxiety will be the patient himself.

Although the family physician may appreciate the probable childhood origins of a patient's chronic anxiety, generally it should not be his role to make extensive interpretations about those origins. Rarely does the family physician have the time or training to explore a patient's past in such depth. A more reasonable focus is to assist the patient in identifying patterns of behavior that have been prominent throughout his life, patterns of behavior the patient may be able to modify.

All people have a fantasy life. Anxious patients, however, often find their fantasies perplexing and disturbing. By paying particular attention to the words a patient uses, the astute clinician will find clues to the patient's fantasy world. Encouraging the patient to express his fantasies can be beneficial in therapy, but the physician must be prepared to deal with frankly sexual and aggressive themes. Frequently these themes arise from a yearning to return to those times of childhood when one's parents were comforting and protective, or they may arise from a desire to seek revenge on a parent for real or fantasized abuse. The patient should not be encouraged to wallow in his fantasies, but the examination of a fantasy, including some reasonable interpretation, may provide the patient with therapeutic insight into his anxiety.

A relatively new technique for treating anxiety is relaxation training. Relaxation techniques are relatively simple to master, but they do require an investment of time. A number of reputable companies offer tape cassette instructions and brief instruction manuals. These self-instructional programs are advertised in medical journals, and the interested family physician may benefit from becoming familiar with one or more relaxation techniques.

REFERRAL

On occasion, the family physician will wish to refer an anxious patient for psychiatric care. Generally, it is preferable to refer the patient to a psychiatrist rather than to a clinical psychologist or social agency. If financial constraints are a factor, referral can be made to a community mental health center that has a sliding fee scale. These centers have been established across the country.

Psychiatric referral should be considered if:

1. The patient's anxiety increases despite a reasonable course of treatment.

2. The patient enters a panic state.

3. The patient broods about or attempts suicide.

4. The physician feels unduly frustrated by the patient's incessant symptomatology. A chronically anxious and demanding patient, with his frequent office visits and telephone calls, may disrupt a physician's practice. An already overworked physician may find he simply cannot attend to all his patients' needs.

The patient and his family should be informed of the reasons for the referral. To allay any feelings of rejection, the physician should reassure the patient and his family that he will continue to look after their other medical concerns.

COMMUNITY RESOURCES

Anxious patients often seek nonmedical help, and the physician should be familiar with reputable service agencies in the community. Many communities have a family service agency staffed by social workers and other professionals; their resources may be helpful in dealing with various family problems. Many patients turn to their ministers, priests, or rabbis for counseling. Although the quality of counseling by clergymen varies greatly (as it does, indeed, among physicians), the family physician should consider such referral as one option. Other reputable organizations such as Parents Without Partners and Big Brother programs may be helpful for social problems.

There are literally hundreds of organizations that attract anxious patients in search of "an answer" to their anxiety. Some of these organizations provide an important adjunct to the more traditional medical therapy. For example, the structured environment and techniques of meditation groups may be beneficial for patients with mild chronic anxiety. On the other hand, some groups and their therapies prove counterproductive for the anxious patient. Some "sensitivity" groups directed by nonprofessionals actually exacerbate a patient's anxiety and may precipitate a psychosis. In short, some organizations and programs have relatively innocuous "therapeutic" impact, while others prove quite harmful, not only to the patient's psyche, but also to his pocketbook. A physician should not refer a patient to nonprofessional agencies or groups, nor should he encourage a patient to participate in their programs, unless he personally can vouch for the reliability and competence of the personnel.

REFERENCES

1. Cameron, N.: Personality Development and Psychopathology. Boston, Houghton Mifflin Co., 1963.
2. Ford, C., Bray, G., and Swendloff, R.: A psychiatric study of patients referred with a diagnosis of hypoglycemia. Am. J. Psychiatry, *133*:290, 1976.
3. Funkenstein, D.: The learning and personal development of medical students: reconsidered. *In* Graham, R., and Royer, J. (eds.): A Handbook for Change: Recommendations of the Joint Commission on Medical Education. Chicago, Student American Medical Assoc., 1973.
4. Glasscote, R., Raybin, J., Reifen, C., et al.: The Alternate Services, Their Role in Mental Health. Washington, D.C., The American Psychiatric Association, 1975.

5. Graham, R., and Royer, J. (eds.): A Handbook for Change: Recommendations of the Joint Commission on Medical Education. Chicago, Student American Medical Assoc., 1973.

6. Lesse, S.: Anxiety: Its Components, Development, and Treatments. New York, Grune & Stratton, Inc., 1970.

7. May, R.: The Meaning of Anxiety. New York, Donald Press, 1950.

8. Nemiah, J.: Anxiety neurosis. *In* Freedman, A., Kaplan, H., and Sadock, B. (eds.): Comprehensive Textbook of Psychiatry/II. Baltimore, The Williams & Wilkins Co., 1975.

9. Rees, L.: Anxiety Factors in Comprehensive Patient Care. New York, Excerpta Medica, 1973.

10. Slater, E., and Roth, M.: Clinical Psychiatry. Baltimore, The Williams & Wilkins Co., 1969.

11. Spielberger, C.: Anxiety: Current Trends in Theory and Research. New York, Academic Press, Inc., 1972.

Chapter 23

HYSTERIA AND PHOBIAS

by SHERVERT H. FRAZIER,
and NICHOLAS J. PISACANO

Hysteria and phobias are two of the six classified neuroses, or psychoneuroses (the latter two terms are used interchangeably). Neuroses are among the most common disorders in medical practice. Family physicians are reluctant to label patients as neurotic, or psychoneurotic, because of the confusion regarding the specific meanings of these two terms and because they may be used pejoratively. As a first step toward clarification, the World Health Organization's *Glossary of Mental Disorders* has defined neuroses as those mental disorders without any demonstrable organic basis, in which the patient may have considerable insight and unimpaired reality testing (that is, he usually does not confuse his morbid subjective experiences and fantasies with external reality). Behavior may be greatly affected, although usually remaining within socially acceptable limits. However, the personality is not disorganized. The symptoms of neuroses may include anxiety, hysteria, phobias, obsessive and compulsive behavior, and depression. Critical to the diagnosis are the (1) absence of loss of reality testing; (2) absence of delusions, hallucinations, bizarre affects, or unusual behaviors; and (3) presence of considerable personal stress of a nonspecific type or of stress of a situational, family, or life-threatening type. Very often, patients who have a physical disorder also have what has been called an "emotional overlay." This occurs frequently in patients with hysterical neurosis. Numerous theories (which means there is no specific knowledge) exist concerning the etiology of the various types of neurosis.

HYSTERICAL NEUROSIS

Two types of hysterical neuroses are usually described in the literature. However, they may coexist, may become mixed with elements of each other, and may become mixed with physical disorders. These two types are called conversion hysteria and the dissociative type of hysteria.

Conversion Hysteria

There are no objective findings in conversion hysteria. The anatomic distribution of motor or sensory innervation is not followed, and the symptoms exist with intact neurologic findings. This then is said to represent a physiologic manifestation of a psychologic conflict, which means that psychologic conflict is *converted* to physiologic expression. Such psychologic conflict may be symbolic of the anatomic part or organ system affected. Conversion, then, is a general relationship between the mind and the body. It occurs throughout the range of mental disorders and also serves adaptive functions. The American Psychiatric Association's *Glossary of Psychiatric Terms* defines *conversion* as a defense mechanism operating unconsciously (outside conscious control) by which intrapsychic conflicts that would otherwise give rise to anxiety are instead given symbolic external expression. The repressed ideas or impulses, plus the psychologic defenses against them, are converted into a variety of somatic symptoms. The symptoms may include such things as paralysis of a limb, which would prevent its use for aggressive purposes, or pain or loss of sensory function. Very often, the disability caused by a conversion element overlaying a physical illness is the main disability-producing factor and, therefore, needs to be managed and treated in a very specific fashion.

Diagnosis. Conversion hysteria is manifest in many different forms, some of which are readily confused with organic illness. It is necessary to distinguish the protean forms of this psychologically-determined illness from the lesional forms of specific anatomically-determined neurologic or internal medical disorders. One generally considers conversion hysteria as a primary diagnosis when there are clusters of physical symptoms without diagnosable structural lesions and when the attitude of the patient is not appropriate to the general disability that would ordinarily accompany the illness, were it physical in origin. There are also disturbances in the patterns of thinking that the individual exhibits when a careful history is obtained. Present also are unusual personality disorders. The individual personality pattern is usually that of a dependent person. The behavior of the patient or the demonstration of his symptoms may be theatrical and dramatic. The history usually reveals that the onset of such a disorder occurred during adolescence or certainly by the time of early adulthood (the early twenties). When physical disease coexists, the physician must be careful to determine which is a physical process and which is emotional overlay. The latter takes the form of exaggeration of symptoms that goes beyond the scope of lesionally-produced symptoms and signs. The attitude of indifference is not always so easily diagnosable when some physically-determined disability is also present.

The early onset usually occurs in discrete episodes that are related temporally to emotionally significant events or circumstances. The initial phase of anxiety or fear is replaced by a physical symptom that leaves the patient calm and somewhat indifferent to the former anxiety. These episodes soon pass. In such an instance, one often finds that simple suggestion by the physician leads to a dramatic relief of the symptoms, but, unfortunately, recurrences are frequent. It has been said for many years that conversion symptoms occur more frequently in women than in men, but this statement is now being questioned.

The condition of grand hysteria was typically described by Charcot and Janet as being associated with gait disturbances; astasia-abasia; paralysis, sometimes ending in fixed contractures in peculiar positions; paresthesias; and bizarre epileptic-like seizures. Other persons suffered serious anesthesia over large or psychologically significant parts of the body. Today it is known that such persons obviously require careful neurologic and medical examinations and may ultimately require prolonged hospitalization. At the termination of the hospitalization, an exacerbation of symptoms is likely to occur, similar to those that caused the hospitalization in the first place. Careful examination and astute observation are required by the physician. An example is the evaluation of a patient with an apparent board-like abdomen. When the patient is carefully examined, one observes that in the lumbar area the arched back assumes the posture present in opisthotonos, thus causing tightening of the abdominal musculature. Facial expressions also do not coincide with those of a person having lesionally-produced pain.

Dissociative Hysteria

In this type of hysteria, the patient demonstrates an altered state of consciousness. This is sometimes associated with confused identity and with what has been called a fugue state, often accompanied by amnesia, sleep-walking, or both, without evident anxiety. The patient also experiences a secondary gain from being ill, called malingering. Malingering is the deliberate simulation or exaggeration of an illness or a disability that, in fact, is either nonexistent or minor, in order to avoid an unpleasant situation or to obtain some type of personal gain, such as developing a compensation neurosis. Jones and Llewellyn state, "Nothing resembles malingering more than hysteria; nothing resembles hysteria more than malingering." It has been said that malingering can be cured by the application of a "greenback poultice." However, one must remember that persons who need to malinger in conjunction with having an altered behavioral state are indeed operating in a maladaptive fashion. This is often the manifestation of a serious personality disorder, usually seen in the immature or in the chronically-disturbed person with psychopathic or sociopathic tendencies. Anyone who feigns illness or malingers obviously is protecting himself from a potential major emotional breakdown.

Diagnosis. Individuals with amnesic states and dissociative hysteria have a loss of memory for past events, which may be a sequel to a functional or an altered state of consciousness. In such a state, very important and significant ideas and life plans are removed from awareness. The patient may act in an entirely different life style, exhibiting mannerisms and other behaviors not usually associated with his ordinary activities. The patient's behavior while in a dissociated state seems to be aimless, but most physicians have been able to interpret some goal-directed, purposeful behavior of a symbolic type. Another presentation of patients with dissociative hysteria may be peculiar kinds of so-called seizures or convulsive attacks, in which the individual demonstrates very unusual patterns that do not seem to fit any of the lesional states affecting the brain. Seizures often result in the patient's maintaining an extremity in a fixed position long enough to cause an hysterical flexion contracture. The individual with a convulsive hysteria is not seen frequently today, but in the nineteenth century when Briquet studied hysterical patients, he found that 75 per cent of his patients suffered convulsive attacks.

The attacks are not symptomatic epilepsy; they are not idiopathic epilepsy. The episodes can usually be distinguished by the fact that the patient is not completely unconscious during the attack, that the attack occurs only when other persons are present who can directly view the seizure, that the individual does not hurt himself during the fall that occurs, and the patient's corneal, pupillary, and deep reflexes are still present. There is no loss of bowel or bladder sphincter control, and the patient usually has a florid, reddened face rather than a pale or gray or even cyanotic facies. The patient responds with pain to pressure applied at pressure points, such as the superocular ridge, and he may have some involuntary movements, but these do not seem to be organically determined. Subsequent to such

seizures, and independent of them, individuals may develop tremors or locomotive disabilities or even paralysis. Experienced physicians have noted that such patients, more often than not, have known someone who had a similar disorder.

In the course of evaluating the development of such sensory disturbances, one must keep in mind the very difficult differential diagnosis of multiple sclerosis and its associated sensory disturbances. More often than not, the symptoms of hysteria may be manifested by a localized reduction of cutaneous sensation or by hyperesthetic spots over particular areas of the body. Very often there is a contraction in the field of vision (tunnel vision), or a feeling of a lump in the throat that cannot be swallowed (so-called globus hystericus), or other kinds of symptomatology without pathologic structural lesions. There may be an affective disorder in which the patient shows a benign lack of concern about the seemingly serious disability; this has been called "la belle indifférence." Any text concerning the psychopathologic aspects of hysteria is replete with the findings of Breurer's and Freud's investigations into the unconscious.

Without doubt, the intertwining histories of hysterical persons and their ability to talk about their disturbances have greatly helped us to understand, in depth, the nature of the hysterical somatic attitude. There is no difference in frequency of occurrence between men and women.

Treatment. The formation of a good, empathic physician–patient relationship is often very helpful. This kind of relationship allows the patient's dependency at first to be re-experienced with the physician. Then the physician, with sage advice and a long-range perspective, may help the patient grow from the state of an utter infantile kind of dependency to a more productive and more adaptive kind of life. Understanding is the important part of treatment. However, the reduction of anxiety may often be accomplished by administering a benzodiazepine drug in small doses for short periods of time. The more severe cases require a prolonged and intensive psychotherapeutic approach. This kind of treatment, although expensive, is sometimes quite helpful.

PHOBIAS

But now I am cabin'd, cribb'd, confined, bound in to saucy doubts and fears.

William Shakespeare, *Macbeth*, Act III, Scene 2

Phobias have been defined as an obsessive, persistent, unrealistic, intense fear of an object or a situation. The fear is believed to arise through a process of displacing an internal and unconscious conflict onto an external object that is symbolically related to the conflict.

There are numerous phobias. Selected examples include acrophobia (fear of high places), agoraphobia (fear of open places), ailurophobia (fear of cats), algophobia (fear of experiencing or witnessing pain), claustrophobia (fear of confined or closed places), cynophobia (fear of dogs), mysophobia (fear of dirt or contamination), xenophobia (fear of strangers or foreigners), and zoophobia (fear of animals).

A phobia neurosis is a disorder occurring in a patient who has an intense and irrational fear of an object, a situation, a person, or an animal. He can recognize the unrealistic basis for his feelings but cannot explain his lack of ability to master a response to the situation. Approaching the object of the phobia frequently precipitates acute anxiety, bordering on panic, in the person. Most patients have had phobias since childhood, having been encouraged or taught by their parents to fear the specific object. Childhood phobias, however, are considered to be normal. The persistence of a phobia into adulthood usually means that the person grew up in a family in which phobias were common and were very often ignored completely. This attitude leads to avoidance of the real object for which the phobia is a symbol. A truly disabled phobic person may not, for example, be able to leave his room or apartment, walk in the street, enter an elevator, or be in a high place. These mechanisms, by which avoidance and inhibition rule the life and symbolize the inner fears of the person, are often related to events that occur continuously or in close proximity to the state of overt fear. Phobic patients very often are afraid to go anywhere alone and are often accompanied by another person dedicated to their care. Such a person is often called a "phobic companion."

Freud thought phobias were forms of defense and containment against anxiety. The behavior therapists think that phobias are related to learned responses (conditioning), and, hence, are the basis for desensitization therapy (see following section).

Phobia occurs in other neurotic as well as in borderline personality organizational states and creates a very difficult living situation. Long-term psychotherapy has not been able to relieve more than 50 per cent of the patients, to uncover the cause of the phobia, or to relieve its manifestations. Phobic persons often belief in magic and are often given "safety passes," which may work for a period of time. Phobic persons have also been medicated with antianxiety drugs, which can be dangerous if used for a long period of time.

Treatment. The most significant treatment for the garden-variety type of phobia is *behavior modification*, a relatively new technique. Behavior modification is often prescribed for anxiety. Anxiety may best be thought of as a shorthand term for a complex pattern of responses characterized by feelings of apprehension and tension accompanied by or associated with physiologic activation or arousal.

One technique of behavior modification is *systematic desensitization*, which was developed by Joseph Wolpe. Guided by Hull's concept of "conditioned inhibition," Wolpe undertook a series of animal studies that led him to conclude that the most satisfactory way of treating conditioned anxiety was through a gradual counterconditioning approach. Wolpe noted the similarity of these procedures to Mary Cover Jones' treatment of a fearful child. Basing his psychologic theorizing on Hull's concepts, Wolpe offered neurophysiologic speculations for the effectiveness of counterconditioning procedures, by extrapolating from Sharington's concept of "reciprocal inhibition." Wolpe formulated a counterconditioning hypothesis for eliminating maladaptive anxiety, which he termed the "reciprocal inhibition principle." He soon found that in vivo relaxation was often impractical because the anxiety-eliciting stimuli could not be controlled. Jacobson, in 1938, had developed the process of progressive relaxation training, since deep muscle relaxation appeared to produce both a reduction in physiologic arousal and a pleasant affective tone. The two features were combined, and a treatment package for human anxiety was developed by Wolpe, which he called systematic desensitization.

It should be noted that both the gradual approach method and counterconditioning principles had previously been proposed by many writers for treating anxiety and phobic disorders. Such terms as "deconditioning" by Burnham, "graded tasks" and "dosing anxiety" by Dollard and Miller, "reconditioning and hypnotic desensitization" by Wolberg, "paradoxical intention" by Frankl, and "autogenic training" by Schultz and Lutag, all referred to therapeutic procedures that share, in part, either principles or techniques with systematic desensitization therapy.

In behavior modification, hierarchies of anxiety are classified into two areas: thematic and spatial–temporal. Thematic hierarchies are focused upon some cluster of anxiety-eliciting stimulus configurations that indicate a common defined mediational feature or theme. Spatial–temporal hierarchies, on the other hand, are focused upon a target event that can be fixed in time and space with atoms of the hierarchy, consisting of points along the approach radiating to the target. The so-called hierarchies are carefully elicited according to their anxiety-arousing potential and are graded on a scale from minimal (least anxiety) themes to the most intense or maximal (panic) themes. Combined hierarchies may also be formed.

The desensitization proper consists of bringing about a deep state of relaxation, induced usually by a much briefer method than that used during the initial training. Instructions are given to signal even the slightest degree of tension, discomfort, or anxiety. The lowest item in the hierarchy is then presented by verbal instructions from the therapist, after which the therapist pauses briefly to allow unimpeded imagination of the item by the patient. After the appropriate exposure time, the patient is instructed to stop visualizing the scene and merely to continue relaxing. When desensi-

tization proper is unimpeded by elicited anxiety, each hierarchy item is repeated at least two times in the same manner, working up the hierarchy from the weakest to the strongest stimulus or stimuli. The therapist thus ensures that higher items are not presented until each lower item can be imagined without disturbance. Should any given item result in disturbing reactions, the client is immediately instructed to stop visualizing the scene, and relaxation is again induced, often aided by instructions to visualize a neutral and pleasant scene. Following the occurrence of anxiety in response to a given item, the same item may again be presented in a diluted form either by shortening the presentation time or by adding factors to the scene that are known to lower the intensity of response, *or* a lower item in the hierarchy may be reintroduced. Each sequence is concluded with a successful item presentation.

When multiple hierarchies are to be desensitized, progress through the hierarchies may be concurrent. Items from different hierarchies are presented during a different session sequentially; one hierarchy is completed before another one is started. Combined sequential and concurrent coverage of hierarchies may also be involved in a single desensitization case. For example, a spatial–temporal hierarchy might first be desensitized alone, followed by concurrent desensitization of two or more thematic hierarchies.

The ultimate questions to be answered concerning behavior modification have been posed by many workers. What treatment, and by whom, is most effective for this individual with that specific problem? Under which set of circumstances is it most effective, and how does this come about? Since systematic desensitization consists of a set of procedures and strategies that are hypothesized to be appropriate for specific problems in which the direct treatment of anxiety is considered of fundamental importance, the basic assessment of its effectiveness, or outcome, is of particular significance. The assessment of the outcome may be viewed as an evaluation of the cause and effect relationship between systematic desensitization as the independent variable (i.e., the treatment) and change in distressing target behaviors related to anxiety as a dependent variable (i.e., the specific problem). Failure has to do with difficulties with imagery or with the patient terminating because he feels a lack of progress. There appear to be no reliable differences in types of distressing behavior, personal characteristics, or anything else that differentiate the failures from the successes. Lazarus reported that the great majority of distressing behaviors that he treated were characterized by high states of anxiety and inhibition of adaptive behaviors, including interpersonal and social anxiety; generalized anxiety; and numerous phobias, such as agoraphobia and claustrophobia. Several patients with panic and pervasive anxiety were also treated. In no instance was desensitization applied to patients who were later diagnosed as psychotic. Persons with panic and pervasive anxiety had relatively lower percentages of success rates than did persons with other problems, presumably the result of inability to construct adequate hierarchies.

In summary, one would say that with moderate and workable anxiety, behavior modification techniques make the eradication of phobic anxiety possible. When pervasive anxiety exists, the prognosis is more serious.

REFERENCES

1. Anton, W. D.: An evaluation of outcome variables in the systematic desensitization of test anxiety. Behav. Res. Ther., 14:217, 1976.
2. Frazier, S. H. (ed.): A Psychiatric Glossary. 4th Ed. Washington, D.C.: American Psychiatric Assoc., 1975.
3. Frazier, S. H.: Phobias and phobic reactions. In Frazier, S. H., and Carr, A. C.: Introduction to Psychopathology. New York, Jason Aronson, Inc., 1974.
4. Frazier, S. H.: Bodily expressions of psychological difficulties for conversion reaction. In Frazier, S. H., and Carr, A. C.: Introduction to Psychopathology. New York, Jason Aronson, Inc., 1974.
5. Frazier, S. H., and Carr, A. C.: Phobic reaction. In Freedman, A. M., and Kaplan, H. I. (eds.). Comprehensive Textbook of Psychiatry. 1st Ed. Baltimore, The Williams & Wilkins Co., 1967.
6. Keltner, A., and Marshall, W. L.: Attribution and subject control factors in experimental desensitization. Behav. Ther., 7:626, 1976.
7. Kolb, L. C.: Modern Clinical Psychiatry. 9th Ed. Philadelphia, W. B. Saunders Co., 1973.
8. Paul, G. L.: Outcome of systematic desensitization. 63–159. In Franks, C. M. (ed.): Behavior Therapy: Appraisal and Status. New York, McGraw-Hill Book Co., 1969.
9. Reich, P., and Kelly, M. J.: Introduction to mental disorders. In Wintrobe, Thorn, Adams, et al. (eds.): Harrison's Principles of Internal Medicine. 7th Ed. New York, McGraw-Hill Book Co., 1974.
10. Reich, P., and Kelly, M. J.: The neuroses. In Wintrobe, Thorn, Adams, et al. (eds.): Harrison's Principles of Internal Medicine. 7th Ed. New York, McGraw-Hill Book Co., 1969.
11. Rosen, G. M.: Subjects' initial therapeutic expectancies and subjects' awareness of therapeutic goals in systematic desensitization: a review. Behav. Ther., 7:14, 1976.
12. Wright, J. C.: A comparison of systematic desensitization and social skill acquisition in the modification of a social fear. Behav. Ther., 7:205, 1976.

Chapter 24

DEPRESSION

by REMI CADORET,
and R. J. COBLE

Depression is one of the commonest conditions encountered in primary care. In a statewide study in Virginia of the content of family practice involving 88,000 patients in whom 526,196 health care problems were noted, depression occurred in 8.9 per cent of the patients, ranking twelfth in the order of frequency in a total of 527 diagnoses.[10] In the United Kingdom, where the general practitioner is truly the first contact in virtually all cases, depression ranks fourth in frequency.[8] Some of the difference in the prevalence of depression between British and American practices could well represent disagreement in diagnosis. Recent cross-national studies of diagnostic practices have shown that in Britain psychiatrists are more likely to diagnose affective disorders than are their American colleagues.[1, 2, 7]

DIAGNOSIS OF DEPRESSION

In private practice, as well as in the cross-national studies, the diagnosis becomes more exact if certain objective criteria are followed.

Affective disorders are syndromes characterized by marked and sustained changes of mood. In depression, the prevailing mood is low, being described as "blue," "down in the dumps," or apathetic. Part of the low mood consists of a decreased ability to enjoy activities that usually were a source of pleasure. The diagnosis of depressive syndrome requires a history of at least 1 month of depressed mood and of at least four of the following eight symptoms: (1) poor appetite with or without weight loss; (2) sleep problems—increased need for sleep, sleep not refreshing, or, more commonly, initial or terminal insomnia; (3) loss of energy—fatigability or tiredness; (4) agitation—anxiety, restlessness; or retardation—slowed movements; (5) loss of interest in usual activities or decreased sex drive; (6) feelings of self-reproach or guilt; (7) diminished ability to think or concentrate—slowed thinking or confused thoughts; and (8) recurrent thoughts of death or suicide or wishing one were dead. The aggregate of these symptoms indicates a significant clinical depression instead of common transient feelings of normal mood shifts.[5] These symptoms should represent a *change* in functioning for the patient. It is useful in asking questions about symptoms to determine which are changes for the patient and when the patient or family first noted them.

Presenting complaints are commonly those of sleep disturbance and those related to diminished energy—"tired all the time," "can't get going." In primary care, somatic complaints are often the presenting symptoms, since 50 to 75 per cent of depressives have been shown to have somatic complaints such as headache, muscle weakness, dizziness, gastrointestinal irritability, heart palpitations, and low back pain.[3] Indeed, full-blown anxiety attacks occur for the first time in about 30 per cent of patients with serious depressions. The anxiety attacks are classic, with palpitations, chest pain, difficulty breathing or hyperventilation, and a feeling of fear. The patient may present with several apparently unrelated complaints (i.e., low back pain, tiredness, headache), each of which may seem insignificant, but the sum of these problems may spell hopelessness to the patient. The physician might try to diagnose and treat each symptom separately or seek in vain for a pathophysiologic explanation for the set of symptoms unless the diagnosis of depression is considered.

Depression is so common that it is a useful practice to screen patients routinely for this condition. A few questions about changes in mood, sleep, and energy are often sufficient.

CLASSIFICATION OF DEPRESSIVE DISORDERS

Depressive syndromes can be divided into several groups of disorders, each with a different prognosis. These are shown in Table 24–1, and their definitions follow:

1. Primary depression—depression that occurs by itself without a *pre-existing* psychiatric condition or physical illness.

2. Secondary depression—depression that occurs in the presence of a pre-existing psychiatric condition or a severe or life-threatening physical illness.

Primary affective disorders are classified as unipolar or bipolar. Unipolar illness is manifested by depression only. Bipolar disease is manifested by episodes of both depression and mania or hypomania (a milder form of mania). The distinction between unipolar and bipolar depression is based on a number of biologic differences that have become apparent in the last decade or two. There is evidence that the clinical courses of unipolar and bipolar disorders are different, and family histories and genetic studies have shown different types of inheritance for these classifications (see Table 24–1).

In family practice, secondary depression is relatively common, occurring in individuals with alcoholism, severe personality disorders (especially antisocial), and the neuroses (anxiety, hysterical, and obsessive-compulsive). Secondary depression as a concomitant of a severe or terminal illness is also common in primary care.

The usefulness of this dichotomy between primary and secondary depression is twofold. First, it encourages the physician to seek other important psychiatric and medical conditions; second, it is a first step toward assessment of suicide potential. Primary depressives have a high risk of suicide (15 per cent lifetime risk of death by suicide), whereas secondary depressives

TABLE 24–1. CLASSIFICATION OF DEPRESSIVE DISORDERS

	Primary Depression		Secondary Depression
	Unipolar Depression	*Bipolar Depression*	**Secondary Depression**
Pre-existing psychiatric condition	None	None	Many conditions common in primary care: alcoholism, antisocial personality, anxiety neurosis, hysterical neurosis, chronic organic brain syndrome
Course of depression Common age of onset	30–40	20–30	Depends on primary illness
Duration	Long	Short	Not clear
Lifetime number of episodes	Few	Many	Not clear
Remission	Generally good	Frequently residual mild mood swings and few symptoms (e.g., sleep disturbance)	Not clear
Family history	High incidence of depression and in some families alcoholism	Condition transmitted as X-linked dominant in *some* families	Usually higher incidence of primary psychiatric condition (e.g., alcoholism, neurosis, etc.)
	No mania in family	High incidence of depression *and* mania	

generally do not (with the one notable exception of alcoholics).

COURSE OF DEPRESSION

Depression is a spontaneously remitting episodic condition. The average length of depressive episodes in primary depression is approximately 2 to 3 months. However, individuals vary greatly, with some being depressed for 1 or 2 years or even longer. The general outlook is for over 90 per cent of episodes to clear spontaneously. The onset of depression is usually datable by the patient by changes in psychosocial functioning. This is especially true in bipolar depression, in which change may be abrupt and dramatic, but is less true in secondary depression, in which onset may be more insidious and more difficult to detect because of confusion with the symptoms of the already present primary psychiatric condition, such as alcoholism.

Symptoms

Symptoms may vary widely within episodes but usually consist of those mentioned in the criteria for diagnosis. In any individual, certain symptoms will be more prominent. For example, students in college might be more likely to complain about lack of concentration, whereas individuals who are not in a situation requiring use of their concentrative faculties might complain of other symptoms, such as somatic disorders. Generally, during a depression, symptoms occur most of the time. However, some are rather episodic. For example, anxiety attacks which are very common during depression, may occur only a few times over the course of several weeks or months of depression, but when they do occur, the attacks are usually so dramatic that the individual consults a physician.

In general, mood is also uniformly lowered during a depression. However, it is important to note that many individuals may experience occasional days when mood and other symptoms are much improved. This is important for the physician and the patient to appreciate, since improvement must be measured by changes in mood average over a period of several days or weeks, rather than momentary feelings that occur at the time the patient is

seen in the office. The fluctuating quality of depression is important to patients, and they should be taught to expect a certain amount of variability. This is especially true in bipolar depression in which marked mood swings occur dramatically, often without warning. Toward the end of a depression, when the individual is experiencing more good days than bad, these mood swings may be especially troublesome and discouraging because of the contrast afforded by the alternating good days. In most individuals, depressions remit over a period of time, but in some, especially the bipolar, the swing back to normal may be more sudden and dramatic and even swing over into a manic or hypomanic episode.

Age and Sex Incidence

In general, there seem to be more women than men affected by depression. This is especially true for the unipolar type of depression but is somewhat less true for the bipolar type. Sex incidences for various secondary depressions have yet to be worked out, but, again, in general, more women than men are affected, especially in conditions such as hysterical neurosis. This is important from a psychosocial point of view, since depressed women generally have severe difficulties in areas of the home and family, and thus much family disruption can be expected in the presence of depression. Age of onset for the different types of depression varies, and the duration of different episodes and the free intervals between them also vary according to the type of depression, as shown in Table 24–1.

The family histories of patients with depression are quite characteristic for a number of features. First, there is generally more depression in other family members than in the general population. In certain types of depression, notably early onset unipolar depression, patients frequently have family members with alcoholism as well as depression. The rate of suicides is also significantly increased in families of depressives, especially those with primary depression. Occasionally, the family history is of importance in suggesting a diagnosis of depression in a patient who presents with a picture of atypical, vague complaints. Family history is also important in that there is evidence that the types of depression (unipolar or bipolar) run in families, and there is some evidence for a genetic factor in depression. This can be used for diagnostic help. For example, given an individual with a depression who has a family member with a clear-cut case of bipolar depression, one should strongly consider a diagnosis of bipolar depression in the patient in spite of that individual's not having had a prior episode of mania.

Complications

No discussion of the course of depression would be complete without mentioning some of the complications that beset depressives. Suicide is the most drastic. Studies have shown that depressives account for close to half of completed suicides. Most of these suicidal patients had visited a physician in the month prior to their death, yet few were treated for depression. Failure to detect depression was the apparent error. This emphasizes the important role of primary physicians in suicide prevention.

Psychosocial problems are marked during depressions, and people tend to make significant and far-reaching changes in their lives, such as dropping out of school, obtaining a divorce, or changing jobs. Self-medication is an important complication with some depressives, the commonest forms being alcohol and diet pills of the amphetamine type. The latter are used because of their effect on energy, and the patient may become habituated to amphetamines as a result. Alcohol is often employed for its effect on general nervousness and is used as a hypnotic at bedtime. Some studies of alcoholics have revealed that many are really primary depressives who have become alcoholic during the course of their depressive illness. This is especially true of women, and primary depression should be considered in those who present with an alcoholism problem.

Correlation with Life Events

Life events have long been noted to be associated with the depressive syndromes. While there is inconclusive evidence of the importance of such events in all kinds of depression, studies have shown that disturbing life events, such as the death of a loved one or another loss situation, often precede the onset of depressive symptoms by a few weeks or months. The clearest example of this type of grief reaction is the depressive syndrome that occurs in large numbers of widows and widowers following the deaths of their spouses. Over half of these individuals will have a significant depressive syndrome, and 1 year following the death of the spouse, approximately a quarter of such individuals will have significant depressive symptomatology. The role of such losses in other types of depressive syndromes is by no means as clear-cut. Many individuals who report precipitating events are actually found to have suffered from depressive symptoms prior to the reported events. Indeed, in some cases it is clear that the altered behavior brought on by the depression may even have caused the so-called precipitating event.

DIFFERENTIAL DIAGNOSIS

Physical Disorders

Once a diagnosis of depressive syndrome is made, it is important to seek out and treat serious physical conditions that can cause depression.

Endocrine disturbances can be associated with mental changes. The commonest is hypothyroidism. Far rarer are hypoparathyroidism and hyperadrenalism (Cushing's syndrome). Exogenous sources of hormone should also be considered. Potent adrenal hormones are commonly given for some conditions (i.e., allergies, collagen diseases), and the hormones in oral contraceptives have been implicated in causing significant mood changes.

Among the infectious diseases, brucellosis is perhaps the one most prone to present as vague aches and pains, fatigue, depression, and a low-grade fever that may escape notice. The depression following a bout of influenza or hepatitis is often difficult to differentiate from primary depression.

Depression is a prominent part of the symptomatology caused by certain toxic chemicals. Bromism and iodism are certainly less common than formerly, but may still occur. Excessive ingestion of vitamin D can produce muscular weakness, paresthesias, anorexia, weight loss, lethargy or depression, headache, and exfoliative dermatitis, as well as urologic changes and calcific deposits in the kidneys, bronchi, blood vessels, and periarticular and subcutaneous tissues.

Many commonly prescribed drugs may also produce depression as a side effect of usually therapeutic doses. Some of the more common are (1) diuretics, e.g., acetazolamide; (2) steroids; (3) atropine, belladonna, and hyoscyamine; (4) estrogens; (5) antipsychotics, e.g., haloperidol; (6) levodopa; (7) antihypertensives, e.g., reserpine, methyldopa, and hydralazine; and (8) antineoplastic drugs, e.g., vinblastine sulfate, vincristine sulfate, and others.

Some of these drugs are used for symptomatic treatment of vague, undifferentiated somatic complaints of the patient with depression. Thus, the treatment may needlessly complicate and delay the discovery of the true diagnosis of depression.

Perhaps the most difficult differentiation arises when the patient's complaints of malaise, vague abdominal discomfort, and weight loss raise the suspicion of an occult malignancy in the mind of the physician. (Perhaps the same suspicion in the mind of the patient accounts for his presence in the examining room at this time.) In this instance, the physician must, of course, take all reasonable measures to rule out such a diagnosis and at the same time avoid allowing the patient to become hopelessly discouraged by the possibility of finding such a malignancy. The physician must maintain the most optimistic attitude his conscience will allow, while providing psychotherapeutic support and perhaps antidepressant medication. Patients have become suicidal during the diagnostic search for a nonexistent cancer.

With most patients in whom a diagnosis of depressive syndrome is made, there may be some question in the physician's mind of ruling out one or more of the physical conditions just mentioned. This does not mean that supportive psychologic treatment for the depressive syndrome, including more definitive treatment with antidepressant medication, cannot be started while the medical work-up is progressing. Generally, current antidepressive treatment causes little interference with medical diagnostic tests. Patients may languish for weeks with an untreated depression while a myriad of diagnostic procedures

are scheduled, run, and interpreted. It is our usual practice to start treatment of the depression while conducting further indicated diagnostic studies.

Other Psychiatric Disorders

There are several important psychiatric conditions that are often confused with primary depression. The commonest of these are conditions in which anxiety attacks are prominent, namely anxiety neurosis, phobic neurosis, hysterical neurosis, and, to a lesser extent, obsessive neurosis. Because anxiety attacks can and do occur in primary depression, there is understandable confusion. One of the commonest errors in primary care is overlooking a depression in someone with an "anxiety-tension" state. However, the most important distinguishing point is that individuals with the neurotic conditions just listed usually have a history of symptoms diagnostic of these conditions going back in time. Primary depressives, on the other hand, usually have developed anxiety attacks only during depressive episodes.

The second differential diagnosis of importance occurs in elderly patients. Depression in the elderly frequently has the appearance of a mild or moderate dementia, with agitation, memory problems, confusion in thinking, and even disorientation. A history of previous depressive episodes and a normal electroencephalogram (EEG) are helpful. Psychiatric consultations might be considered in these difficult cases.

A third important differentiation for the patient with a depressive syndrome is determining whether or not some other psychiatric condition is also present. In primary care, these conditions are likely to be alcoholism and the various neuroses, especially hysterical neurosis. (See Chapter 23 for diagnosis of these conditions.)

The final psychiatric differentiation of some importance to the patient's prognosis and management is in primary depression. Does the individual have unipolar or bipolar disease? Determination of the type of primary affective disorder on the basis of clinical criteria in a given episode of depression may be inexact. Patients may present to the physician or even be hospitalized several times for depression before an episode of manic behavior occurs. Thus, what appears to be unipolar depression early in the course of illness may evolve into, or later manifest itself as, bipolar disease. Sometimes careful history-gathering is required to learn of previous episodes of depression. Families and friends of the patient appear to be quite tolerant of the behavioral changes in the person who is depressed. Interestingly, they are far less tolerant of the flamboyance, various excesses of activity, and financial extravagances of the person in a manic episode. If the first contact with the physician is precipitated by mania, careful history-taking will often reveal one or more preceding episodes of depression. However, in long-term follow-up of a group of patients with diagnosed unipolar affective disorder, less than 5 per cent subsequently developed bipolar disease.[4]

The distinction can be of considerable importance to the patient and the physician, especially in selecting medications for the prevention of a recurrence. As discussed later in this chapter, the tricyclic antidepressants work well in the treatment of depressives with either unipolar or bipolar affective disease. Treatment with lithium salts as long-range prophylactic measures has proved to be of benefit, especially in bipolar patients.

A bipolar diagnosis can be made on the basis of an episode of mania in the patient or can be inferred from a family history, when a relative such as a parent, sibling, or child has had a proven manic episode. The criteria for the diagnosis of manic syndrome are at least 2 weeks of euphoria or high mood or irritability and at least three of the following: (1) hyperactivity, including motor, social, and sexual activity; (2) push of speech, i.e., pressure to keep talking; (3) flight of ideas, i.e., racing thoughts; (4) gandiosity; (5) decreased need for sleep; and (6) distractibility.[5]

Some of these symptoms can only be identified by a mental status examination. In patients presenting with depression, obviously a history of a manic episode must be sought. Useful questions to determine previous manic episodes are directed at periods of decreased need for sleep, increased energy, excessive social activity, increased or unwise spending, and grandiose ideas, such as excessive interest in religion or saving the world. Friends or relatives are often helpful sources of information about prior manic episodes, since they are often made very uncomfortable or embarrassed by the patient's manic behavior.

MANAGEMENT OF DEPRESSION

Hospitalization

Most depressed patients seen in family practice can be managed as outpatients. Some, however, will require hospitalization. Criteria for hospitalization of depressed patients are relatively few. First and foremost is the consideration of the danger of suicide or self-injury. Long-term studies of depressives have shown that over a lifetime approximately 15 per cent of them will die by their own hand. Depressives who are at considerable risk for suicidal behavior are those with primary affective disorders (both unipolar and bipolar) and alcoholics. These diagnoses carry significantly more risk of suicide than does secondary depression in individuals with personality disorders or neuroses.

In assessing a patient's suicide potential, evaluate the patient's suicidal ideation and plans for suicide. These topics should be discussed as part of the assessment of each depressed patient. The physician should not be fearful that discussing suicide with the patient may lead to suicidal behavior, because it is not unusual for the idea to have already crossed the patient's mind. Individuals who admit to considerable suicidal ideation, who have thought of a plan to carry out self-injury, and who furthermore have such means at their disposal should be considered serious suicidal risks. Men are more likely than women to make a successful suicide attempt. This is especially true of individuals over 40 years of age. Individuals who live alone or who have just been separated from a family living situation are more prone to suicide (a characteristic of alcoholics, in whom the risk of suicide is high soon after being separated or divorced). Individuals who have made previous unsuccessful suicide attempts are also much more likely to kill themselves.

If several of the criteria just mentioned are present, the individual should be considered a serious suicidal risk and appropriate measures, such as hospitalization, taken. In the hospital, suitable suicide precautions can be implemented and immediate therapy instituted. It is also important to continue to assess suicidal potential throughout the course of any treatment, since individuals may change their attitudes towards suicide, especially when faced with long treatment that to them appears to be hopeless or unsuccessful.

While suicidal potential is probably the greatest cause for hospitalization, there are other cogent reasons. For example, very depressed individuals are often unable to function in their usual roles. If the poor functioning is such as to interfere with the individual's ability to carry out essential activities, such as eating and clothing oneself, then serious consideration must be given to hospitalization, especially if such a patient does not have good social support to supply the necessities of life.

Assuring cooperation with treatment is also an important reason for considering hospitalization. If an individual is so depressed or has personality traits that militate against cooperation in taking medications and following other instructions as an outpatient, then hospitalization must be considered. As with determination of suicidal potential, reassessment of these other factors should be continued throughout outpatient treatment, since depressions may fluctuate markedly, and significant deterioration in psychosocial adjustment may occur after the initial assessment.

Outpatient Management

Outpatient management may be considered whenever suicidal potential and the other factors just mentioned are low or nonexistent. In addition, a most important consideration is the ability and willingness of the patient to carry out the regimen as prescribed by the physician. A frank discussion of what outpatient treatment will entail is essential. How the patient reacts to information that medication must be taken and that certain duties or jobs may be curtailed should be carefully evaluated. Individuals who might benefit from antidepressant medications but who indicate considerable reluctance about taking them are a special problem. If such patients are not depressed enough to warrant hospitalization, one might explore the patient's reasons for not wishing to take medication. Often a reason is found that the physician can deal with. In negotiating with such reluctant patients, it is important not to close the door to further treatment.

Medication

Antidepressant medication of some type will probably be an important part of treatment of depressives, whether managed as outpatients or inpatients. Medication is helpful in primary and secondary depressions. Medications, however, should not be given without appropriate psychologic management, which will be discussed in the following sections.

Tricyclic Antidepressants. Since both unipolar and bipolar depressions respond to tricyclic medication, this is the usual drug of choice in treating depression. Some of the more commonly used tricyclics are presented in Table 24–2. It is important to note that some of the side effects of these tricyclics are useful in controlling the symptoms of depression. For example, somnolence, which is more marked with some of the tricyclics, can be used to ad-

TABLE 24–2. COMMONLY USED ANTIDEPRESSANTS

Antidepressant	Outpatient Dosage (mg./24 hrs.)	Hypnotic Effect	Anticholinergic Potency	Important Drug Interactions
Tricyclics				
Imipramine	75–250	Mild	Moderate	MAOI's
Amitriptyline	75–250	Marked	Marked	MAOI's
Protriptyline	15–60	Very little	Marked	MAOI's
Doxepin	75–300	Marked	Moderate	MAOI's
MAOI's				
Tranylcypromine	20–40	Very little	Marked	Severe reactions with
Phenelzine	45–75	Very little	Marked	sympathomimetics and foods with tyramine

vantage when initial or terminal sleep disturbance is a special problem by giving the antidepressant in one large dose at bedtime. Individuals who have hypersomnia as a problem of depression may have increased difficulty with oversleeping if given an antidepressant such as amitriptyline and might better be started on some tricyclic with very little hypnotic effect, such as protriptyline.

One of the commonest problems encountered in management of depressives is failure to use adequate doses of antidepressant medication. It is important to try to reach an adequate dosage level for each patient, so that if response does not occur, appropriate action can be taken, such as switching to another antidepressant. Since improvement with tricyclics generally does not occur until 1 or 2 weeks after starting the medication, an optimum dosage is not easy to arrive at. It is our custom to try to have adults take at least 150 mg. daily of such common tricyclics as imipramine, amitriptyline, or desipramine for a 2 week period. If improvement does not follow this regimen, medication can be increased until improvement follows or significant side effects occur. Our custom is to increase the dose a total of 50 to 100 mg. per day over a

TABLE 24–3. TYRAMINE-RESTRICTED DIET

Description

Foods containing tyramine should be avoided in the diet of patients who are receiving monoamine oxidase inhibiting (MAOI) drugs. Abnormally elevated blood pressures have been found to occur after the ingestion of tyramine by persons receiving MAOI's.

Approximate Composition

Calories	2,364	Sodium, mg.	4,225
Protein, gm.	94	Potassium, mg.	3,325
Fat, gm.	92		
Carbohydrate, gm.	290		

Foods Allowed and Foods to Avoid

Food Group	Foods Allowed	Foods to Avoid
Beverages	All except those to be avoided	Coffee, beer, wine, and liquors (ethanol)
Breads	All others	Bread or crackers containing cheese
Cereals	All	None
Desserts	Desserts made with foods allowed	Desserts containing items that must be avoided
Eggs	All	None
Fats	All	None
Fruits and fruit juices	All except those to be avoided	Figs, raisins
Meat, fish, poultry, and cheese	Cottage cheese, cream cheese, and all meats except those to be avoided	Aged cheeses such as Cheddar, Gruyère, Stilton, Swiss, and the like; beef and chicken livers; smoked or pickled fish
Potatoes and substitutes	All	None
Soups	Soups made with foods allowed	Soups containing items that must be avoided
Sugar and sweets	All except those to be avoided	Sweets containing items that must be avoided
Vegetables and vegetable juices	All except those to be avoided	Broad beans, Chinese peas, Italian green beans
Condiments	All except those to be avoided	Chocolate, soy sauce
Miscellaneous	All except items to be avoided	Yeast concentrates, yogurt, and sour cream

TABLE 24–4. SAMPLE MENU FOR TYRAMINE-RESTRICTED DIET

Breakfast
1/2 cup frozen orange juice
1/2 cup Cream of Wheat cereal
1 egg, soft cooked
1 slice toast, white enriched
1 tsp. butter
1 tbsp. grape jelly
1 cup milk
2 tsp. sugar
Tea

Luncheon
3/4 cup creamed chicken on 1 biscuit
1/2 cup green beans
1/2 sliced tomato on lettuce
2 tsp. mayonnaise
1 slice bread, white enriched
1 tsp. butter
1/2 cup canned peaches
1 slice angel cake
1 cup milk
1 tsp. sugar
Tea

Dinner
3 oz. roast beef sirloin
1/2 cup cubed white potato
1/4 cup beef broth gravy
1/2 cup cooked carrots
3/4 cup tossed lettuce salad
1 tbsp. French dressing
1 slice bread, white enriched
1 tsp. butter
1/2 cup sherbet
3 vanilla wafers
1 cup milk
1 tsp. sugar
Tea

week's time and then maintain that dosage level for a period of at least 1 week to 10 days.

Monoamine Oxidase Inhibitors. If improvement does not follow what appears to be an adequate dosage of a tricyclic, the physician has the option of switching to a different medication. A different tricyclic is a possibility, or the physician can elect to stop the tricyclics and after a period of a week start a monoamine oxidase inhibitor (MAOI). Use of an MAOI requires a patient who is reliable in taking medication and in following instructions regarding dietary limitations. If an MAOI is given, the patient should be instructed to avoid foods rich in tyramine and to avoid medications with any sympathomimetic activity. Because of the greater seriousness of side effects, MAOI's have recently been in relative disfavor but nevertheless are effective in treating some patients who do not respond to tricyclic medication. Diet sheets that we give patients who are to be started on MAOI's are shown in Tables 24–3 and 24–4. Such sheets should be given to the patient and the diet thoroughly discussed at the time the medication is prescribed. The patient should be warned to report imme-

diately to the physician serious side effects such as headache, flushing, or diaphoresis.

Lithium. In individuals who have bipolar depressions, lithium can sometimes be used effectively. Before starting the patient on lithium, it is our custom first to obtain some measures of kidney function, such as creatinine clearance, an electrocardiogram (ECG) for older individuals, and a measure of thyroid function, since long-term lithium treatment has been shown to produce goiter and hypothyroidism in some patients. Usually in treating depression a serum lithium level of 1.0 to 1.2 mEq. per liter will be adequate. To reach this level it will be necessary to give the average adult about 1200 mg. of lithium carbonate by mouth in a daily divided dosage. We start patients on two 300 mg. tablets the first day, increase the dosage to four tablets on the second day, and obtain a serum lithium determination on the morning of the third day prior to giving that day's dose of lithium. This early measurement of the lithium level will help detect individuals who, in spite of normal kidney function, reach high and potentially toxic levels of lithium on relatively low doses. We then follow the serum lithium levels at approximately 5 day intervals, since after a change in lithium dosage, time is needed to stabilize lithium in the blood and body fluids.

A physician who feels uncomfortable about managing lithium or has had no experience with this drug may certainly elect to refer his patient to a physician or psychiatrist who can carry out this form of treatment. If a patient is maintained at a serum lithium level of 1.0 to 1.2 mEq. per liter for a week to 10 days and does not improve, then lithium may be cautiously increased, but the physician must keep in mind that the threshold of toxicity may be quite low in some individuals. Patients on long-term lithium therapy should be reassessed at 3 to 6 month intervals for goiter and hypothyroidism.

Combining Antidepressants. Combinations of antidepressants should be considered in many situations. For example, most tricyclic antidepressants or MAOI's may be given along with lithium, and patients who have not responded adequately to lithium might be given a small dose of either an MAOI or a tricyclic antidepressant. Combinations of medications that are not recommended are those involving MAOI's and tricyclic medication or MAOI's and stimulants such as amphetamines or methylphenidate. Such combinations have been associated with severe and even fatal reactions, and their use has been expressly and specifically forbidden by the Food and Drug Administration.

Tranquilizers. Although tricyclics, MAOI's, and lithium constitute the most specific and effective medications for managing depression, other medications have a limited place in the general management of this disorder. One of the commoner symptoms of depression is anxiety, with restlessness and agitation, sometimes bordering on panic. Such marked anxiety may respond to the addition of a minor tranquilizer or small doses of a major tranquilizer. For example, perphenazine and amitriptyline are available in a combination tablet. It is not necessary for the physician to use such a combination tablet, since by prescribing such medications separately, he can give his patient the benefit of a wider variety and range of dosage that might more nearly match the patient's needs. However, the convenience of taking one tablet as opposed to two must also be considered.

Hypnotics. Sleep disturbance, a very prominent symptom, may be so marked that even a strongly hypnotic antidepressant given at bedtime does not suffice. Under these conditions, other hypnotics might be prescribed, generally for short periods of time, until the antidepressant itself is effective. Because an overdose of many of the barbiturates is an extremely efficient means of suicide, it is important that the physician consider this when prescribing such medications. More recent drugs, such as flurazepam, with relatively low suicide potential, might be prescribed in place of the more toxic preparations. In general, we do not advocate prescribing large amounts of tricyclic or MAOI antidepressants at one time, since tricyclic antidepressants and MAOI's are also toxic in large amounts. Weekly prescriptions can minimize the quantity of drugs available for impulsive suicide attempts. It is our custom to prescribe no more than 2.5 gm. total of a tricyclic at any one time.

SIDE EFFECTS OF MEDICATION. Side effects should be dealt with in a positive fashion. The patient should be told that common side effects such as dry mouth, temporary sleepiness, and so forth will occur but are not potentially serious and that their occurrence means that the drug is working. The physician should ask about side effects at each visit and assess their seriousness. A common result of simple side effects is that patients stop taking their antidepressants. Further encouraging information about side effects can be imparted to patients: many of the anticholinergic effects and the somnolence become less marked with time. In general, however, it is the side effects that militate against higher doses of antidepressants. Postural hypotension is probably the commonest reaction, and potentially the most serious. Side effects also severely limit the use of antidepressants in individuals who have had recent myocardial infarctions or have narrow angle glaucoma or prostatism.

In dealing with side effects, the physician must distinguish between symptoms of depression and symptoms caused by the antidepressant. If a drug is strongly suspected of producing a symptom, then altering a dosage is a fairly effective way of determining cause and effect. The initial side effects can be minimized by low starting doses of antidepressants (e.g., 25 mg.

imipramine h.s.) and increasing the drug by increments of 25 mg. every day or two until 150 mg. a day is reached.

DURATION OF PRESCRIBING MEDICATION. The length of time that treatment must be continued with depressives is extremely variable. One of the still unsolved questions is how long to keep people on antidepressant medication once depressive symptoms have resolved. It is our practice to keep them on such medication for at least 3 months after symptoms seem to have resolved and then gradually taper off the medications over a period of several weeks or a month. Should depressive symptoms recur at this time, it is always possible to increase the dosage again until symptoms remit and try tapering off 4 to 6 weeks later.

Psychologic Management

Counseling the individual with depression and members of his family and associates is an essential part of the proper management of depression. Patients frequently do not appreciate the magnitude or the all-pervasiveness of changes associated with depression. Accordingly, one of the most valuable steps that a physician may take is to summarize for the patient those signs and symptoms of depression that are present. As part of this summary, it is important to point out to the patient how these symptoms may significantly interfere with his life. This is especially important, because patients frequently do not see difficulties with personal interactions or difficulties at work in terms of depression. They more often see these events in terms of other people causing problems or the circumstances at work being more than they can handle. Pointing out to the patient that depression makes one more irritable and, as a result, affects interpersonal relationships can be helpful in enabling an individual to get along better with others during a period of depression.

Similarly, students who have lost interest in schoolwork as a result of a depression may be relieved to know that their loss of interest does not mean that a long-cherished vocational goal need be abandoned or that there is something morally wrong with them for not showing more interest in studies. In conducting this type of educational therapy, it is useful to find out which of the symptoms are most trouble-some and then to begin to explain these to the patient in terms of his depression. Many individuals are relieved to learn that all of these strange and upsetting things that have been happening to them are part of a transient mood disturbance.

Another very important part of the education of the patient is imparting information about the natural history of the affective disorder. In the depths of a depression, most individuals are quite willing to believe that they will never get better and that the future is dreary and hopeless. It is useful to point out to patients that although they may feel this way, this is part of the depressive perception and will improve with time, along with other depressive symptoms. Indeed, practically every depression improves spontaneously with time. If an individual has had previous depressive episodes from which recovery was complete, it can be pointed out that past experience should demonstrate to the individual that recovery can and does occur. The *element of hope,* an important ingredient in any cure, should thus be injected early into the therapeutic alliance.[11] It can also be pointed out that the efficacy of various chemical antidepressants lies in their amelioration of depressive symptoms within a very short time. Thus, the patient can see what role antidepressant medication might play in the treatment of the depressive disorder and can be encouraged to watch for the amelioration of his symptom complex.

In addition to education of the patient in the scope and nature of his affective disorder, the physician should obtain as clear an idea as possible of the patient's current adjustment at home, school, or work. The physician can then be in a position to appreciate to what extent the depression is interfering with normal social functioning and to impart to the patient support and advice concerning these very important aspects of his life. Often the physician can talk with the spouse, family, friends, or other significant individuals and obtain an outside view of how the patient's functioning has been affected. Such information should, of course, be solicited only after obtaining the permission of the patient to do so. Most patients are quite willing to have the physician speak to a spouse or other member of the family. In speaking to coworkers or work supervisors, more circumspection is needed. In dealing with any outside informant, whether family member or otherwise, the physician should always be cautious about revealing any confidential information.

The complications of depression in everyday living are incalculable. In general, depression interferes with functioning in such a way that job loss may result, marriages may be terminated, or school and education may be given up for other less demanding activities. One generally useful step in management is to encourage the paitent to postpone any significant major decision regarding change in lifestyle while in the throes of a depression. This includes such decisions as divorce, quitting a job or school, or some other potentially self-destructive step. It should be pointed out that since a depression is a self-limiting process, at some future time not too far in the distance, the individual will be able to get a better perspective of the problem and deal with it more effectively. At the same time this postponement of a major decision gives the individual time to discuss the various aspects of the decision with a counselor, such as the physician (or should the physician elect not to carry out such procedures as marital counseling, these can be undertaken by suitably prepared professionals as part of the program for treatment of the depressive episode).

Having the patient refrain from making decisions can be considered part of a larger principle of management, namely, that of allowing the individual to reduce the current responsibilities that might be extremely difficult to meet in view of the depressive symptomatology. For example, a housewife who is unable to carry out usual functions in the home might be given assistance by either members of her family or hired help, if such is available and the family can afford it. It can be pointed out that reducing social obligations is reasonable and is merely a temporary measure. Young individuals attending school can be encouraged to study only up to their ability and perhaps reduce their course load, postpone examinations, or use other techniques to reduce their work load. In the same vein, short leaves of absence from jobs may be suggested when there is objective evidence that performance on the job is really poor and that continued inferior job performance might lead to serious repercussions.

One of the ubiquitous and most distressing phenomena of depression is the subjective self-deprecatory and nihilistic ideation that leads to conclusions such as "I am worthless," "life is hopeless, or "there is no future." Recently, practical counseling techniques have been devised to encourage the patient to successfully attack this type of thinking. This technique is relatively simple and is clearly described by its originator, Aaron Beck.[2]

Thus, management of individual patients involves (1) educating patients about the natural history of their condition, (2) pointing out areas in which their condition is affecting their everyday adjustment, and (3) trying to manage the environment so as to relieve the individual of some responsibilities that the depression has made it difficult, if not impossible, to fulfill.

In managing patients on an outpatient basis, they must be seen frequently enough for monitoring of significant changes in psychosocial functioning, for compliance in taking medicaton, and for giving the individual sufficient psychologic support. It is our practice to see patients initially on a weekly basis. Between visits, patients can always report by telephone as to the effects of changes in medication or new symptoms or side effects. Each office visit need not be an hour long. While the initial interview might be longer, in order to make all of the assessments previously noted, in follow-up 10 to 15 minute visits are usually all that is required. During this time, symptoms can be evaluated, drug side effects noted, dosages adjusted, and some guidance given regarding social adjustment. If further special counseling is indicated, either extra time can be set aside or the patient can be referred to suitable professionals or paraprofessionals. As control of the depression improves, the interval between visits to the physician can be increased to 2 or 3 weeks. It is important to note, however, that until the individual is completely depression-free, the risk of suicide remains very real. Numbers of patients can and do commit suicide toward the termination of a depression. In part, this may be related to the fact that during depressions marked mood swings are very common, and severe down swings can occur after several days of feeling good. If the patient is prepared by the physician to accept such fluctuations as part of the natural history of the disorder, such mood swings are better tolerated.

In the management of depressives, the major difficulty often lies with the problem of recurrent depressive episodes. There is evidence that for some patients lithium carbonate maintenance treatment may be effective in preventing recurrences, especially of bipolar affective episodes. For individuals who have had frequent serious depressive episodes, the use of lithium prophylaxis might be considered. Also of some value in prophylaxis are tricyclic antidepressants administered in low doses, for example, 75 to 100 mg. daily over an extended period of time. However, the latter medications are more expensive than lithium, which might be a factor in the physician's consideration.

Electroconvulsive Therapy

Most depressions seen in general practice will undoubtedly respond to the measures just outlined. However, there are always a certain number of patients who do not respond well to medication or who cannot tolerate antidepressant medications for various reasons. For such individuals, help is available in the form of electroconvulsive therapy (ECT). Although there has been considerable deprecatory discussion in recent years about ECT, especially in the lay press, it still remains one of the most effective treatments for depression. In essence, ECT consists of passing through the motor cortex a small current of electricity sufficient to cause a grand mal seizure. When first used, ECT was given without anesthetic or muscle relaxants, and the procedure was not only distasteful to those who witnessed it but frightening and occasionally physically injurious to the patients. However, modern techniques of administering ECT have made it a relatively harmless procedure. Generally, following premedication with atropine or a similar drug, the patient is anesthetized with a rapidly acting intravenous anesthetic such as sodium methohexital. A muscle relaxant is administered, followed by the electric current, resulting in a greatly modified grand mal seizure. Usually the tonic and clonic contractions are so slight that it is difficult to detect that a seizure is actually occurring.

As a result of this modified treatment, complications arising from severe tonic muscle contraction very rarely occur. The risk added by being given an anesthetic is very small. The usual course of ECT treatments is a series of three treatments per week for a total of eight to twelve treatments. One of the most disturbing side effects of ECT is its effect on recent and remote memory, which subsides within a short time after cessation of treatments. However, the individual and his family are usually quite concerned about such side effects and require a great deal of support until the brain syndrome subsides and memory returns. ECT treatments are generally given in a hospital setting, although they can be administered to outpatients and are often effective in individuals who have failed to improve on adequate doses of tricyclics or other antidepressants.

Patient Referral

In dealing with the many psychosocial problems that depressives, their families, and their associates face, it is sometimes helpful to consider referral for marriage counseling or for more extensive supportive treatment, if these cannot be provided by the physician. Patients who represent serious suicidal risks may also require referral if the physician lacks access to an adequate local facility for their hospitalization. For individuals who are still depressed after adequate trials of tricyclics or other antidepressants, the option of ECT should be considered. Other patients who may require referral are individuals who suffer repeated depressive episodes and for whom there may be a question of the use of lithium prophylaxis, both to manage the current depression and to prevent future episodes. Of course, if the physician or patient is dissatisfied with diagnosis or progress, then consultation would be a wise recourse. One of the commonest reasons for referral arises in patients with secondary depression for management of their underlying condition, e.g., alcoholism.

REFERENCES

1. Ayd, J. F., Jr.: Symposium on depression. Dis. Nerv. Syst., 37:1, 1976.
2. Beck, A. T.: Cognitive Therapy and the Emotional Disorders. New York, International Universities Press, Inc., 1976.
3. Cadoret, R. J., and King, L. J.: Psychiatry in Primary Care. St. Louis, The C. V. Mosby Co., 1974.

4. Dunner, D. L., Fleiss, J. L., and Fieve, R. R.: The course of development of mania in patients with recurrent depression. Am. J. Psychiatry, *133*:8, 1976.

5. Feighner, J. P., Robins, E., Guze, S. B., et al.: Diagnostic criteria for use in psychiatric research. Arch. Gen. Psychiatry, *25*:57, 1972.

6. Flach, R., and Draghi, S.: The Nature and Treatment of Depression. New York, John Wiley & Sons, Inc., 1975.

7. Gurland, B. J.: The comparative frequency of depression in various adult age groups. J. Gerontol., *31*:3, 1976.

8. Hodgkins, K.: Educational implications of the Virginia study. J. Fam. Pract., *3*:1, 1976.

9. Ketai, R.: Family practitioners' knowledge about treatment of depressive illness. J.A.M.A., *235*:24, 1976.

10. Marsland, D. W., Wood, M., and Mayo, F.: Content of family practice. J. Fam. Pract., *3*:1, 1976.

11. Wetzel, R. D.: Hopelessness, depression and suicide intent. Arch. Gen. Psychiatry, *33*:106, 1976.

Chapter 25

SCHIZOPHRENIA

by HARRIS S. GOLDSTEIN,
and FRANK C. SNOPE

INTRODUCTION

DEFINITION

Schizophrenia is classified as a functional psychosis along with the major affective disorders (depression and mania) and the paranoid states. It is functional, since psychosocial rather than physiologic factors are thought to be dominant in its etiology. The term *psychosis* refers to the severe degree of impairment generally (but not always) characteristic of the illness. Paradoxically, a patient with schizophrenia in remission may still be considered suffering from a schizophrenic psychosis but may not be considered psychotic. The term *psychotic* refers to impairment of mental functioning severe enough to make an individual unable to carry out the usual requirements of daily living. These involve maintaining self-care, retaining the ability to judge what is real and what is imaginary, distinguishing between right and wrong, caring for one's daily needs, and controlling one's impulses within a socially accepted range. Thus, a patient preoccupied with his delusional fears may fail to eat adequately or to care for his personal hygiene, and may be unable to go to work for fear that his "enemies are going to get him."

What distinguishes schizophrenia from the other functional psychoses is that the schizophrenic patient suffers from disturbances in thinking as well as of mood and behavior. The presence of a thought disorder is the central symptom and is necessary, although not sufficient, for establishing the diagnosis. The affective disorders, in contrast, have as their primary characteristic a disorder of mood, either marked depression or elation, while paranoid states primarily have a delusion from which the psychotic process is elaborated.

Of the functional mental disorders, schizophrenia is the most disabling. Although the number of schizophrenic patients occupying hospital beds has dropped dramatically in recent years, schizophrenia remains the major nonorganic reason for hospitalization.

RECENT TRENDS

In the past two decades, the movement toward deinstitutionalization of the mentally ill has had a major impact on the care of schizophrenic patients.[1] The effect on the family physician is correspondingly great. In 1955, the daily inpatient census of state and county mental hospitals reached a peak of 559,000 patients. Half the hospital beds in the United States were occupied by mental patients, of whom the majority were diagnosed as schizophrenic. Even before the advent of the major tranquilizers, it was recognized that the underfunded and understaffed public institutions could not effectively serve this patient population. The Joint Commission on Mental Illness and Mental Health established in 1955 by the American Medical Association (AMA) and the American Psychiatric Association (APA) to study the mental health services delivery system recommended community-oriented care. This policy of community-oriented care has meant the reduction in public hospital inpatients from 559,000 in 1955 to 215,000 in 1974, a drop of 62 per cent. A major consequence of this marked reduction in the public mental hospital census is that many more patients with a schizophrenic disturbance are living in their home communities.

As part of the policy of deinstitutionalization, community mental health centers were to have provided care for the seriously disturbed patient. In practice, this shift in care most often has not been successfully implemented, even where such centers have been established. In many other communities such centers do not exist. In many communities, therefore, seriously and chronically disturbed patients rely increasingly on the family physician for continued and definitive treatment.

CLINICAL FEATURES

ONSET

Schizophrenia most commonly has its onset in adolescence or early adult life. Later onset does occasionally occur, with the first psychotic episode appearing in the 40's or later.

Childhood schizophrenia is, by definition, a psychosis with onset prior to adolescence. Etiologically, childhood schizophrenia is probably a different disorder than the classic postpubertal schizophrenia and is only loosely grouped with the adolescent and adult-onset illnesses.

COURSE

There are patients who have had an acute psychotic episode with disturbance in thinking, have been diagnosed as schizophrenic, but have recovered completely without recurrence. These acute single episode illnesses have all the characteristics of schizophrenia, but the prognosis is favorable. However, such is not the typical course. It would appear that in spite of progress in treatment, specifically psychopharmacologic treatment, the patient afflicted with schizophrenia has a chronic illness, much as a patient with a systemic illness, such as rheumatoid arthritis. Similar to the rheumatoid patient, the course of the schizophrenic patient's illness may take several forms: (1) acute onset with periodic exacerbations and increasing impairment, (2) gradual onset with progressive impairment, or (3) gradual onset with episodic exacerbations and chronic impairment. The analogy to rheumatoid arthritis is useful to keep in mind. When a rheumatoid patient is first examined, there may be some clinical indicators as to likely course, but one cannot prognosticate with any great certainty. In following the patient over time, the pattern that emerges predicts more clearly what is to be expected. Similarly, in treating a patient with schizophrenia over time, seeing him through several exacerbations will provide the knowledge as to the pattern the illness is taking.

SYMPTOMS

Cognition

The symptoms of schizophrenia are multitudinous, perplexing, and often frightening to family and friends. The fear engendered is, in large part, due to the irrationality of the patient. Irrationality, or disturbance in thought processes, is the central symptom of this complex syndrome. The thought disorder of schizophrenia manifests itself in a variety of ways.[8] The most common is *looseness of associations.* This disorder of thinking, although often subtle, may be observed in the patient's responses to questions. The patient will begin to reply to a question but will go off on a tangent, having difficulty maintaining a thematic focus.

A patient was asked what his father was like. He replied: "My father, he was a carpenter. He built houses. Houses are expensive these days, and expensive things are hard to come by. What kind of car do you drive, doctor?"

Perceptual disturbances are another disorder of thought processes. Perceptual disturbances seem to arise from difficulties in sorting out what are inner experiences and what are experiences in the real world. This failure to be able to "test reality" is extremely disabling and limits the ability to cope. It is akin to living a nightmare. The world is distorted and peopled by fears and shapes that are not perceived by others. These distortions take the form of delusions or hallucinations.

Delusions are beliefs that are not only false but which the patient maintains in spite of reasonable proof to the contrary.

Suspicions and concerns are common to all of us. However, suspicions become gross distortions of reality for the patient (e.g., there is a worldwide conspiracy to poison him), and he becomes paralyzed with fear. Radio commentators may seem to be sending messages to the patient, or the patient may feel that his thoughts are under the control of some outside force. The intensity with which a patient suffering from paranoid delusions is convinced that what he perceives is real may lead the observer to believe the patient's perception of events. At times, detailed review of the basis of his beliefs is required for it to become apparent that the patient is truly delusional.

Along with the paranoid delusions there may be delusions of grandeur. The patient believes himself to be a messenger of God or to possess some secret knowledge of great value.

Hallucinations are defined as hearing or seeing something that does not exist. In schizophrenia, they are most often auditory, although they may also be visual. Most frequently, the voices heard are derogatory, calling the patient names. The names called vary with the historical period and culture. At an earlier time, patients might have heard voices telling them that they had sinned and were in league with the devil. More recently, the voices may call out to the patient that he is a "faggot." On occasion, the voices take the form of command hallucinations, which can be especially ominous. The command hallucination is one in which a voice is heard telling the individual to do something. The act being commanded may include harming himself or others.

Interpersonal Relationships

There is inevitably a marked disturbance in relationships with others. Most characteristic is a general social withdrawal, although this usually is not total. There may be a strong dependence on family members, with major reliance being placed on the one member of the family who has assumed responsibility for the disturbed relative. This special attachment to one person may be a great burden for that individual. The patient's social withdrawal is prompted by intense anxiety that he will be rejected or thought peculiar.

Bizarre Behavior

Because the patient, at least in the acute state, is responding to internal cues, i.e., thoughts, delusions, hallucinations, he may engage in behavior that marks him as unusual. Behavior such as smiling and grimacing to himself, talking to someone who is not there, carrying a myriad of old newspapers in a bag, and the like occurs.

Inappropriate Affect

The observer may sense that the affect displayed by the schizophrenic patient is not appropriate to the events or experiences. For instance, he may relate the death of a parent as an event that is of little moment. Or he may be upset and very anxious over what appears to others as innocuous.

Flat Affect

There is a general sense of impoverishment of emotional life. The patient's voice is monotonous, and his face shows little expression. When one knows such patients closely, one feels that their constricted range of response is a defense against overwhelming anxiety. It's as if they protect themselves from overpowering fears by limiting how much they will let themselves feel.

Motor Disturbance

The patient's behavior may vary from marked agitation with extreme pacing and excitement to immobility. Immobility is not very common, but the rigid postures and waxy flexibility (if the patient's arm is raised by someone, the arm will remain raised) of such patients are dramatic when they occur.

SUBTYPES OF SCHIZOPHRENIA

The classification of the schizophrenic syndrome into subtypes is a useful descriptive device. But it is just that, a descriptive classification without etiologic implications. The subtypes are classified by *predominant* symptoms. They are useful in that they provide an idea of major symptoms and probable course.

Simple

There is a slow withdrawal from social contacts that continues to a state of almost total interpersonal isolation. Apathy is marked, and neglect of personal hygiene usually occurs. Neither hallucinations nor delusions occur, and a thought disorder may be difficult to elicit.

Hebephrenic

Silly and regressive behavior is prominent, with much giggling and other child-like actions being common. Personal hygiene may be neglected, and thought processes are grossly disturbed.

Catatonic

Motor activity disturbance is the most obvious symptom. Two types are distinguished, excited and withdrawn. In the excited type, marked agitation occurs that requires measures to protect the patient. In the withdrawn type, there is a general inhibition of motor activity to the point of stupor at times. Mutism is common in the withdrawn type.

Latent

These patients have many of the classic symptoms — thought disorder, marked difficulties in relationships — but their functioning has not been interfered with to the point of being psychotic.

Residual

This subtype includes individuals who have had a psychotic episode and are now no longer psychotic, but who show signs of schizophrenia, such as restricted affect and thought disorder.

Paranoid

Patients of the paranoid subtype are characteristically hostile and aggressive. They suffer from delusions of persecution, grandeur, or both. Paranoid patients, when acutely ill, are often the most difficult to treat because of their suspiciousness and hostility.

Schizoaffective

In this category are those patients whose symptoms are a mixture of schizophrenia and an affective (either depressive or manic) disorder. Many, if not most, schizophrenic patients may be characterized as depressed, but in patients in the schizoaffective category, the depression or elation is a dominant symptom.

Chronic Undifferentiated

Patients of this subtype have the classic symptoms of the illness, but there is not sufficient predominance of symptoms to classify them under one or the other subtype. Being a mixed-symptom category, it ends up being used more than the others, since often the patient's symptoms are shifting and unclear in their eventual direction.

Childhood

This is an even more heterogeneous group than the adult types and includes all psychoses of childhood, i.e., psychosis with onset before puberty. A label of schizophrenia for most of these disorders is probably not appropriate, as a true thought disorder is not frequently seen. Within this category are several types of childhood psychoses classified on the basis of age at onset.

A psychosis of childhood with onset before 2 years of age is called *infantile autism.* These pathetic children are the most severely disturbed of all psychotic patients. They are not even able to relate to their parents and display little interest in human contact. Autistic children are often preoccupied with inanimate objects, such as record players, and may stare at them for hours. Speech is frequently delayed in development or may be absent. When speech is present, it may not be used for communication with others but as a "talking with oneself." There is also an intense need to maintain a sameness in the environment that leads to panic reactions when changes occur. Some view this most serious of the psychoses as a reaction to parental rejection. Others believe that basic to the psychosis is a central language processing deficit, a type of aphasia, that secondarily leads to withdrawal and psychotic behavior.

When the onset of the psychosis is between 3 and 5 years of age, it usually takes the form of an intense clinging to the mother. The intensity is overwhelming and excludes relating to anyone else. This childhood psychosis is termed a *symbiotic psychosis.*

Psychosis with onset before puberty but after 5 years of age is variously called schizophreniform psychosis, childhood schizophrenia, or, simply, childhood psychosis. The primary symptom is overwhelming anxiety that prevents normal socioemotional development. Hallucinations and delusions are rare before 8 years of age, possibly because fantasy may be mixed with reality as a normal event in that age group. Stereotyped and bizarre behavior may be present, but thought disorders are not often seen in the prepubertal years.

ETIOLOGY

Although schizophrenia is classified as a functional disorder, that is, one for which no organic basis is present, there is considerable controversy as to the extent to which biologic or environmental factors are the major determinants of the illness. The genetic studies of the last few years have shifted the balance in favor of a biologic basis. At the same time, environment, in the form of family and social circumstances, is acknowledged as playing an important role, probably acting on a genetically determined substratum. What remains obscure, but the object of much study, is the mechanism by which a genetic anlage would produce a schizophrenic phenotype.

HEREDITY

The first important evidence for the genetic transmission of schizophrenia was a group of studies reporting a high concordance rate in monozygotic twins. The early twin studies were fraught with methodologic problems. Nonetheless, they focused important attention on the possibility of genetic transmission of a schizophrenic disposition.[4] They were inconclusive because the twins studied not only had a common

inheritance but also a common environment. It was also impossible to have blind controls, since one twin had already been diagnosed as schizophrenic before the study of the other twin was attempted.

Studies of adopted children with schizophrenic biologic parents and of separately raised twins have more recently confirmed the role of genetic make-up.[5] In these studies it was possible to separate environmental and genetic influence. In general, the studies indicate that in approximately 50 per cent of monozygotic twins living apart, if one twin develops the illness, eventually the other will too. The risk of schizophrenia with two schizophrenic parents is about 40 per cent and with one parent about 10 per cent.

If simple genetic transmission were involved, then monozygotic twins would both be schizophrenic in 100 per cent of the cases in which one twin was schizophrenic. That that is not the case points up the large role nongenetic factors must play. One set of factors has to do with birth. Studies have found that when only one twin is afflicted, it is most likely to be the lower birth weight infant, who may have had more complications at delivery. Another set of factors is the emotional environment of the family and of the society.

BIOCHEMICAL FACTORS

Given that there are genetic factors in schizophrenia, *what* is inherited is not clear. Is it an enzyme deficiency or a supersensitivity to stimuli? For some time, work on biochemical neurotransmitters has been prominent in the search for the pathogenic mechanisms, but, as yet, a specific biochemical abnormality has not been found in human subjects. Two pathways that are currently of most interest and promise are the dopamine hypothesis and the schizotoxic hypothesis.

The dopamine hypothesis proposes that the abnormal accumulation of dopamine, a central nervous system neurotransmitter, causes the schizophrenic symptoms. It is known that antischizophrenic medications (such as chlorpromazine) block dopamine receptors and that the administration of amphetamines, which enhance the release of dopamines, exacerbates schizophrenic symptoms.[12] (For this reason amphetamines and antidepressants may precipitate a schizophrenic reaction in a vulnerable individual.) However, schizophrenics on antischizophrenic medication are not cured of all symptoms, which would be expected if dopamine is the causal agent and is blocked by the medication. Further, no clear proof is yet at hand that schizophrenics have abnormal concentrations or utilization of dopamine.

The schizotoxic hypothesis suggests that some abnormal metabolite exists in the brain that induces schizophrenic symptomatology. One agent, dimethyltryptamine, which causes hallucinations in normal subjects, has its tryptamine precursors present in man. As an in vivo metabolite it has yet to be isolated. However, the possibility exists that it may be produced by an abnormal metabolic pathway and induce hallucinatory states in patients.[2]

ENVIRONMENTAL FACTORS

Social Class. Schizophrenia has been demonstrated to be more frequent in lower socioeconomic classes. The reasons for this greater incidence are not clear. The most probable reason is the greater stress experienced by those in the lower socioeconomic classes. If a predisposition to schizophrenia diminishes an individual's ability to cope with life stresses, then increased severity of such stresses in poverty environments would increase the incidence. Another factor is the drift of some schizophrenics into the lower socioeconomic level because of their diminished ability to work.[6]

Family. Without doubt the family plays a major role in the etiology and, most importantly, in the treatment of the schizophrenic.[9] However, the specific etiologic factors in family dynamics remain obscure in spite of much effort to elucidate them. Early work suggested certain family types, e.g., a dominant, hostile mother and a passive father, as promoting schizophrenia. Controlled studies have not confirmed these findings. One difficulty such research faces is that it is hard to ascertain what is reaction and what is cause in the behavior of the schizophrenic's family. The area that shows the most promise is that of communication within the family.[10] Studies indicate that clarity of communication and flexibility of communication patterns promote cog-

nitive growth in children and that the contrary experience (i.e., unclear parental communication) makes the development of logical thought processes difficult. It is possible that the family induces the cognitive abnormality of schizophrenia by its mode of communication.[14] If this is the case, then early intervention in families of susceptible children may prevent the illness.

What we are likely to find is that whatever the biologic basis for schizophrenia, the psychosocial environment can either facilitate the disease process or substantially inhibit it.

THE DIAGNOSTIC PROCESS

Since a disturbance in thought process is central to the diagnosis of schizophrenia, it is essential to see other members of the patient's environment at the initial examination. One must check the historical data and the perception of reality that the patient discloses with others in his household.

Most patients have a history of longstanding emotional problems before the process reaches psychotic proportions. There is usually a marked difficulty in forming close relationships that can be traced back to childhood. Typically, the patient is described as having been a quiet, obedient child who was excessively shy and sensitive. This sensitivity is an abiding trait, and as an adolescent or young adult the patient is easily overwhelmed by anticipated or actual rejection.

A history of psychotic disorders in other relatives increases the likelihood of schizophrenia in the patient. Of course, as in all diagnostic considerations, we are speaking of probability. The presence of a psychotic relative should not weigh too heavily, or it may restrict consideration of other disease processes.

The age at onset is also significant. Schizophrenia is largely an illness with onset in adolescence and young adulthood. Late onset, even in the 50's or 60's, does occur and is most likely to take the paranoid form.

Mental Status

The current mental state of the patient requires careful assessment. Schizophrenia is a syndrome, and no one symptom or sign is truly pathognomonic. The finding of psychosis plus a grouping of signs and symptoms establishes the diagnosis.

General Appearance and Attitude

As part of any psychosis, if the disturbance is profound enough, the patient may show lack of care in his appearance. There may also be a lack of cooperation on the part of the patient with a reluctance to answer the interviewer's questions. This reluctance may stem from the basic mistrust and fearfulness characteristic of schizophrenic patients or may be the guarded suspiciousness of the paranoid subtype.

Speech

Speech may be incoherent, pressured, or slowed. Mutism is seen at times. Made-up words or neologisms may occasionally be employed. In extreme forms of disorganization, speech may take on a "word salad" character in which it seems to the listener that there is no meaningful connection between the words spoken.

Affect

Expression of feelings may be quite limited, although the acutely psychotic patient is commonly in a state of panic (overwhelming anxiety). Flatness of affect with little reaction or little variation in expression ("poker face") is common. Affect may also be inappropriate, with laughing or crying for no apparent reason, or may not be consonant with the content of the interview.

Family Interview

Of utmost importance is an interview with the patient and all members of the household. By means of such an interview, one's ability to help the patient, including resources to tap and vulnerabilities to overcome, is ascertained. Since diagnosis is oftentimes difficult and no one member of a family has all the facts, a family interview can rapidly provide clarification of the patient's problems.

Physical Examination

Since a number of psychotic conditions arise from organic causes, the physical examination is crucial in the diagnostic process. Organic psychoses and schizophrenia are usually readily differentiated. However, this is not always the case, and physical findings may prevent misdiagnosis. Also, while environmental stresses may point strongly to the precipitation of functional disorders, they may be coincidental with the onset of a physical illness. For instance, three cases of herpes encephalitis have been reported as initially being diagnosed as schizophrenia because the early course of the encephalitis was afebrile.[13]

Psychologic Tests

There are no specific tests helpful for defining schizophrenia as there are for defining organic brain dysfunctions. Projective tests can be useful in elucidating a thought disorder and in estimating impulse control, but the diagnosis cannot be made definitively by testing.

DIFFERENTIAL DIAGNOSIS

Drug-induced Psychoses

The widespread use of drugs such as LSD and amphetamines and medications such as steroids requires that the possibility of drug-induced psychosis always be entertained in the acutely psychotic patient. Of prime importance, of course, is a history of drug use or abuse. As a rule, the hallucinations induced by LSD are visual, whereas those of schizophrenia are primarily, though not exclusively, auditory. The psychosis induced by excess amphetamine use is more difficult to distinguish from a paranoid schizophrenic reaction. Both may present with acute agitation and paranoid delusions. Here a history of drug intake and a relatively good premorbid adjustment are especially important in ascertaining that one is dealing with an amphetamine psychosis.

Affective Psychoses

The excitement of the manic patient does not usually have the panic character of the schizophrenic. The flight of ideas of a manic patient is also to be distinguished from the looseness of associations of the schizophrenic. In the manic patient, it is as if the stream of thought is racing at a faster than controllable pace, whereas the schizophrenic has associational looseness without the same sense of racing thoughts.

The manic patient also generates a sense of empathy in the observer that the schizophrenic is unable to do. The manic individual is often able to reach out in a very appealing way. The schizophrenic's lack of trust in his ability to be valued by others causes him to maintain an interpersonal distance that makes empathy difficult.

The psychotically depressed patient may suffer from delusions, especially of the somatic variety. As an example, he may feel that his body is decaying. The absence of a looseness of associations coupled with a history of prior adequate interpersonal relationships usually makes the differential diagnosis clear.

Organic Psychoses

Organic psychoses such as those due to degenerative, metabolic, or infectious diseases of the central nervous system (CNS) are characterized by a number of symptoms including memory loss, neurologic signs of CNS impairment, and fever. Typically the sensorium (orientation as to time, place, and person) is more affected in organic psychosis than in schizophrenia, although in an acute psychotic phase the sensorium of the schizophrenic patient may be equally clouded. *Nonetheless*, organic conditions can present as psychotic disturbances without, at first, showing clear evidence of neurologic disease, as in the previously cited example of herpes encephalitis. Careful history-taking, repeated neurologic evaluations, and continued alertness for signs of CNS impairment are necessary in following any patient with schizophrenia, unless history, signs, and symptomatology are present in the classic manner.

Paranoid States

The presence of a thought disorder and shifting delusional content distinguishes the paranoid schizophrenic from a purely paranoid psychotic in whom a single, fixed delusion is the rule.

MANAGEMENT

THE ACUTELY DISTURBED PATIENT

The acutely disturbed schizophrenic patient is an emergency. The patient is in a state of panic, and the longer the panic endures, the more deleterious will be the impact for the patient and his family. However, an acutely disturbed patient does not necessarily require hospitalization. Studies have shown that quite seriously and acutely disturbed patients can be maintained out of the hospital during an acute episode if the family receives intense professional guidance and support.[7] Whether or not to hospitalize will depend on family and community resources as well as patient status.

A schizophrenic presenting with suicidal or homicidal thoughts, especially when coupled with command hallucinations, usually needs hospitalization. Of course, if the patient has become violent, is unable to cooperate in his daily care, is refusing all food, or is totally withdrawn, hospitalization will also be needed. The majority of patients do not display this degree of social incompetence, nor do they display a lack of impulse control. However, when these symptoms are present, prompt hospitalization will be necessary.

THE VIOLENT PATIENT

The individual who has become violent or who appears about to act in a dangerous, destructive manner poses a special emergency. The physician called to intervene with such a patient needs to have a clear plan of management worked out before meeting the patient. First of all, it can be assumed that the patient is extremely frightened and dominated by irrational convictions. If he is paranoid, everyone may be seen as a potential source of harm and not to be trusted. If he is hallucinating, the agitated response to auditory or visual percepts may result in harm to others.

The first and most important rule of management is safety. For safety to be established there must be enough people present to physically restrain the individual with a minimum of fighting. With an adult patient this often means four people, one for each limb. The presence of sufficient assistance to guarantee safety frequently has a calming effect on the individual and permits treatment without physical restraint. However, this should not lull the physician into prematurely seeing the patient in an unsafe environment, e.g., permitting the patient to speak with him alone while the others remain outside a closed door. A key to whether the patient's violent impulses are under control is when being alone with him no longer induces anxiety in the physician. The presence of anxiety in the clinician is an invaluable signal that must be attended to when treating impulsive patients. It almost always means that the patient needs more external controls.

If restraint is required, then sedation is often needed; and for rapid action, intravenous sodium amobarbital or diazepam may be used. When conditions either permit or require intramuscular medication, both the phenothiazines (e.g., chlorpromazine) and haloperidol have been used effectively in the combative patient. In a psychiatric hospital, combative patients may be treated without medication, making use of protective seclusion rooms for times of agitation.

Once a safe environment has been established, the physician can intervene verbally by encouraging the patient to express what he fears or what necessitates his outbursts. Then providing the patient with assurance or helping him test reality will reduce the panic state. Arguing is, of course, of no value and merely serves to increase agitation.

If continued danger exists, hospitalization is indicated. Should hospitalization not be available, fairly high doses of antipsychotic medication may be effective in rapidly achieving a stable condition, following which long-term treatment may proceed.

PHARMACOTHERAPY

The major tranquilizers are the primary therapeutic approach to the acutely disturbed schizophrenic patient.[11] These medications have specific antipsychotic properties even though their mechanism of action is still poorly understood. Chlorpromazine is the prototypical major tranquilizer. Actual choice of which of the many major tranquilizers to use depends as much on the physician's in-depth knowledge of the therapeutic and side effects of the specific medications as on the often minor differences in antipsychotic properties. Of the phenothiazines, chlorpromazine, thioridazine, and trifluoperazine are most widely used. Of the nonphenothiazines, haloperidol is most frequently employed.

For the acutely agitated patient intramuscular medication (e.g., 50 mg. of chlorpromazine) may be needed. For the less acutely agitated patient, chlorpromazine or its equivalent in doses of 2 to 4 mg. per kg. per day in four to five doses may be administered orally. The first effect of chlorpromazine is its sedative action. The antipsychotic effects may not be perceived for 2 days to several weeks. The sedative effect is, of course, very desirable in the panicked patient who cannot sleep and needs sedation as well as tranquilization. After the dosage has been regulated and the sedation is to some extent lessened, a single bedtime dose or a twice-a-day schedule may be employed, since the phenothiazines are metabolized slowly, and no loss of tranquilizing effect will occur. This is true unless continued sedation is needed. The sedative properties of the phenothiazines are relatively short-lived in contrast to their antipsychotic tranquilizing properties.

Medical Side Effects

There are numerous side effects to be reckoned with in using the major tranquilizers. That is one of the reasons it is best to use only a few of the many major tranquilizers, so that the side effects of each are fully recalled. Here we will only consider some of the most frequently seen reactions.

Sedation. While sedation is useful for the acutely agitated patient, it is often troublesome after the acute phase has passed. Patients vary greatly as to how much sedative effect they experience. If drowsiness is a problem, consideration can be given to use of a medication with less sedative effect at an equivalent dose to the medication being taken. Thus, a patient taking chlorpromazine who is too sedated at a dose level required for its antipsychotic properties might be switched to a piperazine phenothiazine (e.g., fluphenazine), a butyrophenone (haloperidol [Haldol]), or a thioxanthene (thiothixene [Navane], all of which produce less sedation.

Extrapyramidal Symptoms. All the major

tranquilizers can produce parkinsonian symptoms: masklike face, cogwheel rigidity, and tremor. As with sedation, it is difficult to predict who will develop these unpleasant side effects, so that *routine* administration of antiparkinsonian medication is not recommended. However, the symptoms may be alleviated if necessary by giving an antiparkinsonian medication such as benztropine (Cogentin) or biperiden (Akineton).

Acute dystonic reactions also occur. These may appear as painful neck or trunk spasms or oculogyric crises. Treatment may require intravenous administration of benztropine or diphenhydramine (Benadryl), providing immediate relief of symptoms.

Another extrapyramidal symptom that may mislead the clinician is akathisia. This symptom consists of motor restlessness, mainly in the legs, so that the patient feels he can't sit still. Akathisia may be confused with agitation, but there is no anxiety associated with it. This symptom also responds to antiparkinsonian agents.

Tardive Dyskinesia. A syndrome of major and increasing concern is that characterized by involuntary tic-like movements of the face. These movements commonly include tongue thrusting, lip smacking, chewing and sucking motions, and grimacing. They usually appear only after long-term treatment (hence the name). Tardive dyskinesia often appears when antipsychotic medications are discontinued or dosages are lowered and will disappear with increased dosages. However, the symptoms eventually reappear at the increased dosage level. It now seems that damage to the substantia nigra occurs, and continued medication will likely exacerbate the process. Patient and physician need to weigh whether continued medication is justified despite these symptoms. Informed consent (in writing) for prolonged use of major tranquilizers in the face of this syndrome is advisable, since there is no known treatment, although when symptoms are recognized early and medication discontinued, spontaneous disappearance can occur.

Polypharmacy. While combining tranquilizers is extremely common, it is recognized today that this is not a good practice and only increases the possibility of undesirable side effects.

PSYCHOTHERAPY

There is a great need for the patient and family to have regular and frequent personal contact with the treating physician. The support, reality testing, and assistance in mobilizing family resources provided by the physician are crucial to the patient's weathering of the acute stage. Insight-oriented therapy has not been shown to be effective in the treatment of schizophrenic patients in spite of the brilliant phenomenologic accounts of the experiences of treating schizophrenics that have appeared in the psychoanalytic literature. However, in the acute phase, the physician must be available to patient and family for the supportive treatment that will stabilize and make possible the patient's extrahospital treatment. Only if such a commitment can be made should one undertake the ambulatory treatment of the acutely psychotic patient of any diagnostic type.

While insight-oriented psychotherapy will not be pursued, a psychotherapeutic relationship is important in the management of the schizophrenic patient. The physician needs to develop a rapport based on an understanding of the special needs of the patient and to promote the patient's recovery within the context of the doctor–patient relationship. Establishing a relationship with the schizophrenic often requires the greatest patience and professional discipline. The patient is fearful, has a basic mistrust that often makes him hostile to those who want to help him, and distorts what is said to him. It is important for the physician to establish an appropriate professional distance, because schizophrenics mistrust relationships that they also greatly desire. An early show of great warmth by the physician may, paradoxically, increase the patient's fear and distrust. Most helpful is to communicate a desire to understand the patient's fears and to accept that, for him, the nightmare he describes is real. While accepting the personal reality of the psychotic experience for the patient, it is equally important not to pretend to understand the meaning of irrational or obscure communications.

In treating the schizophrenic, every physician faces the dilemma of having the patient arouse uncomfortable feelings in the clinician. Feelings of anxiety, frustration, anger, and embarrassment are common. Such emotions become a problem only when they interfere with the physician's willingness to treat the patient. Schizophrenics are difficult patients, but they are also the most needful. That they create discomfort should not be a basis for refusing them treatment.

While the physician will see the patient primarily on an individual, one-to-one basis, family therapy (seeing the entire family together) may be extremely useful. The family of the schizophrenic patient is under a great deal of stress. They need help in mobilizing their resources to assist their ill child, husband, or wife. Often, feelings of hostility, despair, and guilt overwhelm these families and paralyze their functioning. The physician can assist in clarifying their responsibilities to the patient and supporting their role in the therapeutic process. The stress on parents of a seriously disturbed young adult or child frequently leads to splits in the parental relationship. Helping the parents work together will greatly strengthen the family's ability to help their child.

THE CHRONIC PATIENT

The chronic patient is one who exhibits continuing disability over long periods of time. He may not be psychotic but does require continued treatment in order to function optimally.

The continued treatment will often include medication. The needs of the patient will be relatively stable, but as stresses or life changes occur, medication will have to be adjusted. However, medication alone will not suffice. A supportive relationship with the physician will be as crucial as the medication being dispensed. These patients have great difficulty in forming and acknowledging the importance of a relationship. The physician from whom they receive their medication or to whom they go for checkups becomes an island of nonthreatening help in a world of anxiety. Often without the patient's showing the degree of dependence felt, the physician becomes the almost magical source of strength that the patient will grasp through times of panic.

Many patients will not need medication but will need to make periodic contacts with the physician to ensure that an early return of symptoms is recognized and treatment instituted.

Rehabilitation

The goal of rehabilitation for the schizophrenic patient is the same as it is for any handicapped individual—to reach the optimal level of functioning that his handicap permits. Although the physician will play an important role in the rehabilitative process, other professionals will be the primary implementers of this phase of treatment. The family physician will need to know what rehabilitation resources are available locally and how to help the chronic patient make the best use of these resources.

The handicaps of the schizophrenic patient may be of several types. The most common is a persistent difficulty in relations with other people. This difficulty usually takes the form of marked social anxiety leading to aloofness and reluctance to speak to others. However, even with maintenance medication, delusions and auditory hallucinations may also be present. Their presence will not necessarily prevent a satisfactory extrahospital adjustment. Employment may still be possible if the patient can perform a job, ignoring or limiting his response to the voices he may be hearing.

Not all patients will need rehabilitation, and not all will benefit by it. If one believes the oft-cited statistics that one-third of schizophrenic patients recover fully, one-third are mildly to moderately impaired, and one-third are severely impaired, then it is the middle third who will probably benefit most from rehabilitation. However, even the more severely impaired may gain, and if the resources are available, attempts at rehabilitation of all disabled schizophrenic patients would be desirable.

Those patients who return to the role of husband or wife in their families seem to do the best.[14] The reasons are probably twofold. First, they have a clear role in which to function and rewards for functioning well. Secondly, they have already achieved a more advanced level of interpersonal growth and hence are able to return to this premorbid level of functioning.

For the hospitalized patient the first step in adjustment to community living may be in a transitional residential setting. A setting such as a halfway house may be very helpful. Halfway houses provide community-based, group living for former hospital patients. They are supervised by house parents and are usually supported by state vocational rehabilitation or social service departments. The advantages of such residences are that they provide group support to the patient at a time when he is feeling most vulnerable and doubtful about his ability to live independently.

Other aids to community living are social centers or clubs for expatients. The club or social center offers help in a number of areas: developing social skills, receiving support from a group experiencing similar stresses, and, above all, providing acceptance as an individual. The availability of social centers or clubs varies greatly with the development of mental health services in a given area. Inquiry at the local or state social service agencies will provide information as to location and criteria for participation.

Vocational Rehabilitation

Training for employment is an important component of the rehabilitative process. The development of good work habits, care of personal appearance, and skills in relating to others in an employment situation are fostered in programs for schizophrenic patients. Patients can often learn skills that will enable them to earn a living. Even though the employment may be at a level below that at which they were previously functioning, it at least will provide a measure of independence. Such vocational programs, when they exist, are provided by public agencies, and patients can be referred to them by the physician.

Besides training in specific job skills, some patients need a supervised work experience to gain confidence. For them a sheltered workshop provides an environment where they can develop work-related skills while not facing the potential rejection or failure that may be their lot in a regular employment situation.

SUMMARY

Schizophrenia is a functional psychosis classified with the major affective disorders and the paranoid states, but distinguished by its disturbances in thinking as well as in mood and behavior. It usually begins in late adolescence or early adult life with the appearance of an acute psychotic episode. Progression to chronicity with periodic exacerbations and increasing impairment is usual. Exact etiology is undetermined but is probably a combination of genetic, chemical, and environmental disturbances. The advent of the phenothiazines and related antipsychotic drugs has had the effect of permitting most schizophrenics to be treated in an ambulatory setting with hospitalization reserved for only the most severely disturbed. As a consequence, the family physician's role in the treatment of schizophrenia is similar to that in the treatment of other chronic diseases, i.e., establishment of a supportive relationship, control of medication, guidance to the patient and the family, and advocacy for the patient in his relationship with the health care system and with other elements of his environment.

REFERENCES

1. Beckne, A. B., and Schulberg, H. C.: Phasing out mental hospitals—a psychiatric dilemma. New Engl. J. Med., 294:255, 1976.
2. Gillin, J. C., Kaplan, J., Stillman, R., et al.: The psychedelic model of schizophrenia: the case of N,N-dimethyltryptamine. Am. J. Psychiatry, 133:203, 1976.
3. Gittleman-Klein, R., and Klein, D. F.: Marital status as a prognostic indicator in schizophrenia. J. Nerv. Ment. Dis., 147:289, 1968.
4. Kallman, F. J.: The genetic theory of schizophrenia. Am. J. Psychiatry, 103:309, 1946.
5. Kety, S. S., Rosenthal, D., Wenden, P. H., et al.: Mental illness in the biological and adoptive families of adopted schizophrenics. Am. J. Psychiatry, 128:302, 1971.
6. Kohn, M. L.: Social class and schizophrenia: a critical review and reformulation. Schizophrenia Bull., 7:60, 1973.
7. Langsley, D. G., Pittman, F., and Swank, G.: Family crisis in schizophrenics and other mental patients. J. Nerv. Ment. Dis., 149:270, 1969.
8. Lehman, N. E.: Schizophrenia: clinical features. In Freedman, A. M., Kaplan, H. I., and Sadock, B. J. (eds.): Comprehensive Textbook of Psychiatry/II. Baltimore, The Williams & Wilkins Co., 1975, Vol. I.

9. Lidz, T.: The Origin and Treatment of Schizo-phrenic Disorders. New York, Basic Books, 1973.
10. Reiss, D.: The family and schizophrenia. Am. J. Psychiatry, *133*:181, 1976.
11. Shader, R. I., and Jackson, A. H.: Approaches to schizophrenia. *In* Shader, R. I. (ed.): Manual of Psychiatric Therapeutics. Boston, Little, Brown & Co., 1975.
12. Snyder, S. H.: Amphetamine psychosis: A "model" schizophrenia mediated by catechola-mines. Am. J. Psychiatry, *133*:203, 1976.
13. Wilson, F. G.: Viral encephalopathy mimicking functional psychosis. Am. J. Psychiatry, *133*:165, 1976.
14. Wynne, F. C., and Singer, M. T.: Thought dis-order and family relations of schizophrenics. II. A classification of forms of thinking. Arch. Gen. Psychiatry, *9*:199, 1963.

Chapter 26

ALCOHOLISM

by HAROLD A. MULFORD,
and HAROLD MOESSNER

TREATING THE ALCOHOLIC

PHYSICAL COMPLICATIONS OF ALCOHOL ABUSE

Ethyl alcohol (ethanol) is the most widely used and abused drug in our present-day society. Few other drugs have such a variety of harmful effects on nearly all of the organ systems of the human body. Because ethyl alcohol is a relatively simple chemical compound, it rapidly invades all parts of the body. Recent studies have demonstrated that this drug has a direct toxic effect on cells in a wide variety of organ systems and that adequate nutrition does not protect the body from these toxic effects.

The family physician is often involved in the early identification, diagnosis, treatment, and rehabilitation of patients who abuse ethyl alcohol. Given the current emphasis on health maintenance, the family physician is also responsible for educating his patients about the hazards of abusing all drugs, especially our society's soporific—ethyl alcohol.

Following ingestion, ethanol is rapidly absorbed from the upper gastrointestinal tract and can easily be detected in the blood stream. Thus, the blood alcohol level (BAL), or blood alcohol concentration (BAC), is easily measured. This chemical test can be performed by most clinical laboratories and is a useful diagnostic procedure. Unfortunately, many physicians avoid utilizing this test.

Ethanol has a local irritating effect on the mucosa of the upper gastrointestinal tract, frequently resulting in alcoholic gastritis. With higher concentrations of ethanol over longer periods of time hemorrhage from superficial ulcerations may occur, resulting in hematemesis or melena. Also, the inflamed mucosa of the stomach and small intestine does not properly absorb nutrients, therapeutic drugs, and so forth. This complicates the medical management of patients on drugs such as anticoagulants, anticonvulsants, antidiabetic agents, and others.

After alcohol is absorbed, it is carried to the liver via the portal venous system. The drug is metabolized mainly in the liver by a series of oxidative reactions. Approximately 5 per cent of the ethanol is excreted unchanged in the breath, sweat, and urine. This provides the physiologic basis for the Breathalyzer test, which is used in the apprehension and prosecution of drunken drivers.

The ethanol that is not immediately metabolized in the liver is transported to the heart via the hepatic vein and thereby enters the general circulation. Since alcohol is very miscible in water, it easily crosses cellular and vascular barriers and reaches highest concentrations in those organs of the body that have a significant fluid content.

Nervous System

Everyone is familiar with the acute effects of ethyl alcohol on the brain that are due to its depressant effect on the cells of the nervous system. By interfering with such normal cerebral functions as reasoning, judgment, memory, intelligence, sensation, motor function, and neuromuscular coordination, ethanol produces the syndrome of acute intoxication, or drunkenness, that was so vividly described by Henry Voltan Morton:

One drink of wine and you act like a monkey; two drinks and you strut like a peacock; three drinks and you roar like a lion; and four drinks—you behave like a pig.

The chronic effects of ethyl alcohol on the nervous system are well illustrated in such conditions as (1) alcoholic cerebral atrophy, (2) tobacco–alcohol amblyopia, (3) cerebellar degeneration, (4) Marchiafava-Bignami disease, (5) Morel's laminar corticosclerosis, (6) peripheral polyneuropathy, (7) pontine myelinolysis, and (8) Wernicke-Korsakoff syndrome. Many of these conditions may be the result of poor nutrition plus heavy consumption of ethanol over long periods of time. The prognosis for recovery from these chronic nervous system disorders is guarded in spite of abstinence from ethanol, adequate nutrition, and vitamin supplementation. Such conditions are most commonly seen in the lower socioeconomic alcoholic or the "skid row" drunk. Most physicians are exposed to this type of alcoholic in their medical school experience or in residency training. Although less than 5 per cent of persons with a drinking problem fit this description, this stereotype often prevents the young physician from recognizing that the vice-president of the local bank has developed early symptoms of ethanol abuse.

Cardiovascular System

The acute ingestion of ethanol depresses cardiac function and is contraindicated in a patient with angina or congestive heart failure. However, if there is a great deal of anxiety associated with the heart disease, the sedative effect of ethanol may be beneficial. Among the clinical signs of acute alcohol abuse are tachycardia with an irregular rhythm, increased blood pressure, and nonspecific changes in the T wave on the electrocardiogram.

Chronic alcohol consumption may produce a cardiomyopathy with decreased contractility and lipid deposition in the myocardium that leads to congestive heart failure. Abstinence from ethanol is the only beneficial therapy at present, and recovery is a matter of months.

Hyperlipidemia, especially elevated triglyceride levels, has been frequently associated with alcohol abuse. Whether hyperlipidemia is an etiologic factor in atherosclerosis is still open to debate, but it does result in such clinical findings as premature arcus senilis, xanthomas, and a creamy supernatant serum in the patient's blood sample.

Pell and D'Alonzo[19] have demonstrated an increased incidence of cerebrovascular disease in alcoholics. Whether hyperlipidemia and the increase in blood pressure are causative factors remains to be determined.

If ethyl alcohol has any medical indications for use as a drug, it is in its use as a sedative and as a dilator of peripheral blood vessels. But the numerous negative effects and the ever-present danger of addiction should lead the family physician to search for a better drug.

Respiratory System

The patient who abuses alcohol also frequently abuses other drugs and tobacco. Therefore, chronic obstructive pulmonary disease, carcinoma of the lung, tuberculosis, pneumonia, and bronchitis are frequently found in the chronic alcoholic. Aspiration pneumonitis and lung abscess frequently occur as a result of a severe episode of acute alcohol intoxication.

Hematopoietic System

The hematopoietic effects of ethanol are multifarious (malnutrition; liver disease; decreased absorption of folic acid, iron, pyridoxine, and so forth; and abnormal utilization of these nutrients by the bone marrow). Clinically, these effects result in anemia, leukopenia, thrombocytopenia, and a depressed immune response. These findings may explain the increased frequency of infections and of certain types of carcinomas that are found so frequently in the chronic alcoholic.

Gastrointestinal System

Most of the common medical problems encountered in the gastrointestinal tract, from carcinoma of the oropharynx to hemorrhoids, are frequently associated with alcohol abuse. In the preceding pages we have briefly discussed alcoholic gastritis and problems of abnormal absorption of nutrients, therapeutic drugs, and so forth in

TABLE 26–1.   UPPER GASTROINTESTINAL HEMORRHAGE IN THE ALCOHOLIC PATIENT*

Diagnosis	History	Physical Examination	Type of Surgery	Remarks
Mallory-Weiss syndrome	Forceful vomiting precedes hematemesis	Negative	Source of laceration	Majority of patients with this lesion are alcoholics
Esophageal varices	Long history of alcoholism	Signs suggest cirrhosis of liver	Portacaval shunt	Approximately 50 per cent of patients with varices bleed from a different lesion
Peptic ulcer	Previous epigastric pain	Negative	Many operations available; timing of surgery just as important as choice	Increased incidence of gastric ulcers, but not duodenal ulcers, in alcoholics
Gastritis	Recent alcoholic "binge"	Negative	Vagotomy and drainage procedure	Aspirin potentiates this lesion. Bleeding usually stops without surgery

*From Lowenfels, A. B.: The Alcoholic Patient in Surgery, p. 131. © 1971, The Williams & Wilkins Co., Baltimore.

the upper gastrointestinal tract. The association between ethanol ingestion and peptic ulcer disease and between ethanol ingestion and cirrhosis of the liver with esophageal varices is well documented. If the Mallory-Weiss syndrome is added to this list, it is easy to understand why the alcoholic patient who presents with an upper gastrointestinal hemorrhage is such a difficult diagnostic and therapeutic problem (Table 26–1).

Both acute and chronic pancreatitis plus carcinoma of the pancreas seem to be statistically related to alcohol abuse.

Alcoholic Liver Disease

The relationship between cirrhosis of the liver and ethanol abuse has been recognized for many years, but more recent studies have demonstrated that an acute fatty liver and alcoholic hepatitis are earlier stages of alcoholic liver disease. In addition, there is now scientific evidence that good nutrition does not prevent this liver damage and that ethyl alcohol is cytotoxic to the cells of the liver. Recognition of the patient with an acute fatty liver depends on finding a nontender hepatomegaly with elevated liver enzymes. Alcoholic hepatitis has all of the symptoms of infectious hepatitis (fever, nausea and vomiting, anorexia, jaundice, leukocytosis, and so forth) without evidence of a viral infection. Cirrhosis is the end-stage of alcoholic liver disease, with scar tissue replacing the inflammatory response. A liver biopsy is helpful in determining the degree of damage and in assessing the prognosis.

Musculoskeletal System

Numerous studies have demonstrated that acute ethanol ingestion is frequently related to accidental injuries, such as automobile accidents, private airplane accidents, home accidents, pedestrian accidents, industrial accidents, drownings, burns, and so forth. Also, ethanol consumption and poor nutrition contribute to osteoporosis of the skeletal system, which is then more susceptible to fractures. Therefore, the family physician will frequently encounter the alcoholic patient in the hospital emergency room.

Excessive ethanol consumption over prolonged periods of time results in an acute or chronic form of skeletal myopathy. This eventually produces an atrophy of the skeletal muscles, especially of the shoulder and pelvic girdle that leads to a distinctive appearance in the patient. With the wasting of the muscles of the upper and lower trunk and a typical "pot belly" due to cirrhosis with ascites or to excessive fat (ethanol contains 7 calories per gm.), the chronic alcoholic has a physique that is easily recognized.

Several investigators have demonstrated that the alcoholic patient seems to be found more frequently among those patients with aseptic necrosis of the head of the femur. The mechanism for this association is not clear.

Miscellaneous

Glucose.   By depleting hepatic glycogen and interfering with gluconeogenesis, withdrawal from alcohol can produce an acute episode of hypoglycemia. In the alcoholic patient who is stuporous or comatose as a result of hypoglycemia, intravenous administration of glucose may be a life-saving measure.

In the patient with a steady and chronic ingestion of ethyl alcohol, the physician may find a diabetic-type glucose tolerance curve. In order to prevent the misdiagnosis of diabetes, the family physician should instruct his patient not to ingest ethanol for at least 2 weeks prior to performing the glucose tolerance test.

Magnesium. The urinary excretion of magnesium is increased after alcohol ingestion. Therefore, the administration of magnesium sulfate may be useful in treating the withdrawal symptoms if the serum magnesium level is below normal.

Uric Acid. Ethanol produces an increase in the serum uric acid level and thereby aggravates gouty arthritis.

Sexual Problems. Although the sedative effect of ethyl alcohol may relieve anxieties about sexual performance, a large amount of the drug will interfere with the neuromuscular performance of the sex act. In addition, ethanol seems to be an important factor in acute or chronic episodes of impotence. The gynecomastia that is frequently found in the chronic alcoholic with liver disease has been explained by the failure of the poorly functioning liver to detoxify the estrogens produced by all males. More recent studies of testicular biopsies and androgen levels in chronic alcoholics suggest that ethanol has a direct toxic effect on the cells of the testes. This leads to decreased androgen production and diminished spermatogenesis.

THE ALCOHOL WITHDRAWAL SYNDROME

Patients who are withdrawing from ethanol are frequently found in the physician's office or the emergency room or as in-patients in the hospital. Their symptoms may vary from a minor tremor and irritability to full-blown delirium tremens. The early recognition and proper treatment of this condition not only reduce the duration and severity of the withdrawal syndrome but also decrease the morbidity and mortality. The severity of withdrawal is increased by larger amounts and longer duration of eth-

anol consumption. Also, the greater the period of time since the patient's last drink, the more severe the withdrawal symptoms will be.

The symptoms of withdrawal may consist of any or all of the following: (1) tremors—usually generalized but most easily recognized in the upper extremities; (2) irritability and agitation—associated with a generalized restlessness and insomnia; (3) autonomic hyperactivity—increased blood pressure, pulse, and respiration and elevated temperature with excessive sweating; (4) hallucinations—frequently very frightening in nature; (5) delusions and disorientation; and (6) seizures—usually of the grand mal type. Similar symptomatology is seen in withdrawal from other sedatives or stimulant drugs, but such symptoms tend to occur 7 to 10 days after cessation of drug ingestion, compared with 2 to 4 days after abstinence from ethanol.

In the past, the medical literature has stated that the withdrawal syndrome from ethyl alcohol has a mortality of 10 to 15 per cent. In our experience, the modern medical management of withdrawal reduces that mortality figure to less than 1 per cent.

Treatment of Withdrawal

The hallmark of therapy of all drug withdrawal syndromes is a concerned and caring group of medical and nursing personnel. The patients must be repeatedly reassured about their medical condition, their delusions, and their hallucinations and reoriented to time, place, and person. Physical restraints should be avoided at all costs, since they only produce more anxiety. The patient should be placed in a quiet but lighted room where he can be observed closely and can interact frequently with the attending staff.

Sedation. The minor tranquilizers are effective in reducing psychomotor and autonomic hyperactivity. At the University of Iowa Alcoholism Center, the drug of choice is diazepam (Valium) because of its safety, ease of administration, and anticonvulsant properties. It is administered orally, intramuscularly or intravenously in a dose sufficient to produce sleep. The sleep must be light enough so that the patient's vital signs and mental status may be measured and oral fluids or nourishment may be administered. The sedation is gradually reduced after 24 to 48 hours and is never continued for more than a week. We have been pleasantly surprised by the lack of serious complications with the use of this type of sedation.

Anticonvulsants. Phenytoin (Dilantin), 100 mg. three times a day, is given to all patients who have a history of seizures. Since oral or intramuscular phenytoin does not reach an adequate level in the blood for 72 hours, diazepam should be given during this time to prevent seizures.

Fluids. The vast majority of patients can be managed with oral fluids and routine nourishment. Intravenous fluids are required if severe vomiting, diarrhea, electrolyte abnormalities, or hypoglycemia is present.

Infection. The patient in withdrawal is more susceptible to infection, and its presence increases the severity of the withdrawal. The sites most commonly involved are the respiratory tract, the soft tissues, and the urinary tract.

Comatose Patient. A BAC test will identify the patient whose central nervous system is depressed from ethanol, and a blood glucose determination will alert the physician to the problem of hypoglycemia. Other complications such as craniocerebral trauma, diabetic acidosis, renal failure, and so forth may be present and may need to be considered in the differential diagnosis.

Nutrition. Many patients who abuse ethanol do not eat well, and therefore good nutrition with vitamin supplementation is an important factor in recovery. Most of our patients are able to start on a liquid diet shortly after admission and rapidly progress to a regular diet. Avoiding excessive coffee ingestion and cigarette smoking plus the use of antacids quickly controls the alcoholic gastritis and improves the appetite.

Activity. Within 36 to 48 hours, patients will benefit from some activity. At this time, they are filled with feelings of guilt and remorse and are most receptive to counseling about alcohol and alcoholism. During this stage, a well trained staff of paraprofessional counselors can assume the major responsibility for helping the patient with his drinking problems, while the physician continues treating the patient's medical needs.

Follow-up Therapy

Medications. The continuing use of sedatives or stimulants by the patient who has abused alcohol is to be condemned. This same patient frequently transfers his abuse to the new drug, which really doesn't solve the basic problem. The small number of alcoholic patients who have a true psychosis or depression will benefit from the use of phenothiazines or the tricyclic antidepressants, but these patients are the exception. The vast majority of patients need to establish an alcohol-free and drug-free life style.

Disulfiram (Antabuse) can be a valuable drug in the long-term management of the patient who is willing to use it in overcoming his drinking problem. With the present dosage of this medication, the seriousness of the ethanol–disulfiram reaction has been reduced. The drug should be started at a dose of 500 mg. daily, preferably taken in the morning, and at the end of 10 days the dose should be decreased to 250 mg. daily. Side effects of drowsiness, metallic taste, and so forth are minimal. A period of 4 days should separate the ingestion of ethanol and the institution of disulfiram therapy. This form of therapy provides the patient and his family with a period of time in which to make some significant changes from the previous alcoholic existence. In addition, the daily use of disulfiram demonstrates to the physician, the spouse, the employer, the court, and other involved parties the patient's sincerity in his attempt to lead a sober life.

Referral. After the family physician has treated the alcoholic's physical complications, there may well be someone "across the street"—a paraprofessional alcoholism counselor, a drug abuse counselor, an Alcoholics Anonymous (AA) sponsor, or perhaps a pastoral counselor—who is more capable and more willing to give the long-term assistance and support necessary to help the patient with his alcoholism. Prompt and appropriate referral is indicated. Certainly the traditional advice from the authority figure, the physician, such as "Don't drink" or "Join AA" is not sufficient. It is the physician's responsibility to know the helping agencies in his community and to use them for his patients' welfare.

ATTENDING TO THE ALCOHOLISM

Treating the alcoholic's physical complications is not the same as treating his "alcoholism." Physicians hardly need to be reminded that alcoholism does not fit neatly into the classic medical model. Approaching the patient's drinking problem from this perspective only generates frustration for the physician, with little benefit to the patient.

Let us turn then to another model, one that requires a shift in thinking from a single cause and point in time to multiple, weak, interacting causes and an extended period of time. In this model, becoming alcoholic and becoming a recovered alcoholic are viewed as dynamic, progressive, and prolonged processes. The two processes are not sequential, as in Jellinek's phases model. Instead, the individual simultaneously progresses in both of them. Even as he becomes more alcoholic, forces are building toward recovery. Advancement in both processes is influenced by numerous social, psychologic, and physiologic factors, with no single factor being either necessary or sufficient for the development of either alcoholism or recovery. The effect of one variable often depends upon the presence and strength of one or more other variables. Whether the person is an "alcoholic" or a "recovered alcoholic" at any given time depends upon the balance of forces affecting the two processes. The natural course of the alcoholic and the recovery processes and the variables affecting them are poorly understood. However, the fact that some 90 per cent of all drinkers do not become alcoholics suggests that there are natural forces that somehow prevent the alcoholic process from getting started or from progressing very far in most drinkers. The fact that most alcoholics eventually recover, many of them without formal treatment, suggests that the recovery process is also influenced by many natural forces.

The alcoholic process typically begins in the late teens and continues through late middle age. The process starts when the young drinker, having learned of the psychologic effects of alcohol (in addition to its more common social functions) begins to rely on it to cope with an ever wider range of situations. Having learned that taking a few drinks releases inhibitions and reduces the psychologic discomfort of, for example, asking a girl to dance, it is easy for him to gradually generalize such use of alcohol to more and more everyday stressful situations. It is especially easy for young males in our society to drift into frequent heavy drinking. Our drinking norms permit, certainly tolerate, and in many ways even encourage heavy drinking by young men, who are viewed as merely "sowing their wild oats." However, by the time their roles change to that of "responsible citizens" and their habitual heavy drinking is no longer condoned, it has already become a way of life. What's more, they are poorly prepared to cope with life's problems in socially acceptable ways, because each time they used alcohol to cope with a stressful situation, they denied themselves the experience of learning a more socially acceptable response. If they are to recover, they need help beyond physical restoration. They also need assistance to deal with all of their other drinking related troubles and need help to learn a new way of life, free of dependence on alcohol.

Women alcoholics are less likely than men to have learned to use alcohol as a life style to the exclusion of conventional alternatives. The alcoholic process is different for women, especially in the early stages. Our drinking norms not only discourage women from drinking but the start of alcohol use and the onset of heavy drinking, as well as the onset of alcoholic drinking, are all delayed. Whereas men tend to drift into it, women tend to begin heavy drinking to obtain emotional relief more suddenly and at a later age. Heavy drinking by women is more often a response to the build-up of emotional stress and is more often precipitated by a crisis. Thus, the woman alcoholic less likely needs help to learn a new way of life and more likely needs help to learn how to deal with crises and the accumulated stresses that trigger her drinking. She also needs help to regain acceptance as a "respectable" member of the community.

The recovery process begins with an awareness that "I am drinking more and enjoying it less" and that "the kick is going out of the booze." Habitual heavy consumption to relieve tension and anxiety and to solve problems is, in the long run, self-defeating. Eventually, a point is reached when the drinking itself generates tension, anxiety, and guilt. It creates more problems than it solves, all of which call for more drinking. At the same time, this vicious circle also moves the alcoholic toward recovery, as the futility of his life style slowly dawns on him. Among the many factors contributing to this growing awareness is the aging process. The body is becoming less tolerant of the abuse it is receiving, and it is slower to recuperate from a drinking bout. The alcoholic becomes "sick and tired of being sick and tired," which many AA members say is what prompted them to join the group. Although in its natural course, recovery is a prolonged process extending over many years, the AA experience indicates that it can be accelerated by the helping hand of an understanding friend. In fact, as yet there is no medical or other formal treatment proven to be superior to this empathic person-to-person help. Given the limits of present knowledge, helping the alcoholic toward recovery is more of an art than a science. The family physician, by treating the alcoholic's physical complications and by approaching the drinking problem with empathy and firmness, can be an added constructive force in initiating or accelerating the natural recovery process and halting or decelerating the alcoholic process.

NONBIOLOGIC SIGNS

The physician can best meet the needs of his alcoholic patient if he knows how far the patient has progressed in the alcoholic process. There is much consensus among alcoholism experts, community service professionals, and the general public that four signs indicate the presence of a drinking problem: (1) *trouble due to drinking*, (2) *personal effects drinking* (i.e., drinking for psychologic relief), (3) *preoccupied drinking* (i.e., extreme deviant drinking), and (4) *uncontrolled drinking*. These four dimensions of the alcoholism phenomena are incorporated into the Stages Index shown in Table 26–2.

STAGES IN THE ALCOHOLIC PROCESS

While other scales that have been developed for identifying alcoholics and measuring the severity of their alcoholism are based on a unitary, sequential model, the present Index relies on the assumption that the alcoholic phenomena are multidimensional and cumulative, but nonsequential. The Stages Index is based on the concept that while each of the four signs, i.e., each of the four subscales of the Index, indicates

a drinking problem, no single one of them is necessary for a positive diagnosis. However, the *number* of signs the patient manifests, *regardless of their sequential order of appearance*, is a measure of how far he has advanced in the alcoholic process. In other words, the patient's stage in the alcoholic process is indicated by how many of the four subscales in Table 26–2 he qualifies for, according to the following criteria:

Trouble Due to Drinking. A patient qualifies for this subscale by responding "yes" to two or more of ten items, each asking whether a particular drinking-related problem has been experienced during the past 12 months. Five life areas—jobs, family, health, finances, and police—are tapped by the items.

Personal Effects Drinking. The person is defined as using alcohol for psychologic relief, or personal effects, if he responds "yes" to three or more of the six items of this subscale.

Preoccupied Drinking. The qualifying score is a "frequently" or "sometimes" response to three or more of these nine extremely deviant drinking items.

Uncontrolled Drinking. Drinking is uncontrolled if the patient reports "frequently" drinking more than planned or "frequently" finding it difficult to stop. Notice that one of the two items constituting this subscale is also one of the items (item 4) of the Preoccupied Drinking subscale.

A patient who qualifies for only one (any one) of the subscales is classified as being in the early stage (Stage 1) of the alcoholic process. If he qualifies for any two subscales, he is in Stage 2, and so on.

THE ALCOHOLIC STAGES INDEX AS A CLINICAL TOOL

There has been little progress toward classifying alcoholics and specifying their differential needs. Persons with drinking-related problems, even those who have been through the selection process for entering an alcoholism center, are so heterogeneous that it is little wonder that no set of helping techniques, let alone a specific treatment effective for all, has been found. Moreover, as the definition of who is an alcoholic broadens and as an ever wider range of people appears for help with a drinking problem, their heterogeneity in-

TABLE 26-2.   ALCOHOLIC STAGES INDEX SUBCALES°

Trouble Due to Drinking Scale
(Qualifying score = 2 or more "yes" responses)

Yes	No	*During Past 12 Months:*
_____	_____	Has your employer fired or threatened to fire you because of your drinking?
_____	_____	Has your spouse left or threatened to leave you because of your drinking?
_____	_____	Has a family member complained you spend too much money on alcohol?
_____	_____	Have you been picked up by the police because of your drinking?
_____	_____	Has a physician told you drinking was injuring your health?
_____	_____	Have you had any illness due to drinking?
_____	_____	Have you had difficulty meeting bills because too much money was spent on liquor?
_____	_____	Have you quit or changed jobs because you were in trouble or likely to get into difficulty due to drinking?
_____	_____	Have you had any accidents or injuries due to drinking?
_____	_____	Have you failed to do some of the things you should—keeping appointments, getting things done around the house, or attending to your job—because of drinking?

Personal Effects Drinking Scale
(Qualifying score = 3 or more "yes" responses)

Yes	No	*Would You Say These Things About Your Drinking:*
_____	_____	Drinking helps me forget I am not the kind of person I really want to be.
_____	_____	Drinking helps me get along better with other people.
_____	_____	Drinking helps me feel more satisfied with myself.
_____	_____	Drinking gives me more confidence in myself.
_____	_____	Drinking helps me overcome shyness.
_____	_____	Drinking makes me less self-conscious.

Preoccupied Drinking Scale
(Qualifying score = 3 or more positive responses)

Frequently	Sometimes	Never	
_____	_____	_____	I stay intoxicated for several days at a time.
_____	_____	_____	I worry about not being able to get a drink when I need one.
_____	_____	_____	I sneak drinks when no one is looking.
_____	_____	_____	Once I start drinking, it is difficult for me to stop before I become completely intoxicated.
_____	_____	_____	I get intoxicated on work days.
_____	_____	_____	I take a drink the first thing when I get up in the morning.
_____	_____	_____	I awaken next day not being able to remember some of the things I had done while I was drinking.
_____	_____	_____	I take a few quick ones before going to a party to make sure I have enough.
_____	_____	_____	I neglect my regular meals when I am drinking.

Uncontrolled Drinking Scale
(Qualifying score = "Frequently" response to either item)

_____	_____	_____	Without realizing it, I end up drinking more than I had planned to.
_____	_____	_____	Item "4" of Preoccupied Scale above.

°From Mulford, H. A.: Stages in the alcoholic process: toward a cumulative nonsequential index. J. Stud. Alcohol, 38:565, 1977. (Reprinted by permission from Journal of Studies on Alcohol, Vol. 38, No. 3, Mar. 1977. Copyright by Journal of Studies on Alcohol, Inc., New Brunswick, N.J. 08903.)

creases, as does the need for a useful classification scheme.

Persons in the same stage of the alcoholic process should be more homogeneous with respect to the forces affecting their progress in both the alcoholic and the recovery processes. Those in the same stage can be expected to share many distinguishing characteristics, such as their motivation to drink, their motivation to stop drinking, their relationships with others, their self-attitudes, and their views of what alcohol is doing both to and for them, as well as their physical health, their treatment history, and many other factors related to their needs and to the kinds of help that would be most beneficial.

The patient who completes the Stages Index and discusses its implications with his physician may realize for the first time just how pervasive and troublesome alcohol has become in his life. The Trouble Due to Drinking Subscale indicates specific life areas being affected by drinking and suggests specific types of help that might be needed. Higher scores on the Personal Effects Subscale suggest that the person is seeking to satisfy more goals with alcohol and, therefore, has stronger motivation to continue drinking. A higher score also suggests the patient's need for help in dealing with low self-esteem. In other words, the patient's score on each of the subscales should be studied. A high score on a particular subscale would suggest different patient needs than would a low score.

Although the physician may find the Stages Index a useful tool for the alcoholic patient, no paper and pencil test or other mechanical device can substitute for a skilled, empathic interviewer. Such a test is an aid to, not a substitute for, clinical judgment and interpretation. It is recommended that the physician lead up to asking the patient to complete the Index with a few general questions, beginning with the common one about how much the patient drinks. It is no accident that the Index contains no such question. Although prolonged heavy drinking is likely to lead to physical complications, the level of consumption is a poor indicator of the presence of other drinking-related problems, their severity, the patient's stage in the alcoholic process, or how difficult it will be for him to abstain. The next question the

physician might ask is what the patient feels drinking does for him; what he gets out of it. Then one might ask about the frequency of intoxication, whether "blackouts" have been experienced, and whether the patient is having any problems related to drinking. At any point that seems appropriate, the patient can be asked to complete the Stages Index—either by the patient himself or by the physician's systematically asking the questions. With this information available, the family physician can better judge what the nature of his own involvement in the patient's recovery should be and what referrals would be appropriate.

Viewing the alcoholic patient as moving toward recovery even as his drinking problem simultaneously becomes more severe, the physician is provided with a rationale, and some hope, that his efforts to give the patient a helping hand will not be in vain. His efforts can hasten the day when the patient is a recovered alcoholic and, thereby, can benefit not only the patient but also his family and the entire community. In most cases, positive results will not be immediately apparent, and the physician will not be rewarded by a "cure." However, even if the patient returns to drinking, this doesn't necessarily mean that the physician's efforts have failed. It is likely that he has given the patient a boost toward recovery and has shortened the natural course of his drinking career. If the patient is in the early stages of the alcoholic process, there is the potential for shortening it by years. If he is in the later stages and near recovery in the natural course of events, the physician's contribution may be all that is needed to complete the recovery process.

There is much controversy as to whether alcoholics can return to normal social drinking. We recommend abstinence as the goal. While many studies have reported a small percentage of alcoholics returning to social drinking, the chances for this are slight. Our own research shows that while the probability of achieving abstinence *increases* following exposure to help, the chance of achieving regained social drinking *decreases* with advancement in the alcoholic process. However, even in the earliest stage, the probability that an alcoholic can return to acceptable social drinking is only one in three—or about half that of winning at Russian roulette played with a "six-shooter." Only 6 per cent of those beyond Stage 1 return to social drinking, and among Stage 4 cases the rate of regained social drinking is only 2 per cent. The steep decline in rates of social drinking beyond Stage 1 argues strongly for early intervention and secondary prevention efforts, with abstinence as the ultimate treatment goal. Even if abstinence cannot be attained immediately, improvement in the form of reduced consumption can be achieved.

MOTIVATING THE ALCOHOLIC

The physician can expect that for about 20 per cent of the cases identified by the Stages Index as having progressed beyond Stage 1, physical restoration and a frank discussion with the patient and his spouse about the consequences of continued heavy drinking will result in immediate recovery (abstinence). That is, some patients are so near the end of the recovery process that a little added reinforcement of their motivation to do something about their drinking is all that is needed. Still, about 75 per cent of these more advanced patients, and even more of the Stage 1 cases, will resume drinking again. For them, the forces influencing the alcoholic process have not yet been overbalanced by recovery forces. They need long-term support and assistance of the type more appropriately provided by AA, a community alcoholism counselor, or both, than by a physician. However, the physician should not be surprised if his medical services are again required at a later date. For the very early stage alcoholic, the immediate goal is to overcome the patient's denial and initiate the recovery process.

The family physician should be especially alert for signs of alcohol abuse, as well as other drug abuse, among his female patients. As compared with men, the woman alcoholic's drinking is more often associated with emotional stress and precipitating crises. However, alcohol abuse among women is often not as obvious because it is less likely to result in job problems or trouble with the police. Often, it doesn't even generate negative reactions by her spouse. Since the woman alcoholic's husband is likely to be a heavy drinker, if not an alcoholic himself, he does not object to her heavy drinking. He may even encourage it.

All too often, her physician may inadvertently be a negative rather than a positive force in the woman alcoholic's recovery process. The female alcoholic is quite adept at using her physician to justify and continue, rather than to correct, her alcoholic drinking. When her family does insist that she do something about her drinking, she may respond by promising to visit her physician. She presents the physician with vague complaints, but she "forgets" to mention her heavy drinking. If the subject does arise, she denies or understates her consumption. The physician, unable to identify a physical problem and failing to detect the alcohol abuse, gives her a prescription for a drug for her "nerves"—a drug that she will soon abuse in place of, or in addition to, the alcohol.

Awareness of a drinking problem by patients and by those around them comes about gradually. The physician who recognizes early signs can hasten early awareness. Early involvement of the spouse in any efforts to help the alcoholic patient is highly recommended, bearing in mind that the spouse of the woman alcoholic may not be a dependable source of support for her recovery efforts. A frank discussion with both partners may be the first time they have faced the problem or have had a sensible, unemotional discussion of it. Alcoholics tend to be pragmatic and to live very much in the present. Talking to the early stage alcoholic about possible long-range consequences of his drinking will generate little motivation because he believes, of course, that he is "going to quit before it reaches that point." Moreover, it is probably futile to moralize with him. Rather, he should be confronted with any here-and-now physical, psychologic, or social problems attributable to his drinking.

The chances are that the patient in the more advanced stages has been working to correct his problem for some time. Building on these earlier efforts, the physician can accelerate the recovery process, not only through physical restoration but also by reminding the patient of the already existing consequences of his drinking and those that are imminent. Concern about ill health, job loss, family problems, and trouble with the police, in that order, can be powerful motivating levers, as witnessed by the high recovery rate of individuals participating in industrial alcoholism programs in which job security is at stake.

The family physician might go beyond efforts to motivate the alcoholic by helping him to decide what to do next and even by helping him to do it. The physician who is willing to spend the time helping the alcoholic sort out his problems, referring him for needed professional services, helping him follow through on the referrals, and giving him long-term support is encouraged to do so. Otherwise, the physician should know where in the community to refer the alcoholic for this kind of extended support and assistance. Most communities have an AA chapter, and many now have special alcoholism centers offering both in-patient and out-patient services. The family physician should visit these local facilities, become acquainted with their services, and also become acquainted with some of their successful cases.

The physician who prefers not to work with alcoholics probably should do little more than restore the patient physically and make an appropriate referral. However, even those who dislike alcoholics will develop a more favorable attitude as they learn to know them and gain experience working with them and their families.

REFERENCES

1. Cahalan, D.: Problem Drinkers. San Francisco, Jossey-Bass, Inc., Publishers, 1970.
2. Chafetz, M. E., and Demone, H. W., Jr.: Alcoholism and Society. New York, Oxford University Press, 1962.
3. Dietz, P. E., and Baker, S. P.: Drowning epidemiology and prevention. Am. J. Public Health, 64:303, 1974.
4. Drew, L. R. H.: Alcoholism as a self-limiting disease. Q. J. Stud. Alcohol, 29:956, 1968.
5. Galbraith, S., Murray, W. R., Patel, A. R., et al.: The relationship between alcohol and head injury and its effect on the conscious level. Br. J. Surg., 63:128, 1976.
6. Gordon, G. G., Altman, K., Southern, A. L., et al.: Effect of alcohol (ethanol) administration on sex hormone metabolism in normal men. N. Engl. J. Med., 295:793, 1976.
7. Honkanen, R., Visuri, T., and Kilpio, J.: Blood alcohol levels in accident victims. Ann. Chir. Gynaecol. fenn., 64:365, 1975.
8. Jellinek, E. M.: Phases of alcohol addiction. Q. J. Stud. Alcohol, 13:673, 1952.
9. Keller, M.: On the loss of control phenomenon in alcoholism. Br. J. Addict., 67:153, 1972.
10. Lemere, F., and Smith, J. W.: Alcohol-induced sexual impotence. Am. J. Psychiatry, 130:212, 1973.
11. Lieber, C. S.: Alcohol and malnutrition in the pathogenesis of liver disease. J.A.M.A., 233:1077, 1975.
12. MacArthur, J. D., and Moore, F. D.: Epidemiology of burns. J.A.M.A., 231:259, 1975.
13. Mulford, H. A.: Stages in the alcoholic process: toward a cumulative, nonsequential index. J. Stud. Alcohol, 38:563, 1977.
14. Mulford, H. A.: Women and men problem drinkers. Sex differences of clients served by Iowa's community alcoholism programs. J. Stud. Alcohol. In press.
15. Mulford, H. A., and Miller, D. E.: Drinking in Iowa. III. A scale of definitions of alcohol related to drinking behavior. Q. J. Stud. Alcohol, 21:267, 1960.
16. Myerson, R. M., and LaFair, J. S.: Alcoholic muscle disease. Med. Clin. North Am., 54:723, 1970.
17. Packard, R. C.: The neurological complications of alcoholism. Am. Fam. Physician, 14:111, 1976.
18. Patterson, R. J., Bickel, W. H., and Kahlin, D. C.: Idiopathic avascular necrosis of the head of the femur. J. Bone Joint Surg. (Amer.), 46:267, 1964.
19. Pell, S., and D'Alonzo, C. A.: The prevalence of chronic disease among problem drinkers. Arch. Environ. Health, 16:679, 1968.
20. U.S. Dept. of Health, Education, and Welfare: Alcohol and health: New knowledge. Second special report to the U.S. Congress. U.S. Dept. of H.E.W., Washington, D.C., Govt. Printing Office, Preprint Edition, 1974.

Chapter 27

DRUG ABUSE

by KENNETH F. KESSEL,
and MARVIN J. SCHWARZ

GENERAL ASPECTS

The term *drug abuse* is a misnomer. When considering the problem to be discussed in this chapter in its broadest aspects, the term *chemical abuse* would seem to be more applicable because it would include the wide variety of substances currently used that cannot be categorized as "drugs." The word *abuse* also is unfortunate, as it implies an illegal act or a judgmental stance, an attitude that may have contributed to the fostering of an antiestablishment culture or at least to an impairment in communication between users and nonusers. Using chemicals has become a very acceptable way of life for our society and indeed has been looked on by some as an indicator of progress.

Chemical use pervades almost every aspect of our daily living. Acceptable chemical methods used in agribusiness and most industries that are lauded as technologic advances today become the incredible problems of environmental contamination tomorrow. What we condemn in individual chemical users for the injuries they incur to their minds and bodies, we accept, or even defend, in industry's public contamination of air, soil, water, and, consequently, food.

Chemical use is therefore a broad and complex issue. The definition of misuse or abuse is often an arbitrary one. Adherence to this outlook helps increase the physician's judgmental or moralistic posture, which has been detrimental in the past in communicating with and treating the acutely or chronically ill users. The scope of this chapter will be limited to the problems involved in the intentional use of chemicals for the purpose of altering self-perception, or environmental perception, or both. The chapter will not address itself to the socially accepted (and therefore legal) forms of chemical use that are currently in vogue, such as tobacco, alcohol, inappropriate prescribing (iatrogenesis), all forms of the preventable industrial pollution, or the effects of pesticides and other chemical practices on agriculture. Nor will the chapter deal specifically with the use of nonphysician-prescribed medications or household chemicals accidentally ingested by children or intentionally ingested by individuals for the purpose of self-destruction. These matters are covered in other chapters. Hopefully, physicians will develop attitudes that prove to be more effective in dealing with chemical users.

TYPE AND FREQUENCY

There are no adequate demographic data on the frequency of chemical use as defined previously. Various surveys have been done that include "experimental users" as well as chronic users. The estimated number of users of marihuana in the United States according to the Department of Health, Education and Welfare varies from 4 million to 20 million people. The major chemicals used are the central nervous system depressants — narcotics, barbiturates, "sleeping" medications of all varieties, tranquilizers, alcohol, and various admixtures of these. The patterns of chemical use are ever-changing, and the very nature of the subculture involved and the illegality of possession and use make it impossible to derive adequate demographic studies. The financial loss due to narcotic addiction alone is estimated to be 1 billion dollars annually in the United States. Hallucinogenic agents such as dimethoxymethylamphetamine (STP), methyldioxyamphetamine (MDA), lysergic acid diethylamide (LSD), and belladonna alkaloids are still in vogue and present special diagnostic and management problems in acute situations. A common cause of coma in patients between the ages of 15 and 30 presenting in emergency rooms is an overdose of a central nervous system depressant and should be thought of in all adolescent and adult cases of coma.

BEHAVIORAL COMPONENTS

No system has been developed that will predict who will become a compulsive user of chemicals. Experimental or intermittent use of chemicals does not necessarily indicate psychopathology. The use of chemicals seems more related to the following factors: (1) the limited opportunities to experience pride, satisfaction, and pleasure; (2) the social meaning attributed to use by the peer group; (3) the initial attractiveness of the aggressive, goal-oriented life of the user; and (4) the availability of certain chemicals. Originally, white middle-class groups leaned toward cannabis and psychedelic chemical use, while inner city ghetto users favored heroin. These stereotypes no longer apply, and chemical misuse has expanded and continues to be very changeable.

The adolescent or young adult using chemicals generally does not see this as a problem. There is no desire to stop and little conflict about using chemicals. Therefore, there is no motivation to change. Chemical users often assume that professionals cannot really understand them. Contact that does exist with professionals is of a pretended nature or is simply noncommunicative.

Of great importance to the physician is the need to deal realistically with the fantasies about the reversibility of drug use. The adolescent's fantasy is that death is not real, that one's body cannot be hurt, or that one can allow things that are reversible. In addition, there is the evangelic, seductive

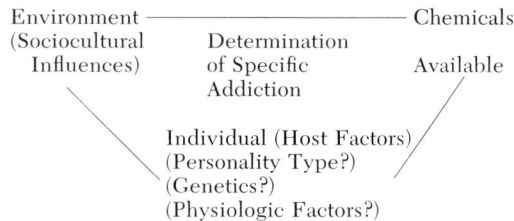

Figure 27–1. Determinants of addiction.

behavior of the peer group that conveys the message that chemical use is both safe and "cool." The concept of incurable disease is not part of the adolescent's vocabulary.

The reality is that many of the biologic effects of chemical use appear to be irreversible. Equally important, the addictive interpersonal relationships and addictive life style to a major degree are irreversible. It would be well for the family physician to thoroughly understand addictive relationships as an important concept, not only relating to chemical addiction but also relevant to many other counseling situations. The book *Love and Addiction* by Stanton Peele and Archie Brodsky[14] gives useful insight in this area.

Adolescence as a stage of the growth process cannot be repeated, and if this time is spent in a "stoned-out," noncontact narcissistic addictive state, this represents an irreplaceable loss. Chemical use then substitutes resolution of problems by avoidance and withdrawal for resolution of conflict and identity problems by mastery. Even in the event of adequate intervention (i.e., disuse of chemicals), it is difficult to do in young adult life what has not previously been done in adolescence (Fig. 27–1).

SOCIAL AND FAMILY IMPLICATIONS

The studies that have been made concerning the impact of chemical misuse on society probably represent the tip of the iceberg. The cost to the nation's economy, industry, courts, prisons, and so forth and the cost in highway mortality, sudden deaths, and accidents at home and at work are only part of the statistic and can only be surmised.

The relationship of supporting "the habit" to committing crime has been studied. Males tend to engage in armed robbery, females in prostitution. Extensive adulteration of street drugs occurs, and every user is a potential dealer. The entire underground industry of acquisition, transportation, control, distribution, and use of chemicals is a complex multibillion dollar business involving thousands of nonusers as well as millions of users. The principal people who benefit from this industry are a handful of nonusers (or users who can easily maintain their habit) who are in control of the "merchandising" of the chemicals.

No one can quantitate the human suffering involved. Specific effects of chemical use by pregnant women have been documented. Sudden deaths in infants born to methadone-maintained addicts, heroin and barbiturate withdrawal syndromes in passively addicted infants, chromosome abnormalities in offspring of LSD users (trisomy D with D/D translocation), and the issue of chemical agents causing chromosome breaks are some examples of direct physiologic and anatomic effects on the children of chemical users. The use of chemicals to rebel against parental authority or to withdraw from family life may have long-range effects on future family cohesion. The effect of the adolescent "drug culture" on the family foundation of the next generation is still an unwritten chapter.

VOCABULARY OF CHEMICAL USE

Frederick Hoffman[8] in his excellent book on drug and alcohol abuse feels that the use of street names by health professionals is self-defeating. This attempt to bridge the generation gap by using words peculiar to adolescent users' vocabulary is viewed by the adolescent as further evidence of adult hypocrisy and dishonesty because the principal purpose of the street name is largely to confuse the nonuser. We have found a difference, however, in the communication that exists between family practice residents and chemical user patients, in whom the generation gap seems less evident. We also feel that some knowledge of street vocabulary as well as professional vocabulary that has evolved around chemical use is very helpful in understanding and caring for the user.

Many street words come and go or change their meaning in different geographic areas or changing subcultures, so the following brief list of terms is by no means considered a comprehensive or permanent document.

Professional Terms

Abstinence syndrome (withdrawal): physiologic effects that occur when the chemically dependent individual is deprived of the specific chemical for a given period of time.

Addiction: physiologic dependence on a chemical.

Cross-dependence: the ability of one chemical agent to suppress abstinence symptoms produced by withdrawal of another agent—may be complete or partial.

Habituation: a psychologic dependence on a chemical.

Tolerance: The decreased effect obtained by repeated administration of a chemical.

> *Metabolic tolerance:* chemical disposition due to an increased rapidity of inactivation, or secretion, or both.

> *Pharmacodynamic tolerance:* cellular adaptation to a chemical agent, requiring more of the agent to produce the same level of response.

Street Terms

Bag: an amount of heroin costing from $2 to $20 for 3 to 30 mg.

Downers: barbiturates, any sedative or sleeping pill.

Fix: sufficient amount of drug to prevent withdrawal.

Joint or Roach: marihuana cigarette.

Junk: street heroin (usually adulterated with quinine, lactose, or maltose).

Junkie: a narcotics peddler or addict.

Kick: orgasmic effect of intravenous heroin.

Mainlining: taking chemicals intravenously.

Mickey Finn: chloral hydrate in alcohol.

Pothead: chronic marihuana user.

Pusher: seller of heroin and other chemicals.

Reefer: marihuana cigarette.

Roach clip: device to hold small marihuana cigarette.

Rush: orgasmic effect of intravenous heroin.

Skin popping: heroin or other chemicals given subcutaneously.

Sniffing: chemical inhalation (glue, cocaine, and so forth).

Speedball: cocaine with heroin.

Tracks: visible remnants of occluded veins used for mainlining.

Uppers: amphetamines, other stimulants, most weight-reducing medications.

Table 27–1 lists specific chemicals, their trade names, street names, and desired effects.

TABLE 27–1. TERMINOLOGY OF CHEMICAL USE

Chemical	Trade Name	Street Name	Desired Effect
Illusionogenics		*Psychedelics*	
Atropine		Belladonna	Flush, hallucinations, excited feeling (signs—tachycardia, flushed dry skin, dilated pupils)
Diethyltryptamine	DET	DET	Similar to DMT, but longer acting
Dimethoxymethylamphetamine		STP, DOM	Prolonged illusionogenic experience or consciousness expansion
Dimethyltryptamine	DMT	DMT, businessman's high	Shortened (1 to 2 hour) illusionogenic experience
Hydroxydimethyltryptamine		Psilocybin, magic mushrooms	Similar to LSD, but quality of experience said to differ from LSD
Lysergic acid diethylamide	LSD	Acid, pearly gates, heavenly blue	Consciousness expansion, self-exploration, experiential
Marihuana, hashish		Grass, weed, pot, smoke, dope reefer, maryjane, tea, Acapulco gold, gold leaf special	Relaxation, disinhibition, decreased threshold to various stimuli, increased sociability
Phencyclidine	Sernyl	PCP, peace pill, angel dust	Not actively sought—often sold as other drug or used to alter effects of base substance
Trimethoxyphenylethylamine		Mescaline, mesc, peyote, buttons	Similar to LSD, but quality of experience said to differ from LSD
Stimulants		*Uppers*	
Amphetamine	Benzedrine	Uppers, speed, whites, bennies, pep pills	Stimulation, motor as well as psychologic; false bravado; creative ideation; increased physical performance
Cocaine		Snow, coke, snort, C	Short-acting mood elevation and cortical stimulation
Methamphetamine		Meth, speed, crystal	Stimulation, motor as well as psychologic; false bravado; creative ideation; increased physical performance
Methylphenidate	Ritalin	Cibas	
Depressants		*Downers*	
Amobarbital	Amytal, Dexamyl	Blue heavens, blues	
Amobarbital/secobarbital	Tuinal	Tooies, rainbows, Christmas trees	Disinhibition, relief of tension, euphoria, alternate drug when opiate addict cannot "score"
Barbiturates		Barbs, downs	
Pentobarbital	Nembutal	Yellow jackets, yellows	
Phenobarbital	Luminal	Whites, purple hearts	
Secobarbital	Seconal	Reds, R.D.'s, red devils	
Nonbarbiturates			
Ethchlorvynol	Placidyl		
Glutethimide	Doriden	Candy, sleeping pills, peanuts	Similar to barbiturates, several members of group known for "aphrodisiac" properties
Methaqualone	Quaalude		
Methyprylon	Noludar		
Alcohol			
Ethanol		Sauce, hooch, booze	Similar to barbiturates, easy availability and social acceptability promote drug as practical alternate
Opiates			
Codeine			
Diacetylmorphine (heroin)		Smack, H, junk, horse, stuff, scag	Initially, euphoria and tranquilization (decreased tension); after physical independence, avoidance or withdrawal syndrome
Dihydromorphinone	Dilaudid	Lords	
Meperidine	Demerol		
Morphine		M., morph	
Paregoric		P.g., blue-velvet°	

TABLE 27–1. TERMINOLOGY OF CHEMICAL USE (*Continued*)

Chemical	Trade Name	Street Name	Desired Effect
Minor tranquilizers		*Tranks*	Occasional disinhibition (when used with alcohol), usually tension relief and self-treatment of dysphoric reactions to other drugs
Chlordiazepoxide	Librium		
Diazepam	Valium		
Meprobamate	Miltown		
Solvents			Unsophisticate's depressants, often used when other drug availability or accessibility restricted
Gasoline			
Glue			
Lighter fluid			
Nail polish, nail polish remover			
Paint			
Miscellaneous			Fad drug, often associated with local peer folklore, often used in combination with other drug experiences
Amyl nitrite		Poppers, snappers	
Asthmador (belladonna alkaloids) tea			
Catnip			
Cough syrups			
Nitrous oxide			
Nutmeg		DDMT	

°Combination of paregoric and tripelennamine.

MANAGEMENT OF ACUTE INTOXICATION

CENTRAL NERVOUS SYSTEM DEPRESSANTS

There are several important principles in managing the acutely intoxicated patient. Often, priorities dictate the order of events.

1. Life support must precede history-taking or complete physical examination.

2. During the initial activity or confusion, the friends or peers who brought the patient in often leave. The history they are able to give may be crucial to the outcome of the patient. Therefore, every effort should be made to delay their departure until time is available to obtain whatever relevant information they may have.

3. There are very few antidotes or specific antagonists to any of the chemicals used, and, furthermore, most hospitals cannot provide emergency drug analysis of urine and blood.

4. Life support measures such as airway-assisted respiration (if needed), intravenous fluids administration, urethral catheterization (usually not needed immediately), or cardiac monitoring should be instituted as required.

5. Look for needle tracks and ask about heroin use. No harm can come from giving 1 or 2 cc. of naloxone (Narcan) while the support measures just listed are being performed. The response will occur in 2 minutes or less. If there is no response and there is no history of chemical abuse but needle marks are present, give 50 cc. of 50 per cent intravenous glucose, as another possible cause of coma in the young person with needle marks is hyperinsulinism. If there is no response to either of these interventions by this time (2 to 3 minutes), the following basic life support systems should be functioning. Nothing has been lost, and two important causes of coma have been ruled out. The usual order of life support events in overdose is:

 a. Respiratory assistance.

 b. Intravenous fluids administration.

 c. Cardiac monitoring.

A flow sheet must be created for monitoring vital signs, intravenous fluids, medications, laboratory tests, and continuous neurologic evaluation. Obviously this requires a team effort, usually managed by the physician in charge.

Therapy

Therapy is adjusted in response to signs and symptoms and laboratory findings. Assuming that the patient is still unconscious and that there is no history or evidence of hypodermic administration of chemicals, no oral evidence of ingestion of corrosive substances, and no olfactory evidence of hydrocarbon ingestion, a nasogastric tube or an oral (Ewald) tube may be inserted for aspiration of gastric contents. This is both for analysis of the aspirate and for prevention of future absorption and aspiration. After the sample is collected, it is customary to administer a slurry of activated charcoal (2 tbsp. of activated charcoal in 8 oz. of warm, one-half normal saline solution) to adsorb chemical substances, especially plant alkaloids (belladonna alkaloids) and glycosides. Blood and urine samples are obtained for chemical analysis (drug screen). (At this point a Foley catheter is inserted.) A complete blood count, urinalysis, blood glucose determination, and electrolyte studies should also be done. Blood gas determinations should also be obtained as a base line. Accurate intake and output measurements are made, and treatment is adjusted to the changing values of physical findings and laboratory studies (determined every 30 to 60 minutes). All of this is unnecessary if the patient responds to naloxone. However, in this case there is one caution—the duration of action of naloxone is usually less than the duration of action of most narcotics. It is therefore dangerous to discharge a patient after a good response to a single dose. These patients must be kept hospitalized or in a holding area for 6 to 8 hours because of the potential danger of relapse into coma.

History. At this point (within the first 30 to 45 minutes), whether the patient has responded or not, a careful history should be taken from the patient's friends. The value of this is to discern the admixture of chemicals used in order to anticipate other complications or reactions or to avoid the use of certain agents that may have an additive effect. Frequently the historical details have great significance. For example, knowing the sequence of events is important in the case of a prolonged alcohol–drug binge, during which methanol products are ingested later in the evening. Therefore, latecomers to the party are subjected to the full toxic effects of methanol without the protection of ethanol that the early partygoers had. If acute methanolism can be detected early, ethanol can be given intravenously as the competitive antidote in a dose of 5 per cent ethyl alcohol in saline. This minimizes the catastrophic effects, especially blindness, on the central nervous system. Hemodialysis is necessary in severe cases.

Drug Medications. Except for the use of naloxone or glucose as diagnostic agents,

other medication is rarely needed. Seizures may be treated with intravenous diazepam (Valium), 5 to 10 mg., repeated every 5 to 10 minutes until the seizures are controlled. Hypotension may be titrated with levarterenol (4 ml. in 1000 cc. of 5 per cent dextrose in water) or phenylephrine (10 mg. in 500 ml. dextrose in water). *Do not give* central nervous system stimulants.

Dialysis. Peritoneal dialysis is of benefit in some cases of prolonged coma (24 hours or more), especially coma due to barbiturates and other nonnarcotic central nervous system depressants.

Clinical Monitoring

Bilateral Pupil Size. Beware of the possibility of head injuries in the chemical user. Disparity in pupil size means subdural hematoma until proved otherwise! Bilateral pupil size is often of little or confusing value in cases involving drug mixtures of narcotics and atropine alkaloids or phenothiazines.

Cardiovascular Status. Monitoring the electrocardiogram (ECG), pulse rate, and blood pressure is essential in the first few hours, when the chemical reaches its peak pharmacologic effect. Central nervous system depressants may cause hypotension. Antidepressants may cause cardiac arrhythmias, especially tricyclic agents such as imipramine (Tofranil).

Level of Consciousness. Record the following signs at 15 minute intervals for the first 2 hours or until patient is responding adequately:

1. Corneal reflex.
2. Response to painful stimuli.
3. Deep tendon reflexes. (Do these bilaterally and be on guard for injury to the central nervous system or for cerebral vascular accidents, which occur at all ages.)
4. Response to verbal commands.

OTHER ACUTE INTOXICATIONS

Every well-equipped hospital emergency room or physician's office should contain an adequate toxicology informational resource. Several of these sources are listed in the references at the end of this chapter.

Special mention should be made of belladonna derivatives, as these commonly occur in combinations of street or commercial drugs. Patients presenting with red skin; dry mouth; dilated pupils; often a nonspecific rash of the face, neck, and upper trunk; fever; tachycardia; and confusion, especially of recent and rapid onset, are probably victims of atropinism. A partial antidote is physostigmine salicylate, 1 to 2 mg. intramuscularly. Avoid phenothiazine tranquilizers because they also have atropine-like effects. The concomitant agitation can be counteracted with small doses of pentobarbital or chlordiazepoxide (Librium).

HALLUCINOGENIC AGENTS

Patients using hallucinogenic agents present with marked alterations of perception, both of themselves and of their surroundings.

An 18 year old boy pushed his way into the emergency room with an obviously injured left arm. He paced up and down, excitedly repeating the phrase, "I know the way to heaven." He refused to sit down and give a coherent history. His friend described the patient's ingesting LSD in a hamburger and shortly thereafter trying to ride his motorcycle up a telephone pole, which he described as the "ladder to heaven."

Patients with hallucinogenic reactions require a quiet, safe environment with a minimal amount of external stimuli. This cannot be achieved in an ordinary emergency room setting. Special rooms need to be available, and a calm attendant capable of "talking down" the patient through the bad trip should be present. Patients should not be left alone or left with angry, judgmental attendants. Restraints should be used only as a last resort. Chlorpromazine (Thorazine), 50 mg. orally, may also be used for LSD intoxication, but only with caution, as it has been known to prolong the hallucinogenic effects of STP or MDA.

CHRONIC CHEMICAL USE AND THE FAMILY PHYSICIAN

Unfortunately, many physicians are unaware of chemical use (drug abuse) in their practice until a patient presents with an acute episode or overdose. As difficult as these are to manage, the physician's work really begins after the patient recovers from the acute episode or overdose. The astute physician may be alerted to chronic chemical users in his practice prior to an overdose incident by increasing his sensitivity to certain behavioral and physiologic changes in his patients. In contrast to other patients, chemical users frequently know more about practical pharmacology and disabilities resulting from long-term chemical use than do their physicians. They can accurately describe the dosage, appearance, and cost of certain agents. Certain clues may alert the physician to chemical use, such as the constipated, sweet-toothed, miotic individual who makes the rounds at local drugstores to obtain paregoric. The experienced pharmacist may know these patients, who often buy candy and laxatives along with their paregoric.

The young chronic sinusitis patient may also be a possible sniffer. In addition, patients with frequent minor trauma may be more than just accident-prone and may actually have sufficient alterations in judgment or chemically induced ataxia to account for their frequent injuries. Significant character changes, especially in adolescents, may indicate chemical experimentation or early repetitive use.

Patient demands for medication to alleviate pain or "nerves" are often given into by the well-meaning physician in the absence of documented need. Chemical misusers often present as just passing through town and as consulting the physician for some chronic or recurring malady, which they act out with amazing expertise. Iatrogenesis has been indicted as a major cause of chronic chemical misuse.

If the physician's suspicions are aroused, his attitude is crucial if he is to be of therapeutic help to his patient. A nonjudgmental and compassionate but firm attitude is essential as a first step toward patient rehabilitation. Even in the best hands, early intervention is difficult, and the physician must tactfully use resources available to the patient that are viewed as "safe" and acceptable.

Once the chemical user has been identified, a treatment plan needs to be formulated. The referring family physician's role is likely to be similar to that of a supportive family member or peer. Unfortunately, most communities do not have treatment resources for chronic chemical users. In general, two treatment modalities exist: professional and peer groups. It is impossible to generalize about the effectiveness of one modality over another because of the variability encountered. Many professionals have limited interest in or training for dealing with the chronic user, and at times their fees are prohibitively expensive. Some peer groups tout evangelistic programs with high cure rates but with little documented evidence of long-term success. Social programs that substitute one addiction for another have the distinct social advantage of patient behavior control. Methadone and equivalent programs have often failed to prove themselves and have been seen as having major cultural and social side effects. They continue to be a potential source of street drugs and an alternate, albeit controlled, chemical way of life.

It is the responsibility of each family physician to identify the best and most available resources for treatment, even if these facilities are at a great distance from and expensive for his patient. The expense is usually no more than that of other catastrophic physical illnesses, such as those requiring cardiac surgery or organ transplantation. Examples of some of these peer or combined professional and peer programs in the United States are listed at the end of this chapter.

The family working together as a unit may be available to help the patient. It is therefore important that the family physician learn supportive techniques to facilitate communication and problem-solving within the family. These techniques are to be used simultaneously with the treatment of the chemical-using family member.

HEROIN DETOXIFICATION IN A GENERAL HOSPITAL

Heroin detoxification has become an increasing problem for many physicians. Often the heroin-addicted patient presents with a traumatic condition that requires orthopedic or general surgery, or the patient may be in labor. Physicians who accept patients primarily for detoxification without associated rehabilitation programs become well known to the narcotic-using community, particularly the heroin-using community. A special license must be obtained by

physicians who use methadone for prolonged detoxification. It is wise to detoxify patients only if there is a reasonable commitment to an adequate rehabilitation program by the patient, and there is an assurance of follow-up by the physician. The difficulties in achieving these are enormous, but not impossible.

We have found the following detoxification regime useful. This regime is a method used by Martin G. Johnson at MacNeal Memorial Hospital in Berwyn, Illinois.

The patient is placed on an every hour dose of methadone on demand. On the first day he may request from 10 to 40 mg. of methadone every 4 hours, based on his previous habit. The overall dose is reduced by 20 per cent each day until the patient is narcotic-free for at least 2 days prior to discharge. During the last 3 days, the patient is placed on Valium, 10 mg. four times a day. For pains, cramps, and headache, Darvocet-N 100, 100 mg. every four hours, is used. Dolophine is used intramuscularly if the patient is nauseated or vomits.

The advantage of this regime seems to be that the patient is allowed to have some control of his daily dosage, reducing it in proportion to his motivation to cut short his hospital stay. Several days prior to discharge, where to send the patient for follow-up care is determined. Ideally, this contact is made while the patient is still in the hospital. Follow-up statistics are poor. Some physicians claim that one can expect favorable results for the first year in about 10 to 15 per cent of cases.

PREVENTION OF CHEMICAL MISUSE

The methods of prevention of addictive chemical use need to be as innovative and assertive as the methods of indoctrination by the chemical culture itself.

The family physician can participate in a number of ways. Educational programs at the grade school and high school levels are potentially beneficial if they are factual. False or exaggerated information usually has a very negative outcome. Popular student leaders should be coplanners and presentors with the teacher and the physician. Field trips to treatment programs often reinforce didactic material and make this material very real. These programs should be part of the regular curriculum and should be repeated annually in each grade, with attention being paid to the appropriateness of content. It must be remembered that by the time a child begins school he has had 5 years of television indoctrination and possibly many hours of advertisements for chemicals as the cure-all for man's common problems.

Possibly even more important and influential is the family physician's preventive "mind set" during his routine day's work in the office and hospital. Drugs must be prescribed judiciously and must never be used as a substitute for the physician's most effective therapeutic tool—himself. The physician's role as a health educator is essential, and much patient and physician unlearning needs to be done. Alternate modes of therapy without drugs must be found for the day-to-day stresses of living. The bereaved must be allowed to mourn, minor discomforts must be tolerated, and insomnia and anxiety can be helped—all without drugs. Counseling, special exercise programs, meditation, or new activities can be prescribed as alternatives. Weight can be lost and smoking can be stopped without drugs. If special groups or clinics are not available for these problems, the physician should be instrumental in starting them. The treatment for alcoholism is not the use of another chemical. It is incumbent upon every physician to reflect upon his own prescribing practices and to weigh to what extent he contributes to the culture of chemical misuse.

It is gratifying to discover the number of community, family, and individual resources available when the physician shifts his focus from pharmacopoeia to himself as his most precious and powerful therapeutic agent for the common behavioral problems he encounters.

SELECTED LIST OF REHABILITATION AND DETOXIFICATION PROGRAMS

Arizona Foundation Mental Health Center
5055 N. 34th Street
Phoenix, Arizona 85018
(602) 955–6200, Ext. 38

St. Luke's-Jane Wayland Comprehensive Community Mental Health Center
525 N. 18th Street
Phoenix, Arizona 85006
(602) 258–7373, Ext. 366

Los Angeles County Mental Health Department
1102 S. Crenshaw
Los Angeles, California 90019
(213) 937–2380

Federal Narcotic Addict Rehabilitation Program
Catholic Family Service
349 Cedar Street
San Diego, California 92101
(714) 235–6481

Mesa Vista Hospital
7850 Vista Hill Avenue
San Diego, California 92123
(714) 278–4110, Exts. 242, 249

San Diego County Mental Health Services
P. O. Box 3067
San Diego, California 92103

Acute Detoxification Unit
San Francisco General Hospital
22 Potrero Avenue
San Francisco, California 94103
(415) 648–6016

Fort Logan Mental Health Center
3520 W. Oxford Avenue
Denver, Colorado 80236
(303) 761–0220

Methadone Maintenance Program
Denver General Hospital, Ward 18
West 6th Avenue at Cherokee
Denver, Colorado 80204
(303) 893–6206

Narcotics Treatment Administration
122 C Street, N.W.
Washington, D.C. 20001

Veterans Administration Hospital
50 Irving Street, N.W.
Washington, D.C. 20422
(202) 483–6666, Exts. 6847, 6848

Youth in Crisis
6737 W. 34th Street
Berwyn, Illinois 60402
(312) 484–7400

Substance Abuse Program
1440 S. Indiana
Chicago, Illinois 60605
(312) 633–0935

Northwest Youth Outreach
7032 W. Belmont
Chicago, Illinois 60634
(312) 777–7112

Dangerous Drug Commission
300 N. State
Chicago, Illinois
(312) 822–9860

Forest Hospital
555 Wilson Lane
Des Plaines, Illinois
(312) 827–8811

Open Door
202 S. 21st
Maywood, Illinois 60153
(312) 865-2796

Hip House
1908 St. Charles Road
Maywood, Illinois 60153
(312) 345-1275

Veterans Administration Hospital
Hines, Illinois 60141
(312) 343-7200

Oak Park Drug Team
1024 N. Boulevard
Oak Park, Illinois 60302
(312) 383-7500

Substance Abuse Program
7400 W. 183rd Street
Tinley Park, Illinois 60477
(312) 532-5550

DuPage Outreach
207 S. Villa, Suite 210
Villa Park, Illinois 60181
(312) 834-8900

Midtown Community Mental Health Center
Marion County General Hospital
960 Locke Street
Indianapolis, Indiana 46204
(317) 630-7606

Elan
RFD Box 33
Poland Springs, Maine 04274
(207) 998-4666

Northwest Drug ALERT
Sinai Hospital
Greenspring and Belvedere
Baltimore, Maryland 21215

Provident Hospital
Project ADAPT
550 Mosher Street
Baltimore, Maryland 21217
(301) 523-3230

Center for Attitude Change
Drug Addiction Rehabilitation Center
591 Morton Street
Boston, Massachusetts 02124
(617) 287-1510

Project Turn-Off
City of Boston Drug Addiction
Treatment and Rehabilitation Program
Psychiatry Service
Boston City Hospital
818 Harrison Avenue
Boston, Massachusetts 02118

Street Youth Program
Children's Service, Behavior Unit
Massachusetts General Hospital

Fruit Street
Boston, Massachusetts 02114
(617) 726-2907, 2994

Tufts Mental Health Center
260 Tremont Street, Metro 7
Boston, Massachusetts 02116
(617) 482-2800, Ext. 2824

Washington Hospital
41 Morton Street, Jamaica Plain
Boston, Massachusetts 01230
(617) 524-1540

Herman Kiefer Hospital Drug Abuse Program
8809 John C. Lodge Freeway, Building 4
Detroit, Michigan 48202
(313) 224-3984, 3985

Lafayette Clinic Methadone Program
951 East Lafayette
Detroit, Michigan 48207
(313) 963-5400

NARA Title II
Federal Program
352 City-County Building
Detroit, Michigan 48226
(313) 224-3826

Department of Psychiatry
Jewish Hospital of St. Louis
216 South Kingshighway
St. Louis, Missouri 63110
(314) 367-8060, Ext. 561

St. Louis Drug Dependency Treatment Center
5400 Arsenal Street
St. Louis, Missouri 63139
(314) 644-2400, Ext. 2100

Fordham Methadone Maintenance Program
Fordham Hospital
Southern Boulevard and Crotona Avenue
Bronx, New York 10458
(212) 583-6244

Kings County Addictive Disease Hospital
600 Albany Avenue
Brooklyn, New York 11203
Drug Detoxification Unit
(212) 462-4000, Exts. 6584, 6115
(212) 270-3130

Edward J. Meyer Memorial Hospital
Department of Psychiatry
462 Grider Street
Buffalo, New York 14215
(716) 894-1212, Ext. 552

Daytop Village
54 W. 40th Street
New York, New York 10018
(212) 354-6000

Daytop Village
Staten Island
New York, New York
(212) 981-3136

Division of Biological Psychiatry
Department of Psychiatry
New York Medical College

Metropolitan Hospital Medical Center
5 E. 102nd Street
New York, New York 10029
(212) 360–6769

Harlem Ambulatory Detoxification Unit
Harlem Hospital Center, K Building
New York, New York 10037
(212) 621–4183, 4184, 4185
(212) 621–3553

Methadone Maintenance Program
Gracie Square Hospital
420 E. 76th Street
New York, New York 10021
(212) 988–4400

Methadone Maintenance Treatment Program
Beth Israel Medical Center
245 E. 17th Street
New York, New York 10003
(212) 673–3000, Exts. 2951, 2952, 2953

Methadone Maintenance Treatment Program
Department of Psychiatry
Jewish Memorial Hospital
196th Street and Broadway
New York, New York 10040
(212) 569–4700, Ext. 16

Methadone Maintenance Treatment Program
Roosevelt Hospital
882–884 Tenth Avenue
New York, New York 10019
(212) 489–8792, 8791, 8790

Mt. Sinai Medical Center
Department of Psychiatry
Individual Drug Abuse Treatment
Fifth Avenue and 100th Street
New York, New York 10029
(212) 876–1000, Exts. 6265, 6268

Mt. Sinai School of Medicine
Methadone Program
Fifth Avenue and 100th Street
New York, New York 10029
(212) 876–1000, Exts. 6267, 6268

New York City Methadone Maintenance Treatment Program
377 Broadway
New York, New York 10013
(212) 966–6308

Roosevelt Hospital City Methadone Maintenance Treatment Program
882 Tenth Avenue
New York, New York 10019
(212) 247–9702

Roosevelt Hospital
Drug Abuse Program

882–884 Tenth Avenue
New York, New York 10019
(212) 247–9702

United Harlem Drug Fighters
Harlem Hospital, Pediatric Building
Fourth and Fifth Floors
530 Lenox Avenue
New York, New York 10037
(212) 621–3219

Veterans Administration Hospital
First Avenue and 24th Street
New York, New York 10010
(212) 686–7500, Exts. 638, 639

Cleveland Metropolitan General Hospital
Methadone Program
3395 Scranton Road
Cleveland, Ohio 44109
(216) 398–6000, Exts. 536, 210

Fairhill Mental Health Center
Drug Abuse Program
12200 Fairhill Road
Cleveland, Ohio 44120
(216) 421–1340

Drug Addiction Clinic
St. Luke's and Children's Medical Center
Eighth Street and Girard Avenue
Philadelphia, Pennsylvania 19122
(215) 684–3900, Ext. 502

Fairmount Farm
561 Fairthorne Street
Philadelphia, Pennsylvania 19128
(215) 483–0735, Ext. 61

The Institute of the Pennsylvania Hospital
111 North 49th Street
Philadelphia, Pennsylvania 19139
(215) 829–2237

Veterans Administration Hospital
2002 Holcombe Boulevard
Houston, Texas 77031
(713) 747–3000, Exts. 522, 476

Vocational Guidance Service
Drug Abuse and Addiction Control Programs
2525 San Jacinto Street, Suite 206
Houston, Texas 77002
(713) 225–0688

Bexar County Drug Dependence Center
Robert B. Green Hospital
527 North Leona
San Antonio, Texas 78207
(512) 233–1838

Seattle Treatment Center
500 17th Avenue
Seattle, Washington 98122
(206) 329–9198

Mount Sinai Medical Center
Psychiatry Clinic

948 N. 12th Street
Milwaukee, Wisconsin 53206
(414) 271–2174, Ext. 766

Wood Veterans Administration Center
Milwaukee, Wisconsin 53193
(414) 384–2000, Ext. 2161

REFERENCES

1. Beeson, P. E., and McDermott, W.: Textbook of Medicine, 14th ed. Philadelphia, W. B. Saunders Co., 1975.
2. Bleyer, W. A., and Marshall, R. E.: Barbiturate withdrawal syndrome in a passively addicted infant. J.A.M.A., 221:185, 1972.
3. Casriel, D. H.: The family physician and the narcotics addict. Sandoz Panorama, 1970.
4. Chatton, M. J., and Krupp, M. A.: Current Medical Diagnosis and Treatment. Los Altos, Cal., Lange Medical Publishers, 1976.
5. Evans, L. E., Swainson, C. P., Roscoe, P., et al.: Treatment of drug overdosage with naloxone, a specific narcotic antagonist. Lancet, 1:452, 1973.
6. Gleason, M. N., Gosselin, R. E., Hodge, H. C., et al.: Clinical Toxicology of Commercial Products, 3rd ed. New York, The Williams & Wilkins Co., 1969.
7. Gottheil, E., Caddy, G., and Austin, D.: Fallibility of urine drug screens in monitoring methadone programs. J.A.M.A., 236:1035, 1976.
8. Hofmann, F. G.: A Handbook on Drug and Alcohol Abuse. New York, Oxford University Press, 1975.
9. House of Representatives: Hearings before the Select Committee on Crime: Crime in America—The Heroin Paraphernalia Trade. 91st Congress, 2nd Session, Washington, D.C., October 5 and 6, 1970.
10. Hsu L. Y., Strauss, L., and Hirschhorn, K.: Chromosome abnormality in offspring of LSD user. J.A.M.A., 211:987, 1970.
11. Judd, L. L., Brandkamp, W. W., and McClothin, W. H.: Comparison of chromosomal patterns obtained from groups of continued users, former users, and nonusers of LSD-25. Am. J. Psychiatry, 126:626, 1969.
12. Litt, I. S., and Schonberg, S. K.: Medical complications of drug abuse in adolescents. Med. Clin. North Am., 59:1445, 1975.
13. MacKenzie, R. G.: Caring for the adolescent drug user. Med. Clin. North Am., 59:1439, 1975.
14. Peele, S., and Bordsky, A.: Love and Addiction. New York, Signet Books, 1976.
15. Pierson, P. S., Howard, P., and Kleber, H. D.: Sudden deaths in infants born to methadone-maintained addicts. J.Å.M.A., 220:472, 1972.
16. United States Department of Health, Education and Welfare: Marihuana, Some Questions and Answers. Public Health Service Publication No. 1829, March, 1969.
17. Wikler, A.: Clinical and social aspects of Marihuana intoxication. Arch. Gen. Psychiatry, 23:320, 1970.

Chapter 28

ORGANIC BRAIN SYNDROME

*by DONALD G. LANGSLEY,
and GABRIEL SMILKSTEIN*

The family physician is apt to be consulted when a family member's behavior or thinking is apparently deviating from normal. When the onset is rapid, the patient himself may realize it and seek help. On the other hand, slow and gradual change may remain unnoticed by anyone for some time. Only when behavior starts to embarrass or frighten family members, or interferes with family function, do the relatives become alarmed. Such disturbances frequently result from an organic brain syndrome.

DEFINITIONS

The organic brain syndrome results from a diffuse impairment of brain function. The process, which has multiple etiologies, may be acute or chronic, reversible or irreversible, and is manifested by the impairment of orientation, memory, judgment, and intellectual function, and by emotional lability (Table 28–1). Patients may also demonstrate secondary physical dysfunction and psychologic disorder.

Organic brain syndrome is most often classified as acute or chronic. Acute brain syndrome results from a temporary, gener-

ally reversible, diffuse disturbance of brain function and is usually characterized by sudden onset with rapid development of the basic disorders noted in Table 28–1. If the etiologic process is identified and treated successfully, the symptoms will disappear, but if the process is untreated or inadequately treated, the symptoms may progress and become chronic, resulting in a relatively irreversible diffuse disturbance of brain function.

Sometimes chronic brain syndrome is erroneously considered permanent and irreversible. Though complete rehabilitation to a symptom-free state is not possible in diagnosed cases of diffuse permanent brain damage, a definite improvement is possible by carefully monitoring those conditions that tend to impair brain function, e.g., hypoxia and drug intoxication. Often developing slowly and insidiously, chronic brain syndrome may have a clinical course that can progress over months or years and has been estimated to afflict 10 per cent of the over-65 age group. Detection of onset is difficult.

The history of patients with chronic brain syndrome usually reveals a gradual loss of intellectual functions and memory. The initial changes are often subtle. Friends or family may notice that the patient has difficulty in thinking through projects, in understanding messages, and in making decisions. The oft-cited example is the successful businessman who becomes repetitious and circumstantial in speech. His diminished capacity to perform his business activities may be hidden for a long time by a tendency to make no changes. However, there are many variations to this story. (See the following case illustrations.)

TABLE 28–1. BASIC IMPAIRMENTS IN BRAIN FUNCTION IN ORGANIC BRAIN SYNDROME

Orientation. Time, place, person, situation
Memory. Registration, retention, recall
Intellectual Function. Calculation, comprehension, general forms of information, ability to learn new tasks
Judgment. Ability to solve situational problems
Affect. Emotional blunting or inappropriateness

TABLE 28–2. CHARACTERISTICS OF ACUTE AND CHRONIC ORGANIC BRAIN SYNDROMES

Acute Brain Syndrome	Chronic Brain Syndrome
1. Onset sudden with rapid development of the five basic impairments. (See Table 28–1.)	1. Onset often (but not always) slow and insidious. Takes several weeks or more.
2. Delirium, stupor, or coma may be present. There may be release of underlying psychotic or neurotic reactions.	2. Clinical course gradual with stupor or coma. Release of underlying functional impairment coexists.
3. Caused by temporary, usually reversible, diffuse disturbance of brain function.	3. Caused by diffuse alteration of brain function that is often (but not always) permanent and irreversible.
4. Thinking, memory, perception, and attention disturbed, usually with rapid onset.	4. Gradual loss of intellectual function. Recent memory impaired first and remote memory later.
5. Diminished cognitive function.	5. Retention of social behavior obscures declining cognitive abilities early in course.
6. Labile mood, but anxiety and fear frequently present.	6. Depression a common component, or may be confused with depression.

Delirium and dementia are terms that have been used synonymously with acute and chronic brain syndrome respectively; however, they have also been considered as components of the classification of organic brain syndrome (Table 28–2).

Organic brain syndrome may be confused with functional psychoses or neuroses due to a release of underlying coexistent psychologic functional impairment. Paranoid delusions, loss of reality, mania, and hallucinations, all of which resemble schizophrenia, have been observed in patients who have an organic brain syndrome. This observation should alert the family physician to the value of an organic work-up for the patient who manifests neurotic or psychotic symptomatology.

The following case histories illustrate some of the varied ways in which a patient with an acute or chronic organic brain syndrome may present.

CASE I

Acute brain syndrome. Etiology—myocardial infarction with cerebral ischemia due to decreased blood supply to brain.

J. K., a 51 year old businessman, experienced an acute onset of severe chest pain radiating down the left arm. The onset occurred at work, and he immediately telephoned his physician, who advised him to come to the emergency room of a nearby hospital. An electrocardiogram (ECG) in the emergency room showed changes suggestive of acute myocardial infarction. J. K. was immediately admitted to the coronary care unit. There he was attached to a variety of monitoring apparatus, including an alarm system that was not operating well and that gave three false

alarms in the first 24 hours. With a history of no prior cardiac illness, it was not surprising that J. K. became anxious and fearful during his first few days in the coronary care unit. This gave way to a sense of sadness and loss of hope when his physician indicated that the coronary occlusion had been a serious one and recommended a surgical bypass procedure. Cardiac catheterization demonstrated sufficient impairment of circulation so that J. K. was taken from the coronary care unit to surgery on the fourth day after the initial onset of pain. His surgery was uneventful from a technical point of view, and he did well during the first few hours postoperatively. However, on the second day he became agitated and resisted attention from the nursing staff. He was clearly disoriented as to place, person, and situation, and his speech indicated that he was experiencing frightening auditory and visual hallucinations. The staff had to restrain him physically because he attempted to strike out at them and to remove his intravenous lines.

CASE II

Chronic brain syndrome with superimposed acute component. Etiology—chronic ischemia due to decreased blood flow to brain resulting from cerebral arteriosclerosis; acute ischemia due to congestive heart failure and failure to develop adequate cerebral perfusion pressure.

A. B., a 71 year old retired government clerk, suffered from progressive memory loss and disorientation. His family brought him to a hospital emergency room because he had become confused and agitated over the past 2 days. In the busy emergency room situation, the physician prescribed diazepam but did not do a thorough evaluation. The patient was advised to see his family physician, who discovered that A. B. had congestive heart failure. When cardiac function was compensated, he was no longer agitated or confused. He continued to demonstrate some recent memory loss and was clinically depressed. Antidepressants resulted in an improvement in the depression, and A. B. was able to continue living in his apartment without apparent behavioral disturbance or undue concern on the part of his children.

Such cases will be familiar to the family physician. J. K. reacted to his heart attack and treatment in the coronary care unit with anxiety and sadness. His postoperative course was complicated by an organic brain syndrome, a change in intellectual functioning accompanied by psychotic behavior that seriously complicated his medical care. The case of A. B. is less dramatic. Because of his age, the progressive memory loss and disorientation did not surprise his family. Only after a period of confusion and agitation did they seek help, and although the congestive heart failure was missed in the emergency room examination, it was diagnosed by his family physician. Correcting the congestive heart failure improved circulation to the brain and oxygenation of its tissue. This resulted in improved mental functioning. An underlying depression then became apparent and probably played a role in the neglect of his health that delayed the request for medical help.

CASE III

Chronic brain syndrome due to multiple sclerosis.

N. O. initially sought help from his family physician because of diplopia over a period of several days. Approximately a month later he described weakness in both legs, but the symptoms disappeared over the next few months. Six months later he returned because of a right hemiplegia associated with ataxia. His wife reported that he showed a lack of ability to control his emotions. Neurologic evaluation and laboratory studies resulted in a diagnosis of multiple sclerosis. Mr. O. recovered from this episode and returned to productive work, but his wife described his thinking as slowed. He continued to experience ataxia. Memory problems gradually became more severe, and thinking and judgment also became increasingly impaired. Several years later he was seen because of difficulty with bladder control. At that time he had ataxic eye movements, pallor of both optic discs, and scanning speech. He was unable to stand and demonstrated hyperactive reflexes with bilateral positive Babinski's signs. He was oriented as to time and place but was unable to tell who the President was and often confabulated answers in response to questioning.

CASE IV

Acute brain syndrome due to drug intoxication.

T. U. was a 35 year old registered nurse who recognized that she was having difficulty because of the increasing amounts of pain medication she required. Back and leg pain had been present for 5 years, and 2 years ago she had had a laminectomy and spinal fusion without significant relief. Medications included a variety of analgesics, including codeine and glutethimide. She complained tearfully and bitterly about her pain, was alert and oriented, and intellectual functions were intact, but she demonstrated slurred speech, dilated pupils, nystagmus on lateral gaze, and slowed thinking.

The cases of N. O. and T. U. suggest other aspects of organic brain syndrome. Mr. O. turned out to have multiple sclerosis, which is caused by structural changes in the brain. Along with the focal changes due to this degenerative disorder, he showed mental symptoms that began with slowing of his higher intellectual functions and a recent memory disturbance. The initial mental changes were followed by further intellectual deterioration. With Miss U. the clinical picture was one of acute rather than slow onset, and only her thinking and problem-solving capacities were involved. She was oriented and did not show the disturbance of intellectual function seen in the other case illustrations.

CAUSES OF ORGANIC BRAIN SYNDROME

Organic brain syndrome can be caused by infectious disease, oxygen deprivation, systemic (metabolic) disease, toxic effect of drugs, and structural brain damage. Plum and Posner have termed all of these causes except the structural brain damage as secondary metabolic encephalopathies (SME). Table 28–3 offers a list of some of the processes that may produce an organic brain syndrome. SME are processes extrinsic to the neurons and glia that may induce an organic brain syndrome. Primary metabolic encephalopathies are intrinsic diseases of the brain cells, such as Huntington's chorea.

Both acute and chronic brain syndromes

TABLE 28-3. SOME CAUSES OF ORGANIC BRAIN SYNDROME

Infectious Diseases
1. Bacterial (abscess, meningitis)
2. Viral (viral encephalitides including the arthropod-borne viruses, enteroviruses, herpes, rubeola, rubella, mumps, infectious mononucleosis, and postvaccinal encephalitis)
3. Spirochetal (syphilis)
4. Protozoan (malaria, amebiasis)
5. Metazoan (trichinosis)
6. Fungal (histoplasmosis)

Oxygen Deprivation
1. Hypoxia—cerebral blood flow normal
   a. Decreased oxygen tension and content in blood, as in obstructive pulmonary disease, pulmonary embolus, or diminished atmospheric oxygen tension
   b. Decreased oxygen content with normal oxygen tension, as in anemia or CO poisoning
   c. Increased oxygen need, as in fever
2. Ischemia—decreased blood supply to brain
   a. Decreased cardiac output, as in arrhythmia, myocardial infarction, congestive heart failure
   b. Imbalance of blood volume and peripheral resistance, as in orthostatic hypotension, hemorrhage, or excessive fluid loss
   c. Increased cerebrovascular resistance, as in hypertensive encephalopathy, dehydration hemoconcentration, cerebral arteriosclerosis, or cerebral embolus

Metabolic Disorders
1. Hypoglycemia
2. Nutritional deficiency (thiamine, niacin, pyridoxine)

Systemic Disease
1. Nonendocrine (hepatic coma, uremic coma, CO_2 narcosis)
2. Endocrinopathies—disorders of pituitary, thyroid, adrenal, pancreas, or parathyroid glands
3. Other systemic diseases (porphyria, lupus erythematosus, cancer)
4. Nutritional deficiencies (thiamine, niacin, pyridoxine, and B_{12})

Exogenous Substances (Toxins)
1. Sedatives, psychoactive drugs, anticonvulsants (barbiturates, tranquilizers, anticholinergics, opiates, phenytoin)
2. Acid poisons (methyl alcohol, ethylene glycol)
3. Enzyme inhibitors (heavy metals, organic phosphates, salicylates)

Acid–Base Imbalance
1. Sodium deficiency or excess
2. Acidosis
3. Alkalosis
4. Potassium deficiency or excess
5. Magnesium or calcium deficiency or excess

Body Temperature Abnormalities
1. Hypothermia
2. Hyperthermia

Brain Trauma or Tumors
1. Nonoperative (concussion, skull fracture, anomalies of blood vessels)
2. Operative (epi- or subdural hematoma, hemorrhage, aneurysm, meningioma)

---

may be caused by SME and structural brain damage, but in chronic brain syndrome the processes tend to be severe, prolonged, untreated, or associated with a delay in treatment. The end result is frequently diffuse brain damage that is permanent and relatively irreversible. The chronic brain syndrome is also found in certain diseases of unknown etiology, such as senile dementia (Alzheimer's disease), and multiple sclerosis.

DIAGNOSTIC EVALUATION

Organic brain syndromes are variable in their clinical picture. It is not always possible to relate specific behavior with etiology. However, there are features that suggest a diffuse brain disturbance rather than a localized lesion. Just as tuberculosis or syphilis can produce varied clinical syndromes, the clinical manifestations of organic brain syndrome will depend on the type and location of brain impairment as well as on the personality and strengths of the individual involved.

The most critical elements in the management of the patient with organic brain syndrome are early recognition and localization of cerebral dysfunction and the establishment of a specific etiology. Many patients with acute illnesses are found to be quietly delirious in a hospital bed. Failure to establish a specific etiology is likely to delay appropriate therapy; consequently, the "golden" period for therapy may be lost, and permanent brain damage and possible death may result from the disease or injury causing the organic brain syndrome.

Suspicion of an organic brain syndrome should alert the physician to take an especially careful history. Information should be obtained about medications, drug abuse, and exposure to toxins. The general medical history should focus on cardiopulmonary and renal functioning, head trauma, seizures, metabolic or endocrine conditions, as well as other systemic diseases and dietary habits.

The brain is so sensitive that even minimal insult may alter its function. Some of the earliest symptoms of brain dysfunction may be anxiety, irritability, restlessness, insomnia, personality change, shortened attention span, loss of memory for recent events, lethargy, and depression. These early symptoms may be fleeting or prolonged, according to the etiology of the acute brain syndrome. Hypoxia resulting from an acute asthmatic attack may produce transient anxiety and restlessness until the reversible airway obstruction is corrected with bronchodilators. Chronic hypoxia caused by chronic obstructive pulmonary disease may result in an extended period of confusion, memory defect, and personality change.

As a disease or injury process involves a greater portion of the cerebral cortex and sometimes the facilitating pathways of consciousness of the brain stem, disorientation as to time, place, and person may be combined with an advancing stupor, thus preventing the investigator from developing a reasonable history. Under these circumstances the physical examination becomes a major diagnostic factor. A complete physical examination may reveal signs of extracerebral disease responsible for an organic brain syndrome. Attention should be directed especially to the patient's gait, the Romberg sign, evidence of tremor or asterixis, neck flexibility, thyroid enlargement, funduscopic findings, cardiorespiratory status, hepatomegaly, cranial nerve integrity, deep tendon reflexes, and any pathologic reflexes.

Structural brain damage may be localized by examination of vital signs, motor activity, pupillary reactions, respiratory pattern, oculovestibular reflex, and level of con-

sciousness. Vital signs may vary considerably with the intracranial pathology. In most cases of increased cerebrospinal fluid pressure, the pulse will decrease, the breathing pattern will change, the blood pressure will increase, and the pulse pressure will widen.

Physical findings in acute brain syndrome will, of course, be significantly influenced by the disease process that is inducing the response. Findings resulting from structural brain damage are anatomically specific for the level of destruction; furthermore, in an enlarging supratentorial lesion due to tumor or bleeding, the progression of brain damage will be in a caudal–rostral direction. In metabolic disease, however, various levels of dysfunction may be identified. For example, in barbiturate intoxication the patient may be flaccid and unconscious with depressed respirations and still retain a pupillary reflex.

The earliest physical findings in acute brain syndrome will vary somewhat according to the etiology. In children especially, a slowing of the pulse should be viewed with suspicion of increasing intracranial pressure. Early symptoms of meningitis and encephalitis may include nuchal rigidity, hyperirritability, and, in some cases, focal upper motor neuron signs. Ataxia and nystagmus resulting from cerebellar and brain stem involvement may be early findings in drug intoxication. In SME resulting from hypoxia secondary to a pulmonary embolus, neurologic defects such as focal motor abnormalities have been reported in 5 per cent of cases studied. Chronic pulmonary disease with right-sided heart failure has been associated with findings of papilledema, focal neurologic defects, and bilateral extensor plantar responses. The investigator may anticipate an impending hypertensive encephalopathic crisis if early symptoms of SME are accompanied by physical findings of a markedly elevated diastolic blood pressure, papilledema, hypertensive retinopathy, and focal neurologic abnormalities. Many neurologic abnormalities have been reported to be associated with the SME of nonketotic hyperosmolar coma. These include aphasia, homonymous hemianopia, nuchal rigidity, and peripheral neuropathy. Myoclonus, asterixis, tetany, and peripheral neuropathy have been reported as components of uremic SME.

Severe hypoglycemia and oxygen deprivation may result in very rapid and dramatic changes in physical findings. The patient may demonstrate unconsciousness, convulsions, dilated pupils, and bilateral extensor plantar responses. The investigator alert to the possible etiology of these changes will immediately initiate glucose and oxygen therapy to prevent irreversible brain damage and to preserve life.

LABORATORY AND SPECIAL STUDIES

Laboratory data will contribute to the identification of major causes of SME — hypoxia, infection, systemic metabolic disorders (e.g., hypoglycemia), and drug intoxication. For the patient who presents as a diagnostic dilemma, the following studies are indicated as soon as possible: arterial blood gases, complete blood count, urinalysis, blood glucose, basic electrolyte panel (CO_2, CL, K, Na), blood urea nitrogen

(BUN), and a drug toxicity panel. Since occult infections may be a factor in SME, cultures of blood, sputum, urine, and cerebrospinal fluid should be considered. Cerebrospinal fluid should also be evaluated for protein, glucose, pH, and chloride levels and for presence of cells, bacteria, and fungi.

X-ray studies and radioactive scanning should be specific for the area of pathologic abnormality under investigation. ECG's are mandatory for any cardiac or pulmonary disease. The electroencephalogram (EEG) can contribute to clarification of various diagnoses. Table 28–4 indicates the distinctions that may exist in the EEG between metabolic, structural, and psychogenic causes for obtunded consciousness. Specialized studies, especially those that are invasive, should be initiated only after carefully weighing the value of the information that will be obtained against the potential hazards to the patient.

TABLE 28–4. DISTINCTIONS BETWEEN METABOLIC, STRUCTURAL, AND PSYCHOGENIC CAUSES OF OBTUNDED CONSCIOUSNESS

	Metabolic	Structural	Psychogenic
Mental State	Confused Disoriented (especially to time) Abstract thinking defective Difficulty concentrating Difficulty retaining new information	Alert → stuporous according to the extent of supratentorial lesion Comatose if both hemispheres and/or facilitating pathways of brain stem involved	If cooperative, not disoriented, can retain information
Motor Signs	Diffuse abnormal motor signs that may include tremor, myoclonus, asterixis, and ataxia May demonstrate dysfunction affecting different levels of the brain, yet retain other functions that originate at or above levels of identified dysfunction	Abnormal focal motor signs — lacks asterixis Expanding supratentorial lesions demonstrate a sequential rostral–caudal progression of dysfunction Subtentorial defects show uniform regional dysfunction from the initial insult	Lacks abnormal reflexes or adventitious movements
Breathing Patterns	Hypoventilation, posthyperventilation apnea	Supratentorial lesions show rostral–caudal progression of breathing from normal → sigh or yawn → Cheyne-Stokes respiration Subtentorial lesions show rostral–caudal progression of breathing from hyperventilation → cluster → irregularly irregular → apnea (ataxic breathing)	Usually normal with the exception of psychogenic hyperventilation
EEG	Generally slow, diffuse changes° (diffuse theta and delta-wave slowing very common)	May be slow, but focal lesion usually seen with supratentorial insult to brain	Normal

° Minimal intoxication with a fast-acting sedative may cause high-frequency background waves.

MANAGEMENT

Obviously, management depends on accurate diagnosis. In the milder forms of SME and structural brain damage, time favors the investigator, but the recognition of etiology is difficult. In the more severe forms of SME and structural brain damage, time is at a premium, so a "shotgun" approach to diagnosis and therapy is often required.

Table 28–4 offers some basic distinctions between metabolic, structural, and psychogenic causes of obtunded consciousness in a patient and suggests several items that require evaluation. A data base that includes information about the patient's mental state, motor signs, breathing patterns, eye signs, oculovestibular reflex, vital signs, and EEG will do much to clarify the etiology of the patient's organic brain syndrome state and to allow the investigator to establish a disease-specific plan for therapy.

The patient with the most critical forms of SME or structural brain damage may present with seizures or be in a comatose state. Seizures may result from any of a variety of causes that include hypoglycemia, uremia, hypoxia, hypertension, drug toxicity, head injuries, and a pre-existent convulsive disorder.

Management of seizures due to SME or structural brain damage presents an exceedingly difficult challenge. The underlying pathologic disorder must be dealt with, while giving careful thought to the detriments of using anticonvulsants. Seizures due to drug toxicity, for example, would be compounded by the use of sedatives. Sedation resulting from barbiturates or diazepam therapy for seizures would eliminate the investigator's ability to evaluate the patient's state of consciousness, an essential component in the diagnosis of brain damage. To avoid sedation, phenytoin is an ideal anticonvulsant; 150 to 250 mg. is given intravenously at a rate not to exceed 50 mg. per minute. Pediatric dosage is calculated at 250 mg. per square meter of body surface.

Other considerations in the management of seizures should include maintenance of an adequate airway (giving 100 per cent oxygen), intravenous dexamethasone to reduce cerebral edema, and if all else fails, complete muscle relaxation and sedation by anesthesia.

Clinical improvement in the patient with an acute brain syndrome may be dramatic, for example, when 50 per cent glucose is given intravenously to the acutely hypoglycemic patient. However, management is complicated and prolonged for patients whose recovery is delayed for days or weeks after severe drug toxicity or structural brain damage. It is necessary to give careful support to vital functions and strictly monitor vital signs, fluids, and electrolytes.

Adequate follow-up of patients who have apparently been cleared of acute brain syndrome caused by SME is essential in order to anticipate occurrences such as delayed postanoxic encephalopathy, an unexplained phenomenon characterized by rapid neurologic deterioration and sometimes death 7 to 21 days after apparent recovery from an episode of anoxia or hypoxia.

In addition to the steps taken to manage the etiology of organic brain syndrome, certain approaches in the management of the hospitalized patient will be helpful. When it is necessary to hospitalize a patient with organic brain syndrome, the physician must remember that the strange surroundings, personnel, and procedures will further confuse the already impaired patient. Familiar people should be available to the patient and family members should be permitted to stay or to visit frequently. The hospital room should have a quiet and unambiguous environment with simple furnishings. It helps to keep a light on at night. Nursing personnel should be constant insofar as possible.

Agitation and anxiety are manifestations of organic brain syndrome. At times medication may be necessary to manage the patient who cannot be otherwise controlled. The agitated behavior that is more characteristic of the acute rather than the chronic brain syndrome may be managed with low doses of chlorpromazine (25 to 50 mg. t.i.d or q.i.d) or similar medications. Dose must be adjusted to the individual response. Anxiety can also be controlled with diazepam (usually 5 mg. t.i.d or q.i.d). For the patient who has difficulty sleeping, paraldehyde is still a useful drug. Barbiturates should be avoided. It is obvious (but probably worth noting) that nutrition and hydration should be carefully watched and that diet and fluids should be adjusted to the patient's needs.

An attitude of therapeutic optimism and of careful consideration of all possible etiologies is especially important. The family physician should remember that many organic brain syndromes are considered hopeless or untreatable when, in fact, considerable improvement is possible. Table 28–5 highlights several examples of treatable chronic brain syndromes. Since this is the group that is most likely to be overlooked, such etiologies should be carefully considered in the presence of a case of chronic brain syndrome.

CONSULTATION

The family physician who has adequately investigated *both* organic and functional factors and still fails to establish an etiology for the patient's disorientation or abnormal behavior should seek consultation to clarify etiology. Referral may also be necessary once a diagnosis has been established to obtain specialized procedures or long-term observation for the patient.

TABLE 28–5. EXAMPLES OF TREATABLE CHRONIC BRAIN SYNDROMES*

Toxins
  Prolonged use of drugs (barbiturates, bromides)
  Heavy metals
Deficiency States
  Pellagra
  Wernicke-Korsakoff syndrome
  B_{12} deficiency (prolonged)
Trauma
  Subdural hematoma, chronic
  Communicating hydrocephalus
Circulatory
  Subarachnoid hemorrhage
  Systemic lupus erythematosus
Infection
  Brain abscess
  Syphilis
Tumor
  Benign tumors
  Treatable malignancies
Endocrine
  Hypoglycemia
  Thyroid, adrenal disorders
Metabolic
  Chronic electrolyte imbalance
  Renal, hepatic, pulmonary insufficiency (chronic)
  Porphyria
  Wilson's disease
Psychogenic
  Depression mimicking chronic brain syndrome

*Adopted from Sandok. *In* Freedman, A. M., Kaplan, H. I., and Sadock, B. J. (eds.): Comprehensive Textbooks of Psychiatry/II, Baltimore, The Williams & Wilkins Co., 1975.

FAMILY

Because acute brain syndrome may appear dramatically and suddenly, a family crisis may result if members fail to react appropriately to initiate health care for the patient. When the etiology of acute brain syndrome is occult and the patient manifests disorientation or behavior problems that challenge normal family intercourse, family dysfunction may be significant. The physician must be willing to speak with family members to gain an understanding of the stability of the family system. This should be common practice for family physicians. By using data bases gained from interviewing various family members, and by offering supportive counseling, the family physician may serve as a major resource to a family by improving communication among members and by relieving family members of fears, guilt, and anger that may be associated with caring for a patient with organic brain syndrome.

SUMMARY

Organic brain syndrome is characterized by various symptoms that include disturbance in orientation, memory, intellectual function, judgment and affect, or abnormal behavior. The cerebral dysfunction may be due to SME or to structural brain damage. Acute brain syndrome reflects cerebral dysfunction of an acute and reversible nature; whereas chronic brain syndrome is associated with relatively irreversible cerebral dysfunction.

Therapy should be etiologically specific whenever possible. Early diagnosis and therapy are critical to arrest disease processes that may advance to chronic and irreversible forms.

The major etiologies of organic brain syndrome are infection, oxygen deprivation, drug intoxication, fluid–electrolyte imbalance, hypoglycemia, and head trauma. When a patient's condition appears to be deteriorating rapidly, a broad spectrum therapeutic program should be initiated while diagnostic studies are under way.

When a patient with organic brain syndrome is experiencing disorientation or behavioral problems, members of the family may require supportive counseling to deal with their fears, guilt, or anger. The recognition of family dysfunction related to the patient's illness may allow the physician to offer supportive counseling to family members that not only will improve the care of the patient but also will improve the status of the family system.

REFERENCES

1. American Psychiatric Association. Diagnostic and Statistical Manual of Mental Disorders. 2nd ed., Washington, D. C., Amer. Psychiatric Assoc., 1968.
2. Arieff, A. I., and Carroll, H. J.: Nonketotic hyperosmolar coma with hyperglycemia: clinical features, pathophysiology, renal function, acid-base balance, plasma-cerebrospinal fluid equilibria and the effects of therapy in 37 cases. Medicine, 51:73, 1972.
3. Benson, D. F., LeMay, M., Patten, D. H. et al.: Diagnosis of normal pressure hydrocephalus. N. Engl. J. Med., 283:609, 1970.
4. Bird, T. D., and Plum, F.: Recovery from barbiturate overdose coma with a prolonged isoelectric electroencephalogram. Neurology, 18:456, 1968.
5. Brown, J. K., and Habel, A. H.: Toxic encephalopathy and acute brain-swelling in children. Dev. Med. Child. Neurol., 17:659, 1975.
6. Busse, E. W., and Pfeiffer, E.: Mental Illness in Later Life. Washington, D. C., Amer. Psychiatric Assoc., 1973.
7. Carroll, B. J.: Barbiturate overdosage: presentation with focal neurological signs. Med. J. Aust., 56:1133, 1969.
8. Devereaux, M. W., and Partnow, M. J.: Delayed hypoxic encephalopathy without cognitive dysfunction. Arch. Neurol., 32:704, 1975.
9. Dooling, E. C., Richardson, E. P.: Delayed encephalopathy after strangling. Arch. Neurol., 33:196, March, 1976.
10. Engel, G. L., and Romano, J.: Delirium, a syndrome of cerebral insufficiency. J. Chronic Dis., 9:260, 1959.
11. Finnerty, F. A., Jr.: Hypertensive encephalopathy. Am. J. Med., 52:672, 1972.
12. Fred, H. L., Willerson, J. T., and Alexander, J. K.: Neurological manifestations of pulmonary thromboembolism. Arch. Intern. Med., 120:33, 1967.
13. Gerich, J. E., Martin, M. M., and Recant, L.: Clinical and metabolic characteristics of hyperosmolar nonketotic coma. Diabetes, 20:228, 1971.
14. Goldstein, G. W., Asbury, A. K., and Diamond, I.: Pathogenesis of lead encephalopathy. Uptake of lead and reaction of brain capillaries. Arch. Neurol., 31:382, 1974.
15. Gorham, L. W.: A study of pulmonary embolism. Arch. Intern. Med., 108:8, 1961.
16. Grant, I., and Mohns, L.: Chronic cerebral effects of alcohol and drug abuse. Int. J. Addict, 10:883, 1975.
17. Hadden, J., Johnson, J., Smith, S., et. al.: Acute barbiturate intoxication. J.A.M.A., 209:893, 1969.
18. Locke, S., Merrill, J. P., and Tyler, H. R.: Neurologic complications of acute uremia. Arch. Intern. Med., 108:519, 1961.
19. Lopez, R. I., and Collins, G. H.: Wernicke's encephalopathy. Arch. Neurol., 18:248, 1968.
20. Maccario, M., Messis, C. P., and Vastola, E. F.: Focal seizures as a manifestation of hyperglycemia without ketoacidosis. Neurology, 15:195, 1965.
21. Mettler, F. A.: Burn encephalopathy as a "diagnosis". J. Med. Soc. NJ, 71:817, 1974.
22. Needleman, H. L.: Lead poisoning in children: neurologic implications of widespread subclinical intoxication. Semin. Psychiatry, 5:47, 1973.
23. Newmark, S. R., Himathongkam, T., and Shane, J. M.: Hyperglycemic and hypoglycemic crises. J.A.M.A., 231:185, 1975.
24. Nicholson, A. N.: Considerations of vision and cerebral function during hypotension. Aviat. Space Environ. Med., 46:996, 1975.
25. Peterson, H., and Swanson, A. G.: Acute encephalopathy occurring during hemodialysis. Arch. Intern. Med., 113:877, 1964.
26. Rosenblum, W. I.: A renewed look at hypertensive encephalopathy. Am. Heart J., 91:264, 1976.
27. Plum, F., and Posner, J. B. (eds.) The Diagnosis of Stupor and Coma. 2nd ed., Philadelphia, F. A. Davis Co., 1972.
28. Roubicek, J., and Matescek, M.: Computer analysed EEG and behavioral changes after psychoactive drugs. Int. J. Neurol., 10:33, 1975.
29. Rubinstein, J. L., Stermann, M. M., Long, T. F., et. al.: Leukoencephalopathy following combined therapy of central nervous system leukemia and lymphoma. Acta Neuropathol. (Suppl.), 6:251, 1975.
30. Sandok, B. A.: Organic brain syndromes: Introduction. In Freedman, A. M., Kaplan, H. I., and Sadock, B. J. (eds.): Comprehensive Textbook of Psychiatry /II. Baltimore, The Williams & Wilkins Co., 1975.
31. Saper, J. R., and Yosselson, S.: Raised intracranial pressure diagnosis and management. Postgrad. Med., 57:89, 1975.
32. Saper, J. R.: Secondary metabolic encephalopathy. Postgrad. Med., 59:122, 1976.
33. Schomerus, H., Buchta, I., and Arndt, T.: Pulmonary function studies and oxygen transfer in patients with liver cirrhosis and different degree of portasystemic encephalopathy. Respiration, 32:1, 1975.
34. Shannon, D. C., De Long, R., Bercu, B., et al.: Studies on the pathophysiology of encephalopathy in Reye's syndrome, hyperammonemia in Reye's syndrome. Pediatrics, 56:999, 1975.
35. Singh, B. M., Gupta, D. R., and Strobos, R. J.: Nonketotic hyperglycemia and epilepsia partialis continua. Arch. Neurol., 29:187, 1973.
36. Tyler, H. R.: Neurologic disorders in renal failure. Am. J. Med., 44:734, 1968.
37. Tyler, H. R.: Neurologic disorders seen in the uremic patient. Arch. Intern. Med., 126:781, 1970.
38. Warren, W. D., Rudman, D., and Millikan, W.: The metabolic basis of portasystemic encephalopathy and the effect of selective vs. nonselective shunts. Ann. Surg., 180:573, 1974.
39. Wilson, L. M. Intensive care delirium: the effect of outside deprivation in a windowless unit. Arch. Intern. Med., 130:225, 1971.
40. Ziegler, D. K., Zosa, A., and Zileli, T.: Hypertensive encephalopathy. Arch. Neurol., 12:472, 1965.

Chapter 29

SEXUAL ASSAULT, SEXUAL VARIATION, AND SEXUAL DEVIATION*

by GENE G. ABEL,
JUDITH V. BECKER,
and THORNTON BRYAN

In family practice, one encounters patients with specific sex or sex-related problems. They include the victims of sexual assaults (rape and child molestation), patients with sexual variations (male or female homosexuals), and patients whose sexual behavior leads to their arrest, i.e., sexual deviations such as exhibitionism, incest, and voyeurism. These three groups are discussed in order to identify the specific problems involved and to explain how family physicians might help their patients having such problems.

VICTIMS OF SEXUAL ASSAULT

Rape has recently become a topic of greater societal concern, as the incidence of rape has increased 165 per cent in the past 15 years.[12] Until recently, there has been a lack of understanding regarding the crime of rape. Myths were prevalent, and even talking about rape was taboo. This situation has changed remarkably in the past 5 years. Books, journal articles, and television programs are discussing the topic more openly; laws pertaining to rape are being reformed; police departments are developing specially trained sex crime squads; hospitals are implementing special treatment programs for the rape victims; and physicians are becoming even more aware of the rape victim's unique treatment needs. A National Center for the Control and Prevention of Rape has been established to research all aspects of treating the rape victim and the rapist. The feminist movement has taken the lead in calling society's attention to the problem of rape and has been instrumental in bringing about legal reforms and establishing rape crisis centers throughout the country.

The objectives of this section are to provide the family physician with general information about rape; to discuss the legal, medical, and psychologic needs of rape victims; and to offer a treatment format for meeting their needs.

GENERAL INFORMATION

Definition of Rape

The definitions of rape found in the literature are as varied as are its victims. Historically, rape has been defined as (1) the victim is female, (2) the rapist is male, (3) there is a lack of consent by the victim, implying either verbal or physical coercion on the part of the rapist, and (4) vaginal penetration must occur. This traditional definition of rape is in a state of transition. The current trend is to broaden the definition of rape to include male victims and to

*Preparation of this chapter was supported in part by the Center for the Prevention and Control of Rape, Grant No. MH-28051.

extend the categories of sexual abuses forced on the victim, such as anal or oral sodomy.

These changes have led to the establishment of model rape laws. Wisconsin, for example, has revised its rape laws to distinguish three degrees of sexual assault. First degree sexual assault includes sexual intercourse or contact without consent, perpetrated by *inflicting injury* on the victim. Second degree sexual assault includes sexual intercourse or contact completed by the *threat of violence* against the victim. Third degree sexual assault includes sexual intercourse accomplished *with a victim who is unable to provide consent* (e.g., children below the age of consent, the mentally ill or deficient, or the unconscious victim). Wisconsin's definition of rape is nongender specific; that is, males or females can be designated as victims or assailants. Since most states are in the process of revising their older rape laws, the family physician needs to review such laws to become familiar with any newer definitions of rape as well as with the evidence needed to document a victim's charge of sexual assault. Such information can usually be obtained from the police department's sex crime squad.

Characteristics of Victims

Any woman may become the victim of a sexual attack. A widely held myth is that only young, attractive women are raped, yet the data indicate that rape victims can range in age from 15 months to 81 years of age.[19] Another misconception is that the rapist usually preselects his victim. Although Amir[4] found that 80 per cent of rapists in the Philadelphia area planned a rape, victims were selected on the basis of their availability, not their physical attributes. Thus, there is no typical rape victim. She is any age, any race, and from any socioeconomic level. She is married, single, divorced, or widowed and may be physically homely or attractive.

Since rape is a crime of availability, women of the lower socioeconomic classes and those living in urban ghetto neighborhoods with high crime rates are especially vulnerable. Since blacks constitute an especially high proportion of such lower socioeconomic environments, it is not surprising that 70 to 90 per cent of rape victims are black, and a similar percentage of rapes are intraracial.[9, 27] The vast majority of victims are relatively young (78 per cent are 11 to 30 years old), while 13 per cent are 1 to 10 years old and 5 per cent are over 70.[27]

Incidence of Rape

Although the incidence of reported rape has increased 165 per cent in the past 15 years, the actual number of rapes committed is unknown because a very high percentage go unreported. Curtis estimates the actual incidence of rape is 2.2 to 5.0 times greater than that reported to the police.[11] Hicks and Platt likewise suspect that only one in four to one in ten rapes are reported.[20] Even with more conservative estimates, however, a rape occurs approximately every 12 to 14 minutes in the United States, and one out of every 30 women will be the victim of rape or attempted rape at some time in her life. At a time when rapes are increasing steadily, successful prosecutions are surprisingly low. The Federal Bureau of Investigation reports that only 79 per cent of rapists are prosecuted, and of these, 49 per cent are acquitted or have the charges dismissed.[12]

Rape Crisis Centers

Adding to the issues of rising rape rates and low conviction rates has been the problem of delivering appropriate care to rape victims. Prior to 1972, although adequate physical care was usually provided, many victims complained that their emotional, social, and legal needs were inadequately attended to. In some situations, victims were left alone and unattended for hours while waiting for treatment. Emergency room staff referred to them as "the rape," and some police questioned victims as if to infer that their behavior may have actually provoked the attack. The techniques of gathering evidence were likewise misunderstood, with the result that many cases of attempted prosecution were thrown out of court for lack of evidence. Some victims felt they were being victimized by the health care system, which led to the development of self-help programs and rape crisis centers.

These centers, strongly supported by the National Organization for Women, provide total treatment for rape victims. Staffed by former victims and by nonvictims, most rape crisis centers provide medical, legal, and psychologic support. Following the crisis intervention model, hotline, individual, and group counseling are offered to victims and their families. Escort services are also provided to hospitals, police stations, and courts.[25] More than 100 such centers are currently operating in the United States and can usually be located through the local chapter of the National Organization for Women.

TREATING RAPE VICTIMS WITH ACUTE SYMPTOMATOLOGY

When a victim presents for treatment, she is usually in a state of emotional and physical crisis. Burgess and Holmstrom,[10] after counseling rape victims in the emergency room of Boston City Hospital, have described a cluster of symptoms typically experienced by most individuals being treated for rape. A victim's initial reaction may be either expressed or controlled. If expressed, she may be crying, hostile, highly anxious, and talking constantly about the rape. Many victims, by contrast, react in a controlled manner. They show little or no emotion and outwardly appear to have been emotionally unaffected by the rape. Such a controlled reaction should be identified as an inappropriate response to a highly charged, emotional experience. In either type of presentation, the victim is out of control regardless of how she presents herself. The family physician's role is to aid her in once again *regaining the control* she had over her life before the assault. To accomplish this, she needs information and medical, legal, and psychologic guidance.

Patients with most other medical problems present themselves with various symptoms to be diagnosed and treated by the physician. In this traditional role, patients relinquish control of their symptoms to the physician. The most effective treatment of the rape victim, however, requires a reversal of this role. The physician's goal should be to give as much control as possible to the victim so that she can determine what actions will relieve her crisis situation. Thus, the victim directs what needs to be done, and the physician facilitates her reaching these goals. If she wishes to talk about the experience, it is the physician's responsibility to discuss the rape with her or, if he cannot, to bring her into contact with a rape counselor who can. If she chooses to report the rape to legal authorities, the physician prepares her for potential problems associated with this. The victim should be asked about her needs, rather than the physician's dictating these needs. The physician's role should be facilitative, so that the victim can regain control over her own integrity. Re-establishing control prevents the sequelae that frequently occur if the victim continues to be manipulated by others after the rape.

Each rape victim presents individual treatment needs. The physician can use the following guidelines to explore possible areas of concern that most victims have.

Immediate Physical and Emotional Protection

A woman should be placed in a private examining room as soon as she identifies herself as a rape victim to the physician's receptionist or the emergency room admissions clerk. If friends or family members have accompanied her, they should be allowed to stay in the room if they appear to be providing support. If no friends or family members are accessible, a nurse, social worker, or female aide should stay with her. While waiting to be examined, a victim often inadvertently destroys valuable evidence by washing or by altering her appearance. Staff members should therefore explain to the victim the necessity of her not doing this. *After* the examination is completed, the staff should do everything possible to ensure her physical comfort and autonomy. A shower, douche, mouthwash (following oral sodomy), the repair of torn clothes, and the application of facial make-up are all potential objectives. The guiding principle should once again be to provide the victim with what she asks for, so as to allow her to regain control over her body.

Before it is begun, explain thoroughly the necessity of doing the examination, i.e., to ascertain the extent of her injuries, to gather medical evidence should she wish to prosecute, and to guard against venereal disease and pregnancy that may result from the rape. This detailed explanation should be provided and all questions answered to her satisfaction before proceeding with the examination.

History-taking

A brief history should include the circumstances surrounding the rape, its physical elements (to help guide the physical examination), and the victim's physical and emotional condition before, during, and after the rape.

Physical Examination

Consent forms should be obtained for photographs and specimen collections before proceeding with the examination. Remember that the extent of the physical examination is determined by the victim, not by the physician. This may well be the first time the victim has related to a male (if the physician is male) since her rape, and it is an ideal opportunity for her to experience an interaction with a male who is sensitive, empathic, and caring toward the victim, in contrast to the rapist. Two cc. of saline should be placed in the vagina and the washings examined for viable sperm and acid phosphatase before proceeding to the bimanual examination. A cervical culture for *N. gonorrhoeae* is also obtained, as is a smear for a Papanicolaou test (if the latter is indicated). The bimanual examination should focus especially on the evidence of trauma to vaginal, pelvic, and rectal tissues. The remaining procedures should particularly include examination of the breasts, torso, and legs for injuries and an examination of the mouth in cases of oral sodomy. Additional laboratory tests should include a blood serology determination and a saliva sample study for typing the victim's blood and secretor substance for the police.

On completion of the physical examination, the physician should discuss the issues of preventive treatment for venereal disease and pregnancy. Benzathine penicillin G, 2.4 million units intramuscularly, or spectinomycin if allergic, should be administered to prevent syphilis, and ampicillin, 3.5 gm. with 1 gm. of probenecid orally, should be given to prevent gonorrhea. If exposure has occurred within 24 hours, pregnancy can be prevented by the administration of diethylstilbestrol. Once again, the victim should be allowed to make the decisions regarding these treatment interventions.

Crisis Intervention Counseling

When and by whom crisis intervention counseling is provided depend on the physician's competency and available time. If the physician lacks training in counseling rape victims or has insufficient time to do this adequately, he should refer the patient to the appropriate counselor as soon as possible so that supportive measures can be begun immediately. Appropriate counseling will markedly enhance the ease and success of the physician's physical examination.

How a victim responds to rape results from an interaction between her emotional development and her current knowledge about rape.[10] The meaning of a sexual assault to a young child will differ markedly from that of an adult victim and will significantly influence the counseling methods provided.

Stages of Response to Rape

Although there is considerable variability among victims, a number of common responses have been observed. Fox and Scherl describe three sequential phases of a victim's emotional response to rape.[13]

The first stage, lasting from a few hours to a week, is characterized by a feeling of numbness and *shock*; the victim appears bewildered by the rape. She may express fear, terror, disgust, vulnerability, powerlessness, anxiety, and shame at being humiliated and despoiled by the rape.

The second state involves a period of *outward adjustment* during which she attempts to reorganize her life and appears to be adjusting to the assault. This period is characterized by denial. She may deny her emotions and feelings regarding the rape and may not care to discuss it. This stage appears to be self-protective and allows the victim to deal with everday life functions, such as preparing meals and going to the hospital for medical care. Should she completely inhibit all expression of feelings regarding the rape, she is very likely to have difficulty at a later date. A similar consequence of denial is seen in individuals who have not accepted a loved one's death. Subsequent emotional dysfunction surrounds the issue of death.[24] Following rape, emotional dysfunction usually surrounds the area of sex.

The third stage is termed *integration*. The victim becomes sensitive to any stimuli that remind her of the assault. She may experience depression and excessive ruminations about the attack, may worry about seeing the rapist again, may fear his returning to rape her again, and may withdraw from stimuli associated with the rapist, such as contact with unknown males, close male friends, or even people in general.

Alternatively Burgess and Holmstrom have divided the rape victim's responses into two stages.[10] The first is the acute stage in which the majority of the victim's coping and life functioning processes are disrupted. She is overwhelmed by the immediate response to the trauma and undergoes strong physical and emotional reactions. Stage two, in which the victim tries to reorganize her life, is often filled with nightmares about the assault as well as with strong avoidance responses to situations and people that take the form of phobias. Drastic changes in life styles are evidenced during this stage.

Counseling Methods

Irrespective of which model the physician may follow, both require a crisis counseling approach in which the physician aids the victim in regaining control of her life. This is accomplished by offering emotional support, providing information to ward off fears, permitting the victim to ventilate her feelings and fears, letting her know that you understand and sympathize, and above all, treating her with dignity.

The victim's social support system is extremely important in treating her. Husbands, boyfriends, fathers, and other relatives frequently need to be included in the counseling process and to be provided with information and emotional support. They need to be made aware of the stages the victim will go through so that they can anticipate and prepare for potential problems. Relatives are often emotionally traumatized by their loved one's being assaulted, and they must be made aware of the services available to them should they develop extensive psychologic sequelae. This is especially true when the victim is a child. An equal amount of time needs to be provided for the parents as well as for the child. Parental attitudes and emotional responses will strongly determine how the child handles this crisis. Parents experience a wide range of emotional responses varying from a realistic, logical approach to anger at the child (because she was raped) to a pathologic sense of seeking revenge or to embarrassment and wanting to conceal the rape.

As with the adult victim, the nature and purpose of the physical examination should be explained to both the parents and the child. Unless the mother is so emotionally upset that her presence would be disruptive to the child, she should be allowed to remain in the examining room. Involve the child as much as possible in the examination. Let her observe, touch, and inquire about all instruments to be used. As with the adult victim, parents should receive information regarding reporting procedures and their consequences.

The psychologic adjustment that the child makes to the rape depends primarily on the response of her parents.[18] If the parents show marked emotional reactions, these are easily picked up by the child. The child manifests symptoms identical to those displayed by adult victims. She will need adults who will listen when and if she wants to talk about the rape. Thus, it is crucial that the parents be supportive and empathic but not overly emotional in their response.

Many parents believe that their child will become promiscuous if sexually assaulted. They need reassurance that this is unlikely, again stressing the importance of their attitudes and the effect these will have on the child. If the parents treat the child as if she were different because of the rape, detrimental behaviors are more likely to be expressed.

Other categories of sexual assault, including homosexual rape, incest, and wives being raped by their husbands, have not been elaborated. However, the victims' response to these assaults and their subsequent needs are similar to those just described.

Medical Follow-up

Arrangements for follow-up should be completed before the victim leaves the office. These will include further crisis counseling sessions, evaluating the results of the culture for gonococci and serology studies, and a repeat pelvic examination to check for possible pregnancy. Since the victim can be expected to deny the rape and its potential sequelae, the physician should make extra efforts to accomplish these follow-up procedures.

Finally, before discharging the victim, be certain that she has a "plan of action." For example, determine where she will go when she leaves your office, if she has transportation, and if there are sources of emotional support in her environment. The victim needs information as to whom she can contact should she need further emergency psychologic care.

Legal Considerations

The victim's legal problems concern whether she wishes to report the crime and to prosecute. Some victims initially believe they will prosecute but then change their minds. The opposite also occurs. In any event, it is to the victim's advantage that the physician be thorough in gathering medical evidence, whether she plans to report and prosecute or not. If she reports the crime, she will have to go to the police station to file charges, to look at mug shots, and to assist in the identification of the possible rapist. She also needs to know that there are different levels of legal intervention. For example, she may want to file a civil rather than a criminal suit. It is also important that she knows that legal action can take months to complete.

Since the victim's records may eventually appear in court, the physician should document results of his examination in clear, concise, readable fashion in the chart. Reference to the *alleged* crime is also applicable, since the determination of whether a rape did or did not occur is a legal matter and not the prerogative of the examining physician.

TREATING RAPE VICTIMS WITH SUSTAINED SYMPTOMATOLOGY

Some rape victims will need more than the crisis counseling just described. The purpose of this section is to alert physicians to those signs and symptoms that indicate that the victim needs more in-depth counseling or psychotherapy.

Those victims with prior psychiatric illness or emotional problems are at higher risk of developing more serious reactions to rape. Individuals with such histories should be followed more closely to be certain that the rape does not exacerbate their pre-existing psychopathology. If this does occur, psychiatric consultation is indicated. Should the victim verbalize suicidal or homicidal ideation, such as, "I'll kill myself if my family finds out," or "I got a good look at him, and I'll see that justice is done,"

consultation is also indicated. Victims manifesting a severely depressed affect, psychomotor retardation, hallucinations, or delusions or those showing very poor emotional control during the examination need referral. The person who is new to the community with few social contacts or family and social support systems will need additional support. Finally, all victims who specifically request to talk with a mental health professional should be aided in making that contact.

Since 2.2 to 10 times as many women are raped as those who report rape, numerous victims fail to report their assault or to seek treatment. Some women feel extremely embarrassed and want to conceal their rape from friends and family, while others believe the myth that if they were raped, their actions in some way precipitated the attack. They incorrectly believe that reporting the rape only draws the incident to the attention of others. In actuality, less than 4 per cent of rapes are victim-precipitated.[12] Other victims have been raped by boyfriends, husbands, or relatives and cannot bear to disclose this, since they believe such information might reflect unfavorably on them or their family. Thus, there are a significant number of women who for various reasons do not seek out medical or psychologic treatment immediately following an assault. The emotional and physical trauma experienced by this group does not disappear; in fact, in many cases symptoms are magnified because these women fail to seek treatment. Later on, these victims may present with somatic or emotional complaints that are not always immediately attributable to the rape.

Somatic Symptoms

Burgess and Holmstrom describe four frequent categories of somatic symptoms manifested by victims in the weeks and months following sexual attack.[10] These are physical trauma, skeletal muscle tension, gastrointestinal irritability, and genitourinary disturbance. A woman who presents with multiple bruises, especially of the thighs, breasts, arms, and neck, should be considered a probable sexual assault victim. Women forced to have oral sex occasionally complain of throat irritation without mentioning the rape. For example, one of our patients was unable to swallow following an oral sexual assault and had to be fed intravenously for 1 week until she had resolved some of the emotional aspects of her assault.

Patients who experience disturbed patterns of eating or sleeping, who show a startle reaction, or who have violent nightmares are generally reacting to some form of trauma, and rape should be considered. Gastrointestinal symptoms include stomach pain, loss of appetite, and feelings of nausea when thinking about the attack. Genitourinary symptoms include vaginal irritation and pelvic pain. Rectal bleeding and pain frequently result from anal rape.

Sexual Symptoms

Bart studied 1,000 rape victims and found that one-third experienced specific sexual consequences of the rape, such as vaginismus, secondary nonorgasmia, decrease in sexual drive, and fear of any type of sexual involvement.[8] These sexual symptoms are especially troublesome for women with an ongoing sexual relationship who chose not to tell their partner about their assault. Their partner frequently feels rejected by the victim's loss of sexual responsiveness and sometimes terminates the relationship, being unaware that it was not the relationship but the rape that caused the changed sexual response.

The following case typifies the consequences of an unresolved reaction to rape.

The patient, now 23 years old, had been raped at age 13. She had chosen not to tell anyone about the assault by five males and consequently received no treatment. Months after the rape, she was hospitalized with fever and abdominal pain and was diagnosed as having gonorrhea of the fallopian tube as a result of the attack. Treatment eventually led to removal of one tube and one ovary. Prior to the rape, the patient had been sexually active and orgasmic. Immediately following the assault, she developed dyspareunia and nonorgasmia. She remained nonorgasmic throughout a subsequent marriage of 5 years. She also developed depressive symptoms with persistent ruminations about the rape and fears that the rapists would return again and eventually developed strong homicidal thoughts regarding the rapists.

Sexual problems such as these occur frequently following a rape. Their severity and duration depend on whether the victim seeks treatment, her previous sexual experiences, and the support and understanding given her by family, friends, and professionals.

Phobias and Nightmares

Long-term emotional reactions also include phobic elements, e.g., a victim raped in a car might avoid riding in cars. Women attacked in their home or apartment often immediately relocate to avoid those physical stimuli that remind them of the rape and also to escape being assaulted again, should the rapist return. Some victims raped out of doors withdraw to the confinement of their home, once again to avoid those stimuli associated with the rape. One of our patients was raped outside the library of the school she was attending. She had only one month of classes remaining before graduation, but she was unable to return to the campus following the attack. Consequently, she would not have graduated had she not been desensitized to returning to the university setting.

Finally, persistent nightmares are a common complaint of victims. They either relive the experience over and over or have violent dreams in which they are either the victim or the aggressor. Obsessive thoughts during the day can also plague these women and interfere with their normal functioning.

Counseling

If the physician suspects that the patient's report of any of the symptoms just mentioned might be related to either an emotional or physical trauma, it is important to gently explore and acquaint the patient with these suspicions rather than glossing over the problem. Some physicians, however, feel that it is better to "leave well enough alone," assuming that once something has been uncovered, the physician will not know what to do next. What the patient wants and needs is to have someone listen to her. Allow her to abreact, then reassure her that her feelings are not absurd. Be supportive and help her divulge the troublesome event. If she appears to distort what has happened, clarify what you think the reality of the situation was.

In summary, those victims who present for treatment in the acute stage of the rape crisis, i.e., the rape has occurred several hours to several weeks before, can be aided by the physician who is knowledgeable about the stages of the rape trauma syndrome. He can then anticipate "what comes next," can be supportive, and can take time to listen to the patient and her family and will behave in a nonjudgmental manner regarding the rape. Those victims who present for treatment with sustained symptomatology can be aided by the physician who has skills in the area in which the symptoms are manifest. For example, if the woman is nonorgasmic secondary to the rape and the physician has skill in sexual dysfunction counseling, he should treat the patient. If the physician lacks the specific skills required, then consultation is indicated. Finally, rape crisis centers can be of valuable assistance to rape victims, and physicians should feel comfortable in referring patients to these centers for consultation or treatment.

SEXUAL VARIATIONS AND DEVIATIONS

DEFINITION AND TERMINOLOGY

A variety of patients are seen in medical practice whose sexual behavior differs from that of the general population. Included in this category are those with sexual variations (such as homosexuals and lesbians) as well as those with sexual deviations (such as individuals whose target of sexual arousal not only differs from the norm but also leads to their arrest, e.g., exhibitionists, voyeurs, pedophiles). Although such patients are seen infrequently, they often pose difficult evaluation and treatment decisions for the family physician because of a lack of appreciation of what the patient's problems are and which of these problems should become the focus of treatment.

Sexual variations and deviations have traditionally been diagnosed on the basis of their sexual arousal patterns, which appear to be qualitatively different from the rest of the population. Recent studies, however, have revealed that such qualitative arousal patterns are also seen in the so-called "normal population." Thus, the major differences between the arousal patterns seen in people with sexual variations and deviations and the arousal patterns seen in the general population may be quantitative rather than qualitative.[14, 15]

It is nevertheless possible to categorize sexual variations and deviations on the basis of their "deviant" arousal pattern to either deviant objects or deviant acts. Some sexual variations and deviations involve arousal to inappropriate objects, i.e., pedophilia (child molestation), fetishism, or bestiality. Others involve being attracted to appropriate objects but manifest inappropriate sexual behavior with that object, e.g., exhibitionism, sadomasochism, and voyeurism. Table 29–1 outlines such categorizations and the general prevalence of these classifications.

Patients can be diagnosed on the sole component of their preferred sexual object or sexual behavior, but this system fails to consider the full breadth of a patient's possible problem areas. Three other components may or may not also be dysfunctional, including insufficient sexual arousal to adults of the opposite sex, inadequate heterosocial skills, and inappropriate gender role–motor behavior.[1, 7]

After the first component, that of deviant object or behavior preference, has been explored, the male patient should be questioned about the adequacy of his sexual arousal to adult women—can he get erections to adult women? Pedophiles, for example, are by definition aroused by male or female children, or both, but a second component of their problem may be insufficient arousal to an adult woman. Pedophiles without such adult arousal will need treatment not only to decrease their pedophilic preferences but also to increase nondeviant arousal. Without adult arousal, the patient's prognosis is definitely more guarded, since treatment may decrease his pedophilic arousal, but he may be left without an appropriate adult sexual outlet.

A third and equally critical potential deficit is the patient's heterosocial skills. He may have adequate erections to adult women but may never have acquired the social skills necessary to talk with a woman or to ask her to go out for a drink, to the movies, or up to his apartment. The result would be that although his sexual arousal might be adequate to perform intercourse, his inadequate heterosocial skills would not provide him with sufficient opportunity to establish a personal relationship with a woman that might lead to sexual inter-

TABLE 29–1.   CLASSIFICATION SYSTEM OF SEXUAL VARIATIONS AND DEVIATIONS

Traditional Diagnostic Category	Preferred Sexual Objects	Preferred Sexual Behavior	Prevalence
Exhibitionism	Adult women, occasionally female child	Exposing genitalia, usually while masturbating	Common
Fetishism	Inanimate objects, e.g., bras, panties	Masturbation while touching objects	Rare
Homosexuality (male)	Male sex partner	Oral or anal intercourse or mutual masturbation	Very common, at least 10 per cent of population
Lesbianism	Female sex partner	Oral–genital intercourse or mutual masturbation	Common, at least 5 per cent of population
Pedophilia	Child, usually female	Oral–genital intercourse	Common
Rape	Adult women, occasionally female or male child	Oral, genital, or anal intercourse	Common
Sadomasochism	Usually adult women, occasionally men	To injure or be injured by partner	Infrequent
Transsexualism	Partner of same biologic sex	Normal, assuming sexual identity is opposite that of biologic sex	Very rare
Transvestism (male)	Adult women	Crossdressing in women's clothes	Infrequent
Voyeurism	Adult women	Watching adult women or watching sex acts performed by others	Common

course. The patient should be asked if he can communicate with women, ask them out, and so forth, and what the extent of his anxiety is while doing so. Either deficit skills or excessive anxiety suggests the need for treatment in this area.

The fourth component needing assessment is the patient's gender role–motor behavior.[1] In any society, individuals acquire gender-specific patterns of sitting, standing, and walking. Typical feminine gender motor behaviors include speaking in a high pitched voice, sitting with buttocks close to the back of the chair with legs crossed knee on knee, standing with the feet close together, and walking with short steps and arms swinging from the elbows. Masculine gender motor behavior, by contrast, includes speaking in a low pitched voice, sitting with buttocks far from the back of the chair with legs crossed ankle on knee, standing with feet far apart, and walking with long steps and arms swinging from the shoulders. Problems occur when the patient's gender role-motor behavior is inconsistent with his gender identity. A male who views himself as a male "inside" may have acquired feminine sitting, standing, and walking behaviors. Treatment would require specific training so that he could acquire a more masculine gender role-

motor behavior consistent with his sexual identity, which is "I am a man."

Traditionally, each of these four components has been viewed as interrelated. For example, male homosexuals were assumed to be aroused to men, have no arousal to women, display appropriate heterosocial skills, and always reveal feminine gender role–motor behavior. In actuality, although all male homosexuals are aroused to men, they may or may not have adequate arousal to women, adequate heterosocial skills, and feminine motor behavior. The physician's evaluation of each of these four specific components will provide a more complete understanding of what assets and deficits any one patient has and, therefore, what his total treatment needs might include.

IDENTIFYING THERAPEUTIC GOALS

A frequent error in aiding individuals with sexual variations or deviations is to ignore why the patient has come for help. Physicians sometime fail to listen to such patients for various reasons including (1) the physician's discomfort in discussing sexual matters, misperceptions about sexual variations or deviations, or belief that such patients are vastly different from his other patients and (2) the patient's discomfort about talking with an authority figure who may react with hostility and anger on learning of the patient's sexual behavior.

A number of conflicts frequently bring patients with sexual variations or deviations to the physician, including:

1. Alteration of a long-standing relationship. As do heterosexuals, patients with sexual variations or deviations have close, meaningful relationships with their sexual partners. Disruptions of these relationships caused by termination by the partner, or in the case of sexual deviations, caused by the patient's arrest, lead to emotional turmoil and the need to discuss these issues with someone the patient can trust.

2. A desire to become more functional within the sphere of the patient's sexual variations. As our society has become more accepting of the rights of others, greater numbers of patients seek treatment to better adjust to their sexual variations. For example, some homosexuals living in a predominantly heterosexual society have not had the opportunity to learn the social and sexual skills necessary to meet and date homosexual partners. As he or she attempts to "come out," the patient fails socially, with the resultant anxiety and discomfort that one would expect from any individual, homosexual or heterosexual.

3. Arrest. In most sexual deviations, the deviate sees his sexual behavior as very much a part of himself. Self-insight regarding the need for change is thus not a common motivation for his seeking evaluation or treatment. Instead, the patient's arrest leads him to seek treatment at the insistence of the police, judge, family, neighbors, or victim.

4. A desire to change. Some patients see their deviant behavior (sadomasochism, exhibitionism, pedophilia, and rape) as self-defeating. Repeated arrests, trauma to their victim, or disruption of their marriage or occupation sometimes lead the patients (as with any nondeviant) to seek treatment. In some patients with sexual variations, societal pressures or their own ambivalent feelings toward homosexuality lead to their seeking treatment in order to become bisexual and, in a few cases, exclusively heterosexual.

5. Sexual problems as a "ticket" to therapy. Not infrequently, patients with sexual variations or deviations seek treatment by identifying their sexual behavior as their problem when other difficulties are the primary reason for their seeking help. The male homosexual with a hysterical personality is a frequent example. Such individuals are anxious to label themselves as homosexual, but questioning reveals that their problems result from a failure of their personality functioning, not from their homosexual arousal pattern.

It is important to remember that there are numerous reasons for patients with variations or deviations seeking help. The physician should be aware of the most common reasons, but, more importantly, *the patient should be allowed to identify his or her problem*, and questions should focus on this issue. The physician should not let preconceived opinions as to what the patient is seeking determine therapy needs. This should be the prerogative of the patient.

COUNSELING SKILLS OF THE PHYSICIAN

The following approach is predicated on the assumption that the family physician will not provide extensive, in-depth therapy to the patient with a sexual variation or deviation but will assist the patient in identifying treatment goals, provide supportive therapy when indicated, and determine the need for consultation and the urgency of the consultation. The following guidelines are suggested:

The first and most critical guideline is to approach the patient as if he or she were heterosexual and without a sexual variation or deviation. This involves empathic listening in order to understand what the patient wants from treatment. Many sexual deviates are acutely aware of their inappropriate sexual behavior and feel quite guilty about it. The physician, as an authority figure, is in a unique position in talking with such patients. If the primary physician is harsh, unempathic, and demanding in attitude, the patient will most likely expect a similar attitude from other physicians as well. Treatment by the physician or referral to a consultant may not occur, and the patient returns to the environment unchanged. If patients with sexual problems meet an empathic physician who does not reject them simply on the basis of their sexual preference, it will be much easier for these patients to accept themselves — a vital step in therapy.

It may be that the physician, due to prior life experiences and background, is unable to accept such patients as individuals, is unable to empathize, and so forth. Under these circumstances, there is nothing wrong with referral to a physician who is less uncomfortable with these patients. The referral might be made by saying, "Well, Mr. Smith, now that you've told me about your attraction to men, I believe I understand more about the type of difficulties you're experiencing. Dr. Jones, a friend of mine, has talked with me about men he's helped with similar difficulties. How would you feel about my talking with him about you and finding out if he could see you? I have a lot of faith in his expertise in this area." In this fashion, rather than rejecting the patient, the physician has assisted him by referring him to someone with more appropriate skills who will probably be more successful in working with the patient.

Another issue is the physician's knowledge about sex. It has only been in the last 10 years that physicians have received adequate sex education in medical schools, and even now the level of sexual knowledge of the average physician is limited.[17] Many myths and misconceptions exist regarding sex, including sexual variations and deviations. These same myths tend to nullify the helping potential of the physician. Further education in the area of sex will clarify some of these myths and improve one's effectiveness with patients. A number of excellent books are currently available.[5, 6, 16, 21, 22, 26]

A final source of sex education is the patient himself. Some physicians, because of their authoritative position, are reluctant to allow patients to discuss their sexual difficulties. This is unfortunate since it prevents the physician from obtaining a potential source of information that will correct many of his misperceptions about this area.

A further concern is the extent to which the physician needs to intrude in the patient's life. This is a difficult decision, because no matter what one does, criticism is possible from a variety of sources. Our own decision about how actively to intervene depends on the degree to which the patient's sexual behavior conflicts with the consent of his adult partner or is injurious to his partner. For the homosexual involved with a mutually consenting adult

partner, the physician's intrusion should be nil. As a patient's sexual behavior becomes more aggressive (rape, sadomasochism) or involves a partner who is unable to consent (pedophilia), our practice is to become more vigorous in outlining to the patient the consequences of his behavior and the need for treatment. When the patient can identify his non-consenting victim (e.g., in cases of incest), it is best for the physician to obtain additional psychiatric and legal consultation, especially in light of the recent Tarasoff decision.[23]

Some sexual problems warrant immediate consultation and, in some cases, hospitalization. Patients seeking sex reassignment surgery, transvestites, and effeminate homosexuals usually pose difficult diagnostic problems, and psychiatric consultation is needed. Sexual deviates whose chronic deviant behavior has become known to their significant others who then reject the patient (such as pedophiles, rapists, homosexuals, and those who commit incest) and those whose socioeconomic status is in acute jeopardy as a result of public disclosure of their deviant sexual behavior should be considered for brief hospitalization until such situations have stabilized. Deviates whose control over their sexual drive is breaking down (such as pedophiles) frequently need brief hospitalization and reduction of their sexual drive with tranquilizers until their control is stabilized and consultation is obtained.

Hospitalization is not required for most individuals reporting good control over their sexual behavior. In our experience, even some aggressive rapists, pedophiles, and sadomasochists can be treated as outpatients when the therapeutic relationship is good and communications remain open between patient and therapist regarding the patient's control.

Finally, various clinical findings can help the physician predict the outcome of therapy. These findings are irrespective of the specific type of therapy undertaken to control or alter a patient's deviant behavior in any of the four components of behavior needing treatment. Favorable prognostic factors include (1) the patient admits that he has a sexual problem and that he wants to do something about it, (2) deviant masturbatory fantasies and deviant behavior occur at a low frequency, (3) deviant behavior has been present for only a short period of time, (4) some degree of heterosexual arousal is or has been present, (5) the patient is not a transsexual, and (6) he does not have a hysterical or antisocial personality.

SPECIALIZED TREATMENTS

It is beyond the scope of this chapter to review the numerous treatments available for the sexual deviations just reviewed. However, one should be aware that major breakthroughs have occurred in the evaluation and treatment of sexual variations and deviations in the past 5 years. First has been the development of objective methods to assess each of the four component areas of sexual behavior either by direct observation of the patient or by physiologic methods to objectify his or her arousal patterns.[1, 2, 3] Secondly, breaking down a patient's sexual behavior into its components has allowed specific treatments to be applied to each component, as opposed to a global treatment approach to all four areas at once. Specific treatments now include methods to reduce excessive arousal to deviant cues, generate or increase adequate heterosexual arousal, teach appropriate heterosocial skills, and help the patient develop gender role-motor behavior consistent with his or her sexual identity.[3] With an enlightened public, better evaluative methods, and a greater repertoire of treatment modalities, the prognosis for these conditions has improved markedly. The family physician's greater knowledge of the assessment and treatment of sexual assault victims and of patients with sexual variations and sexual deviations will hopefully assist in providing additional treatment for these difficult areas of our patients' sexual behavior.

REFERENCES

1. Abel, G. G.: Assessment of sexual deviation in the male. *In* Hersen, M., and Bellack, A. S. (eds.): Behavioral Assessment: A Practical Handbook. New York, Pergamon Press, Inc., 1976.
2. Abel, G. G., and Blanchard, E.: The measurement and generation of sexual arousal. *In* Hersen, M., Eisler, R., and Miller, P. M. (eds.): Progress in Behavior Modification. Vol. II. New York, Academic Press, Inc., 1976.
3. Abel, G. G., Blanchard, E., and Becker, J.: The psychological treatment of rapists. *In* Rada, R. (ed.): Clinical Aspects of the Rapist. New York, Grune & Stratton, Inc., in press.
4. Amir, R. M.: Patterns in Forcible Rape. Chicago, University of Chicago Press, 1971.
5. Annon, J. S.: The Behavioral Treatment of Sexual Problems. Vol. 1. Brief Therapy. Hawaii, Kapiolani Health Services, 1974.
6. Annon, J. S.: The Behavioral Treatment of Sexual Problems. Vol. 2. Intensive Therapy. Hawaii, Mercantile Printing, Inc., 1975.
7. Barlow, D. H., and Abel, G.: Recent developments in assessment and treatment of sexual deviation. *In* Craighead, E., Kazdin, A., and Mahoney, M. (eds.): Behavior Modification: Principles, Issues and Applications. Atlanta, Houghton-Mifflin Co., 1976.
8. Bart: Rape Alert. Newsweek, November 10, 1975.
9. Brownmiller, S.: Against Our Will. Men, Women and Rape. New York, Simon & Shuster, Inc., 1975.
10. Burgess, A. W., and Holmstrom, L.: Rape: Victims of Crisis. Bowie, Md., Robert J. Brady Co., 1974.
11. Curtis, L.: Victimization: present and future measures of victimization in forcible rape. *In* Rape: Research, Action, Prevention. Proceedings of the Sixth Symposium on Justice and the Behavioral Sciences, University of Alabama Report # 29, 1975.
12. Federal Bureau of Investigation: Uniform Crime Reports 1974. Washington, D.C., U.S. Government Printing Office, 1974.
13. Fox, S. S., and Scherl, D.: Patterns of response among victims of rape. Am. J. Orthopsychiatry, *40*:503, 1970.
14. Freund, K., and Costell, R.: The structure of erotic preference in the non-deviant male. Behav. Res. Ther., *8*:15, 1970.
15. Freund, K., McKnight, C., Langevin, R., et al.: The female child as a surrogate object. Arch. Sex Behav., *2*:119, 1972.
16. Gagnon, J. H., and Simon, W.: Sexual Deviance. New York, Harper & Row, Publishers, 1967.
17. Green, R.: Human Sexuality: A Health Practitioner's Text. Baltimore, The Williams & Wilkins Co., 1975.
18. Halleck, S.: The physician's role in management of victims of sexual offenses. J.A.M.A., *180*·273, 1962.
19. Hayman, C., and Lanza, C.: Sexual assault on women and girls. Am. J. Obstet. Gynecol., *109*:480, 1971.
20. Hicks, D., and Platt, C.: Medical treatment for the victim: The development of a rape treatment center. *In* Walker, M. J., and Brodsky, S. L. (eds.): Sexual Assault. Lexington, Mass., D.C. Heath & Co., 1976.
21. Hoffman, M.: The Gay World. New York, Basic Books, Inc., 1968.
22. Hooker, E.: The adjustment of the male overt homosexual. J. Project Tech., *21*:18, 1957.
23. Hospital and Community Psychiatry, *27*:744, 1976.
24. Kubler-Ross, E.: On Death and Dying. New York, The Macmillan Co., 1969.
25. Largen, M. A.: History of women's movement in changing attitudes, law, and treatment toward rape victims. *In* Rape: Research, Action, Prevention. Proceedings of the Sixth Symposium on Justice and the Behavioral Sciences, University of Alabama Report # 29, 1975.
26. McCary, J.: Sexual Myths and Fallacies. New York, Van Nostrand Reinhold Co., 1971.
27. Nevil, L. G.: Memphis Police Department Rape Study Report, 1975.

Chapter 30

PSYCHOPHARMACOLOGIC THERAPY

by CARMEN A. DELCIOPPO,
and L. THOMAS WOLFF

Psychopharmacologic agents have become the most commonly prescribed drugs in the pharmacopoeia. The plethora of drugs in this expanding field of pharmacology often makes the choice of an appropriate agent confusing and difficult. This chapter presents a practical guide for the family physician to assist in making a definitive diagnosis and in selecting a drug of maximal benefit to the patient. It is designed to be a quick, accurate desk reference rather than a complete discourse on psychotropic medications. The chapter has two sections: first, an outline of general principles and specific mental states to act as diagnostic aides to the use of these drugs and, second, an outline of pharmacologic agents by category, including symptoms affected, nonpsychiatric uses, side effects, complications, and dosage regimens.

GENERAL PRINCIPLES

The most potent drug the physician has is himself. The effectiveness of any therapy is influenced by the personality of both the physician and the patient, the rapport and communication between them, the establishment of a definitive diagnosis, and the selection of the appropriate drug.

Definitive Diagnosis

Since psychotropic drugs have specific therapeutic actions, accurate and definitive diagnosis is a must for effective therapy. The greatest failures of drug therapy are due to inappropriate diagnosis, selection of wrong drugs, and lack of patient compliance. Too often, symptoms are treated, and underlying causes are ignored. Differentiation of psychotic from nonpsychotic states is essential. An understanding of anxiety, fear, stresses of living, personality structures, and psychosomatic disorders is crucial. Our pill conscious society seeks panaceas to deal with even the most common of stresses in our daily lives. The vicissitudes of everyday living are the most common causes of stress and anxiety seen by the family physician and are the least affected by drug therapy. Basic personality structures must be recognized so that the individual's "normal" pattern can be established. Drug therapy is often futile if the problems being treated are part of the patient's basic personality.

Drug Selection

There are too many drugs for any given physician to learn to use all of them well. Because of this, it is best to select one or two drugs from each therapeutic category and become thoroughly familiar with them. Know indications, contraindications, dosages, side effects, and complications. Avoid routine use of multiple drugs or drug combinations. If such drugs are necessary, know the specific actions, indications, side effects, and complications for each agent, alone and in combination. Keep accurate records of drugs prescribed and amounts ordered. Do not give open-ended prescriptions. Toxic side effects and self-overdosing are common problems. Warn patients of side effects and explain particularly the potentiation of side effects by other drugs, especially alcohol.

If the patient is not doing well on a certain drug regimen, reassess the entire situation. Review the diagnosis, specificity of the drug, and patient compliance. Lack of compliance is often the cause of poor results, since the patient's underlying problem or personality may cause him not to take the medication as prescribed.

Precautions

The physician should gain an understanding of the overall physical and emotional state of the patient before embarking on a therapeutic drug regimen. A history of any previous psychotropic drug therapy and of the results of such therapy is important. The nature of these agents requires at the very least certain laboratory data (including a complete blood count and an assessment of liver and renal function) be obtained before initiating therapy. If a history or suspicion of heart disease is evident, an electrocardiogram should be included. Depending on the drug, dosage, and duration of therapy, periodic re-examinations, including blood and liver function studies, should be done. New symptoms during therapy should be suspected of being drug-induced. For example, an infectious process necessitates a blood count to check for drug-induced leukopenia. The side effects and complications resulting from the use of psychotropic agents must always be kept in mind.

DIAGNOSTIC AIDS TO MENTAL STATES

The Vicissitudes of Everyday Life

"Life is a mystery to be lived, not a problem to be solved." "There is only one way to live life, live it, all of it, good and bad." "Into each life a little rain must fall, sometimes even a downpour, but it doesn't last forever." These philosophies embrace the concept that much of our emotionality is best "treated" by the understanding, support, and encouragement borne of kindness, wisdom, and experience. Patients come to us with any number of emotional states that are neither truly excessive nor severely over-reactive but occur in direct relationship to real events in the person's present life situation. A wife may be bored, bitter, and tense because her husband is presently maintaining a very irreg-

ular job schedule and is away from home for varying periods of time. The husband himself may be tense and fatigued and may be having difficulty falling asleep because his business is going sour. A person experiencing a grief reaction to a recent self-felt loss, such as the moving away of a loved one, a death, or a divorce, is sad, reminiscent, and ruminative but is quite functional and not pessimistic. A spouse who discovers infidelity in a mate is angry, depressed, and guilty or temporarily "overwhelmed." An adolescent is distressed when his "steady" deserts him.

These are the vicissitudes of everyday life that make up a significant portion of the stresses that bring patients to their family physician. Although drugs are expedient, they seldom help. There is a risk of side effects and habituation. If drugs do work, the patient may develop confidence and respect only for the drug and not for himself and his own capacity to take charge of his own life, especially his emotional life. On occasion, medications will be necessary for a few of the people just referred to, but certainly not to the extent that these are currently being prescribed.

Basic Personality Structure

"A person begins with the person he is," or "everyone has to be some way." There is no such entity or concept as a "normal" personality or psychologic make-up. A person's lifelong personality patterns are "normal" for him, and only negative variations from that "normal" are potentially treatable with drugs. The lifelong paranoid personality who reacts to any criticism with hurt, anger, attacking self-righteousness, and retreat will get over this reaction without drugs, as he has on previous occasions. The manipulative person who has headaches with alarming frequency and convenience will probably obtain relief as soon as he gets what he wants. The lifelong "stomachache to stay home expert" has to go to school or work in spite of his supposed agony. Remember, the older we get, the more we tend to entrench our personality structure! We become more paranoid, more manipulative, and more prone to headaches.

The family physician can have a steady, sensitive finger on the pulse of the characterologic make-up of most of his patients, if he takes the time to do so.

Psychosomatic Disorders
(Psychophysiologic Reactions)

"If the eyes do not cry, other organs will." Crying and blushing are perhaps the two most common psychosomatic reactions the world over. In the simplest sense, psychosomatic reactions can be defined as the "mind" affecting the "body." The American Psychiatric Association defines psychophysiologic autonomic and visceral disorders as "the symptoms due to a chronic exaggerated state of the normal physiological expression of emotion... which may eventually lead to structural changes." This diagnostic category is synonymous with terms such as "organ neurosis," "gastric neurosis," and "cardiac neurosis." As distinguished from the neuroses, psychosomatic disorders are not a direct defense against anxiety but rather a failure of defenses against excessive affective arousal accompanied by autonomic nervous system and other hormonal shifts, especially of a sympathetic type. Sustained muscular tension, both smooth and striated, is included in this concept. Major psychologic conflicts tend to center upon constellations of hate–guilt, dependence versus independence, and, less often, psychosexual conflicts or events. The consensus is that psychosomatic reactions and disorders are neither symbolic nor personality- or organ-specific. More than one psychosomatic disorder can exist concurrently in the same person. One psychosomatic disorder can, and often does, give way to another psychosomatic disorder in the same person at different times.

Psychotherapy alone is ineffective. Ideal treatment should include medical, psychologic, and psychopharmacologic approaches. All psychiatric disorders can be accompanied by some degree of psychophysiologic reaction. For example, sociopathy very often is associated with migraines or gastrointestinal disturbances. Psychophysiologic reactions occur with alarming frequency in the affective disorders, especially in depressions. Theoretically, these psychophysiologic reactions can be seen as depressive or affective equivalents or as a means of masking affective disorders. Clinically, this appears to be so in many people with psychophysiologic disorders, occasionally with even such severe disorders as peptic ulcer, ulcerative colitis, or female sterility.

In the treatment of psychosomatic disorders, antidepressants and low doses of aliphatic and piperazine phenothiazines (e.g., chlorpromazine, flupromazine, thioridazine) are clinically more effective than are other ataractics or barbiturates. The benzodiazepines continue to be quite effective when chronic striated muscular tension and pain or overt anxiety exist. Stimulants such as amphetamines and methylphenidate are not effective. Much clinical research continues to be necessary to confirm these more contemporary impressions.

Depressions

Depressions are the most common and ubiquitous of the emotional disorders. Table 30–1 is a sign and symptom checklist for depressions, and Table 30–2 provides an easy reference guide for selecting antidepressant therapies.

These tables leave many questions unanswered concerning depressions and their many variations. Four problematic areas do deserve special mention. These are the so-called depressive personality, success depression, depression subsequent to an acute schizophrenic episode, and depression following grief.

Depressive personality is a recognized diagnostic characterologic style. It is characterized by a usually likable, placid individual, who tends to bring out the parenting instincts in others. This person is invariably blue or sad and never really happy. He is a follower rather than a leader, tends to be obsessive-compulsive, sees only shades of dimness in life, smiles but sadly, and never really seems to succeed at anything. Drugs and psychotherapy are both ineffective.

Success depression is a peculiar entity that can take any form, psychotic, neurotic, or grief-induced. It usually occurs in an individual who has made a lifelong obsessional project out of attaining some particular self-felt goal (e.g., executive of a company, chairperson of a department), such that the process itself becomes the way of life. Once the goal is attained, the individual experiences an exquisite sense of loss, namely that obsessional project that had become a way of life. These reactions are to be taken seriously and should be treated for whatever category of depression they fall into.

TABLE 30–1. DEPRESSIONS—DIAGNOSTIC AIDES

Signs and Symptoms	Psychotic Depression	Neurotic Depression	"Normal" (Grief Reaction)
Autonomic nervous system complaints (xerostomia, palpitations, constipation or diarrhea, menstrual disorders, diaphoresis)	Prominent and often extreme	Mild, if present	Mild, if present
Psychosomatic complaints (insomnia, fatigue, chest pain, any variety of aches and pains, nausea, cramps, weakness—especially of legs, anorexia, weight loss)	Prominent and often extreme	More hypochondriacal complaint of fatigue, vague complaint of "not feeling well," whine	Rare
Diurnal variation	Early A.M. awakening and feels worse in A.M.	Initial insomnia, feels worse in P.M.	No diurnal variation, restless sleep
Suicidal risk	Can be serious	Threats and gestures, but rarely serious	Very rare, if at all
Age of onset	Aged 40 or over (rare before)	Any age	Any age
Duration of depression	Less than 1 year	Variable, but often more than 1 year	Variable, but almost always quite recent
Precipitating factor(s)	Vague, if at all	Often clear and discoverable	Quite obvious
Loss of interest, apathy, lack of motivation (functioning not at all or poorly)	Marked	Mild to not present	Variable, but almost always mild to not present
Nihilism	Can be present	Rare, if ever	Not present
Depersonalization and feelings or ideas of unreality	Present	Rare	Rare
Positive family history of depression	Frequent	Rare	Not applicable
Concentration and attention span impaired, recent memory difficulty	Frequent	Rare	Rare
Phobias	Frequent	Rare	Not applicable
Paucity of ideation, rumination (especially about past transgressions—real, imagined, or overdetermined), morbid thinking	Severe to profound	Mild to moderate	If present, degree variable
Psychomotor retardation	Moderate to stupor to seeming dementia	Mild to moderate	Mild, if at all
Pessimism, hopelessness, feeling "all black" or bleak	Severe to profound	Moderate	Infrequent
Sadness	Severe to profound	Moderate to severe	Mild to moderate
Somatic delusions ("insides rotting" or "brain has holes") or xoophilic delusions ("covered with vermin" or "cause of all venereal disease in world")	Can be present (very dramatic sign)	Not present	Not present

Table continued on following page

TABLE 30–1.   DEPRESSIONS—DIAGNOSTIC AIDES (*Continued*)

Signs and Symptoms	Psychotic Depression	Neurotic Depression	"Normal" (Grief Reaction)
Kinetics negative (wrinkled brow, worried look, stooped posture, flattened expression)	Moderate to profound	Mild to moderate	Mild to moderate
Indecisiveness	Severe to profound	Mild to moderate	Not present to mild
Aversion to positive influence, obstinate, irritable, dissatisfied, angry, hostile, fault-finding	Moderate to profound	Moderate	Not present to mild
Agitation, anxiety	Severe, if present	Frequent and moderate	Rarely present
Loss of contact with reality	Present	Not present	Not present
Placement of "blame" for present status	Self	Usually others	Not present

TABLE 30–2.   DEPRESSIONS—MEDICAL TREATMENT*

Agent	Psychotic Depression	Neurotic Depression	"Normal" (Grief Reaction)
Ataractics (benzodiazepines, propanediols, hydroxyzines)	(−) to 1	0 to 2	(−) to 2
Amphetamines and methylphenidate	(−) to 0	(_) to 0	2
Alcohol, barbiturates, narcotics, analgesics	(−)	(−)	(−)
Lithium carbonate	† 0 to 1 (but appears to have preventive value in manic-depressive illness)	0	0
Aliphatic or piperidine phenothiazines in low doses (chlorpromazine, thioridazine, etc.)	2 to 3	(−) to 2	(−) to 0
Thioxanthenes—low dose	3	0 to 1	0
Piperazine phenothiazines—low dose (trifluoperazine, fluphenazine, etc.)	2 to 3	0	(−) to 0
Monoamine oxidase inhibitors (those currently available)	2	0 to 2	0
Tricyclic antidepressants (imipramine, amitriptyline, protriptyline, doxepin, etc.)	2 to 4	†0 to 2 (should be tried, but rarely as effective as in psychosis)	0
Electroconvulsive therapy	2 to 4	(−) to 1	(−) to 0
Placebo† (compare with other treatments!)	0 to 1	0 to 2	0 to 1

*Scale: Scale ranges from 0 (no effect) to 4 (very effective); (−) indicates that agent exacerbates condition.
†Please check drug effect against placebo effect before prescribing.

Depression, usually reactive and frequently psychotic in nature, is common subsequent to the encapsulation of an acute schizophrenic episode.

Grief is a form of depression if the grief fits the diagnostic parameters of depression initially or at any subsequent time. However, there are those individuals who seem to grieve for inordinate periods of time. As a general rule, any grief or mourning process that has shown no positive change after 6 months to 1 year should be diagnosed and treated as depression. This is usually a neurotic depression.

Anxiety States and the Psychoneuroses

Anxiety is the common denominator of psychiatry. This state may be unaltered (free-floating anxiety) or altered by psychologic defenses against the anxiety (resulting in the symptoms of the other neuroses). Autonomic nervous system symptoms are a prominent expression of anxiety. Hyperventilation, gastrointestinal visceral spasm or hypermotility, palpitations, tachycardia, premature ventricular contractions, and so on lead to the signs and symptoms of weakness, fainting, diaphoresis, nausea, vomiting, diarrhea, and so forth so frequently seen. Subjectively, the individual is in an agonized state of impending doom, apprehension, fear, and dread, having no discernible basis. Anxiety can, and does, occur under any circumstance, including sleeping, just relaxing, or thinking of nothing in particular. The most extreme anxiety state is the very dramatic problem of panic. Suicidal risk is quite high in panic states. The differential diagnosis of anxiety and fear is shown in Table 30–3.

It is also crucial to rule out toxic states in the differential diagnosis of anxiety.

The ataractic drugs, especially the benzodiazepines, hydroxyzines, and propanediols have their greatest usefulness in

these disorders. However, they should not be prescribed in lieu of some nonpharmacologic approach to resolve the neurosis, such as psychotherapy. Where beta-adrenergic symptoms predominate, propranolol affords much symptomatic relief. Antipsychotic agents are not the drugs of first choice in treating anxiety, but if cautiously prescribed, such medications often help when ataractics fail. Barbiturates, bromides, narcotics, and analgesics are not indicated.

Organic Conditions

"If I'm senile, I'm really dead. I just have a heart beat and my eyes open." An alert and active mind as well as a calm and composed nature as preventives for senility are as old as Plato and Cicero. If only it were so simple!

The five "soft signs" of an organic brain syndrome (OBS) are varying degrees of impairment in orientation, memory, affect, intellectual functioning, and judgment. Unfortunately, the soft signs and symptoms of OBS are usually attributed to senility or cerebral atherosclerosis in the aged or to some form of retardation or functional psychosis in younger patients. When the soft signs are present, regardless of age, a detailed and diligent complete medical, neurologic, and frequently psychologic work-up must be done until an etiologic basis is positively ascertained. The wide variety of neurotic and psychotic problems resulting from OBS are "breakthrough symptoms" not directly ascribable to this syndrome. They are a product of the person's basic personality and conflicts, or an individual way of reacting to present stress, not the least of which is the OBS.

The five "soft signs" of OBS may be outlined as follows:

1. *Orientation:* Orientation to time is affected first, to place second, and to person not at all, unless the patient is delirious or in coma.

2. *Memory:* Recent memory is always impaired; remote memory may or may not be impaired. Simple questions of recent events (what did you have for your last meal?) and tests of immediate recall (a name and address) are usually all that are required to ascertain a defect. Confabulation (filling in a memory gap by a fictional story) is a restitutive function.

3. *Affect:* Affect is shallow, or labile, or

TABLE 30–3. DIFFERENTIAL DIAGNOSIS OF ANXIETY AND FEAR

Parameter	Anxiety	Fear
Object	Unknown	Known
Threat	Internal	External
Definition	Vague	Distinct
Conflict	Present	Absent
Duration	Chronic	Acute

both, with no connection to external or apparent internal events. The patient may cry or laugh suddenly, unexplainably, and for no discernible reason, or the affect, although steady, is vacuous.

4. *Intellectual Functioning:* This is reduced when compared with the individual's previous level of intellectual functioning. Meanings of words, simple calculations, new learning, abstraction, and simple general knowledge are impaired.

5. *Judgment:* Poor judgment is shown through inaccurate interpretation of events and lack of coherence or logic in approach to situations. Solutions tend to be concrete and irresponsible.

Acute OBS either reverses or becomes chronic. Chronic OBS may have acute epi-

TABLE 30–4. DIAGNOSTIC GUIDE TO SCHIZOPHRENIA*

Findings	Diagnostic Significance	Comments
Ambivalence, autism, looseness of association, inappropriate or flat affect (all four concurrently)	4	Possible, but not probable, in hysteria, OBS, depression, or mania
Derealization, desocialization, depersonalization (all three concurrently)	3 to 4	Same as above plus ataractic toxic drug states (alcohol), sociopathy, LSD, etc.
Catatonia (waxy flexibility, posturing, stupor, or excitement)	3 to 4	Not likely, but rule out OBS, mania, hysteria, depression, malingering
Delusions of influence (being controlled by outside forces, e.g., radiowaves, television, etc.)	4	Evaluate patients' seriousness and conviction about delusions
Neologisms	3 to 4	Especially if patient is not concerned about being misunderstood
Delusions that one's thoughts are known to everyone, of hallucinating hearing one's thoughts being publicly revealed or broadcast	4	Occurs in no other disorder
Apathy—total	2 to 3	Must rule out OBS and depression
Bodily delusions or hallucinations (e.g., electricity being sent through body)	3 to 4	Especially diagnostic if associated with other delusions
Other delusions (grandiose, persecutory, erotomanic, etc.)	1 to 3	Rule out paranoia without psychosis, OBS, mania, depression, sociopathy, hysteria
Other hallucinations	1 to 3	Rule out OBS, mania, depression, hysteria
Ideas of reference (e.g., way a person flicks cigarette ash is a special message to patient)	2	Rule out mania, sociopathy, hysteria, paranoia without psychosis
Extremes of bodily concern, unawareness of compulsions	2 to 3	The more extreme or the more bizarre, the more probable schizophrenia. Rule out depression, hypochondriasis, hysteria, drug addiction
Eccentricity, strained to total lack of personal relationships, criminality, poor vocational record, polymorphous sexuality, panic states	0 to 1	Not likely schizophrenia unless associated with more diagnostically significant findings above. Consider sociopathy, schizoid state, hysteria, retardation, criminality, rarely mania or depression

*Scale ranges from 0 (no diagnostic significance) to 4 (very significant).

sodes but never reverses. Rather, there is a variable but progressively deteriorating course. Eighteen to 24 months without complete reversal are needed to diagnose chronic OBS.

For OBS of unknown etiology, such as senility and certain types of mental retardation, there is no known therapy to reverse the signs and symptoms just outlined. Vasodilators are ineffective. However, breakthrough symptoms such as irritability, agitation, assaultiveness, and worsening of symptoms at night can be treated with haloperidol, thioridazine, or sedatives such as chloral hydrate or paraldehyde in divided doses. Other psychotropics must be used with caution. The use of lithium carbonate, although apparently effective for breakthrough hyperactive excited states, hypomania, or mania, is not well documented.

Schizophrenia

"A method to their madness," as paraphrased from Shakespeare, certainly is a noble, compassionate sentiment, but not really applicable to schizophrenic illness. It is applicable to that part of the personality that functions aside from the schizophrenic illness, but not to the illness itself. There is a growing consensus in the medical literature that the majority of cases of schizophrenia are mainly biochemical disorders, whether of affect or effect. Thus, the use of antipsychotic drugs is the cornerstone, but not the only treatment, of schizophrenia. Diagnostic guidelines for schizophrenia are outlined in Table 30–4.

The more acute, florid schizophrenic symptoms usually respond well to aliphatic or piperidine phenothiazines, haloperidol, dihydroindolones, and dibenzoxazepine. Maintenance medications, and potentially useful agents for chronic cases, include the thioxanthenes, piperazine phenothiazines, depot fluphenazine, and, less frequently, other antipsychotic neuroleptics.

Mania and Other Excitement States

It is the authors' subjective impression that there is a mania about diagnosing mania and prescribing lithium. The manic phase of the manic-depressive illness is synonymous with irritability, hyperactivity, and excitement, but the converse is not true. Table 30–5 provides clinical diagnostic assistance.

All the types of mania are associated with some degree of incessant talking and activity (purposeful or not), easy distractibility, impulsivity, and a disregard for manners, the rights of others, propriety, and discretion. The manic rarely finishes anything he starts. He frequently is uninvitingly and inappropriately overly personal and overly "friendly." Promiscuity and embarrassing flirtations are frequent, as are gambling, spending sprees, and drinking binges. Mischievous, boisterous, facetious, teasing, and unrelenting, the manic infects those around him. Uncommon behaviors are haughtiness, cynicalness, revengefulness, abusiveness, sarcasm, and marked paranoid trends. Extremes include deprecating oneself or another with childish abandon yet with a marked tone of underlying hostility. The manic leaves a rather remarkable and usually lasting impression.

Text continued on p. 389

TABLE 30–5. MANIC-DEPRESSIVE STATES*

Findings	Diagnostic Significance	Comments
Strong family history of manic-depressive illness	4	Vast majority of cases are probably genetic
Prior history of manic or depressive episodes	4	Is a chronic, recurring illness in most instances
Triad of high spirits interspersed with moments of anger or crying, hyperactivity, and pressure of thought and speech	4	Depending on degree of severity is hypomanic, manic, or delirious mania
Age of onset, 35 to 45 years	2	—

*Scale ranges from 0 (no diagnostic significance) to 4 (very significant).

TABLE 30-6.   PSYCHOPHARMACOLOGIC AGENTS

Drug Group	Dose	Therapeutic Indications	Side Effects, Adverse Reactions, and Dangers
BENZODIAZEPINES AND HYDROXYZINES		*Psychoneuroses/Anxiety States:* Wide usage in each of their total dose ranges, with low to medium doses being sufficient in the majority of cases. The symptoms, rather than the neurosis itself, very often respond to medication. The target symptoms affected include anxiety, peripheral striated muscular tension, the visceral autonomic nervous system concomitants of anxiety, agitation, irritability, restlessness, and the milder forms of insomnia or restless sleep.	*Side Effects and Adverse Reactions:* Most commonly encountered are sleepiness, fatigue, and ataxia. Less common, but not infrequent, are confusion, perplexity, "clouding," depression, blurred vision, and paradoxical reactions. Adjusting dosage is usually all that is required to relieve these side effects. Allergic reactions are infrequent; discontinuance is recommended when these are encountered.
Benzodiazepines			
Chlordiazepoxide (Librium)	10 mg.–100 mg./day		
Clorazepate (Tranxene)	7.5 mg.–35 mg./day		
Diazepam (Valium)	5 mg.–40 mg./day	*Psychosomatic Disorders:* Useful in total dosage range for the anxiety, tension, or apprehension associated with both psychosomatic and somatic disorders. Musculoskeletal spasm is particularly affected. The disorder itself is not affected.	*Dangers:* Potentiation of adverse effects in conjunction with narcotics, barbiturates, analgesics, sedatives, antihistamines, antipsychotics, and antidepressants. Contraindications include moderate to severe depressions, coma, shock, and renal or hepatic dysfunction.
Oxazepam (Serax)	30 mg.–150 mg./day		
Hydroxyzines			
Hydroxyzine hydrochloride (Atarax)	50 mg.–400 mg./day	*Organic Brain Syndromes (Including Retardation and Senility):* These drugs rarely affect the brain syndrome itself, exceptions being epileptic states and delirium tremens. Target symptoms affected are irritability, agitation, assaultiveness, restlessness, and milder forms of insomnia. The lower dosage range is advisable. Paradoxical effects are not uncommon. With severe confusion, perplexity, and the senile syndromes, caution and close observation are a must. Shock and coma are contraindications.	
Hydroxyzine pamoate (Vistaril)	50 mg.–400 mg./day		
		Personality Disorders: The same target symptoms as previously listed are affected, but usually to a much lesser extent. The disorder itself is not affected. Habituation is more common in this group; therefore, lower dosages of shorter duration are recommended.	
		Alcoholism: Widely used in all categories of alcoholism, the benzodiazepines have in large part replaced paraldehyde in the treatment or prevention of delirium tremens and are on a par with certain phenothiazines in respect to alcoholic hallucinosis. The efficacy of these agents as an adjunct to sobriety and psychotherapy is well accepted. Habituation is a common problem.	
		Drug Addiction: Occasional usefulness for the aforementioned symptoms. Habituation a problem.	

Psychoses: These are not drugs of first choice.

Other Useful Indications: Almost any musculoskeletal spasm, adjunctive anticonvulsant therapy, status epilepticus, "personality changes" associated with epilepsy (slowness, restlessness, perseveration, etc.), certain toxic drug states (LSD, mescaline, amphetamines, etc.), preoperative medication, precardioversion procedures, gastroscopy, sigmoidoscopy, etc. (but not bronchoscopy or laryngoscopy):

Psychoneuroses/Anxiety States: The beta-adrenergic symptoms of anxiety–tension states, in particular cardiac symptoms, are highly affected by the beta-adrenergic blocking properties of the propranolols. Only this symptomatic relief is afforded, no other. These compounds are not to be used indiscriminately. They should only be used in anxiety–tension states in which beta-adrenergic symptoms are severe or particularly disturbing.

Dangers: The risks of these drugs are serious, and the reader is advised to become very familiar with them before using these compounds for psychiatric conditions.

Psychotic Depressions: The symptoms of psychotic depressions respond to the tricyclic antidepressants. Some feel that there may be temporary "cure" of the depression itself. Disturbances of sleep, appetite, mood, and bodily function (psychosomatic aspects of depression) are usually affected positively. In the psychotic category, the higher dosage ranges are recommended even upon commencing therapy. Effectiveness above the highest recommended dosages is occasionally seen.

Schizophrenia: Efficacy can be expected in schizoaffective schizophrenia, depressed type; psychotic depressions concomitant with and separate from a schizophrenic reaction; and depression following an acute schizophrenic episode.

Manic-Depressive Psychosis: The depressive phase of this psychosis is affected. Can be combined with lithium carbonate as part of a preventive maintenance program.

Other Psychotic Depressions: Positive results may be seen in psychotic depressions of middle or later life, including "involutional melancholia"; some psychotic depressions associated with organic brain syndrome (OBS) and senility; and situational depressions of severe degree.

Side Effects and Adverse Reactions: A majority of patients taking these drugs suffer temporary, self-reversing side effects before the therapeutic effects of the drug are seen. Reassurance and frequent explanations are necessary to keep the patient from prematurely discontinuing the prescription. Use of adjunctive agents such as Ritalin or triiodothyronine to decrease the time of side effects and hasten the onset of action is still being debated. The more common side effects and adverse reactions include xerostomia, constipation, fatigue, sleepiness, hypotension, dizziness, arrhythmias, confusion, ataxia, extrapyramidal effects, blurred vision, urinary delay and frequency, nausea, and allergic reactions.

Dangers: Risk in pregnancy, history of cardiovascular disease of any type, glaucoma, genitourinary disease, epilepsy, general anesthetics, hyperthyroid diseases, use with antiparkinsonian or other anticholinergic drugs, risk of suicide. Absolute contraindications include prior use of monoamine oxidase inhibiting drugs within at least 2 weeks and the recovery phase of myocardial infarction.

PROPRANOLOL

Propranolol (Inderal)   10 mg.–60 mg./day

TRICYCLIC ANTIDEPRESSANTS

Amitriptyline (Elavil)   50 mg.–300 mg./day
Doxepin (Adapin, Sinequan)   50 mg.–300 mg./day
Imipramine (Imavate, Tofranil)   50 mg.–300 mg./day
Nortriptyline (Aventyl)   50 mg.–300 mg./day
Protriptyline (Vivactil)   10 mg.– 40 mg./day

(Dosage in children and the geriatric group is 25% to 50% of the usual adult dose.)

Table continued on following page

TABLE 30-6. PSYCHOPHARMACOLOGIC AGENTS (Continued)

Drug Group	Dose	Therapeutic Indications	Side Effects, Adverse Reactions, and Dangers
TRICYCLIC ANTIDEPRESSANTS (Continued)		*Psychosomatic Disorders:* Many psychosomatic disorders are either in direct relation to or masking a depression. A trial of tricyclic antidepressants, in the full dosage range, is frequently rewarding to patient and physician alike. In particular, the wide variety of psychosomatic pain syndromes, such as headaches, back pains, etc., are often positively affected.	
		Organic Brain Syndromes (Including Retardation and Senility): Tricyclic antidepressants are useful in the depressions associated with OBS and senility. However, the risks are much greater than usual, especially those of a cardiac nature, delirium, hallucinations, paranoia, and confusion. Caution, observation, and supervision must be assured.	
		Psychoneuroses: Although usually much less effective in neurotic depressions than psychotic depressions, the tricyclic antidepressants should be tried in the more severe cases. The lower dosage range is recommended to start, and increases beyond the mid-range of dosage are rarely effective.	
		Alcoholism and Drug Addiction: No direct value, unless there is an associated depression not due to the alcohol or drug usage. Abstinence is necessary.	
		Other: Enuresis, school phobia, cyclothymia (when combined with lithium), and habit reactions in children may be benefited.	
PROPANEDIOLS Meprobamate (Equanil, Miltown)	800 mg.–2400 mg./day (Dosage in children is 25% of usual adult dose. In general, these drugs are only recommended for exceptional use in psychiatric conditions.)	*Psychosomatic Disorders and Psychoneuroses:* Symptoms of irritability, mild or moderate types of insomnia, anxiety, tension, and hyperactivity are usually responsive. *Organic Brain Syndromes (Including Retardation and Senility):* Same indications as with the psychoneuroses, but unusual caution and supervision are necessary because of the high risk of confusion and excessive sedation. Occasional paradoxical excitement is known to occur. Avoid in acute OBS. *Other Uses:* Adjunct in various dermatologic and allergic problems. May be effective in temper tantrums and extremes of aggressivity in children and in premenstrual tension.	*Side Effects and Adverse Reactions:* Excessive sedation, ataxia, dizziness, nausea, blurred vision, and allergic reactions are common. *Dangers:* Suicide, use in pregnancy, additive effect with other central nervous system (CNS) depressants, impairment of reactivity and ability, and habituation are high risks. Use is contraindicated in acute intermittent porphyria. Avoid use in personality disorders and drug addiction because of high risk of habituation.

PHENOTHIAZINES

(A) Aliphatic and Piperidine
  Chlorpromazine (Thorazine)   30 mg.–1800 mg./day
  Mesoridazine (Serentil)   50 mg.–600 mg./day
  Thioridazine (Mellaril)   30 mg.–1800 mg./day
  Triflupromazine (Vesprin)   10 mg.–300 mg./day
  Numerous others

(B) Piperazine
  Fluphenazine (Prolixin)   4 mg.–30 mg./day
  Perphenazine (Trilafon)   8 mg.–60 mg./day
  Trifluoperazine (Stelazine)   5 mg.–45 mg./day
  Numerous others

Psychoses:

Schizophrenia: Group A drugs are usually more beneficial than group B drugs for the more acute, florid schizophrenic symptoms, such as panic, severe agitation, hyperactivity, catatonia, confusion, disorganization of thought and behavior, extreme restlessness, aggressivity, assaultiveness, fear, blatant anxiety, insomnia, and hallucinations. Group B drugs are usually more beneficial than group A drugs for maintenance, delusional activity, and some of the more chronic forms of schizophrenic disorders. Special mention is made of depot fluphenazine for maintenance and chronic cases.

Manic-Depressive Psychosis: Use in manic phase only. Group A drugs are usually more effective than group B drugs.

Other Psychotic Depressions: In the agitated or anxious psychotic depressions, either group, in the lower dosage range, can be helpful for the the agitated or anxious symptoms.

Hysterical Psychoses: Group A drugs are usually more effective than group B drugs.

Psychoneuroses and Psychosomatic Disorders: In the depersonalization neurosis, low doses of either group of phenothiazines are the drug of first choice. The sufferers of other neuroses frequently report worsening of symptoms with phenothiazines.

Organic Brain Syndromes (Including Retardation and Senility): Therapeutic efficacy in agitation, restlessness, assaultiveness, insomnia, etc., is often reported. Low dosage group A drugs and close supervision are necessary, as hypotension, excessive sedation, severe confusional states, and extrapyramidal symptoms are commonplace.

Alcoholism: May be used with much caution in delirium tremens or alcoholic hallucinosis, as the seizure threshold is lowered. As an adjunct to abstinence, these drugs are of limited value.

Drug Addiction: Because of the variety of additives in "street" hallucinogens that can be deleteriously potentiated with phenothiazines, they are not recommended for treatment of drug abuse.

Side Effects and Adverse Reactions: Common ones are any variety of extrapyramidal symptoms, drowsiness, hypotension, "fogginess," impairment of ability, xerostomia, blurred vision, constipation, allergic reactions, and lactation.

Dangers: Contraindicated in coma, subcortical damage, blood dyscrasias, concomitant large doses of hypnotics, cerebral thrombosis, severe depression, hepatitis, and severe renal insufficiency. Other dangers include pregnancy, known sensitivity to the drug, potentiation of CNS depressants, abrupt withdrawal, cardiovascular disease, respiratory disorders, and impairment of ability.

Table continued on following page

TABLE 30–6. PSYCHOPHARMACOLOGIC AGENTS *(Continued)*

Drug Group	Dose	Therapeutic Indications	Side Effects, Adverse Reactions, and Dangers
PHENOTHIAZINES *(Continued)*		*Other Indications:* May be useful in acute intermittent porphyria, intractable hiccups, potentiation of analgesics, antiemetic (regardless of cause), as part of a "lytic" cocktail, prevention of irreversible shock from blood loss, tetanus, and enhancing hypothermia.	*Side Effects and Adverse Reactions:* Most common are insomnia, extrapyramidal symptoms, including tardive dyskinesia, depression, allergic reactions, nausea, xerostomia, blurred vision, hypotension, arrhythmias.
BUTYROPHENONES		*Psychoses:*	*Dangers:* Pregnancy, impairment of ability, potentiation of CNS depressants. Contraindicated in coma, severe depression, and Parkinson's disease.
Haloperidol (Haldol)	2 mg.–30 mg./day	*Schizophrenia:* Effective in both acute and chronic schizophrenia.	
		Manic-Depressive Psychosis: Very effective in mania but not depression.	
		Hysterical Psychoses: Alternative choice to phenothiazines.	
		Organic Brain Syndromes (Including Retardation and Senility): In low doses is very often very effective in the personality disorders associated with OBS and in decreasing the anxiety, tension, irritability, restlessness, hyperkinesis, assaultiveness, and insomnia of OBS and senility. Very effective in the treatment of Huntington's chorea and Gilles de la Tourette's disease in children.	
		Personality Disorders: Some value in those disorders associated with OBS.	
		Alcoholism: Alternative to drugs already mentioned (benzodiazepines, paraldehyde).	
		Drug Addiction: Occasionally useful as an adjunct in the treatment of a variety of drug addictions.	
		Psychoneuroses and Psychosomatic Disorders: Sometimes helps pavor nocturnus.	
MONOAMINE OXIDASE INHIBITORS		*Psychoses:*	*Side Effects and Adverse Reactions:* Most common are toxic psychoses, precipitation of mania, insomnia, xerostomia, allergic reactions, hypotension, and seizures.
Isocarboxazid (Marplan) Tranylcypromine (Parnate)	10 mg.–30 mg./day 10 mg.–30 mg./day	*Schizophrenia:* Schizoaffective, schizophrenia-depressed type, or the depression following an acute schizophrenic episode may be helped.	*Dangers:* Use in pregnancy, use in children, hypertensive crises, and dietary indiscretion caused by high tyramine content foods. Monoamine oxidase inhibitors are not to be used with sympathomimetics, other neuroleptics, and tricyclic antidepressants. Contraindicated in any cardiovascular or cerebrovascular
		Manic-Depressive Psychosis: Effective in depressive phase and may be of maintenance effectiveness combined with lithium carbonate.	
		Other Psychotic Depressions: Effective in all types, but use with extreme caution, if at all, in depressions associated with OBS.	

disorder, pheochromocytoma, or with any CNS depressants or antiparkinsonian drugs, and in patients with a history of hepatic or renal dysfunction. Initiation of therapy in a hospital setting is advisable.

Drug	Dose	Uses	Side Effects and Dangers
THIOXANTHENES Chlorprothixene (Taractan) Thiothixene (Navane)	50 mg.–600 mg./day 5 mg.–45 mg./day	*Psychoneuroses:* On rare occasion may help in phobias, severe conversion reactions, and dissociative states when other measures fail. *Psychosomatic Disorders:* Same indications as with the tricyclic antidepressants. *Organic Brain Syndromes (Including Retardation and Senility):* Although effective for associated depressions, these drugs should be avoided in OBS. *Psychoses:* *Schizophrenia:* Much more effective in the chronic cases than in the acute cases. Noticeable effect may take several months. *Manic-Depressive Psychosis:* An alternative, in low doses, when other approaches fail. *Other Psychotic Depressions:* Can be an alternative, in low doses, when other drugs fail. *Hysterical Psychoses:* An alternative when other drugs fail. *Psychoneuroses:* Can be a very useful adjunct in some cases of severe obsessive-compulsive neurosis, severe neurotic depressions, and neurasthenia. *Organic Brain Syndromes (Including Retardation and Senility):* Effective in hypoactive, lethargic states, but high incidence of extrapyramidal symptoms.	*Side Effects and Adverse Reactions:* Most common are dizziness, hypotension, impairment of ability, sedation, extrapyramidal effects, fever of undetermined origin, allergic reactions, headaches, constipation, and potentiation of CNS depressants. As with most neuroleptics, epinephrine should not be used as a pressor agent. *Dangers:* Use in pregnancy, use in children, seizures, and cardiovascular disorders. Contraindicated in coma, blood dyscrasias, cerebrovascular disorders, and shock.
LITHIUM Lithium carbonate (Li_2CO_3) (Eskalith, Lithane, Lithonate, others)	1800 mg.–2400 mg/day for 3–5 days to establish therapeutic blood level of 0.5 to 1.5 mEq./l. Then 600 mg.–1200 mg./day maintenance dose.	*Psychoses:* The only indication for Li_2CO_3 is psychotic excitatory states. The most frequent psychotic excitatory state for which Li_2CO_3 is prescribed is the manic phase of the manic-depressive psychosis. However, Li_2CO_3 is not specific for this disorder and can be tried in any state of "mania." There is even recent evidence to suggest its usefulness in psychotic excitatory states associated with OBS, senility, and retardation.	*Side Effects and Adverse Reactions:* With rare exception, the following occur only above blood levels of 1.5 mEq./l. and are blood level-related: tremor, diarrhea, vomiting, sleepiness, ataxia, blurred vision, ringing in the ears, and polyuria. These progress through any variety of organ systems as levels increase and culminate in stupor, coma, and seizures. Unrelated to blood level are decrease in protein-bound iodine, increase in ^{131}I uptake and goiter, diffuse electroencephalographic slowing, nonspecific electrocardiographic changes, headache, elevated fasting blood sugar, itching, foul taste, peripheral swelling, and allergic reactions. *Dangers:* The patient must maintain adequate diet, salt intake, and fluid intake. Caution in use in pregnancy and use in children. Contraindicated in severe brain damage, coma, and severe cardiovascular and renal disorders.
DIHYDROINDOLONES Molindone (Moban)	30 mg.–300 mg./day	This is an entirely new group of neuroleptics, chemically distinct from the other neuroleptics. Indications and uses are similar to those described for	Supposedly, the incidence and severity of adverse reactions are low.

Table continued on following page

TABLE 30-6. PSYCHOPHARMACOLOGIC AGENTS (Concluded)

Drug Group	Dose	Therapeutic Indications	Side Effects, Adverse Reactions, and Dangers
DIHYDROINDOLONES (Continued)		other neuroleptics, and these drugs are to be considered as an equal alternative to them. To date, major efficacy is in acute schizophrenic states, less so in mania and in some severe chronic anxiety neuroses.	
DIBENZOXAZEPINES Loxapine (Loxitane)	30 mg.–250 mg./day	These drugs are in the tricyclic family and, therefore, are distinct from the other neuroleptics. Major usefulness seems to be in both acute and chronic schizophrenia. The remainder of the drug profile is similar to other neuroleptics and the other tricyclics. These drugs are equal alternatives to the other neuroleptics at the time of this writing.	Side effects and adverse reactions seem to be less severe than with certain other neuroleptics at this time.
COMBINATION DRUGS Triavil, Etrafon, Pro-banthine with Dartal, Tranco-Gesic, Librax, Milpath, and a multitude of others.		See separate drug profiles for actions and indications.	See separate drug profiles for side effects, adverse reactions, and dangers.
BARBITURATES		In general, the barbiturates, along with other CNS depressants such as analgesics, narcotics, alcohol, etc., ordinarily will aggravate any psychiatric disorder, despite some subjective "relief" and are, therefore, to be avoided in these conditions.	
ORTHOMOLECULAR THERAPY		This is commonly known as "megavitamin therapy," as the doses of vitamins used exceed the usual therapeutic doses by several times. The most popularized use of this therapy is in the group of schizophrenias, particularly in those patients who had celiac symptoms as children. Megavitamins have also been used in infantile autism, alcoholism, OBS, depressions, manic-depressive psychosis, retardation, severe neuroses, and others. There have been varying reports of the use of vitamin B_{12} in a variety of psychiatric disorders. There are a variety of theories and combinations of vitamins and doses in orthomolecular therapy. The more commonly employed combinations usually include niacin, thiamine, B_{12}, pyridoxine, riboflavin, and vitamin C, and some use vitamin A. Side effects, etc., are those for high dosage of each vitamin. Orthomolecular therapy encompasses much more than vitamins and special diets and may have more usefulness in the future. Although a placebo effect may be part of orthomolecular therapy, this alone cannot explain reported results and usefulness.	

The several effective medical treatments for mania include lithium carbonate, phenothiazines, haloperidol, dihydroindolones, dibenzoxazepine, and electroconvulsive therapy. Maintenance therapy appears effective with lithium carbonate and to a lesser extent with haloperidol and the other neuroleptics.

PSYCHOPHARMACOLOGIC AGENTS

The listing of all agents of each drug group or a comprehensive compendium of all the uses, side effects, and adverse reactions of each agent is not possible here. Therefore, in Table 30–6 the authors have selected those drugs from each group that are more frequently prescribed and have listed their most common uses and side effects.

CONCLUSION

Through the use of an informed, therapeutic understanding (the broadest sense of psychotherapy) and the judicious, honorable use of psychopharmacologic agents, we might take a step away from some of the tragedy (not drama) and stigma of having or being treated for psychiatric conditions. Little attention has been paid to childhood and adolescent disorders in this chapter, and for these the reader is referred elsewhere in the text.

BIBLIOGRAPHY

1. AMA Drug Evaluations. 2nd ed. Acton, Mass., Publishing Sciences Group, Inc., 1973.
2. Ban, T. A.: Psychopharmacology. Baltimore, The Williams & Wilkins Co., 1969.
3. Cole, J. O., and Hollister, L. E.: Schizophrenia. Baltimore, Medcom., Inc., 1970.
4. Davis, J. M.: Overview: maintenance therapy in psychiatry; II. Affective disorders. Am. J. Psychiatry, 133:1, 1976.
5. Freedman, A. M., Kaplan, H., and Sadock, B.: Comprehensive Textbook of Psychiatry/II. Baltimore, The Williams & Wilkins Co., 1975.
6. Goldberg, H. L., and Finnerty, R. J.: The use of doxepin in the treatment of symptoms of anxiety neurosis and accompanying depression: a collaborative controlled study. Am. J. Psychiatry, 129:74, 1972.
7. Greenblatt, D. J., and Shader, R. I.: Benzodiazepines in Clinical Practice. New York, Raven Press, 1974.
8. Heller, A.: Effectiveness of antidepressant drugs: a triple blind study comparing imipramine, desimipramine and placebo. Am. J. Psychiatry, 127:1092, 1971.
9. Jacobsen, E.: Depression. New York, International Universities Press, Inc., 1971.
10. Keeler, M. H., and McCurdy, R. L.: Medical practice without antianxiety drugs. Am. J. Psychiatry, 132:654, 1975.
11. Klerman, G. L., Dimascio, A., Weissman, M., et al.: Treatment of depression by drugs and psychotherapy. Am. J. Psychiatry, 131:186, 1974.
12. Kolb, L. C.: Modern Clinical Psychiatry. 9th ed. Philadelphia, W. B. Saunders Co., 1977.
13. MacKenzie, K. R., and Caffey, E. M., Jr.: The eclectic approach to the treatment of phobias. Am. J. Psychiatry, 129:74, 1972.
14. Physicians Desk Reference. 30th ed. Oradell, N. J., Medical Economics, Inc., 1976.
15. Shader, R. I.: Manual of Psychiatric Therapeutics. Boston, Little, Brown & Co., 1975.
16. Williams, J. B.: Common errors in treatment of depression. Am. Fam. Physician, 2:60, 1976.

Chapter 31

PSYCHOTHERAPY AND BEHAVIOR MODIFICATION

*by LUCY JANE KING,
and L. E. MASTERS*

PSYCHOTHERAPY – DEFINITIONS AND INDICATIONS

In the broadest sense, psychotherapy, or counseling, is a conversation between two people, one of whom has professional training and who seeks to help the other clarify his understanding of his situation and how best to cope with it. In the field of medicine, psychotherapy is an extension and elaboration of the details of an individual's personal and social history.

Psychotherapy is indicated when:

1. The patient asks to talk about a personal problem. Occasionally, a patient comes to his family physician specifically to seek help in dealing with a psychologic or interpersonal problem. He is concerned about his marriage or his teenaged son or is having problems getting along with his boss at work.

2. The chief complaint represents an interpersonal problem. The patient may be having headaches, poor appetite, fatigue, or abdominal pain, but these are usually specifically related to times when the teenaged son comes home at 3:00 A.M. acting drunk. The chief complaint may be sexual dysfunction, but there are a number of other areas of conflict in the marriage.

3. Information about personal problems is elicited in the medical history. In the course of taking a history, personal problems are alluded to. "My wife is really worried about my health." "I don't dare tell my parents about this." There may be nonverbal cues, such as shrugging the shoulders or rolling the eyes. Sometimes real feelings are masked by a flippant response. "Hah, are you kidding!" "She couldn't care less." "My husband says it's all in my head." If the patient seems concerned about a particular area, the physician allows a few moments of silence or asks an open-ended question, such as, "Can you tell me a little more about that?" This often leads a patient to pour out his story. That story may be what he *really* wants to discuss with his physician, or it may provide data about some problem of living that he hadn't realized might be helped by counseling.

4. The personal and social history reveals a problem. Routine questions in the following areas may pinpoint some current problem:

    a. Family background. The patient may have attitudes that interfere with his coping with current problems, because of a broken home, financial difficulties, illness, or suicide or other death in the family.

    b. Education. Perhaps it was necessary for him to stop school early, thus limiting his current opportunities for employment or making it difficult for him to deal with his better-educated wife, children, or friends. Or possibly he is overeducated for the types of jobs now available to him.

    c. Employment. Perhaps he has had difficulty keeping jobs, is dissatisfied with his line of work, or is presently facing retirement. He may be unhappy with a recent promotion or, on the other hand, may feel a lack of fulfillment in a mundane job.

d. Sexual history. Family attitudes toward sex or early sexual experiences may be influencing current sexual function. Exact details of sexual experiences must be elicited. It is best not to assume knowledge on the part of the patient of even the most rudimentary aspects of sexual function because misinformation abounds in this area.

e. Marital history. Separation, divorce, or physical or mental illness in a spouse indicates problem areas. The age of both spouses at marriage, previous marriages of either, and the duration of the marriage are useful sources of information for understanding the situation.

f. Current living circumstances. The patient may be burdened with caring for an aged relative or a large family. There may be an unhappy relationship with a roommate. Perhaps living quarters are smaller or larger than those the patient was previously accustomed to.

g. Financial status. There may be not enough money to meet expenses, high income but many debts, or injudicious planning of the budget.

THE FAMILY PHYSICIAN AS A PSYCHOTHERAPIST

Special Role

The kinds of information just discussed can be elicited in an initial interview or in subsequent office visits. However, the family physician who has lived in a community for some time and has treated several members of the same family has a special advantage in that he already has much of this information at his fingertips. When a patient comes into the office, the physician already knows the setting in which the patient lives and works. He is aware of certain problems and can inquire about them when members of the family consult him. He is likely to see each member several times a year. Patients often regard their family physicians as trusted friends to whom they can talk, in contrast to feeling uncomfortable when first meeting psychiatrists or others who specialize in treating severe psychologic problems.

Special Problems

While knowing patients and their families well and encountering them frequently in community acitivites are advantageous, this can at times also present problems. If physician and patient have many informal contacts outside the office, it may be harder for the patient to see the physician as an objective, dispassionate counselor. The physician may feel that he is in the embarrassing position of having information relevant to a problem but being unable to mention it for reasons of confidentiality. Each physician has to define his role in a particular situation in the light of his practice and the community in which he lives.

When to Utilize Psychotherapy

Psychotherapy proceeds naturally as a series of questions at almost every encounter with a patient. In order to understand what a situation really is, the physician must ask the patient to define the problem in great detail. What is actually happening? What specific things has each person involved in the situation said and done? How does the patient feel about each of these? What did the patient do in return? In subsequent interviews, the patient can provide additional information in terms of what has happened since the previous visit and how he handled the situations that arose. This can be continued as long as both patient and physician feel that the process is accomplishing something in terms of helping the patient to understand and cope with his problems.

Special times can be set aside for patients for whom psychotherapy seems indicated, for example, utilizing a "30 minute hour" as the last appointment of the morning or afternoon. Some physicians set aside an afternoon for such appointments and allow office staff an afternoon off.

Different physicians may have special interests and training in areas such as treating marital and sexual problems, counseling alcoholics or drug abusers, or dealing with adolescents or with geriatric patients and may make a special effort to work with such patients. Other physicians may have had special experience in working with groups and can set aside a few hours for group psychotherapy. Or, a physician may employ trained counselors to work with groups of patients, sitting in with the group from time to time himself.

When to Refer

Consultation with a psychiatrist should be considered when the physician feels that his sessions with the patient are unrewarding, when the patient presents very complicated psychologic problems, or when the physician feels very uncomfortable with the patient and his problems. Such consultations can be requested either to have the psychiatrist offer suggestions about how the family physician should proceed with counseling or to have the psychiatrist, rather than the family physician, continue appropriate psychotherapy.

A patient's needs might seem more appropriately met by someone other than a physician, for example, a pastoral counselor or a social worker. It is invaluable for the primary care physician to be aware of community health centers, counseling centers, social agencies, private groups that focus on a particular problem (for example, Alcoholics Anonymous), and other sources of help in the community. Clergy, nurses, social case workers, and school counselors with training and experience in counseling and psychotherapy can be of help. Referral to these individuals or agencies is made in the same manner as is referral to another physician, that is, by direct contact (usually a telephone call) with discussion of relevant information about the patient and indication of why the referral is being made.

Conversations with individual counselors or with representatives of community agencies can elicit information about the kinds of problems they handle and just how they approach those problems. The physician can evaluate whether or not their approach seems appropriate and whether or not they seem to take on problems beyond their areas of professional competence. Feedback from and about patients who have been referred can be valuable in evaluating referral sources, as can discussions with colleagues about particular referral sources.

THE PATIENT

Perception of Problems

As previously implied, the patient's initial verbalization of a problem may not really express the nature of the situation. It cannot be emphasized too strongly that detailed questions are necessary to find out exactly what is happening. It is also important to ascertain just what specific factors about the situation are of concern to the patient. What would he like to see changed? If he could magically have any possible solution come about, what would he consider to be the ideal outcome? Given the realities of the situation, what possible solutions have occurred to him? The physician may think of other alternatives and may ask "What about . . . ?" "Have you thought about . . . ?" These questions can be presented in an open-ended fashion to allow the patient to express his opinions without feeling that the physician is providing pat answers. What can the patient do to bring about each of the solutions? What must others do? Is it realistic to expect that they will do what the patient wants them to do? Can family members or friends be recruited to help the patient deal with the problems?

Family members or others involved can be interviewed (with the patient's permission) in order to get their perspectives and to get some idea of how likely they are to actually do what the patient wishes. Not infrequently, the patient has the least awareness of the problem, and in these cases information from relatives is invaluable. For example, depressed patients may not realize that they have a syndrome characterized by marked changes in eating habits, sleeping schedules, and psychomotor activity, but rather they see themselves as no good, worthless, and hopelessly sinful.

Long-term Behavior Patterns

All of us have characteristic ways of dealing with problems. A particular problem mentioned by a patient may actually reflect a more chronic underlying behavior pattern. Some patients make decisions impulsively and consider consequences only after they have occurred. Others avoid meeting problems, hoping that someone else will solve them. An individual's ways of trying to cope with problems may indicate insensitivity to the feelings of others. Unilateral decisions may be made without consulting others involved. Some patients feel they have the burden of solving all the family problems without help from others and characteristically set unrealistic expectations for themselves and others. Understanding such patterns can help the physician predict how an individual might behave in certain circumstances and can aid him in finding ways to cope with the problem at hand.

Environmental Factors

An excellent way to get an idea of a patient's level of functioning is to ask for details of how he spends a typical day. What is involved at work? What are the household duties encountered? If not working, what is done all day? What other individuals are encountered, and how much interaction is there with them? When and where are meals eaten and with whom? What is done in the evening? What, if anything, is done for relaxation?

Changes in the environment can also create difficulties. McWhinney[8] has listed seven such changes that can cause significant problems:

1. Loss. People close to the patient have died or have moved away. He has been fired from his job. Financial problems have forced him to give up his home. Chronic illness (loss of good health) will prevent her from caring for her family and home as she would like to do.

2. Conflict. There are troubles with fellow workers, neighbors, or relatives. Too many demands are being made, and the patient cannot meet them all (for example, job, family, community activities). There is conflict between what the individual wants to do and what he thinks ought to be done.

3. Geographic change. Moving to a new environment creates myriad difficulties in coping with life in unfamiliar surroundings without all the people one ordinarily turns to for information and advice. A middle-aged woman, having recently moved, told one of the authors, "There ought to be a law against transferring a 40 year old woman!"

4. Developmental change. Time of life is a major problem (for example, adolescence, menopause, senescence).

5. Maladaptation. Chronic difficulty is experienced in dealing with school, job, or marriage.

6. Stress. Acute changes in life circumstances present new problems.

7. Failure. The patient realizes that he cannot fulfill his life-long goals, or that his expectations (for career, marriage, or children) are frustrated.

THE PSYCHOTHERAPIST'S ATTITUDE

A number of aspects of a counselor's approach to dealing with patients have been outlined by communications analyst Jergen Ruesch.[11]

Discriminate Permissiveness. The patient is encouraged to tell in his own way all the aspects of the situation that are important to him. The physician gives every indication of his interest or lack of interest in whatever the patient has to say.

Bringing up the Unmentionable. The patient can bring up any topic he wishes and can discuss any of his feelings without condemnation from the physician. The physician will not react with shock and horror. Confidentiality will be observed at all times.

Expectant Readiness. The physician is prepared to deal with whatever the patient says and to meet the patient on his own ground.

Cathartic Listening. The patient is given the chance, initially, to say what he has to say without value judgments by the physician.

Conditional Commitment. The physician is committed to helping the patient in whatever way he can. He is willing to try to understand "where the patient is" and, as much as possible, to understand how the patient sees things (even if he doesn't agree with the patient's viewpoint).

Constructive Selectivity. The physician selects particular areas to focus on, for example, aspects of the personal and social history as previously discussed.

Unaggressive Directness. If the patient rambles away from the main topic or starts discussing his philosophy and what *should* happen rather than his feelings and what actually *is* happening, the physician gently brings him back to the important issues.

Taking Things in Hand. As an interview is concluding, a plan of action is formed in the physician's mind, which he explains to the patient. If referral is in order, that is explained. If additional office visits are planned, this is made clear and their purpose is explained.

PSYCHOTHERAPEUTIC TECHNIQUES

GENERAL TECHNIQUES

Several types of discussion involved in psychotherapy are summarized in the following paragraphs. A number of them have been described by Ruesch[11] or by the late German psychiatrist Karl Jaspers.[7]

Pinpointing. Each situation that the patient mentions is clarified step by step. Specific questions are repeatedly asked to get the patient to describe in detail exactly what is happening. The physician might well play the devil's advocate by bringing up perspectives and viewpoints other than those of the patient. This can be done in a nonthreatening way. "Isn't it possible that . . . ?" "Some people might think you meant. . . ." "How do you think your husband would evaluate this?" Is it possible that your neighbor thinks . . . ?"

A number of specific possible solutions can be brought up for the patient's consideration. These might even be made extreme in order to focus his attention on other alternatives. "What keeps you from just going ahead and getting a divorce?" "What would happen if you quit working?"

Documentation. Effort is made to see how the patient has arrived at particular conclusions and whether or not these seem realistic. "Did she say that in so many words, or is it more a feeling you have?" "What *did* she say that made you think that's what she meant?" "This reminds me of what you said about . . . ."

Translation. The patient is repeatedly encouraged to define exactly what he means. "What things has your neighbor done that make you think he's unfriendly?" "What evidence do you have that your boss goes out of his way to make trouble for you?"

Amplification. Because the patient can discuss any topic he likes and because he is constantly encouraged to evaluate how he feels, what he thinks, and why he feels and thinks as he does, he is made aware of things that hadn't occurred to him, that is, he develops insight into his feelings and behavior.

Confrontation. If there are discrepancies in what the patient says or between what the patient says and the facts known to the physician, these are pointed out. "How does this fit with what you said last week?"

Explanation and Education. At all points, the patient can be informed of the physician's formulation of his diagnosis and his impression of the patient's problems in living. The prolonged plan of action can be outlined, and alternative treatments or approaches can be discussed.

Persuasion. As part of explaining the treatment he feels is best, the physician makes every effort to help the patient see the importance of following through with the outlined plan. He presents his formulation of the situation as convincingly as possible.

Encouragement. Most people are embarrassed to discuss psychologic, interpersonal, or family problems because they feel difficulties in dealing with such problems represent weakness on their part. Frequently, it is useful to interject honest comments such as, "You are really doing a good job of keeping going in spite of all these difficulties confronting you," or "It really is tough to have to face the decisions you must make."

Promoting Awareness of Feelings. Many people avoid facing problems directly by speculating about "why" either they themselves or others are behaving as they do, rather than by considering *what* they are doing and how they *feel* about it. It is often useful to encourage patients to allow themselves to perceive the strong positive or negative feelings they have about particular persons or situations and to see how these feelings are influencing what they do. For example, a patient described an argument with his girlfriend and asked whether his viewpoint or hers was "correct" or "right." The physician replied, "Loss of your friendship with her would really make you feel bad, wouldn't it? Maybe that's why you're upset when you disagree with her."

BEHAVIOR THERAPY

Some general applications of the principles of psychologic conditioning can be made in many kinds of counseling, although the use of specific procedures requires specialized training. Learning theory, which has been formulated to explain the results of experiments in conditioning behavior in animals and humans, can be summarized very simply by saying that individuals continue doing those things for which they receive a reward, or positive reinforcement, and stop doing those things for which they receive punishment, or negative reinforcement. In addition, behaviors for which there is no reinforcement, either positive or negative, tend to disappear, or to become extinguished, over a period of time.

By showing interest in some topics mentioned by the patient but not in others, a counselor rewards, or reinforces, discussion of those topics. Topics that are ignored are brought up by the patient less and less often, that is, become extinguished. Sometimes what appears to be a negative reinforcer is actually a positive reinforcement. For example, a scolding might actually reward the child who is seeking attention of any kind. In such cases, extinction may be preferable to punishment. For example, thumb-sucking or nail-biting in children may disappear if ignored, rather than if attention is constantly focused on these habits by demanding that they be stopped.

In marriage counseling, partners are often asked to describe specifically what things their spouse does that they like and to reward those behaviors with compliments and other encouragements to continue. Sometimes a habit that is irritating to the spouse is decreased more readily by ignoring it (extinction) than by nagging about it (negative reinforcement).

The technique of *implosion* involves having patients with phobias or obsessions imagine vividly the things they fear most. This idea can be applied in a more general way by asking patients to describe the worst possible thing that could happen in a particular situation and to examine what such an outcome would mean to them and to others involved. Thus, patients can gain a better perspective of what consequences might occur and what they might do to prevent these consequences or to cope with them if they can't be prevented.

Frankl's technique of *paradoxical intention*[4] can be illustrated by the case of a patient with writer's cramp who was urged to write with the worst possible scrawl rather than to try to be neat. When he tried to scrawl, he couldn't. Patients can be asked to try to feel as angry as possible or to set aside a specific time each day during which they must worry as much as possible about a particular problem. All of this demonstrates to them that they *do* have some control over their behavior.

Another behavioral technique involves relaxation or *desensitization*. Wolpe[12] and others have used this method in treating obsessions, compulsions, phobias, or anxiety in specific situations. Patients list their fears or anxiety-provoking situations in hierarchies ranging from most to least upsetting. For example, with fears of heights such a list might include: flying, being on the top floor of a tall building, looking out the window of the fourth or fifth floor of a building, and looking over the railing of a porch a few steps above the ground. During the first few sessions, the patient is taught to relax and to imagine pleasant scenes. Then, session by session, he is asked to imagine feared situations, starting with the least upsetting and gradually working up each hierarchy until he can remain relaxed while imagining the most feared situations. Hopefully, feeling relaxed while imagining the situations makes the patient more relaxed while actually experiencing the situations.

TRANSACTIONAL ANALYSIS

Transactional analysis was first developed by Eric Berne, author of the well-known books *Games People Play*[1] and *Transactional Analysis in Psychotherapy*[2] and made even more popular by Harris in *I'm Okay, You're Okay*.[6] Transactional analysis is concerned with four kinds of analyses: structural analysis, transactional analysis, game analysis, and script analysis.

Structural Analysis. Structural analysis examines an individual's personality. Simply put, it is a way of analyzing a person's thoughts, feelings, and behavior based on the phenomenon of ego states. Berne de-

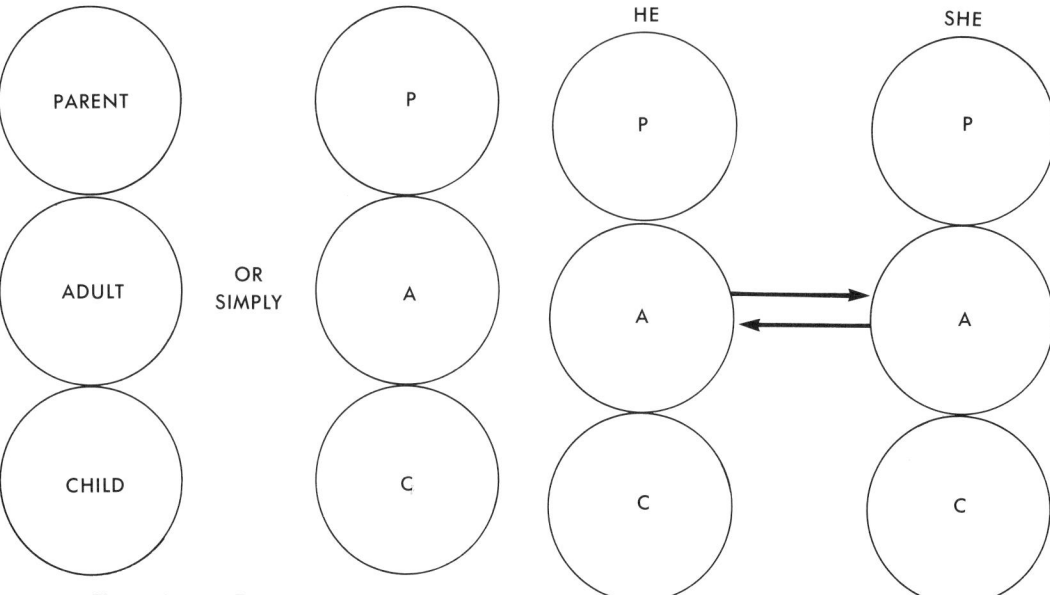

Figure 31-1. *Ego state structure.*

Figure 31-2. *Complementary transaction.*

scribes three ego states: the parent, the adult, and the child (Fig. 31-1).

The parent (P) ego state contains attitudes and behaviors incorporated from external sources, primarily from the individual's own parents. It is expressed outwardly toward others as prejudicial, critical, or nurturing behavior. Inwardly, it is expressed as parental messages influencing behavior, frequently without being tested. The adult (A) ego state is oriented toward current reality and objective gathering of information. It is an organized, adaptable, intelligent ego state; that is, it tests reality, estimates probability, and computes dispassionately. The child (C) ego state is the feeling ego state. No single ego state is better than the other two. The ideal is a proper mix of the three.

Transactional Analysis. Transactional analysis is the analysis of what people say and do to each other. There are basically three types of transactions that occur between the ego states. They are complementary transactions, crossed transactions, and ulterior transactions. Transactions can occur between any two ego states, either at the same level or at different levels.

As long as transactions remain complementary (Fig. 31-2), communication is open and transactions may proceed. For example:

He: I left the tickets at home.
She: Maybe we could go home to get them.

Crossed transactions (Fig. 31-3) occur when a stimulus draws an unexpected response. For example:

He: What time is it?
She: What's the matter, do you have a date somewhere?

Crossed transactions frequently cause trouble between people. The person who initiates transactions but receives an unex-

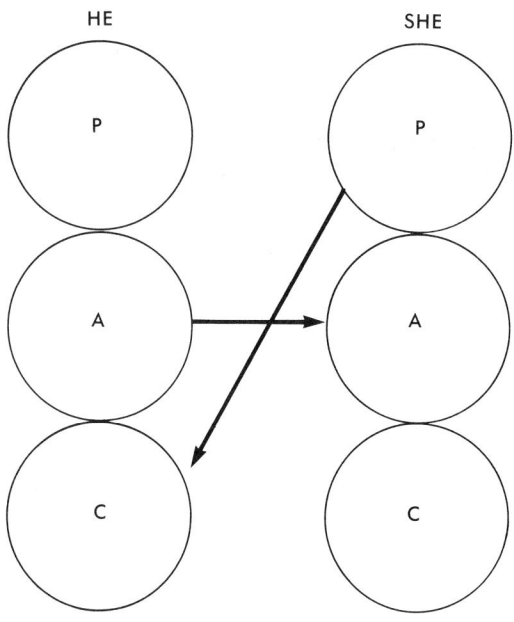

Figure 31-3. *Crossed transaction.*

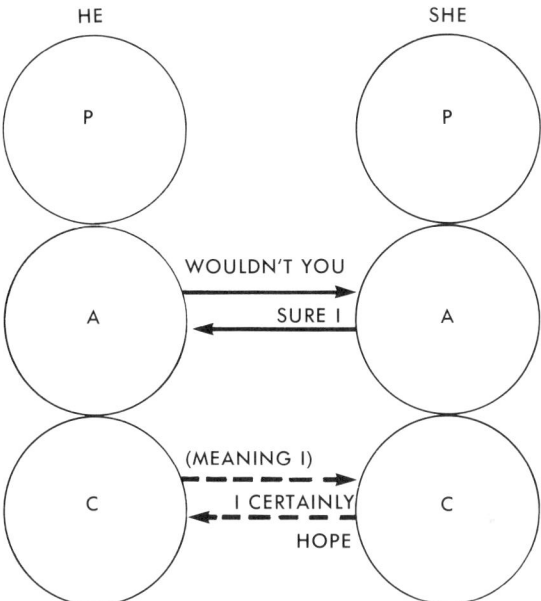

Figure 31-4. *Ulterior transaction.*

pected response feels crossed, tends to withdraw, and often feels discounted.

Ulterior transactions (Fig. 31-4) can be good or bad. They are more difficult to understand because they usually involve more than two ego states and are frequently disguised as more acceptable transactions. For example:

He: Wouldn't you like to come up to see my etchings? (Meaning—I would like to have you come up to my apartment for you know what!)

She: Sure, I love artistic people! (Meaning—I certainly hope he doesn't have looking at art in mind.)

Game Analysis. Game analysis is the analysis of ulterior transactions that lead to a payoff. Berne defines a psychologic game as a recurring set of transactions, often repetitive and superficially rational but with a concealed motivation, or, more colloquially, as a series of transactions with a gimmick. Three elements present in games are (1) an ongoing series of complementary transactions that are plausible on the social level, (2) an ulterior transaction that is the underlying message of the game, and (3) a predictable payoff that concludes the game and is the real purpose for playing.

Games prevent honest, intimate, and open relationships between the players. Some examples of games are: Kick Me,

Uproar, Ain't It Awful, and Nigyysob (Now I Got You, You Son of a Bitch).

Games are often played according to ego state. Players may copy their parents' games that come from their parents' ego states. They may consciously play a game from their adult ego state, and they may also play from their child ego state if this is based on early life experiences, decisions, and the "positions" that a child takes about himself and others.

Berne felt that before a child is 8 years old, he has developed concepts about himself, and although these ideas may be quite unrealistic, they determine what games he will play. These decisions are likely to be quite distorted, as they were formulated during a very early period of life and, as such, can cause a varying degree of pathology.

Position One: I'm OK, You're OK—A person with this perspective about himself and others is generally mentally healthy and can accept himself and others.

Position Two: I'm OK, You're Not OK—This is often the position of delinquents and criminals who feel persecuted and victimized and who feel that any action they take against others is justified.

Position Three: I'm Not OK, You're OK—This is often the first experience a person has to deal with in life—feeling powerless compared with others, ineffective, weak, and perhaps withdrawn.

Position Four: I'm Not OK, You're Not OK—People in this position have little to live for and may even commit suicide or homicide.

Script Analysis. Script analysis examines specific life dramas that individuals compulsively play out. Basically, the script is a life plan. As in a drama, the player is compelled to follow the script. The script is written by the child ego state and is a result of the transactions between a child and his parents. The games played are part of the script. When the positions and games are identified, the player can become more aware of his script; that is, he develops insight into his feelings and behavior. An example given by Berne is that of a woman raised by an alcoholic father. She develops a rescue fantasy and marries one alcoholic after another. Her script calls for a magical cure of the alcoholic husband. When this is not forthcoming, a divorce results and she tries again.

GESTALT PSYCHOTHERAPY

Gestalt psychology started with the experiments of a number of German psychophysiologists at the turn of the century who studied perception (experiential behavior) in addition to the observable (apparent) behavior studied by behavioral psychologists. *Gestalt* is the German word for shape or form. We perceive things as wholes, not just as collections of parts. The mind organizes what is perceived (seen, heard, felt) into overall impressions, or gestalts, so that we are aware of a number of things in the environment at any given time. The perception can be inaccurate, as in the case of optical illusions.

At any given moment, an individual exists in a particular environment, or *field,* that includes all aspects of his environment (social, physical, and the like). The field constantly changes via the many forces acting on one another (for example, what people say or do, the physical aspects such as weather, or changes in inanimate objects).

Each individual exists in his own particular *life space* that includes himself and the environment (field) as it exists for him, including needs, goals, beliefs, other persons, and so on. The boundaries of his life space include the political, legal, social, economic, psychologic, physical, and other processes that modify his behavior. The individual ego, or self, can develop only in the presence of others. Only as a member of a group with whom he interacts can an individual's personality develop.

Psychotherapy based on principles of gestalt psychology has been developed much more recently (for example, at the Esalen Institute in California).[9] Interpersonal problems are thought to develop when an individual is unable to perceive that his life situation, or field, is constantly changing. The gestalts he perceives are those of past experiences and are inappropriate in his current situation. He reacts to people he deals with in the present as if they were just like important people in his past. For example, his employer may be unconsciously seen by him as being just like his harsh father. He reacts by being submissive, although, in reality, his employer wants him to be aggressive and to speak out frankly. Or, he may perceive of his wife as being like his easily upset mother. Subsequently, he deals with his wife passively rather than "acting like a man," which is what she really wants.

In gestalt psychotherapy, the patient is encouraged to become aware of what he actually feels and to recognize all his emotions in a given situation or about a particular person. The therapist may confront him vociferously with critical observations about his behavior in order to provoke anger or other emotions, so that the patient is forced to note his own feelings. Nonverbal communications (gestures, posture, facial expression, tone of voice) are pointed out as communicating just as much (if not more!) as verbal comments. Humor can be used effectively to joke with (but not about) the patient regarding his misperceptions.

Individuals or groups in gestalt psychotherapy might be asked to do certain exercises to enhance their awareness of their perceptions and to learn how those perceptions can change. Examples of such activities are: stare at a single object for several minutes, noting all you perceive; select a recent memory and note what thoughts come to mind; or imagine that you're shorter, fatter, or thinner than you are or that you're a member of the opposite sex and describe how you would feel. At all points, patients are urged to be aware of their bodily feelings (tension, relaxation, and the like). They are encouraged to suspend value judgments for the moment and to realize that they have the capacity to make their own evaluations about a particular person or event.

Gestalt therapy has emphasized a very basic aspect of psychotherapy. There are always *alternative explanations* for events in a person's life and *alternative behaviors* for coping with those events. The suggestion can always be made that there are other possible explanations, such as, "Maybe instead of being angry at you she was just frustrated by something that happened at work." Once the patient sees that alternative ways of looking at things are possible, he may well come up with other perceptions on his own and may attempt to assess his ideas on the basis of what is really occurring in his interactions with others. Whenever a patient says, "There are no alternatives, I have to do this," it can be pointed out that there are always alternatives. The physician can suggest some ("You could change jobs") and can encourage the patient to think of others. When many alternatives are envisioned, more realistic choices of what to do can be made.

CLIENT-CENTERED PSYCHOTHERAPY

The clinical psychologist Carl Rogers[10] introduced client-centered or person-centered psychotherapy, emphasizing understanding how the patient really feels. The physician must make every effort to feel *empathy* for the patient and also feel a deep respect for the significance of each patient. He must try to assume, as much as he is able, the internal frame of reference of the patient, to perceive the world as the patient sees it, and to see the patient as the patient sees himself. How does this person really feel right now? What would it be like to be in his shoes? The physician does not have to agree with what the patient feels but should genuinely try to understand how the patient feels about the things that are important to him. The patient is encouraged step by step to understand himself and others. Questions and comments should reflect what he has said. "I can certainly see how upsetting that must have been for you." "How did you feel about the whole situation at that point?" "What was the most important thing to you about that relationship?" "Can you tell me some more about that?"

The physician acts upon the hypothesis that the patient has the capacity to deal constructively with all aspects of his life of which he can potentially be made aware. A doctor patient relationship is created in which important aspects of the patient's feelings and behavior of which he had not been aware can now come into his awareness. This is possible because the physician accepts unconditionally the patient's feelings and demonstrates to him the belief that he is competent to direct his own life. The physician is not judgmental; thus, the patient feels free to discuss anything. This makes it possible for the patient to become aware of things about himself and his relationships to others that he had not realized previously; that is, he develops insight into his feelings and behavior.

Like gestalt psychotherapy, client-centered psychotherapy sees the individual as existing in a continually changing world of experience of which he is the center. He reacts as an organized whole to the environment as he perceives it. His behavior is *goal-directed,* attempting to satisfy the needs he experiences in that environment. Emotion accompanies and, in general, facilitates goal-directed behavior. The patient's internal frame of reference provides the best vantage point for understanding his behavior. The physician's empathy, in turn, allows him to comprehend the patient's frame of reference.

Both self-concept and changes in self-concept are important. During client-centered psychotherapy, the patient perceives himself as being a more adequate person than he had thought himself to be and permits more data to enter his awareness that he previously ignored or distorted. Thus, he arrives at a more realistic appraisal of himself, his relationships with others, and his environment in general. After client-centered therapy, adaptation to any life situation is improved because fewer experiences are distorted or denied. The patient feels more in control of himself. Most important is greater self-acceptance. The physician's demonstration of empathy for how the patient really feels and his accepting, non-judgmental attitude have made it possible for the patient to become more aware of his attitudes and behaviors. Consequently, more of his actions are subjected to rational examination and meaningful choice. He has independently arrived at mature ways of dealing with problems, which probably would not have occurred to him if the physician had merely scolded him about his selfish behavior in the past.

EXISTENTIAL PSYCHOTHERAPY

Existential philosophy includes many diverse and often complicated theories that arose out of the pessimism of nineteenth century philosophy and intellectual and artistic trends that saw life as meaningless. Existentialism recognizes that, in spite of the horrors of modern existence, there is in the very nature of human beings the will to live and the wish to find meaning in life. Thus, existential psychotherapy focuses on determining the meaning in life.

The Viennese psychiatrist Viktor Frankl[4] has developed an existential psychotherapy that he calls "logotherapy." His theories are related, in part, to his experiences in a

Nazi concentration camp. Even in the most horrible psychologic and physical circumstances imaginable, it was possible to find *meaning*. Prisoners still had some *choice*. For example, there were those who treated fellow sufferers kindly and others who treated fellow prisoners like swine.

Human existence necessitates coping with the triad of *pain* (suffering), *death* (mortality), and *guilt* (fallibility). Social environment, hereditary endowment, and instinctual drives can limit the scope of an individual's freedom, but they can never totally destroy the human capacity to take a stand against pain, death, and guilt. Human freedom is the freedom to take a stand, that is, to make choices. Responsibility in making choices is the essence of human existence but, of course, always includes the risk of error (fallibility). Choices must be made, nevertheless. When a patient says "There's absolutely nothing I can do (about my job, my marriage, my children)," it can be pointed out that doing nothing is in itself a choice.

Meaning can be found not only through acting or through experiencing but also through suffering. There is no ideal answer to "What is the meaning of life?" Each individual has to deal with meaning in terms of his own life. The task of existential psychotherapy is to examine the phenomena of everyday experience. This discipline restricts itself to determining the facts of what actually happens but leaves it to the patient to decide (choose) how to understand (give meaning to) his own responsibilities in his own life situation.

Psychotherapy is a dialogue in which the physician leads the patient through a series of questions to find his own (the patient's) answers; that is, he develops insight into his feelings and behavior. The patient is encouraged to consider all possible alternatives until the one that seems best to him is reached. ("What are you really saying?" "What does that which you just said mean to you?" "Given all that, what can you do about it?") Psychotherapy is an attempt to make the patient aware of what he really longs for in the depth of his being and to realize the best that is within him.

The physician doesn't necessarily know what the final answers will be for a particular patient. This demands humility on the part of the therapist. The pomposity of assuming to know all the answers for a given

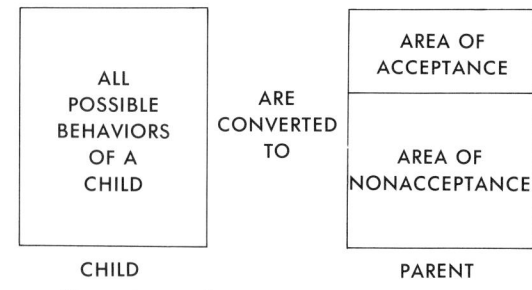

Figure 31–5. *Parent's acceptance diagram.*

patient can be harmful and contrary to the purposes of psychotherapy. This doesn't mean that the physician takes no stands or has no opinions about what is ethical or moral but rather that he endeavors to work together with the patient to help him come to his own decisions about the ethical implications of his daily life. There is emphasis on self-realization and the freedom to express one's self while at the same time dealing with other people with acceptance and compassion. Each individual must develop his own value system and make his own choices in the social and ethical context of his own life.

PARENT EFFECTIVENESS TRAINING

Thomas Gordon has included a number of the concepts just discussed in his book *Parent Effectiveness Training.*[5] In the "parent's acceptance diagram" (Fig. 31–5), the relative size of the areas of acceptance and nonacceptance is different for different parents and different children. The diagram is not static. The child's behavior changes, each parent's feeling about the child's behavior changes, and the feelings of both parents of a child might well be different (Fig. 31–6).

Gordon urges parents to accept that they

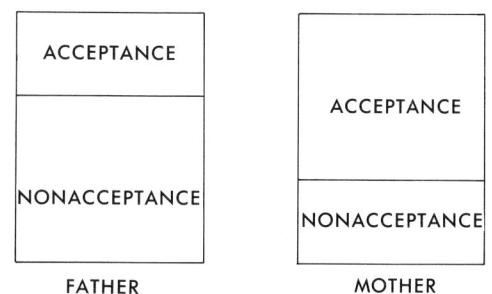

Figure 31–6. *Parents differ in acceptance of child's behavior.*

are human and therefore inconsistent and that two parents may well disagree. He cautions against a false front of parental unity or false acceptance of something the child does that the parent doesn't like. Needless to say, children see through false acceptance.

In contrast, Gordon suggests that parents should employ "the language of acceptance." Like all other language, acceptance can be nonverbal. The parent does not intervene in the child's activities, even if, for example, he knows a better way to build what the child is constructing. Thus, the child's privacy is respected. In other words, doing nothing and saying nothing as the child is "doing his thing" can be reassuring. The child feels he can continue at his own play with parental acceptance.

Nondirective discussions similar to those of client-centered therapy are used. For example:

Child: I got sent to the principal's office today.
Parent: Oh? (rather than "You were sent to the principal!")

The child is allowed to discuss the entire situation until what has happened and how he feels is made clear. For example, if it turns out that he dislikes the particular teacher who sent him to the principal, the parent might say, "I see," or "You really can't stand the way he talks on endlessly." Ultimately, using this method rather than a lecture or sermon, the child is more likely to conclude that life is difficult and that he'll have to put up with the teacher for the time being.

Gordon calls this "active listening." The parent listens to what the child has to say, encourages him to continue, and gives appropriate feedback. For example:

Child: Bob won't ever do what I want to do.
Parent: You're angry with Bob.
Child: I sure am. I don't ever want to play with him again.
Parent: You're so angry you feel like never seeing him again.
Child: Right. But then, there wouldn't be anyone to play with.
Parent: You'd hate to be left with no one.
Child: I guess I'll have to learn to get along with him.

In these situations, the child is allowed to state what he feels and what specifically bothers him, and the real issue is dealt with. For example, a child who makes a fuss every morning about not wanting to go to school is allowed to discuss this with his mother. As it turns out, the mother has afternoon and evening activities away from home, so the child wants to stay home in the morning to be with her. She therefore arranges to be with the child at the same time each day, and the child goes to school without fuss. Eventually, the child volunteers to give up the extra time with his mother.

Gordon advises "I-messages" rather than "you-messages." For example, "I don't feel like playing with you when I'm tired" rather than "You stop trying to get attention," or "I'm really worried about scratching that antique chair" rather than "You get your feet off the chair rungs."

Parent Effectiveness Training ultimately involves giving up all the familiar parent-child power struggles and using the "no-lose method" of resolving conflicts. When parents and children disagree, the pros and cons are discussed; everyone contributes possible solutions; and mutual agreement is reached about a solution. For example, a boy seems interested in learning to play the trumpet but refuses to practice his music lesson when his mother calls him. Discussion reveals that the mother always calls when he is playing football with his friends after school. He is asked about possible alternatives and decides that he could practice his trumpet playing for a half hour every morning before school. His mother agrees that if he does so, she won't interrupt his football playing after school.

Gordon points out that many different solutions to the same problem may be reached by many different families. The specific solution is not as important as the problem-solving process itself. Parents and children each express their concerns calmly, without an argument. Every member of the family makes an effort to think of solutions, and the contributions of each are respected. The six steps of problem-solving are:

1. Identifying and defining the conflict.
2. Generating possible alternative solutions.
3. Evaluating the alternative solutions.
4. Deciding on the most acceptable solution (to all the participants).

5. Working out ways of implementing the solution.

6. Following up to evaluate how it worked.

As the last step implies, solutions are neither perfect nor immutable. If something isn't working out, it can be reassessed and changed. But each participant is allowed his own say, and the comments of each are respected.

FAMILY THERAPY

Family therapy often involves a team of therapists (psychiatrist or other physician, psychologist, social worker, or nurse) and may involve a triad (parents and one child), a nuclear family (parents and all children), extended family (nuclear family plus other relatives and generations), or a social network (nuclear family plus relatives, friends, and neighbors). As in any other form of therapy, it is important to establish initially and repeatedly that no one is "to blame." Therapists and family members are really all on the same side. No one person should be made the scapegoat for all the family's problems (for example, the hyperkinetic child or the alcoholic father). It is especially important to avoid saying that the ill member of the family is "wrong" in his perceptions, while the others are "right" in what they think. On the other hand, the ill member should not be allowed to have his own way about everything just because he is suffering.

Although the family physician may not wish to get involved in complicated long-term family therapy, he may often find it useful to bring all the members of a family together, especially if he has been receiving disparate messages from different family members when seen individually. If there is a great deal of hostility expressed, it is probably best to see family members individually for the time being. However, when there seems to be some willingness to compromise and to work together, seeing the family as a unit can be valuable. The whole is often different from the sum of its parts (as any gestalt psychotherapist would agree). When family members disagree, utilizing the types of compromises discussed previously under Parent Effectiveness Training can be helpful.

GROUP THERAPY

A wide variety of professionals use group techniques in many settings, such as educational workshops or programs in business and industry that help people understand themselves in the context of relating to others. When evaluating any group as a referral source for patients, it is useful to know something about the leader and his training, what he tries to accomplish, and whether these goals are appropriate to his background and experience.

A person who does not gain insight into his problems in individual counseling may understand himself better in a group in which the other members, on the one hand, support him in his weak moments but, on the other hand, confront him with the realities of his undesirable behavior. With the encouragement and support of others in the group, individual members can develop better self-images. Conversely, comments by a number of peers about one's shortcomings are often easier to accept and to assimilate than are interpretations made by a psychotherapist in a one-to-one relationship.

In general, group techniques emphasize the here and now. Participants are encouraged to note and express their feelings, both positive and negative, about others in the group and to examine carefully the opinions others in the group express about them. While candor is encouraged, confrontation solely for the purpose of expressing hostility toward another is not. Although the group is similar to many social settings, it is unique in that emphasis is placed on frankness about feelings that would not ordinarily be expressed in everyday life. The group is seen as a laboratory in which an individual can get training in interpersonal relationships and can experiment with various behaviors in order to learn firsthand how such behaviors might affect those around him.

SUMMARY

Psychotherapy involves a conversation that is confidential and is focused on the patient's problems in living. Often the patient does much of the talking, with occasional questions, comments, and explanations from the physician. At the beginning, neither physician nor patient knows what the problems are, much less the solutions. They work together to define the problems. Using step-by-step questions and comments, the patient is led to understand aspects of his feelings and behavior and what he communicates to others of which he had not previously been aware. The patient is encouraged to define the problems he must confront daily and to conceptualize choices available to him for dealing with his problems. Determination of choices necessitates definition of goals for the future and assessment of how realistic these goals are.

The major accomplishment of psychotherapy is that it suggests, repeatedly, that there are alternative perceptions of situations and alternative behaviors that the patient can choose. One of the most important areas of perception is self-image. Psychotherapy helps a patient to recognize his useful qualities and abilities and to develop them to the fullest while at the same time understanding his shortcomings, correcting them if possible, or accepting them if change is unlikely. In addition, misperceptions about current situations based on memories of important people and events in the past are identified and corrected.

Ultimately, what he does in his daily life with the insights learned in psychotherapy is up to the patient. The crucial work of psychotherapy is always the creative work of the patient himself.

REFERENCES

1. Berne, E.: Games People Play. New York, Ballantine Books, Inc., 1976.
2. Berne, E.: Transactional Analysis in Psychotherapy: A Systematic Individual and Social Psychiatry. New York, Ballantine Books, Inc., 1975.
3. Cadoret, R. J., and King, L. J.: Psychiatry in Primary Care. St. Louis, The C. V. Mosby Co., 1974.
4. Frankl, V. E.: Psychotherapy and Existentialism. New York, Simon & Schuster, Inc., 1968.
5. Gordon, T.: P. E. T. Parent Effectiveness Training. New York, New American Library, 1975.
6. Harris, T. A.: I'm Okay, You're Okay: A Practical Guide to Transactional Analysis. New York, Avon Books, 1973.
7. Jaspers, K.: The Nature of Psychotherapy. Chicago, University of Chicago Press, 1965.
8. McWhinney, I. R.: Beyond diagnosis: an approach to the integration of behavioral science and clinical medicine. N. Engl. J. Med., 287:384, 1972.
9. Perls, F. S.: Gestalt Therapy Verbatim. Stevens, J. D. (ed.), LaFayette, Real People Press, 1969.
10. Rogers, C. R.: Client-Centered Therapy. Boston, Houghton-Mifflin Co., 1963.
11. Ruesch, J. Therapeutic Communication. New York, W. W. Norton & Co., Inc., 1973.
12. Wolpe, J.: The Practice of Behavior Therapy. New York, Pergamon Press, 1973.

Chapter 32

GROUP PSYCHOTHERAPY

by EUGENE F. GAURON,
and ROBERT E. RAKEL

INTRODUCTION

Objectives

The objective of group psychotherapy is the same as that of all other psychotherapy forms: to enable people to make fuller use of their human capabilities for a more personally gratifying and rewarding life. In group psychotherapy, a number of people (usually five to eight, assisted by one or more trained therapists) agree to meet together on a regular basis to help each other. It is important that all members collaborate in the group process. The function of a group member is twofold. Each has come for help related to some personally defined problem or problems. It is anticipated that each member will work toward understanding his own difficulties. In addition, however, everyone is a potential helper for each of the others. All may contribute attentive listening; empathic understanding; feedback, with particular reference to communicating feeling reactions to other members' behavior; support; and encouragement, as well as suggesting options or alternatives to present ways of behaving. A basic focus is that all knowledge gained inside the group will be applied toward improving interpersonal relationships outside the group.

Differentiation from Other Group Processes

Group psychotherapy should be distinguished from the other group-based change processes currently operating in our society.[16]

First, there are a variety of self-help movements—Alcoholics Anonymous, Syn-anon, Recovery, Inc., and so forth—all of which utilize lay leaders to some extent. The choice of appropriate members for self-help groups is much more narrowly defined than for members in group psychotherapy. The self-help groups are limited to individuals who have a common symptom, problem, or life predicament, e.g., alcoholism, drug abuse, or child abuse.

A second set of healing groups evolved as part of the human potential movement and includes such activities as sensitivity training, encounter groups, T-groups, growth groups, and human relations laboratories. These activities usually do involve professional persons as leaders, but this is not necessary, and the group may even be leaderless. A major characteristic of these activities is their universal applicability and relevance to all who want to change, grow, or develop.

A third set of groups includes consciousness-raising groups, which share with self-help groups a commitment to peer control but have broader criteria for inclusion of members. Consciousness-raising groups are formed on the basis of very general demographic similarities: sex, race, age, or ethnic characteristics, e.g., groups concerned about women's rights. The common thread among group members is a shared social characteristic.

A final group-based change process different from group psychotherapy is assertion training. As with self-help groups, individuals possess a similar common characteristic, in this instance passivity or lack of assertiveness. Participants in assertion training come together to acquire a specific skill through practice in changing behavior and role playing of problem situations.

Role of Group Members

There are rarely set topics or prearranged agendas for a group session. Group members are free to participate as much or as little as they wish, while working toward their respective goals in treatment. New members often feel uneasy when they first join a group (Table 32–1). Sooner or later this feeling of apprehension and strangeness is overcome, as they develop feelings of interest and trust in the others. Members discover their communality with others and begin to share thoughts and experiences that had previously been kept to themselves. Through interpersonal interactions with others, members develop a sense of belonging and understanding and thereby overcome feelings of isolation and aloneness. Increased self-disclosure aids in breaking down barriers between people and facilitates the development of effective working relationships and feelings of closeness among members. An open exchange of feedback during group sessions provides increased self-understanding and illuminates previously puzzling behavior.[17]

REFERRAL GUIDELINES

Group psychotherapy can be of value to a variety of persons—from those who simply want to develop emotional freedom and interpersonal skills to those with serious emotional problems, which may range from personal discomfort, tension, anxiety, and depression to feelings of being depleted, alienated, confused, overwhelmed, or, in general, so bewildered thay they feel unable to cope. However, group psychotherapy is not for all people. Not all members do equally well, nor do all members have good outcomes in group psychotherapy. Although the majority of members who enter a group receive positive benefits, recent literature pertaining to outcome studies contains strong indications that some members may emerge harmed or with impaired adjustment from an experience in group psychotherapy.[23] Types of negative effects that might occur include the exacerbation of presenting symptoms, the appearance of new symptoms, a loss of faith and a sense of disillusionment with therapy, or the employment of more maladaptive mechanisms of defense.[12] The establishment of careful

TABLE 32–1. RIGHTS OF PARTICIPANTS IN THERAPY GROUPS°

All groups members possess these basic rights *at all times.*

1. You have the right to express your opinion.
2. You have the right to feel however you want.
3. You have the right to express your feelings in your personal way.
4. You have the right to question anything you do not understand.
5. You have the right to refuse to carry out any suggestion, attempt any homework assignment, or participate in any group exercise, whether initiated by the leader or by a fellow group member.
6. You have the right to at least ask for what you want, while realizing that you may not always get it.
7. You have the right to be irrational and illogical.
8. You have the right to be inconsistent and unpredictable.
9. You have the right to be left alone.
10. You have the right to make mistakes.
11. You have the right to say "I don't know."
12. You have the right to make your own choices.
13. You have the right to relate to whom you want, when you want.
14. You have the right to say "no" to requests that attempt to limit your rights.
15. You have the right to not like everyone in your group.
16. You have the right to expect confidentiality from all other group members.
17. You have the right to inquire about or discuss the therapist's treatment program for you at any time.
18. You do not have the right to physically or emotionally intrude upon someone else in group without that person's permission.
19. You do not have the right to blame someone else for the way you behave, i.e., you are responsible for your own behavior.
20. You do not have the right to demand that you get what you want, unless it is in defense of your rights.

°From Gauron, E. F., Steinmark, S. W., and Jamieson, J. C.: A Community Guide to the Group Psychotherapy Program, Iowa City, Goodfellow Co., 1975, p. 5–6.

selection criteria and evaluation procedures to weed out those who might be harmed would therefore seem to be in order. In accepting a referral, the group therapist must feel that a positive outcome is likely in group psychotherapy, i.e., that this individual possesses the attributes of those who respond to therapy; that a "good fit" appears to exist between patient and therapist and between patient and group members; that the therapist genuinely wants to work with this particular person, has a positive liking for the person,[11] and believes that the person can add to the group and be helped by the group; and, finally, that other treatment methods seem less applicable. The family physician might make use of the following guidelines when evaluating a prospective member's suitability for group psychotherapy:

1. Neurotic individuals are more likely to benefit from group psychotherapy than those who are severely disturbed. Most group leaders prefer not to have actively psychotic members in their groups, but some leaders will treat psychotics who are in remission on a long-term basis.

2. Individuals with personality disorders appear to benefit more from group psychotherapy than those with neuroses. Exceptions include schizoid personalities, who may have difficulty in overcoming their usual pattern of withdrawal from interpersonal relationships.

3. Group psychotherapy is indicated for those who define their problem as interpersonal or who emphasize its interpersonal aspects. These difficulties may take the form of withdrawal from relationships, repetitive transient relationships, difficulty forming close or intimate relationships, or generally unsatisfactory relationships.

4. Group psychotherapy is indicated for those who are committed to a change in interpersonal behavior. Most group leaders place greater emphasis on change in behavior than on the development of insight. Many group leaders attempt to foster a safe, supportive climate that will encourage the patient to risk engaging in and practicing new behavior. Individuals who are able to specify problem areas that they wish to work on will usually experience greater benefit from group psychotherapy than those whose complaints or problems are vague or generalized.

5. Group psychotherapy is indicated for those individuals who already have or who are willing to develop a concern for others. In a group setting, everyone has something to work on, and members have to show willingness to develop and work on their own personal goals, as well as to facilitate the goal attainment of the others.

6. Group psychotherapy is contraindicated for highly independent individuals who resist influence from others, who will not allow themselves to be dependent on others, or who are indifferent to the opinions of others.

7. Group psychotherapy is contraindicated for those individuals who are excessively suspicious and who have difficulty trusting others.

8. Group psychotherapy is contraindicated for those individuals who are overly preoccupied with hypochondriacal concerns and with physical symptomatology.

9. Group psychotherapy is contraindicated for those individuals with organic brain syndromes and other neurologic conditions.

CURATIVE FACTORS

A working knowledge of the essential elements required for the process of change provides a sound basis upon which the group therapist may formulate tactics and strategy. Yalom[20] has presented an inventory of tentative curative factors derived from his own clinical experience, the clinical experience of other therapists, the viewpoints of successfully-treated group members, and the conclusions of systematic outcome research. Presumably, these curative factors operate in any group psychotherapy system, although the relative emphasis given each will vary from one system to the next.

1. Instillation of hope.
2. Universality.
3. Imparting of information.
4. Altruism.
5. Corrective recapitulation of the primary family group.
6. Development of socializing techniques.
7. Imitative behavior.
8. Interpersonal learning.
9. Group cohesiveness.
10. Catharsis.
11. Existential factors.

Instillation of Hope. Several research studies have demonstrated that a high pretherapy expectation of help is significantly related to positive therapy outcome.[10, 15] Belief in the potential effectiveness of the treatment modality, whether group psychotherapy or any other method, can in itself be therapeutically effective. In any group, instillation of hope results from a multitude of inputs. Different members are at different points along the successful-coping continuum. Members who have experienced the group process for a period of time and consider it beneficial will serve as a source of encouragement to the newly joined or the uncertain member. Likewise, a member's personal observation of change in other group members will aid in convincing him of the efficacy of the group. No less important are such factors as the therapist's reputation, optimistic outlook, belief in self and in the efficacy of group, and conviction that, given a mutual commitment to each other, he can be of assistance in overcoming the patient's emotional difficulties.

Universality. Many patients enter therapy with the belief that their problems are unique, that no one else is struggling with the same issues, and that they have a private misery all their own. The encouragement to self-disclose in group psychotherapy assures that members will reveal their worries, concerns, fears, and preoccupations. Members quickly discover that they are not alone and that others are "in the same boat." This is usually a relieving and reassuring discovery.

Imparting of Information. This curative factor involves imparting didactic information about mental health, interpersonal relationships, methods of coping, interpersonal skills, and, in general, a variety of "how to's," as well as suggestions or guidance about life problems offered either by the therapist or by any group member. One aspect of membership in a group is exposure to an ideologic belief system about ways of viewing oneself, ways of viewing others, ways of regarding interpersonal relationships, and ways of learning what one can and cannot get from others, all of which may be somewhat new to the group member.[14]

Altruism. Each group member hopefully learns the process of how to give and how to get in relationships with others and of how to balance giving and getting. Sometimes, the surprising but welcome discovery is made that he has something to offer others and that he can be of importance to others. A system which emphasizes each member's helping every other member depends on the members' offering one another support, encouragement, reinforcement, mutual sharing of common problems, and exchange of feedback. The discovery that one can be of assistance in another's personal development can go a long way toward improving one's low self-esteem and poor self-concept. A possible out-of-group consequence is that a life of self-absorption and preoccupation with one's own problems might be modified to include greater concern for and interest in others.

Corrective Recapitulation of the Primary Family Group. Members come to group with a history of unsatisfactory relationships in their first and most long-lasting group, the primary family. It is in the primary family that attitudes about how to behave and how not to behave have been acquired; viewpoints for looking at oneself, at people, and at life have been presented and adopted; and a set of assumptions about people has been solidified. The group resembles the family in many respects, even to the point that a male and female team may be coleading it. By utilizing relationships with the leaders and with other group members, the patient in group psychotherapy can overcome barriers to growth and can modify some of the early training received in the family. The member is presented with the opportunity to sort out his set of assumptions about life and people acquired from significant others in the past and can decide which assumptions to retain and which to discard.

Development of Socializing Techniques. Many group members are lacking in the basic social skills necessary for satisfactory relationships with others. Apropos of Carkhuff's[4] dictum that training is the best form of treatment, many group therapy programs place emphasis on interpersonal skills training. Skills training can be carried out both in short-term pretherapy or orientation groups designed to prepare patients for the therapeutic experience[8] or through teaching and training exercises in the actual therapy sessions. Research literature suggests that systematic training in such interpersonal skills as listening, awareness, expression and recognition of feelings, mutual communication, empathy, problem-solving, goal-setting, and risk-taking has pay-offs both in terms of positive outcome in group psychotherapy and in improved functioning outside the group.[3]

Imitative Behavior. Bandura and colleagues[1] have adequately demonstrated that imitation is an effective therapeutic force. It is not uncommon for a group member to model behavior after a group leader or an admired group member. This form of imitation is particularly prevalent among new group members, when they are looking to others for indications about the normative structure of the group and for clues about how to behave in this unusual environment. It is also not uncommon for a member to attend closely to another's work in group and to profit vicariously from the exposure to and the solving of another's problem. This is one major advantage of group psychotherapy in comparison to individual psychotherapy. The significance of imitative behavior is that it allows a person to consider options for different ways of behaving, which can be adopted if they seem consistent with the person's own style.

Interpersonal Learning. A key assumption underlying the conduct of group psychotherapy is that the group will develop into a social microcosm for each member. Each person, in the process of behaving spontaneously in group, will give a representative sample of interpersonal behavior and will demonstrate the kinds of problems that typically arise in such interpersonal relations. Consequently, the kinds of maladaptive behavior patterns or interpersonal difficulties that usually occur in the individual's life will be evident in the interactions in the group. A major function of the therapist and the group is to make explicit each member's typical interpersonal style by use of feedback and pattern analysis (demonstrating similarities in how the person behaves over time in a variety of relationships).

Group Cohesiveness. Cohesiveness has been defined as the attraction of the members to each other and to the group itself and is reflected in a group feeling or sense of "we-ness." Many group therapists have concluded that the cohesiveness of the group has assumed a stature similar to the transference occurring in the patient–therapist relationship in individual therapy. There is considerable literature concerning group dynamics that adds support to the value of group cohesion in group psychotherapy.[13, 22] It has been demonstrated that members of cohesive groups (1) are more productive, (2) are more open to influence by other group members, (3) experience more security, (4) are more able to express hostility and adhere more closely to group norms, (5) attempt to influence others more frequently, and (6) continue membership in group longer.[5] The value of cohesiveness is that the individual member of a cohesive group will be likely to make a personal commitment to remain in the group. This collective commitment by the members will assure that the group will continue to function. It also assures that the member will remain long enough to feel the impact of the group and increases the likelihood that the individual member will accept influence from the group. Both stability of the group and influenceability of the members are crucial to effective group psychotherapy.

Catharsis. The open expression of feelings, "letting off steam," or "getting things off one's chest" has always been regarded as a necessary component of a therapeutic experience. However, most group therapy leaders feel that expression of feelings alone is not enough. In the study by Lieberman, Yalom, and Miles,[18] those participants whose critical in-group experiences consisted only of strong emotional expressions had a greater likelihood of having a negative, rather than a positive, growth experience. Catharsis, then, is only part of an interpersonal curative process. Feeling expression must be accompanied by subsequent cognitive work for increased self-understanding or change to occur.

Existential Factors. In his discussion of existential factors in group psychotherapy, Yalom[20] targeted such issues as personal responsibility, freedom, our basic isolation or aloneness, recognition of our time-limited mortality, the capriciousness of our existence, and the fact that we cannot avoid making choices that have consequences. One consequence of being exposed to the existential point of view in group therapy is that members realize that there are limits to the guidance and direction they can receive from others and that the ultimate responsibility for conducting one's life lies with each individual. The patient in group therapy finds that there is no all-wise, all-knowing guru who can provide all the answers to life's problems. After struggling with his expectations, the patient ultimately comes to learn what can legitimately be expected from others and what must be done for oneself. The patient also learns that, although others cannot be used to find out what to do, there is plenty of company from fellow pilgrims along life's wandering way.

THE CONTRIBUTION OF THE GROUP LEADER

Establishing Norms

If group members are to be taught to rely on themselves, what contributions can they expect from the group leader? Or, even more basic, why have group leaders at all? The thrust of the previous discussion has been that the psychotherapy group is a social influence situation, in which members attempt to exert influence on one another in favorable directions.[14] One of the important functions of the group therapist is to assure that the group climate provides a therapeutic atmosphere and to keep the group focused on its therapeutic task. One danger of a leaderless group is that it may behave in nonhelpful ways or may go off on a nonproductive tangent. It is the responsibility of the therapist to assure that the group functions as an effective change agent[11] and that members are influenced only when they want to be and in directions that they deem desirable. All groups are guided by norms that provide guidelines or standards for member behavior. Norms derive from member expectations and preferences, discussions among the members about ways to behave, explicit statements from the leader, and implicit directions inherent in the leader's behavior. It is essential that the leader take seriously his function as a role model–norm setter, so that he is aware of shaping the norms of the group. Which norms are developed will depend, to some extent, upon the group leader's therapeutic approach, but the following are representative examples of frequently occurring norms in therapy groups:

1. Group members, group meetings, and the group itself are to be assigned a high priority in each member's life.
2. Member self-disclosure is a highly important group activity for getting to know the other members and for building trust.
3. The group assumes responsibility to monitor its own functioning.
4. Members agree to keep each other aware of the impact of their behavior by providing frequent feedback.
5. The optimal format of the group emphasizes unrehearsed, spontaneous, free-flowing interaction.
6. Each group member decides upon a personal set of goals to be pursued in therapy. These goals will be evaluated and updated at regular intervals.
7. Group members can be a valuable source of help to each other.
8. Open expression and exploration of feelings, both positive and negative, is encouraged.

Providing Focus

A second important contribution of the group leader is that of providing a focus for the group's activity and illuminating the process of the group. Admittedly, in a group consisting of five to eight members, a great deal is happening at any one point. The group process consists of the sum total of what is happening, of who is doing what to whom, of the explicit and the hidden agendas, of the implications of what is happening in terms of each person's interpersonal style, of the role being played by each member, and of the value to the group of what each individual is doing. The thrust of the group leader's interventions, either on behalf of the individual or toward the entire group, is to indicate, "Of all the things that are happening now, I think it would be profitable for you(us) to look at this in greater detail." Perhaps an example from an actual group session will illustrate group process and the possible directions in which the group leader could focus the group:

Ben, a professed homosexual, had not divulged his homosexuality to the group in a session even though he had been a member of the group for 4 months. One day he decided to do so. Sally was disappointed in him and hurt because he had delayed so long. Mildred was highly supportive of Ben's lack of self-disclosure and pointed out to all that society is very prejudiced against homosexuals. Jane was unmoved by the disclosure because she and a few other members knew of Ben's sexual preference from other sources. The ensuing interaction developed around the issue of the extent to which Ben felt trust in the group and the members' reactions to Ben's apparent low trust level.

From a process point of view, the therapist might be considering the following:
1. Why did Ben delay telling something so important to the group for so long? Is the issue one of lack of sufficient trust in the group or is it concern about what the others would think of him if they knew this about him? Does he fear lack of acceptance or, conversely, being accepted? The therapist could focus on Ben and his relationship to the group.
2. Why did Sally feel hurt because of what Ben did? Is her hurt a result of feeling that Ben is depriving her? The therapist could focus on Sally's reaction to not feeling trusted and being deprived of something to which she feels entitled.
3. Why was Mildred so supportive of

Ben, even to the point of defending his actions to the others? Why did she not personalize his lack of self-disclosure to herself and feel the reaction to not being trusted that the other group members did? The therapist could focus on the Mildred–Ben relationship or on Mildred's willingness to defend Ben against the rest of the group.

4. Since Jane knew of Ben's homosexuality, why had she not confronted him before regarding his not disclosing significant information? Has she been an active or a passive accomplice to Ben's "keeping a secret" from the group? To what extent have other members, or even the entire group, colluded with Ben by not confronting or pressing him? Have keeping secrets and not disclosing material that is difficult to reveal become normative behavior for the group? The therapist could focus on the group's apparent collusion with Ben, by their permitting his low level of self-disclosure, and could use the opportunity to explore group norms.

It is most likely that there is a similar richness of material contained in most interactions in any group. The group leader must keep in mind implications or inferences about the initiator of any sequence (e.g., Ben in this illustration), implications about the responder or responders to the initiator, and implications about the group as a whole. There is no ready-made guideline that tells the leader exactly where to focus. To some extent, this decision is what might be termed the art of doing therapy and is a result of (1) the leader's style (e.g., some leaders will deal with the individual; others will deal with the group as a whole), (2) goals and contracts of particular members that relate to the present interactions, (3) the leader's theoretical orientation, or (4) considerations such as which member has not had group time for a while. It is possible to explore the various aspects of a group interaction by refocusing on a different perspective when one aspect has been sufficiently explored. In addition, some work may have to be put off to another time, if not indefinitely, as the group moves along with spontaneous interaction.

Basic Function of a Group Leader

The outcome study concerning encounter groups by Lieberman, Yalom, and Miles[18]

telescoped all leader behaviors into four basic functions: emotional stimulation, caring, meaning-attribution, and executive function. They presented these factors as an empirically derived taxonomy for examining leader behavior in any form of group aimed at personal change. Presumably, any group leader can be rated or profiled on these four factors.

Emotional stimulation, as a leader behavior, involves the leader's participating as a member of the group—revealing feelings and disclosing personal values, attitudes and beliefs, as well as challenging, confronting, and exhorting. The leader engages in a liberal demonstration of emotional release through personal example. Leaders who favor emotional stimulation are perceived as charismatic, inspiring, believing in themselves, and possessing a sense of mission.

Caring, as a leader style,[19] involves protecting members and offering them friendship, love, affection, and frequent invitations to seek feedback, as well as providing support, praise, and encouragement. Stylistically, such a leader expresses considerable warmth, acceptance, genuineness, and a real concern for others in the group as human beings.

Meaning-attribution involves cognitizing behavior—providing concepts for understanding behavior by explaining, clarifying, interpreting, and providing frameworks for change. A leader utilizing meaning-attribution offers explanations for consideration and is concerned with making sense out of what is happening for the people involved. When engaging in this type of behavior, the leader may choose to focus on the group, or on the individual, or both.

Executive function of a leader involves behavior such as setting limits, suggesting or establishing rules, setting norms, managing time, sequencing, pacing, stopping, blocking, interceding, inviting, eliciting, and questioning.

All group leaders exhibit each of these four dimensions in varying degrees. The study referred to earlier related outcome in the encounter groups to each of these leader dimensions.[18] The most effective leaders were those who showed a moderate amount of emotional stimulation, displayed a high degree of caring, utilized meaning-attribution to a considerable extent, and were moderate in their expression of executive function. Conversely, the less effective leaders were those who utilized either very low or very high degrees of emotional stimulation, showed low degrees of caring, did very little meaning-attribution, and displayed too little or too much executive function. In terms of contributions of the therapist, it appears crucial that the therapist cares about the people he treats and that he provides some cognitive framework for understanding what is happening in therapy.

PREPARING A PATIENT FOR GROUP PSYCHOTHERAPY

It is quite likely that from time to time the family physician will want to refer a patient for group psychotherapy. One of the themes of this chapter has been that adequate preparation, both by the referring physician and by the group leader, or leaders, facilitates and contributes to positive therapy outcome.[7, 21] The referring physician might find the following steps useful when preparing patients for group therapy.

1. Explain some of the fundamentals of how group therapy works, as well as the reasons for considering this recommendation. This might include clearing up any confusion concerning the difference between group psychotherapy and other group methods. Frequently, patients come to a group therapist with the attitude, "I'm doing this because my doctor told me to come, but I really don't know why I am here." Obviously, such an attitude does not lead to active collaboration with the therapist or to commitment to treatment.

2. Encourage the person to shop for a therapist in a somewhat informed manner. The patient should consider (a) What expectations do I have of a therapist, i.e., how do I want him to behave and what do I want him to do for me? (b) Does this therapist match my expectations of how I want my therapist to be? and (c) Do I like the therapist to whom I've been sent, or would I prefer another? Too frequently, patients enter into or continue in a nonproductive therapy relationship because they fail to recognize that they have the right to choose who treats them.

3. Encourage the person to investigate the credentials, training, and ethics of the group therapist. Unfortunately, there are incompetent, ineffective, and poorly trained group leaders from whom patients need protection. This is particularly important since the possibility exists that the patient could be harmed by a poor group experience. Most reputable group psychotherapists (whether psychiatrist, psychologist, social worker, or nurse) are members of the American Group Psychotherapy Association (AGPA), as well as members in good standing of their own professional associations. The AGPA has issued guidelines for training group leaders that include coursework in psychopathology and in group dynamics, supervision from qualified supervisors, personal experience as a member of a group, a training background in the helping skills, and ongoing peer supervision. Any reputable group leader will be most willing to talk about the professional training that has prepared him to lead a group competently.

4. Advise the person to be wary of any group leader who promises or who guarantees results. No one can definitely say that a particular treatment modality will be effective.

5. Check with people in the community to determine the professional reputation and "track record" of a particular group leader. Other professionals will probably have sent this group leader referrals or know of his work. Ideal persons to consult would be those who might have been treated by this therapist. This latter course may be difficult to pursue because of the limitations imposed by confidentiality.

6. Consider group psychotherapy as a method of obtaining help, but also consider other treatment alternatives. The best referral is one in which group therapy is seen as the treatment of choice for a particular individual.

REFERENCES

1. Bandura, A., Blanchard, E. G., and Ritter, B.: The relative efficacy of desensitization and modeling approaches for inducing behavioral affective and attitudinal changes. J. Pers. Soc. Psychol. (in press).
2. Bergin, A. E., and Garfield, S. L. (eds.): Handbook of Psychotherapy and Behavior Change: Empirical Research in Group Psychotherapy. New York, John Wiley & Sons, Inc., 1971.
3. Carkhuff, R. R.: Helping and Human Relations. Vols. 1 and 2. New York, Holt, Rinehart & Winston, Inc., 1969.

4. Carkhuff, R. R.: New directions in training. Counsel. Psychol., 3:4, 1972.

5. Frank, J. D.: Determinants, manifestations and effects of cohesiveness in therapy groups. Int. J. Group Psychother., 7:53, 1957.

6. Friedman, W. H.: Referring patients for group psychotherapy: some guidelines. Hosp. Community Psychiatry, 27:121, 1976.

7. Gauron, E. F., and Rawlings, E. I.: A procedure for orienting new members to group psychotherapy. Small Group Behav., 6:293, 1975.

8. Gauron, E. F., Steinmark, S. W., and Gersh, F. S.: The orientation group in pre-therapy training. Perspect. Psychiatr. Care, 15:32, 1977.

9. Gauron, E. F., Steinmark, S. W., and Jamieson, J. C.: A Community Guide to the Group Psychotherapy Program. Iowa City, Goodfellow Co., 1975.

10. Goldstein, A. P.: Therapist Patient Expectancies in Psychotherapy. New York, Pergamon Press, Inc., 1962.

11. Grunebaum, H.: A soft-hearted review of hard-nosed research on groups. Int. J. Group Psychother., 25:185, 1975.

12. Hadley, S. W., and Strupp, H. D.: Contemporary views of negative effects in psychotherapy. Arch. Gen. Psychiatry, 33:1291, 1976.

13. Kapp, F. T., Gleser, G., Brissenden, A., et al.: Group participation and self-perceived personality change. J. Nerv. Ment. Dis., 139:255, 1964.

14. Kelman, H. C.: The role of the group in the induction of therapeutic change. Int. J. Group Psychother., 13:399, 1963.

15. Korner, I. N.: Hope as a method of coping. J. Consult. Clin. Psychol., 34:134, 1970.

16. Lieberman, M. A.: Problems in integrating traditional group therapies with new group forms. Int. J. Group Psychother., 27:19, 1977.

17. Lieberman, M. A., Lakin, M., and Whitaker, D. S.: The group as a unique context for therapy. Psychother: Theory, Res. Pract., 5:29, 1968.

18. Lieberman, M. A., Yalom, I. D., and Miles, M. B.: Encounter Groups: First Facts. New York, Basic Books, Inc., Publishers, 1973.

19. Mayeroff, M. M.: On Caring. New York, Harper & Row, Inc., 1971.

20. Yalom, I. D.: The Theory and Practice of Group Psychotherapy. New York, Basic Books, Inc., Publishers, 1975.

21. Yalom, I. D., Houts, P. S., Newell, G., et al.: Preparation of patients for group therapy. A controlled study. Arch. Gen. Psychiatry, 17:416, 1967.

22. Yalom, I. D., Houts, P. S., Zimerberg, S. M., et al.: Prediction of improvement in group therapy. Arch. Gen. Psychiatry, 17:159, 1967.

23. Yalom, I. D., and Lieberman, M. A.: A study of encounter group casualties. Arch. Gen. Psychiatry, 25:16, 1971.

PART V

COUNSELING

Chapter 33

MARRIAGE AND FAMILY COUNSELING WITHIN THE CONTEXT OF FAMILY PRACTICE

by WILLIAM M. CLEMENTS, and JIM L. WILSON

WHAT IS MARRIAGE AND FAMILY COUNSELING?

Broadly speaking, marriage and family counseling consists of any single intervention or series of interventions in a familial or marital system intended to bring about a change in the way its members relate to each other and to their system. Individual family members not only have thoughts and feelings about other members of the family but also about the family itself. Family communication styles are seen as one of the forces that help shape individual personality, in addition to merely expressing the needs of family members. Older cause and effect theories are giving way to a more dynamic interactional understanding of the family process. In fact, many modern theorists in the field of family therapy tend to see the family system as one of the creative forces in the shaping of individual personality as distinct from the view that sees the family as nothing more than an accretion of individual personality styles.

WHO IS THE PATIENT?

As a result of this contemporary view derived from the discipline of marriage and family counseling, the family system is not instinctively atomized into merely a group of individual patients to be diagnosed and treated sequentially. Instead, the family system now becomes the unit of both diag-

nosis and treatment—in effect the family system is the patient. While the practice of marriage and family counseling by the family physician may range from brief episodic intervention in conjunction with more conventional medical treatment to formal counseling sessions in which various combinations of family members participate, the perspective that the family system is the patient remains relevant across the entire range of treatment modalities.

Not only does such a perspective allow more than one person to be seen as the patient, but it also allows the family physician to organize previously inchoate and "irrelevant" information into a highly meaningful data bank that feeds into the diagnostic and treatment plan. Multiple contacts with individual patients who are members of the same family thus become a valuable asset instead of a sociologic accident.

WHY MARRIAGE AND FAMILY COUNSELING WITHIN FAMILY PRACTICE?

The Intersection Between Organic Medicine and Family Dynamics

Organic medicine and family dynamics are not mutually exclusive. Each has a correlative effect on health and thereby on each other. The provision of effective medical treatment may dramatically influence family dynamics when, for example, an individual patient regains health and re-

Marriage & Family Counseling Need

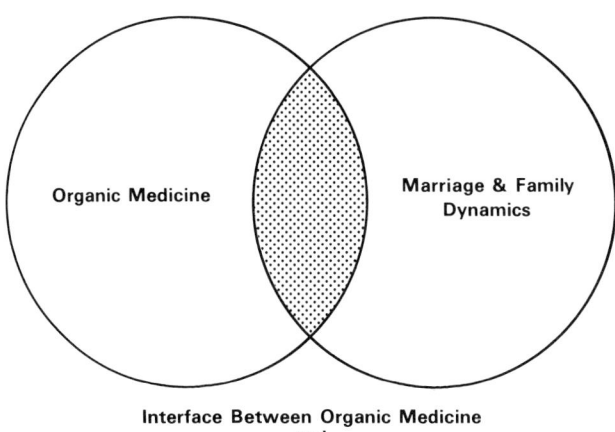

Organic Medicine

Marriage & Family
Dynamics

Interface Between Organic Medicine
and
Marriage & Family Dynamics

Figure 33–1.   Marriage and family counseling needs.

sumes a normative role within the family. So, while the practice of medicine frequently changes familial interactions, it usually does so in ways that are outside the scope of the physician's regular field of awareness. The reverse is equally true. Family dynamics affects health, although this also is usually outside one's field of awareness. When organic medicine intersects with family dynamics in such a way that diagnosis and prognosis are affected, then this inter-section itself becomes an area of particular focus or intervention. It is within this juncture between organic medicine and family dynamics that the methods of marriage and family counseling are most likely to be helpful (Fig. 33–1).

The following case description compiled by a family physician is an example of one such intersection between medicine and family dynamics in which the perspectives of family counseling proved helpful.

George W., a 45 year old high school principal who had experienced a mild myocardial infarction 14 months previously, asked during the course of a routine office examination whether his heart attack could be related to his current loss of sexual appetite and diminished pleasure during intercourse with Anne, his wife of 22 years. When asked why he thought the two might be related, he replied that things had never seemed to get back to normal sexually after his return from the hospital and, in fact, seemed to be gradually deteriorating.

He had followed a standard regimen for post-coronary rehabilitation and was now engaged in a program of regular exercise suitable for a person of his age and physical condition. He met none of the other standard criteria for depression, showed no symptoms of diabetes, drank only moderately, denied undue stress at school, and reported that other than his sexual concern he had a fairly typical relationship with his wife and three children. Following a careful review of the data, I reassured him that the two were probably unrelated and asked him if he and Anne had talked the situation over. He responded that he had tried, but Anne seemed to want to avoid the subject.

At this point in the visit I began to feel pressed for time and asked his permission to give Anne a call later in the day to discuss the situation and perhaps arrange a conjoint visit. He seemed relieved at my interest and said this would be fine.

About 10 days later the three of us sat down for an extended office visit (30 minutes in my practice). I began the session by asking what had happened since George's visit and my call to Anne. George started to say something and then began to laugh. Anne, who was grinning a little sheepishly, said that they "no longer had a problem." I asked what had happened, and George said that after talking for a good part of one night he finally "heard" that Anne was fearful of his having another heart attack and therefore felt reluctant to engage in sex. Anne reported that she now understood why George had felt rejected and hurt and that now he could appreciate the depth of her misplaced concern. About all that I did was reiterate that sexual intercourse was probably less strenuous than George's exercise program and wished them well.

This example reveals an intersection between traditional medicine and family dynamics. Within this juncture the family physician utilized the perspectives and methods of marriage and family counseling to help a basically healthy couple successfully resolve a presenting problem prior to engaging in formal counseling sessions. Medical misinformation coupled with inadequate communication helped produce a less than satisfying sexual relationship.

It seems obvious in retrospect that the couple had not reached a point of mutual problem definition. Each of them correctly felt that medical issues were related to their problem, although, as it turned out, the relationship was not causative in an organic sense. While George and Anne both "knew" that something was wrong between them sexually, neither had reached a sophisticated relational or psychodynamic diagnosis of the problem. Moreover, without an appreciation of the subtle complexity of their problem, they might never have considered consulting a professional marriage and family counselor and, in fact, might have rejected an attempted referral by the family physician if such a suggestion had been made prior to their concurrence with the diagnosis.

The Presence of One Complaint

Unlike George and Anne, who were indeed fortunate, many other couples and families unknowingly deny themselves significant help at an early stage of problem formation. Without overwhelming relational pathology or a tremendous amount of relational "savvy," many would not consider themselves as having the proper "ticket" needed to see a professional marriage and family counselor. In contrast, however, the only "ticket" needed to see a family physician is a complaint that the patient thinks requires attention. Initially, this complaint may or may not relate to family dynamics in either the patient's or the physician's mind. What it does provide is entry into a system that has the potential for early diagnosis and treatment.

Continuity, Accessibility, and Rapport

As a result of patient continuity and accessibility, the family physician has several built-in advantages that may be utilized for the patient's benefit if and when the methods of marriage and family counseling are applied in treatment. Presumably, preliminary history-taking and psychosocial exploration, for example, can be kept to a minimum in view of the data bank already at the family physician's disposal. In addition, time does not have to be spent in the laborious process of establishing patient rapport. Hopefully, this process has taken place long before there is an interface of importance between medicine and family dynamics. The treatment can flow naturally in a holistic context and is seen as one more treatment modality alongside a host of others. Early diagnosis and treatment can always lead to either prompt resolution or referral to a specialist for care in consultation with the family physician.

With approximately a 5 per cent professional time commitment by a family physician, whose education and training experiences also reflect a 5 per cent concentration in marriage and family counseling, about 85 per cent of the patients who would benefit are able to receive help appropriate to their needs. The converse is that much more education and training and a greater professional time commitment are required to help fewer and fewer patients whose relational pathologies are more firmly ingrained into habitual styles of thinking and behaving. Thus, the family physician is the professional *of choice* for a large number of people who would benefit from marriage and family counseling and would not receive help otherwise (Fig. 33–2).

Patient Expectations

In addition to the factors of efficiency, availability, continuity, treatment in a holistic context, and early detection and treatment, patient expectations play a role in securing and maintaining a vital place for marriage and family counseling within family practice. Surveys indicate that among a cross section of the American population, people are more likely to discuss an emotional or relational problem with their family physician than with any other medical specialist. In fact, from the vast panoply of available professional help, the family physician is one of the two most trusted sources of initial counsel.[16] It appears,

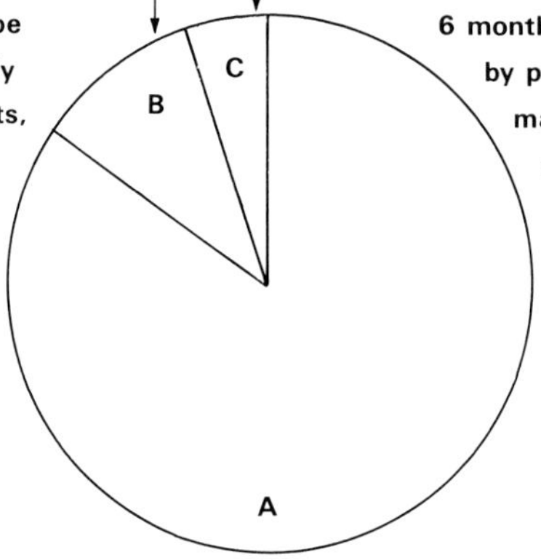

10% of population need more extensive therapy and a longer time to respond. 6+ sessions. These services may be provided by specially trained family physicians, clergymen, psychiatrists, psychologists etc.

5% of population benefit from extensive individual, conjoint and family psychotherapy. 6 months or longer. Services may be provided by professionals who limit their practice to marriage and family counseling from the following groups: pastoral counseling, psychiatry, psychology, psychiatric social work or generic marriage and family counseling.

85% of population able to benefit from short term, crisis intervention, BMT or communication models. 6 sessions or less. By virtue of their primary care role and education, plus accessibility to early problems, many family physicians, clergymen and school counselors are able to help with the majority of those who benefit from intervention.

Figure 33–2. *Total identified population who would benefit from marriage or family counseling.*

therefore, that patients look to their family physician as a viable source of initial diagnosis and treatment regardless of the physician's self-image or lack of formal academic training in the area.

PRESENTING COMPLAINTS AND DIAGNOSTIC CONSIDERATIONS

PRESENTING COMPLAINTS

Stress and Anxiety Related to Illness or Treatment

Probably the single most prevalent and identifiable complaint encountered by the family physician centers around the marital and familial stress resulting from illness, treatment, or both. Families quite predictably react to the illness or incapacity of one member with a variety of coping behaviors until a new dynamic equilibrium is established. Sensitivity to this phenomenon enables the family physician to provide counsel appropriate to the nature of the stress by opening up channels of communication within the family and learning of idiosyncratic fears and emotional needs exacerbated or caused by the illness of a particular family member. Such familial concerns may be verbalized in half-disguised form, making them difficult to assess. Questions about diagnosis, prognosis, and treatment,

in addition to requests for factual information, may also serve as the only means available for the expression of anxiety and stress, in which case more factual data from the physician deals with only part of the issue.

Chronic Fatigue, Anxiety, and Exogenous Depression

Additional complaints indicative of chronic fatigue, chronic anxiety, and situational depression may at times be traced to relational stress. When the stressful conditions are alleviated, one can expect a diminution in the number and severity of such complaints. Quite obviously, a careful diagnostic work-up is in order with special attention being given to the social history, which, along with all additional data, serves to illuminate likely diagnostic possibilities.

Sexual Adjustment

Sexual complaints may be expected to yield not only information of a purely sexual nature but also to provide valuable information about a couple's patterns of communication, power relationships, and so forth, keeping in mind that what started out as a relational problem may now have become focused on sex as the chief symptom in a complex equation involving psyche and soma. Or, what started out as a sexual dysfunction may have, with the passage of time, come to symbolize additional aspects of the relationship beyond the sexual.

Direct Statement of Relational Stress

In addition to the types of complaints in which particular patients disguise relational problems, the family physician needs to be alert to direct statements of relational stress. Utilizing a vague physical "ticket of admission," a patient may wish to talk about the pain of a disintegrating marriage or the feelings of parental inadequacy when faced with a difficult period in adolescent development. All of the obvious symptoms of familial distress may be communicated once the dam of reticence breaks and the physician responds with an attentive ear and appropriate questions. Hopefully, he would not dismiss such concerns as "irrelevant" but would see them as *real* complaints that stem from *real* distress that may be effectively dealt with in the course of his practice.

DIAGNOSTIC CONSIDERATIONS

Within the new and evolving field of marriage and family counseling, there are yet to emerge broadly accepted categories of diagnosis that refer explicitly to marriage and family pathology. Without diagnostic categories that distinguish between syn dromes, clear-cut, objective criteria are also lacking for assisting in the task of identification and differentiation. As a consequence, there is a deficit of specific methods of treatment for particular diagnoses that enjoy applicability and acceptance among a majority of marriage and family counselors.

This is not to say that diagnosis is not important or that diagnostic considerations are secondary. Rather, it is intended to emphasize that diagnostic considerations are still largely idiosyncratic to the individual therapist, as are the treatment modalities utilized. Personality styles and criteria for treatment selection continue to play a significant role in outcome success, regardless of diagnosis or treatment modality.

Problem-Solving Capacity

Nevertheless, there are certain diagnostic inquiries to be considered once an issue has been identified as a potential symptom worthy of further exploration. The first area of consideration is the development of an understanding of the family's or couple's *problem-solving capacity.* Given a problem that requires a decision involving all family members, what process is followed? Does one family member make a unilateral decision without consultation? If so, how do other family members respond to such a decision? With relief? Enthusiastic cooperation? Sullen acceptance? Hostile rejection? One way to obtain this information is to ask how the decision to seek counseling was made. One might ask what procedure is followed when someone feels sick and a decision about a visit to the physician is considered. Who first broached the subject, and what was the response? Who made the call for an appointment? One might also consider inquiring about a recent large purchase, such as a house or automobile, or about a vacation decision. What constellation of family members coalesces for what types of decisions? Do some members tacitly decide on a major purchase before talking with the others? How do certain family members feel about finding out something after the basic goal is set and all that is left to decide is how to attain the objective? Do father and son get together on vacation plans, leaving the mother and daughter only to make the tactical decisions of how to accomplish their goal? The way decisions are really made and executed in a family can reveal much about family communication patterns, power relationships, and self-awareness.

Child-Rearing

A second area of diagnostic inquiry involves child-rearing policies within the home. Each spouse was socialized in a different environment and could therefore be expected to have internalized a multitude of "right" ways to raise children, which might at times be in conflict with the other spouse's divergent ways. Are they *aware* of the differences in their approach to the "right" way to raise children? Do they predominantly accommodate, negotiate, capitulate, or fight when differences emerge?

(It is assumed that *all* couples do all of the above from time to time. The question is one of the presence of a *habitual* style.) How do the children attempt to manipulate these differences, or do the parents feel a false "united front" must be projected to the children at all times? How have each spouse's ideas about the "right" way mellowed and matured with a growing family? Are they aware of their own changes?

Roles

A third area of diagnostic inquiry relates to the roles occupied by family members and the roles expected of each family member. What vocational roles do the adult family members fill? What about familial roles? What are the expectations? Have they ever been verbalized? Are they realistic? Is there conflict between role expectation and performance that seems to center on one or two family members?

Does the wife try to work at the bank all day and keep house as her own mother did (with two servants, which is usually forgotten) without active assistance from other family members? Does the husband really expect that of her? Or, does he work hard all day and even into the night and on weekends, only to disappear on holidays to play golf, forgetting that he has a family who hardly knows him? Or, to take another approach, are responsibilities for family life equitably distributed so that it *really* matters to others whether the children do their chores? What does each family member think is expected of him? How did they learn this expectation? What are the unverbalized expectations floating around that cause conflict? In the physician's presence, can the family get together and talk about roles and expectations without the discussion deteriorating into a sullen confrontation or escalating into World War III? Can they also do this at home alone? Why not? What is there about the physician's office and presence that changes things?

Recreation

Another area for diagnostic inquiry lies in the general field of a family's total recreational experience. Does there seem to be a discernible family ethos in regard to leisure-time pursuits? Is play, for example, a self-validating experience, or must there be "serious" objectives in mind that confirm the presence of "frivolous" activities? Does the family appear to enjoy each other's company, or is a holiday together an event that is merely endured? What are each individual's solo recreational activities? Are there some recreational activities that each individual engages in that involve him in play with persons outside the family?

Who makes the decisions in regard to recreation? Is the decisional person or constellation different from the decisional unit that decided on major purchases? If such differences exist, can the family verbalize them? Does everyone actually *know* what leisure-time activities bring pleasure to other family members? Consider asking each person to write down a list of such activities, and have the family compare notes, discussing differences between lists and ways in which similarities can be maximized in similar or parallel activities.

Try to get some concrete ideas about the amount or distribution of family income spent in leisure-time pursuits. For example, it might be informative to learn that a family spent the bulk of its recreational money on an annual Alaskan hunting trip for the husband, as distinct from a family that spends its money camping together, or one that spends its money supporting each person's solo recreational pursuits, such as the father's photography, the daughter's horse, the son's stamp collection, and the mother's antique collection. What is important is whether or not they enjoy activities together on occasion. Also consider using a time continuum for a different slant on how a particular family manages its recreational "time budget." Flexibility in scheduling, which maximizes both solo and family play, becomes a crucial issue in family life as children mature into adolescents, and peer group play becomes more significant.

Inquiries into the way money and time are spent in the pursuit of recreational activities can provide a gold mine of data in an area that is often not too controversial. Communication patterns, financial planning, power relationships, and areas of personal autonomy can all be explicated with a few simple questions about play.

Religious Beliefs, Practices, and Affiliations

Inquiries in this area can frequently provide a wealth of cultural and religious background information. Do both spouses regularly attend the same church or synagogue? If there are differences in affiliation or participation, are both happy with the arrangements and content with the way in which their children are being reared? If one or both spouses have abandoned the religious identity of their youth, are there occasional feelings of regret or guilt attached to the decision? If present, have these feelings been discussed? What purpose does a family's religious affiliation seem to meet? Does it help provide a sense of identity for all members of the family or does it serve to isolate a few? Is there room for healthy autonomy and diversity, or do even minutiae become matters of anxiety and "ultimate" concern? Are there unhealthy gaps between verbalized religious beliefs and the actual practices of day-to-day living? Does the religious tradition in a family seem inclusive and productive of maturity or exclusive and counterproductive? Does it draw together or separate the nuclear family? Why? The extended family? Why? Are there traditions within a family's particular religious affiliation that lend themselves to wholeness and reconciliation? What are they? Or, are there conflicts between what a tradition says is right and proper and the way a family synthesizes that tradition in the modern world?

Autonomy

Another matter for overall diagnostic consideration is the issue of autonomy. Who has tacit permission to do what? Does each person's level of autonomy seem appropriate for his age and responsibilities? Who grants permission for what activities? To whom? The following vignettes from different families help illustrate possible polarities where autonomy is a significant issue.

Thomas B., the "identified patient," was seen for an initial interview following solo interviews with his mother, father, and older brother. Yet to be interviewed were his younger brother (by 15 months) and sister.
During the course of the interview, he gradually became more relaxed and talkative, typically verbal for one of his background and educational level. He was dressed casually with rather mussed-up hair and had greasy hands from working on a friend's motorcycle. His concerns seemed to center on "getting the folks off my back. Geez, you wouldn't believe the hassle!" Thomas claimed that his parents objected to

"everything" he did. They wanted him to be in bed by 11:00 P.M. on school nights and insisted on a midnight curfew on Friday and Saturday evenings. Thomas rarely made his curfew, usually being from $1/2$ to 1 hour late. The police had called his parents "once or twice" about a few minor things. School grades were only low average—passing but not suitable for college preparatory courses in high school. Thomas wanted very much to be accepted by his older brother's circle of friends; he emulated their language and behavior whenever possible.

This case doesn't seem too unusual for a 16 year old adolescent who is struggling for an identity, recognition, autonomy, and so forth. Thomas, however, was just barely 13 years old and unable to utilize maturely the autonomy he already had.

Maggie S. and her parents came in for an initial family interview. It seemed that her parents were becoming concerned about her frequent minor illnesses, which caused her to miss large blocks of school time, and even threatened her promotion to a high school senior. She was the youngest (by 8 years) of five children. Her parents were in their early 60's. The interview opened with the physician's asking general questions, such as "Well, why are you here today?" directed at no one in particular. After a brief silence, her mother began talking, complaining, and even crying about "poor Maggie." During her mother's outburst, Maggie looked out the window with a feigned, almost regal disinterest. Next her father joined in and spoke to Maggie directly, saying, "All we want is for you to grow up and be happy in life, Maggie." Maggie remained silent until the physician asked her opinion. Then she started to respond somewhat haltingly. Before a sentence was scarcely out of her mouth, Mother was elaborating on and correcting her speech.

It turned out that, among other things, Maggie had very limited autonomy. Her mother filled her plate with food, even denying Maggie a choice of what and how much she ate! Both parents watched her throughout life as if she were a toddler, about to fall down a treacherous flight of steps. Maggie, who was soon to be 18 years old, didn't even select her own clothes for school!

Jeffrey came to the first visit alone. It was difficult to hear him talk because he spoke so softly. He was employed locally and liked his job a lot. His family physician had referred him to the counselor because of gastric distress—Jeffrey called it a knot in his stomach—that was not indicative of any identifiable syndrome. Jeffrey's history was hard to believe, but unfortunately true. Both his parents had been alcoholics, frequently fighting and drunk. One night, 15 years ago, he remembered grabbing his infant brother and running out of the house to call the police because his father had a butcher knife and was threatening everyone. At present, his father had been dead for many years, and his mother was a "permanent" patient at a state hospital. Jeffrey started to work at a dairy when he was underaged, loading milk bottles into cartons for home delivery. He made good money and also could consume all the milk, ice cream, and cheese he wanted. When he was 14 years old, he was living at the YMCA, working at odd jobs and attending school while his younger brother was living with an aged grandmother in another city.

When Jeffrey came for counseling, he was a college graduate, with his first full-time job (working a late afternoon and evening shift) in a professional capacity. The "knot" in his stomach first developed after his younger brother had been living with him a month or so. Jeffrey (who understandably abhorred alcohol) had discovered an empty vodka bottle in the trash one morning. The knot had become progressively worse in the few months since then. While Jeffrey was only 21 years old, he had apparently always functioned more responsibly than either of his parents and was even now trying to "parent" his younger brother under trying circumstances.

Economic Issues

In the course of gaining general diagnostic information, it is often helpful to give a family several opportunities to discuss financial matters. Given the professional setting and rationale for inquiry, almost without exception a family will cooperate and discuss their finances, probably more extensively than they have at home alone.

For adults particularly, feelings of self-esteem and adequacy may be intertwined with success in the area of family finances. If there seems to be a spirit of teamwork present, then each person may gain some measure of satisfaction from having contributed to the attainment of family financial objectives, however limited those objectives may appear. On the other hand, with chronic financial chaos, family morale suffers, and aggression is turned inward, leading to blaming and bitter accusations instead of outward, leading to problem solving. What started out as a minor finan-

cial problem may become ammunition in a "family war," if other interpersonal problems predominate. Regardless of a particular family's style of adjustment to its income level, economic issues allow the physician an opportunity to gain additional information about interpersonal patterns of communication, child-rearing policies, power relationships, autonomy, and problem-solving capacities. An open-ended question, such as "How are your family finances getting along these days?", may provide valuable information about the husband's job, the mother's role in money matters, and whom the children turn to for money if there is no provision for earning their own spending money.

Money worries can be the primary problem area in a family, though in middle class families they often tend to mask other problems. Occasionally, however, in times of unemployment and rampant inflation, money matters *are* the problem and are not merely symptomatic of other problems. In such cases it is helpful for the physician to have a good referral relationship with a successful financial counselor.

Many large banks have a counselor on their staffs who is well-versed in helping families disentangle themselves from a plethora of financial problems by establishing systematic record keeping and planning short-term goals to help re-establish morale and nurture the capacity for creative change. Smaller banks may have an informal service available through a sympathetic officer who is himself a successful family financial manager. Local social service agencies often can assist a family in gaining access to job retraining programs, or income supplementation benefits (e.g., disability assistance), to help them get moving again. Clergymen and others who live successfully on limited incomes might be a potential referral resource when other, more obvious, resources are either unavailable or inappropriate.

Referrals

Within a family practice there are a few contraindications to counseling worthy of note. Cases requiring long-term or in-depth intervention should be screened out for referral to other professionals whose practice and education equip them for the most efficient treatment of such families. The decisive factor in such a referral is one of time effectiveness from the standpoint of the family physician.

Problems that require massive amounts of time and energy for resolution can usually be recognized when one spouse is seriously involved emotionally with a third party, a compulsive gambler, a wet alcoholic, a habitual drug abuser, a grossly immature person, someone in need of individual psychotherapy prior to marriage or family counseling, or a psychotic individual. Also excluded would be those persons normally referred for psychiatric care. A final category contraindicating counseling by the family physician would be those family units lacking sufficient interest in or motivation for the efforts necessary for successful change. Such referrals allow the family physician to concentrate on the majority of cases in which he is the most effective agent of change available to the family unit.

Referrals should typically be made in those instances when another professional can reasonably be expected to do a better job than the job the family physician's interests or training would allow him to perform. A referral would also be in order if the physician is uncomfortable dealing with a particular situation because it reminds him too strongly of unresolved problems within his own family or marriage. Occasionally, even the most adequately trained counselor will find himself in a situation causing him undue anxiety for a variety of perfectly natural, though unknown, reasons. A referral should also be considered if a couple or family expresses a continued desire for interaction, even after a prolonged course of counseling. One good way for the physician to handle referrals is to state explicitly at the outset of counseling that he is available for a specific number of sessions, and at that terminal point, if additional help is needed, a referral will be made. Or if there is a lack of response to counseling efforts, coupled with a verbalized desire for continued counseling, a referral might be appreciated. Even with a referral, however, patient continuity should be assured because the family physician remains the primary physician.

MARITAL, SEXUAL, AND FAMILY COUNSELING AS A PROFESSION

The historical development of marital, sexual, and family counseling began in the mid-1930's when a conglomeration of specialists trained in a variety of disciplines focused their attention on strategies of marital, sexual, and family treatment. The unifying force of this heterogeneous group was their concern in developing clinical techniques for the treatment of marital, sexual, and family dysfunction. While numerous organizations support the study of the family and the individuals in it, the physician in family practice should be aware of the professional and clinical resources available to assist in his work with families. In the field of marital, sexual, and family treatment, the American Association of Marriage and Family Counselors (AAMFC), 225 Yale Avenue, Claremont, California, 91711, can be especially helpful.

The AAMFC is an organization founded in 1942, composed exclusively of clinically trained professionals in the fields of marital, sexual, and family therapy. Membership includes more than 4000 people throughout the United States and Canada whose training backgrounds are in psychiatry, psychology, sociology, social work, pastoral counseling, or education. Each member is trained in the clinical treatment of marital, sexual, and family dysfunction. The AAMFC executive offices are located in Claremont, California with regional divisions throughout the United States and Canada. The organization performs many functions important to its members, to the profession of marital, family, and sexual counseling, to the public that such counseling serves, and to the physician in family practice. These functions include (1) setting rigorous membership standards for marital, family, and sexual therapists, (2) establishing specialized training centers, (3) holding professional meetings at regional and national levels, (4) cosponsoring clinical meetings with other professional associations in the health field, such as the American Academy of Family Physicians, and (5) planning intensive informational programs to help the public understand marital, sexual, and family problems and the value of clinical counseling as a treatment option.

Physicians were among the founders and early members of the AAMFC. Notable among these were Robert L. Dickinson, Abraham Stone, Robert Laidlaw, Sophia Kleegman, and Walter R. Stokes. Increasing numbers of physicians with specialized training in marital, sexual, and family therapy are members of the AAMFC. Recent publications by physicians indicate the growing interest within the medical profession in the development of marital, sexual, and family counseling skills.

METHODS OF SHORT-TERM MARRIAGE AND FAMILY COUNSELING UNIQUELY SUITED FOR A FAMILY PRACTICE

Research into therapeutic outcome in the field of marriage and family counseling has turned up some interesting results having direct applicability to family practice. One study, which investigated a variety of treatment modalities utilized by numerous therapists in disparate settings for varying lengths of time, found that improvement, as defined by the therapist who provided treatment, was positively correlated with a relatively few number of counseling sessions.[17] This means that, among other things, improvement is probably not correlated with length of treatment alone. Other factors, such as treatment effectiveness, are probably more important. While there are numerous ways to interpret (and rationalize) such rudimentary data, one observation is that perhaps short-term treatment is a more aggressive method of intervention, requiring a greater degree of patient–physician involvement in the attainment of clearly delineated goals within a predetermined time frame. Maybe *everybody* works harder, and thereby more improvement is noted.

Early problem detection, pre-existing patient rapport, and greater initial efficiency place the physician in a good position to practice the most successful methods of short-term treatment available. While there are many such treatment designs in existence, some are difficult to learn and practice, and others are rarely utilized. Three have been selected for inclusion here because of their widespread usefulness and successful applicability to problems frequently seen in family practice.

EFFECTIVE COMMUNICATION PATTERN

Applicability

The first method has particular applicability to interpersonal relationships within the family in which basic, straightforward communication is disrupted, rarely practiced, or an unknown art. When utilizing the methods of *effective communication pattern* (ECP), the family physician adopts the attitudes and position of a "coach" who instructs actively by clear example and tactful correction. He does not get involved in the "contest" but remains on the sidelines, calling out instructions, providing encouragement in a dispirited moment, and rewarding his charges when new behaviors bring success.

Procedures

When a family is being counseled using the methods of ECP, only a single dyad (husband–wife), (mother–daughter), (brother–sister) should be allowed in the "ring" at one time. Everyone else is to observe and learn all that they can about what contributes to and detracts from effective communication. Besides, a threesome is more than one can handle and complicates the method beyond belief! The therapist may have the dyad place their chairs squarely facing each other to maximize eye contact between them and minimize distractions and "tuning out" behaviors.

The dyad is then simultaneously instructed in the methods of ECP, and each individual partner is given explicit initial instruction about his particular role in communication during the first interchange. Following the first *successful* interchange, communication roles are reversed, with role reversal following each successful interchange thereafter. (The "coach" determines success.) Such instruction in ECP might be presented as follows:

The object of this exercise, Pat and John, is to provide a laboratory experience for you in effective communication. In this laboratory we try to observe carefully *what* we communicate so that our efforts can lead to faster learning and a more effective exchange of thoughts and feelings. Each of you will have an important role as a partner to the other. After successful completion of one interchange, you will trade communication roles, but not before.

Don't be surprised at old habits of communication that reassert themselves from time to time. Just correct yourselves and continue. As your coach, I will occasionally point out ways in which you may be more helpful to your partner or can better accomplish your objective of effective communication.

Good communication does not guarantee agreement about the matter under discussion. The object of this laboratory experiment is not to produce agreement but instead to teach an effective way to communicate that you will practice at home on your own. It is okay to be different, to think differently, and to remember facts differently. You each have a right to your own opinion. However, the principal rule is that genuine communication must precede either disagreement or agreement. Without accurate communication, we may only *think* we agree and should actually still be talking.

For communication to take place, a message must be sent to another person and understood by that person. Today we will deal with verbal messages primarily. Unlike written messages, verbal messages must be *short* and to the point.

Pat, I want you to be responsible for being the "talker." (Usually this gets a laugh from the partner.) You are to say about three sentences on a subject and then stop.

John, I want you to be the "listener." Your sole objective is to *understand* what Pat has just said. Your first responsibility is simply to comprehend what Pat said, *not* what you think she *ought* to have said. After listening carefully, you are to put into your own words those three sentences and check your communication by asking her if this is what she meant.

Pat, if John's paraphrase of your three sentences seems inaccurate, perhaps he didn't understand what you said. If this is the case, simply tell him that there has apparently been miscommunication. Don't call him a "blockhead" or get angry. Repeat that portion that he misunderstood, using different words this time. It is not fair to enlarge what you originally said but simply restate the troublesome part in different words.

You are to continue this cycle until there is agreement, Pat, that John understands what you have said by accurately translating your message into his own words. Until this happens, communication does not take place.

Now let's see if you understand the instructions. Pat, what are you to do as the "talker"? . . . John, what does the "listener" do? . . . Good. Now that you understand the instructions, let's get into communication positions. (Here the therapist usually rearranges the chairs as mentioned previously.) By the way, John, after you understand Pat, you get to be the "talker." Then you can state your views on the matter or even change the subject if you wish, and it's Pat's turn to listen.

Generally the therapist picks out the first topic of discussion, choosing an event from the local newspaper that all are familiar with but that might be controversial. The aim is to *avoid* one of those exquisitely sensitive areas between the participants that their present skills do not allow them to discuss fruitfully. *After* they have mastered the method, they may discuss personally controversial topics (Table 33–1).

TABLE 33–1. EFFECTIVE COMMUNICATION PATTERN

Time and Place:	Must be done initially during a counseling session with the couple forming a communication team.
Follow-up:	After several counseling sessions may be practiced at home for brief periods of time.
Attitude:	It's okay to disagree *after* you know what the spouse said.
Couple Response:	"We never really listened before today."
Danger:	Couple will spontaneously slide into "deaf" arguing without careful coaching.

Procedure:	1. Explain to couple that two-way communication is a multifaceted process requiring hard work and attention.
	  a. Wife sends message to husband.
	  b. Husband *understands* or comprehends both content and affect levels. This does not mean he has to *agree*.
	  c. Husband repeats in his own different vocabulary what he understood wife to say.
	  d. Wife agrees with his understanding or steps *a* through *c* are repeated, using different words.
	  e. Avoid questions in wife's statements.
	2. Following one complete exchange, the "understander" gets the floor and can change the subject or respond to the first exchange.
	3. Keep all exchanges brief (no more than three simple sentences).

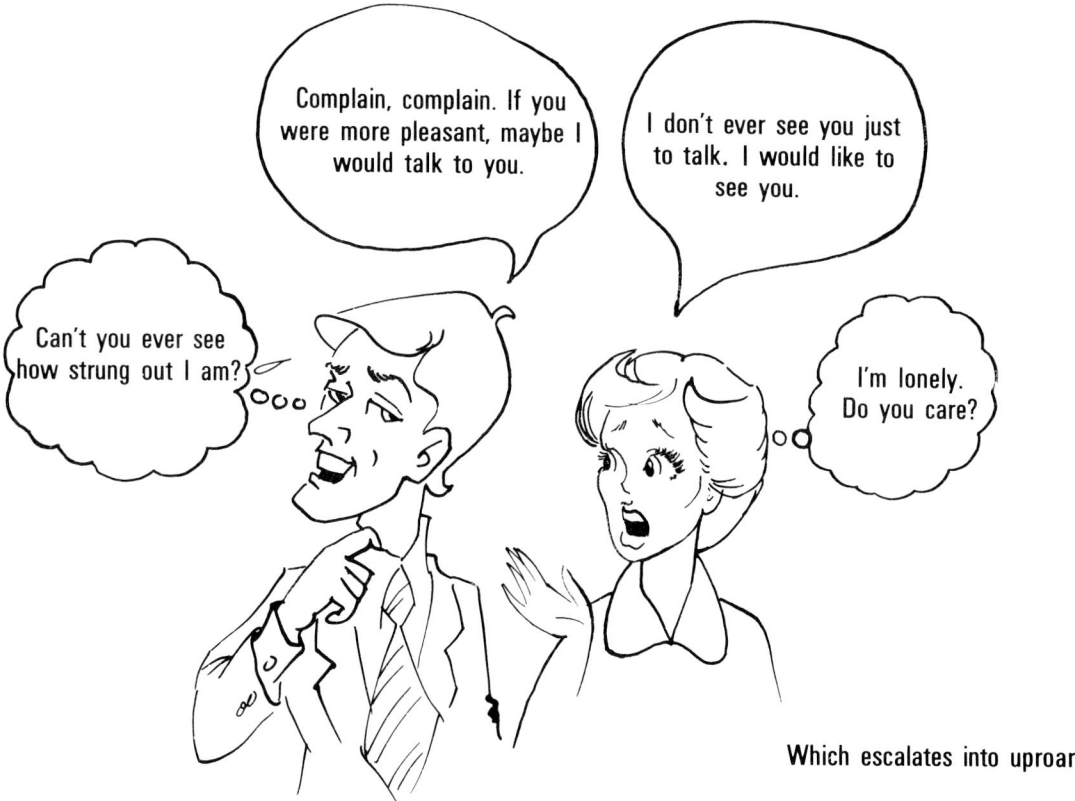

Figure 33-3. Example of interchange before establishment of effective communication pattern (ECP).

Between counseling sessions, they are instructed to spend 15 minutes a day talking about current events, using the method of ECP and alternating the person who is the first talker from day to day. Some couples are pleased to find that they can actually have good conversations again! Practicing ECP between parent and child can also break up destructive patterns of communication. The parent is forced to listen to the child, who struggles to state clearly what he means in an adult fashion.

Before ECP is established, an interchange between Pat and John would be similar to that shown in Figure 33-3. After they are proficient, the same interchange might look like that shown in Figures 33-4 and 33-5.

POSITIVE STROKING

Applicability

Occasionally the physician will become aware of the presence of a hostile, demoralized marriage in which both partners desire a better relationship and have tried (perhaps heroically) on their own to straighten things out. For reasons unknown to them, they just can't seem to bring about creative change. If the couple reports a history of a better relationship at some earlier point in their marriage but now seem to have lost the positive nature of their interaction, they are likely candidates for the method called *positive stroking.* Remember to look for a "golden age" in the marriage when everything was better. Otherwise, the physician may find himself dealing with a pair of professional "guerrilla fighters" who gleefully turn their verbal guns on him, instead of each other.

Positive stroking does not require one to engage in a tricky, triple reverse psychodynamic explanation of "why this couple continues to choose to inflict pain on each other." Instead of dealing with the *why* issue, ask *what* can be done behaviorally to change creatively the manner in which interaction takes place. Instead of trying to change hostile, demoralized *feelings,* focus

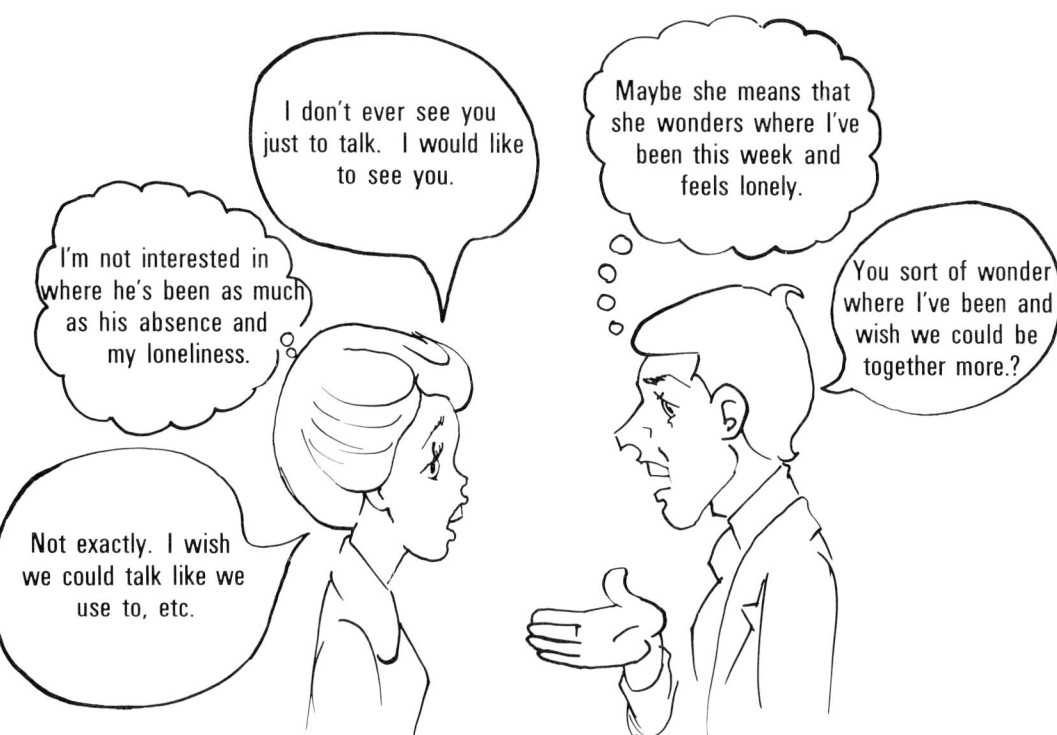

Figure 33-4. *Example of interchange after establishment of ECP.*

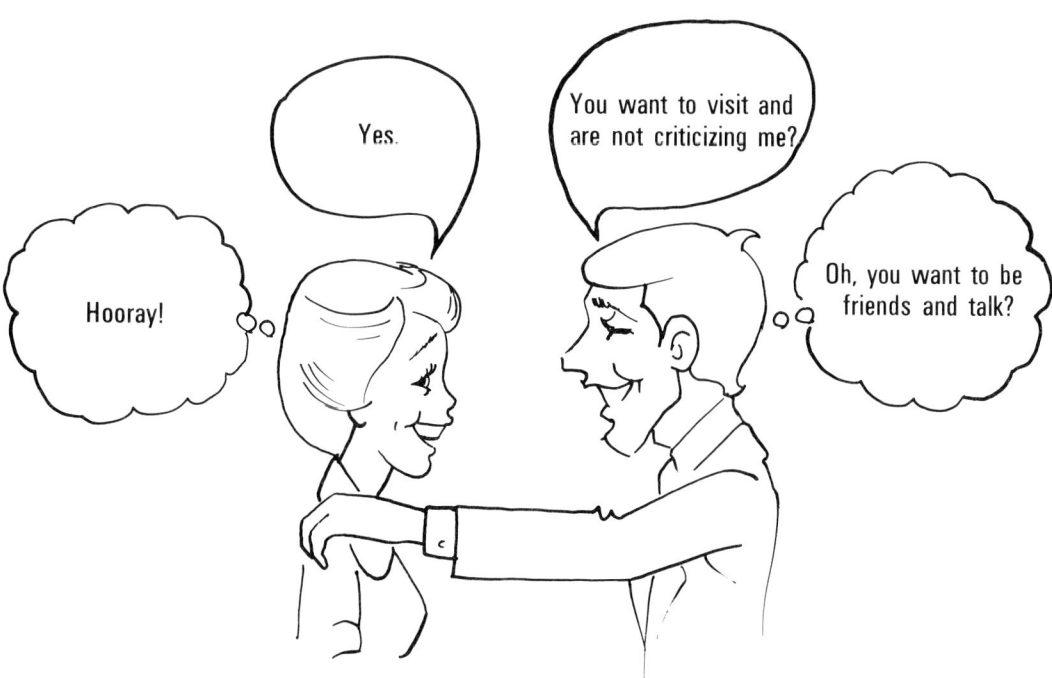

Figure 33-5. *Further interchange after establishment of ECP.*

instead on changing concrete *behaviors,* trusting that different feelings will occur naturally as a result of new behaviors.

Procedures

The first step, that of diagnosis and patient selection, has been mentioned previously. The next procedure is to elicit from each spouse a list containing behavioral complaints that refer to the mate. The wife's list might contain items such as, "He never spends time with the children; the only time he touches me is when he wants sex; he never attends PTA meetings with me," and so forth. The husband's list might contain items such as, "She only cooks TV dinners; I never have clean shirts in the morning; she doesn't like to attend parties," and so forth. Get about ten items on each list.

From these lists of complaints, the couple and the physician should draw up *target behavior changes* (TBC's) such as "Cook three complete dinners per week" for the wife, and "Spend a half hour with children daily" for the husband. *Target behaviors* are discrete units of *observable* action and do not refer to attitudes, feelings, or desires. Try to "coach" the couple so that a written TBC corresponds to each complaint. A list of ten TBC's is developed for each spouse.

Next, allow each spouse to choose about six TBC's that each is willing to make. Allow each spouse to omit three or four TBC's from their final list for reasons of compliance and equity, for example, "I won't trim the hedges for anybody. She knows I *hate* that" and "Our lists aren't equal. It'll take me 4 hours a day and only one half hour for him."

TABLE 33–2. POSITIVE STROKING

Time and Place:	Marriage counseling session.
Follow-up:	At home on daily basis.
Attitude:	Feelings can change as a result of new reciprocal behavior.
Couple Response:	Initial skepticism and fear of additional emotional pain, later enthusiastic cooperation.
Procedure:	Problem behaviors are analyzed into concrete behavioral components. Attitudes and feelings are not programmed. Wife complains, "He never spends time with the children." Husband complains, "She only cooks TV dinners."

1. A list containing behavior complaints is elicited from each partner, and target behavior changes are listed.

   Target behavior for husband—spend $\frac{1}{2}$ hour daily with children (H).
   Target behavior for wife—cook 3 complete dinners per week (W).

2. A list of spousal behavior rewards (R) is elicited:

   R_H = backrub by wife
   R_W = husband washes dishes

3. A list of sanctions is also drawn up. Frequently money provides the "token." Penalty tokens (T−) go to charity; reward tokens (T+) are freely spent.

   Formula is as follows:

   If H, then R_H and T+.   (If husband spends $\frac{1}{2}$ hour daily with children, then wife rubs his back and $1.00 is awarded husband for spending.)

   If not H, then no R_H and T−.   (If husband does not spend $\frac{1}{2}$ hour daily with children, he gets no backrub from wife and gives $1.00 to charity.)

   If W, then R_W and T+.   (If wife cooks 3 complete dinners per week, then husband washes dishes that evening, and $1.00 is awarded wife for spending.)

   If not W, then no R_W and T−.   (If wife does not cook 3 complete dinners per week, husband does not wash dishes and wife gives $1.00 to charity.)

This step is followed by having each spouse draw up a list of approximately ten *behavior rewards* each is willing to perform when the spouse completes a TBC. Behavior rewards should, like the TBC's be discrete, observable units of action, such as the wife's providing a 10 minute backrub or the husband's doing the dishes one evening. Be sure that there is *no cross linkage* between one person's TBC's and that person's behavior rewards for the spouse. Thus, the husband should not have to keep the children a half hour per day as one of his target behaviors, as well as have to provide a behavior reward to the wife of one evening of babysitting. He should choose one or the other, but under no circumstances both. The rewards and behavior changes should be different, depending on each person's schedule. Cross linkage failure is something they have already tried to resolve unsuccessfully on their own. The intent is to have them experience success and not *more* failure; they need positive strokes instead of additional negative strokes. Continued supervision of this process is important.

The final step involves a list of sanctions. Money frequently provides a good "token" reward or punishment. Completion of a TBC brings a predetermined behavior reward from the spouse plus a certain amount of money, for example, one dollar, for free spending purposes (the amount of monetary reward can be adjusted according to a couple's budgetary requirements). Failure to perform a TBC results in missing a behavior reward and also paying a penalty "token" (equal in amount to the "token" reward) to a predetermined charity.

The entire procedure is presented in outline form for review and reference (Table 33–2).

STRUCTURING

Applicability

The chaotic family seems to be falling apart at the seams. One or more family members may have health problems in which anxiety and stress appear to be significant components. This anxiety and stress seem to relate to the difficulties surrounding survival in the midst of chaos. The father may have recently changed jobs, the son is a behavior problem at school and failing a subject or two, the daughter just wants to be left alone (and catered to), and the mother is worried sick about the daughter, who "is much too involved" with a young man. Family responsibilities and chores haven't been defined in years (if ever). There is definitely a lot of bickering and confusion. Almost everyone has an angry attitude that probably relates to the repeated failures of family members to meet inadequately verbalized expectations. Neither parent exerts positive leadership by setting an example for responsible family life. The only "stroking" which takes place is negative, and there is an abundance of this. Oftentimes, one or more adolescents are members of such a chaotic family. Frequently they are presented as the problem by the parents, while the teenagers feel just the opposite—a new set of parents would solve everything!

Procedures

When the family physician becomes aware of the chaotic family, he should think of *structuring* as the most appropriate method of counseling. The chaotic family lacks a realistic, consistent structure. To an outsider, rewards and punishment seem capricious. It's more or less "every man for himself." The first step is to gather the entire family together for a meeting. Such an experience will probably be a new one and may be resisted by one or more persons by remaining away from the conference. *Everyone* who lives in the same home, including parents, children, and relatives, must be present at *all* family meetings. Do not proceed unless the entire family attends.

A long, undifferentiated list should be developed of *what* tasks need to be done for the family to thrive. After such a list is compiled (with a family member serving as secretary on a rotating basis), ask each person to make a separate list of tasks that he sometimes performs that did not appear on the master list. Put these on the master list.

Each person then lists separately ten rewards for himself. Criteria for rewards include things that are inexpensive, not detrimental to health, and not dependent on another person's behavior (i.e., a reward for the son does not include having his mother do one of his chores). Encourage pleasurable activities and positive, self-rewarding behaviors. Each person then rank orders these rewards, going from the *least* significant to the most significant.

The next step involves having each person list ten punishments that he thinks will be effective deprivations, or, instead of deprivations, positive behaviors not particularly enjoyed.

Now, as a family unit, each person's responsibilities are to be delineated in clear behavioral terms. Family members are *not responsible* for failure to comply with behavioral responsibilities that do not appear on their lists. If it doesn't appear on the father's (or child's) list, he does not receive a punishment for lack of compliance. If a person does not choose to participate in the selection process for his responsibilities, it is understood that the remaining family members will complete the task while he silently observes. All tasks appearing on the common list of ideal family responsibilities have to be done by *someone* or crossed off the list. There are no free-floating responsibilities for "someone" to complete. Each person now has a complete list of responsibilities arrived at by a democratic process of negotiation.

Next, individual lists of rewards are drawn up by the entire family, using the previously completed rank order list for each person as a guideline and following the same democratic process of negotiation. Likewise, the same procedures are used to complete a list of punishments for each family member. The last item of business is to set the next family meeting date. (The physician's office should be the site of at least one additional follow-up meeting.)

The family is then instructed to post each person's completed schedule containing duties, rewards, and punishments in a common gathering place in the house.

If each person's schedule is properly drawn up, there will be an escalation of rewards so that the *longer* a person is successful, the more he is rewarded. Similarly, there is an escalation of punishments so that the longer a person fails to learn these behaviors, the more costly it becomes. A synergistic effect usually becomes operative (Tables 33–3 and 33–4). For many families, simply discussing and working out schedules provide enough "structure" so that new equilibrium is established, and the chaos disappears. Other families will find three or four office visits helpful, as they allow new behavioral habits to emerge. Maximum benefit should be attained within six counseling sessions.

TABLE 33–3. STRUCTURING

Time and Place:	Usually done during a family counseling session with *all* members present and participating.
Follow-up:	At home during regular family meeting.
Attitude:	Matter-of-fact (no harassment, nagging, reminding, or evasion of consequences through an appeal to special circumstances).
Family Response:	Resistance, sabotage turning into enthusiastic cooperation. Child—likes getting capricious parents off his back . . . he knows where he stands. Mother (or father)—is relieved at the structuring bearing some of the burden. Father (or mother)—struggles to become a more responsible family member and parent.

Steps to Successful Structuring:
1. As a family unit, members draw up a common list of ideal tasks for successful family life.
2. Each person then lists tasks or responsibilities that he occasionally performs not appearing above.
3. Each person lists ten rewards for himself.
   a. rank order rewards.
4. Each person lists ten punishments for himself.
   a. rank order punishments.
5. As a family unit, members draw up each person's list of responsibilities using steps *1* and *2* as guidelines.
6. As a family unit, members draw up each person's list of rewards using step *3* as a guideline.
7. As a family unit, members draw up each person's list of punishments using step *4* as a guideline.
8. Members set the time for the next weekly family meeting.

TABLE 33-4. ILLUSTRATED STRUCTURING FOR ONE FAMILY MEMBER
(Thomas, 14 year old, 8th grade student, commitment for April 14–21)

Duties	Rewards	Punishments
Daily	A. 1 hour tv time	1 day – do evening dishes, plus
	B. 1 dessert	2 days – 1/2 hour early bedtime, plus
Clean room (specified)	C. 1 free movie	3 days – wash windows for 1/2 hour, plus
Empty all trash recepticles		4 days – loss of allowance for 1 week, plus
Get self up in morning	1 day – A (1 hour tv time)	5 days – 1 hour unpleasant but utilitarian work
Attend school	3 days – A + B	
Do lessons	Week – A + B + C	
1/2 hour unspecified chores		On sixth day of consecutive failure, he:
	i.e., on seventh consecutive day	1. Gets no rewards
Weekly	of success, Thomas gets:	2. Does evening dishes
	A. 1 hour tv time	3. Goes to bed 1/2 hour early
Wash car	B. 1 dessert	4. Washes windows for 1/2 hour
Yard work (2 hours)	C. 1 free movie	5. Loses allowance for 1 week
Write letter to friend		6. Performs 1 hour unpleasant but
(1 to 2 pages long)		utilitarian work

PRACTICAL CONSIDERATIONS

Appointments

Following the detection of a problem calling for marriage and family counseling, many family physicians have found it more realistic to schedule the "patient" (meaning the recipient of treatment) for another interview, at which point more time is allowed for the subsequent visit. This avoids unnecessary delays in succeeding patients' appointments on the day of discovery or presentation of the initial problem. There is no reliable evidence that the *length* of a counseling appointment is at all correlated with a higher incidence of successful treatment outcome or patient satisfaction. Patients want to be *understood* and treated *effectively* and *efficiently,* which can take place in a 30 minute appointment just as well as in the traditionally "sacrosanct" 50 minute hour. In fact, utilizing a shorter appointment time might well help to educate the patient to use his interview time efficiently.

As each physician discovers and establishes his own rhythm of office practice, a natural time slot for scheduling counseling appointments will probably emerge. Some have chosen to schedule all counseling sessions for a single morning each week. Others enjoy a change of pace and schedule counseling appointments in the middle of the morning on successive days. Still others like to close out several afternoons a week with a single counseling appointment. It is best to do what is most comfortable and convenient in order to be the most proficient and experience the greatest degree of satisfaction.

Charges

A good way to *avoid* counseling is to charge for only a single office visit! This will cause a physician to hurry the counseling appointment or to ignore (by not becoming aware of) problems that need attention.

Charging for counseling services on the basis of *time* seems to be the most equitable method for both physician and "patient." The physician is compensated adequately, and the patient is encouraged to solve the problem and get on with life. If an average of five patients are seen in the office in 1 hour, then a 30 minute appointment for family counseling should cost the patient at the rate of 2.5 regular office visits.

Consultation

Having a good consultant available for marriage and family counseling can go a long way toward making a practice educationally rewarding, while enabling the physician to keep in touch with the best methods of treatment in current use, as well as providing a back-up in case of unexpected difficulties.

REFERENCES

1. Ackerman, W.: Treating the Troubled Family. New York, Basic Books, Inc., Publishers, 1966.
2. Addario, D., and Rogers, T. A.: Some techniques

for the initial interview in couples therapy. Hosp. Community Psychiatry, 25:799, 1974.

3. Azrin, N. H., Naster, B. J., and Jones, R.: Reciprocity counseling: A rapid learning-based procedure for marital counseling. Behav. Res. Ther., 11:365, 1973.

4. Bach, G. R., and Wyden, P.: Marital fighting: A guide to love. In Ard, B. N., and Ard, C. C. (eds.): Handbook of Marriage Counseling. Palo Alto, Cal., Science & Behavior Books, Inc., 1969.

5. Boszormenyi-Nagy, I., and Sparks, G. M.: Invisible Loyalties: Reciprocity in Intergenerational Family Therapy. New York, Harper & Row, Publishers, 1973.

6. Clinebell, C. H.: Meet Me in the Middle: On Becoming Human Together. New York, Harper & Row, Publishers, 1973.

7. Clinebell, H. J., and Clinebell, C. H.: Crisis and Growth: Helping your Troubled Child. Philadelphia, Fortress Press, 1971.

8. Clinebell, H. J., and Clinebell, C. H.: The Intimate Marriage. New York, Harper & Row, Publishers, 1970.

9. Committee on Adolescence, Group for the Advancement of Psychiatry: Normal Adolescence. New York, Charles Scribner's Sons, 1968.

10. Eisler, R. M., and Hersen, M.: Behavioral techniques in family-oriented crisis intervention. Arch. Gen. Psychiatry, 28:111, 1973.

11. Fine, S.: Troubled families: Parameters for diagnosis and strategies for change. Compr. Psychiatry, 15:73, 1974.

12. Fisher, E. O.: A guide to divorce counseling. The Family Coordinator, 22:55, 1973.

13. Friedman, P. H.: Outline (alphabet) of 26 techniques of family and marital therapy: A through Z. Psychother.: Ther., Res., Prac., 11:259, 1974.

14. Greer, S. E., and D'Zurilla, T. J.: Behavioral approaches to marital discord and conflict. J. Marr. Fam. Coun., 1:299, 1975.

15. Grace, P. C.: Bargaining: A system of marital counseling for the family practitioner. J. Maine Med. Assoc., 64:224, 1973.

16. Gurin, G., Veroff, J., and Feld, S.: Americans View their Mental Health: A Nationwide Interview Survey. New York, Basic Books, Inc., Publishers, 1970.

17. Gurman, A. S.: The effects and effectiveness of marital therapy: A review of outcome research. Family Process, 12:145, 1973.

18. Hadley, T. R., Jacob, T. Milliones, J., et al.: The relationships between family developmental crisis and the appearance of symptoms in a family member. Family Process, 13:209, 1974.

19. Haley, J.: Changing Families: A Family Therapy Reader. New York, Grune & Stratton, 1971.

20. Haley, J., and Hoffman, L. (eds.): Techniques of Family Therapy. New York, Basic Books, Inc., Publishers, 1967.

21. Hollender, M. H.: Selection of therapy for marital problems. Current Therapies, 11:119, 1971.

22. Landis, J. T., and Landis, M. G.: Marriage under special circumstances, In Landis, J. T., and Landis, M. G. (eds.): Building a Successful Marriage. Englewood Cliffs, New Jersey, Prentice-Hall, Inc., 1963.

23. Neuhaus, R. H., and Neuhaus, R. H.: Common crises in the life cycle. In Neuhaus, R. H., and Neuhaus, R. H. Family Crisis. Columbus, Ohio, Charles E. Merrill, Publishing Co., 1974.

24. Parsons, B. V., and Alexander, J. F.: Short term family intervention: A therapy outcome study. J. Consult. Clin. Psychol., 41:195, 1973.

25. Redmount, R. S. : Marriage problems and the medical professional. Conn. Med., 38:489, 1974.

26. Revitch, E.: The problem of conjugal paranoia. Dis. Nerv. Syst. 25:2, 1954.

27. Satir, V.: Conjoint Family Therapy. Palo Alto, Cal., Science & Behavior Books, Inc., 1967.

28. Satir, V.: Peoplemaking. Palo Alto, Cal., Science & Behavior Books, Inc., 1972.

29. Stuart, R.: Operant-interpersonal treatment for marital discord. J. Consult. Clin. Psychol., 33:675, 1969.

30. Stuart, R.: Token reinforcement in marital treatment. In Rubin, R., and Francks, C. M. (eds.): Advances in Behavior Therapy. New York, Academic Press, Inc., 1969.

31. Trainer, J. B.: The physician as marriage counselor. The Family Coordinator, 22:73, 1973.

32. Weiss, R. L., Birchler, G. R., and Vincent, J. P.: Contractual models for negotiation training in marital dyads. J. Marr. Fam., 36:321, 1974.

33. Weiss, R. L., Hops, H., and Patterson, G. R.: A framework for conceptualizing marital conflict: A technology for altering it, some data for evaluating it. In Hamerlynck, L. A., Handy, L. C., and Mash, E. J. (eds.): Behavior Change: Methodology, Concepts and Practice. Champaign, Ill., Research Press, 1973.

Chapter 34

SEXUAL COUNSELING

by LIBBY A. TANNER,
and LYNN P. CARMICHAEL

INTRODUCTION

Today's family physicians face a special challenge. The current "sexplosion" and openness in social attitudes have increased patients' expectations that family physicians be qualified and willing to help them with sexual concerns. Patients who desire sex education and counseling run the gamut from young mothers wishing advice for their toddlers through aging couples concerned about sexual inadequacy.

Do family physicians need to become sex educators and counselors in addition to all the other demands on their time? The answer is that sexual health or dysfunction must be considered in treating the whole person for any problem. Sexuality is an integral aspect of the total personality and aids in determining a person's sense of femininity or masculinity, self-concept, and sense of self-esteem. Sexual counseling occupies an essential place in the preventive care and health maintenance of the individual and family.

The clinical approach to sexual problems has changed considerably in the last decade. Sexual problems are no longer the sole responsibility of psychiatrists. Sex therapy, which combines behavioral modification with psychotherapeutic techniques, is now being practiced by individual and dual team therapists from a variety of counseling and medical backgrounds. Much scientific information regarding sexual physiology and behavior has become available, and some has been widely disseminated through the popular media. Many traditional health care organizations have recognized the need for improved sexual health, including the World Health Organization,

the American Medical Association, the American Public Health Association, the American Bar Association, the Sex Information and Education Council of the United States (SIECUS), and the National Council of Churches.[19] Many support the SIECUS position statement: "Sexual health care is a valid concern of the total health care to which everyone is entitled, and therefore, provision must be made for it in health care planning, with relation to mental and social, as well as physical well-being."[18]

This chapter will provide information about and an approach to working with sexual problems. The early part of the chapter offers a model for levels of physician intervention and details of obtaining a full or partial sex history. The next section is devoted to sexuality in the family life cycle and gives examples of sex education and counseling provided by the physician. The content and etiology of and current treatment methods for male and female sexual dysfunctions conclude the chapter.

THE PHYSICIAN AS SEX EDUCATOR AND COUNSELOR

Once the physician has accepted the philosophy that sexual health and sexual problems are in his domain, he needs to address himself to ways in which he can be effective with patients in this capacity. There are three major areas in which the physician must prepare himself to deal with sexual problems:

1. He must build up a broad base of knowledge concerning the wide range of human sexual behavior.

2. He must develop comfort with his

own sexuality and sexual value system, so he is not discomfited by his patients' sexuality. Burnap and Golden,[4] in their 1967 study, concluded that the personal comfort of the physician and the degree of initiative he took in asking sexual questions directly influenced the frequency of explicit sexual problems found in medical practice. The Sexual Attitude Restructuring (SAR) Workshop method,[24] utilizing explicit sexual media and discussions, has been used extensively in medical and other settings to help professionals work through sexual taboos that block communications with patients.

3. The physician must develop skills in evaluating and treating a variety of sexual problems. This may be accomplished by working with simple problems presented in his practice, attending continuing education seminars for further training, and working jointly with a skilled sex therapist on a per case basis.

The Plissit Model

Having a conceptual scheme by which the physician can organize his approach to patients assists him in meeting the demands of the three areas just discussed. One such conceptual scheme is the P–LI–SS–IT (permission–limited information–specific suggestion–intensive therapy) model offered by Jack S. Annon.[2] This model focuses on the easiest to the most difficult levels at which the busy physician can address himself to patients' sexual concerns.

Permission. At the first and most simple level, *P* stands for *permission*, which the physician gives by facilitating patients' abilities to express their sexual problems. It also means that the doctor, through his authoritative role, is implicitly giving the patient permission to *be* sexual. When the patient's problem is based (as it often is) on too strict societal and parental taboos about sexuality, the physician's permission becomes infinitely meaningful. Many patients are concerned about the normality of their sexual thoughts and behaviors. Some examples in which the clinician gives permission that the patient's behavior is acceptable are:

1. "The woman who has read that foreplay should be long, involved, and extended to at least 20 minutes, yet she re-

sponds quickly and experiences orgasm in a realtively short period of time. She is very satisfied with her response but worries that she is a 'nymphomaniac.'

2. The couple who have read or heard that simultaneous orgasm is the ideal goal in all sexual relationships. They usually have mutually enjoyable tandem orgasms, but they are worried because they are unable to achieve the 'ideal' goal of all 'normal' people.

3. The young couple who 'secretly' enjoys mutual oral–genital contact, but they have read or heard somewhere that this is considered 'perverted' or 'abnormal' or the symptoms of 'latent homosexual tendencies.'"[2]

Limited Information. At the second level, *LI* means *limited information*. Much of this approach focuses on correcting misinformation and myths and teaching sexual physiology and technique. A common example is the physician's coping with the male adolescent's worry about penis size. By stressing that erect penis sizes do not vary as much as flaccid ones and sharing the fact that this is something most young men do worry about, the young patient may be extremely relieved. Many sexual difficulties, such as discrepancies between partners' sexual interest levels, respond positively to simple reassurance, explanation of causes, and understanding of the patient's fears. We believe that much of the primary physician's role in sexual counseling is educational and permission-giving.

Specific Suggestion. A third, more complex level of patient care, utilizes SS, or *specific suggestion*, enabling patients to make certain adjustments in their sexual behavior. Proper attention to timing and readiness on the part of the patient determines when these suggestions can be made. The physician must be certain to obtain the proper sexual information to assure the appropriateness of his suggestions.

An example of specific suggestion occurs in some cases of secondary impotence when the patient and his partner are advised not to have intercourse for 1 or 2 weeks, but to engage in caressing, massage, and other variants of what might be termed foreplay (see Sensate Focus in later part of chapter). Often, when the man's anxiety is relieved by this nondemand sexual pleasuring, his erections return, and the couple may already have gone on to intercourse by the time they return for follow-up with the physician. This prescription of no intercourse, repeated for 2 more weeks, is often enough to turn the tide of anxiety to one of optimism.

Intensive Therapy. Finally, *IT* represents the highest level of skilled *intensive therapy*. Not only skill but time is necessary to do intensive sex therapy. Usually 10 or more sessions of about 1/2 to 1 hour in length are needed. In many cases the sex problem is only masking deeper problems of the individual or couple, necessitating help from a sex therapist, marriage counselor, or family therapist.

Attending seminars and training courses to reach this level of skill is easier now that many more continuing education opportunities are offered. However, most physicians will not have the time or inclination to undertake the necessary training for sex therapy. Referral outlets are still limited; therefore, the physician needs to explore community resources for the availability of psychiatrists, clinical psychologists, psychiatric social workers, or nurses who have taken this special training. The American Association of Sex Educators, Counselors and Therapists (AASECT)* has developed criteria for and a roster of certified sex therapists.

OBTAINING SEXUAL INFORMATION

For all patients during the full general medical check-up, the physician should be prepared to assess at least three areas: (1) the form or style of sex preference, (2) the frequency of sexual outlets, and (3) the patient's satisfaction with his sexual behavior. In addition, the physician who decides to help patients achieve sexual health must develop a comfortable interviewing style. Some opening questions he can use during the review of systems or afterward, when the patient returns to his office to discuss the findings, are: "Do you have any questions or problems regarding sex? Do you have any sexual difficulties you would like to talk about? Is your sexual functioning satisfactory to you? Do you have any questions about sexual response in yourself or your partner? Tell me about your sexual

---

*AASECT, 5010 Wisconsin Avenue, Washington, D.C. 20016.

behavior or functioning." The physician's attitude of interest and concern will go far toward making up any deficit in verbal skill.

The benefits of the above approach are manifold. Such questioning will facilitate the patient's expressing his present concern. It will also tell the patient that this is, indeed, a service the physician offers, now or at a later time, when and if needed.

The Sex History

When the patient comes in with a sexual dysfunction or if the physician uncovers one and plans to treat it, a complete sex history of each partner must be taken. Since this is a time-consuming effort and explores very private areas, it is recommended that a full sex history never be taken unless the physician plans to give the time necessary to treat the problem. If the physician plans to refer or if the problem does not appear serious, he will not need to take an in-depth history. All that is usually needed is a fuller understanding of the current situation.

Charles Wahl[29] suggests use of the ubiquity question, e.g., "Many people experience problems and concerns in their sexual lives. What kind have you had? Most men and women have masturbated or stimulated themselves at some time in their lives. When did you begin?" He also suggests going from the least sensitive to the most sensitive areas when obtaining sexual information.

The following is an abbreviated sex history that physicians may find useful.

A Sex History Outline

I. Description of presenting problem
  A. Person's label for and description of problem
  B. Under what circumstances the condition improves or what couple have tried to do about it
  C. Person's idea of normality
  D. Partner's reaction to problem
II. General history of problem
  A. Onset and progression
    1. Reactions
    2. Level of anxiety
  B. History of relationship between partners

1. What attracted couple to each other
2. Satisfaction and quality of the relationship
3. Areas of agreement and disagreement (sexual preferences)
4. Levels of individual sexual drive
5. Frequency of sexual outlets (sex play, masturbation, extramarital sex
6. Contraception
7. Pregnancies, abortions

C. Other factors
   1. Illness and operations, medications, alcohol and drug abuse
   2. Fatigue, stress, emotional problems
   3. Other family problems: children, money, in-laws, other

III. General background history of each partner
   A. Earliest experiences or childhood sexuality
      1. Sex play with siblings, other children; playing doctor
      2. How did patient learn about sex
      3. Self-stimulation: when and how often, was it disapproved or approved of
      4. Childhood fantasies and myths
   B. Parental atmosphere
      1. How parents felt about nudity and sex
      2. Parents' sexuality or affection
      3. Religion, discipline, and atmosphere in the home
   C. Adolescence
      1. Girls: menstruation, mother's communication to her, feelings, breast and body development, self-stimulation
      2. Boys: nocturnal emissions, masturbation, body changes
   D. Dating, petting, intercourse, orgasm
   E. Premarital sex, other relationships, other marriages
   F. Homosexual experiences, fantasies, wishes
   G. Sexual variations or deviations: fetishes, cross dressing, incest, molestation, prostitution, venereal disease, voyeurism, sadomasochism, rape, others

H. Erotic values: response to explicit sexual literature, movies, pictures and usage; use of erotic fantasies; sexual dreams, what works for patient

Other reference sources for complete sex histories can be found in Masters and Johnson's *Human Sexual Inadequacy*,[20] Richard Green's *Human Sexuality*,[9] and the Group for the Advancement of Psychiatry's report on *Assessment of Sexual Function: A Guide to Interviewing*.[10]

SEXUALITY AND THE FAMILY CYCLE

The concept of the family developmental life cycle aids the family physician in preparing to manage the multiple sex-related needs of the family. The following is an overview of some developmental stages with examples of areas in which patients have needs for sex education and counseling.

INFANCY AND CHILDHOOD

Human sexualization begins at birth and continues throughout life. The most powerful influence on the child's future sense of himself as a sexual being comes from early impressions, attitudes, and behavior learned in the family. By the age of three, the child's gender identity and sense of individual femininity or masculinity will be relatively fixed. Children particularly receive their values and feelings about sexuality from the way they are physically and emotionally handled by their parents.

The family physician can stress the importance of breast-feeding as a way of developing a close, touching bond between mother and child. Infants need much physical touching and fondling to become well-nourished and mentally healthy. A few mothers will be alarmed by the arousal of some sensual or sexual feelings during breast-feeding and need to be reassured that this is natural. Suggestions to the parents that the infant be allowed opportunities to explore his own nude body will result in the baby's finding pleasure in touching his mouth and genitals. If the parents become concerned about the latter, the physician can use this opportunity to point out that genital pleasuring and masturbation are normal, natural, self-affirming behaviors.

Parents often ask their family physician how to teach sex education to their children. The physician must first ascertain from the parents what their own values and beliefs are by asking how they themselves learned about sexuality and how they would like their children to learn about it. The physician may want to be ready for this kind of question by building up a small library of books, such as Wardell Pomeroy's *Boys and Sex*[22] and *Girls and Sex*,[23] The Child Study Association of America's *What to Tell Your Children About Sex*,[6] and Sol Gordon's books for children and parents.* SIECUS** also offers a bibliography of books that are useful for parents and children at various levels. In addition to recommending these books or articles to his patients, the physician may suggest methods or even phrases to assist the parents in this task.

The normal curiosity of children about sex, sex differences, and their own bodies is usually manifested in early sex play with children of the same and opposite sex. Some people remember these incidents, and many have repressed them, particularly if they have been severely punished for them. It is important that the physician reaffirm with the parents that this is natural curiosity and such early sex play does not lead to abnormality in the child or young adult. Physicians are often asked about the youngster who seems to be "in love" with the parent of the opposite sex. Freud referred to these syndromes as the Oedipus and Electra complexes. It is not uncommon to have a 3 year old girl throw herself upon her father bodily, trying to push the mother away from the father. These actions should be handled as normal manifestations of interest in the opposite sex. An open attitude by the family physician may have far-reaching preventive consequences in helping parents learn to deal with sexuality in less repressed ways than their own parents may have.

---

*Ed-U Press, 760 Ostrom Avenue, Syracuse, N.Y. 13210, has a complete listing of these and other books from the Institute of Family Research and Education.
**National Headquarters, Sex Information and Education Council of the United States (SIECUS), 137–155 North Franklin Street, Hempstead, N.Y. 11550.

PUBERTY AND EARLY ADOLESCENCE

There is an increase in erotic feelings and sexual activity after puberty. Usually this leads to beginning or increased masturbation. Many parents are extremely worried about the effects of masturbation and are concerned that they cannot control this usually secretive behavior. To quote from Mary Calderone, a foremost expert in the field of sex education,

The reassurance of the physician that masturbation is so universal as to be considered entirely normal, that indeed it is a valid and quite harmless way of expressing bodily pleasure and of releasing sexual tension, will do a great deal to offset whatever negative attitudes the parents have communicated. It will also lay the groundwork for a readiness on the part of the adolescent to seek medical help about more serious problems as they emerge in early and later sexual life, including such troubled and troubling questions as premarital sexual activity, contraceptive and pregnancy counseling and venereal disease.[5]

We know that adolescents worry a great deal about their body changes, secondary sexual characteristics, and growth patterns and have many misconceptions about the normality of menstruation, "wet dreams," masturbation, and other areas. The young person may be afraid of rejection by his parents or simply may not be able to transcend the bounds of privacy or secrecy often existing in families. The physician should initiate discussion alone with the youngster to allow response to such questions as, "Most young people are concerned about changes in their bodies. Have you ever wondered whether your body (or breasts, or penis) are normal for your age?" Sometimes the physician may have to speak *for* the patient, using any comfortable manner that allows the young person to open up about his underlying worries. The physician is then in a position to give some sex education in a short, nonlecturing approach, relieving the youngster of guilt and reassuring him of his normalcy.

Sol Gordon, Director of the Marriage and Family Counseling Program at Syracuse University, makes the following statement: "Sex education is a life-long process that begins in the home and continues in the schools, the media, and the community.... If parents wanted to be the only sex educators of their children they would have to prevent them from going to any public school bathroom, having any friends, watching television, or reading virtually anything (including the Bible)."[8] He goes on to state that extremist opposition to sex education is often based on the irrational idea that if you tell children about sex, they will do it. According to research studies, the fact is that mature, responsible sexual behavior is positively correlated with sexual knowledge.

LATE ADOLESCENCE

One does not have to be an expert in sexual counseling to know there has been an increase in both expectations and sexual behavior among young people today. A Michigan State University survey[28] over a 3 year period from 1970 to 1973 found significant increases in coitus for 14 and 15 year olds. They also found that by age 17, rates of sexual behavior were almost as high for females as for males, which is a departure from the past.

The question, "Are you now or have you become sexually active?" must be included in health care for the late adolescent. Issues of morals, ethics, and law plague many a physician when he decides whether or not to prescribe an oral contraceptive or intrauterine device for a 12 to 17 year old or refer her for requested abortion. The physician in these situations needs to adopt a nonjudgmental approach in permitting the patient to tell what behavior is being engaged in so that the physician can make a rational determination of the best medical advice to give.

There are a variety of other problems of a sexual nature that troubled families bring to the family physician. One family with 11 children was distraught upon discovering their eldest son (aged 17) had been sexually involved with his sisters. This family had never been able to discuss sexual matters with their children.

Other problems may include cross dressing, voyeurism, sexual fetishes, and a host of sexual behaviors. Alex Comfort[7] suggests that professionals should be less concerned with what is normal or abnormal behavior and more interested in finding out what meaning the behavior has for the patient, as well as society. Treatment for the more

compulsive disorders may be outside the purview of the family physician, but he must be able to help manage the family's solution to the crisis.

YOUNG ADULT

Homosexual Concerns

Another concern that often appears in the adolescent or young adult years has to do with homosexuality and bisexuality. It is not unusual to find patients who become depressed or even suicidal because they believe one or more casual adolescent homosexual experiences brand them a homosexual for life. One college student, experiencing difficulties with his heterosexual life, panicked because he found himself physically attracted to his roommate. He wondered if this meant he was a homosexual. In giving information, the physician can utilize the Kinsey[16] zero to six continuum, which indicates that none of us is born either heterosexual or homosexual, but all are subject to experiences, fantasies, and thoughts that sometime include members of the same sex. Kinsey found that one-third to one-half of American men had had some overt homosexual experience during adolescence but only 4 to 8 per cent became exclusive homosexuals. For the patient who is comfortably "gay," the physician needs to demonstrate willingness to give good medical care nonjudgmentally.

Cohabitation

Many young people of college age are now using cohabitation to test their own sexuality and commitment to their boy- or girlfriend. This behavior does not appear to reflect promiscuous behavior. Generally, these young persons tend to be serially monogamous and are more comfortable with a commitment accompanied by affection. The phenomenon of living together, either before or instead of marriage, apparently has become relatively fixed in our society at this point in time. Many parents are very concerned about their sons and daughters' living with others outside of marriage and may need the physician to be a good listener and counselor. Hunt's study of sexual behavior in the 1970's indicates that the figures may rise as high as 75 per cent for young women who are not virgins at the time of marriage.[11] It would be inappropriate for the physician to indicate any moral judgment about this behavior, but, instead, he should be prepared to deal with any problems it might bring.

MARRIAGE — PREMARITAL AND EARLY STAGES

At a recent marital health workshop sponsored by the Bowman-Gray School of Medicine, there were some suggestions about approaches by the family physician. The relatively uncommon premarital examination or other office visits are cited as opportunities to open a frank discussion relative to sexuality, as well as other possible sources of conflict in the marriage. Many times couples may be too embarrassed or afraid to show sexual ignorance by asking questions. The physician should initiate discussion concerning previous sexual experience together, different positions and techniques, male and female and individual differences in frequency of desire and sexual capacity.

A yearly marital check-up was suggested as a good time to take a calm, objective appraisal of the strengths and weaknesses of the marital bond. There are at least three transitional periods at which the couple should be helped to see how the marriage is going — 4 months after marriage; 7 months after conception, anticipating the changes the new baby will bring the marital dyad; and 4 months after the birth of a baby — as well as the annual check-up. The early years of raising children are often particularly stressful times for married couples. The physician can help prevent future serious strains by questioning how the marital and sexual relationship is going.

Pregnancy

It has been traditional to prohibit coitus during the 6 weeks prior to and following delivery. This has often caused needless disruption of marital relations leading, in some instances, to the onset of extramarital relations by a disgruntled husband. Current data[12, 27] indicate that unless there are medical contraindications (such as a history of spontaneous abortions) the patient and her partner should be encouraged to have relations whenever they wish during the pregnancy and as soon thereafter as the patient has healed and has no perineal discomfort.

THE MIDDLE AND LATER YEARS

After the child-rearing years are over, the couple have 25 or more years of marriage. The middle years, a period much neglected by writers and educators, are a source of much marital and sexual discord. Aging patients are very concerned about their health and its relation to sexual activity.

The Middle-Aged and Aging Female

In terms of her self-esteem and sexual functioning, the menopause or a hysterectomy has often signified to the woman that her sexual life is, or should be, over. Physicians may have contributed inadvertently to this pessimistic view. The woman needs to be reassured that she will be able to function as well as or better than before. Her sexual response will depend on her relationship to her partner and her interest in continuing to be a sexual person. There is no time limit to female sexuality. It is important for her to know: (1) the uterus is only minimally involved in the orgasmic response and is not necessary for orgasm, (2) changes in estrogen levels some years after menopause may affect her total well-being but will have little or nothing to do directly with her physiologic sexual response, and (3) as she gets older, the walls of the vagina may become thin and inelastic, and there may be a drying of the vaginal mucosa. Estrogen cream topically applied is very effective.

Levels of female masturbation increase up to the middle years, after which time its frequency remains constant.[21] Some older women begin to utilize self-stimulation to meet their sexual needs when they have lost a partner or the partner no longer satisfies them sexually. Masturbation as a viable outlet for older persons must be included in a discussion of healthy functioning.

The Middle-Aged and Aging Male

The male does not experience a physiologic climacteric in the same way that the female experiences menopause. However, even 40 and 50 year old males begin to have fears of losing their sexual powers. The male often experiences some actual physiologic changes in his middle years that, although minor, may be viewed by him with alarm and anxiety, impeding his potency. Depression is not uncommon, with lowered libido as a concomitant. Explaining that lack of libido or erectile difficulty is tied to the depression may be the first step in managing the depressed patient.

The physician needs to be prepared to give information about the physiologic effects of the aging process on sexual response. Middle-aged or aging males should be told: (1) as time goes by, erections will occur less frequently and vigorously and may not always be as firm as before, (2) direct stimulation of the penis may be needed for an erection, (3) it may take longer to achieve an erection, (4) the time between one erection and the next may be longer, (5) the prostate and seminal vesicles do not contract with the same frequency, and the ejaculate is not as forceful, (6) an ejaculation may not occur every time he has sexual activity, or the ejaculation may be delayed, (7) the ejaculation is thinner and scantier, and the seminal fluid gradually diminishes, (8) because the need for ejaculation is reduced, an erection may be maintained longer than in the past, permitting a longer intromission time, (9) sexual interest will not die; in fact, it will continue almost unabated until well into the seventh or eighth decade, and (10) even after necessary prostate surgery, the patient's potency may not be affected.

The physician can inform and reassure by stressing the possibility of sexual longevity if regular sexual activity is continued. Couples need to understand there is a lot more to their sexual activity than just intercourse and should be encouraged to continue caressing, massaging, and touching each other and allowing for alternate ways of making love without the emphasis on orgasm and intercourse that may have been a prime object of their concern during their earlier years.

ILLNESS AND DISEASE

Our society has tended to desexualize the mentally or physically handicapped person. We no longer believe that a mentally retarded person or one with cerebral palsy or a spinal cord injury is not interested in sex or capable of it.

The physician must discuss sexual functioning with the ill person as soon as possible after the critical stages of the illness have passed, whether this be a myocardial infarction, surgery, or whatever, since the patient will already be concerned about permissible future activity, including sexual relations. The physician must, by his demeanor and verbalizations, express belief in this person as a sexual being who may have to modify his activity for the time being, but who will certainly not have to terminate it unless he wishes to. Both partners should discuss with the physician the level of functioning they wish or can be encouraged to reach following an illness or surgery. It is essential that the physician determine what the couple's level of activity was prior to the illness, as there are instances in which a couple's sex life was so unsatisfactory that it would be a real relief to both if it were abandoned.

For many couples a discussion with the family physician following an illness may be the first time they communicate openly about sex. As in pregnancy, more serious harm can be done to patients' emotional and marital life by overly severe restrictions than by permitting sexual relations desired by the couple. Space does not allow a thorough discussion of the effect of specific illness and disease on sexuality. Additional information can be found in studies by the American Medical Association Committee on Human Sexuality,[1] Israel and Rubin,[12] and Kaplan.[13]

THE MAJOR SEXUAL DYSFUNCTIONS

The content and etiology of current treatment methods for the six major sexual dysfunctions will be discussed in the following order: for the male, impotence, premature ejaculation, and retarded ejaculation; for the female, general sexual dysfunction (erroneously called frigidity), orgasmic dysfunction, and vaginismus. Retrograde ejaculation and dyspareunia will also be evaluated briefly.

Let us review briefly the sexual response of both the male and female to understand how these problems may occur. Helen

Singer Kaplan, author of *The New Sex Therapy*,[13] describes a biphasic physiologic sexual response: "It consists of two distinct and relatively independent components: a genital vasocongestive reaction which produces penile erection in the male and vaginal lubrication and swelling in the female; and the reflex clonic muscular contractions which constitute orgasm in both genders." For the male, erectile problems can occur during the excitement or vasocongestive phase; for the female, the corresponding problem is lack of arousal or lubrication. It is possible for one component of this biphasic response to become inhibited or impaired while the other remains normal. In the second, or orgasmic, phase the man can have problems such as premature, retarded, or retrograde ejaculation. For the woman, the comparable impairment is anorgasmia, or inability to have orgasm.

GENERAL DISCUSSION OF TREATMENT

To facilitate the discussion of treatment of the various male and female sexual dysfunctions, first we will outline the therapy that is common to most of them.

Sensate Focus

Essentially there are three steps in the behavioral treatment of most sexual problems. Variations in treatment are tailored to the individual's or couple's problem. (Patients are asked to refrain from intercourse throughout the total treatment period.)

1. During the first phase the couple are instructed to find time to be alone, nude, in a lighted room, with no interruptions. They are to take turns slowly caressing and exploring all parts of each other's bodies, leaving out the breasts, nipples, and genital area. The emphasis is on communicating the various sensations evoked in response to this nondemand pleasuring. Each is to tell the other what kind of touch is desired and what "feels good." The demand for sexual performance is removed, and mutual enjoyment is stressed, regardless of the presenting symptom. They are to use "I language," speaking only for the self, trying not to mind-read the partner's feelings or desires. They are required to spend at least 1 hour three or four times during the

week repeating these exercises until no anxiety is aroused. When they return to the physician or therapist, a determination of their ease and lack of anxiety is made, and the second phase is discussed with them. This phase may continue for several weeks.

2. In the second phase, genital and breast stimulation is added to the nondemand touch-and-tell technique. Usually for male problems, the female is told to position herself facing him between his legs to give her easy access to his body and genitalia. She is asked to stimulate the penis and scrotal area by hand or mouth for as long as it is comfortable for them both. Use of the stop-start method—stopping stimulation when an erection or too much excitement occurs and then resuming stimulation when the erection goes down—reinforces the patient's belief that he can have erections that may come and go. Both partners take turns caressing each other, regardless of which partner has the presenting complaint.

3. The third phase uses the woman superior position, which is less demanding for the male and puts the female in control of the situation. The female will stimulate the male to erection and lower herself upon his penis. (In some cases, "stuffing" the limp penis into the vagina may create a nondemand situation in which erection may occur.) They will lie quietly together, experiencing the sensations of vaginal containment. The female or male may use rolling pelvic motions, but there will be no thrusting for intercourse or ejaculation. When this phase has been completed successfully, the couple can go on to coitus when ready. However, noncoital sex is always continued as a vital part of their total sexual involvement.

In addition to the sensate focus exercises, the couple are given much reinforcement to lessen anxiety and fears. The patient is urged to use a favorite sexual fantasy (or make one up) to distract obsessive thinking and "spectatoring." The dysfunctional partner is encouraged to "be selfish" and focus exclusively on self-gratification, to give up fear of rejection or guilt, and to abandon one's self to sexual feelings. If the nondysfunctional partner becomes excited by the exercises, the other is encouraged to caress and bring the partner to orgasm by manual or oral means after the session is concluded. This is often essential in keeping the nondysfunctional partner from sabotaging treatment.

The fact that both partners must be involved in the genesis and treatment of the problem and that the relationship is the focus of treatment alleviates unnecessary guilt on the part of the affected individual. They take turns pleasuring each other to encourage mutuality. Open communication is stressed. Sex therapy allows couples to "start all over again" and learn new ways of relating to each other.

It is not unusual to find couples resisting the treatment by overt or covert means. A common resistance is insisting they cannot find the time for homework exercises. Some of this is due to the work ethic and upward mobility of many couples, or it may be resistance to moving into intimacy and giving up power struggles in the relationship. It may be necessary for the physician to refer the couple to a marital or sex therapist when the methods he recommends are not sufficient to work through these obstacles.

MALE DYSFUNCTION

ERECTILE DYSFUNCTION (IMPOTENCE)

The term *impotence*, meaning powerlessness, should rarely be used directly with the patient. If the patient states he is impotent, the physician should not simply accept this self-labeling but should obtain an accurate description of the problem. To avoid reinforcing the concept "impotent," he should say something like, "How often do you have erectile difficulty?" A number of other questions must be asked in order to delineate the problem. "Does this occur during all sexual encounters? Do you have difficulty in erecting, or only in maintaining the erection, or both? Is the problem different at different times of day or night or with different partners? Has this problem been of recent onset, or has it gradually come upon you? Is it related to specific instances of stress, such as after a party, a drinking bout, or a fight with your spouse? Do you still have erections on awakening and when masturbating?"

In the past, both the literature and the patient population tended to call any male sexual problem "impotence." Now we realize there are several distinct syndromes, of which erectile difficulty is just one.

Masters and Johnson, in *Human Sexual Inadequacy*,[20] divide sexual dysfunction into two types: primary and secondary. A man who is *primarily* impotent is "never able to achieve and/or maintain an erection of quality sufficient to accomplish successful coital connection." This condition is found relatively infrequently in the population.

The more common type is *secondary* impotence, in which the male previously functioned well but then developed sexual difficulty. In these cases, the male may feel aroused and excited or may wish to feel aroused, but his penis simply does not erect, or it erects only to lose its hardness when he is ready to penetrate. It is possible for some impotent men to ejaculate with a flaccid penis. Some estimate that about half the male population has had occasional transient episodes of impotence, for example, young men just beginning their sexual life, men with new partners or in stressful situations, men in their middle years who begin to fear the effects of aging, and older men from time to time also. Too much alcohol commonly causes transient impotence.

A male who has had some episodes of impotence can become incredibly anxious and frustrated and may feel his masculinity is on the line. He needs all the immediate help the physician can muster: information, reassurance, permission-giving, and specific suggestions.

Etiology

Physical Causes. Depression, diabetes, vascular diseases, alcoholism, stress and fatigue, some medications, and certain types of prostatic surgical procedures are among the most common physical causes. The way in which chronic illness, heart attacks, and prostatic surgery are handled with the patient may induce secondary psychologic impotence because of fear of future failure. In ruling out physical causes of primary and secondary impotence, the physician should look for all signs of potency, such as nocturnal and morning erections and masturbatory activity. Some sleep laboratories and urologists utilize a nocturnal penile tumescence monitor to assist in determining potency.[14] Masters and Johnson[20] state, "Among the 213 men referred to the Foundation for treatment of secondary impotence, there have only been seven cases in which physiological dysfunction overtly influenced the onset of the sexual inadequacy."

Psychologic Causes. It has been estimated that at least 95 per cent of impotence is psychogenic. It is obvious that emotional or psychogenic problems rarely can be attributed to a single cause. In both male and female sexual dysfunction, causation is usually multifarious and may include immediate performance anxiety, restrictive upbringing, ignorance about sexuality, intrapsychic problems, and severe interpersonal conflict.

Relationship problems are among the most prominent causes of all sexual inadequacy. If the relationship is too dishonest or destructive, sex therapy will not be helpful, and there may be questionable success even in long-term marital therapy.

Poor communication contributes to sexual failure, since most couples have not learned an effective language for sex and are not comfortable asking for what they want or do not want in sexual behavior. Additionally, women have been reluctant to express themselves about sexual needs because of what they believed to be the fragility of the male ego, since the male was supposed to be the experienced sexual partner. The husband, on the other hand, often fears his wife's rejection if he were to ask for certain types of sexual behavior from her or is unable or unwilling to have sex when she wants it.

The most common immediate cause of impotence is performance anxiety. Usually this occurs after the patient has had one or more episodes of impotence or failure to maintain his erection. The person involved in "spectatoring" (a Masters-Johnson term) is constantly watching his own performance, wondering when and if it will be successful. Since erections cannot be willed, the attendant anxiety assures another failure, and a spiral of anxiety and failure ensues.

Treatment

Following history-taking and delineation of the problem with the couple, it is appropriate first to suggest to the male that he begin masturbating, if he has not already done so. This will demonstrate that he can stimulate himself, come to a full erection, and ejaculate. It is reassuring to the patient and may condition him to more successful behavior with his partner. The couple are instructed in the sensate focus tasks, tailored to their particular defenses and needs. (The treatment is thoroughly discussed under the section on Sensate Focus.)

PREMATURE EJACULATION

Premature ejaculation is considered to be one of the most common male sexual dysfunctions and occurs at all socioeconomic levels and degrees of mental health. There are many definitions of premature ejaculation. One that is not dependent on female response, but gets to the core of the problem, is that premature ejaculation results when a man is unable to exert voluntary control over his ejaculatory reflex. This may be a long-standing problem occurring after a minimal amount of sexual stimulation, regardless of the partner or situation, or may be a milder disorder connected with other male or female dysfunctions or relationship problems.

Etiology

A number of causes of premature ejaculation have been postulated. Very rarely have physical causes been considered a problem, although prostatitis can be a possibility, as can multiple sclerosis and other degenerative neurologic disorders. Some psychologic causes may be basic ambivalence toward women or interpersonal problems, such as a man who does not wish to satisfy his wife or may be acting out some hostility toward her. The most common theory of causation by Masters and Johnson and others is that during the young male's initial sexual experience he was under stress, such as hurried masturbation or pressured intercourse in a car or on a girlfriend's couch, thereby reinforcing a pattern of rapid ejaculation. Use of withdrawal for contraception can intensify this problem. Performance anxiety, guilt, and fear are basic problems in premature ejaculation. Kaplan[13] believes the man is distracted by anxiety from perceiving the sensations preliminary to orgasm, thus losing sensory feedback that is necessary to bring this reflex function under control. Some authorities call these few seconds before orgasm "aura" or "ejaculatory inevitability."

Treatment

Treatment was instituted in 1956 by James Semans, a urologist who suggested the stop-start technique.[25] The female partner stimulates the penis manually or orally until the patient experiences "aura." She then stops all stimulation until the sensation disappears, resuming it again until the patient reaches the same point. The male is to concentrate on his erotic sensations, allowing no distracting thoughts about his partner or possible failure to interfere with his attention.

The squeeze technique is essentially the same, and both methods are used by various sex therapists. The female stimulates the male until he experiences "aura," then squeezes the penis with her fingers just below the rim of the glans with enough force to cause the patient to lose his erection partially. Stimulation is then resumed and the squeeze repeated several times, alternating stimulation and squeeze. The male can also use the squeeze himself or put his hand over the female's to demonstrate how hard she can press. This is continued until the male controls ejaculation at least four times during each encounter, after which he may ejaculate. Use of a lubricant or petrolatum is introduced along with manual stimulation.

At a later stage, the couple are allowed to go on to nondemand penetration with the woman-above position. The female stimulates, then mounts the penis, gets off, and squeezes the penis when "aura" is reached. Alternatively, she can use a bulbar squeeze at the base of the penis or simply remain motionless until the preorgastic sensation disappears. As ejaculatory control is being achieved, intercourse in the male-superior position is suggested, but the stop-start or squeeze exercises should be continued on some regular basis even after treatment is terminated.

We have suggested for single men without partners, as well as in treatment with couples, that the man stimulate himself and apply the squeeze at home alone, in private. He becomes more sensitive to his own "aura" and in some situations may learn much control by himself before involving his partner. Sometimes it is best to begin with couple treatment, if masturbation by her spouse is unacceptable to the wife.

Other aspects of sensate focus are used in conjunction with the squeeze or stop-start techniques to give the couple an opportunity to relearn a sensuous and sexual approach to each other that does not focus solely on rapid intercourse and orgasm.

RETARDED EJACULATION

The third major male dysfunction is termed retarded ejaculation, or ejaculatory incompetence. It is the least frequent male problem. The problem may be primary, i.e., a male's never having ejaculated intravaginally or never having ejaculated at all by any means. A secondary case of retarded ejaculation usually occurs after a period of normal ejaculatory functioning when the patient either begins to exhibit either occasional inhibition of ejaculation or is never able to reach orgasm during intercourse. Some of these patients can masturbate after withdrawal from the vagina or will respond to manual or oral stimulation by the partner. Some are able to do this with certain partners but not with others. In many ways, retarded ejaculators resemble nonorgastic women who respond sexually to stimulation and reach a high plateau of excitement but are unable to effect orgastic release. In cases of infertility, the physician should question the male closely about ejaculation into the vagina, as some men have concealed this problem from their wives.

Etiology

Retarded ejaculation is rarely due to physical causes, but the use of antipsychotic or antihypertensive drugs, as well as any severe neurologic condition, should be explored, particularly in secondary cases in which this dysfunction occurs with self-stimulation as well as with a partner. Aging has been suggested as a common cause of an intermittent inability to ejaculate as the male approaches his sixth decade. The following psychologic causes have been suggested: conflict over strict religious upbringing; unconscious fears of castration or injury by the female vagina; a destructive interactional pattern, such as an involuntary holding back as an act of rebellion; anger or hostility toward a dominating wife; fears of impregnation; problems of intimacy with women; a specific traumatic event, such as discovering a wife's infidelity; or guilt over a sexual encounter.

Treatment

Treatment consists, essentially, of providing a series of desensitizing experiences along with sensate focus. Usually the couple first engage in nongenital pleasuring and move on to oral and manual genital stimulation, while intercourse and ejaculation are forbidden. In the next stage the male is instructed to ejaculate in his wife's presence when he is sufficiently aroused by any means, such as masturbation. If successful, he goes on to stimulation by his wife and ejaculation. In each succeeding experience, he is told to move closer and closer to the vaginal entrance, later entering the vagina just as he is about to ejaculate. If penetration retards his ejaculation, he withdraws to be stimulated by his partner. In the final stage, manual stimulation and intercourse are combined until the male is able to enter the vagina at lower levels of excitement and still reach orgasm by vaginal penetration.

Treatment usually has to be combined with psychotherapeutic techniques aimed at focusing on resistance or sabotage of treatment by either partner. The female may resist providing for her husband's needs with little attention to her own, and the male may find himself distracted or too anxious to continue.

RETROGRADE EJACULATION

Retrograde ejaculation is not one of the major dysfunctions but may cause a good deal of worry when discovered by a patient. It is characterized by orgasm without ejaculation, or rather, ejaculation occurs into the bladder due to failure of the internal sphincter of the bladder to close. It is almost always due to organic factors—"interference with the integrity of the bladder neck or its sympathetic nerve supply...post ganglionic sympathetic blocking agents and diabetes may also cause ejaculation into the bladder."[17]

FEMALE DYSFUNCTIONS

In the past, the term *frigidity* had been used to describe all kinds of female dysfunctions. Sexual counseling experts today are using this term sparingly, as many feel it is pejorative, implying that a woman who has a sexual problem is cold and hostile toward men.

Masters and Johnson[20] categorize female dysfunctions into orgasmic dysfunctions, vaginismus, and dyspareunia. We prefer Kaplan's[13] three major categories of female dysfunction:

1. *General sexual dysfunction*, which could be termed frigidity, refers to lack of arousal, lack of erotic feelings, and an absence of lubrication or other vaginal changes. This symptom is analogous to impotence in that both lubrication and erection are the first signs of vasocongestion and early sexual excitement.

2. *Orgastic dysfunction*, which is the most common female sexual complaint, is exemplified by a woman who arouses easily, lubricates, has genital swelling, and reaches plateau but has difficulty reaching orgasm.

3. *Vaginismus*, which has nothing to do with the physiologic biphasic sexual response, but is a special instance of an involuntary spastic contraction of the vaginal musculature that prevents penetration. It may be partial or so severe as to cause an unconsummated marriage. Dyspareunia will also be briefly discussed.

ETIOLOGY OF FEMALE DYSFUNCTION

Physical causes of female dysfunction are relatively rare. The female sexual response appears to be more stable in the face of physical disease. Diabetes and aging are two examples in which the male's response is much more vulnerable than the female's. Although rare, physical factors such as endocrine diseases and those affecting muscle tone or neurologic function must be considered.

It is important to remember that women generally need sufficient physical stimulation to be aroused enough for orgasm. Women are usually slower to respond than men, with an average of about 20 minutes of a slow, steady build-up being required. If the stimulation ceases, or if the female is distracted, she generally drops down to a nonexcited state. Obviously, the stereotyped lover who provides little or no foreplay and then "dives for the vagina" is not providing sufficient stimulation for any but the most highly responsive woman.

To really understand female sexuality and the etiology of female dysfunction, one must look at the developmental and cultural components as well as psychologic factors. From their earliest years, many little girls are valued for being pretty, clean, passive, and compliant, not for being sexually responsive. Even their bathroom habits militate against finding and stimulating their genitals. Little boys have much easier access to their genitalia and more societal permission to touch. This appears to have implications for women's sexuality, since only 60 to 70 per cent of women learn to masturbate at some time in their lives. Those women who have never masturbated tend to have the most difficulty becoming orgasmic in later years. (The figures for male masturbation range from 95 to almost 100 per cent.) As the teenage girl begins dating, she receives mostly negative messages from parents, school, and church, emphasizing sex as something dirty, sinful, and bad or to be saved for marriage and reproduction. Even if such negative connotations are avoided, young girls are often given almost no sex education, with the exception of limited information about menstruation. The natural consequence of the dating game is that the girl is given responsibility for "keeping the brakes on." She is encouraged to act sexy to get dates and be popular, but not to *be* sexual. She constantly shuts down her natural sexual responsivity during petting, so it is no surprise that after she marries she often cannot go beyond the excitement phase. Sometimes, as in the case of the woman who has general sexual dysfunction, she cannot give herself permission to receive sexual stimulation.

Studies have disclosed an appalling ignorance by females of their own anatomy and physiology. This is a factor in a number of teenage illegitimate pregnancies. Ignorance also figures heavily in the female's lack of understanding of what she needs or can permit in terms of sexual stimulation.

Women have been programmed to be dependent on men for getting things done, getting married, and being supported economically. This dependency often results in a woman who assumes no responsibility for her own sexual pleasure, is not sexually assertive on her own behalf, and is profoundly afraid of rejection by her lover or husband, were she to reveal any sexual needs. Even women with high sex drives believe they should not initiate sex, since this is a male prerogative. Indeed, some men are threatened by women who become sexually assertive, believing their sexual adequacy is being questioned.

Other factors inhibiting the female response are certain myths that have assumed the power of truths. The freudian myth that a vaginal orgasm is more mature and non-neurotic than a clitoral one has done much damage to women's self-esteem. Masters and Johnson's physiologic data refute this myth, demonstrating that all orgasms, regardless of source of stimulation (from breast, clitoris, or intercourse), are physiologically the same. The clitoris is the most important female sexual organ in terms of triggering sexual response, but orgasm consists of rhythmic spasms of the perivaginal musculature. Women experience orgasms differently at different times and generally have placed much value on having orgasm during coitus. Kaplan and others estimate that 40 to 50 per cent of women cannot achieve orgasm through coitus alone due to insufficient clitoral stimulation.

Other general factors that influence female responsiveness and can cause dysfunction as well as dyspareunia can be a pathologic love of father, fear and anger toward men, shame, fear, and guilt due to repressive upbringing, a fear of losing control, power struggles, and a hostile and dependent relationship with her partner.

GENERAL SEXUAL DYSFUNCTION

General sexual dysfunction is the most severe female inhibition. This problem varies considerably from someone with a minor problem who passively accepts her lack of response to a woman who uses any subterfuge to refuse having sexual relations (sexual aversion).

Treatment

Treatment consists of following the sensate focus tasks: having no intercourse and caressing and touching the partner's body with the woman giving first so she can receive unrestrictedly and without concern for the man's needs. After this is accepted without anxiety, the man, using a light touch, caresses the woman's nipples, breasts, clitoris, and vaginal entrance in a nondemanding atmosphere, following the woman's directions. Any position is acceptable but one that has been suggested has the man's back to the headboard with the woman between his legs facing in the same direction, making it possible for his hands to caress all parts of her body. At the third stage, nondemand coitus is at the woman's initiation. She uses the woman-superior position and sets the pace, concentrating on vaginal containment and sensation and using slow, rotating pelvic movements. As she now has coital thrusting under her control, she can decide when to proceed. If the male must ejaculate, they separate, but the male continues to stimulate the female. The crucial aspect of these low-pressure homework tasks is to allow the female a nonthreatening erotic ambiance in which to abandon herself and get in touch with erotic feelings.

ORGASTIC DYSFUNCTION

Problems in reaching orgasm are the most prevalent sexual complaints of women. If a woman has never experienced orgasm by any means, she may be considered "preorgasmic" or suffering from a primary orgastic dysfunction. The disorder is secondary if it developed after she had previously been orgastic. Some women can reach a climax only under specific situations, such as with a special lover, or a specific position, or alone using a vibrator.

Treatment

There are a number of treatment approaches. One method, developed in California by Lonnie Barbach[3] (described in her book, *For Yourself*) focuses on preorgasmic women in groups, meeting for educational and therapeutic purposes. They are taught to look at, touch, and appreciate their bodies and talk through their ambivalent feelings about becoming orgasmic. Masturbation in a step-wise sequence is taught as one way to find out what is stimulating to the individual woman and to help her reach orgasm. The women are encouraged to think erotically, indulge in sexual fantasies, and read erotic literature before or during masturbation exercises. They may begin with mildly erotic scenes and move on to more erotic ones as anxiety is lessened. Films, slides, and reading material are used extensively in the groups. Usually ten sessions of education and encouragement are needed in addition to the women's homework exercises. A vibrator may be suggested as an adjunct if she does not respond to her own or her partner's stimulation. After concentrating on self, the woman is helped to share her new knowledge with her partner.

Kegel's[15] exercises to strengthen the pubococcygeal muscle are introduced to help women become aware of this muscle and its contractibility. They are instructed to practice stopping and starting when urinating and then to continue the practice of squeezing these muscles and holding the contraction for about 6 seconds, up to 50 times per day. During masturbation or coitus, the woman is encouraged to tighten her abdominal and perineal muscles to encourage orgasm.

Barbach's method can be used with a patient alone but is more dependent on the therapist's or physician's own personality and supportiveness. A masturbation film from Multi Media* entitled *Margo* and a three-section Focus International** film, *Becoming Orgasmic: A Sexual Growth Program for Women*, are extremely useful for the busy physician's office and relieve any problems of constraint between male physician and female patient. A booklet, "Masturbation Techniques for Women—The Yes Book," is also available from Multi Media.

The female masturbation techniques can be combined with couple treatment using the sensate focus series previously outlined.

Many couples, aware that the woman cannot achieve orgasm with coitus alone, pro-

---

*Sex education films may be obtained from Multi Media Resource Center, Inc., 1525 Franklin Street, San Francisco, Cal. 94109.

**Focus International, Inc., 505 West End Avenue, New York, N.Y. 10024.

vide concurrent clitoral stimulation or help her climax by manual or oral stimulation before or after intercourse. However, this is not acceptable to some women who want to achieve a so-called "vaginal" orgasm. The couple are instructed to use rear-entry positions or side-by-side positions to allow the man to continue stimulating the clitoral area during intromission. He should begin to withdraw clitoral stimulation as the woman reaches climax—in later sessions progressively decreasing the amount of clitoral stimulation as intercourse proceeds. In time, she may learn to thrust in her own rhythm to orgasm.

VAGINISMUS

Vaginismus is a relatively uncommon sexual dysfunction. It may be presented along with any of the other female dysfunctions, or the condition may be specific. Usually the patient has associated physical or psychologic pain with vaginal penetration and becomes increasingly afraid of intercourse. Any etiology previously outlined can be causative, including severe or strict religious background, rape, ignorance about sex, and guilt over sexual conflicts.

Treatment

The treatment of vaginismus should begin with a thorough pelvic examination during which the patient can be encouraged to learn about her genital anatomy with the aid of a mirror. If her husband is cooperative, he can observe the examination, becoming more aware of what may be happening to his wife. Of course, pelvic disease and pathology must be ruled out at this time.

Continuing treatment provides the patient with psychologic help and support, while encouraging her to try progressive sexual exercises to relieve the muscular spasm. Deep breathing and relaxation exercises are useful adjuncts to the process. She should be encouraged to try using her own fingers to examine her genitals, inserting one finger when ready. This progresses to the use of two or more fingers, then moving the fingers around in the vagina, attempting to stretch it gently. Some women may be able to do this with the husband present and participating, but others may be able to

bring him into the exercises only after they have become more relaxed. Learning to insert a tampon or graduated objects such as catheters or dilators may be useful for women who are uncomfortable about touching themselves. Some therapists suggest sleeping with a dilator inserted.

One young woman, quite childlike in appearance and manner, presented with vaginismus and a history of all the women in her extended family having had a similar disorder. While she required lengthy treatment, another young married woman responded in three sessions as soon as we had given her permission to set the sexual pace and be in control of intercourse when she was physiologically and psychologically ready.

DYSPAREUNIA

Pain with intercourse is not one of the major female sexual dysfunctions. However, in a recent study, 40 per cent of women attending an outpatient gynecologic clinic stated this was a major complaint, although they presented for routine care.[26] Obviously this problem requires a physician's careful work-up to rule out all reasonable organic causes, including endometriosis, adhered ovarian cysts, vaginismus, genital trauma, rigid hymen, localized and deep lesions, vaginal or pelvic infection and irritation, and others.

If organic causes are ruled out, the physician will have to explain the psychosomatic nature of the ailment. After a thorough history of the origin of the complaint and the relationship between the partners, one can begin a process of therapy including both partners. Examination of the female in the presence of the male as an educational adjunct is extremely useful and facilitates a better understanding of the female sexual response.

SUMMARY

Whether he wishes to or not, the family physician will be called upon to cope with sex-related concerns of patients and families. By giving permission to patients to ventilate their concerns, limited information and, in some cases, specific suggestions may be sufficient to prevent more serious problems.

The physician may choose to take a full sex history and treat sexual dysfunction or to refer the more complicated problems to sex therapists or marriage counselors. In any case, he must prepare himself for the new role of sex educator and counselor by obtaining knowledge, comfort, and skills in this essential area of human personality and health care.

REFERENCES

1. American Medical Association Committee on Human Sexuality: Human Sexuality. 2nd Printing. Chicago, AMA, 1972.
2. Annon, J. S.: The Behavioral Treatment of Sexual Problems: Brief Therapy. Hagerstown, Md., Harper & Row Publishers, Inc., 1976.
3. Barbach, L. G.: For Yourself: The Fulfillment of Female Sexuality. Garden City, N.Y., Doubleday & Co., Inc., 1975.
4. Burnap, D. W., and Golden, J. S.: Sexual problems in medical practice. J. Med. Educ., 42:673, 1967.
5. Calderone, M. S.: Sex education and education for sexuality: The physician's role. In Abse, D. W., Nash, E. M., and Louden, L. M. R. (eds.): Marital and Sexual Counseling in Medical Practice. Hagerstown, Md., Harper & Row Publishers, Inc., 1974.
6. Child Study Association of America: What to Tell Your Children About Sex. New York, Pocket Books Inc., Division of Simon & Schuster, Inc., 1970.
7. Comfort, A.: The "normal" in sexual behavior. J. Sex Educ. Ther., 2:1, 1975.
8. Gordon, S.: Counselors and changing sexual values. Personnel & Guidance J., 54:362, 1976.
9. Green, R. (ed.): Human Sexuality: A Health Practitioner's Text. Baltimore, The Williams & Wilkins Co., 1975.
10. Group for the Advancement of Psychiatry: Assessment of Sexual Function. A Guide to Interviewing. New York, Jason Aronson, Inc., 1974.
11. Hunt, M.: Sexual Behavior in the 1970's. New York, Dell Publishing Co., Inc., 1974.
12. Israel, S., and Rubin, I.: Sexual relations during pregnancy and the post delivery period. Rubin, I.: Sexual adjustments in relation to pregnancy, illness, surgery, physical handicaps, and other unusual circumstances. In Vincent, E. (ed.): Human Sexuality in Medical Education and Practice. Springfield, Ill., Charles C Thomas, Publisher, 1968.
13. Kaplan, H. S.: The New Sex Therapy. New York, Brunner/Mazel, Inc., 1974.
14. Karacan, I., Hursch, C. J., Williams, R. L., et al.: Some characteristics of nocturnal penile tumescence in young adults. Arch. Gen. Psychiatry, 26:351, 1972.
15. Kegel, A. H.: Sexual functions of the pubococcygeus muscle. West. J. Surg., 60:521, 1952.
16. Kinsey, A. C., Pomeroy, W. B., and Martin, C. E.: Sexual Behavior in the Human Male. Philadelphia, W. B. Saunders Co., 1948.
17. Levine, S. B.: Marital sexual dysfunction: Ejaculation disturbances. Ann. Int. Med., 84:575, 1976.
18. Long, R. C.: Sexual Health Care. SIECUS Report, 3:1, 1974.
19. Maddock, J. W.: Sexual health and health care. Postgrad. Med., 58:52, 1975.
20. Masters, W. H., and Johnson, V. E.: Human Sexual Inadequacy. Boston, Little, Brown & Co., 1970.
21. McCary, J. L.: Human Sexuality. New York, Van Nostrand Reinhold Co., 1967.
22. Pomeroy, W. B.: Boys and Sex. New York, Delacorte Press, 1968.
23. Pomeroy, W. B.: Girls and Sex. New York, Delacorte Press, 1969.
24. Rosenberg, P., and Chilgren, R.: Sex education discussion groups in a medical setting. Int. J. Group Psychother., 23:23, 1973.
25. Semans, J. H.: Premature ejaculation: A new approach. South. Med. J., 49:353, 1956.
26. Semmens, J. P., and Semmens, F. J.: Dyspareunia. Med. Aspects Human Sex., 8(7):85, 1974.
27. SIECUS: Sexuality and Man. New York, Charles Scribner's Sons, 1970.
28. Vener, A. M., and Stewart, C. S.: Adolescent sexual behavior in middle America revisited: 1970–1973. J. Marr. Fam. Life, 36:728, 1974.
29. Wahl, C. W.: The Art of Taking the Sex History. Ortho Panel 7. Ortho Pharmaceutical Corporation, Raritan, N.J., 1971.

Chapter 35

CONTRACEPTIVE COUNSELING

by PAUL BRUCKER,
and F. K. CHAPLER

INTRODUCTION

Contraception, a technique that prevents successful fertilization, must be individualized for sexually active individuals capable of reproduction. The physiology of reproduction, the various contraceptive techniques, their efficacy, and their advantages and disadvantages are discussed in this chapter, which can be reviewed by the patient and the physician simultaneously.

It should be emphasized that an adequate history should always be taken concerning the patient's contraceptive needs and expectations. Such a history should consider emotional, social, and motivational factors. It might include such things as the number of children wanted, the ages and general health of the couple and their offspring, the stability or lability of the union, religious and economic considerations, emotional stability, expectations of contraceptive efficacy, amount and type of sexual activity, previous contraceptive procedures employed, and whether or not the decisions for choosing a particular contraceptive technique are unilateral or shared.

PHYSIOLOGY OF FEMALE REPRODUCTION

The physiology of reproduction is complex, but to better understand how various contraceptive techniques work requires knowledge of hormonal relationships, ovum transport and implantation in the endometrium, and the effect that the vagina and cervical mucus can have on sperm motility.

The hypothalamus, influenced by the cerebral cortex and by various emotional stimuli, initiates the hormonal cycle by secreting releasing factors that enter the circulation and cause the pituitary gland to secrete two gonadotropins, follicle-stimulating hormone (FSH) and luteinizing hormone (LH). These two hormones are transported by the blood stream to the ovary, where they exert their influence on the ovarian follicles.

The quantitative, cyclic secretion of each of the gonadotropins and their relationship to each other are critical for ovulation to take place. FSH levels rise just before the menstrual period; continue to rise until just before ovulation, when they drop briefly; and then peak at the time of ovulation, after which the levels decrease gradually until just before the next menstrual period. LH levels rise gradually before ovulation, peak at the time of ovulation, drop abruptly, and then gradually decrease throughout the postovulatory cycle.

The gonadotropins control and direct the ovaries' production of estrogen and progesterone. Starting about the eighth day of the menstrual cycle, the ovarian follicle manufactures fairly large amounts of estrogen and relatively small amounts of progesterone. The amount of estrogen increases until just before ovulation, when it drops abruptly, but in the postovulatory period it again increases as a result of formation of the corpus luteum. On the other hand, the corpus luteum, under the influence of LH, manufactures large amounts of progesterone, beginning at the time of ovulation and reaching a peak just before menstruation, when both estrogen and progesterone fall to a base level. If pregnancy occurs, human chorionic gonadotropin stimulates the corpus luteum to continue to manufacture estrogen and progesterone until such time as the placenta can take over this function.

A feedback mechanism exists between the pituitary gland and the ovary. Large amounts of estrogen suppress the release of FSH by the pituitary, and small amounts of estrogen increase the release of FSH by this gland.

Once the egg is released, it is fertilized in the fallopian tube, after which 2 to 3 days are required for its transport to the endometrial surface. A critical quantitative relationship between estrogen and progesterone levels must exist in order to allow such transportation. Such a balance allows for an appropriate proliferation of the tubal epithelium and for the secretory-like activity and cilia-like action of the tube. The endometrium is prepared for implantation of the fertilized egg by the action of both estrogen and progesterone. Estrogen stimulates proliferation and progesterone stimulates secretory activity.

The cervical mucus serves as an important "gatekeeper" that either facilitates or impairs the transport of sperm. It, too, is under the influence of estrogen and progesterone. Estrogen makes the cervical mucus thin and watery and allows sperm to penetrate. Progesterone makes it thick and tenacious and difficult for the sperm to penetrate.

A knowledge of these principles will allow the physician to better understand some of the more recent contraceptive techniques that interfere with normal reproductive physiology.

EFFICACY

The efficacy of contraceptive methods is dependent upon many variables. Some of these include compliance, age, frequency of intercourse, and fertility of the couple. Table 35–1 classifies efficacy based on consistent and average use.

RHYTHM METHOD

The rhythm method is based on the assumption that one can calculate "safe" and "fertile" periods for conception. When estimating the "fertile" period, one should consider (1) the time of ovulation, estimated to be approximately 14 days (plus or minus 2 days) prior to the onset of menses occurring during the shortest menstrual period, (2) that sperm can survive as long as a week, and (3) that the ovum survives for 24 hours. The remaining time of the menstrual cycle

TABLE 35–1. EFFICACY OF VARIOUS CONTRACEPTIVE METHODS. (Approximate Number of Pregnancies During the First Year of Use Per 100 Nonsterile Women Initiating Method)*

Method	Used Correctly and Consistently	Average
Avoidance		
Rhythm	15	25–40
Coitus Interruptus	9	20–25
Interference with Ovulation		
Oral contraceptives (combined)	0.34	4–10
Interference with Endometrium		
"Mini-pill" (progestin)	1.5–3.0	5–10
Intrauterine device	1–3	5
Mechanical Interferences with Transportation of Ovum and/or Sperm		
Ovum		
Tubal Ligation	0.04	0.04
Sperm		
Condom	3	10
Spermicidal agent (alone)	3	20–30
Diaphragm with spermicidal agent	3	20–25
Vasectomy	0.15	0.15

*Adapted from Hatcher, R. A., Stewart, G. Guest, F., Finkelstein, R., and Godwin, C.: Contraceptive Technology 1976–1977. New York, Irvington Publishers, Inc., 1976, p. 25. With permission of Irvington Publishers, Inc.

is assumed to be "safe." Many elaborate methods are available to calculate the "safe" and "fertile" periods, based on the menstrual calendar, determination of basal body temperature, and evaluation of changes in the character of cervical secretions.

One of the most frequently used calendar methods is to have the patient keep an accurate account of her menstrual cycle for at least 8 months. The "fertile" period is estimated by having her subtract 18 days from the start of the shortest menstrual cycle and 11 days from the longest menstrual cycle. The resulting interval constitutes the time that she should avoid intercourse in order to attempt to prevent pregnancy. The rhythm method is fraught with many inaccuracies, particularly for the individual with irregular menses.

A record of the basal body temperature is obtained by having the patient accurately determine her early-waking basal temperature. Use of this method is based on the assumption that just before ovulation the basal temperature drops and remains low for some 24 to 72 hours, after which time a rise in temperature occurs. The "safe period" theoretically occurs 3 days after such a rise. Such factors as emotional tension, infections, hours of irregular sleep, and basal metabolism affect the temperature determination. There is a higher failure rate in the preovulatory period than in the postovulatory period. Many of the temperature curve recordings are difficult to interpret because of "peaks and valleys" throughout the entire menstrual cycle.

The evaluation of cervical mucus is based on the fact that pre- and postovulatory mucus is yellow and viscous. Just before and during ovulation it frequently becomes more copious, thin, and clear, and this change is frequently accompanied by the "mittelschmerz" of ovulation.

Individuals who practice the rhythm method can take all three considerations (calendar, temperature, and cervical secretions) into account. Unfortunately, the effectiveness of this method is as low as 15 pregnancies per 100 woman-years, and the overall failure rate can be between 25 and 40 pregnancies per 100 woman-years. In addition to the nuisance of the calculations, the rhythm method can lead to frustration during the long periods of required abstinence. However, it is esthetically sound,

frequently complies with religious beliefs, does not have systemic side effects, and does not interfere with sensitivity.

COITUS INTERRUPTUS OR WITHDRAWAL

This is the oldest and one of the least effective methods of contraception available. It is accomplished by the male's withdrawing his penis from the vagina just before ejaculation takes place, and it requires no chemical or mechanical devices. Unfortunately, some preliminary ejaculatory secretions from the male glands can unknowingly "wash out" spermatozoa, which results in contraceptive failure. In addition, the technique is frequently emotionally unacceptable, for it acts against the male's strong desire to penetrate deeply at the time of ejaculation, rather than to withdraw. At times, orgasm occurs before withdrawal has taken place. Coital positions can be limited. This method causes considerable anxiety for both partners, for they must focus on the "ejaculatory moment." Some individuals use a complementary contraceptive method along with the withdrawal technique during the period approximating ovulation. Males who cannot control ejaculation prohibit consideration of this technique. The failure rate in actual users per 100 woman-years is 20 to 25 pregnancies.

ORAL CONTRACEPTIVE STEROIDS

The most frequently used method of birth control in the United States is the oral contraceptive steroid "pill." The popularity of this method reflects patient acceptance, ease of administration, convenience, and a high degree of effectiveness. However, these benefits are not enjoyed without the cost of certain risks and problems, and the patient should be willing to accept this risk–benefit ratio before using this form of contraception. In order to provide the patient with current knowledgeable advice, the physician must try to keep abreast of new developments regarding the pill—no small task when one realizes that each month more than 30 medical articles plus numerous lay press articles are published. Basic information about the pill includes types of pills available, how they are taken and how they are taken and how they work, their potency, guidelines for initiation of use and follow-up of patients, contraindications, and some familiarity with the more serious and common side effects associated with their use.

Choice of Oral Contraceptive

Two types of oral contraceptive steroids are available. The standard combination pill consists of at least 50 micrograms of one of the two synthetic estrogens plus one of the five different progestogens (Fig. 35–1). A new type of combination pill has been produced that contains less than 50 micrograms of estrogen and is called the "low-dose estrogen pill."[29] Combination pills are taken daily for 20 to 21 days, followed by a 7 day rest period. Their mode of action is to prevent ovulation by hypothalamic-pitu-

itary suppression, with subsequent diminished production of gonadotropins and failure of ovarian follicular development. Their failure rate is less than one per cent.[24]

The second type of pill contains only a small amount of one of the progestogens and is called the "mini-pill." It is taken on a strict daily basis with no intervening rest period. Its contraceptive mechanism involves making the cervical mucus and the endometrium unfavorable for sperm migration and for blastocyst implantation. The failure rate ranges from 1.5 per cent to 3 per cent.[3]

The numerous different preparations on the market make it difficult for the physician to choose which pill to prescribe (Table 35–2). When making a selection, it is helpful to understand that the pills do have different potencies. This is a complex problem, involving identifying the target tissue

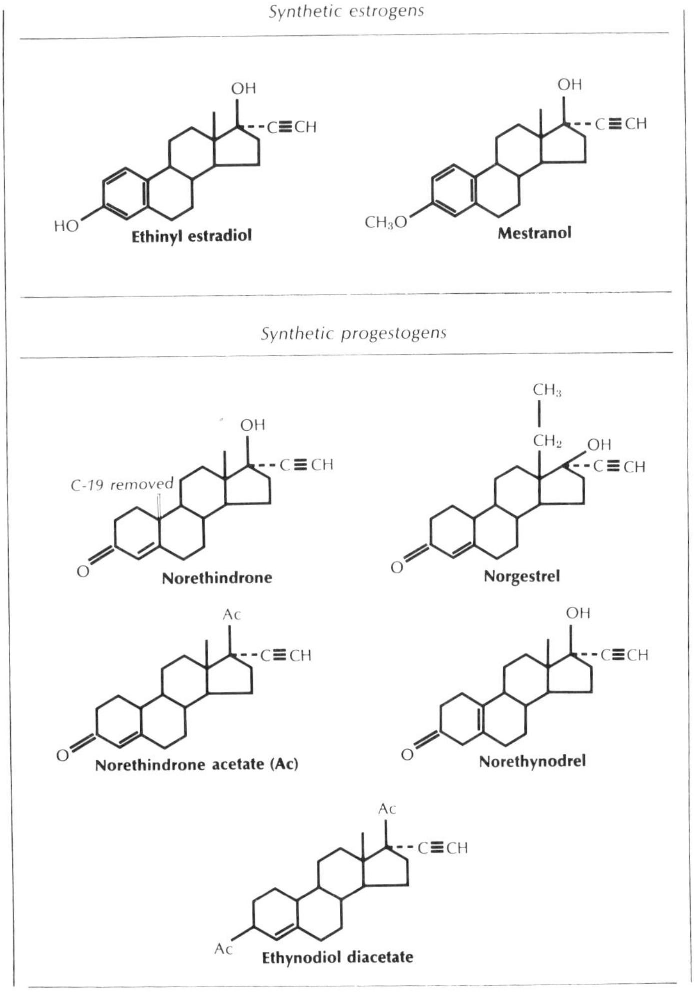

Figure 35–1. Standard oral contraceptive steroid combinations. (From Chapler, F.: Therapeutics. 4:4, 1975.)

TABLE 35-2.   AVAILABLE PREPARATIONS OF ORAL CONTRACEPTIVES *

Trade Name	Progestogen (mg.)	Estrogen (μg.)
Combination Pills		
Demulen	Ethynodiol diacetate 1	EE† 50
Enovid 10 mg.	Norethynodrel 10	M‡ 150
Enovid 5 mg.	Norethynodrel 5	M 75
Enovid-E	Norethynodrel 2	M 100
Norinyl 2 mg.	Norethindrone 2	M 100
Norinyl 1 + 80	Norethindrone 1	M 80
Norinyl 1 + 50	Norethindrone 1	M 50
Norlestrin 2.5 mg.	Norethindrone acetate 2.5	EE 50
Norlestrin 1 mg.	Norethindrone acetate 1	EE 50
Ortho-Novum 10 mg.	Norethindrone 10	M 60
Ortho-Novum 2 mg.	Norethindrone 2	M 100
Ortho-Novum 1/80	Norethindrone 1	M 80
Ortho-Novum 1/50	Norethindrone 1	M 50
Ovcon-50	Norethindrone 1	EE 50
Ovral	Norgestrel 0.5	EE 50
Ovulen	Ethynodiol diacetate 1	M 100
Zorane 1/50	Norethindrone acetate 1	EE 50
Combination "Low-estrogen" Pills		
Brevicon	Norethindrone 0.5	EE 35
Loestrin 1.5/30	Norethindrone acetate 1.5	EE 30
Loestrin 1/20	Norethindrone acetate 1	EE 20
Lo/Ovral	Norgestrel 0.3	EE 30
Modicon	Norethindrone 0.5	EE 35
Ovcon-35	Norethindrone 0.4	EE 35
Zorane 1.5/30	Norethindrone acetate 1.5	EE 30
Zorane 1/20	Norethindrone acetate 1	EE 20
Progestogen (Mini-pills)		
Micronor	Norethindrone 0.35	
Nor-Q.D.	Norethindrone 0.35	
Ovrette	Norgestrel 0.075	

*Adapted from Chapler, F.: Therapeutics, *4*:7, 1975.
†EE = Ethinyl estradiol
‡M = Mestranol

used to measure effect; comparing the differences in milligram weight with the biologic effect; and taking into consideration the total effect of the estrogenic, the antiestrogenic, and the androgenic effects of the progestogen, the necessary conversion of mestranol to ethinyl estradiol, and the synergistic effects of the two components.[7] Table 35-3 ranks the progestational and estrogenic potency of the compounds based on a clinical test.[10] Newer methods assessing the potency of these preparations may alter this list slightly.[6]

In addition to their different potencies, the bioavailability of these steroids is just beginning to be understood. It is known that they are absorbed in the small gut, metabolized in the liver, and excreted in the bile and feces and have a half-life of 24 hours.[3] Since the contraceptive effectiveness of the standard combination pills is the same[8] and the effectiveness of the low-dose estrogen combination pills is only slightly less (not well documented), the choice is made based upon experience with clinical side effects, such as those listed in Table 35-4. In order to select the oral contraceptive with the lowest effective dose and an acceptable level of side effects, a choice of one of the standard combination pills containing 50 micrograms of an estrogen seems reasonable. (The Food and Drug Administration also recommends this.) Changes are then made depending upon the patient's response, or need, or both. If a patient cannot or should not take estrogen-containing pills, the "mini-pill" offers an alternative. However, she must be willing to accept the higher failure rate and the 20 to 30 per cent incidence of breakthrough bleeding.

Guidelines governing the initiation of an

TABLE 35-3. COMPARISON OF ESTROGEN POTENCY AND PROGESTATIONAL ACTIVITY OF ORAL CONTRACEPTIVES*

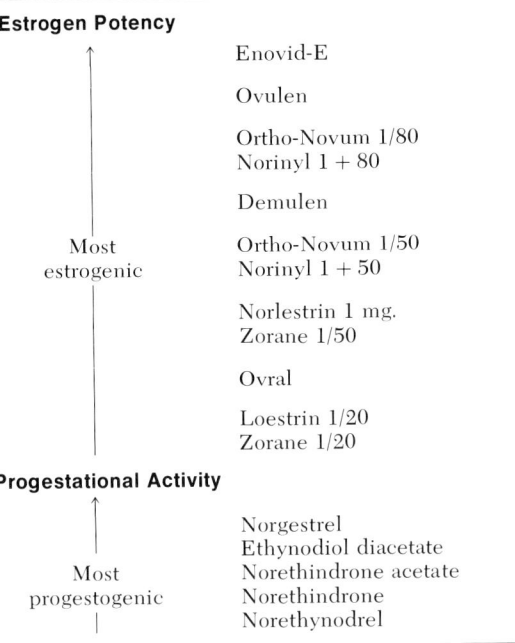

Estrogen Potency

Most estrogenic

Enovid-E

Ovulen

Ortho-Novum 1/80
Norinyl 1 + 80

Demulen

Ortho-Novum 1/50
Norinyl 1 + 50

Norlestrin 1 mg.
Zorane 1/50

Ovral

Loestrin 1/20
Zorane 1/20

Progestational Activity

Most progestogenic

Norgestrel
Ethynodiol diacetate
Norethindrone acetate
Norethindrone
Norethynodrel

*Adapted from Chapler, F.: Therapeutics, 4:5, 1975.

oral steroid contraceptive and further patient follow-up include taking a complete medical history and doing a physical and pelvic examination (including cervical cytology) before starting the pill. Recom-

TABLE 35-4. CLINICAL SIDE EFFECTS OF ORAL CONTRACEPTIVES*

Estrogenic

Nausea
Edema
Chloasma
Headache
Depression
Mucorrhea
Breast tenderness
Weight gain

Progestogenic

Hypomenorrhea
Monilial vaginitis
?Depression

Androgenic

Acne
Hirsutism
Weight gain

*From Chapler, F.: Therapeutics. 4:9, 1975.

mended initial laboratory tests include complete blood count (CBC), urinalysis, sequential multiple analysis (SMA 12/60), and venereal screening tests when indicated. A three-month return visit for a discussion and blood pressure check, followed by at least an annual visit thereafter, seems appropriate for most patients. Certain patients may require more frequent visits.

Absolute contraindications to the pill are relatively few and center around the estrogen component (Table 35–5). There are several relative contraindications that will be discussed along with other systemic and metabolic side effects.

Systemic and Metabolic Side Effects[3]

Cancer. Contrary to previous concern, there is no evidence supporting an increased incidence of cancer of the cervix, ovaries, or breasts in patients taking oral contraceptives. Cervical changes such as erosion, hypersecretion, and glandular hyperplasia have been reported, but these are reversible and can be controlled by changing or stopping the pill. Benign breast disease is encountered less frequently in patients taking the pill. Fibrocystic changes and fibroadenomas are not contraindications to the use of the pill. The incidence of benign ovarian cysts is reduced in oral contraceptive users, most probably due to the suppressed gonadotropin level. A recognized association between the development of endometrial carcinoma and the use of sequential pills in a few patients resulted in this type of oral contraceptive preparation's being removed from the market.[19] Patients who are taking sequential pills should discontinue them and have them replaced with a combination pill. Of current interest is the increase in hepatic adenomas

TABLE 35-5. CONTRAINDICATIONS TO ORAL CONTRACEPTIVES

Thromboembolic disease
Undiagnosed genital bleeding
Estrogen-dependent tumors (uterine, breast)
Hyperlipidemia (relative)
Markedly impaired liver function
Pregnancy (VACTERL)*
? Over 40 age group (relative)

*VACTERL: Acronym for teratogenic-induced anomalies involving the vertebrae, anus, heart (cardia), trachea, esophagus, renal system, and limbs. See also page 458.

among young women taking oral contraceptives. Although the actual incidence is very low (only 71 cases recorded by the Central Registry of the University of California, Irvine) physicians should be on the alert for this finding. These benign liver tumors may be difficult to recognize, as many are asymptomatic, and laboratory tests are not helpful. These tumors are dangerous because of the potential for hepatic rupture and hemorrhage. Early diagnosis is crucial to prevent this catastrophe. Young women who have right upper quadrant pain, or a mass, or both, and a history of having taken oral contraceptives for longer than 4 years are prime candidates and should be adequately evaluated. Diagnostic studies may involve ultrasonography, liver scan, and, if indicated, celiac angiography. Evidence that these tumors are malignant is lacking at present.[21]

Cardiovascular. The most serious systemic side effect is the added risk of thromboembolic disease. This four- to sevenfold increase still represents only a small absolute risk to the individual patient. The most often quoted rates of death from this disease are 0.2 deaths per 100,000 women for nonusers and 1.5 deaths per 100,000 women for pill users below the age of 34. The incidence increases gradually with age. This risk factor is also present in deaths reported from cerebrovascular disease.[5] Attempts to show a definite response relationship between these risk factors and the dose of estrogen have not been successful, but, as previously mentioned, the accepted recommendation is to use 50 micrograms of an estrogen as an initial dose. A strong family history of early death from cerebrovascular disease or conditions predisposing to embolic formation, such as prosthetic heart valves or hyperlipidemia, are relative contraindications to the combination pill. In spite of this increased risk of death reported with the use of the pill, a patient still has a higher risk of loss of life by being in an automobile accident, giving birth, or having an abortion.

Hypertension develops in 2 to 5 per cent of the patients taking estrogen-containing pills.[17] Estrogen-induced activation of the renin angiotensin–aldosterone system explains the elevation of blood pressure. Hepatic production of angiotensinogen (renin substrate) is increased, resulting in excess synthesis of angiotensin, a potent vasoconstrictor. Most women maintain a normotensive state because of a feedback inhibition system that controls the renin production and the subsequent production of angiotensin. In hypertensive women, this regulatory mechanism is blocked, and the kidneys continue to produce renin, with subsequent elevation of the angiotensin and a concomitant elevation of blood pressure. Increased amounts of aldosterone and sodium retention also play a part in the pathophysiology. A woman who develops hypertension while taking the pill should discontinue its use. While pre-existing hypertension is not an absolute contraindication to the pill, such patients require close observation, and other types of contraception should be considered.

Of current interest has been the observation that women over the age of 40 seem to have a higher incidence of coronary heart disease if they take estrogen-containing combination pills.[27] Additional etiologic factors influence the incidence of this disease, but it does seem reasonable to suggest that a patient over the age or 40 who is hypertensive and obese and has increased cholesterol levels, or mild diabetes, or both, should not take the pill. Certainly, if the patient smokes, this should always be the rule, as it has been shown that smoking works synergistically with these other risk factors in the reported association of coronary disease and use of estrogen-containing oral contraceptives.[14] In fact, smoking more than two packs of cigarettes a day should be considered a relative, if not an absolute, contraindication to taking estrogen-containing contraceptive pills.

Lipid and Carbohydrate Metabolism. There is an increase in serum lipids caused by the estrogenic component of the pill. Triglycerides are increased in most patients. Fatty acids, phospholipids, and serum cholesterol are also increased, but with less consistency. The changes are due to an increased lipid synthesis and decreased turnover. Related to this is the observed twofold increase in gallbladder disease in patients taking estrogen-containing pills.[2]

Contraceptive steroids also have the capacity to alter normal carbohydrate metabolism.[28] This change is more apparent in those patients who are predisposed to developing diabetes mellitus. Such patients are characterized by having a family history of diabetes; previous abnormalities in glucose metabolism, as indicated by glucose tolerance studies; obesity; a history of delivering an infant over 10 pounds; and by being in the older age group. Whether or not steroids are clearly diabetogenic has not been established, but women should have their carbohydrate metabolism monitored periodically for as long as they are taking the pill. Although not specifically recommended, patients with diabetes mellitus can take oral contraceptives. Studies have been unable to show a detrimental effect on the patient or an acceleration of the disease process. Control of blood glucose levels may be more difficult, and insulin doses may have to be adjusted. Both the estrogen and the progestogen component affect carbohydrate metabolism, although the estrogen effect is the prodominant one. Since the adverse effect on carbohydrate metabolism may be one of the changes that are related to the length of time a patient takes oral contraceptives, it is important to monitor her periodically, especially if she has been taking the pill for more than 5 years. Ten to 20 per cent of all pill users will have an abnormal glucose tolerance curve, but its exact clinical significance has not been established.

Hepatic Function. The liver plays a central role in the metabolism of oral contraceptives, and many hepatic functions, such as those used for excretion, are altered. Bromsulphalein (BSP) retention is increased, and there is an increased cholestatic potential. Varying degrees of hepatocellular degeneration and stasis have been observed. Estrogen increases hepatic synthesis of the globulins that bind several of the hormones and alter blood coagulation factors and haptoglobin. The increase in heme protein and porphyrins is a result of a steroid-induced increase in enzymatic action. The clinical significance of this is shown by an occasional exacerbation of porphyria in patients taking oral contraceptives. Hepatic metabolism of the pill can be altered by other drugs, such as rifampin. This is important to recognize, as it alters the effectiveness of the oral contraceptives.

Hematology. Changes in the blood clotting mechanisms are estrogen-related. Most clotting factors, as well as platelet numbers and aggregation, increase. An alteration in blood viscosity and flow properties toward a so-called hypercoagulable state has been noted. There is also an increase in activity in the fibrinolytic system. These changes have been measured in vitro and do not necessarily reflect a so-called thrombogenic state in the individual patient. Other hematologic effects consist of folic acid deficiency, megaloblastic anemia, and slight alterations in serum iron and iron binding capacity.

Results of Laboratory Tests. Results of more than 100 commonly used laboratory tests are altered in different ways by steroid contraceptives.[20] Table 35–6 lists some of the more common laboratory tests and how they are altered. It is important to know which patients are taking estrogen-containing pills for proper interpretation of laboratory data. For example, the serum thyroxine level (T_4 test) is elevated in women taking combination pills. This does not represent a hyperthyroid state, but rather an increase in thyroxine-binding globulin, which results in more bound and less free thyroxine. To maintain a euthyroid state, more thyroxine is produced, but the actual level of the free or active thyroxine is normal.

Post-Pill Amenorrhea (Fig. 35–2). This condition develops in 1 to 2 per cent of patients when they discontinue taking the combination pill. There are two explanations for this: endometrial atrophy, which should last no longer than 3 months, and hypothalamic-pituitary axis suppression, which should last no longer than 6 months. A patient who has not resumed normal menstrual function after this allotted time should be evaluated for a secondary amen-

TABLE 35–6. COMMON LABORATORY TESTS ALTERED BY STEROID CONTRACEPTIVES

Albumin	↓
Glucose	↑
Lipids	↑
Cortisol	↑
T_4	↑
T_3 uptake	↓
Iron binding capacity	↑
Hematocrit	↑
Copper	↑
Liver function (Bromsulphalein, enzymes)	↑

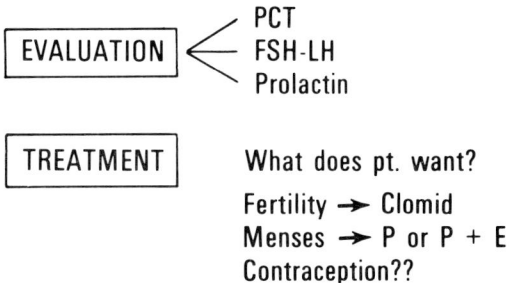

POST-PILL AMENORRHEA

2 mechanisms:

Endometrial Atrophy - 3 mos.
Hypothalamic Suppression - 6 mos.

EVALUATION ⟵ PCT / FSH-LH / Prolactin

TREATMENT   What does pt. want?

Fertility → Clomid
Menses → P or P + E
Contraception??

Figure 35–2. Schema for post-pill amenorrhea management. P = Progesterone. E = Estrogen. Contraceptive choice debatable.

orrhea. Minimal evaluation should include a progesterone challenge test (PCT), blood gonadotropin determinations, and a serum prolactin level. The latter test is very important because many patients with hyperprolactinemia, amenorrhea, and galactorrhea have a small microadenoma (prolactinoma) in the pituitary gland that develops while taking oral contraceptives or is found after the patient has discontinued the pill. Treatment of post-pill amenorrhea will depend upon the patient's desire for children, regular menses, and so forth. If no abnormalities of the sella turcica are found and the patient wants children, ovulation can be induced with clomiphene citrate (Clomid). Hypomenorrhea or occasional skipped menses while taking the pill is usually caused by a progesterone-induced endometrial atrophy and can be treated by increasing the estrogenic component of the pill.

Teratology. Controversial evidence indicates a possible teratogenic effect caused by inadvertently taking synthetic steroids during early embryogenesis (the first 2 to 8 weeks of pregnancy). This is why pregnancy is listed as a contraindication to a patient taking the pill. The types of anomalies reported involve many body parts, including the vertebrae, anus, heart (cardia), trachea, and esophagus and the renal system, as well as causing limb reduction problems. These have been put together to

form an acronym VACTERL.[22] (See Table 35–5.) A carefully obtained menstrual history, pelvic examination, and, when indicated, an HCG beta subunit pregnancy test can help rule out an early pregnancy and avoid this problem. Combination pills should no longer be used as a type of pregnancy test to induce a withdrawal period in a patient who has gone beyond her expected date of menstruation.

Breakthrough Bleeding. One of the most troublesome clinical problems is the breakthrough bleeding that occurs during the time that the patient is taking the pill. Most often, this can be controlled by supplementing the oral contraceptive with a small dose of estrogen for 5 to 7 days or by increasing the amount of estrogen in the pill by changing preparations. Taking two pills a day may solve the problem temporarily, but this frequently results in further breakthrough bleeding later in the cycle. A useful plan for this problem is: no treatment during the first cycle in which breakthrough bleeding occurs; a short course of increased estrogen and, if absolutely necessary, doubling the dosage of pills temporarily during the second cycle in which this occurs; and, finally, a change in oral contraceptive selection. Obtaining the correct progestogen-estrogen ratio for a particular patient to prevent this troublesome problem is difficult because of the differing potencies of the compounds, differences in bioavailability, and individual metabolism of the medications.

Miscellaneous Side Effects. Although *depression* seems to be a clinically frequent complaint of patients taking the pill, most studies do not bear this out. Most depressions are caused by life situational problems or by other stresses. Some scientific basis has been given to the theory of estrogen-related depression, as estrogen does lower brain serotonin concentrations by interfering with tryptophan metabolism and pyridoxine utilization. Patients whose depression seems to be related to interference with serotonin synthesis may be helped by pyridoxine supplementation.

Libido has been reported as both increasing and decreasing in selected patients. No definite conclusions have been reached.

Patients with documented *migraine headaches* are usually advised against taking estrogen-containing pills. Estrogen does cause vascular changes as well as alterations in the electrolyte and water balance. Since there are nonestrogen-containing contraceptives, as well as other methods available, these alternatives should be utilized in patients with migraine headaches. This advice is also usually given to patients with *epilepsy.*

Melasma (chloasma), facial hyperpigmentation, is the most common dermatologic complaint, with an incidence of 5 per cent. The cause is uncertain, but estrogen stimulation of melanocytes with some additional progestational effect has been suggested. Melasma is aggravated by sunlight and seems to occur more frequently with high-dose estrogen pills.

Hair loss is sometimes a reflection of a temporary increase in resting phase hair follicles, with subsequent shedding, and usually returns to normal within 3 to 6 months. *Acne* may be improved by proper use of high-potency estrogen pills. *Facial hirsutism* may occur with some androgenic-type oral contraceptives and can be treated by substituting the more estrogenic-type pills.

Exacerbations of *systemic lupus erythematosus, erythema nodosum,* and *rheumatic symptoms* are rare but necessitate withdrawal of the pill if they should occur.

Monilial vaginitis has been related to a progestogen effect and can often be relieved by increasing the estrogen content of the pill. *Galactorrhea* that develops while the patient is taking the pill should be carefully evaluated, so as not to overlook the presence of a prolactinoma. Discontinuation of the pill will often bring about cessation of the inappropriate milk production. If in doubt, serum prolactin levels and skull films may be in order.

Changes in *vitamin* and *essential trace metal levels* have also been noted, but they have unclear clinical significance. *Increase in body sodium* and *water retention* are related to the estrogen component of the pill and help explain the development of weight gain. Since most progestogens are anabolic, they also cause some tendency toward weight gain. One of the more complete ongoing studies evaluating all aspects of oral contraceptive steroids can be found in the report by the Royal College of General Practitioners, first published in 1974.[25] Updated and more current data will be published periodically.

INTRAUTERINE DEVICES[13, 30]

The intrauterine device (IUD) serves as an effective method of contraception and provides an alternative for the woman who cannot, or who does not wish to, take oral contraceptives or use other mechanical contraceptive devices. Changes in structural design and methods of insertion have improved the effectiveness of this device. There are two types of IUD's currently in use, nonmedicated (Lippes Loop, Saf-T-Coil) and medicated (Copper T, Copper 7, and Progesterone-T or Progestasert). A disadvantage of the newer medicated types of IUD's is that they require replacement every 2 or 3 years, depending on the particular device. The mechanism of action of the IUD remains unclear, but apparently the underlying effect is to render the endometrium hostile for implantation or for proper growth after nidation. There is a mobilization of leukocytes that results in an embryotoxic effect, as well as adversely affecting sperm transport. The medicated IUD's have additional cytotoxic effects resulting from the toxic enzymes liberated from endometrial cells that have been in contact with copper salts. Copper also alters the mitochondria in endometrial cells so that normal metabolic functions are impaired, thus creating a poor environment for the development of the fertilized egg.[9] The progesterone-containing devices maintain a progestational endometrium that is incompatible with implantation. Additional biochemical changes involving the endometrium have been reported, but their role in providing contraceptive effects is not conclusive.

The failure rate of IUD's varies between 1 and 3 per cent; thus, their effectiveness approximates that of the "mini-pill." Twenty-five per cent of women will require removal of the IUD because of bleeding or cramping, or both, or they will have a spontaneous expulsion of the device during the first year. If the device is retained for a year, it has one of the highest continuation rates of any of the currently prescribed methods of contraception.

Contraindications to its insertion include pregnancy, suspicion of gynecologic malignancy, pelvic inflammatory disease, endometritis, an abnormally shaped endometrial cavity, acute cervicitis, and a history of a previous ectopic pregnancy. Complications of inserting the device include bleeding, cramping, infection, and uterine perforation. The latter has an incidence of 1 per 1500 insertions. Perforations are less frequent with those devices that work on the withdrawal technique rather than on the push-out principle. Proper placement of the device high in the fundus is necessary to minimize accidental pregnancy. If a pregnancy should occur with the device in place, serious potential complications can occur. Most pregnancies occurring with an IUD in place eventually abort, but the potential for a septic process exists, and the current recommendation is to have the IUD removed when the pregnancy is detected. This decision requires the participation and approval of the patient. The pregnant patient going to term with an IUD left in place should be assured that there is no evidence of a higher risk of congenital anomalies in the child. Although there is an association between tubal ectopic pregnancies and the IUD, the exact cause is unknown at this time.

Management of the so-called "lost" IUD includes careful assessment and a thorough search. Pregnancy and unnoticed expulsion should be ruled out. Hysteroscopy can often locate an IUD lost in the uterus. IUD's are radiopaque and can frequently be located, if extrauterine, by taking a flat film of the abdomen. Ultrasonography has also been used to locate "lost" IUD's. More often, determining their exact location requires comparison with a second IUD or with a uterine sound placed in the uterine cavity. Hysterosalpingography can also be used to demonstrate an extrauterine placement of an IUD. If the IUD is found to be located in the abdomen outside the uterus, it should be removed by laparoscopy or laparotomy.

POST-COITAL CONTRACEPTION

The administration of high doses of estrogen in the immediate post-coital period should be used as an emergency method of contraception only. This should not be relied upon as a continual method of protection against pregnancy. Before receiving the treatment, the patient should be prepared to make a decision to terminate her pregnancy, if it should ensue, because of the potential effects of the estrogen on the fetus. At the present time, the only estrogen approved by the Food and Drug Administration for this use is diethylstilbestrol (DES). It is given in doses of 25 mg., twice a day for 5 days, starting within 72 hours of exposure. This may cause nausea, and an antiemetic agent may have to be prescribed. The effectiveness of this so-called "morning after pill" method to prevent pregnancy is very high, but it should again be stressed that this is an emergency-only measure.[11, 15]

SURGICAL STERILIZATION

Introduction

For information regarding surgical sterilization, as with all contraceptive advice, the physician should recognize the important and invaluable role that he can play as a counselor. He should be aware of his own attitudes about the surgical sterilization of either the male or the female and should not allow them to interfere with or bias the decision that only the patient or the couple can make. He should discuss and consider with the couple a minimally acceptable age for undergoing the procedure, the number of living children, their general health, and the satisfaction of the couple with that number; the stability of the union; the emotional stability of both partners; the understanding of probable irreversibility; and the potential medical conditions that may affect either the partners' or their offsprings' health or well-being.

Social considerations can be important. The educational level of the couple should be investigated. In general, there is evidence to suggest that the higher the educational level of the couple, the more likely they are to consider and successfully accept surgical sterilization. Religious beliefs about contraceptive sterilization should also be considered. In addition, the economic status and pressures that might lead the couple to consider sterilization should be discussed, and a history of previously used contraceptive techniques and the couples' satisfaction or dissatisfaction with them should be obtained. If feasible, it is helpful to decide whether one partner is a dominant individual or whether there is a true role-sharing process in the couple's decision-making. All of these factors should be investigated by the physician, and there should be a time interval of several weeks after the initial discussion for the couple to consider their decision.

Fallopian Tubal Ligation

Sterilization by fallopian tubal occlusion is rapidly increasing as a method of contraception for those women who have finished their childbearing or who do not want any children. With the advent of the use of the laparoscope and the resultant shortened hospital stay, this trend will undoubtedly continue. Although tubal occlusion can be accomplished by both the abdominal and the vaginal route, more patients are choosing the laparoscopic method. It has less morbidity and mortality and requires a shorter surgical time and hospital stay. Recent estimates reveal a complication rate of 3 per 1000 cases and a death rate of 2.5 per 100,000 cases caused by laparoscopic coagulation of the fallopian tubes.[26] The more frequent complications include hem-

orrhage; bowel perforation; electric burns to the skin or bowel or both; emphysema; cardiorespiratory problems; and accidents caused by anesthesia.[18] Developments in technique, including bipolar coagulation and use of metal clips and Silastic rings placed on the tubes, have helped reduce these complications.

Figure 35–3 shows a laparoscope and grasping forceps used during tubal sterilization by coagulation. Most of these procedures are done in a hospital setting with 1 or 2 days of hospitalization, but there are clinics that offer laparoscopic tubal sterilization, using local anesthesia, as an outpatient procedure. Facilities should be available for immediate abdominal surgery if an accident does occur. The failure rate is less than 1 per cent.

Contraindications to laparoscopic sterilization include abdominal hernia, multiple previous abdominal surgeries (relative), obesity (relative), and any contraindications

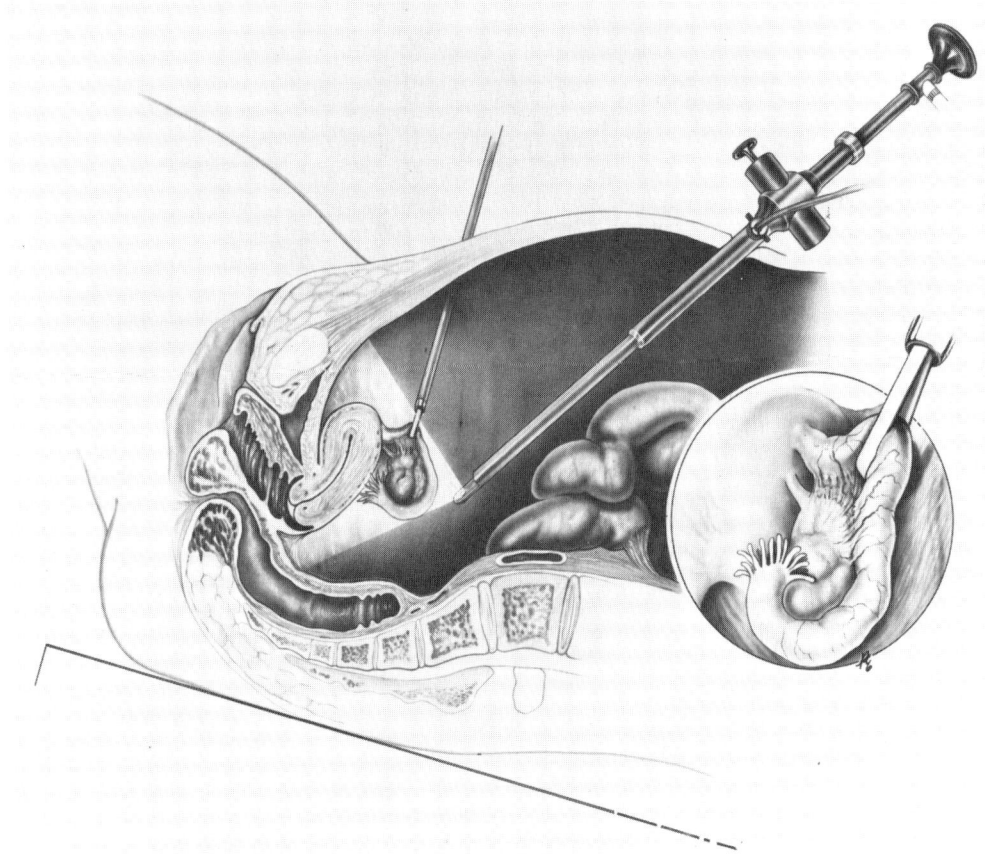

Figure 35–3. *Laparoscopic tubal coagulation. (From Buchsbaum, H. J., and Chapler, F. K.: Gynecology. In Liechty, R. D., and Soper, R. T.: Synopsis of Surgery. Ed. 3, St. Louis, The C. V. Mosby Co., 1976.)*

to general anesthesia, if used. This type of contraceptive method should be considered permanent, as attempts to repair coagulated tubes have not been very successful. Although there is an increased success rate for repair of previous surgical ligation procedures by the abdominal or the vaginal route, ligation should still be presented to the patient as a permanent form of sterilization. Use of the metallic clips and Silastic rings on the tubes, which serve as transient tubal obstructive devices, evidently will leave fertility potential preserved, although this may be slightly diminished.

Vasectomy

Vasectomy, a procedure that mechanically interrupts the delivery of sperm, is a rapidly growing and widespread technique of contraception in the United States. In 1974, vasectomy, or male sterilization, for couples of reproductive age not wanting additional children was as prevalent as female sterilization. Some of the reasons for its increasing acceptance include the fact that it is simpler, cheaper, and safer than female sterilization. In addition, many of the historical myths associated with the use of the procedure have been dispelled. These include the erroneous beliefs that it is indicated only for eugenic purposes and that it is equated with castration. Many of the psychologic and physical concerns about the procedure have been reduced by appropriate education and counseling.

Candidates for the procedure should be informed about the function of the male reproductive organs. A simple approach includes acquainting the patient with the fact that the testes manufacture hormones and spermatozoa and that the accessory sexual glands (such as the prostate, Cowper's glands, and the seminal vesicles) make semen, the vehicle for the transport of spermatozoa. The vessels that transport the spermatozoa include the vas deferens and the seminal tracts. The hormones are transported by both of these vessels, plus the blood vessels. Interruption of all three—the blood vessels, the vas deferens, and the seminal tracts—would result in castration. In vasectomy only one of these, the vas deferens, is divided in its course through the scrotal sac, and the hormones continue to be transported by the blood vessels.

After shaving the area and adequate cleansing of the skin surface, the procedure usually takes only 10 minutes. It can be performed in the physician's office in a completely painless fashion with the use of a local anesthetic. Urologists, general surgeons, and many family physicians can perform the procedure. Following the operation, the patient should be advised to refrain from vigorous exercise for 48 hours, to wear a suspensory, and to expect some discomfort that can usually be relieved by a mild analgesic. He should be advised that he is not immediately sterile and that the residual spermatozoa in the reproductive delivery system can be responsible for an unwanted pregnancy. Usually, follow-up evaluation, by examining a fresh sample of ejaculate, should take place after six ejaculations or after 6 to 8 weeks, or both, to make sure that the procedure was complete and that no residual sperm are present. Less than 0.4 per cent of the patients will be found to have spermatozoa present. This may be due to spontaneous recanalization or to overlooking a third vas deferens at the end of the operation.

In addition to questions concerning the immediate procedure and follow-up, the physician should anticipate and discuss some of the following points with the patient. In the vast majority of patients, there is no change in sexual satisfaction. The degree of libido, volume of ejaculate, strength of erection, degree of orgasm, and control over ejaculation should remain the same. Some individuals claim that their sex life improves greatly once the fear of pregnancy is eliminated. Except for minor soreness experienced immediately after the operation, there is no reason to delay resuming normal sexual activity.

Although there is some evidence to indicate the formation of sperm-agglutinating and sperm-immobilizing antibodies in approximately 25 to 50 per cent of the patients who have had a vasectomy,[1] there is no firm evidence to indicate impairment of general health. Some initial reports indicate that formation of such antibodies may result in systemic conditions such as glomerulonephritis, thrombophlebitis, liver dysfunction, recurrent infections, and multiple sclerosis. There is very little evidence to confirm these reports, and they should be de-emphasized if they are of any concern to the patient. Such antibodies may interfere with the fertilizing capability of spermatozoa and may maintain sterility, even if successful surgical reconstruction of the vas deferens is performed later. For all practical purposes, the irreversibility of the sterilization procedure should be emphasized. There may be an increase in the mean plasma levels of testosterone and luteinizing hormone in patients who have had a vasectomy, but such a change will not cause the mean levels to fall outside the normal ranges for adult males.

CONDOMS

Condoms, or penile sheaths, are made principally from synthetic materials. A small percentage are made from an animal's cecum or intestine. Various types are available, and more recently they have been widely and openly marketed. They require no prescription or physician participation, and they allow the male to share in the contraceptive decision-making. Users' complaints include a lack of sensitivity and the interruption of the sexual act to put the condom on. Patients should be aware of the facts that an old condom may be faulty, that the use of a lubricated condom minimizes tearing, and that the condom should be held on the penis during the act of withdrawal in order to prevent spillage. Condoms should be used only once. Should spillage occur, patients should be instructed in the technique of having the female partner insert either contraceptive jelly or foam. The condom does help protect against some of the venereal diseases, such as syphilis, gonorrhea, and trichomoniasis. The failure rate in extremely compliant patients is approximately three pregnancies per 100 woman-years. In actual use, it is probably closer to 15 to 20 pregnancies per 100 woman-years.

SPERMICIDAL AGENTS

Spermicidal agents consist of jellies, creams, suppositories, or foam-like mediums that are designed to be placed deep in the vagina, close to the cervix, in order to kill spermatozoa before they enter the cervix.

The user of foam should be instructed to insert an adequate amount just prior to intercourse. If this substance is allowed to remain too long in the vagina, it loses its foam-like nature and becomes less effective. Unfortunately, it is impossible to determine when the foam container will become empty, so it is wise to always have an extra dispenser available. The woman should not douche for at least 6 to 8 hours after intercourse. The efficacy in the compliant user is about three pregnancies per 100 woman-years. The average failure rate, however, is approximately 30 pregnancies per 100 woman-years. The efficacy of foam can be increased by the associated use of a condom, particularly during the "fertile" period. Those who object to the "messy" discharge after intercourse should be instructed to insert a tampon. If contact irritation occurs with either partner, a different brand of spermicidal agent should be tried.

DIAPHRAGMS

The diaphragm is a rubber cup-like device supported by a metal spring that, when inserted properly in the vagina, covers the cervix. A spermicidal jelly or cream is used concomitantly around the rim and on the cervical side, so as to be close to the cervical opening and thus provide the principal insurance against sperm entering the cervix. The diaphragm's main advantage is the absence of systemic effects and the lack of subsequent effect on wanted pregnancies. It does require time for proper adjustment, so that it fits snugly between the posterior fornix and behind the symphysis pubis. The patient must be able to understand how to insert the diaphragm properly, and she must insert it no more than 1 or 2 hours before intercourse. Diaphragms come in various shapes and sizes. The All-Flex or arc-spring type diaphragm is used most widely. Nulliparous women usually require a cup with a 65 to 75 mm. ring size, whereas multiparous women require one in the range of 75 to 90 mm. The actual range of sizes available varies from 55 to 95 mm. Flat-spring type diaphragms are occasionally used for the patient with a significant rectocele or cystocele.

REFERENCES

1. Ansbacher, R.: Sperm-agglutinating and sperm-immobilizing antibodies in vasectomized men. Fertil. Steril., 22:629, 1971.

2. Boston Collaborative Drug Surveillance Program: Contraceptives, and venous thromboembolic disease, surgically confirmed gallbladder disease and breast tumors. Lancet, *1*:1399, 1973.

3. Chapler, F.: Oral contraceptive steroids. Therapeutics, *4*:3, 1975.

4. Chihal, H., Peppler, R., and Dickey, R.: Estrogen potency of oral contraceptive pills. Am. J. Obstet. Gynecol., *121*:75, 1975.

5. Collaborative Group for the Study of Stroke in Young Women: Oral contraceptives and stroke in young women, associated risk factors. J.A.M.A., *231*:718, 1975.

6. Dickey, R., and Stone, S.: Progestational potency of oral contraceptives. Obstet. Gynecol., *47*:106, 1976.

7. Edgren, R., and Sturtevant, F.: Potencies of oral contraceptives. Am. J. Obstet. Gynecol., *125*:1029, 1976.

8. Goldzieher, J., Pena, A., Chenault, C. B., et al.: Comparative studies of the ethynyl estrogens used in oral contraceptives. Am. J. Obstet. Gynecol., *122*:615, 1975.

9. Gonzalez-Angelo, A., and Aznar-Ramos, R.: Ultrastructural studies on the endometrium of women wearing T Cu-2000 intrauterine devices by means of transmission and scanning electron microscopy and x-ray dispersive analysis. Am. J. Obstet. Gynecol., *125*:170, 1976.

10. Greenblatt, R.: A new clinical test for the efficacy of progesterone compounds. Am. J. Obstet. Gynecol., *76*:626, 1958.

11. Hatcher, R. A., Stewart, G., Guest, F., et al.: Contraceptive Technology 1976–1977, New York, Irvington Publishers, Inc., 1976.

12. Hubbard, C. W.: Family Planning Education. 2nd Ed. St. Louis, The C. V. Mosby Co., 1977.

13. IUD. ACOG Technical Bull., No. 40, June, 1976.

14. Jain, A.: Cigarette smoking, use of oral contraceptives, and myocardial infarction. Am. J. Obstet. Gynecol., *126*:301, 1976.

15. Kuchera, L. K.: Postcoital contraception with diethylstilbestrol—Updated. Contraception, *10*:47, 1974.

16. Langer, A., Devanesan, M., Pelosi, M., et al.: Choice of an oral contraceptive. Amer. J. Obstet. Gynecol., *126*:153, 1976.

17. Laragh, J.: Oral contraceptive-induced hypertension—nine years later. Am. J. Obstet. Gynecol., *126*:141, 1976.

18. Loffer, P.: Indications, contraindications, and complications of laparoscopy. Obstet. Gynecol. Surv., *30*:407, 1975.

19. Lyon, F.: The development of adenocarcinoma of the endometrium in young women receiving long-term sequential oral contraception: Report of 4 cases. Am. J. Obstet. Gynecol., *123*:299, 1975.

20. Miale, J., and Kent, J.: The effects of oral contraceptives on the results of laboratory tests. Am. J. Obstet. Gynecol., *120*:264, 1974.

21. Nissen, E., Kent, D., and Nissen, S.: Liver tumors and the pill: analyzing the data. Contemp. Obstet., Gynecol., *8*:103, 1976.

22. Nora, J., and Nora, A.: Editorial, Can the pill cause birth defects? N. Engl. J. Med., *291*:731, 1974.

23. Oldershaw, K. L.: Contraception, Abortion and Sterilization. Chicago, Year Book Medical Publishers, Inc., 1975.

24. Oral contraception. ACOG Technical Bull.,: No. 41, 1976.

25. Oral Contraceptives and Health, an Interim Report from the Oral Contraception Study of the Royal College of General Practitioners. Manchester, England, Pitman Medical Publishers, 1974.

26. Phillips, J. M., Keith, D. M., Hulka, J. F., et al.: Gynecologic laparoscopy in 1975. J. Reprod. Med., *16*:105, 1976.

27. Shapiro, S.: Editorial, Oral contraceptives and myocardial infarction. N. Engl. J. Med., *293*:195, 1975.

28. Spellacy, W.: Carbohydrate metabolism in male infertility and female fertility-control patients. Fertil. Steril., *27*:1132, 1976.

29. Speroff, L.: Which birth control pill should be prescribed? Fertil. Steril., *27*:997, 1976.

30. Tatum, H. J.: Clinical aspects of intrauterine contraception: circumspection 1976. Fertil. Steril., *28*:3, 1977.

Chapter 36

GENETIC COUNSELING

by F. CLARKE FRASER, and E. BRUCE CHALLIS

Genetics impinges on the practice of medicine at many points. The family history may be useful both for diagnosis and for preventive medicine if one is alert to the possible significance of diseases in the patient's near relatives.[1] The fact that responses to drugs are often modified by the patient's genes (pharmacogenetics) should be kept in mind when prescribing. A person's racial background puts him at increased risk for certain diseases, for example, the occurrence of thalassemia in those of Italian or Greek origin. Perhaps genetics most often comes into the picture when a patient asks about the cause of a disease and its implications for the family. This falls into the domain of genetic counseling.[2] Some of the problems raised are complex and deserve referral to a genetic counselor. Many are comparatively simple and can be handled by the well-informed family physician. Certainly, the family physician is likely to be in the best position to help with the emotional and other problems that are sometimes caused by the genetic information given.

This chapter does not aim to turn the reader into a genetic counselor. Instead, it will present a selection of basic information that may help family physicians learn how to deal with some of the genetic concerns their patients may have and when to refer to a genetic counselor.

THE BASIC FACTS

In the following pages, a number of basic facts are presented that will aid the physician in evaluating and advising families with genetic problems. The underlying principles may be found in any one of the many textbooks of medical genetics.[6, 9, 10, 11]

Disorders that give rise to genetic counseling problems fall into four major etiologic categories, according to whether they are caused by a *chromosomal* aberration, a major *mutant gene*, a major *environmental* agent, or a combination of genetic and environmental factors *(multifactorial)*.

CHROMOSOMAL ABERRATIONS

The *chromosomes* are the structures that carry the genes. The normal somatic cell contains two sets of 23 chromosomes each (diploid state), one complete set having come from each parent. They can be seen best at metaphase, when they are condensed and doubled, having just replicated. A *karyotype* is prepared by photographing a mitotic spread, making a print, cutting out the individual chromosomes, and arranging them in pairs in order of decreasing size so that they can easily be examined for irregularities. Chromosomes can be classified into groups according to their length and position of the centromere. Thus, the three longest pairs of chromosomes are in group A, and the two shortest pairs, 21 and 22, are in group G. Recently improved staining techniques have made it possible to identify each chromosome by its characteristic pattern of transverse bands (Fig. 36–1). Females have two X chromosomes and males one X and one Y. The Y chromosome carries male-determining factors. Chromosomes other than the X and Y are called *autosomes*.

At meiosis each chromosome is attracted to the other member of its pair, and the

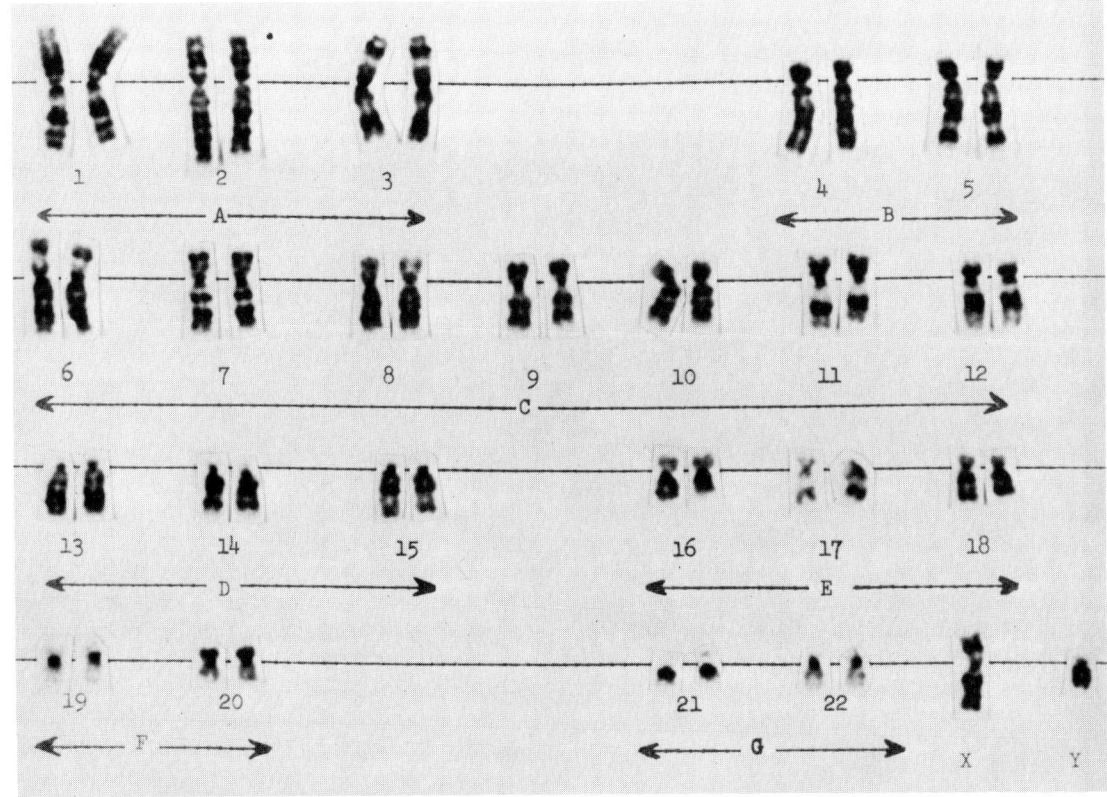

Figure 36-1. A normal human karyotype illustrating the Giemsa banding technique.

pairs line up on the metaphase plate. At anaphase each member of a pair goes to the opposite pole of the cell from the other member (disjunction) so that the two daughter cells each get one set of chromosomes — a reduction division. Thus, the sperm and egg are haploid, i.e., contain only one set of 23 chromosomes. When they combine at fertilization, the diploid state (46 chromosomes) is restored.

Types of Aberrations

Errors in Number (Aneuploidy). Occasionally, the pairing process goes wrong, and the two chromosomes of a pair go to the same pole, resulting in a cell with one extra chromosome and a cell with no chromosome of that particular pair. This is known as *nondisjunction*. If the cell with the extra chromosome differentiated into a sperm and fertilized a normal egg, the resulting zygote would have three members of that pair, or be *trisomic*. Down syndrome, for example, results from trisomy 21. The corresponding cell with none of that pair would result in monosomy, which is

usually lethal. However, in the presence of a single X chromosome, monosomy results in Turner syndrome (XO). A chromosome number other than some multiple of the basic set is called *aneuploid*. For reasons not yet understood, nondisjunction occurs more often in older than in younger mothers. The risk of having an aneuploid child (particularly one with trisomy 21) begins to increase sharply at about age 35 and reaches about 2 to 3 per cent by the age of 40. The recurrence risk is low (see example 1 later in this chapter).

Sometimes nondisjunction occurs at an early cleavage division in the fertilized egg rather than during meiosis, and the resulting individual may then have two or more cell lines, causing a mixture of normal, trisomic, or monosomic cells. This is known as *mosaicism*. Depending on the numbers and locations of the abnormal cell lines, the individual may be normal, may resemble an individual with the corresponding syndrome, or may be intermediate between these two states.

Duplications and Deletions. Sometimes a segment of a chromosome may be repeated, resulting in partial trisomies and monosomies respectively. An increasing number of syndromes of this kind are being recognized.[3]

Rearrangements. Finally, there may be rearrangements of the chromosomal material. A piece of one chromosome may become attached to another (*translocation*), or a segment of the chromosome may be reversed (*inversion*). These rearrangements usually do not have any effect on the individual, since they do not involve an excess or a deficiency of chromosomal material. However, a translocation carrier may produce gametes that are unbalanced. For instance, if a person carries a translocation of chromosome 21 to chromosome 13, the chromosome 13 carrying the translocated 21 may go to the same pole at meiosis as would the normal 21. The resulting gamete will thus have an extra 21 chromosome, and the resulting egg will be trisomic for 21. Other possibilities are that the gamete will be *normal* (receiving the normal 13 chromosome and 21 chromosome) or *balanced* (carrying the 13/21 translocation but no other 13 or 21 chromosome). Thus, translocation carriers are at increased risk for having chromosomally abnormal children but may also have normal children, some of whom will be carriers (see example 1).

Inversions may also occasionally give rise to unbalanced gametes by a somewhat more complicated mechanism. The proportions of normal and abnormal offspring depend on the nature and location of the chromosomal rearrangements, and precise estimates are not yet available. The cytogeneticist can be consulted for information about individual cases.

Indications for Cytogenetic Evaluation

Since karyotyping is a time-consuming and expensive procedure, some discrimination should be used in requesting a cytogenetic examination. This is partially a matter of judgment and partially dependent upon the availability of cytogenetic services. Reasonable indications for cytogenetic evaluation are:

1. Multiple malformations or dysmorphic features such as low-set ears, wide-set eyes, and dermatoglyphic irregularities, with or without mental retardation.

2. Infertility or anomalous genitalia.

3. Unexplained shortness in females, or excessive height together with behavior problems in males.

4. Several otherwise unexplained spontaneous abortions or miscarriages.

5. For prenatal diagnosis in cases in which:

   a. The mother is over 35 years old (40 years old at some medical centers).

   b. The mother has had a previous aneuploid child.

   c. The mother is likely to be a carrier of an X-linked gene for a serious disease and would be willing to have an abortion if the baby were a boy.

Diseases known to result from mutant genes, and simple malformations, are *not* indications for karyotyping.

Procedure. The most convenient material for cytogenetic studies is blood, from which lymphocytes are cultured and mitotic preparations are stained by a variety of techniques. Heparinized blood can be sent to the cytogenetics laboratory by mail (do not freeze or warm), but preferably cultures are prepared when the blood is drawn. In some cases in which the lymphocytes are difficult to grow or there is a question of mosaicism, fibroblasts can be cultured from skin or other tissue, or cells from the bone marrow may be examined directly.

DISEASES CAUSED BY MUTANT GENES

The *genes* are sequences of deoxyribonucleic acid (DNA) in the chromosome. They contain the genetic information that determines the amino acid sequences of the polypeptides that form the proteins. Thus, for every polypeptide there is a corresponding gene that codes the polypeptide's structure. A change in a DNA nucleotide (i.e., a mutation) will cause a change in the corresponding amino acid in the polypeptide controlled by that gene and therefore may result in a change in function of that protein. Other mutations may result in failure to synthesize the polypeptides. Whether or not a disease results depends upon which protein is altered.

Since the fertilized egg receives one set of chromosomes, and therefore one set of genes, from each parent, *each individual has two of each kind of gene, one from each parent, and, in turn, will give one or the other of these two to each child.* This is the essence of mendelian genetics.

Autosomal Dominant Diseases

If a deleterious mutant gene produces a disease when present in a single dose—that is, when in combination with its normal counterpart (heterozygosity)—the disease it produces is said to show *dominant* inheritance. If the mutant gene is inherited from a parent, the parent also should have the disease. Thus, *dominantly inherited diseases characteristically occur in one parent of each affected person* and can be traced back through the direct line of ancestry for many generations. There are two exceptions to this, mutation and reduced penetrance (see following discussion).

The second characteristic of autosomal dominant inheritance is that *each child of an affected parent has an equal chance of being affected or unaffected.* Since the affected parent is carrying one mutant and one normal member of that pair of genes and passes either one or the other to the child, the child will have one chance in two, or a 50:50 chance, of being affected (see example 3). As a corollary to this, those offspring who do not have the disease will not transmit it to their children (except if the condition is one that shows reduced penetrance).

The Sporadic Case. A deleterious gene for a dominant trait may arise by fresh mutation, in which case there will be no affected ancestors (see example 4), and the case will be "sporadic." The more severely the disease limits reproduction of the affected person, the greater the proportion of cases that arises by fresh mutation. For example, in the case of a disease that virtually sterilizes the individual, such as Apert syndrome, almost all patients will have a negative family history, since their condition must almost always result from a fresh mutation, whereas in diseases that do not limit reproduction very much, such as Huntington chorea, sporadic cases are very rare. Since the diseases that limit reproduction most (or have the lowest *fitness* in the darwinian sense) are most rare, it also follows that, for dominant disorders, the more frequent the disease, the lower the proportion of sporadic cases.

Reduced Penetrance. The other exception to the rule that every patient with a domin-

antly inherited disease has an affected parent is reduced penetrance. For one reason or another, some genes for dominantly inherited diseases may not be expressed in a detectable form in some carriers of the gene. This is referred to as lack of penetrance—the effects of the mutant gene have, so to speak, failed to "penetrate" to the clinical surface. This means that the disease may occasionally "skip" a generation, the gene being transmitted through an unaffected carrier (see examples 10 and 11).

Autosomal Recessive Diseases

Some mutant genes do not have any deleterious effect when present in a single dose, presumably because the normal member of the pair produces enough of the corresponding protein (usually an enzyme) to do the job. Thus, these genes can be carried through many generations without being detected and only cause disease when a child receives the mutant form of the gene from *both* parents. When two parents both carry the mutant gene, along with a normal gene of the same kind (heterozygosity), they each have one chance in two of passing the mutant gene to the child, so the chance that the child receives the mutant gene from both parents is $1/2 \times 1/2 = 1/4$. Such a child is said to be *homozygous* for the mutant gene and will have the disease. This is the basis for the pattern of inheritance typical of autosomal recessive diseases. The disease *usually does not appear in the ancestors or collateral relatives* and does appear in one in four children (on the average) of carrier parents. Because of the small size of the average family, most cases will be the only one in the family. The birth of an affected child indicates that the parents are both carriers (heterozygotes) and that *any child of these parents will have one chance in four of being affected* (see example 5).

An affected person will have affected children only if the spouse is a carrier. Since the probability of this is usually quite low (it is calculated as twice the square root of the disease incidence), affected individuals usually do not have affected children.

Relatives are more likely to carry the same mutant gene than are nonrelatives, which is why recessively inherited diseases occur more frequently in the off-spring of related (consanguineous) parents than of nonrelated parents. Conversely, if the parents of a child with a rare disease are related, this suggests that the disease is recessively inherited.

X-linked Diseases

If a gene for a recessive disease is on the X chromosome, it will behave as recessive in females (who have two X chromosomes) but will always be expressed when present in males, since there is no second X to carry the normal allele. The typical pattern of X-linked recessive inheritance is transmission through unaffected females, who carry the mutant gene on one X and the normal member of that pair on the other. Since the son inherits either one X chromosome or the other, he has a 50:50 chance, or one chance in two, of inheriting the mutant gene and of being affected. Thus, the disease characteristically appears in the patient's brothers and maternal uncles and in the sons of some of his sisters (see example 7). All the daughters of affected males will be carriers, and the daughters of carrier females each have a 50:50 chance of being carriers.

The Sporadic Case. The situation becomes a little more complicated in the case of an affected male who has no affected relatives. (1) He may represent a fresh mutation, in which case his brothers are at very low risk, or (2) his mother may be a carrier who has not had any affected male relatives just by chance, and his brothers will have a 50:50 chance of being affected. Therefore, one must not assume that a case with a negative family history is the result of a fresh mutation. As with autosomal dominant conditions, the more severe (and therefore the more rare) the disease, the more likely it is to represent a fresh mutation. It can be calculated from the principles of population genetics that in the case of a fully lethal X-linked condition, such as Duchenne muscular dystrophy, about one-third of the sporadic cases represent fresh mutations, and in two-thirds of the cases, the mother is a carrier. For more frequent, less severe diseases such as hemophilia, the percentage of fresh mutations is correspondingly lower, probably less than 10 per cent. The more unaffected brothers and sons there are in the family, the less chance

there is that the mother is a carrier. The probabilities can be calculated by bayesian algebra[5], but further discussion is beyond the scope of this chapter. For a number of X-linked conditions carrier tests are available, with varying powers of discrimination.[7] (See example 7.)

"Multifactorial" Conditions

A number of diseases and malformations, particularly the common (about 1 case in 1000) familial ones, are clearly not due to single mutant genes with high penetrance, or to a chromosomal aberration, or to a primarily environmental cause, but are the result of the interaction of genetic and environmental factors. These are loosely referred to as multifactorial conditions. Recurrence risks are derived primarily from empiric data, supplemented when necessary by extrapolations from the principles of quantitative genetics.[8] As a rule of thumb, the recurrence risk for first-degree relatives (sibs and children) is roughly the square root of the population incidence (usually approximately 2 to 5 per cent) and increases with the number of affected relatives. Thus, the risk for the sib of a child with an uncomplicated cleft lip and palate being similarly affected is about 4 per cent and increases to about 9 per cent if there are two affected sibs (see examples 13 and 14).

Let us emphasize that a group of patients with any common familial disease is likely to have within it examples of various etiologies. In a series of children with cleft lip, for example, one may find a number of syndromes, some showing mendelian inheritance and some being nonrecurrent, e.g., chromosomal aberrations (trisomy D) or major environmental causes (maternal use of phenytoin, maternal alcoholism). It is only by exclusion that the child is classified in the multifactorial category. The same is true for cases of hereditary hypercholesterolemia among those with early coronary disease, of dominantly inherited maturity–onset-type diabetes among juvenile diabetics, of the mutant or chromosomal forms of excessive tallness or shortness among the overly tall or overly short otherwise normal individuals at the extremes of the height distribution, and of autosomal dominant myoclonic epilepsy among the "idiopathic" epileptics.

THE GENETIC COUNSELING PROCESS

WHO DOES THE COUNSELING?

A physician who refers his problems relative to genetic counseling routinely to the geneticist fails in his role as a family physician. There is no doubt that his training may often be inadequate in an area that has so many emotional, statistical, and judgmental ramifications. In such instances he must therefore seek help, but he must not abrogate responsiblity for his patients by failing to respond to their needs.

The family physician is the only one who has adequate knowledge of his patients and, thus, has the background necessary to offer them genetic counseling. Genetic disease creates unique problems. Any genetic abnormality may not only affect the patient but may put the patient's offspring, sibs, or other relatives at risk and, hence, directly or indirectly, may affect the total family complex. The counseling process must take this into account and should be not only person-oriented but people-oriented. The physician must keep in mind the psychologic, medical, and treatment needs of the patient and must utilize all the resources available to achieve fulfillment of these needs.

Many of the problems encountered will require very difficult decisions on the part of the patient involved. Questions may include "Do I marry?" "Do I have a family?" "Do I risk getting pregnant?" "Do I have an abortion?" "Do I adopt a child?" "Do I consider artificial insemination or sterilization?" "What is the future for me?" "Was it my fault?" The guilt, anguish, and concern for the future may indeed be great and cannot be treated lightly. In order to help patients the most, the counselor must be aware of the psychologic structures of those involved. The family physician is therefore the logical person to turn to.

ESTABLISHING THE DIAGNOSIS

Prior to becoming involved in the process of genetic counseling, the family physician–counselor must be sure of his diagnosis. This may seem to be a cliché, but it is worth emphasizing—because of *genetic heterogeneity*, two clinically similar entities may show different modes of inheritance. For example, there are several superficially similar forms of chondrodystrophy that are often lethal during the newborn period. Some are nonrecurrent, and others recur with a 25 per cent probability for each subsequent child. Without x-rays and photographs (and, ideally, cartilage biopsies), it is usually impossible to distinguish between them and thus to estimate the probability of recurrence. Genetic heterogeneity is present in virtually all classes of genetic diseases, whether it be the muscular dystrophies, albinisms, clotting disorders, chondrodystrophies, retinitis pigmentosas, or cataracts, to say nothing of the commoner "familial" disorders such as the epilepsies, schizophrenias, depressive psychoses, diabetes, hyperlipidemias, neural tube defects, and cleft lips. The geneticist may be able to assist the family physician in advising about possible genetic heterogeneity and about what further diagnostic measures might be useful.

All too frequently, particularly in cases of children with dysmorphic features and mental retardation, it is not possible to make a specific diagnosis. However, every effort should be made to do so before proceeding to the first step in genetic counseling, i.e., establishing the probability of occurrence in the relatives at risk.

ESTABLISHING THE PROBABILITY

To estimate the probability of a given family member's being affected, one must first evaluate the genetic component of the condition in question. One should not shirk this by simply referring the patient to a geneticist. A complete history and physical examination must be done. The history includes that of the near relatives (first, second, and third degree) in an effort to ascertain any possible links to the problem at hand (Fig. 36–2). Specifically, one should inquire about any conditions in the family similar to that of the patient, other "constitutional" disorders in the family, and parental consanguinity. Sometimes the mode of inheritance can be inferred from the family history, although (paradoxically perhaps) most patients with diseases due to single mutant genes do not have affected relatives. Usually the mode of inheritance must be determined from previous observations recorded in the literature.

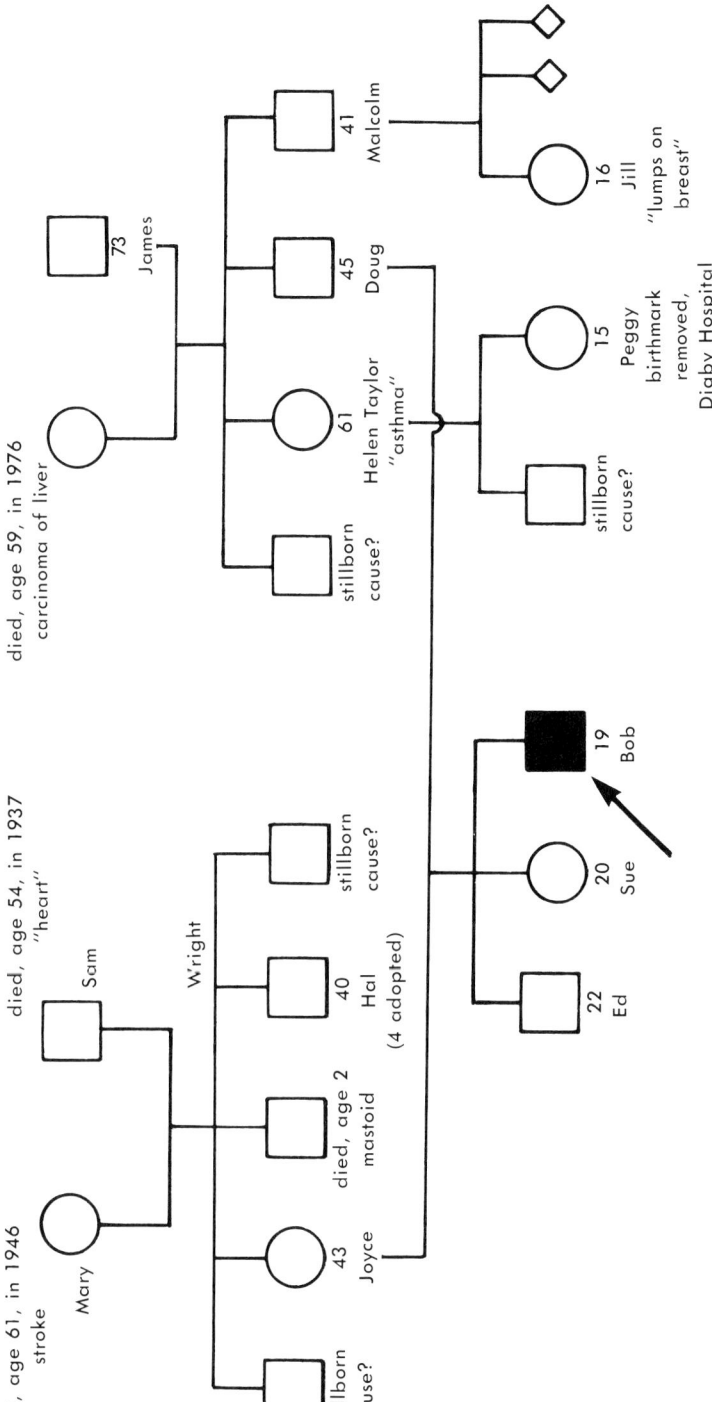

HARRIS FAMILY, January, 1977

Figure 36–2. *A pedigree of a patient with neurofibromatosis, illustrating how family information can be rapidly recorded. Females are represented as circles and males as squares. It is important to record ages when the patient has a condition of postnatal onset. Married names of females are useful for tracking down relatives. The patient (or proband) is designated by an arrow and miscarriages by small diamonds. Having established that Peggy's birthmark and Jill's "lumps" are not neurofibromatous and that there are no café-au-lait spots or other stigmata of neurofibromatosis in the family, one can assume that Bob probably represents a fresh mutation, so his sibs will have a low risk but his children will each have a 50:50 chance of inheriting this dominant gene.*

The physical examination itself may permit decisions relative to the probability of the patient's having a specific problem, but physical examination of other family members may also be required.

With the information garnered from the adequate history, physical examination, and references from genetic literature, the physician may, on his own, establish the mode of inheritance and apply it to the specific situation, using mendelian principles if the condition is caused by a major mutant gene or empiric estimates if not. In other cases, the situation may be sufficiently complex to warrant referral to a medical geneticist. Illustrative examples of the kinds of situations that may arise are provided at the end of this chapter.

INFORMATIVE COUNSELING

Once the probability of recurrence has been estimated, the next step in the counseling process is to impart this information to the counselee, along with relevant facts about the causes of the disease in question, its management and prognosis, its physical and emotional burdens, and its implications for the future family. Depending on the situation, one might wish to consider prenatal diagnosis, abortion, long-term contraception, sterilization, artificial insemination, adoption, and, of course, the prospect of having healthy babies, which, happily, is often good. It may take some time for the parents to grasp the significance of a recurrence risk, particularly if they are not familiar with the concept of probability, and to put the various options into perspective. The counselor should try not to be directive, since the decisions the parents have to make are very individual ones that should take into consideration the family's unique social setting and values. In particular, one should not directly advise parents not to have further children, although one should be sure that they understand fully the consequences of doing or not doing so. The physician–counselor must be prepared to answer many uncomfortable questions relative to the patient's feelings and should not hesitate to seek help from the geneticist who assisted with the diagnostic process as well as from other associated medical people, social workers, clergy, or other trained counselors who might be able to offer assistance in any particular area of family concern.

SUPPORTIVE COUNSELING

The counselor should be aware that the information he is imparting may be highly charged emotionally and that the family may be in the process of coming to grips with the problem of a diseased or defective family member, which may be of more urgent concern to them now than the prospects for the future family. The informative counseling is therefore likely to become interspersed with what can be termed supportive counseling, i.e., the process of helping the family resolve the emotional conflicts generated by such an event. These conflicts need to be dealt with just as much when the condition is nongenetic as when it is. There may be degradation of the self-image, guilt, anger, hostility, fear, rejection, and other potentially damaging feelings to be overcome. The counselor can help by being aware of these responses, by recognizing them when they occur, and by encouraging discussion. This may take a good deal of time. If the family physician is doing the counseling, he should be prepared to set aside such time or to refer the family to an appropriate counselor. The family physician is often in the best position to provide supportive counseling, since he is likely to know the family and its individual characteristics better than a professional counselor does.

FOLLOW-UP

The final stage in the counseling process is the follow-up. The counselees should be followed, since they may need reinforcement of the information given, new questions or sources of conflict may appear, or attitudes may change. Also, the information given may have implications for the extended family. Various relatives may be at high risk without being aware of it and would therefore benefit from genetic counseling. Other relatives may be worried about themselves or their children's developing the disease when, in fact, they are at low risk. The family physician is the most logical person to carry the benefits of genetic counseling to the extended family.

ILLUSTRATIVE EXAMPLES

The following series of cases will illustrate both the kinds of problems that may arise in practice and the approaches to their management.

1. CHROMOSOMAL ABERRATION: DOWN SYNDROME

A 36 year old mother gives birth to a baby suspected of having Down syndrome. The diagnosis can usually be made on clinical grounds, and with a high degree of confidence, on the basis of the dermatoglyphics. Nevertheless, a karyotype should be requested; it will usually report trisomy 21, indicating that a nondisjunction occurred during the formation of either sperm or egg. The chance of recurrence is low, about 2 per cent. This is considered high enough however to *warrant prenatal diagnosis in any subsequent pregnancy.* The parents may need help in handling their anxiety, lowered self-image, guilt, hostility, and other painful feelings that they are undoubtedly experiencing. In about 5 per cent of cases, the karyotype will report a translocation (higher incidence in younger mothers, lower in older ones). If so, the parental karyotypes should be done. They may be normal, in which case the baby's translocation arose de novo, and the chance of recurrence is very small. If one parent carries the translocation in balanced form, the chance of recurrence of a chromosomal aberration in the children is increased. Referral to a genetic counselor may be helpful. The risk of recurrence is not likely to be greater than 10 per cent (except in the rare case of a 21/21 translocation, in which it is 100 per cent). The parents should understand that they have a good chance of having a normal baby and that the pregnancy can be monitored by amniocentesis, with the option of abortion if the baby's karyotype is unbalanced. Key members of the family of the carrier parent should be investigated to detect relatives at increased risk for having a chromosomally unbalanced baby.

2. CHROMOSOMAL ABERRATION: RECURRENT ABORTION

With the use of modern banding techniques, a parental balanced chromosomal translocation has been identified in an appreciable proportion of "habitual" aborters, and a karyotype on *both* parents is warranted in cases in which a woman has had three or more abortions without demonstrable cause. A balanced translocation or inversion may be found in either the husband or wife and provides a reasonable explanation (unbalanced translocations) for the abortions, but not necessarily the correct one. Obtaining a karyotype on one of the abortuses can clarify the picture; if it has a normal or balanced karyotype, some other explanation must be found for the infertility. (The abortus should be kept cool and moist until delivered to the cytogeneticist.) If the translocation is carried by the husband, artificial insemination by a donor may be suggested. Again, the parents should understand that if the translocation is the cause of the reduced fertility, they are capable of producing chromosomally normal or balanced gametes. Prenatal diagnosis should be offered, and discussion with a genetic counselor may be useful. Supportive counseling may be indicated to help the parents deal with the feelings raised by the fact that one of them carries a trait that they are likely to regard as a defect.

3. AUTOSOMAL DOMINANT, POSITIVE FAMILY HISTORY: CATARACT

A couple requests information about the chances of their child's developing cataract. The father, one of his three sisters, his father, and his grandmother all had congenital cataracts.

Here the pattern is clearly autosomal dominant. The father is heterozygous for the mutant gene, and the chance for each child's developing cataract is one in two. Incidentally, it is not safe to assume that if the parents do not inquire, they already know the odds. Many individuals appear unaware of the overwhelming evidence of a strongly positive family history and express surprise when they find that their child is at risk. Note that the affected sister may also benefit from counseling, since her children are at risk. Also the unaffected family members, who may be needlessly worried about having affected children, may be helped by such guidance.

If the cataract is "sporadic" (that is, there is no similarly affected relative) counseling is very difficult, since cataract is highly heterogeneous and could be the result of a fresh dominant mutation, homozygosity for a recessive mutant gene, an X-linked mutant (if in a male), or an environmental agent.

4. AUTOSOMAL DOMINANT, NEGATIVE FAMILY HISTORY: ACHONDROPLASIA

Recurrence in offspring. An achondroplastic male with an unaffected wife wants to know the chances of his children's being affected. He has no affected relatives. He may have been told that since the family history is negative, the condition is not hereditary or that it is recessive.

First make sure that the condition really is achondroplasia and not another kind of chondrodystrophy with another mode of inheritance. Since "classic" achondroplasia always shows autosomal inheritance, the first case in a family is presumably the result of a fresh mutation. The counselee is therefore heterozygous, and each of his children will have a one in two, or 50 per cent, chance of being affected.

Note that many other rare conditions with dominant inheritance may occur as sporadic cases and be transmitted to the offspring, including craniosynostosis with digital webbing (Apert syndrome), the lobster-claw deformity, retinoblastoma, and many others. Do not assume that because a condition is rare and "sporadic" it is not hereditary. When in doubt, check with a genetic counselor.

5. AUTOSOMAL RECESSIVE: CYSTIC FIBROSIS OF THE PANCREAS

The 1 year old second child of nonconsanguineous parents is found to have cystic fibrosis of the pancreas (CF). The parents want to know what the chances would be for their next baby. Since CF shows autosomal recessive inheritance, the parents are both carriers (heterozygotes), and the chance of being affected (homozygous for the mutant gene) is one in four for each subsequent child. Prenatal diagnosis is not yet useful, since homozygotes cannot be distinguished from heterozygotes in cell cultures. Artificial insemination (by an unrelated donor) would reduce the risk to less than 1 per cent. If the parents wish to restrict their family, make sure that they have proper instruction about contraceptive methods, permanent or otherwise.

They also want to know if their normal child will have affected children. The carrier (heterzygote) rate in the general population is roughly 1 in 30 (twice the square root of the disease frequency), and the normal child has two chances in three of being a carrier. Therefore, if the child marries an unrelated person, the chance of both being carriers is about $2/3 \times 1/30 = 1/45$, and the risk for their first child is approximately $1/45 \times 1/4 = 1/180$, considerably higher than the population frequency (roughly 1 in 3600), but reassuringly low to most people. Note that if the disease is Tay-Sachs disease, glycogen storage disease, a mucopolysaccharidosis, or one of the more than 70 other *rare recessively inherited inborn errors of metabolism that can be identified in cell cultures*, prenatal diagnosis can be offered.[4]

6. AUTOSOMAL RECESSIVE WITH GENETIC HETEROGENEITY: CONGENITAL DEAFNESS

The second child of nonconsanguineous parents is found to have severe "congenital" nerve deafness. The parents want to know what the chances would be for their next child. Here the problem is more difficult, as there are many possible causes. Begin by trying to rule out as many causes as you can.

1. Does the child have a significant associated anomaly that may suggest one of the many syndromes of which deafness is a component? Look for such things as hematuria (Alport syndrome), laterally displaced inner canthi and white forelock (Waardenburg syndrome), preauricular pits or branchial clefts, cataracts or myopia, mandibular dysostosis (Treacher Collins syndrome), and retinitis pigmentosa (Usher syndrome). If a syndrome is identified, the counseling depends on the mode of inheritance of the syndrome.

2. Are there near relatives with congenital deafness or with features suggestive of a relevant syndrome? If so, further evaluation of the family is indicated.

3. Is there any evidence of an environmental cause, such as maternal prenatal

rubella, maternal–fetal Rh incompatibility, brain trauma at birth, early meningitis, or exposure to ototoxic drugs? If so, this reduces the likelihood that the deafness is inherited.

4. If no syndrome is identified and there are no significant features of the family, prenatal, or postnatal history, it is probable that the cause is homozygosity for one of the several recessive mutant genes that cause nerve deafness. However, one must take into account the existence of undetected nongenetic causes, and the chance of recurrence is therefore estimated as being somewhat lower than one in four. In summary:

  a. If the parents are related (first or second cousins) or if there are two affected children, the chance of the next child's being affected is very probably one in four, or 25 per cent.
  b. If there are no affected relatives and if the parents are unrelated, the empiric risk is less than one in four, and probably between 10 and 15 per cent.[9]
  c. The empiric risk for the child's children with an unaffected spouse is about 3 per cent.[9]

7. X-LINKED RECESSIVE, POSITIVE FAMILY HISTORY: HEMOPHILIA

A woman whose brother and maternal uncle have hemophilia A wants to know the chances of her son's being a hemophiliac. Her own mother must carry the gene on one of her X chromosomes, since the mother has both a hemophiliac brother and son. The counselee therefore has a 1:1 or 1/2 chance of inheriting the X chromosome carrying the mutant gene and being a carrier. If she *is* a carrier, each son has a 1/2 chance of inheriting the mutant gene and being affected, so the son's probability is $1/2 \times 1/2 = 1/4$.

About 80 per cent of known carriers can be identified by a combination of assay for physiologic activity and radioimmune assay. Consult a hematologist or genetic counselor to find out where such testing is available in the community. If the counselee has a test result in the carrier range, she is almost certainly a carrier. If she falls within the normal range, she has about an 80 per cent probability of not being a car-

rier. If she already has unaffected sons, her chances of being a carrier are proportionally lower and can be calculated by bayesian algebra.[5] Prenatal diagnosis is not available, but prenatal karyotyping can be done to establish the sex of the unborn baby (if the parents are willing to consider abortion should the baby be a male).

8. X-LINKED RECESSIVE, NEGATIVE FAMILY HISTORY

The child has an X-linked disease, and there are no affected relatives. There are two possibilities—either the child is a fresh mutation and the mother is not a carrier, or the mother is a carrier and by chance has had no affected brothers or maternal uncles.

If the disease is lethal, such as Duchenne muscular dystrophy, the a priori odds are 2/3 that the mother *is* a carrier.[5, 9] If the disease is not lethal, and therefore more common, the chances of the mother's being a carrier are still higher—greater than 90 per cent for hemophilia. Tests for carrier detection may provide an answer or at least change the odds. Also, the greater the number of normal sons, brothers, and maternal uncles, the less likely the mother is to be a carrier. A genetic counselor will be able to calculate the odds for each individual case.

9. AUTOSOMAL DOMINANT WITH ADULT ONSET: HUNTINGTON'S CHOREA

A 20 year old girl, about to be married, wants to know whether the fact that her father developed Huntington chorea at the age of 45 implies any risk for her children. This represents one of the most difficult counseling situations because the counselee may not even know that she herself is at risk for developing the disease. This, then, is the first problem. In this case, the counselee, at conception, had a 50:50 chance of inheriting the gene, which will manifest itself sometime between puberty and old age. At age 20, she has already passed through some of the risk period, and since she is still unaffected, her chances of having inherited the gene are somewhat less—about 44 per cent as calculated from the age-of-onset curve.[2] The longer she remains unaffected, the less likely she is to have inherited the gene. By the time she is 35 years old, her risk has decreased to 25 per cent. A genetic counselor can provide appropriate figures for the disease in question. The second problem is the risk for the child, which will be 1/2 the risk for the counselee, and will also decrease as she gets older. If the parent at risk is the father, artificial insemination can be considered. If the mother is at risk and she wishes to have a child, she may wish to wait as long as possible before taking the chance.

In this disease, and in other disorders with dominant inheritance and adult onset, the family physician may want to extend the counseling to other members of the family. Relatives are sometimes quite reluctant to recognize the implications of the family history and even the appearance of early signs of the disease in their near relatives. So, occasionally, are physicians. Sympathetic and tactful explanation by the family physician may do a great deal to improve understanding and to help the family respond constructively to a disastrous situation.

10. AUTOSOMAL DOMINANT, REDUCED PENETRANCE: RETINOBLASTOMA

The unaffected daughter of a blind woman who had both eyes removed because of retinoblastoma wants to know whether her children are at risk. This highly malignant infantile neoplasm typically shows autosomal dominant inheritance. Because it is (or was) highly lethal, most cases represent fresh mutations. However, the gene shows roughly 80 per cent penetrance, that is, about one-fifth of those who inherit the gene do not manifest the disease. Thus, the counselee has a 1/2 (= 5/10) chance of not inheriting the gene and therefore being unaffected and a $1/2 \times 1/5$ = 1/10 chance of inheriting the gene but nevertheless being unaffected. Her chances of being a carrier are therefore 1:5 or 1/6. Her child's chance of being affected is therefore $1/12 \times 80$ per cent = 1/15. The recent improvement in the results of treatment, following early diagnosis, has made the burden of the disease less formidable than it used to be.

For these and other diseases that show reduced penetrance, the situation is complex enough that those who do not feel comfortable with the algebra may prefer to consult a genetic counselor.

11. AUTOSOMAL DOMINANT, REDUCED PENETRANCE, CARRIER DETECTION POSSIBLE: EARLY CORONARY HEART DISEASE

A man, aged 25, whose father, father's brother, and father's mother died of coronary occlusion in their late 30's wants to know whether he should worry about being similarly affected.

Coronary heart disease is a highly heterogeneous disease category: a positive family history suggests that the patient may have an increased risk. An appreciable percentage of early coronary disease results from hereditary hypercholesterolemia, which shows autosomal dominant inheritance. If the patient falls into this class, his risk is appreciably increased, although precise figures are still not available. Other relatives should be screened, even though it is not yet clear how effective preventive regimes may be. Homozygotes are much more severely affected and often have coronary attacks before the age of 30.

The genetic basis for other types of hyperlipidemia is not yet clear, but most of these disorders also carry an increased risk of coronary disease. Data are lacking on life expectancy and other aspects of the disease process important to the patient.

12. MULTIFACTORIAL INHERITANCE: DIABETES MELLITUS

A young, newly married woman with juvenile diabetes mellitus wants to know whether she should have children.

Of the common familial diseases, none is genetically more puzzling than diabetes mellitus (DM). There are a large number of rare syndromes that include DM as a feature. Even after these syndromes have been excluded, the remainder form a heterogeneous category. It is becoming clear that juvenile DM is genetically different from maturity-onset DM, the latter having the higher heritability. It is also clear that neither type is autosomal recessive, contrary to the statement in many textbooks. The etiology is best described as multifactorial. Finally, a minority of patients have maturity–onset-type DM with juvenile onset and benign course that shows autosomal dominant inheritance. A recently recognized association between juvenile DM (but not adult DM) and certain histocompatibility antigens (HLA) may help to clarify the picture.

To return to the counselee, of course she must make up her own mind as to whether she should have children, but the physician can supply some facts for her guidance. The empiric risk that a child of a parent with juvenile DM will develop this disease is estimated as 5 to 10 per cent. The risk of a malformation is about double that of the population level (i.e., from 5 to 10 per cent rather than 2 to 5 per cent). Prenatal diagnosis is still not feasible. Possible obstetric complications should be taken into account.

13. MULTIFACTORIAL, THRESHOLD CHARACTER: ANENCEPHALY–SPINA BIFIDA

The parents of a baby with anencephaly want to know the chances of recurrence in future children. First, the possibility that the baby had a syndrome should be considered—in particular Meckel syndrome in which anencephaly–spina bifida (AN–SB) is often associated with polydactyly and polycystic kidneys. Otherwise, the empiric risk for the sibs of an anencephalic baby having anencephaly or spina bifida aperta, or both, is about 5 per cent. After two such children, the risk increases to 10 per cent. Hydrocephalus with spina bifida is regarded as part of the neural tube defect complex. Hydrocephalus without spina bifida is almost always nonrecurrent, although there are several rare recessive and one X-linked form.

Prenatal diagnosis should be offered. Measurement of alpha-fetoprotein in the amniotic fluid in the second trimester, combined with ultrasound examination, is able to detect more than 90 per cent of neural tube defects. Incidentally, the risk for second-degree relatives (offspring of the patient's normal sibs) is about 2 per cent, so prenatal diagnosis may be considered here also.

If, instead, the baby had cleft lip, with or without cleft palate, the chance of recurrence would also be about 5 per cent if both parents are unaffected, increasing to 10 per cent after having two affected children. Again, careful note should be taken of associated malformations that might indicate the presence of a syndrome. For instance, about 1 per cent of children with cleft lip have pits in the lower lip that are the openings of accessory salivary glands. This association is caused by a dominant gene that causes cleft lip or cleft palate in about half the carriers. Thus, if the patient had lip pits, the risk for the next sib would be 25 per cent, rather than 5 per cent.

14. MULTIPLE MALFORMATIONS, DYSMORPHOGENIC FEATURES, MENTAL RETARDATION

Parents of a child with multiple malformations usually want to know what the chances of recurrence are. It is important to identify the syndrome, if present, since many syndromes show mendelian inheritance, and others do not recur. Most are so rare, and there are so many of them, that it is difficult to be familiar with them all. The same is true for retarded children with minor anomalies (dysmorphogenic features) such as low-set ears and webbed toes. Consultation with a syndromologist may be helpful. If the child dies, it is most important to have as good a description as possible, including photographs and x-rays, if there is to be any chance of fitting the child to a syndrome. Without adequate documentation, the counselor is unable to say whether the risk is very low or quite high. Similarly, it is desirable to have good documentation on stillbirths and late miscarriages.

15. NONSPECIFIC MENTAL RETARDATION

Parents of a boy who is retarded, without known cause, want to know about the prospects for future children. Again, this is probably a genetically heterogeneous category. First, try to rule out known syndromes or identifiable causes for the problem, such a sex chromosome anomaly, birth trauma, or other brain damage. Otherwise, the child is placed in the "multifactorial" category by exclusion. Empiric risks are difficult to determine, but as a rough guide, and considering an IQ of 70 or lower as the criterion for retardation, one can provide the following approximations:

For unaffected parents with one affected child, the chance of the next child's being affected is about 5 per cent. This would increase fairly sharply with each subsequent affected child. For the offspring of one affected and one unaffected parent, the risk is about 10 per cent for each child, increasing to about 20 per cent if there is already an affected child.

REFERENCES

1. Fraser, F. C.: Taking the family history. Am. J. Med., 34:585, 1963.
2. Fraser, F. C.: Genetic counseling. Am. J. Hum. Genet., 26:636, 1974.
3. Lewandowski, R. C., and Yunis, J. J.: New chromosomal syndromes. Am. J. Dis. Child., 129:515, 1975.
4. Milunsky, A., and Atkins, L.: Prenatal diagnosis of genetic disorders. In Milunsky, A. (ed.): The Prevention of Genetic Disease and Mental Retardation. Philadelphia, W. B. Saunders Co., 1975.
5. Murphy, E. A., and Chase, G. A.: Principles of Genetic Counseling. Chicago, Year Book Medical Publishers, Inc., 1975.
6. Nora, J. J., and Fraser, F. C.: Medical Genetics: Principles and Practice. Philadelphia, Lea & Febiger, 1974.
7. Pinsky, L.: Carrier detection in X-linked disease. In Milunsky, A. (ed.): The Prevention of Genetic Disease and Mental Retardation. Philadelphia, W. B. Saunders Co., 1975.
8. Smith, C.: Recurrence risks for multifactorial inheritance. Am. J. Hum. Genet., 23:578, 1971.
9. Stevenson, A. C., and Davison, B. C. C.: Genetic Counselling. London, Heinemann Ltd., 1970.
10. Sutton, H. E.: An Introduction to Human Genetics. 2nd ed. New York, Holt, Rinehart & Winston, Inc., 1975.
11. Thompson, J. S., and Thompson, M. W.: Genetics in Medicine. 2nd ed. Philadelphia, W. B. Saunders Co., 1973.

PART VI

CLINICAL SPECIALTIES

Chapter 37

SURGERY

by RICHARD A. CURRIE

SURGERY IN FAMILY PRACTICE

Family practice is a specialty that provides a very comprehensive type of medical care to patients of various ages within the family group. Surgical illness constitutes a small but significant part of the everyday experience of a family physician. In his role as the physician of first contact, he provides the initial detection or diagnosis, and often the initial care, for a variety of surgical emergencies including acute abdominal disorders, trauma, infection, and acute vascular occlusions. He can also offer care for a number of less urgent office and outpatient surgical problems not requiring hospitalization, as well as assure the essential continuity in the care of surgical patients requiring long-term follow-up.

The demanding nature of his job requires that he work with a group of consultants, among whom are one or more competent general surgeons. An effective arrangement between the family physician and the surgeons requires both easy communication among these individuals and teamwork in the management of surgical problems. The family physician acts as a guide and counselor to the patient on entry into the secondary level of the health care system. As such, the job requires not only skill but tact and diplomacy in dealing with the needs of sick persons and good judgment in referring them, when necessary, to the appropriate consultant. Major operative surgery is clearly not a part of family practice except in unusual circumstances involving physicians with special experience and training.

From the surgeon's standpoint, there should be great satisfaction in working closely with a family physician who is well informed about surgical diagnosis and fully aware of the possibility of operative relief for a variety of conditions. He should feel that he was chosen as the one who was best suited for the patient and that the selection was made by the family physician on an objective basis and without economic or political considerations. The surgeon should clearly have primary responsibility for the care of patients undergoing major surgery. His efforts, however, can be made more effective by the support and help of the dedicated family physician, whose insight into the patient's problems may be of considerable help in making surgical decisions. The family physician's knowledge of the patient from past clinical experience or from laboratory examinations may be of real value to the surgeon in difficult diagnostic situations. Also, in a consultant's role, the family physician can provide support and helpful advice regarding the care of complicated illness in his patients and can serve as an important liaison with other members of the family in time of need.

This chapter presents information concerning some of the surgical problems commonly seen in the practice of family medicine. An effort has been made to relate the subject to the needs of family physicians in the care of patients in the office, emergency room, and hospital. When curiosity is aroused or when more detailed information is required, the reader is directed to the selected references listed at the end of the chapter.

PREOPERATIVE ASSESSMENT OF PATIENTS

The concept of risk in surgery should always be assessed, however briefly, when

TABLE 37–1. BASIC PREOPERATIVE TESTS

Urinalysis (glucose, protein, and sediment)
White blood cell count and differential
Examination of stained blood film
Hematocrit
Chest x-ray
Blood urea nitrogen
Fasting blood glucose
Electrocardiogram (for patients over age 45)

TABLE 37–2. CLASSIFICATION OF PREOPERATIVE PHYSICAL STATUS*

I Good Risk
  Surgical disorder without systemic effects (e.g., early acute appendicitis, hernia, or gallstones in otherwise healthy persons).

II Fair Risk
  Surgical disorder with mild to moderate systemic disturbance or with a significant associated disease (e.g., simple small bowel obstruction, duodenal ulcer with hypertension or mild diabetes).

III Poor Risk
  Severe systemic disturbance or disease with a related or unrelated surgical disorder (e.g., perforated sigmoid diverticulitis with generalized peritonitis, groin hernia with severe chronic obstructive pulmonary disease).

IV Extreme Risk
  Life-threatening disturbance with a surgical disorder, the former not always being correctable by surgery (e.g., organic heart disease with intractable myocardial failure or angina, together with surgical disorder).

V Moribund Patient
  (e.g., ruptured abdominal aortic aneurysm with profound shock.)

*After Dripps, R. D., Eckenhoff, J. E., and Vandam, L. D.: Introduction to Anesthesia. 5th Ed Philadelphia, W. B. Saunders Co., 1976.

patients are considered as candidates for operation. The wise physician considers all operative procedures, however minor, as having some kind of inherent risk for the patient. A successful outcome should never be guaranteed or implied to the patient, and all factors should be considered when the decision for surgery is being made. As in any other therapy, the results of surgical treatment for the individual person are unpredictable. The skill and judgment of the surgeon, the conduct of anesthesia, and the quality of postoperative care rendered are certainly some of the major factors influencing outcome.

However, from the standpoint of objective evaluation, the most important factor that the physician can evaluate carefully is the preoperative physical status of the patient. This can be assessed chiefly by the use of the history and physical examination, with additional information provided by a well-selected group of laboratory tests listed in Table 37–1. The family physician is in an enviable position regarding his familiarity with the patient's history and physical examination, and he should use this knowledge to classify the patient's status as to physical fitness for operation. To do this properly, he should base the information on a knowledge of the systemic effects of the underlying surgical disorder on the patient, together with those effects contributed by any other significant associated disease. A classification of preoperative physical status, as used by most anesthesiologists, serves as a useful guide in evaluating patients as candidates for surgical procedures (Table 37–2).

The discipline enforced by the attempt to classify patients preoperatively along these lines implies recognition of those factors that contribute to the morbidity and mortality of surgery, both in elective and emergency situations. In light of this classification, measures can sometimes be taken to improve the physical status of the patient and thus minimize the risk of a planned operative procedure.

PREPARATION OF THE PATIENT FOR SURGERY

The family physician has a part to play in preparing the patient for surgery. His explanations give the patient some understanding of his illness, and long before the actual decision to employ surgery is made, the patient may have gained the necessary insight to accept the surgeon's recommendations willingly.

When referring the patient to the surgeon, the physician clearly leaves the matter of obtaining an informed consent to the surgeon. During his subsequent discussions with the patient and family, it is the surgeon's duty to offer in simple and understandable terms the description of the operation proposed, the rationale for this procedure, the risk of possible complications, and, in addition, the alternative modes of treatment. This is, of course, the basis of a properly conceived informed consent. Only the operating surgeon can properly present it to the patient. The psychological support of the patient for the coming surgery can be shared by the surgeon and the family physician. The inevitable tension and anxiety created by the prospect of an operation can be much reduced by offering simple explanations and calm reassurance during the preoperative period.

Early identification should be made of those patients who need special attention paid to the psychologic aspects of their illness or planned operation. These, of course, include children, the elderly, those with malignant disease, and those facing the loss of organs or members, such as breast, uterus, or extremity. Special efforts to allay fear, to provide simple explanations, and to encourage open discussions can be shared with the surgeon preoperatively. The recognition of patients with serious emotional overlay, unusual neurotic fears, or psychotic tendencies should be made quite early, and the implications regarding postoperative management should be discussed fully with the surgeon and, in some instances, with a psychiatrist.

OBESITY

The high incidence of obesity in our population makes it easy to overlook this risk factor, which often contributes significantly to surgical complications. A moderately obese patient is one who weighs more than 25 per cent of his ideal weight. A massively or morbidly obese patient weighs two or more times his ideal weight. Most of our clinical problems occur in the former category, and only this group provides candidates for preoperative dietary measures designed to produce weight reduction.

The excessively fat person is generally conceded to be a difficult candidate for surgery from several standpoints. There are difficulties for the surgeon in exposing the operative site as well as problems for the anesthetist in maintaining the airway and in providing a comfortable position for the patient on the operating table. Muscular re-

laxation is generally hard to achieve in obese patients, and the superficial veins are often inadequate for infusions. The physiologic factors associated with obesity are probably of more importance, however, and these include the frequent occurrence of diabetes mellitus; arteriosclerosis; hypertension; and pulmonary problems involving hypoventilation, emphysema, atelectasis, and an enhanced risk of postoperative thromboembolism.

The patient's weight should be compared with the normal weight of persons of various ages and heights as given by standard tables. Purely elective surgery should often be postponed while a program of weight reduction is instituted. The minimum goal for weight reduction must be clearly defined for the patient. The family physician can offer close supervision and constant encouragement while this is being achieved. Even a 5 or 10 pound weight loss accomplished over several months by a patient with a surgical lesion, such as a reducible incisional hernia or mildly symptomatic cholelithiasis, represents an achievement that significantly reduces the risk of surgical complications.

NUTRITION

Recognizing malnutrition in patients is often a matter of guess-work until an accurate nutritional history is obtained. A weight loss of 25 per cent or more of the patient's normal weight should suggest this diagnosis, especially when associated with conditions interfering with adequate intake, incomplete absorption, or inefficient utilization of nutrients. The chronically malnourished patient coming to surgery is faced with certain serious handicaps. Not only are his reserve fuel stores exhausted but there is significant weakness of muscular effort because of wasting with associated loss of muscle mass. Ventilation may be impaired, and coughing is often weakened to a dangerous degree. In addition, protein depletion will be reflected in impaired wound healing and in lowered resistance to infection. A high incidence of stomal malfunction may be expected following gastrointestinal operations in such patients.

When time allows, the nutritional deficit should be corrected by preoperative oral administration of food or specially prepared formulas. Tube feedings and liquid elemental diets may be helpful in restoring positive nitrogen balance in patients who are otherwise unable to take standard oral feedings. The seriously ill patient with gastrointestinal obstruction, enterocutaneous fistula, peritonitis, or other disease preventing the oral administration of food may be a good candidate for parenteral hyperalimentation, which involves the administration through a central venous catheter of hyperosmolar solutions containing a mixture of glucose, protein, minerals, vitamins, and trace elements. Long-term use of intravenous hyperalimentation has significantly reduced the mortality from a variety of gastrointestinal diseases in which a standard nutritional intake is impossible to achieve.

The generally accepted view is that underlying disorders associated with malnutrition require surgical correction without long delay. Preoperative nutritional improvement is designed to restore positive nitrogen balance within a period of 1 or 2 weeks, especially in those patients with underlying malignant disease. In such cases, the operation itself is part of the treatment designed to restore normal nutrition.

DIABETES MELLITUS

Utilization of the screening test for glycosuria and the fasting blood glucose determination in preoperative patients should greatly eliminate the possibility of performing elective surgery in persons with unrecognized diabetes mellitus. When patients are newly discovered to be diabetics, it is best to pause and evaluate the diabetes before proceeding with the planned surgery. The hazard of surgery in unrecognized diabetics is, of course, the sudden development of ketoacidosis.

In the known diabetic patient, dates for hospital admission and elective surgery should be scheduled so that assessment of the diabetic state can be made preoperatively, with fasting blood glucose determinations performed on several successive days, including the morning of surgery. The family physician, when acting as the consultant for patients with diabetes, should keep in mind that the stressful nature of the patient's disease and surgery

may require the administration of additional insulin to counteract the effect of hyperglycemia produced by release of epinephrine. In addition, he should remember that vascular disease in diabetic patients is generally more advanced than it would be in nondiabetic patients of the same chronologic age and is associated with the possibility of significant impairment of cardiac, renal, and cerebral function in such patients.

When diabetic patients taking insulin are having major surgery, it is acceptable practice to give about one-third the daily dose of insulin preoperatively and one-third after surgery and to give additional supplements in the form of regular insulin on a sliding scale, if needed. Blood glucose determinations can be repeated on the afternoon of the day of surgery, and if the blood glucose level is recorded as being greater than 250 mg. per dl. (100 ml.), additional regular insulin may be given. The fasting diabetic patient is given a continuous slow intravenous infusion of 5 per cent dextrose in saline or water. After oral intake is resumed, the standard daily insulin injection can be given once again. Avoidance of both ketoacidosis and hypoglycemia is best achieved by frequent observations and adjustments through the day, utilizing blood glucose determinations as needed and the traditional sliding scale technique of regular insulin administration as indicated by urine testing.

Certain surgical emergencies occurring in conjunction with ketoacidosis in diabetic patients require that the operative procedure be deferred for a few hours while diabetic treatment is initiated. Surgical conditions in this category might include large soft tissue abscesses in need of incision and drainage, gangrene in the extremity, strangulating intestinal obstruction, and suppurative cholangitis. Treatment in the initial phase should include provision of adequate amounts of insulin, antibiotic administration, and fluid and electrolyte therapy.

It is important for the physician to recognize that diabetic ketoacidosis itself can mimic the surgical abdomen. In the diabetic patient, acute abdominal pain and tenderness associated with nausea, vomiting, tachycardia, and leukocytosis can be caused by diabetic ketoacidosis rather than by a specific acute abdominal disorder.

PULMONARY PROBLEMS

Certain factors can be identified that predispose patients to the development of atelectasis and pneumonia in the postoperative period. The most important of these is the presence of pre-existing lung disease, particularly obstructive emphysema and chronic bronchitis. Other significant factors include old age, obesity, malnutrition, mental retardation, heavy cigarette smoking, and untreated oral infections. The presence of a full stomach before induction of anesthesia represents a serious hazard in regard to aspiration pneumonia. Length and depth of anesthesia seem to affect the occurrence of pulmonary complications. Incisions located in the upper abdomen also appear to be associated with a higher risk of pulmonary complications.

Routine measures to prevent pulmonary complications begin in the preoperative period. Cigarette smoking should be stopped 1 or 2 weeks prior to scheduled surgery. The hospitalized patient should be instructed in the methods of effective coughing during a bedside session with a properly trained respiratory therapy technician or nurse. Showing the patient a teaching filmstrip concerned with prophylactic measures may be very helpful in preparing him for surgery.

Older patients, and particularly those with evidence of pre-existing pulmonary disease, may require more intensive measures during the preoperative phase. Baseline examination of such patients, using pulmonary function tests, including timed vital capacity, other ventilatory function studies, and arterial blood gas determinations, may be helpful in determining the degree of functional impairment. Several days spent in clearing up existing pulmonary infection, carrying out postural drainage, and instituting intermittent positive pressure breathing may assist in achieving maximum improvement in the pulmonary status of patients prior to elective surgery.

HEART DISEASE

Detection of heart disease in candidates for surgery is achieved by the evaluation of the history, physical examination, and chest x-ray studies and, in patients over the age of 45, by the use of a routine electrocardiographic (ECG) examination. In patients with known heart disease, the degree of functional impairment can certainly be assessed by the family physician's knowledge of the status of the patient in regard to exercise and the usual physical activities. It is the ability of the patient to increase his cardiac output in response to an increased venous return that represents the basic homeostatic response that is of survival value during and after large-scale surgical procedures. ECG evidence of old myocardial infarction, auricular premature beats, auricular fibrillation, or bundle-branch block indicates the need for careful preoperative evaluation. Other factors to be considered when evaluating the cardiac patient include adequacy of digitalization, a history of recent congestive failure, and clinical or x-ray evidence of cardiac enlargement.

Arteriosclerotic heart disease is the most frequent and serious cardiac disorder enhancing the surgical risk of patients, particularly of those over the age of 50. In its stable and asymptomatic form, it involves little, if any, additional risk in the performance of standard elective or emergency surgery. However, in the presence of shock or other factors predisposing to hypoxemia and hypotension with diminished coronary artery flow, even minor degrees of coronary artery narrowing may become significant. A history or ECG evidence of recent myocardial infarction indicates an unacceptably high risk of mortality and morbidity in elective surgery. The longer the surgery can be postponed in a patient with a fresh infarct, the more the operative risk can be significantly reduced. Diseases of a life-threatening nature, however, should be treated by the appropriate operation, even though a recent infarct is present.

Patients with evidence of congestive failure should be carefully treated during the preoperative period with bedrest, digitalis, restriction of sodium intake, and appropriate diuretics. Careful avoidance of digitalis toxicity at the time of surgery is essential. Use of diuretics should be monitored by electrolyte determinations, and hypokalemia should be corrected prior to surgery. When patients require preoperative transfusions because of blood loss or pre-existing anemia, packed red cells should be used rather than whole blood transfusions in order to restore red cell mass and to avoid overexpansion of the circulating blood volume. Measures to prevent poor oxygenation and the occurrence of hypotension, both preoperatively and postoperatively, include the use of monitoring devices recording pulse, ECG changes, arterial blood pressure, and central venous pressure.

Cardiac patients in general, and those with recent congestive failure in particular, should be considered to be in a high risk category concerning the occurrence of postoperative thromboembolic complications. Prophylactic routines include the selective use of low-dose anticoagulation therapy as well as measures to reduce venous stasis in the lower extremities during all phases of hospital care. When elective surgery is anticipated for patients who are on prophylactic anticoagulant drugs such as warfarin, the dose of the anticoagulant should be tapered and the patient's prothrombin time should be returned to a normal range before surgery is undertaken. Emergency surgery in such patients should be done only after the anticoagulant effect has been neutralized in part by vitamin K given intravenously.

In most patients, antihypertensive drug therapy should pose no major obstacle to the safe performance of both elective and emergency surgery. The opinion of most anesthesiologists seems to be that patients who have been brought to a normotensive range by the use of drug therapy are better candidates for surgery than are those with uncontrolled hypertension. There is no specific reason to stop the antihypertensive medication before patients are hospitalized for elective surgery. Even when hypotension occurs during or after the operative procedure, effective and rational use can be made of vasopressor drugs when the pharmacologic action of the antihypertensive drug is known. Serum electrolyte levels should always be determined preoperatively when the drug regimen has included diuretics. Monoamine oxidase inhibitors are particularly prone to cause adverse drug interactions in conjunction with a number of narcotics, hypnotics, and analgesics. These particular drugs should be stopped when possible well in advance of the admission of patients for elective surgery, and the history of their use by such patients should be made clearly known to the anesthesiologist and surgeon.

ABDOMINAL PAIN

The primary physician who sees patients with acute illness involving abdominal pain must always be aware of the possibility that the disease will require surgery and of the importance attached to its early diagnosis. Sir Zachary Cope's rule that severe abdominal pain of 6 hours' or more duration suggests a surgical abdomen is a very useful one. Recognition of the underlying cause of abdominal pain often may not be possible when the patient is first examined

TABLE 37–3. SUMMARY OF CLASSIC SYMPTOMS AND SIGNS
IN THE ACUTE SURGICAL ABDOMEN

Diagnosis	Symptoms	Signs
Acute appendicitis	Shifting of pain from epigastrium to right lower quadrant Loss of appetite Nausea and vomiting	Right lower quadrant abdominal tenderness
Perforated peptic ulcer	Sudden onset Severe generalized abdominal pain	Board-like rigidity on abdominal palpation Free air on upright x-ray
Intestinal obstruction	Crampy abdominal pain Nausea and vomiting Constipation	High-pitched peristaltic sounds Abdominal distention
Acute cholecystitis	History of biliary colic Right upper quadrant abdominal pain with radiation to right subscapular area	Right upper quadrant abdominal tenderness and guarding Murphy's sign
Acute pancreatitis	History of alcoholism or biliary colic Diffuse upper abdominal pain Persistent nausea and vomiting	Upper abdominal tenderness Elevation of serum or urinary amylase

soon after the onset of this symptom (Table 37–3).

The opportunity to make comparisons between the initial and the later developments in doubtful cases makes prompt contact with the patient a definite advantage in diagnosis. This requires that the physician see the patient on short notice and at rather awkward times of the day or night. A family physician should be willing to fit the patient with this urgent complaint into his daytime office schedule or to find time to see him in the emergency room of the hospital. The information obtained from the history and physical examination, together with the results of a few simple laboratory and x-ray examinations, should in most instances suggest a tentative diagnosis and a course of action. The history and physical examination should be carefully and thoroughly accomplished. Surgical consultation should be obtained promptly, giving the surgeon the advantage of becoming familiar with the presenting physical findings if a period of observation of the patient is elected. A decision to watch the patient closely, with re-evaluation at intervals after the patient has been hospitalized, is justified if the findings on initial examination are equivocal. This must, of course, involve a coordinated effort, with one responsible person following the patient closely in the hospital setting. Use of analgesics and sedatives should be deliberately avoided during this period while the cause of the patient's abdominal pain is being sought.

A special effort must be made when evaluating abdominal pain in patients in the pediatric age group if physical examination is to be rewarding. A calm, unhurried approach with both child and parent is indicated. One should deliberately avoid the prolonged or repetitious palpation of the child's abdomen. A fussy, crying, uncooperative infant can be held by the mother during physical examination. This will aid in relaxing a taut and guarded abdominal wall, especially after sedation has been given (pentobarbital, 1.5 mg. per kg. of body weight intramuscularly). Gentle exploration of the abdomen with the patient's own hand held under the examiner's hand is useful in the older child in localizing the tender area. The wider spectrum of underlying causes of abdominal pain in children, as compared with adults, suggests a need for extreme thoroughness and accuracy in the evaluation of abdominal pain in youngsters. Although only about 10 per cent of children presenting with abdominal pain will eventually need surgical exploration, this small group includes a high proportion of children with diseases that have serious or even life-threatening consequences if overlooked. These chiefly include acute appendicitis, intestinal obstruction caused by hernia, intussusception, Meckel's diverticulum, congenital bands, mesenteric defects, and malrotation.

Proper evaluation of abdominal pain occurring during pregnancy involves awareness on the part of the examiner that the usual acute abdominal conditions occurring in nonpregnant women can also occur in pregnant women. Acute appendicitis is by far the most commonly encountered problem but rupture or torsion of an ovarian cyst, acute cholecystitis, incarcerated external hernia, and intestinal obstruction caused by adhesive bands are also occasionally seen. An association of these disorders with pregnancy should not subtantially change the examiner's approach to diagnosis and treatment of such urgent problems. Abdominal signs may be altered somewhat by the presence of the gravid uterus, causing displacement of organs from their usual location. Appendicitis, for example, may involve a higher and more laterally placed point of maximum tenderness in the third trimester of pregnancy. In addition, the lack of muscle guarding due to the relaxation of the abdominal wall and the normal elevation of the white blood cell count during pregnancy may give rise to some difficulty in recognizing appendicitis and other acute abdominal conditions.

ACUTE APPENDICITIS

By far the most common acute abdominal condition of a surgical nature encountered in family practice is acute appendicitis. Its peak incidence is in adolescence, but it furnishes the most frequent reason for laparotomy in both children and young adults. Acute appendicitis is relatively uncommon in children under the age of 5 years and is quite rare in those younger than 2 years of age. Perhaps because of the thinner wall of the appendix and the meager size of the omentum, the disease progresses to perforation and peritonitis more rapidly in young children. The complication of perforation, which is ultimately due to delay in diagnosis and treatment, provides the basis for almost all the deaths from this disease. Largely stemming from difficulties in early diagnosis, the mortality rate is highest in patients over the age of 50, but it is also relatively high in young children.

Acute appendicitis is notorious for its tendency to be mistaken for other acute abdominal conditions. It should always remain high on the list of possible diagnoses when patients with acute abdominal complaints are seen. The anatomic differences in the location of the appendix, together with the variations in rate of progression and severity of inflammation involving the appendix, largely account for the problems in diagnosis. The family physician is urged to avoid having too rigid a view of the basic features of the history and physical findings thought to be typical of the disease.

It is fairly commonly observed that patients with acute appendicitis subsequently proved at operation may give a history of previous attacks that subsided spontaneously. Acute appendicitis in the western world, however, has a reputation for progressing to perforation and peritonitis in a high proportion of cases. At present, there is no sound basis for the belief that antibiotics and expectant treatment can abort this disease in its early form, nor is there any place in standard practice for temporizing once the diagnosis of uncomplicated acute appendicitis is established.

The term "chronic appendicitis" has been effectively eliminated from the surgical vocabulary. It was often used to justify appendectomy for chronic right lower abdominal pain. In such patients, careful study is recommended to identify underlying causes such as regional enteritis, colonic tumors, adnexal disorders in women, or renal or ureteral lesions. In some patients, however, closely linked episodes of acute right lower quadrant abdominal pain may indeed be caused by repeated bouts of appendiceal inflammation. A diagnosis of recurrent acute appendicitis is appropriate for such patients, and when the other diagnoses have been more or less ruled out, it seems sensible to proceed with appendectomy.

Diagnosis

Recognition of the classic case of acute appendicitis in the young, otherwise healthy adult is usually a straightforward matter. The history is that of sudden appearance of steady epigastric or periumbilical pain, followed in a few hours by a shifting of the pain into the right lower quadrant, accompanied usually, but not invariably, by anorexia, nausea, and vomiting. The concomitant objective findings include abdominal tenderness localized at McBurney's point, voluntary guarding in the right lower quadrant of the abdomen, low-grade fever, and moderate leukocytosis. Rigidity of the abdominal wall and rectal or pelvic tenderness are not typical of early acute appendicitis. By far the most reliable physical sign of early acute appendicitis is well-localized tenderness in the right lower quadrant. In the absence of right lower quadrant localization, the finding of flank or loin tenderness, a positive psoas sign, or pronounced rectal tenderness should bring the possibilities of retrocecal or pelvic appendicitis to mind. Pelvic appendicitis may be associated with little in the way of abdominal pain, but may give rise to diarrhea, tenesmus, or urinary frequency and dysuria. Recognition of the true nature of the process prior to perforation depends upon early and possibly repeated pelvic and rectal examinations. Increasing cul-de-sac tenderness may offer a clue to the diagnosis when abdominal signs are lacking. In the perforated phase of pelvic appendicitis, both the iliopsoas and obturator signs may be present.

In young children, helpful diagnostic clues include loss of appetite, a tendency to become quiet and want to lie down, unusual irritability, or any complaint of abdominal pain. Vomiting is usually prominent in acute appendicitis in children, and diarrhea is part of the mode of presentation in roughly 10 per cent of cases. The finding of localized right lower quadrant abdominal tenderness in a child with abdominal pain and fever amply justifies diagnosing acute appendicitis.

In the elderly and debilitated person, this disease may be associated with strikingly few symptoms. Complaints of indigestion or of right lower quadrant abdominal pain, a mild degree of distention, or perhaps a poorly localized mass in the right lower abdominal quadrant may be the presenting findings. These will often be unaccompanied by a major change in pulse or temperature and will often not be associated with a significant leukocytosis.

There are few laboratory aids for the identification of early acute appendicitis, which is a diagnosis that must be made largely on clinical grounds. X-ray examination of the abdomen by plain films is used chiefly in atypical cases to rule out other causes of abdominal pain, such as ureteral colic or intestinal obstruction, or in complicated cases to identify the features of perforation and peritonitis. About 12 per cent of patients with acute appendicitis may have a visible calcified fecalith located in the right lower quadrant by x-ray examination.

The clinical findings that indicate that perforation has occurred will depend on the degree of containment of the infection provided by the walling-off process. Acute diffuse peritonitis may be expected to be present in a significant number of perforations, particularly in children and young adults in whom the disease has been fulminant or in whom there has been significant delay in establishing the diagnosis.

The signs include tachycardia, fever, and shallow respirations. Palpation will reveal some degree of muscular guarding or reflex spasm in the abdominal wall. Tenderness may be diffuse in all quadrants with rebound phenomenon referred to the point of pressure. There may be abdominal distention, and on auscultation, there will be a diminution or absence of peristaltic sounds. Rectal examination may show impressive tenderness and a sense of fullness in the cul-de-sac. When the perforation is more localized and walled off, the signs may include diffuse right lower quadrant tenderness and spasm with a mass palpable in the iliac fossa. Retrocecal or pelvic perforations will be associated with tenderness, a sense of fullness, or a palpable mass in the flank or true pelvis respectively.

Treatment

In acute appendicitis without evidence of perforation, operation is performed without delay after completion of routine studies. When recent ingestion of food suggests the possibility of a full stomach, emptying of the stomach by introduction of a large caliber nasogastric tube and lavage are indicated before induction of anesthesia. In cases complicated by perforation, there should be a period of preoperative preparation to ensure that the patient is in optimum condition for surgery. Toxicity, which is manifested by high fever, tachycardia, dehydration, and electrolyte imbalance, must be actively treated during this interval. Appropriate amounts of balanced salt solution are given by vein. Broad-spectrum antimicrobial drugs, such as ampicillin, one of the cephalosporins, or penicillin-G, are given intravenously in combination with an aminoglycoside such as gentamicin or kanamycin intramuscularly. A cooling blanket may be used to reduce the fever. Nasogastric suction is begun, using a Levin tube, and urine output is monitored by measurement of hourly volume and specific gravity. Such preparation of patients for operation may require periods of as long as 8 to 12 hours for maximum response to be obtained.

Operation in the usual patient with perforated appendicitis is best accomplished through an appropriately placed gridiron incision. Removal of the appendix and closure of the wound without intraperitoneal drainage are the essential features of the modern operation for cases without abscess formation. Wound infections are common in patients with perforated appendicitis. These can be reduced to a minimum, although not entirely eliminated, by the use of systemic antibiotics, by careful drainage of the subcutaneous layer of the incision, or by appropriate use of delayed primary wound closure.

Postoperative care of patients with perforated appendicitis includes continuation of nasogastric suction, anti-infective measures, and careful fluid and electrolyte therapy. The most common explanation for prolonged fever is wound infection, but signs of hidden sepsis should prompt a thorough search for subphrenic, subhepatic, or pelvic abscess.

In the unusual situation in which the diagnosis has been long delayed, the patient may present with a well-localized periappendiceal abscess without signs of toxicity or of generalized peritonitis. The inflammation is actively treated with antibiotics and allowed to subside without immediate operative interference or drainage. In adults, the overall results of this type of treatment are good if careful choice of the patient is made on the basis of localization of inflammation in the absence of pointing. An interval appendectomy is accomplished after a period of 4 to 6 weeks or before recurrent inflammation of the appendix can occur.

PERFORATED PEPTIC ULCER

Acute perforation, as a complication of either gastric or duodenal ulcer, should be considered a true surgical emergency. It is more commonly associated with duodenal ulcer disease and may occur in some patients without an antecedent history of ulcer symptoms. At least a third of such unheralded perforations, when treated by simple surgical closure, are followed by complete ulcer healing and freedom from further symptoms.

Diagnosis

The diagnosis of perforation is usually suggested by the characteristic history of sudden onset of pain, which is severe and generalized almost from the time of occurrence and tends to worsen with movement or coughing. Typical physical findings include generalized tenderness and a board-like abdominal wall rigidity. In such patients, a Levin tube should be introduced quickly and the gastric contents completely aspirated. Upright or lateral decubitus x-ray films of the abdomen will demonstrate free air between the diaphragm in three-quarters of the cases. Water-soluble contrast medium may be used to confirm the presence of perforation if free air is not seen.

Occasionally, physical findings will be somewhat misleading, especially in patients who are elderly or debilitated or in those who have been on steroid therapy for an extended period. White blood cell count and differential, hematocrit level, and the serum amylase determination may aid in the differential diagnosis. Acute pancreatitis is probably the other most important diagnostic consideration in this regard. The history of more insidious onset, the presence of more persistent nausea and vomiting, the finding of less marked abdominal

rigidity, and the absence of free air in the peritoneal cavity will help to differentiate acute pancreatitis from perforated ulcer. Localization of pain in the lower right abdominal quadrant as a result of the tracking of fluid down the paravertebral gutter may also lead to difficulty in the diagnosis of perforated ulcer. The physical finding of tenderness on one-finger palpation in both the right upper and right lower quadrants is characteristic of perforated ulcer and helps to distinguish this from the otherwise similar findings of acute appendicitis.

Treatment

In general, it is widely agreed that early surgical intervention and closure of the perforation are indicated in most patients. Operation has several advantages—the opportunity for confirmation of the diagnosis; the removal of spilled gastric or duodenal contents, which affords the opportunity for bacteriologic studies; and, finally, prompt cessation of further peritoneal soiling. In selected instances, a definitive operation for peptic ulcer disease may be simply and safely performed at the same time that the perforation is closed. For gastric ulcers, this usually involves the use of a partial distal gastrectomy or, alternatively, an adequate biopsy of the entire ulcer together with vagotomy and pyloroplasty. For duodenal ulcer with perforation, pyloroplasty and truncal vagotomy may be the best therapy. Patients suitable for this definitive approach are, of course, in the younger age group, have a limited degree of peritoneal soilage, and, most importantly, have a documented history of previous ulcer or previous ulcer complications.

In some patients in whom there was a prolonged delay in diagnosis, a nonoperative approach may be elected. In these few patients, spontaneous closure of the perforation may be sought by the use of careful nasogastric suction, parenteral fluid therapy, sedation, and appropriate antibiotics.

Postoperative follow-up of all patients who have sustained a perforation of a duodenal ulcer and who are treated by a simple closure involves the use of a suitable medical treatment regimen, performance of an upper gastrointestinal series or fiberoptic endoscopy at an early date, and observation at suitable intervals to determine if the duodenal ulcer is healing.

TABLE 37–4. COMMON CAUSES OF MECHANICAL INTESTINAL OBSTRUCTION

	Small Bowel	Large Bowel
Adults	°Adhesive bands °External hernia Metastatic cancer °Operative complications	Colorectal cancer Diverticulitis °Sigmoid and cecal volvulus
Children	°Incarcerated hernia °Intussusception °Meckel's diverticulum °Volvulus	Hirschsprung's disease
Neonates	Intestinal atresia °Midgut volvulus Meconium ileus	Imperforate anus Hirschsprung's disease

°Risk of strangulation present.

INTESTINAL OBSTRUCTION

Mechanical intestinal obstruction is found in about 10 per cent of the patients seen with an acute surgical abdomen. About 25 per cent of these cases are large bowel obstructions, while the rest involve the small bowel. About half of the latter are caused by adhesive bands. More than 70 per cent of large bowel obstructions are due to primary colorectal cancer. Although the majority of mechanical obstructions are classed as simple obstructions and involve no interference with mesenteric blood supply, about 10 per cent will be complicated by strangulation of the intestine. These chiefly involve adhesive bands, external hernia, and volvulus as the underlying mechanisms (Table 37–4).

The dangerous effects of simple intestinal obstruction are caused by an outpouring of fluid and electrolytes into the bowel lumen above the point of obstruction. Added sources of loss result from bowel wall edema, peritoneal transudate, and fluid lost by suction or by vomiting. In strangulation obstruction, there is an even more rapid and serious translocation of fluid and electrolytes into the bowel lumen and peritoneal cavity, to which is added a sequestration of blood volume due to blockage of veins and lymphatics in the wall and mesenteries of the obstructed loop of bowel. The progression from strangulation obstruction to peritonitis involves the passage of intestinal contents through the damaged bowel wall into the peritoneal cavity, with subsequent absorption of toxic products of bacterial action into the systemic circulation. While the mortality in mechanical intestinal obstruction is about 10 per cent today, the mortality in strangulation obstruction is greater than 30 per cent, even when cases of acute mesenteric vascular occlusion are excluded.

The four cardinal symptoms of mechanical intestinal obstruction are pain, distention, constipation, and vomiting. The pain is usually crampy or colicky, occurring with a frequency of approximately 3 to 5 minutes in small bowel obstruction and 5 to 15 minutes in large bowel obstruction. The pain in high small bowel obstruction is usually localized in the epigastrium, whereas that from lower ileum or proximal large bowel obstruction may be distributed across the middle of the abdomen. Pain caused by obstruction in the left colon tends to occur in the hypogastric and suprapubic areas. In postoperative patients, the pain may be obtunded by the effects of analgesics and may easily be confused with incisional discomfort. Abdominal distention is more typical of a low-lying obstruction of long duration. It is most marked in obstruction of the left colon in which the ileocecal valve is incompetent and allows free upward reflux of intestinal contents into the small bowel. Obstipation is the usual accompaniment of acute and complete mechanical obstruction. However, passage of gas or a small amount of stool after the pain begins may be due to emptying of the lower bowel beyond the point of obstruction. The vomiting caused by intestinal obstruction usually starts soon after the pain appears and is essentially a reflex emptying of the stomach. High small bowel obstructions, however, tend to cause persistent vomiting with profuse fluid and electrolyte losses. However, vomiting may appear late in low small bowel or large bowel obstruction, in which the character of the vomitus becomes foul-smelling and feculent because of bacterial decomposition of the bowel contents.

Diagnosis

Examination of the patient with a suspected mechanical obstruction should include a careful initial inspection for the presence of scars and evidence of external hernia. In early simple mechanical obstruction, the temperature, pulse, and state of hydration are generally normal. Palpation of the abdomen in the intervals between colicky pains may be notable for the lack of tenderness and guarding. However, localized tenderness may be noted over a dilated bowel loop or mass representing an intussusception or a volvulus. Diverticulitis or cancer of the left colon may also be palpable in some patients. The most important part of the examination in early obstruction is auscultation, and it is the finding of hyperactive and high-pitched bowel sounds synchronous with the patient's colicky pain that is most suggestive of the diagnosis.

The possibility of a strangulation obstruction should be considered most strongly in patients suspected of having closed loop obstruction, such as an incarcerated hernia, a volvulus, or an intussusception. Suspicion of possible strangulation is based largely on clinical findings, and it must be emphasized that signs and symptoms of strangulation are not always clearly present, even in established cases of bowel ischemia. The pain in strangulation obstruction tends to be more constant and more severe than that experienced in simple obstruction. The patient also appears more toxic and dehydrated and may have significant fever and tachycardia as well. Tenderness is more marked on abdominal palpation, and other signs of peritoneal irritation are often present. Evidence of rebound tenderness, rigidity, or an abdominal mass should suggest the possibility

of strangulation. A leukocytosis in the range of 15,000 to 25,000 per cu. mm. is most suggestive of strangulation, while elevations above this level may be thought to be more typical of acute mesenteric vascular occlusion.

The hematocrit level, white blood cell count, and serum electrolyte determinations are routine laboratory examinations that are obtained initially and at regular intervals following the patient's admission to the hospital. Hematocrit levels and urine specific gravity determinations may reflect the degree of dehydration present. The white blood cell count may be particularly useful in patients suspected of having strangulation obstruction. Serum amylase elevations are regularly found in patients with acute intestinal obstruction of both simple and strangulating types.

Most helpful in the diagnosis of intestinal obstruction, however, are the plain x-ray films taken with the patient supine and upright or in the lateral decubitus position (Fig. 37–1). These films, when interpreted in relationship to the history and physical findings, may also serve to identify the level of the obstruction and may help to differentiate simple from strangulation obstruction and mechanical obstruction from paralytic ileus. Additional help may be sought from the radiologist when the findings of plain films are inconclusive. A barium enema may be revealing if large bowel obstruction or intussusception is a possibility. Occasionally, oral administration of barium or meglumine diatrizoate (Gastrografin) may help to identify the type and level of the obstruction. Intravenous pyelography may occasionally be useful in obscure clinical situations involving a paralytic ileus due to ureteral stone. In patients in whom there is a suspicion of strangulation obstruction and particularly in those in whom there is no marked degree of abdominal distention, a peritoneal tap may be of some diagnostic help. Using local anesthesia, a four-quadrant paracentesis or lower midline peritoneal lavage may allow examination of a sample of peritoneal fluid. The fluid obtained from patients with strangulation obstruction characteristically is hemorrhagic in appearance, has a fetid odor, and frequently shows the presence of gram-negative rods on Gram's stain.

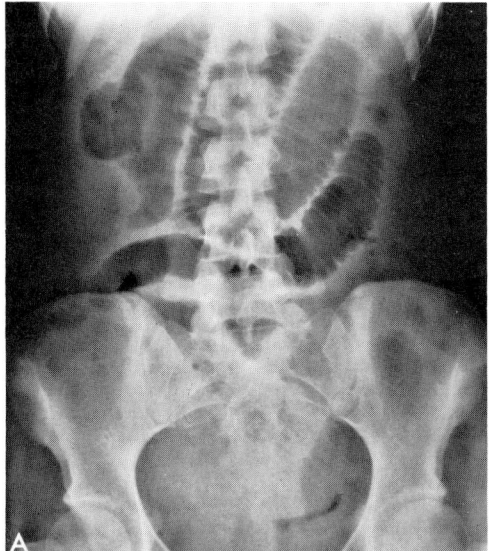

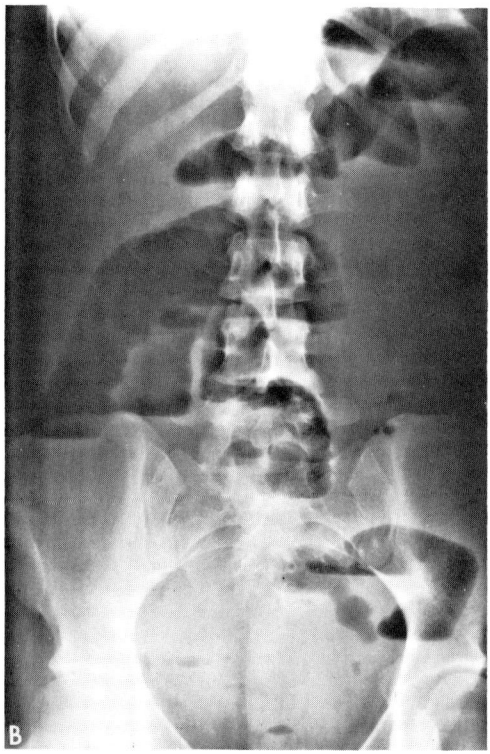

Figure 37-1. A. *Flat film of the abdomen, showing dilated small bowel, haziness suggestive of peritoneal fluid, and minimal gas in large bowel.*

B. Upright film of same patient, showing air-fluid levels. The patient, a 22 year old man with signs of mechanical small bowel obstruction, developed fever, leukocytosis, and a palpable tender abdominal mass over the course of 12 hours of observation. At operation he was found to have a volvulus of the distal ileum with strangulation, caused by adhesions secondary to a previous appendectomy.

Treatment

The general principles of treatment of intestinal obstruction include (1) intestinal decompression, (2) fluid and electrolyte therapy, and (3) timed surgical intervention.

Patients having simple small bowel obstruction of relatively short duration can be prepared for operation within a period of 4 to 6 hours after hospitalization. Insertion of a Levin tube and establishment of nasogastric suction, together with administration of a balanced salt solution by the intravenous route, begin during the period of diagnostic study soon after admission to the hospital. If there are minimal signs of dehydration and no serious associated cardiovascular, pulmonary or renal disease, the patient can be operated on promptly and with a low risk of mortality. In those patients with simple obstruction of several days' duration, longer periods of preparation are required because of the greater degree of fluid and electrolyte depletion, as well as the presence of more severe abdominal distention. In elderly patients or in those with impairment of vital organ function, even more importance may be attached to preoperative restoration of fluid and electrolyte balance, establishment of good urinary output, and improvement in myocardial function. In such patients, it is advisable to decompress the bowel by suction after insertion of a long intestinal tube, such as a Cantor tube. Fluoroscopy may be useful in positioning the mercury-weighted tube and in manipulating its passage through the distal stomach and pylorus. Appropriate repair solutions and potassium supplements should be given, according to the degree of electrolyte losses measured in the suction returns and to the results of serial serum electrolyte determinations.

Recognition of the possibility of strangulation obstruction should lead to a decision for an emergency operation to be performed within 2 hours following hospital admission. Administration of broad-spectrum antibiotics, replacement of fluid and blood as guided by central venous pressure determinations, and monitoring of hourly urinary output are essential parts of the crash program of preoperative preparation of such patients.

Operations for simple small bowel obstruction usually consist of division of obstructing adhesive bands or reduction and repair of an incarcerated hernia. Strangulation obstructions are managed by resection of the damaged segment of small intestine with an end-to-end anastomosis. In occasional instances of obstruction of the lower small bowel caused by Crohn's disease, a bypass procedure such as an ileotransverse colostomy may be chosen. In patients with typical left-sided colonic obstruction, a preliminary proximal transverse colostomy may be performed, followed by a definitive resection of the obstructing lesion somewhat later. In certain cases of volvulus of the sigmoid colon with strangulation, exteriorization of the loop with an obstructive resection may be elected. In right-sided colonic obstructions, immediate resection of the lesion with ileotransverse colostomy is usually chosen, but in debilitated, poor-risk patients, a preliminary bypass operation involving an ileotransverse colostomy followed later by resection of the obstruction may be preferable.

Nonoperative treatment of intestinal obstruction should be limited to a number of well-defined situations. The indiscriminate use of tube decompression and supportive therapy as a definitive treatment carries more risk of overlooking a strangulating mechanism and of causing prolonged morbidity than does the use of a planned operation. The nonoperative approach is usually preferred in patients with early postoperative obstruction, in patients with proven dissemination of intra-abdominal cancer, in babies with ileocecal intussusception when this may be treated by barium enema reduction, and in patients with sigmoid volvulus when decompression of the obstructed loop can be obtained by insertion of a rectal tube via the proctoscope. A case can also be made for nonoperative management of selected patients who have had repeated episodes of small bowel obstruction caused by adhesions and in whom the avoidance of another surgical operation is much desired. Prompt surgical exploration is clearly indicated for any patient being managed conservatively when, under observation, pain is noted to increase in severity or to become steady or generalized or when there is an increase in abdominal tenderness or other indications of possible strangulation.

ACUTE CHOLECYSTITIS

The incidence of symptomatic gallstone disease increases steadily in each decade of life. Acute cholecystitis, which is primarily associated with obstruction due to cholelithiasis, is one of the more serious complications of gallbladder disease, especially since it is most frequent in patients who are 60 to 80 years of age.

The occurrence of acute cholecystitis following surgical procedures that have not directly affected the biliary tree is not rare. This is a particularly difficult diagnosis to make, and the disease has a substantial risk of gangrene and perforation of the wall of the gallbladder. The dehydration, fasting, and higher-than-normal biliary pressure may promote stasis and may encourage obstruction of the gallbladder by stones in the preoperative and early postoperative periods.

The pain of acute cholecystitis is best regarded as simply an extension of biliary colic. Thus, it is usually of sudden onset, reaches its maximal severity quickly, and does not vary much in intensity. Its location is in the right upper abdominal quadrant or in the epigastrium, with radiation to the right costal margin and to the back below the right scapula. The pain is often worse on deep inspiration and infrequently may be associated with much nausea and vomiting.

The usual initiating event both in biliary colic and in acute cholecystitis is blockage of the cystic duct or ampullary end of the gallbladder by a stone. The subsequent distention of the gallbladder in conjunction with transmural inflammation of its wall, infection, and ischemia gives rise to the more severe pain and peritoneal signs that are characteristic of acute cholecystitis.

In a small but significant number of patients, the pathologic process may proceed quickly to gangrene of the gallbladder wall and perforation, usually with localization by a walling-off process in the vicinity of the gallbladder and, rather rarely, with the development of generalized peritonitis.

Diagnosis

There often is a mild degree of abdominal distention caused mainly by swallowed air within the stomach. Respirations may be rapid and shallow, and deep inspiration is inhibited by pain in the right upper quadrant. Peristalsis is usually audible. Palpation reveals maximal tenderness in the right upper quadrant of the abdomen, often accompanied by voluntary guarding and a Murphy's sign of inspiratory arrest. Careful palpation will frequently reveal the outline of a somewhat globular mass in the right subcostal region representing a tensely distended and inflamed gallbladder.

Differential diagnosis chiefly includes acute pancreatitis, perforated peptic ulcer, and strangulating small bowel obstruction. Lesions above the diaphragm should be considered as well. These include pneumonia, myocardial infarction, congestive failure, and pulmonary embolism. Leukocytosis is often present in acute cholecystitis, as are moderate elevations of serum bilirubin, alkaline phosphatase, and serum amylase levels. Chest x-ray films and flat and upright films of the abdomen should be obtained for diagnostic purposes in most instances. Films of the abdomen will reveal radiopaque gallstones in about 10 per cent of patients and a soft tissue mass representing the enlarged gallbladder in a few others. In selected patients, intravenous cholangiography may be useful for diagnostic purposes, and in patients with typical acute cholecystitis, this test reveals an unobstructed common bile duct with nonvisualization of the gallbladder.

Treatment

Preliminary treatment of acute cholecystitis includes the usual measures such as nasogastric suction, analgesics, and parenteral administration of fluids. Intravenous administration of ampicillin, tetracycline, or a cephalosporin is currently recommended. A surgeon should be called to see the patient if symptoms persist for more than 3 or 4 hours from time of onset.

Early surgical intervention appears to be the preferred treatment. Such intervention can be defined as a scheduled operation during daylight hours within the first 2 or 3 days after the onset of illness. Deliberate choice of an early operation effectively reduces the hospital stay of many patients and eliminates the considerable risk of overlooking a perforation. If there is doubt concerning the diagnosis or if the patient

makes a very prompt response to supportive measures during the first 48 hours of hospitalization, the acute inflammation is allowed to subside, and the patient is brought back several weeks later for oral cholecystography. When a diagnosis of cholelithiasis is supported by the x-ray findings, an interval operation can be performed about 6 to 8 weeks following the acute episode.

Acute cholecystitis in an elderly, debilitated, or extremely obese patient has special problems in regard to risk. The operation of cholecystostomy, or drainage of the gallbladder after removal of all visible and palpable stones, can be done with local anesthesia. Cholecystostomy continues to offer a safe and effective way of handling the obstructed and inflamed gallbladder when patients are too sick to tolerate cholecystectomy or when technical factors make removal of the gallbladder risky. This procedure involves draining the gallbladder by means of a catheter, which can be used for cholangiograms postoperatively and which is usually removed within 2 weeks following surgery. In poor risk patients, cholecystostomy can be regarded as a definitive operation. Because of the eventual recurrence of stones in the gallbladder, however, patients with reasonable life expectancy should have an elective cholecystectomy within a few months after recovery from the initial illness.

ACUTE PANCREATITIS

At least half of the patients with acute pancreatitis seen by physicians appear to have associated chronic alcoholism and about a quarter appear to have associated biliary tract disease. Blunt and penetrating abdominal trauma rather infrequently causes acute pancreatitis, as do operative manipulations about the pancreas and the biliary tree. A small number of cases may be associated with primary hyperparathyroidism, hyperlipemia, and other metabolic defects. Ten per cent of the total number of cases have no apparent association with a background disorder. The severity of pancreatitis ranges from mild interstitial inflammation of a transient sort to a fulminating hemorrhagic and necrotizing form of the disease.

Diagnosis

In typical acute pancreatitis, the pain is located in the epigastrium, often with radiation straight through to the back, and is accompanied by a marked degree of nausea and persistent vomiting. There is usually impressive upper abdominal tenderness accompanied by voluntary guarding of the abdominal wall. Peristaltic sounds are hypoactive or absent, and fever and leukocytosis usually occur. In the acute hemorrhagic variety of pancreatitis, there often is evidence of hypovolemia, manifested by tachycardia, hypotension, and other signs of shock. Elevation of the serum amylase level occurs early in the course of the illness and is usually observed to be at a higher and more sustained level than in other acute conditions associated with hyperamylasemia, such as perforated ulcer, strangulation obstruction, or acute cholecystitis. In the milder forms of the disease, however, elevation of the serum amylase level may be transient; thus, the finding of an elevation of amylase output in the urine may be useful in formulating a diagnosis. Elevations of urinary amylase levels greater than 300 Somogyi units in 1 hour should suggest the diagnosis. Hyperglycemia and depression of serum calcium levels are other common laboratory findings.

In patients with abdominal pain and jaundice who are found to have an elevated serum amylase level, the degree of elevation is helpful in differentiating the type of pancreatitis present. Those with elevations of 1000 Somogyi units or greater are usually found to have biliary tract disease. It is wise also to assume that alcoholic patients with abdominal pain have acute pancreatitis until this is ruled out.

Other helpful laboratory examinations for patients suspected of having acute pancreatitis include flat and upright films of the abdomen and, when feasible, films of the upper gastrointestinal tract with use of a contrast material such as barium or Gastrografin. The plain abdominal films serve to identify the characteristic pattern of paralytic ileus associated with acute inflammation of the pancreas, calcifications of the pancreas, and radiopaque calculi seen in the location of the gallbladder or the common duct. Contrast studies serve to show characteristic displacements of the stomach or duodenum caused by swelling of the pancreas and to identify the typical changes in the duodenal mucosa induced by inflammation in the adjacent portions of the pancreas. Occasionally, a paracentesis or peritoneal lavage may help to identify an otherwise obscure process within the abdomen by determining the elevations of amylase levels within the fluid obtained from the abdominal cavity. Sequential measurement of electrolytes and of serum calcium and hematocrit levels may be of great value for patients with more severe acute pancreatitis in gauging the response to therapy and in assessing the severity of the underlying inflammation.

Treatment

The treatment of acute pancreatitis, which is nonsurgical when the diagnosis is well established, involves supportive measures such as gastrointestinal suction and the administration of appropriate amounts of parenteral fluids. Suction is designed to keep the pancreas at rest and the stomach decompressed. Parenteral fluids are given to replace the third-space losses associated with inflammation or hemorrhage in the retroperitoneal area and peritoneal cavity, as well as those incurred by suction and vomiting. Central venous pressure monitoring, by means of a catheter in the superior vena cava introduced through the jugular or subclavian veins, is helpful in guiding fluid administration in elderly patients, particularly in those with the fulminating forms of the disease. Laparotomy is generally recommended at an early stage when the diagnosis is doubtful or when acute cholecystitis or common duct obstruction appears to be the primary problem. Later on in the course of the acute hemorrhagic form of the disease, there may be urgent indications for the drainage of abscesses or collections of necrotic material in the lesser peritoneal sac. In certain patients who fail to improve despite all supportive measures, a more aggressive surgical approach is justified. This includes biliary tract decompression by cholecystostomy, drainage of the lesser peritoneal sac with sump catheters, peritoneal lavage, and establishment of a gastrostomy and feeding jejunostomy.

Relief of pain is achieved by judicious administration of analgesics such as meperidine or morphine. Antimicrobial agents are usually given as prophylaxis against gram-negative enteric organisms in the severe forms of the disease. Calcium salts are administered intravenously if the serum calcium level is markedly depressed or if the patient develops tetany.

Serious pulmonary complications are commonly seen in the more toxic patients with fulminating pancreatitis. Pleural effusions, when present, should be relieved by thoracentesis. Patients with serious ventilatory impairment may require tracheal intubation or tracheostomy with respiratory support. When biliary tract disease is suspected of being associated with acute pancreatitis, it is usual to employ oral cholecystography or intravenous cholangiography several weeks following hospital discharge in order to determine if stones are present in the gallbladder or biliary tree. When gallstones are found, cholecystectomy with common duct exploration and operative cholangiography is performed 1 or 2 months following the subsidence of pancreatitis.

Patients may present with upper abdominal masses either during an attack of acute pancreatitis or during the convalescent phase. These frequently prove to be pancreatic pseudocysts and are seen predominantly in alcoholic patients. Such pseudocysts also occur after trauma and are usually associated with tenderness, fever, and ileus. The displacement of the stomach or other parts of the upper gastrointestinal tract seen with barium studies aids in the localization of these lesions, which most commonly are in the lesser omental bursa. Diagnostic ultrasonography may be of some additional value in differentiating pancreatic pseudocysts from other masses in the pancreas or retroperitoneal tissues. Surgical intervention is reserved for patients who have evidence of sepsis or hemorrhage within the cyst or for those who have chronic pseudocysts as a method of preventing these serious complications from occurring. Operation usually involves anastomosis of the cyst to the posterior wall of the stomach or to a defunctionalized loop of proximal jejunum.

UPPER GASTROINTESTINAL BLEEDING

A presumptive diagnosis of upper gastrointestinal bleeding can be made in patients with a history of hematemesis or melena. Passage of bright red blood by rectum is most often associated with a source of bleeding below the ligament of Treitz, although in occasional instances of massive bleeding from a duodenal ulcer, there may be bright red blood mixed with clots in the bowel movement.

At least two-thirds of patients with upper gastrointestinal bleeding have a duodenal or a gastric ulcer. Hemorrhagic gastritis and esophageal varices are also seen in a significant number of patients. Less common causes include gastric neoplasm, hiatal hernia, leiomyoma of the stomach, gastric erosions, and mucosal tears at the esophagogastric junction.

Management of upper gastrointestinal bleeding includes three sequential and overlapping steps:

1. Treatment of hemorrhage and prevention of shock.

2. Diagnostic measures to determine the source of the bleeding.

3. Choice of surgical or nonsurgical measures for treatment of the patient.

Diagnosis and Early Management

While the history is being taken, a dependable vein is cannulated, and blood is drawn for baseline chemical and hematologic studies and for crossmatching. Appropriate intravenous fluids (usually Ringer's lactate solution initially) are started, and a nasogastric tube is inserted. The stomach is emptied, and the aspirated material is examined for blood. A positive test for blood is proof of a source of bleeding above the ligament of Treitz. A clear aspirate, however, does not rule out the possibility of hemorrhage from a duodenal ulcer. Ice-cold isotonic saline should be used to irrigate the stomach if there is evidence of active bleeding, and lavage should be continued aggressively in the presence of persistent bleeding. Continuous suction with intermittent irrigation is used to keep the stomach empty and to monitor the rate of hemorrhage.

A central venous line is inserted in most situations involving evidence of major bleeding. Requirements for whole blood are gauged on the basis of evidence of hypotension, tachycardia, pallor, and other signs of shock and by measurements of blood pressure, pulse rate, and central venous pressure. The urine output should be monitored on an hourly basis, using an indwelling catheter. The rate of fluid administration is adjusted to maintain a urine flow of at least 30 ml. per hour if myocardial function is judged to be normal and if there is no unusual rise in central venous pressure. The history from the patient, family, or friends should be completely and accurately recorded. Symptoms of peptic ulcer or chronic alcoholism are sought. Questions are asked concerning the possible ingestion of aspirin, phenylbutazone, anticoagulants, or steroids. Careful consideration is given to a history of previous bleeding, the possibility of a hemorrhagic diathesis, and the significance of previous operations.

Physical examination should include a careful search for the stigmata of liver disease. The presence of abdominal tenderness, masses, or fluid; liver enlargement; and splenomegaly should be looked for. Surgical consultation should be sought promptly, and subsequent major decisions concerning therapy should be made jointly with the surgeon. As soon as the patient's situation has stabilized, a fiberoptic endoscopy should be performed. Subsequent to that, if necessary, an upper gastrointestinal x-ray examination should be done.

Estimates of the severity of blood loss are based on observations concerning the patient's vital signs, the amount of fresh bleeding in the suction returns, and the patient's response to blood replacement. The term "massive hemorrhage" is used to describe clinical situations in which signs of shock are present, and, in an adult, this usually indicates a loss of 1500 ml. or more of blood. Signs of continued active bleeding include the frequent passage of tarry or grossly bloody stools accompanied by peristaltic rushes, with a rising blood urea nitrogen level and increasing leukocytosis. Serial hematocrit determinations, together with knowledge of the amounts of fluid and blood given, furnish additional help in gauging the extent and rate of bleeding. Determination of central venous pressure in sequence is useful in following the response to transfusion therapy and will give warning of impending myocardial failure in the elderly patient or in those with significant associated cardiovascular disease.

Triage and Treatment

When peptic ulcer is established as the probable underlying cause of bleeding, the choice of treatment will be based on the age of the patient, a history of previous hemorrhage, the location of the ulcer, and the response of the patient to supportive measures. Other considerations include the adequacy of the reserve supply of blood for the patient and the availability of a competent surgical team if operation is elected. Certain general guidelines for decisions about the need for early operative intervention can be given as follows:

1. Patients over 50 years of age, especially those with significant arteriosclerotic cardiovascular disease, are candidates for an early operation.

2. A history of previous massive hemorrhage in a patient with a proven peptic ulcer is evidence in favor of operation.

3. Gastric ulcer and postbulbar duodenal ulcer, in general, require prompt operation because of their tendency to be associated with massive and recurrent hemorrhage and their predictably poor response to medical therapy. Massive bleeding from a duodenal ulcer that stops for a brief interval and then starts again or, alternatively, evidence of bleeding that requires more than 500 ml. of blood every 8 hours to maintain normal hemodynamics during the first 24 hour period suggests the need for early surgery.

The family physician and his surgical consultant should work together as closely as possible and should try always to avoid making the mistake of hesitating too long about surgical intervention. Choice of operative procedure will of course be made by the surgeon on the basis of accurate identification of the source of bleeding, the patient's age and physical status, and the severity of the hemorrhage. In good-risk patients with duodenal ulcers, antrectomy and vagotomy may be elected, whereas in older patients, suture ligation of the bleeding point, together with pyloroplasty and vagotomy, may be preferred. Gastric ulcer, in most instances, will be best managed by some form of resection with vagotomy, which allows careful pathologic examination of the entire ulcer.

Management of the patient with hemorrhage from esophageal varices includes an initial attempt to verify the diagnosis by esophagogastroscopy. It should be kept in mind that a sizable number of patients with cirrhosis and portal hypertension bleed from causes other than varices, including peptic ulcer and gastritis. When hemorrhage from varices is massive, a Sengstaken-Blakemore tube is inserted, and a trial of tamponade is made with the balloon inflated. Approximately 300 mm. of air is introduced into the gastric balloon, and the tube is placed on gentle traction. The esophageal balloon should then be inflated and its pressure (35 to 40 mm. Hg) monitored continuously with an attached blood pressure manometer. Supportive measures include blood transfusions, iced saline lavage of the stomach, administration of neomycin, 1 gram every 4 hours by tube, and intravenous infusion of posterior pituitary extract (Pituitrin), 20 units in 200 ml. of 5 per cent dextrose and water over a 30 minute period, repeated at 2 hour intervals. Vitamin K_1 should be given intravenously.

After surgical consultation, an emergency portal-systemic shunt should be considered early in the treatment of variceal hemorrhage, when a diagnosis of cirrhosis can be made confidently and when bleeding fails to stop using these measures. In expert hands, an emergency shunt carries an operative mortality that is distinctly less than the mortality resulting from conservative treatment in patients in whom hemorrhage fails to stop with tamponade and other nonoperative measures.

CHOLELITHIASIS

The high incidence of symptomatic cholelithiasis in our population has made cholecystectomy the most commonly performed intra-abdominal procedure in the United States. Cholecystectomy clearly is the treatment of choice for symptomatic individuals with cholelithiasis, and it carries a low risk of mortality and complications when performed as an elective procedure by competent surgeons. There is enormous interest and importance attached to current efforts to evaluate the potential for preventing or dissolving cholesterol gallstones by dietary measures or by the administration of bile salts. Primary physicians should support these national clinical trials whenever possible by referring appropriate patients for study.

Diagnosis

The great majority of patients with calculous biliary tract disease are symptomatic, the clinical manifestations being biliary colic and dyspepsia. The latter symptom includes postprandial fullness and flatulence, belching, nausea, and anorexia. A few patients with gallstones develop acute cholecystitis or obstructive jaundice due to cystic or common duct obstruction by stones. Relatively rare complications of cholelithiasis are suppurative cholangitis, gallstone ileus, and carcinoma of the gallbladder.

The diagnosis of cholelithiasis is made with considerable precision by radiologic methods (Figs. 37–2 and 37–3). Plain x-ray films of the abdomen reveal calcified gallstones in about 10 to 15 per cent of patients. On oral cholecystography, approximately 75 per cent of patients with cholelithiasis will show radiolucent filling defects in the contrast medium within the

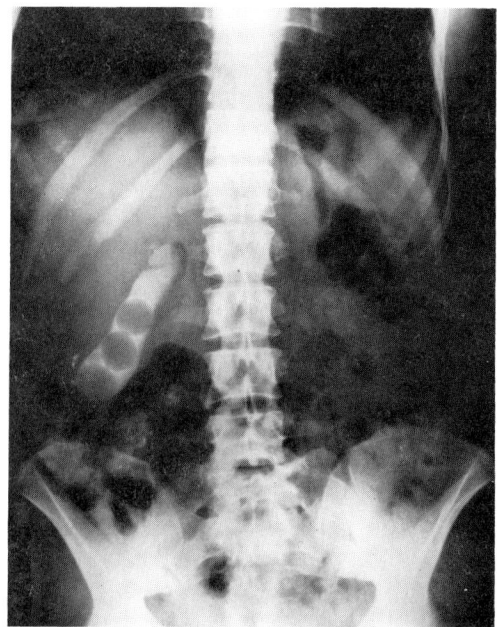

Figure 37–2. *Oral cholecystogram, showing filling defects in the gallbladder caused by nonopaque calculi. The patient, a 39 year old man, gave a history of postprandial fullness, flatulence, and intolerance to fatty foods. He denied biliary colic and was not jaundiced. The gallstones were confirmed at operation, and a cholecystectomy performed. Operative cholangiography showed the common duct to be normal. His symptoms have persisted following surgery.*

Biliary colic is the only symptom of cholelithiasis that can reliably be relieved by cholecystectomy.

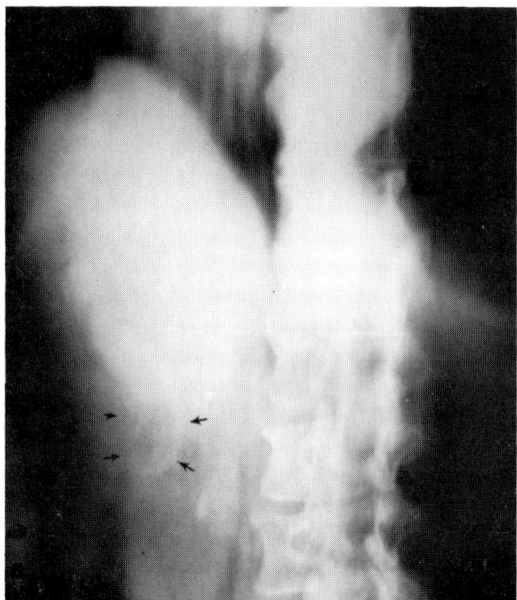

Figure 37–3. Intravenous cholangiogram showing a filling defect within a markedly dilated common duct (arrows). The patient, a 67 year old female, had a 10 year history of intermittent epigastric pain radiating to the right subscapular region, postprandial dyspepsia, and excessive flatulence. There was no jaundice. Symptoms had begun following a cholecystectomy for gallstone disease. At operation, a single large stone was removed from the common duct. Her "postcholecystectomy syndrome" was completely relieved.

gallbladder. The incidence of false positive results in cholecystography is very low. In the great majority of patients, nonvisualization is indicative of bile duct obstruction or of disease within the gallbladder wall resulting in the inability of the gallbladder to concentrate the dye. Other causes of nonvisualization should be considered, however, and these include failure of absorption of the dye and inadequate excretion of the dye by the liver due to disease. Cholecystography is unsatisfactory in patients having bilirubin levels greater than 1.8 mg. per 100 ml. Further accuracy in evaluating patients with nonvisualization may be achieved by repeating the dose of oral dye the following day or, alternatively, by performing ultrasonic cholecystography. The latter method is finding increasing application in the diagnosis of cholelithiasis, especially in emergencies, when acute cholecystitis or pancreatitis is suspected and in pregnancies, when x-ray exposure should be avoided if possible.

Treatment

Although most physicians would concede that cholecystectomy is indicated in symptomatic patients, the place of surgery in the treatment of patients with asymptomatic cholelithiasis is less well established. The majority of instances of truly silent gallstones appear to occur in elderly patients, and in this group, it is probably wise to await the appearance of the first symptoms before recommending cholecystectomy. The association of gallstones with diabetes mellitus or their presence in patients who live in areas remote from hospital facilities should suggest the need for planned removal of the gallbladder. Prophylactic operations can also be urged for patients in good physical condition who have a long life expectancy, on the basis of the likelihood of symptoms appearing sooner or later. During the performance of elective cholecystectomy, most surgeons now use operative cholangiography routinely to visualize the biliary tree during surgery. Use of this procedure helps in an important way to reduce the incidence of stones in the common duct being overlooked at the time of cholecystectomy. The overall frequency of common duct stones in patients with cholelithiasis is judged to be nearly 10 per cent. The standard indications for common duct exploration at the time of cholecystectomy are:

1. Jaundice, or a history of jaundice.
2. Palpable stone within the common bile duct.
3. Finding of a dilated or thickened common bile duct.
4. Presence of multiple small stones in the gallbladder.
5. History of cholangitis or pancreatitis.
6. Filling defect in the bile ducts seen by operative cholangiography.

Postoperative care following cholecystectomy is usually simple and straightforward. Nasogastric suction is seldom needed, and oral intake of fluids is usually resumed 1 or 2 days following operation. The gallbladder bed is usually drained with a Penrose drain, and drainage from this site usually ceases within a few days. The drain is removed 3 or 4 days postoperatively. A hospitalization period of about 6 or 7 days is usually required for cholecystectomy. In the follow-up period, no special diet is prescribed, and the patient is allowed to

resume normal activity after a convalescence of about 3 weeks.

Persistence of pain following cholecystectomy is unusual and should focus attention on the possibility of an alternative
diagnosis such as pancreatitis, peptic ulcer,
or hiatus hernia. An intravenous cholangiogram may show abnormalities such as a
large residual cystic duct stump, stenosis of
the sphincter of Oddi, a retained common
duct stone, or a biliary stricture. Postcholecystectomy problems are remarkably few in
patients whose symptoms are carefully
evaluated and whose gallbladder disease is
proved accurately before biliary tract
surgery is undertaken.

HERNIA

HERNIA IN CHILDREN

The common hernias of infants and children are those in the inguinal and umbilical locations. Direct inguinal and femoral
hernias are almost unknown in infants and
are rare in children. The majority of hernias in infants are indirect inguinal in type.
They are usually discovered by the parent
in the first few months of life, and greater
than 90 per cent of them occur in males.
The diagnosis rests on the physician's examining the infant at the time the hernia is
present. Differential diagnosis of a mass in
a baby's groin includes hernia, hydrocele
of the cord, and inguinal lymph node enlargement. Incarceration is fairly common,
and the majority of these occur in the first
year of life. Prompt reduction of the contents of the incarcerated hernia should be
sought, using sedation and the head-low
position soon after hospital admission with
elective repair delayed for 1 or 2 days to
allow the edema in the peritoneal sac to
subside. Complications of incarceration of
hernias in babies include not only intestinal obstruction and strangulation of the
bowel but damage to the testicle in male infants caused by compression of the pampiniform plexus in the spermatic cord.

In older children, inguinal hernia should
also be surgically corrected when first discovered. The operation involves little risk
in the otherwise healthy child.

Repair is accomplished rather simply by
high ligation and excision of the peritoneal
sac and seldom requires reinforcement of
supporting structures with sutures. The
operation is done under general anesthesia
as an outpatient procedure. Hospitalization
is seldom required, complications are few,
and recurrences are rare, which is in considerable contrast to the situation as it pertains to adults.

Statistics relating to the incidence of bilateral inguinal hernias are somewhat confusing. In children less than 5 years of age,
justification can be made for bilateral
inguinal exploration when only one side
clinically appears to involve a hernia. The
use of an x-ray picture of the hernia sac
obtained by intraperitoneal injection of a
radiopaque dye has proved helpful in selecting patients for bilateral inguinal exploration (Figs. 37–4 and 37–5).

Umbilical hernias in infants include the
very common ones identified at birth,
which seldom become incarcerated. These
can be confidently managed simply by
being followed, in the belief that most of
them will be obliterated by spontaneous
closure of the umbilical ring before the age
of 3 or 4 years. However, the larger umbilical hernias with rings wider than 1.5 cm.
are probably best repaired in early childhood.

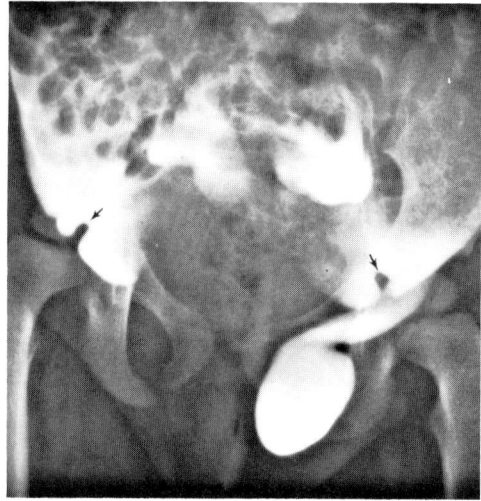

Figure 37–4. *Inguinal herniogram in a 14 month
old female infant with clinical evidence of a left inguinal hernia. X-ray confirmed the absence of a
right-sided peritoneal process. Arrows mark the
notches in the peritoneum caused by the deep epigastric vessels. Film represents an adequate herniogram. (Courtesy Dr. J. J. White.)*

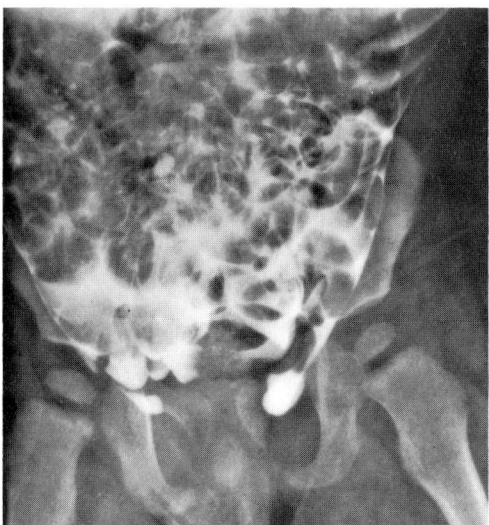

Figure 37–5. *Inguinal herniogram in a 3 month old male infant who had clinical findings of a unilateral inguinal hernia. X-ray, taken 45 minutes following injection of 15 ml. of diatrizoate into the peritoneal cavity, showed filling of both the left-sided hernial sac and an open peritoneal sac on the right. Bilateral exploration subsequently confirmed this finding.*

Another less common hernia of childhood is the epigastric hernia, which appears in or near the midline of the upper abdomen and presents as a small, tender, button-like mass in the subcutaneous fat about halfway between the xiphoid process and the umbilicus. It usually consists of a small incarcerated protrusion of fat or omentum through a slit-like opening in the linea alba or the rectus sheath. Repair is accomplished under general anesthesia in an outpatient setting.

HERNIA IN ADULTS

Inguinal and Femoral Hernia. In adult patients, a greater variety of hernias are seen, many of them first detected at the time of a careful physical examination done by the primary physician. Groin hernias, which include the direct and indirect hernias and the femoral hernia, involve abdominal wall defects that allow protrusion of properitoneal fat and, in most patients, a protrusion of a peritoneal sac. Indirect inguinal hernia, which is the most common type, involves a peritoneal sac protruding through the internal inguinal ring, with the sac having the

same coverings as the investments of the spermatic cord. It develops in males because of failure of the obliteration of the processus vaginalis testis in the descent of the testicle to the scrotum. Direct hernia is more likely to be found in middle-aged males and represents a protrusion through the posterior inguinal wall medial to the internal ring and the inferior epigastric vessels. Clinical identification of the exact anatomic type of groin hernia is not important.

Examination of the inguinal and femoral regions in the adult precedes the abdominal examination. The patient should stand in front of the seated examiner while the inguinal and femoral canals are palpated carefully with the patient straining gently. An actual protrusion must be felt by the examining finger to be sure of the diagnosis of hernia. A marked cough impulse or a patulous external ring is not considered adequate clinical evidence for the diagnosis of hernia. The most difficult hernia to identify on physical examination, especially in obese patients, is the femoral hernia, which may easily be confused with an enlarged femoral lymph node or a thrombosed saphenous varix.

Sudden incarceration of femoral or inguinal hernias is usually associated with hernias passing through narrow internal inguinal or femoral rings and is more commonly seen in hernias that are difficult to reduce in normal circumstances. Prompt operation is recommended for all incarcerated groin hernias in adults because of the risk of intestinal strangulation. Exception might be made in the case of certain incarcerated inguinal hernias detected in patients who show no evidence of peritoneal irritation, fever, or leukocytosis. After surgical consultation has been obtained, a single attempt at gentle manual reduction may be made after the patient has been given sedation and placed in the Trendelenburg position.

It has been a real accomplishment of modern-day surgery that intestinal obstruction, particularly of the strangulation variety, has been markedly reduced by widespread adoption of surgical repair of hernias in all age groups. Early repair of groin hernias is also encouraged based on the observation that the young adult known to have a hernia may have difficulty in finding employment. In addition, most neglected hernias tend to enlarge steadily over the years and become more and more difficult to repair as they get larger. Exceptions to the rule that most hernias should be repaired electively include the few patients with marked obesity, uncontrolled cough, severe cardiovascular or renal disease, or other conditions associated with limited life expectancy and high risk of operation. However, even the very elderly patient can be properly considered a candidate for operation when the hernia is small and symptomatic, and has potential for incarceration. The use of local anesthesia for this type of surgery has proved very satisfactory and is the preferred method for repair in the high-risk patient.

Umbilical Hernia.   The adult type of umbilical hernia, which is more common in the female, also has potential for incarceration. Pregnancy tends to enlarge such hernias, and when neglected, they can become enormous with the advancing years. In the unusual situation involving the presence of an umbilical hernia in a patient with uncontrolled ascites due to underlying cirrhosis, spontaneous rupture of the hernia may occur, with lethal consequences.

Incisional Hernia.   Incisional hernias are the classic example of hernias occurring through an acquired defect in the abdominal wall. These may be largely attributed to failure of wound healing at the time of a previous operation, often associated with wound dehiscence. The underlying causative factors include obesity, increased intra-abdominal pressure caused by cough or distention, wound infection, and error in technique of wound closure. Vertical scars, especially those in the midline, are most frequently involved. The fascial defect underlying the scar can best be felt with the patient lying in the supine position and straining gently against the examiner's hand. Incarceration is a very present danger in those hernias involving narrow defects or multiple fenestrations at the fascial level.

The selection of patients for incisional hernia repair is based on numerous factors, including the size of the defect, the quality of tissues available for repair, and any associated conditions in the patient that might predispose to early recurrence. A period of intensive preoperative preparation may be required when the volume of hernia contents is large and the defect is a broad one. Reduction of weight, control of the factors producing increased intra-abdominal pressure, and occasional resort to progressive pneumoperitoneum may be of help in obtaining optimum conditions for repair of this challenging type of hernia (Fig. 37–6).

Clearly, the best time to repair a hernia

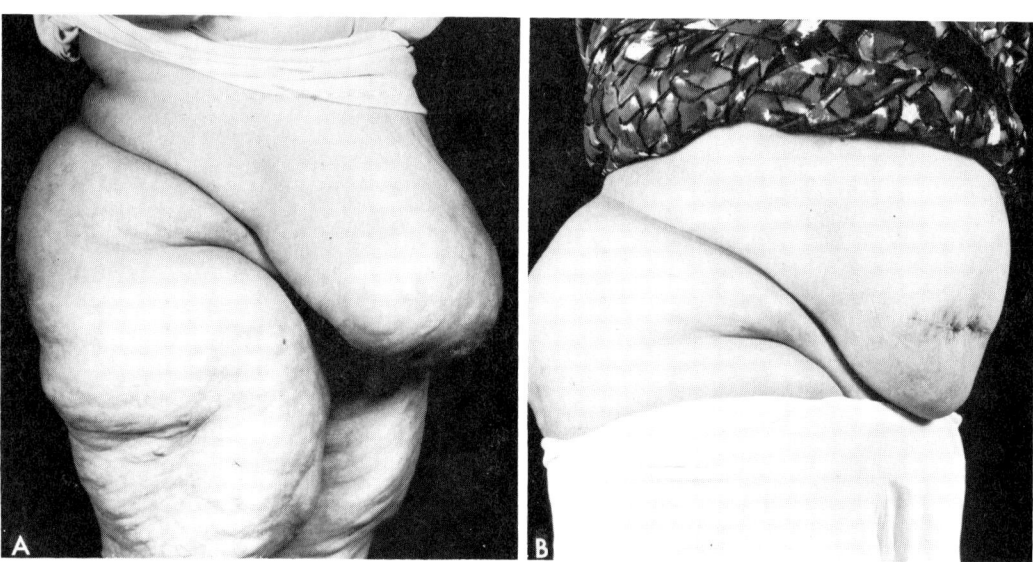

Figure 37–6. A. A large irreducible incisional hernia in an obese woman of middle age. Preoperative measures included weight reduction and use of progressive pneumoperitoneum over a 3 week period.
B. The same patient, following successful surgical repair of the hernia, which did not require the use of prosthetic mesh or autogenous fascial grafts.

is in infancy or in childhood when a simple technical procedure can be done in an out-patient setting and when the recovery period is very short indeed. The operation and postoperative recovery become poten-tially more complicated in adults but still usually require only a brief hospitalization. Early mobilization is recommended, and there is no evidence to confirm that avoid-ance of mild exercise following surgery in any way reduces the possibility of recur-rence. Adult men with sedentary occupa-tions often require a period of about 3 weeks from the time of surgery for convalescence. In those patients resuming heavy physical activity, a convalescence of 4 to 6 weeks is usually recommended. Sutures are removed after a week at the time of the first office visit. The patient is cautioned to avoid all heavy lifting, sports, or activities that might put a heavy strain on the abdominal wall repair.

The majority of recurrences are detected within a period of approximately 2 to 3 years following surgery. The direct inguinal hernias and the larger incisional hernias have the highest rates of recur-rence. While some recurrences are un-doubtedly caused by errors in operative technique, the majority appear to be asso-ciated with persistence of factors tending to increase the intra-abdominal wall pressure, such as obesity or chronic pulmonary dis-ease, as well as to the tissue changes as-sociated with aging, to strains caused by lifting, or to direct trauma.

ARTERIAL DISORDERS

ACUTE ARTERIAL OCCLUSIONS

Arterial Trauma. Certain wounds of the arm and leg, particularly those caused by gunshot or stabbing, may involve trauma to major arteries. Brisk bleeding from wounds in the limb or the location of a wound in proximity to a major vessel should always suggest the possibility of vascular injury. Fractures of the humerus or femur at the supracondylar level, certain femoral shaft fractures, and dislocations of the knee or elbow joint can also be complicated by ar-terial injury.

A familiarity with the signs and symp-toms of ischemia in the extremity is abso-lutely essential for the physician dealing

with trauma. Failure to restore arterial flow in an ischemic extremity within a period of about 6 hours usually results in gangrene and loss of the injured part. Ischemia in a muscle causes pain initially, whereas is-chemia in a nerve causes sensory loss and paralysis in the extremity. The classic physical findings of ischemia are coldness, pallor, and loss of peripheral pulses. In cer-tain instances of occult injury to major arte-ries, the persistence of palpable peripheral pulses or, more rarely, the complete ab-sence of signs of peripheral arterial insuf-ficiency will be misleading, and later oc-currence of arterial occlusion may go unrecognized, particularly if the limb has been bandaged or wrapped in a plaster splint.

Since most of the injuries to arteries in the extremity are manifested by severe ini-tial external bleeding or by formation of a large visible and palpable hematoma, shock will be a frequent finding. Control of hemorrhage should be obtained by applica-tion of a sterile pressure dressing to the ex-ternal wound, and measures should be taken to replace the blood loss rapidly. Ar-terial tourniquets should be avoided when-ever possible.

Obliteration of major blood vessels may also result from hemorrhage or from muscle swelling within a closed fascial space, as in the anterior tibial compartment syndrome. Arteriography is of major help in some doubtful cases, especially those involving fractures, dislocations, and soft tissue inju-ries in which the level and nature of the ar-terial injury is not clearly visualized. Since delay in restoring blood flow to the limb increases the risk of gangrene, all such in-juries involving the possibility of arterial trauma should be considered to be of high priority. Arrangements for prompt surgical exploration should be made at the earliest possible time after hospital admission. Pro-phylactic administration of antibiotics should commence by the intravenous route, using a penicillinase-resistant peni-cillin or a cephalosporin. When control of hemorrhage is obtained, a full restoration of blood volume using blood or plasma ex-panders should be completed before the patient is taken to the operating room for arterial repair.

Arterial Embolism. Embolic occlusion of a major artery is another surgical emergency in which delay in institution of treatment may cause loss of limb or life. It is most frequently seen in patients with arteriosclerotic heart disease and atrial fibrillation. A small percentage of patients will have a history of rheumatic heart disease. The majority of emboli come from the left atrium, but some may also originate from mural thrombus within the left ventricle as a result of recent myocardial infarction. A very small number may come from prosthetic heart valves or from thrombus or atherosclerotic plaques within the abdominal aorta.

Nearly three-fourths of such thrombi lodge in the arteries of the leg or arm, usually at points of bifurcation of vessels where the caliber decreases sharply. Distal thrombosis progressively occludes the collateral circulation and results in irreversible ischemia. The threat of propagation of thrombus distal to the embolus justifies the immediate use of heparin once the diagnosis is made and prior to the performance of surgical embolectomy.

The physician should suspect arterial embolism in patients with known heart disease who complain of pain, numbness, or weakness in the arm or leg, especially when this is of sudden, rather than insidious, onset. A history of suddenness of onset is particularly suggestive of embolism rather than of thrombosis as a cause of acute arterial occlusion.

Physical examination will usually demonstrate marked pallor in the distal part of the extremity in association with coldness and loss of peripheral pulses. When embolization to the bifurcation of the aorta occurs, these signs will be apparent in both legs, and no pulsation will be felt in either groin. When the embolus is lodged in the iliac bifurcation, signs will be unilateral in the lower extremity, and the pulse will be absent in the groin on the affected side. Common femoral artery obstruction will be indicated by a palpable pulse being present in the region of the inguinal ligament and disappearing several centimeters distal to this point. If the pulse can be felt in the common femoral artery but not in the popliteal area or in the foot, the embolus is presumed to be in the region of the bifurcation of the popliteal artery. In the presence of established ischemia, a rapid investigation of the cardiac status of the patient should be made. In the absence of atrial fibrillation or evidence of rheumatic

heart disease, myocardial infarction of recent origin should be suspected in a high proportion of these patients. Preoperative delays should be brief, especially for those patients manifesting severe ischemia. Arteriography is not justified when the diagnosis of embolism can be made with confidence by history and physical examination.

Most of the patients who require embolectomy are critically ill, so that this procedure is best carried out under local anesthesia using the Fogarty balloon catheter for retrieval of the distal or proximal thrombus. Even in the presence of severe heart disease, patients whose limbs are in jeopardy should almost invariably be considered candidates for surgery because of the fairly low operative risks involved.

Initial anticoagulant therapy using 5000 to 10,000 units of heparin intravenously should be instituted as soon as the diagnosis is established and is usually continued postoperatively, beginning 6 to 12 hours following operation. An average of 5000 units of heparin is given every 6 hours through an intravenous catheter placed in a forearm vein. Lee-White clotting time is used to monitor the therapy and is checked once daily, 5 hours after the last injection of heparin. The dose is adjusted downward and is omitted altogether if the clotting time is over 30 minutes. Oral use of anticoagulants such as warfarin sodium is usually recommended if fibrillation persists.

In the absence of prolonged ischemia, excellent results from operative removal of the embolus can be expected in most patients. The golden period for retrieval of thrombi is approximately 6 to 8 hours following embolism, and thereafter the results of embolectomy become progressively poorer owing to the occlusion of collateral arterial branches by extensive distal propagating clot.

Arterial Thrombosis. Arterial thrombosis is a somewhat less frequent cause of acute occlusion of limb arteries than is embolism. Since arterial thrombosis represents a sudden, total obstruction of a previously stenotic or narrowed artery involved in an arteriosclerotic process, it usually has a more insidious onset than does arterial embolism. The first symptom noted in the extremity is frequently that of numbness and is often of gradual onset. Thrombosis can also be associated with peripheral aneurysms or with chronic injury associated, for example, with mechanical compression of an artery, as in the case of the subclavian artery in the thoracic outlet compression syndrome. Diagnosis may be aided by finding evidence of pre-existing arterial disease, including trophic changes in the feet, a history of intermittent claudication, and the presence of other stigmata of chronic arterial insufficiency in the opposite extremity. Absence of evidence of a cardiac source for an embolus is another point in favor of the diagnosis of thrombosis. The skin pallor seen in arterial thrombosis is usually much less impressive than that seen in arterial embolism.

Arteriographic study in these patients is usually essential to evaluate the extent of collateral development, the distal runoff, and the possibility of additional stenotic lesions at other sites. Initial heparinization is begun (as in arterial embolism) while studies are in progress. Patients with potentially salvageable limbs are considered candidates for an early attempt at arterial reconstruction.

CHRONIC PERIPHERAL ARTERIAL OCCLUSIVE DISEASE

Chronic peripheral arterial occlusive disease (PAOD) is practically synonymous with obliterative arterial disease of the lower extremity. The lesions are often initially located at the bifurcation of vessels and are distributed in segmental fashion in the distal arterial tree. They begin as stenosing lesions and progress through various degrees of narrowing to complete thrombotic occlusion. The disease thus progresses in a stepwise fashion with a series of acute arterial thromboses occurring in vessels narrowed by atheromatous plaques. Predilection of the disease for special sites, including the terminal aorta, the iliac vessels, and the superficial femoral artery at the adductor canal, provides characteristic patterns of limb ischemia. PAOD is a disease that predominates in males, and symptoms appear to be aggravated by smoking, presumably by effecting vasoconstriction. An accelerated clinical course and a much higher rate of amputation are seen in the patient with diabetes mellitus.

Diagnosis

The characteristic symptoms of PAOD are intermittent claudication and ischemic rest pain.

The primary physican must learn to recognize these two clear-cut symptoms in order to avoid errors in diagnosis. Intermittent claudication refers to the pain or fatigue in a muscle or muscle group that is apparent to the patient upon use of the affected part in exercise. The pain or fatigue is quickly relieved by rest. In many instances, the patient can measure the distance that it takes to produce the symptom of claudication and can note that this is quickly relieved by standing still. Pain is more apparent when the patient is walking faster, up a hill, or on a hard, unyielding surface. In aortoiliac obstructions, the pain or fatigue is usually experienced in the hip or thigh; whereas, in femoropopliteal obstructions, the symptoms are more commonly localized in the calf. Ischemic rest pain occurring at night in bed is indicative of a far-advanced stage of the disease. Rest pain occurs in the area of the toes or metatarsals of the foot when the limb is in its normal horizontal position. Pain is usually relieved or modified somewhat by putting the leg in the dependent position. Ischemic rest pain is not felt in the calf or thigh and clearly is not a response to exercise. In the presence of ischemic ulcers, pain is often most severe in the area of the ulceration. Ulcerations on the foot or the lateral aspect of the ankle are more commonly due to arterial insufficiency than to venous stasis. The depth of the ischemic ulcer is often greater and results in exposure of tendons and periosteum. Other recognizable characteristics of ischemic feet include numbness, coldness, and lack of any evidence of edema.

Treatment

A small proportion of patients with PAOD will have occlusive disease that is confined entirely to the aortoiliac segment. Even this location gives rise to intermittent claudication in the thigh or hip and occasionally to impotence. Isolated lesions in this area seldom create a threat of gangrene in the lower extremity. Physical findings include diminution or loss of the femoral pulses associated with the obliteration of the lower segment of the aorta as well as wasting in the muscles of the lower limbs and pallor and coolness in the legs and feet. Appropriate diagnostic studies include aortography, which aids in exact localization of the disease when reconstructive surgery is being considered. When occlusive disease is confined to the aorta or to the iliac arteries, endarterectomy may be indicated.

More distal involvement of the external iliac artery or the presence of terminal aortic disease may require the use of a bypass from the aorta to the common femoral arteries. More distal disease in the extremity often localizes in the region of the adductor canal in the form of a stenotic lesion that later goes on to a complete occlusion. Subsequent development of signs of severe ischemia in the extremity is usually due to occlusion of the collateral blood flow or to extension of the disease to involve the entire superficial femoral and popliteal vessels. Symptoms include intermittent claudication, chiefly in the calf of the lower extremity, and, in more severe cases, rest pain, trophic changes, or frank gangrene in the distal portion of the extremity.

As in aortoiliac disease, the presence of obstruction in the femoropopliteal area requires the use of bypass surgery if the claudication is incapacitating. The occurrence of rest pain, trophic changes, or incipient gangrene provides more urgent indications for the need for reconstructive surgery. Preoperative arteriographic studies are needed for planning reconstructive surgery, if such a procedure is thought to be feasible. Femoropopliteal occlusions carry a greater risk of loss of limb than do aortoiliac obstructions. Exploration of the popliteal area is frequently undertaken despite a relatively unfavorable arteriographic picture. When available, the saphenous vein is used as a bypass graft in its reversed position to bridge the gap between the femoral artery and the distal circulation. In those patients in whom the saphenous vein is not available, endarterectomy may be tried, or, alternatively, a synthetic graft may be used. Follow-up studies of the use of synthetic grafts suggest that about three-quarters are occluded by thrombosis during the first year following surgery. Patency of saphenous

vein grafts, however, is 80 per cent at 2 years and greater than 70 per cent at 5 years.

Supportive measures are extremely important in the long-term management of patients with occlusive arterial disease. In those with claudication or rest pain, reasonable physical activity should be encouraged. Walking is the best exercise and, when extended to the point of tolerance, will tend to encourage the development of maximal collateral blood flow to the extremity. Smoking should be prohibited, and the patient should be instructed in a program of foot care designed to protect the extremities from trauma, infection, and extremes of temperature. The obese patient should be made to lose weight, and diabetes mellitus, when present, should be carefully controlled. Treatment of corns and calluses should be carried out by competent persons under a physician's direction. In cases involving severe degrees of ischemia, the temptation to use vasodilator drugs is great. This should be resisted, however, as it has been shown that drugs such as tolazoline (Priscoline), alcohol, and tetraethylammonium chloride are ineffective in producing a significant increase in blood flow in patients with severe obliterative arterial disease. On the other hand, the physician should always remember the beneficial effects of bedrest during a short hospital stay for the healing of ischemic ulcers. At this time, the ischemic extremity is exposed to air, and the ulcer is treated with wet-to-dry, room temperature saline compresses changed 3 to 4 times a day. Appropriate antibiotics and analgesics are also administered.

Lumbar sympathectomy at times has a useful place in the management of patients with lesions not amenable to direct reconstructive surgery. This operation should be considered especially in those with occlusive disease below the level of the popliteal artery associated with trophic changes or skin ulceration. Distal small vessel disease in the young patient is perhaps the prime indication for the use of this operation. Lumbar sympathectomy does occasionally have a place, however, in the treatment of localized blocks in the aorta or in the femoral artery when direct arterial reconstruction is not necessary. Its effect, in general, is to increase blood flow to the integument rather than to relieve claudication by increasing blood flow to the muscle.

AORTIC ANEURYSMS

Aneurysms of the lower portion of the abdominal aorta are almost exclusively due to arteriosclerosis. They occur predominantly in patients over 65 years of age, and their natural history in the overwhelming majority of patients involves progressive enlargement and ultimate rupture. Only a few rather small and heavily calcified aneurysms in this location remain unchanged in size and asymptomatic for long periods of time. Aortic aneurysms are almost invariably located below the level of the renal arteries and above the level of the external iliac vessels, making even the largest of them usually capable of being excised and replaced with a Y-shaped prosthesis.

Diagnosis

Pain is the most important and frequent symptom and is usually indicative of expansion of the aneurysm. Such pain is most typically felt in the back or flank. However, abdominal pain in almost any location has been described as occurring in conjunction with abdominal aortic aneurysm. The iliac aneurysms may be associated with severe sciatica due to pressure of the aneurysm on the pelvic nerve trunks. The majority of iliac or abdominal aortic aneurysms are easily felt as pulsatile masses. Plain x-ray films of the abdomen in the lateral or oblique projections are often of help in demonstrating a characteristic rim of calcification in the outer wall of the aneurysm and also are of help in allowing rough measurement of its dimensions. In some thin persons, the finding of a pulsatile mass may give rise to difficulty in distinguishing an aneurysm from solid or cystic masses with transmitted pulsation or from a prominent or tortuous aorta. Aortography has limited application in the diagnosis of most aortic aneurysms but is most applicable to these doubtful cases. Diagnostic ultrasonography is also quite effective in the identification of aneurysms.

Treatment

Operative treatment of all aneurysms larger than 7 cm. in their widest diameter is recommended because of the threat of rupture, except in the very few patients with cardiovascular or other disease of such severity as to preclude all major surgery because of high risk. In the minority of patients in whom the lesion is small and asymptomatic, clinical examination should be carried out at intervals, using palpation and repeated x-ray films to follow the course of these lesions. Generally, aneurysmectomy with graft replacement doubles the life expectancy of the patient and extends the life span even in the presence of significant coronary artery disease. Operative mortality in such circumstances is now generally less than 10 per cent.

The risk of rupture of aneurysms is clearly related, in an important way, to their size. Those larger than 7 cm. have a 50 per cent or greater chance of rupturing within a span of 5 years, even though they are asymptomatic. In aneurysms larger than 7 cm. that are also symptomatic, the risk of rupture is even greater. Rupture is usually heralded by onset of abdominal, back, or flank pain radiating into the groin with early appearance of signs of shock. In a disturbingly high number of patients with this complication, the initial clinical appearance is frequently mistaken for renal or ureteral colic, pancreatitis, or some other acute intra-abdominal catastrophe. The usual rupture occurs into the retroperitoneum; less commonly, it will be directly into the peritoneal cavity or into a portion of the gastrointestinal tract or vena cava. Early recognition depends on finding a flank or abdominal mass, which is usually both tender and pulsatile. Bleeding may be stopped temporarily by tamponade and thus provides a fleeting opportunity for diagnosis and appropriate treatment to be carried out. Peripheral pulses are usually present until the onset of deep shock, in contrast to those in dissecting aneurysms.

In all patients with suspected rupture of an aneurysm, rapid preparation must be made for hospital admission and emergency surgery. The operation for ruptured aortic aneurysm carries a risk of mortality that is 30 per cent or more. The chief causes of death are shock and renal failure, and their incidence is directly related to the length of the interval between rupture and operation. There is no more urgent operation in the field of abdominal surgery than that involving the ruptured aortic aneurysm. Reduction in the incidence of rupture can be achieved by liberal application of indications for elective repair of aneurysm, together with wide recognition of the presence of pulsatile abdominal masses, which are either asymptomatic or associated with the characteristic symptoms of expansion of the aneurysm.

DEEP VENOUS THROMBOSIS

The initiating events in acute venous thrombosis of the deep veins of the lower extremity and pelvis remain elusive. The importance of background and contributing factors such as trauma, pregnancy, heart disease, contraceptive medication, a postoperative state, or underlying malignancy is widely accepted. Common clinical settings for the occurrence of deep venous thrombosis often involve the older patient in an immobilized or bedfast state or a patient with a history and findings suggestive of previous attacks of thrombophlebitis or with pre-existing varicose veins. The chief complications are pulmonary embolization and massive extension of thrombosis. Both of these can, to some extent, be limited by the use of early and adequate anticoagulant therapy, but direct removal of the occluding thrombus from the deep vein by surgery or by the use of thrombolytic agents is seldom feasible. A devastating consequence of deep venous thrombosis in the lower extremity is the development of chronic venous stasis, resulting from damage to the valves in the veins of the deep venous system. The frequency of this complication of phlebitis is not known with certainty, nor is the role of therapy of phlebitis in limiting or preventing the postphlebitic syndrome capable of exact definition.

Diagnosis

Clinical diagnosis of deep venous thrombosis is often fraught with difficulty. There is startling lack of correlation between signs and symptoms and the proven occurrence of this condition. It is also evident that the disease goes unrecognized in the majority of patients. The clinical diagnosis of deep venous thrombosis rests on the findings of symptoms and signs in the lower extremity that are related to the presence of inflammation in the involved venous segment and to obstruction of venous return caused by the thrombus. The process is apparently so bland and localized in so many instances as to give no clinical warning before pulmonary embolism occurs. Suggestive symptoms include aching pain in the calf or thigh aggravated by muscular activity and a feeling of heaviness in the extremity brought on by putting it in the dependent position. Signs of deep venous obstruction include swelling, with associated calf or thigh tenderness; increased warmth; and, occasionally, visible engorgement of the superficial veins of the leg. Color changes may include a dusky cyanosis in the distal part of the extremity, especially when it is in the dependent position, or, alternatively, a rather marked pallor when it is in the elevated position. Of these signs, the finding of localized tenderness by careful palpation along the course of the involved vein is the most helpful and accurate. Circumferential measurements of the thigh and calf from a fixed point of reference on the edge of the patella are also helpful in detecting subtle changes in limb size.

The site of primary occlusion in the deep venous system can be identified to some extent on the basis of the physical findings. Rather minimal swelling in conjunction with calf tenderness suggests a process confined to the deep calf veins. Extensive swelling of the entire leg to the level of the groin in conjunction with tenderness along the femoral canal indicates an iliofemoral occlusion—the so-called phlegmasia alba dolens. With massive extension of thrombosis from the iliofemoral level upward to the inferior vena cava and downward to involve venous collateral pathways in the limb, there is cyanosis, a cool skin temperature, loss of arterial pulses, and, often, systemic signs of hypovolemia. This is the description of "blue phlebitis," or phlegmasia cerulea dolens. The signs of ischemia allow this clinical syndrome to be frequently confused with acute arterial occlusion. The point to remember is that the nontraumatic arterial occlusions almost never are associated with a major degree of limb edema.

In a number of clinical situations, phlebography is recommended as a useful diagnostic aid that can be performed rather simply in the hospital x-ray department.

Patency of the main veins of the lower extremity can also be tested at the bedside with the Doppler flow meter.

Treatment

The treatment of established deep venous thrombosis is aimed primarily at limiting the extension of the process and preventing pulmonary embolism. Measures include bedrest, elevation of the extremity, application of continuous moist heat to the limb, and the use of anticoagulants. Elevation of the extremity is effected by raising the foot of the bed on 6 inch blocks and by supporting the extremity on pillows. Heat is applied to the leg by hot moist towels covered with plastic, with the surface of the skin protected by a light film of petroleum jelly. Heparin is chosen for initial anticoagulation by the intermittent intravenous injection technique, using a pediatric scalp vein needle or an indwelling catheter in a forearm vein through which the heparin is administered at regular intervals. In adults, an average daily dose of 30,000 USP units is given in divided dosages every 4 to 6 hours. In one accepted method, the Lee-White coagulation time is determined once daily 5 1/2 hours after an injection. The dose of heparin is adjusted to maintain the clotting time at a level between 1 1/2 and 3 times normal. In an emergency, heparin can be neutralized with protamine sulfate. Used intravenously, 1 to 1.5 mg. of protamine sulfate can be expected to neutralize 100 USP units of heparin.

After several days of heparin therapy, as the signs of active phlebitis begin to wane, an oral anticoagulant such as warfarin sodium is started in anticipation of the need for long-term anticoagulation therapy, especially in patients who may be immobilized or bedfast for prolonged periods of time. Warfarin sodium can be begun using doses averaging 10 to 15 mg. a day, with modification according to the patient's response. Therapeutic effect is considered to be achieved when the prothrombin time is 2 to 2 1/2 times the control. The average maintenance dose is 5 to 7.5 mg. daily, but the variability of response suggests that the patient should be observed for several days to be sure that an adequate and stable response has been obtained. It should be remembered that the prothrombin time may be unduly prolonged in the presence of both warfarin sodium and heparin effects.

If anticoagulation with warfarin sodium is complicated by bleeding, Vitamin K_1 (AquaMephyton) should be given intramuscularly, usually in doses of 2.5 mg. to 10 mg. initially. This will cause the prothrombin time to return to safe levels, in most instances in 6 to 8 hours. Use of any anticoagulant substance is contraindicated in patients who are actively bleeding or in whom bleeding is strongly suspected. Active peptic ulcer, recent intracranial hemorrhage, and the immediate postoperative state represent situations in which anticoagulants are unduly dangerous. In patients with anticoagulant effects, venipuncture should be performed with extreme care. Neck and groin veins should be avoided. Arterial punctures, lumbar punctures, and intramuscular injections should be completely avoided in patients undergoing heparin therapy because of the danger of local hemorrhage.

The occurrence of pulmonary embolism in a patient on adequate anticoagulant therapy is cause for alarm, as it points to the presence of an unstable or nonadherent thrombus. Surgical opinion should be sought promptly, emergency plication or ligation of the inferior vena cava being of life-saving value in this critical situation. Excellent results have also been obtained using the umbrella filter, which is implanted in the inferior vena cava through the jugular vein.

The operative removal of venous thrombi is particularly applicable for patients with deep venous thrombosis who show signs and symptoms of extensive obstruction in the main veins. This includes the majority of the patients with phlegmasia cerulea dolens in whom the surgical objective is not only to relieve the venous obstruction but to preserve a viable limb by relieving the ischemia as well. The operation can be done with local anesthesia and carries a rather low risk, even in very sick patients. The Fogarty catheter is used to remove proximal and distal clots through a superficial femoral phlebotomy. In some situations in which extension of clot into the inferior vena cava has occurred, a plication or ligation of that vessel may be combined with thrombectomy. Direct operative removal of thrombi is more successful when carried out within the first 24 to 48 hours following the appearance of signs of iliofemoral thrombosis. However, there is no clearly established upper limit, and the operation should be considered for all patients who have massive swelling or ischemic changes. Anticoagulant therapy should be continued during the postoperative period, and elastic support of the extremities should be maintained for a prolonged period to control edema.

THE POSTPHLEBITIC SYNDROME

The follow-up of patients who have sustained deep venous thrombosis should be thorough and painstaking. Signs of chronic venous insufficiency often take several years to appear. A characteristic feature of the postphlebitic syndrome is the daily appearance of swelling in the lower extremity. This is believed to be secondary to venous hypertension in the distal part of the limb, resulting from incompetence of the deep veins. The incompetence is clearly due to the destruction of the cusps of the valves in the wake of the original thrombotic episode. Symptoms often associated with the swelling include a feeling of tiredness and heaviness after prolonged sitting or standing, nocturnal muscular cramps, and the appearance of a brownish discoloration of the skin of the lower leg. In advanced disease associated with extreme venous stasis about the ankle, the skin becomes scaly and atrophic, and chronic ulceration supervenes.

Persistent edema in the postphlebitic leg must be actively controlled by the use of a well-fitted, two-way-stretch elastic stocking, usually of the knee-length variety. To further reduce swelling, 4 inch blocks under the foot of the patient's bed should be used. Prolonged motionless standing and the use of constricting garments or girdles should be discouraged. Ulceration associated with the postphlebitic syndrome should be treated with pressure bandaging. If the elastic support has been faithfully used but there is recurrence of ulceration, subfascial interruption of the communicating veins, together with removal of the long and short saphenous veins and all visible varicosities, may be indicated.

All patients with established postphlebitic syndrome should be considered to be in the high-risk group as far as recurrence of deep venous thrombosis is concerned. If such patients are hospitalized for elective operations or require immobilization because of injury, the use of prophylactic measures, including anticoagulants, should be strongly considered. A minidose heparin regimen has been highly recommended by investigators participating in several clinical trials. This begins with the administration of 5000 units of heparin subcutaneously 2 hours prior to operation, followed by a twice-daily dose of 5000 units of heparin subcutaneously beginning 12 hours after the 2 hour preoperative dose. This program is continued in hemostatically competent adults for 5 to 7 days following operation. No laboratory control or routine coagulation tests are needed, and the risk of bleeding is low. As the protection offered by minidose heparin administration is not complete, prophylactic use of warfarin sodium may be preferable for patients having a very high risk of thromboembolic complications. This includes patients with a history of previous embolism or phlebitis who are having operations involving large-scale soft tissue trauma or major orthopedic procedures and those with the same history who will be immobilized or bedridden for long periods.

DISEASES OF THE BREAST

Patient History and Breast Examination. The three most common symptoms of breast disease are a lump, a nipple discharge, and pain in the breast. The history should include facts about the onset and duration of the symptom, its relationship to the menstrual cycle and to trauma, and whether there is a prior history of similar complaints. The patient's status in regard to parity, the menses, a history of breast-feeding, ingestion of drugs and hormones, and the use of contraceptive medications should be recorded. Careful questioning concerning a family incidence of breast cancer should be made.

A reliable technique of breast examination should be completely familiar to the family physician. It begins in a private, well-lighted examining room with the inspection of the breasts with the patient in the sitting position. The effects on the appearance of the breasts of the patient's placing her hands on her hips and tensing the pectoral muscles, as well as of raising her arms above her head, should be noted. The neck and axillae are palpated with the patient in the upright position. The breasts are then examined methodically with the patient in a supine position. The flat surfaces of the examiner's fingers palpate each quadrant and the axillary extension of the breast with the patient's arm first at the side and then abducted at right angles. The patient's hand may be used to find the lump in question. Surgical lubricant on the examiner's fingers may assist in finding small areas of thickening or lumps of soft consistency. The examination should conclude with instruction and encouragement to new patients concerning self-examination. Findings can be recorded in a simple sketch or diagram in the patient's record for future reference.

Mammographic and xeromammographic screening for breast cancer in asymptomatic women is appropriate for those over 50 years of age and should always be used in conjunction with careful physical examination of the breasts. When symptoms of breast disease are present, however, it is appropriate to obtain mammography in any patient over 35 years of age when breast cancer is a possibility and when the history and physical examination can be correlated with the films. Other indications for the use of mammography include follow-up examination of the remaining breast after the diagnosis of breast cancer has been established and in the surveillance of female patients over 35 years of age who have a family history of breast cancer, florid cystic disease, or other factors enhancing the risk of breast cancer.

CHRONIC FIBROCYSTIC DISEASE

The pathologic changes constituting cystic disease include both hyperplastic and involutional alterations in the ductal epithelium and stroma. Some of these changes, particularly those producing nodules and cysts, are so common in the breasts of women past 30 years of age that they are best regarded as evidence of aging changes rather than of disease. One-third or more of women from 25 years of age onward have clinical evidence of this disorder. The occurrence of cysts and gross nodularity

together with pain and tenderness all seem to be more frequent as the patient approaches the menopause. The lesions predominate in the upper outer quadrant but may be found in any location. They are frequently multiple and are often associated with local tenderness and diffuse nodularity rather than with a discrete or dominant mass. A few patients may present with a serous or serosanguineous nipple discharge.

Patients often ask about the relationship of cystic disease to carcinoma of the breast. As the true frequency of fibrocystic disease is not clearly known, the relationship of this group of lesions to cancer is still debatable. It does seem apparent, however, that patients with florid cystic disease of the proliferative type beginning in the late 20's and continuing toward the menopause have at least 3 to 5 times the expected incidence of breast cancer.

The management of patients with tender, painful, nodular breasts in the absence of a discrete or dominant mass should include reassurance and advice to the patient, as well as a description of the process in its simplest terms. The usual recommendations include the wearing of a well-fitted brassiere, the application of heat to the painful area of the breast, and the use of simple analgesics. Daily doses of diuretics during the premenstrual phase of the menstrual cycle are sometimes helpful. When pain and distress are severe, one may try the use of an androgenic hormone such as fluoxymesterone, 5 mg. daily, for the first 3 weeks of the cycle.

When a dominant mass is discovered in an accessible position and its characteristics suggest a cyst, aspiration should be carried out. This is done by using a syringe of appropriate size attached to a 20 or 22 gauge needle after prepping the skin with alcohol and trapping the suspected lesion between the fingers of the opposite hand. Complete evacuation of the fluid within the cyst provides both relief of pain and reassurance about the diagnosis. If a mass persists after complete evacuation of the cyst or if the fluid is bloody, the patient should be referred to a surgeon for possible biopsy of the lesion. The paucity of cells in the aspirated fluid in most patients makes an examination of the fluid by the Papanicolaou smear technique uninformative.

In patients with a history of a previous

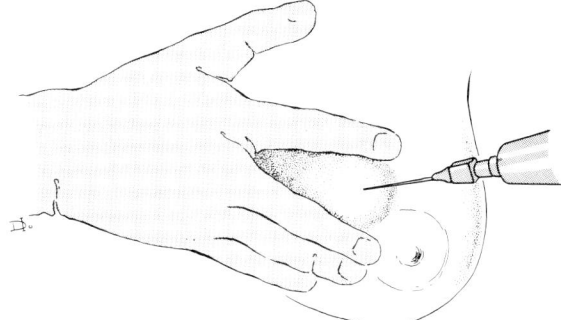

Figure 37–7. *Aspiration of breast cyst. The cyst is identified, stabilized, and evacuated by light finger pressure while syringe barrel is withdrawn.*

biopsy and proof of fibrocystic disease, the appearance of new lumps from time to time requires the exercise of judgment in deciding when to perform another biopsy. Observation over a course of a full menstrual cycle may be helpful in making this decision. Aspiration of these lesions can be done repeatedly (Fig. 37–7).

Most patients with fibrocystic disease are in need of continuing surveillance by regular breast examination. In addition to the patient's monthly self-examination, it seems justified that such women between the ages of 25 and 45 years should have an examination by a physician at least annually. Selective use of mammography, aspiration of breast cysts, and occasional consultation with a surgeon should help to avoid errors in diagnosis and serve to reduce apprehension in the patient concerning breast cancer. Recourse to simple mastectomy in patients with extensive nodularity or multiple cysts would seldom seem to be indicated, except in the unusual situation in which additional high risk factors predisposing to the occurrence of breast cancer can be identified.

FIBROADENOMA

The classic mass lesion occurring within the breast of a young woman in her teens or twenties is the benign tumor known as fibroadenoma. It is usually manifested as a solitary and painless lump, although occasionally it may be multiple. Fibroadenoma is a smooth, somewhat lobulated mass with rubbery consistency that is freely movable within the adjacent normal breast tissue. Such lesions, despite their benign nature, are usually best removed by surgery. The

arguments against their being left alone are their tendency toward slow but definite enlargement and the lack of certainty regarding diagnosis without biopsy.

NIPPLE DISCHARGE

The occurrence of a serous or bloody nipple discharge in a nonpregnant or nonlactating woman needs careful evaluation. The history of the complaint in relation to the taking of contraceptive medication or of other drugs is important. At examination, aided perhaps by a magnifying glass, the distinction between a single duct discharge and multiple duct discharges should be made. A specimen of the fluid should be obtained for a Papanicolaou smear, and the affected breast should be carefully searched for an underlying mass. In the absence of a palpable tumor, the location of the quadrant about the nipple that is the source of the discharge may be established by finger

TABLE 37–5. GUIDELINES FOR SURGERY IN PATIENTS WITH NIPPLE DISCHARGE

1. Discharge should be *spontaneous* and *persistent.*

2. Single duct discharge with or without a palpable mass—biopsy to rule out cancer. (Lesions include intraductal papilloma and intraductal papillary carcinoma.)

3. Multiple duct discharge—biopsy only if mass is palpable or if mammogram shows a localized lesion. (Lesions include fibrocystic disease, papillomatosis, and ductal ectasia.)

4. Pseudodischarge (nipple erosion or eczema)—biopsy to rule out Paget's disease.

pressure. This is helpful to the surgeon for guiding his excision of the involved duct system. A classification of the causes of single and multiple duct discharges is given in Table 37–5. Mammography may be of further help in identifying the source of a nipple discharge.

A weeping, eczematous, or ulcerated nipple, with or without an underlying mass, should suggest Paget's disease until proved otherwise. These characteristically unilateral lesions occur in middle-aged and elderly women and are associated with a carcinoma of the underlying ductal system. Such patients need mammography and prompt referral to a surgeon for consideration of open biopsy.

GYNECOMASTIA

Enlargement of the breast is common both in pubertal males and in men past 50 years of age. Unilateral enlargement in the adolescent is more common than bilateral involvement and is usually transitory. The lesion is felt as a conical, firm mass behind the nipple. Persistence of the swelling over the course of 1 or 2 years of observation is usually an indication for surgical removal by subcutaneous mastectomy. Hormonal treatment is not recommended. Gynecomastia in older men should suggest a rather wide differential diagnosis that includes the ingestion of estrogens, cirrhosis of the liver, tumor or atrophy of the testis, pituitary adenoma, or adrenocortical lesions. Attention should be paid also to the possibility of the association of gynecomastia with a bronchogenic tumor. When a discrete mass can be felt within the male breast, there is a need for surgical opinion concerning biopsy. Carcinoma of the breast in men is rare in patients under 30 years of age. It should be considered in the differential diagnosis of breast enlargement or masses occurring in men chiefly past 50 years of age.

BREAST CANCER

Diagnosis

Clinically detectable breast cancer presents in the majority of patients in the form of a painless lump in the breast. For those patients without a palpable lump, the initial clue is furnished by nipple discharge, enlargement of axillary lymph nodes, eczema or ulceration of the nipple, a positive finding on mammography, or the discovery of distant metastases. The great majority of breast cancers are discovered by the patient herself, thus underlining the importance of self-examination as a routine for all patients over 25 years of age. There are simply not enough contacts between patients and those physicians who can perform a breast examination in a competent manner to allow early diagnosis of breast cancer to be achieved in this way for a significant number of patients. Family physicians should take time to instruct their patients in the method of self-examination and to explain the importance of regular performance of this diagnostic procedure. A minimum frequency of every 3 months for the performance of self-examination is recommended. In premenopausal women, the best time for performance of self-examination is in the immediate postmenstrual phase of the cycle. Ths physician should make a special effort to see the patient promptly when an abnormality is discovered by the patient herself.

Family physicians also have a responsibility to conduct thorough breast examinations in patients with unrelated complaints who have no specific indications of breast disease. Including the breast examination in the routine of the examination of the chest and recording the physical findings in a simple sketch or diagram are recommended. In the presence of equivocal findings, repeated examination at regular intervals is a sound policy. The importance of surveillance by regular breast examination for the patient beyond 45 years of age should be emphasized. At least an annual breast examination of women in the postmenopausal age group is amply justified. Even closer attention should be paid to high-risk patients—those who have a mother or sister with breast cancer, those with a history of cancer in the opposite breast, and those who have borne children for the first time after 35 years of age. Enhancement of the risk of developing cancer may also be seen in other special clinical situations, such as florid cystic disease, histologically proven lobular carcinoma-in-situ, and intraductal papillomatosis. Up to three or four examinations per year should be recommended for such high-risk patients.

The selective use of mammography or

TABLE 37–6. INDICATIONS FOR
BREAST BIOPSY

1. Overt malignant tumor
2. A dominant nodule
3. Nipple discharge
4. Ulcer or eczema of the nipple
5. Positive findings on mammography
6. Axillary lymphadenopathy

xeromammography to complement findings of physical examination has an important place in the surveillance of these patients. In no instance should a mammogram be considered as a substitute for the physical examination of the breast or as reliable evidence that a given lump or another positive physical finding is due to an underlying benign lesion. The indications for breast biopsy should be kept clearly in mind when positive findings of mammograms, or physical examination, or both are being evaluated (Table 37–6). The mammogram clearly cannot provide a histologic diagnosis in any case and can be dangerously deceiving, particularly in premenopausal women, when it is used to forestall or delay the performance of a biopsy.

Biopsy remains the basic required procedure for making the diagnosis of breast cancer. Because of the frequent need for breast biopsy, surgeons in recent years have tended more and more to use outpatient facilities for these procedures. The use of local anesthesia for open biopsy and the technique of needle biopsy with direct filming of the aspirated material on specially prepared slides have both contributed to a containment of cost and a reduction in worry and anxiety for the patient.

It is the surgeon's responsibility to decide about the need for excision of the suspicious lesion. After biopsy, assessment of the probable extent of the malignant disease is accomplished on clinical grounds as follows:

Stage I. Disease apparently limited to the breast.

Stage II. Disease apparently confined to the breast and regional axillary lymph nodes.

Stage III. Disease with signs of a locally advanced nature, e.g., skin infiltration, ulceration, peau d'orange, edema, or pectoral muscle or chest wall attachment.

Stage IV. Disease with signs of distant metastases.

Careful history and physical examination, together with the selective application of certain laboratory examinations, serve to place the patient in the appropriate clinical category. In selected patients, the ^{99m}Tc-phosphate bone scan serves as a sensitive method of detecting occult bone metastases. Appropriate use of lymph node biopsy, liver–spleen scans, liver function tests, bone survey films, liver and pleural biopsies, and a few other diagnostic tests should serve to detect other soft tissue disease.

Treatment for Stages I and II

At this time, surgical therapy for the operable stages of breast cancer is undergoing major re-evaluation. A certain dilemma exists concerning the appropriate least extensive treatment for patients with operable tumors. The surgeon may choose a particular procedure on the basis of his personal views in such cases, but clinical trials, now under way, will ultimately prove what constitutes optimum treatment for early breast cancer. Radical mastectomy of either the traditional or the modified type is still the most frequently selected therapy for early breast cancer in the United States. Radical mastectomy offers at least the advantage of an opportunity for pathologic examination of the axillary lymph nodes. This has an important bearing on the decision to use adjuvant chemotherapy, as well as on the prognosis. Recent reports have suggested that the use of prophylactic systemic chemotherapy in the postmastectomy patient with metastases to axillary nodes serves to prolong the disease-free interval in a significant proportion of premenopausal patients. One current adjuvant chemotherapy regimen involves the use of the drug melphalan (Alkeran) in a cyclic administration for a prolonged period. Another regimen uses three drugs, cyclophosphamide, 5-fluorouracil, and methotrexate, again in a cyclic mode of administration for long intervals.

Because of the uncertainty surrounding the choice of optimal treatment in early breast cancer, the physician should, in general, support the involvement of his patients in clinical therapeutic trials, since controlled comparisons offer help in solving the dilemmas now evident in the treatment of breast cancer.

Prognosis and Follow-up. The outcome of treatment of breast cancer in patients with operable lesions is very similar in many reported series. Patients in both Stage I and Stage II appear to be at risk of recurrence for a period of approximately 7 years following initial therapy, after which time the survival curve tends to approach that of the normal population. At 10 years, the survival rate for patients in Stage I is about 50 per cent and for those in Stage II, 30 per cent.

It is recommended that in the first 2 years after mastectomy, the patient should be seen at 3 or 4 month intervals. Semiannual visits can be arranged from the third to the seventh year and annual visits thereafter. Chest films should be taken on regular occasions—more frequently in the earlier years following mastectomy. The ^{99m}Tc-phosphate bone scan lends itself well to use in postoperative surveillance of patients for skeletal metastases. Mammography or xeromammography should be used at yearly intervals to observe the status of the remaining breast. Complex and expensive examinations should be avoided on a routine basis, but bone survey films, liver–spleen scans, and appropriate biopsies should be used in the presence of symptoms or other clinical or laboratory findings suggestive of tumor spread.

Treatment for Stages III and IV

Initial treatment for patients in the inoperable groups usually begins with a course of radiation therapy to the breast, chest wall, and adjacent node-bearing areas. Radical operations for the locally advanced tumors of Stage III patients are avoided.

Further palliative therapy can be undertaken for patients in the inoperable groups based on the concept that some breast cancers are hormone-dependent (Table 37–7). Use of the estrogen receptor (ER) assay can help determine which patients can be chosen for hormone administration or withdrawal. The test can be performed on as little as 1 gram of tumor submitted at the time of biopsy. Patients with positive assays are candidates for ablative or additive maneuvers. In the case of premenopausal patients with a positive ER assay, the usual recommendation is surgical castration, and this offers about a 60 per cent chance of remission. In postmenopausal patients with a positive ER assay, the first choice is that of administration of an estrogen such as diethylstilbestrol, 5 mg. by mouth, three times daily. In patients with skeletal metastases, it is advisable to watch the serum calcium levels closely during the initiation of estrogen therapy to avoid dangerous hypercalcemia.

TABLE 37–7. SEQUENCE OF PALLIATIVE SYSTEMIC THERAPY IN FEMALES WITH INOPERABLE OR RECURRENT BREAST CANCER

	Premenopausal and up to 5 Years Postmenopausal	
	Estrogen Receptor (ER) Positive	
	Castration	
REMISSION Androgens Adrenalectomy or hypophysectomy Chemotherapy		NO REMISSION Chemotherapy
	ER Negative	
	Chemotherapy	
	Postmenopausal	
	ER Positive	
	Estrogens	
REMISSION Androgens Adrenalectomy or hypophysectomy Chemotherapy		NO REMISSION Chemotherapy
	ER Negative	
	Chemotherapy	

The usual duration of response to endocrine additive or ablative therapy is about 1 to 2 years. Further remission may sometimes be obtained in premenopausal patients by the use of androgens, particularly in patients with metastases to skin or bone. Relatively nonmasculinizing drugs such as fluoxymesterone (Halotestin) and testolactone (Teslac) are available. Combination chemotherapy is generally introduced when first or second line endocrine alterations fail, especially in premenopausal patients (Table 37–8). In certain instances, hypophysectomy or adrenalectomy may be performed when remission ends in patients who have had responses to oophorectomy or estrogen therapy.

TABLE 37–8. COMBINATION CHEMOTHERAPY FOR DISSEMINATED BREAST CANCER

C.M.F.
Cyclophosphamide (PO) 100 mg./m²/days 1 to 14 inclusive
Methotrexate (IV) 40 mg./m²/days 1 and 8
5-Fluorouracil (IV) 600 mg./m²/days 1 and 8 } Repeat every 28 days

C.M.F.V.P. (Cooper Regimen)
Cyclophosphamide – 2 mg./kg./day
Methotrexate – 0.75 mg./kg./wk.
5-Fluorouracil – 12 mg./kg./wk.
Vincristine – 0.25 mg./kg./wk.
Prednisone – 0.75 mg./kg./day ×21, then taper

A.C.
Doxorubicin (Adriamycin) – 40 mg./m²
Cyclophosphamide – 500 mg./m² } Repeat every 28 days

Treatment for Recurrent Breast Cancer

Greater than 85 per cent of recurrences are seen within the first 5 years of follow-up after the primary treatment of breast cancer. Patterns of recurrence are fairly predictable. Soft tissue metastases usually take the form of axillary or cervical lymph node enlargements or lumps in the opposite breast or in the chest wall in the vicinity of the operative scar. Visceral metastases are most common in the pleura, lungs, liver, retroperitoneum, and central nervous system. The pelvis, lumbar spine, ribs, and femur are the common sites of metastatic disease in the skeleton. Early identification of recurrent tumor provides the best opportunity for palliative treatment. Few remissions will be seen in situations involving overwhelming tumor recurrence, especially in patients with liver or central nervous system lesions. The relative rate of tumor progression, as reflected in the duration of the tumor-free interval from the time of primary treatment to recurrence, will help to predict the response to treatment.

In general, patients with long free intervals will make the best response to palliative measures. The quality of survival, rather than the actual duration of life, is usually more important in determining the choices. Local radiotherapy is advisable in treating chest wall and lymph node recurrences, as well as in the management of painful osseous metastases. Pathologic fractures can be treated by a combination of radiotherapy and internal skeletal fixation in conjunction with systemic hormonal treatment or chemotherapy. Pleural effu-sions can be treated by instillation of agents such as nitrogen mustard or quinacrine intrapleurally. A sequence of possible choices in the programs available for systemic therapy is given in Tables 37–7 and 37–8. Guidance offered by the results of estrogen receptor assay is now important in the choice of hormonal therapy. The recent emergence of more effective combination chemotherapy has improved the outlook for palliation in the majority of patients with recurrent breast cancer.

MINOR OFFICE SURGERY

There is frequent need for the performance of minor surgical procedures in an office setting in family practice. Convenience for the patient, containment of cost, and efficient use of physician time are obvious advantages in the choice of office rather than hospital facilities for certain simple surgical procedures. Beside the suture of minor lacerations and the drainage of small abscesses, the physician can carry out the surgical excision of a variety of small skin and subcutaneous lesions. With a reasonable understanding of the principles of wound healing, together with the use of local anesthesia and simple surgical techniques, the physician can have confidence in the outcome and effectiveness of such office procedures. The personnel who help in accomplishing this should be carefully chosen. The presence of an experienced nurse or a physician's assistant with knowledge of operating room routines and a certain reassuring and helpful way with patients would be most valuable in making this phase of office care a success.

A rather simple surgical treatment room can be furnished with a sturdy examining table, good lighting, a scrub sink, and a small autoclave. The instruments required are few, but they should be carefully chosen to make these small-scale procedures easy to perform and to have the resulting incisional scars acceptable to the patient. A typical surgical kit should include a scalpel with a size 15 blade, a toothed Adson forceps, several Halsted mosquito hemostats, a small curved iris scissors, skin hooks, and a lightweight needle holder, all placed on a sterile tray upon a small movable table or Mayo stand. One per cent lidocaine solution is recommended for local infiltration about the operative site, using a small control syringe and a fine gauge needle for this purpose. An additional instrument found to be useful in the office or treatment room is one that provides a damped spark gap current suitable for electrodesiccation, fulguration, or coagulation of small surface lesions such as warts or keratoses.*

Instructions concerning change of dressing and care of the surgical wound should be given to the patient in the office. Limitations in physical activity, if any, should be explained to the patient and provision made for the patient to obtain analgesic drugs if necessary.

Follow-up visits should be arranged, and plans for drain or suture removal should be described to the patient. The neck and face are sites where sutures can be removed in 4 or 5 days. Sutures in the scalp, anterior trunk, and upper extremities can be removed in 1 week. Sutures in the back and lower extremities are usually taken out in 10 days.

SKIN CANCER

Basal Cell Carcinoma. The basal cell carcinomas of the skin are the most frequent malignant skin tumors, and the most common presenting form of this tumor is the nodular lesion that frequently has a central dell or ulcer surrounded by a rolled, pearly

---

*The Birtcher Hyfrecator, The Birtcher Corporation, Medical Division, Los Angeles, Cal.

edge. Another well-localized form is the cystic lesion reminiscent of an inclusion cyst, and there are occasional pigmented forms that are quite easily confused with a nevus or a melanoma. Rarer varieties of this tumor include flat lesions that may have a spreading border surrounding a central scarred area and the so-called rodent ulcer, which has little external bulk but does have a deep projection and undermined edges.

When small lesions are encountered, excision with a 3 or 4 mm. normal skin margin can readily be carried out with local anesthesia (Fig. 37–8). The elliptical incision should usually be directed transversely in locations about the eyes and eyebrows and on the nose and neck. A more vertical orientation, however, is best in the region of the lips, cheeks, and preauricular skin in order to follow the tension lines of the face. The length of the ellipse to be excised should be between 2 and 3 times its width in order to avoid dog-ear deformities at either end of the linear closure. A narrow but adequate margin should also be obtained in the subcutaneous fat deep to the lesion. After removal of the specimen, active bleeding in the subcutaneous plane should be controlled with hemostats and fine plain catgut ties. The skin edges should be united with fine, nonabsorbable suture or, when applicable, with sterile adhesive strips. The margins of the pathologic speci-

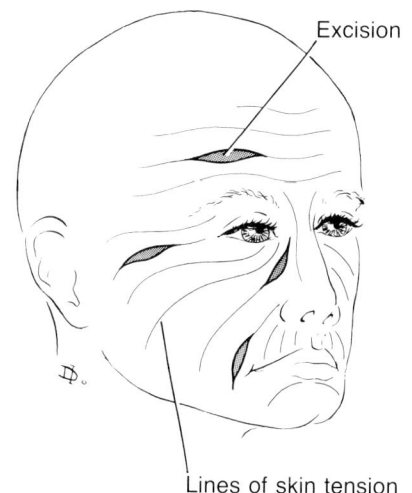

Figure 37–8. *Elliptical excisions of facial lesions are made with their long axes in the direction of wrinkles in the aged or lines of tension in the younger patient.*

men should be marked and oriented, so that the pathologist can accurately identify the areas where margins appear inadequate. In the case of larger lesions not suitable for excision and primary closure as an office procedure, a diagnostic biopsy should be performed under local anesthesia. The specimen should include a small wedge of tumor margin and adjacent skin for pathologic examination. When applicable, a punch biopsy can be simpler than a wedge biopsy and just as useful. If such large lesions prove to be skin cancer, the patient should be referred to a surgeon for appropriate treatment.

Squamous Cell Carcinoma. The squamous cell carcinomas characteristically occur in the skin of the hands, forearms, and face in areas that have been exposed to sunlight, wind, and weather for many years. These lesions can also occur in old burn scars, in the skin of irradiated areas, and in close proximity to chronic draining sinuses. Squamous cell carcinomas do not significantly differ enough in gross appearance from basal cell carcinomas to make a clinical distinction possible. For accurate identification, small marginal biopsies of the larger of these lesions should be obtained under local anesthesia. Definitive treatment may require somewhat wider excision than in the case of basal cell carcinomas of similar size or location and may require skin grafting or skin flaps for closure of the defect. Regional node dissections are generally reserved for patients with clinical evidence of lymph node involvement.

PIGMENTED NEVI

The common pigmented lesions include freckles, lentigines, and a variety of moles. These benign lesions usually exhibit an orderly pattern of color and form. The basic shades seen in benign lesions vary from tan to dark brown. The major exceptions to this are the blue nevi and the Spitz nevi. The distinction between these lesions and malignant melanoma, however, cannot always be made without benefit of a biopsy. Nodular melanoma usually has a uniform bluish-black or gray color, whereas a mixture of colors is characteristic of superficial spreading malignant melanoma and the lentigo maligna melanoma. The variegation of col-

ors usually involves shades of red, white, or blue seen in a basic tan or brown lesion. The presence of shades of blue is considered most significant in regard to the diagnosis of malignant melanoma. The border that is characteristic of malignancy involves an angular indentation or notch at the margin of the lesion. The uneven topography, which is characteristic of malignant melanoma, may be either seen or felt and is emphasized by side lighting as well as by palpation of the surface of these lesions with the fingertip. With the use of guidelines (Table 37–9) for excision or biopsy, there will always be a certain number of lesions that will not turn out to be malignant melanoma, including the usual benign nevi as well as keratoses, vascular nevi, pigmented basal cell carcinomas, and the lesions of Bowen's disease. The fact is that most of these would be quite properly treated by excision in any case.

The type of biopsy chosen in evaluating pigmented lesions should always tend to give the pathologist the best opportunity for accurate identification of the lesion. Total excision, when feasible, has the advantage of allowing a determination of the level of invasion, if the lesion proves to be a malignant melanoma. A punch biopsy or wedge biopsy will be quite appropriate if the lesion is large or is in such a location that primary closure of the incision might be difficult. The physician should have no concern that such procedures would cause the lesion to metastasize if it is a malignant melanoma. In no case should the biopsy involve destruction of the lesion or make later pathologic examination of the total lesion difficult. A preliminary color photograph of the suspicious lesion may sometimes prove to be of considerable value.

In recent years it has become evident that the diagnosis of malignant melanoma in a preinvasive phase rests in large part on the diagnostic skills of the primary care physician. Physical examination of the skin in asymptomatic patients over the age of 20 years offers the best opportunity to make an early diagnosis. Special attention should be paid to the sites of frequent occurrence of malignant melanoma, such as the lower legs in women and the upper back in both sexes. The areas of skin exposed to the sun should be inspected with special care in older individuals. Special attention should be paid to congenital, raised, and pigmented lesions larger than 1.5 cm. in diameter in children and young adults. Pigmented lesions in the palms and soles and those in sites of repeated trauma, such as the scalp, should also usually be removed or biopsied.

It is now generally believed that malignant melanoma seldom arises from the so-called junction nevi. It is also conceded that signs such as rapid growth, bleeding, and ulceration in a malignant melanoma are not early or favorable signs, but are those of a late, incurable, and deeply invasive lesion. The most fortunate patients have small skin lesions without associated symptoms.

Early diagnosis of superficial spreading melanomas, the most frequent type of malignant melanoma, has resulted in a marked improvement in prognosis for this lesion in recent years.

MISCELLANEOUS SKIN LESIONS

Skin tags or squamous papillomas are common tan or flesh-colored lesions attached by a narrow pedicle to the skin in the region of flexion creases, such as the neck and axillae. They are often traumatized and frequently undergo torsion. Such lesions can be removed rather simply in the office, using an alcohol wipe to clean the skin and iris scissors to snip them off at a level flush with the surrounding skin. The resulting bleeding can be controlled by the application of small spot bandages. Unusually large

skin papillomas can be excised using local anesthesia and sutures to control the bleeding at the site of the excision. The specimen is then sent for routine pathologic examination.

Seborrheic keratoses can be recognized by their scaly or greasy consistency. They are frequently pigmented and are often multiple. A simple method of removal is to scrape them off with a scalpel or a dermal curet, using an infiltration of 1 per cent lidocaine for local anesthesia. The bleeding base of the skin is then lightly fulgurated with a high frequency electric current. The specimen can be sent to the pathologist if histologic confirmation of the diagnosis is needed.

Common warts in many areas of the body can be managed with electrodesiccation, using a 30 gauge needle for infiltration of the base of the wart with 1 per cent lidocaine. The wart, after being heated, then comes off easily, using the dermal curet, and the base can then be lightly fulgurated with the high frequency needle.

Plantar warts of a small and localized form occurring in the sole of the foot can often be successfully managed by enucleation of the wart, using local anesthesia. The plane between the plantar wart and the surrounding callus can be defined with a sharp hemostat point, and the lesion can be removed by blunt dissection, using a scoop or dermal curet and avoiding injury to adjacent normal tissue. The surrounding

TABLE 37–9.   GUIDELINES FOR EXCISION OR DIAGNOSTIC BIOPSY OF PIGMENTED LESIONS

History

1. Recent change in size or color.
2. Symptoms such as bleeding, itching, and tenderness.
3. Congenital raised and pigmented lesions.
4. Family history of malignant melanoma.

Appearance

1. Color
    a. Uniform blue, "thunder-cloud" gray, or black.
    b. Mixtures of red, white, or blue seen in brown or black lesions.
2. Irregular border or notching.
3. Uneven surface contour.

callus can be beveled with scissors around the edge of the base of the lesion, and the latter can be cauterized lightly with the high frequency current. There should be very few situations involving the need for surgical excision of these lesions, although the rate of recurrence is about 10 to 15 per cent. It is most important to avoid producing a permanent scar at the site of the wart in the plantar surface of the foot.

SEBACEOUS CYSTS

Epidermal inclusion cysts in young patients are common office surgical problems. They occur most frequently on the face and the upper back and in the neck and post-auricular areas. Their tendency to become infected offers the best reason for excising them at a stage when they are small and quiescent. This can usually be accomplished by using local anesthesia with the excision of a narrow ellipse of adherent skin attached to the apex of the cyst, thus removing the entire wall of the cyst with its cheesy contents intact. In the face of obvious inflammation with local redness and tenderness or a purulent discharge, incision and drainage should be done initially. A definitive excision follows after signs of inflammation have subsided after 1 or 2 weeks.

PILONIDAL CYSTS AND SINUSES

Pilonidal disease may often be conveniently and appropriately handled in the office. This is almost exclusively a disease of young and physically active persons, especially of men. The effects of local trauma, poor hygiene, and a breaking off of hairs in the midline cleft definitely contribute to the development of this lesion. It is often first seen as an acute inflammation manifested by midline swelling, tenderness, and erythema in the coccygeal area. The skin about the pilonidal process is usually quite hairy. One or more sinuses communicating from the skin level to a subcutaneous collection of purulent material containing hair and debris can frequently be demonstrated.

In the presence of such findings, these lesions require incision and drainage followed by a trial of conservative measures, which include taking frequent hot sitz baths, shaving the hair from the edges of the sinuses for a distance of several centimeters in all directions, and avoiding the trauma produced by prolonged sitting and by exercise. These measures are frequently effective in controlling symptoms and avoiding further infection. In instances in which a palpable cyst persists or the sinuses continue to drain and the area remains tender, there may be a need for surgical excision of the lesion. Smaller pilonidal cysts are usually excised and closed primarily, while those of larger size or with extension into the fat of the buttock may be better managed by excision with only partial skin closure. When large defects are left to granulate and epithelialize, there may be rather prolonged postoperative disability. Recurrence rates are highest in those patients with large sinuses and widespread inflammation. The postoperative routine of keeping the area shaved and clean and of avoiding local trauma usually helps to minimize the possibility of local recurrence.

MANAGEMENT OF TRAUMA

In the care of emergencies, the family physician is frequently expected to provide the initial assessment and therapy for patients of various ages, usually in the setting of the community hospital emergency department. The physician's response to this challenge may strongly influence both the patient's subsequent course in the hospital and his ultimate recovery. It is a role that requires the family physician to be quite familiar with emergency surgical care and to be capable, when necessary, of carrying out the basic life-supporting procedures, such as cardiopulmonary resuscitation, relief of airway obstruction, and treatment of shock (Figs. 37–9 and 37–10). In assuming responsibility for such care, he must also be able to mobilize the resources around him for the team effort required in the treatment of major injuries. He is also expected to exercise responsible judgment in requesting early consultation with other physicians, to understand the strengths and weaknesses of locally available personnel and facilities, and to know how and when to transport the injured patient to other treatment centers.

First-contact physicians dealing with

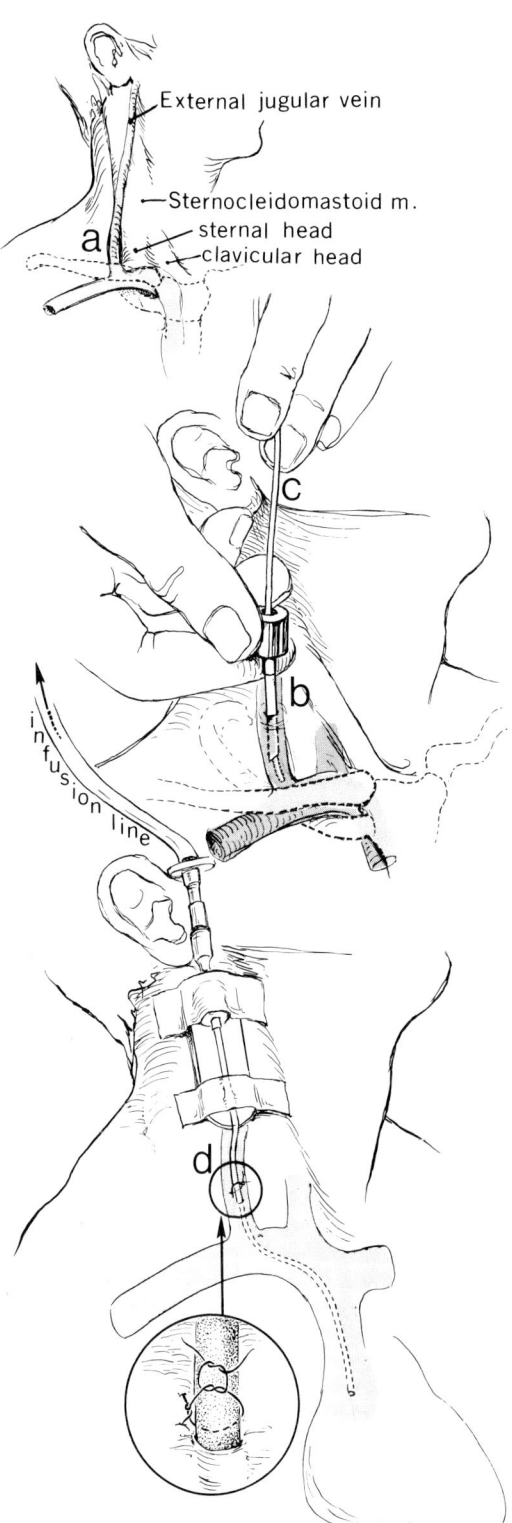

trauma must follow an almost instinctive routine in looking for life-threatening problems. Airway patency should be assured and adequate ventilation established, serious hemorrhage controlled, and circulatory stability restored before other problems are attended to. Knowledge of the priorities in patients with serious or multiple injuries is of vital importance in directing initial treatment efforts.

AIRWAY PATENCY

The most common type of airway obstruction encountered in the unconscious patient is that caused by relaxation of the tongue and pharyngeal musculature. This can be quickly corrected by tilting the head backward and moving the jaw into the jutting position, thus displacing the tongue out of the pharynx. Insertion of an oropharyngeal airway will thereafter maintain patency. Mechanical obstruction from mucus, blood, or vomitus should quickly be cleared from the mouth and pharynx by wiping or suctioning. Early efforts at inser-

---

Figure 37–9. *Central venous catheterization: External jugular vein cannulation.*

Insertion of a central venous catheter through an external jugular vein puncture is recommended in most emergencies requiring large volume fluid infusions and monitoring of central venous pressure. It has fewer complications than subclavian venipuncture and is easier to accomplish successfully without practice, especially in normotensive patients.

Technique: *The patient is supine with the bed tilted downward in 20° Trendelenburg position and the head turned to the opposite (left) side.*

The external jugular vein is located over the lateral edge of the sternocleidomastoid muscle (a). With the operator standing above the head, the 14 gauge needle with attached catheter is introduced into the vein at a point about 3 cm. above the clavicle (b). Once the needle is in the vein, the 20 cm. plastic catheter is threaded into the superior vena cava (c). By turning the patient's head or moving the shoulder, the catheter can be kept from entering the internal jugular vein or from curling back into the subclavian vein in a distal direction. The catheter should not be pulled back until the needle is withdrawn from the vein in order to avoid accidentally severing the catheter with the edge of the needle tip.

The catheter should be secured on the skin of the neck with a suture and taped firmly in place to prevent dislodgement (d). Position of the catheter should be promptly checked by x-ray.

tion of an endotracheal tube should be attempted only by experienced persons, after good ventilation has been established through a patent airway using mouth-to-mouth breathing or a bag and mask system.

Recognition of a bolus of food obstructing the airway, the so-called "café coronary," should be made promptly. In this frightening situation, the patient can make no sound and has absolutely no ventilatory exchange. Heimlich has devised a life-saving maneuver that should be tried in all situations in which this type of airway obstruction is suspected. Making use of the fact that the patient has some residual air in the lungs, compression of the upper abdomen and rib cage with a bear-hug maneuver done sharply will use the air trapped below the

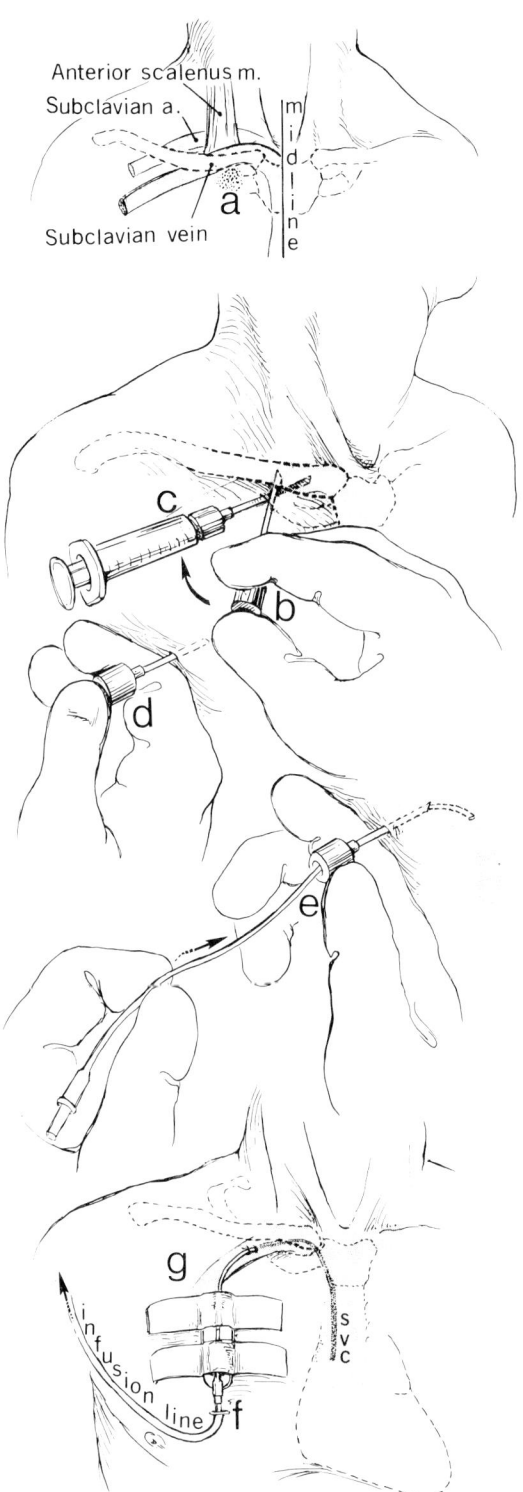

Figure 37–10. *Central venous catheterization: Subclavian vein cannulation.*

Advantages of the use of the subclavian vein for introduction of a central venous catheter are several: It is easy to find, even in patients in whom peripheral veins are collapsed due to hypovolemia. Cannulas in this vein are hard to dislodge by arm or head movements. The use of this vein over prolonged periods of time is associated with a low incidence of infectious or thromboembolic complications.

Technique: The patient is placed in slight Trendelenburg position with the head turned to the left side. The right side is selected to avoid the hazard of trauma to the thoracic duct. The procedure is done with full aseptic precautions, including gloves and drapes after skin preparation.

Local anesthetic is infiltrated into the skin just below the clavicle at a point about 6.4 cm. from the midline (a). A 20 cm. Intracath is detached from its 14 gauge needle and set aside on the sterile drapes. The needle is introduced through the skin wheal and is "walked" down the clavicle to the under surface of the clavicle (b). With a 10 ml. syringe attached, its direction is changed so that it is aimed at the opposite shoulder (c). It is then advanced with the syringe, during which gentle suction is applied so that its tip enters the vein under the surface of the overlying clavicle. When blood is aspirated freely, the syringe is removed and the hub covered with a thumb as it is steadied (d). The catheter is then introduced into the needle and threaded into the vein (e). After again checking for aspiration of blood, the needle is pulled out of the vein, and the hub is attached to the infusion line or venous manometer (f). The external assembly is implanted with a tongue blade and taped to patient's chest. If the catheter appears to be in satisfactory position, it can be secured to the skin with a suture (g). Soon after the catheter's introduction, its position should be checked by chest x-ray.

point of obstruction to dislodge the bolus, the latter usually proving to be a large chunk of meat or other solid food. Wiping and suctioning can then clear the airway further, and ventilation can thus be re-established prior to the onset of cardiac arrest.

VENTILATION

Adequacy of gas exchange in the injured patient should be checked as soon as a patent airway has been established. Inadequate exchange should be corrected immediately by artificial respiration, using mouth-to-mouth or mouth-to-nose techniques. When available, a suitably sized face mask and a self-inflating Ambu bag should be immediately substituted for the expired air technique, and a source of oxygen should be attached. In the event that exchange cannot be established after insertion of an oropharyngeal airway and the use of positive pressure breathing, one must consider the possibility of a retained foreign body in the airway or a crushing injury at the level of the larynx or trachea. This requires immediate action—either the quick mechanical dislodgment of the foreign body by suction or by forceps extraction or the establishment of a temporary vent into the airway through the cricothyroid membrane. Again, only when skilled assistance is available and adequate instruments are at hand should oral endotracheal intubation be attempted.

If the equipment and skills required for oral endotracheal intubation are not immediately available, a coniotomy, or incision in the space between the cricoid and the thyroid cartilages, represents the best choice of procedure for relieving the airway obstruction (Fig. 37–11). In the face of acute airway obstruction and a deteriorating situation, tracheostomy is simply too time-consuming and difficult to undertake in these circumstances. Coniotomy can be done with minimal anesthesia, formal skin preparation, or draping. It involves making a vertical incision over the space between the cricoid and thyroid cartilages and extending the incision through the membrane connecting these structures. The opening is held open with a blunt instrument until a formal tracheostomy can be carried out. The procedure involves minimal risk of permanent damage to the larynx or to the cricoid cartilage, and incisions in this area usually heal without major scarring.

Whenever possible, tracheostomy should be done as a planned procedure without undue haste and under optimal circumstances and with a good airway allowing adequate ventilation of the patient throughout the procedure. A suggested technique for tracheostomy is illustrated in Figure 37–12.

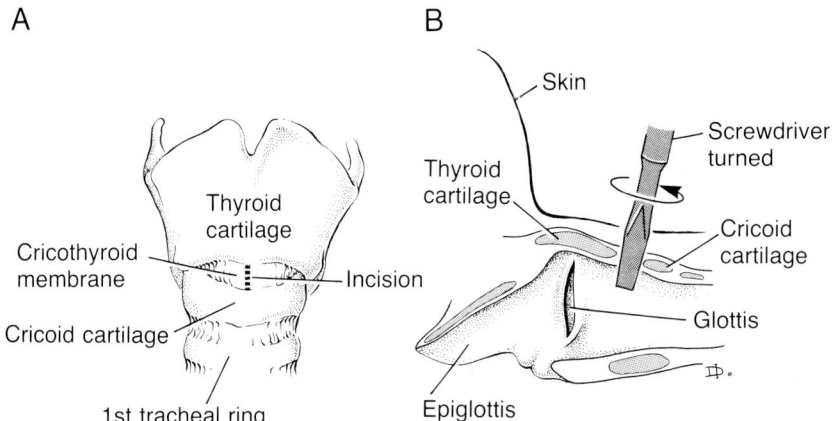

Figure 37–11. *Coniotomy. Coniotomy or cricothyroidotomy is used to establish an airway quickly when a tracheostomy is not possible. The cricothyroid membrane is located by palpating the thyroid and cricoid cartilages. A sharp object is then guided between these two structures to perforate the membrane into the upper trachea. This simple procedure will provide an adequate airway until tracheostomy can be performed.*

The potential threat of invasive infection gaining entrance through a poorly managed tracheostomy is great after performance of this deceptively simple surgical procedure. All efforts must be made to maintain the highest standards of care of tracheostomies, using aseptic techniques in suctioning and paying careful attention to the accumulation of fibrinous crusts in the tube and adjacent parts of the tracheobronchial tree that inevitably accompanies a tracheostomy. Frequent changes of the tracheostomy tube, good humidification of inspired gases, close observation of the fit of the tube within the trachea, and use of the atraumatic, soft, inflatable cuffs are essential in the aftercare of patients who have undergone tracheostomy.

CARDIOPULMONARY RESUSCITATION

Diagnosis of cardiac arrest is made by the detection of pulselessness in the femoral or carotid vessels, usually at the same time that ventilatory failure is recognized. The patient is rapidly placed on a hard surface, such as the floor or a plywood bed board. A sharp blow is delivered to the lower sternum and repeated several times. If this is ineffective in starting the heart beat within a minute, closed-chest cardiac massage is begun, using rhythmic compression over the lower third of the sternum with the heel of the hand at the rate of about 60 strokes per minute. Ventilatory assistance must be given at the same time, preferably by another person. If both are done by the same person, mouth-to-mouth breathing is given after each dozen compressions of the chest. The patient's legs should be elevated to assist in venous return, and an intravenous cannula or needle should be inserted in a suitable vein for administration of fluids and drugs. Skin color and pupil diameter are the best indicators of the effectiveness of cardiac massage.

An electrocardiogram (ECG) is obtained, and if ventricular fibrillation is present, defibrillation can be done at any time after effective resuscitation has begun. The paddles are placed so that the upper one centers over the right third costal cartilage and the lower one is just lateral to the anterior axillary line in the left fifth intercostal space. Intravenous injections of

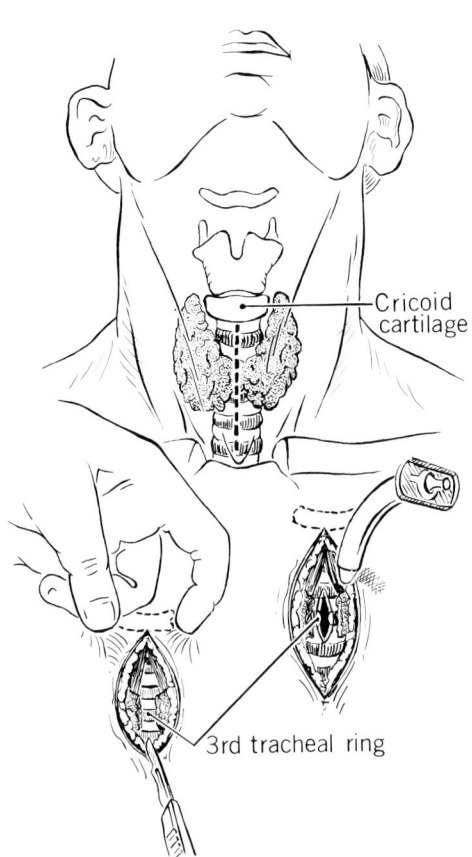

Figure 37–12. *Emergency tracheostomy. An assistant holds the patient's head in extension with the jaw forward in the midline and the shoulders flattened backwards. Rapid preparation of the neck is made with antiseptic, and the pretracheal skin and subcutaneous tissues infiltrated with local anesthetic.*

With the operator's fingers identifying the cricoid cartilage, a vertical midline skin incision is made from a point below this landmark to a level about a fingerbreadth above the suprasternal notch. Strap muscles and fat are incised and the thyroid isthmus divided to expose the upper trachea. The trachea is grasped and stabilized with a hook or towel clip. The position of the cricoid is again checked and a vertical incision is made in the trachea at the level of the second and third tracheal ring. A standard-sized tracheostomy tube is quickly inserted, opened, and suctioned. All bleeders are then secured with catgut ties. A few loosely applied silk sutures are used to approximate the skin edges at the upper and lower ends of the incision. A bib dressing is applied and the tapes are tied after the patient's head has been returned to a normal position.

epinephrine are given at intervals to improve myocardial perfusion and venous return. Direct intracardiac administration of this drug can be made via puncture of the left ventricle in the left fourth interspace if an intravenous line is not available. To combat acidosis, sodium bicarbonate is administered at 5 or 6 minute intervals throughout the period of resuscitation. This is given in individual doses containing 44 mEq. of sodium bicarbonate for an average-sized adult. Calcium chloride, in a 10 per cent solution, is sometimes given to improve myocardial contractility after successful defibrillation has been carried out.

An aggressive and optimistic approach to cardiopulmonary resuscitation is mandatory for all persons when a diagnosis of cardiac arrest has been made. Preparation and practice in the emergency room with a manikin are recommended, and training to achieve coordination of the efforts of all members of the team is essential.

The possibility of success in salvaging patients after cardiac arrest depends on the underlying cause of the arrest and its inciting factors. The physician involved in this type of effort must know something of these causes, as well as of the associated diseases and injuries and the approximate duration of arrest before he can properly abandon the effort. Signs of central nervous system damage, such as widely dilated, nonreactive pupils and absence of spontaneous respiration, together with an ECG showing refractory ventricular fibrillation or continued asystole, should be taken as evidence of failure of the resuscitative efforts.

Care of a patient following successful resuscitation requires the use of careful monitoring of vital organ function. A need for close attention to airway and ventilatory support is suggested by the presence of copious secretions or by the finding of abnormal blood gas values. Support with an endotracheal tube and respirator may be required in some of these patients. A vigilant attitude in regard to the occurrence of arrhythmias and the possibility of recurrent arrest should be maintained. Establishment of adequate renal function and the repair of fluid and electrolyte abnormalities, as well as support of a stable blood pressure level, should also be major concerns in the postresuscitative period.

CONTROL OF HEMORRHAGE

Serious external hemorrhage can usually be controlled by direct pressure over the wound, using a hand protected by a sterile dressing. Elevation of the bleeding extremity is also helpful, but the application of arterial tourniquets should be avoided whenever possible because of the hazard of their causing ischemic damage in the distal extremity, as well as their tendency to cause increased bleeding by interfering with venous return.

Hemorrhage associated with long bone fractures, hemothorax, or hemoperitoneum must be recognized and whole blood administration begun promptly. A selected few patients with very rapid and severe hemorrhage should be identified early in the triage of emergencies and taken promptly to the operating room for immediate surgery. These may include patients with ruptured aortic aneurysms, severe upper gastrointestinal hemorrhage, or penetrating wounds of the chest and abdomen associated with great vessel injury.

CHEST TRAUMA

Serious consequences of blunt and penetrating injuries to the chest include pneumothorax, airway obstruction, hemothorax, flail chest, and cardiac tamponade. Initial assessment of the patient's injuries should first include a rapid evaluation of airway patency and adequacy of ventilation and the detection of signs of shock.

Pneumothorax

An open chest wound with pneumothorax, as seen in some stab or gunshot injuries, is usually associated with a side-to-side movement of the mediastinum associated with free ingress and egress of air at atmospheric pressure into the open pleural cavity. This type of wound must be immediately covered with a sterile compression dressing to seal the wound and stabilize the mediastinum. The pneumothorax is controlled by inserting a chest tube at an appropriate interspace and attaching it to a water-seal bottle or to a chest suction apparatus.

The simple pneumothorax associated

with rib fractures caused by blunt trauma should be promptly detected by the presence of the resonant percussion note and the absence of breath sounds over the affected side of the thorax. Diagnosis should be confirmed, if the patient's condition allows, by a promptly performed chest x-ray examination. A closed pneumothorax, with or without an associated hemothorax, is usually managed by insertion of a chest tube in the appropriate interspace.

A tension pneumothorax may be caused by a persistent air leak from a laceration of lung or bronchus involving a check-valve action that allows leakage of air into the pleural space during inspiration. Its life-threatening effects include compression of the opposite lung by shifting of the mediastinum and compression of the great veins in the mediastinum, resulting in interference with cardiac return. The finding of subcutaneous emphysema, tracheal shift to the opposite side, neck vein distention, or hyperresonance on the affected side in a patient with dyspnea, cyanosis, or signs of shock should serve to identify this dangerous situation. Prompt action without benefit of time-consuming x-ray studies is required. A preliminary puncture of the anterior second interspace with a large bore needle

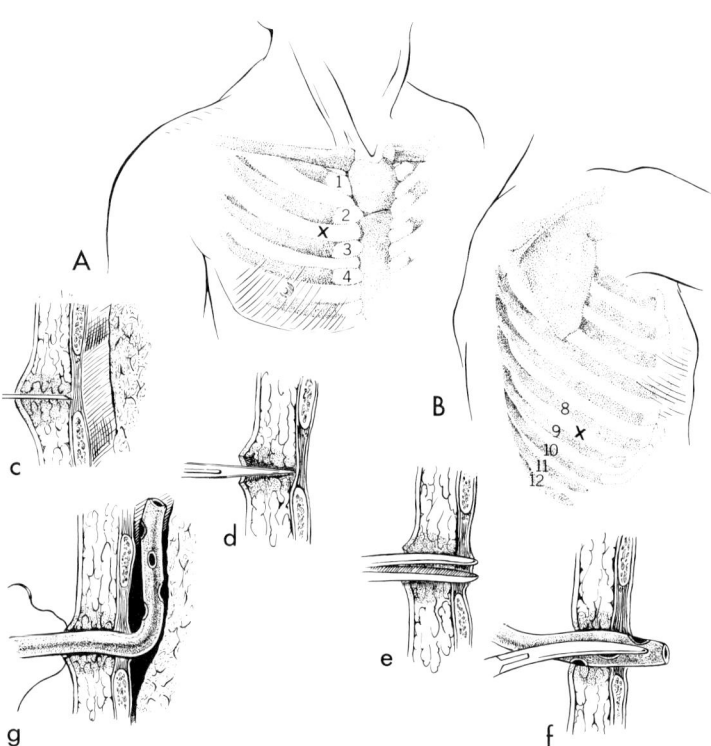

Figure 37–13. *Introduction of chest tubes. A. For treatment of pneumothorax, the anterior aspect of the second intercostal space is selected for chest tube insertion (x). The angle of Louis is the landmark for identifying this interspace. A point about 2 fingerbreadths lateral to the edge of the sternum is infiltrated with local anesthetic, through skin, subcutaneous tissue, and intercostal muscle (c). A small skin incision is made (d). A curved Kelly clamp is used, by pushing and spreading, to develop an opening over the superior edge of the third rib into the pleural cavity (e). The chest tube is introduced into the passage between the blades of the clamp and the tip put into the pleural space (f). The catheter is then threaded in past the most distal suction hole, and secured at the skin level with a suture (g).*

Larger caliber tubes (32 to 36 French) are best employed in patients with active air leaks. The smaller size tubes (20 to 28 French) may be appropriate for treatment of spontaneous pneumothorax with moderate air leaks.

B. For pleural effusion or hemothorax, chest tube insertion in a dependent costal interspace such as the eighth (x) is recommended. The level is identified by counting upward from the twelfth rib. The posterior axillary line is selected, and the patient should be placed in the semierect position if possible. A large caliber chest tube (32 French) is inserted through a small skin incision after preliminary aspiration of the space with a needle and syringe, and the patient may then be returned to the supine position.

will vent the pleural cavity and reduce the pressure to atmospheric level. Subsequent insertion of a chest tube through an anterior or midaxillary intercostal space will relieve the pneumothorax and encourage re-expansion of the collapsed lung when the chest tube is attached to a chest suction apparatus. Details of the procedure of tube thoracostomy are given in Figure 37–13. A simple three bottle trap system is recommended for chest tube suction in most emergency situations, using negative intrapleural pressures of −10 to −20 cm. of water.

Hemothorax

Significant collections of blood in the pleural space are more often associated with penetrating wounds than with blunt injuries accompanied by rib fractures and simple pneumothorax. The source of bleeding is usually from a laceration of the lung or of the intercostal vessels in the chest wall but occasionally is from the heart or great vessels. In most cases, the bleeding stops spontaneously. It is characteristic of hemothorax that the blood in the pleural cavity becomes defibrinated and remains liquefied for long periods of time. Although small volumes of blood in the pleural space can be evacuated by thoracocentesis on one or more occasions, a tube thoracostomy in a dependent interspace, performed under local anesthesia, tends to allow more accurate monitoring of continuing blood loss as well as more thorough evacuation of the pleural space, thus accomplishing early re-expansion of the lung. In the presence of a combined hemothorax and pneumothorax, an additional tube may be required in a more superior location on the affected side to control active air leakage. Persistent bleeding may furnish a sound indication for early performance of an exploratory thoracotomy, which is generally required in only about 10 per cent of instances of traumatic hemothorax.

Flail Chest

These are potentially serious injuries involving severe blunt trauma to the chest wall that usually result from automobile accidents or falls. Fractures of the ribs or sternum in multiple locations may give rise to severe instability of the chest wall, thus causing major ventilatory insufficiency that may be compounded further by underlying lung contusions or lacerations. First aid treatment of flail chest may require the temporary use of sterile towel clips applied to the affected ribs with gentle traction to stabilize the chest wall and minimize paradoxical movement, while an endotracheal tube is inserted and associated pneumothorax or hemothorax is attended to. More definitive treatment of flail chest requires stabilization of the chest wall by mechanical ventilation of the lungs, using positive pressure. Because of the prolonged period required for achievement of healing in the chest wall, it may be necessary to perform a tracheostomy to replace the endotracheal tube. Subsequent treatment of this type of injury can best be accomplished in an intensive care unit equipped for providing respiratory care, with blood gas analysis readily available and a trained team of nursing and other personnel in attendance. Prognosis has been shown to be closely related to the severity of the underlying damage to the lung, as well as to the extent and severity of associated head, abdominal, and extremity injuries.

Cardiac Tamponade

This serious complication of chest trauma is chiefly associated with penetrating wounds and results from the accumulation of blood in the closed space of the pericardial sac. Even a volume of blood less than 100 ml. can produce impairment of venous return and diastolic filling of the heart, resulting in a concomitant rise in venous pressure and fall in stroke volume and systolic arterial pressure. This diagnosis should be suggested by the presence of shock in the absence of external bleeding in cases of penetrating chest trauma. Differential diagnosis rests between hemothorax and cardiac tamponade. The measurement of central venous pressure with an inlying cannula in the superior vena cava is helpful. The detection of a high or rising venous pressure in conjunction with shock, paradoxical pulse, and muffled heart sounds should confirm the diagnosis of tamponade. X-ray studies of the chest often fail to show significant changes in the cardiac silhouette, but in the presence of clinical findings, a normal or slightly larger than normal heart size should suggest tamponade.

When indications for immediate thoracotomy are not present, an emergency pericardial aspiration is indicated, using an 18 gauge needle attached to a three-way stopcock and a 50 ml. syringe (Fig. 37–14). The needle can be introduced into the pericardial sac just to the left of the xiphoid process. Blood is aspirated, and the pericardial sac is drained until dry. The procedure may be repeated at intervals as necessary. The indications for thoracotomy in a patient with cardiac tamponade are usually based on the patient's response to repeated pericardial taps as well as to the rate and severity of bleeding.

ABDOMINAL INJURIES

Blunt Abdominal Trauma

Blunt injuries involving the abdominal wall and the viscera are usually due to vehicular accidents, falls, or fights. They range from simple abdominal wall contusions to rather complex injuries involving multiple organs. Such injuries have a well-deserved reputation for creating diagnostic difficulty, since a good number of them occur in unconscious or inebriated patients and also occur in association with other more obvious injuries to the chest, spine, head, or long bones. The risk of overlooking

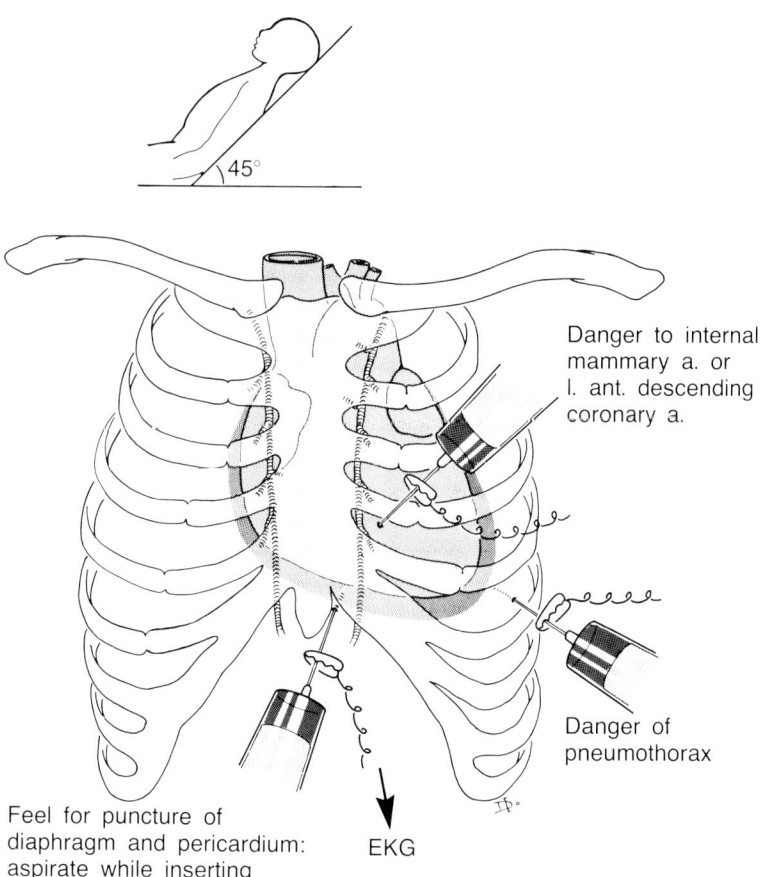

Figure 37–14. *Pericardiocentesis. A needle may be passed into the pericardium via the three routes indicated. Each route has some disadvantages. An electrocardiogram lead is clipped to the needle to monitor contact between needle and myocardium.*

an occult blunt abdominal injury is serious, and it should be remembered that delay in diagnosis of these high-priority injuries is one of the causes for their relatively high mortality.

In the conscious and cooperative patient, diagnosis is aided by the presence of abdominal pain, tenderness, or guarding. A collection of blood under the diaphragm will usually cause the characteristic referred pain in the left shoulder. Bowel sounds will be hypoactive or absent in the presence of a major degree of hemoperitoneum or of soilage by bowel contents. In the comatose patient, clues will include the presence of bruises or contusions in the abdominal wall, lower chest, or flanks. Certain fractures, notably those of the lower ribs, the lumbar vertebrae, or the pelvic girdle, may also suggest the possibility of abdominal injury. The presence of shock should always bring to mind the possibility of intra-abdominal bleeding. The patient's response to blood volume replacement, together with the results of careful re-examination of the abdomen at intervals, may help in identifying those patients with continued intra-abdominal bleeding.

Other useful diagnostic measures include abdominal x-ray studies, a four-quadrant tap, or a peritoneal lavage with an inlying catheter (Fig. 37–15). X-ray findings may include pneumoperitoneum, displacement of hollow organs, masses, loss of psoas shadows, and fractures of ribs, spine, or pelvis. Peritoneal lavage has achieved a high degree of accuracy of diagnosis for patients in whom doubt exists as to whether shock is caused by hemoperitoneum or by some other injury. Identification of blood, bile, and fecal material can be made easily. The question of how much blood in the peritoneal lavage fluid constitutes an indication for laparotomy has not been settled. Most physicians would agree that the finding of 100,000 red blood cells per ml. in the fluid is an indication of the need for laparotomy.

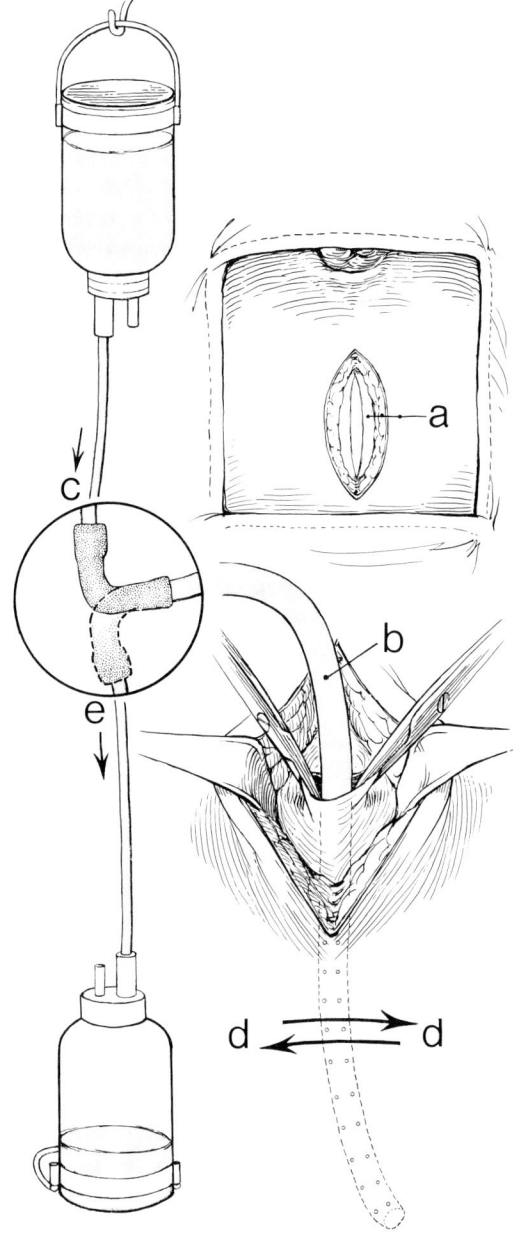

Figure 37–15. Peritoneal lavage in blunt abdominal trauma. The urinary bladder having been catheterized and emptied, the abdomen is prepared with antiseptic, and sterile drapes are arranged. Through a small wheal made with anesthetic agent combined with epinephrine, at a point 2 fingerbreadths below the umbilicus, a small incision is made through skin, fat, and midline fascia (a). It is kept dry by securing all bleeders. The peritoneum is opened between clamps and an adult-sized peritoneal dialysis catheter is introduced (b).

Lavage is carried out with a liter of isotonic saline or Ringer's lactate solution, which runs in by gravity through an intravenous infusion set attaching the bottle to the catheter (c). The fluid is distributed within the abdomen by shifting the patient's position on the table (d). It is immediately withdrawn by suction or siphonage (e) and examined for the presence of gross blood. Clear fluid may be examined under the microscope for red blood cells. Amylase determinations may be done in selected patients.

Blunt abdominal trauma most commonly involves injury to the spleen. In most patients, the resulting hemoperitoneum gives clear-cut symptoms and signs, including left upper quadrant pain and Kehr's sign. Other suggestive findings include localized upper abdominal tenderness, shock, and a palpable left upper quadrant abdominal mass. Fairly frequently, the slow rate of blood loss seen with small capsular tears or with subcapsular hematomas may fail to give immediate and clear-cut abdominal findings. The difficulty may be compounded if the patient is unconscious or has other serious injuries. In this situation, close observation and an aggressive diagnostic approach, including peritoneal lavage, are necessary. A rising white blood cell count may be associated with continuing hemorrhage from splenic rupture. X-ray evidence of fractures of the lower left ribs, an enlarged splenic shadow, displacement of the stomach bubble, or obliteration of the outline of the left kidney, psoas muscle, or properitoneal fat line are radiologic signs suggestive of splenic injury. In doubtful cases in which indication for exploration is lacking but clinical suspicion of splenic injury is high, the use of abdominal angiography and splenic scanning may be of help in identifying occult splenic injury. Delayed rupture of a subcapsular hematoma of the spleen is a potentially fatal complication of such injuries. The majority of these occur within 2 weeks following the original trauma. In selected patients, minor occult injuries may be treated conservatively. This is especially so in children, in whom the spleen's protective role against infection is recognized as being particularly important.

A variety of injuries may involve other intra-abdominal organs, such as the liver, kidneys, mesenteries, and bowel. Hemoperitoneum or leakage of intestinal contents usually explains the presenting signs and symptoms. The diagnosis is usually suggested by the presence of abdominal pain, tenderness, or a palpable mass. Shock is a frequent concomitant finding. X-ray evidence of pneumoperitoneum on upright or lateral decubitus films will confirm the diagnosis of rupture of a hollow viscus. Contrast studies of the urinary bladder after passage of a catheter will be essential in the detection of bladder and urethral injuries. Intravenous pyelography should be done early when renal injury is suspected. Peritoneal lavage may be of assistance when the diagnosis is doubtful. Repeated abdominal examinations by one person during an interval of close observation of the patient offer the best help in the identification of slowly developing signs of intra-abdominal injury. In such patients, the use of narcotics during the period of study should be avoided in order to prevent confusion in regard to the results of abdominal examination.

Penetrating Injuries

Penetrating abdominal injuries are less common in civilian experience than are blunt injuries, but they also require prompt diagnosis and treatment. Obvious gunshot wounds of the abdomen are treated by immediate operation. In the case of an abdominal stab wound, a more selective policy of management may be justified, unless there is clear-cut evidence of intraperitoneal injury. Brief intervals of observing patients with stab wounds of uncertain depth may eliminate some unnecessary laparotomies. Use of sinograms obtained by injection of radiopaque medium into the wound to determine if the peritoneal cavity has been entered may also be helpful in this regard. Exploratory laparotomy is generally indicated when penetration of the peritoneum can be demonstrated by x-ray studies or shown by direct inspection.

SOFT TISSUE INJURIES

Uncomplicated soft tissue wounds are of low priority in the treatment of injured patients. The patient should first be thoroughly examined before such surface lesions as burns, lacerations, abrasions, or contusions are treated. Further contamination of the wound is prevented by covering it with sterile dressings while resuscitation and other diagnostic procedures are carried out.

There are certain soft tissue injuries, however, that do require prompt surgical treatment because of their potential for infection or for risk of loss of function. Wounds of the extremity involving major vascular injury are in this category, as are wounds involving disruption of tendons or major somatic nerves. Recognition of these special wounds must be made early, and definitive treatment must be carried out as soon as the patient's general condition will allow it.

The essential feature of good treatment of soft tissue injuries is performance of adequate debridement, which means the thorough removal of dead or devitalized tissue. This is usually accomplished by a combination of sharp excision of the margins of the wound and the flushing of its surfaces with copious amounts of sterile isotonic saline solution. Most wounds in areas of good blood supply, such as the scalp and face, require minimal excision of margins prior to closure. There is little time restriction placed on the planned closure of wounds in these areas of optimal healing, and careful layer closure with fine suture material is justified even in neglected cases, unless there is evidence of established infection (Fig. 37–16).

Heavily contaminated wounds in other less favorable locations may require quite different handling. A period of 6 to 8 hours is the interval between the receipt of wounds and the time of treatment during which primary closure can be accomplished safely. Beyond this period, heavily contaminated wounds are best left open after debridement. The same approach should be used in most wounds in which all devitalized tissue and foreign bodies cannot be eliminated. If periosteum, cartilage, tendons, vessels, or abdominal viscera are exposed, these structures should be covered by a protective layer of tissue such as muscle, fascia, or peritoneum, using sutures. The fat and skin may be left open in such wounds in the presence of heavy contamination. Delayed primary closure of the superficial portions of the wound is appropriate in certain contaminated wounds of the trunk or extremities. This consists of closure of the wound by suture at an interval of 3 to 7 days following the initial debridement. Some particularly dirty wounds should be allowed to close by second intention or, after delays of 10 to 14 days, should be closed by skin grafts or by secondary suture.

Special anti-infective precautions are required in certain types of soft tissue wounds that are prone to infection. Human and animal bites must be carefully managed. Those of the face or neck may be closed primarily if this is done early after injury, although those located elsewhere are better left open to ensure adequate drainage. Power mower injuries of the foot should be carefully cleaned and debrided and all exposed tendons or bones covered with soft tissue. The superficial portions of these wounds should usually be left open for later closure by suture or by skin grafts. The common puncture wound in the foot or hand must be carefully inspected, and after local infiltration with an anesthetic agent, it must be thoroughly irrigated with sterile saline solution. Enlargement of the skin opening is often effective in providing better drainage of such wounds. On no account should these wounds be closed by suture. The possibility of the presence of a foreign body in puncture wounds or deep lacerations should be kept in mind. In case of doubt, an x-ray examination of the area may localize radiopaque foreign bodies. In any event, whenever the possibility exists, a careful local exploration of the wound is advisable.

TETANUS PROPHYLAXIS

Certain measures to protect the patient from tetanus should be automatically considered by the family physician at the time of initial treatment of soft tissue injuries. Wound surgery with thorough debridement is the first logical step in such prophylaxis. Special importance is attached to debridement of tetanus-prone wounds, which include those involving injury to muscle, those with heavy contamination or retained foreign bodies, and those being treated after a long delay. Debridement converts such wounds to clean wounds with margins having normal blood supply and creates an environment in which growth and proliferation of *Clostridium tetani* are unlikely to occur.

The additional protection from tetanus afforded by active or passive immunization should also be considered in every patient, no matter how trivial the wound. An accurate history of the patient's past tetanus immunizations should be sought. Since the majority of patients will have had adequate primary immunization against tetanus, the most frequent question will concern the need for a booster dose of toxoid. Current

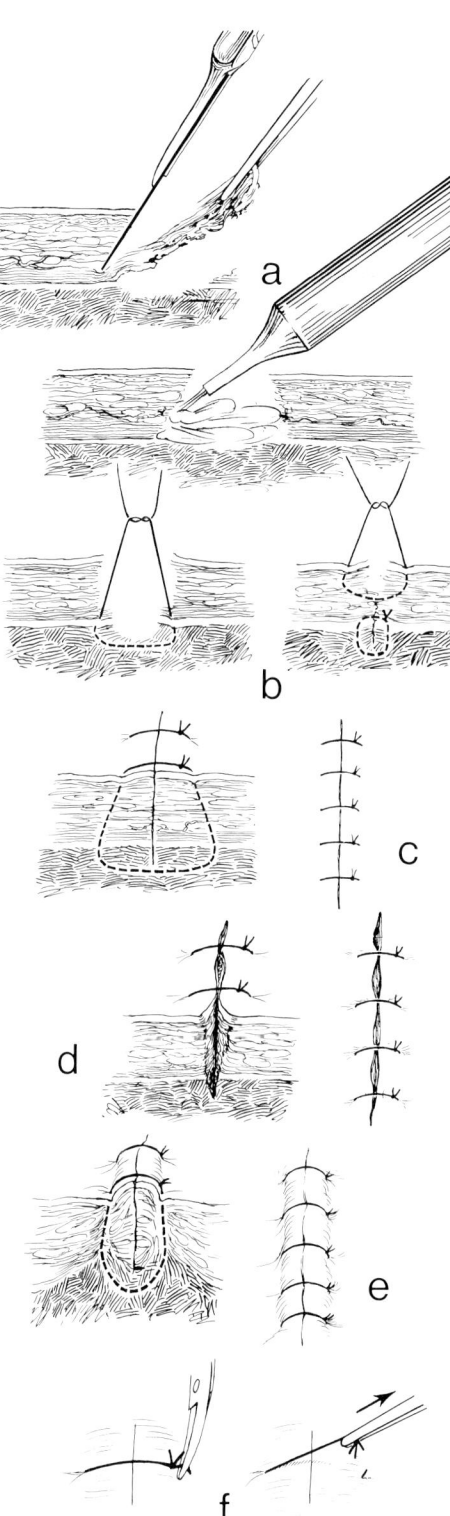

Figure 37–16. *Management of simple lacerations. The surrounding skin should be shaved and washed with soap and water. After sterile drapes have been arranged, the margins of the wound are infiltrated with 1 per cent lidocaine.*

(a) Necessary debridement is accomplished by scalpel excision of devitalized wound edges, undercutting slightly by angling the blade. Bleeders are secured with hemostats and fine ties of catgut (4–0 plain). The wound is thoroughly irrigated with sterile isotonic saline solution.

(b) Closure of the subcutaneous layer by interrupted sutures (4–0 chromic catgut) should be used to eliminate dead space in deep wounds. A minimal number of buried sutures should be employed. They should be tied gently and cut close to their knots.

(c) Fine skin sutures (5–0 nylon) on atraumatic curved needles are applied in an everting fashion, encircling a larger amount of tissue in the lower depths than near the surface. They are spaced and tied to appose the skin edges accurately.

Gaps between sutures creating dead space (d), and undue tension (e), with compromise of blood supply, should be avoided. Knots should be located to one side of the line of closure.

(f) Removal of sutures after about 7 or 8 days should be accomplished by cutting the loop close to the skin surface and drawing the suture across the wound to avoid distraction of the edges.

recommendation is that a booster dose for tetanus prophylaxis in the management of contaminated wounds is needed no more often than once every 5 years. For patients who have had adequate primary immunization and whose wounds are clean and of minor extent, this period can now be safely extended to 10 years. In addition, elective administration of toxoid boosters to maintain a level of immunity in healthy persons should be spaced at 10 year intervals.

Those adult patients who have not had a full primary immunization against tetanus and whose wounds are clean and minor should be given 0.5 ml. of adsorbed tetanus toxoid intramuscularly. Arrangements should be made to complete the immunization by giving a second dose 4 to 6 weeks later, followed by a third dose 6 to 12 months after the second. In the same situation, but this time involving a contaminated wound, primary immunization should also be begun. However, additional protection should be given by the intramuscular injection in a separate site of 250 units of tetanus immune globulin (human). When tetanus immune globulin is unavailable within a 24 hour period, such tetanus-prone wounds should be protected with equine or bovine antitoxin (3000 to 5000 units intramuscularly) after careful testing of the patient for sensitivity. When this treatment is contraindicated because of sensitivity reactions, penicillin or tetracycline should be given for 7 to 10 days or until the immune globulin can be obtained.

SURGICAL INFECTIONS

Prevention of Wound Sepsis

The use of the term "contaminated" to describe a traumatic wound is redundant, since at the time of injury, bacteria are always introduced into a traumatic wound. However, for practical purposes, a contaminated wound can be defined as one involving either the introduction of gross dirt at the time of injury or the presence of devitalized tissue at the site of injury. Wounds seen later than 6 or 8 hours after injury or those contaminated by probing or other meddlesome acts prior to treatment also fall into this category. In addition, wounds involving the opening of a viscus or

those incurred through a dirty surface, such as the mouth or the perineum, should be considered contaminated. Most patients with contaminated wounds should have the protection of prophylactic antibiotics given early and in adequate doses for a period of several days following injury.

Infection of soft tissue wounds should be a rather infrequent occurrence if sound principles are followed at the time of their initial treatment. Aseptic technique with adequate debridement, good hemostasis, and intelligent choice of either primary closure or open methods of wound care leave the local defenses intact and make infection unlikely. Other measures of a prophylactic nature should be considered as well. These include rest for the patient, immobilization of the injured part, and, in the case of an extremity wound, elevation of the limb to promote resolution of swelling and to assist in venous return. In major injuries, shock and hypovolemia should be actively treated. In diabetic patients, careful management is required to avoid keto-acidosis or hypoglycemia.

Although the use of antibiotics offers no substitute for good wound care, this does have a place in the early management of certain types of trauma. The objective is to protect the patient from specific organisms rather than from the entire spectrum of pathogens. Use of antibiotics is tempered by the knowledge of the risk of serious side effects, as well as by the risk of such drugs influencing the appearance of resistant organisms in the host. The use of prophylactic antibiotic therapy is also based on an awareness of the consequences of major infection at the site of injury. Patients with missile wounds; compound fractures; penetrating wounds of the head, pleural cavity or abdomen; and extremity wounds with tendon, nerve, or major vascular injury are candidates for such an approach. A case can also be made for prophylaxis in patients having soft tissue wounds with associated muscle injury; heavy contamination; or unretrievable foreign bodies such as metallic fragments, clothing, or pieces of wadding. Wounds resulting from human or animal bites are included in this category, as are wounds in diabetics or in patients taking corticosteroids or immunosuppressive drugs.

Antimicrobial prophylaxis, when indicated, should be given as soon as possible after hospital admission. In major injuries, such prophylaxis should be given by the intravenous or intramuscular route. It should probably be continued for at least 3 days following the original injury. The choice of antibiotic is based on a consideration of which pathogen would be the most dangerous in a given wound. Infection caused by clostridia, streptococci, and staphylococci would be the major concern in skin and soft tissue injuries with heavy contamination and muscle damage. Penicillin G, erythromycin, or a cephalothin would furnish reasonable protection in this instance, if given early and in adequate dosage parenterally. Patients with wounds involving contamination from the gastrointestinal tract with the possibility of infection by coliform organisms should be given an aminoglycoside such as gentamicin in addition to penicillin or cephalothin. When infection by anaerobic organisms (*Bacteroides*) is likely, as in wounds of the small bowel or colon, clindamycin or chloramphenicol should be added to the regimen. Protection from the mixed pathogens involved in human or animal bites is afforded by the administration of penicillin G and tetracycline. Severely burned patients should be protected from streptococcal and pneumococcal infection in the early phase of their treatment by the intravenous administration of large doses of penicillin G.

Swab specimens taken from the edges of traumatic wounds at the time of their initial treatment should be sent for smear and culture. The results of such bacteriologic studies can be of value in guiding the choice of antibiotics early in the course of wound management.

Treatment of Wound Infections

Recognition of an infection developing in a soft tissue wound should be made early. This can be done by establishing a follow-up routine of inspection of healing wounds within the first 48 to 72 hours after initial care. Unusual pain in the area, erythema around the edges, significant local tenderness, or purulent exudate is evidence of infection. In closed wounds, a few sutures should be removed and the skin edges spread slightly with a sterile hemostat. Cultures should be taken from a swab

specimen of the wound discharge. In situations in which the infection seems poorly localized, as in cellulitis or lymphangitis, local heat, rest, and elevation are begun, and appropriate antibiotics given. Choice of antibiotics is often best made after a Gram's stain of the exudate has been done. Well-localized abscess formation should indicate the need for drainage. Aspiration with a needle through a wheal of local anesthesia may provide further proof of the existence of suppuration in the wound. An abscess occurring in a sutured wound will only require complete removal of sutures and spreading of the wound edges to allow free drainage of pus. The cavity resulting from release of pus from the depths of the wound is lightly packed with gauze. Tight packing, which may interfere with proper wound drainage, is to be avoided. Again, cultures are taken, and local measures such as heat, elevation, and splinting are instituted. If the infection is well-contained, no antibiotic therapy is required.

Response to such local measures for the therapy of wound infections is usually prompt. Most of these patients will not require hospitalization. Indeed, the management of soft tissue trauma complicated by wound sepsis can, in the majority of cases, be accomplished easily and effectively in an outpatient setting, particularly when the patient is cooperative and intelligent and when parenteral administration of antibiotics, general anesthesia, or care of associated disorders such as diabetes mellitus is not necessary.

When wound infections are more severe or when response to initial therapeutic measures has been slow, surgical consultation should be sought and hospital care arranged for the patient. A careful review of the bacteriologic data and antibiotic sensitivities must be made. The need for adjunctive surgical procedures, such as a wider drainage of an abscess or exploration for a hidden foreign body or necrotic tissue, should be considered. Also to be reviewed are systemic factors predisposing to infection, such as diabetes, steroid therapy, administration of immunosuppressive drugs, neoplastic disease, malnutrition, or anemia.

In the presence of evidence of invasive infection or septicemia, rapid institution of treatment is required. Administration of parenteral fluids and high doses of appropriate antibiotics, careful monitoring of vital signs, and maintenance of an adequate airway and ventilation are some of the more essential measures to be initiated promptly. Attention to the primary site of infection and the use of appropriate measures to provide free drainage of pus are essential. Support of the circulation with volume replacement, appropriate use of pressor drugs, and in some instances, administration of large doses of corticosteroids must be continued. Elevation of central venous pressure in the presence of hypotension must be countered by administration of digitalis.

Septic shock is currently a serious problem, particularly when it involves gram-negative invasive infections occurring as the result of major trauma or surgery in elderly or debilitated patients. Even with excellent therapy, the mortality is high in established cases. Early recognition of invasive infection and institution of surgical measures before the appearance of shock seem, at the present time, to offer the best chance for a successful outcome for these patients.

THERMAL BURNS

Provision of initial care for the patient with a thermal burn lies well within the scope and functions of the family physician. The objectives are:

1. Control of life-threatening early complications such as airway obstruction and shock.

2. Full assessment of the extent and severity of the injuries at the time of the first examination.

3. Initiation of general supportive measures and care of local burn wounds.

4. Triage decision concerning the need to transport the patient to another facility for definitive treatment.

Minor Burns

First degree or superficial burns can be easily recognized and treated on an outpatient basis. They are usually caused by brief exposure to flash or hot liquids or by longer exposure to ultraviolet light. Uncomplicated healing can be expected to occur within a week without specific treatment.

Pain can be relieved and swelling reduced by early application of ice water. Dressings should be avoided, and use of topical anesthetic or analgesic ointments should be restricted to small first degree burns of minor extent.

Partial-thickness burns of less than 10 per cent of body surface may also be considered minor burns. These are usually recognized by the presence of blistering and exudation, local edema, and good tactile sensation. They can be expected to heal within a 2 or 3 week period. Such burns are caused in most cases by spills of hot liquids or by brief exposure to flash. Treatment consists of initial cleaning of the wound with soap and water, trimming of blisters, and application of a fine mesh petrolatum gauze occlusive dressing. The object of the dressing is to prevent infection and to immobilize the part. Dressings should be changed at 3 or 4 day intervals, using sterile technique. Prophylactic penicillin should be administered by the oral route for 5 to 7 days to prevent streptococcal infection.

Major Burns

Major burns can be defined as those burns involving partial-thickness injury greater than 10 per cent of body surface area in an adult or greater than 5 per cent in a small child or old person, or those burns with full-thickness injury greater than 2 per cent of body surface area. Other factors to be considered in defining the severity of burns are their anatomic location, the nature of the agent causing the burn, and the presence of other injuries or associated diseases.

Plan of Initial Care of Major Burns

EXAMINATION OF THE PATIENT. Evaluation of the patient begins with attention to the airway. Smoke inhalation or asphyxiation caused by carbon monoxide inhalation are the major causes of respiratory distress in burn patients seen soon after injury. The presence of deep burns about the neck or face, together with dyspnea, cyanosis, hoarseness, and labored respirations, suggests the additional possibility of upper airway injury caused by hot gas or by steam inhalation. Initial treatment should involve the administration of high concentrations of humidified oxygen by mask and, in some patients, the insertion of an oropharyngeal airway and the use of assisted respiration with a mask and bag. If gas exchange

TABLE 37–10. SURFACE AREA BY THE RULE OF NINES

	Per Cent
Head and Neck	9
Upper Extremity (1)	9
Lower Extremity (1)	18
Anterior Trunk	18
Posterior Trunk	18
Perineum	1

TABLE 37–11. BROOKE FORMULA, UPDATED, FOR FLUID THERAPY IN ADULTS

First 24 Hours

Lactated Ringer's solution – 3 ml./kg. body weight times per cent of burn

Urine output – 50 ml./hr.

Second 24 Hours

Glucose in water
Plasmanate

Urine output – 50 ml./hr.

remains inadequate because of secretions or glottic edema, insertion of an oral endotracheal tube should be carried out by an expert, and ventilatory assistance should be continued with a bag or anesthesia machine attached to the endotracheal tube. In most patients, an initial tracheostomy should be avoided because of the high incidence of serious respiratory complications following its use in burned patients. Evidence of carbon particles in the sputum or tracheobronchial secretions should be considered an indicator of smoke inhalation damage. Blood gas determinations and administration of large doses of steroids may be helpful in the management of this problem.

While the general examination of the patient is being carried out, a history of the incident is taken. The presence of other significant injuries or diseases is determined, and the patient's status in regard to tetanus immunization is ascertained.

The burn wound is surveyed, and an initial estimate of its extent and depth is made using the rule of nines (Table 37–10). All of the patient's clothing is removed, and an accurate body weight is obtained if possible. The patient is then placed on a sterile sheet on an examining table. Body heat is conserved by covering the patient with several layers of sterile sheets and blankets.

INITIAL THERAPY. An intravenous cannula is inserted through unburned skin, if possible, into the jugular or subclavian veins, and its tip is positioned in the superior vena cava. Acceptable alternative routes for fluid administration include a cut-down in the cephalic vein at the shoulder or in the long saphenous vein at the ankle. Blood samples should be drawn for baseline determination of serum electrolytes, blood urea nitrogen, blood glucose,

and a complete blood count. Intravenous administration of 5 per cent dextrose in Ringer's lactate solution should be started. A plan for instituting further fluid therapy should be developed, using a simple calculation based on an acceptable formula (Table 37–11).

An indwelling urinary catheter is inserted. Urine volume and specific gravity are determined and a specimen sent for urinalysis. Hourly urinary output and specific gravity are monitored thereafter. A tetanus booster or human immune globulin injection is given as indicated.

A nasogastric tube is inserted and attached to suction if the patient is nauseated or if a full stomach is suspected. Small doses of narcotics can be given intravenously for the relief of pain. Application of cool sterile saline compresses may help to relieve pain, particularly in the patient with a partial-thickness burn.

CARE OF THE WOUND. The physician dons cap, mask, and sterile gloves and, using sterile instruments, removes blisters, debris, and foreign material. The wound is then cleaned with cool saline and topical ointments are removed by gentle sponging with a mild detergent soap. Topical application of antibacterial agents should not be made at the time of the initial dressing without the surgeon's advice and consent. If transfer of the patient to another facility is planned, a simple occlusive dressing, using fine mesh petrolatum gauze, sterile absorbent pads, and nonelastic bandages, can be applied on the extremities of the lower trunk. Circular dressings about the chest or neck are avoided. If the patient is to remain in the same hospital for subsequent treatment, the burn can be covered with sterile sheets to await the first inspection and the choice of definitive wound care by the surgeon-in-charge.

Because of their tendency to restrict respiration, deep circumferential burns of the thorax may require emergency incision. Such escharotomies are usually done with aseptic technique, using a sterile scalpel to make vertical incisions in the midline over the sternum and in the midaxillary areas.

TRIAGE OF BURN PATIENTS. After full evaluation of the patient and his injury, a decision must be made concerning the advisability of transfer to another hospital for definitive care. Consultation with a surgeon should be obtained, and careful assessment should be made of the available means of transportation, the time required, and the need for further treatment prior to moving the patient. In the absence of shock or severe respiratory difficulty, and with initial care under way, the proper time to move the patient with severe burns is best described as early in the course of treatment and should occur sometime within the first 24 hours after receipt of injury.

Optimum treatment for the extensively burned patient requires a team effort and facilities of a specialized kind seldom available in community hospitals or even in most general hospitals. Knowledge of the location and accessibility of centers specializing in burn care is important for the physician who provides the initial service for burn patients in outlying communities.

BIBLIOGRAPHY

General

Condon, R. E., and Nyhus, L. M. (eds.): Manual of Surgical Therapeutics. 2nd Ed. Boston, Little, Brown & Co., 1972.

Dunphy, J. E., and Botsford, T. W.: Physical Examination of the Surgical Patient. 4th Ed. Philadelphia, W. B. Saunders Co., 1975.

Hill, G. J., II (ed.): Outpatient Surgery. Philadelphia, W. B. Saunders Co., 1973.

Kinney, J. M., Egdahl, R. H., and Zuidema, G. D. (eds.): Manual of Preoperative and Postoperative Care. Philadelphia, W. B. Saunders Co., 1971.

Schwartz, S. I. (ed.): Principles of Surgery. 2nd Ed. New York, McGraw-Hill Book Co., 1974.

Swenson, O.: Pediatric Surgery. 3rd Ed. New York, Appleton-Century-Crofts, 1969.

Wells, C., Kyle, J., and Dunphy, J. E.: Scientific Foundations of Surgery. 2nd Ed. Philadelphia, W. B. Saunders Co., 1974.

Preoperative Assessment and Preparation of Patients

Alexander, S.: Surgical risk in the patient with arteriosclerotic heart disease. Surg. Clin. North Am., 48:513, 1968.

Arkins, R., Smessaert, A. A., and Hicks, R. G.: Mortality and morbidity in surgical patients with coronary artery disease. J.A.M.A., 190:485, 1964.

Clowes, G. H. A., Jr., Del Guercio, L. R., and Barwinsky, J.: The cardiac output in response to surgical trauma. A comparison between those who survived and those who died. Arch. Surg., 81:212, 1960.

Dripps, R. D., Eckenhoff, J. E., and Vandam, L. D.: Introduction to Anesthesia. 4th Ed. Philadelphia, W. B. Saunders Co., 1972.

Dudrick, S. J., and Rhoads, J. E.: Long term parenteral nutrition with growth and positive nitrogen balance. Surgery, 64:134, 1968.

Gilmore, H. R.: Preoperative responsibilities of the family physician. Consultant, 165:30, 1976.

Meng, H. C.: Principles of parenteral nutrition. Hosp. Med., 7:102, 1971.

Stein, M., and Cassara, E. L.: Preoperative pulmonary evaluation and therapy for surgical patients. J.A.M.A., 211:787, 1970.

Steinke, J.: Management of diabetes mellitus and surgery. N. Engl. J. Med., 282:1472, 1970.

Webb, R. S., Jr.: Correction of malnutrition in surgical patients. Surg. Clin. North Am., 44:141, 1964.

The Acute Abdomen

Ayala, L. A., Williams, L. F., and Wildrich, R. C.: Occult rupture of the spleen. Ann. Surg., 179:472, 1974.

Botsford, T. W., and Wilson, R. E.: The Acute Abdomen, 2nd Ed. Philadelphia, W. B. Saunders Co., 1977.

Cope, Z.: The Early Diagnosis of the Acute Abdomen. 14th Ed. New York, Oxford University Press, 1972.

Fraser, G. M., and Fraser, I. D.: Gastrografin in perforated duodenal ulcer and acute pancreatitis. Clin. Radiol., 25:397, 1974.

Glenn, F.: Acute cholecystitis. Surg. Gynecol. Obstet., 143:56, 1976.

Griffen, W. O., Jr., Dilts, P. V., Jr., and Roddick, J. W., Jr.: Non-obstetric surgery during pregnancy. Curr. Probl. Surg., November, 1969.

Nadrowski, L. F.: Pathophysiology and current treatment of intestinal obstruction. Rev. Surg., 31:381, 1974.

Naylor, R., Coln, D., and Shires, G. T.: Morbidity, mortality and injuries of the spleen. J. Trauma, 14:773, 1974.

Spiro, H. M: Clinical Gastroenterology. 2nd Ed. New York, The Macmillan Co., 1977.

Warshaw, A. L., Imbembo, A. L., Ciretta, J. M., et al: Surgical intervention in acute necrotizing pancreatitis. Am. J. Surg., 127:484, 1974.

Upper Gastrointestinal Bleeding

Bauer, J. J., Kreel, I., and Kark, A. E.: The use of the Sengstaken-Blakemore tube for immediate control of bleeding esophageal varices. Ann. Surg., 179:293, 1974.

Crook, J. N., Gray, L. W., Jr., Nance, F. C., et al: Upper gastrointestinal bleeding. Ann. Surg., 175:771, 1972.

Finley, J. W., and Paulson, P. S.: Selective arteriography and infusion in diagnosis and treatment of acute gastrointestinal bleeding. Am. Surg., 39:448, 1973.

Franken, E. A., Jr.: Gastrointestinal bleeding in infants and children. Radiologic investigations. J.A.M.A., 229:1339, 1974.

Malt, R. A.: Control of massive upper gastrointestinal hemorrhage. N. Engl. J. Med., 286:1043, 1972.

Orloff, M. J., Chandler, J. G., Charter, A. C., III, et al: Emergency portacaval shunt treatment for bleeding esophageal varices. Prospective study in unselected patients with alcoholic cirrhosis. Arch. Surg., 108: 293, 1974.

Stanley, R. J., and Wise, L.: Arteriography in diagnosis of acute gastrointestinal tract bleeding. Arch. Surg., 107:138, 1973.

Welch, C. E., and Hedberg, S.: Gastrointestinal hemorrhage I. General considerations of diagnosis and therapy. Adv. Surg., 7:95, 1973.

Cholelithiasis

Colcock, B. P., Killen, R. B., and Leach, N. G.: The asymptomatic patient with gallstones. Am. J. Surg., 113:44, 1967.

Colcock, B. P., and McManas, J. R.: Experience with 1,356 cases of cholecystitis and cholelithiasis. Surg. Gynecol. Obstet., 101:161, 1955.

Glenn, F., and McSherry, C. K.: Secondary abdominal operations for symptoms following operations upon the biliary tract. Ann. Surg., 157:979, 1965.

Isselbacher, K. J.: A medical treatment for gallstones? N. Engl. J. Med., 286:40, 1972.

Mundth, E. D., : Cholecystitis and diabetes mellitus. N. Engl. J. Med., 267:642, 1962.

Munster, A. M., and Brown, J. R.: Acalculous cholecystitis. Am. J. Surg., 113:730, 1967.

Small, D. M.: Gallstones. N. Engl. J. Med., 279:588, 1968.

Hernia

Bucy, R. S.: A comprehensive study of incarcerated and strangulated hernias. Am. Surg., 26:476, 1960.

Gaster, J.: Hernia: One Day Repair. Darien, Conn., Hafner Publishing Co., 1970.

Nyhus, L. M., and Harkins, H. N. (eds.): Hernia. Philadelphia, J. B. Lippincott Co., 1964.

Usher, F. C.: The repair of incisional and inguinal hernias. Surg. Gynecol. Obstet., 131:525, 1970.

White, J. J., Haller, J. A., Jr., and Dorst, J. P., Congenital inguinal hernia and inguinal herniography. Surg. Clin. North Am., 50:823, 1970.

Williams, J. S., and Hule, H. W.: The advisability of inguinal herniorrhaphy in the elderly. Surg. Gynecol. Obstet., 122:100, 1966.

Zimmerman, L. M., and Anson, B. J.: The Anatomy and Surgery of Hernia. 2nd. Ed. Baltimore, The Williams & Wilkins Co., 1967.

Vascular Disease

Baker, A. G., and Roberts, B.: Long-term survival following abdominal aortic aneurysmectomy. J.A.M.A., 212:455, 1970.

Baker, W. G.: Surgical Treatment of Peripheral Vascular Disease. New York, Blakiston Div., McGraw-Hill Book Co., 1962.

Cranley, J. J.: Vascular Surgery. Hagerstown, Md., Medical Dept., Harper & Row, Publishers, Inc., 1972.

Darling, R. C.,: Medical progress. Peripheral arterial surgery. N. Engl. J. Med., 280:141, 1969.

Drapanas, T., Hewitt, R. L., Weichert, R. F., III, et al: Civilian vascular injuries: A critical appraisal of three decades of management. Ann. Surg., 172:351, 1970.

Fairbairn, J. F., II, Juergens, J. L., and Spittell, J. A., Jr. (eds.): Allen-Barker-Hines Peripheral Vascular Diseases. 4th Ed. Philadelphia, W. B. Saunders Co., 1972.

Kakkar, W. V., Corrigan, T., Spindler, J., et al: Efficacy of low doses of heparin in prevention of deep-vein thrombosis after major surgery. Lancet, 2:101, 1972.

Linton, R. R.: Post-thrombotic ulceration of the lower extremity. Ann. Surg., 138:415, 1953.

Salzman, E. W., and Clagett, G. P.: Prevention of venous thromboembolism in surgical patients. N. Engl. J. Med., 290:93, 1974.

Shuck, J. M., Omer, G. E., Jr., and Lewis, C. E., Jr.: Arterial obstruction due to intimal disruption in extremity fractures. J. Trauma, 12:481, 1972.

Szilagyl, D. E., Smith, R. F., DeRusso, F. J., et al: Contribution of abdominal aneurysmectomy to prolongation of life. Ann. Surg., 164:678, 1966.

Diseases of the Breast

Anderson, W.: Boyd's Pathology for the Surgeon. 8th Ed. Philadelphia, W. B. Saunders Co., 1967.

Barnes, W. C.: Management of cystic disease of the breast. Am. J. Surg., 129:324, 1965.

Bonnadonna, G., Brusamolina, E., Valagusa, P., et al: Combination chemotherapy as an adjuvant treatment in operable breast cancer. N. Engl. J. Med., 294:405, 1976.

Fisher, B.: The surgical dilemma in the primary therapy of invasive breast cancer. Curr. Probl. Surg., Oct., 1970.

Fisher, B., Fisher E. R., and Gregario, R. M.: Pathology of invasive breast cancer: Syllabus derived from findings of the National Surgical Adjuvant Breast Project. Cancer, 36:1, 1975.

Haagensen, C. D.: Diseases of the Breast. 2nd Ed. Philadelphia, W. B. Saunders Co., 1971.

Handley, R. S.: Benign breast diseases: surgical aspects. Proc. R. Soc. Med., 62:722, 1969.

Rosemond, G. P., Maier, W. P., and Brobyn, T. J.: Needle aspiration of breast cysts. Surg. Gynecol. Obstet., 128:351, 1969.

Spratt, J. S., Jr., and Donegan, W. L.: Cancer of the Breast. Philadelphia, W. B. Saunders Co., 1967.

Minor Office Surgery

Clark, W. H., Jr., Schoenfeld, R. J., and Walton, R. G.: Skin cancer—Spotting changes that signal melanoma. Patient Care, Aug. 1, 1974.

Conway, H.: Tumors of the Skin. Springfield, Ill., Charles C Thomas, Publisher, 1956.

Davis, N. C., McLeod, G. R., Beardmore, G. L., et al: Primary cutaneous melanoma: A report from the Queensland Melanoma Project. CA, 26:80, 1976.

Mihm, M. C., Fitzpatrick, T. B., Lane Brown, M. M., et al: Early detection of primary cutaneous malignant melanoma. A color atlas. N. Engl. J. Med., 289:989, 1973.

Rickles, J. A.: Ambulatory surgical management of pilonidal sinus. Am. Surg., 40:237, 1974.

Sanders, B. B., Jr., and Stretcher, G. S.: Warts. Diagnosis and treatment. J.A.M.A., 235:2859, 1976.

Wolcott, M. W.: Ferguson's Surgery of the ambulatory Patient. Philadelphia, J. B. Lippincott Co., 1974.

Trauma

Ballinger, W. F., II, Rutherford, R. B., and Zuidema, G. D. (eds.): The Management of Trauma. Philadelphia, W. B. Saunders Co., 1973.

Beall, A. C., Patrick, T. A., Okies, J. E., et al:

Penetrating wounds of the heart: Changing patterns of surgical management. J. Trauma, *12*:468, 1972.

Blair, E., Topuzlu, C., and Deane, R. S.: Major blunt chest trauma. *In* Ravitch, M. M. (ed.): Current Problems in Surgery. Chicago, Year Book Medical Publishers, 1969.

Freeark, R. J.: Penetrating wounds of the abdomen. N. Engl. J. Med., *291*:185, 1974.

Parvin, S., Smith, D. E., Asher, W. M., et al: Effectiveness of peritoneal lavage in blunt abdominal trauma. Ann. Surg., *18*:255, 1974.

Shires, G. T., and Jones, R. C.: Initial management of the severely injured patient. J.A.M.A., *213*:1872, 1970.

Walt, A. J., and Wilson, R. F.: Management of Trauma: Pitfalls and Practice. Philadelphia, Lea & Febiger, 1975.

Resuscitation

Ad Hoc Committee on Cardiopulmonary Resuscitation of the Division of Medical Sciences, National Academy of Sciences — National Research Council: Cardiopulmonary resuscitation. J.A.M.A., *194*:373, 1966.

Heimlich, H. J.: A life-saving maneuver to prevent food choking. J.A.M.A., *234*:398, 1975.

Newman, M. M.: Tracheostomy. Surg. Clin. North Am. *49*:1365, 1969.

Northfield, T. C., and Smith, T.: Physiologic significance of central venous pressure in patients with hemorrhage. Surg. Gynecol. Obstet., *135*:267, 1972.

Safar, P.: Recognition and management of airway obstruction. J.A.M.A., *209*:1722, 1969.

Zoll, P. M.: Rational use of drugs for cardiac arrest and after cardiac resuscitation. Am. J. Cardiol., *27*:645, 1971.

Wound Healing and Infection

Alexander, J. W.: Emerging concepts in control of surgical infections. Surgery, 75:934, 1974.

Altemeier, W. A., Burke, J. F., Pruitt, B. A., Jr., et al (ed. subcommittee): Manual on Control of Infection in Surgical Patients. American College of Surgeons. Philadelphia, J. B. Lippincott Co., 1976.

Bane, A. E.: The treatment of septic shock: A problem intensified by advancing science. Surgery, *65*:850, 1969.

Bartlett, R. H., Galzaniga, A. B., and Geraghty, T. R.: Respiratory maneuvers to prevent post-operative pulmonary complications. J.A.M.A., *224*:1017, 1973.

Douglas, D. M.: Wound Healing and Management: A Monograph for Surgeons. Baltimore, The Williams & Wilkins Co., 1963.

Peacock, E. E., and Van Winkle, W.: Surgery and Biology of Wound Repair. 2nd ed. Philadelphia, W. B. Saunders Co., 1976.

Polk, H. C., Fry, D., and Flint, L. M.: Dissemination and causes of infection. Surg. Clin. North Am., *56*:817, 1976.

Ryan, G. B.: Inflammation and localization of infection. Surg. Clin. North Am., *56*:831, 1976.

Siegel, M. E., Giargiana, F. A., Jr., Rhodes, B. A., et al: Perfusion of ischemic ulcers of the extremity: A prognostic indicator of healing. Arch. Surg., *110*:265, 1975.

Thermal Burns

Artz, C. P.: Burns updated. J. Trauma, *16*:3, 1976.

Ayvazian, V. H., and Monafo, W. W.: Initial management of the burned patient. Emerg. Med. Svcs., 5:6, 1976.

Ballin, J. C.: Evaluation of a new topical agent for burn therapy, silver sulfadiazine (Silvadene). J.A.M.A., *230*:1184, 1974.

Moncrief, J. A.: Burns. N. Engl. J. Med., *288*:444, 1973.

Polk, H. C., Jr., and Stone, H. H.: Contemporary Burn Management. Boston, Little, Brown, & Co., 1971.

Pruitt, B. A., and Curreri, S.: The burn wound and its care. Arch. Surg., *103*:461, 1971.

Chapter 38

ORTHOPEDICS

by WILLIAM J. MITCHELL

The advice "Study principles rather than methods—the mind that grasps principles will devise its own methods" succinctly summarizes the approach that will be followed throughout this manual in dealing with problems of the musculoskeletal system.

Toward that end, only that type of information that can be put to concrete use by the family physician is included. Brevity is intentional. This basic material is programmed to be of immediate assistance to the physician who has not studied in depth in the field of orthopedics. Sufficient coverage of each orthopedic topic is presented in a manner designed to provide recognition of problems that can be adequately treated by the nonspecialist.

Although good history taking is essential, emphasis is placed on the comprehensive physical examination. This approach requires the examining physician to *look at, feel,* and *move about* the affected part. Careful palpation of the entire area of difficulty is necessary, so that the exact location of the tender or pain-originating area is identified.

Use of this "anatomic" approach reduces the number of differential diagnostic possibilities. Thus, by narrowing the area of concern during physical examination, only a few basic disease processes have to be considered. A comprehensive review of anatomy is not necessary, but a few simple diagrammatic anatomic pamphlets at hand will be helpful.

As an example of this approach, if the knee were being examined, the physician would first palpate the skin overlying the area of pain to determine whether the pain arose from this tissue or at a deeper level. Next, the examiner would penetrate to deeper layers, such as to the level of the patella and the neighboring soft tissues. Following this, he would carefully feel structures such as the medial or lateral ligaments and other tissues at this level. Finally, the physician would palpate the innermost aspects of the knee at the level of the knee cartilages, and the margins of the femur and tibia themselves (Fig. 38–1). This is what is meant by exact site identification and localization of the pain source. If, for example, the pain arose exclusively from the patella, the physician would then be concerned mainly with lesions that affect this bone rather than with diseases that affect the other components of the knee.

With this in mind, the text presents only the more common pain-producing lesions that the family physician would expect to encounter in his office. If he comes across something that cannot be reconciled with the material in the text, then he is encountering some type of problem that will require either much more in-depth study on his part or, more appropriately, a referral to a specialist.

One final note: for a musculoskeletal examination the patient must be suitably undressed. If the knee or ankle is to be exposed, the opposite one must be exposed as well, so that the two may be compared.

GROWING PAINS

Physicians who provide care for children are frequently asked by parents about "growing pains." Most physicians have learned that children really do not have "growing pains" as such. Pains so described are more often the first symptoms of serious orthopedic disease. Much less commonly

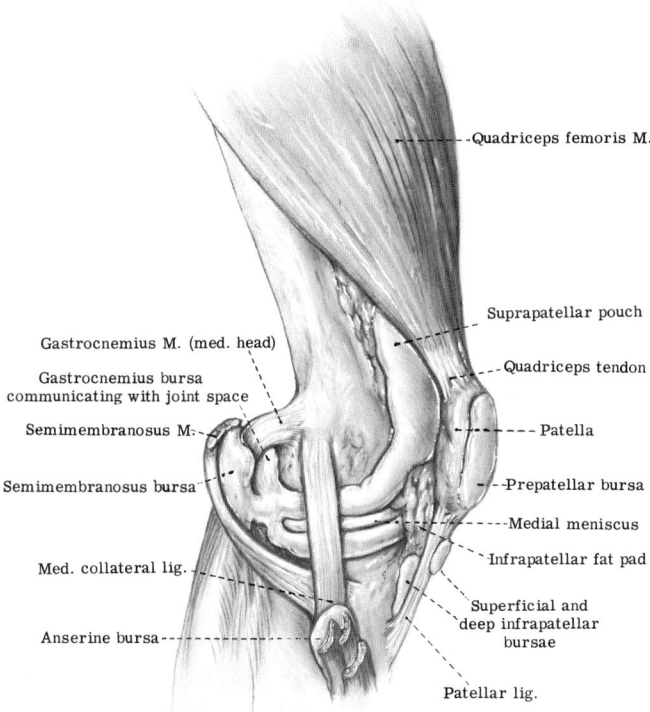

Quadriceps femoris M.

Suprapatellar pouch

Gastrocnemius M. (med. head)

Gastrocnemius bursa
communicating with joint space

Quadriceps tendon

Semimembranosus M.

Patella

Semimembranosus bursa

Prepatellar bursa

Medial meniscus

Infrapatellar fat pad

Med. collateral lig.

Superficial and
deep infrapatellar
bursae

Anserine bursa

Patellar lig.

Figure 38–1. Medial aspect of the knee. (From Beetham, W.P., Polley, H. F., Slocumb, C.H., et al.: Physical Examination of the Joints. Philadelphia, W. B. Saunders Co., 1965, p. 145.)

do these complaints arise from simple fatigue.

Examination of the child who is experiencing so-called growing pains should be considered incomplete without a roentgenogram of the part involved. In spite of a very thorough physical examination, this type of diagnosis is elusive, and the child is frequently labeled "neurotic" by the parents or teachers because a physician states he can find nothing wrong.

A typical history is presented by a 15 year old girl. Her mother stated that at age 10 the child experienced considerable pain in the right knee and began walking with a limp. She consulted a physician who examined the knee but who did not take a roentgenogram. She was told that her daughter had growing pains and that the problem would soon resolve itself.

The daughter continued to limp for at least another year or two, but the mother was fortified with the original diagnosis of "growing pains" and did nothing. When the girl was about 13, the mother took her to another physician who examined the knee, confirmed that it was abnormal, but stated that growing pains could produce these changes. Again, no roentgenograms were taken.

The mother was almost apologetic when

she again brought the child to another orthopedist. The examining physician found that the knee *lacked at least 25 degrees of complete extension.* There was evidence of muscle wasting as well. X-rays showed a radiolucent defect in the right medial femoral condyle. A tiny fragment of bone was seen within the defect. The diagnosis of *osteochondritis dissecans* was easily established by roentgenogram (Fig. 38–2).

Osteochondritis dissecans is not a very common lesion, but it is detectable by radiographic examination. Basically, this disease is a type of epiphyseal ischemic necrosis in which only a peripheral segment of the bone epiphysis is involved. It causes mild to severe pain in the affected joint. There is usually some limitation of motion and disuse atrophy. The treatment varies from casting to surgery. The pain and disability persist until satisfactory treatment is rendered.

In the case of this young girl, it was too late to restore a normal knee. *She was left with a permanent limp because an x-ray examination had not been made.*

In any type of joint complaint in children, roentgenograms must be taken since physical findings are often minimal.

A similar situation deserves attention in

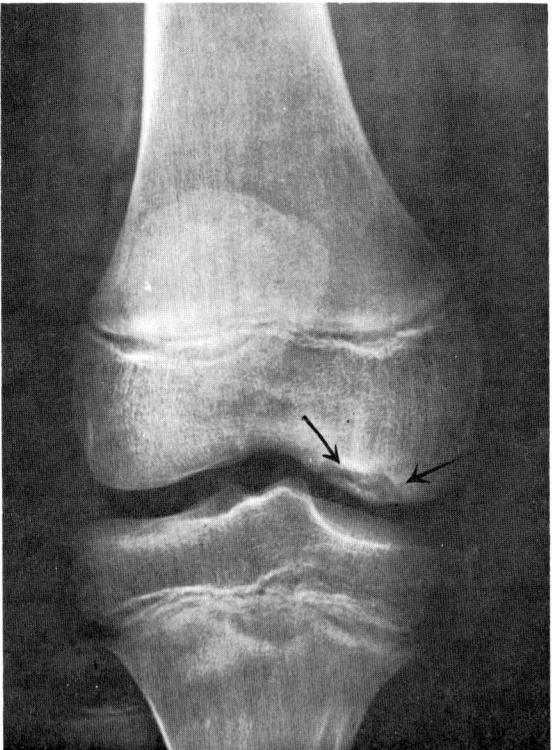

Figure 38-2. Osteochondritis of the medial femoral condyle. Arrows point to edge of radiolucent zone which contains tiny fragment of bone. (From Gartland, J.J.: Fundamentals of Orthopaedics. 1st Ed. Philadelphia, W. B. Saunders Co., 1965, p. 295.)

patients between the ages of 8 and 15. Complaints of pain and tenderness on the medial side of the foot may bring the patient to the office. The examining physician can usually find no specific anomaly. The area may be tender when pressure is applied. Quite often, this is described as "growing pains," and the child has to suffer for a varying period of time until the lesion heals itself.

If a radiologic examination is made of the foot, a typical change of increased density in the tarsal navicular bone with areas of rarefaction will be found, to which the descriptive term fragmentation is given. The bone appears narrower than normal when compared with that of the opposite foot. This is an osteochondritic process involving the navicular bone (Fig. 38-3).

With this painful condition, children do not wish to participate in physical activities. They are labeled "crocks" by their parents or teachers because the examining physician fails to take an x-ray and on the basis of physical findings alone calls the condition "growing pains."

Another typical history of a chubby 11 year old boy is illustrative. Six weeks after starting a paper route, he began complain-

ing of knee pain. His parents took him to a physician who examined the knee. They were told that it was a mild sprain. The child's symptoms persisted. Finally, he had to ride in the family car to deliver newspapers because of the pain.

His parents felt that he was lazy and that his obesity was causing the knee strain. A brief examination of the leg established that there was some restriction of hip motion and roentgenograms of the hip showed upward displacement of the shaft and neck of the femur with angulation and slipping of the head. The diagnosis of *slipped capital femoral epiphysis* was obvious, and the patient was immediately hospitalized for surgery.

In this condition, a high percentage of complaints are first of knee pain, and a hip limp subsequently develops. Children with the problem suffer needless torment when the physician fails to request a radiologic examination of the knee and hip. Classification of such problems as "growing pains" does a disservice to the patient and to his parents as well.

In that small group of children who show no physical abnormality, who also have normal roentgenograms of the areas in-

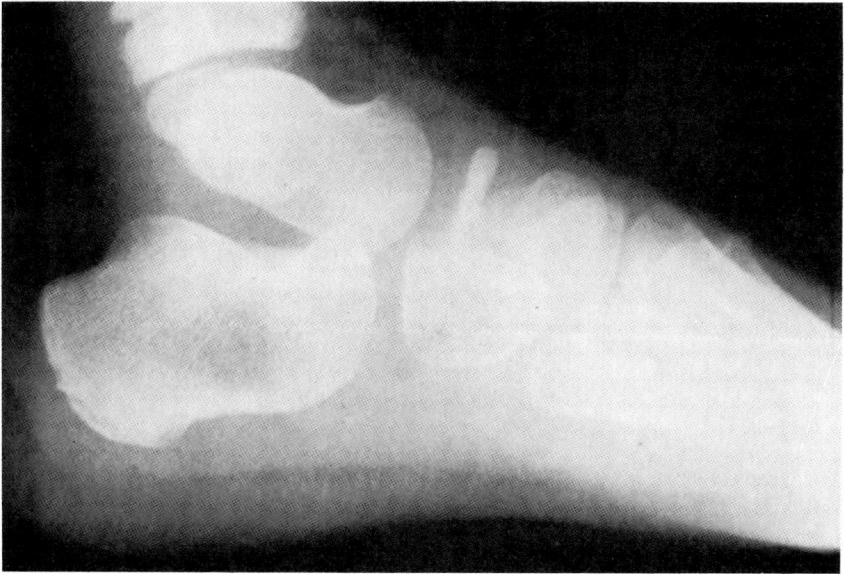

Figure 38–3.   *Osteochondritis of the tarsal navicular bone. (From Ferguson, A. B.: Orthopaedic Surgery in Infancy and Childhood. 3rd Ed. Baltimore, The Williams & Wilkins Co., © 1968, p. 81.)*

volved, and who thus have no demonstrable cause for their pain, the only treatment indicated is extra rest. Children, because of their extreme activity, develop fatigue, and this is often a cause of fleeting pain. Fatigue is an acceptable diagnosis only after all else has been ruled out.

FOOT AND ANKLE DISORDERS (NONTRAUMATIC)

Some background information will be helpful at this point before proceeding with clinical details. The average foot posture in a standing position is one of out-toeing about 15 degrees. Inasmuch as the talus is

rigidly held in the ankle mortise, the direction of the long axis of the normal foot is determined by the rotation of the femur at the hip. Thus, out-toeing means some degree of external rotation and in-toeing some degree of internal rotation at the hip joint. The position of the patella can be taken as an indicator of the limb rotation.

Weight is supported in the foot by the heel (os calcis), the two sesamoids under the first metatarsal, and the head of the two lateral (fourth and fifth) metatarsals in tripod fashion (Fig. 38–4). When shoes are worn, the proportion of weight borne by the forefoot (metatarsal area) increases as the level of the heel is raised.

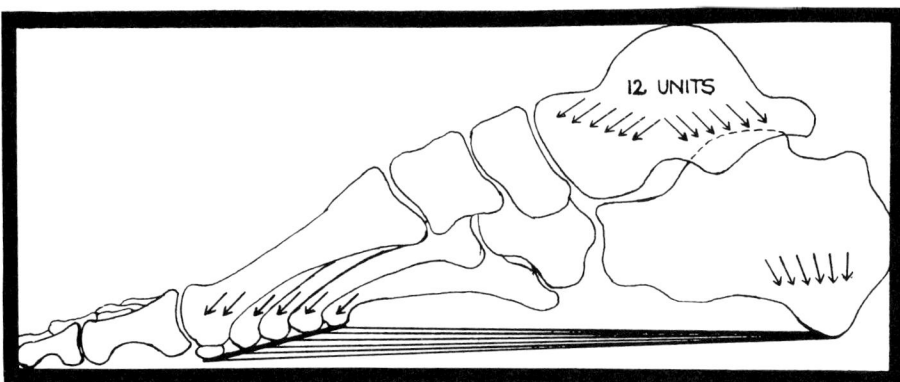

Figure 38–4.   *Modern concept of weight distribution. (From Kelikian, A. B.: Hallux Valgus, Allied Deformities of the Forefoot and Metatarsalgia. Philadelphia, W. B. Saunders Co., 1965, p. 23.)*

Flat Feet (Adult)

The concept that an adult foot with a low arch needs some type of treatment must be rejected. It lends confusion to the diagnosis and management of real foot disorders. The low arch is compatible with normal foot function. Only when symptoms arise or when there is loss of function associated with the low arch are diagnosis and treatment required.

Acute foot strain may be superimposed on a low arch. (Strain and sprain are used interchangeably throughout this chapter. There are some technical points of difference noted by the pathologist, but there is no real value in making this differentiation in clinical practice.) This type of strain can follow unaccustomed standing on concrete floors, unusual walking habits of recent origin, or the excessive carrying of heavy weights. Likewise, prolonged bed rest followed by excessive ambulation can be incriminated. In all these conditions, however, the fault does not lie with the low arch.

Physical examination discloses only a foot with a low arch. The examiner will not be able to localize a specific area of tenderness. The foot is diffusely tender.

X-rays should be made only to eliminate the possibility of some unsuspected disease. Standing anteroposterior, standing posteroanterior, and lateral views are requested.

Diagnosis of acute foot strain rests on a positive history of precipitating factors as well as a negative radiologic examination. The presence or absence of a flat foot (low arch) should be disregarded.

Treatment must be directed to the cause—reduction of weight, rest periods when standing on concrete, avoidance of carrying heavy loads, and so forth. Feet will recuperate more quickly if a program of whirlpool treatment for 4 to 5 days is coupled with a physical-therapy-directed exercise for the anterior tibial muscle group.

The prescription sent to the therapist should specify anterior tibial (muscle-setting routine) exercises for the involved foot. The patient should continue this program at home for several weeks. Unless the precipitating factors are eliminated, however, the benefits of therapy will be short-lived. Orthopedic shoes and appliances directed toward the flat foot are not indicated for adults with this problem.

Flat Feet (Child)

By age 2, most children lose the so-called fat pad from the undersurface of the mid-

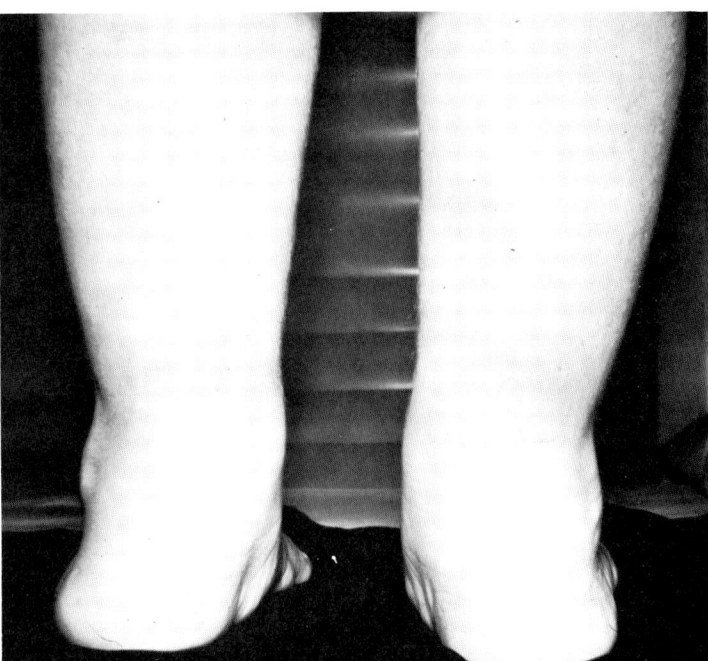

Figure 38–5. *Child with flat feet.* (From Gartland, J. J.: *Fundamentals of Orthopaedics.* 2nd Ed. Philadelphia, W. B. Saunders Co., 1974, p. 395.)

foot. Until its disappearance, this pad gives the foot the look of a flat foot. With the exception of that small group of individuals who later develop knock knees and associated low arches, only those who continue to show a low arch after age 2 should be regarded as having a true flat foot (Fig. 38–5). One should be aware that black children have a large fat pad in the arch area that tends to persist even after age 2. An observation of their instep in a standing position tends to indicate a flat foot. However, when the foot is raised and palpated, a well-formed arch is present.

Once the parent becomes aware of the flat foot, the child is usually taken to a store for special shoes. The majority of these children with flat feet do quite well even if not treated. However, from experience, one learns that the innocuous Thomas heel added to a pair of normal shoes by the shoe repairman is reassuring to the mother and other concerned members of the family. *No amount of explanation that treatment is not necessary will accomplish the same purpose.*

The parents should be given a prescription blank with the words "Thomas heels" on it. Any shoe repairman will be able to attach this to the shoe. The child should wear these shoes until about age 7. The physician should explain to the parents that this is a form of support and not a correction. Low arches cannot be corrected. There is a degree of pes planus, however, that deserves serious effort at support with a Thomas heel and a medial arch support, usually about ⅛ inch. This is the type in which the heel is in valgus, or displaced at least 10 degrees outward or greater from a direct line drawn down the Achilles tendon when the child is in a weight-bearing position.

On occasion, a 5 year old child will be brought to the office accompanied by a tearful mother who states that she buys the best shoes but her child will not wear them. The child indicates that the shoes hurt his feet. Examination of the shoes reveals a steel-arched shoe with rigid counters and other corrective elevations. These have been prescribed by a shoestore proprietor who specializes in orthopedic shoes. Experience has shown that this type of shoe does produce foot pain. Immediate cessation of using this type of shoe will relieve the pain

and solve the problem. When parents ask for recommendations, they should be told that the best shoes for growing children are not the hard-soled shoes advocated by shoe salesman, but rather tennis shoes or moccasins, which are more supple and permit a more normal gait pattern while providing good traction and foot protection.

If the family physician should ever see a patient with a pair of what he considers to be really disabling flat feet, he should not hesitate to request a specialist's opinion.

Foreleg, Ankle, and Foot Pain

Inflammation of the synovial-like tissue around the anterior tibial tendon, the posterior tibial tendon, the Achilles tendon, or other less commonly involved tendons resulting from overuse and only rarely from gout or rheumatoid involvement produces the particular syndrome of tenosynovitis.

The patient complains of pain over the area of the involved tendon on standing or walking. It is a constant pain and grows worse with time.

Physical examination elicits palpable crepitus over the path of the involved tendon, especially at any point where the tendon twists around bones or lies adjacent to bony surfaces. Palpation of the tendon with the index or middle finger while the foot is dorsiflexed and plantarflexed will elicit tenderness in the early stages of this condition. In advanced stages, the tendon and surrounding tissues have a watery feel beneath the skin's surface.

X-rays taken of patients with this condition are reported as normal.

Diagnosis rests on the physical findings just listed.

Treatment consists of the application of an icepack to the inflamed area for 24 hours. Rest from all activity is prescribed for 2 to 3 days. Recovery is speeded with the use of an anti-inflammatory medication such as prednisone, which is prescribed for 7 days only: 10 mg. is to be taken after meals 3 times a day during this period.

If ambulation is a must, a Medicopaste or Dome Paste Bandage is applied for 7 days to the foot, ankle, and foreleg. A 7 day course of anti-inflammatory medication is also given.

If there is no response to this program within 3 days, an injection of a corticoid solution (such as betamethasone acetate) is given into the tendon sheath at the site of maximal involvement. A description of the technique for intra-articular and intra-synovial injection can be found in reference 22 cited in the bibliography.

Ultrasonic therapy treatments prescribed for intervals of 3 days for a total of about 11 treatments and dispensed in the physical therapy department will also prove helpful. The treatment is prescribed as follows: 2.5 microwatts per cm.[2] for a 3 minute interval. This treatment may be substituted for the injection if so desired. Treatment response to ultrasound therapy is not as rapid as it is to injection.

Foot Pain (General)

Except for reference to the unsightly deformity found in women with bunions (hallux valgus), adults are rarely concerned with the appearance of their feet. They visit the physician's office only because of pain.

To help diagnose complaints of pain, the following descriptions will be based on the anatomic location of the complaint and listed in order of frequency of encounter in the average family practice situation.

Heel Pain (Adult). This complaint is common to adults between ages 55 and 70. On arising in the morning, the patient usually finds it unbearable to place weight on the foot. The real problem is a "myositis" of the plantar muscle group at its attachment to the os calcis. Recent stress, such as increased weight gain or excessive standing on concrete surfaces, precipitates the condition suddenly.

Physical findings consist of local tenderness over the undersurface of the heel — at the site of the calcaneal attachment of the plantar fascia. Deep pressure with the thumb or forefinger, especially over the medial side of the heel at this level, will produce exquisite pain.

X-rays are usually reported as negative. Occasionally, a plantar spur is described by the radiologist. This is rarely the pain-producing mechanism. Uric acid and blood glucose determinations should be requested for completeness of the work-up.

Treatment consists of a course of anti-inflammatory medication. Prednisone is prescribed in a dose of 10 mg. to be taken after meals 3 times a day for period of 7 days.

This can be combined with a course of ultrasonic therapy over the heel area given by the physical therapist. This is given every 3 days for a total of 11 treatments.

An alternative to this program is the injection of 1 cc. of betamethasone acetate into the site of maximal tenderness. A family physician can readily acquire expertise in this technique.[22]

Supportive devices, such as heel cups, cork heels, and so forth, are rarely helpful in this condition. Should these be used and relief not obtained, the patient is doubly upset because of the cost of the device as well as its failure.

Heel Cord Pain. Those presenting with this type of complaint — heel pain at the insertion of the Achilles tendon into the os calcis — are obese women with a history of swelling at this site that has been present for many years. The pain is aggravated by standing and walking, especially in a new pair of high-heeled shoes.

The rigid posterior counter touches this critical swollen area (there is a subcutaneous bursa located here) and produces sufficient friction so that each step re-aggravates the swelling and pain. Redness is only occasionally present.

Physical examination discloses a varying sized area of tender thickening at the level of the Achilles tendon insertion into the os calcis. The superficial skin is caloused and may be reddened.

X-rays are not readily required for diagnosis. It is wise to take one of the foot and ankle area, however, for the sake of completeness.

Treatment consists of sending a marked diagram to the shoe repairman so that he will cut an appropriate wedge out of the posterior counter of the offending shoes and sew a piece of soft leather in its place (Fig. 38–6).

Patients occasionally inquire about surgery rather than "bothersome" shoe repairs. The scar following such procedures, however, is often so located that it becomes irritated by the rigid shoe counter just as the previous bursa did, and a new pain syndrome is produced that is difficult to eliminate. Shoe alteration is the best form of treatment for this condition.

Heel Pain (Child). Children between the ages of 4 and 14 may complain of pain over the posterior aspect of the heel following a

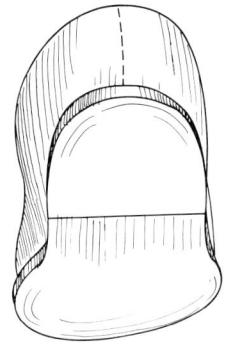

Before Posterior Heel Cut Out

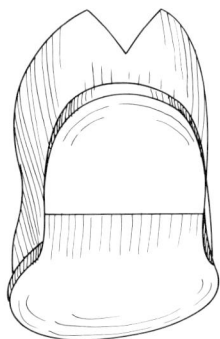

After Posterior Heel Cut Out

Figure 38-6. *Shoe with posterior counter cut out.*

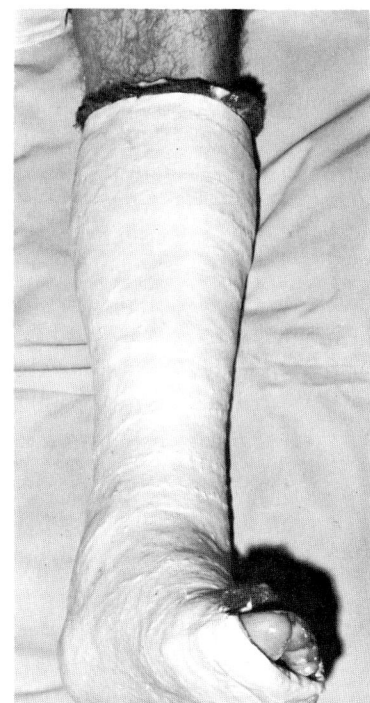

Figure 38-7. *Short leg cast. (From Gartland, J. J.: Fundamentals of Orthopaedics. 2nd Ed. Philadelphia, W. B. Saunders Co., 1974, p. 15.)*

strain or blow. The course of this painful condition is self-limiting, but usually spans 3 to 6 months.

Physical examination discloses marked tenderness over the posterior surface of the os calcis on palpation. Often, there is associated swelling.

X-rays disclose increased density of the epiphysis of the calcaneus, with some appearance of fragmentation *(osteochondritis).*

Diagnosis is made by the localized tenderness found on physical examination over the posterior surface of the os calcis and by the accompanying radiologic changes.

Treatment consists of the application of a below-knee walking cast for a period of 6 weeks, especially if the discomfort is severe (Fig. 38–7). If it is not, an overall heel lift of ³⁄₁₆ of an inch may be worn on the affected side to reduce the symptoms. Restriction of extracurricular activity is indicated until the pain disappears. X-ray changes may persist for 2 to 3 years.

Midfoot Pain. Adults rarely complain of foot pain unless there has been prior injury with subsequent arthritic change in the joints of the midfoot.

One most commonly encounters complaints of pain in this area in children between the ages of 5 and 12. The pain is usually due to an *osteochondritic process* involving the *navicular bone.*

Physical examination discloses marked pain and tenderness on the dorsum of the medial side of the midfoot area, specifically at the location of the navicular bone.

X-rays show typical changes of increased density with areas of what appear to be fragmentation confined to the navicular bone. This bone is definitely narrower than its opposite member, and this change persists for at least a year (Fig. 38–8). It must be remembered, however, that radiologic changes may not be apparent for many months after the onset of pain.

Diagnosis is made by finding localized pain and tenderness over the navicular bone in the 5 to 12 year old age group.

Treatment: Six weeks or more in a short-

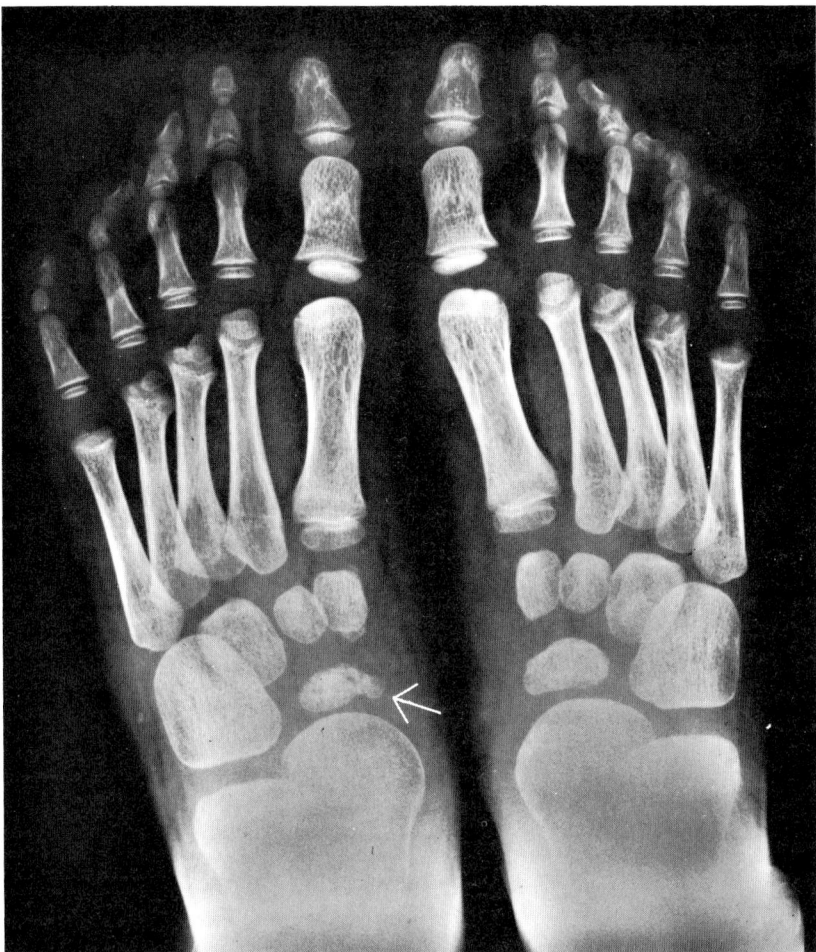

Figure 38-8. Roentgenogram of osteochondrosis of the tarsal navicular bone. (From Gartland, J. J.: Fundamentals of Orthopaedics. 1st Ed. Philadelphia, W. B. Saunders Co., 1965, p. 67.)

leg, walking plaster cast will relieve the symptoms, if severe. If symptoms are milder, restriction of extracurricular activity will prove satisfactory.

Special arch shoes or corrective shoes have no place in the treatment of this condition. The course of this disease is self-limiting and usually lasts for about 4 to 6 months.

Forefoot Pain (Adult). Pain arising from the level of the ball of the foot is most common in middle-aged female patients (*metatarsalgia*). It is thought that relaxation of the interosseous and lumbrical muscles occurs, producing a forefoot splay (flattening and widening of the transverse arch) with secondary dorsiflexion of the proximal phalanges of the four lateral toes. The second, third, and fourth metatarsal heads are depressed, and later the plantar skin underlying the heads of these bones becomes hypertrophied, calloused, and very painful (Fig. 38-9). High-heeled shoes aggravate the problem.

Patients complain of pain in the forefoot area initially localized to the area of the plantar callus but later radiating widely up the foot and leg.

Physical examination discloses a plantar callus extremely tender to the touch. This is located under the head of the second or third metatarsal bone. There is an associated splay-foot. In patients in whom this problem has existed for some time, dorsal subluxation of the proximal phalanges occurs at the metatarsophalangeal joint level. This involves the second, third, fourth, and fifth toes.

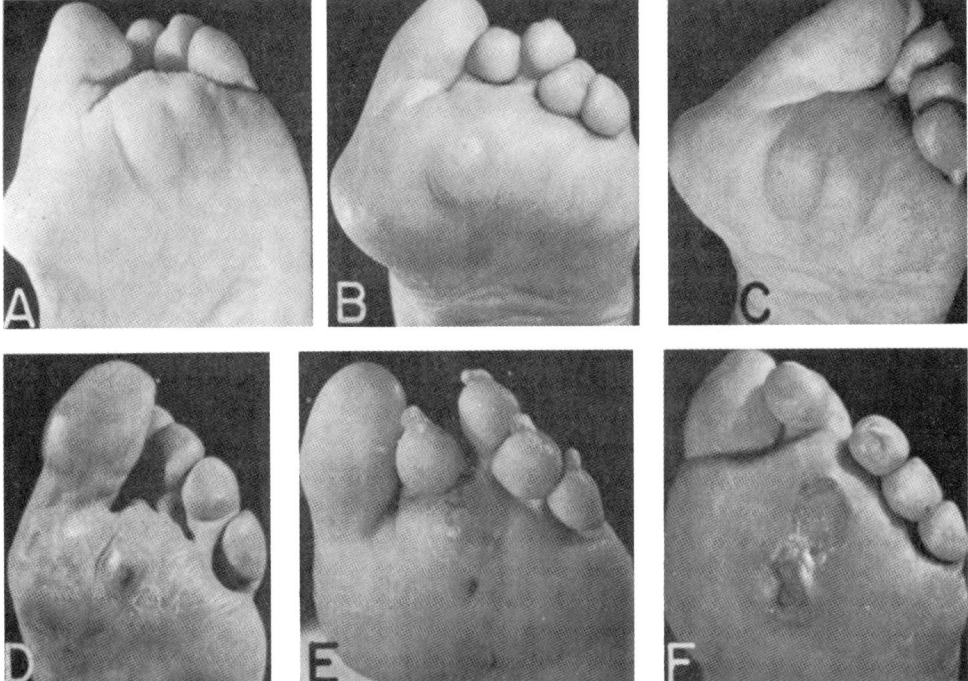

Figure 38–9. *Splayed forefeet seen from plantar aspect. Varying degrees of collapse and plantar callus development from simplest (A) to most advanced (F) with skin ulceration. (From Kelikian, A. B.: Hallux Valgus, Allied Deformities of the Forefoot and Metatarsalgia. Philadelphia, W. B. Saunders Co., 1965, p. 70.)*

X-rays should be routinely requested, but in this disorder they will not be diagnostic.

Treatment consists of the application of a metatarsal bar, usually ¼ inch in thickness, to the undersurface of both shoes (Fig. 38–10). A diagram is given to the patient to take to the shoe repairman, who will attach the bar to the pair of shoes that the patient wears throughout the day.

It is important that the bar be positioned behind the metatarsal heads to give "a lift." This bar should be worn for 1 month.

If during this time the patient notices continued improvement, he should be instructed to have the bar replaced on the shoes at monthly intervals. Additionally, hot footbaths are recommended at the end of each day for about 5 to 10 minutes.

Likewise, a series of foot intrinsic muscle exercises is prescribed by sending the patient to the physical therapist with the

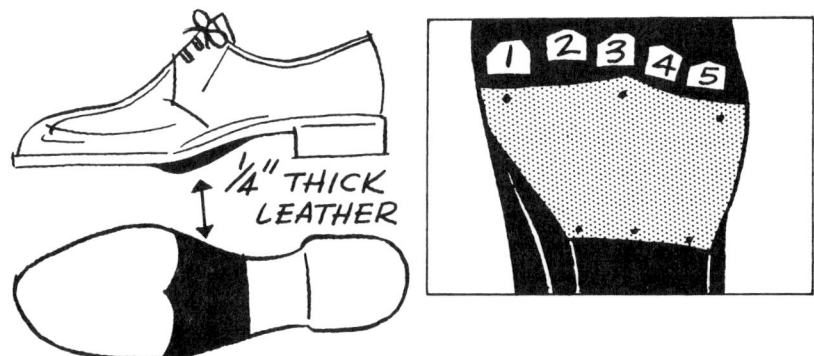

Figure 38–10. *Metatarsal bar. (From Ishmael, W. K.: Care of the Feet. Philadelphia, J. B. Lippincott Co., 1967, p. 13.)*

following directions: Instruct the patient in muscle-setting exercises for the gastrocnemius and soleus muscle group and the foot intrinsic group.

Occasionally, patients prefer special built-in metatarsal arches, which, if properly placed, will serve as well as the metatarsal bars. However, the placement of these is critical and should the patient be disappointed initially, he will usually abandon all treatment.

For the patient who does not respond to the metatarsal bar, referral can be made to any nearby special-shoe center that builds custom shoes. These shoes will be constructed to conform to the patient's individual foot characteristics and usually the only prescription necessary is to indicate that the patient needs a pair of custom-made shoes. The individual who offers this service is an expert and will install all corrections necessary without specific direction.

It is important that the physician emphasize to the patient that this is the final alternative for relief of foot pain. Use of the shoes at least during working hours will produce maximal improvement.

Lateral Forefoot Pain. The patient typically complains of sharp, spasmodic, burning pain radiating up adjacent sides of the third and fourth toes. The pain occurs first while walking and, later, while in bed at night. There may be some dull, throbbing pain in the adjacent metatarsal regions as well.

Frequently, there is difficulty in localizing the pain to one or the other toe. This pain often lacks objective confirmation and is at times so persistent that many patients have been referred to psychiatrists.

The source of this difficulty is a *neuroma* formed *on the digital nerve* just proximal to the head of the metatarsals. It is most frequently localized to the third-fourth interspace (Fig. 38–11). The friction and pressure between the metatarsal heads as the result of degenerative changes precipitate the onset of the pain. Careful questioning usually elicits a history of some type of trauma that antedates the onset of the symptoms for an indefinite period.

Physical findings are elicited by compressing the forefoot transversely in the palm of the examiner's hand so that the neuroma is caught between the two metatarsal heads. This maneuver causes pain to

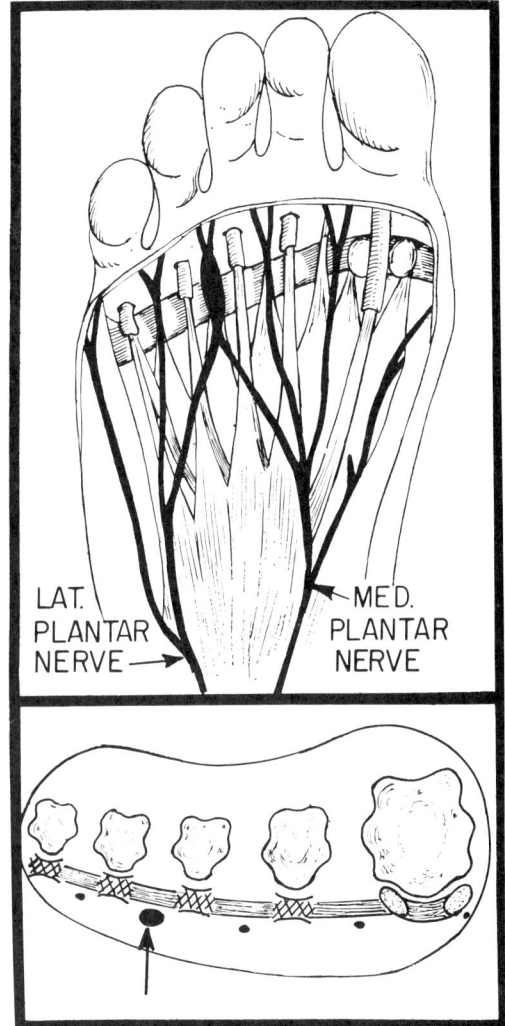

Figure 38–11. *Formation of neuroma by contributions from medial and lateral plantar nerves. (From Kelikian, A. B.: Hallux Valgus, Allied Deformities of the Forefoot and Metatarsalgia. Philadelphia, W. B. Saunders Co., 1965, p. 363.)*

shoot into the affected toes and often to the ankle.

X-ray films are not helpful.

Diagnosis is made by the typical physical findings and history. Further confirmation and often relief can be produced by infiltrating a local anesthetic agent such as 1 per cent procaine (5 cc.) into the third-fourth interspace level.

Treatment is afforded by an injection of 1 cc. of betamethasone acetate. The relief produced is not long-lasting. For more permanent benefit, a ¼ inch metatarsal bar should be used on the outside of the shoe for 1 month. If the patient accepts this and

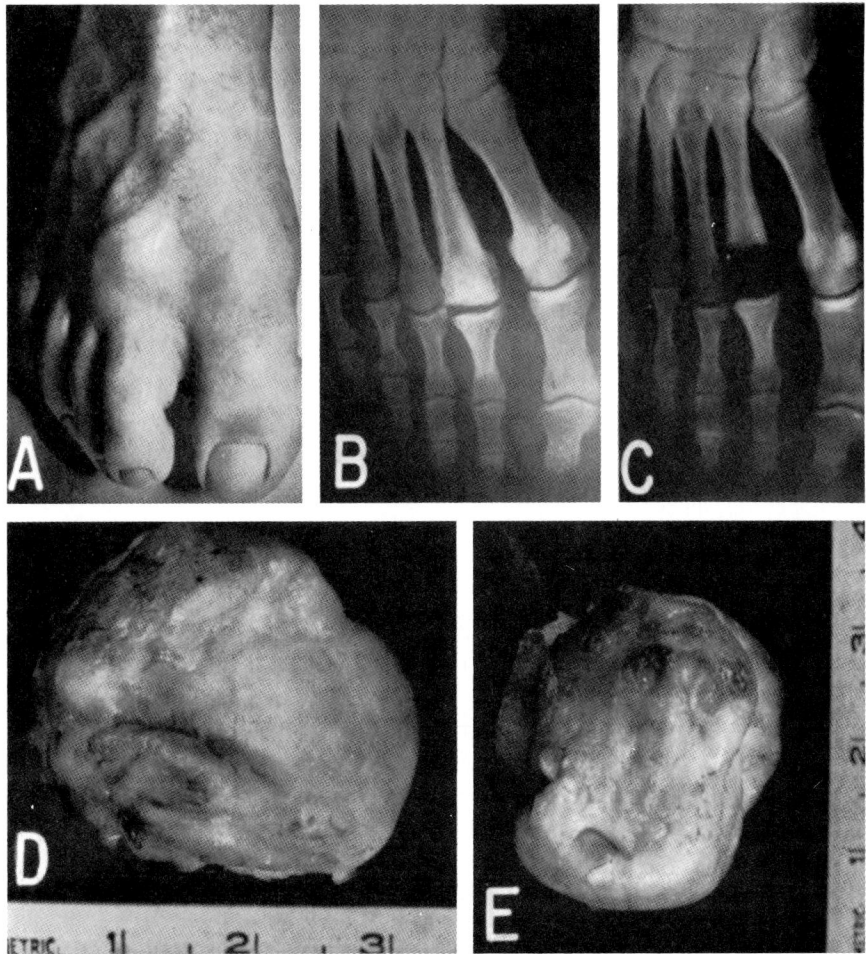

Figure 38–12. *Metatarsalgia of second metatarsal head. A. Clinical appearance. B, X-ray changes. C, Post-surgical. D and E, View of pathologic specimen. (From Kelikian, A. B.: Hallux Valgus, Allied Deformities of the Forefoot and Metatarsalgia. Philadelphia, W. B. Saunders Co., 1965, p. 376.)*

gains partial relief, a more exact-fitting metatarsal pad can be substituted on the inside of the shoe. Its placement is very important and should be done by an experienced shoe repairman. If one is not available, it would be wise to refer this patient elsewhere.

If symptoms do not improve within a reasonable period (3 months), referral for surgical excision of the neuroma is indicated. This is usually performed through a dorsal incision, and no special care is necessary postoperatively. Relief will be obtained by this method, but there is a permanent area of decreased sensation on the inner surface of the third and fourth toes.

Second Toe Pain—Metatarsophalangeal Joint. In late adolescence, the patient be-

comes aware of growing discomfort localized to the area of the metatarsophalangeal joint of the second toe.

Physical examination discloses marked tenderness on compression of the second metatarsophalangeal joint. Pain is produced in this joint by either active or passive plantar flexion of the toe.

X-ray changes show flattening of the head of the second metatarsal with narrowing and sometimes obliteration of the joint (Fig. 38–12).

Diagnosis of metatarsalgia is made by the suggestive physical findings. X-ray confirmation is necessary in order to rule out the possibility of a slow-healing sprain.

Treatment consists of the use of a metatarsal bar for at least 1 month. If this fails to provide relief, the injection of 0.5 cc. (3 mg.)

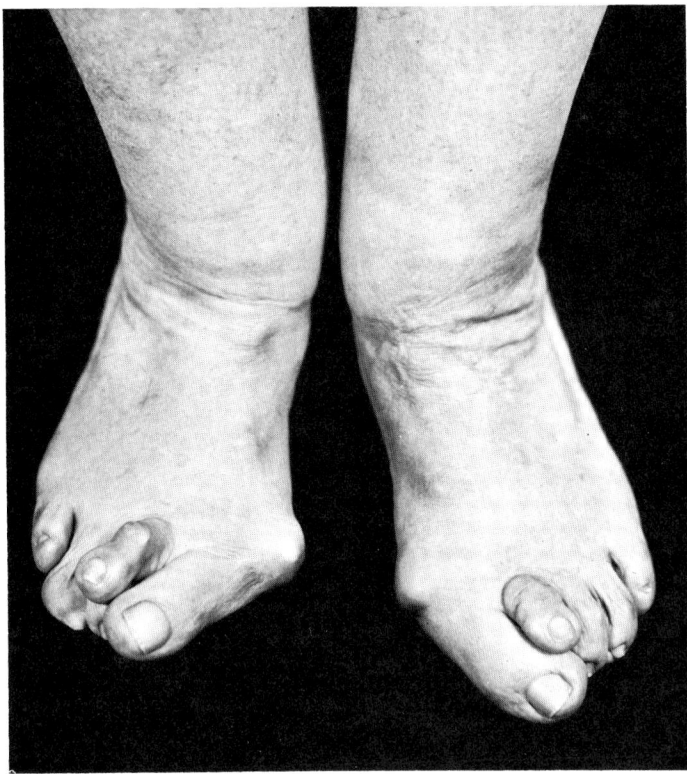

Figure 38-13. Bilateral hallux valgus with subluxation of second toes.

of betamethasone acetate into the joint will often produce marked improvement. If neither of the these treatments is successful, referral to a specialist is indicated, since this particular condition may require surgery for ultimate relief.

Great Toe Pain. Hallux valgus may be difficult for the family physician to treat. It is the most frequent source of pain in the great toe, and it requires surgery when the pain reaches a significant level (Fig. 38-13). Some help is obtained by wearing widened shoes. These are not stylish and are rejected outright by most women.

Uric acid tests as well as determination of blood glucose levels should be done to rule out the possibility of either gout or diabetes mellitus. If the laboratory studies are normal, the patient should be referred to a specialist for appropriate surgery.

Also listed as disorders that will require surgery for their correction are the following: clawtoes, hammertoes, mallet toes, bunionette, and overlapping of the fifth and fourth toes. Popularly advertised gadgets do not really work. If the patient is serious in

desiring cosmetic improvement or relief of local pain due to these conditions, he should be referred for surgery.

Ingrown Toenail. Most often, the great toe is involved but occasionally other toes may be affected. The cause of this disorder is improper paring of the corners of the nails. The nail, with subsequent growth, then becomes too wide for the space, and ulceration occurs with cutting of the flesh by the sharp corner of the nail. Infection usually ensues followed by sharp pain.

Physical examination reveals a granulomatous mass of tissue with reddening and evident infection. This mass projects over one end of the nail.

X-rays should be taken to rule out underlying infection of the distal phalanx.

Treatment consists of hot soaks, usually in moderately warm water, for about 5 to 10 minutes 3 times a day. Antibiotics are indicated if there appears to be a spreading infection.

When the acute episode is under control, the offending half of the nail can be incised by anesthetizing the toe with a local anes-

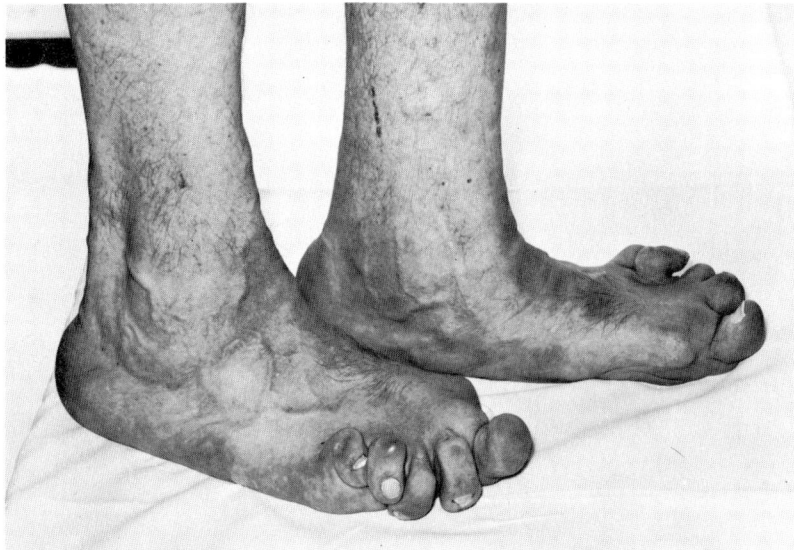

Figure 38-14. *Broken-down feet. (From Beetham, W. P., Polley, H. F., Slocumb, C. H., et al.: Physical Examination of the Joints. Philadelphia, W. B. Saunders Co., 1965, p. 182.)*

thetic such as 1 per cent procaine. Three cc. of this material injected into either side of the toe produces satisfactory anesthesia.

Following removal of the nail, a bacitracin type of ointment is applied in a small amount daily until normal healing occurs. The patient is then instructed in correct nail care. In recurrent cases, it may be necessary to excise the nail and its bed as well. Consult reference 9 in the bibliography for further detailed information.

Broken-Down Foot Pain. Patients who have severe rheumatoid arthritis or who undergo crushing injuries to the foot or who have combinations of diseases such as diabetes and arthritis will often be left with a severely deformed foot and generalized foot pain (Fig. 38–14). The diagnosis is usually obvious at first inspection, and the history indicates that the condition has been present for many years.

Treatment consists of emphasizing to the patient that no one specific medication or operation or treatment modality will produce the relief he seeks. It must be explained in detail that only a shoe that compensates for all of the multiple incongruities will produce any type of weight-bearing relief. When the patient accepts this, he should be referred to a special-shoe center or to the individual in the area who will make appropriate molds of the feet and custom-build shoes to the necessary specifications. Many patients reject this suggestion, but it is the only realistic approach to the problem.

Foot and Ankle Sprain

The ankle sprain is probably the most common athletic injury. It will be described in detail and everything that is said about it applies in a general way to foot sprains, which are treated in the same manner.

The ankle is a hinge joint permitting only dorsal and plantar flexion. Injuries are due to lateral stresses that force the ankle through a range of motion that it does not normally possess. Ligaments surrounding the ankle that are injured as a result of overstress are called "sprained ligaments." Should the force be sufficient to cause one of the attachments of the ligament to give way and pull loose with a fragment of bone, it is then classified as a type of fracture and requires treatment entirely different from that for the more common sprain.

Physical examination of the sprained ankle indicates restricted motion because of pain or edema, and occasionally there is surrounding soft tissue hemorrhage. Careful palpation will disclose one or more areas of localized tenderness in the region of the ankle ligamentous apparatus.

Diagnosis of a sprain is made by the presence of a negative radiologic examination of the ankle area and localized tenderness over the ligaments.

Treatment consists of the immediate application of icepacks to reduce further swelling.

The next step, whether or not ice has been used, is the application of a Medicopaste or Dome Paste Bandage. This is wrapped slightly loose in a contoured figure-of-eight manner to include the foot and ankle. An Ace elastic bandage is then applied over this, and the patient is given a pair of crutches. He is advised to remain off the ankle for 24 hours. He may be given aspirin or propoxyphene hydrochloride for the soreness.

Following this initial 24 hour period, the patient is advised to remove the Ace bandage, since the paste bandage will then be dry. He may put on his stocking and shoe. If there is still too much swelling, a stocking and slipper can be used.

The patient is instructed to begin walking with a normal gait, using the crutches initially and then discarding them as he gains confidence. He is advised to resume his normal ambulatory pattern within the limits of pain during the next few days.

This patient should be re-examined approximately 9 days after the initial sprain. The paste bandage can be removed by soaking it in hot water for $1/2$ hour and then cutting it with a pair of scissors. The patient could do this at home the night before his examination.

Should there be any significant residuals of edema or pain remaining, a new paste bandage is applied and worn for another 9 day period. Only about 10 per cent of the persons so treated will require a second paste bandage. The final test, applying moderate stress as the ankle is moved passively through a range of motion by the examiner, should indicate freedom from pain and laxity. The paste bandage is preferred to plaster because it eliminates the stiffness frequently associated with plaster casts and does not necessitate further rehabilitation following its removal.

Weak Ankles

Patients (more commonly athletes) complain of insecurity, weakness, and giving-way of the ankle joint. On uneven surfaces, a sudden twist may actually throw the patient to the ground.

Physical examination shows no abnormality.

Routine radiographic examination likewise shows no abnormality.

Treatment consists of the development of strong quadriceps, hamstring, and gastroc-nemius muscle groups through a progressive resistance-exercise program.

This would include muscle contraction against a static object, movement against spring resistance, movement against forceful resistance of another person, or movement against weight-loading resistance.

This type of rehabilitation program should be discussed with the physical therapist so that he is cognizant of the goal.

Taping the ankle or foot will not prevent injuries to the ankle or foot. Actually, because taping restricts inversion and eversion of the subtalar joint, it may produce harm. This joint often acts as a safety valve in twisting injuries.

Athletes in high school and college who cannot participate in sports without a brace of some sort because of a weak joint should be denied the right to play by the family physician until the joint is repaired. Taping may have some psychological value, but the physician's emphasis should be on building a strong muscle that can protect the joint rather than on any type of support.

KNEE DISORDERS

Diagnosis of knee problems is facilitated by considering the most prominent physical features first. Examination is always begun with the patient lying flat on the examination table with both lower extremities exposed to hip level.

Locked Knee (Adult)

Most normal knees lie completely flat against the table. With the locked knee, the examiner will be able to place his hand between the posterior aspect of the knee and the examination table. The locked knee lacks the last 15 or less degrees of motion that would permit it to lie flat against the table in complete extension (Fig. 38–15).

The locked knee is usually the result of a torn cartilage that is sufficiently displaced to prevent the femur and tibia from reaching their normal positions of complete extension. Only rarely does a loose body, such as an osteophyte, initiate this locking mechanism.

A glance at an anatomic picture of the

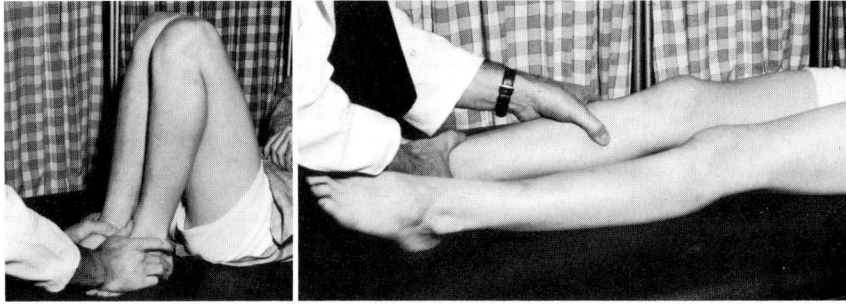

Figure 38–15. *Locked knee flexes fully, but lacks full extension. (Reproduced from A System of Orthopaedics and Fractures, 3rd Ed. by A. Graham Apley, published by Butterworths, London.)*

knee illustrates that the medial semilunar cartilage is C-shaped and the lateral cartilage is almost circular. The difference is that the medial cartilage has a peripheral attachment to the adjacent collateral ligament and is less mobile than the lateral cartilage. As a result of the lateral cartilage's greater mobility, it is 10 times less likely to be torn than the medial one.

When examining a young patient, the physician should consider disorders of the knee cartilage. Middle-aged and elderly patients must also be thought of in this category. The knee bears the body's weight and because it does so, it is vulnerable to the stress of obesity and to the degeneration of aging.

In eliciting the history, the physician must remember that acute cartilage tears usually occur when the knee suddenly twists inward while the outward-turned foot remains firmly planted on the ground. In the young, this happens during athletic activities such as football and skiing. In the middle-aged or older patients, such simple activities as gardening done in the kneeling position can cause cartilage derangement with change of position. This is because elderly, overweight patients already have knee cartilages that are somewhat degenerated.

Physical examination indicates that the involved knee will not lie flat against the examining table. The inability of the knee to reach normal extension may range from as little as 5 degrees to as much as 45 degrees. There may or may not be effusion. The torn cartilage, whether it be medial or lateral, produces pain only at the joint line.

To locate the joint, find the depression just below the lower borders of the patella and above the flare of the medial tibial surface. Move the fingers, usually the index and third fingers, slowly from anterior to posterior along this line (Fig. 38–16).

A significant degree of pressure is applied. The patient will then inform the examiner of the site of maximum pain on palpation. This gives a clue as to whether

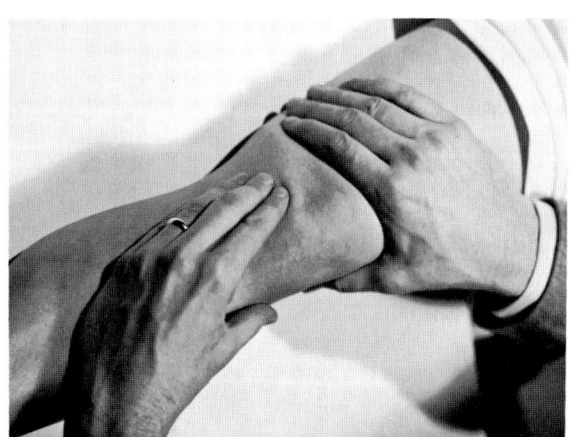

Figure 38–16. *Palpation of medial aspect of joint space of left knee with left index finger. (From Beetham, W. P., Polley, H. F., Slocumb, C. H., et al.: Physical Examination of the Joints. Philadelphia, W. B. Saunders Co., 1965, p. 158.)*

the cartilage is detached anteriorly or along its middle third or its posterior component. If the medial side of the knee is examined first, the lateral side is examined next. The findings of lack of complete extension with pain located at the level of the semilunar cartilage are sufficient to confirm the diagnosis of a locked knee.

There are many additional findings that are helpful. In knee cartilage disorders of any duration, such as 10 days, the quadriceps muscle group (especially the vastus medialis component) wastes rapidly. Measurement of the circumference of the thigh about an inch or two above the patella will detect this wasting when compared with the circumference of the unaffected side. Elderly patients may show a wasting from gradual disuse; thus, this sign is not diagnostic.

Effusion and extracapsular swelling may or may not be present. This is a general finding and merely indicates knee trauma.

X-rays taken in anteroposterior, lateral, and oblique planes are always reported as within normal limits unless, on rare occasions, a loose body is present; the roentgenogram then would be diagnostically helpful. Special studies (such as arthrograms) are rarely indicated.

Diagnosis of a locked knee rests on a lack of complete extension and palpable localizing pain over the medial or lateral joint lines.

Treatment for the locked knee consists of placing the individual at rest and applying icepacks while arrangements are made for referral to an orthopedic specialist. The patient can be provided with a pair of crutches and allowed to ambulate only if necessary.

This is a very serious injury, and immediate surgical excision of the detached joint cartilage is undertaken to prevent erosion of the articular cartilage and further degenerative change on the knee surface.

A younger, fibrous type of cartilage is thought to form approximately a year or so following surgery. During the postsurgery convalescent phase a rehabilitation program is undertaken.

Trick Knee (Adult)

This type of disorder lends itself more readily to management by the family physi-

cian. It is more often found in late adolescence or in middle-aged former athletes. It develops following a specific injury that the patient can usually remember. Occasionally, there is no real history except for a minor traumatic incident.

The distinguishing feature is that this type of knee never locks irreversibly. There may be many episodes of pseudolocking, but the patient is always able to shake the knee or work it loose himself.

When the patient attempts to descend stairs, the knee frequently pops or clicks, and often this is accompanied by swelling that remains for 2 to 3 days. In between these episodes, the knee is basically normal and trouble-free.

Patients with this problem usually have learned to protect themselves by restricting their athletic endeavors. Often the patient will use a support for the knee that permits limited participation in athletics.

Physical examination is made with the patient lying on his back. The examiner grasps the involved leg, flexes the knee as much as possible, and rotates the foot outward to test the medial cartilage, and inward to test the lateral cartilage.

Next, he palpates the medial joint line with the index finger as the knee is slowly extended. A painful click will occur. The greater the degree of flexion at the time the click occurs, the more posterior the portion of the cartilage that is torn.

X-rays will occasionally disclose slight narrowing of the medial joint component if the lesion has been present for 10 years or more. Otherwise, the films are reported as within normal limits.

Diagnosis is made by means of the history of frequent pseudolocking, which the patient can readily reverse himself, and of a painful click localized to the joint line on physical examination.

Treatment consists primarily of a course of rehabilitative exercises. The patient is instructed in quadriceps-setting exercises by the physician, or he can be referred to the physical therapist with a specific prescription. Once the patient masters this muscle-setting routine, he is started on progressive resistance exercises. Initially, a limit of 10 pounds of weight should be prescribed. Once the patient has reached this level under the guidance of the therapist, he is usually sufficiently versed in the procedure to continue the progressive resistance program on a daily basis at home until he is able to lift 35 to 40 pounds (15 pounds is sufficient for a female patient).

An analysis of the role of specific activities in producing temporary giving-way of the knee is then offered to the patient, and it is left to him to practice prevention.

For the temporary episodes of pain and swelling, the patient is advised to rest the knee completely and to apply icebags for 6 to 8 hours. Following this, he should resume the quadriceps-setting routine and continue this every hour during the day for 5-minute periods.

The following day, ambulation with crutches is permitted. The next step is referral to a physical therapist for the progressive resistive exercise routine. If the patient is familiar with this, he is then advised to begin the routine at home until the prescribed 10 to 30 pound limit is reached, according to the indications.

Aspiration of fluid from these traumatic knees with a syringe and needle is not routinely performed because the knee reabsorbs the effusion quite satisfactorily when the patient is following the rehabilitative program just outlined. The introduction of possible infection into a receptive culture medium of knee fluid is thus avoided. The value of fluid analysis in the differential diagnosis of traumatic knee conditions is minimal and is far outweighed by the risk of introducing infection. This synovial fluid analysis is far more helpful in chronically swollen knee conditions, such as are discussed in the section on rheumatoid arthritis. Steroid injections have no place in the treatment of either the locked or the trick knee.

Unstable Knee

The diagnosis is quite evident at first glance (Fig. 38–17). This condition is often due to old trauma, severe enough to involve multiple ligaments and cartilages.

The unstable knee is frequently incompatible with routine activities of daily living. Since this problem is usually due to advanced osteoarthritis or previous extensive traumatic injury, the patient has pronounced restrictions unless ancillary supports such as crutches or long leg-braces are available. The unstable type of knee varies from the mildly unstable to the extremely

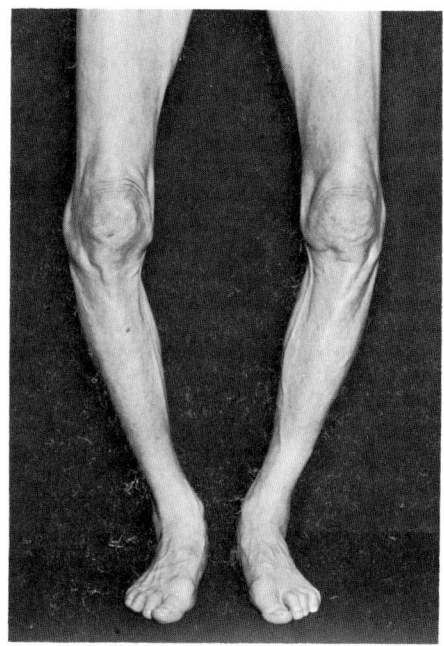

Figure 38–17.   *Unstable knees caused by degenerative changes. (From Beetham, W. P., Polley, H. F., Slocumb, C. H., et al.: Physical Examination of the Joints. Philadelphia, W. B. Saunders Co., 1965, p. 148.)*

wobbly knee. It gives the patient an uneasy sense of discomfort when he attempts ambulation. The patient voluntarily restricts activities and avoids situations that would place him at a disadvantage.

Physical examination is performed with the patient flat on the table and the knee flexed to a right angle. Both of the examiner's hands are placed behind the tibia just below the knee joint, and the tibia is gently pushed forward and pushed backward (Fig. 38–18). Increased mobility, compared with the opposite knee, indicates ligamentous instability (cruciate ligaments).

The examiner similarly tests medial and lateral stability by placing his hands on the medial and lateral aspects of the tibia and carefully moving it toward the opposite leg and then away from the opposite leg. Increased mobility of these movements when compared with those of the opposite knee denotes ligamentous damage. The knee often has the appearance of a severe bowleg.

X-rays are reported as showing varying degrees of osteoarthritic change, usually with associated varus or valgus displacement of the femur on the tibia.

Treatment consists of an appropriate re-

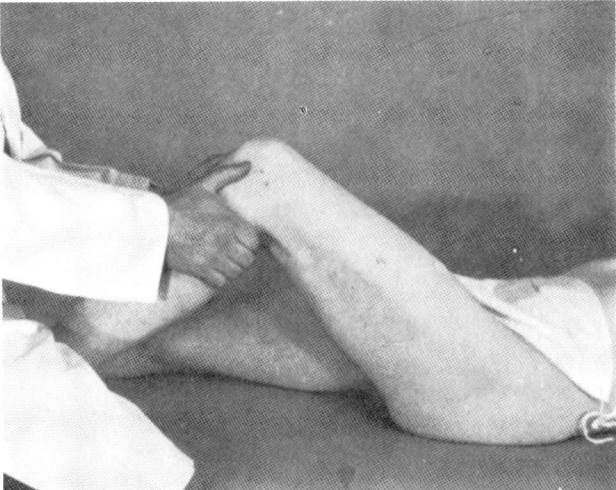

Figure 38-18. *Examination of cruciate ligaments of the knee for laxity. (From Wiles, P.: Essentials of Orthopaedics. 2nd Ed., Boston, Little, Brown & Co., 1956, p. 189.)*

habilitative routine. These patients are referred for physical therapy for a progressive resistance program until 30 pounds of weight can be lifted by a male, and about 10 pounds by a female.

Additional support is often wisely prescribed in the form of a knee-cage brace, usually purchased from a drugstore or an orthopedic appliance manufacturer. For severe cases, a long leg-brace with rigid steel support is required. This has to be obtained by making prior arrangements with a prosthetist. A list of certified companies can be found in the Yellow Pages of any large city telephone directory.

For many patients, the pain factor is of more concern than the instability. In these instances, the physician might well consider the use of daily doses of aspirin or aspirin-like compounds titrated to the level of the patient's comfort.

Since this type of knee already exhibits advanced destructive and degenerative changes, occasional injections of steroids are indicated to decrease the pain and improve the function. The concern about neuropathic changes following steroid injection should be disregarded, since little further damage can be produced and the benefits to the patient of successful pain relief are considerable. Canes and crutches should not be overlooked in these conditions. The use of this supplemental support considerably decreases the amount of weight placed on the damaged joint.

Occasionally, there is an indication for surgery, such as the insertion of a total knee prosthesis or an arthrodesis of the knee, especially if the patient is in relatively good health and if the other knee is not involved.

Acute Knee Injury (Adult)

A variety of clinical pictures may be present following an acute knee injury. The previously described conditions—locked knee, trick knee, and unstable knee—are excluded from this discussion.

The patient presenting with a history of a recent knee injury may often have an effusion. There may or may not be ecchymosis, and the knee may be held in a flexed or extended position.

The distinguishing characteristic is that although the cartilage might be torn, it is not displaced sufficiently to lock the knee.

The injury may consist of a *sprain* of the *medial* or *lateral collateral ligaments* or of a *partial detachment* or *sprain* of the *cruciate ligaments*. It is possible that only a *tear of the retinacular apparatus* is sustained. The diagnosis is usually apparent following physical examination.

Physical examination may or may not reveal an effusion. Ecchymosis is often present over the area of greatest injury. The knee may be held in the flexed position because of an effusion that fills the joint compartment with about 70 cc. of blood or synovial fluid. Pain frequently prevents the patient from extending the knee, but it is apparent that this is not a locked knee. Usually, with careful coaxing, the patient can be induced to straighten the knee to the degree that indicates that if it were not for pain and swelling, there would be no problem in extending the knee completely.

The most important step in exact diagnosis, then, is careful palpation. If the most severe pain is localized to the medial or lateral knee joint on palpation, then a *diagnosis of torn joint cartilage* is entertained (Fig. 38–19). It is obvious that the cartilage is not displaced since the knee is not locked.

If palpation is carefully conducted over the area of the insertion and origin of the *medial* or *lateral collateral ligaments*, localizing pain and tenderness in this area indicate a sprain of this structure. Careful palpation just above the joint line indicates whether the superior pole of the ligament is damaged, while careful palpation below the knee joint line over the tibia indicates whether the inferior pole of this ligament is sprained.

Pain only at the joint line is difficult to differentiate from a semilunar cartilage tear at this same level. Fortunately, however, this distinction is not necessary.

A similar palpatory examination should be carried out on the lateral aspect of the knee. If no localizing pain is found over the joint line or over the contour of the medial and lateral collateral ligaments, palpation then should be carried out around the patella. If there is localizing tenderness medial or lateral to the patella (this is the area of the *retinacular apparatus*), a small tear or sprain in this area should be suspected. Likewise, pain detected below the patella indicates a *sprain of the infrapatellar ligament*. Pain detected above the patella indicates a *sprain of the quadriceps tendon* as it inserts into the patella.

Localized tenderness over any of the tendons posterior to the knee indicates a *sprain* of these structures, such as the *hamstring tendon* or the *biceps femoris tendon*. By palpation of these structures and brief referral to an anatomic text, the examiner can readily diagnose the exact structure

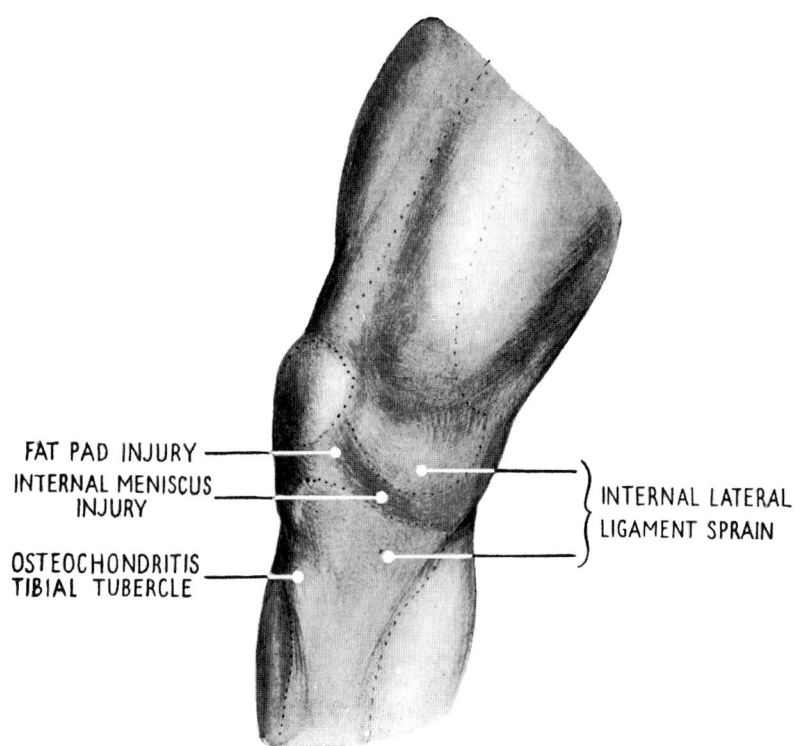

FAT PAD INJURY

INTERNAL MENISCUS INJURY

OSTEOCHONDRITIS TIBIAL TUBERCLE

INTERNAL LATERAL LIGAMENT SPRAIN

Figure 38–19. *Points of tenderness on inner side of knee used in diagnosing acute knee injury.* (From Wiles, P.: Essentials of Orthopaedics. 2nd Ed. Boston, Little, Brown & Co., 1956, p. 190.)

involved. Once familiarity is obtained with these structures, their identification is quite easy.

The two cruciate ligaments are deep in the center of the joint and cannot be readily palpated. They are tested by the following set of maneuvers.

Injuries of the cruciate ligaments can be diagnosed with the knee flexed to a right angle. The tibia is then pulled forward and pushed backward. Increased anterior mobility denotes a rupture of the anterior cruciate ligament; increased posterior mobility indicates a rupture of the posterior cruciate ligament. Increased anterior and posterior mobility is present when both cruciates have been avulsed.

In *complete tears* of the *medial or lateral collateral ligaments,* the gap in the ligament often may be felt. In the case of the lateral ligament, it can be felt by adducting the tibia on the femur with the knee flexed to about 15 degrees. In the case of the medial collateral ligament, it can be felt by abducting the tibia on the femur, again with the knee flexed at 15 degrees. If a gap is not felt but increased mobility is present, it often indicates a partial tear.

X-rays fail to disclose abnormalities in most of these cases unless one of the ligaments has avulsed a small flake of bone with it. This would be diagnostic.

Diagnosis rests on localization of the area of significant pain. The absence of the previously described pathologic lesions, such as locking of the knee, and so forth, also lends emphasis to the diagnosis of a sprain or ligamentous injury.

Treatment of the patient with really severe pain or significant effusion consists of placing him at bed rest for 3 days. Bathroom privileges are allowed if the patient can ambulate with crutches. The knee can be supported on pillows for comfort, if desired. Icebags should be applied for the initial 24 hour period and quadriceps-setting exercises initiated as described previously.

Aspiration of the knee joint can validly be sanctioned in this instance as a pain-relieving technique. Experience will indicate, however, that the only two materials found will be blood or synovial fluid. Following an acute injury, early aspiration of these materials results in recurrent effusions, especially in the 24 to 72 hour period

postinjury. The introduction of infection by frequent aspiration must be considered.

The application of ice and the institution of the quadriceps-setting routine usually control the effusion quite satisfactorily and produce a more rapid disappearance than that effected by any other method of treatment.

As the effusion fades, many small areas of tenderness will gradually disappear. A reevaluation of the knee in 3 to 4 days will usually result in more exact localization of the injury site.

If the *diagnosis* is a *nondisplaced semilunar cartilage,* the patient should be continued on the rehabilitative program and progressive resistance exercises begun. These should be carried out until prescribed limits (10 to 15 pounds for females and 30 to 35 pounds for males) are reached. At this stage, usually only minimal symptoms are present, and if the cartilage has not been sufficiently dislodged, there will usually be a peripheral attachment remaining that will continue to receive blood from the adjoining capsule, permitting the cartilage to heal satisfactorily. The overall time required for this program varies from 4 to 8 weeks.

Immobilization in any type of plaster cast is rarely indicated, since it frequently produces adhesions, restriction of motion, and wasting of the musculature from disuse.

If the main brunt of the *injury* is to the *collateral ligaments* either on the inside or the outside of the knee, a program similar to that just described is followed. The patient may use crutches with full weight-bearing on the involved extremity in the early stages of recuperation, as early as 72 hours following injury. When the patient is able to lift 10 pounds of weight by the progressive resistive-exercise methods, the crutches can be safely discarded.

Resumption of any type of athletic activity, such as wrestling, basketball, football, and so forth, should be forbidden for at least 3 months following a serious injury to the knee structures.

Injuries to the *retinacular apparatus* or the *inferior* or *superior patella ligaments* usually heal more rapidly than the injuries just described. They are treated with an identical regimen.

Finally, *injuries* to the *collateral ligaments* or the *cruciate ligaments* that result in instability and increased mobility, as detected on physical examination, are serious enough to require surgery. These injuries can be treated temporarily with rest and ice applications while arrangements are being made for referral to an appropriate specialist.

Tibial-Prominence Pain (Adolescent)

The tibial tubercle is located just at the lower border of the knee and is prominent in most individuals. It is the site of insertion of the infrapatellar ligament. In individuals between ages 10 and 16, this site can become the source of pain, limp, and often persistent swelling. An *osteochondritic process* involves this zone of the tibia, and it more frequently affects males than females.

Flexion movements of the knee are painless, but any activity requiring active extension, especially with stress, is quite painful. This condition is self-limiting and complete anatomic and functional recovery usually takes place once growth ceases, by age 16 at the latest.

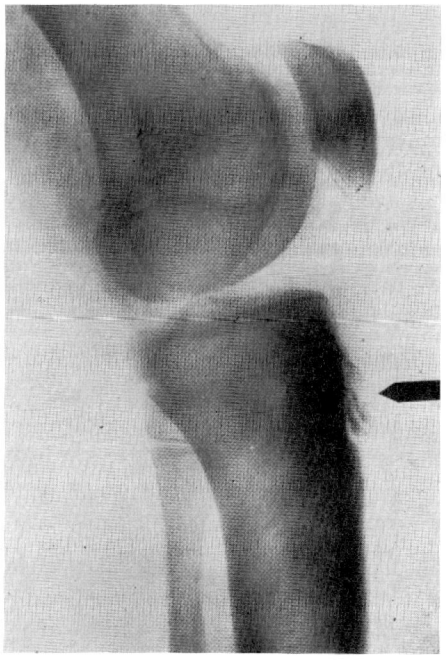

Figure 38–20. *Lateral roentgenogram showing osteochondritis of the tibial tuberosity. (From Shands, A. R., Jr., and Raney, R. B., Sr. (with collaboration of Brashear, H. R.): Handbook of Orthopaedic Surgery. 7th Ed., St. Louis, The C. V. Mosby Co., 1967.)*

Physical examination reveals that pressure by the examiner's finger or thumb over the tibial tubercle always produces slight to exquisite pain. Similar pressure exerted over the opposite tibial tubercle produces no reaction. The painful area is usually surrounded by a more or less permanent swelling that increases the prominence when compared with the tubercle of the opposite knee.

X-rays show irregularity in the ossification zone of the tibial tubercle (Fig. 38–20).

Diagnosis is never based on radiologic findings unless accompanied by localized pain over the tibial tubercle.

Treatment consists of restriction of strenuous activity, especially of all games that place stress on the knee, such as running, jumping, bicycling, climbing steps, and so forth. This should be enforced for a period of from 2 to 6 months.

Immobilization in a plaster cast or other apparatus is not necessary. In most instances, the pain disappears as soon as activities are restricted. It is important that both the parent and the young patient understand the reason for this restriction.

If activities are not curtailed and the pain and swelling persist past age 16, a permanent change occurs. In these patients, surgical excision of the ossicle often becomes necessary at a later date. With sufficient understanding on the part of all involved, the condition should not progress to this stage.

An especially acute episode can be dramatically relieved by the injection of 1 cc. of betamethasone directly under the patellar ligament at the site of the tibial tubercle.

If a patient past age 16 complains of this problem, surgical excision of the ossific particle and snug suturing of the infrapatellar ligament will relieve the symptoms.

Locked Knee (Child)

An adolescent, following a severe injury, could show the typical locked knee as described previously for the adult, and it could be due to an identical type of injury to the knee cartilage. There is another entity, however, that is just as common in the youngster. The type of locking that occurs in this condition is secondary to a discoid meniscus.

The joint cartilages during their development usually undergo absorption of the central zone at a special time. When this fails to occur (and it usually involves the lateral cartilage) it leaves a complete disc, referred to as the discoid cartilage. This becomes symptomatic between the ages of 6 and 14.

Prior to the irreversible locking episode, the adolescent often notices an audible or palpable click during certain movements. If the patient is examined at this phase, the snap or click will be found to take place when the flexed knee is being extended and just lacks a few degrees of complete extension. It also occurs when the joint is being flexed and is approaching the position of complete flexion. This type of cartilage is more susceptible to trauma than is the normal lateral cartilage in any type of injury.

Physical examination indicates the presence of a locked knee that has been described previously under the section on the adult locked knee. The causation, as already explained, can be different in a child, but the end result is still the same. When the knee finally locks, it is irreversible.

X-rays fail to disclose any abnormalities.

Diagnosis rests primarily on the presence of the physical findings indicative of a locked knee (lack of complete extension).

Treatment in the young child is bed rest for 3 days and the application of icepacks to the knee. Often this will produce spontaneous remission. The child can then be given a brief course of rehabilitative exercises for the knee.

In adolescents, spontaneous recovery is less probable, and following initial treatment with rest and icepacks, referral should be considered because it is more likely than not that surgery will be required. If, however, spontaneous recovery should occur, the family physician should proceed with the usual rehabilitation program described earlier in the text.

Trick Knee (Child)

Between the ages of 11 and 15 years, many children encounter this condition for the first time. There may or may not be an episode of initial trauma. Usually the child notices that on climbing steps or suddenly squatting or participating in some athletic activity, such as basketball, the knee gives way spontaneously, often causing the individual to drop to the floor.

Upon wiggling the knee for a moment or two, the temporary weakness is corrected, but there is often associated pain and swelling at the time of the first episode. Subsequent episodes of giving-way are readily recognized by the patient, and he temporarily restricts activity until the symptoms disappear.

Physical examination often reveals knock-knees. To the experienced examiner, the patella might appear to be placed abnormally high. At most, the only positive physical finding is that the patella can be made to ride over the outer condyle of the femur as the examiner presses it outward while passively flexing the knee. This maneuver is basic to the diagnosis.

If the patient is examined immediately after the first episode, there may be enough swelling to confuse the situation. However, when he is examined after the swelling subsides, the clinical findings are usually unmistakable.

X-rays occasionally demonstrate flattening of the outer condyle of the femur. Failure of the outer femoral condyle to develop may be reported.

Diagnosis rests on the history of repeated giving-way and the positive patellar displacement maneuver. Likewise, the absence of any other significant findings, such as cartilage displacement or weakness of the ligaments, is helpful.

Treatment for this condition is first begun with the quadriceps muscle-setting routine and followed with the progressive-resistance rehabilitative routine as outlined previously. For adolescent females the weight limit is about 10 pounds, and for adolescent males the limit is about 25 pounds.

If the individual perseveres in these programs and eliminates excessive athletic activity, he usually will reach adult life with a normal knee joint. If, however, the subluxations continue to occur, surgical repair is indicated for this type of *congenital dislocation of the patella* (Fig. 38–21). It is extremely rare to find any other condition in a child or adolescent producing a recurrent giving-way of the knee.

Acute Knee Injury (Child)

Any severe knee injury in a child or adolescent will usually produce swelling, pain, ecchymosis, and temporary restriction of motion. As outlined for all of the previously described conditions, a roentgeno-

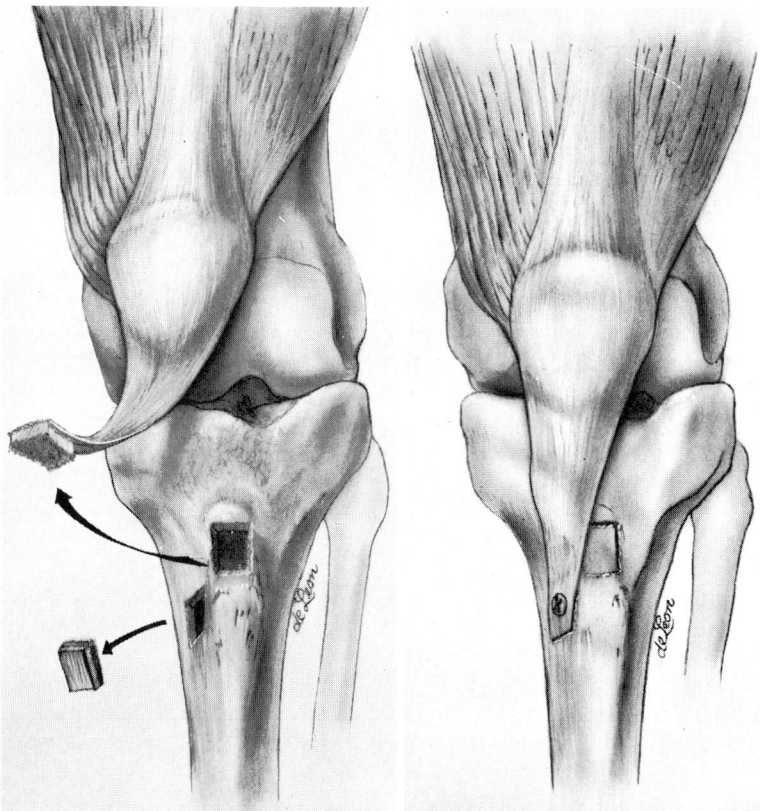

Figure 38–21. *Operation for recurrent dislocation of the patella. The tibial attachment is transplanted medially. (From Raney, R. B., Sr., and Brashear, H. R., Jr.: Shand's Handbook of Orthopaedic Surgery. 8th Ed. St. Louis, The C. V. Mosby Co., 1971.)*

gram should be taken to rule out the possibility of fracture. Following this, one may proceed with the examination to attempt to localize the areas of most significant tenderness. In the absence of any locking, one should proceed as in the adult, with similar diagnostic considerations.

The likelihood of a torn semilunar cartilage is just as great in the child as in the adult. The possibility of sprain of the medial or collateral ligaments should be entertained.

Diagnosis of an injured ligament or cartilage, of course, rests on localizing the tenderness to the specific anatomic location as well as on the absence of the other major disorders previously discussed.

Treatment for sprain of the ligaments or retinacular apparatus or for injury to the cartilage in a child is similar to that described previously. Initially, ice is applied and then the child is started on a quadriceps-setting routine to be followed by a progressive-resistance routine. Crutches

and rest are indicated according to the degree of response. Usually, it will be found that in a child the total recovery time from a knee injury takes less than 2 weeks, in contrast to the adult, who may well require 3 to 4 months.

Painful Knee (Adolescent)

Often, the child will give a history of intermittent pain that seems to arise deep in the knee joint, comes and goes without any specific aggravation, and occasionally is related to changes in the weather.

Physical examination is usually unrewarding. However, if the examiner displaces the patella either medially or laterally and presses against the undersurface with his thumbs, he will often produce marked pain when compared with the opposite, normal patella (Fig. 38–22).

X-rays are within normal limits.

The *diagnosis* suggested by these findings is *chondromalacia of the patella* and is

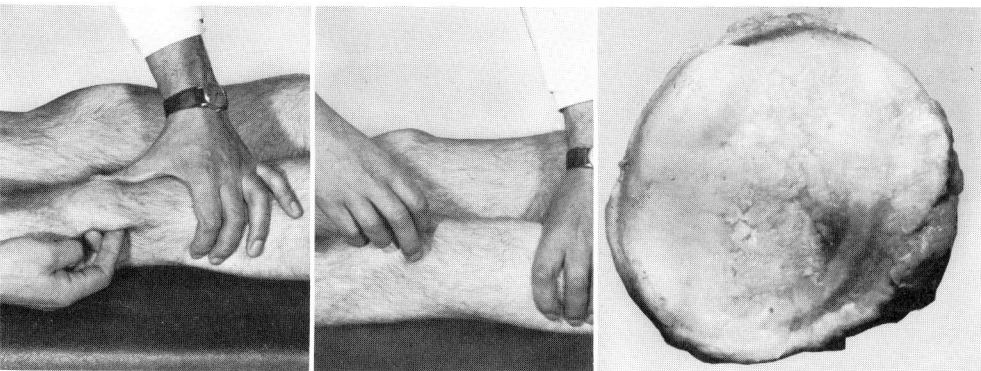

Figure 38-22. *Tenderness under patella, and appearance of the bony lesion (chondromalacia). (Reproduced from A System of Orthopaedics and Fractures, 3rd Ed. by A. Graham Apley, published by Butterworths, London.)*

a very difficult condition to treat. The family physician would be wise to refer the patient to a specialist.

Swollen, Painful Knee (Child)

These two symptoms will appear quite commonly in many knee disorders. They are only listed here as a general catch-all for any condition not already indicated. The findings of swollen, painful knee are supplemental to most of these conditions. For instance, if in an evaluation of swelling of the knee the physical examination indicates localized tenderness at a particular anatomic site and a diagnosis of a locked knee is made, the swelling would merely be considered a secondary accompanying finding and not a diagnostic possibility.

If, however, the knee is examined and no areas of localized tenderness or pain are found—only localized swelling—other possibilities might be suggested, such as Baker's cyst, popliteal aneurysm, and so forth, conditions that the family physician

would not be expected to be familiar with or to treat (Fig. 38-23). This type of finding would indicate that a referral is necessary unless the family physician intends to become as deeply involved in orthopedics as the specialist.

The possibility of infection in a swollen, painful knee joint in children must never be overlooked. An early diagnosis of this condition is possible only with aspiration of the knee fluid. When changes in the bones are detectable on x-ray, serious damage has already taken place. Every knee that is swollen is not aspirated. There are, however, several criteria that are helpful in determining whether to aspirate or not. The first is fever, the second is an elevated white blood count, and the third is an elevated sedimentation rate. If any one of these three is positive, aspiration of the knee is recommended. The fluid so obtained should be sent immediately to the laboratory for culture and antibiotic sensitivity studies.

Likewise, as has been suggested earlier, with almost every examination a roentgen-

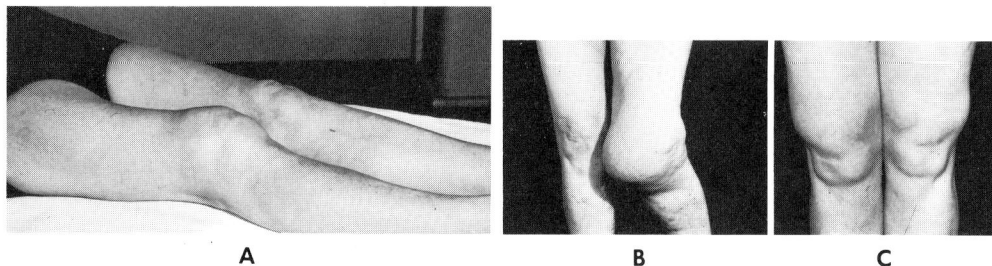

A   B   C

Figure 38-23. *Swollen knees, A, Rheumatoid arthritis. B, Charcot knee. C, Villous synovitis. (Reproduced from A System of Orthopaedics and Fractures, 3rd Ed. by A. Graham Apley, published by Butterworths, London.)*

ogram is required. Therefore, if the family physician encounters a patient with a history of repeated giving-way of the knee and occasional swelling, but on physical examination can find nothing, he should not be discouraged. When the x-ray is ordered and the radiologist reports an osteochondritis dissecans, a completely unfamiliar condition to the family physician, he should refer the patient for in-depth studies by the specialist.

Since conditions such as these are not very common, one could not expect the family physician to devote a large percentage of his time attempting to diagnose them. They more correctly belong in the province of the specialist. Using the approach previously outlined, the family physician can expect to diagnose and treat with confidence the more common disorders of the knee in both the adult and the child.

THIGH DISORDERS

Thigh Injuries

Muscles in general will tolerate a certain amount of stress without rupture. If, however, a muscle is already maximally stressed and a sharp increase in tension is produced, the muscle will infrequently give way somewhere along its length. In an athlete who is moving rapidly in one direction and who suddenly reverses his direction, this additional unexpected force can cause the muscle to give way.

The most frequent sites of rupture are in the quadriceps muscle group, especially the attachment of the rectus at the hip and the hamstrings at the ischial spine.

Usually the condition is diagnosed as a contusion or hematoma because of marked swelling and ecchymosis. When the local reaction subsides and the true nature of the injury is apparent, it is usually too late for any type of surgical treatment.

Attempts at repair several weeks after injury are not worthwhile because it is impossible to suture the muscle firmly enough to maintain the desired length.

The patient usually presents himself with a history of a swollen, painful thigh or calf and localized tenderness. After several weeks, the swelling disappears, the soreness remains, and the muscle mass appears.

At this stage, all that can be done is to explain to the athlete that the pain will eventually disappear but the bunched-up muscle mass will remain.

It should be emphasized that there will be no real disability. If some persistent pain should remain because of chronic myositis in the area involved, this tissue can be carefully removed surgically later.

Initially, however, the patient should be given a trial of physical therapy, which includes heat, followed by setting exercises of the muscle group involved, and, ultimately, progressive-resistance exercises to the same group. The weight limit for the quadriceps muscle in the average person is about 10 pounds for a period of a month or so following the injury. Similar limits are set for other muscles, such as the gastrocnemius and soleus group, but these limits are from 4 to 6 pounds.

It must be emphasized that during the acute period no active use of the extremity should be permitted. The individual should get about on crutches or remain in a nonstressful type of situation. The best criteria for resumption of activity lie with the patient, since once pain is gone he can resume activity without any harm. He can also determine which activities are pain-free. The estimated healing time is about 6 weeks. Such injuries occur not only in sports such as track or football but also in snow skiing, water skiing, and other sports. They involve the well-conditioned athlete as well as the amateur.

Mass in the Thigh

Myositis Ossificans. A young person may complain of swelling and pain in the thigh. The swelling usually does not disappear. The patient frequently cannot participate in athletic activities because of pain. However, if there is no concern on the part of the patient, the physician may not see the lesion until it is 2 to 3 months old, at which time there is a prominent mass of bony consistency without significant pain.

This can occur in any muscle. The adductor muscle group of the thigh is a frequent site of myositis ossificans.

Physical findings include a tender mass, but it is somewhat rubbery instead of soft and is usually prominent. It is localized primarily in the adductor region of the thigh. After 4 to 8 weeks it increases in size and acquires a hard, bony consistency.

X-rays taken in the anteroposterior and lateral planes within the first 2 weeks after injury are reported as negative. However, beyond the 2-week period x-rays usually show faint calcification, which gradually increases in density until an amorphous tumor-like mass is visible.

The size of this lesion causes interference with muscle function, and quite often this is the first time the athlete seeks attention. Only in rare cases does the mass attach to the bone.

Diagnosis is made principally by roentgenogram, although clinical findings are highly suggestive, especially if correlated with a positive history. The trauma need not be severe.

During the early stages, the diagnosis may evade even the most experienced physician. However, a period of watchful waiting is justified with repeat radiographic examinations. Usually by 4 to 6 weeks the nature of the lesion is evident.

Treatment consists of resting the part and allowing the disorder to take its course. No other treatment is required.

Excision of the mass, if it is sufficiently large and bothersome, may be performed late in the course of the disease after it has reached its maturity. It is not wise to take a biopsy or to attempt to remove the mass during its early stage, since considerable confusion can result from the interpretation of the biopsy material. In its early growth phase, myositis ossificans can be misinterpreted as a malignant lesion by the pathologist. Some recommend that a bone scan be performed as proof of the maturity of the lesion. When the bone scan is no longer "hot", the myositis ossificans can be resected safely.

HIP DISORDERS

Although there are many conditions that affect the hip from birth through maturity, these can be conveniently grouped into two broad categories: those that are readily treated in the family practice situation and those that must be referred to the specialist.

By using such designations, the family physician is spared the effort of becoming familiar with many subtle manifestations of the multitude of pathologic processes that can involve the hip joint.

The following material is organized and presented with this in mind. Clinical syndromes are listed in the order in which the family physician would expect to encounter them in his office practice. For example, hip afflictions in the 60 to 75 year age group are listed first because they will be more common in the average population group. The afflictions in the 10 to 15 year old group are equally serious but are not as common or as apt to be seen in the family practice office. Hip problems in the 1 to 2 year old age group are listed last because these are usually screened at birth and referred early to specialty centers.

The first part of the examination of the hip must be conducted so as to afford the examiner the opportunity of observing gait as the patient walks toward and away from him. The hallway between examining rooms may be an ideal area for this analysis. After minimal experience, the examiner will be able to determine at a glance whether a limp is originating in the hip, knee, or ankle.

The second part of the examination is conducted with the patient on the examination table. An appropriate gown must be used, which exposes the patient at least from the level of the umbilicus to the toes.

Hip Pain and Limp (Ages 50 to 80)

Complaints of hip pain and limp are primarily a manifestation of degenerative disease (arthritis), which is part of the aging process, or of increased static abnormality such as overweight, prior hip disorder, and, occasionally, a constitutional predisposition.

When analyzing the complaint of pain, the examiner should ask the patient to point to the area of pain with the index finger. Many patients consider the sacroiliac area as the hip joint and the real hip area as belonging to the thigh. This can result in considerable confusion.

With the pain there is often a complaint of stiffness that is worse on arising in the morning but improves after several hours of activity. However, excessive activity appears to have a cumulative effect and tends to incite pain and spasm in the hip area.

Changes in position from sitting to stand-

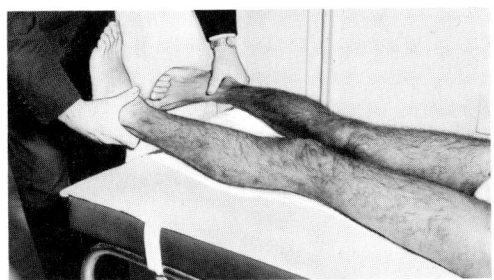

Figure 38–24. *Internal rotation of the hip. (Reproduced from A System of Orthopaedics and Fractures, 3rd Ed. by A. Graham Apley, published by Butterworths, London.)*

ing will often produce sudden pain that may last beyond the moment of activity but will fade with further limited movement.

Gait changes vary from mild awkwardness to a pronounced limp. Also, inability to cross the leg while putting on a shoe and similar types of restriction of activity will gradually be noted by the patient.

Physical examination includes moving the sound limb through its various ranges of motion and repeating this on the side of the involvement. In this way, the examiner can obtain a good idea of all the limitations of motion in the affected hip.

Specifically, most of the common types of hip disorders will manifest a loss of internal rotation of the affected hip joint first. With the patient flat on his back on the examination table, request that he point the toes of both feet to the ceiling. This is regarded as neutral position. Then ask the patient to turn the toes of the normal leg inward (toward the opposite leg as far as possible without lifting the leg from the table). Then ask the patient to perform this same maneuver with the involved hip.

A normal range (which is really just estimated) is about 10 to 15 degrees (Fig. 38–24). The involved hip will show some restriction, which may vary from no internal rotation to as much as 5 to 10 degrees. In any serious hip disease, the hip tends to lie in an externally rotated position with little or no internal rotation.

The second movement restricted is extension. This is detected by testing for fixed flexion in the unsound hip. With the patient supine, both thighs are flexed completely on the abdomen. With the examiner's hand under the patient's lumbar spine, the nor-

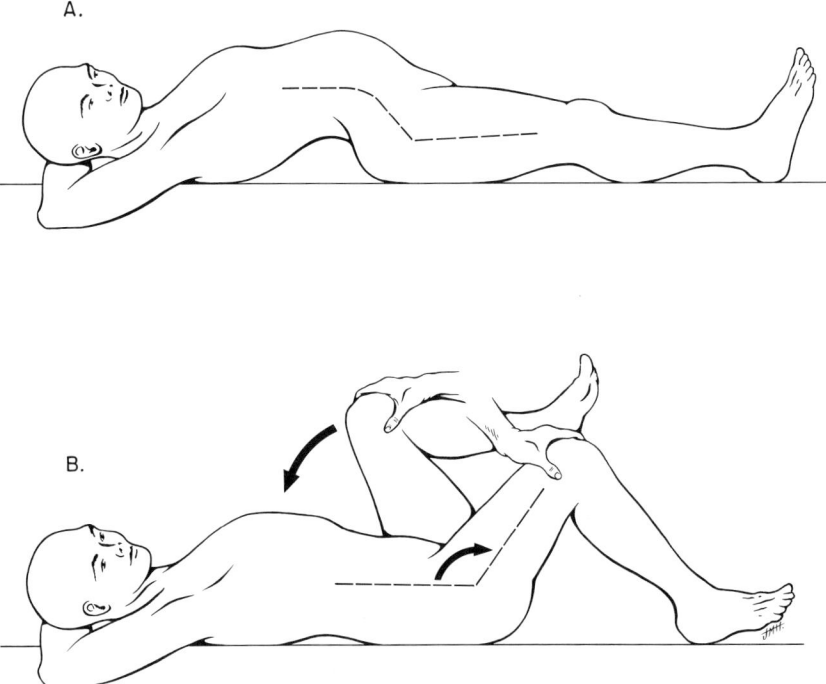

A.

B.

Figure 38–25. *Detection of flexion deformity of the hip. (From Beetham, W. P., Polley, H. F., Slocumb, C. H., et al.: Physical Examination of the Joints. Philadelphia, W. B. Saunders Co., 1965, p. 129.)*

mal lordotic curve is felt to be obliterated (Fig. 38-25). The patient is instructed to hold the normal limb manually with this flexed position.

The affected limb is then lowered toward the examination table until it reaches the position from which it can progress no further.

In this position, the angle of the leg with the table can be measured, and it indicates the angle of the fixed flexion deformity in degrees. For the purpose of the family physician, it should only be necessary to detect the presence or absence of such a flexion deformity.

The final movement tested is abduction, since this is the last to show limitation of movement. This deformity is detected by testing the range of abduction when both hips are extended and both feet are side by side. As the knees are pushed apart, any limitation of abduction on the side of the unsound hip will become apparent (Fig. 38-26).

Leg lengths should be measured routinely during any hip examination. This is accomplished with the patient lying supine and the pelvis in a level position. Measurements are then taken from the anterior superior iliac spine to the lower margin of the internal malleolus on one lower extremity and then the other (Fig. 38-27). Significant shortening can be detected.

In summary, a deranged hip in this age group lies in varying degrees of external rotation, flexion, and abduction, usually with some shortening. Muscle spasm is not present routinely unless there has been some recent episode of stress. Muscle wasting is often detectable but is secondary to loss of motion.

X-rays may be reported as negative in the early stages. As the disease progresses, roentgenograms show narrowing of the joint space, subcortical cysts near the joint surfaces, and, later, marginal proliferation of bone. A radiologist typically categorizes these findings with the term "*hypertrophic osteoarthritis*" (Fig. 38-28).

Diagnosis of degenerative joint disease is best reserved for those patients who exhibit some loss of hip joint motion, however minimal, with accompanying x-ray changes of some degree.

Treatment in the acute phase should include instructing the patient to rest on a firm mattress. If spasm or flexion deformity is marked, a pillow should be placed under the knee to relieve the discomfort. Heat should be applied over the affected hip (anterolaterally). The heating pad can be used at home, or moist heat in the physical therapy department can be prescribed.

Local injections of 5 cc. of 1 per cent procaine or 1 to 2 cc. of hydrocortisone solution may prove effective for the relief of

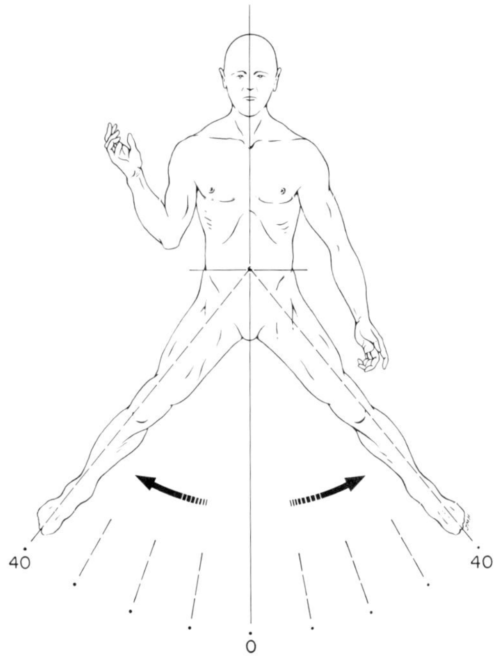

Figure 38-26. Range of hip abduction. (From Beetham, W. P., Polley, H. F., Slocumb, C. H., et al.: Physical Examination of the Joints. Philadelphia, W. B. Saunders Co., 1965, p. 135.)

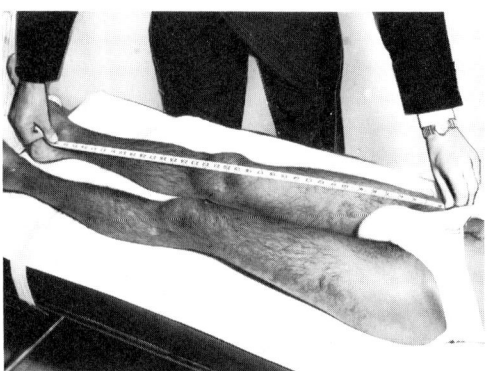

Figure 38-27. Measurement of leg length. (Reproduced from A System of Orthopaedics and Fractures, 3rd Ed. by A. Graham Apley, published by Butterworths, London.)

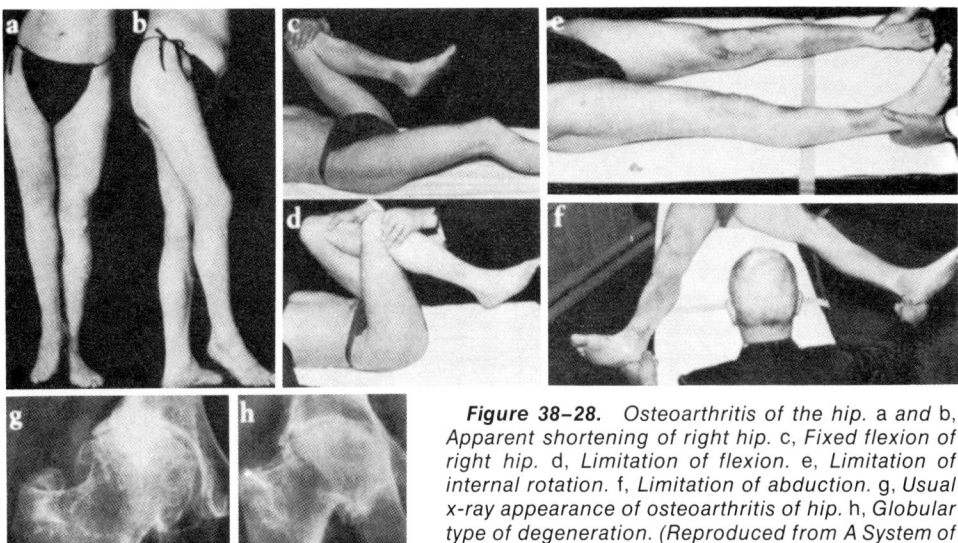

Figure 38-28. *Osteoarthritis of the hip. a and b, Apparent shortening of right hip. c, Fixed flexion of right hip. d, Limitation of flexion. e, Limitation of internal rotation. f, Limitation of abduction. g, Usual x-ray appearance of osteoarthritis of hip. h, Globular type of degeneration. (Reproduced from A System of Orthopaedics and Fractures, 3rd Ed. by A. Graham Apley, published by Butterworths, London.)*

acute pain. Aspiration of synovial fluid and subsequent analysis should be performed if it is possible to obtain fluid. This is not as easy in the hip as in the knee. Analgesics should also be prescribed for the first 24 to 48 hours, depending on the severity of the pain.

After the acute phase has subsided, the patient should be referred to a physical therapist for instruction in "active setting exercises for the gluteal musculature and passive stretching exercises for the iliopsoas muscle on the involved side." If both hips are involved, the same treatment program would apply.

Enteric-coated sodium salicylate tablets (5 grains) can be given 3 to 6 times a day or less for aching discomfort or continuous nagging pain. Ideally, these should be taken after meals.

Patients with this problem should be instructed to restrict activity to the limits the joint can accept gracefully. This will keep symptoms to the minimum. It should be emphasized that excesses of physical activity appear to be cumulative in effect and produce further irritation, which in turn produces pain and muscle spasm.

Support in the form of a cane in the hand opposite to the involved hip should be recommended. If the disease is bilateral, a quadripod cane can be used in both hands or crutches should be recommended.

All patients with unilateral disease and extensive malformations of the femoral head and acetabulum, especially if they are in good overall health, should have the benefit of an orthopedic consultation.

Surgical management ranges from removal of spurs to displacement osteotomy. Total hip replacement offers dramatic results for the appropriately selected patient.

Hip Pain, Limp, and Knee Pain (Ages 10 to 16)

Knee pain and hip limp is described as occurring in tall, thin individuals with a history of recent rapid growth. It is also associated with overweight adolescent boys with undeveloped sexual characteristics. There is often precipitating trauma present.

The problem is basically that the capital femoral epiphysis undergoes varying degrees of displacement either acutely or gradually. This displacement produces the clinical picture. A capital epiphysis rarely fuses with the neck of the femur before age 18. It must be remembered that although one hip is involved, the other hip may suffer the same fate.

Knee pain on the side of the involved hip is often the only complaint. X-rays made of the knee are reported as normal, and little subsequent attention is given to the patient until the disastrous "slip" takes place. In this age group, therefore, an evaluation of knee pain is not adequate unless the hip on the same side as the knee pain is x-rayed and reported as normal.

Physical examination in early cases

shows a mild hip limp with the leg held in external rotation, flexion, and abduction. Later the limp is more pronounced. There is an increased loss of motion at the hip, especially in the range of internal rotation and abduction in that order. There may be only a mild loss of the flexion unless the displacement is of a very significant degree.

Anteroposterior x-ray views are not adequate to demonstrate early displacement. *Lateral x-ray views* are essential to show the backward projection of the capital epiphysis.

Diagnosis is strongly suggested by the clinical findings. X-rays are needed to confirm the borderline cases.

Treatment at first involves immediate hospitalization and bed rest as soon as the diagnosis is made. Further degrees of slippage are thus protected against while tentative treatment is being undertaken. Treatment consists of operative reduction and insertion of some type of metallic pins across the epiphyseal plate to prevent further slippage and to promote early fusion of the epiphyseal plate (Fig. 38–29).

In patients in which the deformity is marked and the situation has existed for a considerable amount of time, reconstructive surgery is necessary.

Avoidance of weight bearing on the affected side is essential during the period of waiting for the epiphyseal plate to fuse.

Hip Pain and Limp (Ages 3 to 10)

Hip pain and limp is a very common condition affecting the hip, especially of males, in this age range. In many of the patients, there is a history of recent upper respiratory infection, which suggests an infectious origin of the hip disorder. Likewise, there are an equal number of children who give a history of some minor trauma shortly before the onset of symptoms.

Physical examination reveals the characteristic limp with the leg in slight external rotation. There may be a temperature elevation of 101° F. (38.3° C.). Occasionally, an elevated white blood count will be noted. Some general limitation of motion will be present, but it will usually be obvious on examination that this is due more to spasm than to real blockage of hip motion.

X-rays in some cases reveal capsular swelling. However, most of the films are normal.

Diagnosis rests on the absence of real restriction of hip motion and on negative x-ray reports.

Treatment consists of bed rest until pain

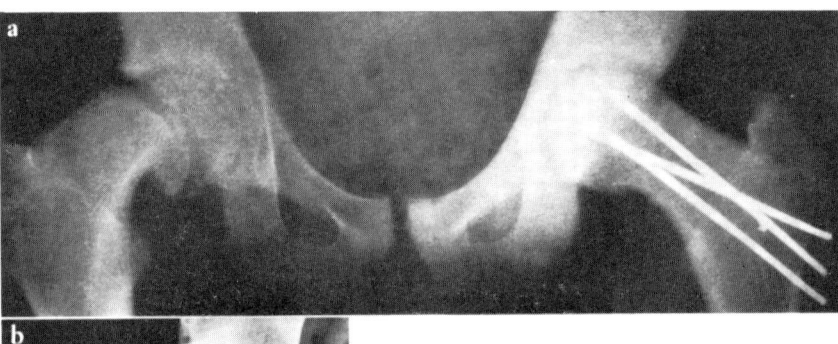
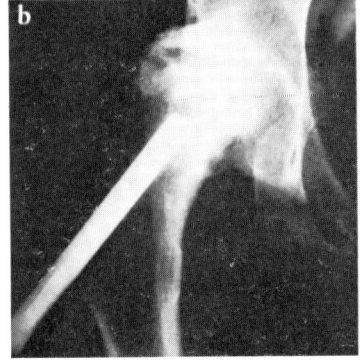

Figure 38–29. *Slipped epiphysis* (a) *before and* (b) *after treatment. (Reproduced from A System of Orthopaedics and Fractures, 3rd Ed. by A. Graham Apley, published by Butterworths, London.)*

disappears. This may require 3 to 10 days. Some therapists empirically prescribe broad-spectrum antibiotics for 7 days.

The limp may persist for a week to several months after the pain disappears. This is a frequent concern to parents. However, in the absence of positive x-ray findings in this age group, the physician can safely reassure the parents that while there is some abnormality present, it is not serious and usually self-limiting. A full range of hip motion may return within a week, but the limp often persists longer.

This condition, diagnosed as *transient synovitis*, will finally clear. It may test the patience of the physician on occasion, but with negative x-ray examination and periodic follow-up he can confidently reassure the parents that it will disappear without a trace.

Hip Pain and Limp (Ages 5 to 10)

A condition that occurs predominantly in males is called Perthes' disease. It is an aseptic necrosis of the proximal femoral epiphysis and is also referred to as osteochondrosis.

The basic disease process is thought to be obliteration of the blood supply to the femoral epiphysis. This results in a crushing or flattening of the femoral head with some thickening of the femoral neck.

Physical examination shows a hip limp on the affected side. There is a protective limitation of motion. Internal rotation is first lost, and then abduction, and finally flexion is limited.

X-ray findings depend on the stage of the disease. In the first 3 months there is an increase in the density of the capital femoral epiphysis. Some authorities suggest that a bone scan would be positive long before x-ray changes are noted in this condition. During the next 15 months, there is fragmentation of the epiphysis and thinning and absorption of the dense portion. The healing stage, which may last up to 3 years, shows regeneration and reossification of the epiphyseal zone.

Diagnosis is suggested by the clinical signs and symptoms but rests primarily on the appearance of x-ray changes.

Treatment is prolonged bed rest with traction according to some physicians. This can mean bed rest for as long as 2 years. In some specialty centers, there are entire programs built around these patients, beginning with custom-made wheelchairs and continuing with special educational programs in a complete hospital environment.

Other physicians with equal conviction feel that ambulation with avoidance of weight on the involved leg is the treatment of choice. They utilize special braces that elevate the involved side and thus prevent

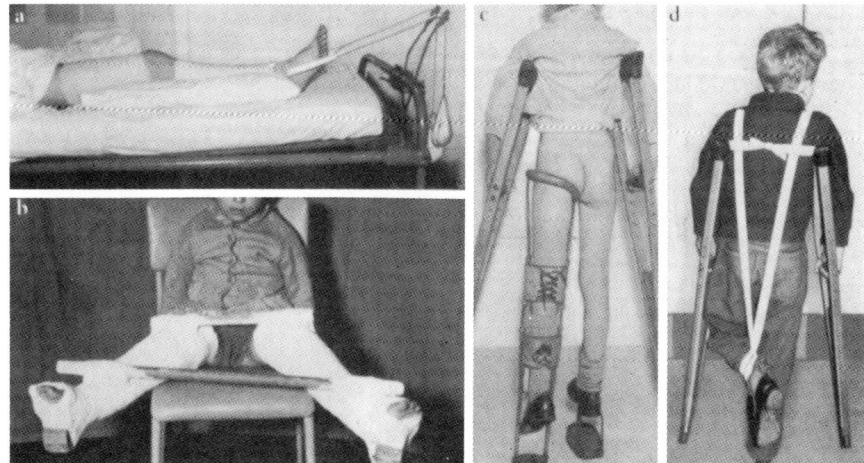

Figure 38–30. *Various methods of treating Perthes' disease. a, Traction needed when hip is painful. b, Hips held abducted in plaster cast which permits patient to get out of bed. Weight bearing on involved hip prevented by (c) special brace and crutches or (d) sling and crutches. (Reproduced from A System of Orthopaedics and Fractures, 3rd Ed. by A. Graham Apley, published by Butterworths, London.)*

normal weight bearing (Fig. 38–30). The family physician will wisely refer this type of patient to the specialty center.

Hip Limp (Ages 1 to 3)

A hip limp, though always painless at this age, is a tragedy because it means that the diagnosis of the congenital hip dislocation had been missed at an earlier age when it would have been much more responsive to treatment and without the complications that follow late detection and treatment.

Although there is considerable speculation regarding the cause of dislocation of the hip, there is little difference of opinion regarding its progressive evolution.

There is a presubluxation stage, during which the hip is vulnerable, followed by the subluxation stage, and, eventually, by the stage of dislocation.

The physician who examines newborn infants should be well read on the physical findings and x-ray changes that accompany this condition. This will require extra reading in highly specialized texts. The physician who does not perform newborn hip examinations very often should consider immediate referral when confronted with a child who displays a limp.

With early diagnosis and early management, a predictably normal result can be expected. With delay, regardless of the cause, a child is usually condemned to periods of prolonged treatment with variable results and perhaps a lifetime of partial disability. Emphasis therefore is placed on early diagnosis.

Clinical signs of the *presubluxation stage* indicate some slight external rotation, flex-ion, and abduction of the affected limb. There is apparent shortening of the affected leg. Gluteal folds are asymmetrical, and thigh folds are increased in number (Fig. 38–31).

A medial and upward pressure applied in the region of the hip as the thigh is abducted and externally rotated produces a click that is both felt and heard. This is called Ortolani's sign.

X-rays at this stage may show an increase in the acetabular index beyond 30 degrees. Retardation of the normal appearance of the bony nucleus is detectable as early as the fourth to fifth month.

The patient should be referred to a specialist for appropriate management.

If the child is not seen until the *subluxation stage*, the clinical signs will be similar, but the infant is usually 6 months or so of age.

X-ray findings are also similar but a greater degree of dysplastic change may be reported along with irregular maturation of the capital epiphysis with some displacement.

This patient also should be referred to the orthopedic specialist.

In the *dislocation* stage, the only significant finding that the family physician need appreciate is that the child walks with a hip limp.

X-ray findings, in addition to the ones mentioned previously, indicate a broken Shenton's line and widening of the teardrop shadow.

Management again consists of quick referral without hesitation, since a tragedy has already occurred when the condition has reached this stage without detection.

Figure 38–31. Unilateral dislocation—left hip. Note asymmetry of skin creases: a, Back view. b, Front view. c, Head palpated out of socket. d, X-ray confirms hip not in socket and shows delayed development of ossific nucleus. (Reproduced from A System of Orthopaedics and Fractures, 3rd Ed. by A. Graham Apley, published by Butterworths, London.)

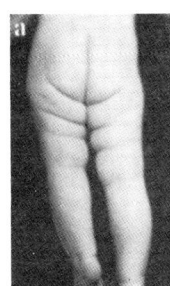
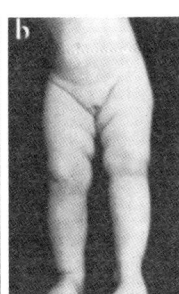
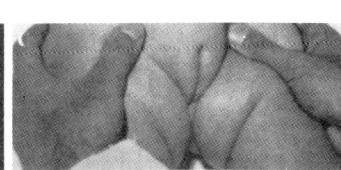
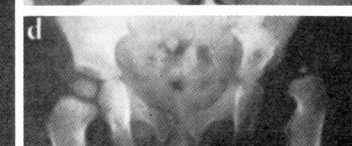

Hip Pain

Exclusive of the conditions just mentioned, most other hip complaints occur in adults. These are usually not accompanied by a limp. They exhibit subtle changes and require careful diagnosis and knowledge, which is usually only available to the specialist. X-rays can be taken but are often reported as negative (in cases of trochanteric bursitis and early aseptic necrosis of the femoral head).

The average family physician will not find it rewarding to spend the considerable time necessary to make this type of diagnosis. Any of these conditions or other conditions that have not been mentioned are therefore considered to fall into that category in which patients should be referred for both diagnosis and treatment unless the family physician is interested to the degree that he wishes to make orthopedics his subspecialty.

LOW-BACK DISORDERS

The approach used throughout this chapter will permit the family physician to become adept in the diagnosis and management of low-back disorders. It is based on the premise that the "skeletonized" physical examination introduced here will force the examiner to decide at its conclusion whether the clinical findings justify a diagnosis of either *low-back syndrome* or *disc-like syndrome.*

Regardless of the cause, there are a great many signs and symptoms that patients with back problems exhibit in common. By encompassing the myriad of complaints and clinical findings under these two headings, the physician is relieved of the necessity of pursuing a multitude of diagnostic possibilities. Freed from this burden, he can then concentrate and become proficient in the management of that group of low-back disorders of which he is quite capable of treating (those that fall into the category of *low-back syndrome*). He will wisely refer any patients whose symptoms and findings indicate a diagnosis of disc-like syndrome to either the orthopedic or neurosurgical specialist.

In addition, a program of phased management is described for the low-back syn-

TABLE 38–1. SCHEME OF EXAMINATION

Back		Right	Left
Symmetrical	Leg lengths		
Asymmetrical	Thigh circumferences		
	Calf circumferences		
Motion	Straight-leg raising test		
Complete	Patellar reflex		
Restriction	Achilles reflex		
	Great toe extensor strength		
Spasm	Sensation		
Yes			
No	Areas of palpable tenderness		
Gait			
Normal	Digital rectal examination		
Cautious			
Limp			
List			
Heels			
Right			
Left			
Toes			
Right			
Left			

drome disorders. Reliance on this system will permit the physician to treat and help most of the patients whose clinical findings place them in this category. As his experience grows, he will find that he develops confidence in his own ability to manage these disorders.

Physical Examination

The patient must be completely disrobed for this examination. Disposable paper gowns that open down the back are ideally suited for this purpose.

A glance at Table 38–1 will indicate the outline of the routine that is followed. With a copy of this list kept at hand during the examination, the physician will find that he has only to circle the findings that apply.

Symmetrical versus Asymmetrical. The patient is first examined while standing erect with his back to the examiner. Either the overall spine and back area has a balanced (symmetrical) appearance or it does not (Fig. 38–32). The examiner records his opinion by circling the correct designation and moves on to the next item.

Motion (Restricted versus Complete). Motion is determined next. The patient is

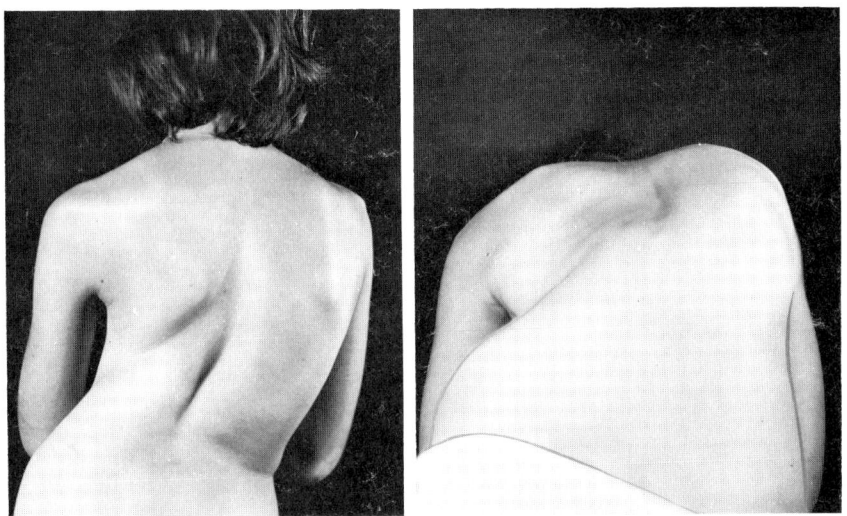

Figure 38-32. *Asymmetry of the spine accentuated in the posterior thorax with patient flexed. (From Gartland, J. J.: Fundamentals of Orthopaedics, 2nd Ed. Philadelphia, W. B. Saunders Co., 1974, p. 303.)*

asked to bend as far to the right and left (lateral bending) as he can. In addition, he is requested to touch his toes (flexion) and bend backwards as far as possible (hyper-extension) (Fig. 38–33). A rough estimate of restriction of motion is made and recorded.

Spasm. Next, the presence or absence of spasm is determined. It may have already

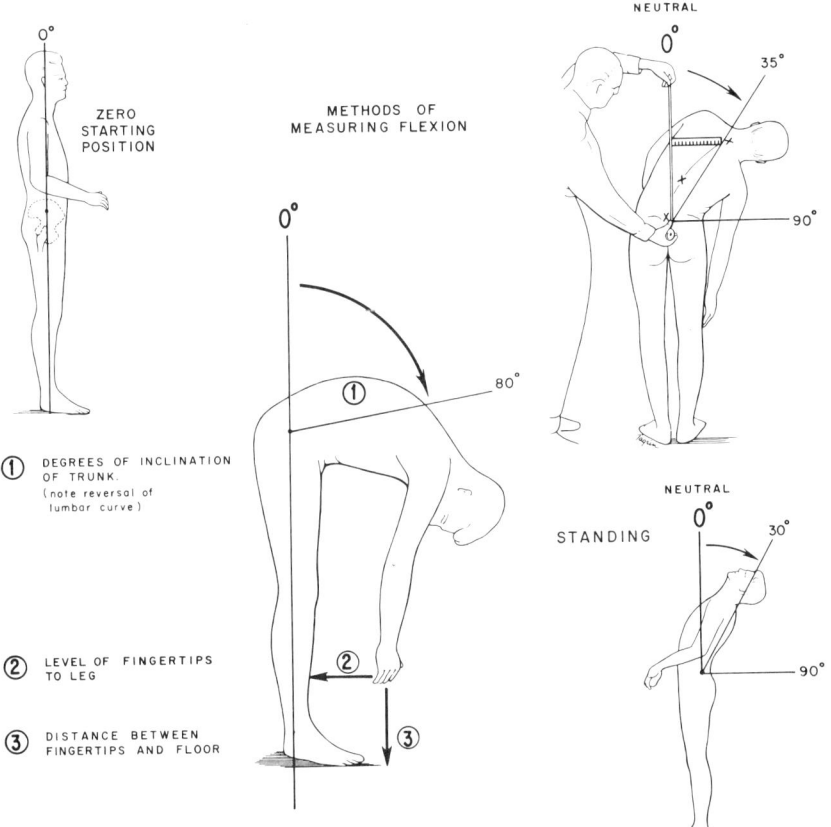

Figure 38-33. *Movements of the spine. (Courtesy of American Academy of Orthopaedic Surgeons.)*

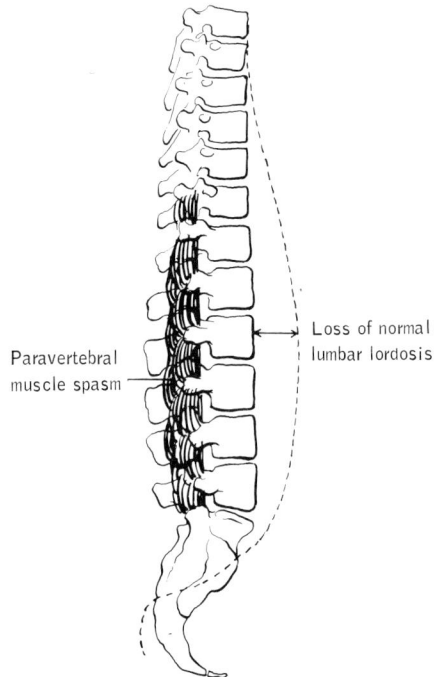

Figure 38–34. *Paravertebral muscles in spasm. (From Gartland, J. J.: Fundamentals of Orthopaedics. 2nd Ed. Philadelphia, W. B. Saunders Co., 1974, p. 311.)*

been detected during the evaluation of the symmetry of the back or during the analysis of motion of the spine. Muscle (paravertebral) spasm obliterates the lumbar lordosis and often elevates the side of the pelvis, thus producing a list to either side (Figs. 38–34 and 38–35). It may also force the back into a fixed flexion attitude. Muscle spasm is recorded as being present or absent. It is completely involuntary in nature.

The paravertebral muscles act as "guy wires" in holding the trunk erect. The upright position of the spine provides a normal stimulus for their postural tone. In the prone position they are completely flaccid. They also act protectively in that a painful stimulus will initiate paravertebral muscle spasm, which restricts motion of the low-back area, preventing further damage.

Gait. Evaluation of gait is important in adding information to the total picture. A patient with a "foot drop" due to nerve root compression will exhibit a limp entirely different from that of a patient who walks with a list to one side as a result of acute back pain with secondary paravertebral muscle spasm. Some experience with these

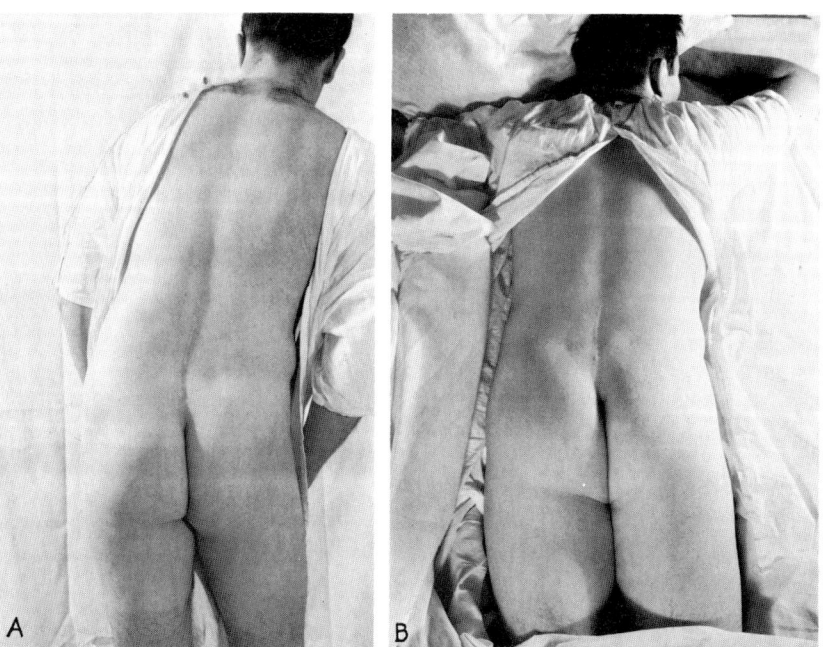

Figure 38–35. *A, Paravertebral muscle spasm obliterates normal lordosis and tilts pelvis. B, Spasm is absent in relaxed prone position. (From Gartland, J. J.: Fundamentals of Orthopaedics. 2nd Ed. Philadelphia, W. B. Saunders Co., 1974, p. 319.)*

conditions will quickly enable the physician to decide what type of gait the patient demonstrates.

Heels and Toes. Heel-toe gait is tested to search for weakness of muscle groups. Thus, a patient who could walk on the toes of the right foot but not on the heel would be demonstrating weakness of the right dorsiflexor muscle group. If the reverse were true for the left lower extremity, it would indicate weakness of the plantar-flexor muscle group of the left lower extremity.

Leg Lengths. Leg lengths are measured as described earlier (page 569). The patient is asked to climb onto the examination table, and he remains there until the conclusion of the examination. Inequality of leg lengths may be related to pelvic tilt, curvature of the spine, and other conditions.

Thigh and Calf Circumferences. These are determined with the measuring tape and recorded in inches. A position is selected about midthigh level and the measurement taken. The opposite thigh is measured by sliding the tape directly across at the same level and again measuring its circumference. Similar measurements are made of the calf.

In the absence of prior poliomyelitis or knee disease, a loss of circumference indicates muscle wasting, usually attributable to long-standing nerve root compression, especially in the L4–L5 interspace level if the thigh alone is involved. In L5–S1 disc herniation there is often some atrophy of the calf muscles on the same side.

Straight-Leg Raising Test. This is one of the pivotal determinations in the entire examination. When positive, it is an unfailing sign of nerve root compression, and when negative, it almost completely eliminates this entity from consideration.

It is performed with the patient lying supine. The extended leg is gradually flexed on the trunk at the hip by the examiner. One of the examiner's hands should stabilize the knee in complete extension throughout the test (Fig. 38–36). This maneuver stretches the sciatic nerve of the leg being tested. The test is positive if it reproduces or aggravates the pain in the anatomic distribution of the sciatic nerve. It is negative if it produces pure back pain or discomfort due to hamstring muscle tightness. When the disc is herniated, the

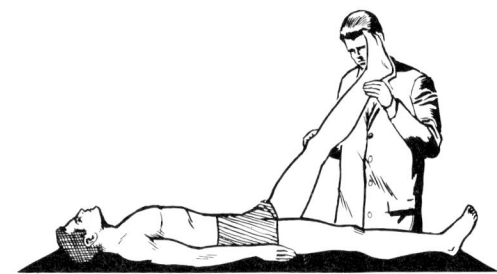

Figure 38–36. *Straight-leg raising test.* (From Gartland, J. J.: Fundamentals of Orthopaedics. 2nd Ed. Philadelphia, W. B. Saunders Co., 1974, p. 317.)

straight-leg raising test tenses the nerve root over the disc protrusion and causes the pain.

An intervertebral disc is composed of a central mucoid gel (the nucleus pulposus) and a tough fibrocartilaginous outer shell (the anulus fibrosus). It functions as a shock absorber. When the disc becomes herniated, it is nothing more than a fibrogranular mass compressing the nerve root.

Patellar and Achilles Reflexes. These reflexes are tested bilaterally with the standard reflex hammer and the results compared. With sufficient compression of the first sacral nerve root, for example, the Achilles reflex will be decreased or absent. The reflexes are never increased in any nerve root compression syndrome.

Great Toe Extensor Strength. This is determined bilaterally by having the patient simultaneously move the great toes in the direction of his head as vigorously as possible. The examiner then attempts to push the toes in the opposite direction by placing his thumb nails against the nails of the great toes and applying force.

Any significant weakness is immediately evident. If the result is borderline, consider the test as negative. Record the weakness as present or absent and ignore any degrees of strength between these determinants. Weakness of the great toe extensor muscle points to a nerve root compression at the level of the fifth lumbar nerve root on the involved side.

Sensation. Sensation to pinprick is tested completely over both lower extremities, and comparisons are made one with the other.

Decreased pinprick sensation over the great toe would incriminate the fifth lumbar nerve root on the involved side. Decreased

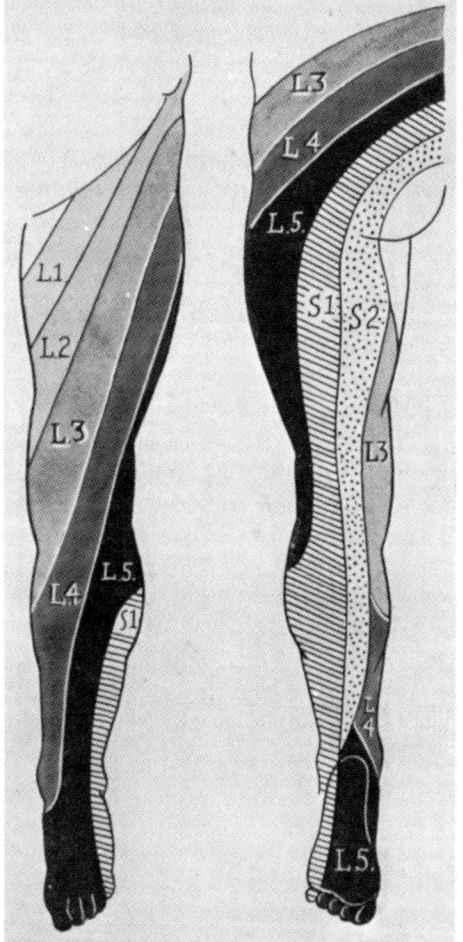

Figure 38–37. *The dermatomes of the leg. (Modified from Keegan, In Wiles, P.: Essentials of Orthopaedics. 2nd Ed. Boston, Little, Brown & Co., 1956, p. 88.)*

sensation over the heel or lateral aspect of the foot or the fifth toe would point to the first sacral nerve root as the site of compression. Normal pinprick sensation would help rule out nerve root compression syndromes. In addition, in L5–S1 herniation, sensory loss may be detected over the anterior aspect of the involved lower leg as well as of the outer three toes (Fig. 38–37).

Areas of Palpable Tenderness. These are determined with the patient lying prone. The examiner then proceeds to press upon the spinous processes and the intervertebral disc spaces. The L4–L5 disc lies at the level of the iliac crest. Incidentally, the two dimples in the skin over the sacroiliac joints help to locate the level of the L5–S1

interspace. More than 80 per cent of disc disorders occur in the L4–L5 area.

To complete the evaluation, the examiner should palpate the course of the sciatic nerve through the buttocks, trochanteric region, posterior thigh, popliteal space, calf, and over any other remaining points of pain reference indicated by the patient. Naturally, tenderness over the sciatic nerve root and its distributions indicates the presence of some nerve root compression.

Digital Rectal Examination. This is the final portion of the physical examination and should never be omitted in low-back disorders. Its importance in detecting carcinoma of the bowel or prostate cannot be overemphasized.

DISC DIAGNOSIS

Refer to Table 38–2. If the majority of the findings listed in this table are detected during the physical examination, the examiner is justified in concluding that he is dealing with a ruptured lumbar disc. He may then ask further leading questions (examples of which follow) to sketch in the history. *However, based on these physical findings alone, he can make a diagnosis of disc-like syndrome.*

When the diagnosis is made, the patient should be referred quickly to an orthopedic or neurosurgical specialist for further, definitive treatment.

The following findings are supplemental and may be present in many other conditions and therefore are not diagnostically helpful in the disc-like syndrome: inequality of leg length, asymmetry of the back, restriction of lumbar spine motion, gait disturbances, and so forth.

TABLE 38–2. SKELETONIZED FORMAT IN DISC DIAGNOSIS

1. Positive straight-leg raising test.
2. Weakness of great toe extensor strength.
3. Decreased pinprick sensation over the L4, L5, or S1 skin dermatomes.
4. Diminished or absent Achilles or patellar tendon reflexes.
5. Palpable tenderness over the course of the sciatic nerve.
6. Loss of thigh or calf circumference in the absence of other disease.

Additional History in Disc Syndromes

The following types of questions will prove helpful in adding to the understanding of the condition being diagnosed. They are not essential to the diagnosis or management of disc-like syndromes, however.

How far down your leg does the pain travel? Does the pain travel into the heel? As far as the fifth toe? Does it travel down to the toe exclusively? Is there a "pins and needles" feeling (paresthesia) that travels with the pain? Is there any paresthesia present at all? Is there any numbness (absence of feeling)? Are there any shock-like or electric sensations in the leg? Has the leg ever dragged or does the foot slap the pavement when you walk? Has the voiding pattern changed with the onset of pain? Is there increased frequency or difficulty in voiding? Does coughing or sneezing aggravate the leg pain?

LOW-BACK SYNDROME

Classification of the remaining variety of back disorders under the low-back syndrome category is necessary for orderly discussion. It is of necessity a clinical classification because there is insufficient knowledge to formulate as broad a classification based entirely on etiology or pathology. The distinctions that follow are made for convenience in treatment because there is often considerable overlap in the symptoms and clinical findings.

1. Acute lumbosacral sprain.
2. Unstable lumbosacral mechanism.
3. Degenerative lumbosacral change.

Acute Lumbosacral Sprain

This is the most common cause of low-back pain. Traumatic force applied in the lumbosacral area may cause a sprain, fracture, or dislocation. It is important to remember that the forces that are acting in this region are different from those acting on other joints because of the weight-bearing role of this structure. For example, a lifting force applied with the spine bent forward would concentrate its effect exclusively at the lumbosacral junction. Likewise, a force applied with the spine twisted or rotated would produce partial tearing of the paravertebral muscles, lumbar fascia, and in-

terspinous ligaments in a more oblique manner.

Whatever the force application and direction, the end result has to be "soft tissue injury" by definition.

Pain may be of rapid onset. However, there is frequently a lag, varying from hours to days, between the time of the trauma and the clinical symptoms, and therefore the cause is often quite unknown. Occasionally, in retrospect it is determined that there was some type of twisting or lifting injury to the low back.

The symptoms may seem unusually severe in relation to the clinical findings. This is because of the intense paravertebral muscle spasm that is initiated by the stimulus of pain in this area.

Following the "skeletonized" physical examination described in Table 38–1, if the examiner's results closely parallel those in Table 38–3, he is justified in making a diagnosis of acute lumbosacral sprain.

To document his records and add to his personal knowledge, the physician may wish to ask the following types of questions: Was there a lifting or twisting injury? How many days or hours passed between the stress and the onset of symptoms? Does lying completely flat and motionless relieve the symptoms? Is there a history of prior "sprained back," "sacroiliac sprain," "subluxation," or "slipped vertebra"? Does coughing or sneezing aggravate the pain? (If it does, it does not necessarily imply the presence of a disc-like lesion.) Does the pain radiate? (It often radiates upward toward the neck with a severe degree of paravertebral muscle spasm.)

TABLE 38–3. ACUTE LUMBOSACRAL SPRAIN

1. Asymmetry due to paravertebral muscle spasm.
2. Restricted lumbosacral motion (proportional to spasm present).
3. "List" type of gait, often present with unilateral elevation of pelvis.
4. Negative neurologic examination.
5. Negative x-rays. Occasionally a congenital defect is noted, but it is of no consequence.
6. All findings disappear with the patient prone and relaxed on the examination table.
7. Straight-leg raising test produces back pain, not sciatic pain.

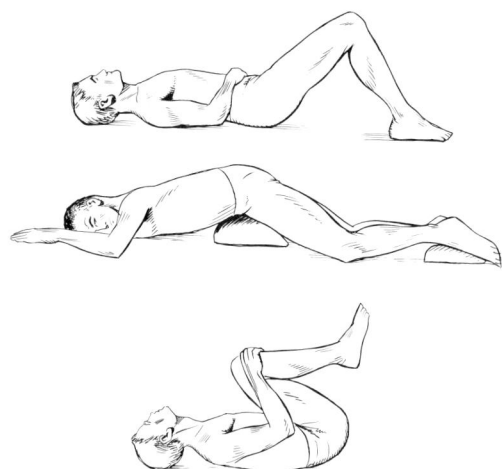

Figure 38–38. Initial exercises for acute lumbo-sacral sprain. Assume each illustrated position in sequence for periods of 3 minutes each, 4 times a day.

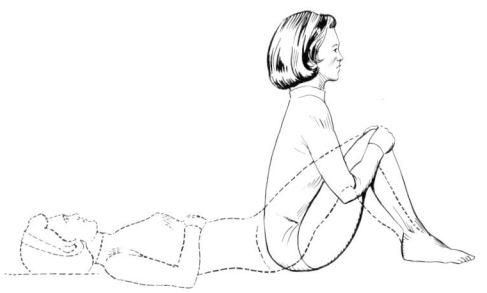

Figure 38–39. Exercise to prevent recurrence of acute lumbosacral sprain. Lie on floor. Keep knees bent throughout. Have someone, or a weighted object, put pressure on top of feet to stabilize. Come to erect position. Repeat for total of five situps once daily.

Treatment during the acute phase consists of removing the stimulus for paravertebral muscle spasm. Since the upright posture produces the normal physiologic stimulus for paravertebral muscle tone, it must be removed when a disorder causes increase in the intensity of this tone. Thus, the patient must be placed at complete and strict bed rest.

Propoxyphene hydrochloride, aspirin, phenacetin, and caffeine (Darvon Compound-65) or a similar analgesic is given every 6 hours during the first 48 to 72 hours unless the pain is relieved earlier.

During the second day, if the patient is able to move freely in bed, he may be permitted limited bathroom privileges.

By the third day, the exercises shown in Figure 38–38 are begun in bed. Each one is performed in sequence 3 times a day.

A daily, hot soaking tub bath of about 15 minutes' duration is begun at this time and is continued for the following 7 days.

At about the third or fourth day, muscle relaxants are substituted for analgesics. Such compounds as meprobamate, 400 mg., or chlordiazepoxide, 5 mg., 3 times a day are appropriate for at least 5 to 7 days.

As the pain and spasm fade, the patient is permitted to resume full activity.

For future prophylaxis as well as maintenance of improvement, on the tenth day the patient is started on the exercise shown in Figure 38–39. He is instructed to perform this daily at one sitting and is advised to continue it indefinitely.

Hospitalization is not necessary for the treatment of this problem, but if the patient happens to be hospitalized, the program just outlined can be accomplished by referring the patient to the physical therapy department. The prescription reads as follows: Moist heat and Williams' flexion exercise program twice daily for 5 days. The predictable results will be the same as those obtained at home.

In treating this condition it is essential to remember that the normal stimulus for paravertebral muscle tone is the erect position. Normal paravertebral muscle tone is present, then, only in the standing position. Spasm is merely a marked exaggeration of normal tone initiated by the stimulus of painful trauma and maintained by the stimulus of the upright position. Thus, ambulation activities prolong the pain and, alternatively, absolute bed rest promotes the rapid remission of the symptoms.

Unstable Lumbosacral Mechanism

This is a condition in which there is a "structural" weakness at the lumbosacral junction that gives rise to acute or chronic low-back pain because the paravertebral muscles have decompensated.

This joint must be able to meet the mechanical demands placed upon it. In the presence of one or more of the many types of congenital anomalies, it is structurally weakened to the point that it is unable to fulfill this role.

To understand this condition better, consider it first as an instability resulting from movement taking place between the fourth and fifth lumbar vertebrae or the fifth lumbar vertebra and the sacrum. This type of displacement usually occurs in a forward direction during flexion of the spine. The normal position is restored by extension of the spine. When displacement occurs in the backwards direction, it is referred to as a "reverse spondylolisthesis."

There is no defect of the pars interarticularis, as occurs in true spondylolisthesis, but a combination of some type of disc derangement and an abnormality of the neural arch is held responsible for the shearing movement that occurs.

Another condition is this category that deserves consideration is the "sprung back." It is due to a forgotten injury that produced a partial or complete rupture of the supra- and interspinous ligaments. These partial tears often heal with scar tissue that is painful when placed under tension. Complete rupture leaves an attenuated ligament that remains as a permanent weakness. This permits recurrence of the low-back pain at frequent intervals.

The lumbosacral joint is also potentially weak. When functional demands placed on it exceed its strength, the patient becomes symptomatic and presents with an acute or chronic low-back condition.

The precipitating factors that cause paravertebral muscle decompensation may be increasing age, sedentary occupation, prolonged bed rest, gradual loss of muscle tone due to overweight and underactivity, and unexpected temporary overexertion involving the low-back muscles.

Whether the patient with these unstable mechanisms will present to the examiner with acute back symptoms or chronic back symptoms depends on the state of the paravertebral muscles. If the paravertebral muscles still retain enough tone to go into a good spasm, then the finding will be compatible with those described previously under acute lumbosacral sprain.

However, if the paravertebral muscles have become weakened by constant effort to stabilize the lumbosacral joint, they will have become flat and wasted in appearance, and the presenting symptoms will then be those of a chronic back sprain. There will be a constant low-back pain of comparatively low intensity relieved by rest but recurring at frequent intervals.

The pain in this type of syndrome is annoying rather than severe. It is described as a dull or nagging ache. It is made worse by bending or lifting or working in a stooped position, as is necessary with much housework. Likewise, sitting or standing for long periods with the back unsupported will aggravate the symptoms.

Myofascial pain is common in the chronic phase of this condition. This type of pain develops at places where muscle fibers arise from bone or fascia without intervening tendon. The common sites are in relationship to the extensor muscles of the back especially at the origins of the glutei muscles from the dorsum of the ilium and the margins of the sacrum. Also involved are the origins of the paravertebral muscles from the dorsum of the sacrum and the iliac crests.

Myofascial pain accounts for the complaints of pain spreading to the buttocks, anterior thigh, and groin and along the lateral aspects of the thigh to the knee. This radiation is along muscular and ligamentous distributions and does not follow true nerve pathways.

At the conclusion of the examination, if the majority of findings concur with those listed in Table 38–4 the examiner should consider that he is dealing with an unstable lumbosacral mechanism.

Further questioning to clarify details might include the following: Is there a history of chronic low-back pain or repeated episodes of acute low-back pain? Is there a

TABLE 38–4. UNSTABLE LUMBOSACRAL MECHANISM (Ages 15 to 45)

1. Asymmetry, restricted lumbosacral motion, "list" type of gait if paravertebral muscle spasm is present in *the acute phase.*
2. Normal symmetry and gait and a functional range of motion are present, but the paravertebral muscles are flat and atrophic in *the chronic phase.*
3. Constant tenderness over the supraspinous ligament between the fifth lumbar vertebra and sacrum.
4. Negative neurologic examination.
5. X-ray evidence of congenital anomaly or of signs of undue pressure, such as thinning of the disc space.
6. Myofascial pain radiation more common. Does not follow true nerve pathways.

history of an asymptomatic back with the addition of some recent precipitating stress such as increased weight, gradual loss of muscle tone due to sedentary habits, and so forth? Is there a history of weakness, pain, and fatigue following periods of standing or sitting? Is there constant aching or soreness localized to the lumbosacral junction?

Treatment consists of two phases. It is directed first toward relieving the spasm syndrome if present and, second, toward strengthening the unstable joint mechanism.

The acute phase is treated as described in detail in the prior section, Acute Lumbosacral Sprain. In addition, one other element of treatment might be added. If there is a significant area of palpable tenderness at the level of the fifth lumbar vertebra and sacral areas with the patient lying prone, the examiner might consider the injection of 10 cc. of 1 per cent procaine into this area. The injection is made into the site of maximal palpable tenderness, which is the interspinous ligament area between the fifth lumbar vertebra and the sacrum. This often relieves the local pain temporarily and promotes more rapid recovery.

When the spasm has subsided, it is often not practical to do more than give advice as to how sprain may be avoided. Reference 14 in the bibliography lists a pamphlet covering this topic.

Treatment of the chronic phase is directed toward strengthening the low-back area. This assumes that the spasm, if once present, is completely gone. It consists of the performance of hyperextension spinal exercises directed toward strengthening the paravertebral muscles to the point that they can act as an internal brace (Fig. 38–40). These exercises should be performed intensively for a period of 6 months and then tapered to a minimum, as directed. They are performed 3 times a day for periods of 3 to 5 minutes total time.

A small group of patients will not get complete relief from the exercise program. Some cannot or will not stay with the program. A firm lumbosacral support will be found helpful for these particular patients. More rigid types of braces that prevent all motion in this area are not indicated. It must be remembered that extrinsic support of the back muscles weakens them, and a brace is therefore a poor compromise at best.

Patients not adequately controlled by any of the measures just described should be referred for evaluation for possible lumbosacral fusion.

Degenerative Lumbosacral Change

The lumbar spine is a common site of degenerative change (osteoarthritis). This process may be part of a generalized disease or localized to one spinal segment (usually the area between the fifth lumbar vertebra and the sacrum) as the result of repeated local trauma or occupational stresses over long periods of time.

Complaints are of stiffness in the morning upon arising or of pain and stiffness following inactivity, such as prolonged sitting. Motion relieves the stiffness and discomfort. In the early stages of the syndrome, these patients prefer actual work. With the passage of time, however, they find that prolonged activity reproduces the pain.

Pain does not usually interfere with sleep, but with progression of the disease, it might be troublesome. Cold, damp weather frequently aggravates the discomfort.

Many of these patients have the myofascial pain radiation described for the unstable lumbosacral mechanism syndrome. Occasionally a troublesome trochanteric bursitis may also be present. Rarely, true nerve pathway radiation is present. This occurs only when one of the degenerative spurs impinges directly on an adjacent nerve root.

Based on the presence of the findings in Table 38–5, the examining physician is

TABLE 38–5. DEGENERATIVE LUMBOSACRAL CHANGE (Ages 55 to 80)

1. Paravertebral muscle spasm is rare.
2. Lumbosacral motion decreased by stiff, tight lumbar spine; paravertebral muscles flat and atrophic.
3. Cautious type of gait may be present owing to presence of generalized osteoarthritis (affecting knees and so forth).
4. Negative neurologic examination unless spur impinges on nerve root.
5. X-ray shows narrowing of lumbar spaces, dense sclerotic vertebral body margins, spur formation, and often some osteoporosis of the entire lumbar spine.
6. Myofascial pain radiation often present but not as intense or as involved as that found in an unstable lumbosacral mechanism syndrome.

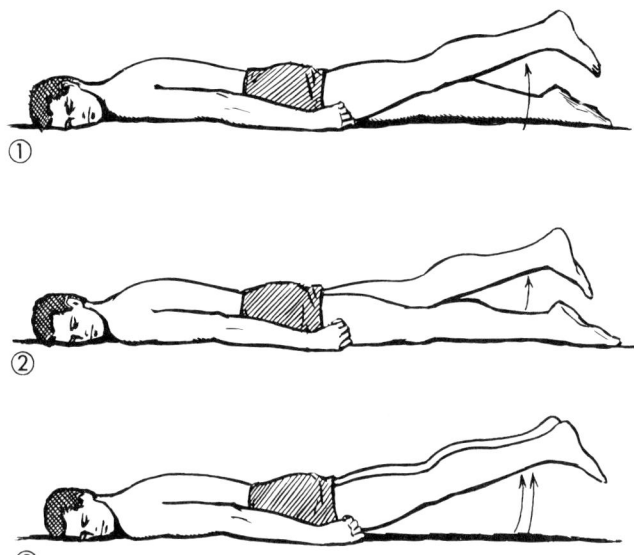

Figure 38-40. *Muscle-strengthening back exercises. Perform this sequence for 3 minutes 3 times a day for 6 months. (From Gartland, J. J.: Fundamentals of Orthopaedics. 2nd Ed. Philadelphia, W. B. Saunders Co., 1974, p. 322.)*

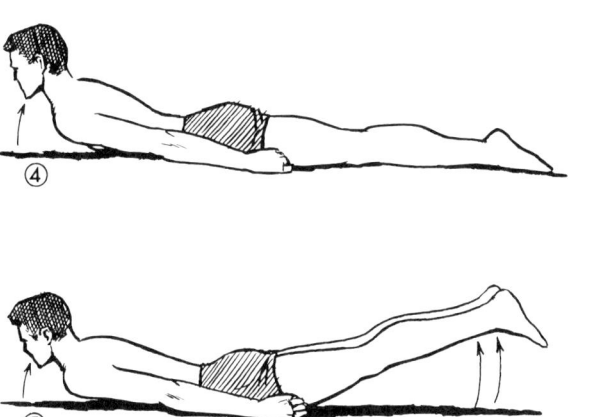

justified in making the diagnosis of degenerative disease of the lumbosacral spine.

Treatment is primarily directed toward the stiffness, if this appears to be the major component of the syndrome. For this, medication such as indomethacin is prescribed in doses of 25 to 50 mg. given 3 times a day after meals and at bedtime with some milk or other food. See official package insert for precautions in using indomethacin.

Once improvement is noted, the drug should be reduced to a maintenance level, which is that amount just necessary to maintain the improvement. This does not mean that all symptoms will disappear, but a reasonable amelioration of symptoms can be expected.

Enteric-coated sodium salicylate in doses of 0.3 to 0.6 gram (5 to 10 grains) may be given 3 times a day if the pain component bothers the patient more than the stiffness. Again, this dosage should be reduced to maintenance levels once improvement has been achieved.

Judicious exercise such as that shown in Figure 38-41 should be performed on a daily basis to maintain muscle tone and mobility. Local measures such as hot tub baths and massage will be beneficial during periods of prolonged stiffness.

Bracing should be avoided unless absolutely necessary. If the pain and stiffness are of such magnitude as to prevent the patient from participating in the activities of daily

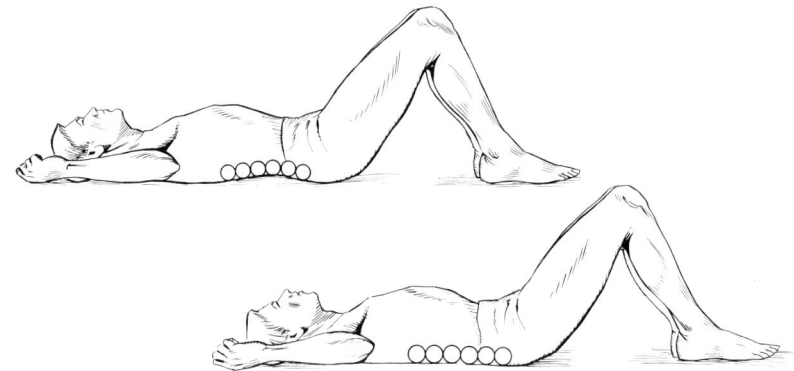

Figure 38–41. *Exercise for degenerative lumbosacral change. Relax with your arms above your head and your knees bent. Now tighten the muscles of your lower abdomen and your buttocks at the same time so as to flatten your back against the mat. This is the* **flat back position.** *Hold the position for a count of 10. Relax and repeat the exercise.*

living, a specially prescribed "chair back" brace should be considered. This brace is made from light aluminum and will provide sufficient rigid fixation of the lumbosacral spine to permit ambulation.

Surgery is rarely necessary in this condition unless nerve root impingement is present, and removal of the offending spur or decompression of the bony exit canal will eliminate the source of discomfort.

DISORDERS OF THE NECK AND THORAX

The use of the "skeletonized" physical examination, outlined in Table 38–6, is recommended for evaluation of neck and thorax disorders. Based on the positive findings, the physician can decide whether

TABLE 38–6. SCHEME OF EXAMINATION

		Right	Left
Neck	Arm circumference		
Symmetrical	Forearm circumference		
Asymmetrical	Biceps reflex		
	Brachioradialis reflex		
Motion	Triceps reflex		
Complete	Grip strength (hand)		
Restricted	Interosseous muscle function (hand)		
	Interosseous muscle wasting (hand)		
Spasm	Pinprick sensation (upper extremities)		
Yes			
No			

to classify the problem as *acute neck sprain, chronic neck sprain,* or *cervical disc rupture.* Once the problem is classified, the physician can then delve for further details with appropriate tests, or he can refer the patient, depending on his particular training and interests.

Pain is the symptom that brings the patient to the physician's office. Treatment must be designed for its relief, as well as for restoration of function. An attempt should be made especially in these cases to explain the situation to the patient in simple language and on the basis of mechanical derangement. It should be emphasized that relief can be given but that there will be recurrences from time to time.

In all of these disorders, the patient should be taught how to protect his neck to reduce exacerbation of his symptoms. It is true that some patients resist teaching and that some cannot learn, but the attempt must be made by the physician.

Acute Cervical Sprain (Stiff Neck)

Frequently, an acute cervical sprain starts insidiously. It is often noted on awakening in the morning as slight stiffness and pain. The patient usually attributes it to "sleeping in a draft." Symptoms then progress during the next few hours, and the pain becomes so severe that there is difficulty in even turning over in bed. The onset may also follow an auto accident in which the patient's vehicle is struck unexpectedly from the rear. It may also follow some routine but abrupt movement of the neck.

TABLE 38-7. ACUTE CERVICAL SPRAIN
(Stiff Neck)

1. Very often asymmetrical.
2. Motion severely restricted (early stages).
3. Spasm of all neck muscles (severe).
4. No change in arm girth, reflexes, or grip strength of hand.
5. Negative neurologic examination.
6. X-rays are negative except in children, in which they may reveal "ragging."

In children it often follows a minor injury such as might occur in wrestling or diving, and occasionally it develops in conjunction with acute tonsillitis or other febrile illnesses.

Examination (see Tables 38–6 and 38–7) shows the head and neck to be held more to one side than to the other (asymmetry). This finding is readily apparent at a glance.

Cervical motion shows varying restriction (Fig. 38–42). Most of the loss will be in the direction of right or left bending. Flexion usually causes pain but if the patient is coaxed carefully by the physician, the motion will be found unrestricted. Extension likewise is usually not restricted in this condition. The patient often has to turn his whole trunk while looking to either side.

Involuntary neck muscle spasm affects all of the muscles of both sides and will be present in severe cases. In mild disorders

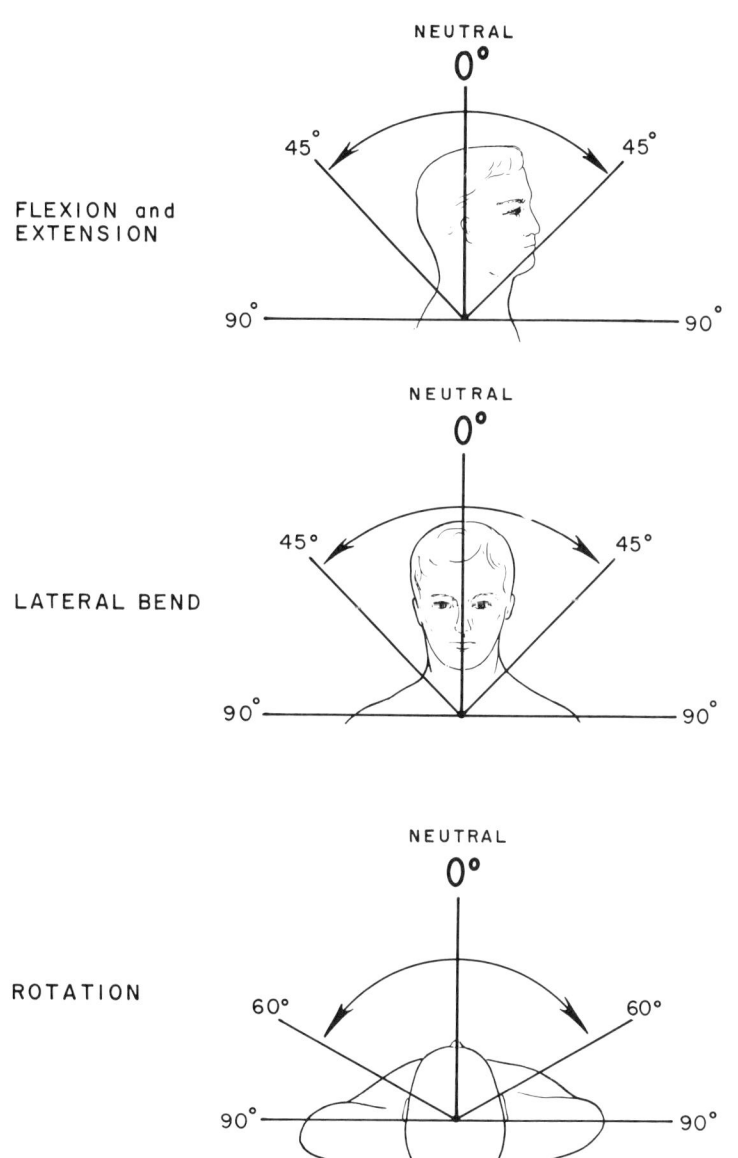

Figure 38–42. Motions of the cervical spine. (Courtesy of American Academy of Orthopaedic Surgeons.)

spasm may be limited to a small area. The stimulus for this spasm is pain, and the mechanism is similar to that previously described in the section dealing with low-back disorders.

Although pain is occasionally referred to the arms, the neurologic examination is negative, indicating that this is a subjective finding. Major protrusion of the cervical intervertebral disc is excluded by the negative neurologic findings.

X-rays exclude diseases of the vertebra. However, this acute sprain syndrome can be present in a rather alarming form in children. The onset is abrupt, often from a minor injury. The clinical picture, however, suggests a serious fracture or dislocation of the spine. X-ray films show only an alteration in the normal curvature of the spine. The x-ray changes routinely return to normal with the use of constant cervical traction with 5 pounds of weight for about 48 hours (Fig. 38–43).

Since this type of injury often occurs following wrestling or some type of child-hood activity, it was called "ragging" by some British orthopedists, and the name has been popular enough to remain attached to the x-ray picture of this condition in children.

In children, one must also be concerned with the dislocation of the atlas on the axis, which sometimes occurs after tonsillitis. X-ray studies will, of course, reveal this bony change. Therefore, an x-ray examination is an essential part of evaluation of cervical disorders.

Treatment may involve heat for relief of the pain. It increases the blood supply and relieves some of the muscle ischemia and spasm. Moist pads (Hydrocollator Packs) are most gratifying to the patient. These can be given in the office or in the physical therapy department.

Heat is applied for periods of 15 minutes on a daily basis for 1 week. If the patient has some difficulty getting to therapy or the office, this treatment can be given at home. A large towel is placed around the neck and shoulder and hot water from a shower is

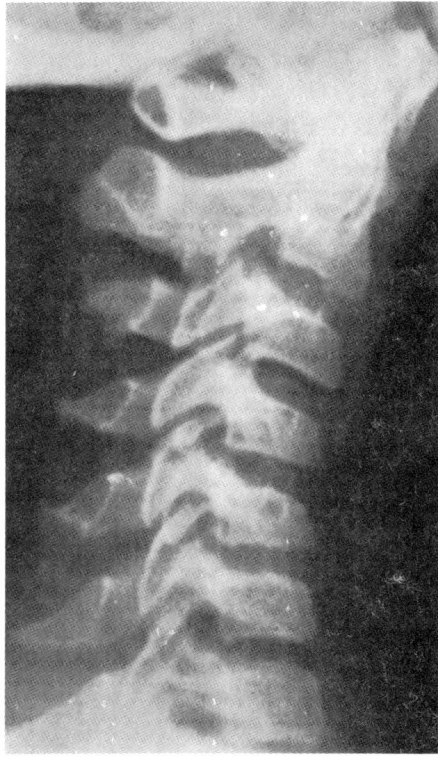 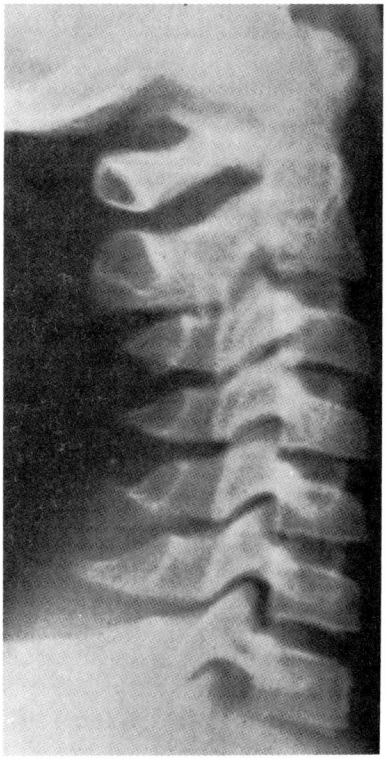

A   **B**

Figure 38–43. *Roentgenograms of "ragging injury." A, At admission. B, Following traction for 48 hours. (From Wiles, P.: Essentials of Orthopaedics. 2nd Ed. Boston, Little, Brown & Co., 1956, p. 46.)*

allowed to run over the towel for 10 minutes. Massage can be added to the treatment with moist heat if an experienced therapist is available.

Intermittent traction also relieves muscle spasm. It has a massage-like effect and prevents formation of adhesions between the nerve roots and adjacent capsular structures. A prescription for this should read as follows: 20 minute intermittent traction treatments daily for 7 days, then 3 times a week for 2 weeks, then 1 treatment weekly for 3 weeks. The range of weight is 12 to 16 pounds for females and 14 to 20 for males. For children the weight should not exceed 8 pounds. For children under age 10, continuous traction in a hospital setting is preferred. Only 5 pounds of weight is used for this type of treatment.

Immobilization in the form of a padded foam rubber cervical collar is recommended for continuous use between traction and heat treatments. It holds the neck in the optimum position for healing of the sprained ligaments and capsular structures. The neck must be held straight with the chin "tucked in" (Fig. 38–44). Hyperextension is definitely not recommended. These cervical collars can usually be purchased from local pharmacies or drug supply houses. The cervical collar is used until all symptoms subside. It is then gradually

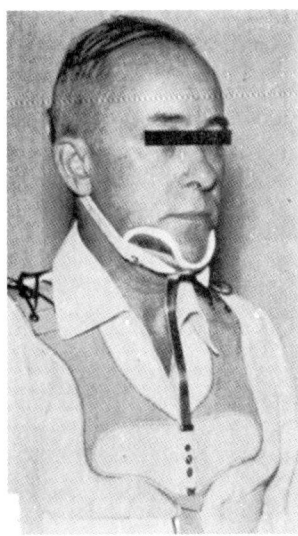

Figure 38–44. *Excellent support position for acute cervical sprain. (From Jackson, Ruth: The Cervical Syndrome, 2nd Ed., 1958. Courtesy Charles C Thomas, Publisher, Springfield, Illinois.)*

discontinued until the patient can do completely without it. It is not necessary to use the collar while sleeping.

Analgesic medication such as propoxyphene, 65 mg. given every 6 hours, is suggested for the first 72 hours. After this, a combination muscle relaxant-tranquilizer such as chlordiazepoxide can be given in the dosage of 5 mg. 3 times a day and at bedtime for the following 7 to 10 days.

Chronic Neck Sprain (Spondylosis)

Persistent pain in the neck, shoulder girdle, arm, and hand is due more often to a lesion of the cervical spine than to any other condition. It is often an intractable complaint of middle-aged and elderly people. Chronic neck sprain is a common cause of headache. It is likewise the most common cause of pain over the upper and midthoracic areas of the back.

Spondylosis is not a single, well-defined entity but a term used to described the end results of a number of different pathologic processes taking place in the intervertebral discs. It is a condition in which degeneration of the intervertebral discs is associated with changes in the bodies of adjacent vertebrae. X-ray films show narrowing of the intervertebral disc spaces with reactive lipping of the bodies and, often, sclerosis. This is quite distinct from osteoarthritis, which affects the joints and is not synonymous with disc degeneration.

Symptoms are not always related to pathologic findings. Gross x-ray changes are often present without symptoms. Likewise, symptoms may be severe when x-ray changes are slight. Correlation is often difficult because the degenerative changes develop gradually, but there may be an abrupt onset of symptoms as the result of an auto accident or other type of injury that disrupts the relationship of the nerve roots in the cervical area.

The first complaints are of pain, "paresthesia" (pins and needles or electric feelings), and weakness, occurring in that order.

Pain is often the ordinary "stiff neck" variety at first. Later, it radiates more widely to the trapezius, latissimus dorsi, or the pectoralis major muscles. It often travels from the shoulder tip down the outer side of the arm to the elbow or hand.

Myofascial pain areas are often present

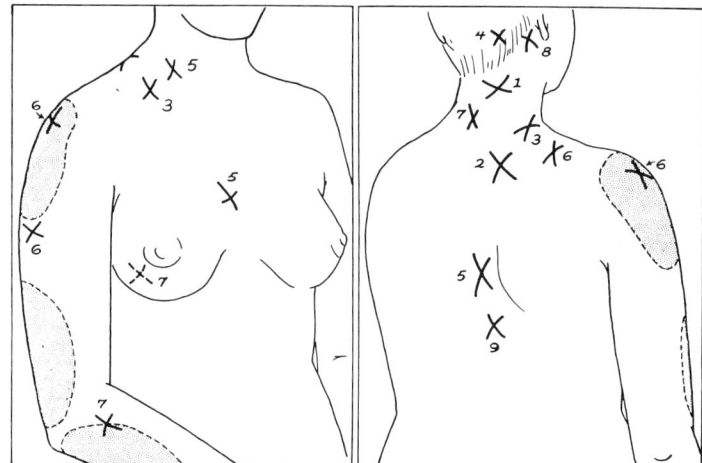

Figure 38-45. *Sites of myofascial pain in spondylosis. (From Jackson, Ruth: The Cervical Syndrome, 2nd Ed., 1958. Courtesy Charles C Thomas, Publisher, Springfield, Illinois.)*

with this syndrome (Fig. 38-45). These are mostly in the trapezius muscle and the muscles of the upper and lower thorax. Occasionally there are some areas located along the occipital ridge. Pain in these areas is continuous and made worse by worry and fatigue.

Numbness and tingling are often described in the fingers, hand, and occasionally the forearm over one or both upper extremities. There may be a constant feeling of coldness. The difficulty may be worse during the day, but it is also bothersome at night. It is often present on awakening in the morning.

Weakness is often described as "clumsiness" of the hands. Inadvertent dropping of small objects that previously produced no difficulty is also a frequent complaint. If the cervical cord becomes involved, there may be unexpected falling or difficulty in walking straight, associated with dizziness. This is not a very frequent finding, fortunately.

Patients who have been "rear-ended" in auto mishaps will often complain of "ringing in the ears," "unilateral blurring of vision," and unilateral headaches. Evaluation by a competent specialist in these fields will fail to disclose true eye or ear disorders. These complaints arise from the cervical derangement, and they will respond to treatment of the basic condition. Too often these complaints are described as "neurotic."

If the majority of findings listed in Table 38-8 are positive, the examiner has es-tablished the diagnosis of chronic neck sprain and should begin immediate treatment by placing the neck at rest.

Treatment begins with the cervical collar. Its use has been explained in the previous section. The collar is rather unpleasant to wear, but it must be worn, except for sleep, for several months. It is given up gradually as the pain subsides.

Propoxyphene, 65 mg., and chlordiazepoxide, 5 mg., may be given as outlined in the previous section.

If the collar fails to give relief or is not

**TABLE 38-8.   CHRONIC NECK SPRAIN
(Spondylosis)**

1. Neck usually symmetrical.
2. Motion moderately restricted; restricted right and left lateral bending (occasional loss of flexion and hyperextension).
3. Spasm rare unless acute injury present.
4. Reflexes may be exaggerated or decreased. If cord pressure is present, leg reflexes are increased and an extensor type of plantar response is present.
5. Grip strength may be weaker if the disorder has been present for a considerable period of time.
6. Borderline sensory changes (decreased pinprick sensation) are only occasionally present.
7. Anteroposterior, lateral, and right and left oblique x-ray films of the neck in extension and flexion show narrowing of intervertebral disc spaces: new bone encroachment on the intervertebral foramina and, often, forward shift of a vertebra on the one below it during flexion.

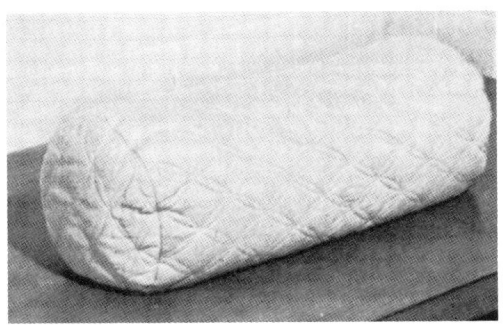

Figure 38–46. Cervical contour pillow. (From Jackson, Ruth: The Cervical Syndrome, 2nd Ed., 1958. Courtesy Charles C Thomas, Publisher, Springfield, Illinois.)

tolerated by the patient, rest in bed is then indicated. A "cervical contour" pillow is recommended (Fig. 38–46). These can be purchased from local pharmacies or drug supply houses.

Home traction kits are advised if the cervical collar cannot be used, and rest for the neck area is essential. The patient is instructed to use continuous traction with 5 pounds of weight. The head-halter type of traction is used for periods of about 2 hours, and then its use is omitted for approximately 1 hour and then resumed. The treatment is conducted basically during the day; it is not necessary during night hours. Usually, bed rest combined with the home traction program is recommended for a 2 week period unless the symptoms are relieved earlier. If some of the symptoms persist, the traction may be continued on a once-daily basis for an hour or so for several months.

These patients may also get additional relief with the application of moist heat. This can be self-administered by using a towel and a hot shower as described previously (page 586).

If the patient has shown moderate but incomplete relief following the home program and if it is not too inconvenient, he can be referred to the physical therapy department. There, intermittent cervical traction combined with moist heat can be given, using the directions listed in the prior section. However, it must be remembered that in these chronic conditions intermittent traction may aggravate the symptoms, especially when nerve roots are adherent as they often are at this phase of the disorder.

Myofascial pain areas are treated by injection. At each point of maximal tenderness, a local anesthetic agent is injected. Only monocaine solutions are recommended. The concentration of the solution should be no more than 0.5 per cent. The inadvertent injection of a 1 or 2 per cent solution into the blood stream can produce convulsions and even a fatal reaction. Inquiry should be made prior to the injection regarding sensitivity to local anesthetic agents.

The patient should be lying in a prone position for the injections. The area is cleansed with an alcohol swab. The needle is then placed into the tender area and must momentarily reproduce the pain if the procedure is to be of some help.

If the needle insertion does not reproduce or aggravate the original pain, then the injection will be of little benefit. Once the radicular or referred pain is reproduced, 5 cc. of the solution is injected in a stellate fashion. The total dosage limitations recommended by the manufacturers for the particular solution being used should not be exceeded.

Deep massage may follow these injections if an experienced therapist is available. During the recovery phase the patient may be referred to physical therapy for ultrasonic applications to the myofascial areas in preference to local anesthetic injections. This treatment is prescribed as follows: Apply ultrasound, 1 microwatt per cm², over the sites of maximal tenderness (extra spinal areas only) for 5 minute periods. Give 1 treatment every third day for a total of 11 treatments.

These myofascial areas are more difficult to clear when they are the result of pressure on the nerve roots. They should, however, be treated along with the basic disorder pathology because much relief and benefit will be derived from their elimination.

Severe pain that fails to respond to the conservative management just outlined is often an indication for surgery. Patients who reach this stage without benefit should be given a referral to an orthopedic surgeon for further evaluation.

Younger patients and those with only slight to moderate degenerative changes on x-ray examination should be instructed in proper posture and given a simple exer-

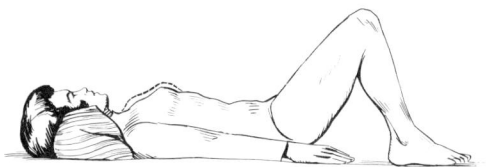

Figure 38–47. *Exercise 1, for chronic neck sprain.*

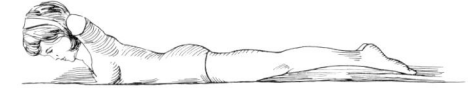

Figure 38–48. *Exercise 2, for chronic neck sprain.*

cise program that will help to prevent further episodes of either the acute or chronic disorders.

A pamphlet[15] that will prove quite helpful in explaining these disorders and their postural associations is listed in the bibliography at the end of the chapter.

Exercises should be performed on a weekly basis. *Exercise 1*, shown in Figure 38–47, should be performed for about 5 minutes every day for about 1 week. *Exercise 2*, Figure 38–48, is performed for 5 minutes of each day the following week. These exercises are then alternated week in and week out indefinitely.

Rupture of Cervical Disc

Symptoms of disc protrusion in the cervical spine frequently follow trauma and are localized most commonly at the C5–C6 and C6–C7 interspace levels, because maximal movement occurs there.

Grip strength is tested by the examiner's placing the index and middle fingers of his left hand in the patient's right hand and the index and the middle fingers of his right hand in the patient's left hand. The patient is asked to squeeze as hard as possible simultaneously with both hands. Weakness is readily discernible with this test. Any result that is questionable or borderline is disregarded. The weakness has to be obvious to be listed as a finding.

The state of the interosseous muscles is evaluated by looking at the dorsum of the hand. These muscles lie between the metacarpals and also between the thumb and index finger. When the metacarpal shafts are unusually prominent and these interosseous muscles appear to be shrunken, they are considered to be wasted.

To the experienced examiner, wasting is more readily detectable in the web space between the thumb and index finger. When

the muscles are noted to be deficient on sight, they are considered to be wasted and this is a positive finding. This atrophy is a result of interference with the C8 nerve root. Interosseous muscle function is tested by having the individual hold both hands outstretched with the dorsum of the hand facing the examiner. The patient is then asked to abduct and adduct the fingers. Any weakness or difficulty here is readily detectable.

When the findings conform to those listed in Table 38-9, the diagnosis is a ruptured disc. Many of these discs will require surgical treatment, although some will respond to cervical traction. Because of the problem of neurologic deficits such as paralysis, however, the family physician will be wise to refer this type of problem once the diagnosis has been made.

TABLE 38-9. RUPTURE OF CERVICAL DISC

1. Asymmetry. Restriction of motion and involuntary spasm are present.
2. Decrease in arm or forearm circumference present if condition present for 2 or 3 months.
3. Reflex changes as follows: Decreased biceps jerk—indicates pressure on C6 nerve root from herniation between C5 and C6. Triceps jerk absent—pressure on C7 from rupture between C6 and C7. No reflex change (pressure on C8 from rupture between C7 and T1).
4. Grip strength weaker on involved side (50 per cent).
5. Interosseous muscles wasted in hand and loss of abduction and adduction in fourth and fifth fingers (pressure on C8 nerve root from C7–T1 disc rupture).
6. Decreased to absent pinprick sensation over involved dermatome: Numbness in thumb—C6 root pressure. Numbness in index and middle fingers—C7 root pressure. Numbness in ulnar border hand and fifth finger—C8 root pressure.

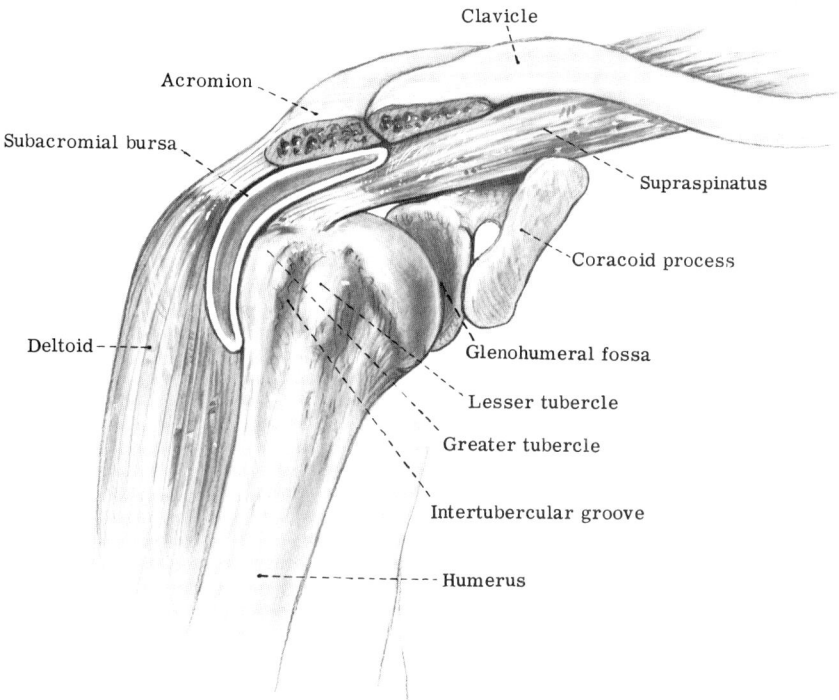

Clavicle

Acromion

Subacromial bursa

Supraspinatus

Coracoid process

Deltoid

Glenohumeral fossa

Lesser tubercle

Greater tubercle

Intertubercular groove

Humerus

Figure 38–49. Anterior aspect of shoulder joint, showing palpable landmarks and their relationship to the subacromial bursa. (From Beetham, W. P., Polley, H. F., Slocumb, C. H., et al.: Physical Examination of the Joints. Philadelphia, W. B. Saunders Co., 1965, p. 28.)

SHOULDER DISORDERS

Shoulder disorders are discussed in the order of frequency in which they will be encountered in the family physician's office. The necessary information is given for diagnosing these conditions, and additional references are listed at the end of the chapter.

The glenohumeral joint (shoulder joint) suffers from few diseases. It is a shallow ball and socket joint with a loose capsule and a wide range of movements. No part of the capsule is tense within ordinary functional range. *Sprains are therefore rare.* The multiple forces operating on the joint are usually such as to distract rather than compress it. This may explain why the shoulder joint is *rarely affected by osteoarthritis.*

Movement at the glenohumeral joint is necessarily accompanied by movement of the head of the humerus relative to the acromial process. This takes place at the "bursal joint" (Fig. 38–49). For practical purposes, then, the shoulder is a double joint, and any condition preventing movement in

one part must also prevent movement at the other part. Pain and stiffness are nearly always caused by afflictions of the bursal joint and very seldom by disorders of the glenohumeral joint.

The Stiff Shoulder (Adult)

This syndrome is more common in the fifth and sixth decades. There are a large variety of causes, and rather than attempt to isolate the individual entities it makes more sense to categorize them with one term, such as the "frozen" or "stiff" shoulder. This grouping appropriately encompasses all of these lesions because the end point of this large variety of diseases and conditions is identical.

Regardless of cause, the individual patient complains of inability to move the shoulder away from the side of the body and of severe shoulder pain. There is, in effect, an adhesion of the layers of tissue around the shoulder joint (arthrofibrosis). Any attempt by the patient to move the shoulder results in a tearing of these adhesions with additional pain. Further attempts at motion

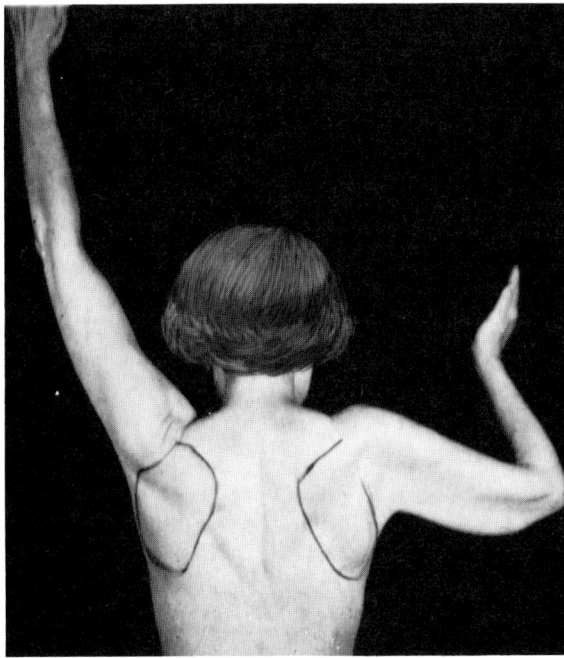

Figure 38–50. *Frozen shoulder deformity of the right shoulder. (From DePalma, A. F.: Surgery of the Shoulder. Philadelphia, J. B. Lippincott Co., 1950.)*

are then abandoned and the adhesions quickly re-form. The fact that the shoulder cannot glide through its complete range of motion is also a pain-producing factor that helps to perpetuate the cycle.

The causative factor might have been early bursitis, a partially healed rotator cuff injury, bicipital tendinitis, or any other of the variety of shoulder-joint lesions.

Physical examination establishes the fact that the patient cannot actively abduct the arm more than 15 to 20 degrees away from the side in the most severe type of case (Fig. 38–50). In more moderate conditions the patient can abduct as far as 80 degrees but no further.

This range is confirmed by the examiner, who holds one of his hands on top of the acromioclavicular joint as he faces the patient and passively lifts the involved arm. Whenever the fixation point is reached, the examiner will not be able to push the arm further because of blockage of motion and severe pain.

It is important to remember that scapulothoracic movement can be substituted for shoulder movement. Therefore, if the patient is requested to elevate the arm, motion of more than 90 degrees may take place, but this is scapulothoracic motion, not really glenohumeral (shoulder) motion. Since

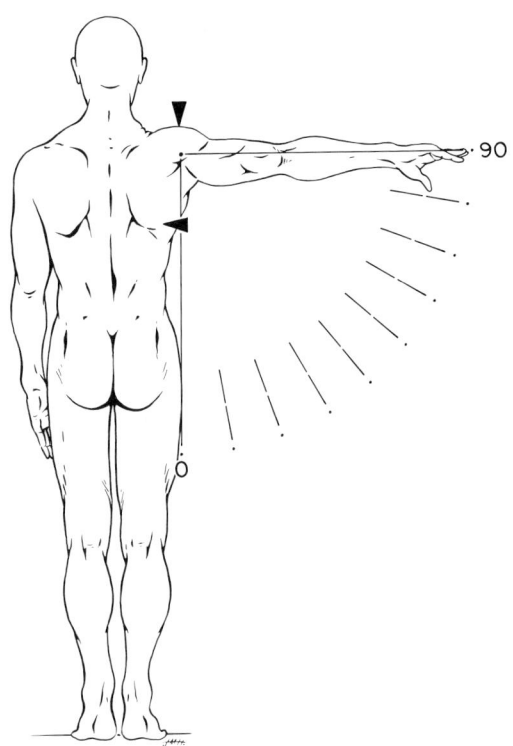

Figure 38–51. *Physical range of abduction of glenohumeral joint, with acromioclavicular and scapulothoracic joints stabilized at black triangles. (From Beetham, W. P., Polley, H. F., Slocumb, C. H., et al.: Physical Examination of the Joints. Philadelphia, W. B. Saunders Co., 1965, p. 40.)*

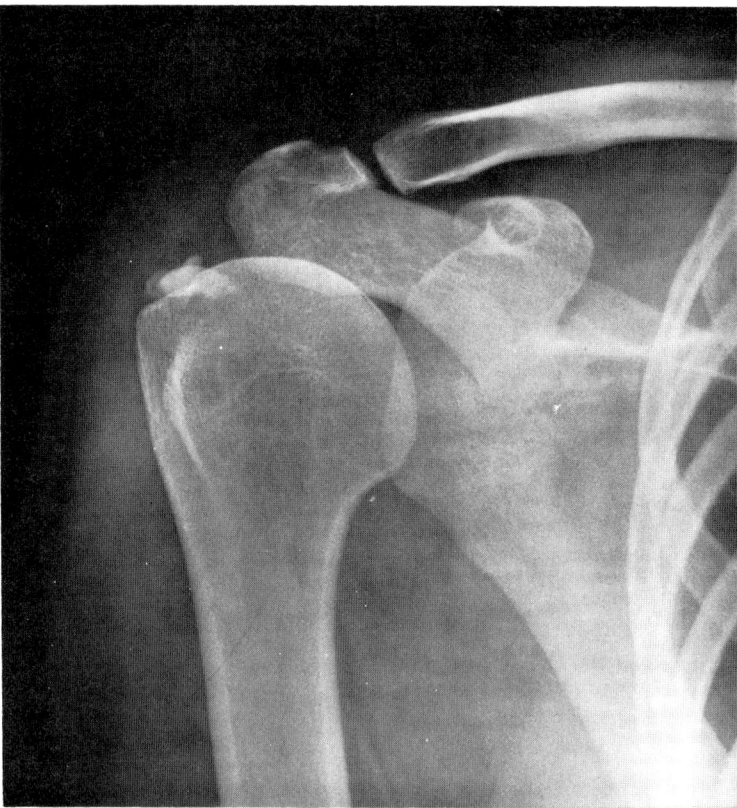

Figure 38–52. Calcium deposit in rotator cuff. (From Gartland, J. J.: Fundamentals of Orthopaedics. 2nd Ed. Philadelphia, W. B. Saunders Co., 1974, p. 230.)

these areas are rarely involved in this syndrome, the examiner must differentiate carefully to make the correct diagnosis (Fig. 38–51).

As a second finding, the patient lacks external rotation, especially in severe cases. An attempt to passively externally rotate the shoulder with the elbow fixed at 90 degrees results in exquisite pain and blockage of further motion at this point of restriction in the shoulder.

These two findings, lack of abduction and external rotation, are sufficient to make the diagnosis of a stiff shoulder. Other movements, such as flexion, adduction, and so forth, can be tested but changes here are not really diagnostic. The shoulder joint may also show local changes such as thickening, edema, and even mild wasting of the musculature, but again these findings are not of diagnostic value in this syndrome.

X-ray studies should be requested and should include internal and external rotational views of the shoulder joint. These films may show the presence of early

calcific bursitis; they may reveal some attritional changes at the insertion of the rotator cuff group; or they may even demonstrate calcification in the bicipital groove (Fig. 38–52).

Regardless of the abnormality found on the x-ray studies, treatment must be directed first to the stiffness and pain. Further refinements, such as treatment for incompletely healed rotator cuff lesions or bicipital tendinitis, can be undertaken later if need be, but they must not pre-empt treatment for the patient's central problem, which is the frozen shoulder.

Treatment consists of phased management. During *Phase I*, the patient is taught active exercises by the examiner or by the physical therapist if one is available (Fig. 38–53). It must be emphasized that the patient has to perform these maneuvers actively even when pain is encountered. These exercises must be performed at least 3 times a day for 15 minute periods until a normal or near normal range of motion is achieved. Prescription of propoxyphene, 65

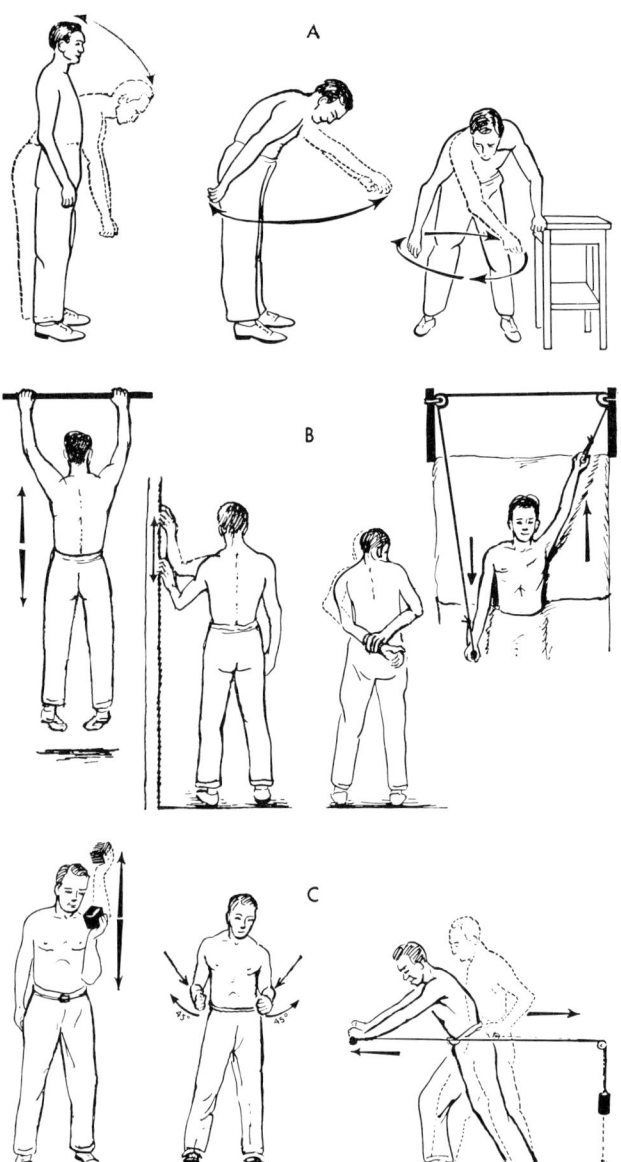

A

B

C

mg., is sufficient for the anticipated pain related to the exercise program.

If the physician is adept at giving intra-articular injections, he can inject some steroid medication into the glenohumeral joint at this time (1 cc. of betamethasone). This is not really essential to the treatment. In many cases it will produce marked reduction of the pain, but this is not completely predictable, and there may be little or no pain relief.

Many patients with shoulder pain state that they have had a "shot" many years ago for bursitis and that this is all they really require. Occasionally, rather than arguing the merits, it is easier to give the injection if one is adept at doing so.

Nothing, however, must be allowed to detract from the emphasis on the daily range of motion exercises. It may be wise to explain to the patient that the active exercise program produces tearing of the adhesions around the shoulder joint. If these range of movement exercises are not continued on a daily basis, the adhesions will re-form within a 24 hour period, and the next time the exercises are undertaken the adhesions will again have to be torn. The patient must accept the idea that only the daily performance of these exercises will prevent the adhesions from re-forming and allow the shoulder to obtain a permanent improvement in motion which, of itself, will decrease the pain.

If there is no improvement when the patient returns within 10 days for a re-evaluation, *Phase II* of the treatment program is begun. This consists of referring the patient to a physical therapy facility for ultrasound treatment. The prescription should read as follows: Apply ultrasound to the involved shoulder at the rate of 1 or 1.5 microwatts per cm² for 3 to 5 minutes. Administer this treatment every 3 days for approximately 11 treatments unless relief is obtained sooner.

At this time the patient is also started on a home program that consists basically of the "broomstick" exercise. To perform this, the patient must lie flat on the floor. A broom is placed across the front of the thighs. This broom is then picked up in both hands with the elbows locked in a straight "extended" position. The broom is lifted into the air over the patient's head and must touch the floor above the patient's head. The normal shoulder guides or pulls the diseased shoulder with it during this maneuver. Patients often require 1 to 6 weeks before they are able to touch the floor with the broom. This maneuver improves abduction and external rotation.

In addition to this exercise, it must be emphasized that the patient should continue with all normal activities, such as washing walls, reaching overhead to wash windows, and so forth. In other words, the emphasis is on activity rather than rest.

The patient is then given a follow-up appointment in 2 to 3 weeks. On the return visit, if the patient volunteers that improvement has been made and that the pain is decreasing, Phase II of the treatment program is continued for several more weeks. If there is no improvement as manifested by an incomplete recovery of motion or if the patient is not satisfied, he should be referred to an orthopedic specialist.

Usually 90 per cent of patients will respond to either Phase I or Phase II of treatment. Those patients that do not respond will require a manipulation under general anesthesia and perhaps even surgical intervention.

Deformity and Pain of the Shoulder Joint (Ages 12 to 50)

Lesions of the acromioclavicular joint are frequently found in patients between ages 12 and 50, although they are possible at older ages. They usually occur with youth and athletic activity. Although the family physician will encounter this disorder more commonly than other lesions, emphasis is only on diagnosis rather than treatment, since these are rather difficult to treat without surgical intervention.

Physical examination discloses that the acromion is pulled downward by the weight of the arm and that there is an obvious step-up of about one-half inch at the site of the joint. The distal end of the clavicle is elevated under the skin (Fig. 38–54). In less serious cases this characteristic appearance is not present, especially if only a partial rupture of the acromioclavicular joint has occurred. Usually there is pain with motion of the shoulder. Often swelling and perhaps even ecchymosis or bruising occurs.

X-ray studies will not reveal the defect when taken with the patient lying prone unless the arm is pulled downward. Should this lesion be suspected, even in mild cases, the radiologist should be requested to

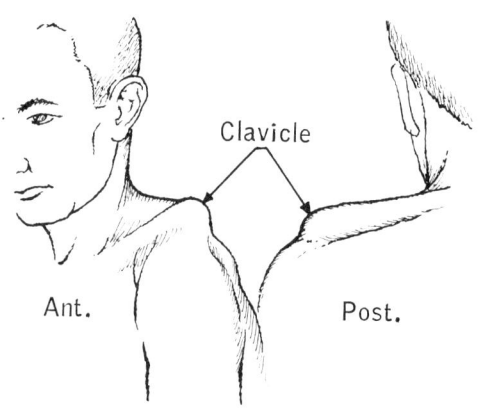

Figure 38–54. *Diagrammatic illustration of complete acromioclavicular dislocation. (Modified from DePalma, A. F.: The Management of Fractures and Dislocations: An Atlas. 2nd Ed. Philadelphia, W. B. Saunders Co., 1970, Vol. 1, p. 519.)*

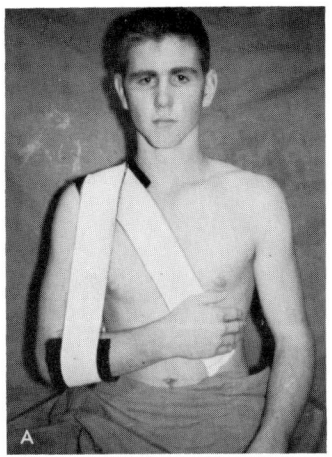 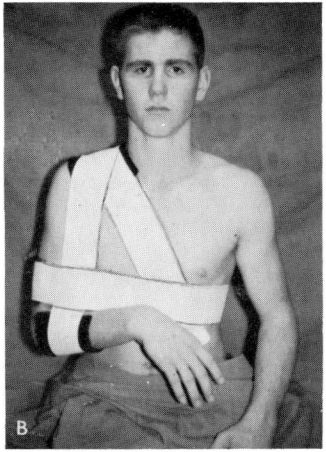 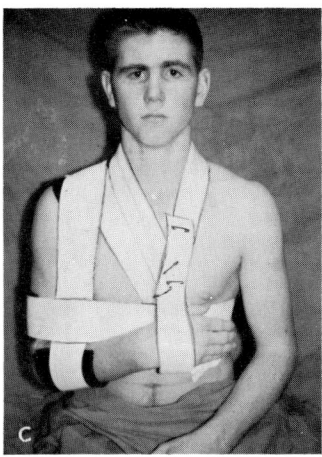

Figure 38–55. *Application of acromioclavicular dressing for mild cases.* (From O'Donoghue, D. H.: Treatment of Injuries to Athletes. 3rd Ed. Philadelphia, W. B. Saunders Co., 1976, p. 166.)

secure a standing view on both acromioclavicular joints without weight. The patient then gradually is instructed to hold 10 pounds of weight in each hand and a second x-ray film is taken. This second x-ray will demonstrate any mild subluxation. Complete dislocation does not occur unless both the coracoclavicular and coracoacromial ligaments are disrupted.

Conservative treatment consists of appropriate collar and cuff apparatus (Fig. 38–55). It is difficult to keep the young person in this apparatus and, frequently, after about 6 weeks there is little or no improvement. The pain usually subsides within a few days. In cases of mild subluxation no further treatment is needed.

When there is an obvious deformity, it is good practice to reduce the deformity during surgery and hold it transfixed with Kirschner wires while the ligaments are repaired. The wires are usually removed in 6 weeks, and the youthful patient obtains a completely functional and normal joint.

If the condition is allowed to go untreated for more than 8 to 10 weeks, repair is usually unsuccessful because there is accompanying stiffness and pain. Other reconstructive procedures may then be needed.

Too often, patients with this problem are advised that the joint is sprained and that the deformity will go away. It does not go away, and the condition becomes more symptomatic with the passage of time.

Reconstructive rather than reparative surgery is then needed. Unless the family physician is particularly interested in this aspect of orthopedics, he is urged to establish the diagnosis and then quickly refer the patient for treatment.

Painful Upper Extremity (Ages 1 to 7)

A painful upper extremity is often seen in children. The "pulled elbow" is produced by a jerk on the child's upraised arm, usually by the mother or some playmate. This results in subluxation of the radial head under the annular ligament. At this age the radial head is no greater in diameter than the shaft and can subluxate easily.

The subluxation is extremely painful and often mistaken for a more serious injury. The elbow is held stiffly in moderate flexion and the forearm in midpronation. The child screams and resists all attempts at examination.

X-ray examinations of the elbow are negative. Occasionally, the radiologic technician in attempting to get appropriate views will manipulate the elbow and reduce the subluxation.

Diagnosis is made by the fact that supination is limited. For example, if the examiner gently holds the patient's right elbow in his left hand and attempts to complete passive supination with his right hand, he will find restriction near the extreme limit of supination.

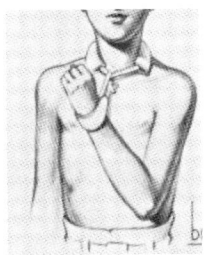

Figure 38–56. Collar and cuff in position. (From Blount, W. P.: Fractures in Children. Baltimore, The Williams & Wilkins Co., © 1955, p. 34.)

Treatment is accomplished by maneuvering the child's arm into full supination. A palpable click will be felt by the examiner's thumb if it is placed over the head of the radius. There is often an audible click associated with this maneuver. The child gives one last scream as the pain subsides.

The elbow should be immobilized in a collar and cuff for about a week or more to prevent recurrence (Fig. 38–56). Motion, however, is normal from the very minute that the subluxation is reduced, and the pain does not return.

The parents must be informed that the elbow may be easily subluxated before the child reaches age 7 if rough play or other precipitating trauma is applied to the elbow. It is important to teach the mother to perform the reduction maneuver, for, depending on circumstances, the child may go from 2 to 3 days without appropriate treatment.

Pain and Pseudoparalysis of the Arm (Child)

The common symptom of a fractured clavicle in the young child is pseudoparalysis of the arm with pain. This can easily be confused with a pulled elbow since the child tends to hold the arm at the side and will not move it. It often baffles the physician who is not certain whether the lesion is in the shoulder, the elbow, or the wrist.

The fact that the clavicle is the most frequently fractured bone in the body during childhood should help in making the diagnosis. Inasmuch as it is the only bony connection between the shoulder girdle and the trunk, any medially directed blow on the shoulder is transmitted to the clavicle. Likewise, any force applied to the outstretched hand, elbow, or shoulder summates in the clavicle.

Physical findings include pseudoparalysis or the lack of ability to move the affected arm. In addition, there is tenderness and pain on palpation of the clavicle by the examiner's fingers. By simply running the index finger of the right hand over the right clavicle and the index finger of the left hand over the left clavicle along the outline of its contour, the examiner will note that the child winces sharply with pain when the fracture site is encountered. This is diagnostic because sprains never occur in this area. X-ray studies confirm the diagnosis (Fig. 38–57).

In the young child a greenstick fracture (incomplete) may occur, and the child will be unusually fussy, especially when the clavicle is touched. Motion of the arm is good, however. Oftentimes this type of fracture is not discovered until a large lump (callus) appears. The mother then becomes worried and seeks help because of the growth.

Treatment: Reduction is rarely necessary in a child under 6 years of age. Usually a figure-of-eight stockinette is sufficient. This is tightened every morning by the mother.

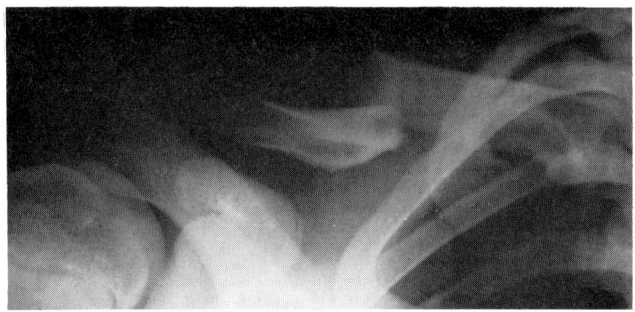

Figure 38–57. Displaced fracture of the clavicle. (From O'Donoghue, D. H.: Treatment of Injuries to Athletes. 3rd Ed. Philadelphia, W. B. Saunders Co., 1976, p. 161.)

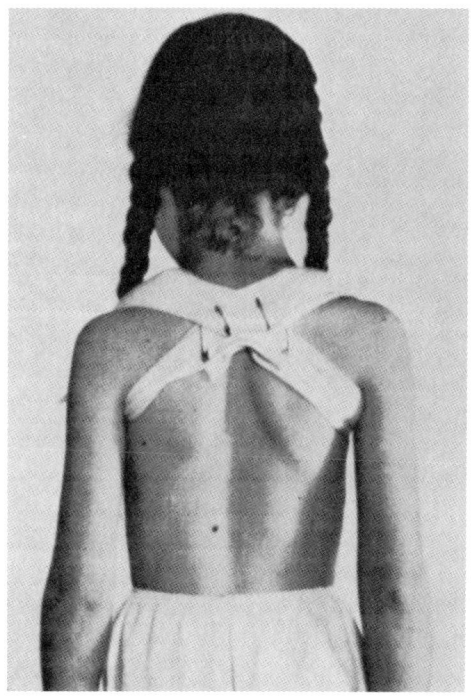

Figure 38–58. *Nondisplaced fracture of the clavicle treated with simple figure-of-eight bandage. (From Blount, W. P.: Fractures in Children. Baltimore, The Williams & Wilkins Co., © 1955, p. 14.)*

It is left in place for approximately 6 weeks.

In an adult with a nondisplaced fracture, the identical treatment is acceptable (Fig. 38–58). However, the examiner must be certain that x-ray films show the presence of abundant callus before discharging the adult from treatment. Iatrogenic nonunion of the clavicle is very embarrassing.

Athletic Trauma to the Shoulder (Sprain)

Twisting the upper extremity or shoulder region can produce a stretching of the capsule or muscles about the shoulder joint. This may cause temporary painful disability. The shoulder will have a swollen appearance if hemarthrosis is present.

X-ray examination will be negative.

Treatment consists of a simple sling support for a week to 10 days with the application of ice or cold compresses for 24 hours. Motion is encouraged as soon as the discomfort subsides.

Sprains in the area of the acromioclavicular joint usually result from direct blows

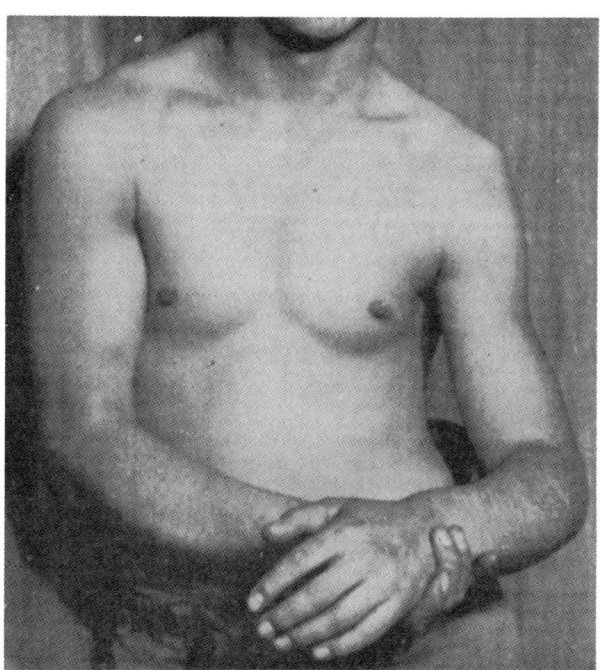

Figure 38–59. *Dislocation of the shoulder. Note the flattening in the region of the deltoid, indicative of the absence of the humeral head. (From McLaughlin, H. L.: Trauma. Philadelphia, W. B. Saunders Co., 1959, p. 246.)*

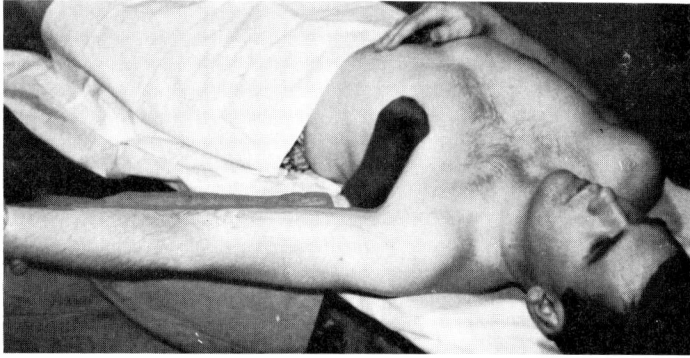

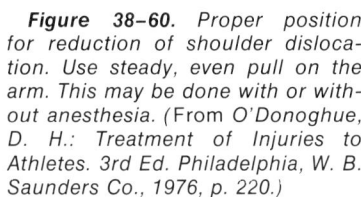

Figure 38–60. Proper position for reduction of shoulder dislocation. Use steady, even pull on the arm. This may be done with or without anesthesia. (From O'Donoghue, D. H.: Treatment of Injuries to Athletes. 3rd Ed. Philadelphia, W. B. Saunders Co., 1976, p. 220.)

on this area. There is very severe pain and inability to move the shoulder area. The x-ray films are negative. Treatment is the same as for any other sprain in the area: the use of a sling along with ice and oral analgesics until the discomfort subsides to permit normal recovery of motion. Needless to say, participation in all athletic activities is discouraged until normal, pain-free movement returns.

Dislocation of the Shoulder

Force applied to the upper extremity may result in an abnormal degree of elevation and external rotation to the humerus and force the humeral head to tear out of the joint and lodge in some position outside the joint. This is usually in an anterior and inferior position.

Physical examination demonstrates severe deformity and inability to use the shoulder because of pain and restriction of motion. With a little experience the examiner can readily detect the flattening of the shoulder when the normal, rounded humeral head is dislocated (Fig. 38–59).

Prior to any treatment, the examiner should carefully check the extremity distal to the shoulder joint with a sharp pin to determine the integrity of the nerves of the upper extremity.

X-rays should always be taken to confirm the diagnosis and to establish the absence of a fracture. Otherwise, the physician who manipulates the shoulder may be credited with producing the fracture.

In spite of the urge to "do something" in crowded sports arenas, the physician must refrain from definitive treatment until he has an x-ray film to clearly indicate the

absence of a fracture. Once this is established, the dislocation can be reduced by manipulation of the arm and shoulder (Fig. 38–60). The shoulder is then immobilized in a soft bandage or occasionally a plaster cast for 3 weeks. This is essential at the time of the first dislocation to prevent recurrence. It is not as important in the habitual dislocation.

ELBOW DISORDERS

Many complications follow injury or disease of the elbow joint. This is because of its unusual anatomic relationships (Fig. 38–61). Most elbow disorders are characterized by pain and stiffness deformity and only occasionally by locking. Numbness and weakness of the hand may also be a result of elbow disorders.

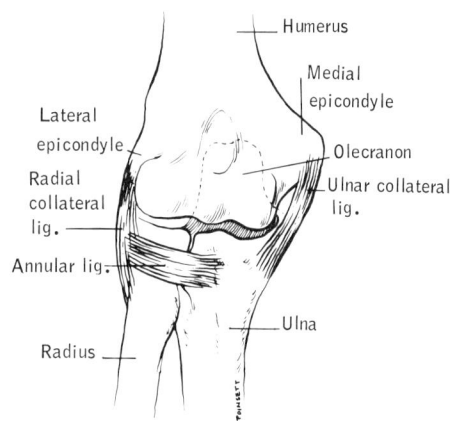

Figure 38–61. Skeletal anatomy of the elbow. (From Gartland, J. J.: Fundamentals of Orthopaedics. 2nd Ed. Philadelphia, W. B. Saunders Co., 1974, p. 239.)

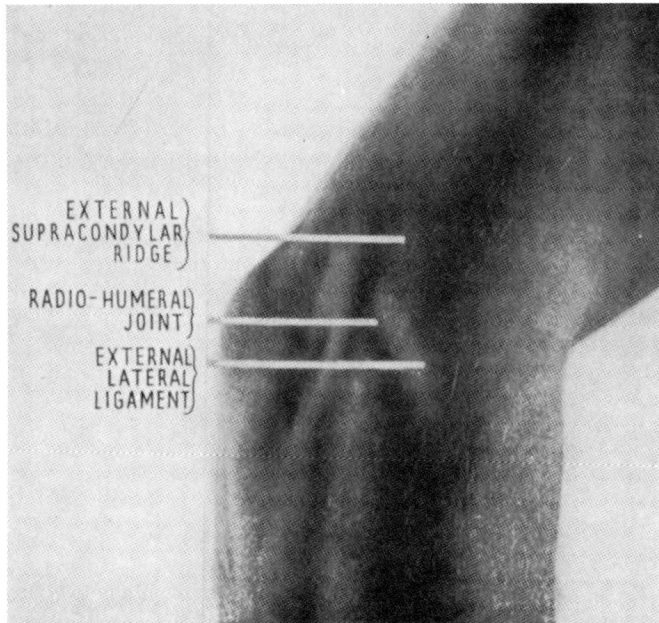

EXTERNAL
SUPRACONDYLAR
RIDGE

RADIO-HUMERAL
JOINT

EXTERNAL
LATERAL
LIGAMENT

Figure 38–62. Outer side of elbow, showing sites of pain in epicondylitis. (From Wiles, P.: Essentials of Orthopaedics. 2nd Ed. Boston, Little, Brown & Co., 1956, p. 349.)

Lateral Epicondylic Pain (Adults)

Lateral epicondylic pain is the most common disorder of the elbow (Fig. 38–62). It is referred to as epicondylitis. The cause is probably unrecognized trauma to the common origin of the extensor muscle of the forearm at the outer side of the elbow. There is subsequent adherence of the torn fibers to the untorn fibers and to the joint capsule as well.

The onset of symptoms usually follows a minor strain or energetic use of the arm. Though gradual at first, the intensity of pain increases and may radiate widely over the forearm to the wrist. It is associated with activities that will require pronation and supination of the forearm, such as the use of a screwdriver, clipping the garden hedge,

playing tennis, or even lifting a cup of coffee (Fig. 38–63). In early cases the pain is improved by rest but returns immediately when the arm is used.

Physical examination discloses an apparently normal-looking elbow. Flexion and extension movements are complete and painless. There is an area of acute tenderness that can be localized accurately to the lateral epicondyle. Pain can be characteristically aggravated by forced dorsiflexion of the wrist against resistance because tension is put on the common extensor origin (Fig. 38–64).

X-ray studies of the elbow are normal.

Diagnosis rests on localizing tenderness over the lateral epicondyle and on a positive wrist-flexion test against resistance.

Treatment consists of injecting 0.5 cc. (3

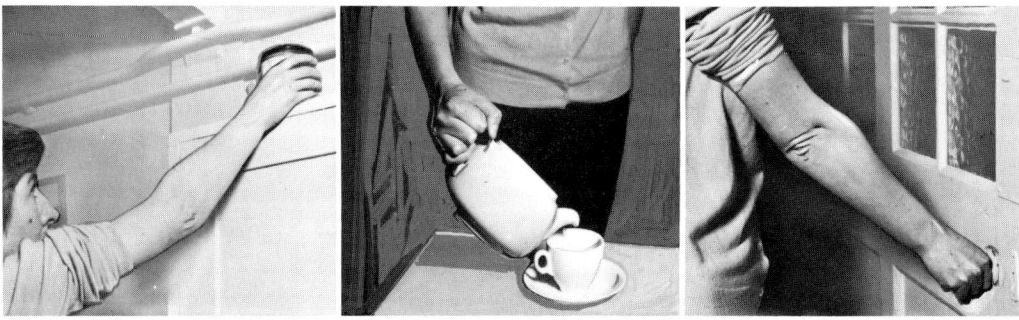

Figure 38–63. Movements that produce epicondylic pain. (Reproduced from A System of Orthopaedics and Fractures. 3rd Ed. by A. Graham Apley, published by Butterworths, London.)

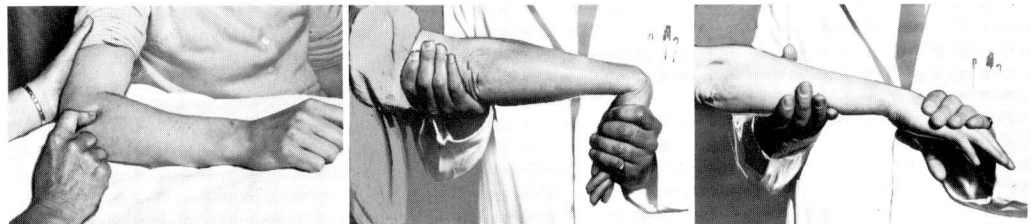

Figure 38–64. Tenderness on passive stretching. Pain on resistive dorsiflexion. (Reproduced from A System of Orthopaedics and Fractures, 3rd Ed. by A. Graham Apley, published by Butterworths, London.)

mg.) of betamethasone acetate into the site of acute tenderness. In addition, all activity requiring pronation and supination of the forearm should be avoided for a minimum of 3 weeks. If after 3 weeks the symptoms still persist, another injection is given.

This condition is very resistant to treatment and even when recovery is apparent, the symptoms will return with vigorous use of the arm. Therefore, some physicians recommend as additional treatment a course of ultrasonic therapy, which is prescribed as follows: Apply ultrasound at the rate of 1.5 microwatts per cm^2 for a 3 minute interval over the lateral epicondylar area. This treatment is to be given every 3 days for a total of 11 treatments unless the disorder is relieved sooner.

Operation is occasionally desirable when conservative methods have failed. The origin of the common extensor muscle is detached from the lateral epicondyle or, alternatively, the tendon of the extensor carpi radialis brevis is lengthened in the lower half of the forearm.

Elbow Stiffness (Adult)

Permanent limitation of motion follows severe fractures into the joint or osteo- or rheumatoid arthritis in adults. Symptoms are few. Until the stiffness is considerable it often passes unnoticed. There is rarely much pain, and infrequently the joint will lock.

Physical examination discloses varying degrees of motion. The joint may look slightly enlarged, but there is no localizing tenderness.

X-ray films show decreased joint space with osteophytes and occasionally loose bodies.

Diagnosis is confirmed by the combination of limitation of movement and positive x-ray changes.

Treatment is conservative. Heat and massage given in the physical therapy department will afford some relief from symptoms provided excessive use of the arm can be avoided. Should pain become a factor, aspirin can be given daily in doses to provide sufficient relief.

Operation is recommended only for removal of loose bodies or when there is much pain and disability, especially in young people.

Acute Elbow Injuries (Contusion)

Acute injuries to the elbow are common. There are many subcutaneous areas about the elbow, and a fall on the flexed elbow will crush skin against the underlying hard bone (olecranon) with resulting abrasion or contusion. Since this area is relatively insensible, the injury may be overlooked.

X-ray examination is indicated to rule out a fracture.

Treatment will depend on the degree of injury. If a hematoma is present or developing, an icepack should be applied for 24 hours. Following this, proteolytic enzyme tablets are prescribed 3 times a day after meals for a period of 5 days. A sling may be worn for the first 2 to 3 days, if indicated.

Contusions of the Ulnar Nerve

Traumatic ulnar neuritis and even ulnar palsy can develop from contusion of the ulnar nerve. Contusion occurs more readily at the elbow because of the anatomic position of the nerve. It is in a vulnerable position in the ulnar groove behind the epicondyle of the humerus. Because it is subcutaneous, a direct blow can produce damage.

The patient may complain of numbness, tingling, and pain along the ulnar distribution, particularly in the fourth and fifth fingers. There may also be a feeling of clumsiness in the hand if palsy ensues. Ultimately, there may be paralysis and wasting of all of the interosseous muscles of the hand.

Physical examination will elicit no objective findings if only ulnar neuritis is present. Palsy, however, will present an early loss of the ability to adduct the little finger against the ring finger. The metacarpal shafts become more prominent on the dorsum of the hand because of interosseous muscle wasting. Pinprick sensation is also decreased or absent over the ulnar distribution, especially in the fifth and fourth fingers.

X-ray studies will be unrevealing. Occasionally the presence of an osteoarthritic spur may be detected in the ulnar groove in noninjury types of cases.

Diagnosis rests completely on clinical findings in the late cases. Often, however, early cases can be detected by nerve conduction–velocity studies.

Treatment for contusion and subsequent neuritis of the ulnar nerve consists of administering 1000 micrograms of vitamin B_{12} intramuscularly daily for 30 days or more.

If the signs of ulnar palsy are emerging, surgical transposition of the nerve must be considered. Neurolysis is performed and the nerve transferred forward to pass in front of the condyle rather than behind it. Should surgery be delayed too long, recovery is not promising.

Tendon Strain and Rupture (Adult)

Extremely forceful action is required at the elbow joint in many work activities as well as in sports. This accounts for the frequency of strain of the musculotendinous units about the elbow joint.

A rather common strain is that of the biceps tendon where it attaches in front of the elbow joint to the neck of the radius. There is also an extensive aponeurosis called the lacertus fibrosus, which spreads the attachment of the biceps to the fascia of the forearm. Strain may occur at any point in this complex.

The triceps is a powerful muscle that attaches posteriorly to the olecranon. It can be strained from its attachment all the way to its musculotendinous junction.

Physical examination will elicit localized tenderness over the area. Pain on forced motion of the muscle against resistance will also be detected. If the triceps muscle is being evaluated, the elbow should be placed in forceful extension with the forearm against resistance. This will produce pain over the area of the insertion of the triceps. If the biceps muscle is being tested, the elbow should be forcefully flexed against resistance, and pain will be reproduced over the anterior aspect of the elbow in the region of the biceps complex.

X-ray films will show no significant changes.

Diagnosis is made by the history and by the physical findings of tenderness and pain against resistance in the appropriate anatomic areas.

Treatment will depend on the degree of injury. If severe, ice should be applied for 24 hours. The arm must be rested in a sling for several days until the pain subsides. Forceful movements of the elbow joint should be avoided for at least 2 to 3 weeks.

Biceps Rupture. A severe strain can avulse the biceps from the radius. Under usual circumstances the biceps shortens and bunches itself so that an abnormal mass is

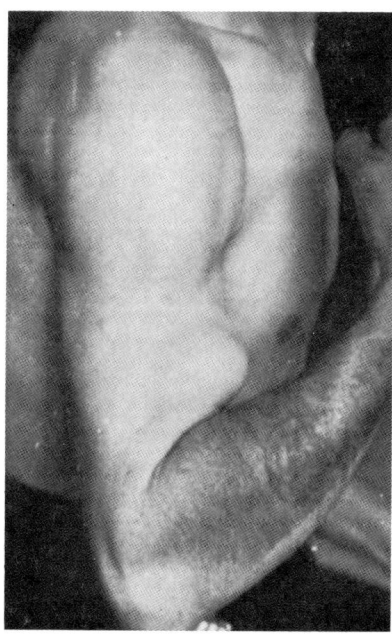

Figure 38–65. *Rupture of the biceps.* (From Wiles, P.: *Essentials of Orthopaedics.* 2nd Ed. Boston, Little, Brown & Co., 1956, p. 359.)

present in the lower arm area if the injury has been at the elbow level. Occasionally the biceps will rupture the tendon of the long head at the shoulder level and this will retract to the mid- or lower arm area, giving the appearance of a bulge in the lower arm (Fig. 38–65).

Treatment consists of surgical reattachment when complete rupture is present. This is more important at the elbow than it is at the shoulder. For this reason, when the condition is diagnosed, immediate referral should be made for appropriate surgery.

Elbow Sprain

Elbow sprain usually occurs in patients who have a history of sudden hyperextension of the elbow followed by severe pain on the medial and sometimes lateral side of the elbow. This pain is relieved by holding the elbow flexed. This patient prefers to keep the elbow flexed and suspended in a sling to relieve the pain.

The elbow is a rather stable joint, and ligament injury here is not common. The elbow can really be sprained only by excessive extension. This results in injury to the anterior portion of the collateral ligaments, especially on the medial side. Instability, regardless of the type of sprain, is extremely infrequent.

Physical examination demonstrates localized tenderness at the site of the tear, either along the ulna on the medial side or along the epicondyle. Attempts to extend the arm cause pain. Motion in the normal arc of extension is prevented by muscle spasm.

X-ray films are of little value except to rule out fracture.

Diagnosis is made by the history of injury as well as by the localized areas of tenderness, especially along the medial joint ligaments.

Treatment consists of ice applications in the early acute stage for 24 to 48 hours. A protective sling should be worn for at least 2 to 3 days. When the joint is asymptomatic, activity may be initiated. Stressful sports or work activities should be avoided for 4 weeks.

Painful Swelling of the Posterior Elbow Joint

Varying degrees of trauma to the elbow at its posterior aspect produce marked swell-

ing in the olecranon bursa, which is located between the skin and the olecranon bone in this area.

The swelling frequently consists of blood. As a result, the walls of the bursa become permanently thickened. This condition often occurs without precipitating injury. The usual complaint is one of pain and swelling behind the elbow area (Fig. 38–66).

Physical examination will reveal erythema around the olecranon bursal area with marked tenderness on palpation and restriction of extension of the elbow. When the bursa is palpated, it is felt to be thickened but distensible, indicating that fluid is present. Usually it is adherent to the underlying olecranon and cannot be displaced.

X-ray films occasionally will show some small fragmentation or flake-like appearance along the posterior margin of the olecranon.

Diagnosis is made by the presence of the distended bursa and the signs and symptoms of local inflammation.

Treatment consists of the aspiration of the bursal fluid, which may be bloody in the early stages and straw-colored in later stages. Fluid that is withdrawn should be sent to the laboratory for analysis of crystalline content. Occasionally, gout masks as a traumatic incident. Following this, 0.5 cc. (3 mg.) of betamethasone is injected. The patient is then advised to apply ice to the area for 48 hours and to avoid further trauma to the bursa.

If initial treatment does not completely clear the condition, recurrence is inevitable. Usually only a slight bump of the elbow is required to reproduce the signs and symptoms at a later date.

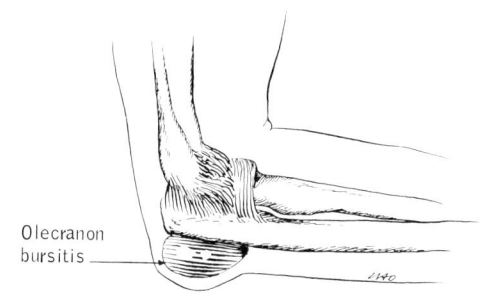

Olecranon bursitis

Figure 38–66. *Olecranon bursitis. (From O'Donoghue, D. H.: Treatment of Injuries to Athletes. 3rd Ed. Philadelphia, W. B. Saunders Co., 1976, p. 275.)*

If the initial symptoms persist in spite of adequate treatment or if there is recurrence, it must be explained to the patient that surgical drainage and excision of the bursa are necessary. At least two serum uric acid determinations should be made to rule out the presence of underlying gout prior to undertaking any surgery.

All of the contiguous tentacle-like portions of the bursa must be excised. Failure to do this results in persistent drainage through the wound, which usually necessitates a second surgical procedure.

Fractures and Dislocations of the Elbow

None of the fractures or dislocations of the elbow is simple. The results of treatment are not fully satisfactory even in the best of hands. Therefore, the family physician would be wise to refer these conditions as soon as they are diagnosed.

FOREARM INJURIES

Contusion and strain are very common problems in the forearm area because of the substantial area of subcutaneous bone and because of frequent overstretching of the musculotendinous junctions of the forearm tendons.

The contusion, with its damage to the skin and typical pain, local swelling, and hematoma, presents minimal disability.

Treatment is largely of a local nature: application of ice in the early stages, followed by a small pressure dressing over the hematoma if indicated, and ultimately, protection by a pressure pad if the individual must continue to pursue some competitive activity.

More serious and disabling is the acute injury to the tendons or musculotendinous units of the forearm, especially as they become more superficial just proximal to the wrist joint.

Physical examination detects localized pain along the area of the tendon that has been injured. There may be local swelling (occasionally followed by inflammation and exudation of fluid). As the tendon tends to glide within the irritated sheath, sticky adhesions result, and crepitation is detected by running the finger over the tendon as it moves up and down the sheath.

If the condition progresses, the examiner will find that the tendon ceases to move because of adhesions between it and the sheath.

X-ray films are usually within normal limits.

Diagnosis is made by the presence of the positive physical findings just listed.

Treatment for the acute condition depends on its severity. Early rest and the application of an icepack are indicated in the first 24 hours. If the condition appears extremely unstable, a splint may be used to immobilize the forearm from just distal to the elbow to include the wrist joint. The fingers need not be immobilized in this condition. As soon as unresisted movement of the wrist is pain-free, complete immobilization can be discontinued. If the injury is of moderate severity, 10 days will usually be required. If the condition has progressed to formation of adhesions (tenosynovitis), treatment will be more prolonged. Once tenosynovitis has been established by thickening around the tendon and restriction of motion, a local injection of 0.5 cc. (3 mg.) of betamethasone should be given. Often this will produce marked improvement. If it does not, surgery may be indicated, depending on the location of the tendon.

Pain and Swelling on Thumb Side of the Wrist

This condition is similar to that described previously except that the traumatic factor is not present. It is more frequent in women than in men. Often attempts are made to relate it to special occupations. The causation is not firmly established, however.

The patient complains of pain on the thumb side of the wrist. The pain occasionally radiates up the forearm and down into the thumb. This pain is aggravated by the use of the hand, especially by wringing or typing activities. Ultimately, it may produce disability.

Physical examination often discloses a visible swelling on the outer side of the lower end of the radius (Fig. 38–67). If the examiner causes the patient to abduct the thumb actively against resistance, exquisite pain will be felt in the area of this localized swelling. There is also marked tenderness on local palpation.

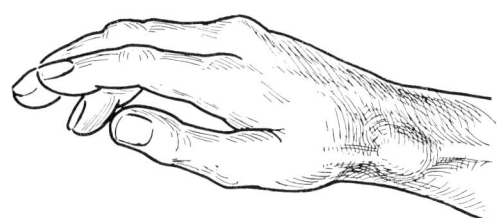

Figure 38-67. *Quervain's disease (stenosing teno-vaginitis).* (From Wiles, P.: Essentials of Orthopaedics. 2nd Ed. Boston, Little, Brown & Co., 1956, p. 363.)

Treatment is usually attempted with conservative modalities at first, such as rest and restriction of activities. This, however, is usually followed by pain when activity is begun again.

The injection of 0.5 cc. (3 mg.) of betamethasone will produce relief in a large percentage of patients. The period of relief may extend from 6 weeks to several years. If relief is not produced by the first injection or if a recurrence of the condition is detected, the ultimate treatment is surgery.

The surgical procedure consists of excising the greatly thickened area of sheath that encompasses and binds three separate tendons at this site. Active movement is begun several days after surgery, and the patient can return to work within a week.

DISORDERS OF THE WRIST AND HAND

Wrist Sprain

Contusions of the wrist are of frequent occurrence and are usually caused by a direct blow. Careful examination will disclose no significant injury to the deeper structures, and if the contusion seems severe, x-rays should be taken to rule out fracture. Treatment is as outlined for contusions in earlier sections.

A sprain is a ligament injury, and it is relatively uncommon in the wrist. Most of the "sprains" are not really sprains but strains of the tendon attachments or injuries to the bone. The ligaments on the volar and dorsal aspects of the wrist are so strong that injury is more likely to be a fracture of the carpal bones than a tearing of the ligaments.

Therefore, if the injury is a dorsiflexion type, one looks for damage on the dorsal aspect of the wrist, especially for a navicular fracture, and if it is a plantar flexion type, one evaluates the volar surface of the wrist.

There are several localized areas of tenderness that indicate specific injuries. Pain and tenderness on the ulnar aspect of the wrist especially in the sulcus between the ulna and the closest carpal bone are indicative of an injury to the triangular cartilage. There is a fibrocartilaginous extension of the radiocarpal joint that lies between the ulna and the carpus. Rupture of these fibers results in hemorrhage and degeneration. Occasionally, calcification occurs much later. Treatment for this condition is the same as for other wrist injuries to be described at the end of this section. There is one exception: if the condition becomes chronic and relief cannot be obtained, an injection of 0.5 cc. (3mg.) of betamethasone should be considered. Should this prove ineffective after 4 to 6 weeks, the patient should be referred for surgical exploration, since the cartilage may have to be excised or the ligament repaired, depending on the findings.

Physical examination will reveal tenderness over the area of injury. The physician should make a determined effort to place localized pressure over the dorsum of the navicular bone by familiarizing himself with its location just distal to the radial styloid process. Tenderness over this area on pressure should make one suspicious of a fracture of the navicular bone.

X-ray films of the wrist bones should be ordered to include "navicular views." In the absence of an outright fracture, the physician can conclude, at least at this stage, that he is more probably dealing with a tendon or ligamentous problem.

Treatment for sprains, strains, and minor subluxations includes immobilization of the wrist in slight dorsiflexion for at least 3 weeks unless the symptoms subside before this time. Ice should be applied for the initial 24 to 48 hours.

Following removal of the splint, physical therapy should consist of whirlpool and range of motion activities of the wrist for 1 or 2 days. Once pain-free motion is achieved, treatment can be discontinued. If heavy work or athletic participation is to be permitted at the end of this period, the wrist should be protected with an elastic wrist support for a period of several more weeks.

Should the patient continue to complain of pain especially over the radial aspect of the wrist in spite of initial negative x-ray films, the examiner must consider the possibility of a fractured carpal navicular bone. The fracture is notoriously missed and is often only detected by repeat x-ray studies taken 10 days to 3 weeks after injury. This is because there is some widening that occurs at the fracture site, disclosing its presence. It is therefore considered good treatment if the physician routinely takes repeat x-ray studies of all wrist injuries that have been diagnosed as sprains approximately 2 to 3 weeks after the injury, especially in the presence of persistent complaints of weakness, soreness, or pain produced by pressure over the area of the carpal navicular bone.

Night Pain and Tingling—Fingers and Hands

A complaint of night pain in the hands is common in middle-aged women, but younger and older people are not exempt. The most troublesome aspects occur at night, since pain and tingling in the hands and fingers often interrupt sleep after a few hours. Hanging the arm over the bedside may give partial relief, as may rubbing the fingers. On awakening in the morning, the patient states that the hand is clumsy and difficult to use for several minutes.

The principal complaint is burning, tingling, numbness, or "pins and needles," especially in the thumb, index, and middle fingers. Occasionally the fingers feel as though they were swollen. There may even be pain in the forearm and the arm above the elbow. These symptoms can be present all the time or only at intervals. In the daytime these complaints are often made worse by energetic use of the hand.

The cause is divided among multiple pathologic conditions that diminish the space in the rigid carpal canal on the volar surface of the wrist. This syndrome develops from the unusual relationships on the volar side of the wrist where the 8 flexor tendons of the fingers pass through the

constricted confine of the carpal tunnel and include in their mass the median nerve.

The median nerve, which is vulnerable and compressible, bears the brunt of damage when constriction occurs in this carpal tunnel. Among the many common conditions known to produce this syndrome are tenosynovitis of the flexor tendons, rheumatoid arthritis, and even fractures of the carpal bones.

Physical examination when the condition is well developed will detect impairment of pinprick sensation over the thumb, forefinger, middle finger, and the radial half of the ring finger. In advanced stages there will be wasting of the outer half of the thenar eminence and weakness of the abductor and opponens muscles of the thumb.

Direct pressure over the median nerve as it passes under the volar ligament will often increase the pain and paresthesia in the median nerve distribution.

If there is any doubt about the diagnosis in the early phase of this syndrome, nerve conduction studies should be performed, since the delay in conduction activity can be detected at the wrist joint.

X-ray examination is mostly unrevealing. Occasionally, in a very rare instance, an osteoarthritic spur will be detected.

Treatment is indicated especially in the stage of night pain. For the individual patient suffering very mild symptoms, reassurance is needed, and often the symptoms disappear spontaneously, especially if they are related to recurrent edema such as occurs in relationship to the menstrual cycle.

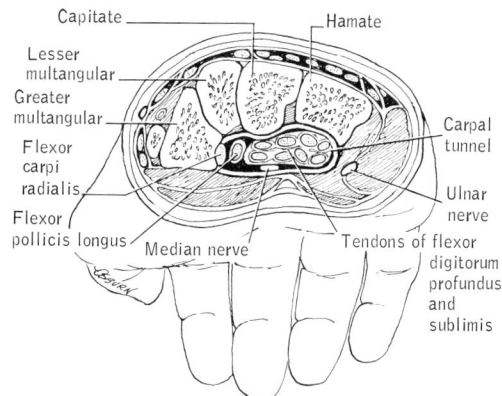

Figure 38–68. *The carpal tunnel. (From O'Donoghue, D. H.: Treatment of Injuries to Athletes. 3rd Ed. Philadelphia, W. B. Saunders Co., 1976, p. 293.)*

In the presence of positive neurologic signs or a report of a nerve conduction lag, surgery to divide the flexor retinaculum is necessary.

Many causative lesions can be diagnosed at the time of surgery, but whether or not a cause is established, improvement follows the release of the tight flexor apparatus.

Although the procedure appears relatively simple, dissection in this area is not for the uninitiated (Fig. 38–68). If irreversible changes of the nerve have not occurred prior to surgery, recovery will be complete.

Painless Mass — Wrist Area

The chief complaint of the patient is of a painless swelling of the wrist (Fig. 38–69). Occasionally the patient complains of associated weakness of grip, but rarely is there pain unless stressful activity is performed on a daily basis.

The most common lesion fitting these

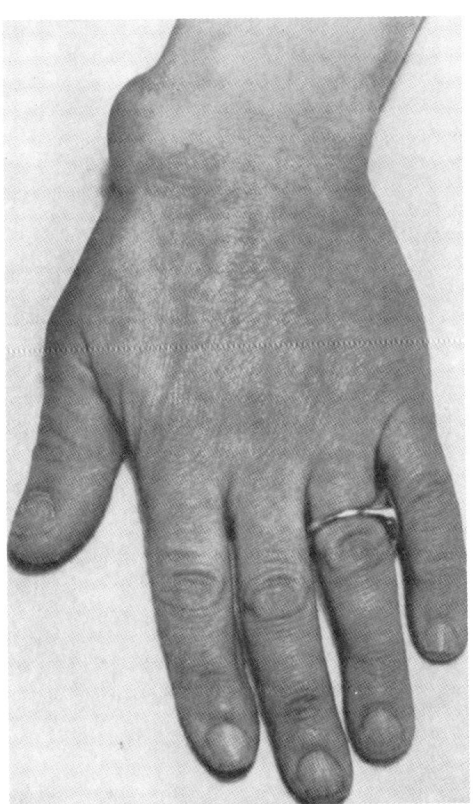

Figure 38–69. Ganglion. (From Wiles, P.: Essentials of Orthopaedics. 2nd Ed. Boston, Little, Brown & Co., 1956, p. 365.)

characteristics is a *ganglion*, which is a cystic swelling that occurs in connection with the lining of a joint or of a tendon sheath. A ganglion itself has a fibrous outer coat and an inner layer of synovial tissue and contains thick gelatinous fluid. Its cause is uncertain.

Diagnosis is made by the presence of this compressible but nondisplaceable swelling around the wrist area. Occasionally pain is associated with increased pressure on palpation. Several other rare lesions have to be considered, such as lipoma, synovioma, and so forth. The ultimate diagnosis is made only on pathologic examination.

Treatment: Occasionally spontaneous disappearance occurs without treatment. However, if the ganglion is burst by direct pressure, it usually seals itself off and reappears in its original form in 4 to 6 months.

Many physicians prefer to puncture the ganglion with multiple needle stabs and occasionally inject some steroid medication. This is usually followed by recurrence.

The only satisfactory way to completely eliminate the ganglion is by surgical excision. This operation must be performed in a bloodless field because the dissection among the tendons is extensive. Unless the "roots" of the ganglion are removed from deep within the joint area with meticulous care, recurrence is possible.

DISORDERS OF THE HANDS AND FINGERS

Almost the entire function of the upper extremity depends on the intact nature of the fingers and thumb.

Pain at the Base of the Thumb (Adult)

Pain at the base of the thumb is quite disabling because it interferes with the use of the thumb and, therefore, with use of the whole hand. The initial cause may be a malunited fracture or repeated minor trauma sustained at work. Often no cause can be found.

Physical examination detects tenderness on palpation over the carpometacarpal joint. Passive anteroposterior and lateral movements to the thumb also produce pain localized to the joint.

X-ray examination shows obvious changes, such as narrowing of the joint, irregularity of the articular margins, and spur formation when the disease is advanced.

Diagnosis of osteoarthritis of this carpometacarpal joint of the thumb is made early by the presence of localized pain over the joint and confirmed by x-ray studies when the disease is advanced.

Treatment consists of restriction of activity. If accepted, particularly by women, this will relieve a great deal of the pain. The activities that are restricted include sewing and other types of repetitive movements. Some benefit has been reported from the use of a removable thumb splint to immobilize the joint while the patient is working.

Occasionally injections of 0.5 cc. (3 mg.) of betamethasone repeated at intervals of 2 to 3 months will produce relief and permit the wage earner to continue necessary activities.

In more severe cases surgical treatment is necessary. Arthrodesis of the first metacarpal in a partly opposed position is one surgical approach. Total replacement of the carpal component of the joint with a silicone implant is another surgical approach that has been achieving increasingly good results during the past few years.

Fixed Flexion Deformity — Fingers

This condition affects middle-aged and older men 10 times more frequently than it affects women in the same age group. The first sign is often a nodule that appears in the skin of the palm of the hand, sometimes in the first phalanx of the ring finger. As the nodule increases in size, other nodules appear, and the skin becomes puckered.

As a result of the underlying fascial changes, the involved finger or fingers flex slowly and inexorably in the direction of the palm. In severe cases the fingertips press against the palm and cause indentations. The rate at which the deformity develops varies considerably.

In the early stages the patient may complain of pain on grasping. Later the condition is painless but the grip is impaired, and there is difficulty in releasing objects as the bent fingers get in the way.

This condition, referred to as *Dupuytren's*

contracture, involves the palmar fascia lying immediately beneath the skin of the palm of the hand. This fascia becomes thickened and contracted and draws one or more of the fingers into a position of flexion.

The cause is not known. Heredity may be a factor, but trauma is oftentimes blamed. There is also an incidence of occupational association.

Physical examination shows the skin to be thick, nodular, and adherent to the deep fascia. The affected fingers are flexed at the knuckle joints and extended at the distal tips. Any attempt to straighten the fingers makes the palm or fascia more tense. The ring or little finger is most often involved (Fig. 38–70).

X-ray films are of no value in this condition.

Diagnosis is made by visual examination, history, and palpation of the nodular lesion.

Treatment is surgical. A variety of conservative treatments have been attempted, including physiotherapy, stretching, and various medicinal preparations. They are quite useless. Once the disease is progressing, early surgery that consists of a fasciotomy or of a fasciectomy is indicated.

If the condition is allowed to progress so that the skin is severely involved, much

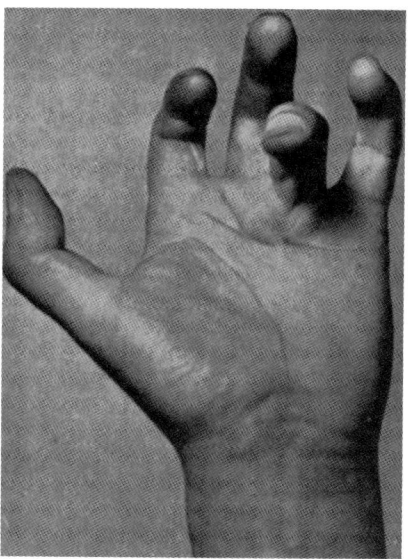

Figure 38–70. *Dupuytren's contracture.* (From Wiles, P.: *Essentials of Orthopaedics.* 2nd Ed. Boston, Little, Brown & Co., 1956, p. 372.)

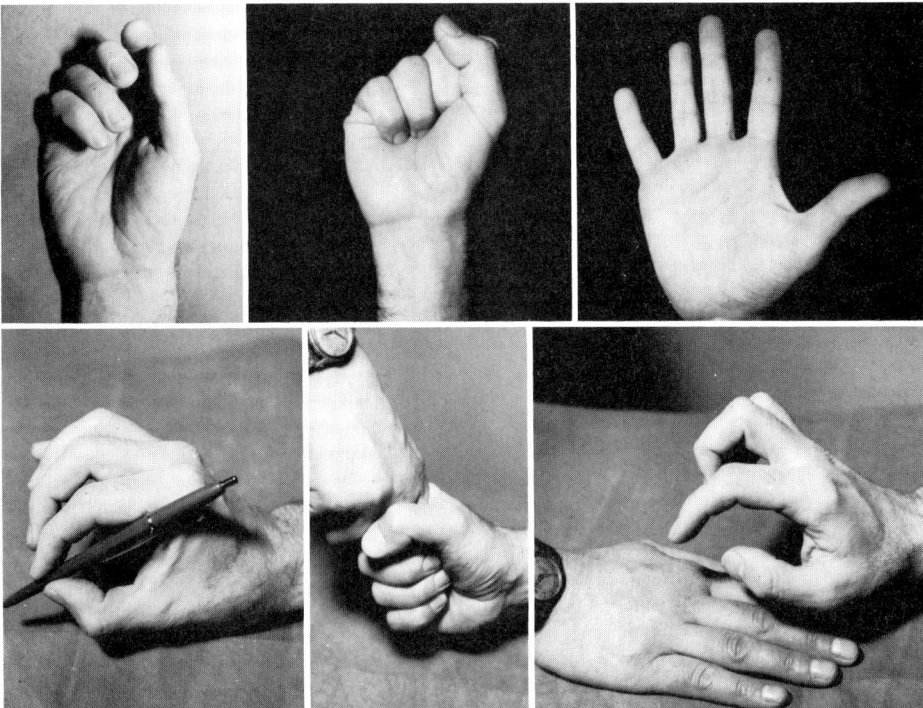

Figure 38-71. Examination of the hand. (Reproduced from A System of Orthopaedics and Fractures, 3rd Ed. by A. Graham Apley, published by Butterworths, London.)

more extensive surgery is necessary, including skin grafting.

Lacerations

A laceration may penetrate the skin with the finger in a fixed position of flexion or extension. When the cut is examined, the finger may be in another position, and a quick glance through the wound opening will reveal only normal tissues. Ignorance of the real damage to the deeper tissues may then have serious consequences.

Treatment must not be initiated until an adequate assessment is made of the function of the lacerated part and the hand as well. All motions, both active and passive, of the involved area must be checked (Fig. 38-71). Nerve function should be assessed as well. It is not necessary to repeatedly remove the dressings in order to perform these tests; they can be readily performed with the wound covering in place. A sterile dressing should be removed only on the occasion of the first hospital examination to permit a thorough inspection of the laceration, which will help determine the type of

anesthetic needed. Disturbances of tendon or nerve function or joint involvement usually require a general anesthetic for their treatment.

X-ray studies are necessary to evaluate the full extent of bone damage. Tetanus antitoxin or toxoid may be given at this time.

Following the preliminary preparation, the patient is taken to the operating room and given a general anesthetic. The wound is then examined in detail and cleansed thoroughly. The area is now ready for definitive treatment.

Unless the family physician has taken advanced training in hand surgery or has considerable previous experience, he would do well to refer these complex injuries when they are of sufficient magnitude to require the use of the operating room.

Puncture Wounds

After a puncture wound, especially to the palmar aspect, the hand should be carefully assessed for disturbance of nerve function.

610 PART VI CLINICAL SPECIALTIES

If the nerves are intact, the wound is meticulously and thoroughly cleansed. A sterile dressing is applied and the wound regularly observed. Routinely, tetanus antitoxin or toxoid should be given.

Wounds of this nature should not be closed. Often they are due to a "human bite" or a contaminated instrument. Closure by suture hinders adequate drainage and promotes infection.

There is often deep soreness in the early days, but this should not be confused with infection. However, if after several days the patient reports fever, malaise, throbbing in the hand, and erythema, infection in the puncture site should be suspected and a broad-spectrum antibiotic administered.

Occasionally, a penetrant carries with it foreign objects such as clothing or glass to the depth of the wound. These objects also contribute to the continuation of infection. X-ray studies may be of help if the penetrant is metallic or possesses some degree of density. If necessary, in special cases the wound may be enlarged to remove foreign objects or devitalized tissue.

Contusions and Abrasions—Hand (Direct Trauma)

The hand is very susceptible to damage. It is exposed to direct blows and crushing types of injuries. Often the injury is a combination abrasion, contusion, and laceration.

The back of the hand is especially subject to rapid swelling. Nerve contusion is not likely to result from direct blows here because most of the nerves are on the volar aspect of the hand and protected.

Tendons and bones, however, lie subcutaneously on the back of the hand, and they may be damaged. These areas are available for careful examination, and simple palpation will usually be sufficient to determine whether there is a fracture of the metacarpals. No examination is complete, however, without an evaluation of tendon and nerve function.

Should the contusion seem unusually severe with marked local tenderness over the bones and pronounced swelling, an x-ray evaluation must be requested.

If the skin is abraded, very careful cleansing is carried out with a bland soap and water. Painting of the area with anti-

septics is not needed. Antibiotic ointment may be used if there is no sensitivity present.

A mild compressive dressing is then applied to the hand, and an icepack is placed over this. The ice may be dicontinued after 24 hours.

If the area remains swollen and stiff, protective dressings are used for several more days until function of the fingers becomes pain-free. The possibility of subsequent tenosynovitis must be kept in mind.

Sprain and Dislocation—Metacarpal and Phalangeal Joints

Because of the vast functional and anatomic differences between the thumb and fingers, injuries to these areas will be discussed separately when appropriate.

Sprain and Subluxation—Fingers (Swelling, Pain, Some Loss of Function). Sprain occurs from forcible lateral angulation or hyperextension. There is considerable swelling and pain, and recovery is slow. These joints permit limited circumduction, so that extremes of motion in any direction can cause injury to the carpal ligaments.

Involvement of the index and fifth fingers is most likely since either of these may be forcibly abducted away from the hand. If the force is limited, the resultant injury does not produce instability. However, if the force continues, subluxation may occur with tearing of the ligament opposing the force, for example, collateral ligaments from a lateral force and the volar capsule from a hyperextension type of force.

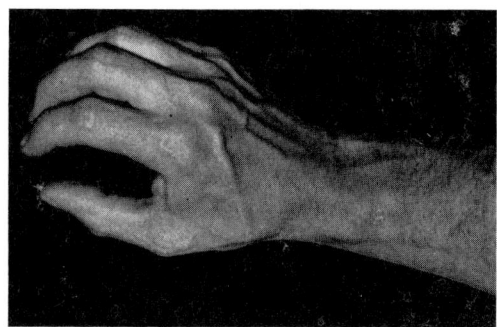

Figure 38–72. Position of function. (From Nichols, H. M.: Manual of Hand Injuries. 2nd Ed. Chicago, Year Book Medical Publishers, Inc., 1960, p. 57.)

With release of the force, the joint falls back into place with no obvious deformity. If the tear is not detected and immobilized, the ligaments may heal with redundancy that permits chronic sprain and recurrent subluxation.

X-ray studies are of no benefit.

Treatment consists of immobilization in the position of function for at least 3 weeks (Fig. 38–72). If any instability is detected after 3 weeks of treatment, 3 more weeks of immobilization are indicated. Icepacks should be applied for 24 hours following the initial injury when moderate to pronounced swelling is present.

The most common damage to the ligament holding the adjacent metacarpal heads together. For example, the ligament binding the third and fourth meracarpal heads together may be torn. It is easily overlooked and results in chronic weakness and disability.

Physical examination will detect the presence of pain with simple separation of the two involved fingers.

X-ray films will not detect the lesion.

Treatment consists of holding the fingers together for at least 6 weeks. A plaster of paris cast extending from the forearm and encompassing the metacarpophalangeal joints but permitting free motion of the digits will be adequate.

Sprain and Subluxation — Thumb. The thumb possesses extensive circumduction mobility, and it is therefore axiomatic that stability must be maintained almost exclusively by ligaments. Forced motion by ligamentous stretching will cause a sprain that can be mild, moderate, or severe, depending on how much force has been applied.

Mild sprain manifests itself by pain around the joint, tenderness to pressure over the area, and pain on reproduction of the motion that caused the injury. The base of the thumb is swollen.

Treatment consists of protecting the joint against stress and immobilizing it in a position of function such as would be assumed by gripping a 2 inch ball. It is not necessary to immobilize the fingers, but the splint should include the hand, the wrist, and the thumb to its distal tip. The period of immobilization varies from 10 days to 3 weeks. A plaster of paris cast is best for this purpose.

Subluxation or moderate sprain due to rupture of the external lateral ligament of the thumb may be very troublesome. The thumb is unstable and weak, and on examination there is painful, unnatural mobility.

Treatment consists of plaster of paris fixation for 6 weeks. If the subluxation cannot be reduced and the joint structures held in their normal relationships, immediate referral is indicated. An old injury inadequately treated may require a fascial graft, and even then some disability will persist.

Dislocation of the Metacarpals — Thumb and Fingers. Simple dislocation of the thumb at the carpometacarpal joint is not common. Usually the injury is more complex and often of the so-called Bennett type of fracture, in which a small portion of the end of the metacarpal fixes to the anterior capsular ligaments and remains in position while the larger portion of the metacarpal bone dislocates.

X-ray evaluation will readily establish the presence of dislocation and Bennett type fracture dislocations.

Treatment of these injuries of the thumb, including fractures, should consist of immediate referral unless the practicing physician is skilled in their management. Considerable disability follows incorrect or inadequate treatment. There is no justification for the inexperienced physician to attempt to treat complex injuries of this nature.

Dislocation of the distal end of the metacarpal at the metacarpophalangeal joint of the fingers occurs as a result of hyperextension and force. The proximal phalanx moves backward over the metacarpal. As the metacarpal head thrusts forward, the anterior capsule tears, and the phalanx dislocates onto the back of the metacarpal and may stand at a 90 degree angle to the metacarpal.

X-ray films will clearly show this deformity.

Treatment consists of reduction by applying pressure directly along the base of the phalanx in the direction of the long axis of the metacarpal while the finger is maintained in hyperextension (Fig. 38–73). This reduction may be performed without anesthesia, provided no earlier traumatic reduction was attempted. If such has been the case, a local anesthetic is injected at the

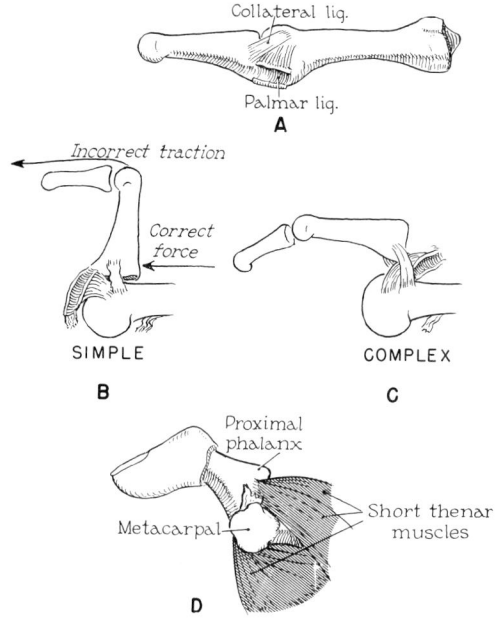

Figure 38–73. *Simple and complex metacarpo-phalangeal dislocations. (From McLaughlin, H. L.: Trauma. Philadelphia, W. B. Saunders Co., 1959, p. 135.)*

base of the metacarpophalangeal joint on either side. When the finger is sufficiently numb, the reduction may be performed.

Should the reduction require undue force, it should be discontinued and arrangement made for open reduction. In these instances, interposed tissue usually prevents the metacarpal head from moving backward under the phalanx. Following reduction, the finger should be immobilized in the position of function for about 10 days.

Sprain and Dislocation — Interphalangeal "Small" Joints, of Fingers and Thumb

Interphalangeal joint sprains are more serious than is generally realized. The delicate capsule and lateral ligaments of these slender joints are readily sprained. Unfortunately, they are often not treated, and the finger remains crippled for many months.

Sprain may be produced by hyperextension of the joint, which causes the anterior capsule to tear, or by excess lateral angulation, which damages the collateral ligaments. These usually occur with the joint in extension.

Physical examination in the presence of a "sprained" anterior capsule will elicit pain on an attempt to completely extend the involved joint. Should the injury be severe, it may be possible to hyperextend the joint.

X-ray studies will be negative in the absence of fracture or dislocation.

Treatment in the presence of pain and instability consists of immobilization of the sprained joint in the position of function for at least 3 weeks (Fig. 38–74). If pain alone is present, only 10 days of immobilization are required. Even after immobilization and return of normal function, some fusiform swelling of the joint may remain permanently.

The collateral ligaments of the interphalangeal joints are tight in flexion and relatively loose in extension. Thus, lateral angulation easily stresses these ligaments. If the damage is severe enough, instability is produced.

Careful physical examination will establish the presence or absence of instability.

Treatment, if there is instability, is immobilization of the joint in extension with appropriate lateral deviation to close the joint on the involved side. This is maintained for 2 weeks. Some motion may then be permitted, but flexion beyond 90 degrees is avoided for at least 6 weeks.

With old injuries — and many patients will not consult a physician for some months — little can be done to promote

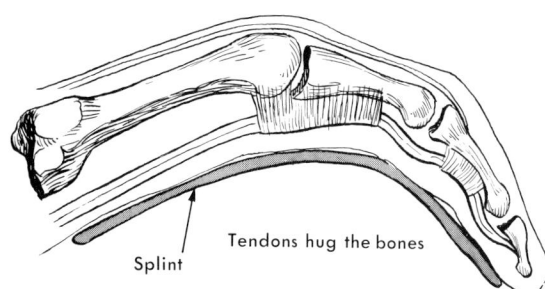

Figure 38–74. *Aluminum splint supporting the finger in functional position.*

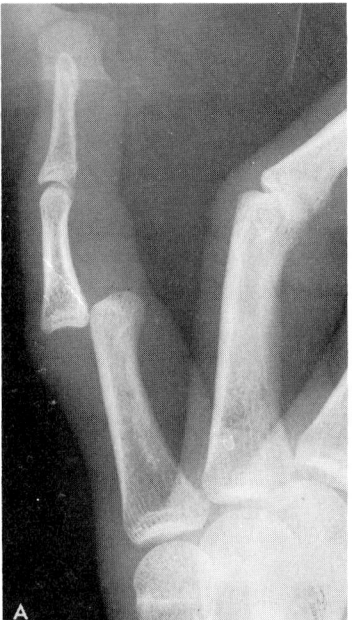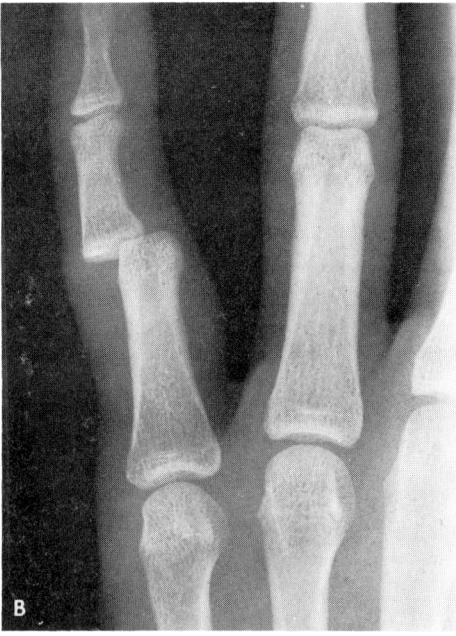

Figure 38-75. *Dislocation of interphalangeal joint of the fifth finger. A, Lateral view of dislocation. B, Posteroanterior view of dislocation. (*From *O'Donoghue, D. H.: Treatment of Injuries to Athletes. 3rd Ed. Philadelphia, W. B. Saunders Co., 1976, p. 355.)*

recovery. Assurance can be given that even though some swelling and perhaps instability will remain, the pain will disappear. Operation is not recommended except for a really gross deformity.

Interphalangeal joint dislocations of the fingers and thumb are caused by the same type of force that "sprains" the anterior joint capsule. Continued hyperextension tears the capsule, and the head of the more proximal phalanx thrusts forward through the palmar surface.

If the tear is incomplete, the dislocation often spontaneously reduces itself. If complete, however, it may require reduction.

X-ray examination will indicate the degree of severity (Fig. 38-75).

Treatment is reduction by manipulation if the injury is seen immediately after it has occurred. Anesthesia is not required at this time. The manipulative movement entails reproduction of the hyperextension to unlock the dislocation. Then, by traction along the line of the dislocated phalanx, the base of the bone can readily be pushed down into contact with the head of the more proximal phalanx.

Should treatment be delayed or difficulty encountered in performing a smooth reduction of the dislocation, 1 per cent procaine solution is infiltrated under sterile conditions into the base of the finger along both sides. The injection is in the area of the neurovascular bundles. Epinephrine solution is *never* used. Once anesthesia is established, the manipulative movements are then repeated.

Following reduction, immobilization is carried out with an aluminum splint in the position of function for about 7 days. Alternatively, the immobilization may be achieved with the apparatus shown in Figure 38-76.

If the dislocation is an open one or if the physician is not able to reduce it, the patient

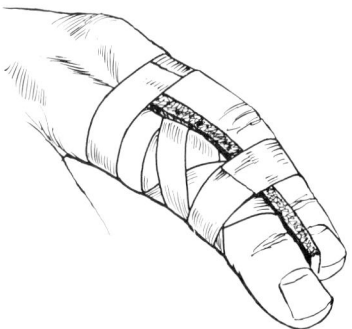

Figure 38-76. *Taping for a sprained or dislocated finger.*

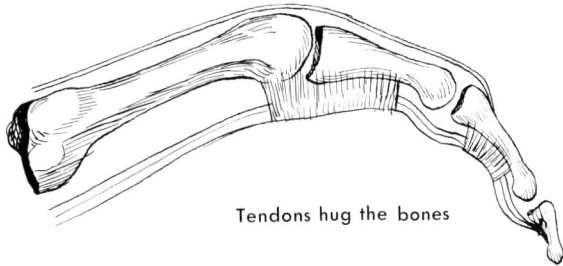

Tendons hug the bones

Figure 38-77.   Skeletal mechanics.

should be referred to someone experienced in hand surgery, since this type of injury is quite complex.

Fractures of the Finger and Hand Bones

Fractures of the bones of the fingers and hand get less attention than fractures of large bones. However, improper management of finger fractures results in disabilities that do not improve spontaneously and that are difficult to correct surgically.

All of the general principles of fracture treatment apply to the hand, but the small size of the bones makes technical application of these procedures more difficult. Restoration of anatomic alignment is the most important element in maintenance of function. Most poor results are due to acceptance of "less than the best" on the part of the treating physician.

No single method can always be correct for every situation, but principles of treatment are consistently applicable. These are as follows:

The mechanics of the skeleton establish the tenet that tendons closely hug the bones (Fig. 38–77). The collateral ligaments are loose during extension and tight during flexion (Fig. 38–78).

Reduction of displaced fractures should be accomplished as a positive maneuver in order to correct alignment and rotation at the fracture site. Do not rely on splints, traction, and so forth to perform the reduction; do it yourself (Fig. 38–79).

Following reduction, position the part in "muscle balance," referred to as the position of function (Fig. 38–80).

Almost all fractures of the digits, with few exceptions, should be immobilized in flexion. Minor irregularities can be overcome because the finger will work when the support is removed. Splinting in full extension (for example, on a tongue blade) must be condemned because this produces permanent stiffness of the joints and less function of the involved finger and the hand as well (Figs. 38–81 and 38–82).

The average period of healing is about 4 to 5 weeks for all closed phalangeal fractures.

Local anesthesia can be injected under sterile conditions at the fracture site, but distention of the finger should be avoided. One to 2 per cent lidocaine solution can be used. Epinephrine solutions must *not* be

Metacarpophalangeal
extended

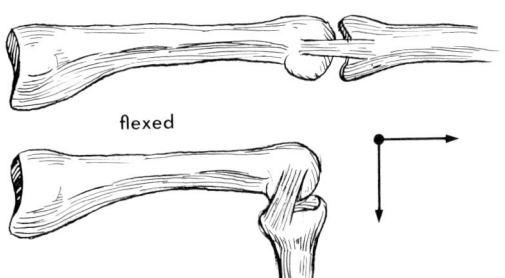

flexed

Figure 38-78.   Dynamics of ligamentous function.

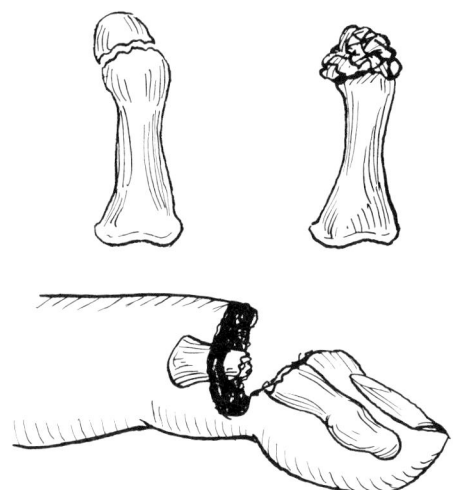

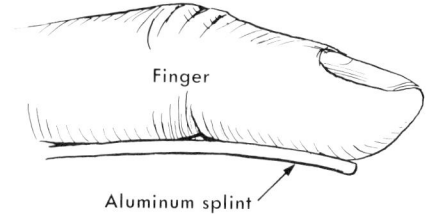

Figure 38–85. Immobilization of dropped distal joint or fracture of distal phalanx of finger.

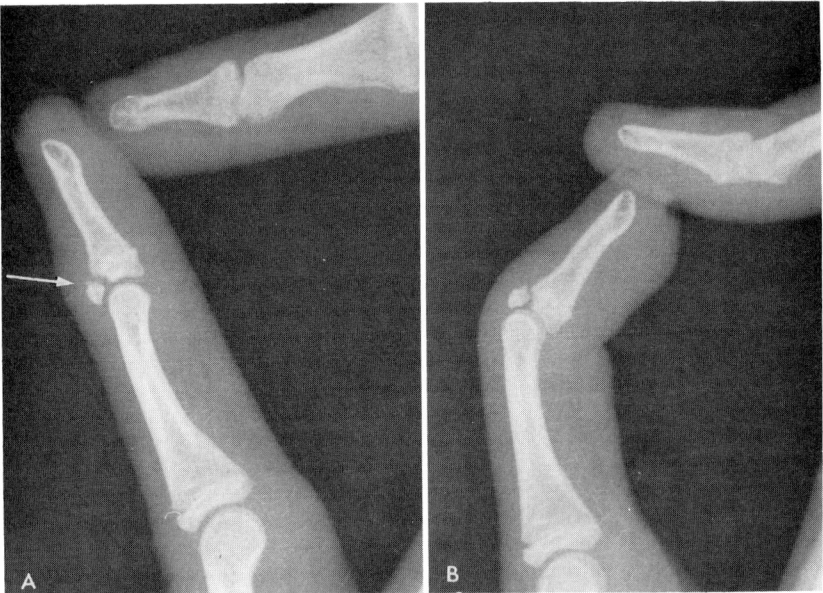

Figure 38–84. Compound fractures of the distal phalanx.

should be relieved by penetrating the base of the nail with a number 25 hypodermic needle. This is performed under sterile conditions. With the hematoma evacuated, the physician can then proceed with reduction and splinting of the finger (Fig. 38–85).

Dropped Distal Fingertip. This traumatic deformity, often calletl "baseball" or "mal-

let" finger, is caused by avulsion of the extensor tendon from its insertion into the base of the terminal phalanx, either with or without an attached fragment of the distal phalanx.

It is usually due to a blow (baseball) forcibly flexing the fingertip at the moment the extensor tendon is contracting, as when attempting to catch a ball.

X-ray films demonstrate the loose fragment to which the extensor tendon is attached (Fig. 38–86).

Diagnosis can also be made by the position of the distal phalanx of the involved finger. It will hang in flexion but can passively be restored to full extension. Several weeks after injury, the deformity, if untreated, will still persist, but the pain

Figure 38–86. Detached fragment and dropping of the distal joint. A, Unstable joint supported firmly by examiner's finger. B, Dropping of fingertip into flexed position when support withdrawn. (From O'Donoghue, D. H.: Treatment of Injuries to Athletes. 3rd Ed. Philadelphia, W. B. Saunders Co., 1976, p. 379.)

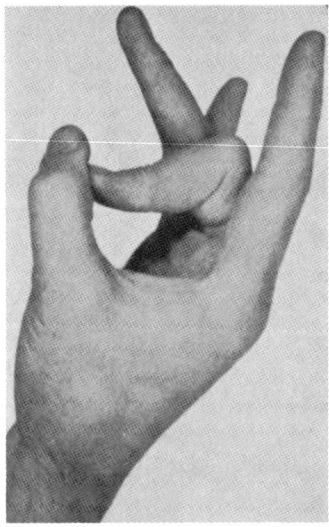

Figure 38–87. *Extensor tendon injury. Immobilization position for distal joint. (From Wiles, P.: Essentials of Orthopaedics. 2nd Ed. Boston, Little, Brown & Co., 1956, p. 369.)*

associated with it will gradually disappear.

Treatment by nonoperative methods is adequate but difficult. It often tests the patience of the treating physician. The most commonly recommended position is that with the terminal joint extended but not hyperextended. Figure 38–87 demonstrates this very well.

Plaster of paris is used to maintain the position for a minimum of 6 weeks or longer. If there is slight weakness in extension following removal of the cast, the finger should be immobilized for an additional 2 to 4 weeks.

The use of metallic splints and tape is also an acceptable method of treatment, provided the same position of immobilization is used. Frequently, perspiration loosens the tape and, in spite of explicit instructions, the patient will remove the splint and

reapply it himself. This disrupts the healing that has taken place up to that time.

To overcome this problem, some physicians prefer to insert a Kirschner wire across the joint, or use a stainless steel pull-out suture, or employ other types of surgical treatment. These methods are not for the inexperienced, however, because of the possibility of serious infection, and also because at times the end result is either a finger with permanent extension or permanent flexion rather than active flexion and active extension. To treat or not to treat is best left to the judgment of the family physician, with the added comment that this particular injury poses many difficulties even in the hands of "experts."

Metacarpal Head Fractures (Boxer's Fracture). Fractures in this region of the metacarpal are usually caused by the knuckle of the clenched fist forcibly contacting some object. It is called a boxer's fracture because it is most usually associated with this type of activity, whether in or out of the ring. The result is a flexion deformity of the metacarpal head rotated over the neck, so that the head presents itself in the palm of the hand (Fig. 38–88).

Treatment is achieved with adequate reduction. Anesthesia is usually required. Figure 38–89 demonstrates the maneuvers essential for reduction.

Immobilization is then carried out with a carefully molded plaster splint to just beyond the distal portion of the metacarpophalangeal joint (Figs. 38–90 and 38–91). The plaster cast is left in position for 4 to 5 weeks. At this time, x-ray studies will usually demonstrate early callus and the cast can be removed, and early motion begun.

Open Finger Fractures and Basilar Thumb Fractures. These types of injury most often are complex and require debridement or

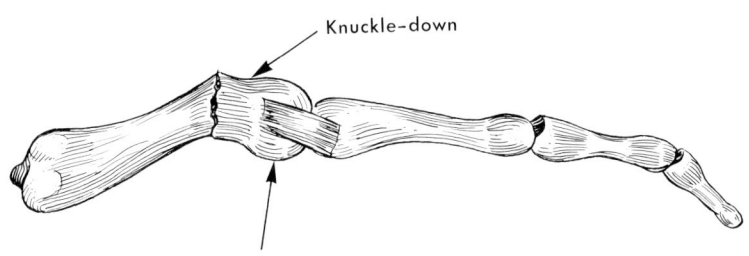

Knuckle-down

Tender in palm

Figure 38–88. *Flexion deformity of the head of the metacarpal.*

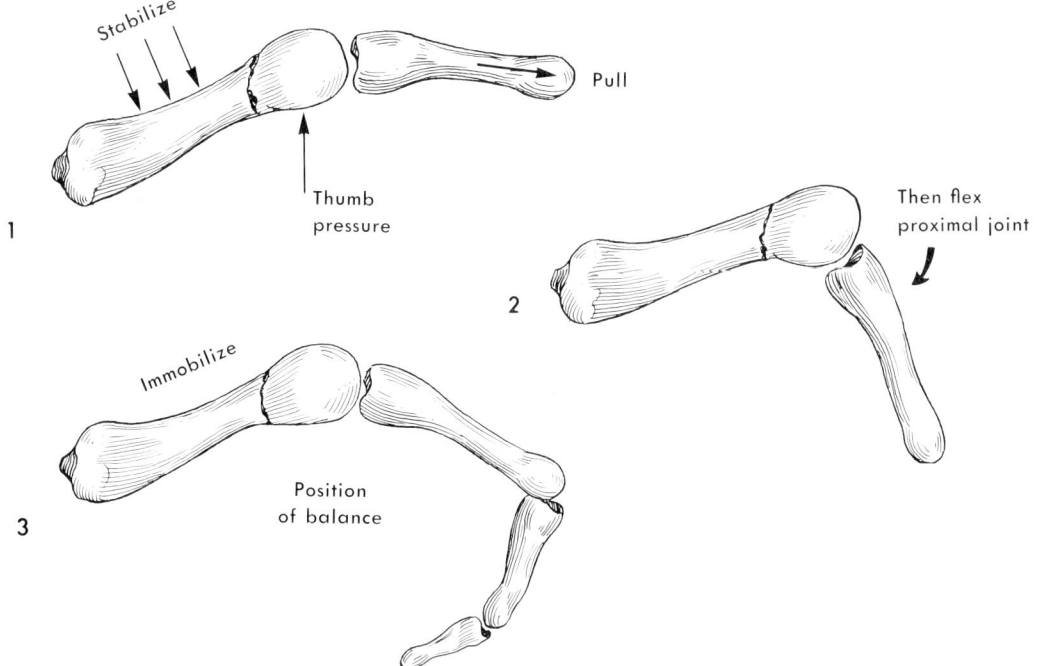

Figure 38–89. *Technique for reduction of metacarpal neck fractures.*

repair or both. If too much initial damage is present, amputation may be the procedure of choice. Often, delayed emergency treatment procedures are used in order that valuable skin and other soft tissues are not sacrificed too early in the management of these injuries.

By their very nature they are complex and are usually handled best by the skilled hand surgeon or by the physician experienced in their management. Unless the reader qualifies as one of these, it is recommended that he refer this type of case and avoid needless difficulties and criticism.

Injuries and Infections About the Fingernails

Contusion of the fingernail is likely to cause hemorrhage, because on the back of

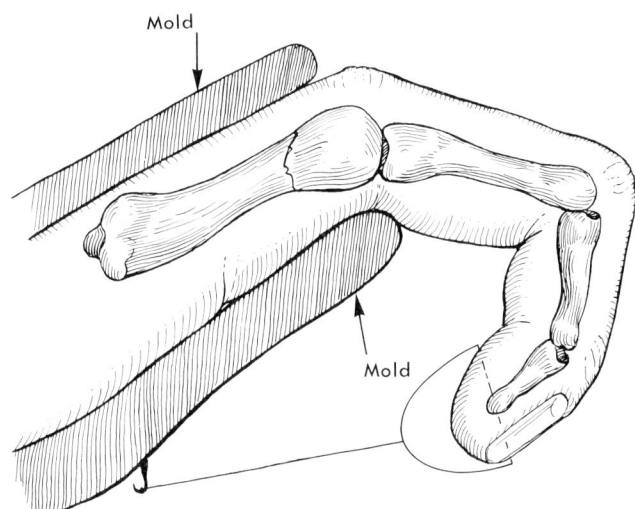

Figure 38–90. *Correct immobilization for metacarpal head fractures.*

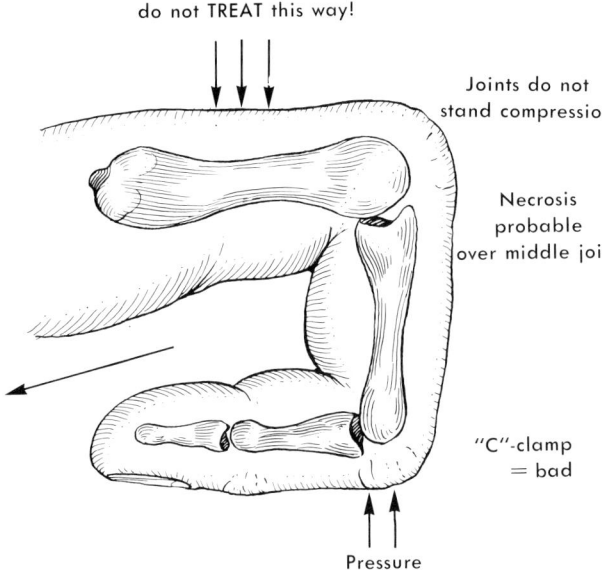

do not TREAT this way!

Joints do not
stand compression

Necrosis
probable
over middle joint

*Figure 38–91. Improper fracture man-
agement.*

"C"-clamp
= bad

Pressure

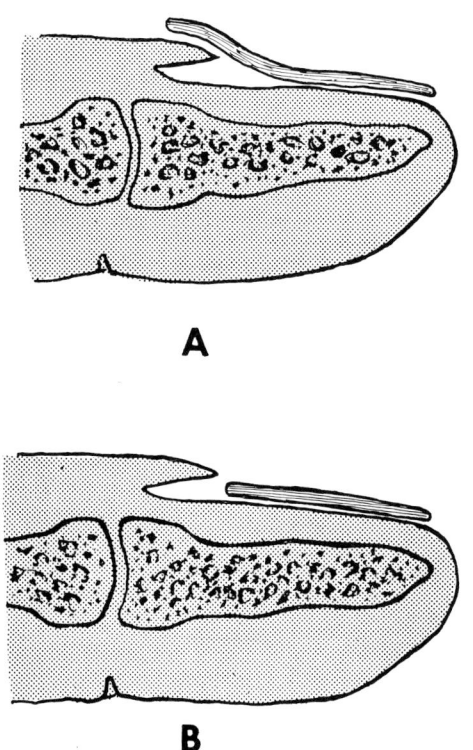

A

B

*Figure 38–92. Correct treatment of avulsed nail.
(From O'Donoghue, D. H.: Treatment of Injuries to
Athletes. 3rd Ed. Philadelphia, W. B. Saunders Co.,
1976, p. 331.)*

the finger the nail is very closely apposed to
the bone. Pressure symptoms and throbbing
pain develop as the hematoma progresses.
As blood accumulates under the nail, the
treatment at this stage consists of drilling
through the nail to evacuate the blood.
There are many methods of accomplishing
this. It is performed with aseptic technique.
Many physicians prefer the use of a sterile
number 25 hypodermic needle. Following
the release of the blood, ice is applied to the
fingertip for several hours.

In the event that the root of the nail is
forced out from under the eponychial fold,
the proximal end of the nail should be cut
away to permit the nail to fall back onto the
nail bed (Fig. 38–92).

Simple contusion of the nail area also can
produce an abrasion with a subsequent
inflammatory reaction with erythema. In the
early stages the application of local heat
several times a day is recommended.

Should treatment be delayed and suppuration occur, a knife blade should be
passed between the paronychial fold and
the nail, and the proximal end of the nail
should be lifted and trimmed to permit the
pus to exit (Fig. 38–93). Local anesthesia (1
per cent procaine *without epinephrine*) is

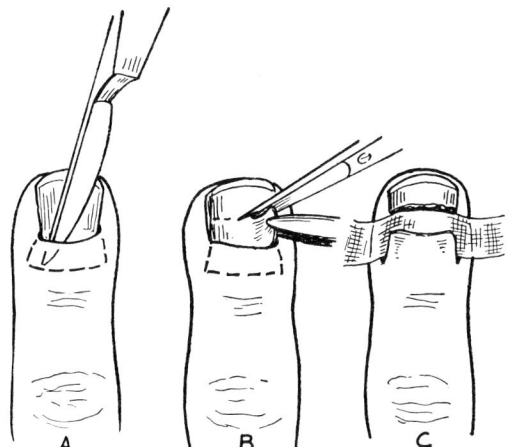

Figure 38–93. *Incisions for paronychia. (From Wiles, P.: Essentials of Orthopaedics. 2nd Ed. Boston, Little, Brown & Co., 1956, p. 385.)*

infiltrated into the base of either side of the finger prior to this procedure.

Following this, hot soaks are recommended for several days until early healing occurs. If drainage is delayed, destruction of the nail root and bed will lead to gross deformities.

X-ray films should be taken in all these conditions, since occasionally the distal phalanx becomes involved with osteomyelitis. Should this occur, the patient should be referred to a specialist.

Snapping Finger

This curious behavior involving the fingers and thumb is caused by a constriction of the flexor sheath at the level of the metacarpal neck. The patient first notices that the finger clicks (often painfully) when flexed. Later, when the hand is unclenched, the affected finger remains bent. It may straighten suddenly with a snap, or it might remain flexed until forced straight with the other hand (Fig. 38–94).

Physical examination will demonstrate the presence of a nodule overlying the flexor tendon. The nodule is palpable under the metacarpal head. The "trigger mechanism" is readily demonstrable by requesting the patient to lock the finger, and the examiner can passively stretch it and feel the nodule on the tendon lock and then pass the point of obstruction.

X-ray films are negative.

Treatment consists of making a transverse incision in the distal palmar crease, or in the crease at the base of the thumb, and incising the fibrous tendon sheath longitudinally until the tendon moves freely.

In children, especially infants, the thumb is affected and it usually cannot be pushed straight. This is often misdiagnosed as a dislocation.

JOINT ASPIRATION

Joint aspiration and analysis of the fluid so obtained are often helpful as an additional diagnostic aid in the conditions listed in Table 38–10. The collection of synovial fluid from any involved joint is not difficult but must be performed under rigid aseptic technique. Skin over the site of the joint to be aspirated is carefully and completely cleansed, using alcohol, and then painted

Figure 38–94. *The adult trigger finger. (Reproduced from A System of Orthopaedics and Fractures, 3rd Ed. by A. Graham Apley, published by Butterworths, London.)*

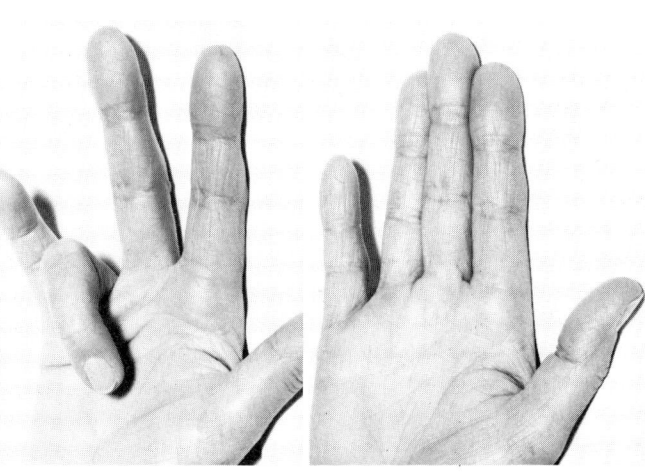

TABLE 38–10. SYNOVIANALYSIS IN ARTHRITIS

Disease	Color	Clarity	Mucin Clot (Viscosity)	Cell WBC/mm³ % Polys	"R.A." Cells	Bact.
Traumatic arthritis	Straw to bloody to xanthochromic	Transparent to turbid	Good	2000 WBC; few to many RBC; 25%	0	0
Osteoarthritis	Yellow	Transparent	Good	1000 WBC; 25%	0	0
Gout	Yellow to milky	Cloudy	Poor	10,000 to 12,000 WBC; 60 to 70%	0	0
Rheumatoid arthritis	Yellow to greenish	Cloudy	Poor	15,000 to 20,000 WBC; 75%	+	0
Septic arthritis	Grayish or bloody	Turbid, purulent	Poor	80 to 200,000 WBC; 75%	0	+

with tincture of iodine, which is allowed to dry for 2 minutes. The site of aspiration is then anesthetized with ethyl chloride spray, and the aspiration of the joint is carried out using sterile disposable or autoclaved 20 gauge needles and sterile syringes. See Figures 38–95 to 38–101 for injection techniques.

Fluid can often be obtained from any swollen joint, but the knee is by far the most frequent site of aspiration and the most accessible joint. At the time of joint aspiration, as much fluid as possible should be removed and placed in sterile test tubes. It then should be forwarded to the laboratory

immediately for the performance of the tests listed in Table 38–10. These findings are not meant to be absolutely diagnostic but merely an additional aid to correlate with the history and clinical findings.

MANAGEMENT OF RHEUMATOID ARTHRITIS

In the management of rheumatoid arthritis, family physicians must use all available treatment methods. Only with this type of approach will the majority of rheumatoid arthritics be able to continue to function

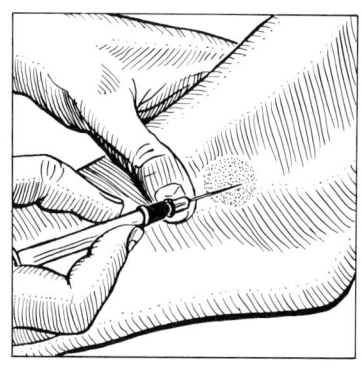
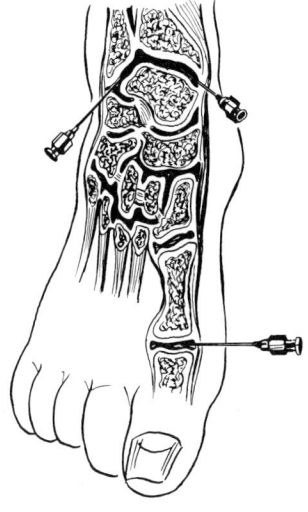

Figure 38–95. *Ankle — technique of joint aspiration. Approach the ankle joint from the front. For landmarks, use the bony prominences of the malleoli. You can enter the joint laterally just inside the fibula or medially just inside the tibial malleolus. In the medial approach, feel inside the tibial malleolus for the depression, and plantarflex the foot to open the ankle. The needle is aimed at the tibiotalar articulation from a point 2 cm. in front of the tip of the internal malleolus. Avoid tendons, and direct the needle parallel to the superior surface of the talus.*

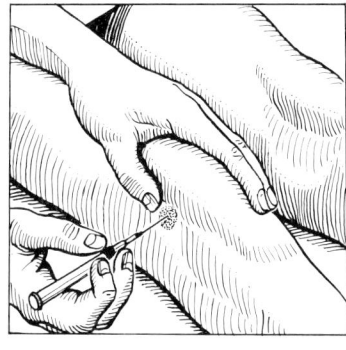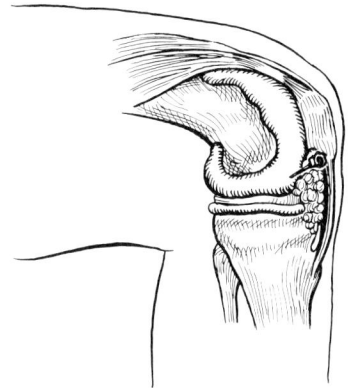

Figure 38–96. *Knee—technique of joint aspiration. The knee is the easiest joint to inject and aspirate. A tightly distended knee joint can be aspirated from any angle without difficulty, but the following technique may be used for ready entrance into the joint space even if there is no excess fluid present: With a single free thrust, introduce the needle parallel to the undersurface of the patella. The entry point is the slight depression under the patella at about the junction of the mid and upper third.*

well, to work, and to lead relatively normal lives.

Too few physicians treat arthritis as a long-term illness. They treat only the acute manifestations. Thus, the patient is unsupervised during periods of remission. With a comprehensive treatment program, this type of management is eliminated. Anyone undertaking the treatment of rheumatoid arthritis must keep this in mind.

Rheumatoid arthritis affects the synovial and other joint structures, but no tissue is exempt. Muscles, spleen, tendons, and central and peripheral nervous systems can be affected.

Serologic testing may be used to classify patients as seropositive or seronegative, depending on whether or not they produce rheumatoid factor. High levels of rheumatoid factor along with subcutaneous rheu-

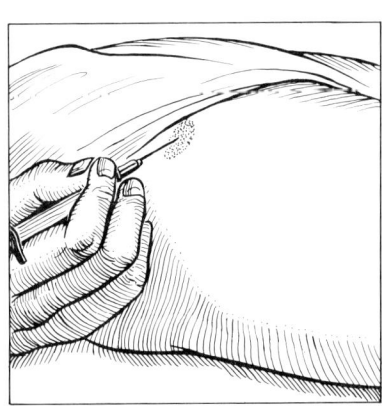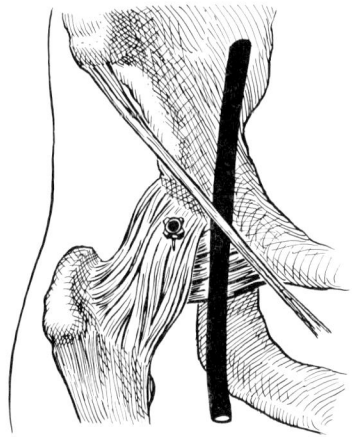

Figure 38–97. *Hip—technique of joint aspiration. The hip is the most difficult joint to inject and aspirate, mainly because of the amount of soft tissue overlying it in all directions. In many cases of osteoarthritis of the hip, it is impossible or nearly so to enter the joint because of bony overhang and adherence of capsule and synovia to the neck and head of the femur.*

In the anterior or lateral approach, the patient lies with the leg in full extension. A 20 gauge needle, 9 cm. long, is employed for either approach. Pay careful attention to landmarks. There are the greater tuberosity of the trochanter, the anterior superior spine of the crest of the ilium, and the symphysis pubis.

Direct the needle just above or anterior to the trochanter and parallel to the femoral neck. Aim for the acetabulum, which lies in the middle-third segment of the line between the symphysis pubis and the anterior superior iliac spine. With the long needle, make the approach. You will probably feel firm resistance as the needle penetrates the thick hip capsule; then you will feel the bone.

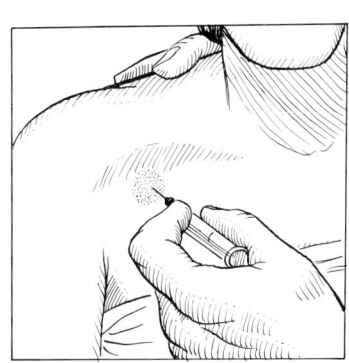

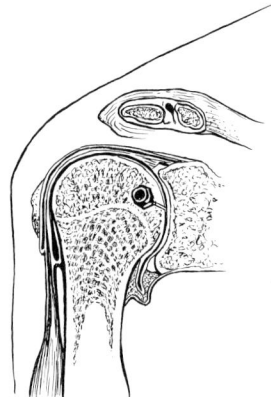

Figure 38–98. *Shoulder—technique of joint aspiration. The tip of the coracoid process is the guide to the anterior approach. You can easily feel this bony landmark. Enter just below the coracoid, with the needle penetrating in an upward and outward direction.*

Aspiration of the shoulder is easily accomplished in the presence of marked effusion by inserting the needle in the space between the head of the humerus and the rim of the glenoid cavity.

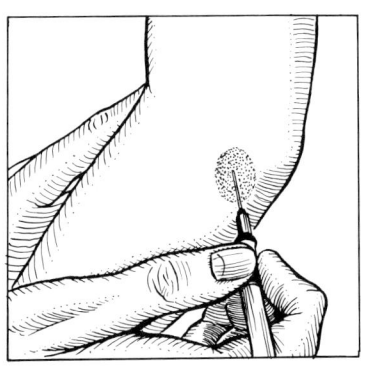

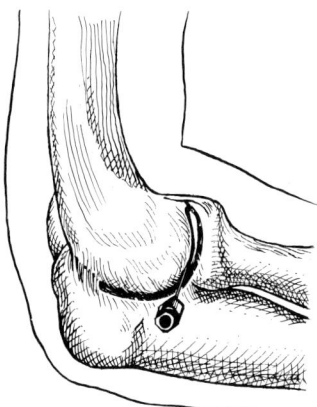

Figure 38–99. *Elbow—technique of joint aspiration. Approach this joint laterally. You can enter the radio-humeral joint area, sliding the needle just above the olecranon of the ulna. The head of the radius is the landmark. Pronating and supinating the forearm will help to identify it.*

The elbow is preferably held at 90°. When effusion is present, the bulging tissue fills the area bounded by the olecranon process, the lateral humeral condyle, and the radial head. The needle should be inserted into this bulging region. Injection should meet little resistance if the needle is properly placed.

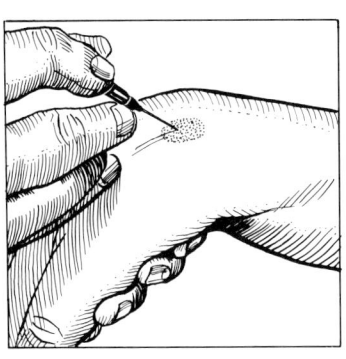

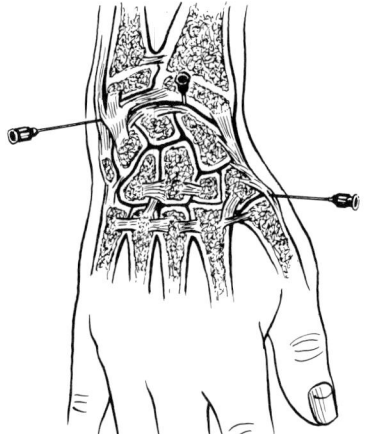

Figure 38–100. *Wrist—technique of joint aspiration. The needle is inserted perpendicularly to the skin at a point just distal to the radius, and just ulnad to the "anatomic snuffbox." The needle is inserted until the point impinges against the carpal bone(s). Most of the small intercarpal joints have connecting synovial spaces. The wrist must be well supported so that it can be properly relaxed. Also shown is a needle in the thumb metacarpophalangeal joint. See also Figure 38–101.*

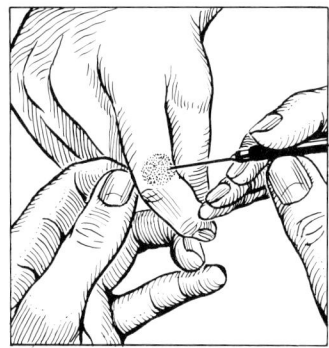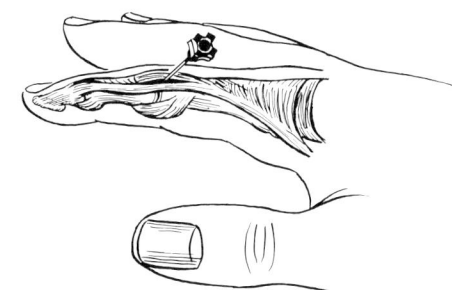

Figure 38–101. *Finger—technique of joint aspiration. Metacarpophalangeal and interphalangeal joints are punctured from the lateral or medial approach on the dorsal surface. A small needle (23 or 24 gauge) is used to avoid undue trauma.*

The tip of the needle is placed beneath the extensor mechanism from either side. About 0.25 ml. is the acceptable volume. It is possible to interpose the needle point between the articular surfaces.

matoid nodules strongly indicate a destructive and less predictable disease course. Serum levels that are low (seronegativity) correlate with milder, more predictable, and more easily manageable disease. It has been estimated that about 70 per cent of patients with rheumatoid arthritis are seropositive, and of these about 25 per cent will have nodules.

Naturally, the management of rheumatoid arthritis varies according to the severity and stage of the disease. The better the patient understands his disease, the more intelligently he can cooperate with the family physician. Therefore, treatment should always begin with a general outline of the nature of rheumatoid arthritis and an explanation of what benefits can be expected from treatment.

It must be explained to the patient why he must take aspirin and how crippling deformities can be prevented; for example, by splinting. Appropriate reading material, such as the Arthritis Foundation booklet *Home Care in Arthritis* and the United States Public Health Service booklet *Strike Back at Arthritis*, should be recommended. It should also be explained that the services of a physical therapist, an occupational therapist, a social service worker, and even occasionally a psychiatrist or an orthopedic surgeon may be required from time to time. The patient must be convinced early of his permanent need for a modified work schedule. He must understand that he can continue to be productive but always on a time schedule that consistently provides enough rest.

Give the patient a prescription for total body rest. Insist that it be followed rigidly. Suggest 9 hours of night-time rest and one-half hour of rest after every 3 hours of activity during the daytime. Ask the patient to elevate his chair and the toilet seat to make them easier to use. Suggest ways to apply heat to joints, such as an infrared light bulb, heating pad, electric blanket, hot tub, or Hydrocollator Packs, which can be obtained from various medical supply houses without too much difficulty. Hot paraffin treatments should be recommended for the hands. All of this can be done at home.

Splints should be provided. There are many types of these on the market today. They are easy to use, and they should be used for acute and persistent joint inflammation that leads to a risk of laxity of the ligaments and secondary subluxation. Rest splints can be used at night but only intermittently during the day. Progressive splints or half-shell splints can be used to overcome deformities. Do not hesitate to use splints, since joint damage and cartilage destruction can occur in as little time as 3 to 4 months. Strict and total immobilization of the joint by means of a splint for 2 to 6 weeks usually prevents such crippling.

Prescribe specific daily exercises for the affected joints. One example is the quadriceps-setting exercise previously mentioned (page 557) to be done 20 times each, 4 times a day.

Insofar as drug treatment is concerned, a careful record of the patient's response to each drug must be recorded. Along with this there should be a list of the laboratory findings that reflect joint changes as well as clinical observations, such as degree of swelling, duration, presence or absence of morning stiffness, sense of well-being or fatigue, and so forth. Also, notes should be made on the presence of rheumatoid nodules, which may appear with flare-ups and disappear with remission. Grip strength (this can be measured with a folded blood pressure cuff) and the number of clinically active joints should be recorded. If all of these facts are kept on a small chart and correlated with the treatment prescribed, the physician can determine which drugs are really helpful and which are not, and when the dosage needs to be adjusted.

Never use more than two anti-inflammatory drugs at the same time. Most authorities suggest that the initial drug be aspirin for its anti-inflammatory and immunosuppressive effects and its effect on connective tissue. The aspirin dosage can range from 4 to 6 grams daily. The usual dosage is 1 gram (3 five grain tablets) every 6 hours. Patients with rheumatoid arthritis may need 4 to 6 grams of aspirin for many years. Serum levels should be monitored, especially the serum salicylate level. To prevent side effects it is recommended that aspirin always be taken with food, milk, or antacids. If side effects such as nausea or tinnitus occur, the dosage should be reduced by decrements of 2 tablets a day to serum levels of 20 to 30 mg. per 100 ml.

Phenylbutazone is prescribed to suppress inflammation during periods of activity. This drug can be used for long periods if necessary. The average dose is 100 mg. 2 to 4 times a day. Side effects are rare at these low dosages. Nevertheless, a urinalysis and complete blood count should be ordered once a week for 2 or 3 weeks when the patient is taking this drug. It should be used, however, only intermittently when aspirin is being taken.

Indomethacin produces analgesic antiinflammatory effects in roughly 30 per cent of patients with rheumatoid arthritis. Start treatment with 25 mg. at bedtime with a glass of milk for 7 to 10 days. Increase to 25 mg. in the morning to be taken after breakfast and at bedtime, again with milk, for another 7 to 10 days. Then increase the dose to 25 mg. after breakfast, after the noon meal, and at bedtime, with milk. Continue to increase the doses in this fashion gradu-

ally until a daily maximum of 100 to 150 mg. is being taken. This gradual increase usually minimizes the side effects such as headache, dizziness, nausea, and vomiting. Indomethacin should be used intermittently with aspirin for weeks or months during acute flare-ups.

Gold salts are used by some physicians, but the side effects of thrombocytopenia, aplastic anemia, and renal toxicity are potentially serious, and for this reason the use of this drug is not as popular as it once was. A similar situation occurs with the hydroxychloroquine type of drug. Side effects here might include pigmentary changes, retinal toxicity, and possible blindness. Therefore, its use is not recommended for the average patient.

Corticosteroids can be prescribed for their anti-inflammatory and immunologic effects and their effect on connective tissue. The effective dose may be as low as 1 mg. of prednisone 2 or 3 times a day. The usual dose schedule is 2 mg. 4 times a day. It is suggested that administration follow the ingestion of meals or be taken with milk to reduce gastric side effects. Steroids should never be used as the primary drug. Prednisone and prednisolone are really the only two steroids recommended for use in rheumatoid arthritis. The recommended low doses rarely cause steroid side effects. If side effects do occur, they may be so mild that they can only be separated with difficulty from the usual clinical manifestations of rheumatoid arthritis. The physician, however, should be cognizant of the manifestations of hypercortisonism, such as extreme fatigue, gross emotional instability with wide mood swings, Cushing's syndrome, steroid myopathy, and water and salt retention.

Therefore, steroids are only recommended when a comprehensive program fails after 6 months of conscientious trial and when severe inflammation persists. They are recommended when the tests show seropositivity for rheumatoid factor and when rheumatoid nodules are present. They are also recommended when studies show vasculitis, serous membrane involvement, extensive tenosynovitis, and generalized rheumatoid disease. Use of steroids must be avoided in patients with peptic ulcer, active infection, tuberculosis, gross emotional instability, renal insufficiency, diabetes mellitus, or congestive heart failure.

When steroid therapy is to be discontinued, it should be done gradually. For instance, if the daily dose is 40 mg., it should be decreased by 2.5 to 5 mg. each day until the level of 10 mg. per day is reached; thereafter it should be reduced by another 1 mg. each 1 or 2 weeks. If reducing the dose causes rheumatoid symptoms to recur, the physician may have to raise the dose to the previous level. Often it is necessary to hold the dose at a certain level for several weeks before reduction can continue. In some instances the total process of withdrawal may take more than a year to complete. After such a withdrawal period advise patients that for up to 2 years afterward they risk adrenocortical deficiency during acute infection, trauma, pregnancy, or surgery. In such situations they will need supportive cortisone acetate therapy given intramuscularly.

Methylprednisolone acetate, because of its anti-inflammatory effect, or a similar product can be injected into joints, especially during acute flare-ups. The usual dose is 25 mg. given intra-articularly for inflamed tendon sheaths or tendons, ligamentous insertions, or bursa. No more than 3 injections should be given in any 6 month period. The technique of joint injection is described elsewhere in this text (page 621).

Finally, never allow a patient with active rheumatoid arthritis to go more than 7 weeks without reassessment of his condition, his drugs, and his overall program.

REFERENCES

1. Aegerter, E., and Kirkpatrick, J.A.: Orthopedic Diseases, 4th Ed. Philadelphia, W. B. Saunders Co., 1975.
2. Apley, A. G.: A System of Orthopaedics and Fractures, 3rd Ed. New York, Appleton-Century-Crofts, 1968.
3. Appleton, A. B., Hamilton, W. J., and Simon, G.: Surface and Radiological Anatomy, 3rd Ed. Baltimore, The Williams & Wilkins Co., 1949.
4. Beetham, W. P., Polley, H. F., Slocumb, C. H., and Weaver, W. F.: Physical Examination of the Joints. Philadelphia, W. B. Saunders Co., 1965.
5. Bleck, E. E.: Atlas of Plaster Cast Techniques. Chicago, Year Book Medical Publishers, Inc., 1956.
6. Blount, W. P.: Fractures in Children. Baltimore, The Williams & Wilkins Co., 1955.
7. Campbell, C. J.: Orthopedic management: Principles and alternative techniques. Surg. Clin. N. Amer. Vol. 41, 1961.
8. Crenshaw, A. H., and Milford, L.: Campbell's Operative Orthopaedics, 4th Ed. St. Louis, The C. V. Mosby Co., 1963, Vol. I.
9. Crenshaw, A. H., and Milford, L.: Campbell's Operative Orthopaedics, 4th Ed. St. Louis, The C. V. Mosby Co., 1963, Vol. II.
10. Ferguson, A. B.: Orthopaedic Surgery in Infancy and Childhood, 3rd Ed. Baltimore, The Williams & Wilkins Co., 1968.
11. Gardner, E., Gray, D. J., and O'Rahilly, R.: Anatomy, 4th Ed. Philadelphia, W. B. Saunders Co., 1975.
12. Gartland, J. J.: Fundamentals of Orthopaedics, 2nd Ed. Philadelphia, W. B. Saunders Co., 1974.
13. Ishmael, W. K.: Care of the Back. Philadelphia, J. B. Lippincott Co., 1962.
14. Ishmael, W. K.: Care of the Neck. Philadelphia, J. B. Lippincott Co., 1966.
15. Jackson, R.: The Cervical Syndrome, 2nd Ed. Illinois, Charles C Thomas, Publisher, 1958.
16. Kopell, H., and Thompson, W. A. L.: Peripheral Entrapment Neuropathies. Baltimore, The Williams & Wilkins Co., 1963.
17. Moseley, H. F.: Clinical Symposia. Static Disorders of the Ankle and Foot. Volume 9, Number 3, Summit, New Jersey, CIBA Pharmaceutical Products Inc., 1957.
18. Moseley, H. F.: Clinical Symposia. Traumatic Disorders of the Ankle and Foot. Volume 7, Number 6, Summit, New Jersey, CIBA Pharmaceutical Products Inc., 1955.
19. O'Donoghue, D. H.: Treatment of Injuries to Athletes, 3rd Ed. Philadelphia, W. B. Saunders Co., 1976.
20. Preston, R. L.: The Surgical Management of Rheumatoid Arthritis. Philadelphia, W. B. Saunders Co., 1968.
21. Pruce, A. M.: Anatomic Landmarks in Joint Paracentesis. Volume 10, Number 1, Summit, New Jersey, CIBA Pharmaceutical Products Inc., 1958.
22. Shands, A. R., Jr., and Raney, R. B., Sr.: Handbook of Orthopaedic Surgery, 6th Ed. St. Louis, The C. V. Mosby Co., 1963.
23. Wiles, P.: Essentials of Orthopaedics, 2nd Ed. Boston, Little, Brown & Co., 1956.
24. Wilkinson, M.: Cervical Spondylosis, 2nd Ed. Philadelphia, W. B. Saunders Co., 1971.

Chapter 39

OTORHINOLARYNGOLOGY

by LOUIS LOWRY

Philip L. Roseberry,
Family Practice Consultant

Otorhinolaryngology is that branch of medicine that encompasses diseases and functions of the ears, nose, paranasal sinuses, mouth, pharynx, larynx, salivary glands, neck, facial skeleton, and upper aerodigestive tract. When seeing a patient with complaints referable to these areas, a history should not be a ritual but should instead be a vital, important source of providing clues for solving the mystery of the patient's complaints. Also while taking the history, the physician should organize his thoughts as to the cause of the patient's disease. The disease will either consciously or unconsciously be placed into some classification. In this chapter, disease processes will be classified as congenital, hereditary, traumatic, infectious, iatrogenic, idiopathic, neoplastic, or drug-induced, and these categories will encompass most otorhinolaryngologic diseases.

This chapter is also divided into nine subsections that are presented in the order in which the author examines patients. These subsections include: (1) Ears, (2) Nose and Paranasal Sinuses, (3) Mouth and Oropharynx, (4) Nasopharynx, (5) Larynx and Hypopharynx, (6) Salivary Glands, (7) Neck, (8) Facial Skeleton, and (9) Upper Aerodigestive Tract. In each of these subsections, embryology, anatomy, and physiology are covered briefly. Instruments used for the examination, diagnostic tests available, review of common problems encountered, and treatment of these problems are listed. Emphasis is placed on the most common disorders, but references for review are listed at the end of the chapter for those wishing to obtain additional information.

EARS

Embryology and Anatomy

The pinna and external auditory canal are derived from the first branchial groove and from small hillocks around the outer edge of the first branchial groove. The middle ear and eustachian tube are derived from an invagination of the first branchial pouch, and the ossicular chain develops from the first branchial arch, second branchial arch, and a portion of the stapes from the otic capsule. The inner ear is derived from an invagination of the ectoderm in the embryo and first forms an otocyst that is carried inward and subsequently is buried beneath the surface. The innervation is derived from the neuroectoderm. The bony ear is thus formed embryologically in the petrous bone. The petrous bone comprises three separate sections—the tympanic plate (the bony external canal), the squamous portion of the temporal bone, and the petrous portion of the temporal bone. These sections are fused, so that in anatomic dissections they are considered to be one unit. The mastoid process is actually a fusion of air cells of the petrous and squamous portions of the temporal bone and is undeveloped at birth, being only a small air cell. Pneumatization of the temporal bone may occur not only in the mastoid process but in the petrous pyramid, zygomatic process, and elsewhere, as shown in Figure 39–1.

Pinna and External Auditory Canal. The examination of the ear requires a knowledge of its structures. Figure 39–2 illustrates the normal configuration of the pinna,

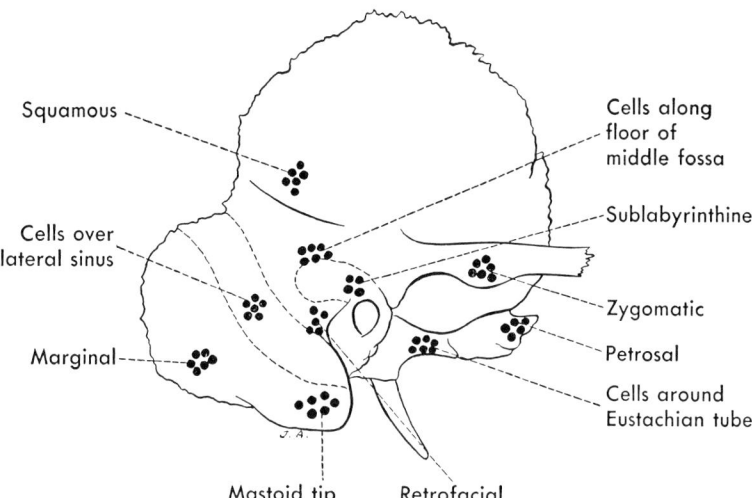

Figure 39-1. *The chief groups of air cells in the temporal bone.* (From Tremble, G. E.: Arch. Otolaryngol., 19:172, 1934. Copyright 1934, American Medical Association.)

which is inspected first. After observation of the pinna, the external auditory canal is the next structure to be examined. The external auditory canal makes a slightly S-shaped curve, which is first angled posteriorly and superiorly, then medially, and finally anteroinferiorly. The length of the external auditory canal is approximately 2.4 cm. (approximately 1 inch) in the adult. The outer one-third consists of the cartilaginous skeleton and the inner two-thirds of the bony skeleton. Hairs and sebaceous and cerumen glands are found only in the cartilaginous portion of the external canal.

Transverse fissures (the fissures of Santorini) are present in the anteroinferior portion of the cartilaginous canal. Lymphatic vessels passing through these fissures are in communication with the parotid compartment and provide access for infections from the ear to the parotid nodes and for infections from the parotid nodes to the external auditory canal.

Tympanic Membrane. The tympanic membrane is placed at an angle of approximately 55° along the axis of the external auditory canal, and the posterosuperior portion of the tympanic membrane is more lateral than its anteroinferior portion. The tympanic membrane has a concavity, and because of this concavity and the placement of the tympanic membrane itself, the portion of the tympanic membrane that is nearly at right angles to the observer is the anteroinferior portion. This position gives the maximum light reflection, which accounts for the light reflex (Fig. 39–3).

The tympanic membrane is covered with a squamous epithelium and is divided into the pars tensa and the pars flaccida. The short process of the malleus is the landmark that divides the pars tensa from the pars flaccida, the pars tensa being inferior to the short process and the pars flaccida being superior to it. The pars tensa has a middle fibrous layer, and on the inner surface the mucous membrane is continuous with the mucous membrane of the middle ear and the pharynx. The pars flaccida also has three layers, but the middle layer is loose areolar elastic tissue and is not readily apparent.

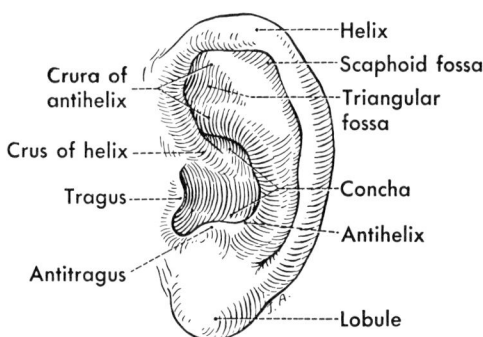

Figure 39-2. *Anatomy of the external ear.* (From Hollinshead, W. H.: Anatomy for Surgeons. Vol. 1, 2nd Ed. Hagerstown, Md., Harper & Row, Publishers, Inc. 1968, p. 184.)

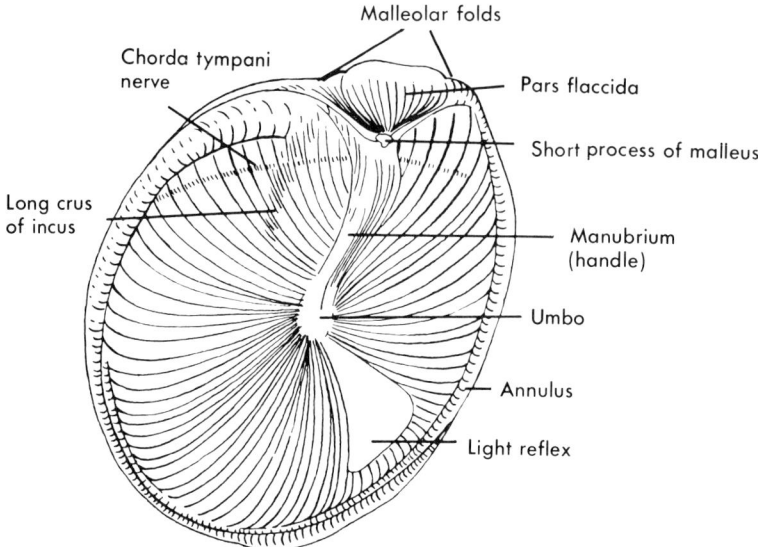

Figure 39-3. *Landmarks of the right tympanic membrane. (From Saunders, W. H.: Ears, nose and throat. In Prior, J. A., and Silberstein, J. S.: Physical Diagnosis. 4th Ed. St. Louis, The C. V. Mosby Co., 1973, p. 137.)*

On observation of the pars tensa, a thickening of the middle fibrous layer around the periphery can often be seen as a fine white line. This thickening forms the annulus tympanicus, which rests in a groove in the most medial aspect of the bony ear canal (the sulcus tympanicus). The pars tensa is classically divided into four quadrants by extending a line through the long process of the malleus and bisecting it with a perpendicular line at the umbo. The long process of the malleus is embedded in the fibrous layer, and the short process of the malleus projects laterally and appears whitened in most instances, as the fibrous layer is deficient in this area.

Physiology

External Ear. The external auditory canal maintains the temperature and humidity of the external environment of the tympanic membrane, and this environment varies very little, regardless of the ambient temperature or humidity. The canal is self-cleaning. Debris is carried by migration of a sheet of desquamating epithelial cells from the center of the tympanic membrane to its periphery and from the medial portion of the canal to its lateral extent.

Middle Ear. The middle ear has the function of allowing sounds in the air to be transmitted to the inner ear, which is fluid-containing. Except for the eustachian tube, the middle ear space is closed to the atmospheric pressure. Malfunctions of the eustachian tube lead to a differential in pressure on both sides of the tympanic membrane, changes in mobility of the tympanic membrane, and hearing loss. During times of nonfunction of the eustachian tube, fluid can accumulate in the middle ear space by two mechanisms—(1) serous effusion with transudate of fluid through the small capillaries of the middle ear space and (2) mucoid production by the small glands in the mucous membrane of the middle ear space.

Inner Ear. The inner ear has two distinct functions, auditory and vestibular, which merit further discussion, as symptoms of disturbance of these functions often bring the patient to you.

AUDITORY FUNCTION OF THE INNER EAR. Sound produces vibrations in an elastic medium. These sound waves are propagated as compressions and rarefactions of the elastic medium and have the ability to cause vibrations in other objects. Sound waves impinging upon the tympanic membrane set the tympanic membrane in motion, and this movement, in turn, causes movement of the malleus,

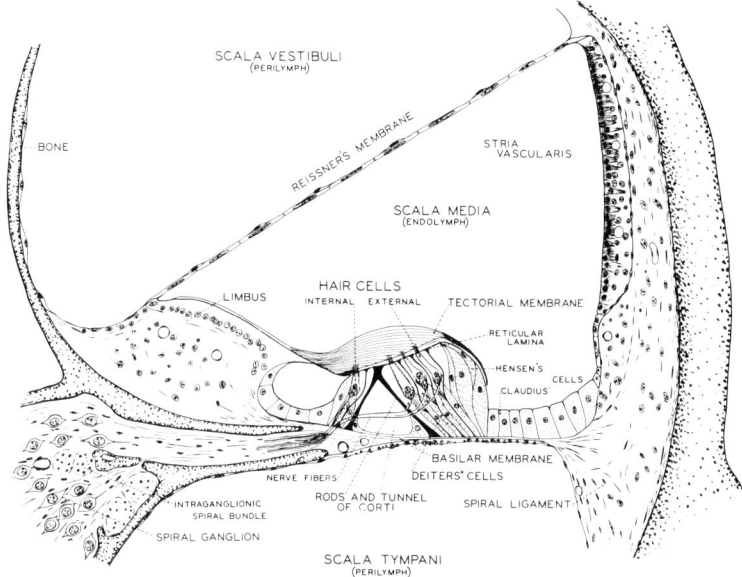

Figure 39–4. *Cross-section of a turn of the cochlea.* (From *Davis, H., et al.: J. Acoustic Soc. Amer., 25:1180, 1953.*)

incus, and stapes. The movement of the stapes results in deformation of the basilar membrane.

A traveling wave is propagated in the basilar membrane from the base of the cochlea to the apex (Fig. 39–4). Along the length of the basilar membrane, a point of maximum displacement occurs with each traveling wave. The location of the point of maximum displacement depends upon the frequency of the stimulating tone. High frequency tones cause displacement in the base of the cochlea, and as the frequency of the stimulating tone is decreased, the point of maximum displacement moves from the base of the cochlea to the apex. The relationship between the frequency of the stimulating tone and the location of maximum displacement appears to depend upon changes in the physical characteristics of the basilar membrane over its length. A traveling wave results in displacement of the basilar membrane, causing movement of the organ of Corti and deformation of the hair cells. As the hairs of the hair cells are bent, depolarization occurs within these cells.

An alternating current potential, known as the cochlear potential, or cochlear microphonic, occurs in response to stimulation of the hair cells. The cochlear potential faithfully reproduces the frequency and intensity of the acoustic stimulation. A chemical transmitter is released in the region of the ends of the afferent VIII nerve fibers, and this chemical transmitter initiates the depolarization of the dendritic terminals of the afferent nerve. At the level of the cochlear nuclei, a single nerve gives a frequency response to tones that is a function of both the intensity and the frequency of the tones. A limited tonal spectrum activates a given neuron at a given intensity. With increasing intensity, other tonal bands may activate the same neuron. At very high intensities, almost all neurons may respond. If the intensity is decreased, a very narrow tonal band activates a given neuron. A frequency that activates a given unit at an intensity at which no other frequencies activate that unit is its *characteristic or best frequency*. This phenomenon of characteristic frequency occurs in all synaptic regions along the auditory pathway.

Individual nerve fibers of the auditory nerve presumably follow the "all or none" principle of nerve excitation and have a refractory period of 1 millisecond. Low and medium frequency acoustic stimulation produces nerve impulses that are synchronous with the frequency of the stimulating tone. At higher frequencies (above

3000 hertz), the refractory period prevents an individual fiber from responding synchronously, but the whole nerve tends to respond synchronously. Synchronous action potentials of the whole nerve at high frequencies probably occur because of the ability of individual nerve fibers to take turns and to respond to every third or fourth sound wave. Each sound wave appears to act as a separate stimulus. Volleys of nerve impulses following one another to a whole fraction of the frequency stimulus have been observed in patterns of nerve impulses in the auditory nerve. This phenomenon has been referred to as the volley principle of coding.

With increasing intensity of the stimulating tone, the rate of discharge of the neural impulses of individual neurons and of the nerve as a whole increases. However, the range over which the frequency of impulses increases with intensity is very limited. It is more likely that the intensity of the acoustic stimulus is more directly represented by the total number of fibers active rather than by the total number of nerve impulses in a single nerve fiber during a given length of time. The threshold for different neurons with the same characteristic frequency may vary by as much 40 to 60 dB. Loudness estimation is probably not based entirely on the rates of discharges of single fibers or groups of fibers but also depends on which fibers are being stimulated.

VESTIBULAR FUNCTION OF THE INNER EAR. The vestibular system plays a role in the organism's ability to maintain balance, posture, and orientation to space; to navigate in the environment; and to respond to acceleration and deceleration. This system functions in conjunction with the systems of vision and proprioception (the other two modalities of the balance triad) to enable a subject to maintain balance and posture and navigate well in his environment, as long as any two of these three modalities remain intact. If two of these systems become impaired, difficulty results. The tabetic patient does well until he is in the dark. The blind person becomes disabled by the impairment of vestibular apparatus caused by streptomycin ototoxicity. The person who has lost his vestibular function because of bilateral basilar skull fractures will become disabled with the onset of peripheral neuropathy.

The peripheral vestibular mechanism, including the saccule, utricle, and semicircular canals, responds to acceleration and deceleration. The macula of the saccule faces laterally. The macula of the utricle is essentially horizontal and faces superiorly. The three semicircular canals (on one side) are in planes at right angles to each other. The six semicircular (on both sides) canals are arranged in three pairs. One member of a pair lies in the plane that is parallel to the plane of the other member of the pair. The two horizontal semicircular canals make one pair. The left superior semicircular canal and the right posterior semicircular canal make another pair. The dilated or ampullated ends of the two canals in each pair are oriented in opposite directions about the axis of rotation of their planes, so that any movement of fluid in the plane of the pair of canals results in movement of fluid toward the ampulla in one and away from the ampulla in the other.

The maculae are composed of hair cells and supporting cells. The hairs of the hair cells extend to a gelatinous mass loaded with tiny, ovoid masses of calcium carbonate. These *otoliths* have a greater density than endolymph and respond differentially to changes in linear acceleration and deceleration in the polar gravity, which can be thought of as linear acceleration.

The semicircular canals respond to angular acceleration and deceleration. Acceleration causes movement of the endolymph relative to the membranous semicircular canal by virtue of the inertia of the endolymph. Continued movement at a steady rate in time allows the endolymph to move at the same velocity as the walls of the canal. During deceleration, the inertia of the endolymph again causes movement of the endolymph relative to the membranous semicircular canal. This movement displaces the cupula and deforms the hair cells of the crista that are in contact with the cupula.

Examination

Instruments for examination of the ear are shown in Figure 39–5 and include equipment for the clinical examination of hearing and of the vestibular apparatus.

Each of the two otoscope heads is used for a specific purpose, that is, (1) the clinical examination of the ear and removal of

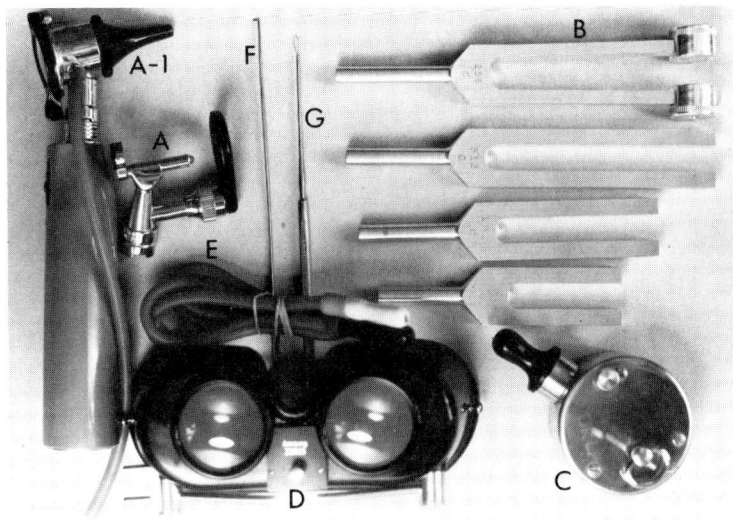

Figure 39–5. *Instruments for examination of the ear.* A, *open and closed otoscope heads;* B, *full set of tuning forks 256, 512, 1024, and 2048 Hz.;* C, *Bárány noise box for masking;* D, *Frenzel glasses for detection of nystagmus;* E, *Toynbee tube to auscultate the ear for objective tinnitus;* F, *ear hook for foreign body removal; and* G, *ear loop for removal of cerumen.*

small pieces of cerumen or foreign bodies that can be retrieved by the use of an ear hook, which pulls the foreign body outward (Fig. 39–5A) and (2) a pneumatic otoscope that should be employed in the clinical examination of each patient (Fig. 39–5A-1). The tympanic membrane should normally have an equal pressure from both sides of the drum and should move when positive as well as negative pressure is applied. Any limitation of the mobility of the drum denotes a pathologic process.

Tuning Fork Tests. Tuning fork tests are of great clinical importance and can be used to estimate the severity of conductive hearing losses or to ascertain a unilateral sensorineural hearing loss. The two specific tests most commonly employed are the Weber test and the Rinne test.

WEBER TEST. The Weber test is performed by striking a tuning fork so that it has a pure tone and by placing it anywhere on the midline of the skull, including the upper teeth. The mandibular teeth are not suitable for placement, as they are not directly connected to the skull. The five possible results are that the sound will be (1) felt but not heard, (2) not felt or heard, (3) heard in the right ear, (4) heard in the left ear, or (5) heard equally bilaterally.

Results of this testing are considered important because a person who does not hear the tuning fork may have a moderate-to-severe sensorineural hearing loss. When the Weber test lateralizes to either ear, there are two diagnostic possibilities. These are a conductive hearing loss in the ear in which the sound was heard or a sensorineural hearing loss in the opposite ear. To ascertain which of these possibilities is correct, it is necessary to perform the Rinne test. The Weber test heard equally in both ears denotes equally good or equally poor hearing function. It should be noted that the Weber test is not completely reliable and that the test results must be integrated with the findings of the physical examination and history.

RINNE TEST. The Rinne test is based on the fact that under normal conditions transmission of sound is heard more loudly by air conduction than by bone conduction. This test can be performed in several ways. The usual description is that of striking the tuning fork and placing its stem on the mastoid. When the patient can no longer hear the sound by bone conduction, he is then asked to listen for the sound by air conduction. It is important that the tines of the tuning fork be placed parallel to the external auditory

canal approximately 1 inch from the opening of the ear canal. If the patient hears
sound by air conduction better than by
bone conduction, the test is considered
Rinne-positive (normal). Variations of this
test include placing the stem of the tuning
fork on the mastoid and then placing the
tines near the external auditory canal and
asking the patient which sound is louder.
The Rinne test was originally performed
by timing the duration of the patient's
hearing by bone conduction and by air
conduction and by noting that normally
the duration of hearing by air conduction
is approximately two times longer than
that by bone conduction.

In patients with a unilateral sensorineural hearing loss, the tuning fork may be
heard in the better ear. When this condition is suspected, the Bárány noise box is
placed in the external auditory canal of the
better ear (without occluding the canal),
and the noise apparatus is activated while
the Rinne test is performed on the ear
with the greater hearing loss. If bone conduction is greater than air conduction in
one ear, a higher frequency tuning fork
should be used. The more severe the conductive deficit, the higher the frequency
must be to obtain air conduction greater
than bone conduction. If bone conduction
remains greater than air conduction using
a tuning fork as high as 2048 Hz., it can be
said that the patient has a maximum conductive hearing loss.

UTILIZING TUNING FORK TESTING. Figure 39–6 diagrams the major findings of
the Weber and Rinne tests. The diagram
shows the possibilities for utilizing the
Weber test and also raises some questions
that may only be defined by audiometric
evaluation. However, when the Weber test
lateralizes to one ear or the other, the
Rinne test is of utmost importance in
ascertaining if a conductive hearing loss is
present. If there is a conductive hearing loss
in the ear to which the sound is lateralized
on the Weber test, the Rinne test should
show bone conduction greater than air conduction. If there is a sensorineural hearing
loss in the opposite ear, air conduction
should be greater than bone conduction.
However, if sensorineural hearing loss in
the opposite ear is severe, bone conduction
by Rinne testing will lateralize to the good
ear, so that the Bárány noise box may be
necessary to mask hearing in the good ear.
Finally, if there is lateralization to one
ear on the Weber test and a normal physical
examination and Rinne test, it would be
well to repeat the Weber test.

**Additional Instruments for Examining the
Ear.** The Toynbee tube is simply a rubber
tube with a small ear adapter at each end
to listen for tinnitus. Approximately 5 per
cent of patients with tinnitus have been
reported to have objective tinnitus, that is,
tinnitus that another person can hear. This
type of tinnitus is nearly always caused by
a vascular abnormality and may be correctable. Subjective tinnitus is presumed to be
due to inner ear disturbances.

The ear loop is used in removing small
amounts of wax and debris from the exter-

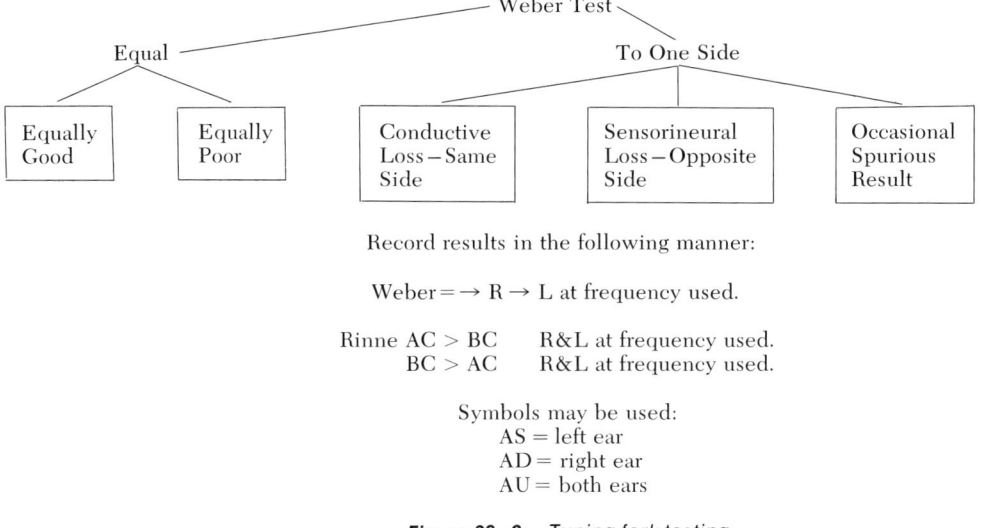

Figure 39–6. *Tuning fork testing.*

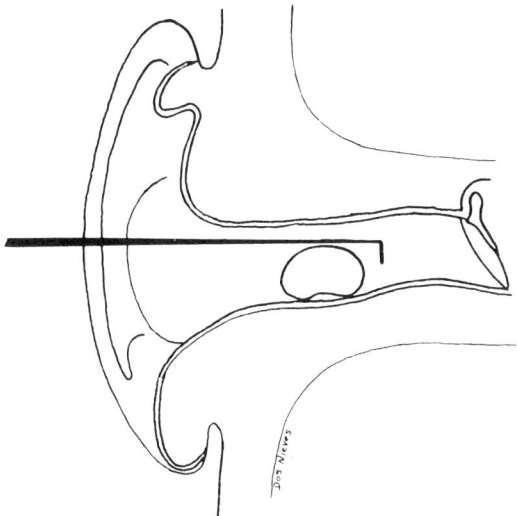

Figure 39-7. *Technique for the removal of foreign bodies in the ear canal. The foreign body is raked out with a blunt Day hook. (From Snow, J. B., Jr.: Surgical disorders of the ears, nose, paranasal sinuses, pharynx and larynx. In Davis–Christopher Textbook of Surgery. 10th Ed. Philadelphia, W. B. Saunders Co., 1972, p. 1207.)*

nal ear canal. The ear hook is used to reach around foreign bodies, and the method of its use is demonstrated in Figure 39–7. It is important to note that a foreign body should be pulled toward the observer and should not be grasped, as this may further push the foreign body into the external ear.

Frenzel glasses are +20 diopter lenses that are placed over the patient's eyes. This facilitates the detection of nystagmus and should be used routinely in the vestibular examination.

Testing of the Peripheral Ear

Should the history or clinical examination reveal an abnormality, further testing procedures may be desirable.

Audiometry. One such procedure is audiometry, and an explanation of the basic audiometric tests is as follows: Figure 39–8 shows an audiogram, which gives several results. Each audiogram has a code listing X's for air conduction in the left ear, O's for air conduction in the right ear, and some form of half-open symbol for bone conduction. The air conduction and bone conduction are recorded in a superimposed fashion, so that an overview of the entire process can be obtained. It should be noted that 0 to 20 dB. is the normal range of hearing that has been determined by testing a large number of normal people.

For the purpose of audiometry, bone conduction is equal to air conduction. Therefore, air conduction and bone conduction should be equal in each ear and should be above 20 dB. to be considered normal. If there is discrepancy between bone conduction and air conduction, a conductive hearing loss is diagnosed. The severity of the conductive hearing loss can be measured, and on the audiogram shown, there is an average of the air conduction and the bone conduction in the speech frequencies. The three frequencies averaged are the 500 Hz., 1000 Hz., and 2000 Hz. After averaging the air conduction and the bone conduction for each ear, these figures are recorded to see if they are indeed equal.

The *Speech Reception Threshold* (SRT) is performed by transmitting words to the patient, which he attempts to repeat, while varying the intensity of the stimulus until he identifies approximately 50 per cent of the words. SRT is important in that this should correlate well with the air conduction-pure tone average. If there is a discrepancy between the SRT and the pure tone average for air, the patient may be unreliable in the test situation. *Discrimination* is the ability of patients to understand and repeat words spoken at a normal conversational level of loudness. Each audiogram will record a discrimination, and the number of decibels above the patient's hearing level will be noted. Discrimination should be 90 per cent or more to be considered normal. In addition, there are special audiometric tests for cochlear and retrocochlear problems, which will not be discussed here.

Electronystagmography. This is the standard test for evaluating the peripheral vestibular apparatus. Basically, electronystagmography consists of detecting eye movements by recording the movement of the corneal-retinal potential and stimulating the vestibular system to cause movements of the eyes. Standard caloric testing is done using water at 30° C. and 44° C. As this is 7° C. warmer and 7° C. cooler than

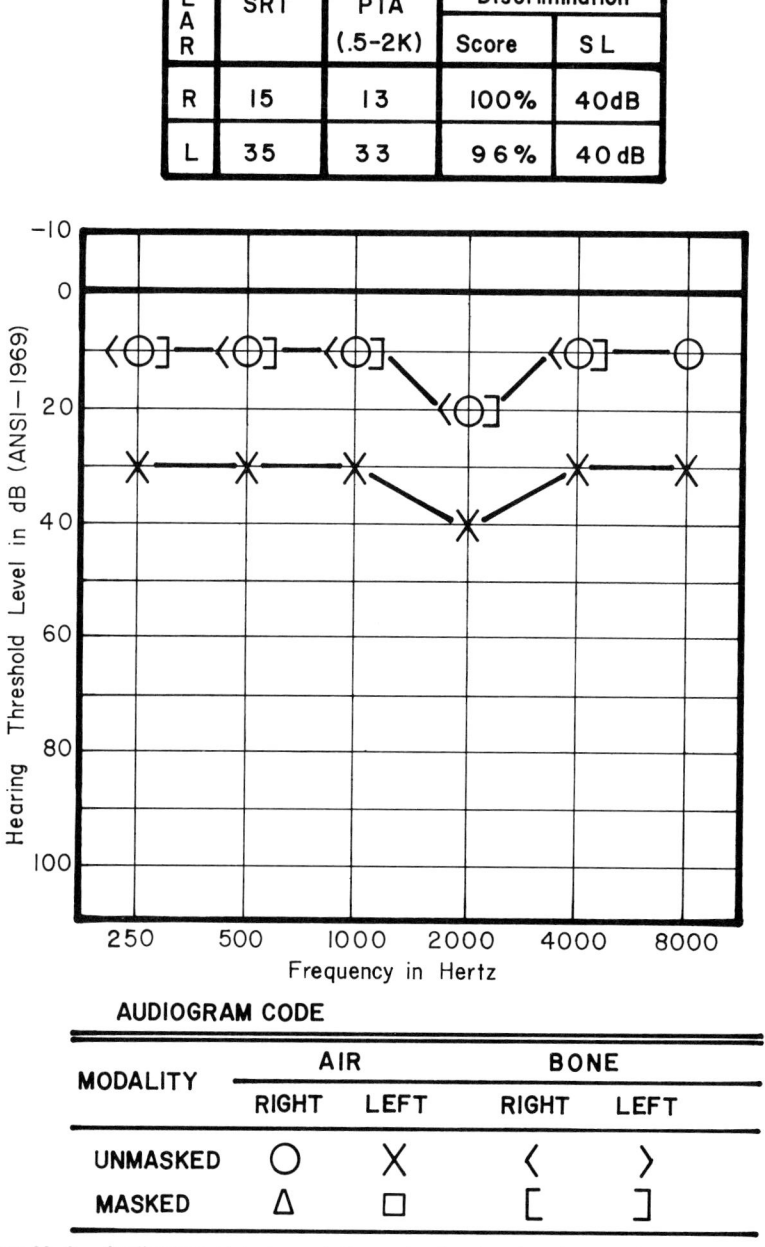

E A R	SRT	PTA (.5-2K)	Discrimination	
			Score	S L
R	15	13	100%	40dB
L	35	33	96%	40 dB

AUDIOGRAM CODE

MODALITY	AIR		BONE	
	RIGHT	LEFT	RIGHT	LEFT
UNMASKED	O	X	⟨	⟩
MASKED	Δ	□	[	]

Figure 39-8. Audiogram showing a left conductive hearing loss and use of masking.

the normal body temperature, it causes convection currents in the endolymph and thus produces a nystagmus. By comparing the right ear with the left ear, an estimation of the patient's normal response can be made. It should be noted that prior to this recording, any spontaneous nystagmus is also noted. Positional testing is performed by placing the patient (with closed eyes) in the supine position with the head hanging, and then in the supine position with the head to the right and to the left. Any positional nystagmus elicited by these maneuvers is thereby recorded, even though the eyes are closed.

Clinical testing, whenever electronystagmography is not possible, may be done with the use of the Frenzel glasses and a small amount of ice water. A blunt needle is placed in the external canal, and 5 ml.

of ice water is used to irrigate the posteroinferior quadrant of the tympanic membrane. The duration of the nystagmus is then recorded. This screening measure can be quite helpful when evaluating someone who may have a peripheral vestibular problem.

Mastoid x-rays and polytomography of the middle and inner ear may be required for the complete evaluation of a patient, and these studies should be reviewed with a radiologist in conjunction with the history and clinical findings.

Congenital Disorders

Lop Ear. The auricle of the ear may protrude too far from the skull. This is termed an outstanding ear, lop ear or protruding ear. The basic deformity is caused by a lack of development of the anthelix (see Fig. 39–2). This deformity can be corrected surgically by weakening the spring of the cartilage of the pinna, so that the anthelic fold can be created. Such surgery is ideally performed at age 5 or 6 years.

Preauricular Cysts and Sinuses. These are fairly common and may be unilateral or bilateral. They are usually asymptomatic but may become infected and require incision and drainage and possible excision. Complete excision is difficult because these sinuses are in close proximity to the branches of the facial nerve. Excision is recommended only if recurrent infection has become a problem.

Microtia. This is a term used to describe the presence of major developmental defects of the pinna, resulting in a relatively small or misshapen external ear. If a major portion of the auricular cartilage is absent, surgical reconstruction rarely produces a satisfactory cosmetic result. Microtia is often associated with stenosis or atresia of the external auditory canal. These deformities are often found in conjunction with developmental anomalies of the middle ear, resulting in profound conductive hearing losses. The course of the facial nerve through the temporal bone may be abnormal, making surgical repair of the sound pressure transformation apparatus of the middle ear hazardous. In unilateral defects with normal hearing in the other ear, middle reconstruction is not recommended because of the danger of facial nerve injury. However, if there is bilateral profound hearing loss, attempts at reconstruction should be made. A bone conduction hearing aid will contribute to the rehabilitation process when surgical reconstruction is not feasible.

Congenital malformations of the inner ear resulting in profound sensorineural hearing losses may or may not be associated with abnormalities of the external and middle ear.

The evaluation of congenital malformations of the ear is facilitated by radiography of the temporal bone, electronystagmography, and audiometric testing.

Hereditary Disorders

Otosclerosis. Otosclerosis is the most common cause of hereditary deafness and has been determined to be due to a dominant gene with variable penetrance. It has been estimated that 10 per cent of the Caucasian population in the United States has histologic otosclerosis and that 10 per cent of persons thus afflicted will have a conductive hearing loss. Otosclerosis produces a progressive conductive hearing loss in the adult. It is a disease of abnormal bone formation in the otic capsule and has a predilection for the anterior part of the oval window. Histologically, foci of otosclerosis show irregularly arranged, new, immature bone interspersed with numerous vascular channels. As these foci of otosclerotic bone enlarge, they cause ankylosis of the foot plate of the stapes and produce a conductive hearing loss. Physical examination will reveal normal tympanic membranes and a conductive hearing loss. The family history is positive for this disorder in approximately 50 per cent of these patients. The conductive hearing loss becomes clinically evident in the late adolescent or early adult years. Fixation of the stapes may progress rapidly during pregnancy. Otosclerosis is rare in blacks, American Indians, and Japanese and is common in Asiatic Indians.

The conductive hearing loss can be corrected surgically in the vast majority of instances by microsurgical techniques. This involves removal of the stapes and placement of a prosthesis extending from the long process of the incus to the oval window. The complication of profound sensorineural hearing loss occurs in 2 to 4 per cent of recorded operative cases.

An alternative to surgery is the placement of a hearing aid. Candidates for this procedure already have excellent discrimination scores and only need an increased loudness.

Sensorineural Hearing Loss. This disorder is transmitted by a large number of syndromes, with approximately 90 per cent of these being transmitted by a recessive gene and 10 per cent by a dominant gene. In recessively transmitted hearing losses, many patients have no other associated anomalies. However, in dominantly transmitted sensorineural hearing losses, many associated syndromes have been found. These include hypothyroidism, retinitis pigmentosa, cardiac anomalies, and renal disease. The article by B. Proctor and C. A. Proctor provides an excellent in-depth look at the problem of hereditary sensorineural deafness.

Infectious Disorders of the External Ear

Infections of the Pinna. Such infections are unusual but are important to diagnose because of the possibility of *perichondritis* and the loss of cartilage, with resulting deformation of the ear. These infections may be treated by antibiotic therapy and by careful observation of the patient. If there appears to be subperichondrial dissection of the infection, incision and drainage are necessary. Infections of the pinna can be quite resistant to treatment once the cartilage is invaded, and consultation with an otorhinolaryngologist should be obtained.

Otitis Externa. There are two forms of otitis externa, which is an infection of the external auditory canal. The *localized form* is due to furunculosis, which is usually caused by *Staphylococcus aureus*. Furuncles of the external auditory canal should be allowed to rupture spontaneously, because incision may lead to a perichondritis of the pinna. Antibiotic treatment with ampicillin or penicillin is helpful in localizing the infection.

The *diffuse form of external otitis* is called otitis externa generalizata and is commonly termed *swimmer's ear*. This infection is usually caused by a gram-negative rod such as *Escherichia coli, Pseudomonas aeruginosa,* or *Bacillus proteus,* or by *Staphylococcus aureus*. Predisposing factors include the patient's cleaning and traumatizing the canal, introducing irritants such as hair spray, or allowing water to accumulate in the canal. Attempts by the patient to clean the canal interrupt its self-cleaning mechanism and cause the accumulation of debris. Debris and cerumen tend to allow retention of water in the canal and to macerate the skin. This maceration sets the stage for invasion by pathogenic bacteria.

Patients with diffuse external otitis complain of itching, pain, foul-smelling discharge, and loss of hearing if the canal becomes swollen or filled with purulent debris. Tenderness after applying traction to the pinna or after applying pressure over the tragus tends to distinguish external otitis from otitis media. The skin of the external canal appears red, swollen, and filled with purulent debris.

Treatment consists of the application of topical antibiotics and corticosteroids. These preparations usually contain neomycin, polymyxin, and steroids and have an acid pH that deters the growth of bacteria. Systemic therapy for external otitis is rarely necessary unless there is spreading cellulitis about the ear. For the topical therapy to succeed, the infected debris must be removed from the canal by suction or by dry wipes of cotton. Often, a narcotic is needed for relief of pain during the first 24 to 48 hours. If the treatment is to be successful, the patient must be cautioned about keeping his ear *absolutely dry*. The reintroduction of water into the external ear will often cause an acute exacerbation of the symptoms.

Infectious Disorders of the Middle Ear

Chronic Otitis Media. This is defined as a perforation of the tympanic membrane. There may or may not be active infection, and the term is presented here only for its definition.

Acute Otitis Media and Serous Otitis Media. Acute otitis media and serous otitis media are presented together, as they commonly present a problem in differential diagnosis.

Acute otitis media is an infectious, inflammatory process of the middle ear, usually secondary to an upper respiratory tract infection. It has been reported to be the most common localized infection in children. Most children between 1 and 5 years of age have two or three episodes of acute otitis media each year. Acute otitis media may be viral or bacterial. Viral otitis media may resolve, or the middle ear may be secondarily invaded by bacteria. Acute suppurative otitis media is caused by group A beta-hemolytic streptococci, *Diplococcus pneumoniae*, *Staphylococcus aureus*, or *Hemophilus influenzae*. Infections caused by *H. influenzae* have a greater incidence in children less than 5 years of age. In older children and adults, streptococcal infections are the most common forms, followed in incidence by pneumococcal and staphylococcal infections.

Serous otitis media is caused by eustachian tube dysfunction that may be due to acute viral upper respiratory infection and edema of the eustachian tube or to secondary blockage of the eustachian tube. Initially, the tympanic membrane is retracted, as the air from the middle ear space is resorbed. Fluid begins to accumulate from a transudate of fluid through the vessel walls and from production of mucus by the small mucous glands in the middle ear mucosa. There may be secondary bacterial invasion of the fluid of the middle ear transforming a serous otitis media to acute suppurative otitis media.

The differential diagnosis between these two disease processes is difficult, as both may have fever, hearing loss, and redness of the tympanic membrane. However, on *pneumatic otoscopy*, the acute suppurative otitis media will cause a bulging tympanic membrane, and the serous otitis media will cause a retracted tympanic membrane that will move only on negative pressure during the pneumatic otoscopic examination. In many instances of serous otitis media, there will be an upper respiratory infection that requires therapy with antibiotics. However, if no bacterial infection is found, treatment with antibiotics is not indicated. Rather, in serous otitis media, the eustachian tube dysfunction should be treated with an antihistamine–decongestant combination, such as triprolidine hydrochloride and pseudoephedrine hydrochloride (Actifed).

When pneumatic otoscopy shows the tympanic membrane to be reddened and bulging, a diagnosis of acute otitis media can be made. Penicillin is the drug of choice in treating patients over 5 years of age. For children under 5 years of age, ampicillin is preferred because of the frequency of *H. influenzae* infections. Treatment should be continued for at least 10 days in order to assure resolution and prevention of recurrent streptococcal infections. In the presence of penicillin allergy, erythromycin for older children and adults and the combination of erythromycin and sulfisoxazole for those children under the age of 5 years may be employed. Pharyngeal cultures may be helpful but generally do not identify the causative agents of acute suppurative otitis media.

A myringotomy is indicated if the tympanic membrane has become discolored and is bulging or if pain, fever, vomiting, and diarrhea are severe. Myringotomy is performed in the anteroinferior quadrant of the tympanic membrane. The material removed from this site should be cultured for identification of the causative organism and for determining antibiotic sensitivities.

If there is a doubt as to whether the patient has an acute middle ear infection or a systemic illness with fever and possible middle ear infection, it is recommended that the patient be treated for acute otitis media.

The *complications of acute otitis media* are numerous and include *acute mastoiditis, petrositis, labyrinthitis, facial paralysis, conductive* and *sensorineural hearing loss, epidural abscess, meningitis, brain abscess, lateral sinus thrombosis, subdural empyema*, and *otitic hydrocephalus*. The most common intracranial complication of acute otitis media is meningitis. Prior to the development of such complications, there may be warning symptoms and signs such as severe headache, sudden profound hearing loss, vertigo, and chills and fever.

Acute Mastoiditis. Acute mastoiditis invariably occurs in conjunction with acute otitis media, the infection extending to the mastoid antrum and to the mastoid air cells. However, the term acute mastoiditis is not used clinically until destruction of the bony partitions between the mastoid air cells has occurred. Progression of an acute infectious process of the mastoid has become rare since the advent of antibiotic therapy. The bacteria causing acute mastoiditis are the same as those causing acute otitis media. Acute coalescent mastoiditis becomes clinically apparent 14 days or more after the onset of acute otitis media, as the cortices of the mastoid process are destroyed. The destruction of the mastoid cortex is usually associated with an exacerbation of aural pain, fever, and otorrhea. The pain tends to be persistent and throbbing, and the discharge is usually purulent and profuse. Increased hearing loss is characteristic of acute mastoiditis.

The lateral mastoid cortex is most frequently the first to be destroyed, and a postauricular subperiosteal abscess develops. The first signs of this development are thickening of the postauricular tissue, reduced mobility of the skin over the mastoid cortex, and a blunting of the postauricular crease. As pus exudes from the mastoid cortex deep into the periosteum, an erythematous, hot, tender, fluctuant postauricular mass develops that displaces the pinna laterally and inferiorly. Less commonly, the coalescence of the air cells and the destruction of the cortex occurring with cellular extension to the zygomatic process result in formation of a preauricular subperiosteal abscess. When destruction of the cortex occurs at the tip of the mastoid process, it produces an abscess (the so-called Bezold's abscess) in the neck deep to the superior one-third of the sternocleidomastoid.

Destruction of bone adjacent to the external auditory canal results in sagging of the posterior canal wall. Destruction of the inner cortices of the mastoid process opposite the middle or posterior cranial fossae may occur, and such destruction results in an epidural abscess.

Radiographs show an increased density of the mastoid air cells in acute otitis media. In coalescent mastoiditis, cell partitions become indistinct, and the individual septa can no longer be seen, as one air cell coalesces with its neighbor.

In early cases of acute mastoiditis in which there are postauricular signs of tenderness and edema but no fluctuation, antibiotic therapy may result in complete resolution of the infectious process.

In the presence of a subperiosteal abscess, a complete mastoidectomy should be performed. The objective of the surgery is to drain the abscess in the mastoid air cells and antrum. Drainage of the middle ear is provided by myringotomy or through the pre-existing perforation. The primary goal of surgery is resolution of the infection.

Petrositis. Petrositis is an infection of the pneumatized petrous bone. Pneumatization of the temporal bone medial to the cochlea in continuity with the middle ear space is common. Infection of these air cells, similar to the infection described in acute mastoiditis, may result in the destruction of the cortex of the petrous pyramid and in the formation of an epidural abscess. An epidural abscess occurring in the apical carotid portion of the petrous pyramid produces Gradenigo's syndrome (suppurative otitis media, headache, diplopia due to VI cranial nerve paralysis, trigeminal neuralgia, and retro-orbital pain). Treatment requires surgical drainage of this area and antibiotic therapy with penicillin for persons over age 5 and with ampicillin for persons under age 5.

Purulent Labyrinthitis. This is defined as invasion of the inner ear by bacterial organisms. This infection may be secondary to acute otitis media or to meningitis. It is characterized by severe vertigo and nystagmus and invariably results in complete loss of hearing. Purulent labyrinthitis is often followed by facial paralysis. Surgical treatment includes a labyrinthectomy for drainage of the inner ear in conjunction with a radical mastoidectomy.

Cholesteatoma. This is a tumor caused by an ingrowth of squamous epithelium into the middle ear space or by the development of a congenital rest of squamous epithelium. Cholesteatomas are classified as congenital, primary acquired, and secondary acquired.

Congenital cholesteatomas are quite rare and are thought to be produced by congenital rests of squamous epithelium in the petrous pyramid.

Primary acquired cholesteatomas are defined as cholesteatomas associated with a perforation of the pars flaccida (the area of the tympanic membrane above the short process of the malleus). Presentation of a patient with an acute otitis media with purulent drainage and a perforation in the area of the pars flaccida is pathognomonic of a cholesteatoma. Cholesteatomas usually extend posteriorly into or invading the mastoid antrum. They cause destruction of bone, which can be seen radiographically, and are prone to recurrent infections.

Treatment involves surgical removal of this benign tumor.

Secondary acquired cholesteatomas are associated with perforations of the pars tensa and are suspected when the margins of the tympanic membrane have been destroyed. Classically, the perforation contains desquamated epithelial debris. The treatment of a secondary acquired cholesteatoma is surgical removal.

Ear Polyps. Polyps in the external auditory canal are uniformly associated with a perforation of the tympanic membrane. These polyps may obscure the perforation and may lead to a chronic infectious process. Local and systemic treatment of the infection may result in a resolution of the polyp. If the polyp does not resolve, surgical exploration of the middle ear space and removal of the polyp are indicated.

Tuberculous Otitis Media. This infection is now rare. Its chronic form is characterized by persistent drainage and multiple perforations of the tympanic membrane. More than one perforation is pathognomonic for tuberculous otitis media. The infection produces a very destructive process in the middle ear and is associated with a profound conductive hearing loss. It is also associated with intracranial complications. Tuberculous otitis media occurs secondary to tuberculosis elsewhere in the body and is most often associated with miliary tuberculosis and hematogenous spread to the middle ear. Unless there is some complication, this disease process is treated with the same chemotherapeutic regimen used for pulmonary tuberculosis.

Infectious Disorders of the Inner Ear

The inner ear can be invaded by bacterial organisms as a complication of acute otitis media or by meningitis organisms via the VIII nerve or the cochlear aqueduct.

Of the several viral infections of the inner ear, the most common disorder occurring after birth is that of the mumps virus. Invasion of the inner ear produces a pathologic process known as viral endolymphatic labyrinthitis. In children and adults, mumps, measles, influenza, and adenoviruses may invade the inner ear and produce sudden deafness. The pathologic process of viral endolymphatic laby-

rinthitis is similar in all cases, regardless of the causative agent. Degenerative changes may cause atrophy of the organ of Corti, which may be missing in the basal turns. Individual hair cells may be missing in the higher turns. The stria vascularis tends to be atrophic. Loss of hearing is frequently profound and permanent. Tinnitus and vertigo may be present initially.

Congenital deafness and deafness acquired in early infancy should be detected during infancy, and amplification of sound by means of a hearing aid should be started as early as 8 or 9 months of age. Deaf children do not develop language skills because they must hear language to learn it.

There is no known treatment for viral inner ear infection, and early detection and rehabilitation are essential.

Viral Neuronitis. This disorder is caused by an invasion of the VIII nerve and its ganglia by a herpes zoster virus, producing hearing loss, vertigo, and paralysis of the facial nerve in association with vesicle formation on the pinna along the distribution of the sensory branch of the facial nerve. This symptom complex is known as the *Ramsey Hunt syndrome or herpes zoster oticus.* Lymphocytes may be present in the cerebrospinal fluid, and the protein content is often increased. Evidence of a mild generalized encephalitis can be found in most patients. Treatment of the facial nerve paralysis is only moderately successful, even with surgical intervention. It is likely that other undocumented viruses invade the VIII nerve and its ganglia without being detected.

Iatrogenic Disorders

Iatrogenic causes of ear injury fall into two categories. The first category is that of surgical trauma, and the second is that of drug-induced changes. Drug-induced changes will be discussed in a separate section on ototoxic drugs.

Surgical causes of hearing loss are usually related to mastoid surgery and the necessity for removing the ossicular chain to prevent recurrence of infection and its complications. Two to 4 per cent of persons undergoing a stapedectomy will have a sensorineural hearing loss. At the present time, the cause of this hearing loss is unknown.

Idiopathic Disorders

Meniere's Disease. This is one of the most overdiagnosed diseases seen in the practice of otorhinolaryngology. Strict adherence must be paid to the diagnostic criteria of vertigo, tinnitus, sensorineural hearing loss, and fullness of the ear, as the patient may have another disease process that will go undetected once the label of Meniere's disease has been given to his illness.

The pathologic change in the inner ear is a generalized dilatation of the membranous labyrinth or endolymphatic hydrops. Only one ear is involved in 85 per cent of the patients with Meniere's disease. Sensorineural hearing losses are initially more severe in the lower than in the higher frequencies. Hearing tends to fluctuate and becomes depressed following an attack of vertigo. The tinnitus has a low-pitched, roaring quality and is worse just before, during, and after an attack of vertigo. Attacks of vertigo occur suddenly, last from a few to 24 hours, and subside gradually. Attacks are typically associated with nausea and vomiting. In the *Lermoyez's variant* of Meniere's disease, the loss of hearing and tinnitus may precede the first attack of vertigo by months or years. Over the course of many years, the hearing becomes progressively worse.

Each patient who presents with the symptoms just described should undergo an extensive work-up to rule out other disease processes. This work-up should include an audiogram with special audiometric tests, polytomograms of the middle and internal ears, electronystagmography with caloric testing, 5 hour glucose tolerance test, thyroid function tests, VDRL serology determination, and lipoprotein electrophoresis.

Documentation of *fluctuating sensorineural hearing loss* narrows the diagnosis to Meniere's disease or to a fistula communicating from the middle ear to the inner ear. Metabolic test results may show hyper- or hypoglycemia, which when treated may lead to relief of the patient's symptoms. Similarly, findings of hyper- or hypothyroidism or syphilis may lead to resolution of the symptoms after treatment of the underlying disease. Discussions in the recent literature have cited hyperlipoproteinemia as a cause of vertigo.

Treatment of Meniere's disease is widely varied and uniformly successful. Since most patients will have spontaneous resolution of their symptoms for a period of time, treatment may be classified as either uniformly successful or uniformly unsuccessful, depending on whichever criterion you wish to use. It is essential that the work-up be complete in order to rule out underlying disease. If no underlying disease is found and the patient is incapacitated by vertigo, ablative surgery may be considered.

Presbycusis. Presbycusis is defined as the hearing loss that occurs as part of the normal aging process. Typically, the high frequencies are affected first. There is progression to the low frequencies and eventually to a difficulty with speech, as the speech frequencies of 500 to 3000 Hz. are affected. Many explanations for presbycusis have been advanced. Among these are stiffening of the basilar membrane, deterioration of the hair cells, atrophy of the stria vascularis, loss of the ganglion cells, and loss of cells in the cochlear nuclei.

At the present time, there is no known treatment for presbycusis unless exposure to noise is associated with the hearing loss. The loss cannot be reversed, but with proper protection of hearing, the loss can be stabilized at that point.

Noise Exposure. Noise exposure is included in this section, as noise is with us all our lives. It is known that noise exposure can cause sensorineural hearing loss. Apparently, persons who have a hereditary predisposition to this disorder may have an accelerated hearing loss caused by a noise exposure that is "safe" for other persons. In evaluating a patient for hearing loss, a history of noise exposure is important. Therefore, not only the patient's occupation but his avocation should be determined. The classic audiogram of such a patient shows a sloping sensorineural hearing loss that is more severe in the high frequencies. Typically, the frequency of 4000 Hz. is the most affected, and there is some recovery at the frequency of 8000 Hz. This classic configuration may be the only difference in the results of an audiogram performed to differentiate between presbycusis and noise-induced hearing loss. Of course, it is most likely that a hearing loss in a person aged 40 or older would be a combination of presbycusis and noise-induced hearing loss.

Vestibular Neuronitis. This is a disease without proven cause, characterized by the sudden onset of vertigo that is at first persistent and then becomes paroxysmal. The attacks are frequent at the onset, gradually become less frequent, and finally disappear after 1 or 2 years. The disease is thought by some to be caused by a virus because of its frequent occurrence in epidemic form, particularly among adolescents and young adults. There is no associated loss of hearing or tinnitus and no relationship of the vertigo to head position. It is thought that this disease represents a viral neuronitis involving the vestibular division of the VIII nerve.

Persons fitting this description should be evaluated by audiometric tests, polytomography, and electronystagmography to rule out other diseases. Treatment is symptomatic after the initial work-up.

Positional Vertigo. Positional vertigo of the benign paroxysmal type is also called *postural vertigo* and, most recently, *cupulolithiasis.* Classically, these patients complain of violent vertigo lasting approximately 30 seconds that is brought on by certain head positions. The attacks may be accompanied by nausea, vomiting, and ataxia. Diagnosis is made by placing the patient in a position that induces this vertigo and then observing him for nystagmus. There should be a short latent period followed by vertigo, which is usually rotatory and fatigable. The important criteria are a period of latency and the fatigability of the response that document this disease. Repetitive testing will lead to a fatigue of this phenomenon.

Positional Nystagmus. This may occur with both peripheral and central nervous system lesions. Central nervous system lesions produce positional nystagmus that is direction-changing. Positional vertigo of the benign paroxysmal type is differentiated from positional nystagmus caused by central nervous system lesions by the latency of response, severe subjective sensation, limited duration, rotatory character of the nystagmus, and fatigability of the response. Baroney attributed the condition to a disorder of the otoliths. Causative factors appear to be spontaneous degeneration of the utricular otolithic membranes, labyrinthine concussion, otitis media, ear surgery, and occlusions of the anterior vestibular artery.

Treatment is usually not successful, but meclizine hydrochloride and diazepam (Valium) have been of some help.

Bell's Palsy. Bell's palsy is included in this section because it is a disorder related to the ear. Bell's palsy is defined as a unilateral, total facial paralysis of peripheral origin and of unknown cause. The fact that all divisions of the nerve are paralyzed distinguishes this disorder from a supranuclear lesion (Fig. 39–9).

The site of injury to the facial nerve may be determined by testing the intratemporal branches of this nerve. The greater superficial petrosal nerve arises at the geniculate ganglion and provides the parasympathetic supply to the lacrimal gland. The integrity of the nerve may be tested by performing the Schirmer tear test. Thin strips of filter paper are placed over the lower lid of both eyes, and the difference in range of wetting of the papers over both eyes is compared. The integrity of the branch of the stapedius muscle is determined subjectively by inquiries concerning the presence of hyperacusis (unusual sensitivity to loudness of sound) and objectively by tympanometry. The integrity of the chorda tympani is determined by testing taste at the anterior two-thirds of the tongue or by comparing the salivary flow from the submandibular glands. By performing these three tests, the site of the lesion can be identified as distal to the chorda tympani, between the stapedius nerve and the chorda tympani, or between the geniculate ganglion and the stapedius nerve. If the greater superficial petrosal nerve is not functioning, the lesion lies medial to the geniculate ganglion.

Nerve excitability testing is performed to determine whether neurapraxia, axonotmesis, or neurotmesis exists. When testing, if a contraction can be induced by peripheral stimulation of equal strength on each side, a complete recovery can be anticipated. Loss of nerve excitability (showing degeneration of the nerve) is an indication for decompression of the facial nerve. Approximately 85 per cent of all patients with idiopathic facial nerve paralysis have spontaneous recovery. If recovery has not begun by 3 weeks after the onset of facial paralysis, the chance of spontaneous recovery is

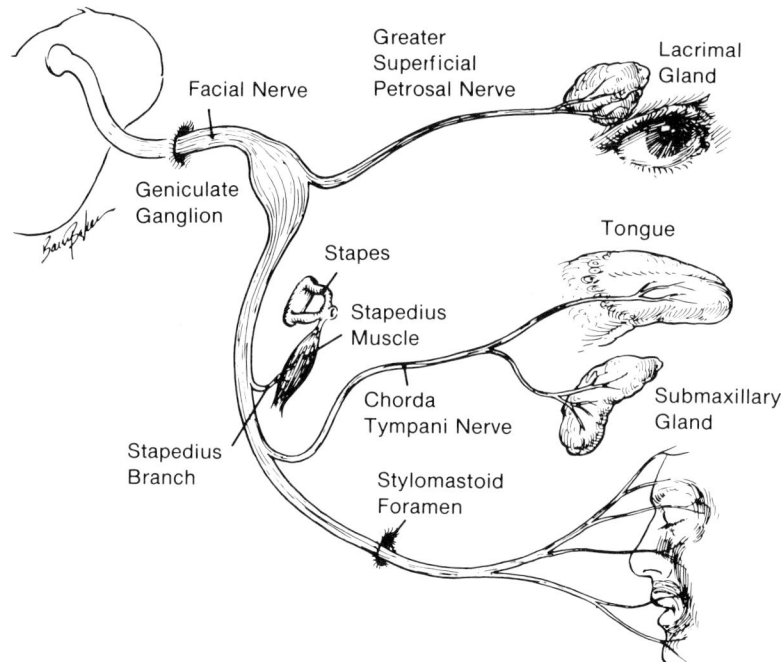

Figure 39–9. *Schematic anatomic illustration of facial nerve and its branches. (From Alford, B. R., Jerger, J. F., Coats, A. C., et al.: Arch. Otolaryngol., 97:214, 1973. Copyright 1973, American Medical Association.)*

greatly reduced. Ordinarily, facial nerve decompression is performed at this time if there has been no recovery or at any time that the nerve excitability deteriorates. If the loss of voluntary facial movement is not total, there should be a complete recovery of facial nerve function.

Neoplasms

Carcinoma. *Squamous cell carcinoma* and *basal cell carcinoma* frequently develop on the pinna of those people who are exposed to the sun. Early lesions can be successfully treated with irradiation therapy or with cautery and curettage. Surgical excision of a V-shaped wedge or, for more advanced lesions, of large amounts of the pinna may be needed. Invasion of cartilage usually contraindicates irradiation therapy and makes surgery the treatment of choice. Squamous cell and basal cell carcinomas also arise in the external auditory canal. These lesions require extensive resection in order to offer the best chance of cure. Block resection of the external auditory canal with sparing of the facial nerve is performed for

those lesions that are limited to the ear canal and have not invaded the middle ear. Squamous cell carcinomas may arise in the middle ear. The persistent otorrhea of chronic otitis media is a predisposing factor in the development of squamous cell carcinomas arising in the middle and external ear and in the external auditory canal. Squamous cell carcinoma involving the middle ear requires resection of the temporal bone in order to obtain an adequate margin around the tumor.

Ceruminomas. Ceruminomas arise in the outer one-third of the external auditory canal. Although these tumors appear to be benign histologically, they behave in a malignant manner and should be widely excised.

Chemodectomas. These are the most common of the tumors that arise in the middle ear. These nonchromaffin paragangliomas are called glomus jugulare or glomus tympanicus tumors, depending on their site of origin. Usually these tumors grow slowly, and the symptoms are not evident until the lesion is quite large. Pulsatile tinnitus, facial nerve paralysis, otorrhea, hemorrhage, vertigo, and paralysis of cranial nerves IX, X, XI, and XII are often presenting symptoms and signs. Typically, a red mass that pulsates and blanches with compression by the pneumatic otoscope can be seen in the ear canal or middle ear. Arteriography or retrograde venography should be performed to ascertain the extent of these tumors. Office biopsy should not be performed. Although the mass may appear to be an ear polyp, pneumatic otoscopy with blanching should alert the physician not to biopsy the lesion, as it bleeds profusely.

Acoustic Neuromas. These lesions account for approximately 7 per cent of all intracranial tumors. They arise most often on the vestibular division of the VIII nerve and are derived from Schwann cells.

The presenting complaint is usually that of a unilateral sensorineural hearing loss. Complaints of unsteadiness and vertigo are rare. The hearing loss is predominantly a high tone loss with greater impairment of speech discrimination than would be expected from a cochlear lesion producing the same amount of pure tone hearing loss. Special audiometric tests may point to a retrocochlear lesion. Electronystagmography with caloric stimulation will show a canal paresis on the involved side.

This benign tumor is initially confined to the internal auditory canal. As it increases in size, it projects into the cerebellar pontine angle and begins to compress the cerebellum and brain stem. With enlargement of the tumor, the V cranial nerve may become involved, causing a decreased or absent corneal reflex on the side of the tumor. The VII cranial nerve is rarely paralyzed. Papilledema is a late sign of acoustic neuroma. Early diagnosis is based on auditory findings suggesting a neural loss of hearing and on findings of hypoactivity on caloric stimulation plus the results of polytomography of the internal auditory canal, computerized axial tomography, and myelography of the posterior cranial fossae.

Smaller tumors may be removed with preservation of auditory function. Larger tumors may be approached from the middle cranial fossae or suboccipital route. Unless the tumor is quite large, the facial nerve can usually be spared.

Ototoxic Drugs

The *salicylates, quinine* and its synthetic substitutes, the *aminoglycoside antibiotics,* and *certain diuretics* are ototoxic. These drugs are primarily toxic to the organ of Corti. Nearly all ototoxic drugs are eliminated through the kidneys, and renal impairment is a predisposing factor in the accumulation of toxic levels of these medications.

Salicylate ototoxicity is reversible with discontinuance of the drug. The onset of tinnitus will usually be associated with a measurable sensorineural hearing loss. An audiogram should be obtained prior to the institution of aspirin therapy.

The *aminoglycoside antibiotics* are concentrated in the inner ear fluids to as much as 3 to 4 times more than the highest blood level. The mechanism of hearing loss is unknown and may be immediate or delayed. Streptomycin causes greater damage to the vestibular portion of the inner ear, but hearing loss has been found in as many as 15 per cent of patients receiving 1 gram per day of streptomycin for more than 1 week. This hearing loss may be of delayed onset.

Neomycin, kanamycin, vancomycin, doxycycline hyclate, and gentamicin have all been known to cause hearing loss.

Monitoring of blood levels of the aminoglycoside antibiotics and following blood urea nitrogen (BUN) levels and creatinine clearance to evaluate renal function are helpful but may not prevent hearing loss because of the concentration of the aminoglycosides in the inner ear fluids.

High frequencies are usually affected first, and a high-pitched tinnitus may develop, although this *cannot* be relied upon as a warning symptom. Older persons and those with pre-existing hearing loss should not be treated with ototoxic drugs if other effective drugs are available. Hearing loss is expected, and therapy with an ototoxic drug should not be initiated until audiometry has been carried out. Hearing should also be monitored by audiometry while the treatment is being continued. Ototoxic antibiotics should be avoided in pregnancy.

Quinine and its derivatives used for the treatment of malaria have been shown to cause hearing loss that is irreversible. Classically, the onset of tinnitus is a warning sign, but the hearing loss may progress even after the medication is discontinued.

Furosemide and *ethacrynic acid* have been associated with sensorineural hearing loss. This loss is usually associated with the administration of a large intravenous bolus of diuretic for the acutely ill patient. The cause of this hearing loss has not been ascertained but has been documented to be reversible on occasion. Prompt discontinuance of the diuretic is indicated, unless the life of the patient is threatened.

Aminoglycoside and diuretic hearing losses are more common in the renal-impaired patient, and creatinine clearance tests should be performed prior to the institution of therapy.

At the present time, there is no known treatment for these hearing losses. Vestibular paralysis may be nearly total and lifelong, with resultant unsteadiness. Such paralysis has been seen by one author on at least three occasions in the last year.

NOSE AND PARANASAL SINUSES

Embryology and Anatomy

Development of the nose occurs simultaneously with development of the face, palate, and sinuses. These structures must be reviewed as a total embryologic unit.

The external nose has a compound origin. The dorsum and apex of the nose are formed by downward continuation of the frontal nasal process. The sides and wings of the nose are formed by the lateral nasal processes of the maxilla. The maxillary processes are derived from the first branchial arches. In the 10 mm. embryo, nasal pits open into the primitive mouth. As development continues, the lateral nasal processes are pushed toward the midline, and the frontal nasal process is pushed upward. The tissue between the two openings is termed the median nasal process. As further development continues, the palatine processes of the maxilla push medially and fuse with the median nasal process, thereby separating the nose from the mouth. Posteriorly, the nose is closed by epithelial plugs during the second through the sixth month of fetal life. The entire nasal passage is derived from the primitive oral cavity and is composed of ectoderm.

Thus, the nose is developed from a midline ectodermal process. Its floor is derived from the palatine processes of the maxilla and the median nasal process, which is in continuity with the frontal nasal process.

The turbinates of the nose arise as a series of elevated folds in the lateral wall of each nasal passage. By birth, they are reduced to three in number. The paranasal sinuses are lodged within the adjoining bones and are in communication with the nasal cavity. All are apparent at approximately the fourth month of fetal life, although at birth only the ethmoid sinuses are well developed.

The development of the sinuses is of clinical importance because the ethmoid sinuses are present at birth and are the largest sinuses during the first 3 years of life. The maxillary sinuses enlarge as the deciduous teeth erupt into the mouth and again as the permanent teeth erupt. The frontal sinus is present at birth, but its development may be delayed until the child is 10 years of age. The sphenoid sinuses also develop in childhood. However, development is variable, and the sinuses may be quite small until puberty.

The skeleton of the nose consists of the nasal bones, ascending processes of the maxilla, upper lateral cartilages, lower lateral cartilages, and septal cartilage (Fig. 39–10). The nasal bones are oblong and

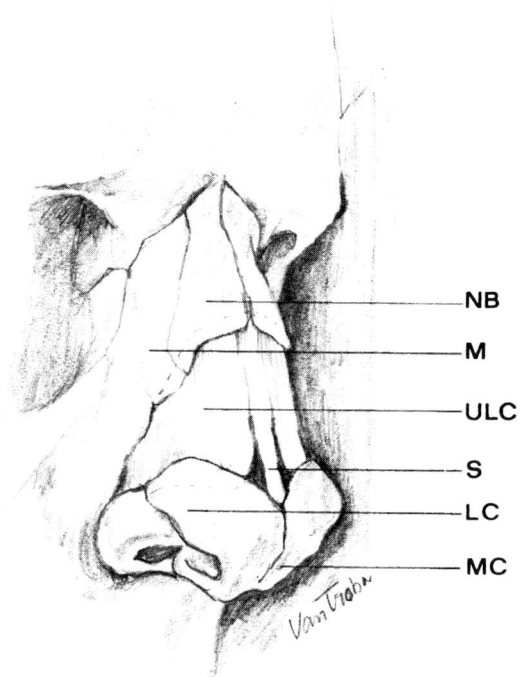

Figure 39–10. *The external nose. NB, nasal bone; M, frontal process of maxilla; ULC, upper lateral cartilage; S, septal cartilage; LC, lateral crus; and MC, medial crus of lower lateral (alar) cartilage. (From Walike, J. W.: Otolaryngol. Clin. North Am., 6:610, 1973.)*

articulate with the frontal bone. The medial borders unite, and the lateral borders articulate with the ascending processes of the maxilla. The upper lateral cartilages are wing-like expansions of the septal cartilage and articulate with the anterior edge of the nasal bones. The lower lateral cartilages are thin, curved, and pliable and form the skeleton of the tip of the nose. They are folded to form a medial and a lateral crus. These crura contribute to the maintenance of the patency of the nares. The nasal septum makes up the medial wall of each nasal cavity. The skeleton of the nasal septum consists of the quadrilateral cartilage, the perpendicular plate of the ethmoid bone, the vomer, the palatine processes of the maxilla, and the horizontal plates of the palatine bones. The lateral wall of each nasal cavity provides for the attachment of the three turbinates.

The turbinates divide the nose into three anatomically defined areas—the superior, inferior, and middle meatuses. The turbinates define these meatuses, and the inferior meatus is located below the inferior turbin-

ate and has the opening of the nasolacrimal duct on its lateral wall. The middle meatus is a space between the middle and inferior turbinates and has openings for the maxillary sinuses, ethmoid sinuses, and the frontal sinus via the nasal frontal duct. The superior meatus has no openings into it (Fig. 39–11).

The ethmoid air cells lie lateral to the superior half of the lateral wall of the nasal cavity. These cells are divided into anterior and posterior air cells by the attachment of the middle turbinate. The ethmoid cells that lie anteroinferior to the attachment are anterior ethmoid cells. The ethmoid cells that are posterosuperior to the attachment are posterior ethmoid cells. There are 4 to 20 cells on each side.

The maxillary sinus lies lateral to the inferior half of the lateral wall in the nasal cavity. The inferior part of the maxillary sinus extends to the alveolar arch and lies at a lower level than the floor of the nasal cavity. The medial wall of the maxillary sinus is the lateral wall of the nasal cavity. The roof of the maxillary sinus is the floor of

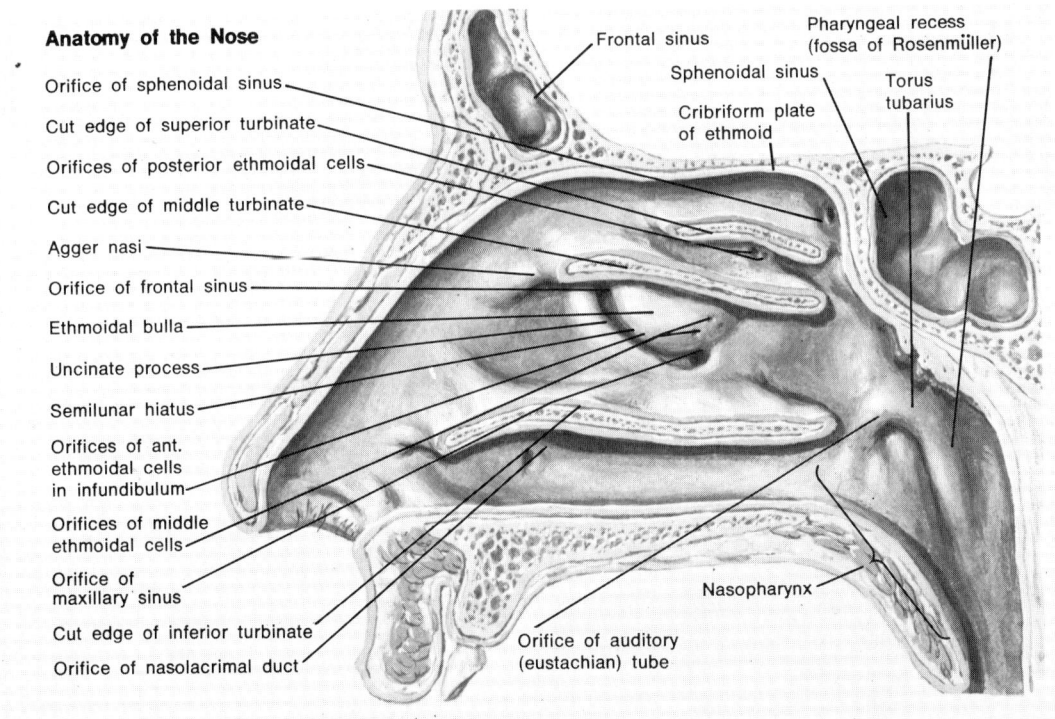

Figure 39–11. *Lateral wall of the nose. (From Jaffe, B. F.: Diseases and Surgery of the Nose. Clinical Symposia. Vol. 26, No. 1, CIBA Pharmaceutical Company, 1974. © Copyright 1974 CIBA Pharmaceutical Company, Division of CIBA–GEIGY Corporation. Reproduced, with permission, from CLINICAL SYMPOSIA. Illustrated by Frank H. Netter, M.D. All rights reserved.)*

the orbit. The medial wall of the ethmoid air cells is the lateral wall of the superior one-half of the nasal cavity. The lateral wall of the ethmoid air cells is the medial wall of the orbit. The posterior wall of the ethmoid air cells is the lateral portion of the anterior wall of the sphenoid sinus. The frontal sinus lies in the frontal bone, and the nasal frontal duct courses through the anterior ethmoid air cells.

The sphenoid sinus lies in the body of the sphenoid bone and opens on its anterior face into the most anterior portion of the nasopharynx in the area of the superior meatus of the nose.

Physiology

The nose humidifies, warms, and cleans the inspired air. The temperature of the inspired air is raised to near body temperature, and the relative humidity of the inspired air is raised to near 100 per cent by the time the air reaches the nasopharynx. Large particulate matter is removed from the inspired air by the vibrissae. Smaller particles are attracted to and retained in the mucous blanket of the nose, which has an electrostatic charge that improves its effi-

ciency in collecting minute particulate matter. Under normal conditions, approximately 1 liter of mucus is produced per day, and approximately 700 ml. of water from this mucus is expired. This constitutes the major portion of the insensible water loss. The mucous blanket moves in a continuous sheet from the anterior parts of the nasal cavity to the nasopharynx, and the residual mucus is swallowed.

The anterior naris is smaller than the choana. A stream of inspired air does not follow a straight path between these two openings but rather passes in a curve in an upward direction, which is more pronounced with deep breathing. With expiration, there are large eddies of the expired air, as the choana is larger than the anterior naris.

The lamina propria of the mucous membranes of the nasal turbinates contains large, thin-walled vascular spaces referred to as sinusoids or blood lakes. These vascular spaces respond to various stimuli. Most prominent among these stimuli are the temperature and humidity of the inspired air.

The olfactory epithelium occupies 2 to 3 cm. square of the superior portion of the

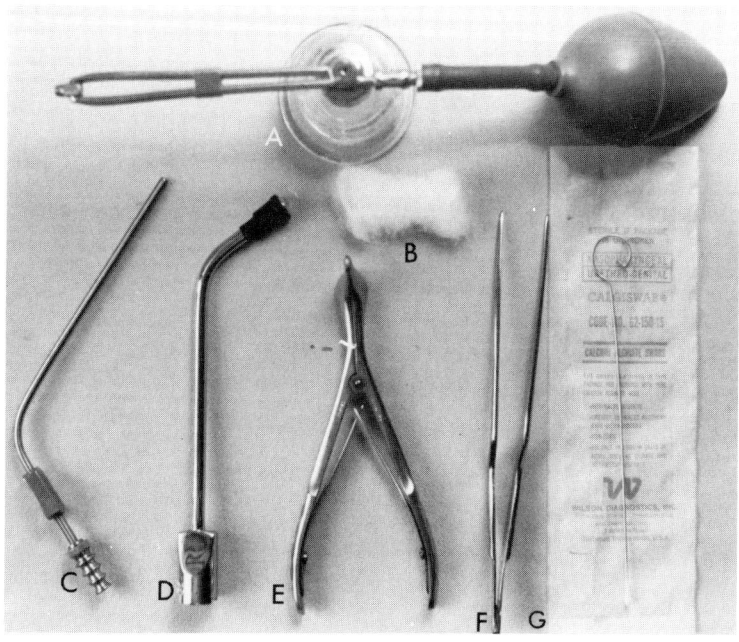

Figure 39–12. *Nasal examination instruments.* A, *atomizer containing 1/4 per cent Neo-Synephrine or 1 per cent ephedrine;* B, *cotton for application of vasoconstrictor or 4 per cent lidocaine;* C, *nasal suction;* D, *sinus light (fits on otoscope);* E, *nasal speculum;* F, *bayonet forceps;* and G, *culture swab. Not shown is light source.*

septum and the lateral wall of the nose. The hairs and the neuroepithelial cells are immersed in a layer of fluid secreted by Bowman's glands. The hairs of the neuro-epithelial cells are composed largely of lipid material. It appears that odorous substances must be soluble in lipids as well as in water. However, mechanisms underlying the sense of smell have not been satisfactorily explained.

Examination

Instruments for use in the nasal examina-tion are shown in Figure 39–12.

For satisfactory use of the nasal speculum, a light source such as a head mirror or a head light is necessary. An otoscope with a nasal attachment or, in small children, one of the larger ear specula can also be used. Bayonet forceps, cotton, and a vasoconstric-tor to shrink the turbinates are often neces-sary to visualize a larger portion of the nose. Suction may also be required, and a small culture swab may be used to take material for cultures from the middle meatus in the area of the maxillary, ethmoid, and frontal sinus ostia. The nasopharyngoscope is a useful adjunct in the examination of the nose (Fig. 39–13).

During the examination, it should be noted that the normal nose has essentially the same coloration as the mucous mem-brane of the lower lip in the gingival buccal sulcus. Secretions should be thin and not stringy and should be nearly clear. As one side of the nose is normally engorged while the other is shrunken, it is necessary to examine the nose before and after the application of vasoconstrictors. Placement of the septum, septal deviation, and types of secretions should be noted. Palpation and visualization of the external nose should be routine.

Congenital Disorders

Congenital Posterior Choanal Atresia. This condition may be unilateral or bilateral. The bilateral disorder should be diagnosed im-mediately after birth, as a newborn infant lacks mouth-breathing reflexes.

If a rubber catheter cannot be passed more than 3 cm. into the infant's nose, a presumptive diagnosis of choanal atresia should be made. An oral airway should be placed, and contrast studies should be done, using an iodized oil (Lipiodol) in the nose after using topical vasoconstrictors.

Unilateral choanal atresia may go unno-ticed for many years and is also diagnosed by placing a catheter into the nose. Anterior nasal atresia is extremely rare, as is a bifid nose.

Cleft Lip and Palate. These malformations are easily identified and result from a failure of fusion of the median nasal process and the palatine processes. The anomaly may be unilateral or bilateral, and anomalies of the

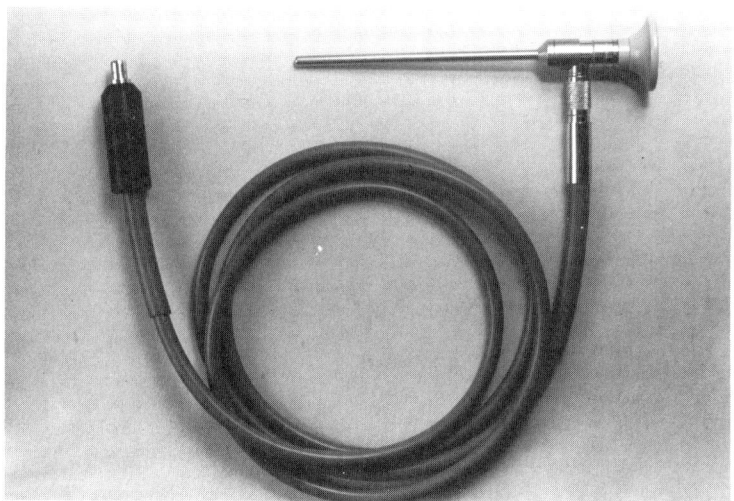

Figure 39–13. *Nasopharyngoscope. This instrument is placed along the floor of the nose and has a right angle lens to view the nasopharynx.*

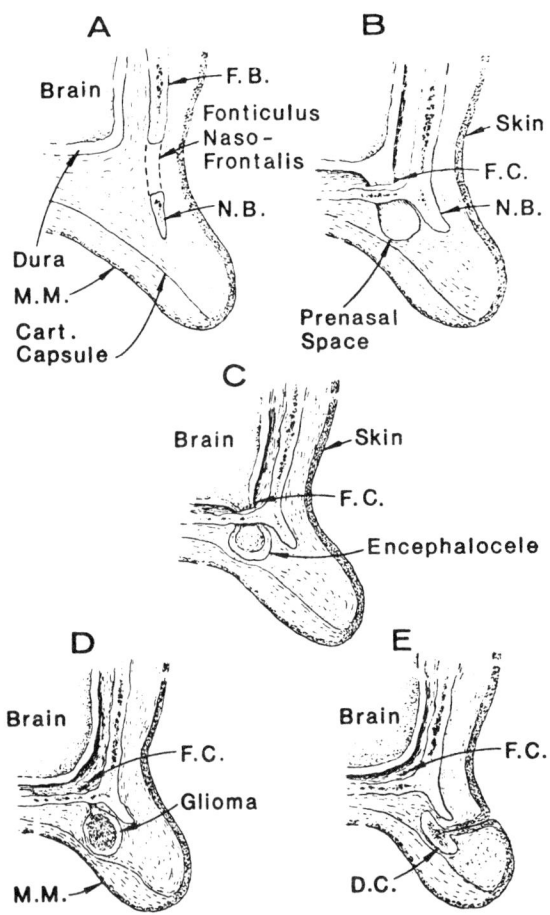

Figure 39-14. Sagittal section of the nose at birth. A, The membranous fonticulus nasofrontalis lies between the frontal bone (FB) and the nasal bone (NB). This is the site for the development of the foramen cecum. Mucous membrane (MM) lines the interior of the nose, and a cartilaginous capsule is well developed. The brain and its dural covering are well formed. This situation is present before birth at an early stage of development. B, Later during development before the foramen cecum is closed, a small extension of dural tissue may extend into the prenasal space through the foramen cecum. C, When the foramen cecum (FC) fails to close, brain and dura may herniate through the foramen to form an encephalocele. D, A glioma is a congenital tumor that is connected by a fibrous stalk to the skull near the foramen cecum. E, When the fonticulus nasofrontalis is replaced by bone, part of the ectoderm may not separate from the dura. This small bit of skin is left in the prenasal space; it is the antecedent of a midline dermoid cyst. These cysts usually lie beneath the nasal bone and are often connected to the external skin by a small sinus tract. (From English, C. M.: Anomalies of the ear, nose, mouth and throat. In Maloney, W. H. (ed.): Otolaryngology. Hagerstown, Md., Harper & Row, Publishers, Inc., 1973, p. 41.)

lip usually extend to the floor of the nose. Diagnosis is made by inspection, and digital palpation of the posterior palate should be done in all infants at birth to determine if a posterior cleft is present. This is particularly important in order to detect the presence of a submucous cleft in which the muscles of the soft palate have not come together.

Congenital Nasal Tumors. Such tumors are classified according to embryologic origin. The neurogenic group consists of gliomas, encephaloceles, and neurofibromas. The ectodermal group consists of dermoid cysts of sinuses, and the mesodermal group consists primarily of meningiomas. Figure 39–14 shows that the differential diagnosis is difficult, as the lesions tend to present in the midline and are the result of improper development of the embryo. Of the aforementioned tumors, dermoid cysts are more common than are other congenital tumors.

Anomalies of the paranasal sinuses are extremely rare, with absence of the paranasal sinuses being reported only once.

Hereditary Disorders

Hereditary Anosmia. This disorder has been described but is extremely rare and has been thought to be caused by agenesis of the olfactory bulb.

Hereditary Telangiectasia and Von Willebrand's Disease. These may present as epistaxis.

Respiratory Allergies. Respiratory allergies include seasonal hay fever, perennial allergic rhinitis, and asthma. Some patients with hay fever will subsequently develop asthma. Often the reverse occurs. Unfortunately, in some persons, asthma and allergic rhinitis coexist throughout their lifetime. Allergic rhinitis is usually the manifestation of a reaction to identifiable inhaled allergens such as pollens, danders, and molds. Some foods may also play a role in allergic reactions. Allergic rhinitis is characterized by nasal obstruction, recurrent sneezing, watery rhinorrhea, and anosmia. The development of nasal polyps is not unusual. The mucous membrane of the nose is pale and swollen, although during acute episodes the membrane may be red.

Seasonal allergic rhinitis is effectively managed by suppression of the allergic manifestations with antihistamine therapy. Depending upon the severity, *perennial allergic rhinitis* may merit desensitization therapy. Evaluation to determine specific allergens is indicated, so that the patient may eliminate these substances from his environment. If the allergens cannot be satisfactorily eliminated from his environment, the decision regarding hyposensitization therapy must be made on the basis of the severity of the patient's symptoms.

Allergic rhinitis predisposes the patient to acute and chronic sinusitis and *nasal polyp formation.* A polyp forms at the site of massive dependent edema of the lamina propria of the mucous membrane. As the polyp matures, it becomes teardrop-shaped and has a relatively narrow stalk. Such a polyp has the appearance of a peeled seedless grape. Most polyps arise from the mucous membrane surrounding the ostia of the maxillary sinuses. Although polyp formation is usually caused by an allergic reaction, polyps also occur in response to acute and chronic infections. Polyps occurring as a result of an acute infection may regress following the resolution of the infection.

Corticosteroid therapy topically and by injection has been effective in eliminating polyps or in reducing their size. However, surgical removal is the more reliable form of therapy. Nasal polyps should be removed if they obstruct the airway or contribute to the development or persistence of sinusitis. Polyps tend to recur unless the underlying allergic or infectious process is controlled.

Trauma

Fractures. Traumatic fractures of the nasal bones and dislocation of the cartilages may be easily recognized by physical examination and x-ray studies. In each person presenting with a history of trauma to the nose and a subsequent epistaxis, a nasal fracture must be ruled out. Since the mucous membrane must have been disrupted for the epistaxis to have occurred, it follows that there probably is a nasal fracture.

The examination begins with visualiza-

tion of the nose. It is important to tilt the patient's head upward and to look down the dorsum of the nose to inspect the tip, the alar cartilages, and the lateral portion of the nasal skeleton. Next, gentle palpation of the nasal bones should detect any fracture. In most instances, the physical examination is a better diagnostic aid than are x-ray studies.

X-ray examinations consist of soft tissue views of the nose. These are obtained by using bilateral projections and by having a small film placed under the chin and directing the x-ray beam down over the dorsum of the nose. Linear radiolucencies parallel to the long axis of the nasal bones are usually nutrient vessels. Radiolucencies transverse to the long axis of the nasal bones are usually fractures. It should be noted that x-ray studies should be taken to confirm the diagnosis.

The nasal speculum should then be inserted into the nose and the nose cleaned of blood. Vasoconstrictors are used to shrink the turbinates. The septum should be closely inspected for the possibility of a subperichondrial hematoma. A septal hematoma presents as a bulge in the nasal septum. This hematoma should be incised and evacuated immediately, as the cartilage of the nose has no direct blood supply and will undergo aseptic necrosis if the perichondrium remains elevated from the cartilage.

Fractures of the nasal complex are often associated with fractures of other facial bones, and x-ray studies of the paranasal sinuses are obtained if there is suspicion of fracture to the other facial bones. Examination of the facial skeleton is reviewed later in this chapter.

Cerebrospinal Fluid Rhinorrhea. Trauma to the facial bones may be associated with cerebrospinal fluid rhinorrhea. Following injury to the central portion of the face, the patient is clinically examined for cerebrospinal fluid rhinorrhea by having him tip his head forward and collecting any drainage from the nose. Any watery fluid is examined for glucose content. Although this test is not an absolute indication of cerebrospinal fluid leak, it gives a presumptive diagnosis if the results are positive. If the patient has cerebrospinal fluid rhinorrhea, he is instructed to avoid blowing his nose and is given prophylactic antibiotic therapy to prevent meningitis. Most cerebrospinal fluid rhinorrheas cease spontaneously. If the rhinorrhea does not cease within 14 to 21 days, the dural leak is repaired through a frontal craniotomy.

Reduction of Fractures. Nasal fractures in adults may be reduced under local anesthesia, but general anesthesia is necessary for reduction of nasal fractures in children. Thorough anesthesia is the key to satisfactory reduction of the nasal bones. The fracture is manipulated into good position by internal traction of the fragments, using a blunt periosteal elevator associated with external digital traction. The need for internal and external splints depends on the postreduction stability of the fracture.

If blunt trauma to the nose is neglected, it results in permanent deformity that ultimately requires septal surgery to improve the airway and rhinoplasty to improve the appearance of the nose.

In summary, a close visual and manual inspection of the nose is necessary in diagnosing fractures, as is x-ray confirmation. Nondisplaced fractures need not be reduced, but displaced fractures should be reduced to prevent later complications.

Infectious Disorders

Coryza. This is a common complaint. Initially after the virus begins to multiply, paralysis of the cilia occurs, and the mucous blanket begins to stagnate. There is secondary edema of the basement membrane area and even sloughing of the superficial cells. During this period, irritation, dryness, and tickling of the nose and nasopharynx occur. If there is secondary bacterial invasion, the nasal discharge becomes purulent. Culture of the normal nasal cavity usually does not demonstrate pathogens. The mucous membrane is erythematous and swollen, and there is frequently slight tenderness over the maxillary and frontal sinuses. Acute sinusitis, exacerbation of chronic sinusitis, acute otitis media, and exacerbation of chronic otitis media are complications that require prompt antibiotic therapy.

Acute Rhinitis. Acute rhinitis may also occur as streptococcal, pneumococcal, and staphylococcal infections. Appropriate therapy is based on demonstration of the causative pathogen by culture. Systemic antibiotic therapy is indicated, as outlined for acute otitis media.

Chronic Rhinitis. Chronic rhinitis may be due to specific diseases such as *syphilis, tuberculosis, rhinoscleroma, rhinosporidiosis, leishmaniasis, blastomycosis, histoplasmosis,* and *leprosy.* Each of these is characterized by the production of granulomatous tissue and the presence of a process that is destructive to soft tissue, cartilage, and bone. Rhinosporidiosis is also characterized by bleeding polyps. Rhinoscleroma is distinguished by progressive nasal obstruction caused by induration and by inflammatory tissue in the lamina propria of the mucous membrane. The diagnosis is made by demonstration of the specific micro-organism either by culture or in biopsy tissue.

Vestibulitis. This is a low-grade infection in the area of the vibrissae of the nose manifesting as a folliculitis with crusting. These infections are effectively treated by the application of an antibiotic ointment to the nose twice a day for a period of 14 days.

Furuncles. Furuncles of the nasal vestibule are usually staphylococcal infections and may develop into a spreading cellulitis at the tip of the nose. Systemic antibiotic therapy should be employed, penicillin being the drug of choice. Hot compresses should also be applied. Incision and drainage are specifically contraindicated because of the possibility of spreading the infection to the nasal cartilages. Furuncles of the central portion of the face should be allowed to drain spontaneously. Operative intervention increases the risk of development of retrograde thrombophlebitis and subsequent cavernous sinus thrombosis.

Acute Sinusitis. This disorder is usually precipitated by an acute respiratory tract infection of viral etiology. The swelling of the nasal mucous membrane produces obstruction of the ostium of the paranasal sinus. The oxygen in the sinus is then absorbed by the blood vessels in the mucous membrane, and a relative negative pressure in the sinus develops, causing pain. This condition is termed vacuum sinusitis. If the vacuum is maintained, a transudate of the blood in the vessels of the mucous membrane occurs and fills the sinus. The transudate serves as a culture medium for bacteria that enter through the ostium or through a spreading cellulitis or thrombophlebitis of the mucous membrane. In response, there is an outpouring of serum and leukocytes to combat the infection, and a painful positive pressure develops in the obstructed sinus.

Acute maxillary sinusitis produces pain in the maxillary area, toothache, and frontal headache. *Frontal sinusitis* produces pain in the frontal area and a frontal headache. *Ethmoid sinusitis* causes pain in the retro-orbital area and between the eyes and a frontal headache, often described as a "splitting" headache. Pain from *sphenoid sinusitis* is less well localized and is referred to the frontal or occipital area. Yellow or green purulent rhinorrhea may be present, and malaise may occur. Fever and chills suggest an extension of the infection beyond the sinus.

The mucous membrane of the nose is red and turgescent. There is seropurulent or mucopurulent exudate in the middle meatus with maxillary sinusitis, anterior ethmoid cells, and frontal sinusitis or exudate medial to the middle turbinate in posterior ethmoid cell and sphenoid sinusitis. There may be tenderness and swelling over the involved sinus. The frontal and maxillary sinuses may be opaque to transillumination. Radiography of the paranasal sinuses is a more reliable method of defining which sinuses are involved and the degree of involvement. Radiopacity of the paranasal sinuses may be produced in acute sinusitis because of swollen mucous membranes or retained pus in the sinus.

The two organisms most commonly causing acute and chronic sinusitis are *Hemophilus influenzae* and *Diplococcus pneumoniae*. Other micro-organisms responsible for acute sinusitis are streptococci, pneumococci, and staphylococci. Treatment is directed toward improvement of the drainage of the infected sinus and control of the infection with systemic antibiotic therapy. Drainage can be improved by topical vasoconstriction. The use of topical vasoconstrictors should be limited to a maximum of 7 days. Prolonged use leads to a state in which the only adequate stimulus for vasoconstriction is reapplication of a topical agent, as the nasal vasculature becomes refractory to the usual stimuli that produce vasoconstriction. Systemic vasoconstrictors such as ephedrine, pseudoephedrine, and phenylpropanolamine improve drainage in most patients, but their effect for any given patient is less reliable than the topical

vasoconstrictors. Steam inhalation very effectively produces vasoconstriction of the nasal mucous membrane and promotes drainage. The antibiotic of choice for treatment of acute sinusitis is ampicillin. Erythromycin is the drug of second choice.

Chronic Sinusitis. The signs and symptoms of chronic sinusitis are similar to those of acute sinusitis. During an exacerbation of chronic sinusitis, the causative micro-organism may be a gram-negative rod. Therefore, a broad-spectrum antibiotic such as ampicillin or tetracycline is more effective. In both acute and chronic sinusitis, the antibiotic treatment should be continued for at least 10 to 12 days. Culture of the exudate from the sinus, determination of the sensitivities of isolated pathogens, and evaluation of the patient's response to treatment guide subsequent therapy.

Approximately 25 per cent of chronic maxillary sinusitis is secondary to a dental infection. In such cases, x-ray studies of the apices of the teeth should be obtained to exclude the possibility of a periapical abscess.

Complications of maxillary sinusitis are rare. In children, *ethmoid sinusitis* is frequently complicated by *orbital cellulitis* and *abscess*. Eighty per cent of all orbital cellulitis is secondary to ethmoid sinusitis. In patients presenting with erythema and swelling of the eyelids, proptosis, and displacement of the globe laterally and inferiorly, the source of the infection is sought by inspection of the nose for mucopus and by radiography of the paranasal sinuses for ethmoid sinusitis. Ethmoid sinusitis and accompanying orbital cellulitis respond well to systemic antibiotic therapy. If the proptosis fails to subside or continues to progress, incision and drainage of the abscess that is between the lamina papyracea and the orbital periosteum are performed through an incision that extends from the lateral aspect of the nose to the eyebrow (Killian incision). In order to reach the abscess cavity, the orbital periosteum is elevated from the medial wall of the orbit. The optic nerve tolerates 11 to 14 mm. of proptosis, and the point at which extraocular motion is lost is also the limit of stretch of the optic nerve. Therefore, incision and drainage of an orbital abscess are performed prior to complete loss of extraocular motion to prevent permanent blindness.

Frontal sinusitis may cause intracranial

complications such as *meningitis, epidural abscess, subdural empyema,* and *brain abscess.* In severe acute frontal sinusitis that fails to respond promptly to systemic antibiotic therapy, the anterior wall of the frontal sinus is trephined through an incision in the medial plane of the eyebrow. An opening of approximately 7 to 8 mm. is made, and a catheter is placed in the sinus to maintain drainage. Trephination is performed in an attempt to prevent the intracranial complications of frontal sinusitis.

Fractures of the frontal sinus lead to the development of *mucoceles.* Mucoceles result from duplication of the mucous membrane. They gradually enlarge and destroy the floor of the frontal sinus, and as they expand into the orbital cavity, they produce proptosis and inferolateral displacement of the eye. Mucoceles and other forms of chronic frontal sinusitis that do not respond to medical management can be managed surgically by using an osteoplastic flap approach for obliteration of the frontal sinus. The incision in the bone is made at the periphery of the frontal sinus, and the anterior wall is rotated inferiorly on the hinge of periosteum at the floor of the sinus. Infected mucous membrane is removed with a motor-driven burr, and the cavity of the frontal sinus is obliterated by the implantation of fat taken from the abdominal wall.

Chronic maxillary sinusitis that does not respond to medical management may be controlled by performing a Caldwell-Luc operation, which is a maxillary sinusotomy performed through an incision in the canine fossa. The bone of the anterior wall of the maxillary sinus is resected in order to gain access to the interior of the sinus so that infected mucous membrane, cysts, and epithelial debris can be removed. The drainage of the maxillary sinus is improved by creating a nasoantral window in the inferior meatus.

Chronic ethmoid sinusitis is usually associated with allergic rhinitis and the formation of nasal polyps. An ethmoidectomy is indicated for those patients in whom the formation of nasal polyps and the symptoms of ethmoid sinusitis cannot be controlled adequately by intranasal polypectomy and medical management, including desensitization. Ethmoidectomies are performed intranasally or through an external approach, utilizing a Killian incision. In the external ethmoidectomy, the orbital periosteum is elevated, and the lamina papyracea is removed to gain access to the ethmoid air cells. Infected mucous membrane, polypoid tissue, and epithelial debris are removed. The anterior half of the middle turbinate is excised to create a large opening between the ethmoid air cells and the nasal cavity.

Chronic sphenoid sinusitis that does not respond to medical management may be controlled by an operation in which the sphenoid sinus is approached through an external ethmoidectomy. After the external ethmoidectomy has been accomplished, the anterior wall of the sphenoid sinus is resected to remove infected mucous membrane, polypoid tissue, and epithelial debris. The anterior and inferior walls of the sphenoid are removed. In this way, the interior of the sphenoid sinus is incorporated in the posterior part of the nasal cavity and the nasopharynx, and, in essence, the sphenoid sinus is eliminated as a separate entity.

The need for sinus surgery has been greatly reduced by the responsiveness of acute and chronic sinusitis to antibiotic therapy.

Iatrogenic Disorders

Rhinitis Medicamentosum. This is one of the most common problems seen in the otorhinolaryngologist's office and appears to afflict many paramedical personnel. Vasoconstrictors applied to the nose on a continual basis cause persistent nasal edema, except during the time of the action of the vasoconstrictor. This becomes a chronic condition because with each subsequent application, small vessels may be coagulated, and eventually fibrosis will ensue. The history is vital in formulating a diagnosis, and patients must be asked if they are using nose drops, nasal sprays, or inhalers. Many times, the symptoms of the acute episode pass without notice, as the symptoms when the vasoconstrictor is not used are similar to the initial symptoms.

The patient must absolutely discontinue all nasal medications. Antihistamine decongestants may be given as a supportive measure, and occasionally a 6 day course of low-dose steroids can be prescribed.

A follow-up evaluation in approximately

30 days is necessary, as the nose of persons using nasal medication will appear abnormal at the time of initial examination.

Idiopathic Disorders

Epistaxis. Epistaxis, or bleeding from the nose, is a common clinical problem. Ninety per cent of episodes of epistaxis occur from a plexus of vessels in the anteroinferior part of the septum. The other 10 per cent of episodes of nasal bleeding occur from the posterior part of the nose, particularly from the far posterior and inferior meatus at the junction of the inferior meatus and the nasopharynx. Patients with arteriosclerosis and hypertension are especially prone to have bleeding from this area. This type of bleeding may be difficult to control and is associated with a 4 to 5 per cent mortality.

Mild epistaxis from the anterior part of the nasal septum is usually effectively controlled by steady pressure applied by squeezing the alar portion of the nose between the index finger and the thumb for 5 to 10 minutes.

Treatment for anterior epistaxis is local. The bleeding point can be controlled temporarily, and anesthesia is achieved by pressure applied over a cotton pledget saturated with a vasoconstrictor and a topical local anesthetic. The bleeding point can be cauterized chemically (with a silver nitrate stick), or electrocautery can be used. Silver nitrate is preferred as the cauterizing agent, as it produces satisfactory intravascular coagulation without causing a severe burn of the mucous membrane. Cautery is applied in a circumferential manner around the bleeding point. Lastly, the cautery is applied to the bleeding point itself. Following this, the patient is advised to use a small amount of antibiotic ointment several times daily to prevent crusting of this area. If the bleeding point cannot be visualized, strips of ½ inch petrolatum gauze are placed in the nose. The packing is layered from the floor of the nose upward, until the anterior nasal cavity is filled (Fig. 39–15).

Posterior epistaxis should be treated as an emergency, as patients with posterior bleeding are often elderly and hypertensive. Figure 39–16 shows the placement of a

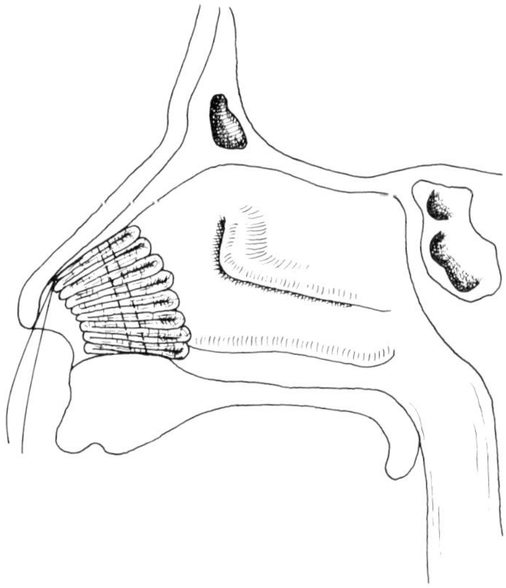

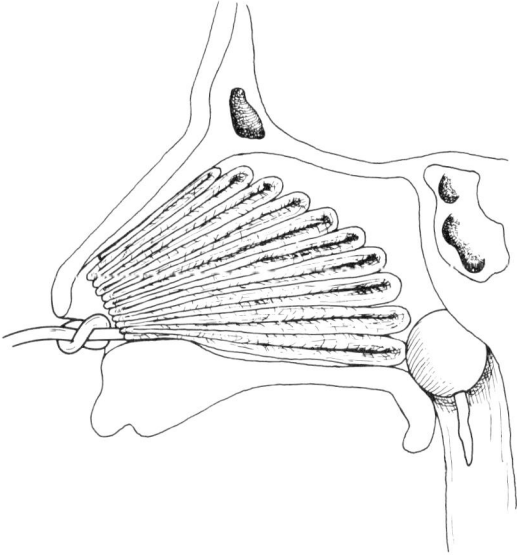

Figure 39–15. Anterior nasal packing. One-half inch petrolatum gauze is used to pack the anterior nasal chamber. If more than one pack is used, they are tied together in a continuous length. The packing is layered from bottom to top. The pharynx should be inspected to ensure that bleeding has been controlled. (Adapted from Hollinshead, W. H.: Anatomy for Surgeons. Vol. 1, 2nd Ed. Hagerstown, Md., Harper & Row, Publishers, Inc., 1968, p. 265.)

Figure 39–16. Posterior nasal packing. A Foley catheter (#14 with a 30 ml. balloon) is pushed through the nose until the tip is seen in the back of the mouth. Bacteriostatic water is used to fill the balloon until a slight bulge is seen in the soft palate. The catheter is then pulled firmly into the choana. The balloon acts as a buttress for the petrolatum gauze packing. A knot is placed inside the nares. The packing and Foley catheter are removed in 4 to 5 days. (Adapted from Hollinshead, W. H.: Anatomy for Surgeons. Vol. 1, 2nd Ed. Hagerstown, Md., Harper & Row, Publishers, Inc., 1968, p. 265.)

posterior pack using a Foley catheter with a 30 ml. balloon. The Foley catheter is inserted in the nose and advanced to the nasopharynx, and the balloon is filled with bacteriostatic water until the soft palate begins to bulge. It is important to visualize the tip of the Foley catheter during this inflation. After the bulging of the soft palate begins, the catheter is then pulled firmly into the posterior choana of the nose. A hemostat is placed across the anterior end of the catheter, and an assistant is asked to hold the catheter firmly against the nose. One-half inch strips of petrolatum gauze are then placed in the nose, until the entire nose is filled from the Foley balloon forward. It should be noted that the Foley catheter usually does not control the bleeding but acts as a buttress for the petrolatum gauze packing.

After the catheter and the packing have been placed, the catheter is stretched to its fullest extent, the hemostat is reapplied near the nose, and a very tight knot is placed firmly against the hemostat. The hemostat is removed, and the knot is placed in the vestibule of the nose to prevent sloughing of the skin of the nose. The catheter is now firmly anchored, putting pressure on the petrolatum gauze both anteriorly and posteriorly. The nasopharynx is then inspected to see that all bleeding has ceased. It is not unusual to find that the opposite nostril begins to bleed after this packing has been placed. Placement of the posterior pack is quite painful, and medication may be required. The patient should be admitted to the hospital and prophylactic antibiotics begun. Such patients have a low arterial PO_2 level while the packing is in place and should have oxygen by face mask. Replacement of blood lost by the epistaxis is carried out as indicated by monitoring the hemoglobin and hematocrit levels and the patient's vital signs.

Patients hospitalized because of posterior packing should be watched closely, as there have been reports of mortality of as high as 5 per cent.

An alternative to nasal packing is ligation of the internal maxillary artery through a Caldwell-Luc approach. This method of controlling posterior epistaxis has been advocated to lessen the mortality and morbidity associated with posterior nasal packing.

Atrophic Rhinitis. Atrophic rhinitis, also known as *ozena*, is characterized by atrophic and sclerotic mucous membranes, abnormal patency of the nasal cavity, crust formation, and a foul nasal odor. The mucous membrane undergoes a metaplasia, changing from ciliated pseudostratified columnar epithelium to stratified squamous epithelium, and the lamina propria is reduced in vascularity. Anosmia results, and epistaxis may be recurrent and severe. Although bacterial infections play a role in the pathogenesis, the cause is unknown, and the treatment is empiric. Treatment is directed toward reducing the crusting and eliminating the odor. Topical antibiotics with a water-soluble base and isotonic saline nasal douches have been employed. Surgical attempts to reduce the patency of the nasal cavity have had some success. Alternatively, occlusion of one nasal cavity either surgically or by insertion of a pledget of lamb's wool is effective in decreasing the crusting caused by the drying effects of air flow over the atrophic mucous membrane.

Vasomotor Rhinitis. Vasomotor rhinitis is characterized by intermittent vascular engorgement of the nasal mucous membrane, sneezing, and watery rhinorrhea. The mucous membrane varies from a bright red to a purplish hue and is turgescent. The cause is uncertain. No allergy can be identified in such patients. Treatment is empiric and is not always satisfactory. Although the condition is chronic, periods of remission and exacerbation occur. Vasomotor rhinitis appears to be aggravated by a dry atmosphere and is improved by humidification of inspired air. Patients with this condition benefit by installing a humidifier in their home's central heating system or by using a vaporizer in their workroom and bedroom. The use of systemic sympathomimetics, such as ephedrine, pseudoephedrine, or phenylpropanolamine, is effective for temporary symptomatic relief but is not recommended for regular long-term use.

Wegener's Granulomatosis. This disorder is characterized by granulomas of the nose and lung and by glomerulitis of the kidney. This disease is fatal, and the pathologic changes encountered are caused by necrotizing vasculitis, similar to that seen in periarteritis nodosum. The patient usually presents with a granulomatous process of the nose that is often mistaken for chronic sinusitis. Subsequently, the patient may develop pulmonary granulomas, and fever, weight loss, anemia, leukocytosis, transient eosinophilia, and a globulinemia occur. Hematuria and urinary casts are found late in the course of the disease. Death is usually due to renal failure. The cause of Wegener's granulomatosis is unknown. Treatment is directed toward immunosuppression, and it appears that immunosuppression with corticosteroids, methotrexate, and azathioprine prolongs life.

Lethal Midline Granuloma. The cause of lethal midline granuloma remains unexplained. This lesion may present as a destructive process of the nasal septum but more usually presents as a destructive process of the hard and soft palate. In addition, destructive lesions of the bone, cartilage, and soft tissue of the nose and paranasal sinuses occur, and ultimately a malignant tumor may be found. A wide biopsy of available tissue is likely to establish the correct diagnosis. At the present time, there is no known effective treatment.

Neoplasms

Papillomas. *Squamous cell papillomas* occur in the nasal cavity and are thought to be caused by papovaviruses. Exophytic papillomas recur after excision but have a benign course. *Inverted papillomas* are invasive and behave in a locally malignant manner. They destroy soft tissue and bone and tend to recur after excision. Inverted papillomas require removal, along with removal of a large margin of normal tissue.

Fibromas. Fibromas, hemangiomas, and neurofibromas occur occasionally in the nasal cavity. Fibromas, neurilemomas, and ossifying fibromas occur in the paranasal sinuses.

Squamous Cell Carcinoma. The most common malignant tumor to occur in the nose and paranasal sinuses is the squamous cell carcinoma. Adenoid cystic carcinomas, adenocarcinomas, mucoepidermoid carcinomas and malignant mixed tumors, lymphomas, fibrous sarcomas, osteosarcomas, chondrosarcomas, and melanomas occur in the nose and paranasal sinuses. Metastatic tumors may involve the paranasal sinuses, and the most common tumor to metastasize

to the paranasal sinuses is the hypernephroma.

Early squamous cell carcinomas and basal cell carcinomas are treated with radiation therapy or with cauterization and curettage. Larger carcinomas involving cartilage require excision. Nasal septal carcinomas often require sacrifice of the columella as well as of the adjacent structures. The combination of irradiation therapy to a tumoricidal dose and of radical resection offers the best survival rate for patients with carcinomas and sarcomas of the nasal cavity and paranasal sinuses. Malignant tumors of the lateral wall of the nose require a lateral rhinotomy.

Neoplasm should be suspected when there is recurrent epistaxis or when a chronic sinus infection does not respond to therapy. Careful visual inspection of the nose is helpful, but radiographic findings of loss of bone should be considered as evidence of a carcinoma until proved otherwise. The best x-ray view for evaluation is the Waters' view, which shows the maxillary sinuses and medial wall of the maxillary sinuses.

Drug-Induced Disorders

Rhinitis. Rhinitis mimicking allergic rhinitis, rhinitis medicamentosum, or vasomotor rhinitis may be induced by treatment of elevated blood pressure with sympatholytic drugs, which cause a relative overaction of the parasympathetic system. This type of rhinitis presents as a nasal obstruction with watery rhinorrhea. There is no history of allergic rhinitis or infection, unless these are coincidental findings.

Treatment is difficult because the patient's symptoms are usually worse at night. A low dose of a sympathomimetic decongestant at bedtime may be tried; however, the use of sympathomimetics in a hypertensive patient should be coordinated with the treatment being given by the physician caring for the hypertension.

MOUTH AND OROPHARYNX

Embryology and Anatomy

The stomadeum is converted into the mouth by the anterior growth of the max-

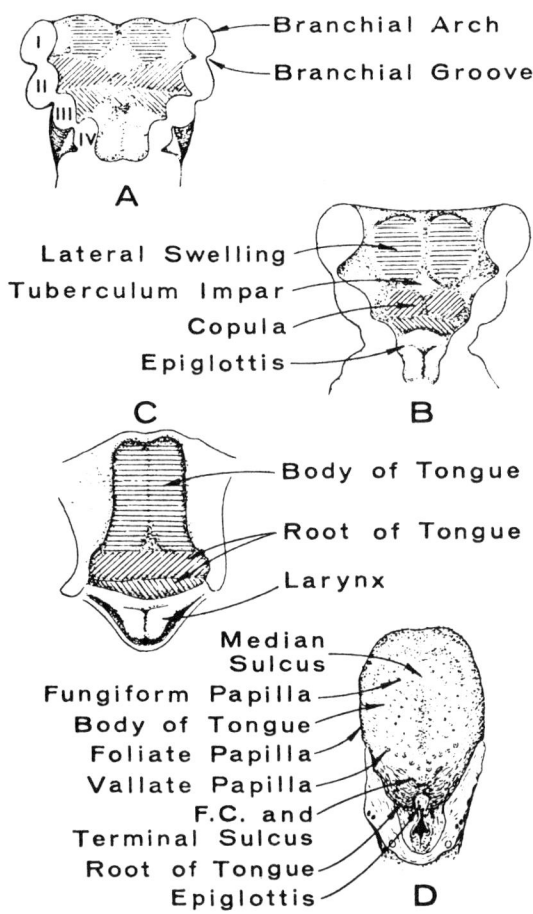

Figure 39–17. Embryology of the tongue. A, At 6 mm. the branchial arches have formed paired lateral swellings that contribute to the development of the tongue, the mandible, and parts of the larynx. B, The tuberculum impar, copula, and lateral swellings of the tongue are well developed in the 9 mm. embryo. C, The body and root of the tongue have developed an adult shape by 15 mm. of growth, and the primitive larynx is apparent. The contributions of the arches to these structures is indicated by appropriate marking. D, The tongue at birth. The locations of the various types of papillae and the area of the terminal sulcus are indicated on this drawing. The foramen cecum (FC) represents the site of origin of the thyroid gland. (From English, G. M.: Anomalies of the ear, nose, mouth and throat. In Maloney, W. H. (ed.): Otolaryngology. Hagerstown, Md., Harper & Row, Publishers, Inc., 1973, p. 41.)

illary and mandibular processes, which fuse in the midline. The foregut ends blindly anteriorly and forms the buccal pharyngeal membrane, which separates the foregut from the stomadeum. The buccal pharyngeal membrane disintegrates, and the palatine processes of the maxilla grow medially, forcing the tongue in a downward position and separating the nasal cavity from the mouth. The line of fusion of the ectodermal derivatives of the stomadeum and of the entodermal derivatives of the foregut disappear and are unidentifiable in the adult. The boundary line normally lies behind that part of the mandibular process from which the teeth are derived. The enamel organs of the teeth and the epithelial lining of the cheeks and parotid gland are derived from ectoderm. The boundary between the entoderm and the ectoderm in the adult can be located at a line approximately between the gums and the attachment of the tongue to the floor of the mouth.

Since the lower lip lies external to the teeth of the lower jaw, its epithelium is also ectodermal. The tongue, the epiglottis, and the submandibular and sublingual glands are derived from entoderm and associated mesoderm of the floor of the primitive buccal cavity.

The tongue develops from the first, second, and third branchial arches, with the greater portion being derived from the first and third arches (Fig. 39–17). The line represented at the junction of these two portions is indicated in the epithelium by the sulcus terminalis. The tongue, therefore, results from a developmental interlocking of pharyngeal entoderm, branchial mesoderm, and occipital myotomes. Its nerve supply is derived from the V, VII, IX, X, and XII cranial nerves (Fig. 39–18).

The thyroid begins to develop in the area of the adult foramen cecum and migrates inferiorly, after proliferation of the two lateral lobes.

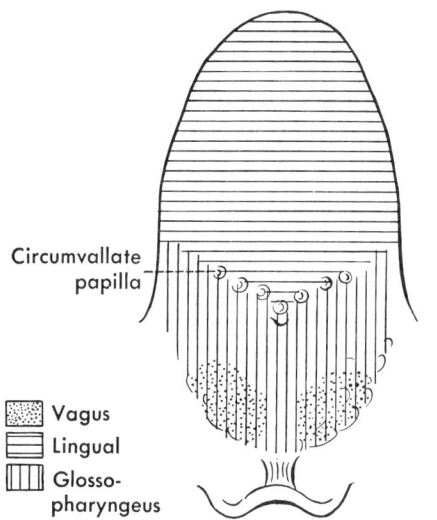

Circumvallate
papilla

Vagus
Lingual
Glosso-
pharyngeus

Figure 39-18. Sensory innervation of the tongue. (From *Hollinshead, W. H.: Anatomy for Surgeons. Vol. 1, 2nd Ed. Hagerstown, Md., Harper & Row, Publishers, Inc., 1968, p. 421.*)

The pharynx represents the embryonic foregut. It extends from the posterior nose (buccal pharyngeal membrane) and is modified by its connection with the primitive stomadeum (the mouth) and more inferiorly is again modified by its division into two separate tubular structures, thus being a tube within a tube (the larynx and the pharynx). The pharynx may be thought of as a tubular muscular structure with striated muscle.

Physiology

The mouth and oropharynx provide an entrance for food. They serve as organs for mastication, salivation, and articulation of speech and are a secondary airway.

Examination

Examination of the mouth and oropharynx requires little instrumentation (Fig. 39-19) but does require the physician to be methodical. Examination begins with visualization of the right parotid duct, the superior gingival buccal sulcus around to the left parotid duct, and the gingival buccal sulcus of the maxillary teeth. The floor of the mouth and the submandibular ducts are then inspected by having the patient elevate his tongue. The soft and hard palate is then visualized, and, lastly, the tongue blade is inserted in the mouth to depress the tongue so that the tonsils, base of the tongue, and the oropharynx can be exam-

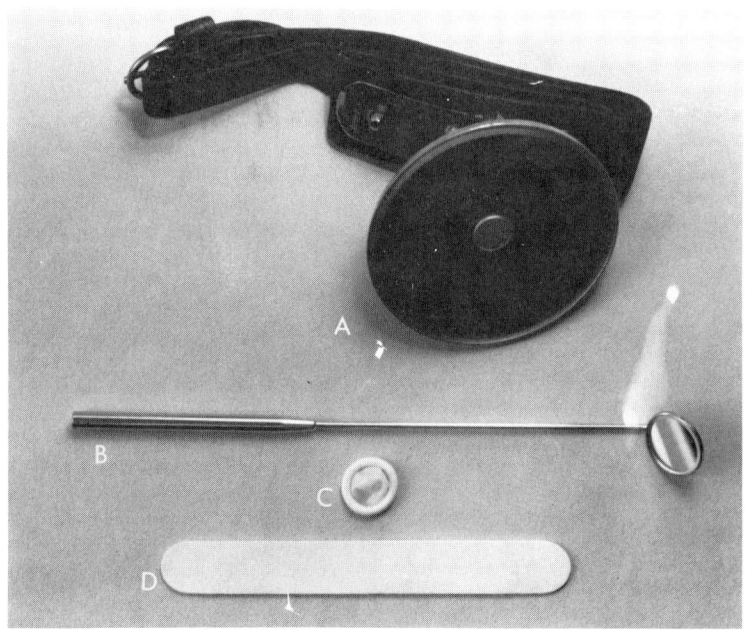

Figure 39-19. Mouth and oropharyngeal instruments. A, *head mirror;* B, *mirror to observe base of tongue;* C, *finger cot for palpation;* and D, *tongue blade.*

ined. The tongue must be kept in the mouth for adequate depression of the tongue musculature.

Use of the finger cot is important, and the floor of the mouth and the base of the tongue should be palpated in each patient. The mirror provides access to the base of the tongue and the area of the vallecula. Any suspicious lesions of the mouth or oropharynx are palpated separately to check for induration.

Radiographic studies of the salivary glands will be discussed in a separate section on the examination of the salivary glands. Radiographs of the mandible and lateral neck are helpful adjuncts in evaluating the mandible and base of the tongue. The xeroradiograph may be helpful in delineating the soft tissue. Cineradiography, in conjunction with running speech and the placement of contrast material in the pharynx, will provide a true picture of palatal and tongue function during articulation.

It should be emphasized that this area can easily be examined by visualization and palpation.

Congenital Disorders

Double Lip. This is a condition of the vermilion border in which the border is divided in two parts by a transverse groove. In most instances, only the upper lip is involved. Double lip may occur together with blepharochalasis and nontoxic thyroid enlargement. This triad constitutes *Ascher's syndrome.*

Cleft Lip. Cleft lip, partial or complete clefts of the upper lip, may be unilateral or bilateral. A cleft may also extend superiorly into the nose, and the maxilla usually shows retrodisplacement.

Clefts of the lip and palate are distributed as follows: 50 per cent involve both the lip and the palate, 25 per cent affect only the lip, and 25 per cent affect only the palate. A unilateral cleft appears in approximately 80 per cent of affected persons. Bilateral cleft lip extends into the palate in 80 per cent of patients.

Aglossodactyly. This is easily recognizable because of the partial or complete absence of the tongue associated with absence of the hands and feet. Both the hands and feet are usually involved, with phocomelia and absence of the nails.

Ankyloglossia. Ankyloglossia (tongue-tie) is a developmental variation of the lingual frenulum of the tongue. There is a restriction of elevation and protrusion of the tongue. With forward protrusion of the tip of the tongue, a central groove is often demonstrable. Speech disorders induced by ankyloglossia are extremely minor. Surgical treatment should be considered *only* when associated dental disorders are apparent or when dental prostheses are required.

Cleft Tongue. This is an unusual anomaly, and when it presents in its isolated form, it does not seem to interfere with longevity.

Geographic Tongue. This congenital disorder is characterized by discrete, reddened, smooth, irregularly shaped patches on the dorsolateral surface of the anterior two-thirds of the tongue. About one-fourth of the affected persons have symptoms of tenderness and burning. The cause of this type of tongue disorder is unknown, and if the patient is asymptomatic, no treatment is indicated.

Macroglossia. Macroglossia is a congenital enlargement of the tongue and is a common sign of cretinism and mongolism.

Median Rhomboid Glossitis. This disorder results from failure of the lateral lingual tubercles to completely overgrow the tuberculum impar during the development of the tongue. This results in a zone of nonpapillated mucosa. Median rhomboid glossitis presents as an ovoid or rhomboid nodule that is either fissured or a smooth red mass or zone in the midline of the dorsum of the tongue. The nodule is located just anterior to the V formed by the circumvallate papillae and is usually somewhat elevated.

Cleft Palate. Except for a *submucous cleft* of the palate, in which muscles of the soft palate are not joined in the midline, palatal clefts are easily identified. Approximately 35 to 50 per cent of patients with cleft palate have an associated anomaly. Most common are umbilical hernia, clubfoot, and deformities of the limbs and ears.

Cleft palate surgery has several objectives that include the establishment of adequate pharyngeal function, normal speech production, normal masticatory apparatus without malocclusion and with minimal interference with underlying bone growth, and the avoidance of facial deformity and interference with nasal physiology. Cleft palate surgery should be undertaken when the patient is approximately 1 year of age, whereas cleft lip should be corrected during the immediate postnatal period.

Palatal Fistula. Palatal fistula results from maldevelopment of the second branchial pouch. Small openings are apparent at the junction of the soft palate and the pharynx. Treatment is usually not indicated unless there is an associated infection.

Cleft Uvula. This malformation results from a failure of complete fusion of the uvular portion of the lateral halves of the soft palate. Cleft uvulae may be associated with other clefts of the palate, and their presence should be a signal to check specifically for submucous clefts, as such patients may develop hypernasality after adenoidectomy. Unless there is another associated cleft of the soft palate, no treatment is indicated.

Torus Palatinus. Torus palatinus is an enlarged mass of bone at the fusion line of the palatine processes. If this bony lesion grows excessively large, there is interference with mastication, speech, or the fitting of dentures. In such cases, it may be surgically removed. Otherwise, no treatment is indicated.

Agnathia. Agnathia is extremely rare and is incompatible with life. This disorder is associated with extremely low-set ears, which may be fused in the midline.

Mandibular Prognathism. This malformation results from excessive anterior mandibular growth. The condition is rarely evident at birth but becomes more apparent with subsequent growth and development. Surgical correction, orthodontic treatment, or both, are indicated when patients are dissatisfied with their physical appearance.

Micrognathia. Micrognathia has no known cause and is associated with torus mandibularis (an enlargement in the area of the genioid tubercle). It is thought to be transmitted by an autosomal dominant gene. Surgical removal is indicated if the growth inteferes with oral function.

Hereditary Disorders

Little has been written about hereditary disorders of the mouth and oropharynx. There is some evidence that cleft palate is caused by recessive genes and that torus mandibularis is a result of an autosomal dominant gene.

Trauma

Fractures of the mandible will be discussed in the section dealing with examination of the facial skeleton.

Lacerations. Even small lacerations of the lip should be sutured, primarily to minimize the cosmetic defect.

Lacerations of the tongue should be repaired, unless the wound is minimal. These lacerations should be sutured primarily with an absorbable material, which provides for satisfactory hemostasis and more rapid healing. Small lacerations that are not bleeding at the time they are seen initially need not be treated but should be observed, as they routinely become infected.

Lacerations of the tonsil and soft palate should be carefully evaluated, as these injuries usually are caused by falling on an object such as a Popsicle stick or a pencil, and they have been reported to cause thrombosis of the internal carotid artery. If there is any suspicion of deeper laceration, the patient should be admitted to the hospital and treated with a systemic antibiotic and possibly with surgical intervention.

Infectious Disorders

Infections of the lip tend to resolve rapidly and should be treated with appropriate antibiotics and soaks. An abscess rarely forms, and resolution of the infection is rapid.

Abscesses of oral structures are usually the result of direct trauma or are related to carious teeth. Systemic antibiotics are helpful, but the offending tooth, or teeth, should be removed.

Vincent's Angina. Vincent's angina presents as gingivitis or inflammation of the gums and may be the first indication of a spirochetal infection of the mouth with secondary bacterial invasion. The interdental papillae have a grayish exudate at their tips, and there may be a necrosis of these papillae. Treatment is directed toward maintaining oral hygiene and taking systemic antibiotics. Gentle brushing from the root of the tooth toward the tip is indicated to remove the necrotic debris. This should be done in a gingerly fashion, as bleeding will often ensue. Mouth rinses with an isotonic saline solution are also helpful.

Ludwig's Angina. This is a diffuse cellulitis of the floor of the mouth and neck that may occur following extraction of an abscessed tooth. Usual causative organisms are streptococci, staphylococci, and pneumococci. The condition is characterized by massive swelling and edema of the floor of the mouth in the submaxillary and suprahyoid regions. Respiratory difficulties may ensue because of the superior and posterior displacement of the tongue. Treatment includes systemic antibiotics and hospitalization for possible tracheotomy. Should the cellulitis become fluctuant, incision and drainage in the submental area should be performed. The abscess cavity will be deep to the mylohyoid muscle.

Acute Pharyngitis. Although acute pharyngitis is usually a viral infection it may be due to group A beta hemolytic streptococci. Both forms of pharyngitis produce soreness of the throat and pain on swallowing. Viral pharyngitis cannot be easily differentiated from bacterial pharyngitis on the basis of the physical examination. Both may demonstrate mild injection, purulent exudate, and membrane formation. With streptococcal pharyngitis, fever may be more prominent, cervical adenopathy may be more severe, and the white blood cell count may be more elevated. Since pharyngitis is usually a viral infection, antibiotic therapy should be withheld until group A beta hemolytic streptococci are obtained on culture. Depending on the course of the illness, treatment for pneumococcal and coagulase-positive staphylococcal pharyngitis is determined on an individual basis.

Acute Tonsillitis. This infection is characterized by sore throat and pain that is more marked on swallowing. Very young children will not complain of sore throat but will refuse to eat. Pain is often referred from the tonsillar fossae to the ears. There is usually a high fever, malaise, headache, and vomiting. The tonsils are edematous and hyperemic. There may be a purulent exudate from the crypts. The membrane seen in nondiphtheritic tonsillitis is white and nonconfluent, and peels away without bleeding but does not extend beyond the tonsil. The diphtheritic membrane is dirty gray, thick, and tough, and bleeding occurs if it is peeled away. It may spread to the mucous membrane of the tonsillar pillars, soft palate, and pharyngeal wall. The breath

in patients with diphtheria has the odor of mouse droppings. A smear for *Corynebacterium diphtheriae* and a culture on Klebs-Löffler media should be performed in patients with membranous tonsillitis and pharyngitis. Tonsillitis is usually a streptococcal infection, and penicillin is the antibiotic of choice, given after a culture of the pharynx is taken. Treatment is continued for 12 days. If streptococci are cultured, another throat culture is done 5 to 6 days after antibiotic therapy is completed. Other members of the family should have throat cultures when the tonsillitis is recurrent, so that carriers are treated at the same time. It should be noted, however, that recent studies have shown that only approximately 70 per cent of pathogenic organisms are recovered with throat swabs for culture.

Lingual tonsillitis follows the same pattern as palatine tonsillitis. The same microorganism is usually responsible, and the treatment is the same.

Infectious Mononucleosis. This disorder may produce a membrane that mimics the membrane described for diphtheria. In general, the patient has marked cervical adenopathy, difficulty swallowing, low-grade fever, and malaise. The patient may have been previously treated with antibiotics without good response, and this should provide a clue for the physician. Diagnosis is made by white blood cell count, differential blood cell count, Mono-Spot test, and heterophil antibody titer. Treatment consists of rest and supportive measures until the heterophil antibody titer is within normal limits. Early return to physical activities may produce a relapse.

Peritonsillar Abscess. Peritonsillar abscess results when infection spreads deep to the tonsillar capsule and produces peritonsillar cellulitis and abscess. The pus is located between the tonsillar capsule and the superior constrictor of the pharynx, and the tonsil is displaced medially. The uvula becomes edematous and is displaced to the opposite side. The soft palate is reddened. There is marked trismus resulting from irritation of the pterygoid muscles, and the head is tilted toward the side of the abscess. Swallowing and talking are painful, and swallowing may become so painful that the patient drools. The breath is foul-smelling, and the temperature is usually between 38 and 40°C. (100.4 to 104°F.). Peritonsillar cellulitis or abscess rarely occurs prior to the age of 10 to 12 years, and it is usually caused by group A hemolytic streptococci. Cellulitis without pus formation may exist and will respond to intensive penicillin therapy in 24 to 48 hours. If pus is present, incision and drainage should be performed. Patients with a diagnosis of peritonsillar cellulitis or abscess are admitted to the hospital, and if no obvious abscess has occurred, intravenous antibiotic therapy consisting of approximately 20,000,000 units of penicillin in the first 24 hours is instituted. Re-examination may show abscess formation, and incision is performed through the mucous membrane of the anterior tonsillar pillar. A hemostat is placed in the incision and gently spread.

These abscesses tend to recur and are an indication for tonsillectomy, which is performed 6 weeks after the acute infection subsides. At the time of tonsillectomy, pus may be encountered between the capsule and the tonsillar fossae.

In summary, patients presenting with trismus, deviation of the uvula to the opposite side, and cellulitis in the area of the tonsil should be diagnosed as having a peritonsillar cellulitis or abscess.

Parapharyngeal Abscess. This abscess usually occurs secondary to pharyngitis or tonsillitis and may appear in all age groups. Pus develops in the parapharyngeal space secondary to breakdown of lymphadenitis. The pus is located lateral to the superior constrictor of the pharynx and adjacent to the carotid sheath. The tonsil and soft palate may be displaced medially, but there is often no inflammatory reaction in the pharynx. There is marked swelling in the anterior cervical triangle. Penicillin is the antibiotic of choice. If fluctuation develops, the abscess is incised and drained. Drainage is performed through the external neck by making an incision along the sternocleidomastoid muscle. Blunt dissection is carried toward the carotid sheath where pus is encountered. A drain is placed in the wound, and antibiotic therapy is continued.

Retropharyngeal Abscess. This abscess occurs in infants and young children but is rare in those over the age of 10 years. Infections are located between the constrictors of the pharynx and the prevertebral fascia. They are secondary to pharyngitis

with breakdown of retropharyngeal lymph nodes. Infants with retropharyngeal abscesses usually present with opisthotonos and hyperextension of the ncek and are toxic and febrile.

A lumbar puncture is an appropriate diagnostic procedure for a toxic infant who presents with opisthotonos. If the lumbar puncture is normal, the possibility of retropharyngeal abscess must be excluded. Diagnosis is made by palpating the posterior pharyngeal wall and obtaining a lateral neck x-ray study. The infant is held in a prone position for the examination, so that if the abscess is ruptured during the examination, the pus will not be aspirated. The abscess has a boggy, fluctuant texture, and the bodies of the cervical vertebrae are not palpable. A lateral neck film should demonstrate the abscess, which is seen as an enlargement between the vertebral bodies and the normal pharyngeal air column. A lateral neck x-ray study is important, as inspection of the pharynx may not demonstrate the abscess because the entire pharyngeal wall may be displaced forward without inflammatory reaction of the mucous membrane. The child should be allowed to hyperextend his neck in order to maintain the airway. Tracheotomy is rarely necessary.

Treatment includes penicillin therapy and incision and drainage under general endotracheal anesthesia with the patient in the Rose position. The mucous membrane of the posterior wall is incised vertically. The incision splits only the mucous membrane, and the pus is obtained by gently spreading the fibers of the constrictor muscle and entering the retropharyngeal space. No drain is necessary because the abscessed cavity tends to be emptied on swallowing.

With proper diagnosis and treatment, there should be no untoward sequelae from this disease process.

Iatrogenic Disorders

Velopharyngeal Insufficiency. This disorder may be seen after tonsillectomy. Speech therapy evaluation is necessary to determine the extent of the nasal air escape. Children who have a submucous cleft are particularly prone to velopharyngeal insufficiency following adenoidectomy.

Idiopathic Disorders

Foreign Bodies. Objects may lodge in the palatine tonsils or in the lingual tonsils. The patient presents with a history of foreign body ingestion and localized pain. Finger palpation will often confirm the diagnosis. Lateral neck films may be helpful in detecting metallic objects. X-ray studies are usually not helpful when radiolucent foreign bodies, such as fish bones, are swallowed. Many foreign bodies are swallowed by persons who wear dentures, as they have a decreased area of sensation of the mouth and thus ingest the foreign body. Foreign bodies of the palatine tonsil may be removed by grasping them with a hemostat. Foreign bodies of the vallecula and base of the tongue are removed by direct laryngoscopy under local or general anesthesia.

Pemphigus. This is a rare condition characterized by formation of bullae that soon break down and leave a superficial membrane, so that the lesion resembles a blister that has burst. The bullae may be widely distributed over the surface of the body, but occasionally they are confined to the buccal mucosa of the pharynx. Any chronic, painful, ulcerative lesions of this area should be considered to be pemphigus until proved otherwise. A diagnosis is made clinically or by biopsy.

Neoplasms

Leukoplakia. Leukoplakia may be the result of chronic irritation. It is defined as a white patch that varies in thickness and extent. Histologic examination reveals thickening of the squamous mucous membrane with hyperkeratinization of the surface and dysplasia. Single, isolated lesions should be biopsied. If the patient has numerous leukoplakic lesions, these should be followed at 2 to 3 month intervals with regular and thorough inspection for ulceration or induration. Any lesion that changes should be biopsied.

Benign Tumors of the Oral Cavity. Such lesions include hemangiomas, lymphangiomas, papillomas, fibromas, and muco-celes. These lesions are often incidental findings discovered during a thorough physical examination. If they are symptomatic, the patient should be referred for appropriate treatment.

Oral Cavity Carcinomas. These neoplasms occur in several distinct anatomic areas that include the lips, tongue, floor of the mouth, buccal mucosa, gingiva, and the hard and soft palate. It is estimated that in 1977, 23,900 new patients with carcinomas of the buccal cavity and oropharynx have been identified. Cancer of this area is nearly always squamous cell carcinoma. Although the true causative factors in carcinomas are unknown, they have been related to smoking, jagged teeth, dental caries, ingestion of spices and hot foods, syphilitic glossitis, malnutrition, alcoholism, psoriasis, and chemical poisoning.

Carcinoma of the Lip. These carcinomas are easily identifiable, and the diagnosis should be confirmed by biopsy and histologic examination. Appropriate treatment may consist of radiation or surgery, radiation being preferred for basal cell carcinomas.

Carcinoma of the Tongue. The overall 5 year survival for patients with carcinoma of the tongue is approximately 45 per cent. Patients presenting with carcinoma of the tongue often complain of a lump in the tongue and some superficial ulceration with pain. They may also present with a lump in the neck and the primary lesion in the tongue. Biopsy for confirmation of the type of lesion should be obtained at the primary lesion.

Carcinoma of the Floor of the Mouth. Squamous cell carcinoma of the floor of the mouth may remain quiet, and the patient presents with a lump in the neck. In my own experience, I have seen three people who had neck node biopsies and who had unidentified carcinomas under the tongue in the area of the frenulum. The emphasis is placed on diagnosis of the primary tumor, which can be biopsied in the office. Treatment is by surgery and irradiation, depending on the location, size, and extent of spread of the tumor.

Carcinoma of the Buccal Mucosa. Lesions of the buccal mucosa are often detected by our dental colleagues. Many of these lesions are detected when they are small and can be excised locally with good control.

Carcinoma of the Gingiva. Squamous cell carcinomas of the gingiva are often diagnosed by a dentist, as the patient may appear in his office with a loose tooth. Once the diagnosis is made, treatment consists of radical surgery and radiation therapy. Early invasion of bone prevents easy local excision of these tumors.

Carcinoma of the Hard and Soft Palates. Fortunately, these tumors are rare, as their removal results in a marked functional deficit with regard to eating and speaking. Again, biopsy and histologic examination are imperative. Referral for thorough evaluation of the extent of the tumor and for subsequent treatment is necessary.

Carcinoma of the Tonsil. Nearly all malignant tumors of the tonsil are squamous cell carcinomas, and the overall survival rate of patients for 5 years is approximately 45 per cent. Many of these tumors present as a node in the neck with very few symptoms. Biopsy is obtained for histologic examination. Treatment consists of preoperative radiation and radical excision of the tonsillar fossa and a portion of the mandible including the mental foramen.

Carcinoma of the Oropharynx. The patient with oropharyngeal carcinoma often presents with a mass in the neck. On physical examination, a fungating exophytic lesion is seen on the pharyngeal mucosa. Biopsy is obtained for histologic examination, and appropriate treatment usually consists of full-course radiotherapy to the oropharynx and neck and surgical resection of the neck if the tumor mass persists.

Drug-Induced Disorders

Black Hairy Tongue. This condition is often associated with prolonged antibiotic therapy and is the result of overgrowth of squamous epithelium. The patient may complain of a bad taste in his mouth but is usually asymptomatic. Brushing gently with a toothbrush and sodium bicarbonate can remove most of this squamous epithelium.

Moniliasis. Moniliasis of the mouth is often the result of antibiotic therapy. The patient may present with thin, atrophic tongue epithelium or, more commonly, with a fine white exudate over the tongue and buccal mucosa. Diagnosis is made by scraping and by using potassium hydroxide (KOH) solution in methylene blue for detection of budding yeast. Treatment of this condition may be prolonged, particularly in patients with dentures. Appropriate treatment includes using a nystatin preparation (Mycostatin oral suspension) three times per day in the mouth and soaking the dentures overnight each night in the suspension of Mycostatin. The treatment should be prolonged for at least 4 weeks. After discontinuance of treatment, moniliasis may recur.

NASOPHARYNX

Embryology and Anatomy

The nasopharynx is the most anterior portion of the embryologic foregut and extends from the posterior choanae to the free edge of the soft palate.

The nasopharynx includes the adenoids, the eustachian cushions, the posterior choanae, and the superior surface of the soft palate.

Examination

Instruments for examination of the nasopharynx include a light source and a tongue blade to depress the tongue in a downward direction (Fig. 39–20). The small mirror is then placed behind the free edge of the soft palate, and the structures of the nasopharynx are inspected. On occasion, a local anesthetic, such as lidocaine (Xylocaine) 4 per cent may be sprayed onto the posterior oropharynx and nasopharynx. The soft palate retractor may be used to pull the soft palate anteriorly for better visualization.

The nasopharyngoscope may be inserted through the anterior nose and placed along the side of the inferior turbinate after a local anesthetic and vasoconstrictors have been applied. This instrument provides an excellent view of the eustachian cushions and the vault of the nasopharynx.

Physiology

The nasopharynx provides a conduit for respiration and access to the nose for resonation of speech during articulation. This organ also provides an airway to the middle ear space via the eustachian tube. The function of adenoids was unknown until recently. It now appears that they assist in the early production of antibodies against viruses. The most useful aid in the examination of the nasopharynx is the lateral neck x-ray study, which provides an outline of

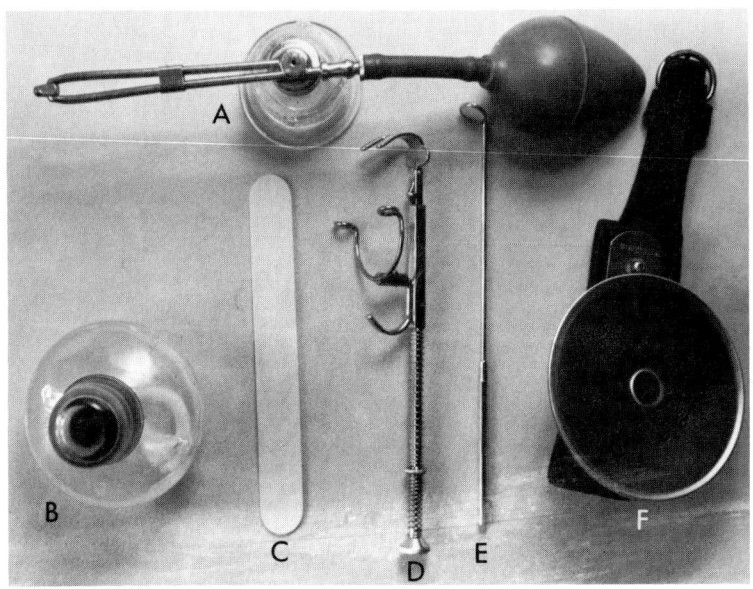

Figure 39-20. *Nasopharyngeal instruments.* A, *local anesthetic (4 per cent lidocaine);* B, *alcohol lamp to warm mirror;* C, *tongue blade;* D, *soft palate retractor;* E, *#0 mirror; and* F, *head mirror.*

the air column. Submental vertex x-ray views may also be of assistance. Contrast cineradiography may be helpful in specific instances.

Congenital Disorders

Cysts of the Nasopharynx. These include branchial cleft cysts, intra-adenoidal cysts, and extra-adenoidal cysts. The usual clinical manifestations of nasopharyngeal cysts include purulent posterior and postnasal discharge, an aching pain behind the throat or base of the skull, and a feeling of pressure or fullness that is periodically relieved by evacuation of the secretions.

Diagnosis is made by lateral neck x-ray studies and cinecontrast studies with examination and removal of the cyst under anesthesia. Intra-adenoidal cysts can easily be removed by adenoidectomy. The other two types of cysts may present difficulties in diagnosis.

Nasopharyngeal Stenosis. This disorder may result from incomplete rupture of the buccal pharyngeal membrane. A diagnosis is made when the soft palate and the posterior nasopharynx are found to be attached to each other. This is a rare condition and is usually diagnosed by physical examination of infants having respiratory distress at birth. Treatment consists of dilatation and occasionally of surgery.

Nasopharyngeal Teratomas. Such tumors are uncommon and may be associated with other cranial deformities such as an encephalocele, hemicrania, and palatal fissures. When there are associated cranial problems, neurosurgical procedures may be necessary for the removal of these tumors.

Nasopharyngeal Choristoma. This lesion is extremely rare and is defined as a tumor of histologically normal tissue for an organ or part of the body other than the site at which the tumor is located. Airway obstruction and displacement of the soft palate are the common presenting complaints.

Nasopharyngeal Encephalocele. This disorder has an unknown cause. A patient with such a malformation presents with nasal obstruction and occasional spinal fluid rhinorrhea. Treatment consists of neurosurgical closure as soon as the condition permits.

Tornwaldt's Bursa. This malformation represents persistence of an embryonic communication between the anterior tip of the notochord and the roof of the pharynx. Symptoms are varied but relate to an infection of the bursa. Treatment includes antibiotic administration and occasionally drainage.

Trauma

Trauma to the nasopharynx is unusual, the most common cause being adenoidectomy that may result in nasopharyngeal stenosis. Such stenosis is treated by surgery.

Foreign Bodies. Such objects occasionally enter the nasopharynx by direct penetration of the soft palate or by coughing up of a foreign body from the pharynx. Foreign bodies of the nasopharynx usually occur in children and should be removed under general anesthesia.

Infectious Disorders

Infections of the nasopharynx are common is childhood but are difficult to evaluate. Lymphoid hyperplasias secondary to infections are associated with obstruction of the eustachian tube and the choanae. Obstruction of the eustachian tube leads to serous or secretory otitis media and to recurrent acute otitis media and exacerbations of chronic otitis media. Obstruction of the choanae produces mouth-breathing, hyponasal voice, and purulent rhinorrhea. Treatment is medical and usually includes penicillin and oral decongestants for relief of secondary edema.

Indications for Adenoidectomy. *The most common indication for removal of the adenoid tissue is persistent serous or secretory otitis media.* In a child, a sterile effusion in the middle ear lasting 6 weeks or longer and occurring de novo or following acute otitis media that does not respond to medical management responds regularly, but not invariably, to adenoidectomy. The use of myringotomies with the insertion of tympanotomy tubes increases the chance of success.

Chronic otitis media in children is another common indication for adenoidectomy. This procedure reduces the severity and frequency of exacerbations of chronic otitis media. Recurrent acute otitis media is a fairly frequent indication for this procedure. Many children between the ages of 1 and 6 years will have two to three episodes of acute otitis media per year that will completely resolve with antibiotic therapy. On the other hand, the child who is on antibiotic therapy for otitis media for more than half of the year should be considered for adenoidectomy. Febrile convulsions in conjunction with acute otitis media weigh heavily in favor of performing an adenoidectomy, since antibiotic therapy ordinarily is not initiated prior to the convulsions.

In treating persistent nasal obstruction caused by *adenoid hyperplasia*, the age of the patient is considered, since lymphoid tissue reaches an absolute maximum size at puberty and a relative maximum size at ages 8 to 10 years. Persistent recurrent purulent rhinorrhea occurring in spite of adequate antibiotic therapy is occasionally encountered on the basis of adenoid hyperplasia and chronic adenoiditis. Sinusitis occurring in children who do not have an underlying immunologic defect, such as hypogammaglobulinemia, is relatively rare but is regularly improved or eliminated by adenoidectomy.

Adenoidectomy is performed under general anesthesia. The lymphoid tissue is removed superficial to the superior constrictor of the pharynx by sharp dissection with an adenotome or a guillotine-type instrument. Iatrogenic velopharyngeal insufficiency or stenosis may result from adenoidectomy. It is thought that nasopharyngeal stenosis with the palate attaching to the nasopharynx is caused by extensive trauma during adenoidectomy.

Palatal Insufficiency. This disorder has a higher incidence in children with a submucous cleft of the soft palate, but may occur in normal children. Treatment of palatal insufficiency is by speech therapy and at times by surgical placement of a superiorly based pharyngeal flap or by implantation of a polytetrafluoroethylene (Teflon) implant in the posterior pharyngeal wall.

Idiopathic Disorders

Foreign Bodies. Objects may occasionally be lodged in the nasopharynx, and the patient may present with signs of purulent rhinorrhea. Other patients may present in the emergency room with a history of foreign body ingestion in which the object cannot be found in the pharynx, larynx, esophagus, or bronchi. In these instances, the foreign body should be suspected of being in the nasopharynx. A preoperative lateral neck x-ray examination is routine and may show the object, if it is radiopaque. The foreign body may be removed under general anesthesia at the time of direct laryngoscopy, and the nasopharynx should be inspected routinely when the foreign body is not found in the upper aerodigestive tract.

Neoplasms

Juvenile Angiofibroma. This is a benign neoplasm of the nasopharynx. The lesion is found only in males and usually presents prior to puberty. Presentation of angiofibroma is usually by epistaxis but may be manifest by obstruction of the nasal cavity or by sinusitis. Histologic examination shows that these tumors are composed of fibrous tissue and numerous thin-walled vessels without contractile elements. Such angiofibromas tend to involute at puberty.

Epistaxis is a major problem in patients with angiofibromas, and bleeding may become life-threatening. Occasionally, when nasal masses mistakenly thought to be nasal polyps are biopsied, the bleeding may be so severe that the patient may need to be given several units of blood. On examination, the masses are red and quite firm. Portions of the tumor that project into the airway may become ulcerated during episodes of upper respiratory tract infections.

Surgical removal is indicated to prevent massive bleeding. The extent of the tumor can be determined by angiography. The tumor is removed through a transpalatal approach, and often a lateral rhinotomy is performed in combination with this procedure. Blood loss during the surgery may amount to several liters. Preoperative estrogen therapy has been advocated by some, and more recently intra-arterial injections of absorbable gelatin into the major feeding vessels prior to surgery have been used. (This use of absorbable gelatin may not be listed in the manufacturer's official directive.) Also, radiation therapy has been used in extensive tumor formations involving the paranasal sinuses, orbit, or base of the skull.

Malignant Tumors of the Nasopharynx. Such tumors are numerous and include squamous cell carcinomas, malignant mixed tumors, melanomas, chordomas, sarcomas, plasmacytomas, and lymphomas. Lymphomas and lymphosarcomas are the most common nasopharyngeal tumors in children. In adults, squamous cell carcinomas and lymphoepitheliomas occur most frequently.

Because of eustachian tube involvement, the patient who presents with a serous otitis media and a posterior neck node on the same side should be suspected of having a nasopharyngeal carcinoma. On physical examination, the tumor may not be apparent, but it may be submucosal and found by blind nasopharyngeal biopsy.

The diagnosis is made by biopsy of the primary tumor under general anesthesia. Biopsy of the metastatic neck node should be avoided, as this may result in implantation of the tumor in the skin and subcutaneous tissue. It is essential that the primary tumor in the nasopharynx be identified before treatment, even if a histologic diagnosis is obtained from biopsy of the cervical metastases.

Treatment of choice for carcinoma of the nasopharynx is radiation with a supervoltage source. The radiation is delivered to the primary tumor and to both sides of the neck. Cervical metastases that remain clinically palpable following radiation therapy may be treated by a radical neck dissection, if the primary tumor has been controlled. The five year survival rate of patients with nasopharyngeal carcinoma has been reported as 30 to 40 per cent. The low survival rate is felt to be related to the late diagnosis.

Drug-Induced Disorders

Occasionally, overuse of nasal sprays or nose drops can cause a chronic eustachian tube irritation that may present as a deep itching in the ear, although the physical examination is normal. Treatment consists of discontinuance of the offending topical vasoconstrictor.

LARYNX AND HYPOPHARYNX

Embryology and Anatomy

The hypopharynx is a portion of the foregut of the embryo and is continuous with the oropharynx as a muscular tube. By approximately the twenty-sixth day after conception, the pulmonary diverticulum begins to arise in the area of the sixth branchial arch. By approximately the twenty-eighth day, differentiation of the larynx can be seen. The larynx develops from the fourth and sixth branchial arches and is formed as a tube within a tube in the midventral wall of the foregut. The foregut caudal to the pulmonary diverticulum develops into the esophagus, the stomach, and the duodenum to the level of the common bile duct.

The skeleton of the larynx consists of the thyroid cartilage, the cricoid cartilage, the epiglottis, the arytenoid cartilages, the corniculate cartilages, and the cuneiform cartilages. Only the cricoid cartilage completely encircles the airway and maintains patency. The arytenoid cartilages articulate with the cricoid cartilages.

The true vocal cords are attached to the vocal processes of the arytenoid cartilages and to the isthmus of the thyroid cartilage anteriorly halfway between the thyroid notch and the lower border of the thyroid cartilage. The superior surfaces of the true vocal cords are flat and are covered with stratified squamous epithelium; the inferior surfaces are concave. The inferior surfaces of the false vocal cords are flat, and the superior surfaces are convex. The true vocal cords and the false vocal cords form a double-layered valve. The configuration of the true vocal cords makes them a good barrier for the ingress of air and a poor barrier for the egress of air. The false vocal cords, because of their configuration, provide a poor barrier for the ingress of air and a good barrier for the egress of air. The true vocal cords can be thought of as an inlet valve, and the false vocal cords can be thought of as an outlet valve.

Physiology

The primary function of the larynx is that of a sphincter (Fig. 39–21). Its sphincter mechanism is used during deglutition, parturition, and defecation. The larynx also serves as a sphincter during coughing. After deep inspiration, the larynx closes as an outlet valve, and the intrathoracic pressure is increased. With coughing, the larynx suddenly opens, resulting in a blast of air that carries with it particulate matter from within the lumen of the tracheobronchial tree.

A secondary function of the larynx is that of voice production. The fundamental tone is produced by the movement of the vocal cords that is brought about by the flow of exhaled air past lightly approximated vocal cords. Loudness of the tone is controlled by increasing intrathoracic pressure by further tensing the cords and increasing the intrathoracic pressure. The fundamental tone and its overtones are modified into speech by the articulators, which include the phayrnx, palate, teeth, tongue, and lips. The fundamental tone varies with the sex and age of the person. Adult males produce a fundamental tone of 125 Hz., and adult females produce a fundamental tone of 250 Hz.

In the normal voice, the overtones of these fundamental tones are whole numbers of the fundamental tones (harmonics). The predominance of harmonic overtones gives the voice a musical quality. The distribution of the harmonics gives the voice a timbre that is characteristic for that person. A healthy voice has frequent changes in the frequency of the fundamental tone, which provides it with a melodious quality. The normal speaker uses changes in frequency for emphasis, rather than changes in intensity. Changes in the mass, configuration, or mobility of the vocal cords cause asynchrony of the vibration of the two

Figure 39–21. Cavity of the larynx and its subdivisions in a frontal section. (From Hollinshead, W. H.: Anatomy for Surgeons. Vol. 1, 2nd Ed. Hagerstown, Md., Harper & Row, Publishers, Inc., 1968, p. 475.)

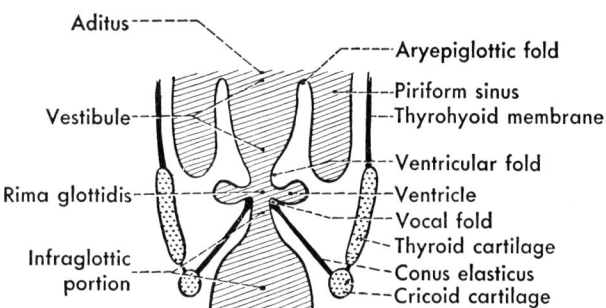

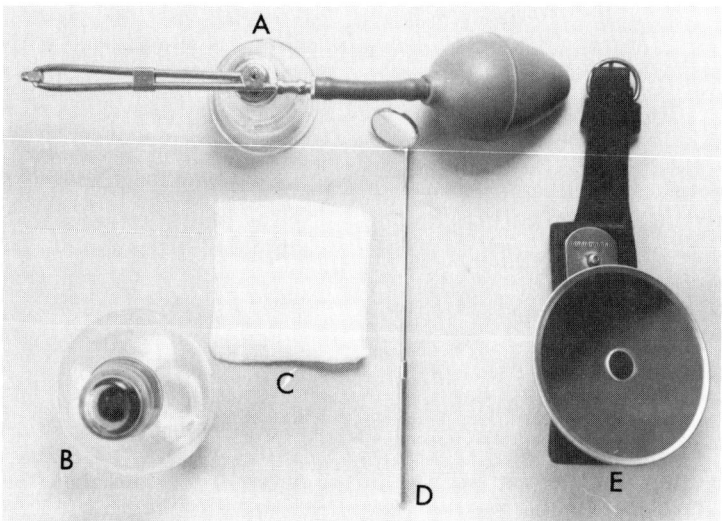

Figure 39-22. *Laryngeal instruments. A, local anesthesia (4 per cent lidocaine); B, alcohol lamp to warm mirror; C, cloth sponge to hold tongue; D, #5 laryngeal mirror; and E, head mirror.*

vocal cords, which results in hoarseness. Abuse and misuse of the voice can result in a structural change in the true vocal cords.

Examination

Instruments for the examination of the larynx and hypopharynx include a light source such as a head mirror, a laryngeal mirror, an alcohol lamp for warming, 4 × 4 cm. gauze sponges for holding the tongue, and a local anesthetic (Fig. 39-22). Indirect mirror examination of the larynx and hypopharynx is not difficult if practiced on a regular basis. Local anesthetic is rarely needed but is occasionally helpful. The mirror is placed against the soft palate and pushed in an upward direction, while the tongue is held anteriorly with a gauze sponge (the tongue should not be pulled). Inspection should include the base of the tongue, valleculae, epiglottis, aryepiglottic folds, pyriform fossae, and true and false vocal cords during inspiration and expiration. The patient should be instructed to say a prolonged "eh," as an "ee" requires lifting of the base of the tongue.

Indirect laryngoscopy is complemented by contrast laryngography, in which the endolarynx and the upper trachea are coated with a radiopaque material. Films are then taken during quiet inspiration, during production of sound in the normal manner and production of sound on inhaling, and during a Valsalva maneuver. Laminagraphy may also be helpful. Patients who have been hoarse for 2 to 3 weeks and whose larynx cannot be visualized by indirect laryngoscopy should have direct laryngoscopy for evaluation of possible carcinoma.

Congenital Disorders

Congenital Laryngeal Atresia.   This anomaly is incompatible with life. At birth, marked respiratory efforts without passage of air or stridor are the first signs of laryngeal atresia. Diagnosis is made by direct laryngoscopy, and unless tracheostomy or dilatation with passage of an endotracheal tube is performed, death ensues. In mild cases with partial stenosis, recurrent episodes of upper respiratory tract infections are common. Associated anomalies are abnormalities of the central nervous system, alimentary tract, kidneys, and skeletal system.

Laryngeal Cysts.   Hoarseness, muffled cry, stridor, and suprasternal and upper gastric retractions are all symptoms and signs of laryngeal cyst. Anyone presenting with these signs and symptoms should have a lateral neck x-ray examination and direct laryngoscopy. Most congenital cysts of the larynx are confined to the area of the ventricular appendix. Treatment generally consists of aspiration or removal of the cyst and possibly of a tracheostomy.

Congenital Laryngeal Webs. Such webs result from failure of normal splitting of the vocal cord primordium. They are more commonly found at the level of the glottis between the interior faces of the vocal cords. Signs and symptoms depend on the severity of the web, varying from complete respiratory obstruction to weakness and hoarseness of the infant's cry.

Diagnosis can be made by direct laryngoscopy, soft tissue x-ray examination of the larynx, or a laryngogram. Extensive webs require emergency treatment at birth. A tracheotomy may be indicated if an endotracheal tube cannot be passed through the web. Thin webs located at the level of the glottis may be treated with repeated laryngeal dilatations.

Bifid Epiglottis. This disorder may be an incidental finding or may present as stridor due to prolapse of the bifid epiglottis into the glottis.

Congenital Laryngeal Hemangioma. These hemangiomas, usually of the cavernous type, tend to occur anteriorly in the infraglottic region of the larynx. They are more common in females than in males and are associated with cutaneous hemangiomas in the majority of patients. Symptoms and signs are those of laryngeal obstruction, which may appear in conjunction with the first upper respiratory tract infection of the newborn.

Diagnosis is made by direct laryngoscopy, which discloses a red or purple subglottic mass covered with normal epithelium. A biopsy is dangerous if a tracheostomy has not been performed. If the symptoms are intermittent, the child may be observed before therapy is instituted, as there are many instances of spontaneous regression during the first few years of life. If there is no spontaneous regression, small doses of radiation may be used.

Laryngocele. This is a saccular dilatation of the appendix of the laryngeal ventricle and may present in the neck, passing between the thyroid cartilage and the hyoid bone at the perforation of the neurovascular bundle.

The cyst may be internal, external, or in combination. The signs and symptoms vary with the extent and location of the lesion. Asymptomatic laryngoceles may be observed. Larger laryngoceles cause hoarseness, dysphagia, aspiration, and potential airway obstruction. Treatment of laryngocele is by surgical excision.

Laryngomalacia. Laryngomalacia is the most common congenital laryngeal anomaly. It is thought to result from exaggerated or persistent infantile features of the larynx together with a longitudinal infolding of the epiglottis. On inspiration, the epiglottis may fall into the glottis, causing varying degrees of obstruction. At this time, the symptoms and signs of retraction are apparent. Signs and symptoms usually present shortly after birth and increase in severity until the age of 6 to 18 months.

Diagnosis is made by indirect laryngoscopy, which reveals flaccidity of all the supraglottic structures. The epiglottis is curled, tubular, and soft. The arytenoids and aryepiglottic folds are soft, and these structures flutter during inspiration.

Treatment consists of placing the infant on his stomach and of giving multiple small feedings. Tracheostomy is indicated only in patients who have severe respiratory difficulty.

Stridor. Stridor that is present at birth should be evaluated by first placing an airway in the mouth. If this provides relief of the airway difficulty, catheters should be placed in the nose, as there is a great possibility of choanal atresia. If the oral airway does not relieve the difficulty, direct laryngoscopy should be performed in the delivery room, with examination of the larynx and possibly the placement of an endotracheal tube. If the origin of the difficulty is still not apparent, a lateral neck film, chest x-ray film, and contrast study of the esophagus should be performed.

Congenital Vocal Cord Paralysis. The cause of congenital vocal cord paralysis is unknown but is thought to be related to birth trauma and presents as a weakened cry. The child may aspirate on feeding. Diagnosis is made by direct laryngoscopy. Treatment consists of thoroughly evaluating the child's airway and esophagus and exercising care during his feeding. A tracheostomy may be needed.

Hereditary Disorders

Achondroplasia may present as a laryngomalacia.

Trauma

Traumatic injuries to the larynx may occur from automobile accidents in which the patient is thrown forward, and the larynx is crushed between the cervical vertebrae and the object against which he decelerates. Children may fracture their larynx by falling against the handlebars of a bicycle.

Laryngeal Fracture. In patients with laryngeal fracture, crepitus is usually present. There may be complaints of pain on swallowing and hoarseness. Progressive dyspnea is a usual finding, and *subcutaneous emphysema* is felt to be diagnostic of fractures of the larynx or the trachea. The laryngeal cartilages may not be directly palpable because of soft tissue swelling. On direct laryngoscopy, the laryngeal lumen appears disrupted or bloody, and there may be exposed cartilage and lacerated mucous membrane.

Initial management of the patient with laryngeal fracture begins with a tracheostomy performed under controlled conditions in the emergency room. X-ray studies of the lateral neck and laminagrams of the larynx may define the type and degree of injury. A careful survey of the cervical vertebrae by x-ray examination may demonstrate associated fractures or dislocations. After initial management, direct laryngoscopy and bronchoscopy are performed. If the patient's condition permits, immediate open reduction of the mucosal tears and wiring of the fragments are performed. Laryngeal stenting may be required when there is extensive soft tissue loss.

Tracheostomy is often necessary in patients with multiple injuries because such injuries may cause upper airway obstruction. This procedure is especially important during management of massive intra-abdominal and intracranial trauma and difficulty with the functioning of the larynx is not discovered until removal of the tracheostomy tube is tried. Failure to recognize laryngeal fractures at the time of injury will routinely lead to laryngeal stenosis. The repair of laryngeal stenosis at a later time is much more difficult and is often unsuccessful.

Infectious Disorders

Although upper respiratory obstruction in a child is often diagnosed as *croup*, the two most common forms of upper respiratory obstruction are *acute epiglottitis* and *laryngotracheobronchitis*, which is classic croup.

Acute Epiglottis. This is a clinical entity that should be distinguished from all other types of laryngeal obstruction because it develops with such great rapidity. Only 4 to 5 hours may elapse from the time of the first symptoms until a tracheostomy is urgently needed. It may occur in children of any age after 5 months old, and up to adulthood. Stridor is chiefly inspiratory, and children with acute epiglottitis appear exhausted but insist on sitting up. They have a pale ashen or gray skin color. Hoarseness is rarely noted, but they have a muffled, thick, guttural voice and have a much higher fever than do children with laryngotracheal bronchitis.

Diagnosis is made by lateral neck x-ray studies or by examining the child in the upright position with direct observation of the epiglottis made possible by depressing the posterior tongue. The normal epiglottis should appear thin, like the edge of the pinna of the ear, but in epiglottitis, it will appear swollen, like a cherry-red mass.

Treatment is tracheostomy, which should be performed in the operating room with either anesthetic intubation or after a bronchoscope has been passed through the larynx. Recently, intubation with a silicone endotracheal tube has been advocated. However, unless a team of physicians is immediately available, tracheostomy appears to be safer if the patient becomes extubated. The underlying causative organism is said to be *Hemophilus influenzae*, type B. However, recent studies have shown that many of these infections have been caused by either viral or other pathogenic organisms. Ampicillin or another appropriate antibiotic is indicated for treatment of epiglottitis, after the tracheostomy is performed.

Croup. The development of laryngotracheobronchitis (croup) begins with an upper respiratory tract infection. If the upper respiratory tract infection continues, it results in edema of the subglottic space and eventual sloughing of the superficial epithelium with crust formation. As the cricoid area is the narrowest portion of the infant's airway, respiratory insufficiency from partial obstruction may develop. Typically, there is a brassy cough and hoarseness that is worse at night. The symptoms may develop over a 2 to 3 day period, and the fever is often elevated only to 38 to 39° C. (100.4 to 102.2° F.). Drying of the mucous membrane is worse during the cold winter months when atmospheric humidity is low.

Treatment consists of placing the patient in a high-humidity, oxygen-enriched atmosphere and administering corticosteroids and an appropriate antibiotic, usually penicillin.

A rule of thumb for performing a tracheostomy is the presence of a continuous pulse rate greater than 140 beats per minute or a respiratory rate greater than 40 per minute lasting 3 hours after the institution of treatment. Steroid therapy consists of giving hydrocortisone phosphate, 100 mg. intramuscularly, on admission and of occasionally repeating this dose after 8 hours. Racemic epinephrine has not been shown to be of benefit.

Laryngeal Diphtheria. Although laryngeal diphtheria is now rare, it should be noted that tracheostomy was perfected for the treatment of diphtheria, and use of this procedure subsequently became widespread. Diagnosis depends upon the recognition of the diphtheritic membrane at the time of laryngoscopy and tracheostomy. Appropriate antibiotic therapy and diphtheria antitoxin should be used for the treatment of the primary infection.

Tuberculosis, Syphilis, and Histoplasmosis. These may present as hoarseness, or, less commonly, as dysphagia, pain, or stridor. Diagnosis is made by biopsy, histologic examination, and fungal cultures.

Juvenile Papillomas. These lesions of the larynx are thought to be of viral etiology and appear as moist, wart-like growths in the larynx. The patient complains of hoarseness, and the diagnosis is made by indirect laryngoscopy. The lesions typically appear during the second or the third year of life but may appear as early as the first year.

Therapy consists of careful removal, using endoscopic procedures and possible tracheostomy if airway obstruction is present and the recurrence is rapid. Typically, these lesions do recur, and endoscopic removal may be required as often as every 1 to 2 months. Regression at puberty is usual,

although not uniformly so. Radiation therapy is mentioned here only in the context of being condemned as poor treatment that is possibly carcinogenic.

Iatrogenic Disorders

Subglottic Stenosis. The classic subglottic stenosis was first described in 1923 as a complication of high tracheostomy. At the present time, subglottic stenosis is more commonly encountered as a complication of prolonged endotracheal intubation, and a tracheostomy should be performed if the patient is to be intubated for longer than 3 days. The classic tracheostomy is performed at the third or fourth tracheal ring to prevent subglottic stenosis.

Subglottic stenosis usually presents as an inability to remove the tracheostomy tube or endotracheal tube, or it may present as a progressive dyspnea after extubation. Evaluation is by mirror laryngoscopy, and the area below the cords is seen to be markedly narrowed. Laminagrams of the larynx are helpful, and pulmonary function tests give information as to the degree of obstruction.

Many methods of treating subglottic stenosis have been tried, but results are poor and no uniformly satisfactory method is known. If granulations are present, injections of steroids into the subglottic area are often helpful. Dilatations of the subglottic larynx may be performed as often as once monthly. A tracheostomy is routinely needed. Numerous surgical procedures for the treatment of subglottic stenosis have been described, and in the young, otherwise healthy patient, surgery should be performed in an effort to allow removal of the tracheostomy tube at a later date.

Idiopathic Disorders

Vocal Cord Polyps. Such polyps develop from misuse and abuse of the voice. A typical patient is someone who must speak loudly over a great deal of background noise or someone who must speak constantly, as is required of a salesman. Similar pathologic changes also occur in persons with chronic allergic manifestations and those who chronically inhale irritants, such as tobacco smoke.

These persons complain of hoarseness

that is secondary to a chronic subepithelial edema in the lamina propria of the true vocal cords. The polypoid swellings of the free edges of the true vocal cords interfere with approximation of these cords.

Diagnosis is made by the mirror examination. The polyps appear as a smooth swelling of the free edges of the vocal cords and may be quite large, so that they fall into the larynx on inspiration and are pushed upward on expiration. The polyps usually extend anteriorly from the vocal process of the vocal cord to the anterior commissure of the larynx.

Treatment consists of speech training, as many of these persons are using their voice improperly. If speech training is unsuccessful, the lesion should be removed under general anesthesia with direct laryngoscopy and microsurgical control.

Vocal Nodules. These growths are also caused by misuse and abuse of the voice, particularly by using the voice too loudly and too long and by using a fundamental frequency that is unnaturally low. Vocal nodules are condensations of connective tissues in the lamina propria at the junction of the anterior one-third and the posterior two-thirds of the true vocal cords. Diagnosis is made by mirror laryngoscopy, and discrete nodules will often be seen that may be likened to calluses on the hands from manual labor.

Treatment consists of the institution of speech training. Singers and actors should also abstain from speaking for a variable period of time, usually for a minimum of 2 weeks. If speech therapy is unsuccessful, the nodules can be removed by microsurgical techniques with the patient under general anesthesia.

Contact Ulcers. Contact ulcers are thought to be a result of misuse of the voice, particularly in the form of a sharp glottal attack (that is, sudden, very loud speech). These ulcerations occur on the vocal processes of the arytenoids and cause mild pain or pain on swallowing. After examination is made by indirect laryngoscopy, a tiny biopsy specimen may be taken to rule out the possibility of carcinoma, but the ulcerations are not biopsied deeply for fear of permanent impairment of the voice.

Treatment consists of prolonged speech therapy, and, in general, surgical removal is contraindicated.

Neoplasms

Benign Neoplasms of the Larynx. These include *papillomas, fibromas, myxomas, chondromas, neurofibromas, and meningiomas* and may involve any part of the larynx, including the true vocal cords. Such lesions may be removed at direct laryngoscopy for histologic examination. These lesions are rare, but any lesion of the larynx should be biopsied for histologic evaluation.

Malignant Neoplasms of the Larynx. Squamous cell carcinoma accounts for more than 95 per cent of malignant neoplasms of the larynx. The number of new cases of carcinoma of the larynx in 1977 was estimated to be 9200. This disease is predominant in males, with the peak incidence occurring in the fifth and sixth decades of life. Carcinoma of the larynx rarely develops in those who do not smoke but has an even higher incidence with smokers who drink excessively.

Carcinoma may arise from the mucous membrane of any part of the larynx or hypopharynx. However, there is a predilection for the true vocal cords, particularly for the anterior two-thirds of the vocal cords. The epiglottis, pyriform sinus, and postcricoid area are also common points of origin.

The presenting symptom is predominantly that of hoarseness, followed by dysphagia, hemoptysis, and airway obstruction. A mass in the neck is also a frequent sign.

Presumptive diagnosis of carcinoma of the larynx or hypopharynx is made by indirect laryngoscopy. Any discrete lesion should be biopsied for histologic evaluation. Patients presenting with a neck mass but with no other lesion being found on the examination should also undergo laryngoscopy, bronchoscopy, and esophagoscopy.

Treatment depends on the size and the location of the tumor, but, in general, except for small lesions of the true vocal cords, which are treated by irradiation, carcinomas of the larynx and hypopharynx are treated by combination therapy consisting of irradiation and surgery.

In some patients, conservation surgery of the larynx can be performed, which will eradicate the carcinoma and save the functions of the larynx.

Drug-Induced Disorders

Hyper- or Hypothyroidism. These disorders may present with hoarseness and edema of the vocal cords. Although unusual, occasional patients treated medically for hyperthyroidism may consequently become hypothyroid and present with hoarseness. Treatment consists of replacement therapy for the hypothyroidism, but often a mild degree of hoarseness persists.

SALIVARY GLANDS

Embryology and Anatomy

The major salivary glands and many of the minor salivary glands are derived from the stomadeum ectoderm. Each of the major salivary glands develops from an ingrowth of oral epithelium into the underlying mesenchyme. As this invagination continues, the primordial cells elongate and undergo budding and branching, resulting in the formation of primordial ducts in the acini. The outer ductal cells differentiate into secretory epithelium, and the ductal lumen is formed by degeneration of the central cells. Serous and mucous acini develop from the terminal buds.

The parotid gland extends from near the arch of the zygoma just anterior to the ear downward approximately 2 cm. below the angle of the mandible, wraps around the angle of the mandible on the anterior portion of the sternocleidomastoid muscle, and extends deep to the stylomandibular ligament. Anteriorly, the parotid gland extends to near the anterior edge of the masseter muscle. The facial nerve transverses the parotid gland. The parotid gland normally is not palpable, and if a discrete parotid gland is felt, we usually look for some pathologic change.

The submandibular gland lies along the floor of the mouth below the mucous membrane. The digastric muscle bounds the gland inferiorly, and it lies deep to the superficial layer of the deep cervical fascia. Anteriorly, the submandibular gland extends under the mylohyoid muscle, and just deep to it the lingual and hypoglossal nerves are found. The facial artery pene-

trates the submandibular gland inferiorly near the digastric muscle, and as the artery exits, it traverses over the mandible. The gland extends posteriorly approximately 2 cm. anterior to the angle of the mandible.

The sublingual gland is the smallest of the three major salivary glands. It is located along the floor of the mouth anteriorly and lies on the genioglossus muscle. Posteriorly, the sublingual gland abuts the deep anterior projection of the submandibular gland. It empties into the mouth by multiple small ducts.

There are several hundred minor salivary glands located on the soft palate, hard palate, buccal mucosa, base of tongue, and epiglottis. These glands empty independently.

Physiology

The primary function of the salivary glands is to generate an adequate volume of saliva, which serves to maintain oral and dental hygiene, to prepare food for mastication, to augment taste sensation and deglutition, and to initiate the preliminary phase of carbohydrate digestion.

The parotid gland is primarily a serous gland, the submandibular gland is primarily serous- and mucous-secreting, and the sublingual and minor salivary glands are primarily mucus-secreting.

Examination

Instruments used in examination of the salivary ducts include a head light, tongue blade, finger cot, and, on occasion, a culture tube (Fig. 39–23). The dilators shown in this illustration can be used to dilate the salivary ducts for cannulation.

The examination should include the inspection of salivary secretions, which normally are clear. Cloudiness of secretions may be due to stasis or infection. If the cloudy secretion appears milky or yellow, it is most likely purulent. Cultures can be obtained by placing a dry sponge in the mouth for absorption, gently massaging the offending gland so that only one drop of purulent secretion is released, and then gently touching this droplet with a culture swab.

An analysis of salivary secretions can be obtained on special occasions, but routine

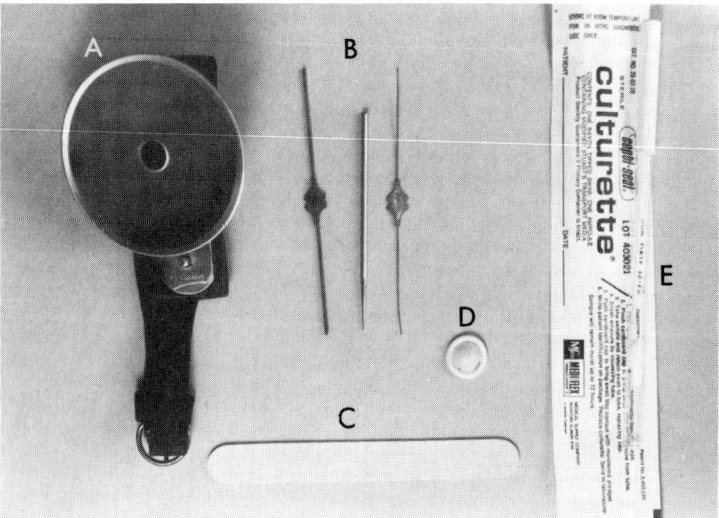

Figure 39-23. *Salivary gland instruments. A, head mirror; B, lacrimal dilators for submandibular duct; C, tongue blade; D, finger cot; and E, culture tube for salivary secretions.*

tests available include plain films of the mandible, sialography, and salivary gland scanning.

Approximately 50 per cent of salivary gland calculi can be seen on plain films and can usually be related to the submandibular gland. It should be cautioned that as only 50 per cent of these calculi are identified on plain films, sialography may be necessary. A sialogram is performed by cannulating the duct of the gland to be studied and injecting a radiopaque dye (iodinated compound) into the gland. Films are taken while the ducts are filled with the dye, in the posteranterior (PA) and lateral positions and after a few minutes to allow egress of the iodinated compound, the x-rays are repeated. The sialogram should appear very much like an oak tree in winter with the ducts becoming smaller in the periphery of the gland. Filling defects can be noted and are indicative of a mass within the gland itself. Stones can be identified by an area of nonfilling. Dilatation and strictures of the ducts can also be seen. Small and large cavities are indicative of infectious processes and can be identified by comparing diagnostic films with normal gland radiograms.

Scanning is performed with technetium-99m approximately 30 minutes after a dose of 0.8 to 1.0 mg. of atropine has been given. Scanning can be used to identify Warthin's tumor and oncocytomas, as these lesions will show areas of increased radioactive uptake. This procedure may also identify areas of occult metastases and may confrm the presence and extent of a neoplasm that has been palpated on physical examination. Care must be taken to compare the normal with the abnormal side, as these scans are sometimes difficult to interpret.

Congenital Disorders

Benign Congenital Hemangiomas. Such growths are the most common cause of parotid swelling in the newborn. It is estimated that most of these lesions will regress in the first 5 years of life, and surgery should therefore be deferred until the child is 5 years of age.

First Branchial Cleft Anomalies. These anomalies may be associated with the parotid glands and may present as an abscess in the neck or as a spontaneously occurring sinus tract. The tract may extend to the external auditory canal.

Treatment for first branchial cleft anomalies is surgical excision, including facial nerve dissection and partial parotidectomy.

Trauma

Because of their protected position, the salivary glands are rarely injured as a result of trauma. An exception to this is a stab wound of the face that transects the parotid duct. This condition is usually recognized early, as there is a concomitant paralysis of the buccal branch of the facial nerve that runs along the parotid duct. However, if the condition is unrecognized, a salivary fistula may develop to the skin or into the mouth. Should the salivary fistula develop into the mouth, further treatment may not be necessary. If the salivary fistula develops to the skin, surgical exploration of the duct is necessary. Cannulation of the duct orally at the time of surgery will locate its cut end and will provide access for the placement of a stent into the duct.

Infectious Disorders

Acute Epidemic Parotitis (Mumps). Mumps is caused by a viral infection and occurs in epidemics. The incubation period is 2 to 3 weeks. Stiffness of the neck and pain in the region of the parotid gland are the first symptoms noted. The degree of malaise varies, but the patient usually suffers a great deal of discomfort. One or both glands may be affected. Secretions in acute parotitis are usually scanty and are sometimes slightly cloudy. If there is suspicion of acute suppurative parotitis, a culture should be taken. Treatment is symptomatic.

Acute Suppurative Parotitis. This disorder occurs generally in elderly hospitalized patients who have a serious primary disease associated with dehydration or oral hygiene deterioration. At the onset, there is acute, painful, and diffuse swelling of one gland and purulent material may be expressed from the parotid duct for culture. Treatment involves the administration of an antibiotic that is effective against penicillinase-producing staphylococci. Most patients will recover following appropriate antibiotic therapy and rehydration.

Patients who do not respond to medical treatment should be considered for an incision and drainage that is done through a modified parotid flap and multiple blunt openings into the parotid.

Chronic Recurrent Sialadenitis. This infection is characterized by a recurrent diffuse or localized salivary gland swelling associated with pain and tenderness. Systemic signs of sepsis are minimal. Pus can be extracted from the duct, and the sialogram shows a normal ductal system. Treatment is conservative and symptomatic.

Chronic Sialectasis. Sialectasis may be compared with a chronic process such as bronchiectasis and is thought to be the end result of chronic recurrent sialadenitis. This disease process usually involves a parotid gland, and partial or total parotidectomy may be indicated.

Iatrogenic Disorders

Stricture of the parotid or submandibular duct can be secondary to previous surgery in this area, but its most common occurrence is secondary to trauma, infection, or neoplasm. Simple dilatation of the duct is usually effective.

Idiopathic Disorders

Benign Lymphoepithelial Sialadenopathy. This disorder, formerly referred to as Mikulicz's disease, has an unknown cause. The most plausible theory of its cause at the present time is that of an autoimmune mechanism similar to that of Hashimoto's thyroiditis. Benign lymphoepithelial sialadenopathy is characterized by symmetric enlargement of the lacrimal and salivary glands that is usually progressive but may be subject to regression. Considerable deformity may be caused by the disease, which is often associated with keratoconjunctivitis sicca and rheumatoid arthritis.

The history is the key to making this diagnosis, and sialography reveals the typical appearance of nonobstructive sialectasis with dilatation of the interlobular ducts and delayed emptying of contrast material.

Treatment is directed toward increasing salivary flow and preventing inspissation of secretions. Daily massage of the salivary glands, increased intake of oral fluids, and use of sialagogues are helpful in maintaining salivary flow and in providing mechanical cleaning of the ductal system.

Salivary Calculi. Approximately 90 per cent of salivary calculi occur in the submandibular gland. These calculi consist of an inorganic crystalline body in an organic matrix with a laminar structure. The cause is not known. Salivary stones can be diagnosed by bimanual palpation and confirmed by sialography. Submandibular stones can often be removed by incision of the duct in the mouth. Occasionally, resection of the offending gland is indicated because of obstruction and repeated infection.

Neoplasms

Neoplasms of the salivary glands are usually benign and include benign mixed tumor, Warthin's tumor (papillary cystadenoma lymphomatosum), acidophilic cell adenoma (oncocytoma), serous cell adenoma (acinic cell adenoma), lymphangioma, hemangioma, lipoma, and neuroma. Malignant tumors include squamous cell carcinoma, adenocarcinoma, acidophilic cell adenocarcinoma, mucoepidermoid carcinoma, and malignant mixed tumor.

In many instances, the differentiation of malignant from benign tumors of the salivary glands is done only by histologic examination. Each tumor of the salivary gland must be approached as a malignancy. Each tumor should be studied by sialography, scanning, and a thorough physical evaluation to determine the possible presence of metastatic disease either to or from the parotid gland.

Tumors are removed by an en bloc dissection.

Drug-Induced Disorders

Chronic intake of heavy metals may lead to parotid hypertrophy, the cause of which is determined by exclusion of underlying processes.

NECK

Embryology and Anatomy

The neck of the adult is composed of a small portion of the first branchial arch and the second, third, fourth, and sixth branchial arches. Innervation is by the fifth cranial nerve for the first arch, the seventh cranial nerve for the second arch, the ninth cranial nerve for the third arch, the tenth cranial nerve for the fourth arch, and the recurrent laryngeal branch of the tenth cranial nerve for the sixth arch.

The neck is divided artificially for anatomic description into the anterior and posterior cervical triangles, the digastric triangle, and the submental triangle. The structures that can be examined in this area are easily defined as the trapezius muscle posteriorly, the sternocleidomastoid muscle anteriorly, and the clavicle inferiorly, forming the posterior cervical triangle. The sternocleidomastoid muscle is the posterior boundary of the anterior cervical triangle, and the midline is the medial boundary. The upper boundary is the digastric muscle. The digastric triangle is outlined by the mandible, and the two bellies of the digastric muscle are attached to the hyoid. The submental triangle is that area overlying the mylohyoid muscle.

Examination

No special equipment other than good illumination is needed to examine the neck. Visualization and palpation of the structures of the neck in a routine manner are important, with particular emphasis on palpation of masses or lymph nodes.

Congenital Disorders

Lateral Cysts of the Neck. These cysts represent the embryonic cervical sinus and persistent embryonic cysts of the neck. These are caused by persistence of the embryonic endodermal pouches and the ectodermal branchial clefts. The connections may be with the second pouch, which opens into the tonsillar fossa, or with the third pouch, which opens into the pyriform fossa. Theoretic connections for the fourth and sixth pouches have been described but have not been seen. Diagnosis is made by physical examination and, if the sinus tract is present, by injection of contrast material into the sinus tract.

Treatment is by surgical excision.

Thyroglossal Duct Cyst. This cyst presents as a midline swelling at any level from the hyoid to the area of the cricoid. Occasionally, a sinus is present, particularly after an infection. Examination will show a cystic structure in the midline or occasionally a sinus tract. If the sinus tract persists, a contrast radiographic study may be performed. A thyroid scan is essential, as there may be no other functioning thyroid tissue. Treatment is by surgical excision.

Cystic Hygroma. Cystic hygroma is a congenital defect. It is thought to be derived from lymphatics that have no efferent connections and therefore contains lymph that cannot drain. These tumor masses present as soft, fluctuant swellings and when enlarged can easily be transilluminated. With marked enlargement, there can be airway embarrassment.

Surgery is indicated, but the surgery is

quite tedious. Treatment with radiation therapy is not indicated.

Infectious Disorders

Deep Neck Abscesses. Such abscesses may occur with breakdown of infected lymph nodes in the jugular chain and present as a mass at the anterior border of the sternocleidomastoid muscle in its upper portion. These abscesses usually present with acute tonsillitis or dental infection and may be life-threatening because of the danger of thrombosis of the internal jugular vein or rupture of the internal carotid artery. The patient usually presents with pain and stiffness of the neck. Fever is variable but is often elevated to 39° C. (102.2° F.).

Treatment consists of administering systemic antibiotics to a hospitalized patient. Penicillin is the antibiotic of choice. If fluctuation is apparent or develops subsequently, surgical incision should be performed. If fluctuation is present at the initial examination, it is recommended that high doses of antibiotics should be given for 12 to 24 hours in an effort to decrease the fever and thereby reduce the anesthetic mortality. An incision is made along the anterior border of the sternocleidomastoid muscle, and by using blunt dissection, the carotid sheath is entered. Once the purulent material has been emptied, a small drain is placed in the depth of the abscess cavity, and the skin is loosely approximated.

Idiopathic Disorders

Torticollis (Wry Neck). Torticollis results from fibrosis of the sternocleidomastoid muscle on the affected side. The cause is unknown. Treatment consists of exercise to lengthen the affected side. If exercise is not successful, surgical transection of the sternocleidomastoid muscle may be performed.

Neoplasms

All neck masses should be considered metastatic disease, and a thorough search of the scalp, ears, nose, throat, mouth, pharynx, and larynx for the primary lesion should be performed. A primary tumor in the cervical esophagus should also be considered. Prior to biopsy of a neck mass, the patient should have a thorough physical examination, lateral neck x-ray study, barium swallow, direct laryngoscopy, bronchoscopy, esophagoscopy, and examination of the nasopharynx under general anesthesia. If the neck mass is near the thyroid, a thyroid scan should be performed.

Except for supraclavicular metastases, thyroid neoplasms, and lymphomas, these examinations should identify the primary tumor. If no primary lesion can be found, a direct biopsy is in order.

FACIAL SKELETON

The examination of the facial skeleton after trauma deserves special mention because once the concept of facial fracture is understood, the examination can be performed in less than 5 minutes, and persons suffering massive trauma will not have fractures of the face overlooked.

Fractures of the Malar Complex. Such fractures must, by necessity, break four separate areas for movement of the malar bone.

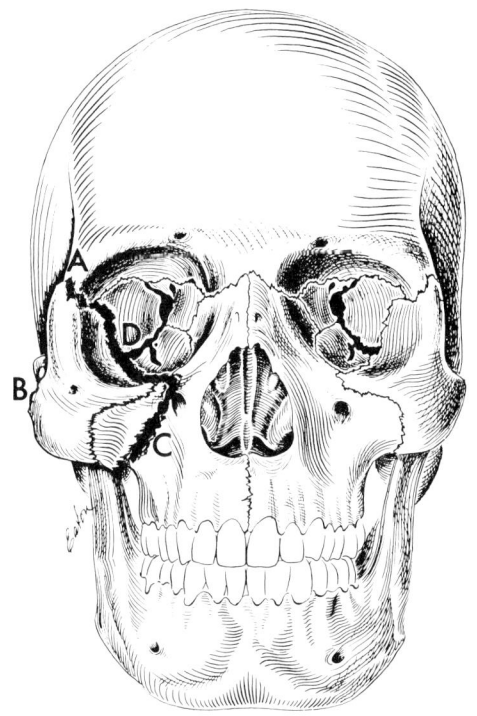

Figure 39–24. *The zygomatic compound fracture. Illustrates the four fracture sites to be palpated. A, frontozygomatic suture; B, arch of zygome; C, face of maxilla; and D, infraorbital rim. (From Hofman, W. E.: Otolaryngol. Clin. North Am., 2:313, 1969.)*

These areas are the frontozygomatic suture, the zygomatic arch, the infraorbital rim, and the face of the maxilla (Fig. 39–24).

Additional inspection should include looking at the patient from the top of the head to see if one malar eminence is more prominent than the other. Typically, the malar eminence on the fractured side is depressed. Palpation of the zygomatic arch is from above and may detect a depression or actual fracture of the zygomatic arch. Palpation of the frontozygomatic sutures will usually *not* reveal the fracture, but if the patient is able to respond, this may elicit tenderness on the affected side. Palpation of the infraorbital rim fracture will reveal a step fracture, and both rims should be palpated by placing the fingertips just inside the orbit and moving them along the rim. It is important that bilateral palpation be done, as there is normally a small notch in the rim.

Infraorbital nerve anesthesia and diplopia on upward gaze are two other physical signs that may be positive. Fractures of the infraorbital rim must extend through the floor of the orbit, and the infraorbital nerve is often trapped or severed. A finding of infraorbital anesthesia is common and should be tested for routinely. Diplopia on upward gaze results from entrapment of the inferior rectus muscle, and occasionally diplopia on lateral gaze may be present because of entrapment of the medial rectus muscle. Palpation of the anterior face of the maxilla may reveal comminution of the anterior maxillary face.

Blowout Fractures. A blowout fracture of the orbit is detected by the presence of infraorbital nerve anesthesia, entrapment, and diplopia on upward gaze. If these physical signs are found without other evidence of fracture, a "true blowout fracture" has been identified (Fig. 39–25).

Mandibular Fractures. If there is suspicion of a fracture of the mandible, the occlusion of the teeth should be visualized by placing a tongue blade lateral to the teeth on each side to hold the cheeks away from the teeth and asking the patient to bite down. The mandible should be palpated for fracture and radiographs taken. The finding of a loose tooth, poor occlusion, pain on biting, or a fracture line confirms the diagnosis of a fractured mandible. Unlike fractures of the malar eminence or blowout fractures, a

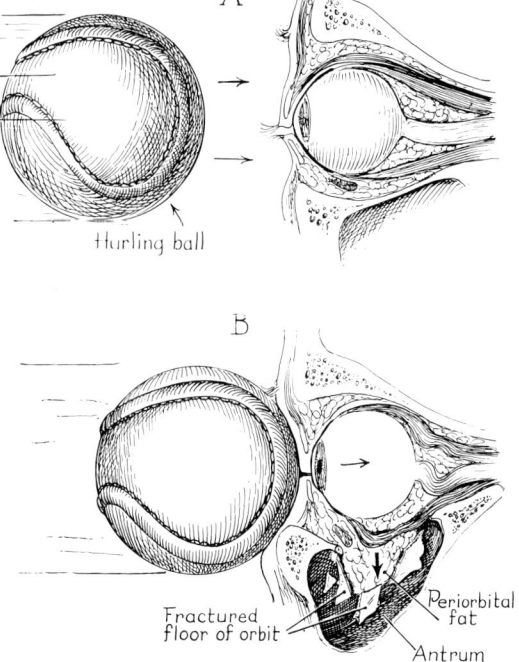

Figure 39–25. *External pressure forcing a blowout fracture of the orbital floor with incarceration of the inferior rectus muscle.* (From *Smith, B., and Regan, W. F., Jr.: Am. J. Ophthalmol., 44:733, 1957.*)

diagnosis of mandibular fracture may be missed on physical examination, as approximately one-third of these fractures occur on the ascending ramus and condyle (Fig. 39–26). These fractures cannot be identified by physical examination, and diagnosis is made by radiographs.

Maxillary Fractures. LeFort fractures are identified by grasping the upper teeth and checking for movement. Figure 39–27 shows the three classic LeFort fractures. For purposes of identification, the LeFort I fracture may be called the false teeth sign, the LeFort II fracture may be called the false nose sign, and the LeFort III fracture the false teeth sign. If by grasping the upper teeth abnormal mobility of the face can be produced, it is important to identify which portion of the face moves.

Table 39–1 outlines the major physical signs found in diagnosing facial trauma. Radiographic confirmation of the facial fractures is mandatory. Radiographs of the cervical spine should be done routinely to rule out cervical spine fracture of subluxation of the cervical spine.

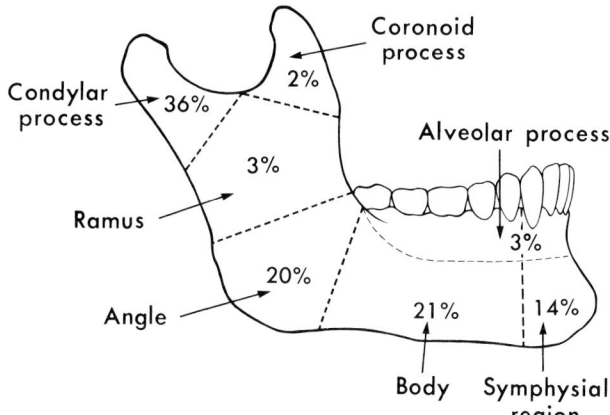

Figure 39-26. *Classification of fractures of the mandible, showing respective incidence. (From Dingman, R. O., and Natvig, P.: Surgery of Facial Fractures. Philadelphia, W. B. Saunders Co., 1964, p. 144.)*

Treatment of these fractures is surgical. Although many patients will present with other trauma that will require immediate attention, careful examination to detect facial fractures must not be neglected. Repair of a facial fracture that has been delayed more than 2 weeks will be a difficult surgical procedure and may result in a cosmetic defect.

AERODIGESTIVE TRACT

Embryology and Anatomy

The esophagus is developed from the primitive foregut. The tracheobronchial tree becomes evident in the embryo approximately 26 days after conception at the time of ventral invagination of the mucosa,

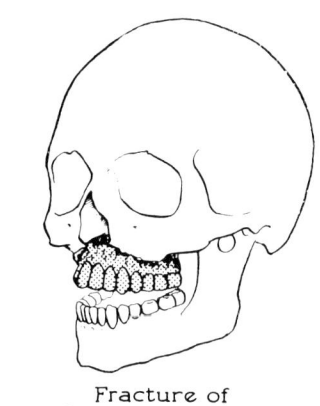

A Fracture of Palatal Segment

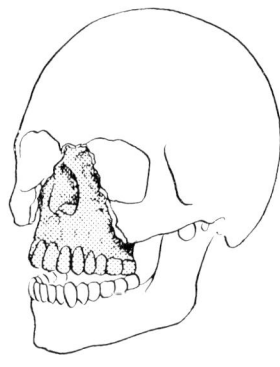

B Fracture of Maxillary Complex

Figure 39-27. *A, The Lefort I or Guérin fracture; B, the LeFort II (pyramidal) fracture; and C, the Le-Fort III fracture, complete craniofacial separation. (From McGregor, J.: Fundamental Techniques of Plastic Surgery. 3rd Ed. Baltimore, The Williams & Wilkins Co., 1965, p. 283.)*

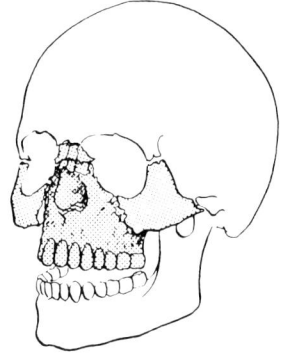

C Middle ⅓ Fracture *(maxillary complex, nose and both malars)*

TABLE 39-1.   MAJOR PHYSICAL FINDINGS IN FACIAL FRACTURES

	Zygomatic Fractures	LeFort Fractures	Blowout Fractures	Zygomatic Arch Fractures
Frontozygomatic suture tenderness or separation	+	+ for LeFort III	−	−
Fracture of infraorbital rim	+	+ for LeFort II	−	−
Fracture of zygomatic arch	+	+ for LeFort III	−	+
Diplopia on upward gaze	+ or −	May be + for LeFort II and III	+	−
Depression of globe	usually +	+ for LeFort II and III	+	−
Infraorbital nerve anesthesia	+ or −	+ or −	+	−
Fracture of anterior face of maxilla (canine fossa area)	+	+ for LeFort I and II	−	−
Pain on opening mouth	+ or −	+ or −	−	+
Maxillary teeth move as separate unit on traction	−	+	−	−
Malocclusion	−	+	−	−

so that a separate tube for respiration is developed. Early in the fifth week of embryonic life, the endodermal lung bud has already developed two branchial buds. Also during the fifth week, each primary bronchus gives rise to two new bronchial buds. These bronchial buds develop into the secondary bronchi. The tertiary (segmental) bronchi (10 in the right lung and 8 or 9 in the left) begin to appear in the seventh week of life.

The esophagus is a muscular tube that extends from the cricoid cartilage to the fundus of the stomach. There are two esophageal sphincters, the cricopharyngeus at the upper end and the cardia at the lower end. The muscles of the upper esophagus are striated, and those of the lower esophagus are smooth. There are two indentations in the esophagus caused by the left main bronchus and the left atrium.

The tracheobronchial tree develops 14 to 21 tracheal cartilages associated with smooth muscle and connective tissue. Transformation of the lung from a glandular structure to a highly vascular alveolar structure is completed by 28 weeks. At birth, the number of alveoli is approximately 24,000,000 and by 8 years approximately 300,000,000.

Examination

Although physical examination of the aerodigestive tract is difficult in the office, the history is the key to the underlying pathology. The use of a stethoscope is helpful in otolaryngologic diagnosis. Cineradiographic techniques, still films using contrast material, esophagoscopy, and esophageal manometrics are the appropriate diagnostic procedures for evaluating the esophagus.

Cineradiographic studies are particularly important when evaluating the action of the entire swallowing mechanism as well as the esophagus. Review of the cineradiographs with the radiologist and comparison with previous films are important. Still films can provide evidence of stricture, foreign body, hiatal hernia, and esophageal reflux.

Esophagoscopy is employed whenever it is necessary to visualize the esophagus for purposes of biopsy, removal of a foreign body, or dilatation of a stricture under direct vision.

Manometry of the esophagus is particularly important in evaluating those patients who suffer from difficulty in swallowing but who show no lesion on radiographic examination.

Examination of the tracheobronchial tree is done by thorough auscultation of the chest, with PA and lateral neck films and chest x-ray as the minimum radiographic studies. Cytologic examination of sputum, cultures for acid-fast bacteria and fungi, contrast radiography, and bronchoscopy are auxiliary studies. Auscultation of the chest may provide clues to underlying diseases.

PA and lateral radiographs of the chest during inspiration and expiration provide numerous diagnostic possibilities and should be performed routinely.

Cytologic examination of sputum is now being recognized as a possible screening test for early carcinoma of the lung and when properly performed provides valuable diagnostic assistance.

Cultures for acid-fast bacteria and fungi should be routine when diagnosing the cause of purulent secretions or hemoptysis.

Contrast radiography, tracheograms, and bronchograms are most helpful for evaluation of solid and cavitary lesions.

Bronchoscopy may be used for diagnostic purposes and is useful in obtaining uncontaminated specimens for cytologic examination and for acid-fast bacteria, fungi, and routine bacterial cultures. Biopsies of neoplasms may be performed and foreign bodies retrieved. Bronchoscopy may also be used for evaluation of the airway below the larynx.

Congenital Disorders

Tracheoesophageal Fistula. The incidence of tracheoesophageal fistula has been estimated to be approximately 1 in 100,000 live births. Symptoms associated with this abnormality are usually present at birth, but the correct diagnosis is often delayed. Coughing or choking when swallowing, especially when swallowing liquids, is the most common complaint. Cyanosis is the next most frequently occurring complaint. Children with this abnormality universally have abdominal distention that is more marked after crying.

Diagnosis is made by cine-esophagogram, visualization of the trachea by the bronchoscope, and instillation of colored dye into the trachea during the esophagoscopy.

Treatment is surgical, and the technique varies, depending on the type and severity of the disorder. Esophageal atresia may occur along with symptoms of tracheoesophageal fistula presenting during the first few hours of life. The most common tracheoesophageal atresia is associated with a distal tracheoesophageal fistula. Procedures for the diagnosis of esophageal atresia are the same as those for tracheoesophageal fistula.

Gastroesophageal Reflux. An infant with typical gastroesophageal reflux vomits when fed from birth, and the majority of these patients are not diagnosed until complications occur. They may be admitted to the hospital with aspiration pneumonitis and failure to thrive. Diagnosis is by cineradiography and esophagoscopy. Manometric studies may be helpful.

Achalasia. Achalasia is a disease of unknown cause characterized by failure of relaxation of the inferior esophageal sphincter. This disorder is associated with megaesophagus. The most common symptom is dysphagia. On x-ray examination, there is a lack of peristalsis and an enlarged esophagus.

Treatment by dilatation may be helpful, but an esophagomyotomy is the operation of choice.

Congenital Esophageal Stenosis. This is an unusual occurrence. Stenosis may present at an early age but is often not manifested until solid foods are added to the infant's diet.

X-ray studies show narrowing of the middle one-third of the esophagus, and treatment consists of dilatation when possible. If dilatation is unsuccessful, esophageal resection may be necessary.

Duplication of the Esophagus and Esophageal Diverticulum. Both of these anomalies are extremely rare.

Primary Tracheomalacia. This disorder is characterized by stridor that is associated with periods of effort, such as crying, exercise, or overcoming pulmonary infection.

Diagnosis is made by laryngoscopy and bronchoscopy when collapse of the airway is noted on inspiration. Fortunately, the obstruction is usually self-limiting, and treatment consists of supportive care and control of recurrent infections.

Congenital and Acquired Tracheal Stenosis. The majority of these cases occur secondary to tracheal intubation but congenital forms include fibrous webs and deformed tracheal cartilage (which may be associated with vascular rings).

Diagnosis is made by the observation of webs and vascular rings during bronchoscopy. In patients with tracheomalacia, the bronchoscopist will see a normal trachea, and the diagnosis will be made by exclusion.

Bronchogenic Cysts. Bronchogenic cysts appear to result from abnormal budding of the fetal tracheal tree. They are usually single but may be multiple or lobulated.

The symptoms depend on the size and location of the cyst.

Diagnosis may be exceedingly difficult, as chest x-ray examinations often fail to show the cyst. Bronchoscopy may not reveal the cyst either, and contrast studies of the trachea and esophagus may be necessary. Diagnosis of bronchogenic cysts has been made on an autopsy table more often than in the operating room. Treatment, once the diagnosis is made, is surgical excision.

Infantile Lobar Emphysema. This disorder may result from bronchial obstruction or from a primary alveolar lesion. In approximately 50 per cent of the patients, no cause is found. As the lobe distends, the other lobes on the same side are compressed. Respiratory distress is the most common finding during the first few days of life. Dyspnea and cyanosis are also common. Cough and wheezing may be present.

The treatment is surgical resection of the affected lobe, as conservative measures are useless.

Vascular Rings. Vascular rings are anomalies of the greater arteries and may be the cause of respiratory difficulties. The anomalies include double aortic arch, right-sided aortic arch, aberrant left pulmonary artery, and aberrant subclavian artery.

The typical history is that of wheezing, recurrent infections, dyspnea, tachypnea, and cyanosis. Some patients may be asymptomatic. Diagnosis is made by cinecontrast radiography and by bronchoscopy. Treatment depends on the severity of the symptoms and is surgical.

Agenesis. Agenesis of a lung segment or of one lung results from an abnormality of the growth and development of the lung bud and may be entirely asymptomatic.

Differential diagnosis includes atelectasis, pneumonia, hydro- or chylothorax on the ipsilateral side, or a lobar emphysema on the contralateral side. Diagnosis is made by chest x-ray examination and bronchoscopy.

Other congenital anomalies may be identified on thorough work-up by chest x-ray studies, cineradiography of the esophagus, tracheobronchogram, bronchoscopy, and esophagoscopy. Suspicion should be aroused if the patient has repeated upper respiratory infections or if there is a failure to thrive. Many of these congenital anomalies are not found until autopsy.

Hereditary Disorders

Hereditary anomalies compatible with life are extremely rare.

Infectious Disorders

Acute subglottic edema is thought to be caused by an allergic phenomenon and is diagnosed at the time of endoscopy while preparing the patient for a tracheostomy.

Other respiratory infections include tracheobronchitis of varying degrees of severity and, of course, pneumonitis.

Except for moniliasis, which affects the mouth, pharynx, trachea, and esophagus, there are few esophageal infections.

Iatrogenic Disorders

Stenosis. *Subglottic stenosis* was discussed in the section on the larynx and hypopharynx. Subglottic stenosis at the present time is usually associated with an indwelling tracheal tube and assisted ventilation. Occasionally, subglottic stenosis still results from tracheostomy. *Tracheal stenosis* is also associated with tracheostomy and trauma. Diagnosis is usually made at the time of extubation, with stridor beginning immediately afterward to 48 hours later. Polytomograms of the larynx and contrast studies of the larynx and trachea will be of assistance in determining the severity, degree, and length of stenosis.

Esophageal Perforation. Perforation of the esophagus has been estimated to occur in approximately 1 in every 200 patients undergoing esophagoscopy and most commonly occurs in the cervical esophagus. Distal esophageal perforations usually occur when there is an esophageal stricture in the area of the cardia. The lower esophageal perforations have a high mortality and can be diagnosed by the early elevation of temperature and the presence of air in the mediastinum, as shown on a chest x-ray film.

Idiopathic Disorders

Foreign Bodies. Patients with foreign bodies of the esophagus and bronchi usually present as emergencies and give a history of the foreign body ingestion. However, unsuspected foreign bodies in the lung may lead to recurrent pneumonia without a foreign body's being diagnosed.

Patients with tracheal and bronchial foreign bodies usually present with a history of aspiration of a foreign body with immediate choking and coughing. A quiet period follows this that may lull the physician into complacency. Thorough auscultation of the chest will detect wheezing when there is an incomplete obstruction or a quiet area of the lung when the obstruction is complete on expiration but incomplete on inspiration. This latter type of obstruction will produce an emphysematous segment or lobe that may be the only clue to the foreign body. Inspiratory and expiratory chest x-ray studies are mandatory. Once the foreign body is suspected hospitalization for bronchoscopy should be routine. Prior to hospitalization, lateral neck films should be obtained for each patient.

Patients with foreign bodies of the esophagus usually present with drooling, and if the patient is old enough, a description of localized pain can be obtained. Lateral neck and chest x-ray studies should be obtained. If a diagnosis still cannot be made, a contrast study obtained by having the patient swallow a cotton ball soaked in barium will delineate the foreign body. In children, however, a foreign body of the esophagus often presents with drooling. The most likely position for a foreign body in children is in the esophagus.

At esophagoscopy, other underlying pathologic disorders should be ruled out, such as a stricture or tumor.

Corrosive Ingestion. Patients with corrosive ingestion should be admitted to the hospital. It must be emphasized that the only way to properly evaluate the extent of damage is by esophagoscopy. Reliance on the severity of oral and mucous membrane lesions is not satisfactory. There is some variation in treatment, but most physicians will hospitalize the patient and begin antibiotic therapy. Esophagoscopy is performed approximately 12 to 24 hours later to delineate the burns. Burns of the esophagus require intensive antibiotic and steroid treatment and close follow-up because of the possibility of a stricture developing later.

Dysfunctions of the Esophagus. Such disorders often require extensive work-up that includes a cineradiographic study, motility studies, and esophagoscopy. Diagnoses such as achalasia and diffuse spasm may be considered. However, metabolic diseases such as scleroderma should be kept in mind, as the presenting complaint in these disorders may be dysfunction of the esophagus. For an in-depth discussion of dysfunction of the esophagus, Andersen's article "Dysfunction of the Esophagus" (listed in the references at the end of this chapter) is recommended.

Neoplasms

Bronchogenic Carcinoma. This tumor is usually diagnosed at a fairly late stage because x-ray changes are not seen in the early stages. However, the new technique of fiberoptic bronchoscopy may lead to an earlier diagnosis and a delineation of segmental involvement. Washings should be taken at each bronchoscopy for cytologic examination. When a lesion is seen, biopsy should be taken for histologic examination.

Metastatic Carcinomas to the Lung. Such lesions will often be negative on cytologic examination. Primary squamous cell carcinomas of the lung will, however, be approximately 80 per cent positive on such examination.

Neoplasms of the Esophagus. Such lesions are often suspected because of abnormalities of the barium swallow or cine-esophagogram. Esophagoscopy will usually reveal the neoplasm by direct visualization or a biopsy will be positive. Patients with esophageal carcinomas have a poor 5 year survival despite treatment, except for those with lesions at the cardia, which may be resected and treated postoperatively with radiation therapy.

REFERENCES

EAR

Embryology:
Anson, B. J.: Developmental anatomy of the ear. *In* Paparella, M. M., and Shumrick, D. A. (eds.): Otolaryngology. Vol. 1, Basic Sciences and Related Disciplines. Philadelphia, W. B. Saunders Co., 1973, pp. 3–74.
Anson, B. J., and Bast, T. H.: Developmental anatomy of the ear. *In* Shambaugh, G. E. (ed.): Surgery of the

Ear. 2nd Ed. Philadelphia, W. B. Saunders Co., 1967, pp. 5–36.

Bast, T. H., and Anson, B. J.: The Temporal Bone and the Ear. Springfield, Ill., Charles C Thomas, Publisher, 1949.

Anatomy:

Donaldson, J. A., and Miller, J. F.: Anatomy of the ear, *In* Paparella, M. M., and Shumrick, D. A. (eds.): Otolaryngology. Vol. 1, Basic Sciences and Related Disciplines. Philadelphia, W. B. Saunders Co., 1973, pp. 75–110.

Physiology:

Cawthorne, T., Dix, W. R., Hallpike, C. S., et al.: The investigation of vestibular function. Br. Med. Bull., *12*:131, 1956.

Kirikae, I.: Physiology of the middle ear including eustachian tube. *In* Paparella, M. M., and Shumrick, D. A. (eds.): Otolaryngology. Vol. 1, Basic Sciences and Related Disciplines. Philadelphia, W. B. Saunders Co., 1973, pp. 261–274.

Lawrence, M.: Inner ear physiology. *In* Paparella, M. M., and Shumrick, D. A. (eds.): Otolaryngology. Vol. 1, Basic Sciences and Related Disciplines. Philadelphia, W. B. Saunders Co., 1973, pp. 275–298.

McCabe, B. F.: Vestibular physiology: its clinical application in understanding the dizzy patient. *In* Paparella, M. M., and Shumrick, D. A. (eds.): Otolaryngology. Vol. 1, Basic Sciences and Related Disciplines. Philadelphia, W. B. Saunders Co., 1973, pp. 318–328.

Rasmussen, G. L., and Windle, W. F.: Neural Mechanisms of the Auditory and Vestibular Systems. Springfield, Ill., Charles C Thomas, Publisher, 1960.

Shambaugh, G. E.: Mechanics of hearing. *In* Shambaugh, G. E. (eds.): Surgery of the Ear. 2nd Ed. Philadelphia, W. B. Saunders Co., 1967, pp. 369–400.

Congenital:

Alford, B. R.: Rubella La Bête Noire de la médecine. Laryngoscope, 78:1623, 1968.

Anthony, W. P.: Congenital and acquired atresia of the external auditory canal. Arch. Otolaryngol., 65:478, 1957.

Bergstrom, L., et al.: A high risk registry to find congenital deafness. Otolaryngol. Clin. North Am., 4(June):369–399, 1971.

Bergstrom, L.: Lop Ear. *In* Bergsma, D. (ed.): Birth Defects Atlas and Compendium. Baltimore, The Williams & Wilkins Co., 1973, p. 584.

Bergstrom, L.: "Macrotia." *In* Bergsma, D. (ed.): Birth Defects Atlas and Compendium. Baltimore, The Williams & Wilkins Co., 1973, p. 592.

Downs, M. P.: The identification of congenital deafness. Trans. Am. Acad. Ophthalmol. Otolaryngol., 74:1208, 1970.

Fraser, G. R.: Profound childhood deafness. J. Med. Genet., *1*:118, 1964.

Lindsay, J. R.: Histopathology of deafness due to postnatal viral disease. Arch. Otolaryngol., 98:258, 1973.

Proctor, B., and Proctor, C. A.: Congenital lesions of the head and neck. Otolaryngol. Clin. North Am., 3(June):221–248, 1970.

Hereditary:

Pearson, R. D., Kurland, L. T., and Cody, D. T.: Incidence of diagnosed clinical otosclerosis. Arch. Otolaryngol., 99:288, 1974.

Proctor, C. A., and Proctor, B.: Understanding hereditary nerve deafness. Arch. Otolaryngol., 85:23, 1967.

Soifer, N., Weaver, K., Endahl, G. L., et al.: Otosclerosis: a review. Acta Otolaryngol. (Suppl.), 269:1, 1970.

Infectious:

Alford, B. R.: Complications of suppurative otitis media and mastoiditis. *In* Paparella, M. M., and Shumrick, D. A. (eds.): Otolaryngology. Vol. 2, Ear. Philadelphia, W. B. Saunders Co., 1973, pp. 153–160.

Armstrong, B. W.: A new treatment for secretory otitis media. Arch. Otolaryngol., 59:653, 1954.

Brookler, K. H., et al.: Etiologic factors in non suppurative otitis media. Laryngoscope, 85:1882, 1975.

Dysart, B. R.: Otitis media and its complications. Arch. Otolaryngol., *80*:587, 1964.

Harbert, F., and Riordon, D.: Tuberculosis of the middle ear. Laryngoscope, 74:198, 1964.

Henneford, G., and Lindsay, J. R.: Deaf mutism due to meningogenic labyrinthitis. Laryngoscope, 78:251, 1968.

McLaurin, J. W.: Trauma and infections of the external ear. *In* Paparella, M. M., and Shumrick, D. A. (eds.): Otolaryngology. Vol. 2, Ear. Philadelphia, W. B. Saunders Co., 1973, pp. 24–32.

Iatrogenic:

Alonso, W. A., and Gill, A. J.: Pneumocephalus following mastoid surgery: a case report. Laryngoscope, 79:2150, 1969.

Shambaugh, G. E.: Facial nerve decompression and repair. *In* Shambaugh, G. E. (ed.): Surgery of the Ear. 2nd Ed. Philadelphia, W. B. Saunders Co., 1967, p. 585.

Shambaugh, G. E.: The simple mastoid operation. *In* Shambaugh, G. E. (ed.): Surgery of the Ear. 2nd Ed. Philadelphia, W. B. Saunders Co., 1967, pp. 262–263.

Idiopathic:

Eichel, B. S., and Landes, B. S.: Sensorineural hearing loss caused by skin diving. Arch. Otolaryngol. 92:128, 1970.

Glorig, A.: Tinnitus. *In* Paparella, M. M., and Shumrick, D. A. (eds.): Otolaryngology. Vol. 2, Ear. Philadelphia, W. B. Saunders Co., 1973, pp. 426–431.

Harker, L. A., and McCabe, B. E.: Meniere's disease and other peripheral labyrinthine disorders. *In* Paparella, M. M., and Shumrick, D. A. (eds.): Otolaryngology. Vol. 2, Ear. Philadelphia, W. B. Saunders Co., 1973, pp. 439–449.

Naunton, R. F.: Presbycusis. *In* Paparella, M. M., and Shumrick, D. A. (eds.): Otolaryngology. Vol. 2, Ear. Philadelphia, W. B. Saunders Co., 1973. pp. 368–376.

Shambaugh, G. E., Jr., and Clemis, J. D.: Facial nerve paralysis. *In* Paparella, M. M., and Shumrick, D. A. (eds.): Otolaryngology. Vol. 2, Ear. Philadelphia, W. B. Saunders Co., 1973, pp. 263–282.

Snow, J. B., Jr.: Sudden deafness. *In* Paparella, M. M., and Shumrick, D. A. (eds.): Otolaryngology. Vol. 2, Ear. Philadelphia, W. B. Saunders Co., 1973, pp. 357–365.

Symposium on Meniere's Disease. Pulec, J. L. (ed.). Otolaryngol. Clin. North Am., *1* (Oct.) 1968.

Neoplastic:

Mathog, R. H.: Otologic manifestations of retrocochlear disease. *In* Paparella, M. M., and Shumrick, D. A. (eds.): Otolaryngology. Vol. 2, Ear. Philadelphia, W. B. Saunders Co., 1973, pp. 450–468.

Paparella, M. M.: Cysts and tumors of the external ear. *In* Paparella, M. M., and Shumrick, D. A. (eds.): Otolaryngology. Vol. 2, Ear. Philadelphia, W. B. Saunders Co., 1973, pp. 36–43.

Rossenwasser, H.: Tumors of the middle ear and mastoid. *In* Paparella, M. M., and Shumrick, D. A.

(eds.): Otolaryngology. Vol. 2, Ear. Philadelphia, W. B. Saunders Co., 1973, pp. 185–204.

Drug-Induced:

Lowry, L. D., and Pastore, P.: Acute histopathologic inner ear changes in deafness due to neomycin: a case report. Ann. Otol. Rhinol. Laryngol., 82:876, 1973.

Meyers, F., and Bernstein, J.: Salicylate ototoxicity: a clinical and experimental study. Arch. Otolaryngol., 82:483, 1965.

Quick, C. A.: Chemical and drug effects on inner ear. *In* Paparella, M. M., and Shumrick, D. A. (eds.): Otolaryngology. Vol. 2, Ear. Philadelphia, W. B. Saunders Co., 1973, pp. 391–406.

NOSE AND PARANASAL SINUSES

Embryology and Anatomy:

Davies, J.: Embryology and anatomy of the face, palate, nose and paranasal sinuses. *In* Paparella, M. M., and Shumrick, D. A. (eds.): Otolaryngology. Vol. 1, Basic Sciences and Related Disciplines. Philadelphia, W. B. Saunders Co., 1973, pp. 150–178.

English, G. M.: Anomalies of the ear, nose, mouth and throat. *In* Maloney, W. H. (ed.): Otolaryngology. Vol. 2. Hagerstown, Md., Harper & Row, Publishers, 1973, Chapter 3, pp. 33–35.

Hollinshead, W. H.: The nose and paranasal sinuses. *In* Hollinshead, W. H. (ed.): Anatomy for Surgeons. Vol. 1, 2nd Ed. New York, Harper & Row, Publishers, 1968, pp. 253–282.

Physiology:

Abramson, M., and Harker, L. A.: Physiology of the nose. Otolaryngol. Clin. North Am., 6:623–636, 1973.

Williams, H. L.: Nasal physiology. *In* Paparella, M. M., and Shumrick, D. A. (eds.): Otolaryngology. Vol. 1, Basic Sciences and Related Disciplines. Philadelphia, W. B. Saunders Co., 1973, pp. 329–346.

Congenital:

Miller, D. R.: Anterior nasal atresia. *In* Bergsma, D. (ed.): Birth Defects Atlas and Compendium. Baltimore, The Williams & Wilkins Co., 1973, p. 177.

Miller, D. R., and Bergstrom, L.: Bifid nose. *In* Bergsma, D. (ed.): Birth Defects Atlas and Compendium. Baltimore, The Williams & Wilkins Co., 1973, pp. 207–208.

Singleton, G. T., and Hardcastle, B.: Congenital choanal atresia. Arch. Otolaryngol., 87:620, 1968.

Walter, C. D.: Congenital defects of the nose. *In* Paparella, M. M., and Shumrick, D. A. (eds.): Otolaryngology. Vol. 3, Head and Neck. Philadelphia, W. B. Saunders Co., 1973, pp. 3–26.

Hereditary:

Bryan, W. T. K., and Bryan, M. P.: Allergy in otolaryngology. *In* Paparella, M. M., and Shumrick, D. A. (eds.): Otolaryngology. Vol. 3, Head and Neck. Philadelphia, W. B. Saunders Co., 1973, pp. 69–74.

Trauma:

Beekhuis, J.: Nasal fractures. *In* Paparella, M. M., and Shumrick, D. A. (eds.): Otolaryngology. Vol. 3, Head and Neck. Philadelphia, W. B. Saunders Co., 1973, pp. 39–74.

Mallen, P. W.: Fractures of the nasofrontal complex. Otolaryngol. Clin. North Am., 2(June):335–361, 1969.

Infectious:

Chapnik, J. S., and Bach, M. C.: Bacterial and fungal infections of the maxillary sinus. Otolaryngol. Clin. North Am., 9(Feb.):43–54, 1976.

Montgomery, W.: Complications of sinus disease. *In* Ballenger, J. J. (ed.): Diseases of the Nose, Throat and Ear. 11th Ed. Philadelphia, Lea & Febiger, 1969, pp. 170–177.

Quick, C. A., and Payne, E.: Complicated acute sinusitis. Laryngoscope, 82:1248, 1972.

Williams, H. L.: Infections and granulomas of the nasal airways and paranasal sinuses. *In* Paparella, M. M., and Shumrick, D. A. (eds.): Otolaryngology. Vol. 3, Head and Neck. Philadelphia, W. B. Saunders Co., 1973, pp. 27–38.

Iatrogenic:

Cassisi, M. D., Biller, H. F., and Ogura, J. H.: Changes in arterial oxygen tension and pulmonary mechanics with the use of posterior packing in epistaxis. Laryngoscope, 79:969, 1969.

Herzon, F. S.: Bacteremia and local infections with nasal packing. Arch. Otolaryngol., 94:317, 1971.

Idiopathic:

Eichel, B. S., and Mabery, T. E.: The enigma of the lethal midline granuloma. Laryngoscope, 78:1367, 1968.

Fahey, J. L., et al.: Wegener's granulomatosis. Am. J. Med., 17:168–179, 1963.

Goodman, W. S., and DeSouza, F. M.: Atrophic rhinitis. Otolaryngol. Clin. North Am., 6(Oct.):773–782, 1973.

Saunders, W. H.: Epistaxis. *In* Paparella, M. M., and Shumrick, D. A. (eds.): Otolaryngology. Vol. 3, Head and Neck. Philadelphia, W. B. Saunders Co., 1973, pp. 39–47.

Taylor, M.: The nasal vasomotor reaction. Otolaryngol. Clin. North Am., 6(Oct.):645–654, 1973.

Neoplastic:

Bortnick, E.: Neoplasms of the nasal cavity. Otolaryngol. Clin. North Am., 6(Oct.):801–802, 1973.

Ogura, J. H., and Schenck, N. L.: Unusual nasal tumors, problems in diagnosis and treatment. Otolaryngol. Clin. North Am., 6(Oct.):813–837, 1973.

Patterson, C. N.: Juvenile nasopharyngeal angiofibromas. Otolaryngol. Clin. North Am., 6:839, 1973.

MOUTH AND OROPHARYNX

Embryology and Anatomy:

Davies, J.: Embryology and anatomy of the face, palate, nose and paranasal sinuses. *In* Paparella, M. M., and Shumrick, D. A. (ed.): Otolaryngology. Vol. 1, Basic Sciences and Related Disciplines. Philadelphia, W. B. Saunders Co., 1973, pp. 150–178.

Physiology:

Bosma, J. F.: Physiology of the mouth, pharynx and esophagus. *In* Paparella, M. M., and Shumrick, D. A. (eds.): Otolaryngology. Vol. 1, Basic Sciences and Related Disciplines. Philadelphia, W. B. Saunders Co., 1973, pp. 356–370.

Congenital:

Bernstein, L.: Congenital malformations of the oral cavity. *In* Paparella, M. M., and Shumrick, D. A. (eds.): Otolaryngology. Vol. 1, Basic Sciences and Related Disciplines. Philadelphia, W. B. Saunders Co., 1973, pp. 177–183.

English, G. M.: Anomalies of the ear, nose, mouth and throat. *In* Maloney, W. H. (ed.): Otolaryngology. Vol. 2. Hagerstown, Md., Harper & Row, Publishers, 1973, Chapter 3, pp. 49–62.

Trauma:

Fitz-Hugh, G. S., and Powell, J. B., II: Acute traumatic injuries of the oropharynx, laryngopharynx and cervical trachea in children. Otolaryngol. Clin. North Am., *3*(June):375–394, 1970.

Infectious:

Everts, E. C., and Echevarria, J.: The pharynx and deep neck infections. *In* Paparella, M. M., and Shumrick, D. A. (eds.): Otolaryngology. Vol. 3, Head and Neck. Philadelphia, W. B. Saunders Co., 1973, pp. 327–340.

Fernbach, D. J., and Starling, K. A.: Infectious mononucleosis. Pediatr. Clin. North Am., *19*(Nov.):957–968, 1972.

Levitt, G. W.: Surgical treatment of deep neck infections. Laryngoscope, *80*:409, 1970.

Paradise, J. L.: Why T and A remains moot. Pediatrics, *49*:648, 1972.

Idiopathic:

Johnson, R. L.: Ulcerative lesions of the oral cavity. Otolaryngol. Clin. North Am.,*5*(June):231–248, 1972.

Nash, H. S., Jr.: Benign lesions of the oral cavity. Otolaryngol. Clin. North Am., *5*(June):207–230, 1972.

Neoplastic:

DiTroia, J. F.: Nodal metastases and prognosis in carcinomas of the oral cavity. Otolaryngol. Clin. North Am., *5*(June):333–342, 1972.

Gates, G. A.: Minor salivary glands of the oral cavity. Otolaryngol. Clin. North Am., *5*(June):283–290, 1972.

Vaughan, C. W.: Carcinogenesis in the oral cavity. Otolaryngol. Clin. North Am., *5*(June):291–300, 1972.

NASOPHARYNX

Embryology and Anatomy:

Davies, J.: Embryology and anatomy of the face, palate, nose and paranasal sinuses. *In* Paparella, M. M., and Shumrick, D. A. (eds.): Otolaryngology. Vol. 1, Basic Sciences and Related Disciplines. Philadelphia, W. B. Saunders Co., 1973. Chapter 3, pp. 161–170.

Physiology:

Bosma, J. F.: Physiology of the mouth, pharynx and esophagus. *In* Paparella, M. M., and Shumrick, D. A. (eds.): Otolaryngology. Vol. 1, Basic Sciences and Related Disciplines. Philadelphia, W. B. Saunders Co., 1973, pp. 356–361.

Congenital:

English, G. M.: Anomalies of the ear, nose, mouth and throat. *In* Maloney, W. H. (ed.): Otolaryngology. Vol. 2. Hagerstown, Md., Harper & Row, Publishers, 1973. Chapter 3, pp. 45–68.

Kornblut, A. D.: Non-neoplastic diseases of the tonsils and adenoids. *In* Paparella, M. M., and Shumrick, D. A. (eds.): Otolaryngology. Vol. 3, Head and Neck. Philadelphia, W. B. Saunders Co., 1973, pp. 277–295.

Infectious:

Kornblut, A. D.: Non-neoplastic diseases of the tonsils and adenoids. *In* Paparella, M. M., and Shumrick, D. A. (eds.): Otolaryngology. Vol. 3, Head and Neck. Philadelphia, W. B. Saunders Co., 1973, pp. 277–295.

Neoplastic:

Hara, H. J.: Cancer of nasopharynx. Review of the literature. Report of 72 cases. Laryngoscope, *79*: 1315, 1969.

Toomey, J. M.: Cysts and tumors of the pharynx. *In* Paparella, M. M., and Shumrick, D. A. (eds.): Otolaryngology. Vol. 3, Head and Neck. Philadelphia, W. B. Saunders Co., 1973, pp. 341–347.

LARYNX AND HYPOPHARYNX

Embryology and Anatomy:

Davies, J.: Embryology and anatomy of the larynx, respiratory apparatus, diaphragm and esophagus. *In* Paparella, M. M., and Shumrick, D. A. (eds.): Otolaryngology. Vol. 1, Basic Sciences and Related Disciplines. Philadelphia, W. B. Saunders Co., 1973, pp. 179–183.

Hast, M. H.: The developmental anatomy of the larynx. Otolaryngol. Clin. North Am., *3*(Oct.):413–438, 1970.

Physiology:

Kirchner, J. A.: Physiology of the larynx. *In* Paparella, M. M., and Shumrick, D. A. (eds.): Otolaryngology. Vol. 1, Basic Sciences and Related Disciplines. Philadelphia, W. B. Saunders Co., 1973, pp. 371–379.

Congenital:

English, G. M.: Anomalies of the ear, nose, mouth and throat. *In* Maloney, W. H. (ed.): Otolaryngology. Vol. 2. Hagerstown, Md., Harper & Row, Publishers, 1973. Chapter 3, pp. 63–66.

Fearon, B.: Respiratory distress in the newborn. Otolaryngol. Clin. North Am., *1*(June):147–160, 1968.

Ferguson, C. F.: Congenital abnormalities of the larynx. Otolaryngol. Clin. North Am., *3*(June):185–200, 1970.

Trauma:

Fitz-High, G. S., and Powell, J. B., II: Acute traumatic injuries of the oropharynx, laryngopharynx and cervical trachea in children. Otolaryngol. Clin. North Am., *3*(June):375–394, 1970.

Shumrick, D. A.: Trauma of the larynx and lower airway. *In* Paparella, M. M., and Shumrick, D. A. (eds.): Otolaryngology. Vol. 3, Head and Neck. Philadelphia, W. B. Saunders Co., 1973, pp. 609–615.

Infectious:

Davison, E. W.: Acute laryngotracheal infections in childhood. Otolaryngol. Clin. North Am., *1*(June): 69–90, 1968.

Friedman, I.: Granulomas of the larynx. *In* Paparella, M. M., and Shumrick, D. A. (eds.): Otolaryngology. Vol. 3, Head and Neck. Philadelphia, W. B. Saunders Co., 1973, pp. 616–630.

Heldtander, P., and Lee, P.: Treatment of acute epiglottitis in children by long-term intubation. Acta Otolaryngol., *75*:379, 1973.

Heller, M. F.: Supralaryngeal and laryngeal cellulitis in adults. Arch. Otolaryngol., *80*:110, 1964.

Jones, R. S.: The management of acute croup. Arch. Dis. Child., *47*:661, 1972.

Rapkin, R. H.: Acute epiglottitis: pitfalls in diagnosis and management. Clin. Pediatr., *10*:312, 1971.

Rapkin, R. H.: The diagnosis of epiglottitis: the simplicity and reliability of radiographs of the neck in the differential diagnosis of the croup syndrome. J. Pediatr., *80*:96, 1972.

Iatrogenic:

Cooper, J. D., and Grillo, H. C.: The evaluation of tracheal injury due to ventilatory assistance through cuffed tubes: a pathologic study. Ann. Surg., *169*:334, 1969.

Ogura, J. H., and Biller, H. F.: Reconstruction of the larynx following blunt trauma. Ann. Otol. Rhinol. Laryngol., *80*:492, 1971.

Idiopathic:

Fisher, H. B., and Logemaun, J. A.: Voice diagnostics and therapy. Otolaryngol. Clin. North Am., *3*(Oct.): 639–663, 1970.

Friedman, I.: Granulomas of the larynx. *In* Paparella,

M. M., and Shumrick, D. A. (eds.): Otolaryngology. Vol. 3, Head and Neck. Philadelphia, W. B. Saunders Co., 1973, pp. 618–630.

Neoplastic:

Ogura, J. H., and Biller, H. F.: Cysts and tumors of the larynx. *In* Paparella, M. M., and Shumrick, D. A. (eds.): Otolaryngology. Vol. 3, Head and Neck. Philadelphia, W. B. Saunders Co., 1973, pp. 658–665.

SALIVARY GLANDS

Embryology and Anatomy:

Gates, G.: Embryology and anatomy of the salivary glands. *In* Paparella, M. M., and Shumrick, D. A. (eds.): Otolaryngology. Vol. 1, Basic Sciences and Related Disciplines. Philadelphia, W. B. Saunders Co., 1973, pp. 233–240.

Physiology:

Gates, G.: Biochemistry of the salivary glands and saliva. *In* Paparella, M. M., and Shumrick, D. A. (eds.): Otolaryngology. Vol. 1, Basic Sciences and Related Disciplines. Philadelphia, W. B. Saunders Co., 1973, pp. 401–410.

Gates, G.: Physiology of the salivary glands. *In* Paparella, M. M., and Shumrick, D. A. (eds.): Otolaryngology. Vol. 1, Basic Sciences and Related Disciplines. Philadelphia, W. B. Saunders Co., 1973, pp. 347–355.

Congenital:

Work, W. P., and Hecht, D. W.: Congenital malformations and trauma of the salivary glands. *In* Paparella, M. M., and Shumrick, D. A. (eds.): Otolaryngology. Vol. 3, Head and Neck. Philadelphia, W. B. Saunders Co., 1973, pp. 253–257.

Trauma:

Work, W. P., and Hecht, D. W.: Congenital malformations and trauma of the salivary glands. *In* Paparella, M. M., and Shumrick, D. A. (eds.): Otolaryngology. Vol. 3, Head and Neck. Philadelphia, W. B. Saunders Co., 1973, pp. 253–257.

Infectious:

Work, W. P., and Hecht, D. W.: Inflammatory diseases of the major salivary glands. *In* Paparella, M. M., and Shumrick, D. A. (eds.): Otolaryngology. Vol. 3, Head and Neck. Philadelphia, W. B. Saunders Co., 1973, pp. 258–265.

Idiopathic:

Blatt, I. M.: On sialectasis and benign lymphosialadenopathy. Laryngoscope, 74:1684, 1964.

Kelly, D. R., Spiegel, J. C., and Maves, M.: Benign lymphoepithelial lesions of the salivary glands. Arch. Otolaryngol., *101*:71, 1975.

Neoplastic:

Work, W. P.: Cysts and tumors of the major salivary glands. *In* Paparella, M. M., and Shumrick, D. A. (eds.): Otolaryngology, Vol. 3, Head and Neck. Philadelphia, W. B. Saunders Co., 1973, pp. 266–274.

NECK

Embryology and Anatomy:

Davies, J.: Embryology and anatomy of the head and neck. *In* Paparella, M. M., and Shumrick, D. A. (eds.): Otolaryngology. Vol. 1, Basic Sciences and Related Disciplines. Philadelphia, W. B. Saunders Co., 1973, pp. 111–149.

Congenital:

Sade, J., and Rosen, G.: Thyroglossal cysts and tracts. Ann. Otol. Rhinol. Laryngol., 77:139, 1968.

Simpson, R. A.: Lateral cervical cysts and fistulas. Laryngoscope, 79:30, 1969.

Hereditary:

McLaurin, J. W., Kloepfer, H. W., Laguite, J. K., et al.: Hereditary branchial anomalies and associated hearing impairment. Laryngoscope, 76:1277, 1966.

Infectious:

Everts, E. C., and Echevarria, J.: The pharynx and deep neck infections. *In* Paparella, M. M., and Shumrick, D. A. (eds.): Otolaryngology. Vol. 3, Head and Neck. Philadelphia, W. B. Saunders Co., 1973, pp. 327–340.

Neoplastic:

See *Neoplastic* in other sections for references.

FACIAL SKELETON

Maxillofacial Trauma. Mathog, R. G. (ed.). Otolaryngolog. Clin. North Am., 9(June):315–553, 1976. (This current symposium has an excellent reference list for further reading.)

AERODIGESTIVE TRACT

Embryology and Anatomy:

Davies, J.: Embryology and anatomy of the larynx, respiratory apparatus, diaphragm and esophagus. *In* Paparella, M. M., and Shumrick, D. A. (eds.): Otolaryngology. Vol. 1, Basic Sciences and Related Disciplines. Philadelphia, W. B. Saunders Co., 1973, p. 185.

Congenital:

English, G. M.: Anomalies of the ear, nose, mouth and throat. *In* Maloney, W. H. (ed.): Otolaryngology. Vol. 2. Hagerstown, Md., Harper & Row, Publishers, 1973, pp. 63–74.

Fearson, B.: Respiratory distress in the newborn. Otolaryngolog. Clin. North Am., *1*(June):147–170, 1968.

Ferguson, C. F.: Congenital abnormalities of the infant larynx. Otolaryngol. Clin. North Am., 3(June):185–200, 1970.

Infectious:

See "Larynx and Hypopharynx."

Iatrogenic:

Silvis, S. E., et al.: Endoscopic complications. Results of 1974 American Society for Gastrointestinal Endoscopy survey. J.A.M.A., 235:928, 1976.

Idiopathic:

Andersen, H. A.: Dysfunction of the esophagus. Otolaryngol. Clin. North Am., *1*(June):195–218, 1968.

Daly, J. F.: Corrosive esophagitis. Otolaryngol. Clin. North Am., *1*(June):119–132, 1968.

Jackson, C.: Observations on the pathology of foreign bodies in the air and food passages (based on an analysis of 628 cases). Otolaryngol. Clin. North Am., *1*(June):3–36, 1968.

Tucker, G. F., Jr.: Foreign bodies in the esophagus or respiratory tract. *In* Paparella, M. M., and Shumrick, D. A. (eds.): Otolaryngology. Vol. 3, Head and Neck. Philadelphia, W. B. Saunders Co., 1973, pp. 753–768.

Neoplastic:

Holinger, P. H.: Benign tumors of the trachea and bronchi. Otolaryngol. Clin. North Am., *1*(June):219–338, 1968.

Norris, C. N.: Tumors of the trachea, bronchi and esophagus. *In* Paparella, M. M., and Shumrick, D. A. (eds.): Otolaryngology. Vol. 3, Head and Neck. Philadelphia, W. B. Saunders Co., 1973, pp. 740–752.

Putney, F. J.: Bronchoscopic aspects of bronchogenic carcinomas. Otolaryngol. Clin. North Am., *1*(June): 239–258, 1968.

Chapter 40

OPHTHALMOLOGY

by YALE SOLOMON,
and MELVILLE G. ROSEN

INTRODUCTION

To appreciate the context of this chapter, it is important to understand the perspective of family practice from which it was written. In our view, it is a misconception to infer that a family physician fulfills his role only by knowing scientific facts, applying them in practice, recognizing problems outside his ken, and referring patients with such problems to the appropriate subspecialist. The family physician should indeed be very aware of scientific facts, but, in addition, he should utilize his distinct advantage that stems from his continual relationship with the entire family under his care. This doctor-family relationship, coupled with the family physician's knowledge of his patients' social and behavioral patterns rarely apparent to the consultant, will undoubtedly be a major contribution to health care in the specialty of ophthalmology, or in any specialty. The family physician and the specialist must act as a team, giving each other the benefit of their respective knowledge. They must be consultants to each other in order to achieve the best results for the third member of the team, the patient.

This mutual consultation constitutes a major innovation in the practice of ophthalmology for the family physician. It is assumed that the family physician will not be involved in active therapy for most medical conditions related to the eye and certainly not in most surgical procedures. This does not imply, however, that he should be unaware of the details of secondary and tertiary ophthalmologic conditions. Some conditions should be treated by him, many should be recognized as requiring referral, and many are in need of associated therapy that only the family physician can provide.

The ophthalmologist and the family physician should never abandon their respective roles of preventing, as well as treating, illness and disease.

This chapter includes two parts: diseases of the external eye, many of which are treatable by the family physician, and diseases of the internal eye, most of which should be referred to the specialist, again, in consultation with the family physician.

VISUAL AND NONVISUAL SYMPTOMS AND SIGNS

It has been estimated that symptoms and signs related to the eye constitute up to 10 per cent of the problems seen in a family practice. As a means of rapid classification, it is useful to present eye disorders in the categories of visual and nonvisual problems.

Visual Problems

Loss of Vision. The patient may complain of simple blurring of vision or of total or partial loss of vision. A blurry image in the eye may be due to uncorrected refractive errors, such as myopia or astigmatism; changes in the media, such as opacities or haziness in the lens or vitreous; inflammatory or degenerative changes in the retina, particularly in the area of the macula, or inflammatory changes in the optic nerve, such as an optic neuritis or papilledema.

When the patient has a partial or total loss of vision, a retinal detachment or an occlusion of a central retinal artery or vein should be considered.

Visual Phenomena. Such phenomena are fairly common symptoms and consist of three major types: light flashes; spots, or so-called floaters; and halos or rainbows around lights. Light flashes are generally of two types. The most common are the arcuate luminescent reflections, typical of migraine. The other is the more significant occurrence of lightning streaks noted in a dark room, suggestive of peripheral retinal degeneration, which may precede a retinal detachment.

Spots, or so-called vitreous floaters, are most often fine vitreous opacities, usually related to a simple degenerative change in the vitreous. There are, however, larger, denser opacities that may be due to a vitreous hemorrhage from a retinal tear.

The occurrence of rainbows or halos seen around lights is most frequently due to the corneal edema related to glaucoma. It may also be caused by cataracts of a nuclear sclerotic type, but this is far less common.

Painful Vision (Asthenopia). Painful vision may be related to the "eye strain" of an uncorrected refractive error or to a muscle imbalance, but this is not nearly as common as is generally thought.

Visual Field Defect. Awareness of a visual field defect may be a presenting complaint. Very simply stated, if the patient is aware of this defect in only one eye, the problem is in the retina or the optic nerve of that eye. If the patient realizes that there is a problem with his ability to see a certain portion of the field in each eye, the lesion is in or behind the optic chiasm.

Nonvisual Problems

Redness. The overall appearance of a diffusely injected conjunctiva may be due to an acute conjunctivitis in which discharge is common and injection is more intense near the conjunctival fornices. In acute iritis, the primary redness is more intense around the cornea and is most often accompanied by a severe photophobia. The redness of acute glaucoma is less intense and more diffuse; the cornea is hazy, and the pupil is moderately dilated.

Pain. This may be classified into three general types: ocular, orbital, and "ocular headache." Ocular pain generally resem-

bles that felt with a foreign body or with any corneal irritation or trauma, but also may be a burning sensation that is frequently associated with conjunctivitis, allergy, or fatigue. Orbital pain is of a deeper type and is commonly noted in iritis or glaucoma. It may also be associated with a sinusitis or a retrobulbar neuritis. The so-called ocular headache is most often not ocular in origin, as eye disorders are an uncommon cause of chronic headaches. Refractive errors do occasionally result in headache, but this is usually associated only with tasks requiring close work.

Discharge. The complaint of discharge can often refer to a thin and watery type of exudate seen with a foreign body or a blocked tear duct. A thicker or purulent discharge is seen with conjunctivitis or tear sac infection, while a dry and flaky form occurs in blepharitis or eyelid margin inflammation.

Masses. The presence of masses should lead one to think of anatomic anomalies. In the eyelids the most common causes would be hordeolum, chalazion, or neoplasm. On the conjunctiva, one would ordinarily suspect pingueculae, pterygia, or nevi. Masses at the inner or outer canthi would lead one to consider disorders of the lacrimal system, as a mass at the outer canthus would possibly indicate a lacrimal gland tumor, whereas a lesion in the inner canthus might be due to a dacryocystitis causing a dilated tear sac. A mass in the orbit would usually present as proptosis, and one should think of hemangiomas and dermoids before considering malignancies of a local or metastatic nature. One must always rule out hyperthyroid exophthalmos, as this is the most common cause of proptosis, even when unilateral.

EXAMINATION OF THE EYES

When diagnosing eye disease, it is vitally important to follow a rigid protocol of examination, as fine detail is easily overlooked. It is not necessary to reiterate the importance of a complete eye examination for patients with or without ocular complaints. However, we would like to emphasize again the advantage that the family physician may have, not only in applying his scientific knowledge, but in having the

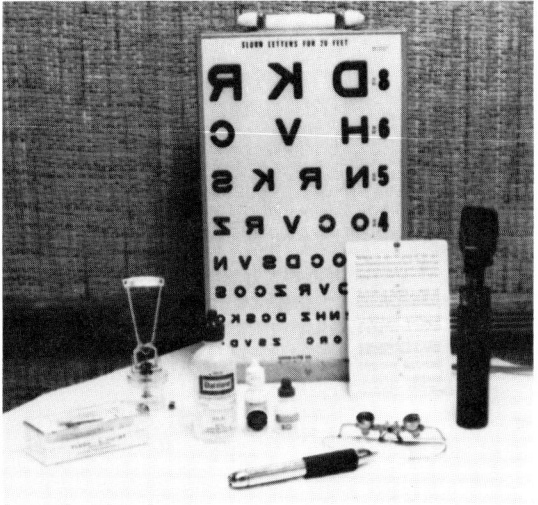

Figure 40–1. Total list of essential equipment for family practice of ophthalmology: clockwise, starting with the Snellen eye chart (Goodlight, with reversed letters for reading in a mirror at 10 feet, giving a 20 foot equivalent distance), Halogen ophthalmoscope, near vision test card, binocular 2 × loupe, penlight, topicamide (Mydriacyl) 0.5 per cent for dilating pupils, proparacaine-chlorobutanol-benzalkonium chloride (Ophthetic) for topical anesthesia, isotonic solution of boric acid-potassium chloride-sodium carbonate with benzalkonium chloride-disodium EDTA (Dacriose) irrigating solution, Schiötz tonometer, Fluor-I-Strips.

distinct advantage of being able to carry out this important examination more frequently and more completely than can the consultant, who is often seeing the patient for the first time. This is especially true with children and the elderly. Because of the trust that has been established and demonstrated by prior encounters, the family physician is often able to put the patient at ease and can thus do a more complete and successful examination.

One should proceed along the lines of establishing a standard physical diagnosis and should include the following procedures in the examination: (1) visual acuity testing, (2) observation, (3) palpation, (4) auscultation, and (5) visual field survey (Fig. 40–1).

VISUAL ACUITY TESTING

Visual acuity should be tested by the physician or his assistant and is a vital preliminary step for every patient. The equipment needed is a cardboard Snellen chart with direct illumination at 20 feet and a near vision testing card, obtainable from

any medical supplier. A self-illuminated distance chart made by the Good-Lite Company is also satisfactory. The vision should be tested in each eye separately and *with glasses if worn.* Both distance and near vision are recorded as a fraction, with the numerator as the distance from the chart, i.e., usually 20 feet for distance and 14 inches for near vision. This examination alone is an excellent preliminary guide to ocular function.

OBSERVATION

The physician then begins his examination of the external eye. It is helpful to think sequentially in terms of ocular anatomy, so that the first thing one would observe is the gross binocular appearance, including eyelid ptosis, proptosis, or any other difference between the two eyes. The lids are then examined for masses, such as chalazia or basal cell carcinoma, and for the discharge and crusting seen in blepharitis.

The conjunctivae are then inspected. Normally, the transparent bulbar conjunctiva reveals the underlying sclera, but an abnormality will cause an increase in vascularity and thickness of the conjunctiva. The palpebral conjunctiva of the lower lid is easily revealed by simple downward traction at the lid margin. The upper lid conjunctiva, however, can be viewed only by everting the upper lid. This is accomplished by pulling downward gently on the lashes while pressing a cotton applicator downward at the edge of the tarsus (4 mm. from the lid margin). At that moment of downward pressure, the lashes are gently pulled upward as the patient continues to look down, and the lid will evert (Fig. 40–2).

The cornea is inspected, and its sparkling, clear appearance is seen best when viewed by oblique illumination from a good pocket flashlight. This type of illumination coming from about 45 degrees is best for demonstrating scars, ulcers, and foreign bodies. The use of fluorescein (sterile Fluor-I-Strips supplied by Ayerst Laboratories) is indispensable in detecting breaks in the corneal epithelium that would otherwise be missed.

The anterior chamber is next viewed by oblique illumination. Here it is useful to estimate the distance between the cornea and the iris near the limbus to determine

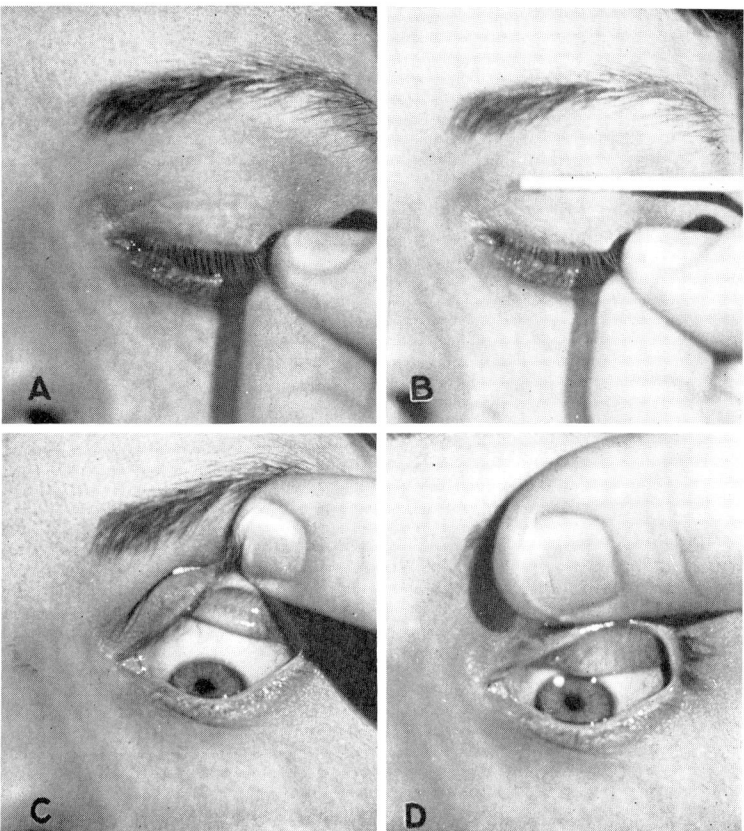

Figure 40–2. *Everting lid. A, First procedure in everting upper lid. B, Second procedure in everting upper lid. C, Third procedure in everting upper lid. D, Maintaining lid in everted position. (From Scheie, H. G., and Albert, D. M.: Textbook of Ophthalmology. 9th Ed. Philadelphia, W. B. Saunders Co., 1977, p. 175.)*

the presence of a narrow angle, which predisposes to glaucoma. The iris is examined primarily for any grossly raised lesions, suggestive of melanomas, or for obvious heterochromia (different colored iris in each eye), which is a possible precursor of a form of iritis. The pupil is then examined for size, shape, and equality (25 per cent of normal people have slightly unequal pupils). The pupillary reaction to light, both direct and consensual (one eye contracting on illumination of the opposite eye), is an important neuro-ophthalmologic test. The pupil should also be tested for its reaction to accommodation. This is done by having the patient shift his gaze from any distant object to focus on his fingernail, while the examiner observes the accommodative contraction, which is normally slight. The lens of the eye is usually best seen with the ophthalmoscope, but gross clouding or opacities may actually be seen by oblique illumination.

Direct Ophthalmoscopy

For the family physician, observation of the remainder of the eye is best accomplished by direct ophthalmoscopy. Many ophthalmologists have found the halogen ophthalmoscope manufactured by Welch-Allyn to be superior in illumination. The lens, the vitreous, and remainder of the fundus are examined after the pupil is dilated with one or two instillations of 10 per cent phenylephrine hydrochloride (Neo-Synephrine) or 0.5 per cent tropicamide (Mydriacyl). Fear of precipitating an attack of acute glaucoma should not be a factor in avoiding dilatation, as the incidence of such attacks is very low. In addition, "unmasking" a patient with glaucoma may be performing a great service to the patient because the attack, which may be inevitable later, has at least occurred under ideal conditions for treatment.

The examination begins with the oph-

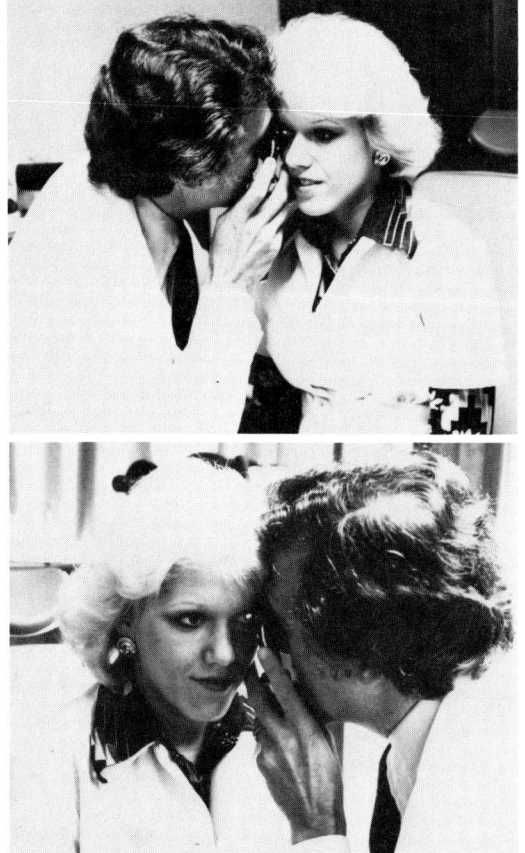

Figure 40–3. *Ophthalmoscopy, showing close position.*

thalmoscope held at about 6 inches from the patient's eye, and the following technical points, although probably well known, warrant review.

1. The patient's and the examiner's heads should be on the same level.

2. The examiner's right hand and eye are used to examine the patient's right eye and are switched to the left to examine the patient's left eye.

3. The patient should fixate at a distance point.

4. The ophthalmoscope should be brought as close to the examiner's eye and to the patient's eye as possible (Fig. 40–3).

5. Starting with a +10 lens in the ophthalmoscope to view the lens of the eye, the power is gradually decreased by keeping the index finger constantly on the lens wheel.

The vitreous is brought into view as both the distance from the patient and the power in the aperture are slowly decreased.

Usually with a + 5 lens held several inches from the patient's eye, floaters or opacities will be seen by having the patient move his eye in horizontal and vertical directions of gaze.

A systematic approach is essential in examining the fundus, and the following routine is suggested:

1. As the patient fixes on a distance point, the examiner directs the ophthalmoscope from about 15° temporal to the visual axis, and the disc will appear in view.

2. The optic nerve head appears as a slightly vertical pinkish oval with a pale central depression, the physiologic cup. The base of this cupped area may be mottled gray, caused by prominent fibers of the sclera (the lamina cribrosa) which the nerve penetrates.

3. The relationship between the diameter of this central cup and the diameter of the disc, called the C/D ratio, is of increasing importance in glaucoma detection. Although a "normal" ratio might be 0.3, i.e., the cup diameter is three-tenths that of the disc diameter, the critical evaluation is that of comparing the C/D ratio of each eye. A significant difference of 0.2 or more should be an indication for frequent re-evaluation of the eye with the greater C/D ratio to detect the possible development of chronic simple glaucoma.

Pathologic variations of the discs include the blurry borders and congested vessels caused by papilledema and the large, sharp-edged cup resulting from glaucoma, with retinal vessels disappearing over its edge.

Each of the retinal vessels must be examined from the disc to the periphery by proceeding clockwise from the superotemporal vessels. They should, in particular, be observed for the AV ratio (the diameter of the brighter, thinner arterioles to that of the darker, thicker venules), the ratio usually being about 3 to 4. The important changes caused by hypertension and arteriosclerosis will be discussed in detail in the section on retinal disease.

The retinal periphery should be examined next and is best seen by having the patient move his eye in the direction desired. Early retinal detachment and small melanomas may be detected by careful examination of this area.

The most uncomfortable and therefore the last part of the examination is visualization of the macula. Located about 2 disc

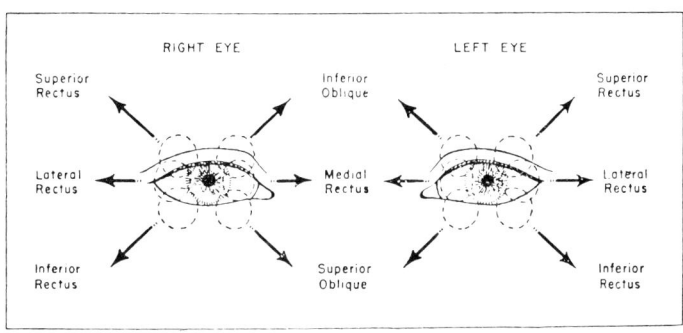

Figure 40–4. *Motility examination —cardinal fields of gaze. (From Allen, J. H.: In Perera, C. A. (ed.): May's Manual of the Diseases of the Eye. Baltimore, The Williams & Wilkins Co., 1968. Reprinted by Robert Krieger Publishing Co., 1974.)*

diameters (DD) temporal to the optic nerve, the macula is a slightly darker, vessel-free area about the size of the nerve head. It is bounded by small branches of the superior and inferior temporal arterioles, and at its center is the fovea centralis. This is the small central "pit" of maximal retinal sensitivity that reflects the ophthalmoscopic light as a bright pinpoint reflex in the darker areola of the macula.

The use of the "disc diameter" and clock positions is recommended as a record-keeping device for locating lesions. The disc, actually about 1.5 mm. in diameter, is the standard reference. If a lesion of 2 DD size (3.0 mm.) is referred to as being 3 DD distance from the disc at 2 o'clock, it can be quickly located by another examiner.

Motility Examination

The careful observation of the movement of the eyes in all directions may elicit very useful information. The motility examination of the eyes consists of the following:

1. The six cardinal fields of gaze are examined to elicit the isolated function of each of the six oculorotary muscles (Fig. 40–4). By asking the patient to fixate on a light held in each of the cardinal fields, the observer can detect a lag of either eye, indicative of a paretic muscle. The subjective response is elicited by asking the patient about the presence of diplopia in each field of gaze, which is significant in detecting minimal paresis.

2. Phoria testing consists of using the so-called "alternate cover test." A *phoria* is a *latent deviation* of an eye, which is ordinarily held in alignment by the fusion capability of the brain. An eye may drift *in* (esophoria) or *out* (exophoria); when the

eye is covered, fusion is broken and the deviation occurs under the cover. Any fixation object, such as a pocketlight or pen, and either an occlusion paddle or the examiner's fingers held tightly together may be used (Fig. 40–5). The patient fixates his

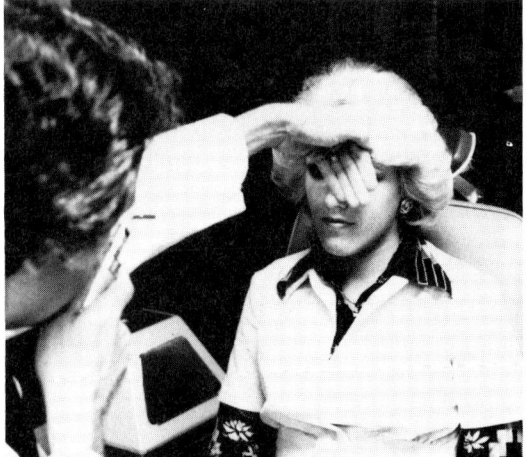

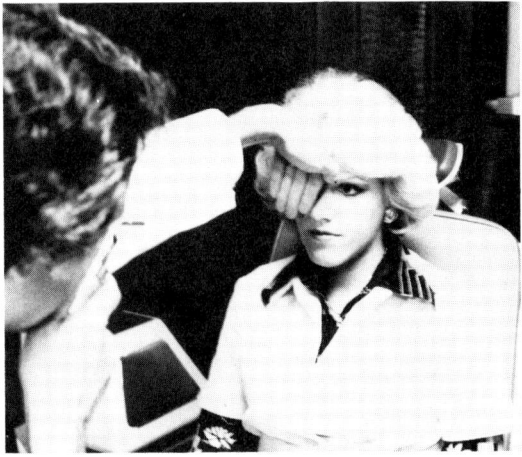

Figure 40–5. *Cover testing.*

eye on the light or object, which is held in the examiner's hand at about a 2 foot (30 cm.) distance, and each eye is alternately and abruptly uncovered. The movement of the eye as the cover is removed is carefully observed. If the eye has deviated under the cover, it must move to fixate on the light again. If the eye seems to move quickly in an inward direction, it was deviated outward (exophoria); if the compensatory fixating movement is outward, the eye was deviated inward (esophoria).

It should be noted that most people have some degree of a phoria and are completely asymptomatic. A large phoria, i.e., one that very obviously swings in when the cover is removed, can be productive of symptoms, particularly when the patient is reading. In this instance, some form of orthoptic or exercise treatment can be very valuable. However, this does not mean that children with reading disabilities or learning disabilities can be helped by the use of so-called "visual exercises." There has been no indication that coordinating cerebral and visual dominance or instituting prolonged courses of visual training for phorias are of any benefit in the treatment of learning disabilities. It is the view of almost all ophthalmologists that therapy for children with learning disabilities should be provided by the educator and that these children are not benefited by various forms of visual and coordinative "exercises."

3. The test for detecting a *tropia* is the "cover-uncover test." A tropia (strabismus) is a constant or manifest deviation of one eye, turned inward (esotropia) or outward (exotropia). After the alternate cover test is done and the compensatory movement is recognized, the occlusion paddle or hand is suddenly removed from the eye *without* occluding the opposite eye. This uncovered eye is carefully observed for any movement to regain fixation. If it does so, the condition is a phoria; if the eye remains deviated in or out, the disorder is a tropia.

PALPATION

Examination by palpation encompasses surface palpation, retropulsion, finger tension, and the technique of tonometry. Palpation of the eyelids for small tumors or chalazia is best done by gliding a finger gently over the upper and lower lids. If too much pressure is applied, however, the presence of small chalazia may be missed.

The technique of retropulsion is accomplished by using the thumb or forefinger to exert backward pressure over the closed lid to determine the relative firmness of the orbital contents. A gross difference of resistance between the two eyes may be indicative of orbital disorders, such as thyroidopathy or orbital tumors.

The use of the fingers to obtain an estimate of intraocular tension has been mentioned in textbooks of physical diagnosis. Placing both forefingers on the upper portion of the globe and applying alternate pressure between the fingers create a ballottement effect that can give the trained observer a very rough estimate of intraocular tension. Use of this technique can result in mistakes in diagnosis and, therefore, is not an alternative to the routine use of tonometry.

Tonometry

Glaucoma testing should be considered part of a complete physical examination. Positive findings are greater in tests for glaucoma detection than in tests for detection of other diseases that are amenable to screening tests, such as diabetes, cervical carcinoma, or tuberculosis. The instrument used for tonometry in a general practice setting is the Schiötz tonometer manufactured by Storz or Sklar at a cost of less than $100.00 It is generally employed with the preattached 5.5 gram weight and should be checked daily on the testplate provided to ensure that is calibrated to zero. After each use the tonometer should be set in an ultraviolet sterilizer stand (manufactured by Storz) or the footplate should be wiped with a 1:5000 solution of benzalkonium chloride (Zephiran). At the end of each day's use, the plunger should be removed, and a pipe cleaner soaked in ether should be run through the barrel to remove any drying secretions.

Technique. The patient reclines on an examining table while one drop of tetracaine (Pontocaine) or, for less stinging effect, one drop of proparacaine (Ophthaine) is instilled in each eye. The patient then raises one arm in order to fixate on his thumb, as the examiner stands to one side or at the head of the table. Holding the tonometer between the thumb and third

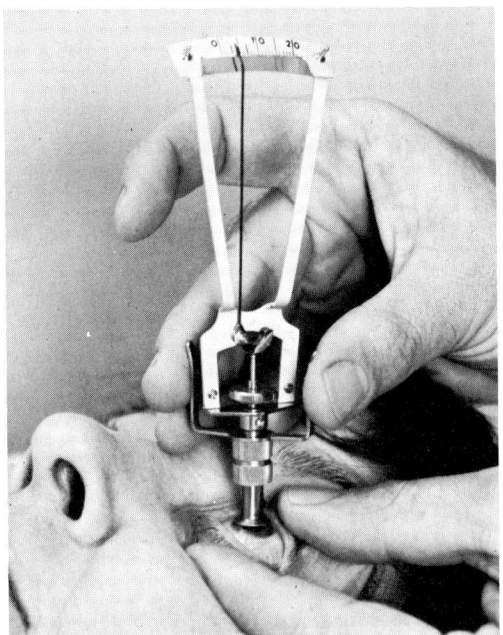

Figure 40–6. Technique of tonometry. (From Demorest, B. H.: In Conn, H. F., Rakel, R. E., and Johnson, T. W. (eds.): Family Practice. 1st Ed. Philadelphia, W. B. Saunders Co., 1973, p. 759.)

finger, the examiner's hand is stabilized by resting the little finger on the patient's cheek. The other hand is used to gently separate the lids, using the thumb and third finger, while the tonometer footplate is placed directly on the cornea and lowered half way until a steady reading is obtained (Fig. 40–6). This should be repeated once or twice to corroborate the reading, which is noted in simple units from the scale markings on the tonometer. These units may be translated into millimeters of mercury pressure by use of the card that is provided with each instrument. For purposes of screening, however, this is not really essential.

A patient with a reading of from 0 to 3 units should certainly be referred to an ophthalmologist; a reading of 3½ to 4 units is borderline and should be rechecked at another time. Any reading of 4½ or more units is considered normal, and the patient should be informed that there is no evidence of an increase in intraocular pressure. The physician should not hesitate to perform this test because of fear of damaging the cornea. If done gently, the patient should experience no damage or discomfort other than a numb feeling in the eyes from the anesthesia, lasting about 15 minutes.

AUSCULTATION

The fourth aspect of physical diagnosis, auscultation, is primarily concerned with the rather limited technique of listening with a stethoscope placed over the closed lids or over the carotids to reveal the presence of an arteriovenous fistula in the orbit or the cavernous sinus. The typical machinery bruit heard over the globe is pathognomonic for this fistula.

VISUAL FIELDS SURVEY

The final procedure for a complete eye examination done by the family physician is a survey of the visual fields. Although a complete visual field study should be done by a specialist, the family physician can evaluate a complaint suggesting a disturbance in the visual field in a very simple manner. The importance of performing a reliable study for detecting neurologic disorders is evidenced from reviewing the diagram analyzing the localization of visual field defects (see Fig. 40–33). Although the specific details of a visual field are elicited only by a tangent screen or a perimeter examination, the so-called "4-point confrontation field" is simple, rapid, and accurate.

With the patient seated comfortably, directly facing the examiner, his left eye is occluded, and he is directed to stare into the examiner's left eye. While ensuring the maintenance of steady fixation, the examiner carries out the following four points.

1. He gradually brings one or two fingers into each visual field quadrant until the patient can correctly identify the number of fingers. This will give the first indication of any quadrantic or hemianopic defect.

2. The examiner then holds fingers of each hand in opposite quadrants, e.g., one finger in the superior temporal quadrant and two fingers in the superior nasal quadrant, and asks the patient to state the total number seen. The technique is repeated for the inferior nasal and inferior temporal quadrants. If the patient shows no field defect in the first point examination and yet in the second point procedure is not able to recognize the total number of fingers on each hand, this is indicative of a relative or less dense scotoma. The basis of this test is

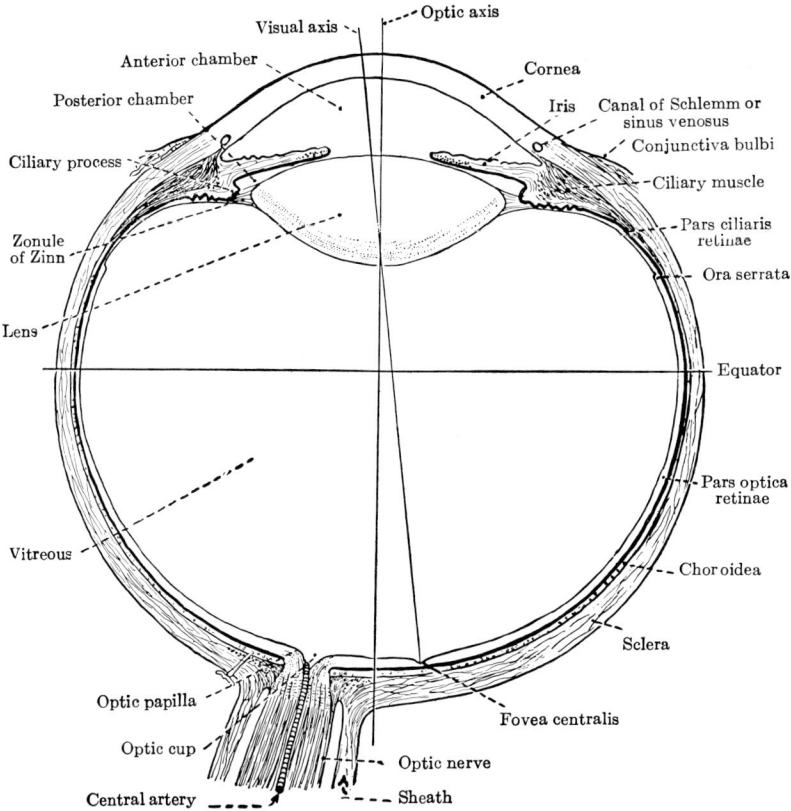

Figure 40–7.   *Anatomy of the right eyeball. (From Scheie, H. G., and Albert, D. M.: Textbook of Ophthalmology. 9th Ed. Philadelphia, W. B. Saunders Co., 1977, p. 57.)*

the phenomenon of simultaneous extinction, in which the stronger visual stimulus coming from the fingers in the normal quadrant will extinguish the weaker visual stimulus that arises from the finger in the affected quadrant.

3. One finger is then presented in each of the upper quadrants, and the patient asked if one appears more distinct than the other. The same question is again asked to compare the intensity of the stimulus of the fingers presented in front of each of the lower quadrants.

4. The same procedure is performed as in point 3, but the patient is asked to compare the intensity of the stimulus as the fingers are presented in the upper nasal quadrant and the lower nasal quadrant; the simultaneous presentation in the upper temporal quadrant and the lower temporal quadrant concludes the test.

This refinement of the simple confrontation fields has been shown to be quite accurate in detecting defects that would otherwise be missed in the simple "wiggling finger confrontation field."

SPECIAL OCULAR ANATOMY AND PHYSIOLOGY

Unfortunately, instruction in the detailed structure or even in the gross anatomy of the eye is often neglected in medical schools. Therefore, two anatomical diagrams (Figs. 40–7 and 40–8) are presented for a brief review of ocular structures.

Our discussion of physiology will be limited to those changes in the eye that are manifested as refractive errors, as these are nonpathologic, physiologic variants. Such changes include myopia, hyperopia, astigmatism and presbyopia. Therapy with use of spectacles or contact lenses is also discussed.

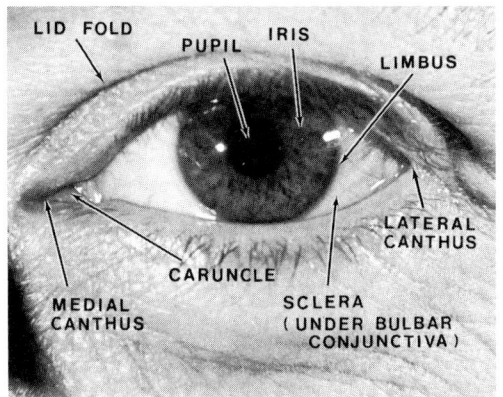

Figure 40–8. The anatomy of the external eye. (From Demorest, B. H.: In Conn, H. F., Rakel, R. E., and Johnson, T. W. (eds.): Family Practice. 1st Ed. Philadelphia, W. B. Saunders Co., 1973, p. 739.)

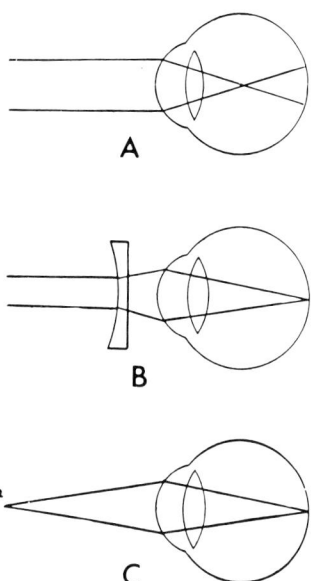

Figure 40–9. Myopia. A, *Parallel rays cross in front of retina.* B, *Effect of concave lens on parallel rays.* C, *Divergent rays from punctum remotum, P^2, focus on retina without use of accommodation. (From Scheie, H. G., and Albert, D. M.: Textbook of Ophthalmology. 9th Ed. Philadelphia, W. B. Saunders Co., 1977, p. 270.)*

Myopia

Myopia, or nearsightedness, occurs when the axial length of the eyeball is too long for the refractive power of the lens and cornea (Fig. 40–9). This disorder is usually hereditary in origin. In myopia, the focal point of light rays will lie in front of the retina, resulting in a blurred image of distant objects. As the eye continues to grow, the degree of myopia increases, particularly during early adolescence, until stability is reached at about age 16 to 18.

The basic treatment consists of prescribing properly measured concave lenses that will diverge the light rays back to the proper point of focus on the retina, enabling the patient to see clearly. The glasses are to be worn when the patient is in need of clear distance vision, i.e., for school work, movies, television, and so forth. It has *never* been demonstrated that constant wearing of glasses will do more than enable the patient to constantly see clearly. It has also never been demonstrated that avoiding reading or close work will help to slow or reverse the progress of myopia. Furthermore it has never been shown that eye drops, exercises, or special contact lenses will reverse or slow the progression of this condition.

Pathologic myopia, on the other hand, is a condition in which the eyes have greater than 5 diopters of myopia, and the elongation, with stretching and thinning of the inner coats of the eye, may continue. One may see patients with "myopic conus" or bare sclera around the disc, atrophic areas

in the macula, and small holes in the retinal periphery. These patients should be referred for frequent ophthalmologic follow-up to monitor the possible development of retinal detachment. This is particularly important because such retinal holes can be simply sealed by laser therapy, and many of these detachments can be prevented. Many ophthalmologists feel that children with pathologic myopia should be advised to avoid violent sports, such as boxing or football, but should not be otherwise restricted.

Hyperopia

Hyperopia, or farsightedness, exists when the axial length of the eyeball is too short for the refractive power of the cornea-lens combination, and light rays are focused at a point behind the retina (Fig. 40–10). The *normal* infant's eye is short and hyperopic and elongates with growth and development until it reaches normal size at age 9 or 10 years. Most young patients with only a small degree of hyperopia have adequate vision for distance and can accommodate (change the shape of the lens in the eye by

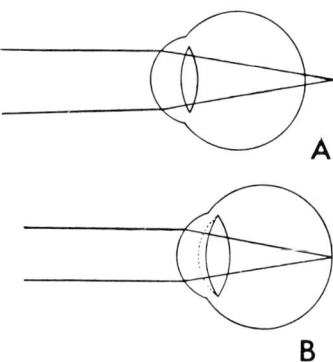

Figure 40-10. *The hyperopic eye.* A, *With accommodation relaxed.* B, *Effect of accommodation on parallel rays. (From Scheie, H. G., and Albert, D. M.: Textbook of Ophthalmology. 9th Ed. Philadelphia, W. B. Saunders Co., 1977, p. 269).*

the action of the ciliary muscle) and focus the light rays for clear near vision. When this accommodative effort becomes symptomatogenic, e.g., blurred print, ocular aching, or fatigue when reading, lenses may be prescribed. Frequently, a very hyperopic child will develop an esotropia caused by the overconvergence associated with constant effort at accommodation. These patients may be dramatically helped with the use of proper glasses.

Hyperopic patients must be examined with the use of cycloplegic drops that eliminate the patient's ability to accommodate, which may give a false refractive measurement.

Astigmatism

Astigmatism, or corneal asphericity, occurs when the curvature in one meridian of the cornea is bent more, i.e., has a shorter radius, than the curvature in the meridian at right angle. This condition is congenital and genetically determined. The normal cornea is spherical in shape, each meridian having the same curvature, and thus is comparable to a hemisphere. The curvature of the astigmatic cornea could be thought of as being similar to the curvature of a spoon. The difference between the two curvatures varies from a slight degree, 0.5 diopter, to a marked difference of 3 to 5 or more diopters.

People with astigmatism cannot achieve a clear retinal image of an object at any distance, so there is a constant reflex stimulus to accommodate. This is futile, since accommodation cannot improve the visual acuity, and the constant effort results in symptoms of eye fatigue. For this reason, most patients with astigmatism should wear glasses at all times and should be examined annually during the period of growth and development to keep up with the corneal anatomic changes.

The treatment involved for such patients is the prescription of cylindrical lenses that bend light in only one meridian and can balance the refractive error produced by the cornea in the same meridian. Astigmatism, however, is rarely an isolated condition, but occurs in patients with varying degrees of myopia or hyperopia. A compound or combined spherical and cylindrical lens is therefore most often prescribed.

Presbyopia

Presbyopia is the condition in which, with increasing age, a loss of ciliary muscle function or a loss of elasticity of the lens fibers, or both, result in the inability to focus on close objects. This usually becomes more apparent in patients over 40 years of age. In the generally accepted theory of accommodation, the contraction of the ring of ciliary muscle releases the normal tension of the lens capsule, allowing the elastic lens fibers to bulge forward and thereby increasing the refractive power of the lens. The decrease in accommodative ability continues gradually until about age 60, at which time virtually no accommodative ability remains. Treatment consists of prescribing a convex lens for the patient for reading, in addition to any refractive correction that he may already have. The power of this lens will vary from 1 diopter for patients in their early 40's to 2½ diopters by age 60.

Contact Lenses

Contact lenses are becoming increasingly popular and are now owned by millions of people in the United States. The family physician should be aware that corneal metabolism is affected by any contact lens and should suggest that his patient be fitted only by someone who has the training and the time to regularly evaluate these metabolic changes. He should also know and tell the patient about the advantages and disadvantages of the various types of lenses.

The two basic lens types available now are the hard lenses and the soft lenses, each giving marked cosmetic improvement and wider range of peripheral vision, particularly for high myopes. They are both particularly useful for patients who participate in sports, for whom spectacles would be inconvenient. Both types are safe if fitted properly, i.e., using biomicroscopic techniques. Care must be taken by the patient to ensure that the lenses are kept sterile during storage and are clean during insertion and removal.

Hard lenses have the disadvantage of a longer, more uncomfortable adaptive period and a longer, blurrier transition period when switching to regular glasses. The usual maximum wearing time for hard lenses is only 10 to 14 hours a day, and it is necessary to wear them regularly to obtain adaptation.

By contrast, the increasingly popular hydrogel or soft lens has a very short and comfortable adaptive period and can be worn from 16 to 18 hours a day. Intermittent wear is also feasible, with no need for readaptation after not wearing the lenses for some time. The major disadvantages of the soft lens are variations in visual acuity caused by the state of hydration of the lens, which may change because of a number of factors. There is also a poor visual correction when the patient has corneal astigmatism. The nightly sterilization process of boiling or chemical disinfection is somewhat more time-consuming than with hard lenses.

In general, the family physician may feel free to recommend contact lenses to his patients with the assurance that most people can wear them comfortably and safely.

PATHOLOGY OF THE OUTER EYE

Ocular pathology will be discussed in terms of diseases of the outer eye and the inner eye. Those conditions that affect the outer eye are strabismus and amblyopia; disorders of the lids and lacrimal apparatus, conjunctiva, and cornea; and trauma.

Strabismus and Amblyopia

Strabismus is an ocular deviation from the normal position of fusion and is an impor-

tant problem for the family physician to detect. Although only about 2 per cent of children develop strabismus, the functional and cosmetic consequences are so great that this condition should be detected at the earliest possible time. Early detection of eye disorders may prevent profound behavioral problems in the child and subsequent difficulties for his family. Learning disabilities and impaired relationships with self and peers are examples of problems facing such children that the family physician must be concerned with and knowledgeable about. An understanding of the intellectual capabilities and personality profiles of those involved is more likely to be apparent to a family physician than to any other member of the health care team. Indeed, the family physician may see patients with a variety of behavioral problems unrelated to the eye problem. He should therefore be of constant supportive help to the family and the ophthalmologist in the frequently prolonged and difficult task of treating amblyopia or visual loss due to cerebral suppression of the vision from a deviating eye.

Strabismus. This disorder may be classified descriptively as a horizontal deviation or "tropia," in which case it will be either an *esotropia* (convergent strabismus or "crossed-eyes") or an *exotropia* (divergent strabismus or "wall-eyes") (Fig. 40–11). Vertical deviations also exist concomitantly with the horizontal abnormalities and are termed *hypertropias*, in which one eye is notably higher in position than the other eye. Strabismus may also be classified in terms of nonparalytic and paralytic forms. In

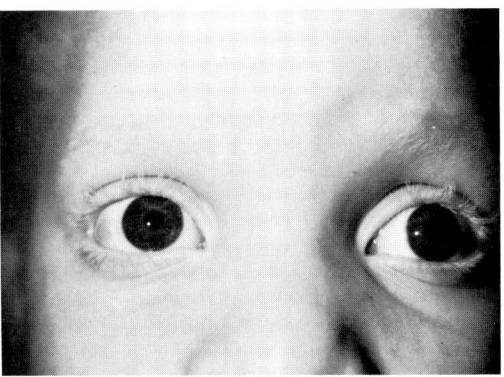

Figure 40–11. *Exotropia. (From Scheie, H. G., and Albert, D. M.: Textbook of Ophthalmology. 9th Ed. Philadelphia, W. B. Saunders Co., 1977, p. 341.)*

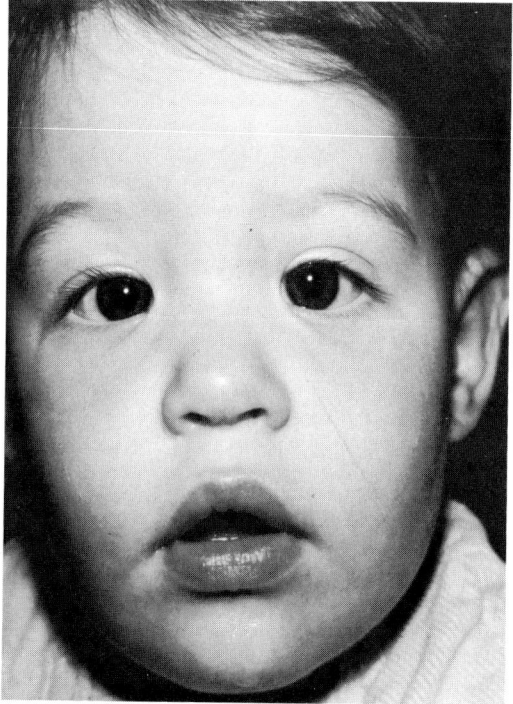

Figure 40–12. *Pseudostrabismus. Marked epicanthal folds cover the medial sclera and give the false impression of esotropia. However, the light reflexes from both corneas can be seen to be in identical positions. (From Scheie, H. G., and Albert, D. M.: Textbook of Ophthalmology. 9th Ed. Philadelphia, W. B. Saunders Co., 1977, p. 337.)*

paralytic disorders, a rectus or oblique muscle will not move the eye in its particular field of action, whereas in the more common nonparalytic forms of strabismus, each eye can be observed to move in all directions of gaze.

Pseudostrabismus is an optical illusion with which the family physician should be acquainted. This is most commonly seen in a young child with a broad epicanthus, whose eyes appear grossly convergent, but in actuality are straight (Fig. 40–12).

The inner portion of the sclera is obscured by the overlying skin fold of the epicanthus and gives the appearance, particularly on lateral gaze, of one eye's being esotropic. The orthophoric or *normal muscle status* can be detected by observing the reflection of a pocketlight in the exact center of each pupil and by obtaining a negative cover test result.

The basic cause of strabismus may be congenital factors, refractive errors, or neurologic disorders.

It should be noted that the intermittent crossing of an infant's eyes until he is about 4 months of age may be considered a normal development of convergence ability. This should *not* be regarded lightly, however, if the crossing is constant or does not disappear by 6 months of age. Other congenital factors include a familial frequency in siblings or parental siblings, or both, which strongly suggests a genetic determinant. There may also be anatomic changes, such as muscular fibrosis or fascial bands, that may account for a small number of cases of strabismus.

The refractive error of hyperopia is a common cause of what is known as accommodative esotropia (Fig. 40–13). This results in a breakdown in the relationship between accommodation and convergence of the eyes and usually occurs between the ages of 2 and 4 years. The uncorrected farsightedness results in a constant demand on the accommodative ability of the lens to bring things into focus for the child. Ordinarily, the act of accommodating is restricted to near vision and is accompanied by the act of convergence of the eyes. The relatively constant stimuli to the medial recti muscles to converge during the process of accommodating eventually results in a constant esotropia.

The opposite condition, that of an uncorrected myopia in a child, may result in the absence of any need to accommodate for near vision, as the myopic eye is in focus only for near objects. In some patients, this will result in the development of an exotropia due to lack of stimulus to the medial recti muscles.

Neurologic disorders, more commonly seen in adults, may affect cranial nerves III, IV, and VI, causing an isolated paralytic strabismus.

TREATMENT. The treatment techniques for strabismus may be refractive, orthoptic, surgical, or a combination of these.

Any refractive errors (myopia, hyperopia, or astigmatism) should be corrected as early as possible. This correction may indeed be curative for patients with accommodative estropia or for some patients with intermittent exotropia, which is related to myopia. Orthoptic treatment, which involves the use of various techniques and training to "exer-

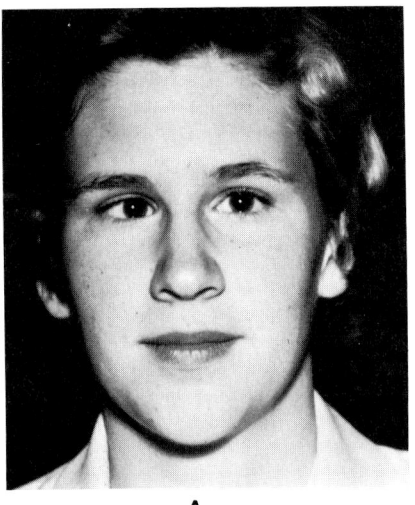
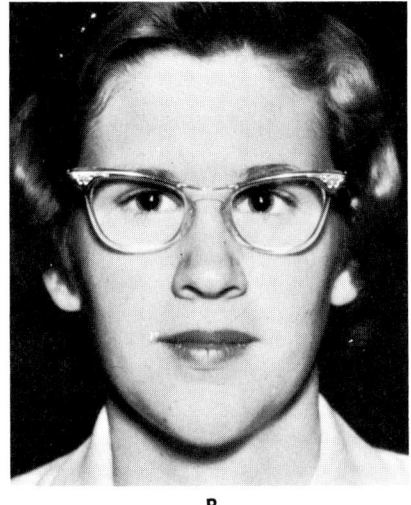

A B

Figure 40-13. A, *Manifest accommodative esotropia, uncorrected.* B, *Corrected accommodative esotropia. (From Scheie, H. G., and Albert, D. M.: Textbook of Ophthalmology. 9th Ed. Philadelphia, W. B. Saunders Co., 1977, pp. 338 and 339.)*

cise" the fusion faculty to bring the eyes into proper alignment, is occasionally helpful. The careful surgical repositioning of properly selected muscles will most often give cosmetic improvement but will far less often effect a functional cure, i.e., re-establishment of normal fusion.

Amblyopia. This emphasis on fusion is relevant to the very important subject of amblyopia, the uncorrectable reduction in visual acuity in an eye that is normal on ophthalmoscopic examination. This condition is found in about 2 per cent of the young adult population. It is primarily due to some form of strabismus, with a small number of cases being caused by other rare disorders. The typical case occurs in a child with monocular esotropia. When one eye is constantly turned in, there is no attempt to alternate the eyes for fixation, and the deviating eye is rarely used. The deviating eye receives a retinal image that, when transmitted to the cerebral cortex, produces such confusion with the image received from the fixing eye that the higher cerebral centers in some way suppress the stimuli from the deviating eye. This cerebral process of maintaining "visual homeostasis" becomes so adaptive that in a very short time the vision in the deviating eye is greatly reduced and cannot be improved unless strenuous retraining is undertaken at the earliest possible age. This is best done

before 4 years of age, and certainly before age 6 if positive results are to be expected.

TREATMENT. The treatment consists of occluding or patching the good eye constantly, literally 24 hours a day, while stimulating the uncovered amblyopic eye by various visual "exercises." This may take months and may have to be continued intermittently for a year or longer.

The need for a positive role by the family physician is mandatory with these patients. The great inconvenience to the child and the psychic trauma involved are bound to be reflected in the entire family situation. The family physician, by reassuring the child and the parents of the value of this difficult therapy in preventing the development of an essentially blind eye, can help ensure bringing the treatment process to a successful conclusion. The family physician can also provide a primary amblyopia detection service by establishing a simple vision test for children when they reach 3 years of age. He can purchase (from Cooper Laboratories) or can easily make a large cut-out cardboard or wood "E" for the child to hold and five cards, each with a printed "E" of different sizes—20/20, 20/40, 20/60, 20/80, and 20/100. The examiner stands at a distance of 20 feet; rotates the largest "E" card up, right, left, or down; and asks the child to match his cut-out "E" to the position on the examiner's card. Proceeding

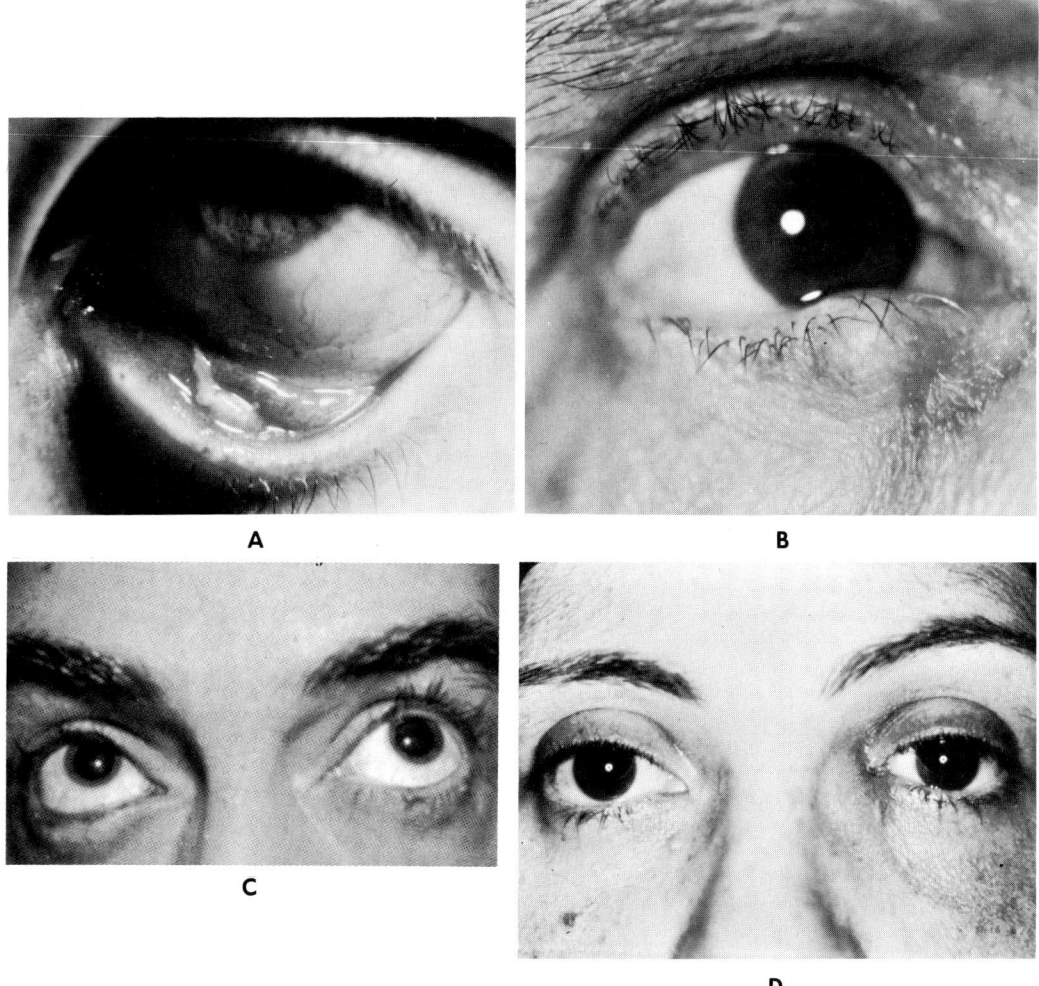

Figure 40-14.   *External disease. A, Stye. B, Chalazion. C, Blepharitis. D, Dacryocystitis. (From Scheie, H. G., and Albert, D. M.: Textbook of Ophthalmology. 9th Ed. Philadelphia, W. B. Saunders Co., 1977, pp. 361, 381, 382, 385.)*

to the smallest-sized cards and comparing one eye with the other, it can easily be determined if there is a substantial difference in vision between the two eyes.

Disorders of the Lids and Lacrimal Apparatus

The common entities of the lids and lacrimal apparatus that will be encountered in a family practice setting are stye, or hordeolum; chalazion; blepharitis, either allergic or infectious; ectropion; entropion; traumatic ecchymosis, or "black-eye"; and lacrimal tract disorders, either congenital or acquired.

Hordeolum.   A hordeolum is an infection in the root of an eyelash or in a sebaceous gland on the lid margin (Fig. 40-14A). It is usually staphylococcal in origin and is introduced by finger contamination. Therapy consists of the application of hot packs three to four times a day and the use of an antibiotic ointment containing neomycin or sulfacetamide. If the lesion is resistant to

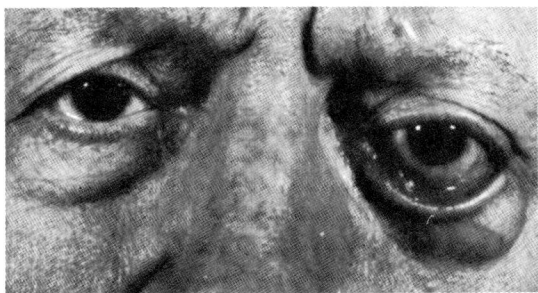

Figure 40–15. Ectropion. (From Fox, S.: Ophthalmic Plastic Surgery. 1st Ed. New York, Grune & Stratton, Inc., 1970, p. 273. By permission.)

this treatment and is well localized, a small incision will facilitate drainage.

Chalazion. A chalazion is a deeper localized nodule in the lid, consisting of a meibomian gland abscess in the tarsus that has progressed to a granuloma and usually bulges on the conjunctival surface (Fig. 40–14B). It may be caused by various bacterial agents and is usually noninflammatory and noninfective when seen. Antibiotics are not of much value. Local heat may result in some regression, but the lesion is best excised totally under local anesthesia through the conjunctival approach. Although not a difficult procedure, excision can result in considerable bleeding and scarring and should be performed by an ophthalmologist.

Blepharitis. The allergic type of blepharitis is usually caused by a form of contact dermatitis related to either medication or cosmetics (Fig. 40–14C). The lids usually appear acutely swollen and erythematous, or thickened reddish patches at the inner half of the upper lids may occur. Treatment consists of eliminating any causative agent and applying cold packs and steroid ointment.

The infectious type of blepharitis is much more common and is usually associated with seborrhea, complicated by staphylococcal infection. The scaling and redness around the lashes seen in large numbers of children and in many adults is usually not related to refractive errors or eye strain. Accordingly, the treatment must be prolonged and recurrent, as the condition is chronic with frequent exacerbations. The

seborrhea of the scalp and brows should be controlled with a shampoo such as selenium sulfide (Selsun). Mechanical removal of the scales by applying hot packs followed by massage with a moistened cotton swab (Q-tip) is an essential step prior to the application of any medication. A steroid antibiotic ointment, such as Ophthocort, Metimyd, or NeoDecadron, is applied after lid massage at least twice daily. If the lids are severely inflamed, a course of systemic antibiotics, such as ampillicin or tetracycline, is indicated.

Ectropion. An ectropion is a relaxation of the muscle along the lid margin, usually occurring with senility, that causes the lower eye lid to droop downward and outward from the globe (Fig. 40–15). A simple oculoplastic procedure can correct the condition and prevent the severe, chronic conjunctivitis that would otherwise accompany it.

Entropion. This is a condition in which the marginal muscle of the lid is tightened or spastic and causes the lid margin and lashes to roll inward, rubbing upon the cornea (Fig. 40–16). Again, a relatively simple oculoplastic procedure will correct the condition and prevent the gross corneal damage that would occur from chronic rubbing by the lashes.

Traumatic Ecchymosis. A "black-eye" or ecchymosis under the skin from trauma is due to a rupture of vessels against the underlying bone of the orbit. The simple type requires only applications of cold compresses for 24 hours followed by warm compresses to hasten the absorption of the

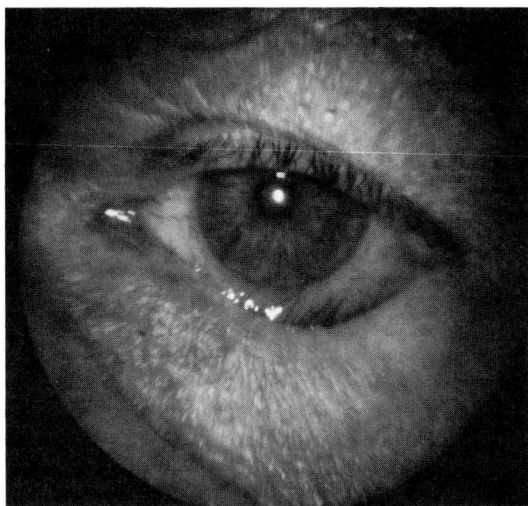

Figure 40–16. *Entropion.*

blood. The eye, however, should always be examined for damage to the cornea or the anterior chamber. A test for diplopia in all fields of gaze should be performed to rule out the possibility of an orbital floor fracture.

Lacrimal Tract Disorders. A common type of lacrimal tract disorder occurs in infants in whom stenosis or an imperforate opening of the nasolacrimal duct into the nose causes a tearing eye. Perhaps 1 per cent of newborns have this to some degree, and treatment should be attempted as follows: After the removal of any discharge with moistened cotton, a solution of polymyxin-B, neomycin, and gramicidin (Neosporin Ophthalmic Solution) should be instilled into the inner canthus of the eye every 2 hours. Following this instillation, pressure should be exerted with the small finger over the sac of the inner canthus, pressing the sac against the nose. If no improvement occurs in the tearing or if a discharge continues by the age of 2 to 3 months, the infant should be referred for probing of the nasolacrimal duct. This is usually done under general anesthesia and is almost always curative.

In older children or adults, a *dacryocystitis,* or infection of the tear sac, may occur, usually secondary to some form of acquired dacryostenosis or narrowing of the nasolacrimal canals (see Fig. 40–14*D*). This will result in a swollen and tender tear sac that is usually filled with pus. If treatment with systemic and local antibiotics does not result in improvement, referral to an oph-

thalmologist should be made for a possible surgical incision of the sac or, if needed, a dacryocystorhinostomy to form a new bony aperture between the lacrimal sac and the nasal cavity.

Disorders of the Conjunctiva

The conjunctival lesions that are commonly encountered are conjunctivitis — bacterial, viral, or allergic; pinguecula; pterygium; and subconjunctival hemorrhage.

Conjunctivitis *Acute bacterial conjunctivitis,* usually referred to as "pink-eye," is most often caused by *Staphylococcus.* One usually sees both bulbar and palpebral conjunctival injection with a mucoid or mucopurulent discharge. A more chronic form exists, which is also caused by *Staphylococcus,* but which may be due to an inadequately treated previous acute phase or to a coexistent meibomitis. There is less injection and discharge in the chronic form, but the infection is quite resistant to treatment. Therapy, in general, consists of frequent irrigation and removal of any discharge formed and the *frequent* use of antibiotic drops. The use of an hourly regimen of neomycin-polymyxin or sulfacetamide is recommended for 2 to 3 days, to be tapered off gradually as the condition improves. A complementary antibiotic ointment, such as chloramphenicol (Chloromycetin) or erythromycin (Ilotycin), is instilled in the lower fornix at bedtime. Neomycin with polymyxin B and bacitracin (Neosporin) is extremely useful, particularly when the presence of *Pseudomonas* is suspected, and is often prescribed by ophthalmologists. However, one should always be aware of the possibility of an allergic reaction to neomycin and should observe the eyelids carefully for any sign of erythema. If an allergic reaction does develop, the patient should be told that a future application of any neomycin product is likely to exacerbate the allergic reaction started by the previous use of neomycin eye drops.

The *viral form of conjunctivitis,* not always distinguishable from the bacterial form, is usually seen as fine follicles on the conjunctiva of the lids and is the lymphoid reaction to the virus. There is generally less redness and less discharge than that seen in bacterial conjunctivitis. In such patients it is very important to stain the cornea with fluorescein to rule out the possibility of either punctate or herpetic lesions. Treatment consists of controlling any secondary infection by use of a topical antibiotic regimen, as just outlined. If one can be certain that there is no herpes infection, topical steroid eye drops may also be used for symptomatic relief.

Allergic conjunctivitis occurs primarily as vernal conjunctivitis and as toxic or drug-induced conjunctivitis. Vernal conjunctivitis is of undetermined origin, affects children in the spring and summer, and is manifested by broad, cobblestone-like follicles on the upper and lower palpebral conjunctivae. The condition gradually subsides as the child reaches adolescence. Treatment is symptomatic for the severe itching and consists of topical steroids (prednisone solution, 0.12 per cent) and vasoconstrictors (naphazoline, 0.1 per cent).

A follicular or velvety reaction of the palpebral conjunctiva is occasionally seen in patients using certain eye medications for long periods of time. A common example is the reaction seen in a number of patients with glaucoma who have used pilocarpine for many years.

Pinguecula. A pinguecula is a small round or triangular yellowish, raised area adjacent to the cornea in the 9 or 3 o'clock position (Fig. 40–17). It is a degenerative, probably hereditary, condition in adults, which is usually not noted until an inflamed conjunctiva causes the lesion to stand out against the reddish background. Although benign, if the pinguecula turns a darker yellow color with age, it may be easily excised for cosmetic reasons.

Pterygium. A pterygium is a vascularized overgrowth of conjunctiva invading the cornea (Fig. 40–18). It is occasionally based

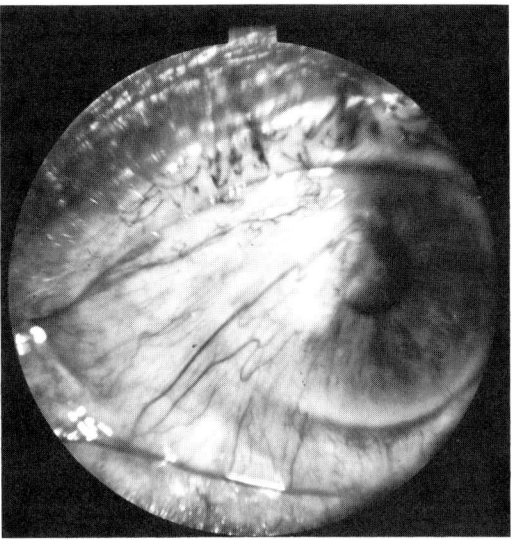

Figure 40–18. A typical nasal pterygium.

in a chronically inflamed pinguecula, grows in a roughly triangular shape, and progresses slowly toward the pupil. This lesion is seen more frequently in tropical areas and is thought to be related to the chronic irritation by wind, dust, and sun. A pterygium is not neoplastic and may be surgically excised if it appears to be growing into the visual area of the cornea.

Subconjunctival Hemorrhage. A subconjunctival hemorrhage is a common occurrence and is responsible for a great deal of anxiety on the part of the patient. The spontaneous rupture of a conjunctival vessel may cause blood to seep between the conjunctiva and sclera that appears as a bright red blotch of blood on the eye. It is usually related to an increase in intravascular pressure in a predisposed sclerotic vessel. Coughing, sneezing, or straining at stool may be some possible causes, but in many instances there appears to be no definitely related causative factor. It is usually *not* due to hypertension or systemic disease, but for assurance, it may be well to measure the blood pressure and perform a blood count to rule out some of these unusual possibilities. The primary treatment consists of reassuring the patient as to its benign nature. Warm compresses and a drop of a vasoconstrictor agent may hasten the absorption, which usually takes approximately 1 or 2 weeks.

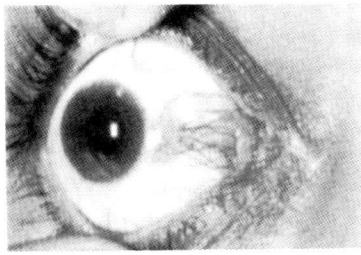

Figure 40–17. Pinguecula. (From Duke-Elder, G.: *System of Ophthalmology. Vol. VIII, Part I. London, Henry Kimpton, Publisher, 1965, p. 570.)*

Disorders of the Cornea

The cornea, 12 mm. in diameter and 0.5 mm. thick, is subject to a wide variety of disorders. Because of the cornea's crucial importance in visual functioning, an attempt will be made to classify these diseases as an aid to diagnosis. One may think of corneal involvement in terms of congenital, inflammatory, metabolic, and traumatic disorders.

Congenital Corneal Disorders. Of the various congenital anomalies, that of megalocornea, a larger corneal diameter than average, and microcornea, a smaller corneal diameter than average, may be observed on gross examination. These abnormalities should be routinely noted in an ophthalmologic examination because of the possible association of each condition with either a severe refractive error or glaucoma.

Inflammatory Corneal Disorders. The inflammatory changes that affect the cornea can be considered in two broad classifications, *keratitis* and *ulceration*. The superficial form of keratitis is usually seen as punctate spots on the cornea that stain with fluorescein. These should be searched for when diagnosing all bacterial and viral infections of the conjunctiva, as the therapy and prognosis would be more involved if they were present than it would be with a simple conjunctivitis. A deeper or interstitial type of keratitis is seen as a deep vascularization of the cornea, which can occur with syphilis or following severe systemic viral disease, such as herpes zoster or mumps.

The most common ulcer of the cornea is

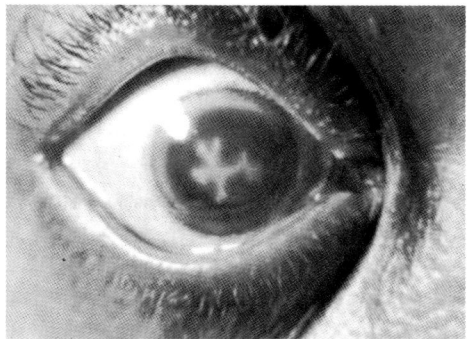

Figure 40–19. Herpes simplex—dendritic keratitis. (From Scheie, H. G., and Albert, D. M.: Textbook of Ophthalmology. 9th Ed. Philadelphia, W. B. Saunders, Co., 1977, p. 361.)'

that caused by the virus of herpes simplex (Fig. 40–19). The herpes virus, which in the dormant or carrier state may be found in the eyes of many patients of all ages, can be triggered by assorted stimuli, such as upper respiratory tract infections, fever, trauma, stress, and so forth to form a dendritic ulcer. The pattern of this ulcer is typically linear and branching. Every inflamed eye should be stained with fluorescein and examined for this lesion because the complications, particularly if exacerbated by the use of topical steroids, can be severe, with possible loss of vision. Therapy consists of the frequent application of the antimetabolite idoxuridine (Stoxil or Herplex) and the possible débridement of the corneal epithelium. Treatment should probably be handled by the ophthalmologist. The role of the family physician in this potentially serious disease should be recognition of the lesion, avoidance of steroids, and counseling the patient as to the potential seriousness of the ulcers.

Bacterial and fungal ulcers appear as circumscribed depressions in a grayish, edematous area of the cornea, which frequently may be caused by pneumococci or staphylococci. A more serious form of the ulcer can be caused by *Pseudomonas* or by various fungi. A severe ulceration, particularly in a debilitated person, may progress to perforation in several days and should be treated intensively by the specialist.

Metabolic Corneal Disorders. Metabolic alterations of the cornea are seen primarily as vascularization, edema, and pigmentary or degenerative changes. Vascularization of the cornea usually occurs secondary to other lesions. It may be seen as the "ciliary flush," or fine vessels at the limbus, e.g., in iritis; as the localized vascularization in acne rosacea, or as the deep vascularization in interstitial keratitis. Gross corneal edema, which is usually seen as a loss of the brilliant clarity of the cornea, may occur as a primary entity, as in disease or degeneration of the corneal endothelium or epithelium. A secondary effect may result from increased intraocular tension.

A degenerative change known as arcus senilis is a bilateral, grayish, ringlike deposit seen in older people (Fig. 40–20). It is about 1 mm. wide and is separated from the limbus by a clear zone. Arcus senilis has no pathologic significance.

The deposits of inflammatory cells on the

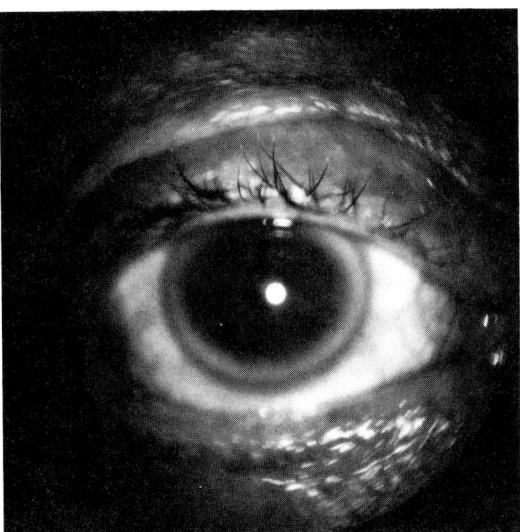

Figure 40-20. *Arcus senilis.*

posterior surface of the cornea, known as keratic precipitates (KP's), indicate the presence of an active or a previous iritis. These deposits may be seen with a loupe but can be best detected with the slit lamp microscope.

Traumatic Corneal Disorders. If a foreign body is present, visual acuity should always be recorded before manipulating the cornea. One should then proceed to instill fluorescein in the eye and examine both the cornea and the upper and lower lids for the presence of other foreign bodies. If the foreign body is not deeply embedded, the physician may instill 0.5 per cent proparacaine into the eye and attempt to lift the foreign body gently off the cornea with a foreign body spud or a 25 gauge hypodermic needle, whose extreme tip has been bent at an angle of approximately 90°. If any rust or discoloration remains, the patient should be referred for removal of the rust ring under the biomicroscope, as this frequently requires the use of a corneal drill. If there is no residual material, an antibiotic ointment (neomycin or chloramphenicol) should be instilled, followed by the use of a *firm* eye pad for 24 hours. At the return visit, if healing is satisfactory, antibiotic drops (sulfacetamide) or a combination of polymyxin B, bacitracin, and neomycin (Neosporin) should be prescribed every 2 hours for 4 to 5 days, and a final examination should be performed at that time to recheck visual acuity.

Abrasions of the corneal epithelium are common from scratches from bushes, fingernails, toys, and paper and may readily be seen after the use of fluorescein (Fluor-I-Strip) staining. The major potential problem, as with a corneal foreign body, is the development of a deep corneal infection once the epithelial protective barrier is damaged. Treatment therefore is similar to that for a foreign body: patching and instillation of an antibiotic ointment for 24 hours followed by use of topical antibiotic drops. The physician should advise the patient, particularly one with a fingernail abrasion, of the possibility of a recurrent erosion. This fairly common complication may result from a spontaneous breakdown of a poorly adherent area of re-epithelialization at some future time. The patient should be informed that he may have the exact symptoms of the original abrasion and that he should consult the physician again.

Laceration into the corneal stroma or into the anterior chamber is an ocular emergency, and the patient should be promptly referred for surgical care.

General Ocular Trauma

The subject of general trauma to the eye or its adnexa deserves special mention, as the sequelae of injury in the orbital region can be so severe and the full extent of the injury so difficult to evaluate that any but obviously minor trauma should be treated by the specialist. The family physician, however, should be aware of several particularly significant factors in ocular trauma.

The severity of *lid lacerations*, for example, depends completely on anatomic position. A superficial laceration parallel to the lid margin may be handled in the usual manner by simply employing fine (6-0 silk) sutures. A laceration, however, that crosses the margin of the upper or lower lid may result in a severe notching deformity if not accurately apposed and so should be handled only by the specialist. If the punctum or canaliculus is severed, a major microsurgical repair is essential to prevent epiphora, or chronic tearing. A deep laceration of the upper lid may injure the levator muscle and result in ptosis if not properly repaired.

Contusion injuries causing a hyphema (blood in the anterior chamber) are of serious import regardless of the amount of blood seen (Fig. 40–21). Complications,

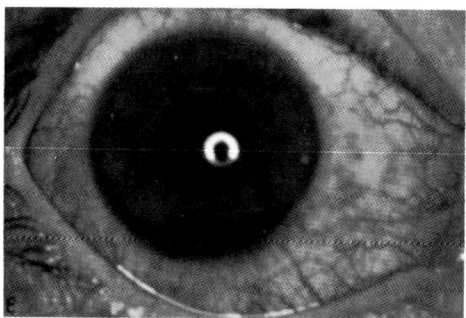

Figure 40–21. *Hyphema. (From Scheie, H. G., and Albert, D. M.: Textbook of Ophthalmology. 9th Ed. Philadelphia, W. B. Saunders Co., 1977, p. 561.)*

such as tears of the iris, traumatic cataract, blood-staining of the cornea, and immediate or long-delayed glaucoma all require intensive operation and care.

The presence of *intraocular foreign bodies* should be considered, even when this is only remotely possible, and x-rays should be ordered. The sequelae of undetected foreign bodies inside the eye are usually disastrous.

Orbital floor fractures of the so-called "blowout" type are seen after direct injury to the orbital rim. A deep subconjunctival hemorrhage following such an injury should lead to suspicion of an orbital floor fracture. Diplopia in any field of gaze is suggestive of fracture, and orbital tomography is essential in diagnosing most floor fractures.

PATHOLOGY OF THE INNER EYE

Glaucoma

Although the cause and pathogenesis of glaucoma are receiving increasing attention and research, many definitive answers are not available.

Glaucoma is a common disease, occurring in about 2 per cent of persons over age 40. In order to understand the importance of screening for this condition in a family practice, it is useful to compare the incidence of other common entities with the incidence of glaucoma. Diabetes is found in 0.8 per cent of the general population, cancer of the cervix in 0.4 per cent of females over 25 years of age, and tuberculosis in 0.1 per cent of the general adult population. It would therefore appear obvious that in a complete physical examination one should include tonometry along with a urinalysis, Papanicolaou smear test, and Tine test.

Glaucoma is manifested by increased intraocular pressure and degenerative changes in the optic nerve, resulting in progressive visual field defects. Physiologically, the continuous formation of aqueous by the ciliary body and the drainage of this fluid via the canal of Schlemm back into the venous system maintain a relatively constant intraocular pressure of less than 20 mm. Hg (Fig. 40–22A). Various neurogenic, hormonal, and mechanical factors control the inflow and outflow of aqueous and determine, when disease occurs, which form of glaucoma may be produced. It is important to note that the physician should be aware of "steroid sensitive" patients. Approximately 25 to 35 per cent of the adult population may react with an increase in intraocular tension to the use of steroid eye drops over a period of more than 1 or 2 weeks.

It is useful to classify glaucoma into the following categories:
1. Primary glaucoma.
   a. Congenital glaucoma.
   b. Adult glaucoma.
      (1) Open angle or chronic simple type, the type most frequently seen.
      (2) Narrow angle or acute angle closure type.
2. Secondary glaucoma.
   a. Increased intraocular tension occurring with trauma, neoplasm, or intraocular inflammation.

Congenital Glaucoma. This is a rare recessive genetic disease, usually with bilateral involvement, characterized by enlarged hazy corneas causing tearing and photophobia. Surgery for these patients is essential to prevent blindness and consists of opening the occluded drainage meshwork by a procedure known as goniotomy.

Open Angle Glaucoma. This form of glaucoma occurs when the obstruction to the aqueous outflow is not caused by the mechanical blockage of the root of the iris, but is located elsewhere within the drainage network (Fig. 40–22B–H). Diagnosis is generally made by routine tonometry, as visual or other subjective symptoms are usually absent. When gross visual field defects or marked cupping of the optic disc

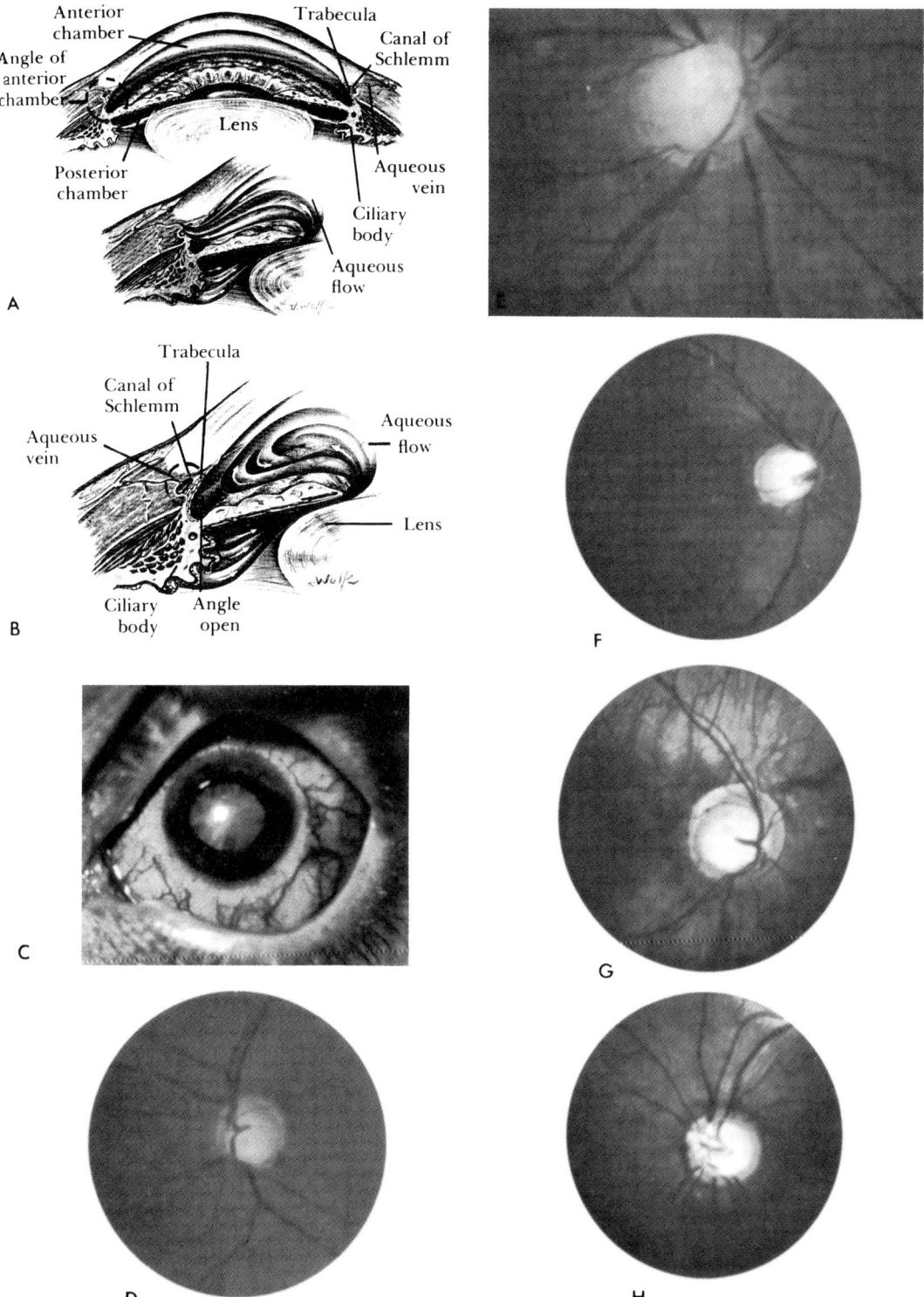

Figure 40-22.   A, *Drawing that shows flow of aqueous from ciliary body leaving eye through the trabecula and canal of Schlemm via a normal open, wide angle. B, Chronic simple glaucoma. Arrows indicate obstruction to aqueous outflow in angle wall. C, Dilated vessels of caput medusa with advanced glaucoma. D, Early glaucoma cupping. E, Moderate glaucoma cupping. F, Moderately advanced glaucoma cupping. G, Advanced glaucoma cupping. H, Very advanced glaucoma cupping with atrophy. (From Scheie, H. G., and Albert, D. M.: Textbook of Ophthalmology. 9th Ed. Philadelphia, W. B. Saunders Co., 1977, p. 523.)*

occurs, the disease is well advanced toward causing blindness.

Treatment is primarily medical, consisting of pilocarpine drops to increase the aqueous outflow, topical epinephrine derivatives to decrease aqueous formation, and systemic carbonic anhydrase inhibitors, e.g., acetazolamide (Diamox), to further decrease aqueous production. If medical therapy does not control the pressure and stabilize the visual fields, an "aqueous filtering" area is formed surgically. This opening in the sclera allows aqueous to seep under and be absorbed by the conjunctiva. The popular procedure currently being used to establish this opening is known as trabeculectomy. It is noteworthy that since the iris does *not* block the angle in this disease, drugs that dilate the pupil are *not* contraindicated. The usual warning against the use of sympathomimetic drugs in patients with glaucoma applies only to narrow angle glaucoma.

Narrow Angle Glaucoma. Narrow angle glaucoma occurs in the anatomic configuration in which the periphery of the iris is very close to the cornea. Contact of the iris root with the trabeculum may occur in predisposed persons, completely blocking the outflow of the aqueous fluid. Although far less common than the open angle type, an angle closure attack can be a dramatic emergency. Typical symptoms include ocular pain radiating to the forehead and cheek, accompanied by blurred vision. Gastrointestinal symptoms are frequent and indeed may occasionally mask the eye complaint and mislead the diagnostician. When the diagnosis is confirmed by the presence of a dilated, fixed pupil, cloudy cornea, and a high tonometric reading, the patient should be immediately referred to a specialist for treatment.

Although intensive medical treatment may terminate an acute attack, the primary therapy is surgical. A peripheral iridectomy acts as a safety valve, preventing the iris diaphragm from being pushed against the trabecular meshwork.

In summary, glaucoma is a relatively common, insidious disease that should be diagnosed by the family physician. Glaucoma is still the cause of 15 per cent of the cases of blindness in adults in the United States, and early diagnosis constitutes the best public health approach toward reducing this percentage.

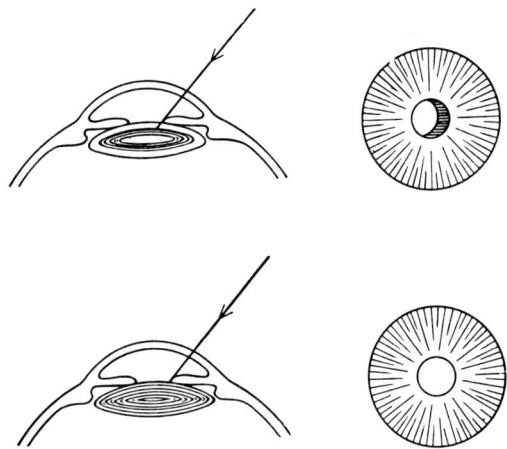

Figure 40–23. Cataract, maturity determination. A, In immature cataract a shadow of the iris appears by oblique illumination. B, Shadow is absent in mature cataract. (From Duke-Elder, G.: System of Ophthalmology. Vol. II. London, Henry Kimpton, Publisher, 1965, p. 146.)

Cataract

A cataract, technically, is any opacity or decreased clarity of the lens or its capsule (Fig. 40–23). With the slit lamp biomicroscope, one can see such change in most adults, but the term is usually reserved for clinically significant, vision-reducing opacities.

The basic cause of cataracts is still unknown, despite a great amount of research. However, it is known that denaturation of the lens fiber protein and imbibition of fluid through the lens capsule play a role.

Diagnosis is readily made by examining a dilated pupil with the ophthalmoscope. The specific location and degree of the opacities can only be seen with the biomicroscope. Cataract formation may be divided into five general categories: congenital, senile, complicated, traumatic, and toxic.

Congenital Cataract. These opacities may be either unilateral or bilateral, can generally be seen at birth, and may remain stationary or progress further. About 25 per cent of congenital cataracts are inherited, and a substantial number are due to intrauterine rubella. In counseling the parents, it is important to be aware of several prognostic factors. If the cataracts are bilateral and dense with no other ocular abnormality, e.g., nystagmus or microphthalmos, surgery should be performed early, at about 6 months of age, to prevent amblyopia. Visual prognosis for such patients should be about 20/70 or better. If there are associated anomalies, the vision will be considerably less, and the prognosis is guarded.

The problem in treating unilateral cataracts in patients with good vision in the other eye is the frequent development of an insurmountable amblyopia after surgery. Many ophthalmologists feel that surgery for monocular cataracts is unwarranted because of difficulties with the essential postoperative contact lens and the poor visual results under the best circumstances. However, if the lens is quite opaque and white, surgery may be performed for cosmetic reasons.

Senile Cataract. Some patients in their 40's may develop senile cataract, but it is seen more often in patients in their 60's, increasing in frequency with advancing age. The cataracts are usually bilateral, with one more advanced than the other; the rate of progression is variable. When the decrease in visual acuity interferes with the patient's ability to function in any desired manner, the cataract should be removed.

When the cataractous lens is surgically removed, the eye is termed "aphakic" (without lens), and the concept of monocular aphakia is important to review. An aphakic eye sees very little unless a strong convex lens, about +12.00 diopters, is placed in front of it to refract light onto the retina. This "cataract spectacle" magnifies the retinal image about 30 per cent more than the image of the other eye, creating a "size" diplopia that is intolerable. This problem had previously been resolved by waiting until both eyes needed surgery, as bilateral image magnification creates little difficulty.

Since fairly recently, monocular aphakia has been successfully overcome by the use of either a hard or a soft contact lens to afford the necessary refractive power without the intolerable image size difference. Very recently, the intraocular lens implant, a plastic insert suspended within the pupil at the time of surgery, was also found to eliminate the problems of monocular aphakia without the need for daily insertion of a contact lens. The long-term result of this advance is not yet available, but it shows great promise.

It would be a service to the elderly patient if the family physician, who is aware of the patient's needs and abilities, would advise him of the ideal time for surgery and the various means available to correct monocular aphakia.

Complicated Cataracts. These are lens opacities resulting from or related to some intraocular or systemic disease process. Some common causes of complicated cataract are chronic iritis, severe glaucoma, retinal detachment, diabetes, pathologic myopia, and certain dermatologic conditions such as atopic dermatitis.

Traumatic Cataracts. Such cataracts can ensue following a blunt contusion to the eye or after a penetrating injury, with or without the presence of an intraocular foreign body. After any such injury, the eye should be examined periodically for several years to observe the possible delayed formation of a lens opacity. Other forms of energy, e.g., heat (glassblowers' cataract), radiation, or high voltage electricity, may induce cataract formation.

Toxic Cataracts. These lesions are formed as a result of the chronic ingestion of certain drugs, especially of steroid preparations. Long-term, high-dosage steroids can create changes in newly forming lens cells, resulting in radiating lines appearing under the posterior capsule of the lens. Other drugs such as the phenothiazines may also be cataractogenic.

Cataract Extraction

The surgical technique of cataract extraction, the most common eye operation, may be of interest to review. Briefly, an incision is made at the limbus, opening the cornea from about the 9 o'clock to the 3 o'clock position. A small peripheral iridectomy, or hole in the iris, is made to prevent any possible postoperative glaucoma. The lens is secured with a cryoprobe; the zonulae, or attachments to the ciliary body, are carefully broken; and the lens is delivered through the pupil and out through the corneoscleral incision. This incision is then sutured with multiple interrupted or running very fine sutures (7–0 to 10–0).

This recent improved suturing technique has allowed very early ambulation, the same or the following day, and hospital discharge from 1 to 4 days postoperatively. The former restrictions on activity have been greatly relaxed, and postoperative care usually consists of steroid-antibiotic drops, often combined with a drop of atropine to relieve any postoperative iritis. Recent publicity about "new" techniques of cataract extraction involving ultrasonic instrumentation to fragment and remove the lens would seem to imply a "breakthrough." In actuality, a modification of technique is all that is involved, and the final decision about choice of procedure should be left to the ophthalmic surgeon.

Knowledge of the surgical technique and postoperative course is imperative for the family physician, so that he may be able to clearly and thoroughly counsel his patients. Although most ophthalmologists are willing and able to prepare the patient emotionally for the surgery, the relationship between patient and family physician, referred to earlier, is more likely to be successful in such preparation. It is, therefore, essential that the family physician have firsthand knowledge of the surgical procedure and postoperative course by observing many such procedures in the operating room and by following the patient in the hospital postoperatively.

More importantly, the present procedures for evaluating patients medically for this and other operative procedures are incomplete. The family physician should be capable of knowing the physical condition of the patient and matching the physical status to the appropriate surgical procedure, but there is much more. The patient with a cataract is a total person with individual capabilities, needs, and desires as well as a person with physical disorders. An elderly patient confined to a wheelchair because of arthritis who is also in congestive heart failure may be easily declared unfit for surgery for medical reasons. The physician must assess more than the physical condition. This same patient who is confined to a severely limited life style may have little reason to live except for those few pleasures that are available only through his ability to see. Reading, watching television, seeing relatives, or just seeing the beauty of nature may be all that the patient wants. Ignoring the possibility of this patient's regaining sight is to deny him the right to live. The ophthalmologist is not looking for computerized assessment preoperatively but for a total consultation to help him make his decision regarding surgery. The primary physician with the scientific knowledge and the capability of understanding and respecting the patient's wishes and behavior is the most qualified consultant.

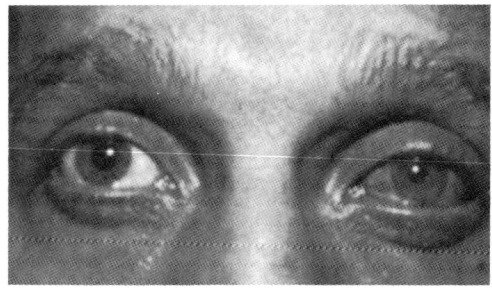

Figure 40-24. Acute iritis. Note size of pupils. (From Scheie, H. G., and Albert, D. M.: Textbook of Ophthalmology. 9th Ed. Philadelphia, W. B. Saunders Co., 1977, p. 13.)

Uveitis

The uveal tract consists of the iris, which continues into the ciliary body, which, in turn, progresses posteriorly into the choroid. These three areas, anatomically, embryologically, and physiologically related, are usually involved in similar inflammatory processes, generally referred to as uveitis. If primarily involving the iris, the inflammation is referred to as iritis (Fig. 40-24). If, less commonly, the ciliary body is the primary site, the process is called a cyclitis. The choroid alone is frequently involved as a choroiditis or as a chorioretinitis when the overlying retina is also usually involved.

Of major interest to the family physician is iritis (anterior uveitis), as this inflammation may pose a diagnostic problem in differentiating it from glaucoma and conjunctivitis (Table 40-1). Anterior uveitis is of unknown cause in many instances. It is felt to be a hypersensitivity reaction to systemic bacteria or to allergenic or toxic agents and may be related to the various collagen diseases. The presenting symptoms of ocular pain and photophobia, with deep redness around the cornea and a small or miotic pupil, should be suggestive of uveitis. The definitive diagnosis can be made only with the slit lamp biomicroscope, which will reveal white blood cells in the aqueous and clumps of cells that have precipitated on the corneal endothelium (KP's). This disease must be treated actively by the ophthalmologist with steroids and atropine to prevent the possible complications of glaucoma and pupillary occlusion.

When an inflammatory lesion affects the choroid specifically, it may be found in three general locations. If the lesion affects the far

TABLE 40-1. THE DIFFERENTIAL DIAGNOSIS OF THE RED EYE*

	Acute Conjunctivitis	Acute Iritis	Acute Glaucoma
Etiology	Usually bacterial (also virus, fungus, or allergy)	Uveal inflammation	Blockage of canal of Schlemm
Symptoms	Irritation—mild foreign body sensation	Eye ache with light sensitivity	Pain and severely blurred vision, nausea, and vomiting
Vision	Normal	Normal to hazy	Markedly impaired
External Signs	Diffuse bright red injection, both palpebral and bulbar conjunctiva Mucopurulent discharge	Purple-red circumcorneal injection of bulbar conjunctiva with tearing	Diffuse injection of bulbar conjunctiva, steamy cornea with tearing, shallow anterior chamber
Pupil	Normal	Constricted	Dilated
Intraocular Pressure	Normal	Normal or low	Very elevated (over 35 mm. Hg)
Prognosis	Usually excellent Rapid response to antibiotics when caused by bacteria.	Slow response to steroids and mydriatics Frequent exacerbations	Needs immediate medical and surgical therapy Good visual result if treated, early

*From Demorest, B.: Ophthalmology. In Conn, H. F., Rakel, R. E., and Johnson, T. W. (eds.): Family Practice. 1st Ed. Philadelphia, W. B. Saunders Co., 1973.

anterior choroid, it is referred to as a *pars planitis*, or peripheral uveitis. This is very difficult to see without indirect ophthalmoscopy and scleral indentation. The family physician may suspect such a lesion if the vitreous is hazy and no other focal signs are seen.

In the posterior choroid, lesions usually involve the overlying retina and appear as puffy white patches of exudate, single or multiple, with varying degrees of vitreous haze. Lesions may also appear adjacent to the disc, appearing as a pseudo-optic neuritis, known as Jensen's juxtapapillary chorioretinitis.

In all instances of chorioretinitis (posterior uveitis), diagnosis and treatment are very difficult, and patients should be immediately referred for specialty care.

RETINAL DISEASE

The retina is not only the site of many common and serious diseases of the eye; it also represents the well-known "mirror" of several systemic entities that are reflected and manifested to the observer by the changes that they create in the retina. Retinal disease may be categorized arbitrarily in order of the most frequently encountered entities:

1. Vascular diseases including sclerotic changes, hypertensive changes, and occlusive disorders.

2. Diabetic retinopathy.
3. Diseases peculiar to the macular area.
4. Detachment of the retina.
5. Tumors of the fundus. To be perfectly correct, all of these do not involve the retinal cells, but they are usually manifested as a mass involving the retina, originating most often in the cells of the choroid.

VASCULAR DISEASES

Perhaps the principal use of the fundus examination by the family physician will be in evaluating the vascular changes of arteriosclerosis and hypertension. At this point, it is important to review some vascular anatomy, particularly retinal vascular structure.

The essential difference between an artery and an arteriole is the presence of an intimal elastic lamina in the former and a patchwork, rather than a continuous, muscle layer in the latter. Most retinal vessels are arterioles; the exception is the central retinal artery and its branches on the disc.

Sclerotic and Hypertensive Changes

Arteriosclerosis is a general term referring to degenerative disease of any part of the arterial system. Some types affect specifically large arteries, e.g., Mönckeberg's sclerosis, senile ectasia; others cause an intimal thickening and thus can affect only true arteries. Therefore, the only type of arteriosclerosis that affects the major part of the retinal vascular tree is arteriolar sclerosis. The central retinal artery is affected by another form of arteriosclerosis, known as intimal atherosclerosis, and these two conditions should be carefully differentiated. They are frequently confused even by the ophthalmologist, and a clear distinction is important, as they represent different disease processes.

Arteriolar sclerosis is a condition caused by the physical stress of hypertension on the vessel wall. It involves all of the body's arterioles uniformly, and the changes seen in the fundus vessels reflect those of other vital areas. The pathologic change that occurs is a diffuse infiltration of hyaline material under the endothelium that gradually involves the rest of the arteriolar wall.

Intimal atherosclerosis, on the other hand, is a disease with a spotty distribution whose appearance in the central retinal artery is not necessarily reflective of disease elsewhere. The primary lesion, occurring most often in males over age 30, is the atheromatous plaque. This area of intimal thickening consists of cholesterol and lipid deposits, with subsequent proliferation of connective tissue. As it thickens, it may ulcerate, form thrombi, and obstruct the lumen. Depending on the organ, this may result in a myocardial infarction, cerebral vascular accident, or an occlusion of the central retinal artery of the eye. An interesting side note is that in the eye the intimal atherosclerosis may result in a *venous* thrombosis. The central retinal artery and vein are encased in a common adventitial coat within the optic nerve and at their crossings. This results in an invasion of the atheromatous process into the vein, with subsequent thrombosis. (A discussion of vascular occlusion will follow the more important topic of differentiating hypertensive from arteriolar sclerotic changes in the fundus.)

Ophthalmologic Differentiation of Hypertension and Arteriolar Sclerosis. The retinal arteriole wall is normally transparent, so that all one sees is a pink column of blood with a thin reflective streak of the ophthalmoscope light coming from the convex surface of the blood column. It should be kept in mind that the ophthalmoscopic changes

due to hypertension all relate to *constriction* of the arterioles and that the changes that are visible from arteriolar sclerosis are caused by thickening and opacification of the vessel wall, secondary to the hypertension.

A simplified system of ophthalmoscopic grading of hypertension should be considered first:

Grade I: Consists only of generalized arteriolar narrowing, less than the average 3:4 ratio (arteriole to vein), and seen best in the smaller branches. These changes may be slight and are easily missed.

Grade II: Focal constriction or irregular narrowing due to local spasm is seen along with the generalized narrowing.

Grade III: The reduced capillary flow from Grade II hypertension interferes with the metabolism of the vessel walls; the resultant damage causes *edema, exudation,* and finally small, irregularly shaped *hemorrhages.*

Grade IV: The degree of anoxia from the Grade I, II, and III changes results in papilledema.

The grading of arteriolar sclerosis should be accomplished ophthalmoscopically by a parallel but separately identifiable system (Plate 1). The degree of change is based upon the severity and intensity of the hypertension, and one should attempt to isolate the grade of hypertension from the grade of sclerosis. The two phenomena in grading are thickening and opacification of the vessel wall, as manifested by changes in the light reflex, and the resultant compression of the vein at the site of arteriovenous crossing. At this point, arterioles and veins are in a common adventitial sheath:

Grade I: The light reflex strip is slightly broader, and there is minimal arteriovenous (AV) compression.

Grade II: Obvious broadening of the light reflex and definite AV compression signs, such as tapering of the vein, occur.

Grade III: When the arteriolar wall becomes so thickened and reflective that the light reflex appears to occupy the entire width of the blood columns, the phenomenon is known as "copper-wire" arteries. This is accompanied by further AV constriction, such as "banking" or dilatation of the vein distal to the crossing.

Grade IV: Occurs when the vessel wall is so thickened by sclerosis that no blood flow

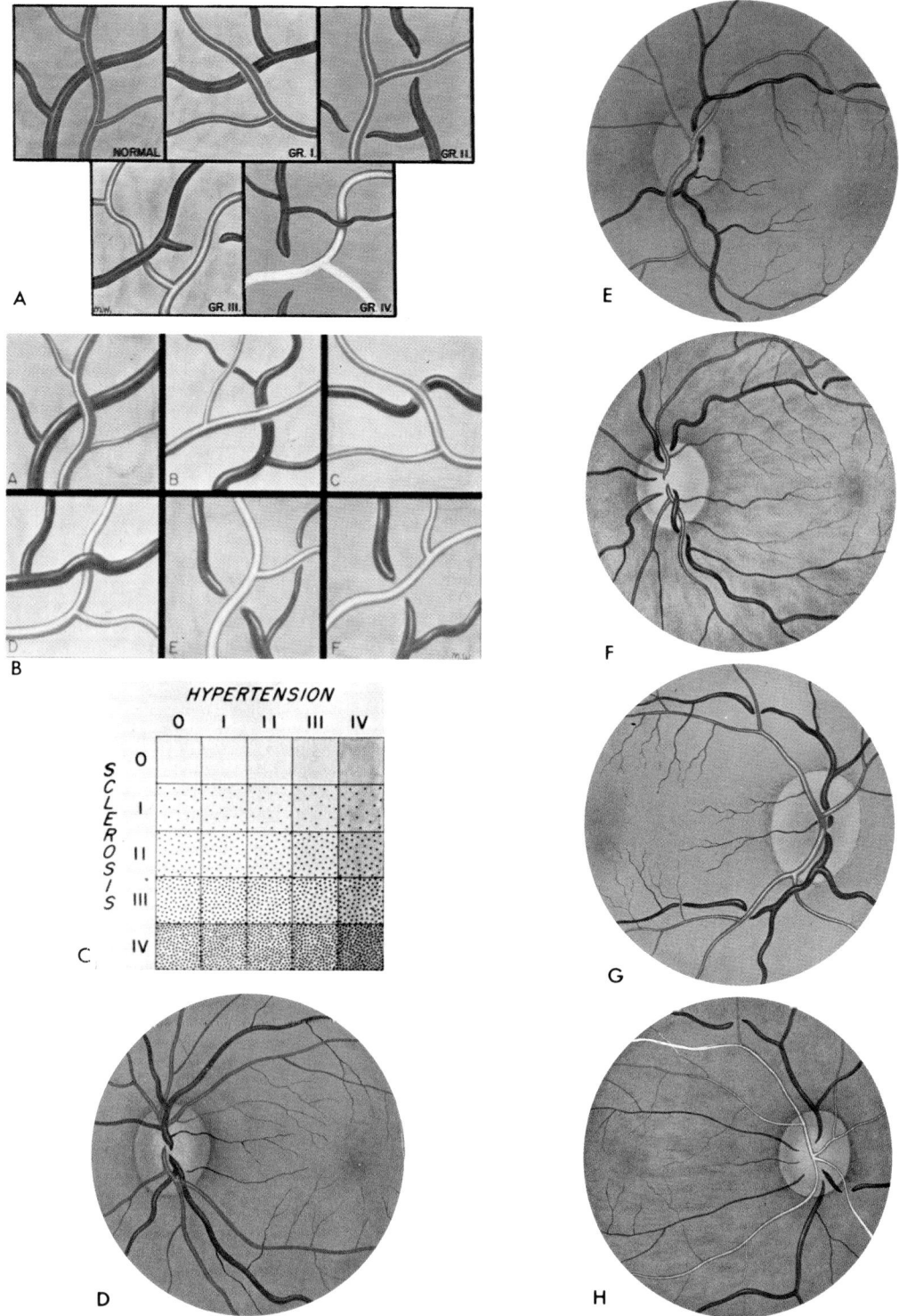

Plate 1. (A) *Schema for ophthalmoscopic classification of arteriolar sclerosis.* (B) *Changes in arteriovenous crossing in arteriolar sclerosis: A, normal crossing; B, early arteriovenous compression; C, deviation of vein; D, humping of vein; E, tapering of vein; F, banking of vein.* (C) *Correlation of degree of retinal changes of hypertension and degree of retinal arteriolar sclerosis.* (D) *Grade 0 hypertension; grade 0 arteriolar sclerosis.* (E) *Grade 0 hypertension; grade I arteriolar sclerosis.* (F) *Grade 0 hypertension; grade II arteriolar sclerosis.* (G) *Grade 0 hypertension; grade III arteriolar sclerosis.* (H) *Grade 0 hypertension; grade IV arteriolar sclerosis. (From Scheie, H. G., and Albert, D. M.: Textbook of Ophthalmology. 9th Ed. Philadelphia, W. B. Saunders Co., 1977, p. 418.)*

is visible, though it may still be present, and the vessel appears as a whitish cord or "silver-wire." The degree of AV compression is as severe or more so than in Grade III arteriolar sclerosis.

The separate grading of hypertensive and sclerotic changes may be of great importance to the family physician. The grade of hypertension is of only moderate importance, since the level of blood pressure is more accurately gauged with a sphygmomanometer. The grade of sclerosis, however, offers the only estimate of the duration or the severity of the hypertension. A patient with mild hypertension for many years may have Grade I hypertensive retinopathy with Grade III arteriolar sclerosis. The picture of the arterioles also gives the primary clue to the effect of the hypertension on the kidneys, heart, and brain. With increasing ability to lower blood pressure therapeutically, it becomes more important for the family physician to study and treat arteriolar sclerosis early in its course.

Vascular Occlusive Disorders

An occlusion of the *central retinal artery* is the primary cause of sudden, total, and painless loss of vision in one eye. It occurs rarely, usually in the elderly, and is caused mainly by an obstructive atheromatous plaque, an embolic occlusion of the carotid artery (Fig. 40–25), or temporal arteritis.

Ophthalmoscopically, one sees a pale disc with markedly attenuated arteries and a milky, edematous retina against which the thin fovea stands out as a cherry-red spot.

Therapy is usually futile, since ischemic infarction occurs in a few minutes, but heroic measures occasionally help. Giving a retrobulbar injection of vasodilators and rapidly decreasing the intraocular pressure by puncturing the anterior chamber may dislodge an embolus. The occasional occurrence of prodromal attacks of transient visual loss should always be investigated by ophthalmodynamometry. This technique of measuring the central retinal artery pressure may reveal an impending occlusion or carotid artery stenosis.

The central retinal vein or its larger branches may be the site of occlusion from constriction in the common adventitial sheath of a sclerotic artery (Fig. 40–26). Venous occlusion is also seen in diabetes and in thrombosis related to hematologic disorders. This form of painless visual loss occurs also in the elderly but is never as complete as in arterial occlusion. The fundus appears splashed with irregular hemorrhages along the course of all engorged veins. The disc is frequently ede-

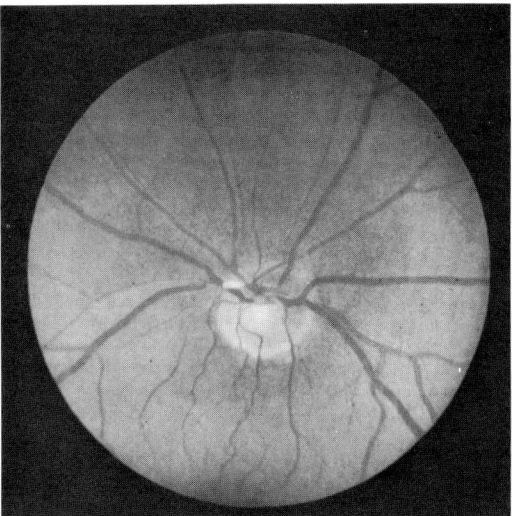

Figure 40–25. *Embolus lodged in the inferior temporal artery on the nerve head. (From Cogan, D. G.: Ophthalmic Manifestations of Systemic Vascular Disease. Philadelphia, W. B. Saunders Co., 1974, p. 121.)*

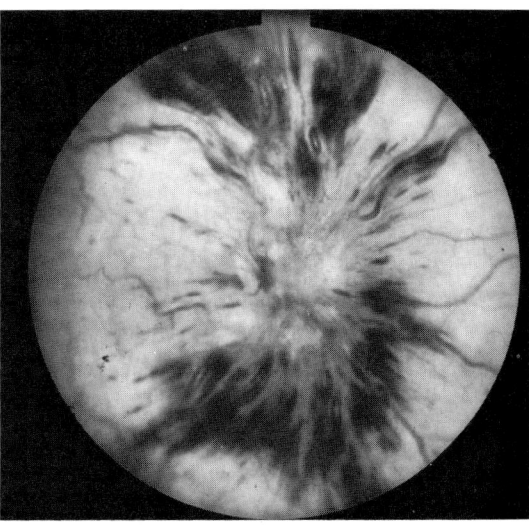

Figure 40–26. *Occlusion of the central retinal vein.*

matous. In the case of a branch vein occlusion, only that part of the visual field will be affected. Treatment of this condition is also rather futile, although some claims have been made for the use of anticoagulants and intravenous fibrinolysin. A significant number of patients, about 10 per cent, may develop a delayed form of glaucoma within 3 to 4 months following the occlusion. This is usually painful and intractable, requiring enucleation.

DIABETIC RETINOPATHY

For the family physician, the control of diabetes is a major problem. The presence or degree of diabetic retinopathy does not appear to correlate enough to the control of the disease to be of any real value. Although it has been therapeutic dogma for years, there is little basis for the belief that careful control of glycemia and glycosuria will prevent or moderate diabetic retinopathy. A

recent study suggests that a great increase in the incidence of retinopathy has occurred since the introduction of insulin therapy. It has been noted that in monkeys a proliferative retinopathy may be induced by an antibody response to the exogenous insulin.

Diabetic retinopathy is a major cause of blindness in American adults, second only to glaucoma, and accounts for from 7 to 20 per cent of the cases of newly reported blindness.

The primary role of the family physician in this regard is to recognize early signs of retinopathy, as laser photocoagulation therapy has recently been demonstrated to reduce the risk of blindness by more than half.

The fundus picture of patients with diabetic retinopathy is classified according to one of three types, with one type usually predominating. The most frequent is the intraretinal or background retinopathy (Fig. 40-27A), and the least common is engorge-

A

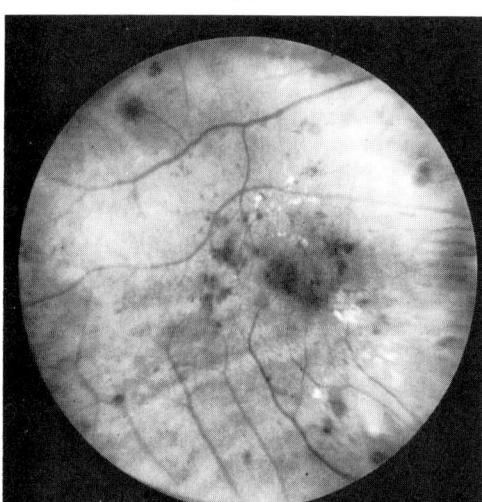

B

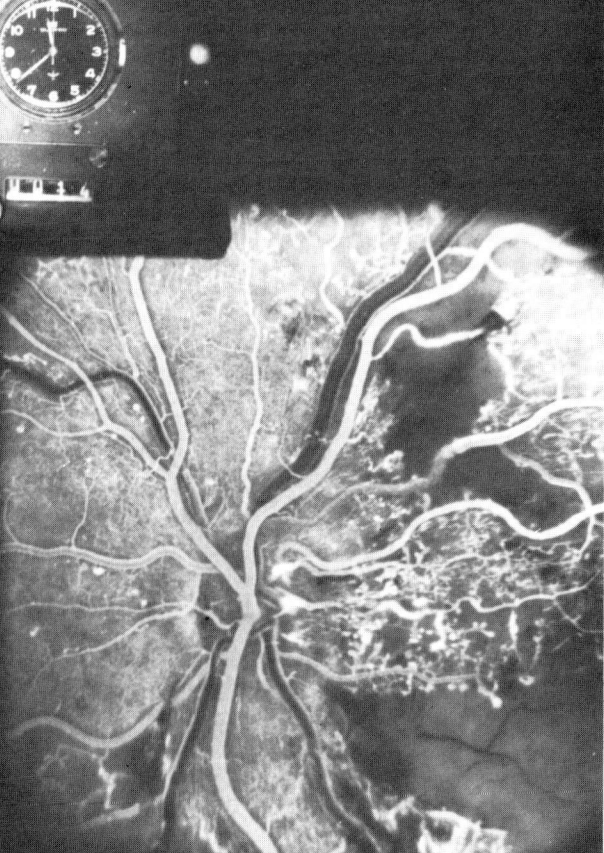

Figure 40-27. Diabetes (intraretinal type). A, Intraretinal type of diabetic retinopathy. Characteristic are the punctate red spots (hemorrhages and microaneurysms) and white spots (exudate) in the central fundus. B, Fluoroangiogram of an eye with moderate diabetic retinopathy. Especially noteworthy are the large avascular areas bordered by microaneurysms and dilated capillaries. The patient was a 31 year old man who had had diabetes since 7 years of age. (From Cogan, D. G.: Ophthalmic Manifestations of Systemic Vascular Disease. Philadelphia, W. B. Saunders Co., 1974, pp. 81 and 83.)

ment or occlusion of the large veins. The most severe is the proliferative type, now occurring with increasing frequency.

The typical picture is that of round microaneurysms or small round hemorrhages seen with discrete or coalescent exudates at the posterior pole. This appears to be related to the pathologic loss of the mural cells (pericytes) of the capillaries. The resultant outpouching causes the microaneurysms and also the stasis ischemia, which is the basis of the exudates.

The proliferative type, often referred to as retinitis proliferans, is characterized by the growth of retinal vessels into the vitreous, usually at the disc. The vessels proliferate in a network pattern, may bleed and cause massive hemorrhage within the vitreous, or may contract in a scar formation that will detach the retina.

It is now felt that patients with any significant degree of retinopathy should be evaluated by fluorescein angiography (Fig. 40–27B), which gives a much clearer and more meaningful view of diabetic change and the possible need for photocoagulation. As mentioned, the ongoing study by the National Institutes of Health appears to validate the therapeutic value of laser photocoagulation in diabetes.

MACULAR DISEASE

The macula, that area of the retina that appears avascular, consists primarily of cones in its central portion, the fovea. Because of its dependence on the choriocapillaries and the basement membrane (Bruch's membrane) for nutritional supply, many degenerative changes occur with age. Perhaps one-quarter of the population over 65 years of age have some degenerative change observable funduscopically (Fig. 40–28). Some of these changes have an hereditary basis, while others are caused by sclerosis of the choriocapillaries or breaks in Bruch's membrane. In any case, as the cones and ganglion cells degenerate, central vision is lost, and the patient has increasing difficulty with reading and fine tasks.

The ophthalmoscopic picture consists of changes varying from a loss of the foveal reflex and increased and irregular pigmentation to atrophic scarring and hemorrhages.

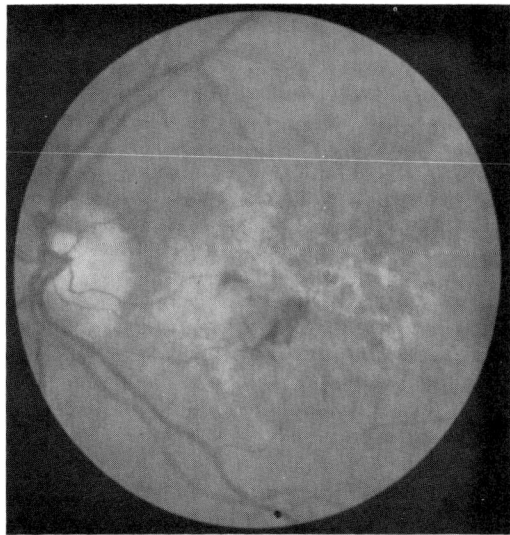

Figure 40–28. Senile macular degeneration.

Although treatment is generally not helpful, the family physician should be aware of two specific concepts in patient referral and counseling. These patients should all be referred for ophthalmologic work-up, particularly for possible fluorescein angiography. There are instances in which a break in Bruch's membrane can be seen angiographically and treated with laser photocoagulation. This has prevented further deterioration in some eyes and may be prophylactic in the fellow eye.

The more important message to impart to patients is the fact that they will not go blind. These people will maintain functional peripheral vision, and their reading ability may be helped by "low vision" aides and special illumination. It is most gratifying to observe the relief expressed by almost every patient with macular disease when they are reassured that they will not be blind.

RETINAL DETACHMENT

Although patients with a retinal detachment will frequently experience the symptoms of "lightning flashes" and "black floaters," these phenomena are by no means pathognomonic, as indicated previously. If such symptoms are followed by a "cloud" or "shadow" over part of the visual field, a detachment should be strongly suspected, and the fundus should be examined after

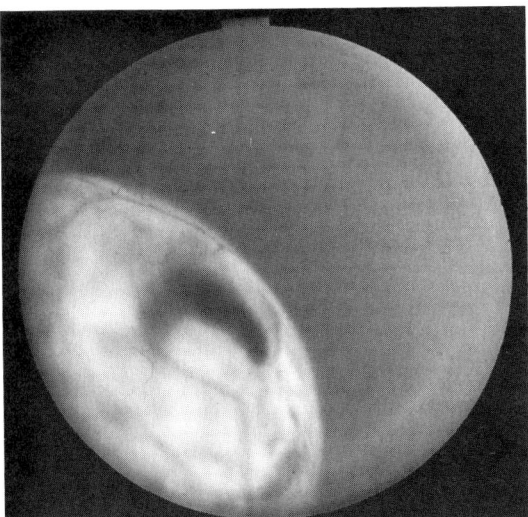

Figure 40–29. Retinal detachment.

complete pupillary dilation (Fig. 40–29).

Retinal detachment occurs most frequently in males over the age of 45 years. It also has a significant association with myopia, related to the retinal thinning in this condition. The sensory retina is attached to its pigment epithelium only at the optic disc and at the ora serrata. There is actually a potential space between these layers held together by the pressure of the vitreous. If a tear occurs in the retina from trauma or disease, fluid from the vitreous seeps through the hole and separates the retina from its pigment epithelium. The visual loss will become permanent because of loss of blood supply from the choroid causing atrophy of the rods and cones. Surgical repair is successful in greater than 86 to 90 per cent of patients.

The ophthalmoscopic appearance may be difficult to evaluate in a flat retinal detachment, but as more fluid accumulates under the retina, a billowy grayish area of the retina is seen, with very dark arteries and veins. The periphery of the retina should be examined closely, as this is where most tears occur and where the detachment process begins.

Obviously, a retinal detachment is a surgical emergency, and the patient should be referred for treatment. This consists primarily of creating an exudative reaction by diathermy or cryothermy in the appropriate area to seal the tear. The choroid is also frequently pressed into the detached retina by use of an encircling band or a localized implant of silicone into the sclera. In some instances, a retinal tear may be sealed by photocoagulation before fluid has seeped behind the retina to detach it.

INTRAOCULAR TUMORS

Although intraocular tumors are rare, even in an ophthalmologic practice, two types are worth discussing because of their notoriety.

Retinoblastoma is the principal tumor of the retina proper and is the most frequent malignant ocular tumor found in children. The disease is congenital and autosomal dominant. The diagnosis is made by noting a mass that creates a white reflex in the pupil. Unfortunately, this often cannot be seen until the child is 1 to 3 years old. Children with this neoplasm may present with a strabismus, as the vision is markedly decreased. This is one reason why every child with early-onset strabismus should have a thorough ophthalmoscopic examination.

Enucleation is still the treatment of choice unless, as in 30 per cent of the patients, the disease is bilateral. In such instances, the eye with the most advanced tumor is removed while the other eye is treated with radiation, chemotherapy, or both. The family physician should emphasize to parents of children with such tumors and to survivors of the neoplasm that in each case the risk of the tumor's appearing in future offspring is 50 per cent.

The most common intraocular tumor, arising from the choroid, *not* the retina, is a *malignant melanoma* (Fig. 40–30). It occurs primarily in the fifth and sixth decades of life as a solitary lesion in one eye. There are usually no symptoms until the neoplasm is large enough to cause a retinal detachment, at which time metastases have usually occurred. Patients with pigmented lesions observed in the fundus, most of which are benign nevi, should be referred for thorough ophthalmologic examination. Most malignant lesions can be differentiated by means of radioactive phosphorus uptake, fluorescein angiography, and ultrasonography. Adequate treatment, usually by enucleation but occasionally by photocoagulation or local resection, can apparently maintain a 5 year survival rate of greater than 50 per cent.

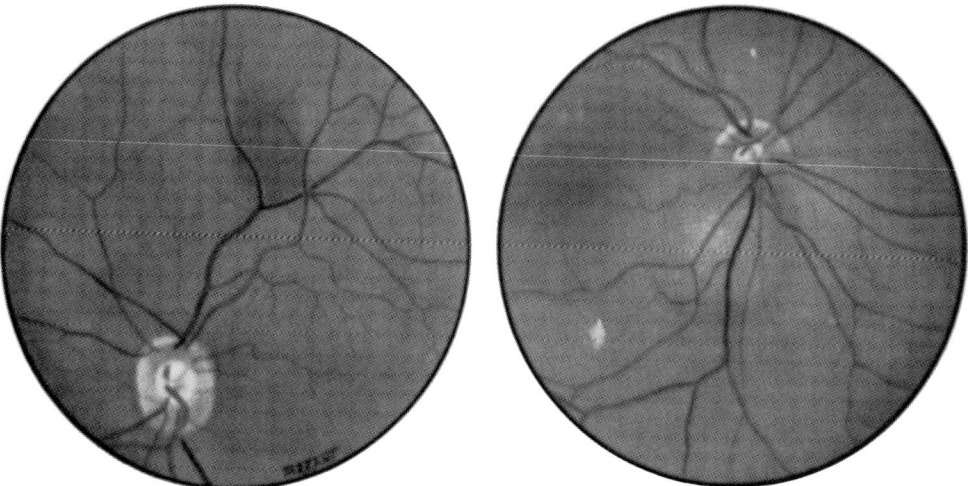

Figure 40–30. *Retinal nevus or melanoma.*

OPTIC NERVE DISEASE AND VISUAL FIELD DEFECTS

Optic Nerve Disease

The optic disc is the area of the fundus most easily observed and consequently is the site of the greatest familiarity for the physician. One should be aware of several physiologic changes in this disc that can be misinterpreted as being abnormal.

Congenital and myopic crescents are areas of white sclera visible around the disc, usually on the temporal side. These occur when the retinal pigment epithelium and choroid do not terminate as usual adjacent to the optic nerve, but leave a crescent of bare sclera visible. They are most often seen in myopic eyes and may be associated with a pigment ring if the pigment epithelium at their terminal edge increases in thickness.

Drusen or hyaline bodies of the optic nerve are seen as waxy, roundish irregularities along the margin of the disc, occasionally simulating papilledema (Fig. 40–31). They usually have no clinical significance.

Myelinated nerve fibers of the optic nerve, which extend beyond the disc margin, may form a whitish bundle radiating into the retina about 1 disc diameter. This may also be confused with papilledema.

"Pits" of the optic disc are discrete, isolated holes near the temporal border of the disc. Although usually benign, they may occasionally result in macular edema.

The primary diseases of the optic nerve are inflammatory or degenerative and depending upon the location of the lesion will cause either a *papillitis* or a *retrobulbar neuritis*. The essential difference between the two is really based on ophthalmoscopic findings. If the lesion is close enough to the nerve head, a swollen disc similar to that seen in papilledema will be visible. There is usually less venous engorgement and less

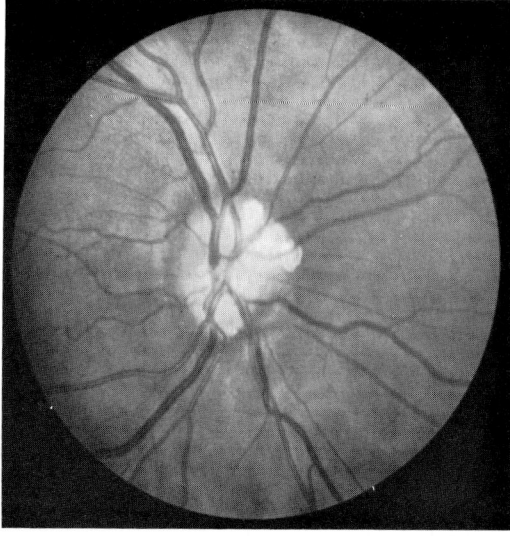

Figure 40–31. *Drusen or hyaline bodies of disc simulating papilledema. (From Scheie, H. G., and Albert, D. M.: Textbook of Ophthalmology. 9th Ed. Philadelphia, W. B. Saunders Co., 1977, p. 489.)*

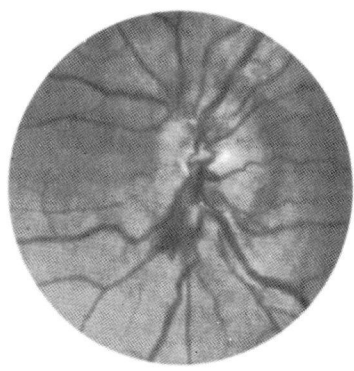

Figure 40-32. *Papilledema. (From Scheie, H. G., and Albert, D. M.: Textbook of Ophthalmology. 9th Ed. Philadelphia, W. B. Saunders Co., 1977, p. 488.)*

hemorrhagic tendency, but differentiation is sometimes difficult.

Retrobulbar neuritis refers to an optic neuritis in which the lesion involves the nerve sufficiently posteriorly to cause no change in the disc detectable by ophthalmoscopy.

In both instances, the presenting symptom is sudden onset of poor vision, frequently accompanied by pain on moving the eye. The pupillary reflex is typically poorly sustained, i.e., slow to react, and contraction is not maintained in the presence of the light. There may be numerous causes for these two disorders, but multiple sclerosis is probably the most common. Other causative factors include sinus infection spreading to the orbit, viral infections, and so-called toxic amblyopias caused by tobacco, alcohol, quinine, or arsenicals.

Papilledema simply describes a condition of the optic nerve head that is associated with increased intracranial pressure. The causative factors are diverse but most frequently include cerebral tumors and subdural hematomas. The ophthalmoscopic examination reveals a bilateral blurring of the disc margins with increased vascularization of the disc (Fig. 40-32). As pressure increases, the veins become engorged and flameshaped hemorrhages appear. The edema of the disc may be measurable ophthalmoscopically by focusing on a small vessel at the disc margin and determining how many diopters of lens power in the ophthalmoscope are needed to focus from the vessel on the retina to the same vessel

on the disc. A key differentiation between papilledema and papillitis is the bilateral occurrence of the former and the decreased visual acuity *only* in the latter.

Optic atrophy may occur from diverse causes—degenerative, from glaucoma; vascular, from central retinal artery occlusion; inflammatory, from postpapillitis; toxic, from obvious poisons such as methyl alcohol; and descending atrophy, from cranial lesions affecting the optic pathway. The fundus picture is similar in all cases, a pale, sharp-edged nerve head with a decreased number of arterioles crossing the disc margin.

Visual Field Changes

Visual field changes are best discovered by using careful perimetric techniques that require a good deal of time and sophisticated equipment. The family physician will be limited to an examination of the visual field by the confrontation method, as previously described. By being aware of the basic neuroanatomic structure of the optic nerve, however, he should gain more insight into neuro-ophthalmologic diagnosis (Fig. 40-33). The optic nerve consists of about 1 million axon fibers connecting the ganglion cells of the retina to the neurons that originate in the lateral geniculate body. Along this course, the fibers exit through the optic foramina. The lateral half of the fibers remain on the outer side of the chiasm and proceed to the geniculate ganglion of the same side. The optic nerve fibers of the nasal half of the retina cross over in the chiasm to the geniculate body of the other side. The portion of the optic pathway from the chiasm to the geniculate body is called the optic tract. The fibers from the geniculate body, after going into the temporal lobe, proceed back along the lateral ventricles as the "optic radiations" to the calcarine fissure in the occipital lobe.

Referring briefly to Figure 40-33 will help clarify the following major simplified points:

1. Monocular field defects result from retinal or optic nerve lesions.

2. Chiasmal lesions cause a bitemporal hemianopsia.

3. Optic tract lesions cause an incongruous (dissimilar) homonymous hemianopsia.

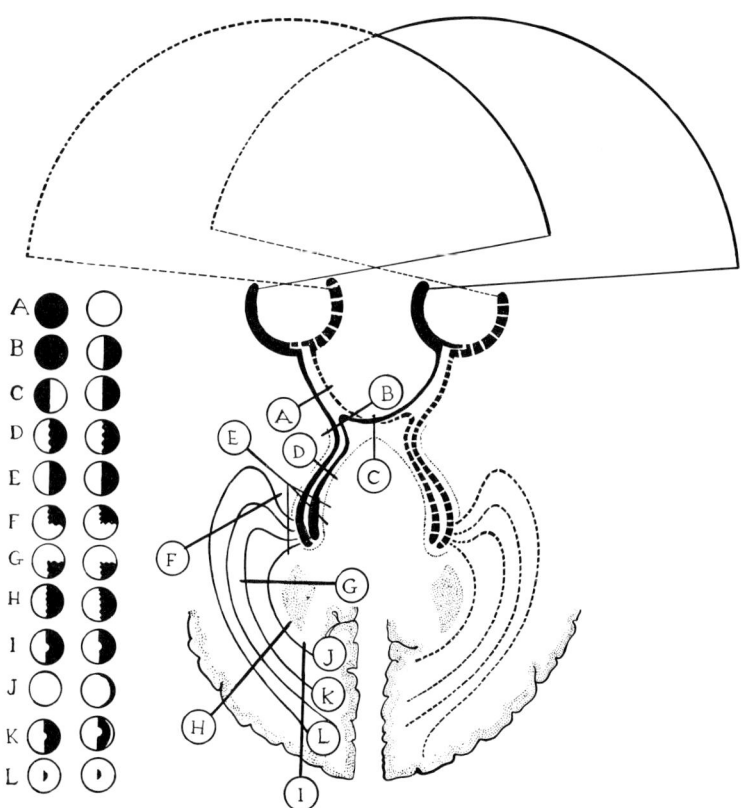

Figure 40–33. *A composite diagram showing type of visual field defect caused by lesions affecting the optic pathways. The solid black lines represent the temporal retina, the cross-hatched lines the nasal retina. On the left are represented the visual field changes with the site of the lesion indicated in the diagram corresponding to the letters as follows:*

A, Lesion behind eyeball, anterior to the chiasm. B, Commencement of optic nerve just anterior to the chiasm (ipsilateral blindness with contralateral temporal hemianopia). C, Chiasmal lesion (bitemporal hemianopia). D, Optic tract (markedly incongruous homonymous hemianopia). E, Beginning of optic tract (clear-cut homonymous hemianopia without sparing of the macula). F, Anterior loop of optic radiations (markedly incongruous superior quadrantopia—right superior hemianopia). G, Inner part of optic radiations (slightly incongruous inferior quadrantopia). H, Middle of optic radiations (slightly incongruous homonymous without macular sparing). I, Posterior part of optic radiations with macular sparing. J, Anterior part of calcarine cortex (contralateral blindness in temporal crescent). K, Middle part of calcarine cortex (congruous homonymous hemianopia with sparing of the macula and contralateral sparing of temporal crescent). L, Occipital pole (congruous homonymous hemianopic central scotoma).

Sometimes a bilateral thrombosis of the posterior calcarine arteries causes complete blindness, or there may be sparing of a small island of vision slightly excentric to the macular area.

Tubular fields of vision are frequently seen in the later stages of glaucoma. The examiner should always make certain that the intraocular tension is normal and that there is no evidence of glaucoma present before attempting to interpret the visual fields. (From Paton, R. T.: Ophthalmology. In Cecil, R. L., and Conn, H. F.: The Specialties in General Practice. Philadelphia, W. B. Saunders Co., 1964, p. 344.)

4. Optic radiation lesions generally cause congruous (similar) homonymous hemianopsia without macular sparing, i.e., poor central vision.

5. Temporal lobe lesions cause quadrantanopsias.

6. Occipital lobe lesions may cause homonymous hemianopsia with macular sparing, i.e., good visual acuity.

Although the family physician will not ordinarily perform specifically detailed field examinations, he will have a better understanding of the pathogenesis of many neurologic symptoms by keeping this schema in mind.

OPHTHALMIC MANIFESTATIONS OF SYSTEMIC DISEASE

The eye, being so readily accessible to both external inspection and thorough examination of the retinal vasculature, is ideally suited for detecting manifestations of systemic disease, particularly of vascular disease, as these diseases also affect the eye. For example, the yellowish sclera indicative of jaundice and the whitish palpebral conjunctiva in anemia are well-known indicators.

SYSTEMIC DISEASES CAUSING CHANGES IN GROSS APPEARANCE OF EYE

In reviewing the major ophthalmic manifestations of systemic disease, it is best to start with diseases causing changes in the gross appearance of the eyes, including:

1. Thyroid disease, manifested by exophthalmos.

2. Intracranial vascular disease, manifested by ocular motor paralysis.

3. Temporal arteritis, suggested by prominent, tender temporal arteries.

4. Various dermatologic and connective tissue disorders seen as external ocular changes.

Thyroid Disease

The dramatic appearance of severe bilateral exophthalmos is obvious to all as suggestive of thyroid disease (Fig. 40–34). There is, however, a graded spectrum of ocular findings that may be related etiologically to the supposed predominance of either thyrotropic or thyrotoxic effects. Although the basic pathogenesis remains unclear, it appears that the sympatheticotonic signs, i.e., upper lid retraction, lid lag on downward gaze, and weakness of convergence, are related to the thyrotoxic state. As the disease progresses, particularly if the basal metabolic rate is lowered suddenly by medical or surgical means, the so-called thyrotropic effect on the orbital contents ensues, causing real proptosis, extraocular muscle involvement, and conjunctival con-

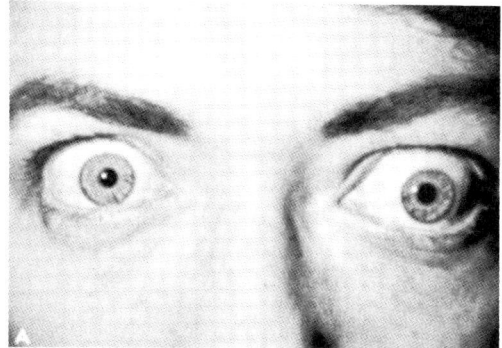
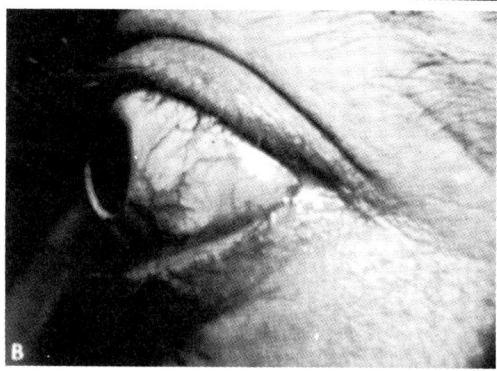
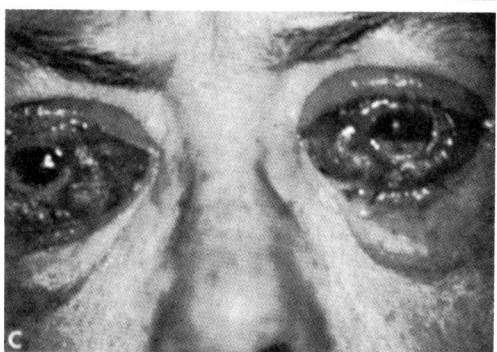

Figure 40–34. *Exophthalmos — thyrotoxic and thyrotropic. A,* Endocrine ophthalmopathy with exophthalmos and lid retraction. B, Endocrine ophthalmopathy with exophthalmos and congestion. C, Endocrine ophthalmopathy with exophthalmos, chemosis, and exposure keratitis. (From Scheie, H. G., and Albert D. M.: Textbook of Ophthalmology. 9th Ed. Philadelphia, W. B. Saunders Co., 1977, p. 427.)

gestion. Although the milder forms of thyroid disease are much more common in females, the severe and occasionally disabling state shows no sex predilection.

It is of particular diagnostic interest that many patients exhibit a *unilateral* lid retraction or mild proptosis as the presenting sign of thyroid disease. The wider lid aperture on one side may be misinterpreted as normal, leading to the mistaken diagnosis of a ptosis on the normal side.

The eye may also reveal evidence of hypothyroidism, although far less commonly than it shows hyperthyroid signs. The ocular signs are part of the myxedematous picture, but the appearance of baggy, swollen lids with loss of the outer half of the eyebrows may be the presenting signs.

Intracranial Vascular Disease

Vascular disease of the brain may affect the function of the ocular motor nerves and cause tropias, ptosis, or nystagmus.

Ocular Motor Paralysis. The three ocular motor nerves—the third (oculomotor), the fourth (trochlear), and the sixth (abducens)—may be affected by many intracranial disorders, but the three major causes of paralysis are *aneurysms, diabetes,* and *trauma.*

Paralysis of the abducens nerve causes an inability to abduct the eye, resulting in an obvious esotropia and subjective diplopia. One will frequently observe that the patient *turns* his head toward the side of the paralyzed muscle. In this way he avoids diplopia by not using the lateral rectus muscle of the affected eye.

When the trochlear nerve is affected, a gross deviation of the eye is not often observed. However, the affected superior oblique muscle will fail to intort the eye, and diplopia will result unless the patient *tilts* his head to the shoulder opposite the affected eye. This eliminates the need for intorsion, and fusion may be maintained.

If the oculomotor nerve is paralyzed, all the other eye muscles are affected, including the levator muscle of the lid and the pupillary muscle. Such a patient often will not complain of diplopia even though the eye is exotropic (paralyzed medial rectus muscle) because the lid droops over the eye (*ptosis*) and occludes the dilated pupil. Although the combination of ocular motor paralysis and pain should suggest aneurysm, diabetes is a frequent cause of this syndrome and particularly involves the oculomotor nerve. One major differentiating point is the sparing of the pupillomotor fibers in diabetes, so that an oculomotor nerve paralysis with an active pupil will usually clear completely in about 2 months.

In summary, the ocular manifestations of head turn, head tilt, or ptosis should suggest the presence of intracranial aneurysm, diabetes, or trauma.

Nystagmus. Nystagmus of the horizontal pendular type is usually congenital, but an acquired horizontal nystagmus of jerklike quality is most characteristic of brain stem lesions, with the fast (jerk) component toward the side of the lesion. The most common cause of acquired horizontal nystagmus is a vascular lesion in the pons; the less commonly seen acquired vertical nystagmus is characteristic of posterior fossa lesions.

Temporal Arteritis

Temporal arteritis is included in this discussion because of the urgency involved in establishing the diagnosis. The ophthalmic manifestations are really not marked until almost too late, that is, not until ischemic optic neuropathy occurs. However, one should look temporal to the eyes to find nodular, tortuous, or tender temporal arteries. If this finding accompanies headache, pain on chewing, malaise, or polymyalgia rheumatica in an elderly female, an elevated sedimentation rate will establish the diagnosis. Prompt treatment with high-dosage steroids appears to significantly prevent the irreversible blindness that occurs in 50 per cent of these patients.

Dermatologic and Connective Tissue Disorders

Various dermatologic disorders may affect the conjunctiva and cornea. Ordinarily, the diagnosis will be made by the appearance of the skin. In some instances, knowledge of accompanying ocular involvement may confirm the diagnosis. Occasionally, the eye signs may be a precursor of the skin eruption.

Rosacea. This is a relatively common disease, and the eye signs, though infrequent, are quite characteristic. The typical eye lesion consists of dilated and thickened conjunctival vessels associated with a blepharoconjunctivitis and frequent marginal corneal ulcers.

Ocular Pemphigus. This disorder may develop as part of the full-blown cutaneous disease or, less commonly, as an independent entity. The eye picture in such patients is that of a chronic conjunctivitis with progressive cicatrization that leads eventually to contraction and obliteration of the conjunctival fornices.

Erythema Multiforme. An acute, self-limited dermatosis, erythema multiforme is occasionally associated with a severe, purulent conjunctivitis, leading to obliteration of the conjunctival fornices and necrosis of the cornea. The variant, known as Stevens-Johnson syndrome, occurs primarily in children and seems to be associated with drug hypersensitivity.

Dermatitis Herpetiformis and Epidermolysis Bullosa. The appearance of a thickened, pseudomembranous formation that is followed by shrinkage and scarring of the conjunctival cul de sac should suggest two other relatively rare skin disorders, namely, dermatitis herpetiformis and epidermolysis bullosa. Both conditions are unusual and are included here for the sake of completeness in the differential diagnosis of the thickened, scarred lower conjunctiva.

Rheumatoid Arthritis. This may cause several specific eye lesions that should be recognized by the family physician. In juvenile rheumatoid arthritis (Still's disease), one of the most frequent complications may be a smoldering, bilateral uveitis. This may occur in 20 per cent of such patients and is often manifested by a horizontal band of opacification across the cornea as a sequela of the chronic inflammation. Any evidence of ocular inflammation in patients with Still's disease should be vigorously treated to prevent possible visual impairment.

In the adult form of the disease, a rheumatoid scleritis may develop, particularly in older women. This may appear as a solitary nodule, which gradually thins out the sclera to leave a punched-out defect through which the darker uveal tissue appears and may actually herniate. This condition, known as *scleromalacia perforans,* is quite pathognomonic of long-standing rheumatoid arthritis.

Sjögren's Syndrome. A deficiency of lacrimal and salivary secretions in older women with polyarthritis, Sjögren's syndrome may be recognized by eye signs. The decreased lacrimation often results in a chronic conjunctivitis with a foamy secretion and corneal erosions that have small filaments of cells visibly adherent to the cornea. Symptoms are aggravated by a dry environment, but treatment is unsatisfactory.

Other Connective Tissue Diseases. Although various connective tissue diseases can affect the external eye, most are rare conditions, such as periarteritis nodosa, scleroderma, and dermatomyositis. These cause nonspecific changes in the conjunctiva, sclera, or cornea.

OTHER EXTERNAL EYE MANIFESTATIONS OF SYSTEMIC DISEASE

There are other changes in the external appearance of the eye that require closer observation and even magnification. In the absence of a slit lamp biomicroscope, which is obviously ideal but not at his disposal, the family physician should utilize a good head loupe (e.g., the Magnifocuser). The loupe has many other uses but is really very rewarding when used to examine the eye at 2× magnification.

Conjunctival Changes

Congestion. The conjunctiva may reveal the presence of either passive or active congestion by a pattern of dilated, thickened congested vessels.

In *passive* congestion, several veins appear prominent. This is most commonly related to early thyroid disease but may also be a consequence of various hyperviscosity syndromes, such as polycythemia and multiple myeloma.

When there is an increased arterial pressure causing *active* congestion of more conjunctival vessels, one should suspect a cavernous sinus fistula or gradual stenosis of the internal carotid artery. In the former, the venous system is subjected to arterial pressure, causing conjunctival vessel engorgement. With internal carotid narrowing, blood is bypassed to the brain via the external carotid, which, by increasing the supply to the conjunctiva, causes the conjunctival vessels to become distended. The conjunctiva may also exhibit a gross form of edema known as *chemosis.* This may be so billowy as to protrude between the lids and is simply related to the very loose structure of the conjunctiva. It usually suggests a severe local allergic reaction, but one must consider whether a more generalized allergic diathesis is an underlying factor. This form of edema is also associated with the orbital congestion of thyroid disease.

Hemorrhage. In the previous discussion

of subconjunctival hemorrhage, it was noted that the gross hemorrhages that appear without cause are usually not related to hypertension or to arteriosclerosis. However, when such hemorrhage is associated with extensive ecchymosis in the lids, one should consider an orbital neoplasm or a hemorrhagic dyscrasia. The presence of small petechiae or splinter hemorrhages in the conjunctiva, though far less common, is suggestive of systemic disease, accompanied by increased capillary fragility, purpura, or subacute bacterial endocarditis.

Arcus Senilis and Arcus Juvenilis

A common eye finding is arcus senilis, the whitish ring found at the periphery of the cornea. Although the popular belief is that this is related to generalized atherosclerosis and is prognostic of premature senility, there is no apparent correlation between these findings. When, however, a similar arcus appears in the young, i.e., arcus juvenilis, it may be associated with familial hypercholesterolemia and may portend a more serious prognosis.

Changes Caused by Hypertension, Arteriolar Sclerosis, and Diabetes

The best known internal eye manifestations of systemic disease relate to hypertension, arteriolar sclerosis, and diabetes. These conditions have been discussed under the section on retinal disease. It may be reassuring to the family physician to know that the ophthalmoscopic signs of these conditions are not easy to discern in many patients, even by the trained ophthalmologist.

In hypertension, a critical factor in the development of typical narrowing or "spasm" is the age of the patient. A younger person may have obvious retinal narrowing with a certain degree of hypertension, while an older patient with more vascular rigidity will have no signs with an equal degree of this disorder. The nasal retinal vessels will show the earliest signs of focal narrowing and should, therefore, be more closely scrutinized in all age groups.

In arteriolar sclerosis, the chief clinical ocular appearance is that of opacification of the arteriolar wall. It is probably impossible to clinically distinguish between the hyalinization secondary to hypertension and the similar ophthalmoscopic changes in senile vasculopathy.

As early diabetic changes occur in the posterior pole of the fundus, around the macula, pupillary contraction will prevent an adequate view of this area unless the pupil is well dilated. Early changes may consist of only a few microaneurysms, and care must be taken in such cases to carefully observe the finer arterioles for evidence of diabetic change. It should be remembered that microaneurysm formation has a pattern of development and decline. Such aneurysms will be seen to "disappear" after a period of time because of the hyalinization of endothelial cells trapped in the lumen. This, of course, does not necessarily indicate an improvement in the course of the disease.

Changes Caused by Anemia

Although changes in the fundus caused by severe anemia are not specific enough to be pathognomonic, the occurrence of blotchy hemorrhages, "cotton-wool" spots, and occasionally of papilledema, in the absence of any vascular abnormality, should suggest a severe anemia. This does not seem to occur in children and apparently requires a reduction of 50 per cent in the hemoglobin level to result in typical changes. Although the pathogenesis is not clear, the result may be severe optic atrophy and blindness, but most patients recover. When acute and severe blood loss (for example, after gastrointestinal bleeding) is followed several days later by blurry vision, one should examine the fundus, as these patients can develop similar changes and an ischemic optic atrophy.

Sickle cell disease can cause retinal changes, particularly in the peripheral temporal vessels. As the sickled cells cannot mold into the small capillaries, they cause obstructive phenomena such as tortuosity of the veins or arteriolar occlusions that may cause hemorrhages into the peripheral retina or vitreous. This may progress to retinal detachments and is an important clue in attempting early diagnosis of sickle cell retinopathy. Laser photocoagulation of the peripheral vessels may not only occlude potential bleeding sites but may also act prophylactically to prevent retinal detachments.

Angioid Streaks

Angioid streaks are an uncommon finding in the fundus but are so dramatic as to be noteworthy. These irregularly branching streaks usually radiate from one streak that partially encircles the disc. They look somewhat like vessels but can be easily distinguished by their jagged course. The streaks are thought to be due to cracks in Bruch's membrane, and although usually asymptomatic, they may occasionally result in a subretinal hemorrhage. They are most often associated with the condition known as pseudoxanthoma elasticum, or Grönblad-Strandberg syndrome. This is a dystrophy of the elastic fibers of the skin, resulting in leathery, redundant skin in the creases of the face, neck, and axilla. Angioid streaks have also been noted in Paget's disease and in sickle cell disease.

Hyperlipemia

A level of hyperlipemia of over 2.5 per cent has been shown to impart a pale, whitish look to the retinal vessels. This appearance results from increased triglyceride levels and may be caused by diseases such as diabetes, cirrhosis, and others. It is reversible when the level of blood lipids returns to normal. There have been recent reports that cholesterol levels of over 400 mg. per 100 ml. may cause whitish deposits, strung along the outside of several retinal vessels.

Occlusive Carotid Arterial Disease

The increasing recognition of occlusive carotid arterial disease as being a major factor in causing cerebral vascular accidents emphasizes the importance of knowing the ophthalmic manifestations of this disease. Over half of the patients with carotid insufficiency will have visual symptoms, primarily transient and recurrent blurring on the side of the occlusion.

Noting certain statistics will be of diagnostic value. For example, the occurrence of occlusions in males is twice as common as in females and left-sided occlusions occur seven times as frequently as right-sided occlusions. Perhaps 25 per cent of cerebrovascular accidents are related to carotid occlusion. The concurrence of a transient crossed hemiplegia with monocular blur-

ring should strongly suggest carotid occlusion. Although only 10 to 15 per cent of such patients will show progressive visual dysfunction leading to blindness, it is vitally important to diagnose this condition early, as carotid artery surgery may cure the disease.

Ophthalmodynamometry. The recognition of even the possibility of carotid occlusion or stenosis should suggest a referral for ophthalmodynamometry. This technique of measuring the blood pressure of the retinal arteries uses an instrument to apply a calibrated pressure to the globe. The Bailliart ophthalmodynamometer has a smooth footplate that is pressed against the sclera at the lateral canthus while the examiner focuses on the central retinal artery through the ophthalmoscope. The pressure on the instrument is gradually increased until the higher vitreous pressure equals the arterial pressure. At this point the artery will suddenly begin abrupt, rhythmic pulsations. The calibrated endpoint is read from the instrument as the diastolic pressure. It is the comparative pressure reading of the two eyes that is of value in diagnosis. A difference of greater than 20 per cent suggests carotid stenosis on the lower side. For this reason, it is usually not necessary, and may even be dangerous, to obtain the systolic pressure, which necessitates increasing the pressure until all pulsation ceases.

Although this test is valuable, a number of patients with stenotic carotids may exhibit equal retinal artery pressure in each eye because of the development of collateral circulation from the homolateral external carotid or the contralateral patent internal carotid.

Aortic Arch Syndrome

Although venous pulsation may be seen normally during a retinal examination, the spontaneous appearance of an arterial pulsation is a sign that the intraocular tension is very high, as in glaucoma, or that the arterial pressure is very low, below the normal intraocular pressure of 20 mm. Hg. Carotid stenosis, as just described, aortic insufficiency, and the aortic arch syndrome are examples that may cause such a phenomenon.

The ophthalmic manifestations of the aortic arch syndrome are those of ischemia.

This syndrome, productive of one of the so-called pulseless diseases, is caused by stenosis of one of the major branches of the aorta, most commonly the carotid, subclavian, innominate, or vertebral artery. The basic cause is atheromatosis, but symptomatology varies, depending upon the branch involved. Generally, there are weak or absent pulses in the arm or neck, accompanied by syncope related to posture. This may also appear as visual blackouts related to postural changes. The fundi may show narrowed arteries and distended veins, "cotton-wool" exudates, and many identical-sized microaneurysms. Cataracts commonly appear after several years.

In the interesting variation known as the *"steal" syndromes,* an occlusion of the subclavian artery on the left or the innominate artery on the right may result in "stealing" blood from the posterior cerebral circulation through the vertebral arteries. This may result in the phenomenon of transient hemianopsia or even in loss of vision precipitated by vigorous use of the arms.

In conclusion, although many other systemic diseases can cause changes in the eye, many of the ophthalmic manifestations are nonspecific. It would not be helpful to the family physician to outline every disease that can cause hemorrhages or exudates. An attempt has been made to demonstrate a method of eliciting signs and symptoms that would suggest specific disease entities. However, it is not to be inferred that such correlation is either easy or definitive, and the family physician should not expect to discover signs that still elude many specialists.

BIBLIOGRAPHY

1. Ballantyne, A. J., and Michaelson, I. C.: Textbook of the Fundus of the Eye. Baltimore, The Williams & Wilkins Co., 1963.
2. Cogan, D. G.: Ophthalmic Manifestations of Systemic Vascular Disease. Philadelphia, W. B. Saunders Co., 1974.
3. Duke-Elder, S.: System of Ophthalmology. Vols. I–XII. St. Louis, The C. V. Mosby Co., 1958–71.
4. Fox, S. A.: Ophthalmic Plastic Surgery. 4th Ed. New York, Grune & Stratton, 1970.
5. King, J. H., and Wadsworth, J. A. C.: An Atlas of Ophthalmic Surgery. 2nd Ed. Philadelphia, J. B. Lippincott Co., 1970.
6. Perkins, E. S., and Hansell, P.: An Atlas of Diseases of the Eye. Boston, Little, Brown & Co., 1957.
7. Reese, A. B.: Tumors of the Eye. 2nd Ed. New York, Harper & Row, Publishers, 1963.
8. Scheie, H. G., and Albert, D. M.: Textbook of Ophthalmology. 9th Ed. Philadelphia, W. B. Saunders Co., 1977.
9. Vaughan, D., Asbury, T., and Cook, R.: General Ophthalmology. 6th Ed. Los Altos, California, Lange Medical Publications, 1971.
10. Walsh, F. B., and Hoyt, W. F.: Clinical Neuro-Ophthalmology. 3rd Ed. Baltimore, The Williams & Wilkins Co., 1969.
11. Warwick, R.: Wolff's Anatomy of the Eye and Orbit. 6th Ed. Philadelphia, W. B. Saunders Co., 1977.

Chapter 41

GYNECOLOGY AND OBSTETRICS

by JOHN T. QUEENAN,
DOUGLAS M. HAYNES,
and WILLIAM P. VONDERHAAR

In discussing the principles of office gynecology and obstetrics, we shall make the basic assumption that the well-trained family physician will take a careful history and perform a thorough physical examination. As a physician develops skills in history-taking, a thorough and comprehensive summary can be obtained in a few minutes. Obviously, more elaboration on certain aspects of the history will be indicated if the patient has a specific problem. The most frequent reason for a history and examination will be in connection with the annual physical check-up. Good medical practice demands that women receive a complete physical examination at least annually after the menarche. When specific clinical situations are present, more frequent routine examinations may be indicated. In the course of the annual examination, the clinician elicits a careful history regarding both the patient's general health and her gynecologic status and then proceeds to perform a physical examination. This includes a general physical survey and a gynecologic examination, with attention to the breasts and the pelvic organs.

In eliciting the gynecologic history, the adept physician can get a patient to define specific problems if he asks questions skillfully, listens carefully, and deftly directs the patient's elaboration of her chief complaint and medical status. Certain basic information is necessary to establish that the patient does not have a problem. For instance, knowing that the patient's menstrual periods are normal and regular without intermenstrual or postcoital bleeding is absolutely essential. Furthermore, knowing that a patient does not have abdominal pain or vaginal discharge is very reassuring when doing the annual physical examination.

Conversely, if the patient has a specific complaint, such as bleeding, pain, or discharge, the physician must obtain more specific information concerning this problem. As the history unfolds, the physician can usually call to mind the differential diagnoses that fit the symptoms. Until the physical examination is coordinated with the history, the total assessment of the gynecologic condition cannot be made.

EXAMINATION

The examination consists first of a general physical examination that includes recording of vital signs; evaluation of the head and neck; auscultation of the heart and lungs; survey of the extremities; palpation of the abdomen; search for costovertebral angle tenderness, ascites, and neurologic abnormalities; and evaluation of the lymph nodes.

In addition, the clinician examines the patient's breasts, beginning with a visual inspection followed by a manual examination of each quadrant of the breast and corresponding axilla, with particular attention to the possible presence of palpable masses. He should note if it is possible to express secretion or blood from the nipples. Self-breast examination should be taught at this point and should be performed by the patient monthly, the week after the menses.

A pelvic examination is then performed. The inspection of the external genitalia in a normal woman would show female distribution of hair, a normal urethra without discharge when stripped, no discharge from the Skene's glands adjacent to the urethra, and the absence of tumors or pigmented moles of the labia majora or minora.

The clinician then checks the vaginal outlet, including urethral and rectal support. It is not uncommon to encounter an isolated prolapse of the bladder or of the urethra without an associated major relaxation of the rectovaginal septum. Conversely, it is possible to have a rectocele in the absence of a cystocele. The most common situation, however, in the multipara is the presence of both a cystocele and a rectocele because of damage to the supporting tissues at the time of childbirth. Having the patient cough may elicit urinary incontinence. Rectoceles may become apparent by asking the patient to "bear down."

A speculum is then inserted into the vagina for examination of the vaginal epithelium, the fornices, and the cervix. Attention is paid to any lesions of the vaginal epithelium and to the presence and nature of any vaginal discharge. Does the vagina have the rugae characteristic of normal estrogen levels or is the epithelium smooth, thin, and atrophic? Does the epithelium bleed easily?

The cervix is then inspected. The nulliparous patient has a pinpoint external os, whereas the parous patient has a cervical os that has had small or large lacerations because of dilatation associated with delivery. The speculum is then removed, and the examiner palpates the labia majora and minora and evaluates vaginal support. The absence of tumor or pus in the periurethral Skene's glands or in the Bartholin duct glands located in the posterior aspect of the labia majora is confirmed by palpation. The evaluation of the support of the vaginal outlet is determined by having the patient bear down or cough. The Papanicolaou smear test is done at this time.

Attention is then turned to the mobility of the cervix. Does the cervix move easily? Does it move without causing the patient pain? The examining fingers of one hand are placed in the vagina behind the cervix and advanced up toward the posterior aspect of the uterus while the other hand is placed on the abdomen to exert pressure, pushing the fundus of the uterus down toward the hand examining the vagina. In this manner, the fundus can generally be felt by the fingers on the abdomen, and the transmission of motion from the fingers in the vagina or the hand examining the abdomen can be perceived. The uterus is moved from side to side gently to see if it is mobile and to determine if motion causes the patient pain or discomfort. It is immaterial whether the left or right hand is used for vaginal palpation, but it is advisable always to use the same one, as expertise is most readily acquired if a consistent routine is followed.

After determining uterine mobility, the fingers examining the vagina sweep out to the adnexal area. The hand examining the abdomen accompanies the sweeping motion, pushing downward in the lower abdomen on the corresponding side to determine if any structures can be brought within reach of the fingers in the vagina. Ovarian enlargement or other adnexal masses would be immediately perceived by this maneuver. The presence of a normal-sized ovary should be detected with ease by this maneuver, particularly on the right side if the examiner is right-handed or on the left side if he is left-handed.

The clinician then performs a rectovaginal examination, first feeling the area behind the uterus to determine if there are any nodules or masses suggestive of endometriosis, myomas, or cancer. The uterus is moved with the fingers performing the rectovaginal examination to determine its mobility. The fingers then sweep out into the adnexal area to determine if any masses are present in the posterior adnexal area or on the pelvic side wall. This procedure is carried out on both sides. Any palpable ovary in a post-menopause woman is abnormal and warrants further investigation. The fingers then are pushed forward to determine if there is good support of the rectovaginal septum. If a rectocele is present, the finger in the rectum will protrude forward into the vagina, and the vaginal mucosa will protrude from the introitus. If stool is present on the glove, a guaiac test can be performed to rule out colon bleeding.

Two situations deserve special attention: gynecologic examination of the obese patient and the adolescent patient.

The Obese Patient

The body configuration of the obese patient defies adequate pelvic examination.

Nonetheless, by using several techniques, the clinician can ascertain that at least gross abnormalities do not go undetected. The physician can usually examine the external genitalia in the same manner as in the nonobese patient. A large speculum, however, must be used for the vaginal examination. The bimanual examination is always difficult in obese patients because of the thickness of the abdominal wall. In this situation, the fingers examining the vagina are used to move the cervix laterally and up and down to gain an appreciation of the mobility and the size of the uterus. If the cervix and the uterus are readily mobile, it is unlikely that the uterus is involved with a large tumor. Next, the examiner presses the hand examining the abdomen toward the promontory of the sacrum. By moving the fingers in the vagina posteriorly and upward, the examiner can be certain that although the uterus may be involved with myomas or other forms of space-occupying lesions, there can be no mass of greater diameter than the distance between the examiner's fingers.

The next procedure is to sweep the fingers examining the vagina laterally toward one adnexal area, at the same time trying to push the hand examining the abdomen toward this area in order to determine if the ovaries are normal. If this adnexal region is free of masses, the examining fingers ought to be able to move freely as they proceed toward the lateral pelvic wall. Then the fingers in the vagina are swept along the pelvic sidewalls and posteriorly toward the sacrum to ascertain that there are no masses on the pelvic side walls. The same procedure is carried out on the opposite side.

The Child or Adolescent Patient

The second clinical situation that warrants special attention is the examination of the child or adolescent gynecologic patient. Since the reason for the visit is frequently the presence of discharge or abnormal bleeding, performing a thorough examination is mandatory. Visualization must be accomplished to rule out a foreign body. Furthermore, although neoplasms are uncommon in this age group, in the presence of abnormal bleeding these must be ruled out. The cooperation of the patient can often be obtained by careful psychologic prepara-

tion and thorough explanation of the mechanics of the examination. Even with the cooperation of the child, the examination may be technically difficult because of an intact hymen. The use of a nasal speculum, test tube, or cystoscope can be very helpful in visualizing the vagina. Rarely, the examination proves impossible in the physician's office. In this circumstance, it may be necessary to perform the procedure in the hospital under general anesthesia.

SCREENING PROCEDURES

Papanicolaou Smear Test

An integral part of any examination is the Papanicolaou smear test (Pap smear). This is performed on all patients beginning at 15 years of age at least annually, or more frequently if indicated. The only two reasons for not doing an annual Pap smear would be a recent negative smear or the absence of the uterus and cervix.

As this test is also performed to measure the hormone responses of the vaginal epithelium (K.P.I.) in addition to detecting early neoplastic changes, there is still a reason to perform a Pap smear in a patient following total hysterectomy. As it takes many years to develop cervical intraepithelial neoplasia, the reward for doing a careful Pap smear is the assurance that the patient with a negative smear is almost completely safe until her next examination and cytologic smear.

The Pap smear should be taken at least once every year. Because of the widespread use of the cytologic smear beginning in the late 1940's, the incidence of early cervical intraepithelial neoplastic lesions detected by this test has risen sharply, and as might be expected, the incidence of advanced carcinoma of the cervix has sharply declined. Nonetheless, today there are still many women who do not receive the Pap smear.

It is best not to use any lubricating jelly prior to the insertion of the speculum for a Pap smear. The speculum may be lubricated by immersing it in warm water. A wooden spatula is used to scrape the exfoliated cells from the squamocolumnar junction. This is the site from which abnormal cells arise when patients have cervical intraepithelial neoplasia. In addition, cells high in the cervical canal, and perhaps from the uterus, may be sampled either by aspirating the vaginal pool in the posterior fornix or by inserting a pipette into the cervical canal for aspiration of the endocervical secretions.

In the past, results of Pap smears were reported on a scale of 1 to 5, with 1 being negative and 5 being frank cancer. A more recent classification proposed by the American Cancer Society states that a Pap smear is negative, positive, or suspicious. The negative smear may indicate that there is metaplastic change. In this instance, the clinician should repeat the smear in 3 months. If the smear is suspicious or positive, the clinician must follow through with a very carefully planned work-up.

An abnormal or suspicious smear must be followed by histologic investigation. In the past, patients with abnormal Pap smears all underwent cone biopsies, which ordinarily necessitated hospitalization and general anesthesia. More recently, colposcopic examination with directed biopsies has obviated the need for conization in many instances.

Colposcopy

This gynecologic advance, recently introduced into American gynecologic practice, is very helpful in decreasing the necessity for conization biopsy of the cervix. The colposcope is an instrument that magnifies the epithelium of the cervix under direct vision. Physicians with proper training are capable of identifying epithelial changes that warrant colposcopically directed biopsies. In this way, the clinican is able to obtain biopsies of all tissues that are potentially malignant. If the cervical canal is long or if the squamocolumnar junction is high up inside the endocervix, colposcopic examination is not adequate. This is often the case in postmenopausal women. In these instances, a conization biopsy of the cervix is essential.

Colposcopy offers the advantage of decreasing the hospitalization and the extent of the operation that would be involved in performing a cone biopsy, an operation that, although generally safe, can cause some serious problems, including hemorrhage, infection, and miscarriage. Decreasing the incidence of hospitalization by systematically screening all patients

with abnormal Pap smears represents a major breakthrough. The physician performing the colposcopy must be well trained, thorough, and systematic. Otherwise, an occult early carcinoma that would have been found in a cone biopsy may go undetected.

The Schiller Test

Staining the cervix with Lugol's iodine solution will delineate areas of abnormal epithelium and facilitate accurate biopsy. The normal cervical epithelium contains glycogen. Lugol's solution combines with glycogen to produce a dark staining of the normal cervical epithelium. When the epithelium undergoes neoplastic change or inflammation, the cells frequently contain a decreased amount of glycogen. The application of Lugol's solution to the cervix may result in a positive Schiller test, which identifies the abnormal epithelium as areas of pale staining or poorly staining cervical epithelium. These areas should be further evaluated by biopsy.

Cervical Biopsy

Any abnormal exfoliative cytologic smear must be followed by a tissue examination. Therefore, the clinician must perform cervical biopsies, colposcopically directed cervical biopsies, or a cone biopsy. The cervical biopsy may be done in the office by taking a Kavorkian-Younge punch biopsy forceps and performing a four quadrant biopsy at 3, 6, 9, and 12 o'clock in the region of the squamocolumnar junction. Any visible lesion should be biopsied.

Endometrial Biopsy

By use of a Novak suction curette, an endometrial biopsy may be performed in the physician's office. A tenaculum is placed on the anterior lip of the cervix, and following sounding of the uterine cavity, the small curette is inserted into the endocervical canal. It is passed up into the uterine cavity, and the endometrium is sampled. Although this technique has been used primarily for detection of ovulation in infertility or endocrine investigations, it is also very helpful in detecting endometrial carcinoma. In addition, more recent endometrial sampling methods have allowed clinicians to aspirate the endometrium. One such method is the use of the Vabra and Gravlee jet aspirators.

CONTRACEPTION

The most common reason for which women during the active menstrual years will vist the family physician is for advice regarding prescription of an effective contraceptive. The numerous methods of contraception in use today clearly indicate that there is no one method that is both effective for and acceptable to all. The proper selection of a contraceptive should be made after a dialogue between the patient and her physician. During this dialogue, the physician should elicit the patient's feelings concerning her sexuality, her own body, and her partner's potential role in the responsibility for contraception. Additional information should be obtained about her menstrual history, past medical history, and her concerns and fears about her body. Following such dialogue between the physician and the patient, a proper choice of a contraceptive can be made.

Oral Contraceptives

The most effective and the most common form of contraception today is the oral contraceptive pill. Basically, at present there are only three choices of oral contraceptives: the 50 μg. estrogen and progesterone pill, the sub-50 μg. estrogen and progesterone pill, and the "mini-pill," which consists only of progesterone. Certainly, the 50 μg. and the sub-50 μg. oral contraceptive pills are effective in preventing pregnancy. The mini-pill is less effective, but may be effective enough to warrant prescribing it for selected individuals. Higher estrogen-containing oral contraceptives are available for specific indications.

Although the vast majority of women in their reproductive years can take the oral contraceptives, there are some women for whom these are contraindicated. The *absolute* contraindications to the prescribing of oral contraceptives are:

1. Thrombophlebitis, thromboembolic disorders, cerebro-vascular disease, or a past history of these conditions.

2. Markedly impaired liver function; cholestatic jaundice during pregnancy.

3. Known or suspected carcinoma of the breast.

4. Known or suspected estrogen-dependent neoplasia.

5. Undiagnosed abnormal genital bleeding.

6. Known or suspected pregnancy.

Additional contraindications include:

1. Congenital hyperlipidemia.

2. Gestational diabetes.

3. Gestational jaundice.

4. Heart disease.

5. Progressive hypertension.

The *relative* contraindications are:

1. Epilepsy.

2. Hypertension.

3. Leiomyoma.

4. Migraine headache.

5. Oligomenorrhea.

6. Severe depression.

The oral contraceptive pills have some definite advantages. The patient with mild acne tends to find that this improves on an estrogen-dominant oral contraceptive. The patient with moderate to severe dysmenorrhea may find that this disappears while she is taking oral contraceptives. Minimal adenomyosis or endometriosis tends to improve, or at least does not progress, while a patient with these lesions is taking contraceptive pills. The patient with irregular menses may have her periods regulated by the oral contraceptives. If menses are irregular, the patient should be evaluated. Oral contraceptives can then be prescribed to regulate the menstrual period.

There are, however, several disadvantages inherent in the use of oral contraceptives. The patient may experience nausea, breakthrough bleeding, weight gain, fluid retention, or breast tenderness.

The *nausea* generally "cycles out," that is, disappears following one or two cycles. If the patient takes oral contraceptives at bedtime, frequently the nausea will be minimized because the symptoms will occur during the sleeping hours.

The *breakthrough bleeding* also tends to "cycle out," often disappearing after two or three cycles. If it persists, the physician should consider prescribing an oral contraceptive with a high estrogen content or one with a different estrogen-progestogen ratio.

Breakthrough bleeding is one of the major clinical problems of managing a patient taking oral contraceptives. As a rule, increasing the estrogen content of the oral contraceptive will stop breakthrough bleeding. The patient in her teens or 20's presents few major clinical problems in this regard. However, the patient in her late 30's or early 40's who is using an oral contraceptive can be having vaginal bleeding because of an early carcinoma. This must be differentiated from persistent breakthrough bleeding and must be investigated. If a clinician were to permit a patient to have intermenstrual bleeding over a prolonged period of time without investigation, he could unwittingly be allowing an undetected cancer to progress.

Weight gain on oral contraceptives occurs because these pills are anabolic steroids. The patient may have 3 to 5 pounds of true weight gain, which may be manifest in breast tissue, hip tissue, and other areas that make up feminine contours.

The *fluid retention* experienced with the oral contraceptives is usually mild and intermittent. Occasionally, a patient may be very sensitive to the fluid-retaining properties of the steroid contraceptives, but in most instances, the fluid retention may be managed by mild salt restriction until the patient becomes adjusted to the oral contraceptive. A diuretic is rarely indicated.

Breast tenderness is a common symptom during the first cycle following the initiation of the oral contraceptive. Generally, this "cycles out" and is rarely experienced subsequent to the second cycle.

Another problem with oral contraceptives is the occurrence of *"silent menses."* This is said to be present when a patient takes oral contraceptives for 3 weeks, discontinues the pills for 1 week, and experiences no withdrawal bleeding. This finding indicates that the oral contraceptive has caused a minimal growth of the endometrium, so that withdrawal of the pills does not cause a shedding of the endometrium. Clinically, this becomes bothersome because the patient fears that she might be pregnant. Indeed, if she is pregnant, the oral contraceptives should be discontinued because of a rare but definite syndrome that may be caused by taking the contraceptive pills during early pregnancy. A report by Nora[6] about the potential teratogenicity of progestin-estrogen combinations describes a disorder called the VACTERL syndrome, as the congenital lesions associated with this syndrome consist of vertebral, anal, cardiac, tracheal, esophageal, renal, and limb malformations (see also Chapter 35, page 458). With the help of today's more sensitive pregnancy tests, the clinician can rule out pregnancy very early. If the patient experiences new episodes of "silent menses," she should have a pregnancy test prior to the resumption of the oral contraceptives. A higher estrogen-dose oral contraceptive may be indicated.

Intrauterine Contraceptive Devices

The intrauterine device (IUD) is the second most common form of contraception. The advantage of this technique is that once the IUD is inserted, the patient does not have further responsibilities in order to achieve effective contraception. The disadvantages are that the patient may have intermenstrual spotting, cramping, and a pregnancy risk of approximately 3 pregnancies per 100 woman-years.

The optimal time for the insertion of the IUD is during the menstrual period. At this time, the cervical os is slightly dilated, there is minimal chance of a pregnancy, and insertion of the device is usually facilitated. The patient should return in 1 to 3 weeks for a follow-up examination to make sure that she has not expelled the intrauterine contraceptive device and that the strings are properly protruding from the cervical os. If the nylon string is too long, it is trimmed off at this time. The patient should be instructed to check for the IUD string periodically.

The recent intrauterine contraceptive devices contain a fine strand of copper wire wrapped around the carrier device. The copper tends to decrease uterine activity and to promote retention.

The use of the Progestasert device has offered an additional form of intrauterine contraception. In this instance, the vehicle contains progesterone that is slowly released over a 1 year period. The T carrier in itself is not a good contraceptive device except when combined with a slow release progesterone. Based on 45,848 woman-months of use with 5495 women, the pregnancy risk of the Progestasert was 1.9 pregnancies in multiparas and 2.5 in nulliparas per 100 woman-years. The Progestasert must be removed each year, as the progesterone will be expended in approximately that time.

Condom

The next most common form of contraception is the condom. The condom has a pregnancy risk of 17 pregnancies per 100-woman years. Failures are usually due to improper use.

Diaphragm

The diaphragm, once very common, became less frequently used following the popularity of the oral contraceptives and the IUD. Because of recent concern about the risks of the oral contraceptives and the intrauterine contraceptive device, there has been an increase in the use of the diaphragm. The diaphragm serves as a barrier. When used with spermicidal cream, it serves as an effective contraceptive with a pregnancy risk of 18 pregnancies per 100 woman-years. The major problem with the diaphragm is that it must be used every time the couple has intercourse. If coitus occurs more than once in a short period of time, an additional application of contraceptive cream must be applied without disturbing the diaphragm. The diaphragm should always remain in place at least 6 to 8 hours after coitus.

Foam

Vaginal foam is the next most common contraceptive. This has a use effectiveness of 25 pregnancies per 100 woman-years. It, too, must be used each time a couple has intercourse.

For a further discussion of contraceptive counseling, see Chapter 35.

PELVIC INFECTIONS

VAGINITIS

Vaginitis is one of the most common complaints encountered in the practice of office gynecology. Although this may be considered a rather routine and mundane sort of problem to treat, it is generally of major concern to the patient and if not treated skillfully will usually recur. The clinician should muster all of his talent to make the correct diagnosis and prescribe the proper treatment so that the patient may overcome this extremely bothersome problem.

Leukorrhea

Anatomically, the vagina is an invagination covered with squamous epithelium. Unless dilated by some structure, the vaginal walls are in apposition. Throughout the menstrual cycle, there is a continual shedding of the epithelial cells. There is also a continual secretion of mucus from the endocervical glands. The combination of the epithelial cells and the endocervical mucus results in a clear, colorless or white discharge called leukorrhea. This discharge generally collects in the vagina and in the normal patient is expelled intermittently. It may be removed by bathing the area of the introitus or by douching. Normal leukorrhea may be increased during pregnancy, sexual excitement, or the use of contraceptive pills. The sequential contraceptive pill, now removed from the market, caused excessive leukorrhea in some women because of stimulation of the endocervical glands by estrogen.

An additional cause of excessive vaginal discharge, or excessive leukorrhea, is cervical erosion. In this condition, the squamocolumnar junction migrates outward on the pars vaginalis. If the squamocolumnar junction moves significantly out onto the portio of the cervix, the increased surface area of columnar epithelium may cause increased mucous discharge and therefore excessive leukorrhea. In addition, if there is increased vascularity of this epithelium when the increased surface area of the columnar epithelium is extensive, there may be frequent inflammation that may cause elaboration of purulent mucous discharge.

Leukorrhea usually does not cause irritations; however, it may cause a sensation of dampness. Treatment for this problem is cryosurgery. The freezing of the cervix causes destruction of the columnar epithelium and subsequent regeneration of squamous epithelium. Electrocautery will work in the same manner.

Monilia Vaginitis

Monilia vaginitis is caused by the *Candida albicans* and related fungi, which are natural inhabitants of the bowel. These fungi may also be found on the skin and in the vagina in the absence of clinical infection.

The character of the discharge is thick,

white or yellow, and curdlike. The amount of discharge may range from minimal to profuse.

The symptoms are generally a mild to moderate discharge with vulvar irritation and itching. The itching may be extremely pronounced. As the organism thrives in moist, warm media, it is more common during the summer months when swimming and sunning are prevalent. It is also associated with use of oral contraceptives and antibiotic therapy. If a patient has recurrent monilia, she should be screened for diabetes.

The diagnosis is made by noting the large, curdlike discharge on speculum examination. Less severe forms of the disease may be diagnosed by making a wet mount preparation at the time of speculum examination. This simple diagnostic test is done by placing a small amount of discharge on a glass slide and adding a drop of saline solution. Occasionally, when looking for *C. albicans*, there is so much debris present that a solution of 10 per cent KOH is required to destroy the blood cells and decrease the amount of debris present. *Candida* may be identified by observing the hyphae and the spores. In those instances in which *C. albicans* cannot be identified on a wet mount preparation, it may be necessary to perform a culture. A cotton swab containing the vaginal secretion is smeared on Nickerson's medium and incubated for 24 to 48 hours. If positive, the brown colonies of *Candida* may be identified on the surface of the medium. This method of diagnosis is rarely needed, however.

The treatment for a *C. albicans* infection is the use of a chlordantoin-benzalkonium (Sporostacin) vaginal cream, nystatin (Mycostatin) vaginal tablets, or an acetic acid-oxyquinoline (Aci-Jel) vaginal jelly.

Trichomonas Vaginalis Vaginitis

This form of vaginitis is caused by *Trichomonas vaginalis,* a motile protozoan with a flagellum. This one-celled organism is slightly larger than a white blood cell. Trichomonas vaginitis is less frequently encountered than monilia vaginitis.

The patient experiences symptoms of moderate to profuse discharge that is generally yellow or greenish and opaque and contains small bubbles. The foamy appearance is highly suggestive of *Trichom-onas*. The patient may also have moderate vulvar irritation and itching.

The detection of *T. vaginalis* is made by a wet mount preparation. The motile trichomonads may be seen moving in relation to other cellular debris. The diagnosis is definitive and relatively easy to make.

The treatment for trichomoniasis is metronidazole (Flagyl), 250 mg. orally, three times a day for 10 days. Generally, only the gynecologic patient is treated. If the infection recurs, both the patient and her partner should be treated. The trichomonads may be harbored in the male urethra and prostate gland without causing symptoms. In such a setting, reinfection will occur unless the male is treated concurrently. Patients who consume ethanol should be warned that one of the side effects of metronidazole is a reaction similar to that occurring in patients being treated with disulfiram (Antabuse).

Hemophilus Vaginalis Vaginitis

Hemophilus vaginalis vaginitis is of less common occurrence. In the past, this infection was frequently called a "nonspecific" vaginitis.

The patient may experience symptoms of profuse discharge, which is usually yellow-green, appears purulent, and has a foul odor. The diagnosis may be made by finding "clue cells," epithelial cells containing the *Hemophilus* bacteria within the cytoplasm in a wet mount preparation. There is usually minimal to moderate vulvar irritation. Although there is usually no itching, the patient may experience a burning soreness.

The treatment for *H. vaginalis* infection is a triple sulfonamide (Sultrin) vaginal cream inserted twice daily for 2 weeks.

General Considerations in Diagnosing Vaginitis

Often there is a discrepancy between the source of infection and the location of symptoms. For instance, a patient often complains of pruritus of the vulva when on examination the clinician can see that the bulk of the infection is actually occurring inside the vagina. The treatment of the local pruritus, therefore, would be only symptomatic. To eradicate the infection, the therapy must be directed at eliminating the vaginitis.

Because the female urethra is short and is traumatized by intercourse, urinary tract infections are relatively frequent in women. Occasionally, a patient will have a mild cystitis or urethritis, which she will confuse with vaginitis. Because of urinary frequency or even of urge incontinence, the patient finds herself with a sensation of moistness and irritation around the vulva. Vaginitis may be excluded by careful examination of the vagina and examination of a wet mount preparation. A urine culture should be performed. Simple lower urinary tract infections will generally respond to a course of antibiotics.

ENDOMETRITIS

In recent years, endometritis has become a relatively common disorder. Although endometritis occurred prior to the use of intrauterine devices (IUD's), it has become much more frequent since the advent of this form of contraception. The most common time for endometritis to occur is immediately following the insertion of an IUD. However, it may occur at any time as long as the IUD is in place. Occasionally, this disorder is accompanied by a unilateral salpingitis. The uterus and cervix are very tender on motion, and there may be a mild to moderate discharge. If an IUD is present, it should be removed. Furthermore, the patient should be treated with an antibiotic such as ampicillin, 250 mg. orally, 4 times a day for 7 days after appropriate cultures are taken.

VENEREAL DISEASE

Because of increased physician awareness and better methods of detection, most venereal disease is now treated on an outpatient basis.

Gonorrhea

Gonorrhea is caused by the *Neisseria gonorrhoeae* organism. In the United States today, gonorrhea is prevalent in epidemic proportion because of increased sexual promiscuity. This has resulted in part because the oral contraceptive pill, which gives almost complete protection against pregnancy but offers no protection against venereal disease. The oral contraceptive has resulted in more premarital promiscuity and has eliminated the use of barrier contraceptive devices that once helped prevent the spread of venereal disease. Unfortunately, much of the spread of gonorrhea occurs before the victim knows she has the disease, and therefore it goes untreated. Even among those who are willing to seek treatment, the situation has become problematic. The strain of the gonococcus that has reached the United States from the Phillipines is resistant to penicillin and is threatening to become widespread.

In 1966, there were 351,738 cases of gonorrhea reported in the United States. In 1975, this figure had risen to 999,937 cases.

The increased frequency of intercourse among young people and the increased incidence of multiple partners have been partial causes of this epidemic. A further problem is that the gonococcal organism may exist in the lower genital tract of the woman without causing symptoms. As long as a woman is unaware of her gonococcal infection, she can potentially be the source for multiple infections.

Female children may become infected by transmitting the gonococci from their hands to their genitalia or even by handling infected bedclothes and linens. Fortunately, in young children the disease is generally limited to the vagina and can be treated effectively with penicillin.

The frequency of asymptomatic carriers of the gonococcal organisms has been as high as 6 per cent in general clinic populations and as high as 9 per cent in the high risk clinic groups. The routine screening of patients for gonorrhea is indicated in young, sexually active patients. Whether this is done for all patients in a private practice must be determined by the frequency of the disease in the particular practice in question. Diagnosis can be made by culturing material from the cervix, vagina, and Skene's glands and by swabbing the material on the Transgrow medium, which assures an anaerobic climate in which to transport it to the laboratory for definitive culture. Of course, a positive culture is the indication for treating a patient, and all of her contacts should be treated as well. The usual regimen of treatment is aqueous procaine penicillin G, 4.8 million units intramuscularly, and probenecid, 1 gram by mouth at least one-half hour before the injection of penicillin. Spectinomycin, 4.0 grams intramuscularly, is prescribed if the patient is allergic to penicillin.

If the culture is negative but the patient has a definite history of exposure, it may be prudent to treat her also. The treatment is relatively inexpensive and simple to administer, provided the patient is not allergic to penicillin. Furthermore, the risk of severe complications from an untreated case of gonorrhea is much greater than the risk of treating a patient unnecessarily. If a patient has a doubtful history of exposure and a negative culture, perhaps treatment need not be administered.

Gonococci spread by direct extension from the vagina and the cervical canal along the endometrial surface. Following a menstrual period, the organisms can pass through the internal os and ascend to the endometrium and to the mucous surface of the fallopian tubes.

Pelvic Inflammatory Disease Caused by Gonorrhea. The major clinical manifestations of acute pelvic inflammatory disease (PID) are fever and extreme tenderness of the fallopian tubes. Tubal infections usually produce folds of endosalpinx that give rise to blind pockets of infection (salpingitis isthmica nodosa). When the infection is caused by the gonococcus alone, the destruction of tissue is usually limited to the endosalpinx. The fallopian tube may become enlarged and distorted if there are secondary invaders. The invasion of the tubes by bacteria such as *Escherichia coli* occurs with an advanced, acute PID.

Because acute PID can mimic appendicitis and ectopic pregnancy, the clinician must be perceptive and astute when making this diagnosis. If a vaginal discharge is present, a Gram's stain may show intracellular diplococci, which would give an immediate indication that the diagnosis is gonorrhea. Furthermore, if the cervix is exquisitely tender on motion and if a purulent discharge is coming from it, gonorrhea is a likely diagnosis. The erythrocyte sedimentation rate rises markedly in the presence of an acute pelvic inflammation but not with an appendicitis.

An ectopic pregnancy may be ruled out if the clinician has facilities for receptor site binding assays available. This sensitive test for detecting early pregnancy is usually positive when an ectopic gestation is present. Nonetheless, because the consequences of missing the diagnosis of appendicitis or ectopic pregnancy would be grave, occasionally a laparoscopy or laparotomy must be performed to rule out these entities.

Complications of Gonorrhea. The major complication in gonorrhea is secondary invasion by coliform organisms. *Escherichia coli* is the most common invader, spreading from the rectum via the lymphatics. An *E. coli* infection causes massive tissue destruction in large collections of pus. The typical tubo-ovarian masses are then formed. The patient becomes febrile, complains of severe pain, and appears acutely ill. Cul-de-sac aspiration is productive of free pus from the peritoneal cavity. A culture of this pus generally will not grow the gonococcus, but will grow the secondary coliform invaders.

Primary Syphilis

Syphilis has become less of a problem than it formerly was, having been brought under control soon after World War II. In 1966, 105,159 cases were reported, whereas only 80,356 cases were recorded in 1975. Testing for syphilis during premarital and initial prenatal examinations has markedly reduced the incidence of congenital syphilis in the United States; nonetheless, this may still occur, and the physician must be aware of this problem.

Syphilis is a venereal disease caused by *Treponema pallidum*, which causes a painless, shallow ulcer or open pustule (chancre) to develop on the epithelium of the vulva, vagina, or cervix, or even on the skin of the fingers, 2 to 4 weeks after sexual exposure. The initial lesion may be small, or it may be large and deep. The typical ulcer is nontender and has a clean base with indurated edges. Generally, there is a discrete inguinal adenopathy.

The primary lesions of chancre, lymphopathia venereum, granuloma inguinale, and herpes progenitalis may resemble the syphilitic chancre. All of these ulcerations must be considered to be syphilitic until proved otherwise. The diagnosis depends upon a darkfield identification of the spirochete in the serous fluid taken from the ulcer. The serologic test for syphilis may remain negative for 1 to 3 weeks after the appearance of a chancre and may remain positive years after treatment.

Gynecologic complications of syphilis are rare. The major clinical implication is that the pregnant woman with an active syphilitic infection may transmit it to her fetus and give birth to an offspring with congenital syphilis.

The treatment of primary syphilis is 2.4 million units of procaine penicillin G injected into the buttocks initially and 1.2 million units of this drug injected intramuscularly every other day for a total dose of 4.8 million units. If the patient is allergic to penicillin, she may be given tetracycline, 1.5 grams orally, followed by 500 mg. four times a day orally for at least 7 days. Tetracycline should not be used for complicated gonococcal infections during pregnancy because of the potential toxic effects for the mother and fetus. Instead, erythromycin, 500 mg. orally four times daily for 15 days, may be given. These are the minimal doses according to recommendations of the Communicable Disease Center. Occasionally, higher doses must be given.

Condylomata Acuminata

Condylomata acuminata may appear on the labia, in the vagina, or on the anal area. They may appear as either single wartlike or cluster growths on the skin. The moist perineum and the perineal area are receptive environments for condylomata, particularly when vaginitis causes a purulent discharge. Condylomata are the result of a venereal infection and therefore are also inoculable.

The treatment of condylomata acuminata is the local application of 25 per cent podophyllum in tincture of benzoin. The treatment of a concurrent vaginitis would be helpful in eliminating the cause of condylomata. If the number of vaginal warts is large, electrocoagulation with local anesthesia or cryosurgery is effective.

Herpesvirus Type I and Type II

Herpesvirus Type I is generally found in and around the mouth, whereas herpesvirus Type II infection is usually found in the genital region. Either type of virus may cause infection of the genital tract. The

patient develops clusters of small vesicles that are filled with clear fluid. She may have shallow vulvar lacerations and leukorrhea. She will generally complain bitterly of vulvar pain. Herpes genitalis is an acute inflammatory disease of the genitalia caused in most cases by the herpes simplex virus Type II. This problem is being encountered with increasing frequency. It is most often seen in the office practice of both the family physician and the gynecologist. Herpes genitalis is perhaps seen more commonly today than is gonococcal infection, which it resembles in the respect that both are venereal diseases.

The symptoms of primary herpes infection usually appear within 3 to 7 days after exposure to the virus. The lesions may be extensive and multiple and may involve the labia majora, labia minora, perineal skin, and vestibule of the vulva as well as the vagina and endocervical mucosa. Vesicles appear early in the course of the disease. These frequently rupture, leaving shallow, painful ulcers.

The treatment is a polymyxin B, neomycin, gramicidin (Neosporin) ointment applied locally three times a day and oral analgesics. The use of ethyl chloride and povidone-iodine (Betadine) on the vesicle also has been suggested.

Recurrence of herpes genitalis, though common, is not seen in all patients. The virus of herpes genitalis is probably harbored in the dorsal nerve root ganglia that receive sensory fibers from the genital tissues. The virus is believed to migrate down the nerve fibers to the affected area when the infection recurs. Causes of reinfection may be emotional stress, premenstrual tension, and severe systemic disease. Recurring lesions are generally not as well defined as the primary lesions. They may be vesicular or ulcerative in type and may vary in size from pinpoints to 5 mm. in diameter. The vesicles generally rupture within 2 days and healing is complete in approximately 10 days. The symptoms of recurrent infection include burning and pain and, frequently, burning on urination.

ABNORMAL VAGINAL BLEEDING

One of the most common complaints of gynecologic patients is abnormal vaginal bleeding. Although there are many causes of such bleeding, these may be broken down into several categories so that the clinicians can make a logical approach to diagnosis and management. First, it is important to ascertain whether the reason for bleeding is obstetric or gynecologic, as these causes have completely different implications. There are times when the patient in early pregnancy presents as a gynecologic patient. The cause of bleeding may be the result of implantation site bleeding, and ectopic pregnancy, or a threatened abortion.

The Normal Menstrual Cycle

To establish that a given bleeding pattern is abnormal, the clinician must have a very definite idea of what normal bleeding is. The normal menstrual cycle consists of sloughing of the secretory endometrium at regular intervals. This implies the occurrence of ovulation and the production of progesterone by the corpus luteum. The onset of the menarche generally begins between ages 11 and 16 years in the United States, the average age being 12 years. If a patient starts to menstruate 1 or 2 years earlier than age 11, this in itself is not abnormal, but the clinician must be on the lookout for other factors, such as precocious puberty or irregular bleeding. If menstruation does not occur by age 18, investigation is definitely indicated. Generally the thelarche precedes the menarche. Siblings in the family tend to experience the menarche at about the same age.

Normal menstrual periods recur at a range of 21 to 36 days, with an average 28 day cycle. The menstrual cycles are always counted from the first day of the menstrual flow to the first day of the subsequent menstrual flow. As a patient ages, or as her metabolism changes, the frequency of her normal menstrual cycle may change; a month-to-month change, however, is abnormal.

The duration of menstrual cycles ranges from 3 to 7 days. On the first day, the flow is often light, becoming heavier thereafter. Bleeding is abnormal when it occurs 1 or 2 days after the end of a menstrual period. A light day of spotting followed by regular menses can be considered normal. A period that exceeds 7 days of flow is considered prolonged.

Character of Menses. The menstrual flow consists of a shedding of the endometrium mixed with blood, vaginal cells, and endocervical mucus. The blood is generally dark red because of its slow passage through the vagina, but if the bleeding is brisk, it may be bright red. The average volume of a single menstruation is 30 to 100 ml., although volumes up to 300 ml. would not be considered excessive for some women. The counting of sanitary menstrual pads or tampons required is an excellent method of determining the amount of bleeding. When patients state that they have heavy menstrual periods, the clinician should ask how many pads are used each day and should multiply this by the number of days of menstruation. Some patients need to wear both a tampon and a pad in order to absorb the flow. A tampon or a pad is generally saturated when it absorbs 25 ml. of menstrual flow.

Frequently a patient will experience premenstrual tension several days prior to a normal menstrual period. She may notice a slight increase in weight, slight bloating of the abdomen, and tenderness and heaviness of the breasts. Some women complain of feelings of tension, headaches, or pressure sensations. On the day prior to menstruation, many women experience mild to moderate menstrual cramps. These are most frequently noted on the first day of menstruation. Generally, there is a decreasing amount of menstrual cramps as the period progresses. When pain with the periods is moderate to severe, it is categorized as *dysmenorrhea* (see page 745).

Metrorrhagia

Metrorrhagia is intermenstrual bleeding, or bleeding that occurs at a time other than the menstrual period. If the bleeding occurs at midcycle, particularly when accompanied by a sharp or dull persisting lower quadrant pain, the patient may be experiencing *mittelschmerz*, which is a manifestation of ovulation. This is one of the major points in the differential diagnosis of intermenstrual bleeding. Often, however, a patient will complain of bleeding between menstrual periods that may bear no cyclic relationship to the periods. In this instance, the patient is experiencing metrorrhagia, and the cause must be determined.

Great emphasis is placed on evaluating intermenstrual bleeding because it is one of the indications of investigation for carcinoma. For instance, women with endometrial carcinoma may have intermenstrual bleeding, while women with advanced cervical epithelial neoplasias may have intermenstrual or postcoital bleeding.

Most of the other causes of intermenstrual bleeding are not clinically as important. Nonetheless, intermenstrual bleeding *must* be investigated until the clinician is satisfied that the patient does not have a malignancy.

The cause of metrorrhagia can be organic or dysfunctional. Among the organic causes are uterine polyps, endometrial hyperplasias, uterine fibroids, cervical erosions, cervical polyps, senile vaginitis, and urethral caruncles, to name a few. The lesions that are located at the introitus, cervix, or vagina can generally be seen by inspection and speculum examination. The lesions that are present in the uterine cavity are often diagnosed only following hysterograms, endometrial biopsies, aspiration biopsies, or dilatation and curettage.

Menorrhagia

Menorrhagia is an excessive menstrual flow. In the extreme situation, a woman may lose as much as 500 to 1000 ml. of blood during the menstrual period. Obviously, blood loss of this magnitude would cause anemia and, eventually, symptoms of blood loss. Nonetheless, many women experience significant menorrhagia without any other major symptoms.

The most common cause of severe menorrhagia is a submucous myoma that is generally diagnosed at the time of dilatation and curettage. There are many other organic and nonorganic causes of menorrhagia. The presence of this symptom demands a thorough work-up and treatment for the same reason that metrorrhagia must be investigated—the patient may have a carcinoma. The clinician *must* perform a thorough investigation to ascertain the cause of the menorrhagia. If a malignancy, such as an endometrial carcinoma, a malignant uterine or cervical polyp, or a carcinoma of the cervix, has been ruled out by cytologic studies, fractional dilatation and curettage, and biopsies of the cervix, the problem

becomes one of the medical management. Frequently, the dilatation and curettage will prevent further menorrhagia. If it does not, the patient may respond to the 50 mg. or the sub-50 mg. dose of an oral contraceptive pill. If menorrhagia is not amenable to medical management, hysterectomy may be indicated.

Menometrorrhagia

Menometrorrhagia presents a problem for the clinician because it also can be a sign of an undetected malignancy. Menometrorrhagia is irregular bleeding during and between menstruation of such a pattern that it is difficult to tell when a period starts and stops. The most common cause is dysfunctional uterine bleeding, and consequently the results of a thorough work-up for cancer are often negative. Nonetheless, the clinician must proceed as if a malignancy could be present. In this instance, a thorough history and physical examination, cytologic smear examinations, and frequently fractional dilatation and curettage are necessary to arrive at the proper diagnosis. The patient may have hyperplasia of the endometrium, an endometrial polyp, submucous myomas, a cervical polyp, cervical erosion, atrophic vaginitis, or one of the numerous other problems that can cause menometrorrhagia.

Postcoital Bleeding

Bleeding following intercourse is a warning sign to the clinician, because postcoital bleeding may be associated with cervical carcinoma. In actual practice today, most women who have had regular smears will not have a lesion of the cervix that is sufficiently advanced to cause postcoital bleeding from a gross cancer. However, as there are still many women who do not have annual Pap smears, the clinician must always suspect that an undetected cervical carcinoma may be the cause. Examination of exfoliated cytologic smears will generally be helpful in such patients, but if there has been a significant amount of postcoital bleeding, fractional dilatation and curettage will be necessary.

Among the other causes of postcoital bleeding are cervical erosion, cervical polyps, and endometrial polyps.

Dysfunctional Uterine Bleeding

During the course of a normal menstrual cycle, the lining of the uterus is growing. At the time of ovulation, the corpus luteum produces progesterone, which causes hypertrophy of the endometrial stroma and secretory changes in the glands, with subsequent sloughing at the time of menstruation. In dysfunctional uterine bleeding, the patient does not ovulate. The endometrium grows to a point at which the vascular supply can no longer meet the demands of the rapidly growing membrane. There is an irregular shedding of the endometrium with concomitant bleeding. The patient may state that she has spotting on and off throughout the month. In dysfunctional uterine bleeding, there is an absence of organic causes such as tumors, pregnancy, or infection.

The patient must be managed by cytologic smear examination and fractional dilatation and curettage. Frequently, the dilatation and curettage corrects the problem. If this fails, hormonal therapy may be employed. The clinician must be aware that dysfunctional uterine bleeding is a diagnosis made by excluding other causes. If bleeding continues to recur despite therapy, the suspicion of an undetected carcinoma must be raised. Obviously, the younger the patient, the less likely that the cause will be carcinoma. Since dysfunctional uterine bleeding has a tendency to recur, a hysterectomy is frequently the choice of management following the patient's reproductive years.

Postmenopausal Bleeding

Postmenopausal bleeding can be defined as any bleeding that occurs 6 months or more after cessation of the menses. The average age for the menopause is 48 years, although many women menstruate on into their 50's. Postmenopausal bleeding is of particular concern because several studies have indicated that the incidence of endometrial or cervical carcinoma is as high as 30 to 50 per cent in patients with such bleeding. When postmenopausal bleeding occurs, a thorough history and physical examination are mandatory. Cytologic smears are taken on the first visit. In spite of a normal examination and a negative Pap smear, the patient must be scheduled for a fractional dilatation and curettage because of the extremely high incidence of carcinoma. Even if an obvious cause for the vaginal bleeding is found, such as senile vaginitis, a dilatation and curettage is still mandatory because of the grave risk of overlooking a life-threatening malignancy.

Another common cause of postmenopausal bleeding today is the use of exogenous estrogen therapy. Conjugated estrogens (Premarin) taken on a regular schedule (for example, either 3 weeks on and 1 week off or the first 25 days of each month) frequently induce withdrawal bleeding in the postmenopausal patient. More recently, clinicians have added medroxyprogesterone acetate (Provera), 10 mg. per day, to the last week of the conjugated estrogens. This regimen ensures a proper slough of the endometrium. It appears logical that if the endometrium builds up and does not properly regress prior to the next course of therapy, bleeding will quite likely occur with the next cycle of therapy. Any other bleeding that occurs while a patient is taking conjugated estrogens should be investigated by performing a fractional dilatation and curettage or at the very least by an endometrial aspiration. The withdrawal bleeding is to be expected, and any investigation will have to be left up to the clinician's judgment.

Bleeding During Pregnancy

First Trimester Bleeding. During the time of implantation, the patient may experience some vaginal spotting. This may occur anywhere from the seventeenth to the twenty-ninth day of the cycle. It is short in duration and small in amount.

Any vaginal bleeding following a missed menstrual period must be considered a possible complication of pregnancy, such as a threatened abortion or an ectopic pregnancy. The work-up for this problem includes a pregnancy test and a careful history and physical examination. *Ectopic pregnancies* are generally unilateral, associated with vaginal spotting, and accompanied by pain. *Threatened abortions* typically start with bleeding, which may be accompanied by midline cramping or pain and tenderness on examination. It is most important to make the proper differential diagnosis, particularly since these abnormal conditions occur at the same time that a patient may be having implantation bleeding or bleeding from decidual shedding. When an abnormal condition occurs, intervention may be necessary; on the other hand, intervention when only implantation bleeding is present would be unfortunate. An ultrasound scan showing an intact gestational sac implanted high in the uterus can be reassuring of a normally progressing pregnancy.

Second Trimester Bleeding. Bleeding during the second trimester may be caused by threatened abortion, hydatidiform mole, or placental complications such as placenta previa or premature separation of the placenta. The history and physical examination usually establish the diagnosis. Today, quantitative pregnancy tests and ultrasound scanning of the pregnant uterus may be useful in determining the cause of the bleeding.

Third Trimester Bleeding. Such bleeding is generally due to placenta previa, premature separation of the placenta, or bloody show. All third trimester bleeding must be considered a placental complication until a work-up rules this out. Of course, there is a possibility that the bleeding could be coming from the cervix or vagina. This too must be considered and ruled out. From a clinical standpoint, however, third trimester bleeding should put the clinician on guard for placenta previa or for a premature separation of the placenta. Diagnostic ultrasound examination is helpful in differentiating these causes. If the bleeding occurs near term and the placenta does not appear to be involved because of the location of its implantation or because of the clinical picture, a diagnosis of bloody show may be made.

Other Bleeding Disorders

In very young or very old patients, a history of vaginal bleeding may actually be caused by rectal or urinary tract bleeding. These patients may be poor historians. An additional work-up must be undertaken to be certain that the clinician does not overlook a malignancy.

PELVIC PAIN

Dysmenorrhea

The term dysmenorrhea refers to pain occurring at the time of the menstrual period.

It is probably the most common of all the gynecologic symptoms, as most women who reach the age of menstruation experience it in some form. Dysmenorrhea is classified as primary, secondary, or membranous. *Primary* or *essential* dysmenorrhea characteristically occurs at the time of the menarche or 1 or 2 years later and is said to be present when the patient complains of painful menstruation but exhibits no evidence of organic disease. *Secondary* or *acquired* dysmenorrhea appears years after the menarche and usually occurs in conjunction with demonstrable disease processes, notably endometriosis. *Membranous* dysmenorrhea is a syndrome in which severe, cramping pain is associated with sloughing of the endometrium, resulting in expulsion of an endometrial cast.

The cause of primary or essential dysmenorrhea is unknown. It is probably related to myometrial contractility, but it is unclear why uterine contractions are painful in some women and not in others. The pain is often relieved by mechanical dilatation of the cervix, whether by dilatation and curettage of the uterus or by childbirth. Emotional disturbances and anxiety increase the severity of the pain in dysmenorrhea, and it may be aggravated by telling the girl beginning her menstrual cycles of the painful experiences remembered by her mother. The pain is cramping in character and is noted as an aching sensation in the suprapubic area or as discomfort in the low back. It usually appears just before the onset of the menstrual flow and lasts for several hours, or sometimes for a whole day.

The treatment of primary dysmenorrhea is symptomatic and begins with the performance of a thorough physical examination, which enables the physician to reassure the patient that no pelvic disease is present. Analgesics are prescribed, and antispasmodics are sometimes helpful. The patient is advised to use local heat in the form of a heating pad or a hot tub bath. If these simple measures are not successful, anovulatory cycles may be induced, using cyclic administration of estrogen-progestogen combinations for 6 months. If the pain continues in the presence of anovulation, one must consider the possibility of a psychoneurosis requiring psychotherapy. In the past, surgical relief was occasionally attempted by performing a presacral neurectomy, but this operation is rarely done today in the absence of organic disease.

Secondary or acquired dysmenorrhea is most characteristically caused by pelvic endometriosis. When this is the basis for the pain, pelvic examination will often show thickening and nodularity of the uterosacral ligaments or fixed retroversion of the uterus. Characteristic peritoneal implants can be observed at laparoscopy. Another cause of secondary dysmenorrhea is an imperforate hymen behind which menstrual blood accumulates and distends the uterus (hematometra) and the vagina (hematocolpos). The same effect can be produced by congenital strictures of the vagina and by anomalies of the uterus. Patients with a history of recurrent attacks of acute salpingitis sometimes complain of acquired dysmenorrhea. A pedunculated submucous leiomyoma may act as a foreign body and be partially extruded through the cervical os, and in such a situation the patient will complain of intermenstrual bleeding accompanied by cramping pain continuing into the menstrual period itself.

The treatment of secondary dysmenorrhea is dictated by the demonstrable cause of the symptom as well as by its severity. If the organic lesion responsible for the pain cannot be identified by ordinary physical examination, endoscopy and hysterosalpingography may be useful diagnostic aids. Surgical extirpation may be required in patients who have severe endometriosis and pelvic inflammatory disease. In early endometriosis with only moderate dysmenorrhea, hormonal induction of anovulation may be sufficient to control this disorder.

Dyspareunia

The underlying cause of dyspareunia may be an organic lesion of the pelvis or vagina, such as trichomonal or monilial vaginitis; congenital vaginal anomalies, such as a septum or band; or an unyielding hymen. Postmenopausal women with atrophic vaginitis may develop dyspareunia, and it also occurs in patients with longstanding chronic pelvic inflammatory disease or when an ovary has prolapsed into the cul-de-sac of Douglas. In the absence of organic disease, women may complain of severe pain on intercourse associated with involuntary spasm of pelvic and paravaginal muscles that is caused by psychosexual

disturbance—so-called "functional" dyspareunia. These women require expert sexual counseling. Yet another recognizable basis for dyspareunia is pelvic congestion occurring in anorgasmic women.

The treatment of organic causes of dyspareunia varies, depending upon the lesion that is present. A painful episiotomy scar can be revised surgically. Congenital bands can be excised, or a rigid hymen incised. Severe chronic pelvic inflammatory disease and extensive endometriosis may require surgical extirpation. Atrophic vaginitis responds to estrogen replacement, both local and systemic. The cure of psychogenic forms of dyspareunia is more difficult to attain and may involve psychiatric consultation.

UTERINE TUMORS

Enlargement of the uterus is detected by pelvic examination and requires careful evaluation as to its nature. It is important to distinguish between the benign and malignant processes that cause enlarged uteri. True neoplasms of the uterus may affect the corpus or the cervix, and, together with tumors of the ovary, are the principal forms of gynecologic cancer.

TUMORS OF THE UTERINE CORPUS

Leiomyoma

In everyday gynecologic practice, the most common neoplasm of the uterus proper is the leiomyoma, often referred to as a "fibroid" tumor. This usually occurs as multiple, irregular, nodular enlargement of the uterus that is readily recognized on bimanual examination. It is estimated that about one-fourth of all women over the age of 35 years will have palpable leiomyomas, although many of them will be free from symptoms. This tumor is characteristically found in women during the fourth and fifth decades of life.

Leiomyoma may be classifed according to its location in the uterus. *Intramural* myomas are those that occupy the wall of the uterus without impinging on either the endometrial or the serosal surfaces. Those that protrude from the external surface and stretch the visceral peritoneal covering are called *subserous* myomas, while the tumors that distort the endometrial cavity are termed *submucous* lesions. Both the subserous and submucous tumors may be either *sessile,* with a broad, flattened base, or *pedunculated,* attached to the uterus by broad or thin pedicles. The tumors are surrounded by a pseudocapsule, and each has a single source of blood supply that enters the myoma at one point. This creates a situation in which varying degrees of acute or chronic ischemia are likely to be present. Consequently, myomas are subject to a number of forms of degeneration, most commonly *hyaline* change, but sometimes *cystic* degeneration and *calcific* generation. During pregnancy, myomas are subject to a form of aseptic necrosis with hemorrhage and hemolysis, producing *carneous* or *red* degeneration, evidenced by softening of the tumor that simulates the gross appearance of sarcoma. Submucous pedunculated tumors are apt to become secondarily infected after compromise of their blood supply has resulted in necrotic changes.

Leiomyomas are almost always benign. The incidence of leiomyosarcoma arising in a myoma is approximately 0.5 per cent, so that this possibility is not a factor influencing management.

Diagnosis. As has been noted, the diagnosis of uterine leiomyomas is most often made with ease by performing pelvic examination, although when the tumors are large, they can be palpated abdominally and may be noticed by the patient herself. Even though symptomatic myomas constitute one of the most frequent indications for hysterectomy, the majority of uterine myomas do not produce symptoms or interfere in any way with the health or well-being of the woman. However, an asymptomatic myoma may cause a problem in differential diagnosis. Thus, pedunculated subserous myomas may be difficult to distinguish from ovarian tumors or adnexal inflammatory masses, while symmetrical enlargement due to myoma can mimic a pregnancy. In the latter event, a pregnancy test is mandatory before undertaking surgical treatment.

When leiomyomas do become symptomatic, they may bring about *uterine bleeding,* usually in the form of menorrhagia. Sometimes the bleeding is sufficiently massive to result in anemia, and in such patients removal of the uterus is clearly indicated. Whenever bleeding of an abnormal pattern

occurs in a patient known to have myomas, other causes of such bleeding must be ruled out by appropriate investigation. For instance, women with adenocarcinoma of the endometrium frequently have coincidental leiomyomas. Another frequently associated condition is endometrial hyperplasia, presumably due to the presence of anovulatory cycles.

Pedunculated submucous myomas may act as foreign bodies and produce cervical dilation with protrusion of necrotic tumor into the vagina. In this case, the patient may have a foul vaginal discharge and irregular spotting, which may be confused with an exophytic carcinoma of the cervix. Another occasional symptom of myomas is urinary frequency brought about by pressure of the tumors on the bladder. Degenerative changes in the tumors can produce dull, aching pain, while torsion of the pedicle of a subserous lesion may result in the picture of an acute abdomen, with nausea, severe local tenderness, and signs of peritoneal irritation.

When the tumors are large, they may produce a feeling of heaviness in the pelvis, often associated with constipation. Myomas tend to increase in size during pregnancy because of edema and degeneration. Submucous tumors may increase the incidence of spontaneous abortion. The previously mentioned "red" degeneration may bring about sudden uterine pain that can be confused with appendicitis or diverticulitis. If degeneration of a myoma is the working diagnosis during pregnancy, conservative treatment is best, as myomectomy increases the change of abortion or premature labor.

Treatment. The definitive treatment of leiomyomas of the uterus is total hysterectomy, but this is indicated only if the tumors produce significant symptoms or if they become very large. A patient with asymptomatic myomas need only have periodic pelvic examinations to detect rapid growth of the tumors or other complications. The tumors will regress after the menopause, and if they have not been troublesome before the perimenopausal period is reached, they will not require active intervention after cessation of the menses.

An occasional patient who is being studied because of infertility will be found to have asymptomatic myomas. Although most patients with fibroids do not have decreased fertility, in a few instances myomas may be associated with inability to conceive, although this is often difficult to prove. If a thorough investigation of an infertile couple fails to demonstrate any cause for the infertility and if the patient has a myomatous uterus, a multiple myomectomy may be performed. This consists of removal of as many of the tumors as possible and reconstruction of the uterus, thus preserving the childbearing potential. Such surgery does not constitute a curative intervention, as once a patient has demonstrated her ability to grow myomas, she is likely to continue to do so. In addition, the operation may give rise to postoperative complications such as intestinal obstruction and pelvic adhesions.

Hysterectomy, when indicated, may be done by the vaginal route if the symptomatic myomas are small, although in most instances in which hysterectomy is indicated, the tumors will be of sufficient size to make the abdominal approach preferable. Particularly when the tumors are large or if the patient is obese, exposure may be difficult, and the operation will often be technically intricate. For this reason, even asymptomatic tumors should be removed, if large, particularly those leiomyomas larger than a uterus of 12 weeks' size.

Adenomyosis (Internal Endometriosis)

Occasionally, uterine enlargement may be caused by adenomyosis or internal endometriosis, a condition in which displaced islands of endometrium occur in the uterine wall, causing hypertrophy of the myometrium. Although symptoms of irregular and profuse bleeding and pelvic discomfort have been attributed to this disease, it does not constitute a significant clinical entity, as the diagnosis is made only upon examination of a specimen taken at hysterectomy.

Endometrial Adenocarcinoma

Of much greater import is adenocarcinoma of the endometrium. This neoplasm occurs most often in women in the postmenopausal age group and is the most important cause of postmenopausal bleeding. As this tumor tends to remain confined to the endometrium for a long time before spreading beyond the confines of the uterus, it is imperative that any woman with a history of postmenopausal bleeding of any

degree whatsoever be thoroughly investigated to rule out endometrial cancer.

Diagnosis. Although a number of methods for sampling the endometrium in the physician's office have been described (notably the Gravlee jet washer and the Vabra suction curette), the most reliable way to screen the endometrium for cancer is to perform a fractional curettage under general anesthesia. In this way, very few endometrial cancers will be missed. It should be noted that the Pap smear, which is the prime tool for the diagnosis of early cervical cancer, is not useful for screening patients with endometrial carcinoma, as the endometrial cells do not reach the ectocervix and the vagina with sufficient regularity to herald the presence of a malignant process in the endometrium.

The peak incidence of endometrial carcinoma in women is between the ages of 50 and 60 years, or some 10 years past the average age for the cessation of the menses. Approximately three-fourths of the cases occur after the menopause, and in the exceptional instances in which this tumor occurs at an earlier age, there is frequently a long history of irregular bleeding associated with anovulatory cycles.

Both endogenous and exogenous estrogen stimulation, unopposed by progesterone, appear to predispose the patient to the development of endometrial cancer. In recent years, statistical evidence has accumulated that suggests that a greater number of women than expected who had been given estrogen for many years as replacement therapy ultimately developed endometrial carcinoma. There are certain other characteristics of women prone to develop this lesion that can serve as criteria of suspicion when postmenopausal bleeding is the presenting complaint. Thus, the triad of obesity, diabetes, and hypertension should alert the physician to the possibility of endometrial carcinoma. More than half the patients with proven endometrial cancer will have at least one feature of the triad. Patients with polycystic ovaries are also more prone to endometrial carcinoma.

Treatment. The treatment of endometrial cancer should be undertaken in a medical center in which the facilities for systematic follow-up and the team approach to cancer therapy are available. In some instances, total hysterectomy and bilateral oophorectomy are all that is required, although with bulky tumors preoperative radium application or external radiation therapy may be indicated. Each patient's treatment should be individualized, and this is best done in an environment in which many patients are seen and multiple specialists are available for consultation. This principle holds true for patients with all forms of genital cancer.

Other Tumors of the Uterine Corpus

Other tumors of the uterine corpus are unusual and will not often be encountered in family practice, but the physician should be alert to their occasional occurrence, so they will not be missed. The *mixed mesodermal tumor* is a highly malignant and usually fatal form of cancer that presents as a uterine enlargement with irregular, usually postmenopausal, bleeding and sometimes with a bulky tumor mass protruding from the partially dilated cervix. A slightly more favorable prognosis is attached to the *leiomyosarcoma*, which may arise either in conjunction with antecedent leiomyomas or de novo. This diagnosis may be thought of when a patient with previously slowly growing leiomyomas exhibits a sudden, rapid growth of one of the tumors; such cases demand prompt surgical exploration. It should be reiterated, however, that the vast majority of fibroid tumors of the uterus are benign, and the possibility of sarcoma is sufficiently remote that this alone does not justify routine hysterectomy in the absence of significant symptoms.

TUMORS OF THE UTERINE CERVIX

Polyps

The uterine cervix is the site of origin of a variety of tumors, both benign and malignant in their clinical behavior. Cervical polyps are benign pedunculated growths seen protruding from the partially dilated cervical os. They are friable, glairy masses that can be treated in the office by twisting them off at the pedicle if the site of attachment is low down in the cervix; if it is higher up, a curettage may be necessary. Although a few polyps have been described as having malignant changes in the base of the pedicle, such changes are extremely unusual. Cervical stenosis may follow operations on the cervix (cryosurgery, cau-

terization, radium therapy) and can produce uterine enlargement caused by the accumulation of blood (hematometra), fluid (hydrometra), or exudate (pyometra). Treatment of these disorders consists of cervical dilatation and insertion of a drain to maintain patency.

Carcinoma

Diagnosis. The most important clinical lesion of the uterine cervix is carcinoma. The routine use of the Pap smear has made possible the diagnosis of this lesion in its earliest stages and has enabled researchers to study the development of cervical cancer in great detail. It is now thought that the earliest recognizable stage in the development of squamous cell carcinoma is *dysplasia*. This lesion cannot be discerned by the naked eye but will be suggested by the appearance of a cervical scraping of cells (Pap smear) that displays certain characteristic features of anaplasia, notably variation in size, shape, and chromatin content of nuclei; multinucleation; abnormal mitoses; and other cytologic abnormalities. Appropriate biopsy sites for exploration of the extent of early cervical cellular abnormalities can be determined by the gynecologist who has the special expertise necessary to employ the colposcope. This technique is now emerging in the United States as a useful adjunct to the cytologic smear in the diagnosis of early cervical cancer.

Cervical dysplasia is often found adjacent to areas of *carcinoma in situ*, in which the anaplastic changes extend throughout the entire thickness of the cervical epithelium but do not penetrate beyond the basement membrane. The definitive diagnosis of intraepithelial or in situ cancer is made only after histologic study of the entire squamocolumnar junction; cytologic studies and colposcopy serve merely as screening methods to indicate which patients require cervical biopsies.

The standard method of biopsy in patients with evidence of carcinoma in situ is conization of the cervix, in which a cone-shaped piece of tissue is removed, incorporating the entire squamocolumnar junction and the lower part of the cervical canal. This rather extensive biopsy is necessary because a cervix with foci of carcinoma in situ may harbor early invasive cancer in another part of the same organ, and the treatment for invasive cancer must be far more aggressive than that of in situ cancer without invasion. It is now recognized that both cervical dysplasia and carcinoma in situ are to be considered progressive stages in the development of frankly invasive cancer, although it is difficult to provide absolute proof of this progression.

The average age of patients who develop invasive carcinoma of the cervix is 48 years, or 8 to 10 years older than the average age for carcinoma in situ. It has not been established that every case of invasive cancer is preceded by an in situ phase; some of these lesions may well be invasive from the beginning. There is evidence that the development of invasive squamous cancer of the cervix is related to early sexual activity and childbearing. This would account for its higher rate among women in less privileged socioeconomic circumstances.

Invasive cancers may be *exophytic*, in which the cervix is replaced by friable, hemorrhagic, necrotic, cauliflower-like masses of tumor tissue, or *endophytic*, in which the tumor develops in the cervical canal and spreads into the parametria without appearing at the cervical os. The extent to which the tumor has spread beyond the cervix is determined by bimanual rectovaginal examination.

Classification. If the biopsy shows invasive cancer, the stage of the tumor is determined by evaluating the base of the broad ligament, which becomes indurated as the result of fibrous tissue proliferation around the tumor cells as they migrate along the lymphatic drainage pathways of the cervix. Carcinoma in situ is classified as Stage 0. If the tumor is confined to the cervix, it is said to be a Stage I lesion. In Stage II carcinoma, there is extension to the vagina, or the parametrium is infiltrated, but the induration does not reach the lateral pelvic wall. Stage III carcinoma involves the lower third of the vagina or reaches the pelvic wall, or there is renal obstruction. In Stage IV the cancer extends outside the reproductive tract (distant metastases, extension to bladder or rectum).

Treatment. The treatment of carcinoma in situ ordinarily is simple total hysterectomy, but some patients can be treated by cryosurgery. The latter is the standard method of managing cervical dysplasia. Invasive cancer requires the attention of the

gynecologic oncologist and the therapeutic radiologist. In early invasive lesions, radical hysterectomy with pelvic lymphadenectomy may be the procedure of choice; in the more advanced stages, radiation therapy is indicated. There is no place in the management of this disease for the occasional surgeon or the inexperienced radiotherapist. Such patients should always be managed in cancer centers in which an experienced team of physicians and ancillary personnel can concentrate on the problem.

ADNEXAL TUMORS

By definition, the adnexa include the fallopian tubes and the ovaries. These structures are not usually palpable as distinct masses unless significant enlargement exists; when this is the case, it is imperative to determine the nature of the enlargement felt. This is of particular importance because ovarian cancer is an insidious disease that produces very little or no symptomatology until it reaches an advanced, incurable stage. One of the principal reasons for routine periodic pelvic examinations in apparently healthy women is the discovery of silent enlargements of the adnexa that could be caused by true neoplasms.

Ovarian Tumors

The ovaries may harbor *physiologic cysts* (cystic corpus luteum, follicular cyst, simple cyst) that are large enough to be detected on pelvic examination. Such cystic enlargements rarely attain the size of 5 or 6 cm. and are characteristically transient, disappearing when the patient returns for re-examination within a few weeks. True neoplasms, on the other hand, grow progressively larger and never regress; thus, progressive enlargement of an adnexal mass demands definitive diagnosis to rule out neoplasm.

When an adnexal mass is felt on bimanual examination, the most essential feature that is to be evaluated is the consistency of the mass, i.e., whether it is felt to be cystic or solid. The reason for the importance of this determination is apparent from referring to Figure 41–1, which indicates the relative risk of cancer in both solid and cystic ovarian neoplastic masses.

As this figure indicates, although the relative risk of malignancy for all ovarian

Ovarian tumors

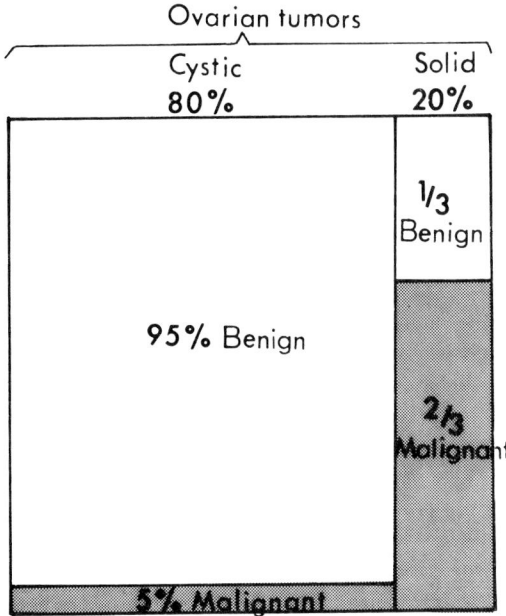

Figure 41–1.   *Relative risk of cancer in cystic and solid ovarian masses.*

neoplasms is approximately 17 per cent, the great majority of the clinically malignant tumors will be solid in consistency. Therefore, although one may temporize with a cystic adnexal enlargement in order to avoid unnecessary surgery for patients who may have physiologic cystic enlargements of the ovaries, every solid adnexal tumor demands immediate exploration, as does a cystic mass greater than 7 cm. in diameter.

Ovarian tumors may occur at any age but are most prevalent during the reproductive years. The clinically malignant neoplasms, however, are most likely to occur in either prepubertal girls or in women past the age of 50 years. They are often entirely asymptomatic; as they grow larger, they may be noticed as palpable abdominal masses.

Pain is not usually present with an uncomplicated ovarian tumor, but torsion of the pedicle of a pedunculated tumor, usually a cyst, produces a typical clinical picture of sudden, exquisite abdominal pain associated with signs of peritoneal irritation (rectus muscle guarding, rebound tenderness) as the result of interference with the blood supply. Sometimes there is a history of repeated episodes of such attacks, with quiescent periods between the acute episodes. This pattern represents the clinical

equivalent of the alternate twisting and untwisting of the cyst. Hemorrhage or torsion into the cavity of an ovarian cyst may result in rupture and spillage of the cyst contents into the free peritoneal cavity, and in some instances the full-blown symptomatology of an acute abdomen is produced, necessitating exploratory laparotomy.

Ovarian neoplasms may also become infected, but this is rare. When infection is present, it may be difficult or impossible to distinguish the resulting clinical picture from that of a tubo-ovarian abscess.

Some varieties of ovarian cysts may attain huge size and be felt abdominally as a tense accumulation of fluid. In such patients, it is important to differentiate between the presence of encapsulated intracystic fluid and ascites or that of free fluid in the peritoneal cavity, since paracentesis, which may be indicated for the treatment of ascites, is contraindicated with an ovarian cyst. This is because puncture of such a cyst may possibly disseminate viable tumor cells into the peritoneal cavity.

A simple test will differentiate encapsulated from free fluid. When the abdomen is percussed with the patient lying supine, encapsulated fluid will yield a dull percussion note anteriorly, and the displaced intestines will produce tympany in the flanks. The opposite would be true with ascites. Ascites is characteristic of advanced inoperable ovarian cancer with spread of implants to the peritoneum. However, ascites may also be present in conjunction with a solid tumor of the ovary, the *benign fibroma*. The presence of a benign fibroma in conjunction with ascites and hydrothorax is called *Meigs's syndrome,* and in this entity simple excision of the fibroma is curative.

Diagnosis. The diagnosis of ovarian tumors is most directly made by pelvic examination. Roentgenography may demonstrate calcification or formed teeth within a benign cystic teratoma (dermoid cyst), while diffuse calcification may denote the psammoma bodies of a potentially malignant serous cystadenoma. Recently, it has been suggested that ultrasound studies may be useful in detecting some ovarian tumors. For those rare ovarian neoplasms that are capable of elaborating hormones, whether male or female in type, hormonal assays may be useful in the preoperative diagnosis.

Whenever an ovarian neoplasm is suspected, exploratory laparotomy is indicated. The rule of thumb is that all adnexal enlargements greater than 7 cm. should be considered as possibly being neoplastic, as physiologic ovarian cysts do not reach these dimensions. Since the incidence of malignant change in definitely cystic ovarian neoplasms is very low, a patient with a cyst of borderline size may safely be re-examined in several weeks for signs of persistent growth of the cyst. Solid tumors, on the other hand, demand immediate exploration since two-thirds of them will prove to be malignant. The extent of the operation is determined by the nature of the tumor and the patient's desires with respect to the preservation of childbearing potential.

Classification. The histogenesis of ovarian neoplasms is one of the most complex subjects in the field of pathology, and a discussion of this subject is beyond the scope of the present work. Although classifications of ovarian neoplasms tend to be long and complicated, in actual practice the great majority of the cystic tumors encountered will be examples of the *cystadenoma group*—mucinous and serous cystadenomas. In the group of *germ cell tumors,* the most frequently encountered

lesion is the benign cystic teratoma or dermoid cyst, in which the tumor reproduces adult tissues of various types, most notably ectodermal tissues (hair, skin, skin appendages). *Gonadal stromal tumors* are rare but are of special interest because of their capacity in some instances to elaborate feminizing hormones (granulosa cell tumor, thecoma) or masculinizing hormones (Sertoli-Leydig cell tumors), which produce appropriate clinical manifestations. Solid *adenocarcinoma* of the ovary may have an endometrioid appearance on histologic examination and tends to produce peritoneal implants, bloody ascites, and large bilateral masses before the patient experiences severe symptoms.

The precise nature of a given ovarian tumor cannot usually be determined prior to surgery, so that the extent of the procedure will depend on the gynecologist's evaluation of the situation during the operation.

Occasionally, enlarged ovaries may present as so-called *"chocolate cysts,"* containing old brownish blood. These are lesions of external endometriosis, and are usually associated with puckered implants of ectopic endometrium in the peritoneal cavity and in the uterosacral ligaments. Endometriosis is not a true neoplasm, but it exhibits locally invasive properties that in some respects resemble those of invasive cancer. In advanced cases, the treatment is also surgical.

Fallopian Tube Tumors

Lesions of the fallopian tubes are relatively rare as clinically significant entities, except for those associated with acute and chronic pelvic inflammatory disease. A variety of cysts and non-neoplastic tumors may arise in the oviducts; they are most often benign and originate from embryonic remnants or from peritoneal inclusions. Pedunculated cysts of the broad ligament may arise from the mesonephric remnants that are frequently seen in this region; these so-called *hydatids of Morgagni* are usually small and are usually found incidentally at laparotomy.

A variety of benign tumors of the fallopian tubes have been described, but these lesions are so rare as to be of little practical consequence. Likewise, cancer arising primarily in the fallopian tubes represents less than 1 per cent of all female genital cancers.

This possibility should, however, be considered in a nulliparous postmenopausal woman with a serosanguinous discharge and an adnexal mass. The treatment is surgical; its extent is determined by the degree to which the lesion is found to have spread, as determined by exploratory laparotomy.

VAGINAL TUMORS

Cystic Lesions

Benign cystic lesions of the vagina are inclusion cysts, cysts of Gartner's duct, endometriosis, adenosis, and vaginitis emphysematosa.

Inclusion cysts of the vagina are common. They are often seen near the introitus in episiotomy scars. Such cysts are often asymptomatic and rarely require incision or excision.

Cysts of Gartner's duct may cause protrusion of the anterolateral wall of the vagina and can easily be confused with cystocele formation. Sometimes these cysts are large enough to be symptomatic and therefore require surgical removal.

Endometriosis may appear in the vagina as bluish lesions in the area of the posterior fornix that are an extension of cul-de-sac involvement. The diagnosis is made by biopsy, and suspicion regarding this diagnosis is aroused by the characteristic history of endometriosis, the finding of nodular induration in the uterosacral ligaments, and the fixation of the uterus to a cul-de-sac mass.

Adenosis refers to the occurrence of subepithelial adenomatous masses involving any part of the vagina, though these lesions are most often encountered in the upper half of the vaginal vault. These islands of glandular tissue arise from aberrant glands of cervical type; they rarely produce symptoms and do not require treatment. Recently, adenosis has been found to occur in the vaginas of young women whose mothers received diethylstilbestrol at the time they were pregnant with the patients in question, and in a few instances a clear-cell adenocarcinoma has developed in these girls.

Vaginitis emphysematosa is characterized by the formation of diffusely scattered submucosal cysts. The patients affected are most often pregnant, or they have severe cardiac decompensation. The blebs have been determined to contain carbon dioxide, but no consistent bacterial flora have been found. There is usually an associated vaginitis, most often caused by *Trichomonas vaginalis.*

Solid Tumors

Solid tumors of the vagina may be fibromas or uterine leiomyomas that have dissected into the paravaginal area. Others are warty growths, the condylomata acuminata, which are viral in origin and may become very extensive. The latter are particularly widespread and troublesome when they occur during pregnancy, but tend to regress during the postpartum period. The treatment is the application of podophyllum if the lesions are not too extensive. Cryosurgery may also be useful, and sometimes excision is necessary.

Primary malignant tumors of the vagina are extremely rare, making up less than 1 per cent of all tumors of the genital canal. Cancer of the vagina may take the form of either in situ or invasive squamous carcinoma, adenocarcinoma, or the so-called *sarcoma botryoides,* a malignant mixed mesodermal tumor that is more likely to occur in prepubertal girls than in adults. Most malignant lesions of the vagina are metastases from a variety of primary sites, such as choriocarcinoma of the uterus, extensions from squamous cancers of the cervix, or lesions arising in the ovary, endometrium, bowel, vulva, or urinary tract. Treatment of malignant lesions of the vagina must be individualized and should be coordinated by members of oncologic teams in cancer centers, as the problems involved can be extremely complex. In any event, the prognosis is always very poor.

AMENORRHEA

Amenorrhea is defined as the absence of menstruation and is divided into primary and secondary types. Primary amenorrhea is defined as the complete absence of menstruation, whereas secondary amenorrhea is the lack of a menstrual period for 3 or more months.

The most common cause of amenorrhea during the reproductive years is pregnancy.

Before any evaluation of amenorrhea is initiated, pregnancy must be ruled out. Primary amenorrhea should be evaluated in the female who reaches 16 years of age without development of secondary sexual characteristics, i.e., pubic and axillary hair and breast development, or in one who reaches 18 years of age with development of secondary characteristics. Prior to a thorough evaluation, radiologic studies to evaluate bone age for comparison of physiologic age with chronologic age is mandatory. If these are in agreement, further evaluation is in order. The initial evaluation of patients with amenorrhea must include assessment of evidence for acute or chronic disease, weight pattern, and general physical habitus.

Evaluation of Primary Amenorrhea

Evidence for gonadal dysgenesis (e.g., Turner's syndrome), testicular feminization (androgen receptor abnormality), true hermaphroditism, and male or female pseudohermaphroditism must be assessed. Examination of the external genitalia and outflow tracts and a pelvic examination will give some insight concerning these entities.

Evaluation of Secondary Amenorrhea

Central nervous system abnormalities, including emotional upset, hypothalamic abnormalities, pituitary gland malfunction, anorexia nervosa, pseudocyesis, depression, schizophrenia, Sheehan's syndrome, or Simmonds' disease, must be evaluated.

Endocrinopathies in the form of thyroid abnormality, diabetes mellitus, or adrenal malfunction must be investigated. Careful evaluations of ovarian function must be made; ovarian neoplasms, premature ovarian senescence, or surgical, irradiation, or infectious castration may be the underlying cause. Additional evaluation is in order to determine if the patient has ovaries.

If a nongenetic etiology is proposed, the evaluation should begin with the administration of medroxyprogesterone acetate (Provera), 10 mg. daily for 5 days. If withdrawal bleeding occurs, this is evidence of anovulation.

If no withdrawal flow occurs, conjugated estrogens (Premarin), 1.25 mg. daily for 28 days, with Provera added the last 7 days may be tried. Lack of response could

indicate an outflow tract failure or a uterine problem. If bleeding does occur, follicle-stimulating hormone (FSH), luteinizing hormone (LH), and prolactin levels must be assayed 6 weeks after administering hormonal therapy. Such assays will evaluate the hypothalamic pituitary axis. High serum FSH and LH levels indicate ovarian failure. A normal FSH level with an elevated LH level is consistent with polycystic ovarian disease. Low gonadotropin levels are evidence of central nervous system abnormalities. Elevated prolactin levels can inhibit FSH and LH secretions, even without abnormal breast discharge, and therefore can account for amenorrhea.

Karyotyping may be indicated if there is evidence of probable chromosome anomaly with secondary ovarian failure.

Post-pill amenorrhea is a more frequently noted entity because of widespread use of oral contraceptives. If amenorrhea persists for 6 to 9 months following discontinuation of oral contraceptives, the patient must have an endocrine work-up.

RELAXATION OF PELVIC SUPPORTS

As the result of stretching of the supporting fasciae of the pelvis, usually by childbirth, women may experience a variety of symptoms for which relief is desired. The symptoms of pelvic relaxation vary with the particular structure that is principally affected. The patient may complain of protrusion or swelling, a sense of pressure, or a low backache. Bulging of the anterior vaginal wall under the floor of the bladder is called a cystocele; if the relaxation involves the urethra as well, a *urethrocele* is said to be present. These conditions may be associated with symptoms of urinary frequency and urgency and of painful urination. Relaxation in the area of the bladder neck produces an obtuse angle at the ureterovesical junction, which is specifically related to the symptom of *stress incontinence,* or involuntary loss of urine when the patient coughs, strains, sneezes, or laughs.

Uterine prolapse occurs when the cardinal ligaments, the primary supports of the uterus, are stretched, resulting in descent of the entire uterus to a lower level in the pelvis. Uterine prolapse is classified as *first degree prolapse,* in which there is some descent but the cervix has not reached the introitus; *second degree prolapse*, in which the cervix and part of the uterus protrude through the introitus; and *third degree prolapse*, in which the entire uterus protrudes beyond the introitus. The symptoms of uterine prolapse include the discomfort of the actual protrusion as well as irritation and ulceration of the exposed cervix and vaginal epithelium, resulting in bleeding, secondary infection, and discharge.

A *rectocele* is a protrusion of the anterior rectal wall through the relaxed or ruptured vaginal fascia and rectovaginal septum. When this defect is present, the patient may find it necessary to place her fingers in her vagina to empty her lower bowel. An *enterocele* is a true hernia of the pouch of Douglas, with dissection of the upper portion of the rectovaginal septum by a sac lined with peritoneum. Loops of bowel or bits of omentum may prolapse into the sac.

Prolapse of the vagina occasionally occurs after hysterectomy and is usually associated with enterocele and cystocele. It tends to become worse as the patient gets older and represents a formidable technical problem for the gynecologic surgeon.

Although minor degrees of prolapse may sometimes be relieved by nonsurgical methods, such as the use of supportive pessaries or exercises to strengthen the perineal muscles, the principal form of curative treatment is surgical. Uterine prolapse can be dealt with by hysterectomy performed by the vaginal route. Cystocele and rectocele repairs require reconstruction of the paravaginal supporting tissues. Asymptomatic prolapse is not an indication for operation, as in such instances the woman's health and well-being are not in jeopardy. However, extensive degrees of prolapse give rise to sufficiently uncomfortable symptoms to require surgical attention.

INFERTILITY

Infertility affects 10 to 15 per cent of all couples. Forty per cent of cases are attributed to male factors. Female factors accounting for infertility are divided as follows: failure to ovulate—10 to 15 per cent, tubal adhesions—20 to 30 per cent, and cervical factors—5 per cent. An infertility work-up is indicated after approximately 1 year of unprotected coitus without conception.

The history for an infertility work-up should include age, previous pregnancies and outcome, length of marriage, prior marriages, menstrual history, methods and duration of birth control, medical and surgical history, history of venereal diseases, medications taken, occupation, family history, frequency of coitus, and postcoital activities. The latter two points should be thoroughly discussed to ensure that the couple is adequately informed about the basis of ovulation, menstruation, sperm survival, and spermatogenesis.

Both the male and female partner must be examined. Special attention should be paid to the male's general nutritional state, height and weight; testicle size; evidence of gynecomastia, phimosis, epispadias, hypospadias, or varicocele (usually on the left) and stigmata of endocrinopathy, i.e., cushingoid, hypothyroid, and so forth.

In the female, care must be paid to general habitus, pubic hair distribution, nutritional state, thyroid gland function, and evidence of galactorrhea. The pelvic examination should include evaluation of the external genitalia; degree of estrogenization of the vagina; cervical abnormalities; and uterine size, shape, consistency, and position. The work-up should also include ovarian evaluation and rectovaginal examination, with attention to the uterosacral ligaments for evidence of nodularity (as noted with endometriosis) or for lack of mobility of the adnexa (suggesting chronic pelvic inflammatory disease). The initial examination provides the opportunity to treat several easily diagnosed and remedied common causes of infertility, such as cervicitis and vaginitis in the female and prostatitis in the male.

The infertility evaluation must include a semen analysis, an endometrial biopsy to check for evidence of ovulation, and a postcoital test to evaluate survival of sperm in the cervical mucus. A basal body temperature (BBT) graph is useful to assess possible ovulation and timing of coitus.

A semen analysis is obtained after 4 days of abstinence. The normal criteria include a volume of 2 to 6 ml. full liquefaction in 1 hour, over 60 million sperm per ml., 60 per cent mobility, and 60 per cent normal forms. Sperm antibodies are implicated in infertility more frequently today, as sophisticated techniques are more readily available for evaluation.

An endometrial biopsy indicating secre-

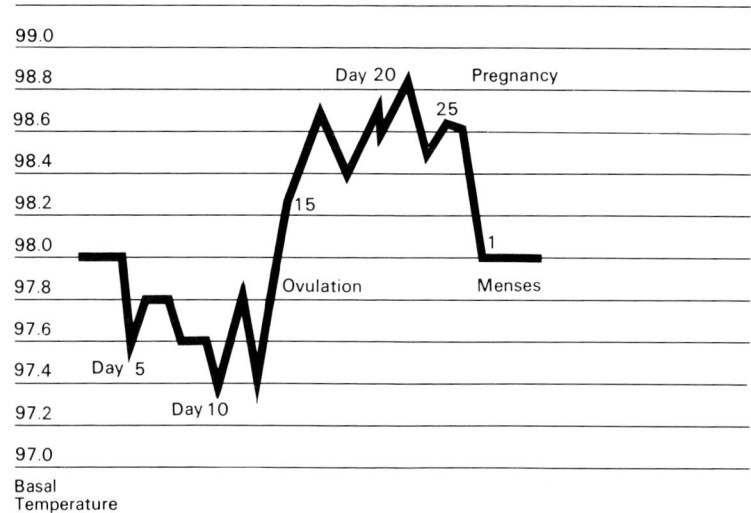

Figure 41-2. Biphasic basal body temperature. (From Speroff, L., Glass, R. H., and Kase, N. G.: Clinical Gynecologic Endocrinology and Infertility. Baltimore, The Williams & Wilkins Co., 1973, p. 181.)

tory endometrium usually is good evidence of ovulation. Luteal phase defects may also be diagnosed if the biopsy indicates a lag of 48 or more hours from the predicted cycle date, based on the next menstrual period.

The Sims-Huhner or postcoital test should evaluate the cervical mucus for spinnbarkeit (stretch of cervical mucus) and should determine the microscopic count of the number of viable sperm per high power field (20 or more is excellent) and the presence of ferning for evidence of progesterone effect. The couple should have coitus the evening before or the morning of the examination.

The basal body temperature is biphasic with ovulation. Temperatures are taken each morning before the patient gets out of bed (Figs. 41–2 and 41–3).

Hysterosalpingography evaluates the endometrial cavity and fallopian tubes. With a history of previous pelvic inflammatory disease, a normal erythrocyte sedimentation rate is a necessary prerequisite for the procedure.

Laparoscopy is a technique used to directly visualize the pelvic organs. It is used as an adjunct to diagnose other possible causes of infertility, such as tubal adhesions, endometriosis, or leiomyomas.

After thorough evaluation, 10 to 20 per cent of couples have no detectable cause for

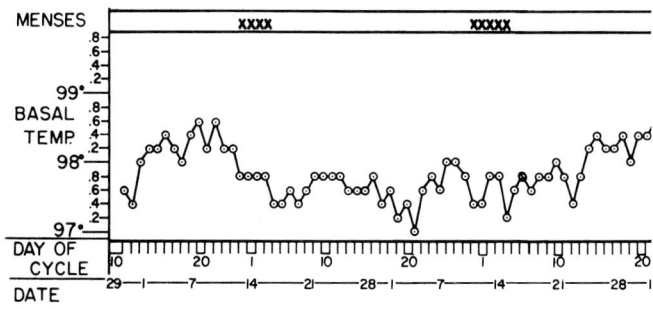

Figure 41-3. Monophasic basal body temperatures. (From Greenblatt, R. B. (ed.): Ovulation. Philadelphia, J. B. Lippincott Co., 1966, p. 140.)

their infertility. At present, artificial insemination, sperm banking, and, in the near future, in vitro fertilization and subsequent intrauterine implantation offer new hope for the infertile couple.

PREGNANCY

Rubella During Pregnancy

Rubella is generally a mild, 3 day childhood disease, but when it occurs in the first trimester of pregnancy, it can cause major congenital malformations and mental retardation. Congenital malformations of the heart and eyes and congenital deafness are particularly common. The risk of congenital malformation is very high if rubella occurs in the first trimester; this risk drops precipitously in the second trimester and is negligible in the third. A major epidemic of rubella in 1964 caused 30,000 stillborns and 20,000 newborns with mental retardation and congenital malformations.

In 1966, there were over 200,000 cases of rubella in the United States. In 1967, a safe antirubella vaccine became available, and by 1974, the number of cases of rubella decreased to 12,000. Since then, however, the incidence of rubella has been increasing slowly. A rubella antibody titer should be performed on all pregnant patients who do not already have a known positive titer or a documented episode of rubella. Rubella immunization must not be done during pregnancy. If a patient is not immunized against rubella prior to her pregnancy, she may be immunized following delivery, provided she is given adequate contraception to protect her from a pregnancy during the subsequent 3 month period. If a significant rise in rubella titer occurs following suspected rubella infection during the first or second trimester of pregnancy, a therapeutic abortion should be offered to the patient. Although the patient, after hearing all of the facts, may choose not to terminate the pregnancy, this information should be presented carefully to her.

Immunizations During Pregnancy

One of the grave considerations in obstetric care is whether or not to immunize pregnant patients against infectious disease. Immunizations against infections such as poliomyelitis, smallpox, and diphtheria

have had excellent results. Immunization against poliomyelitis was begun in 1955 when the Salk vaccine became available. In 1961, the Sabin vaccine was first used. As a result of these immunization methods, the incidence of poliomyelitis decreased from thousands of cases annually a quarter of a century ago to only eight cases in 1975.

Diphtheria was once a major killer of young children. Its occurrence has been reduced sharply because today more children are inoculated against diphtheria than against any other disease. Nonetheless, one in five children is still susceptible, and over the last decade, the incidence of diphtheria has remained between 200 and 275 cases per year.

Immunization against smallpox has met with the greatest success, as there have been no known cases of smallpox in the United States since 1949. Furthermore, vaccinations against this disease are no longer required in this country. After several disastrous epidemics, the long campaign to wipe out smallpox began in 1850 when a number of United States cities began inoculating school children with a smallpox vaccine. The most severe form of smallpox disappeared by 1900, and the last outbreak took place just after World War II.

Because of a comprehensive immunization program, smallpox has been almost completely eliminated. The last known case in the world occurred in Somalia. This individual case has been under surveillance by the World Health Organization.

Patient Instructions

Instructions to the pregnant patient are extremely important, as she has many fears and concerns regarding the bodily changes that she is undergoing. Often the husband also has a great deal of anxiety about the physiologic changes to be expected during pregnancy.

Nutrition.   In the past, the rule that only a 16 to 20 pound weight gain was allowed throughout pregnancy was adhered to rigidly by physicians. This caused undue regimentation of obstetric care. Emphasis was on limited sodium and caloric intake, to the exclusion of other important factors. In 1968, the Committee on Maternal Nutrition, Food and Nutrition Board of the National Academy of Sciences–National Research Council recommended that the pregnant woman consume a diet containing 2400 calories a day. This should include 78 grams of protein, 800 mg. of folic acid, and 18 mg. or more of iron. Today less emphasis is placed on weight gain, with greater emphasis given to meeting nutritional requirements, particularly that of protein. It is recognized that pregnancy causes an increase in dietary needs. There are increased requirements for vitamins A and C because of their known concentrations in the fetal circulation. Intake of folate is needed because of the increased maternal and fetal hemoglobin synthesis. Studies by Niswander and coworkers show that fetal birth weight has a significant relationship to maternal prepregnancy weight. The World War II studies of the effects of starvation on people in Holland and in the Soviet Union during the siege of Leningrad show that the infant born during significant periods of nutritional deprivation is lighter in weight for gestational age than the normal infant.

Exercise. The patient may safely engage in physical exercise similar to that in which she participated before she became pregnant. Generally speaking, she may engage in the same athletic activities she participated in prior to pregnancy. It is unwise, however, to undertake new sports or sports such as skiing that may result in significant blunt abdominal trauma, should an accident occur.

Intercourse. There is no evidence to indicate that intercourse is harmful to the fetus. Yet intercourse may sometimes be associated with premature labor. In instances of ruptured membranes and bleeding, the patient should be instructed to abstain from coitus.

Smoking. Smoking more than one pack of cigarettes a day during pregnancy has been associated with the birth of smaller infants compared with those of nonsmoking mothers. There is some question as to whether the patients who choose to smoke are those who normally would have smaller infants or whether the smoking itself is responsible for this occurrence. More recently, Yerushalmy[12] has reported that mothers who subsequently start smoking give birth to smaller infants than do nonsmoking mothers used as controls.

Douching. Douching should be avoided during pregnancy unless under the specific directions of a physician, as the possibility of injecting air or solution into the venous circulation is increased. Occasionally, the clinician will recommend a very low pressure vaginal douche to treat a vaginal infection.

Dental Care. Routine dental care may be undertaken during pregnancy. If dental x-rays are necessary, the patient should have a lead apron applied to her abdomen to protect the fetus from radiation exposure. Medications associated with dental operations should be avoided, if at all possible. It is therefore unwise to undertake elective dental work that requires medication during pregnancy.

Medications. There is no medication that can be stated to be without potential harm to the fetus or the newborn. The more we learn about medications, the more side effects we find in the fetus and the newborn. Daily, we give prescriptions or patients take over-the-counter preparations that apparently do no harm. Nonetheless, the best policy is that the pregnant patient take no over-the-counter medicine. The physician should limit prescribing to vitamins, iron, and folic acid and only those additional medications that are absolutely essential.

Obviously, there are certain instances in which the risk of a medical problem far exceeds the risk of taking medication. A good example of this is maternal pyelonephritis. If this condition is severe, premature labor may ensue, so this disease should be treated early and adequately.

HIGH RISK PREGNANCIES

Of the obstetrical patients seen by the family physician, probably between 10 and 20 per cent will fall into the high risk pregnancy category. Many of these patients will have some predisposing factor, either in their history or in their examination, that indicates a threat to the mother, fetus, or newborn. Others will develop problems during pregnancy. Basically, the concept of high risk pregnancy management was developed from the model of managing Rh factor pregnancies more than a decade ago. All patients who were Rh-negative were identifiable as a high risk group. Until they developed antibodies, there was no threat to their pregnancy. When an antibody developed, these patients were referred to a high risk pregnancy clinic and were followed throughout their pregnancy with intensive evaluation by physical examination, antibody studies, amniocentesis, and other diagnostic modalities. By following this protocol over a 5 year period, no immunized patients arrived in the hospital for delivery without prior detection of this disorder. The perinatal mortality from Rh disease was decreased from 45 per cent to 8 per cent. This model has since been applied to other forms of high risk pregnancies. During the transition period, patients with numerous unrelated problems were referred to the Rh clinics, such as women with habitual abortion, bicornuate uterus, diabetes, and recurrent hydramnios.

Applying this high risk pregnancy concept to the practice of obstetrics enables the physician to identify patients with a problem and to arrange their referral to a clinic in which special attention may be directed to the high risk situation. This special attention is provided by highly trained health professionals, including obstetricians, neonatologists, internists, nurses, nutritionists, and laboratory personnel. In addition, diagnostic laboratory modalities are readily accessible. The clinics are generally held in the morning. The results of the laboratory data collected at that time are available for a high risk pregnancy conference the next day, during which the history, physical examination, and laboratory data are all presented and total evaluation of the patient is possible.

Basically, high risk pregnancy patients can be divided into two groups. The first group is composed of those patients whose problems can be predicted and managed comprehensively by prenatal examination, discussion, and planning prior to a subsequent pregnancy. These would include such situations as Rh immunization, diabetes, and heart disease. The second group is composed of patients who develop a problem during the pregnancy that could not have been detected in advance. These problems need to be identified during the course of the pregnancy. This group includes those patients with pre-eclampsia, hydramnios, and multiple pregnancy and those who may deliver premature or postmature infants or whose fetuses may die in utero.

HIGH RISK PREGNANCIES PREDICTED IN ADVANCE

Rh Disease

The Rh-negative patient stands a 1 per cent chance of being immunized during her first full term pregnancy and a 10 per cent of becoming immunized with each subsequent term Rh-positive pregnancy. A spontaneous abortion followed by curettage represents a 3 per cent risk of immunization. Rh-immune prophylaxis administered after any exposure to Rh-positive blood will prevent Rh immunization in more than 90 per cent of cases. Nonetheless, there are failures caused by an exposure to a larger antigenic stimulus than anticipated or by an unprotected exposure, such as may occur with a transplacental hemorrhage during pregnancy.

Incidence. Rh-immune globulin is potentially 100 per cent effective, and yet there is a 5 to 10 per cent incidence of failures. These failures are due to (1) an undetected Rh-negative patient who does not receive Rh-immune prophylaxis, (2) a failure to administer Rh-immune prophylaxis, (3) a failure to administer an adequate dose of Rh-immune prophylaxis, (4) a transplacental hemorrhage during pregnancy.

1. The patient typed as Rh-negative who has an abortion or a full term pregnancy may be overlooked as a candidate for Rh-immune prophylaxis. The Rh immune globulin should be administered within 72 hours. It is very important that each patient have an initial Rh type firmly established prior to the time of delivery; otherwise, she may be a candidate for Rh-immune prophylaxis and fail to receive this important drug.

2. Failure to give Rh-immune prophylaxis can occur when a patient has a spontaneous abortion and may or may not see her physician (or when other obstetric events cause an exposure to Rh-positive erythrocytes or the accidental transfusion of Rh-positive erythrocytes). If the patient does not receive Rh-immune prophylaxis, she may become immunized to the Rh factor, and this will jeopardize her future pregnancies.

3. Failure to administer a sufficient dose of Rh-immune prophylaxis can also occur. The patient who has a large, spontaneous

fetomaternal hemorrhage, a placenta previa, a premature separation of the placenta, or a spillage of blood into the peritoneal cavity at the time of cesarean section must receive adequate Rh-immune prophylaxis to counteract the antigenic stimulus. One ampule of Rh-immune globulin will counteract 30 ml. of Rh-positive blood. If the volume of the fetomaternal hemorrhage is in excess of 30 ml., 1 ampule (300 μg.) of Rh-immune prophylaxis will not be adequate to protect the patient against this antigenic stimulus. Rh-immune prophylaxis is only effective when the Rh antibody is administered in excess of the Rh antigen. In instances in which the fetomaternal hemorrhage is massive, *more than one ampule of Rh-immune globulin must be administered.* The Kleihauer-Betke stain technique may indicate how many ampules of Rh-immune globulin to give. The disappearance of fetal erythrocytes on Kleihauer-Betke stain or the presence of anti-D antibodies indicates adequate administration of Rh-immune globulin.

4. Transplacental hemorrhage — Under the present treatment protocols, Rh-immune prophylaxis is administered after an abortion or after a premature or term pregnancy. However, the occurrence of a significant transplacental hemorrhage during pregnancy creates a large antigenic stimulus that is not protected against by antibody prophylaxis. In this circumstance, a patient may become immunized during pregnancy. An exposure to 0.3 ml. of Rh-positive blood is theoretically enough to immunize a patient. During pregnancy, however, some protective mechanisms appear to be in operation that prevent such a small amount of blood from immunizing the mother. Nonetheless, a small number of patients still become immunized in this manner. These patients will have their future childbearing potential jeopardized.

Management. All obstetric patients seen for the first time *must* have blood group and Rh blood type determinations. If a patient is Rh-negative, she must be screened for Rh antibodies. All patients subjected to an induced abortion, a blood transfusion, or a cesarean section should be screened for atypical antibodies regardless of their Rh blood type. During a *first immunized pregnancy*, that is, when the titer was initially negative but became positive during the pregnancy, the patient can usually be managed by antibody titer determinations alone, if performed in a reliable laboratory. However, this is no longer true if the antibody titer rises *above a critical level*, which is determined for each individual laboratory. The critical antibody titer is that titer below which no fetal or neonatal deaths directly due to erythroblastosis fetalis have occurred. During the first immunized pregnancy, factors such as when an antibody appeared, how long it has been present, and how strong it is are known. This thus provides a great deal of information about the fetal condition. Amniocentesis need not be performed during the first immunized pregnancy if the critical antibody titer is not reached.

In a *subsequent immunized pregnancy*, the Rh-antibody titer tells far less about the fetal condition. First, it has been present from the beginning of pregnancy and, second, it is frequently elevated. In the subsequent immunized pregnancy or in the first immunized pregnancy in which the antibody titer surpasses the critical level, the surveillance of the fetal condition must be done by amniocentesis and amniotic fluid analysis.

Amniotic fluid analysis provides direct information about the fetus. Amniocentesis is first performed at 28 to 29 weeks' gestation, unless the antibody titer or the patient's history indicates that it should be performed earlier. The earliest that amniocentesis need be done is at 24 weeks' gestation, because intrauterine transfusions (IUT's) are generally not successful if they must be initiated prior to 25 weeks' gestation. The purpose of amniotic fluid analysis is to allow the severely affected fetus to be delivered before severe deterioration takes place in utero and to allow the Rh-negative, mildly or moderately affected fetus to stay in utero long enough to gain valuable maturity. Thus, the amniotic fluid analysis enables the severely affected infant to be delivered before death in utero, whereas the moderate or mildly involved infant is allowed to stay in utero longer.

Basically, rising amniotic fluid bilirubin levels at 450 mμ indicate that a fetus will deteriorate and even die in utero if left unattended. A decreasing amniotic fluid bilirubin level at 450 mμ indicates a fetus that is Rh-negative, Rh-positive and mildly involved, or Rh-positive and moderately involved. The most important information is that the fetus is not going to die in utero. If monitored carefully by amniotic fluid analysis until the fetal amniotic fluid maturity studies indicate that the fetus is mature enough to deliver, this infant will survive. The infant may require no exchange transfusion, or perhaps may require one or more, but in any event he should survive and develop normally with appropriate neonatal management.

If the amniotic fluid bilirubin level rises prior to 32 weeks' gestation and indicates that the fetus will die in utero, an intrauterine transfusion is required. After 32 weeks' gestation, it is better to allow the fetus to stay in utero as long as possible and to attempt delivery instead of subjecting the fetus to the risks of an intrauterine transfusion.

Heart Disease

Because of the increased cardiac load from 28 to 34 weeks' gestation, maternal heart disease represents a particular threat to the favorable outcome of the pregnancy. Rheumatic heart disease is the most common form of organic cardiac disability encountered in pregnant patients. Congenital heart disease is seen less frequently.

If the patient has a history of congestive heart failure or cyanosis, the successful outcome of pregnancy is endangered. If the patient is maintained successfully through 28 to 34 weeks' gestation, during the time of the peak cardiac load, she should have a favorable outcome of her pregnancy, provided careful attention is paid to the increase in cardiac output during labor and delivery and to the marked decrease during the immediate postpartum period.

The cardiac patient must be seen frequently during her pregnancy. General medications used for cardiac patients have minimal effects on the fetus and may be prescribed. Diuretics may also be used, although the thiazides may sometimes cause thrombocytopenia in the fetus.

The fetal well-being may be monitored by 24 hour urinary estriol determinations. The delivery of the cardiac patient is best performed by the vaginal route. Elective induction of labor at term is usually the method of choice.

Such a delivery requires the cooperation of the obstetrician, anesthesiologist, internist, and neonatologist. A true team approach is essential. The choice of anesthesia for delivery is generally nitrous oxide and local anesthesia. Conduction anesthesia may be employed as a continuous epidural or caudal anesthesia in patients with mitral stenosis and mitral insufficiency, for whom a decrease in venous return to the right side of the heart may be advantageous. Conduction anesthesia is contraindicated, however, in the patient with aortic valvular disease. A sudden drop in the blood pressure would result in a decrease in cardiac output and failure to perfuse the coronary arteries. General anesthesia may be used in these patients.

In the cardiac patient, particular attention must be paid to the avoidance of intravenous fluid overload, to the risk of infection following surgical manipulations, and to postpartum hemorrhage. The second stage of labor should be shortened by forceps extraction when possible. In addition, this will eliminate the need for the patient to bear down to deliver the infant.

Immediately postpartum there is an increase in the amount of blood entering the circulation as the uterus contracts. This is a time when congestive heart failure must be anticipated and forestalled. A diuresis will be observed during the postpartum days if the patient has been retaining fluids.

Diabetes

Prior to the introduction of insulin, pregnancy was rarely encountered in diabetic patients. A juvenile diabetic who reached the childbearing years was usually infertile. If a patient did achieve pregnancy, it often ended in a spontaneous abortion or precipitated severe bouts of diabetic acidosis and coma. The pregnancy frequently ended in stillbirth or produced infants with congenital malformations, severe episodes of neonatal hypoglycemia, or both. Today with the availability of insulin, the number of diabetic patients who became pregnant has increased markedly.

Since diabetes has a pronounced effect on the outcome of pregnancy, it is a model for the high risk pregnancy concept referred to previously. The proper diagnosis and management of this problem will produce a rewarding outcome.

Prior to the intensive management of the diabetic pregnancy, the incidence of preeclampsia was 25 per cent. Hydramnios was

TABLE 41-1. WHITE'S CLASSIFICATION OF DIABETES MELLITUS*

Class A: Glucose tolerance test abnormality only
Class B: Onset after age 20, duration 0–9 years, no vascular disease
Class C: Onset age 10–19, duration 10–19 years, no vascular disease
Class D: Onset under age 10, duration 20+ years, vascular disease, calcification in legs, retinitis
Class E: Calcified pelvic vessels
Class F: Nephritis

*From Nelson, H. B., Gillespie, L., and White, P.: Obstet. Gynecol., 1:219, 1953.

frequently encountered, and urinary tract infections were common. Vascular complications occurred in the severe diabetic. The perinatal mortality rate for newborns of diabetic mothers was 10 to 40 per cent higher than that of infants of nondiabetic mothers, being approximately 25 per cent. Today, high risk pregnancy programs have reduced the mortality rate to approximately 8 per cent.

Table 41–1 divides patients with diabetes mellitus into five classes.

Class A Diabetes. The Class A, or gestational, diabetic may present no history of diabetes; however, many of these patients have gestational diabetes that is recurrent in each pregnancy. The infants of Class A diabetics do not usually die in utero, but can have a significant perinatal mortality if not properly managed. If there is no superimposed pre-eclampsia or other complications, the outcome for the well-managed Class A diabetic pregnancy should be excellent. The usual reason for the perinatal mortality is trauma incurred while delivering the excessively large infant vaginally or problems arising in the newborn nursery, where the infant can develop severe hypoglycemia if proper measures are not taken.

The recognition of Class A diabetes demands careful monitoring of the mother throughout pregnancy. Strict diet is essential in order to keep the blood glucose at a near normal level. It is unlikely that the mother will require insulin. Since intrauterine death is not likely, the need for estriol determination and oxytocin challenge tests is not urgent. The most important areas of management are diet, immediate diagnosis and treatment of urinary tract infection, selection of the proper method

and timing of delivery, and availability of intensive newborn care.

Classes B through F Diabetes. The situation with the Class B through F diabetic is much more guarded. These patients can develop a variety of problems. Urinary tract infections are common and routine cultures should be obtained each trimester. Diabetic acidosis and coma are possible in the more severe form. In patients with vascular involvement, intrauterine growth retardation is possible.

These patients are generally monitored by 24 hour urinary estriol determinations from 28 weeks' gestation to delivery. In addition, the oxytocin challenge test, or contraction stress test, may be used to help avoid an intrauterine death. The adjustment of insulin dosage during these pregnancies is often fraught with problems. Many of these patients (80 per cent) have an increased need for insulin during pregnancy. A sudden decrease in insulin need is an ominous sign, as is the development of hydramnios.

The management of delivery must be selected carefully. Since there is a high incidence of respiratory distress syndrome in these infants, amniocentesis to evaluate fetal maturity should be performed prior to the delivery. The use of ultrasonography to determine biparietal diameters is helpful in evaluating the growth of the fetus; however, the fetus is often large for gestational age, and therefore the head size may give misleading information, indicating that the fetus is more mature than it is. If diabetes is strictly controlled, the head may grow at a normal rate. If significant vascular disease is present, there could be intrauterine growth rate problems.

At the time of delivery, the neonatologist should be present to provide optimal care for the newborn. An immediate inspection for the presence of congenital malformations should be carried out. Infant resuscitation is paramount. The possibility of hypoglycemia, respiratory distress, and asphyxia must all be considered.

HIGH RISK CONDITIONS DETECTED DURING PREGNANCY

Multiple Gestation

The incidence of multiple gestation is 1 in 80 for twins and 1 in 6400 for triplets.

The diagnosis of this phenomenon is frequently met with joy by the potential mother and father. It is not always such an easy situation for the clinician, however. Multiple gestations are fraught with problems. There is an increased incidence of prematurity, pre-eclampsia, congenital malformations, severe maternal anemia, postpartum hemorrhage, and hydramnios.

The early diagnosis of multiple gestation is beneficial because the clinician can instruct the patient to increase her rest periods and decrease her activities. The diagnosis of a twin gestation may be made as early as 8 weeks after conception by ultrasonography. The diagnosis is generally suspected when the uterus is larger than the gestational dates would indicate. Early in pregnancy the presence of marked symptoms of nausea and vomiting accompanied by marked breast tenderness should lead the obstetrician to suspect multiple gestation. Spotting during early pregnancy and uterine cramps are also suggestive of a rapidly growing multiple gestation.

The patient with a twin gestation will have a slightly increased weight gain. The uterus will grow at a more rapid rate, and it may become so large that the patient is rendered extremely uncomfortable. Hospitalization may be required.

The patient with a multiple gestation requires additional iron and folic acid supplementation.

Pre-eclampsia

Pre-eclampsia is more frequent in the primigravida than in the multipara. This disease is unique to the human pregnancy. It consists of a triad of edema, hypertension, and albuminuria, generally occurring after the twentieth week of pregnancy. The only time that pre-eclampsia is known to occur prior to 20 weeks' gestation is when it is associated with a hydatidiform mole.

Because pre-eclampsia is a progressive disease, the clinician must be observant for its occurrence. Generally, the fetus is mature and can be delivered before the disease progresses to the eclamptic stage. This is extremely important because the perinatal mortality for pre-eclampsia is low, whereas the perinatal mortality for eclampsia is as high as 30 per cent. The maternal mortality for eclampsia is as high as 10 per cent.

Pre-eclampsia may be divided into mild and severe forms. Although pre-eclampsia consists of a triad of three signs, only one need be present to establish the diagnosis. *Mild pre-eclampsia* consists of a blood pressure of 140 systolic and 90 diastolic or of a rise of 30 mm. of Hg in the systolic pressure and 15 mm. of Hg in the diastolic pressure. Albuminuria or edema may be present. *Severe pre-eclampsia* consists of a blood pressure of 160 systolic and 110 diastolic or greater. There is marked albuminuria, and in this severe form of the disease, the patient may have dizziness, blurring of vision, spots in front of her eyes, epigastric pain, and hyperreflexia.

If the pre-eclampsia progresses, the patient may develop *eclampsia.* This consists of convulsions, in addition to the hypertension, albuminuria, and edema.

Pre-eclampsia is more common in patients with twin gestations, diabetes mellitus, renal disease, hypertension, hydramnios, and hydatidiform mole. It is also more common in primigravidas. The cause is unknown.

In the United States, pre-eclampsia affects 6 per cent of pregnant patients and progresses to eclampsia in 1 in 500 patients. This is a disease of the arterioles. There is generally impairment of renal function secondary to progressively developing hemoconcentration and decreased renal blood flow. Glomerular capillary endothelial cell swelling is characteristically present in this disease.

When pre-eclampsia is diagnosed in the office, the patient should be admitted to the hospital. Management in the hospital consists of bed rest in the lateral position, which increases renal blood flow. A normal sodium diet is ordered. Even though there is a slight decrease in the sodium metabolism during pre-eclampsia, salt deprivation is not indicated. Diuretics are *contraindicated* because they cause further hemoconcentration and decreased blood flow to the fetus.

The objective of the management of pre-eclampsia is to enable the fetus to mature enough for safe delivery prior to progressive deterioration of the fetus or the mother caused by the pre-eclampsia. Certainly, delivery is desirable prior to the development of eclampsia. The management of the patient with severe pre-eclampsia or with eclampsia includes intravenous administration of magnesium sulfate, stabilization of the vital signs, and delivery. The intravenous infusion of diazepam (Valium) may be useful during a convulsion. Generally, magnesium sulfate, 1 to 4 grams per hour, is given to decrease deep tendon reflexes to hypoactive levels, provided the respiratory rate is not significantly depressed (below 10 breaths per minute.) The patient is stabilized and then delivered. Lactated Ringer's solution is given intravenously to correct the decreased vascular volume and maintain normal sodium levels. If the patient has decreased blood flow, mannitol may be administered.

Even after the successful delivery of the pre-eclamptic patient, there is still the risk of her developing eclampsia. In 25 per cent of patients, eclampsia can develop during the postpartum period. The period must be watched carefully for changes in deep tendon reflexes. If they are hyperactive, additional magnesium sulfate is indicated.

Hydramnios

Hydramnios is an excessive collection of amniotic fluid (usually greater than 2000 ml.). It is generally a disease of the third trimester of pregnancy and occurs in 1 in 328 patients.

If hydramnios is present, the cause must be investigated. As there is a major difference in the clinical outcome depending on the underlying cause, it is very important to investigate the patient's condition thoroughly. For instance, the perinatal mortality for hydramnios is approximately 50 per cent, whereas the perinatal mortality for hydramnios associated with erythroblastosis fetalis is 73 per cent. The investigation for hydramnios can be done in 1 day. A 2 hour postprandial blood glucose can rule out severe diabetes; an antibody screening for atypical antibodies can rule out blood incompatibilities. In addition, an ultrasound B-scan can rule out the presence of a multiple gestation. If diabetes, erythroblastosis fetalis, and multiple gestation can be ruled out, 50 per cent of the causes of hydramnios are eliminated. Of the remaining 50 per cent, ap-

proximately one-half of the causes will be associated with congenital malformation and the other half with idiopathic hydramnios.

The types of congenital malformations generally consist of neurologic and gastrointestinal defects. The neurologic defects, such as anencephaly and spina bifida with meningocele, may be detected by B-scan ultrasonography. Definitely, however, congenital malformations are best detected by amniography. In this procedure, 20 to 30 ml. of diatrizoate meglumine and diatrizoate sodium injection (Hypaque-M, 75%) is injected into the amniotic sac. This renders the fluid radiopaque. The soft tissues of the fetus will then be outlined on the amniogram. An x-ray is taken of the uterus, and attention is paid to the thickness of the scalp, the outline of the fetal head, and the presence of any abnormal structures, such as a meningocele. In addition, attention is directed to the gastrointestinal tract. The normal fetus will have swallowed the opacified amniotic fluid by 1 hour following injection into the amniotic sac. The fluid can usually be seen in the stomach and small intestine. In this way, the presence of esophageal atresia, diaphragmatic hernia, or other congenital malformations that might involve the gastrointestinal tract can be identified.

The remaining patients are those who have idiopathic hydramnios. Provided there is no underlying cause for the hydramnios, the outcome should be good. The patient probably will do well with bed rest. There is no rationale for giving diuretics, as they do not decrease the hydramnios. The likelihood of needing to decrease uterine size by multiple amniocenteses is extremely small. A patient who is developing severe hydramnios should be hospitalized.

Postmaturity

Generally speaking, postmaturity occurs after 42 weeks' gestation. Postmaturity is a relatively rare clinical problem in which the fetus reaches a state of maturity, yet continues to be retained in the uterus. Gradually the placenta begins to fail, and the fetus undergoes progressive deterioration. Fetal deterioration can be detected by oxytocin challenge tests or by decreasing 24 hour urinary estriol levels. A fall is noted in the urinary estrogen levels as the placenta fails.

REFERENCES

1. Current Concepts in Oral Contraceptive Treatment. Health Learning Systems, Bloomfield, N.J., 1975.
2. Greenblatt, R. B.: Induction of ovulation with clomiphene. *In* Greenblatt, R. B. (ed.): Ovulation. Philadelphia, J. B. Lippincott Co., 1966.
3. Mollison, P. L.: Annotation: Suppression of Rh-immunization by passively administered anti-Rh. Brit. J. Haemat., *14*:1, 1968.
4. Moore, C.: Synopsis of Clinical Cancer. St. Louis, C. V. Mosby Co., 1970.
5. Nelson, H. B., Gillespie, L., and White, P.: Pregnancy complicated by diabetes mellitus. Obstet. Gynecol., *1*:219.
6. Nora, F. F., and Nora, A. H.: Birth Defects and Oral Contraceptives. Lancet, *1*:941, 1973.
7. Queenan, J. T.: Modern Management of the Rh Problem. 2nd Ed. Hagerstown, Md., Harper & Row, Publishers, 1977.
8. Queenan, J. T., and Gadow, E. C.: Polyhydramnios: chronic versus acute. Amer. J. Obstet. Gynecol., *108*:349, 1970.
9. Queenan, J. T., Gadow, E. C., and Lopes, C. A.: The role of spontaneous abortions in Rh-sensitization. Amer. J. Obstet. Gynecol., *110*:128, 1971.
10. Romney, S. L., Gray, M. J., Little, A. B., et al.: Gynecology and Obstetrics. The Health Care of Women. New York, McGraw-Hill, 1975.
11. Speroff, L., Glass, R. H., and Kase, N. G.: Clinical Gynecologic Endocrinology and Infertility. Baltimore, The Williams & Wilkins Co., 1973.
12. Yerushalmy, J.: Methodologic problems encountered in investigating the possible teratogenic effects of drugs. Adv. Exp. Med. Bio., *27*:427, 1972.

Chapter 42

UROLOGY

by JOHN D. YOUNG, JR.,
SAID A. KARMI,
and WILLIAM L. STEWART

THE URINE TRANSPORT SYSTEM

NORMAL COLLECTION AND VOIDING OF URINE

The glomerular filtrate is propelled from the glomerulus through the tubules of the nephron into the collecting ducts to the tips of the renal papillae by a secretory pressure of 35 to 50 mm. Hg. The urine enters the calyx, distends it, and causes it to contract and propel the bolus of urine to the renal pelvis, in which the intraluminal pressure is 10 to 20 cm. of water. Urine is then transported to the bladder by rhythmic unidirectional peristalsis (normally 1 to 5 waves per minute) beginning at the calyceal fornix, where the muscle layers are attached around the base of the papilla. Urine is stored temporarily in the bladder. The normal capacity of the adult bladder is 300 to 500 ml. of urine at about 10 cm. of water pressure until the bladder is nearly filled. This pressure increases to 40 to 50 cm. of water during voiding. Voluntary control of interval voiding, which occurs every 4 to 5 hours in the adult, depends upon the proper relationship of the expulsive force of the bladder detrusors, the capacity of the bladder, the resistance of the urethral·sphincter system, and the inhibitory influences of the higher centers of the central nervous system.

There are no motor nerves to the smooth muscle of the calyces, infundibula, pelvis, and ureter. Sympathetic fibers to the ureter control its vascular element. Afferent fibers traveling with the vascular motor fibers carry sensory impulses from the ureter to the spinal segments T11, T12, L1, and L2.

Painful stimuli from the ureter are perceived along the area of distribution of the ilioinguinal, iliohypogastric, and genitofemoral nerves. Since tonicity and peristalsis of the ureter are autonomous, no adrenergic, cholinergic, sympatholytic, or parasympatholytic drugs in a physiologic dose will influence the muscular activity of the ureter.

Normal renal function, sterility of the urine, and absence of urinary tract symptoms depend to a great extent on complete emptying under normal pressures of all parts of the transport system and on maintaining it free from injury.

EVALUATION OF THE URINE TRANSPORT SYSTEM

Symptoms

Symptoms of disorders of the urine transport system include:

1. Urinary frequency—Voiding every 2 hours or more often after the age of 2 years. Frequency may be caused by residual urine, irritation from infection, the presence of a foreign body, or injury. Increased urine volume causes frequency in disorders such as diabetes insipidus, diabetes mellitus, and the diuresis caused by renal failure, as well as during periods of increased fluid intake. Diseases that cause fibrosis of the bladder with decreased bladder capacity are also accompanied by frequency, e.g., tuberculosis, bilharziasis (schistosomiasis), interstitial cystitis, neoplasms, pelvic masses, and neurogenic dysfunction.

2. Nocturia—Awakening to void one or

more times. This is often a symptom of renal disease related to a decrease in the functioning renal parenchyma with loss of concentrating ability. Nocturia occurs with decreased bladder capacity, apparent or real; with increase in nighttime urine output, as in cardiac insufficiency; and with increased fluid intake.

3. Dysuria—Painful voiding. Dysuria is common in acute cystitis and prostatitis. It usually indicates inflammation of the proximal urethra and bladder neck but can also occur with trauma and obstruction. It is usually felt in the distal urethra in the male and can occur at any time during the act of urination.

4. Enuresis—Voiding during sleep. Enuresis is physiologic during the first 2 years of life. After 2 years of age, it may be functional or secondary to delayed neuromuscular maturation of the urethrovesical component. If present with other urologic symptoms, organic disease such as infection, distal urethral stenosis, urethral valves, or neurogenic bladder should be ruled out. When the cause is psychogenic or idiopathic, anticholinergic drugs or imipramine might be of help.

5. Urgency—The inability to control voiding after the desire appears. Urgency usually accompanies irritation and neurologic disorders. It is often an early sign of upper central nervous system disease, such as multiple sclerosis.

6. Change in character of urinary flow during voiding—A decrease in caliber and force of the urinary stream accompanied by hesitancy (difficulty in initiating voiding). These are early symptoms of prostatic enlargement and other types of bladder outlet obstruction.

7. Incontinence—Involuntary loss of urine. True incontinence occurs with vesicovaginal fistulas, epispadias, ectopic ureteral orifice, injury to the urethral sphincter, or neurologic disease with incompetent sphincter. Stress incontinence is loss of urine during physical strain that occurs in persons with weakness of the sphincter mechanism, such as multiparous women with cystocele and urethrocele and patients with neurologic disorders.

8. Anuria—Complete cessation of urine output. Anuria can occur with obstruction, parenchymal renal disease, and decreased renal blood flow (hypovolemic shock, septic shock, acute tubular necrosis).

9. Fever, malaise, weight loss, nausea, pallor, edema, and hypertension are several of the systemic manifestations of disorders of urine transport.

10. Pain—Kidney pain is usually seen with acute obstruction and occurs in the costovertebral angle just below the twelfth rib. It is a dull and constant ache when the obstruction is chronic in nature. Ureteral pain usually radiates from the costovertebral angle down toward the lower anterior abdominal quadrant, along the course of the ureter to the bladder, scrotum, and testicle in the male or to the bladder and vulva in the female. Bladder pain occurs with acute overdistention, trauma, and inflammation. Patients with chronic urinary retention may experience little or no discomfort. Prostatic pain is usually felt as a vague discomfort or fullness in the perineal or rectal area.

Diagnostic Procedures

The following diagnostic procedures are used in evaluating disorders of the urine transport system:

1. *Urinalysis.* Urinalysis is essential when a urologic disorder is suspected. The first urine specimen voided after sleep is best for detecting formed elements and for determining if urinary infection is present, as the overnight incubation of the urine yields higher bacterial counts. The specimen should be examined within 30 minutes after voiding. Culture and colony count of a clean-catch midstream specimen after adequate preparation provide a reasonably accurate determination of the bacteriologic status of the urinary tract. Examination and culture of a catheterized or aspirated specimen may be necessary to provide accurate data about bladder urine. Both microscopic and gross hematuria can occur with infection, nephritis, neoplasm, trauma, and blood disorders. The presence of pyuria, proteinuria, crystalluria, casts, and bacteriuria should be noted.

2. *Renal function tests.* Obtain serum creatinine, blood urea nitrogen, and electrolyte values. Creatinine clearance, phenolsulfonphthalein (PSP) excretion, and urine-plasma ratios of urea or creatinine provide more precise evaluation and are useful in detecting changes during follow-up.

3. *Radiologic examination.* Radiologic studies include excretory urograms, cys-

tourethrograms, and cystometry. The *excretory urogram* (intravenous pyelogram) is the basic x-ray study of the urinary tract. It depends primarily on the urine concentration of the contrast medium that is filtered by the glomerulus and is neither secreted nor absorbed by the tubules. A plain film of the abdomen (kidney-ureter-bladder—KUB) can reveal calcifications, kidney size, bone structure, and soft tissue shadows. The intravenous pyelogram (IVP) reveals the shape and size of the collecting systems, ureters, and bladder. High-dose urography may provide better visualization in patients with renal insufficiency. The sequential (or hypertensive) urogram provides information about renal blood flow. *Cystourethrograms* are used for visualization of vesical and urethral abnormalities. Voiding cystourethrograms are helpful in detecting vesicoureteral reflux. *Cystometry*, and urethral pressure profiles, are used to measure generated intraluminal and sphincter pressures and are helpful in determining neurogenic bladder dysfunction.

4. *Instrumentation.* All instruments must be used with aseptic precautions. *Catheterization* is helpful in collecting clean urine from females, in measuring residual urine, and in decompressing distended bladders. *Endoscopy* is the examination of the interior of the bladder and the urethra with the use of an illuminated lens system to detect tumors, stones, trauma, and abnormal anatomic configurations. Catheterization of the ureteral orifices may be done for evaluation of individual kidney function and instillation of contrast material for more detailed radiographic visualization (retrograde pyelogram).

5. *Scintigraphic studies.* Scintigraphic studies with radioisotopes provide information about renal blood flow, tubular function, and urine transport. Three major isotopes are used: technetium (^{99m}Tc) for blood flow measurements, iodohippurate sodium (^{131}I) (Hippuran) for determination of tubular function and urine transport, and iothalamate (^{125}I) for measurement of glomerular filtration rate.

6. *Angiography.* Arteriography is used to visualize arterial distribution to the kidneys, to determine extent of neoplasms, to differentiate tumors from cysts, and to detect renal artery obstructions as a cause of hypertension. *Phlebography* is used to visualize venous drainage, to determine tumor invasion of veins, and to obtain blood for renin assays on individual kidneys.

7. *Sonography.* This is the evaluation of renal and other masses by use of ultrasound, which helps to differentiate fluid-containing from solid masses.

8. *Measurement of rate of urine flow during voiding.* A uroflowmeter is used to localize the site of obstruction at various parts of the urethra.

DISORDERS OF URINE TRANSPORT

Mechanical Obstructive Uropathy

Obstruction to urine flow first results in increased intraluminal pressure proximal to the site of blockage, without necessarily causing any accumulation or retention of urine. The increased pressure alone might be a contributing cause to development of infection and a threat to the kidney. As the obstruction persists and becomes more severe, the retained urine causes dilatation of the urinary tract and may eventually destroy the kidney. Although the pressure decreases toward normal levels in chronic obstruction, the persistent accumulation of urine in the kidney results in decreased renal blood flow and renal cortical atrophy in proportion to the duration and severity of the obstruction. Also, the accumulated urine predisposes to the growth of pathogenic bacteria that will hasten the destruction of the urinary tract.

Congenital Causes of Obstruction. Obstruction may be due to various forms of congenital anomalies.

Ureteropelvic strictures are the most common form of congenital ureteral obstruction and are evidenced by mechanical narrowing from either intrinsic stenosis or extrinsic compression from a band or blood vessel or by abnormal development of musculature. Treatment of these conditions is surgical and depends on the patient's symptoms and degree of hydronephrosis and kidney damage.

Ureterovesical stenosis is another cause of obstruction. A ureterocele is a ballooning of the submucosal ureter into the bladder, secondary to congenital stenosis of the epithelial lining at the vesical end of the ureter. It is diagnosed by intravenous pyelogram (IVP), which shows a "cobra head" deformity at the distal end of the intramural ureter. Treatment is by meatotomy or by surgical excision and reimplantation of the ureter.

A *bladder neck contracture* is difficult to diagnose by objective findings. Stricture sufficient to cause obstruction to urine flow is rare. The treatment is by surgical excision, but this may lead to retrograde ejaculation in males and urinary incontinence in females.

Posterior urethral valves occur in the prostatic urethra as congenital folds of urothelium. They are a common cause of congenital urethral obstruction in males, usually first diagnosed in childhood, and also cause dilatation of the prostatic urethra, hypertrophy of the detrusors, vesical diverticula, and hydronephrosis. Treatment is by transurethral electrosurgical excision.

Urethral stenosis and stricture may also cause obstruction. Stenosis of the external meatus is common and should be ruled out in all newborn males. It can be so severe as to cause massive dilatation of the entire urinary tract. Treatment is by meatotomy. Congenital urethral stricture occasionally occurs in males. The two most common sites for these anomalies are the fossa navicularis and the membranous urethra. The strictures are treated by urethral dilatation or by surgical repair, depending upon their severity.

Distal urethral stenosis is the most common cause of urinary tract infection in girls during infancy and childhood. The ring is detected by urethral calibration with a bougie. Urethral dilatation relieves symptoms and persistent infection in 80 per cent of patients.

An *ectopic ureter* is another cause of obstruction. Most ureters with ectopic openings are one of a pair attached to a single kidney, and the ectopic ureter almost always drains the upper pole. These ureters are usually obstructed, resulting in a hydroureteronephrosis. Treatment is surgical.

Acquired Disorders of Urine Transport. These diseases will be discussed in more detail in the latter part of this chapter. They include urethral strictures secondary to infection and trauma; benign hyperplasia and cancer of the prostate; tumors of the urethra, bladder, ureters, and kidneys; urinary calculi in the kidneys, ureters, bladder, and urethra; and pelvic and retroperitoneal masses caused by pregnancy, by neoplasms of the cervix, ovaries, or uretus, by lymphomas, and by metastases to retroperitoneal lymph nodes.

Adynamic Disorders of Urine Transport. The term *megaureter* is applied to a dilated ureter in which no overt obstructing lesion is demonstrable. It is usually caused by a functional abnormality in the lower ureter

that interferes with emptying (adynamic segment). Treatment is by surgical excision of the segment, tapering of the ureter, and reimplantation.

Vesicoureteral Reflux. This implies regurgitation of urine from the bladder into the ureter and is never a normal finding. Acute, chronic, or healed pyelonephritis is secondary to vesicoureteral reflux in a high percentage of patients. Primary congenital reflux occurs with attenuation of the trigone and intravesical ureteral musculature and with shortening of the intramural ureter. It is found more commonly with duplicated systems.

Secondary reflux occurs with obstruction, vesical trabeculation, and infection. This reflux will disappear upon relieving the cause.

Primary reflux is found in 50 per cent of children with urinary tract infection, but in only 8 per cent of adults with bacteriuria. All children with urinary tract infection should have a voiding cystogram to rule out reflux. Approximately 10 per cent of renal failure in patients who require kidney transplantation or chronic dialysis is due to reflux. Reimplantation of the ureter into the bladder is required for patients with recurrent infections, or pyelographic changes in the presence of reflux, or both.

Neurogenic Dysfunction of the Bladder and Urethral Sphincters

Normal urine flow depends on an intact nerve supply to the bladder. Parasympathetic motor fibers are responsible for detrusor contraction and expulsion of urine. Sympathetic and somatic motor supply to the sphincters is essential for continence and retention of urine. Somatic innervation is through the pudendal nerve. The centers controlling micturition are located in the spinal cord segments S2, S3, and S4 at the skeletal level of T12–L1. Destruction of these segments causes a hyporesponsive or denervated bladder. Sensation from the bladder is returned through somatic, parasympathetic, and sympathetic nerves and ascends through the lateral spinothalamic tracts and the fasciculus gracilis. Loss of proprioception in the bladder can cause urinary retention in diseases such as tabes dorsalis, diabetes mellitus, and pernicious anemia.

Cerebral innervation is mostly inhibitory, permitting filling of the bladder under low pressure without sensation until it reaches near capacity.

Evaluation of Suspected Neurogenic Bladder Dysfunction. Neurologic or neurosurgical consultation is required to rule out central nervous system lesions. Cystometric examination should be done to evaluate pressure generated in the bladder during filling in order to determine the presence of involuntary contractions and to rule out denervation. A urethral pressure profile is required to measure the sphincter tone. Finally, look for skeletal abnormalities on x-ray (spina bifida, absent sacrum).

Types of Neurogenic Bladder. A *hypertonic bladder* is caused by an upper motor neuron deficit. This lesion occurs above the level of the T12 vertebra. As the bladder is characterized by intermittent, uninhibited contractions with automatic reflex voiding, it is constantly spastic. The causes of hypertonic bladder trauma, cerebral vascular accidents, Parkinson's disease, and multiple sclerosis. Treatment is often unsatisfactory.

A *flaccid* or *atonic bladder* indicates a lower motor neuron deficit at the S2–S4 level of the spinal cord. The most common cause is trauma; other causes are tumors, a herniated intervertebral disc, tabes dorsalis, poliomyelitis, and meningomyelocele. The atonic bladder is characterized by large capacity, no involuntary detrusor contractions, low intravesical pressure, and trabeculation. Treatment is aimed at relieving the distention and accumulation of residual urine. The atonic bladder is easier to manage than the hypertonic bladder.

In patients with a *sensory paralytic bladder*, overdistention occurs because the patient has no sensation of fullness. This causes destruction of the detrusors and loss of expulsive force. A sensory paralytic bladder occurs in patients with diabetes, tabes dorsalis, and pernicious anemia.

Treatment. Treatment in general is aimed at preventing infection and upper urinary tract deterioration. A neurogenic bladder is one of the most serious disorders of urine transport.

UROLITHIASIS

Urolithiasis is one of the most common diseases of the urinary tract, and approximately 0.1 per cent of the population is hospitalized for treatment of this disorder every year. Urinary calculi may occur at any age, but are rare in children less than 10 years of age and in adults over the age of 65 years. Calculi are more common in males and in Caucasians, and there is general agreement that the highest incidence of stone disease in the United States occurs in the Southeast.

Etiology of Stones

No specific cause can be found in 60 per cent of patients. A variety of contributing factors are known:

1. Increase in concentration or total amount, or both, of stone-forming crystalloids in the urine. This is found in disorders such as hypercalciuria, hyperoxaluria, cystinuria, uricosuria, and dehydration. *Hypercalciuria* occurs with increased ingestion of calcium, idiopathic disorders, hyperparathyroidism, vitamin D intoxication, recumbency, high salt intake, and sarcoidosis. *Hyperoxaluria* or *oxalosis* is a rare, often lethal genetic disorder that affects the metabolism of glyoxylic acid, which forms oxalate rather than glycine. Decreasing the intake of certain foods, such as cabbage, spinach, and tomatoes, usually has little effect in preventing this disorder because the majority of oxalates are endogenous in origin. *Cystinuria* is a hereditary disease that is more common in infants and children with a defect in renal tubular absorption. It is manifested by the precipitation of hexagonal cystine crystals in an acid urine. The sodium cyanide test is a simple way of confirming the diagnosis. *Uricosuria* occurs in patients with gout and in those in whom there is rapid breakdown of tissue, such as patients undergoing chemotherapeutic treatment of leukemia, carcinoma, or polycythemia. It also occurs when urine is abnormally acid. Finally, *dehydration* increases the concentration of crystalloids, leading to precipitation and stone formation.

2. Urinary pH changes. Uric acid stones may be found in patients with a persistent pH below 5.5 with no other apparent cause. Calcium phosphate and magnesium ammonium phosphate are least soluble in an alkaline urine with a pH range of between 6.6 and 8.0. Ingestion of alkali, particularly of absorbable forms such as sodium bicarbonate, in the treatment of peptic ulcer produces an alkaline urine that can contribute to inorganic stone formation.

3. Renal tubular acidosis. This disease causes a defect in the ability of the kidney to excrete acid, so the urine is constantly alkaline. The resulting acidosis mobilizes calcium from the bone, causing hypercalciuria that leads to nephrocalcinosis and nephrolithiasis in some patients. However, the cause of the calculi is not known in many patients with this disorder.

4. Mucoprotein matrix. Some mucoproteins found in urine have an unusual affinity for salts and thus produce stones.

5. Urinary stasis and obstruction. These disorders also contribute to formation of stones.

6. Foreign bodies. Catheters, cellular debris, sutures, and so forth may produce stones.

7. Deficiency of solubilizers. Certain solubilizers in the urine are thought to keep salts in solution. Absence of these leads to precipitation and stone formation.

Composition of Stones

The composition of urinary calculi is outlined in Table 42–1.

Symptoms and Signs

Calculi cause obstruction and erosion and harbor bacteria. Pain is severe following acute occlusion of a ureter by a ureteral calculus and results from distention of the renal pelvis and ureter with urine. The pain is relieved if the ureter relaxes and allows drainage of urine around the stone, which is erroneously interpreted as passage of the stone. Such pain is usually felt over the T12–L1 dermatone. With chronic obstruction and renal damage, pain is either mild or absent. Urinary urgency or dysuria is noted if the stone is at the ureterovesical junction. Gross hematuria occurs in 5 to 10 per cent of patients. Microscopic hematuria is found in most patients but might not be present if

TABLE 42–1. COMPOSITION OF URINARY CALCULI

Substance	Per Cent
Calcium oxalate and/or phosphate	75
Calcium phosphate–magnesium ammonia phosphate	15
Uric acid	7
Cystine	2
Miscellaneous	1

obstruction is complete. Pyuria might be the only sign of "staghorn" calculi in patients who have an alkaline-infected urine.

Vomiting may occur with severe pain. Fever is a sign of infected urine above the obstructing stone, and this is an indication for immediate or early drainage. Urinary retention can occur when the stone obstructs the urethra, and anuria can occur when stones obstruct both ureters.

Diagnosis

History. A family history of stone formation is important, especially in patients with cystine and uric acid stones and those with renal tubular acidosis. The intake of foods high in calcium, excessive vitamin D intake, use of drugs such as acetazolamide, climate, geographic location, and the presence of certain diseases are also important in determining the background of stone formation, along with the signs and symptoms mentioned previously.

Radiologic Examination. Scout films of the abdomen (KUB) reveal the presence of calcifications along the genitourinary tract. An intravenous pyelogram (excretory urogram) confirms the location and indicates the degree of obstruction. Delayed films are helpful in visualizing the tract above the stone. This study should be done as early as possible if a calculus is suspected. A ureteral catheterization and retrograde pyelogram study is performed if the stone is nonopaque (uric acid and matrix stones). This study helps in localizing the position of the stone as a nonopaque filling defect in the column of contrast medium.

Laboratory Studies. A urinalysis, particularly for determining red blood cells (RBC), white blood cells (WBC), protein, glucose, crystals, and pH should be done. Blood studies include a hemogram and measurement of blood urea nitrogen (BUN), creatinine, electrolyte, calcium, phosphorus, total protein, fasting blood glucose, uric acid, and alkaline phosphatase levels. Urine culture is also indicated. Examination of a stained sediment for bacteria should be done immediately if the patient is febrile. Obtain a 24 hour urine collection to measure calcium and creatinine excretion. Quantitative measurement of uric acid, cystine, and oxalate levels in the urine should be done as indicated.

Treatment

Symptomatic. As soon as the diagnosis of an acute obstructing ureteral calculus is made, adequate analgesic medication should be given.

Surgical. No early or immediate surgical treatment is indicated unless the stone is causing significant obstruction. If infection is present above the obstructing stone, the stone should be removed immediately, or a catheter should be passed beyond the stone to drain the proximal urinary tract. Even potent antibiotics are not adequate treatment.

Most ureteral stones 5 mm. or less in greatest diameter will pass spontaneously; most stones greater than 5 mm. in diameter will require some type of instrumental or surgical procedure for removal.

Small nonobstructing stones need not be removed until they obstruct. Large renal stones, particularly the branched calculus ("staghorn" calculus) associated with infection, usually should be removed even though they are causing no pain, as they can produce renal destruction by erosion and infection, even with little or no pain.

Medical. The following points are important in the medical management of urinary calculi:

1. To dilute urinary crystalloids, increase the volume of urine.

2. Adequate, vigorous treatment of urinary infections is required, including use of suppressive therapy indefinitely when indicated.

3. Hyperparathyroidism is treated as indicated, such as by the removal of a parathyroid adenoma or hyperplasia.

4. Alkali (citrate mixture or sodium bicarbonate) is administered for stones caused by renal tubular acidosis.

5. Thiazide diuretics are effective in reducing urinary calcium.

6. Orthophosphates decrease urinary calcium and increase the solubilizing property of urine.

7. A low oxalate diet is effective only in treating hyperoxaluria and is usually prescribed in combination with pyridoxine, which also reduces urinary oxalate.

8. Magnesium oxide (200 mg. three times daily) and pyridoxine (25 mg. daily) are reported to be effective in the treatment of patients who form calcium oxalate stone.

9. Methylene blue (65 mg. three times daily) is given for repeated formation of calcium stone and supposedly prevents adherence of crystals.

10. Alkalinization of urine to pH 7.0 every day prevents uric acid calculi, and might dissolve those stones already present, without the addition of allopurinol. Allopurinol is used if the serum uric acid level is elevated in patients with oxalate as well as with uric acid stones. Allopurinol has been used in combination with thiazides for treatment of calcium oxalate stones associated with hypercalciuria and elevated serum uric acid levels.

11. The alkalinization of urine to pH 7.8 or above plus a high fluid-low calcium intake are recommended in patients with cystine stones. A low methionine diet decreases urinary cystine.

12. D-penicillamine and pyridoxine are given if large amounts of cystine are present in the urine.

13. In healthy young persons with a single stone, normal urogram, and normal laboratory studies, no further medical treatment is advised, except for increased fluids, unless the stones recur.

ANOMALIES OF THE GENITOURINARY TRACT

Anomalies of the Kidney

Failure of Development. *Bilateral agenesis* is very rare and incompatible with life and is associated with other congenital anomalies. *Unilateral agenesis* or congenital solitary kidney occurs in 0.1 per cent of the population, with or without absent ureters. If the ureter is absent, the ipsilateral vas deferens also may be absent. *Hypoplasia* refers to subnormal growth of a kidney, the organ being smaller than normal or even infantile, with resultant compensatory hypertrophy of the other kidney. The incidence for hypoplasia is the same as for agenesis. Hypoplasia should be differentiated from vascular or pyelonephritic atrophy. Treatment is nephrectomy when hypertension becomes apparent. A *supernumerary kidney* is the rarest of renal anomalies, as only about 50 cases have been reported. It differs from duplication of the pelvis and the ureter.

Abnormal Location. *Ptosis* occurs in older patients with faulty nutrition and should be differentiated from congenital mobility. It is rare in children. Nephropexy is rarely indicated for relief of pain or infection. *Ectopia* may involve one or both kidneys, and malrotation with anterior calyces and pelves is usually present. This anomaly occurs in 1 of every 800 persons, being more frequent in males than in females, and is treated only when complications occur. In *crossed ectopia* both renal masses are on the same side and are fused. The ureters enter the bladder on both sides.

Vascular Anomalies. Multiple arteries and veins occur commonly, may cause obstruction of the ureter and pelvis, and present a hazard during surgical procedures involving the kidney.

Fusion Anomalies. Contralateral fusion occurs in about 1 of every 400 persons and is most often of the "horseshoe" variety, in which the lower poles of the kidneys are fused. Bipolar fusion results in a "disc" or "doughnut" kidney. The upper pole of one kidney may be fused to the lower pole of the other, producing a "sigmoid" kidney, or the entire renal substance may be fused in one lump, called a "cake" kidney. The horseshoe kidney is the one most commonly encountered (all other forms being rare), and treatment is indicated only for complications such as stones, infection, pain, or stasis.

Cystic Abnormalities. The most common types of cystic abnormality are found in the various forms of adult polycystic disease. Potter[6] classified these diseases and their cause as:

1. Congenital infantile polycystic disease (Potter Type I) is caused by saccular enlargement of the interstitial portion of the collecting ducts; all patients die in the newborn period. The kidneys are large and are studded with 1 to 2 mm. cysts. This is a familial disease, with cysts noted in other organs, and is autosomal recessive.

2. Multicystic kidney (Potter Type II) is characterized by collecting tubules that are inadequately branched and terminate in cysts. This abnormality is almost always unilateral, is nonhereditary, and is also called dysplastic kidney.

3. Adult polycystic disease (Potter Type III) is hereditary, bilateral, and autosomal dominant. Symptoms ordinarily appear when the patient is about 40 years of age. The kidneys are large and studded with cysts because of faulty union between the collecting ducts and the nephron. Treatment is symptomatic, i.e., alleviating pain, fever, infection, hypertension, or anemia, but the result may be end-stage renal disease.

4. Solitary cysts of the kidney usually involve the lower pole. They may cause pressure on the ureter or kidney and lead to pain, infection, or hematuria. Treatment is by excision if the cyst is symptomatic or if a tumor cannot be ruled out.

5. Medullary cystic disease or sponge kidney is due to cystic dilatation of the renal collecting tubules. It is a congenital, autosomal recessive defect and is usually bilateral. Infection and calculi are seen as a result of urinary stasis. Treatment is directed toward alleviating the complications, and the prognosis is good.

Anomalies of the Ureter and Pelvis

Anomalies of Number. Either complete or partial duplication of the ureter is one of the most common congenital ureteral anomalies. The incomplete type is more common, and both types have duplicated pelves. In complete duplication, the upper pole ureter opens distally in the bladder closest to the bladder neck, and ureteroceles usually involve this segment, leading to obstruction. The ureter from the lower segment often has a short intravesical segment, predisposing to reflux.

Anomalies of the Ureteral Orifice. One or more ureteral orifices may open at a point other than the lateral margin of the trigone and may cause incontinence if they open distal to the urethral sphincter in girls. This anomaly occurs four times more often in females than in males, and the incidence is about 1 in 1100 children. It usually occurs with duplicated systems.

Anomalies of the Bladder

Agenesis is extremely rare and is of academic interest only. Duplication of the bladder may be complete or incomplete. Two penises and two urethras usually accompany complete duplication. Exstrophy of the bladder is a defect in fusion of the lower abdominal midline, pelvis, and bladder with eversion of the posterior bladder wall that occurs in 1 in 50,000 births. Early surgical correction is required.

Anomalies of the Genitalia

Anomalies of the Testis. Anorchism and polyorchism are very rare. Anomalies of descent are of three types. The *retractile* testis reaches the scrotal sac but then ascends, owing to a strong cremasteric muscle. This type needs no treatment. The *ectopic* testis has strayed from the path of descent, probably because of an abnormal connection of the distal end of the guberna-culum. The sites for ectopic testes include the superficial inguinal (most common), perineal, femoral, penile, and pelvic areas. *Cryptorchidism* involves arrest at some point in the normal descent of the testis. At the time of birth, following normal gesta-tion, the incidence of maldescent of the testis is 3.4 per cent. In half of these children, the testis descends in the first month of life. The incidence of cryptorchi-dism in the adult is 0.7 to 0.8 per cent. In the premature infant, it is 30 per cent. Three causative factors have been described:

1. Abnormality of the gubernaculum.
2. Intrinsic testicular defect.
3. Deficient gonadotropic hormone stim-ulation.

Cryptorchidism may be unilateral or bi-lateral. Treatment is aimed at bringing the testis down before the patient is 5 years old in order to prevent infertility and neo-plasm.

Anomalies of the Spermatic Cord. A *hy-drocele* is a collection of fluid within the tunica vaginalis around the testis. This disorder is common in the newborn, often disappears during the first few months of life, and should be treated as a congenital inguinal hernia if its persists. A *sperma-tocele* is a painless cystic mass containing spermatozoa that lies above and posterior to the testis. Both the hydrocele and the spermatocele transilluminate. A *varicocele* is caused by dilatation of the pampiniform plexus above the testis. It occurs most often on the left side. Tumor or other types of obstruction to venous return should be suspected if a varicocele is present on the right.

Torsion of the spermatic cord (torsion of the testis) is characterized by the sudden onset of sharp pain in the testis, occurring usually in the prepubertal boys. Torsion is more common in the cryptorchid testis. Treatment is by surgical exploration and fixation of both testes within 5 hours after the onset of symptoms to avoid loss of the testis.

Anomalies of the Phallus. Absence is very rare and few cases of duplication have been reported.

Microphallus is the term used for inade-quate development of the corpora in the penis that may require rearing the patient as a female. This *must* be differentiated from an *apparent* small phallus seen with severe chordee and hypogonadism.

Hypertrophy of the clitoris occurs as a result of the adrenogenital syndrome, ex-ogenous androgen intake by the mother of the newborn, or excess androgen produc-tion in a female of any age.

Hypospadias usually occurs with chordee (ventral curvature of the penis). The meatal opening may be at any point between the glans and the perineum. If the meatus is in the perineum, female gender is often er-roneously assigned to the patient (male pseudohermaphrodite). The foreskin is de-ficient on the ventrum. Circumcision should be avoided, as the prepuce is used later for surgical repair of the anomaly. Chordee may occur without hypospadias.

In *epispadias*, the urethra opens on the dorsum of the penis at some point proximal to the glans. If the epispadias is complete, the patient is incontinent. If the urethra opens to a point under the pubis, incontin-ence may persist after repair.

URINARY TRACT INFECTIONS

Definition

Urinary tract infection (UTI) implies the presence of bacteriuria plus inflammation of the tissues of the urinary tract from bacterial invasion. As inflammation of tissues is difficult to assess clinically, bacteriuria and UTI are considered synonymous, whether or not the patient has symptoms.

Contributing Factors

The factors contributing to UTI can be expressed most simply as Host + Organism = Infection.

When considering host factors, the fol-lowing points should be kept in mind:

1. Bladder defense is affected when the antibacterial mucous layer of the urothe-lium is disrupted by low pH, direct trauma,

high intravesical pressure, or stasis of urine.[5]

2. Urine causes decreased growth of normal urethral flora, especially when the urine has a low pH and a high concentration of urea.

3. Vaginal fluid with a low pH resists the growth of *Proteus* and *Pseudomonas* organisms but supports the growth of *Escherichia coli*.

4. Prostatic fluid contains antibacterial factors.

5. The role of immune defenses in the kidney is questionable.

6. *Urinary tract infection is rare if all parts of urinary tract empty completely under normal pressures and are not injured.*

7. Host defense is affected by diabetes, sickle cell disease, malignancy, chemotherapy, drug abuse (phenacetin), hypokalemia, and hypercalcemia.

8. Local resistance is affected by obstruction, stasis, reflux, trauma, foreign bodies (catheter, calculi, and so forth), sexual activity, and pregnancy.

Of the organisms causing urinary tract infection, *Escherichia coli* organisms (strains 04, 06, 075, 01, 02, 07) are the most common. Other organisms include *Proteus* (frequent urease producer), *Klebsiella*, *Pseudomonas*, enterococcus, *Enterobacter*, *Serratia*, *Staphylococcus* (urease producer), *Citrobacter*, *Candida*, and *Mycobacterium tuberculosis*.

Pathogenesis

Infection ascending from the urethra may be caused by bacteria in the urethra (periurethral glands) and prostate. Catheterization and instrumentation are another frequent cause (2 to 4 per cent of patients have infections following these procedures). A properly inserted and managed catheter is of less risk to the patient than is retained infected urine. The retention catheter should not be clamped for more than 15 minutes.

Lymphatic and hematogenous sources of infection can also occur. Small particles introduced into the bladder under increased pressure can be transmitted to the kidneys by the lymphatics, and infection of kidney can be caused by organisms carried in the blood, particularly in the presence of ureteral obstruction.

Clinical Manifestations

Lower urinary tract infection is manifested by frequency, urgency, dysuria, and hematuria. These are common findings and are caused by irritation from inflammation of the bladder neck and proximal urethra resulting from acute prostatitis and cystitis. Chronic prostatitis and urethritis may cause discomfort in the suprapubic or perineal areas. Fever is not commonly present.

Upper urinary tract infection findings include fever, chills, and flank pain in addition to frequency, dysuria, and urgency in acute infections. Chronic pyelonephritis may cause the loss of renal function with few or no symptoms.

Urinary tract infection in children causes failure to thrive and abdominal symptoms, including pain, diarrhea, and vomiting.

Diagnosis

In addition to the presence of the symptoms just described, the diagnosis is determined by the examination of urine.

Methods of collection include obtaining a clean-catch specimen or performing urethral catheterization or suprapubic aspiration. A clean-catch urine is always reliable in the male and is reliable in the female if 100,000 or more organisms per ml. of urine are found or if the same organism is found on repeat culture. The patient probably does not have an infection if less than 10,000 organisms per ml. of urine are found by this method. Urethral catheterization is the best way to obtain bladder urine in the adult and to verify uncertain results of a clean-catch urine. It is an appropriate procedure when urethral instrumentation is indicated for other purposes. Suprapubic aspiration is the best way to obtain a clean specimen in infants.

When doing a quantitative urine culture, the finding of 100,000 or more organisms per ml. is always significant. Lesser counts are significant if the specimen is collected by catheter or by suprapubic aspiration, if the same organism is demonstrated on consecutive cultures, or if the patient has recurrent infection.

Microscopic findings should be noted. Pyuria may be absent in 50 per cent of neonates and 15 per cent of adults with positive cultures. Bacteria on stain (methylene blue or Gram's stain) of a noncentrifuged drop of urine is predictive of the finding of 100,000 or more organisms per ml. in the culture.

The urine pH is alkaline if urease-producing organisms are present. Another finding is a decrease in maximal concentrating ability with renal infection.

Newer methods of screening include bacteriologic procedures (Dip Slide-Uricult, Clinicult, Oxoid, and so forth) and chemical evaluations utilizing the principle that bacteria reduce nitrate in urine to nitrite (Griess's test).

Epidemiology

Bacteriuria is found in 1 per cent of newborns, two-thirds of whom are males.

In a 10 year study of school children, bacteriuria was found in 1.2 per cent of girls and 0.03 per cent of boys. Each year, 0.3 to 0.4 per cent of girls who were previously uninfected developed bacteriuria. During the first 12 years of school, 4.5 to 6 per cent of girls had one episode of bacteriuria and 20 per cent of these had reflux, while 13 per cent had dilatation of a calyx of the kidney (calicectasis) on intravenous urogram. One-third of the patients said to have "asymptomatic bacteriuria" did admit to having symptoms of urgency, frequency, or dysuria after careful questioning.

The incidence of bacteriuria in young adults is 1.2 per cent in women and 0.5 per cent in men. Bacteriuria in patients over the age of 60 years occurs in 15 per cent of both men and women.

Management

Antimicrobial Treatment. For patients with acute, uncomplicated infection (no fever and no evidence of renal involvement), urine culture is unnecessary. Administer a sulfonamide, nalidixic acid, or nitrofurantoin for 10 days, and culture urine 2 weeks after treatment. If the follow-up culture is positive, treat the infection with a specific antibiotic and find the contributing cause, if not found previously.

Acute, complicated infection (fever, flank pain, and urinary symptoms) is treated by obtaining urine for culture but starting therapy immediately with ampicillin or a sulfamethoxazole-trimethoprim combination. Change to a specific therapy after the organism is identified. Gentamicin and a cephalosporin are given if evidence of systemic sepsis is present. An intravenous urogram is done *early* to rule out obstruction. The relief of obstruction is more important to the survival of the patient than is antibiotic therapy, as infected urine proximal to the obstruction is forced into the renal veins and lymphatics.

Urologic Survey. A urologic survey should be done to find the contributing cause. Do an intravenous urogram, including voiding and post-voiding films (does not rule out all lower urinary tract pathology); cystourethroscopy; calibration of the urethra; cystogram (stat and voiding cinefluorography); and neurologic examination, including cystometry (look for spina bifida). Indications for performing this survey include a first infection in males; infections with flank pain and fever; a persistent infection or an infection causing symptoms, or both; and recurrent infections.

Elimination of Contributing Factors. The following disorders are likely to cause urinary tract infections and should therefore be treated whenever possible.

1. Obstruction (urethra, ureter, bladder neck).
2. Calculi.
3. Vesicoureteral reflux.
4. Neurologic dysfunction.
5. Urethritis in females.
6. Prostatitis in males.
7. Venereal infection. Have subjects void after sexual intercourse.

Recurrent or Persistent Bacteriuria. If the urine can be sterilized, recurrent bacteriuria may be prevented by suppressive therapy using less than therapeutic doses of urinary antiseptics such as nitrofurantoin, the soluble sulfonamides, nalidixic acid, or methenamine preparations with acidifying agents such as ascorbic acid, and so forth. Bacterial counts may be kept at lower levels by use of suppressive therapy in patients in whom contributing factors cannot be eliminated (hydronephrotic kidneys, some stones, some neoplasms). A dose of a urinary antiseptic immediately after sexual intercourse may also be helpful.

Urethral Catheterization. The indications for use of urethral catheterization include the need for immediate catheterization to obtain urine specimens, check post-voiding residual urine, calibrate the urethra, and instill substances in the bladder. Urinary catheterization is also used to monitor hourly urine output in critically ill patients and to treat and prevent urinary retention that is secondary to obstruction or that occurs in paralyzed or comatose patients. It is also indicated to protect the urethra after trauma or surgery and to treat selected patients with incontinence.

The technique of and procedure for urinary catheterization are as follows:

1. Adequate lubrication, preferably instilling water-soluble lubricant into the urethra as well as on catheter, is required.

2. Proper cleansing of the meatus, introitus, and penis is necessary.

3. Use sterile gloves, sterile clamp, sterile catheter, and sterile drainage apparatus.

4. Use a closed drainage system.

5. Irrigate the catheter with a sterile solution, using sterile technique. (Irrigation is necessary only to check patency and to dislodge obstructing blood clots and debris.)

6. The catheter should be fixed with adhesive tape to the thigh or suprapubic area so that there is no traction on the catheter from the patient's movements or from the weight of drainage tubing. It is best to fix the catheter to the suprapubic area in male paraplegics to prevent both erosion of the urethra opposite the suspensory ligament of the penis and the development of a urethral fistula.

7. Either attending personnel or the patient should cleanse the catheter surface at the urethral meatus daily and apply an antiseptic ointment to the catheter at the meatus.

8. The catheter should not be clamped, except when necessary, and then it should not be occluded for more than 15 minutes.

9. Change the catheter only when precipitate or encrustation develops on its inner surface. This can be detected by compressing the catheter between the thumb and finger. A gritty sensation is felt when the inner surfaces are rubbed together.

10. The 5 ml. balloon catheter is preferred for usual straight drainage. The larger the lumen of the catheter, the better the drainage, *but* the catheter must be small enough to fit loosely in the urethra, allowing space for urethral secretions to drain outward through the meatus. If the meatus is small and fits snugly around the catheter, a meatotomy should be done if the patient is to have the catheter in place more than 24 hours. Very small catheters (10 to 14F) tend to twist easily and obstruct. A 16 to 20F catheter is the usual size required for adults.

11. Intermittent self-catheterization or catheterization done by an attendant (family or professional) is useful for keeping the bladder empty at intervals in patients who retain urine but who cannot void (neurogenic bladder).

12. If a catheter has been indwelling more than 24 hours, the bacterial flora of the urine should be determined prior to its removal, and specific antibiotics should be given 12 hours prior to removal and continued for 3 days thereafter. The amount of voiding should be checked frequently after removal of the catheter. Bacteriemia is apt to occur if the bladder becomes distended with infected urine.

Complications from the Urethral Catheterization. Bacteriuria is likely to occur after the catheter has been indwelling for more than 72 hours. This is preventable to some degree by use of a sterile technique of insertion, good catheter care, and sterile closed drainage systems. Antibacterial drugs may delay the bacteriuria but will not prevent or control it. The best protection against deep tissue involvement or ascending infections with an indwelling catheter is to keep the bladder empty at all times in addition to good catheter care.

Periurethral abscess usually occurs because the catheter is too tight or is under tension. These abscesses often result in urethral fistulas.

Septicemia usually occurs because the catheter is obstructed or partly pulled out, allowing the bladder to fill with inoculated urine under pressure and forcing organisms into the lymphatics and blood stream.

Follow-Up. Urine culture should be done at 2 weeks and 3 months after the apparent successful treatment of an acute urinary tract infection. Periodic culture is required in patients with chronic and recurrent bacteriuria. As organisms change, suppressive and therapeutic antimicrobial agents must be changed also.

Potent broad-spectrum antibiotics should be used only in acute exacerbations of urinary tract infection, particularly in pyelonephritis. Use suppressive urinary antiseptics at other times.

Periodic check of renal function, including determination of creatinine clearance, phenolsulfonphthalein (PSP), and blood urea nitrogen (BUN) levels, is required in patients with chronic infection, particularly when associated with chronic uropathy. Toxins from some organisms have been shown to inhibit ureteral peristalsis. Finally, order radiographic evaluation as indicated in patients who have chronic uropathy contributing to infection.

TRAUMA TO THE URINARY AND MALE REPRODUCTIVE TRACTS

Injury to the kidney

Direct injury to the kidney may be caused by blunt trauma (50 to 60 per cent of such trauma results from automobile accidents, 30 per cent from football injuries, falls, and so forth) or by penetrating injuries (stabbing or gunshot wounds). Indirect injury due to inertia occurs if the kidney continues to move following a fall. This causes stretching or tearing of a renal artery or vein, or both, and may result in an intimal tear, causing thrombosis. The term *exercise or athletic pseudonephritis* is used when protein, red blood cells (RBC), and casts are found in the urine following physical stress. The urine clears in 12 hours, but these findings may be mistaken for indications of renal injury or other renal disease.

Diagnosis is based on symptoms and signs and on the results of radiologic examinations. Hematuria is found in 85 to 90 per cent of patients but may be absent if the area of renal damage does not connect with the renal pelvis or ureter or if the ureter is obstructed. Pain and tenderness occur in the kidney region. A mass may be felt in the flank if the perinephric space is filled with blood and may be mistaken for a muscle spasm.

An infusion intravenous urogram should be performed as soon as possible on all patients with hematuria following trauma and on patients suspected of having renal injury, e.g., those with fractured lower ribs or lumbar vertebrae. Visualization of the kidney and any portion of the pelvocalyceal system indicates perfusion of the kidney and no major injury to renal pedicle. In addition, look for hydronephrosis or distortion by a renal or perirenal mass as predis-posing to renal injury. Extravasation of urine and filling defects from clots may also be evident.

Do an arteriogram as soon as possible if there is no visualization of the kidney on the infusion urogram to rule out renal artery obstruction or a tear, which must be repaired early to restore renal perfusion. This study is less urgent if the kidney is visualized on infusion urogram, but should be done on all patients with major renal injuries.

Radioisotope renography may also be used. A scintigram indicates perfusion, and may show the extent of damage. A retrograde urogram may also be required. Ureteral catheterization is occasionally necessary to determine the extent of injury and may be done early if indicated and if needed for diagnosis.

The final study to consider is sonography, which aids in the diagnosis of perirenal collections of blood or urine, or both.

Management may include the need for immediate surgical intervention, delayed surgical intervention, or nonsurgical treatment only.

Indications for immediate surgical intervention are renal artery injury or threatened exsanguination from renal hemorrhage. Bleeding from a kidney is usually contained by Gerota's fascia located in the perinephric space. If the fascia is disrupted, bleeding continues in the retroperitoneal space and may surface as an ecchymosis in the femoral canal or may be evidenced by an expanding flank mass. Immediate surgery is also required for disruption of the renal pelvis or the ureteropelvic junction.

The indication for delayed surgical intervention (5 to 15 days post-trauma) is a transcortical-transcapsular injury connecting the pelvocalyceal system and the perinephric space (evidenced by urinary extravasation).

Nonsurgical treatment is indicated for trauma without evidence of extravasation of urine or for subcapsular injuries or cortical lacerations that do not connect the pelvocalyceal system and the perinephric space.

Follow-up urograms should be done 1 and 5 years later, unless symptoms indicate that additional studies are required.

Finally, it is important to rule out associated intra-abdominal injuries when diagnosing and treating injuries to the kidney.

Injury to the Ureter

Trauma to the ureter may be caused by pelvic, retroperitoneal, or intra-abdominal surgery; penetrating abdominal injuries; or instrumentation.

Symptoms and signs include pain in the kidney from obstruction, abdominal pain from urinary extravasation (urinary ascites), fever, and anuria, if the injury is bilateral.

When diagnosing ureteral injuries, maintain a high index of suspicion regarding symptoms and signs. Pertinent radiologic studies include an intravenous urogram to show obstruction or extravasation, or both; ureteral catherization and retrograde urogram; and a sonogram to localize collections of urine.

Management includes early deligation, ureteral catheter insertion if a partial transection is present, and drainage of extravasated urine. Surgical repair may be required, including ureteral anastomosis, ureteroneocystostomy, transureteroureterostomy, or use of an intestinal segment. Occasional temporary diversion of urine above the site of injury, e.g., by nephrostomy, is sometimes necessary.

Injury to the Bladder

Causes of bladder injuries include blunt trauma to the lower abdomen when the bladder is distended, penetrating injuries, bone fragments from a fractured pelvis, or trauma caused by instrumentation and transurethral surgery or pelvic surgery. Occasionally, spontaneous bladder rupture may occur.

Symptoms and signs of such injuries are suprapubic or abdominal pain, or both, following a blow to the abdomen or a fractured pelvis, hematuria, and inability to void. However, ability to void does not rule out bladder injury. Additional symptoms and signs are abdominal tenderness or rigidity, or both, if there is intraperitoneal extravasation; shock; fever, if urine is infected; and leakage of urine through the vagina.

To establish the diagnosis, catheterize the patient gently and perform a cystogram. The bladder must be filled to capacity to demonstrate smaller lacerations. Leave the catheter in the bladder until it is certain that there is no injury. Cystoscopy is occasionally necessary when a small laceration does not show extravasation on a cystogram. An infusion urogram to evaluate the upper urinary tract may also be required.

When treating bladder injuries, first drain urine from the peritoneal cavity or extraperitoneal space. Treat early, as mortality is higher with delays. Suture the lacerations (smaller, more inaccessible lacerations need not be sutured if the bladder is kept empty until these are healed). Leave the catheter or suprapubic tube in place until the bladder has healed, and leave drains in the perivesical space but not in the peritoneum.

Injury to the Urethra

Fracture of the pelvis may cause urethral injury, as the membranous portion of the urethra is quite vulnerable. The urethra may be sheared off at the apex of the prostate. Additional causes are straddle injuries (injury to the bulbous urethra in the male or the distal urethra in the female), instrumentation trauma (internal laceration or false passage injuries), and penetrating injuries (knife or gunshot wounds).

Bleeding from the urethral meatus, particularly if independent of voiding, is a sign of urethral injury. Extravasation of urine may also occur. This will cause swelling of the scrotum and lower abdominal wall after voiding if the rupture of the urethra is below the urogenital diaphragm. Ecchymosis in the perineum and scrotum may appear following injuries to the bulbous urethra. Pain in the area of injury is a common symptom. If the injury is above the urogenital diaphragm, extravasation of urine into the pelvis and retroperitoneal space may not be apparent but may cause pain and possibly shock.

Diagnosis is made by a urethrogram. In the injured patient with bleeding from the urethral meatus or with other evidence of urethral injury, the physician should attempt to pass a well-lubricated 5 ml. balloon catheter (size 16F in the adult). If the catheter enters the bladder, leave it in place at least 72 hours. If it does not enter the bladder easily, discontinue the attempt and perform the urethrogram by low pressure injection of contrast medium into the urethra, using a plain tip or cone tip syringe. Extravasation of contrast medium indicates the site of injury. If the injury is above the urogenital diaphragm, an intravenous urogram should be done also.

Management of urethral injuries includes the following: If the urethrogram shows an injury, insert a catheter (16 to 20F) if possible and leave it in place for at least 10 days. If the urethral catheter cannot be passed into the bladder, a suprapubic cystostomy tube should be inserted to drain the urine. (Repair of the urethra may be done at the time of cystostomy, or it can be done at a later date.) Drain the extravasated urine.

Permanent follow-up to detect any evidence of stricture at the site of injury or of repair, or both, is required.

Injury to the Penis

Penile injuries may be caused by traumatic sexual activity, including fracture of the erect penis. Fracture also occurs by striking the erect penis against the bed or some other firm object. Contusion and avulsion of the penis may result from by entanglement in machinery. Knife and gunshot wounds, self-mutilation, and burns are also causes of penile injury.

Symptoms and signs include pain and swelling, evidence of the wound, and ecchymosis.

Diagnosis is made by the findings of these symptoms and signs and occasionally by cavernosograms (injection of contrast medium into the corpora cavernosa in some cases of suspected rupture.) However, this procedure usually is not necessary.

The following steps are required in the management of penile injuries: Suture lacerations. A fracture of the corpus may require surgical repair, although some fractures have been successfully managed with compression dressings, with or without the use of a urethral catheter.

An attempt should be made to replace an amputated penis as soon as possible, as this has been successful after several hours' delay. The skin should be replaced also, if present. If this is lost, the penis can be buried in the scrotum or covered with a skin graft. Associated urethral injury is managed as previously outlined.

Injury to the Scrotum

Scrotal trauma may be caused by penetrating wounds or by direct blows (contusion or fracture of the testes).

Symptoms and signs include severe pain if the testis is injured (differentiate from torsion), swelling of the scrotum and its contents, and ecchymosis of the scrotum.

To treat injuries to the scrotum, first control bleeding if it has not already ceased when the patient is seen. Conservative management is preferred. The less the testis is disturbed, the more likely that some blood supply will be retained if there is injury to the spermatic cord. Direct penetrating wounds and lacerations of the testis may require débridement and closure of the tunica albuginea.

DISORDERS OF THE MALE REPRODUCTIVE TRACT

Normal Male Reproductive Organs

Physical examination of the normal reproductive organs of the male will reveal the following:

Penis. No lesions will be seen on the skin of the shaft, glans, or corona or under the side of the prepuce. The prepuce should retract easily if not circumcised. A single meatus should be located at the tip of the glans and should be nearly as large as the urethral lumen. The corpora cavernosa and other structures in the shaft will be uniform in consistency and straight on erection and will contain no indurated areas (plaques).

Urethra. The penile and perineal portions should be palpable, with no induration or masses. Note the presence and character of any urethral discharge.

Scrotum. The skin should be elastic and thin. No masses should be palpable.

Testis. One testis will be in the dependent portion on each side of the scrotum and will have a homogeneous, firm, spongy consistency and a smooth surface. (Palpation is the *only* means of diagnosing early neoplasm.)

Epididymis. The epididymis should be barely palpable as a soft, elongated structure along the posterior surface of the testis. The upper pole (globus major) is slightly larger than the lower pole.

Spermatic cord. The vas deferens is palpable as a cordlike structure the size of the lead in a lead pencil. Other structures including the cremaster muscles, fused processus vaginalis, arteries, and veins (pampiniform plexus) are all softer than the vas. The entire cord is usually about 1 cm. thick.

Prostate. The posterior surfaces of the right and left lateral lobes are palpable through the anterior wall of the lower rectum. Each lateral lobe is 1.5 to 2.0 cm. wide and about 3.0 cm. long. The median furrow (or groove) is felt between the lateral lobes, and palpation of the furrow creates a desire to void, as the prostatic portion of the urethra lies just anterior to this furrow. The base of the prostate is attached to the bladder neck, and the apex is closest to the anal sphincter. The margins of the prostate should be well defined. The consistency is the same as that of the palmar surface of the thenar eminence when the fist is clenched, and the gland is normally slightly movable (not fixed). Palpation is the *only* means of diagnosing early cancer of the prostate.

By compressing the prostate with the tip of the examining finger from the outer margins toward the median furrow and then compressing the median furrow from the above downward, prostatic fluid is expressed. Normal fluid shows many "lecithin granules" and less than 5 white blood cells per high power field. Normal prostatic fluid is reported to be antibacterial.

Seminal vesicles. Although the seminal vesicles are normally not palpable, they are palpable if distended with fluid or if involved by a neoplastic or infectious process.

Disorders of the Penis

Problems with erection include priapism and impotence. *Priapism* is a prolonged, painful erection without sexual desire that is caused by an obstructed venous outlet. It may be associated with blood disorders, neoplasm, neurologic disease, or prostatitis or is often idiopathic. *Impotence,* or absence of erection, may be due to psychogenic causes, prostate infections, neurologic disease, or vascular insufficiency (Leriche's syndrome).

Phimosis is a disorder in which the small opening in the prepuce prevents retraction. This is treated by circumcision or by dorsal slitting. In *paraphimosis* the retracted prepuce cannot be returned to the normal position. Manual reduction should be performed as soon as possible. If impossible, the tight ring or prepuce must be divided.

Balanoposthitis is an infection of the glans (balanitis) and prepuce (posthitis).

Peyronie's disease is characterized by plaques of fibrous dysplasia in the shaft of the penis. The cause is unknown. The disorder is significant only if pain or curvature, or both, occur during erection. Peyronie's disease is treated by vitamin E administration, sometimes by the injection of steroids, by ultrasound therapy, or by surgical excision.

Most cases of *carcinoma* are found in uncircumcised men and rarely develop in males circumcised at birth. They usually occur on the glans or prepuce and metastasize to the inguinal nodes. If the urethra or corpora are involved, lesions are likely to metastasize to higher nodes. These carcinomas are treated by surgical excision, although some are treated by irradiation.

"Precancerous penile lesions" can be determined by histologic diagnosis. Erythroplasia of Queyrat appears as a shiny, red, papular lesion on the glans, and carcinoma in situ (Bowen's disease) is seen as a red papule. Condyloma acuminatum usually appears as a warty growth, but some of these lesions may become malignant.

Skin lesions of the penis include herpes progenitalis, allergies, fungus infections, and so forth. When ulcerative lesions are present, it is important to rule out venereal disorders such as chancre, chancroid, or granuloma inguinale.

Disorders of the Urethra

Stenosis of the meatus appears in both males and females and may cause obstructive symptoms, ulceration around the meatus, and hematuria.

Infection is often associated with a urethral discharge. The infection may be venereal (specific) or nonvenereal (nonspecific). Periurethral gland infections may lead to abscess and fistula formation (some occur after catheter use). Skene's gland abscesses are palpable at the meatus in females.

A *urethral stricture* is the fibrous replacement of normal urethral tissue following trauma or infection. The stricture obstructs urine flow as the fibrous tissue gradually contracts. It is treated with dilation or surgery, or both. Abscesses, pseudodiverticula, or fistulas may develop proximal to the stricture.

Of the *urethral tumors,* condylomas and papillomas are usually benign. Other tumors are the transitional cell carcinomas of the proximal urethra in both males and females, squamous cell carcinomas in the distal urethra in both males and females, and adenocarcinomas, found mostly in the female urethra. These are treated by surgery and by irradiation. A *caruncle* is a granular, red, tender mass on the posterior lip of the urethral meatus in the female that is treated by excision or cauterization. It is important to differentiate caruncles from neoplasms.

Urethral diverticula may be congenital or acquired, the latter being a complication of a periurethral abscess in the male or female. A diverticulum causes leaking of urine after voiding and is treated by surgical excision.

Prolapse of the urethra is caused by eversion of redundant mucosa in the female. This is usually treated by excision of the redundant portion, if severe.

Disorders of the Scrotal Contents

Skin lesions such as sebaceous cysts and hemangiomas occur commonly. *Skin cancer* occurs in the scrotal skin as it does in the skin in other areas of the body.

Cystic lesions include hydroceles, spermatoceles, and varicoceles.

A *hydrocele* is an accumulation of clear, straw-colored fluid between two layers (visceral and parietal) of tunica vaginalis that transmits light. The causes are trauma, inflammation, and hernia or idiopathic. The mass may disappear spontaneously in newborns and infants. If it does not, it should be considered a hernia. Surgical incision should be performed if the hydrocele is large or symptomatic in the adult.

A *spermatocele* is a cystic lesion caused by obstruction of the duct carrying sperm from the testis to the epididymis. It often feels like another testis. A spermatocele also transmits light.

A *varicocele* is a dilation of the pampiniform venous plexus in the spermatic cord and is usually found on the left, where the spermatic vein is longer. The spermatic vein drains into the renal vein, and the venous valves may become incompetent. A varicocele occasionally causes dull pain when the patient is standing and may be a cause of oligospermia. Treatment, when indicated, involves ligating the spermatic vein.

An *abscess of the scrotum* usually originates from the urethra or is caused by extensions from perianal infection.

For a discussion of *undescended testis*, see the section on Anomalies of the Testis.

Torsion of the testis is a twisting of the spermatic cord caused by rotation of the testis that is secondary to an anomalous attachment. The signs are excruciating pain, scrotal swelling, and tenderness to touch or on any movement. Ischemic gangrene of the testis may occur if the torsion is not treated promptly by surgery (5 to 24 hours after the occurrence). No blood flow is heard in the testis with the Doppler stethoscope. A radioisotope scan can be done to determine the absence of blood flow. *Torsion of the appendages* may occur. An appendix testis (hydatid of Morgagni-Müllerian remnant) or an appendix epididymis (Wolffian remnant) may twist, become gangrenous, and cause acute scrotal pain.

Infections of the spermatic cord are uncommon, except when associated with infections of the prostate and epididymis. A beaded vas deferens may indicate tuberculosis. Of the *infections of the testis*, pyogenic orchitis is uncommon, and mumps orchitis usually occurs after puberty.

Epididymitis may result from the passage of urine down the vas deferens during stress (chemical epididymitis) or from inoculation with bacteria through the vas deferens or the blood stream. Tuberculosis is a cause of chronic epididymitis. About 60 per cent of urine samples from these patients produce no organisms on culture. Epididymitis is very common and causes acute pain and swelling. It must be differentiated from torsion. Treatment is symptomatic, including therapy for infection if present. Vasectomy may prevent frequent recurrences.

Tumors of the testis occur in 2.1 per 100,000 males per year and account for 0.64 per cent of cancer deaths in the male. They occur more often in young men and are more common in those who have an undescended testis. Most are malignant seminomas, embryonal carcinomas, teratocarcinomas and choriocarcinomas. A painless nodule or swelling is the most common finding. Treatment includes inguinal orchiectomy, irradiation, chemotherapy, and retroperitoneal lymphadenectomy.

Disorders of the Prostate

Acute infections of the prostate are manifested by dysuria, frequency, fever, perineal pain, and difficulty when voiding. The abscess rarely requires drainage. *Chronic infections* are common, but bacteria frequently are not found on culture or by stain. Such infections are often caused by stasis of fluid (prostatosis). White blood cells are often found in expressed prostatic secretion. The patient may complain of perineal and low back pain or may have urinary tract symptoms. The chronic infection may contribute to impotence and infertility. A sulfonamide-trimethoprim combination is helpful if white blood cells are found in the prostatic fluid. Periodic drainage by prostatic massage is helpful in most patients. The disorder may simulate symptoms of benign prostatic hyperplasia.

Benign prostatic hyperplasia is a benign neoplasm originating in the "inner prostate" or periurethral glands and is a common cause of bladder outlet obstruction in older men. Bladder outlet obstruction is the only indication for treatment. The enlargement may be detected by rectal examination, but some obstructions can be identified only by endoscopy. The obstructing tissue is removed by "prostatectomy," which is a misnomer as the benign neoplasm is removed from the prostate and most of functioning prostate remains. Retrograde ejaculation usually occurs after removal of hyperplastic tissue.

Carcinoma of the prostate is the cause of 17,000 deaths annually in United States. Autopsy studies have identified cancer of the prostate in 20 per cent of men over 50 years of age. The patient has no symptoms in the curable stage, during which the lesion is found only by palpating a hard area or nodule on rectal examination. The carcinoma may later enlarge and obstruct urine flow. Serum acid phosphatase values are elevated with local extension or metastases. Osteoblastic metastases to the bone may be found. Treatment is by surgical excision or by irradiation. Estrogens or castration, or both, are effective for varying periods of time. Other "antiandrogens" and chemotherapeutic agents show promise.

Disorders of the Seminal Vesicles

Infections of the seminal vesicles are associated with prostate infections or stasis. The vesicles are palpable only when distended, and the infection may be the cause of a bloody ejaculate. Primary *neoplasms* are rare, but the seminal vesicles are the first site of local extension from prostatic cancer.

EVALUATION OF THE INFERTILE MALE

The history should include questions pertaining to the duration of sexual relations without use of birth control, use of lubricants (some are spermicidal), and pattern and frequency of intercourse. A history of undescended testes, mumps, urinary infections, prostatitis, venereal disease, febrile illnesses, or exposure to radiation, drugs, or heat should be elicited, and the past marital history, should be recorded.

Physical examination includes determination of habitus and neurologic evaluation. The genitalia and prostate should be examined and the blood pressure and femoral pulses recorded. The presence of a varicocele or hypospadias should be determined.

Laboratory evaluation includes semen analysis, testicular biopsy, vasography, and chromosome karyotype. Determinations of serum luteinizing hormone (LH), follicle-stimulating hormone (FSH), and testosterone levels; urinary hydroxycorticoid and ketosteroid values; and sperm immunity in the patient or his partner should also be carried out.

NEOPLASMS OF THE KIDNEY, URETER, BLADDER, AND URETHRA

Tumors of the Renal Parenchyma

Benign tumors include adenomas, angiomyolipomas, and juxtaglomerular cell adenomas.

An *adenoma* should be examined carefully for signs of malignancy. An *angiomyolipoma* (hamartoma) is a single, unilateral lesion that causes hematuria. Radiographic features differentiate this tumor from carcinoma. Multiple renal hamartomas associated with tumors of the brain, retina, and lungs and with mental retardation are characteristic of tuberous sclerosis. Fetal hamartoma is occasionally found in newborn infants. This must be differentiated from Wilms' tumor. *Juxtaglomerular cell adenoma* (hemangiopericytoma) causes elevated plasma renin values and hypertension.

Malignant tumors of the renal parenchyma are adenocarcinomas and Wilms' tumors.

Adenocarcinoma (hypernephroma, Grawitz's tumor, renal cell carcinoma) constitutes 80 per cent of all renal tumors. These tumors are more common in men, are multiple in Lindau's disease, and produce hematogenous metastases. There are no early symptoms. Gross hematuria is found in less than 50 per cent of patients, 15 per cent have fever, and less than 50 per cent have a palpable mass. Pain often indicates metastases, which are common in the lung, bone, brain, and liver. Adenocarcinomas occasionally secrete erythropoietin and cause secondary polycythemia. Diagnosis is made by intravenous and retrograde urograms, sonograms, and arteriograms. Treatment is surgical, as irradiation and chemotherapy have given disappointing results. The 5 year survival rate is 35 per cent.

Wilms' tumor (embryoma, adenomyosarcoma, nephroblastoma) is a malignant tumor of children and is most frequently found in those under 6 years of age. Ten per cent of the tumors are bilateral, and 6 per cent are present at birth. The incidence is 1 in 10,000 children. The first finding is a painless, palpable mass, and the presence of symptoms usually indicates metastases. Diagnosis is made by intravenous urography and sonography and by the presence of hypertension. Hematuria and fever are uncommon. Treatment is by surgical removal. The tumor is radiosensitive, and chemotherapy with actinomycin and vincristine has increased the survival rate from 35 to 75 per cent.

Tumors of the Renal Pelvis

Tumors of the renal pelvis account for 10 per cent of all kidney tumors. There are two types. Transitional cell tumors (80 per cent incidence) are usually papillary. There is some question of their tendency to "seed" to the ureter and bladder and of whether or not there is a relationship to smoking and to exposure to aromatic amines, including tryptophan metabolites.

Squamous cell tumors (15 per cent incidence) are often associated with chronic infection or stone formation, or both.

Symptoms include hematuria and pain from the tumor or from clots obstructing the ureter. Radiographic examination will show a nonopaque filling defect (differentiate from uric acid stone) on intravenous or retrograde urograms. Cytologic studies of urine should be done. In addition, there may be questionable elevation of plasma or urinary carcinoembryonic antigen. Cystoscopy is necessary to rule out bladder tumor. Finally, it is important to remember that these tumors may mimic renal or ureteral tuberculosis.

Treatment involves surgical excision, preferably of the kidney, ureter, and cuff of the bladder. The prognosis ranges from a 75 per cent 5 year survival rate for patients with low-grade transitional cell tumors to no known 5 year survivors for patients with squamous cell carcinoma.

Tumors of the Ureter

Types of ureteral tumors include benign polyps and squamous cell lesions (both rare) and transitional cell tumors. The latter tumors are usually papillary, may be multiple, and may cause questionable "seeding" to the bladder.

Symptoms are those of hematuria, pain from obstruction of the ureter, and infection secondary to this obstruction. The tumor will appear as a lucent defect on the ureterogram of an intravenous or retrograde urogram, with a hydroureter being seen above the defect. Laboratory studies include a differential blood count and a cytologic study of urine. Cytoscopy should also be done to rule out a bladder tumor.

The preferred treatment is surgical excision of the entire ureter, kidney, and cuff of the bladder if the opposite kidney and ureter are normal. Segmental resection of the ureter or a ureterotomy with excision of the tumor is the second option. The prognosis is excellent with benign tumors, fair with low-grade carcinomas, and poor with high-grade tumors.

Tumors of the Bladder

Types. Transitional cell carcinoma is the most common type of bladder tumor. The incidence is high following prolonged exposure to industrial aromatic amines. Tryptophan metabolites may also be causative. These tumors may be graded, depending on histopathology, and staged, according to the extent of the tumor.

GRADING:

1. *Grade I.* Very well differentiated, called benign papilloma by some pathologists. Usually manageable by cystoscopic resection or fulguration, or both.

2. *Grade II.* Less differentiated papillary tumors. More apt to be invasive, often also treatable by cystoscopic resection. Grade I and II tumors are relatively radioresistant.

3. *Grade III.* Poorly differentiated and tend to be nodular or sessile rather than papillary. Usually invade muscle of bladder and are radiosensitive.

4. *Grade IV.* Anaplastic, often with squamous metaplasia. Tumors are radiosensitive and metastasize early.

STAGING:

1. *Stage 0.* No invasion of tumor below surface.

2. *Stage A.* Invading lamina propria, but not muscle.

3. *Stage B_1.* Invading less than halfway through bladder muscular wall.

4. *Stage B_2.* Invading more than halfway through bladder muscular wall.

5. *Stage C.* Invading through bladder wall to perivesical fat or peritoneum, but no metastases evident.

6. *Stage D.* Demonstrable metastases to lymph nodes, liver, bone, and so forth.

Other types of bladder tumor also occur. Epidermoid neoplasms constitute 5 per cent of all bladder tumors. These are squamous cell, highly malignant lesions that invade and metastasize early. They may be associated with chronic infection or stone formation. Adenocarcinoma is a rare tumor that arises most often at the urachus. Rhabdomyosarcomas and leiomyosarcomas, also rare, are very malignant lesions that metastasize early. The "botryoides" variety may be seen in children. Rare primary lymphomas, carcinosarcomas, neurofibromas, hemangiomas, and pheochromocytomas are occasionally found. Metastatic tumors from other sites and lesions caused by endometriosis are also seen.

Carcinoma in situ mimics cystitis. Cytologic studies and random biopsy are indicated for this tumor.

Diagnosis. Symptoms and signs may include only the finding of hematuria. Urinary frequency will occur if the bladder capacity is diminished. Frequency and dysuria will be present if infection is superimposed or if the tumor is obstructing the bladder outlet. Pain in the flank occurs if the tumor is obstructing a ureter, and a mass can be detected on rectal or vaginal examination if the tumor is invasive.

Diagnostic studies include a cytologic study of the urine and radiographic examinations. Do an intravenous or retrograde urogram, or both, to look for upper urinary tract tumor and obstruction. An arteriogram is sometimes helpful. A metastatic survey (x-rays, bone scan, and so forth) are also required, and cystoscopy, bimanual examination, and biopsy for diagnosis, grading, and staging should also be done.

Treatment. Surgical treatment may involve transurethral resection or fulguration. Irradiation therapy may be used as definitive treatment for higher grades and stages of tumors or as an adjunct to surgical excision of all or part of the bladder. Another form of surgical management is total cystectomy, alone or in conjunction with irradiation. The prostate in the male, vagina and uterus in the female, pelvic lymph nodes, and urethra are removed, as indicated by the type of tumor and the preference of the surgeon. If urinary diversion is required, establishment of an ileal or colon conduit or a ureterosigmoidostomy, ureterostomy, or nephrostomy may be done.

Chemotherapy may also be tried. Thiotepa is occasionally effective intravesically. Administration of 5-fluorouracil intravesically or systemically, or both, may also be attempted, although this form of therapy is not very promising. Systemic platinum (investigational) and doxorubicin (Adriamycin) have also been used. Intravesical triethylene glycol diglycidyl ether (Epodyl), which is investigational in the United States, and trial doses of various chemotherapeutic combinations are currently being evaluated.

Immunotherapy includes administration of bacille Calmette-Guérin (BCG) vaccine and other nonspecific antigens.

Palliative management consists of control of bleeding by use of intravesical formalin, fulguration, and so forth; diversion of urine to control severe bladder symptoms and bleeding; and irradiation.

Finally, transurethral cryosurgery may be attempted.

Prognosis. The prognosis is good for patients with low-grade, low-stage transitional cell tumors, but there is 25 per cent or less survival in those with high-grade, high-stage transitional cell tumors and with other malignant tumors.

Tumors of the Urethra

The two types of benign urethral tumors are polyps and condylomata acuminata. The latter are recurrent but rarely become malignant.

Malignant lesions causing early involvement of the lymph nodes are transitional cell tumors of the proximal urethra in men and women, squamous cell lesions of the distal urethra in men and women, and adenocarcinomas, which are more common in women and seldom found in men.

Symptoms and signs include obstruction to urine flow that mimics urethral stricture, urethral bleeding, and a urethral induration or mass. Diagnosis is confirmed by cytologic study of urethral washings.

The patient may be treated by surgical excision (anterior pelvic exenteration might be required) or by irradiation (reported by some to be as effective as surgery).

The prognosis is poor for patients with malignant tumors.

RENOVASCULAR HYPERTENSION

Renovascular hypertension may be caused by partial occlusion of the renal artery or its branches ("Goldblatt" kidney) or by constricting perirenal fibrosis that follows certain types of trauma and infection. Chronic pyelonephritis and obstructive uropathy (hydronephrosis) are less common causes.

Diagnosis. Persistent or labile hypertension is most common. "Malignant" hypertension is occasionally seen. A sequential (hypertensive) intravenous urogram may show differential renal size (ischemic kidney smaller); delayed visualization of one kidney suggests decreased blood flow to that side. An iodohippurate sodium (Hippuran) gamma camera photoscan provides information about differential kidney function and blood flow. Renal arteriography may also be done.

Catheterization of the renal veins through the vena cava should be done to obtain differential renal vein renin assays. Bilateral ureteral catheterization for determination of differential renal function studies is occasionally helpful; the ischemic kidney excretes a lower volume with decreased sodium concentration and increased creatinine concentration.

Treatment. Initiate therapy by a trial medical regimen if renal function is not significantly impaired by vascular lesions. If medical therapy of hypertension is unsuccessful and the hypertension is a threat to target organs and longevity, arterial repair or bypass is indicated. Partial or total nephrectomy is occasionally required.

REFERENCES

1. Campbell, M., and Harrison, H.: Urology. 3rd Ed. Philadelphia, W. B. Saunders Co. 1970.
2. Hamm, F. C., and Weinberg, S. R.: Introduction to Urology. New York, Dept. of Surgery, University of the State of New York, Down State Medical Center, 1957.
3. Karafin, L., and Kendall, R. A.: Urology. Vol. II. Hagerstown, Md., Harper & Row, Publishers, 1975.
4. Lapides, J.: Fundamentals of Urology. Philadelphia, W. B. Saunders Co., 1976.
5. Mulholland, S. G., Parsons, C. L., and Murphy, J. J.: Urinary bladder antibacterial defense mechanism. J. Am. Assoc. GU Surg, 68:83, 1976.
6. Potter, E. L.: Normal and Abnormal Development of the Kidney. Chicago, Year Book Medical Publishers, 1972.
7. Smith, D. R.: General Urology. Los Altos, Cal., Lange Medical Publications, 1975.
8. Wyker, A. W., and Gillenwater, J. Y.: Method of Urology. Baltimore, The Williams & Wilkins Co., 1975.

Chapter 43

PROCTOLOGY*

by GERALD R. GEHRINGER
and IRVING A. LEVIN

As specialization in medicine progresses, many family physicians may fear that their usefulness and activity are becoming limited. This concept of advancing limitation is far from the truth, and the concern about it should be supplanted by the idea that, through intelligent cooperation, the common aim of all physicians — improvement of medical care — will be promoted. In the field of colon and rectal diseases alone, family physicians have almost unlimited opportunity to widen their scope of activity by diagnosing and treating lesions earlier than would otherwise be done. Afflictions of every system of the body relate to colon and rectal problems in one way or another.

ANORECTAL SURGERY AND THE FAMILY PHYSICIAN

Because of their present degree of training, most family physicians should be able to do anorectal surgery. Techniques, of course, will differ, as each physician combines procedures learned in training and at postgraduate sessions. The family physician should be capable of providing total care for 75 to 85 per cent of all the anorectal problems he encounters and also should be knowledgeable enough to assist in the management of the other 15 to 25 per cent, by working with appropriate consultants and with other members of the health care team. The more examinations and the more surgical procedures performed, the more skilled the physician becomes in recognizing those patients who need referral to surgeons specializing in colon and rectal disorders. The conditions that will present problems for the family physician are:

1. Difficult and complicated fistulas-in-ano, including those that extend around the entire muscle, or are both anterior and posterior, or are horseshoe-shaped, with the external opening lying anteriorly and the internal opening being directly posterior.

2. Anal stenosis found in older patients or in female patients who do not have thick musculature. In these patients, correction of the stenosis may result in some degree of prolapse of the rectal mucosa or incontinence.

3. Prolapsing internal hemorrhoids or combined external and internal hemorrhoids that are circumferential and that might soon recur, unless a radical procedure is done.

The selection of patients for surgery will be discussed separately for each type of anal disease. Surgery itself is important, but the difference between poor, average, and excellent anorectal surgery relates directly to the selection of patients and to their postoperative care.

ANATOMY OF THE ANORECTUM

Knowledge of some basic anatomic principles is also necessary to understand the

*The authors wish to thank Mr. Charles F. Chapman and Ms. Virginia Howard for their editorial assistance. Thanks are also given to the typist, Mrs. Sandra French Maloney, who struggled with the writers' poor handwriting and dictations. The authors would also like to recognize the talents of the illustrator, Mr. Donald Alvarado.

787

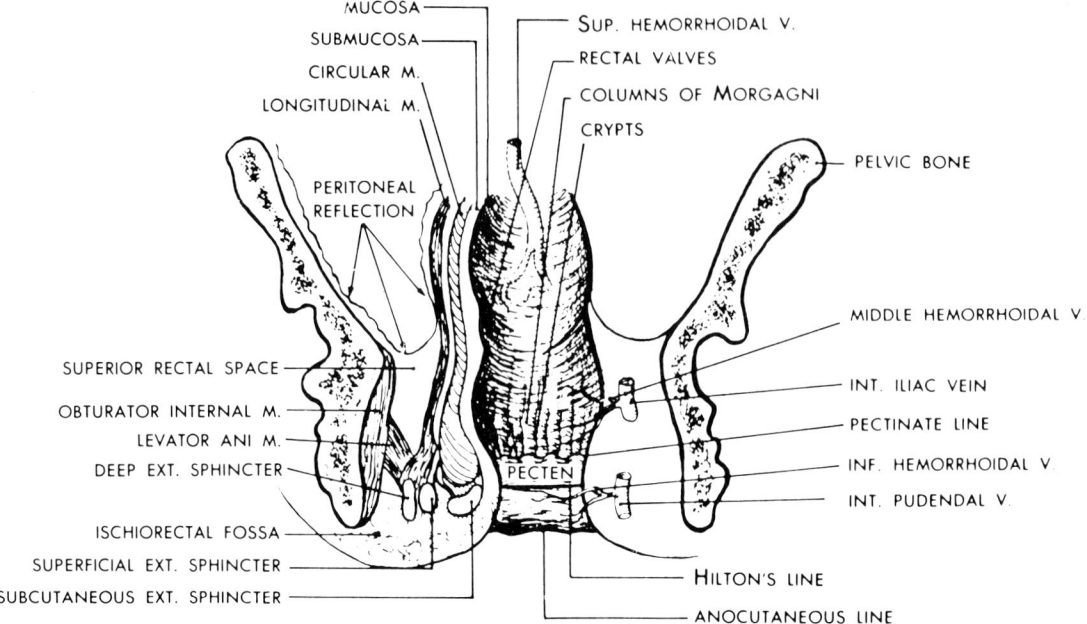

Figure 43–1. *Schematic coronal section of the anorectum. (From Kellogg, C. S.: Diseases of the Anus, Colon, and Rectum. In Conn, H. F., Rakel, R. E., and Johnson, T. W. (eds.): Family Practice. 1st Ed. Philadelphia, W. B. Saunders Co., 1973.)*

rectal complaints of patients. These few facts will make history-taking easier and more meaningful.

From the anatomic point of view, the most important structure in the anorectum is the pectinate line because it is the line of separation of the integumentary, vascular, lymphatic, and nervous systems of the entire area (Fig. 43–1).

The pectinate line consists of five to eight small projections (papillae) pointing upward. The papillae are covered by squamous epithelium and are connected with each other at their bases by thin semilunar folds (the valves of Morgagni). These valves and papillae enclose the anal crypts of Morgagni. Extending upward from each papilla and bordering the crypts are longitudinal folds of mucous membrane (the columns of Morgagni). The pectinate line with its crypts and papillae is easily palpated by the examining finger, and a diagnosis of cryptitis or papillitis may be made by digital examination.

Integumentary System

At the pectinate line, the invaginated squamous epithelium changes to transitional cell epithelium and then to columnar epithelium a short distance farther in the anal canal. This fact is important in predicting the pathologic type of the malignant lesions that occur in these areas. Those lesions below the pectinate line are squamous cell malignancies, those at the line are usually transitional cell malignancies, and those above the line are adenocarcinomas. Thus, prognosis can be determined and treatment can be prescribed according to the position of the lesion.

Blood Supply

The arterial blood supply to the area is likewise divided at the pectinate line. The superior and middle hemorrhoidal arteries originate directly from the aorta via the inferior mesenteric and hypogastric arteries. The inferior hemorrhoidal artery descends below the pectinate line and is a terminal branch of the internal pudendal artery. Likewise, the inferior hemorrhoidal vein drains at the area at and below the pectinate line and empties into the inferior vena cava, which returns the blood to the right heart and lungs. Thus, a malignancy at or below the pectinate line would be expected to spread via the venous system to the lung. The middle and superior hemor-

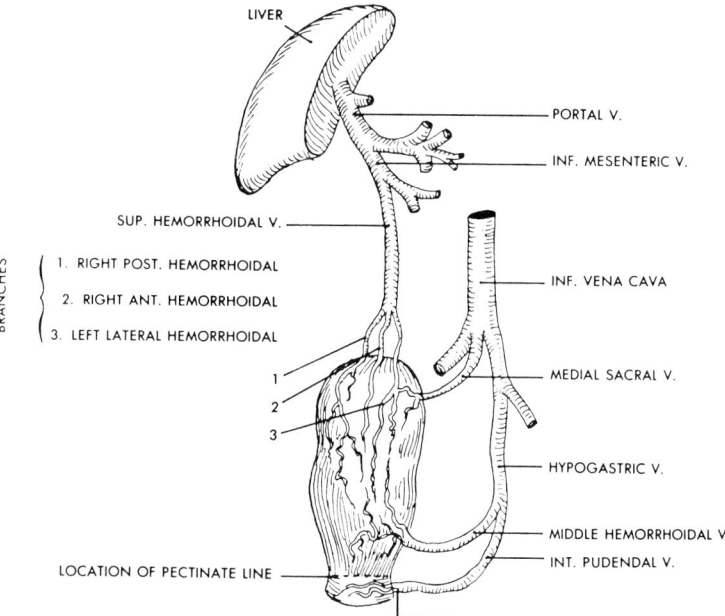

Figure 43–2. *The venous blood supply of the anorectum. (From Kellogg, C. S.: Diseases of the Anus, Colon, and Rectum. In Conn, H. F., Rakel, R. E., and Johnson, T. W. (eds.): Family Practice. 1st Ed. Philadelphia, W. B. Saunders Co., 1973.)*

rhoidal veins drain via the portal system through the liver. Hence, malignancies in the area above the pectinate line would metastasize to the liver (Fig. 43–2).

Lymphatic System

The lymphatic drainage systems are also divided at the pectinate line, so that the lymphatic drainage at or below the pectinate line goes to the inguinal lymph nodes. Therefore, one might expect that the finding of squamous cell malignancies of the anorectum below the pectinate line will necessitate an inguinal node dissection for greater assurance that the tumor will be eradicated. The lymphatic drainage above the pectinate line finds its way to the nodes in the hypogastric glands, the iliac glands, or those glands on the bifurcation of the aorta.

Nerve Supply

The nerve supply of the anorectum is likewise divided at the pectinate line. Above the line only autonomic nerves are present, accounting for the lack of pain following such procedures as the injection of hemorrhoids or the placing of Barron ligatures on internal hemorrhoids above the line. The nerve supply at and below the pectinate line occurs via the inferior hemorrhoidal branch of the internal pudendal nerve, which is composed of fibers of the second, third, and fourth sacral nerves. Surgery in this area causes pain and must be preceded by anesthesia. The superficial sphincter and its three portions are likewise innervated by the second, third, and fourth sacral nerves and are, therefore, under control of the brain and may be contracted at will.

General Anatomic Relationships

The anal canal extends approximately 1 1/2 inches from the anal opening to the pectinate line (Fig. 43–3). The rectum extends about 5 to 7 inches farther to the level of the peritoneal reflection at about the level of the third sacral vertebra. The rectum below the peritoneal reflection consists of four layers: mucosa, submucosa, muscularis, and fascia propria; above the peritoneal reflection, the outer layer is the serosa. The muscular layer is composed of an inner circular layer and an outer longitudinal layer. The circular muscles thicken toward the outlet and form the internal sphincter, and the teniae coli of the colon fuse at the rectum and surround the entire tube. The external sphincter is supplied by the cerebrospinal nerves and is under the

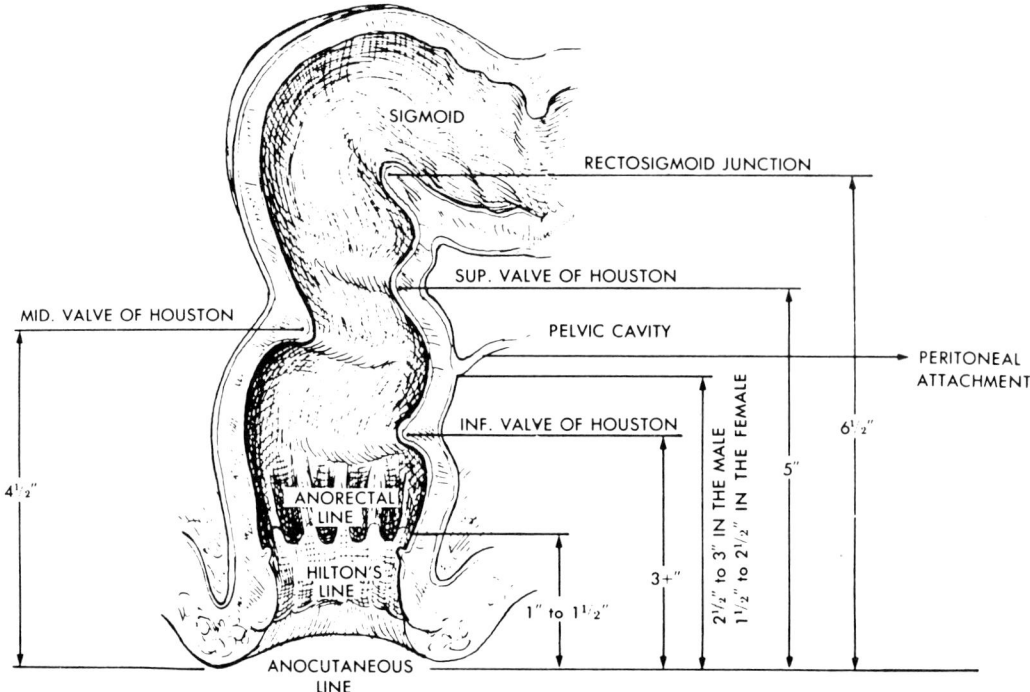

Figure 43–3. *Schematic drawing of the boundaries of the anus, rectum, and rectosigmoid junction. (From Kellogg, C. S.: Diseases of the Anus, Colon, and Rectum. In Conn, H. F., Rakel, R. E., and Johnson, T. W. (eds.): Family Practice. 1st Ed. Philadelphia, W. B. Saunders Co., 1973.)*

direct control of the brain. The internal sphincter is controlled autonomically.

Proceeding from the anal verge up to the rectum, one notes that three crescentic folds project into the lumen of the bowel, first from the patient's right side, then from the left side, and, finally, again from the right side. These folds are known as the valves of Houston, and they sometimes make passage of the sigmoidoscope difficult. The second valve, the one projecting from the left side of the bowel, is usually at or near the peritoneal reflection. The latter anatomic part is a good landmark and should determine the upper level at which polyps are removed in the office. Above this area, bleeding caused by surgery frequently necessitates performing an abdominal celiotomy to control the flow.

Surgical Spaces

Four paired spaces (the supralevator, retrorectal, ischiorectal, and perianal spaces) adjacent to the rectum are important in localizing and treating abscesses.

The supralevator space is bounded in-

feriorly and laterally by the pelvic diaphragm (the levator ani muscle, the short coccygeus muscle, and their fasciae), medially by the rectum, and superiorly by the pelvic peritoneum.

The retrorectal space is located above the pelvic diaphragm and is bounded anteriorly by the rectum, posteriorly by the sacrum, laterally by the lateral ligaments, and inferiorly by the levator ani muscle.

The ischiorectal space is below the pelvic diaphragm, which forms its superior border. It is bounded medially by the external anal sphincter, laterally by the obturator fascia, and inferiorly by the skin of the perineum.

The perianal space may be considered the inferior part of the ischiorectal fossa.

These fossae are of utmost importance when considering the origin of abscesses and when predicting the course they might take to the area of fluctuation or pointing.

PATIENT HISTORY

The most important element in making a correct diagnosis is the taking of a good, careful history. For colon and rectal diseases, as for other conditions, if the physician asks the proper questions and listens carefully, the patient usually provides the diagnosis. The important symptoms of anorectal disease are:

1. Bleeding—The most frequent complaint is bleeding. The amount, color, frequency, and duration of each bleeding episode are vital sources of information but can be difficult to elicit. A successful method for determining the amount is to ask the patient to compare the quantity of blood with a known quantity, such as a teaspoonful or a quart. The relationship of bleeding to bowel movements is also important; whether bleeding occurs before, after, during, or instead of the bowel movement should be noted.

2. Pain—Important aspects to note are severity; relationship to bowel movements; and whether constant or intermittent, recent or chronic, or minor or incapacitating.

3. Presence of a lump or prolapse of internal hemorrhoids—Because patients frequently do not know what is meant by "prolapse," the term must be carefully explained. Knowing whether the prolapse occurs only during a bowel movement or whether it is present at all times and also whether it interferes with work are essential.

4. Pruritus—This is certainly a common symptom and will be discussed in detail later in this chapter.

5. Drainage or discharge—A history of this symptom is best elicited by inquiring about the amount, color, and frequency of soiling of underclothing.

6. Change in bowel habits—Any change in bowel function is an important part of the history and should be discussed thoroughly. Change in bowel habits may be the major symptom and may relate to constipation or to diarrhea. If constipation is involved, an understanding between patient and physician of the definition of constipation is important. If the patient has diarrhea, the frequency, character, color, and number of stools and any relationship to diet or other daily activities need to be known.

7. Tenesmus—This is the cardinal symptom of carcinoma of the rectum or the rectosigmoid colon and should be carefully differentiated from true diarrhea by both physician and patient.

The remainder of the history should review other gastrointestinal symptoms or general diseases. A specific history of abdominal pain and abdominal symptoms can be the key to an easy diagnosis. If a patient, 55 years of age, has a history of increasing constipation for several months, abdominal cramps, and tenesmus, the physician should certainly be alert to the possibility of a malignant neoplasm of the sigmoid or rectum. If the symptoms of fever and lower abdominal pain are also noted, diverticulitis would be a more likely diagnosis. Naturally, a general history should be taken on all patients so that concomitant diseases and the relationship of these diseases to the colon symptoms can be determined. A cardiovascular history and examination are important for assessing patients at operative risk. Because information about previous anorectal or colon operations is imperative, any physician previously involved in this regard should be consulted, if possible, and the original operative report and other pertinent records should be obtained from the physician and hospital.

Any allergic reactions to medications or test materials should be determined.

Because the interaction of medications is also dangerous at times, any medication that the patient is taking, including types of ointments and other medicaments used in the anorectal area, should be recorded in the history to avoid repetitive use and avert possible allergic reactions.

DIAGNOSTIC PROCTOLOGIC PROCEDURES

After taking an accurate history, prepare the patient for examination. First, explain to the patient the procedure to be performed. In any examination, the cooperation of the patient is essential, and most patients are afraid of an anorectal examination. They have heard "it" is "the most terrible thing in the world." Before beginning the examination, reassure the patient that it will be gentle. Tell the patient that the proctologic examination will not be painful but will produce a feeling of wanting to have a bowel movement. The patient who comes to you in pain should be especially assured that the examination will be brief and gentle.

TABLE 43–1. A CLASSIFICATION OF RECTAL LESIONS°

Intraluminal (Intrarectal)
A. Impactions
B. Foreign bodies

Intrinsic (Mucosal and/or Submucosal)

A. Inflammatory
   1. Recently injected or thrombosed internal hemorrhoids
   2. Submucosal abscess
   3. Large, discrete ulcers, including factitial ulcers
   4. Stricture
      a. Venereal lymphogranuloma
      b. Colitides—especially chronic ulcerative colitis
B. Traumatic
   1. Enema tip injuries
   2. Impalement injuries
C. Neoplastic
   1. Polyps
   2. Carcinoid
   3. Carcinoma

Intramural

A. Endometrial deposits—especially in recto-vaginal septum
B. Benign tumors
   1. Lipoma
   2. Leiomyoma
   3. Fibroma
   4. Neuroma
   5. Hemangioma
C. Malignant tumor (sarcoma)
   1. Lymphosarcoma

2. Fibrosarcoma
3. Melanosarcoma

Extrinsic (Extramural or Extrarectal)

A. Anterior (Fig. 43–4)
   1. Prostatic and seminal vesicular enlargement in the male
   2. Progress of first stage of labor in the female
   3. Pelvic masses in the female
   4. Metastases to rectal shelf (cul-de-sac) in both sexes
   5. Pelvic mass in both sexes
      a. Cancer of proximal loop of bowel
      b. Diverticulosis
      c. Inflammatory
         (1) Diverticulitis
         (2) Regional ileitis
         (3) Appendiceal abscess
B. Lateral (Fig. 43–5)
   1. Ischial spine and greater sciatic notch (landmarks)
   2. Pelvirectal abscess
   3. Carcinomatous spread into rectal stalks (from prostatic cancer) with resultant narrowing of rectal lumen
C. Posterior (Fig. 43–6)
   1. Coccyx and attached ligaments (landmarks)
   2. Presacral tumors
      a. Inflammatory—retrorectal abscess
      b. Neoplastic
         (1) Teratoma (including dermoid cyst)
         (2) Chromaffin body cyst
         (3) Chordoma
         (4) Sarcoma (soft tissue)
         (5) Metastatic carcinoma
         (6) Tumor arising from bone or periosteum

°From Nesselrod, J. P.: Clinical Proctology, 3rd Ed., Philadelphia, W. B. Saunders Co., 1964, pp. 43–45.

A tilt table is not essential for examining the rectal area; any examining table may be used. Either the knee–chest or the left lateral (Sims's) position is adequate for a good examination. Regardless of the types of table available, a patient having cardiovascular disease or problems with backaches or with his extremities certainly should not be examined in a kneeling position. Such a patient should be placed in the left lateral position for examination. Most patients over the age of 65 years routinely are examined in the left lateral position. The perianal and scrotal or vulvar areas should be carefully inspected for skin lesions before the rectum itself is examined. The lesions to look for during digital rectal, anoscopic, and proctoscopic examinations are classified in Table 43–1.

THE EXAMINATION

Digital

Digital inspection of the anorectal area for signs of tenderness, masses, strictures, bleeding, and other abnormalities is a necessary part of any physical examination (Figs. 43–4, 43–5, and 43–6). After the digital examination, the anal canal should be inspected with an anoscope.

Anoscopy

The small and the medium-sized Hirschman anoscopes with a beveled end are recommended. The patient should always be advised as to the type of procedure to be performed and the amount of discomfort to

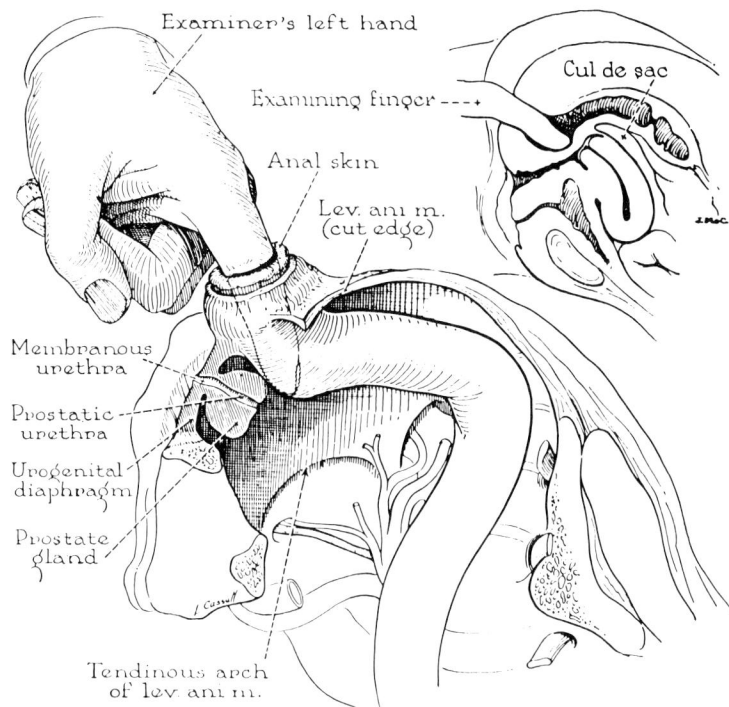

Figure 43–4. *Diagrammatic parasagittal section, inverted position, demonstrating palpation through the anterior rectal wall in male subject. Inset: median sagittal section in female. (From Nesselrod, J. P.: Clinical Proctology. 2nd Ed. Philadelphia, W. B. Saunders Co., 1957.)*

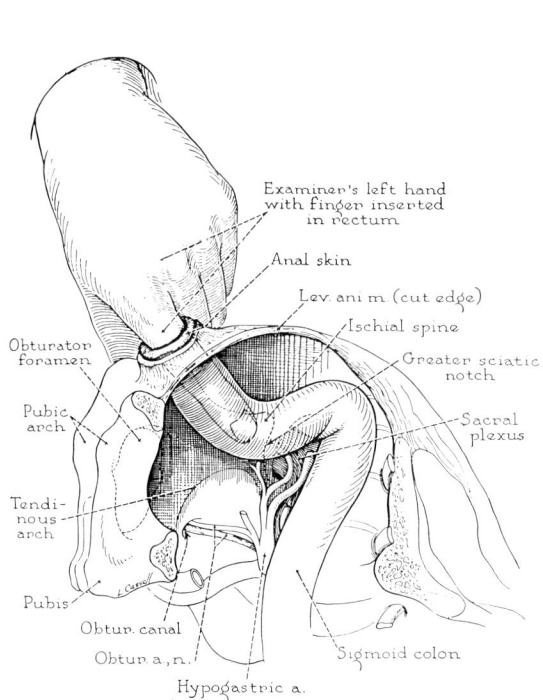

Figure 43–5. *Diagrammatic parasagittal section, inverted position, demonstrating palpation through the lateral rectal wall. (From Nesselrod, J. P.: Clinical Proctology. 2nd Ed. Philadelphia, W. B. Saunders Co., 1957.)*

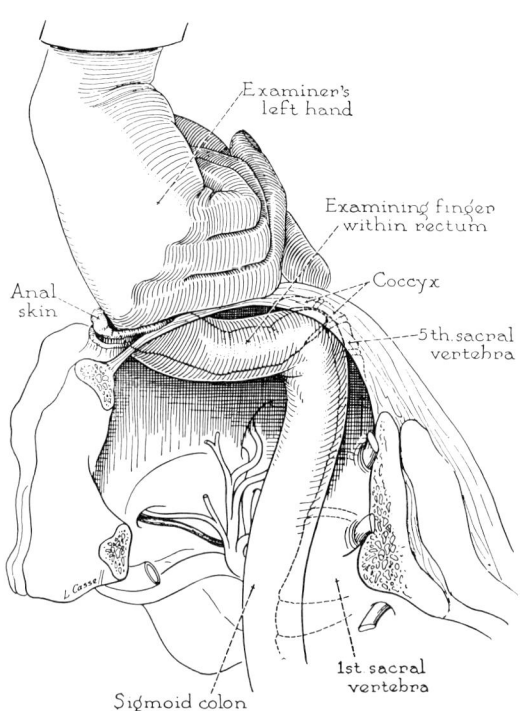

Figure 43–6. *Diagrammatic parasagittal section, inverted position, demonstrating palpation through the posterior rectal wall. (From Nesselrod, J. P.: Clinical Proctology. 2nd Ed. Philadelphia, W. B. Saunders Co., 1957.)*

be expected. Gentleness is important in the examination. Insert the anoscope gently in the anal canal and direct it toward the umbilicus. Each anal area, posterior, anterior, right, and left, must be examined separately. The obturator should be reinserted into the anoscope prior to repositioning the instrument for examining each quadrant separately. During these observations, instruct the patient to strain or to bear down, thus increasing the size of any hemorrhoids by 2 or 3 times. If the anoscope is gently removed while the patient is straining, prolapsed hemorrhoids can be detected. If the diagnosis of prolapsed hemorrhoids is questionable, examining the area while the patient is squatting will confirm the diagnosis. With the patient leaning forward over a toilet or a bedpan, have him bear down or strain while you observe. During the examination on a table, the patient will be reluctant to strain, and a true evaluation of the amount of prolapse is often not obtainable. Treatment is governed by the amount of prolapse. The size of the hemorrhoids when they protrude is huge as compared with their size when seen through the anoscope.

Proctoscopy

Prophylactic medicine is an important part of family practice. Few procedures are as valuable as proctoscopic examination in preventing cancer. Annual or semiannual Papanicolaou smear tests (Pap smears) have become routine and have certainly improved the overall prognosis for cervical malignant neoplasms. Sigmoidoscopy must become as frequent an examination as the Pap smear before the morbidity and mortality from colon cancer will change. Sigmoidoscopy is not the monopoly of any specialist, but rather is a common diagnostic technique, a skill that all competent medical examiners should develop and use. Almost every patient who enters the family physician's office should be examined by sigmoidoscopy, but the following list will help to determine which patients must have this examination:

Sigmoidoscopy should be performed on any patient
1. with bowel or anal symptoms,
2. for whom anal surgery is contemplated,

3. who wants a "complete check-up,"
4. who comes for a cancer detection study,
5. with a family history of gastrointestinal malignant neoplasm,
6. with a family history of rectal or sigmoidal polyps, or
7. who is more than 45 years old. In the fourth decade of life, the incidence of polyps begins to rise, and in the fifth decade, the incidence of cancer has its most dramatic upswing.[8]

A complicated set-up is not necessary for proctoscopic examination. These instruments, however, are essential:
1. Some type of suction—electric, wall suction produced by water, or a simple suction from an attachment to a faucet in a sink.
2. Long cotton-tipped applicators—to clean and wipe the mucous membrane and for use in the diagnosis of colitis of various types. Swabs are also used to obtain stool specimens for examination for occult blood and for detection of ova, cysts, and parasites.
3. Biopsy forceps—the type depending on the physician's preference.
4. The Welch-Allyn disposable scope—which either is easily cleaned or, in a family physician's office where the volume of these examinations is not great, is easily disposed of, thus obviating cleaning.

Test the light before inserting the instrument. Nothing is more embarrassing than to insert the instrument into the anal canal and then find that the light is not functioning. Be familiar with whichever instrument you use, so that its idiosyncrasies are well known to you.

For the average physician, only minimal instruction is necessary before using the sigmoidoscope. Regular use of the instrument is the best way to improve one's technique. Remember that the procedure is disliked by the patient, and any indication of lack of confidence by the physician will increase the difficulty, because the patient will be uncooperative. To perform this examination, it is essential that the patient is relaxed, comfortable, and cooperative. If the patient is not cooperative, the examination should be ended immediately, because certain dangers do exist. The primary danger is perforation, and lacerations and bleeding are also possible. Such mishaps are rare, however, and should not occur if the usual precautions are taken, as described in the following section.

Procedure. After digital examination, the sigmoidoscope is immediately inserted past the anal sphincter (Fig. 43-7, Position A). Once the sphincter is "passed," the obturator is removed, and the remainder of the examination is performed under direct vision. At this point, the proximal, or eye, end of the scope will need to be moved anteriorly to visualize the most inaccessible part of the rectum, that is, the posterior segment (Fig. 7, Position B). As the scope is introduced as far as the rectosigmoid (Fig. 43-7, Position C), a distance of 11 to 14 cm., the bowel angulates sharply anteriorly. As this portion of the rectosigmoid is approached, the physician must tell the patient that he will experience an abdominal cramp. The patient will have a sensation similar to that of having a bowel movement. Advise the patient not to strain, not to push, and not to cough. Pushing, in particular, makes proctoscopy difficult and occasionally impossible. At this point in the proctoscopic examination, gentleness is important. If your patient is a woman who has had a hysterectomy or a man who has had lower abdominal surgery, introduction of the in-

strument beyond the rectosigmoid may be difficult. Remember that a straight instrument is going to be passed into a curved organ. Only if the sigmoid beyond this point is somewhat mobile can the sigmoidoscope be introduced beyond the rectosigmoid into the distal sigmoid. Once this curve is passed, the instrument can usually easily be advanced to 25 cm. (Fig. 43-7, Position D).

You should be able to pass the proctoscope to the full 25 cm. in approximately 65 to 75 per cent of patients. In performing the initial sigmoidoscopy, keeping the patient cooperative and happy, advising him not to push or strain, and making the passage of the instrument beyond the rectosigmoid neither painful nor difficult are important. If you suspect that the patient has a disorder just beyond the rectosigmoid and you are having difficulty passing the sigmoidoscope beyond this junction, stop the procedure and order a barium enema study. If the results of the barium enema examination are negative and you are still suspicious, you should re-examine the patient by sigmoidoscopy while he is sedated. If this fails, refer the patient to a rectal and colon surgeon for colonoscopy. Make it a policy to

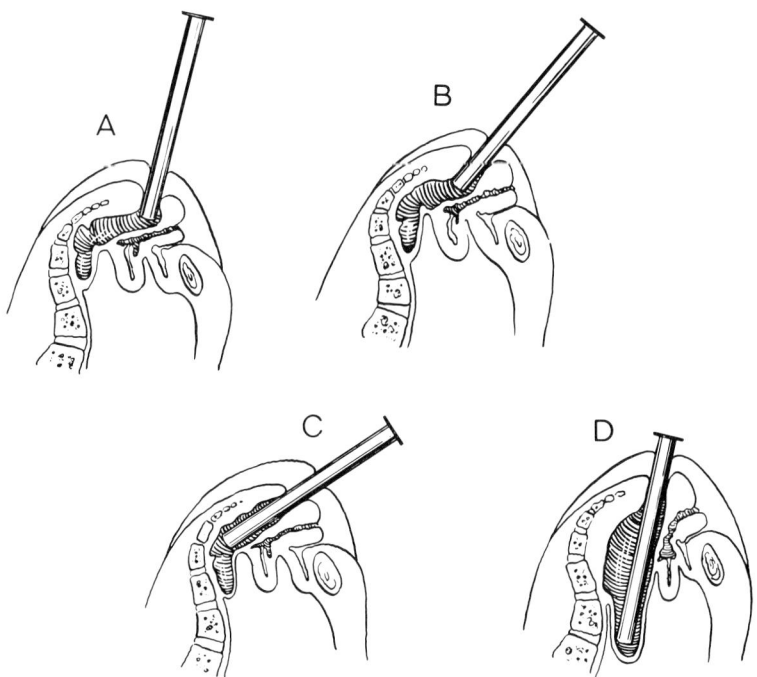

Figure 43-7. *Diagrammatic scheme of maneuvers used during insertion of sigmoidoscope.*

advance the sigmoidoscope as far and as rapidly as possible. Examine the bowel carefully when withdrawing the instrument. Once it reaches the most distal part of the bowel, tell the patient, "I am now removing the instrument." Usually, the patient will relax. During withdrawal, air insufflation may be used to flatten the many folds.

When the anal canal is reached during withdrawal of the proctoscope, do not attempt to visualize the canal, for such maneuvering with a flat-ended instrument is painful. The anal canal should have been examined previously, both digitally and with a tangential-ended anoscope. On completion of the sigmoidoscopic examination, the patient should be returned to a comfortable prone position and allowed to remain so for a few minutes. The patient should then be allowed to sit upright for a few minutes, under observation, before allowing him to stand and dress. This will avoid a possible hypotensive or syncopal episode. After dressing, the patient should be taken to the office or consultation room for a complete discussion of the findings.

Key Points for a Satisfactory and Easy Proctoscopic Examination

1. Positions should be comfortable for both the patient and the physician.

2. Gentle rectal examination should be done prior to proctoscopy.

3. Before and during the examination, explain the sensations that the patient should expect.

4. When the rectosigmoid and higher portions of the rectum and sigmoid are reached, encourage the patient to relax and to breathe deeply and tell him that the procedure will be over soon and that the sensation he will experience is similar to the need for a bowel movement.

5. During the procedure, if the lumen is not visualized, withdraw the proctoscope several centimeters, so that a shadow of the lumen may be seen.

6. Gently use air insufflation, which is essential for passing the proctoscope and for visualizing all of the folds.

7. Patiently examine all abnormal tissue, taking biopsy specimens if necessary.

8. *Gentleness*—For an adequate and accurate proctoscopic examination, gentleness is the keynote.

When the procedure is completed, the patient should say, "That wasn't as bad as I expected after all."

After the proctosigmoidoscopy, you must accurately describe to the patient your findings, both abnormal and normal.

When recording data of digital, anoscopic, or proctoscopic examination, or any combination of these, descriptions should be based on the anatomic quadrants. Do not describe locations as being one o'clock, two o'clock, or three o'clock—we "do not tell time by the anus." Abnormalities or normal areas of the skin, anal canal, or inside the rectum or colon must be described in relation to the various quadrants, such as directly posterior, directly anterior, right posterior, right anterior, right central, left posterior, left anterior, or left central.

Approximate dimensions, by centimeters, are also noted, and an accurate description of the abnormal colon is given in contrast to the normal. Thus, when you or anyone else re-examines the patient, the exact site of the abnormal pathology can be found at a particular level. Because the family physician will refer many of these patients to other physicians, an accurate description of the exact location of any abnormality is a valuable aid for the consultant.

Extent of Endoscopic Procedures by the Family Physician. Procedures done through the anoscope or the proctoscope by the family physician will depend on the manual dexterity of the physician and the number of examinations performed. To set a minimum number of examinations for each physician would be unfair. Some physicians might proctoscope 10 patients and be perfectly competent, whereas others might need to do 25 to 50 examinations to gain the same amount of expertise. Each should have some instruction from a competent physician concerning biopsy and coagulation techniques before attempting such procedures for the first time. Such instruction is necessary not because the procedure is difficult but because of the distinct possibility of two serious complications with both diagnostic and therapeutic proctoscopy: the bowel may be *perforated, serious bleeding* may occur, or both may happen. The patient should be told of the possible complications before the examination, and, at least in the hospital, a consent sheet must be signed before the proctoscopy is undertaken. In the office, a consent sheet is probably not necessary, but this could be valuable and is recommended. Before performing sigmoidoscopy, biopsy, and coagulation and before snaring a polyp, the physician should have had prior training and supervision and should be familiar with the procedure and the instrument. Taking biopsy specimens of either a small adenoma or a large neoplasm is perfectly permissible. Multiple superficial bites provide the same results as those obtained from "deep bites," with less chance of complication. Endoscopic polypectomy, a dangerous procedure that can be difficult, should be left to the anorectal surgeon. Electrosurgical snaring can easily cause perforation of the bowel, particularly if this is done above the level of the rectosigmoid. Patients having pedunculated polyps or large sessile polyps should be referred to a trained colon and rectal surgeon.

SPECIAL DIAGNOSTIC PROCEDURES

Fiberoptic Colonoscopy

Fiberoptic colonoscopes are now available and are useful in visualizing and treating disease areas in the entire colon. Patients requiring this procedure should be referred to those who have had considerable training and experience in fiberoptic colonoscopy as well as in colon and rectal surgery. The following list will assist the family physician in knowing which patients need referral for colonoscopic examination.

Refer patients with:

1. Equivocal and unidentifiable lesions detected on barium enema studies, such as
   a. identified polyps beyond the reach of the proctoscope;
   b. suspicious lesions requiring histologic confirmation beyond the reach of the proctoscope; or
   c. inflammatory bowel disease to
      (1) determine the extent of the disease,
      (2) clarify the diagnosis, or
      (3) detect malignant transformation.
2. Gastrointestinal bleeding of unknown origin, particularly melena.
3. Unexplained chronic diarrhea.
4. Prior surgery for colon cancer, to investigate the possibility of recurrence at the anastomotic site or to detect new diseases.
5. Diverticulitis, to rule out cancer.
6. Lesions of the cecum, to differentiate among
   a. carcinoma,
   b. hypertrophic ileocecal valve,
   c. lipoma,
   d. inverted appendiceal stump, or
   e. ameboma.

Fiberoptic colonoscopy should not be performed on patients with acute inflammatory diseases of the colon, such as ulcerative colitis, abdominal surgery within the past three weeks, peritonitis, any hematologic difficulties, acute cardiorespiratory disease, or acute diverticulitis.

Selective Visceral Angiography

Family physicians do not do selective visceral angiography, but a vascular surgeon or a radiologist should be available who can do this procedure on selected patients.

The procedure, although done infrequently, may be used to localize the site of persistent bleeding in patients having diverticulosis, small tumors, or small telangiectases.

Carcinoembryonic Antigen (CEA) Serum Test

The CEA serum test, which is now available in most laboratories, is important in the follow-up of patients who have had cancer surgery, particularly for gastrointestinal lesions. The procedure was once mistakenly thought to be useful in diagnosis, but its true value is in postoperative follow-up of patients with rectocolon cancer. The procedure should be done preoperatively and then postoperatively every 2 to 4 months during the first year and every 6 months thereafter. Any slight rise in the CEA level should be an indication for referring the patient back to the operating surgeon or to another surgeon to investigate the possibility of recurrent tumor.

ANAL DISEASES

HEMORRHOIDAL DISEASE

Hemorrhoids are vascular tumors made up of varices in the anal canal, usually involving the right posterior, right anterior, and left central quadrants. The affected veins occur as a normal finding in all persons, but symptoms develop only in patients with enlargement, infection, and inflammation of the mucous membrane.

Cause. Many factors contribute to the cause of hemorrhoidal disease, the most important being the erect posture of man, an absence of valves in the veins, straining at stool, pregnancy, parturition, and a constitutional difference in the support of the veins in the anal canal. Nesselrod, in his text, discusses ideas concerning infection as the principal cause of hemorrhoidal disease. He believes that infectious material gains entrance into the anal canal through the anal crypts and the anal ducts. Thus, a periphlebitis and an endophlebitis occur, thinning the venous walls and resulting in the dilatation of the infected portions of the hemorrhoidal plexus and in the development of hemorrhoids, as we know them.[5]

The simplest and easiest classification of hemorrhoids is based on anatomy. External hemorrhoids are those that involve the part of the hemorrhoidal plexus that is distal to the dentate line and is therefore covered with skin. Internal hemorrhoids involve the part of the hemorrhoidal plexus that is proximal to the dentate line and is therefore covered with mucous membrane. The term "mixed hemorrhoids" pertains to a combination of internal and external types. The most common type of hemorrhoid is the mixed type.

Thrombosed External Hemorrhoids

Thrombosed external hemorrhoids are also called perianal hematomas. They are usually caused by excess straining of one sort or another and may occur following diarrhea, constipation, or unusual types of exercise. The usual history is that of a sudden onset of a lump that has "come out." The patient believes that because the hemorrhoid did not exist before, it must have come from the inside. The common symptom is pain, usually constant and usually decreasing in intensity in 2 to 4 days.

Thrombosed hemorrhoids bleed only when they rupture. Examination reveals a swollen, tender area or areas that are usually bluish or bluish-red, depending on the amount of edema and inflammation in the area. All the swollen areas are covered with skin and extend from the dentate line outward. They may occur in any quadrant and may occupy a variable area. Diagnosis is easily made by inspection and gentle digital examination.

Treatment. If the condition is found early, the best therapy is excision under local anesthesia, an easy procedure that all family physicians should be competent in performing. If the patient is seen after 2 to 4 days, when the edema is subsiding and he is feeling better, he can be treated conservatively with bed rest, sitz baths, and analgesic ointments. Stool softeners are advised, and oral sedatives and analgesics containing codeine are usually necessary.

Office Surgery. The patient is placed in a comfortable position, usually face down with the buttocks held spread with adhesive tape. After cleaning with a hexachlorophene detergent (pHisoHex) and water, the entire area is infiltrated with 1 per cent lidocaine. An elliptical skin incision is made, and all hemorrhoidal tissue underneath is excised. Bleeding is controlled with chromic sutures. This procedure is preferred to incision and clot extraction because it is curative and not just palliative. The base of the wound may occasionally bleed, but bleeding is easily controlled with electrocautery or sutures.

If the patient is kept in the office for 10 to 30 minutes for observation after the surgery, any organic or psychologic reaction to the excision or the local anesthetic will be observed in the office and not as the patient is on the way home. Time is thus allowed for any small oozing to be controlled in the office, thereby avoiding having the patient call later for treatment of this minor but often alarming occurrence. The postoperative care consists of the use of ice bags for the first 10 to 12 hours followed by a warm tub bath 3 to 4 times each day until healing is complete. Cotton or a small gauze dressing should be kept on the anal canal, and either benzocaine or lidocaine ointment may be used to control burning. The patient is given an analgesic drug, such as APC with codeine (Empirin No. 3), APC with oxycodone (Percodan), or one of the propoxyphene (Darvon) compounds. He is told to remain in bed during the first 6 to 12 hours, and after this time, normal activity may be resumed, depending on the symptoms. Pain relief is usually rapid and occurs within 6 to 12 hours.

The patient should be followed up twice weekly for the first several weeks. At the end of 10 to 14 days, a complete examination should be performed, including careful digital, anoscopic, and proctoscopic examinations. No patient should be discharged until he has had a complete proctologic re-evaluation. A patient more than 45 years old should be encouraged to return for annual proctoscopic examinations.

Nonthrombosed external hemorrhoids and skin tags can occur without the presence of prolapsing internal hemorrhoids. Such hemorrhoids are only symptomatic when the patient has poor anal hygiene, and they may cause itching, burning, or pain due to inflammation. These are treated by instructing the patient about anal hygiene and about the use of steroid or analgesic ointments, or both. If the patient continues to complain and to have symptoms, external tags can be excised as an office procedure.

Combined External and Internal Hemorrhoids

The most common symptoms caused by combined hemorrhoids are bleeding, drainage, discomfort and pain, prolapse, and itching. The treatment depends on the symptomatology and the size of the hemorrhoids. Bleeding during or after a bowel movement is the most common symptom and usually is relatively minor. Blood may stain the toilet tissue or drip into the bowl. Patients may show no concern when they note a small amount of bleeding on the toilet tissue. However, they become alarmed and immediately report to the physician when the water in the toilet bowl becomes red or when blood appears on their underclothing. Bleeding is bright red and usually is not accompanied by clots. Discomfort may occur initially during a bowel movement and may stop immediately afterward. However, as hemorrhoids increase in size and prolapse more, the discomfort increases and interferes with normal activity. Itching occurs only when hemorrhoids are prolapsing, and the symptom represents poor anal hygiene. Good anal hygiene is impossible for patients with severe prolapse unless the patient wears a

small dressing or a pad over the anal canal at all times to prevent maceration of the skin. Even when patients report having minimal symptoms, careful digital, anoscopic, and proctoscopic examinations must be done, and in some patients, a barium enema study may be advisable.

Once a decision has been made that the bleeding, no matter how minor, is due only to hemorrhoids, the type of treatment is determined by the severity of symptoms and the discomfort they produce.

Selection of Patients for Surgery. Indication for surgery is not based merely on the existence of hemorrhoids, whether symptomatic or asymptomatic. If a person has combined external and internal hemorrhoids that are completely asymptomatic and are discovered on a routine physical examination, such hemorrhoids should be left alone. The patient should be told to avoid constipation and to consult his physician if bleeding, itching, irritation, or other symptoms appear. If the patient has hemorrhoids that do not prolapse but continue to bleed at regular intervals despite all conservative therapy, surgical intervention may be indicated. If, however, the patient bleeds rarely or has moderate-sized hemorrhoids that do not prolapse or that prolapse with infrequent bleeding, he may be treated conservatively by using injection or ligation techniques. All patients with bleeding must have a complete examination, including proctoscopic and barium enema examinations, to rule out malignancy or premalignant disease before conservative therapy is advised. Those who should always be treated surgically and should never be treated conservatively are:

1. Good-risk patients who have internal hemorrhoids that are protruding at all times.

2. Patients who have huge internal hemorrhoids that prolapse and produce difficulty during each bowel movement.

3. Patients who have bleeding hemorrhoids severe enough to produce hypochromic anemia.

Hemorrhoidectomy

Performing a hemorrhoidectomy is within the realm of all family physicians who want to do surgery. Certain principles must be observed, and important factors such as preoperative evaluation, good operative technique, and excellent postoperative care are essential to successful treatment.

Regardless of the particular technique preferred for hemorrhoidectomy, the three essential purposes of the operation are: (1) removal of all diseased tissue, (2) return of the anal canal to as near normal as possible, and (3) prevention of recurrence.

Most operations about the anorectal area are anatomic, and unless anatomic differences are known and are taken into consideration, the best results cannot be obtained. Fansler[3] states that there are variations in the length of the anal canal, from 1/2 to 3 inches; amount and placement of the skin around the canal; diameter of the canal, both resting and in maximum dilatation; position of the dentate line; and texture of the skin, anoderm, rectal mucosa, and other tissues making up the anal canal.

If all these factors are not considered, the results of the procedure are often poor.

Hemorrhoidectomy is a hospital procedure, and the preoperative preparation is not complex. Generally, the usual preoperative work-up is necessary, and a local, general, or spinal anesthetic may be used. The type of anesthetic used will depend on the physician who is operating and the hospital in which the procedure is performed. Most anorectal surgeons prefer to use a general or a spinal anesthetic and to operate on a prone patient. The table is angled slightly, thus making exposure of the anal canal easy. The buttocks are held spread with adhesive tape, and the anal area is prepared and cleaned with a hexachlorophene detergent (pHisoHex) and water. Manual dilatation of the anal canal allows adequate exposure and also helps to relieve some degree of postoperative pain.

Before making any incision, the surgeon should carefully inspect all hemorrhoids to reaffirm the diagnosis. He should also have done an inspection the night before the surgery in order to evaluate the type of treatment necessary. Occasionally, only two quadrants of the hemorrhoids are removed because, although one knows that a third quadrant of hemorrhoidal tissue exists, the stretching of the mucous membrane during excision of the other two quadrants makes the third quadrant seem insignificant and almost nonexistent. However, neglecting the third quadrant is the reason for early recurrence.

The surgeon should use the type of retractor with which he is familiar. The Hill-Ferguson half-moon retractor or the Pratt bivalve speculum, which is self-retaining, is preferred. Electrosurgical units and standard sutures (chromic 0, chromic 00, and chromic 000, and occasionally plain 00 and plain 000) are used. Excisions are done in a radial fashion, an essential part of the technique. If the dissection is kept in a radial fashion, one quadrant will not run into the other one, and a complete hemorrhoidectomy will be performed.

A quadrant is treated in the following fashion. An Allis forceps is placed on the most redundant and distal portion of the external skin. An elliptical incision is made electrosurgically to prevent oozing. External hemorrhoidal tissue is dissected off the muscle. Several arterial "pumpers" are usually exposed in this area and are clamped and either coagulated electrosurgically or ligated with plain 000 catgut. The bleeders are controlled immediately to maintain a clear field, so that an accurate anatomic dissection can be done throughout the procedure. Dissection is directed upward, and at this point an important procedure is carried out. Using blunt dissection, the surgeon holds the scissors on the surface of the muscle and spreads it (Fig. 43–8A). This technique breaks or cuts the tough fibrous bands that have pierced the internal sphincter muscle from the longitudinal fasciculi and that have held the hemorrhoidal tissue and mucous membrane to the muscle. Once this separation is accomplished, the redundant mucosa and hemorrhoidal tissue can easily be delivered out of the anal canal. The extent of this dissection depends on the amount of redundancy. Failure to dissect high enough is one of the errors that should be avoided. The apex of the hemorrhoid is ligated with two transfixing chromic 0 or 00 sutures. The first transfixing suture is placed through the mucous membrane and the apex of the hemorrhoidal tissue (Fig. 43–8B) and is tied and cut. The second transfixing suture is then placed distal to the first and is tied, and, at this point, the redundant hemorrhoidal tissue is excised. Then the second transfixing suture is used in a continuous fashion to completely close the mucous membrane and skin (Fig. 43–8C).

Each patient will present different problems, but each hemorrhoid incision should

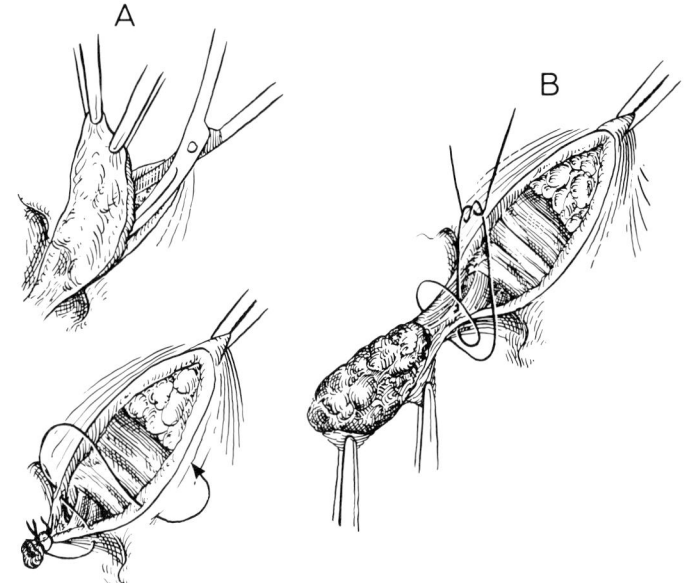

Figure 43–8. *Steps in excision hemorrhoidectomy.*

be completely closed, if possible. Complete closure can be done in about 65 to 75 per cent of all patients. As an alternative, the suture can be ended in all quadrants at the mucocutaneous junction, and the decision as to the management of the skin wounds can be delayed until surgery on all internal quadrants is completed. The skin wounds can then be closed by continuous or interrupted chromic 000 sutures or can be partially closed by marsupialization.

Figure 43–9 illustrates an interesting method of taking care of the angle between the skin and the mucous membrane that

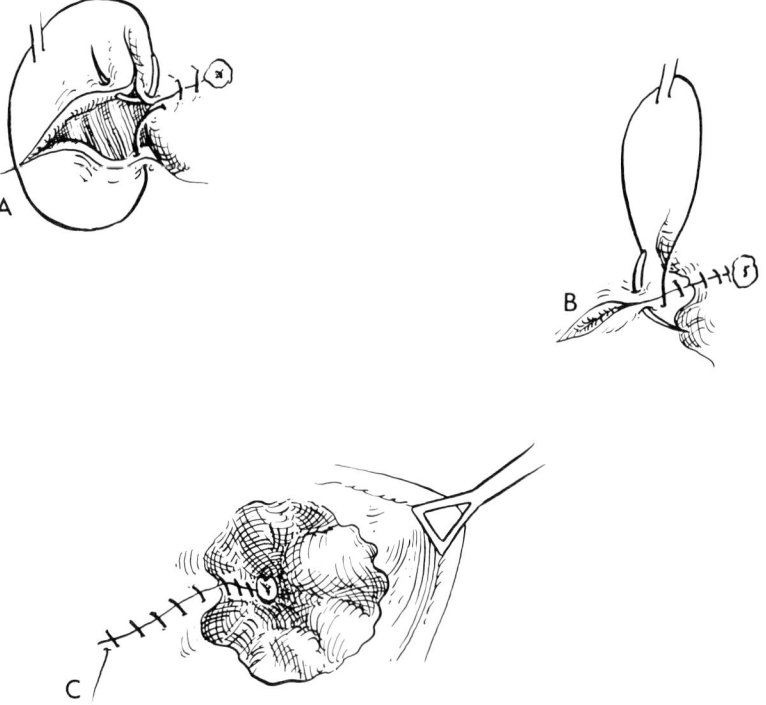

Figure 43–9. *Closure of skin and mucous membrane after hemorrhoidectomy.*

tends to protrude. When the surgeon begins closure of the skin as a continuation of the mucous membrane, the two corners are sutured within the anal canal, thus accomplishing two goals: the ragged edges straighten out, enabling the surgeon to make a straight-line incision for closure, and the anal canal becomes lined with skin that becomes soft and creates a normal canal.

After completion of all three quadrants, the anal canal, the hemorrhoidal stumps, and all other areas are carefully inspected for bleeding. Oozing is controlled at that time and is not delayed. The use of an Asepto syringe, water, and suction is helpful in such situations. Also useful is a small or medium-sized Hirschman anoscope to inspect each quadrant separately. Thus, the wounds are inspected in their most relaxed state. Be certain the patient's blood pressure is within normal limits. If it is not above 100 mm. Hg systolic, it should be raised to that level so that any bleeding points at normal pressure can be seen. All bleeding points should be either sutured or tied with chromic 000 catgut. Electrocoagulation should be avoided at this point because it may melt previously placed sutures. Packing is uncomfortable and is not a reliable method to control bleeding.

A small absorbable gelatin (Gelfoam) wick (not pack) can be used in the canal, or, if the wound is open, a small piece of Gelfoam can be left in the open wound. A small dressing without pressure is then applied with narrow strips of Dermacil, which is preferable to regular tape because it is nonallergenic.

Postoperative care of and complications resulting from all types of anorectal surgery will be discussed later in this chapter.

Nonoperative or Conservative Management of Hemorrhoids

Not all patients should be admitted to the hospital and treated surgically. Other methods of management include instructions concerning anal hygiene and the use of analgesic salves and stool softeners; injection of a sclerosing agent, such as phenol in oil or quinine in urea, into the internal hemorrhoid; ligation, using the rubber band technique for internal hemorrhoids; and the freezing technique.

Self-care. The first of these measures consists of "self-care," to be carried out by the patient who has infrequent bleeding and infrequent hemorrhoidal prolapse. Regulation of the bowel with stool softeners plus adequate anal hygiene can keep these patients asymptomatic for years. Even patients having frequent prolapses may be kept comfortable with simple instructions about anal hygiene.

Injection. The second type of office procedure for treating hemorrhoids is injection with sclerosing solutions. Such injection is done for hemorrhoids causing rectal bleeding of a minimal-to-severe amount, with the hemorrhoids usually divided accurately into three or four quadrants and with minimal or no prolapse. A poor-risk patient, such as older patients who have had cerebrovascular accidents or who have coronary artery disease or severe senility, may be adequately treated in this fashion, even when there is considerable hemorrhoidal prolapse. The injection treatment is safe for the family physician to use only after he receives adequate instruction by a physician well trained in this procedure.

A solution of 5 per cent phenol in cottonseed oil is preferred by the authors. Five per cent quinine in urea is another solution that is useful in this technique. With the patient in a comfortable position, the anoscope is inserted, and each quadrant is carefully exposed at a level varying from 1 to 3 cm. above the dentate line. Amounts of the solution varying from 1 to 3 ml. may be injected into each quadrant, depending upon the size of the quadrant. It is important to inject the solution into the depths of the hemorrhoid and not too close to the mucous membrane. When using phenol, be sure to aspirate before injection. Do not inject into the lumen of the vein. The area is distended until the mucous membrane blanches, and then the other quadrant is approached. All three quadrants may be injected at one time. The injections are done at weekly intervals, and usually three to four visits are necessary to treat the patient satisfactorily.

The injection itself causes a minimal amount of pain, and after the injection, there is some discomfort for several hours. Patients undergoing this procedure can usually return to work immediately, and those who must remain at home overnight will certainly be able to return to work the next morning. This excellent technique has been used by many physicians for years, and complications, residual masses, or "sloughs" are rare when the solution and technique just described are used.

This technique can be used in addition to the ligation technique to treat the hemorrhoidal areas that are not large enough to remove with a rubber band.

Rubber Band Ligation. Another popular conservative method is rubber band ligation. The physician should be familiar with the instrument he is using. Either the Barron or the McGivney ligator is satisfactory. This technique is different from that involving injection because the initial pain is more severe, and in approximately 25 per cent of patients, there will be severe pain for the first 12 to 36 hours, which may require them to stay home. When this procedure is used, the patient should be instructed to bring a friend with him, so that he may be accompanied or driven home. The severe pain does not occur often, but it is frequent enough to take this precaution. The patient should also be told that only one hemorrhoid is treated at a time and that treatments will be 2 to 3 weeks apart. The number of treatments will vary according to the number and size of the hemorrhoidal masses. Ligation is a technique that could be used by family physicians, but, again, they must be trained by a physician who is competent to perform this procedure.

The anoscope is inserted in the selected quadrant, the ligator is passed through the anoscope, the internal hemorrhoid is pulled into the ligator, and the rubber band is easily snapped around it.

The sequence of events is that in 2 to 5 days the hemorrhoid distal to the rubber band will drop off, and at that time, the patient may experience a minimal amount of bleeding. In several days, the type of pain will change from an aching to a burning sensation during bowel movements.

When the ligature sloughs off, a moderate amount of bleeding may occur in 0.5 per cent of the patients, which will require ligation with a rubber band or suturing. For this reason, the patient is told that if he has considerable bleeding occurring 3 to 5 days after ligation, he is to report to his physician immediately. This conservative measure is very successful and is the most permanent type of nonoperative treatment presently available.

Freezing Technique. The freezing technique is one used by specialists all over the world, but, in our opinion, it is not a technique that should be used by family physicians. Complications are more frequent than with the other methods, the technique is difficult to learn, and the results are not as satisfactory.

Nonoperative treatments, as described, will not replace surgical removal of hemmorhoids but are useful in many patients. Only experience will teach a physician which cases are suitable for either conservative or operative treatment.

ANAL INFECTIONS

J. Peerman Nesselrod was certainly not the first physician to describe anal infection of various types. He is, however, to be given credit for presentation of the clearest discussion of anal infection in his book *Clinical Proctology*. His definition states, "The term anal infection pertains to the orderly chain of events occurring in the pathogenesis of anorectal inflammatory disease. The anatomic structures involved are anal crypts, anal ducts, anal glands and adjacent blood vessels and lymphatics. The various ramifications of anal infection are best presented in the diagram."[5] (Fig. 43–10).

As noted in this diagram, Stage I anal infection is a minor one in which the infectious material gets into a crypt or an anal duct and remains in the anal canal itself or in the anal crypt (cryptitis). Such infection can account for various stages of anal burning and pain. In Stage II infection, the invasion of the perianal and perirectal tissues occurs directly or indirectly, either via breaks in the gland–duct structure or via the blood vessels and lymphatics. Stage III infection develops from Stage II, resulting in many of the anal diseases that occur in man. Nesselrod believes that almost all anorectal diseases are a consequence of infection, which is certainly true of anal fistulas, anal abscesses, and probably anal fissures and an enlarged anal papilla. Many hemorrhoids are caused by infections, but not all degrees of chronic hemorrhoidal disease are related to infectious processes.

DIAGRAM OF ANAL INFECTION

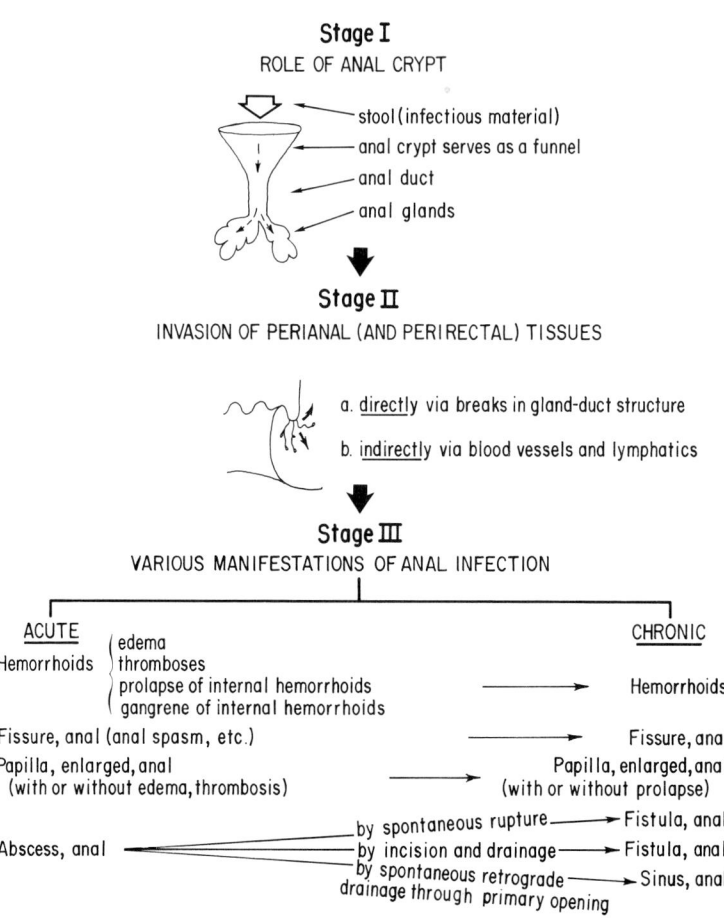

Stage I
ROLE OF ANAL CRYPT

- stool (infectious material)
- anal crypt serves as a funnel
- anal duct
- anal glands

Stage II
INVASION OF PERIANAL (AND PERIRECTAL) TISSUES

a. <u>directly</u> via breaks in gland-duct structure

b. <u>indirectly</u> via blood vessels and lymphatics

Stage III
VARIOUS MANIFESTATIONS OF ANAL INFECTION

ACUTE | | CHRONIC
Hemorrhoids { edema, thromboses, prolapse of internal hemorrhoids, gangrene of internal hemorrhoids } ⟶ Hemorrhoids

Fissure, anal (anal spasm, etc.) ⟶ Fissure, anal

Papilla, enlarged, anal (with or without edema, thrombosis) ⟶ Papilla, enlarged, anal (with or without prolapse)

Abscess, anal — by spontaneous rupture ⟶ Fistula, anal
— by incision and drainage ⟶ Fistula, anal
— by spontaneous retrograde drainage through primary opening ⟶ Sinus, anal

Spasm, anal ⟶ Contracture, anal

Figure 43-10. Diagram of anal infection.

ABSCESSES

Infections and abscesses in the perianal region must be treated early and aggressively. The causative organisms are highly virulent and are generally mixed aerobic and anaerobic gram-negative bacteria. This type of infection will advance rapidly and will produce severe systemic symptoms. The symptoms will depend on the severity of the infection and on how early the patient reports to the physician. Types of abscesses are noted in Figure 43–11. Perianal and ischiorectal abscesses are the most common, submucosal ones are infrequent, and supralevator and retrorectal abscesses are rare.

The characteristic symptoms are pain that begins intermittently and becomes constant, a bearing-down (or "pressure type") pain or both. When the inflammation has been converted to "pus," the patient is unable to walk, sit, or sleep without discomfort—a situation that the patient considers to be "unbearable." The two differential diagnoses are (1) an anal fissure, which is manifested by an intermittent type of pain that gradually improves after a bowel movement, and (2) a thrombosed hemorrhoid, which starts suddenly with severe pain that either remains the same or gradually decreases with treatment. The patient may or may not have a fever when first seen, depending on the size of the abscess.

Diagnosis.   In most patients, the diagnosis should easily be made from the history. Any patient who has an increasing amount of anorectal pain that becomes constant and who has fever must be considered to have

TYPES OF ABSCESSES

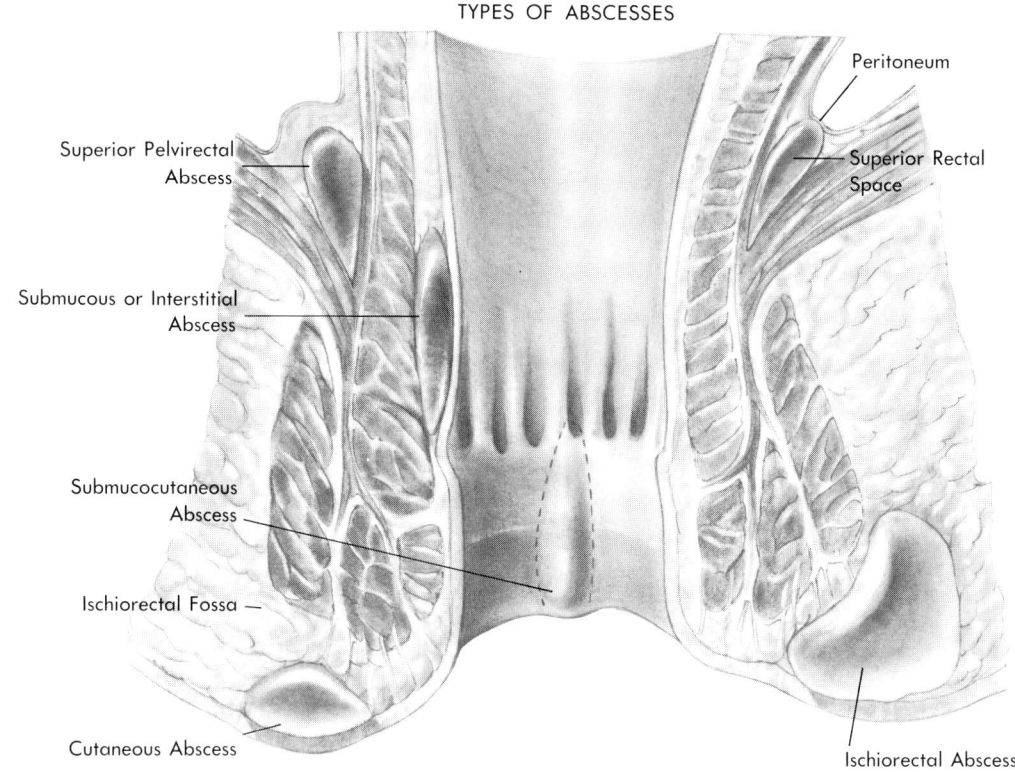

Figure 43-11. *Types of anorectal abscesses. (Adapted from Spiesman, M. G., and Malow, L.: Essentials of Clinical Proctology. New York, Grune & Stratton, 1957.)*

an infection until proved otherwise. Many times, gentle examination and observation will reveal inflamed, reddened, and edematous perianal skin. If such infected tissue is not visible, gentle palpation of the anal canal with the little finger or, in female patients, palpation through the vagina will reveal a tender mass. The mass is soft and warm, and the skin or mucosa is edematous and red.

Treatment. Once a diagnosis of abscess is made, the area should immediately be incised and drained. If the diagnosis is doubtful, do not delay treatment. Using local anesthesia, an incision may be made as a diagnostic procedure or, as in most cases, as a therapeutic measure. If the diagnosis is inflammation and the decision is made not to incise the area or to treat it surgically the patient must be seen daily to make sure that an abscess does not spread or become a supralevator or ischiorectal abscess, or that the patient does not become seriously ill. *It is much better to incise an inflamed area than to delay drainage of an abscess and allow it to spread circumferentially or to cause septicemia.*

The tendency in the treatment of perianal abscesses is to open them in the emergency room or in the office. However, it should be pointed out that using local anesthesia or freezing the skin is totally inadequate preparation for drainage of most abscesses, and the abscess is likely to recur because loculi cannot be adequately treated. Under such circumstances, the procedure is usually too painful for an adequate job to be done. With the patient under general anesthesia, however, incision can be made from the outside to the internal opening, thus saving the patient from developing a fistula in most instances.

Therefore, most patients with perianal abscesses should be admitted to the hospital. If the patient's general condition is satisfactory, incision and drainage is performed on the day of admission.

Patients are usually given general anesthetics and are treated in the lithotomy or the left lateral (Sims's) position, whichever is preferred by the anesthetist or the physician.

The abscess is opened in a radial fashion in the most fluctuant area. Once the abscess is opened, the physician determines the extent of the cavity by inserting his finger into it. If the abscess is only perianal and not ischiorectal or supralevator and only a small amount of muscle is undermined, the incision is carried through the internal opening at the dentate line. Thus, an abscess and fistula are treated in one operation. If the depth or extent of the abscess is in doubt, only incision is performed. Care must be taken not to cut too much muscle and cause incontinence.

If the cavity extends circumferentially in the ischiorectal spaces and involves half of the anal canal, multiple radial incisions are made. These incisions are connected by Penrose drains to keep them open. The cavity is usually irrigated with saline and peroxide. Although antibiotics are not used in treating these abscesses, antibiotics are started intravenously at operation because many bacteria will be released into the bloodstream during the procedure. Either cephalothin sodium (Keflin) or chloramphenicol sodium succinate (Chloromycetin), 1 gram by intravenous push, is given stat, and this level is maintained with intravenous or intramuscular (chloramphenicol given intravenously only) medications for 24 hours. The drug is then given by mouth for another 48 to 72 hours. Antibiotic therapy can be readjusted according to the severity of the infection and the results of culture and sensitivity reports.

Hemostasis is obtained either with sutures or with electrosurgical coagulation. The electrosurgical unit is invaluable for incision as well as for coagulation of the bleeding points in these conditions.

Postoperative orders for these patients are the same as for any patient undergoing anorectal surgery with the following exceptions:

1. Any packs that are left in the wound are removed the morning after surgery.

2. Injectable antibiotics are continued for at least 48 hours.

3. Adequate sedation is essential.

The patients are usually kept in the hospital for 3 to 5 days, and their postoperative care is the same as the routine postoperative care for all patients after anorectal surgery.

In the management of these infections, early surgical intervention and not watchful waiting is the keynote. Early use of antibiotics may mask the condition and delay needed incision and drainage. However, at the time of surgery and for several days postoperatively, antibiotics are important in preventing systemic infections. If the patient has recurrent abscesses or recurrent fistulas, he must be examined carefully for systemic diseases such as diabetes or granulomatous ileocolitis.

FISTULA-IN-ANO

Essentials of Diagnosis
1. History of abscess.
2. History of draining sinus.
3. Underwear soiled with mucus, blood, or pus.
4. External draining wound found on examination.
5. A probe inserted in the external opening should exit in the adjoining crypt.

Cause. As seen in Figure 43–12, anal infection burrows into the perianal tissue, forming an abscess that, if drained or ruptured spontaneously, becomes a fistula-in-ano. The major sign is drainage of purulent, clear, or serosanguineous fecal-type material. A history of drainage, including soiling of underclothes, intermittently associated with periods of anal swelling, pain and tenderness with no drainage, is almost pathognomonic of fistula-in-ano. Occasionally, the patient will give a history of an abscess that drained several years before. Other symptoms are mainly a consequence of drainage. The patient may have chafing, anal itching, or anal skin irritation related to the drainage rather than to the primary disease. Systemic disease must be ruled out. If the patient has an unusual type of fistula that recurs, a history of diarrhea, or any change in bowel habits, investigation by means of a barium enema examination and a gastrointestinal series with small bowel study should be carried out, particularly in children and in adults less than 40 years old. The diagnosis of regional ileitis or of granulomatous ileocolitis is frequently made in patients who have atypical fistulas. *In cases of multiple fistulas-in-ano, recurring anal abscesses,*

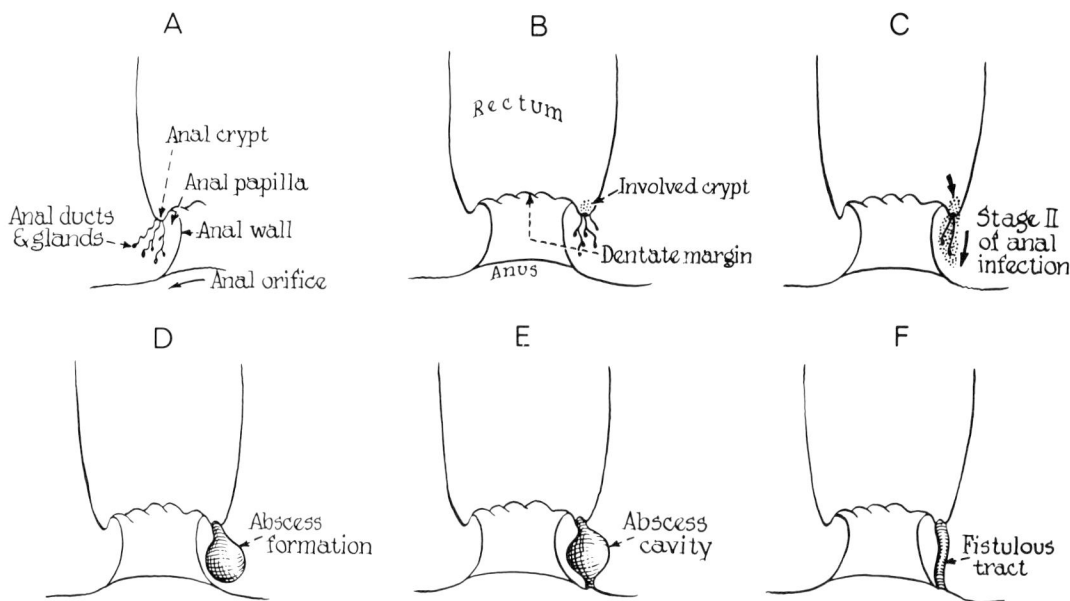

Figure 43–12. *Diagrammatic representation of pathogenesis of anal fissure. (From Nesselrod, J. P.: Clinical Proctology. 2nd Ed. Philadelphia, W. B. Saunders Co., 1957.)*

or unhealed fistulas or fistulas in the younger age group (from childhood through the 30's), the presence of granulomatous ileitis or ileocolitis (Crohn's disease) must be ruled out. Differential diagnosis includes pilonidal cyst, hidradenitis suppurativa, infected sebaceous cyst, infected comedones, retrorectal dermoid cysts, coloperineal fistulas, rectovaginal fistula, fungus infections (such as actinomycosis), and lymphogranuloma venereum.

Diagnosis. Ninety-five per cent of draining sinuses in the perianal area are fistulas-in-ano. Therefore, one can state that a draining sinus in the perianal area is a fistula-in-ano unless proved otherwise. Diagnosis is made by inspection. Usually, a purplish-red edematous area is seen, varying in distance from 0.5 cm. to 6 to 8 cm. from the dentate line. External sinuses are usually single. They may, however, be multiple, either located in the same quadrant or in different quadrants. Gentleness will accomplish much in allowing a careful examination of the perianal area. Palpation in the vicinity of the fistula will generally reveal induration directed toward the anal canal. A small, malleable probe carefully and gently introduced into the external opening can be guided toward the anal canal. In about 30 to 40 per cent of the patients, the probe can easily be carried through the internal opening into the anal canal. If the insertion is difficult, do not force the probe into the anal canal... which would be painful for the patient. Instead, insert an anoscope, palpate the fistula with the probe in place, and look for a drop of pus exuding from the offending crypt. This procedure can be done easily at the time of surgery and confirms the diagnosis. All quadrants of the anal canal should be examined, not just the quadrant containing the anal fistula. Sigmoidoscopic study should be done on all patients with anal fistulas.

Treatment. If a simple fistula-in-ano without evidence of systemic disease has been diagnosed and if the general condition of the patient is satisfactory, surgery is advised. A fistula-in-ano is rarely an emergency. Surgical management of a simple fistula-in-ano with combined external and internal hemorrhoids should certainly be well within the realm of all family physicians. However, because recurrences are frequent, operation for any complicating type of fistula or for any multiple fistulas that require reoperation should certainly be done with the assistance of a qualified colon and rectal surgeon, or the patient should be referred to a specialist.

SURGICAL TREATMENT. Fistulotomy, rather than fistulectomy, is preferred because a similar type of wound is created but less muscle is destroyed. Hemorrhoidectomies and multiple cryptotomies must also be performed to cure the patient and to avoid recurrent disease.

The essentials for cure using surgical treatment are:

1. Find the primary or internal opening.
2. Completely identify the tract from the internal to the external opening.
3. Construct the incision so that the wound is flat with no overhanging edges, which will allow the wound to heal from within outward.
4. Open all other crypts and treat all hemorrhoidal disease.

Postoperative Care. See section on postoperative care.

ANAL FISSURE

Signs and Symptoms. The patient usually complains of having anal pain during bowel movements, a pain that may have been present at various times. The pain is mild at first and in time becomes more severe, but it is not the constant pain that is associated with inflammatory diseases. Often the patient gives a history of chronic discomfort with the pain coming and going over a period of several months or several years, during which time his own self-treatment was felt to result in his being "cured." Diagnosis is easily made by spreading the skin of the anal canal and looking directly posterior; usually a small ulcer will be seen at the dentate line, extending upward as well as outward. The ulcer varies in size and often will be undermined. The base usually consists of the transverse fibers of the underlying muscle. Careful evaluation is necessary to decide whether the tightness of the anal canal is caused by true stenosis or by muscle spasm from pain.

Treatment. If the disease is not chronic and the ulcer is small, the patient can be treated symptomatically with stool softeners, such as mineral oil or Irish moss with mineral oil (Kondremul, plain), and analgesic ointments. Steroid ointment used on a regular basis for 2 to 6 weeks often promotes rapid healing of acute cases. Fifty per cent of all anal fissures will heal using this simple medication. Other conservative methods are dilation of the anal canal (after injecting a local anesthetic to make the procedure pain-free) or excision in the office of the distal undermined edge, which occasionally will promote healing from the outside inward.

Should all conservative measures fail, hospitalization and surgical excision are required.

SURGICAL TREATMENT. Surgical treatment is done on an inpatient basis, with all the usual preoperative preparation. The choice of anesthetic is up to the patient and the physician.

THE SURGICAL TECHNIQUE. Beginning on the outer edge and dissecting upward, excise all diseased skin, mucosa, and adjoining hemorrhoidal tissue. The wound is sutured open in a triangular shape with the base outward. All other adjoining crypts and any hemorrhoidal disease should be treated simultaneously. The family physician should not use elaborate closures, flaps, or grafts to assist in healing. Simple excision and marsupialization are adequate.

The disease is almost always cured by surgical treatment.

Postoperative Care. See section on postoperative care.

POSTOPERATIVE CARE FOR ANORECTAL SURGERY

As stated before, the basic principles of good postoperative care are essentially the same for patients with all types of anorectal surgery. The results of surgery in anorectal disease are related to accurate diagnosis; careful selection of cases; careful, gentle surgery; and good postoperative care.

Postoperative care is the most important consideration and the one in which the family physician is most intimately involved. When the family physician is the operating surgeon, he is totally responsible for the patient's care. When he refers a patient to another physician, he should know what his own role will be both before and after the referral. Complete referral with total care of the patient by the surgeon would amount to the surgeon's operating and treating the patient exclusively for about 3 months, the time needed for complete healing in most patients. If the operating surgeon sees the patient only in the hospital, the family physician will be responsible for the follow-up visits in the office. The responsibility for the patient's care should be determined by the family physician and the surgeon at the time of the referral. Nevertheless, the patient must be seen by either physician the day of surgery after he is returned to his room and has recovered from the anesthetic. Orders should be written and discussed with the nurse caring for the patient. The patient should be seen at least twice each day during hospitalization, twice a week during the first 3 weeks after he leaves the hospital, then every other week for 6 weeks, and finally once a month for 2 months. At the end of 3 months, the patient's anal area should be healed, the exception being the patient with complicated abscesses or fistulas.

During the period of hospital care, the anal wound must be examined daily and must be as carefully cared for as a wound in any other part of the body. The following daily routine and orders are presented for the average patient.

Immediate Postoperative Instructions

The intravenous infusion should be discontinued in the recovery room if the patient is stable and there is no further need for hydration or for intravenous medication. A full liquid diet is allowed following recovery from the anesthesia. The more food the patient eats, the greater the bulk and the earlier a more normal stool will begin to develop. Pain medication is usually given by injection for the first 24 hours, and in the morning following surgery, oral analgesics are prescribed.

In 4 to 6 hours, remove all dressings and apply either an additional dressing or cotton coated with lidocaine (Xylocaine) jelly every 3 hours for the first 24 hours and then 4 times daily thereafter. Usually after the first 24 hours, the patient may apply the lidocaine (Xylocaine) to the dressing and change the dressing himself. Instruct the nurses and the patient that the application of dressings or cotton is an important part of anal wound healing. Instruct them that it is not sufficient to apply a dressing to the buttocks; it must be against the anal canal. The patient should continue the dressings until wound healing is complete. Drainage from the anal canal, whether blood, mucus, or mucopurulent discharge, will collect on the dressing if the dressing is against the canal and will not drain onto the skin. If the discharge is allowed to drain onto the skin, it may cause maceration and inflammation and, as a result, delay healing.

The use of warm or cold compresses immediately after surgery is an individual preference. Warm compresses are preferred for a patient whose pain threshold is low, as these provide an added factor in relieving discomfort. The Aquamatic pad, which is used to apply heat, is effective and is not likely to burn the skin.

Male patients are allowed to stand to void and go to the bathroom; female patients may sit up to void into a bedpan, use a bedside commode, or go to the bathroom on the day of surgery. The greater the degree of pain and the lower the pain threshold of the patient, the more likely that voiding will be difficult. If the patient requires catheterization, a sulfonamide should be given for urinary antisepsis. Once started, the sulfonamide medication should be continued for a minimum of 2 weeks. If the patient needs a second catheterization, a Foley catheter is introduced and is allowed to remain in place until the patient's pain has decreased. The catheter can usually be removed in 24 to 48 hours. The patient rarely has any major problem because of urinary retention. It is better to insert an indwelling catheter to keep the bladder drained than to have the patient "overflowing," maintaining some residual, having continual symptoms from the accumulation of residual urine, and, eventually, developing an infection. The dehydration technique, that is, not allowing the patient to drink during the first 18 to 24 hours until he voids, is unnecessary. Dehydrating the patient is more dangerous than the use of a catheter.

Stool softeners, such as Irish moss with mineral oil (Kondremul, plain) 60 ml. twice a day, are begun either the day before surgery or the day after surgery and are usually continued for 5 to 10 days. However, decreasing doses are administered after the third day because the oil will be "leaking out."

First Postoperative Day

Examine the wounds to be sure that there is no bleeding and that any open wounds are not closing prematurely. Have the patient begin sitz baths 4 times a day.

High-risk patients should not take these baths. Sitz baths should be started *early* following surgery and should be given at regular intervals, and an aide should accompany the patient for the first several times to make sure he does not become weak, faint, or overheated.

The most important part of postoperative care is the relief of pain. Usually, hypodermic medication can be discontinued on the first postoperative day, and oral medication of the physician's preference may then be used, either APC with oxycodone (Percodan), APC with codeine (Empirin No. 3), or acetaminophen (Tylenol) with codeine, one tablet every 3 to 4 hours. The patient must be told that medications for relief of pain are available to him.

Analgesics plus tranquilizers such as propoxyphene-acetaminophen (Wygesic) and aspirin-ethoheptazine-meprobamate (Equagesic) can be used at regular intervals for individual patients. Make sure that the patient has been placed on a regular diet and is ambulatory.

Second Postoperative Day

The same orders as for the first day are followed, with reinforcement concerning the use of sitz baths and examination of wounds. At the second visit (the afternoon visit) on the second postoperative day, this order should be written: "If no bowel movement by 9:00 P.M., give Senokot tablets" (or some other stimulant laxative, such as Modane, Prulet, or milk of magnesia).

Third Postoperative Day

If the patient has not had a bowel movement before your morning visit, instill 4 ounces of mineral oil into his rectum through a No. 18 Foley catheter with a catheter-tipped syringe. Orders are then written: "If no bowel movement within 1 hour, use a No. 18 Foley catheter and give a 500 ml. tap water enema."

This treatment will usually promote a relatively normal bowel movement. The quantity will depend on the volume of food the patient has eaten. When visiting the patient on the evening of the third day, discuss the results of the enemas with him and insert a small cotton-tipped applicator into the rectum to determine if a soft stool still remains or adequate bowel movement has occurred.

Fourth Postoperative Day

The patient is usually discharged in the morning if the physician, after seeing him, is certain that there is no bleeding and no difficulty in voiding and that the patient can be maintained relatively comfortably at home. The following written orders are given to each patient on discharge:

1. Full diet—limit highly seasoned foods.
2. Ambulatory as desired—no heavy lifting for 2 weeks and no automobile driving for 1 week.
3. Warm baths or showers 3 to 4 times per day—particularly after bowel movements.
4. Keep cotton or gauze against anus, change frequently.
5. Medications:
   a. Irish moss with mineral oil (Kondremul, plain), 2 tablespoons nightly.
   b. Pain tablets as needed.
   c. Benzocaine (Americaine) or lidocaine (Xylocaine) ointment applied to anus as needed.
6. Call office for an appointment (first revisit is 2 to 4 days after leaving hospital).

Postoperative Office Visits

The patient is usually seen twice a week for 2 to 3 weeks, depending on the individual case; once a week for an additional 2 to 3 weeks; and then once a month for two visits or until healing is complete.

Persons employed in sedentary occupations may usually return to part-time work at the end of 2 to 3 weeks and to full-time work in 3 to 4 weeks. Patients whose jobs require physical labor usually are able to return to full duty after 4 weeks.

Cardinal Points Concerning Postoperative Treatment in the Office.

1. On the first office visit, the physician usually uses a cotton-tipped applicator to inspect the wounds and the rectum. Beginning on the second visit, which would be about 8 to 10 days postoperatively, the physician should use his little finger to palpate the incisions and to feel the rectum.
2. On the tenth postoperative day, the dosage of Irish moss with mineral oil

(Kondremul, plain) or other stool softeners should be decreased or completely discontinued and bulk laxatives, such as sodium carboxymethylcellulose with dioctyl sodium sulfosuccinate (Dialose) capsules, or psyllium hydrophilic mucilloid (Metamucil or L.A. formula), should be started. At that time, the patient should be informed that the stools will become firmer, which is essential to complete healing and recovery. As the stools become more formed, the patient may have increased pain with bowel movements, but he may continue to use oral or topical analgesics, or both, if needed. If the patient is encouraged to produce normal, formed stools rather than to continue the use of stool softeners, the anal canal should heal to a normal size, and digital dilatation will not be needed.

3. During the patient's ensuing early postoperative visits (second and third week), excessive granulations on indolent or unhealed wounds on the external skin are treated by the application of silver nitrate. Pockets that are distal to or in the anal canal and might represent an area of possible infection either may be incised rapidly without anesthetic or a local anesthetic may be instilled and these areas trimmed. Trimming the areas in the early postoperative period is essential because such a procedure is relatively easy to do at that time and assists the healing process.

4. Use of soap and water and excellent anal hygiene, consisting of the application of dressings and appropriate analgesic ointments, are the only means of improving the anal healing. No antibiotic ointments or scarlet red, gentian violet, or other elaborate salves will help healing. During the third and fourth weeks, a skin or vaginal fungus infection may occur because of the excessive moisture from constant warm baths and perspiration. Monilia, the most common type of fungus, can be treated with appropriate antifungal creams, ointments or vaginal inserts Discontinue analgesic ointments 3 to 4 weeks postoperatively and encourage the use of cotton or dressings covered with starch powders to absorb excess drainage and to aid in keeping the area dry. Tight-fitting or nylon underclothing, or both, worn by either sex can contribute to poor healing, as such garments inhibit evaporation and tend to produce more moisture.

Patients should not be discharged until the following conditions exist:

1. The anal canal has returned to as normal a condition as possible.
2. The patient is asymptomatic, with normal-sized stool.
3. The anal skin is not irritated, and there is little or no evidence of bleeding.

When discharging the patient at the end of the 3 months, remind him that should he have any problems at all you are available for consultation. Once a patient has had anorectal surgery, he should be followed up at annual intervals, with inspection of the anal canal as well as with an annual proctoscopic examination, to detect any evidence of polypoid or malignant disease.

In summary, the following steps are essentials for all types of anorectal surgery:
1. Accurate diagnosis preoperatively.
2. Preoperative and operative evaluation of the exact extent of surgery necessary.
3. Removal of all diseased tissue and removal of all hemorrhoids during hemorrhoidectomy.
4. Promotion of normal, formed bowel movements as soon as possible.
5. Frequent postoperative visits.
6. Instruction during postoperative visits concerning anal hygiene. The most important point of such instruction is to have the patient keep a small dressing on the canal at all times and change it when it becomes soiled.

COMPLICATIONS OF ANORECTAL SURGERY

As with any surgical procedure, certain early and late complications are frequent and must be classified as being almost "normal."

EARLY COMPLICATIONS

Early complications, those occurring on the day of operation or during the period of hospitalization, are primarily: excess pain, hemorrhage, dysuria, and nausea.

Excess Postoperative Pain

The degree of postoperative pain in individual patients is difficult to evaluate. Causes are often obscure, and the interrelationship between functional and true organic elements must be carefully evaluated.

Tolerance to pain will vary among patients, and factors such as fear, insecurity, apprehension, and ignorance about the type of pain experienced are involved. Most people have never experienced severe anorectal pain, and the type of discomfort they will have is difficult for them to realize. Cooperation and confidence on the part of the patient are often of much greater value in relief of pain than is the administration of large doses of opiates or the injection of long-lasting anesthetics. "Tender loving care" by the physician, as well as by the nurse, is important in alleviating postoperative pain. One particular type of anorectal procedure or anorectal surgery is not likely to cause more severe pain than any other type. The pain does not differ in patients whose wounds are closed tightly, left open, or coagulated or in those who have few or many sutures. Pain is relieved by loose dressings, application of analgesic ointments, application of cold or warm compresses, and appropriate use of injectable narcotics for the first 24 hours and oral narcotics thereafter. The use of warm compresses and warm tub baths relaxes both the patient and his anal canal. The application of heat and the administration of sedatives will do more to relieve postoperative pain than will anything else.

Hemorrhage

Patients may bleed in the recovery room or during the first 8 to 12 hours following surgery, and most such bleeding comes from small bleeders on the surface of the skin or over the external sphincter. If the bleeding is early, that is, within minutes after surgery, treatment with ligation without local anesthetic is possible. However, if 30 minutes to 1 hour postoperatively, a local anesthetic should be injected, and the bleeding points should be quickly clamped and sutured or ligated.

Internal bleeding is classified as an early type of hemorrhage because it may occur within the first 6 to 8 hours following surgery, but usually it occurs within the first 2 to 3 days postoperatively. Blood may begin to ooze from the patient's anal canal, or a sudden onset of more excessive bleeding may occur, including the passage of large clots. If the external area is not the site of the bleeding and if this is persistent, profuse or both, the bleeding site should be identified and the bleeding controlled in the operating room under anesthesia. The cause is usually a blood vessel at the apex of the hemorrhoidal group or one on the mucosal surface.

Postoperative bleeding is an unforeseen mishap and should occur only minimally. The maximum rate should probably be one patient in every 200 to 300, or even less. Simple steps can be taken to avoid this complication:

1. The apex of each large hemorrhoidal group should always be ligated separately under direct vision, and if a large pedicle is present, two ligatures are advised. If a wound is closed in the anal area, the running suture should be locked and bleeding controlled in this fashion. If the wound is to be left open and if there is any amount of oozing, a running lock chromic suture to marsupialize the wound is effective in controlling bleeding.

2. If sutures are used at the apex and if the incisions or the wounds are not to be sutured, the bleeding points may be electrosurgically coagulated. Care must be taken to avoid melting the chromic sutures during the coagulating procedure.

3. Never complete an operation if a small amount of oozing continues, assuming that the oozing will stop. It is much easier to observe the wound or the anal canal carefully and to stop the bleeding during the original procedure than it is to do this in the recovery room or later, when the patient is under a second anesthetic.

4. As precautionary measure the operative area is examined carefully by means of a Hirschman anoscope. At the completion of the procedure, use the anoscope for direct vision; irrigate the area, using an Asepto syringe and water; and aspirate by suction. This procedure will aid in identifying all bleeding vessels. Any small bleeding points are controlled by clamping, ligating, or suturing.

5. Blood pressure should be normal (not below normal) during the final inspection of the wound for bleeding.

Dysuria

Urinary difficulty occurs frequently. Rather than being labeled as a complication, dysuria should really be considered a normal or expected difficulty after anorectal surgery. This is because the nerves of both the bladder and the rectum are mediated through the pudendal nerve, and, therefore, pain in the anal canal coincides with reflex spasm of the sphincter muscles of the bladder. Simple methods for avoiding this problem are:

1. Giving adequate sedation to decrease pain.

2. Allowing the male patients to stand and the female patients to sit up while voiding early during the first postoperative day.

3. Beginning warm compresses early to relieve spasm and to enable the patient to void.

4. Judiciously using injectable bethanechol chloride (Urecholine) and catheterization to keep urinary difficulty to a minimum. Early catheterization to avoid overdistention of the bladder is much better than waiting too long to catheterize the patient. Not recommended is dehydrating the patient to prevent his bladder from becoming full and thereby decreasing the need for catheterization. If a patient is catheterized once, he should be given an appropriate sulfonamide such as sulfisoxazole (Gantrisin) or sulfamethoxazole (Gantanol). If a second catheterization is needed, a Foley catheter should be inserted and left in place 48 hours or until the pain has substantially decreased in intensity.

LATE COMPLICATIONS

"Late" means any complication occurring after the patient leaves the hospital. Thus, this may be from 7 days to several months postoperatively.

Hemorrhage

After the patient returns home, is having normal stool function, and is following the usual postoperative routine, severe hemorrhage is a rare development. The usual symptom is rectal bleeding, occurring either immediately after or instead of a bowel movement. The patient feels an urge to go to the toilet and suddenly passes large volumes of maroon-to-bright-red clots or liquid blood. The passage either will be in one large volume or may be a continuous bleeding and draining. When the patient calls his physician with this complaint, he should be told to report immediately to the hospital emergency room. When you see the patient for examination, he will likely

be apprehensive, and his condition will depend on the volume of blood lost.

Blood pressure and pulse rate should be determined and the anal area examined. If much blood is present on the anal skin or on the dressing and the patient is obviously bleeding severely, local examination should be postponed. Blood should be drawn for a complete blood count (CBC), prothrombin time, partial thromboplastin time, and platelet count and should be typed and matched. At the same time, the patient should be given intravenously administered Ringer's lactate solution, and, if any degree of shock exists, include a plasma volume expander. Then, placing the patient on his left side and in the Trendelenburg position, gently examine his anal canal. If continued oozing is observed and there is no obvious external bleeding site, large clots will probably be seen rectally. The easiest method for treating such a patient is to obtain a No. 30, 32, or 34 Foley catheter with a 30 ml. bag. Lubricate it well and insert it into the anal canal above the surgical site. Inflate the balloon with 30 to 40 ml. of water, pull it down firmly against the anus, and tape the catheter on the thigh. In many instances, this procedure will tamponade the bleeding enough to stop it. Once the bleeding stops, sedate the patient and irrigate the rectum thoroughly with cold isotonic saline through the catheter. The irrigation will aid in controlling and following the progress of the bleeding. This method either will stop the bleeding or will tamponade it enough to allow time to have the blood typed and matched and to give the patient a transfusion.

Any further therapy will depend on the severity and continuation of the hemorrhage. In about 75 to 85 per cent of patients, this treatment will result in a cessation of the hemorrhage. The catheter is left in place for at least 24 hours and then removed, and the patient is observed in the hospital for an additional 48 hours.

If this method of tamponade with a catheter and balloon does not stop the hemorrhage, the patient must be brought to surgery immediately and appropriate measures must be taken. The cause of the bleeding will usually be a premature sloughing of the ligature at the apex of the hemorrhoidal excision. Most of the wounds in such situations will be friable, and it will be impossible to clamp the bleeders.

Instead, with either chromic 0 or 00 sutures, control any bleeding point by using trans-fixing and continuous interlocking sutures. In these instances, the authors have avoided using electrosurgical coagulation to control the major bleeders because a larger slough will develop and arterial bleeding cannot be well coagulated.

Severe hemorrhage, sufficient to have the patient return to the hospital for examina-tion or admission, usually occurs in 1 per cent or less of patients. Methods of averting such hemorrhages have been described in this chapter in the section dealing with hemorrhoidal surgery. If severe hemor-rhage does occur, treatment must be rapid.

Anal Contracture

This is an infrequent and avoidable com-plication. The more radical the surgery in the anorectal area, the more likely that some degree of anal stenosis will occur. When using the "flap procedure" that requires transverse incisions or circular incisions, one must be extremely careful about the possibility of anal stenosis. No digital ex-amination is necessary before the 8th or 10th postoperative day; occasionally a little finger may be inserted into the canal before this time to be sure that fecal impaction does not exist. The authors' practice is to decrease the amount of stool softener, such as mineral oil, on about the 7th or 10th day and to increase the amount of both bulk laxatives and high residue foods, so that the patient will begin having a normal, formed stool. The best method of dilating the anal canal and maintaining its size is to have the patient pass normal, formed stools. If on about the 10th or 14th day the patient still has small stools and on digital examination the canal seems to be organically tight, he must be seen twice a week for gentle examination with the index finger. If after an additional 10 days to 2 weeks the anal canal still seems snug or tight, daily self-dilatation by the patient with Young's dila-tors may be necessary, after appropriate instruction by the physician.

Anal contracture should not occur in more than 1 per cent of patients if proper post-operative care is observed. This complica-tion will be averted if simple postoperative dilatations are performed early during the recovery period and if the patient is en-couraged to have a formed stool.

Sloughing of Anal Tissue

Beginning on about the 7th or 10th day after the patient goes home, areas of mucosa that were previously healthy or areas of skin that seemed to be macerated may become necrotic. Carefully observing these areas in the office, debriding them by means of sharp dissection, and instructing the patient about how to keep the area clean with soap and water will help to heal the tissue. If the skin edges of these wounds become under-mined, local injection and trimming of the edges may be necessary.

Impaction

After the patient has had a normal bowel movement in the hospital, he is allowed to return home usually the same day or the next day. However, when visiting the office later, the patient may complain that he has many stools, each of a small amount, every morning and "never quite feels empty." The patient should immediately be exam-ined, first with a cotton-tipped applicator and then, if stool is felt in the rectum, with an index finger. These symptoms may be the first indication of a fecal impaction, or they may mean that the patient is having an incomplete bowel movement because of pain. Early during the postoperative period, when the anal area is still in the healing phase, the sphincter will contract tightly after a small bowel movement because of the pain. Later on, after the patient is relaxed and sedated, he will again have the urge to go and will pass more stool. Usually this happens during the early postoperative period, but it is also a strong indication that the patient has fecal impaction.

Once the diagnosis of fecal impaction is made, the treatment consists of using a No. 20 or 22 soft rubber catheter and a catheter-tipped syringe to instill 4 to 6 ounces of mineral oil into and around the impaction. This fluid should be retained about 1 or 2 hours, and then the patient is given a tap water enema. Usually the enema will pro-mote an excellent bowel movement for most patients. The patient is then instructed to continue using stool softeners and to take analgesic tablets before bowel movements, so that forceful expulsion of stool may occur. If recognized early, this complication is not too uncomfortable. However, if allowed to continue for 2 or 3 days, fecal impaction can be a very distressing symptom.

DIVERTICULAR DISEASE

A frequent abnormal finding in a barium enema test on a patient over 45 years of age is diverticulosis. This disease, which is common and well known to all family physicians, must be managed properly. Just because a patient is shown to have a diverticula on the x-ray film does not mean that the condition is symptomatic. Most patients with diverticula have no symptoms at all. Minor symptoms such as abdominal cramps, nausea, and a bloated feeling are difficult to distinguish from the irritable colon syndrome. True diverticulitis is accompanied by abdominal tenderness and elevated body temperature. Once the diagnosis of diverticulosis is made, giving the patient instructions for maintaining a high residue diet is important. The diet includes foods that are high in fiber content, that is, whole wheat bread and bran flakes and vegetables and fruits that contain much fiber. The diet will assist in preventing symptoms and the possible progression of diverticulosis into diverticulitis or symptomatic diverticular disease. Diverticulosis of the colon usually starts in the sigmoid, and, as repeated observations show, the disease may remain in the sigmoid area or may progress to involve the entire left colon and possibly the entire colon.

Only 10 to 15 per cent of patients with diverticulosis develop complications sufficient to warrant surgical intervention. Reasons for surgery are obstruction, perforation, massive hemorrhage, and intractability.

Obstruction. Obstruction caused by diverticular disease results most commonly from diverticulitis. The typical signs and symptoms are abdominal pain that is mild at first and increases in severity, causing nausea, vomiting, and inability to pass gas. The patient should be admitted to the hospital immediately and a surgeon consulted. Resolving the condition by treating the obstruction with antibiotics is unlikely, but this probably should be tried. The patient is given nothing by mouth (NPO), is given antibiotics intravenously, and is observed hour by hour. A decision about surgery can then be made, contingent upon the progress of the disease.

Perforation. Although it is unusual, perforation of the bowel does occur and is accompanied by all of the catastrophic findings present in free perfortion: acute, severe abdominal pain; elevated body tem-perature; rigid or board-like abdomen; and explicit tenderness with rebound tenderness. X-ray studies usually reveal free air beneath the diaphragm. Such patients should be admitted to the hospital and operated on immediately.

Massive Hemorrhage. The most common cause of massive hemorrhage by rectum in older patients is diverticular disease. These patients have diverticulosis and not diverticulitis. Management of this syndrome is complicated and will not be discussed in this chapter except to state that consultation should be obtained immediately. If no localized area of bleeding is detected by proctoscopy, barium enema examination, or intestinal arteriogram, a subtotal colectomy with ileorectal anastomosis (a common treatment) yields the best response.

Intractability. Patients who have recurrent diverticulitis and who are treated conservatively may eventually reach a point at which they are unable to work and unable to remain out of the hospital or out of bed for more than several months at a time. Such patients are classified as intractable. They should be operated on during a quiescent phase, because at this time the patients are happier and surgery is much easier.

ULCERATIVE COLITIS

Idiopathic ulcerative colitis is a diarrheal disease of severe nature that occurs in young persons and is confined to the colon. The disease is idiopathic, although many causative theories have been evolved. The disease occurs only slightly more commonly in females. Five to 10 per cent of the patients are children, aged 11 to 13 years, and most patients are in their teens or twenties.

The family physician has a great advantage over a consultant or another physician when seeing a patient with ulcerative colitis for the first time. Physicians know that the emotional responses or actions of the patient are important in the development and recurrence of the disease. By knowing the patient and the family, the family physician will be able to treat this aspect of ulcerative colitis in an excellent fashion. Once a diagnosis of ulcerative colitis is made, a gastroenterologist or a colon and rectal surgeon should be consulted. If the family physician does not want to treat the patient, the patient should be referred immediately to either or both of these specialists. However, the family physician should treat those patients whose condition is mild-to-moderately severe and who can be managed medically.

Symptoms of ulcerative colitis are the same as those of any acute diarrheal disease. The initial attack may be of sudden onset, with severe fulminating diarrhea. Proctoscopic examination reveals an "angry red" and bleeding bowel. However, most cases of ulcerative colitis are less severe, with initial symptoms of perhaps slight bleeding and diarrhea. On proctoscopic study, a faint blush or a limited area of inflammation will be noted. Follow-up in the early stages should be made weekly or biweekly, depending on the severity of the symptoms. Repeated proctoscopy will assist in making the diagnosis and following the progress of the disease. Ulcerative colitis must be considered the most likely diagnosis for any patient with persistent bleeding from a granular mucosa of the colon.

The initial treatment of acute ulcerative colitis consists of bedrest and of limiting the diet to liquids at first and then gradually increasing the bulk of the diet. Antispasmodics and the judicious use of sulfasalazine (Azulfidine) may also aid in management. Azulfidine is a sulfonamide that is effective and occasionally, when used alone, may result in an excellent response. Initially, the drug should be used in doses of 1 gram or two EN-tabs (enteric coated) every 4 hours for 48 hours and then 4 times daily. If such treatment is not effective, topical steroids uuch as hydrocortisone (Cortenema), as a retention enema, should be used early. These enemas should be given twice daily for 1 week and then nightly until the desired response is obtained. The patient must be told that these are retention enemas. If the patient is treated with this routine for 2 weeks and little or no response results, oral steroids should be started. In the past, this medication had been initiated as a last resort, and many patients had developed permanent damage to their bowels unnecessarily. Start the patient on a regimen of 40 mg. of prednisone each morning. This dosage is continued for 2 weeks, and if the response is good, the dose is decreased gradually by 5 mg. decrements every 2 weeks to 20 mg. Once prednisone is started, it should be continued for a minimum of 6 weeks and preferably for 12 weeks.

The reasons for surgical intervention in ulcerative colitis are intractability, toxic megacolon, perforation, and suspicion of malignant neoplasm.

Intractability. If the patient is treated adequately on a routine of diet, sufficient rest, antispasmodics, sulfasalazine (Azulfidine), and steroids and he continues to require treatment at home, misses much work or school and continues to lose weight, total colectomy or ileostomy should be considered.

Toxic Megacolon. If a patient treated for ulcerative colitis suddenly develops abdominal distention, constant diarrhea, and elevated temperature, immediate hospitalization is necessary. Once a diagnosis of toxic megacolon is made, the patient should be prepared appropriately, and immediate surgery should be performed. This complication is serious, and the morality is high.

Perforation. The same signs and symptoms occur as with any other abdominal perforation, and this is naturally an indication of the need for immediate surgical exploration and probably total colectomy.

Suspicion of Malignant Neoplasm. Patients with chronic recurrent ulcerative colitis for many years have a higher incidence of malignancy than do persons in the normal population. For this reason, these patients should have frequent proctoscopic, colonoscopic, barium enema, and carcinoembryonic antigen (CEA) examinations. If any questions arise concerning results of these studies, exploratory laparotomy should be performed.

REGIONAL ILEITIS

Regional ileitis, granulomatous ileitis, or Crohn's disease is a common diarrheal disease occurring in young persons. The diagnosis is not difficult if one remembers the existence of the disease. A patient having recurring abdominal cramps and episodes of diarrhea, or fever of undetermined origin, or unusual types of anal fistulas should be studied by barium enema and gastrointestinal series with small bowel visualization. The disease is divided into several types and may involve the ileum, the colon, or both organs. It is characteristic of this disease to find segments of normal bowel interposed between areas of diseased bowel. This is important in the differential diagnosis of Crohn's disease and ulcerative colitis. Regional ileitis may occasionally be diagnosed at the time of exploratory laparotomy after a preoperative diagnosis of appendicitis. If this occurs and the patient is found to have acute regional ileitis not involving the base of the cecum or the appendix, appendectomy should be performed and the abdomen closed. Many of these patients will become completely asymptomatic and will not require further treatment.

Once a diagnosis of regional ileitis is made, the only treatment is an adequate high vitamin, high calorie diet and the use of sulfasalazine (Azulfidine) and steroids The clinical symptoms of progression of the disease are abdominal cramps, recurrent episodes of fever and diarrhea, inability to gain weight, and inability to perform useful work. Steroids can produce dramatic remission, and the remission should be governed by the ability of the patient to perform his normal duties. X-ray evidence of the disease may appear severe, although the patient may be totally asymptomatic.

Recurrences are characterized by progression of the disease, causing obstruction; by progression of the disease, causing fistula formation from the small bowel to the skin, from one loop of the small bowel to the other, and from the small bowel to the colon; and by acute free perforation. The great difference between ulcerative colitis and regional ileitis is that the treatment of ulcerative colitis with total colectomy is curative, whereas treatment of regional ileitis with resection is not. Regional ileitis is treacherous and, regardless of therapy, will recur in 15 to 30 per cent of the patients. Malignant neoplasms are not directly associated with this disorder.

Once a diagnosis of regional ileitis is made, the patient should be treated by the family physician in close cooperation with a competent colon and rectal surgeon or a gastroenterologist.

POLYPS OF THE COLON

Benign tumors of the colon and rectum occupy a prominent position among diseases of the digestive tract because they are being detected with an ever-increasing frequency. As discussed in this section, the term "polyp" applies to any outgrowth from the mucosal surface and has no pathogenic connotation. Many types of polyps exist, but this discussion will be limited to the neoplastic type. Neoplastic polyps may be subdivided into adenomatous, adenovillous, and villous polyps. The familial polyposis syndrome will also be discussed.

On examination with a proctoscope or on viewing the barium enema films, the physician is confronted with a polypoid mass without a histologic diagnosis. Since these masses either are already malignant or may become malignant, all of them should be removed for histologic diagnosis. The only exception to this rule would be if the same physician had repeatedly examined the patient with a proctoscope and had received a previous histologic diagnosis of small, so-called adenomas that are multiple or recurring. These masses may be coagulated without further histologic evaluation. The family physician should seek consultation for all patients diagnosed as having polyps. However, for purposes of follow-up care and counseling the patient and his family, the family physician must have an excellent knowledge of the type of treatment and the continuing care necessary for patients with rectal and colon polyps. It is for this purpose that this section was written.

Adenomatous polyps can be sessile or pedunculated. The great majority will be minute, varying in size from 1 to 6 mm. These small polyps will usually have the same color and texture as the surrounding mucous membrane. As they increase in size, they usually change color, becoming dark red, and begin to contain a villous component followed by development of a stalk. Pathologists have learned more and more about the histologic and developmental anatomy of polyps. We now realize that the adenoma and the villous adenoma can be completely separate entities but that many times villous elements are present in adenomatous polyps. The incidence of villous elements seems to be related to polyp size. It is also true that the larger the polyp, the more likely the presence of carcinomatous changes in its structure. Polyps found to be greater than 1.5 cm. in diameter, either by radiologic or by proctoscopic examination, have a greater propensity for malignant change. One-fourth of polyps having a diameter greater than 2.5 cm. will have carcinomatous changes in the superficial portion, and many of these will show invasion beneath the muscularis mucosa. Thus, patients with lesions that measure less than 1 cm. in diameter in the upper colon beyond the reach of the proctoscope may be followed up by repeated annual examination and should undergo surgery only if the polyps increase in size. However, lesions 1.5 to 2.5 cm. in diameter must be treated aggressively and immediately upon diagnosis.

The demonstration of any pedicle or stalk is an optimistic sign. Carcinoma can exist on a stalk, but this is rare. The longer the stalk, the more optimistic the prognosis. The majority of polyps with stalks are adenomatous or mixed adenomatous and villous types. Although these are premalignant, they do not bear the malignant potential of the villous polyps.

Villous adenomas usually are found in the rectum and present special problems. They are almost always sessile, and, when diagnosed, 25 per cent of these polyps will have malignant changes. Once a diagnosis of villous adenoma is made, the polyp should be completely removed, either by abdominal exploration or by excisional biopsies. Only after the entire lesion is removed and studied by pathologists can a decision as to definitive therapy be made.

The larger villous tumors that are soft and palpable and easily visualized after multiple biopsies may be treated conservatively by using electrosurgical coagulation. After complete eradiction of the polyp, all patients must be followed up every 2 months for the first year and every 4 months thereafter. If, at the end of 2 years, no polyps are seen, such patients may then be followed up annually.

Colonoscopy will certainly broaden the range of nonoperative treatment of polyps above the level reached by the sigmoidoscope. A great majority of polyps that are seen on x-ray films can be easily visualized and removed by the use of a colonoscope.

Familial Adenomatous Polyposis

There is a certain group of patients whose family members for generations have had familial adenomatous polyposis. The genetic history of these patients reveals that 50 per cent of them will develop polyps. All patients who have this disease will develop cancer if not treated appropriately. They are in a very high-risk group and must be treated accordingly. Once a history of familial adenomatous polyposis is obtained by the family physician, he should immediately seek consultation with a colon and rectal surgeon and also should begin to familiarize the patient and his family with this disease. Most of these patients will present with a history of knowing that members of their family have had polyps, or cancer, or both, and will be fairly knowledgeable concerning this disorder. If this is not true, they must be thoroughly instructed immediately. The family physician should inform the patient that all of his siblings should have annual proctoscopic examinations beginning at age 10 to 12 years in order to detect this disease early and to begin appropriate management. The most common and acceptable treatment is subtotal colectomy with ileorectal anastomosis and careful repeated proctoscopic examinations to coagulate any existing or recurring polyps. However, if the patient has the entire rectum completely coated with polyps, making coagulation and proctoscopic management impossible, total colectomy and ileostomy are the best treatment.

Behringer very well states the problem of the patient with polyps: "To consider all such lesions innocent will result in tragic neglect of some malignancy, and yet to treat all as malignant will result in unnecessary morbidity and mortality. If the knowledge that has been gained is carefully applied, both these extremes can be avoided."[1]

CANCER

Cancer of the lower intestinal tract was the second greatest cause of death from cancer in 1976, and its position has remained essentially unchanged during the past 4 decades. Seventy-five per cent of all intestinal cancers arise in the colon, rectum, or anus. In 1977, an estimated 99,000 new cases of colon and rectal cancer will have occurred, resulting in 49,000 deaths. In the male, the three leading sites of malignancy are the lung (22 per cent), prostate gland (17 per cent), and colon and rectum (14 per cent); in the female, the breast is the first site (26 per cent) and the colon and rectum the second (15 per cent). Twelve per cent of deaths from cancer in men and 15 per cent in women will be due to cancer of the rectum and colon. The incidence between men and women is equally distributed, and two-thirds of all patients are more than 50 years of age. The demographic distribution is worldwide, and, like other alimentary tract cancers the incidence of colon and rectal cancer varies from country to country. The prevalence is highest in the United States and lowest in Japan and Finland. The disease is relatively uncommon in Puerto Rico and Africa.[6]

No common cause has been discovered. Some recent articles by Burkitt[2a] and others have begun to scratch the surface, implicating diet and certain carcinogens as playing a role in the origin of colon and rectal malignant neoplasms. This work is in an early stage and is "interesting" but not in any way conclusive.

Spratt and Ackermann[7] are to be congratulated on their work in 1958 concerning the de novo origin of colon and rectal cancer. Their work promoted the huge volume of research that is still in progress and has conclusively proved that all cancers of the colon develop in benign adenomatous, villous, or adenovillous polyps. Therefore, early discovery and eradication of premalignant tumors of the rectum and colon provide an unusual opportunity for preventing a malignancy from developing. Routine proctoscopy annually is essential for all patients 40 years of age or older.

Cancer of the colon must be cured, not tomorrow but today, and it can be if physicians utilize the following methods:

1. Aggressive educational programs for physicians and the general public, pointing out the importance of regular examination of asymptomatic persons older than 40 years of age and the necessity for immediately reporting anorectal and colon symptoms at any age.

2. Early and appropriate use of all available diagnostic tools by the physician, including:

    a. History and physical examination.

    b. Rectal examination.

    c. Proctoscopic examination.

    d. Stool examination for occult blood. If positive, recheck two stools when the patient is on a meat-free diet. If results are still positive, even without symptoms of bleeding, a barium enema examination must be done.

    e. Barium enema examination—plain or with air.

    f. Colonoscopic examination for diagnosis and treatment.

    g. Blood studies:

      (1) CBC.

      (2) Sequential multiple analysis (SMA–12) screening.

      (3) Blood CEA.

    h. Various nuclear scans:

      (1) Liver.

      (2) Bone.

      (3) Lung.

      (4) Total body.

3. Early and appropriate treatment once the diagnosis is made:

    a. Polyps:

      (1) Eradication by use of proctoscopic, colonoscopic, or abdominal surgery.

      (2) Regular follow-up examination once a polyp is found.

    b. Aggressive treatment of cancer by combination therapy with the proper and appropriate use of surgery, x-ray therapy (cobalt or linear accelerator), and chemotherapy.

Treatment of cancer no longer consists of simply surgical removal of the lesion. This is now a multidisciplinary approach and provides not just alleviation of symptoms but a cure in many instances. "It is a whole new ball game," and the family physician, as the "leader of the team," must get in and stay in the ball game from the beginning to the end. He will certainly be expected to seek consultants in the fields of surgery, x-ray therapy, immunotherapy, and chemotherapy. Surgical and medical oncologists are available in most areas to advise about modalities of treatment. Surgeons should be working with these therapists.

Once the diagnosis of cancer of the colon, rectum, or anus is made, the patient is referred to an appropriate surgeon for definitive diagnosis and advice concerning therapy. Never refer a patient without first discussing the patient and his problem with the consultant. This will clear the way for intelligent interpretation of "what to tell the patient and the family." Early in the course of management, the patient and his family must be told the truth concerning the problem. Continuing, honest appraisal and discussion with the patient and his family will provide the type of cooperation needed for long-term management of the problem. Such communication will also lessen the chance for misunderstanding that can lead to a lawsuit. Once the diagnosis is made and the treatment is decided upon, informing the patient and his family as to the exact diagnosis is important. Whether you use the word "tumor," "malignancy," "cancer," or any other term, make sure that the family understands the seriousness of the disease. When using multidisciplinary treatment methods, reassure the patient optimistically rather than being pessimistic concerning the outcome of treatment. Many patients will believe that extra treatment with cobalt or treatment with chemicals is dangerous and that a case involving such treatment is hopeless. A new approach must be made that adds to the optimism rather than to the pessimism of the patient.

The family physician's role will vary according to his degree of involvement. If he assists in the surgery and follows up the patient postoperatively, understandably his role will be different than when the referral is total and the surgeon takes over treatment of the patient. Once surgery is completed, further treatment must be carefully discussed between the surgeon and the family physician, and a follow-up plan must be agreed upon and documented. Each member of the health care team must understand his role and the total approach to the management of the patient. *Surgical treatment is still the best curative treatment for cancer of the colon, rectum, and anus.*

If the surgeon believes the postoperative prognosis is excellent, which should be true in 75 per cent of the patients, no other type of adjunctive therapy is necessary, unless metastatic disease appears. Frequent follow-up visits by these patients during the first 12 to 18 months are essential. Recurrent disease, if diagnosed early, can be re-treated, and a cure can still be obtained. If the lesion was above the level visualized by the proctoscope, examination involving a barium enema study should be done 3 months postoperatively to serve as a base line. The patient should then be followed every 2 to 3 months. Complete physical examination, history, and blood studies (including CEA) should be recorded at every visit.

If the lesion was within range of the proctoscope, the anastomosis can be inspected regularly by proctoscopy. The patient must have a proctoscopic examination every 2 months for the first 12 months and every 4 months for the second 12 months. On each visit during these 2 years, a blood sample for a CEA determination is drawn. Although this blood test certainly is not a good screening test, it will probably prove to be an excellent test in determining recurrences. Any small rise in the CEA level found on these frequent studies should put one on guard.

If the pathology report on a surgically removed specimen reveals either lymph node metastasis or invasion by the tumor through the wall, even without lymph node metastasis, adjunctive therapy must be used. Chemotherapists and x-ray therapists should be consulted. The consultants must decide what the patient should be told. Once the type of therapy is decided, the consultants and the family physician should discuss it thoroughly with the patient and the family.

COLOSTOMY CARE

With the increasing incidence of colon cancer and the increasing use of abdominoperineal resection, the family physician will see more patients who have had colostomies. Although well-trained surgical supply house representatives and enterostomal therapists are available, the physician himself must know and be familiar with the method of colostomy care and with all of its possible complications. There are two important methods of colostomy management. One is the wearing of a bag that allows the patient's functions to be controlled by simply collecting the stool and emptying the bag. The other is the use of self-administered enemas. In a transverse colostomy or any colostomy that is proximal to the left or middle half of the transverse colon, liquid stool and irregular bowel movements will occur. Therefore, a properly fitting bag is the best method of treatment. Different types of bags are available, and the appliance dealer should certainly be allowed to fit the patient. Skin irritation is not uncommon with this type of colostomy. The best method for controlling skin irritation is the use of karaya (either paste or powder), applied liberally, and the wearing of a well-fitted colostomy appliance. A new type of skin protection available is Stomahesive, developed by the Squibb Pharmaceutical Company.

A colostomy in the descending or sigmoid colon is managed by daily or alternate-day enemas. Using appropriate enemas, the patient spends about 20 minutes in the bathroom every other day and does not have to wear any type of a bag at all. Occasionally, a small security pouch might be used. The device most helpful for irrigating the colostomy is one that fits the skin well and does not leak when water is instilled into the colostomy.

The following instructions are given to the patient concerning colostomy irrigation:

1. Maintain a comfortable position on the commode.

2. Hang the colostomy irrigation bag in a convenient location, so that it may be turned off and on easily. Use either a cone or a catheter in the colostomy. Gently instill approximately 1 quart of water into the colostomy.

3. If a cramp occurs, turn the water off and instill it more slowly.

The volume of stool expelled is *not important.* Many patients will state that they are not getting good irrigation when they do not have a large volume of stool. The important part of irrigation is not the quantity of stool but the comfort of the patient and the absence of leakage between enemas. The patient should be told, and it should be reiterated, that only 1 quart of water should be used and that the volume of stool obtained is not important, but rather that the comfort and the lack of leakage between irrigations are what really count.

In your particular city or area, an enterostomy group or an enterostomy therapist is probably available who can help a patient and change his attitude regarding his colostomy completely. This is an important part of postoperative care that must not be neglected. Part of your duty as a physician is to provide the patient with information relative to community resources available to him and his family for any problem that may exist.

ILEOSTOMY CARE

An ileostomy and an ileobladder require different care from that of a colostomy. A bag must be worn at all times, and skin care is important. One-half day of neglect of the skin surrounding an ileostomy can cause much aggravation for the patient. Family physicians who are not familiar with treating ileostomy patients are advised to seek the assistance of an enterostomal therapist or a physician who is knowledgeable about

assisting these patients. Various types of appliances are available, and the greatest improvement in ileostomy care is that in the development of appliances and skin-care products. Once the family physician discovers the ease with which a patient handles his ileostomy, he will be more at ease with the patient and more likely to suggest ileostomy for those with intractable disease somewhat earlier in the disease process

MISCELLANEOUS BOWEL DISORDERS

Bowel function is an important part of the health of all patients from the cradle to the grave. Mothers worry about their children's bowel habits. Such worry may create undue attention to bowel function on the part of the child and may further complicate matters. Adolescents usually do not worry about bowel function because they have other things to be concerned about, such as sexual problems and sexual development. However, somatic complaints do develop during adolescent illnesses, and bowel function is certainly one of the most prominent complaints. For patients over the age of 55 or 60 years who have a decreasing interest in many other pleasures, "a good bowel movement becomes one of the most important things in life."

FUNCTIONAL BOWEL DISORDERS

A great portion of a family physician's time will be spent treating patients with functional bowel disorders. Nothing can be more difficult and more time-consuming than the treatment of this syndrome. For centuries, people have been concerned about bowel disorders, and the 12th century physician Maimonides was said to have advised, "Man should always strive to have his intestines relaxed all the days of his life." We always counsel patients colloquially, "Don't get your bowels in an uproar." There is more truth than poetry in the latter statement, and, because of the frequency of functional bowel complaints, understanding something about their cause is important. "The extent of exact knowledge is inversely proportional to the verbosity of designations and the prolixity of pathogenesis." The present topic fits this rule, as is attested to by the following terms:

colitis, spastic colitis, mucous colitis, cathartic colitis, simple colitis, emotional diarrhea, irritable colon, unstable colon. Obviously none of these terms is entirely satisfactory, and the use of the term "colitis" should cease. The pathogenesis of this syndrome is unknown. Certain stimuli that cause patients to react by having functional bowel complaints are well recognized and occur with different intensity in different patients. These may vary from patient to patient and in the same patient from time to time. Taking an accurate history and listening to the patient are important, because factors such as diet, use of drugs, emotional reactions, allergies, mild congenital differences in the size of the small bowel, and angles of colon attachment could all be contributing influences in this disease.

As mentioned previously, a good portion of the family physician's practice will be concerned with treating the patient having a functional bowel disorder. Fifty per cent of patients seen in a gastroenterology clinic are found to exhibit functional bowel disorders of one type or another. Women outnumber men three to one in having this syndrome. The peak incidence of functional bowel disorders occurs in the fifth and sixth decades. However, children are frequently affected by this disorder as well.

The patient's complaints, in the order of frequency, are usually abdominal distress, erratic frequency of bowel function, and variation in the consistency of stools.

Abdominal distress consists of symptoms such as difficulty in swallowing, belching, flatulence, borborygmus, abdominal cramps, and passing flatus, which the patient will discuss in great detail. These patients are usually long-winded and are able to discuss their symptoms for hours on end. The more intelligent and the more educated the patient, the more long-winded the discussion will be about the various types of abdominal discomforts, and the physician must be prepared to listen and to interject questions concerning possible causes. As older women lose their spouses and become more and more interested in their own physical well-being and less interested in other activities, complaints of bowel disorders become more frequent.

Patients will spend much time in describing the consistency and character of stools, the inability to pass stool, and the relationship of food to the type of bowel movement they have. Bockus[8] provides a classic example in which a patient brought a picture of a toilet bowl containing his stool.[2] In taking a history, the physician must search for the major factors provoking or aggravating the distress. At the top of the list are emotional disturbances. The family physician has a great advantage over other specialists in treating this syndrome, as he is usually familiar with all of the family's problems and can quickly identify the cause of the episodes described by the patient. The physician must be a good listener.

A complete history must be taken of surgical procedures, allergies, and emotional problems, among others. Physical examination is important, but there are no physical findings pathognomonic of functional bowel disorder. In thin patients, tenderness, distention, or both, of the small bowel, resulting from swallowed air, may be noted. When the abdomen is percussed and gas is found, the patient will say, "You see, there it is." Scars from previous abdominal surgery will probably be found in this type of patient. Pelvic, rectal, and proctosigmoidoscopic examinations are necessary to rule out organic disease. It is essential to use x-ray and laboratory aids judiciously. A baseline gastrointestinal series and small bowel, barium enema, and gallbladder x-ray studies are essential. CBC, multiple biochemical survey, and urinalysis must also be done. The x-ray films must be studied carefully by the physician, because small defects such as hiatal hernia or spasm of the duodenum or sigmoid colon frequently may exist. The patient may have a few diverticula and may display some gallbladder dysfunction without stones. Appropriate repeated x-ray examination of the most important areas may be necessary to rule out organic disease.

Treatment. Once organic disease has been ruled out, appropriate sedatives, antispasmodics, and laxatives must be used and "juggled" to relieve the patient's symptoms. Simultaneously, a more in-depth psychosocial history should be undertaken, and if emotional problems are discovered, appropriate therapy should be instituted. Follow-up visits every 2 weeks for the first several visits, then every month, and finally every several months will certainly be necessary to control the patient's symptoms and to work toward an eventual cure. An easy solution is not available. Such patients will certainly take a great deal of time, but that is unavoidable.

CONSTIPATION

Physicians, as well as patients, should understand what is meant by the term "constipation." Constipation is infrequent or difficult evacuation of feces. There are three types of bowel problems that may be interpreted as forms of constipation: (1) when no urge occurs for the bowels to move, (2) when the stool is either too large or too firm, and (3) when, because of insufficient bulk in the diet, an inadequate amount of stool exists to initiate a normal bowel movement.

From the history, one should be able to determine which of the three types of constipation exists. One should also be able to determine whether the possibility of a true organic cause for the constipation is great or small. Make sure the patient understands the question, "Have your bowel habits changed?" Is there any difference from 1 year ago, from 1 month ago, or from 1 week ago is what is meant. Another important question is, "Has any change occurred in your dietary habits?" In the younger age group, the patient diets to reduce weight and consequently eats less bulk and a lesser quantity of food. When he skips bowel movements or goes for days without having a bowel movement, he thinks that the cause is bowel dysfunction rather than a decrease in food intake. Older persons, particularly those living alone or cooking for themselves, usually eat less frequently. Usually they have fewer bowel movements also.

Although there may be scientific data to prove that constipation cannot cause systemic symptoms, the patient may feel bloated or full. If he has a fecal impaction, he may have rectal pressure. However, symptoms such as "toxic feelings," headache, nausea (not related to obstruction), a tired feeling, and an inability to walk around or work are complaints some patients believe are caused by constipation. This misconception has been taught them by their mothers or grandmothers who, in turn, had been told this by physicians in years gone by.

A complete physical examination is necessary. Special attention to anal, rectal, and proctoscopic examinations performed on a well-prepared patient is essential. During such proctoscopic examination, one frequently encounters a dark mahogany color of the colon. This is caused by melanosis coli, a condition resulting from excessive use of laxatives containing methylanthraquinone, which is found in senna, cascara, and aloe. A pigment is deposited in the mononuclear cells in the mucous membrane, causing this coloration. Melanosis coli has no other clinical significance and will disappear in time, when the laxatives are discontinued.

For women, rectovaginal examination is important. A thin rectovaginal septum with a relatively normal anal sphincter is a common cause of constipation.

If the patient has not had a barium enema examination within 12 months, a plain barium enema with good postevacuation films should be done. The history should be supplied to the radiologist to assist him in the interpretation of these studies.

Treatment. Once all organic causes, such as obstructing malignancy, diverticular disease, volvulus or adhesion, and extrarectal tumors are ruled out, treatment can be instituted according to the type of constipation existing. Treatment for patients who have a normal food intake, including normal amounts of bulk, consists of giving stimulant laxatives, such as milk of magnesia, senna concentrate (Senokot), phenolphthalein (Prulets), or danthron (Modane). These should be given at appropriate times, such as every other day or every third day, starting with small doses and then increasing the amounts until the desired results are obtained. If the patient is too busy to have an early morning bowel movement, it is perfectly permissible to give stimulant laxatives in the morning, so that the urge for a bowl movement will be in the evening, after supper or later.

If a normal urge but hard stools exist, stool softeners such as dioctyl calcium sulfosuccinate (Surfak) or mineral oil may be used. Kondremul, which is an emulsion of a bulk product and mineral oil, is also an excellent softener. Prolonged use of such softeners is permissible and will not limit vitamin or protein intake.

Many patients who need bulk should be put on high-residue diets plus the use of bulk laxatives, such as psyllium hydrophilic mucilloid (L.A. formula, Konsyl, or Metamucil) or dioctyl sodium sulfosuccinate (Dialose plain capsules).

A "shotgun" approach, using a combination medicine that contains softeners, bulk, and stimulants all in one capsule or in a one teaspoon dose, should not be used. No remedy is so good that it can be used for every patient, and only by thorough history and proctologic evaluation can most patients having constipation be relieved.

Occasionally, one or more patients—depending on the volume of the geriatric population being treated by the family physician—will require enemas. An occasional tap water or a sodium biphosphate-sodium phosphate (Fleet) enema is satisfactory for the average patient. When a patient who has been taking enemas for many years is seen for the first time, it is not necessary to stop such use. You are required, however, to rule out all organic causes that might necessitate this practice. Once that is done, the patient can be convinced that a small enema is all right, and he will be satisfied.

FECAL IMPACTION

Fecal impaction, which occurs in all types of practices and in all types of patients, is painful and uncomfortable. The patient first complains of having had no bowel movement for many days, and then, before having severe discomfort, he may complain of having diarrhea. If the patient is not examined at that time and only a history is taken, medications such as diphenoxylate with atropine (Lomotil) or paregoric must not be prescribed, as the condition will become worse. The patient will become extremely uncomfortable and will complain of inability to pass any stool but will still have some leakage on his underclothes. Diagnosis is easily made by digital examination of the rectum. The bulk of the fecal impaction will depend on the diet and on the number of days since the patient had a bowel movement. Although most of these patients are in the geriatric age group, the condition may also occur in children. Patients on prolonged bed rest for any reason, those with back pain, and those on antispasmodics and antacids should be watched closely for fecal impaction.

Treatment. Treatment is prophylactic and consists of appropriate measures to keep the stool soft. Also, at the first sign of change in bowel habits, a rectal examination should be done. Once the condition develops, the following measures may become necessary: In mild cases, oil instillations will be all that is needed. The canal becomes lubricated, and the stool passes with difficulty, but the patient obtains immediate relief. In difficult cases, the patient must be treated by digital manipulation and by "breaking up" the firm stool. Should the impaction be higher than the finger can reach, a large Foley catheter (No. 30 to 34) should be inserted and used as an instrument to assist in breaking up the impaction. By means of a large syringe, mineral oil can be instilled through the catheter and around the impacted feces. Digital manipulation of the stool, mineral oil instillation, and, later, a tap water enema usually bring relief. Occasionally, impactions will occur higher than the rectum and will occupy the sigmoid as well. Therefore, the patient should be re-examined daily for several days to be sure that continued impaction does not exist.

The physician must examine the patient and do the initial manipulation of the huge bolus of stool. Later, manipulations with large catheters and enemas may be done by the nurse.

Once the impaction is relieved, the patient must be given stool softeners, such as mineral oil or Kondremul, and possibly stimulant laxatives, so that recurrent impactions do not occur. Proctoscopy should be performed as soon as feasible to rule out the presence of organic disease. The patient should also be observed for several weeks or months to assure that no recurrent impactions occur. Do not neglect these patients; fecal impaction is one of the most uncomfortable feelings that exist. These patients will be eternally grateful for your support and management of this problem.

DIARRHEA

In dealing with this symptom, the patient and the physician must understand and agree on the definition of the term "diarrhea." True diarrhea means the passage of liquid or watery bowel movement from the anal canal. That is simple enough. Many patients will insist that they have diarrhea, but when questioned carefully, they are found to be having semi-solid frequent stools. The condition they describe is certainly urgent and not normal, but it is not true diarrhea. Certain patients with acute and chronic diarrhea will have three to four large liquid stools a day. Others may have 10 to 15 episodes of passing small amounts (a tablespoonful or cupful) of mucus or of liquid stool with or without blood. Such passage is a frequent symptom in true ulcerative colitis or proctitis. A patient may complain of diarrhea occurring 20 times a day, and yet he may come in looking perfectly normal and not appearing dehydrated. The patient is having small amounts of liquid stools frequently or small amounts of mucus frequently. Therefore, the history is probably the most important factor in the diagnosis and treatment of diarrhea.

For this discussion, seven categories of diarrhea will be used, including diarrhea caused by:

1. Viruses.
2. Bacteria.
3. Toxins and endotoxins.
4. Parasites.
5. Intrinsic disease of the gastrointestinal tract.
6. Functional disorders.
7. Pseudomembranous colitis.

In most cases of diarrhea, the history presented by the patient concerning onset, severity, duration, and character of the stools should aid in narrowing down the diagnosis. Viral diarrheas tend to be epidemic. Food poisoning generally involves having more than one person with the same history and symptoms. Patients with true bacterial diarrheas usually present with fever and systemic complaints. Parasitic infections and functional diarrheas are generally recurrent. Pseudomembranous colitis is always preceded by the patient's receiving antibiotic therapy.

Treatment. Simple diarrhea without systemic complaints should be treated with fluids and rest. No attempt should be made to decrease bowel motility, and no antibiotics should be prescribed. Reliable evidence shows that either of these treatments may prolong or increase the severity of the disease, or both.

Any patient who has diarrhea that persists for more than a few days or who develops severe systemic symptoms should be hospitalized for a complete work-up, including proctoscopic examination, stool cultures, Gram's stains, and studies for ova, cysts, and parasites. Barium enema examination may be indicated in some instances. It is important to arrive at a diagnosis before beginning other than supportive therapy.

PROCTALGIA FUGAX

This syndrome is characterized by an excruciating pain high in the rectum or low in the pelvis, usually waking the patient at night from a sound sleep. It is described as a lower abdominal or upper rectal aching, not in the skin and not in the pelvis. The patients try all positions to relieve the pain. Many will take enemas, sit in warm tub baths, and use various suppositories. The duration of the pain varies from 5 seconds to 30 or 40 minutes. It is essential to rule out organic causes in these patients before making this diagnosis. In women, one must rule out pelvic inflammations or tumors, cystitis, urethritis, endometriosis, ureteral stones or disease, and adhesions from previous surgery. In men, prostatitis and diverticulitis are the most common causes of such pain. Once organic disease has been ruled out, a diagnosis of proctalgia fugax is made by elimination. The disease is thought to be caused by spasm of the levator ani muscle, spasm of the rectal musculature, or both. It is not a life-threatening disease and is usually self-limiting. Emotional stress seems to play an important role in this disorder.

Treatment. Treatment is difficult. One must first use appropriate diagnostic studies to rule out organic disease in the mind of both the patient and the physician. Once this is done, if the problem still exists, a more in-depth psychosocial history should be obtained. It is amazing to find how often the patient is totally unaware of any emotional stress that might be associated with this disorder. Forms of treatment that have been helpful include warm baths, nitroglycerin, chlordiazepoxide-clidinium (Librax) or diazepam (Valium), and analgesic suppositories. Once the patient is convinced that he has no organic disease and once the emotional stress is resolved, the problem often disappears.

Although proctalgia fugax can be a distressing and severely painful disease, it occurs infrequently and usually presents no major problem.

PRURITUS ANI

This term, which describes a symptom rather than an organic disease, means anal itching. The symptom is described separately becuuse it is an important complaint that occurs both alone, without any other anal symptoms, and together with all other anal symptoms.

Twenty years ago, about 10 to 20 per cent of anal pruritus was believed to be idiopathic, and all sorts of descriptions and chapters were written about elaborate operations and methods of treatment for the intractable cases. More time and space have been given to the idiopathic and the intractable cases than to the more usual forms. Because cases involving unknown diagnosis and difficult treatment are less than 5 per cent of the total, emphasis will be on the more common causes.

History. The usual complete proctologic and general histories are taken with concentration in the following areas:

1. *Relationship to time:* How long has the itching been present? Is it constant or intermittent? Is it chronic (duration)?

2. *Relationship to season of year:* Whether the condition is worse during the winter or the summer is important, because most fungus diseases are more severe during warm weather, and sensitivity to wool clothes or wool underwear is a cold weather problem.

3. *Relationship to peers, to other family members, or both:* Do his peers or other family members have the same symptoms? Certain contagious diseases such as scabies and pinworms should be suspected in such instances.

4. *Relationship to medical history:* Any history of diabetes mellitus, jaundice, or other diseases that might produce itching should be considered.

5. *Relationship to accompanying anal symptoms:* Is itching a predominant symptom, or does the patient have other complaints, such as bleeding, discharge, or pain that might indicate other pathology?

6. *Relationship to medications:* What medications have been used, and did they relieve the symptoms or make them worse? Mild anal irritation can be aggravated by allergic reactions or by overmedication.

7. *Relationship to treatment by other physicians:* If there is a history of involvement with other physicians, they may be consulted about the patient's previous medications. If the patient has seen another specialist, such as a dermatologist or gynecologist, then certainly a combined regimen established by the family physician and the other specialist is important. The names of physicians who treated the patient previously are essential.

Examination. Examination of the entire body for evidence of scratching in areas other than the anus may produce evidence of conditions such as scabies, body lice, or psoriasis.

For examination of the anal area, the patient must be in a comfortable position. The knee-chest or Sims's position is recommended, or when a woman is undergoing a pelvic examination, the lithotomy position is acceptable. A good light is important for determining the degree of inflammation and for seeing small defects. Before digital examination is performed, inspection is essential. Occasionally, an immediate diagnosis or a partial diagnosis is made by the presence of a small pinworm on the anal skin. The Scotch-tape test for pinworms and a stool analysis for ova, cysts, and parasites should be done. Patients who have acute itching and whose anal and perianal skin is inflamed, edematous, ulcerative, or swollen should not be examined beyond the initial inspection. In such severe cases, nothing is gained by forcing a digital or anoscopic examination, or both. Initial therapy should consist of Burow's solution (Domeboro) compresses, bed rest, application of dressings or soft cotton to the anal area to prevent chafing, and the use of steroid ointments or creams and antibiotic ointments to relieve the acute inflammation. After several days of this therapy, the patient should return for re-evaluation. During the patient's return visit, careful digital, anoscopic, and proctoscopic examinations are performed, and a thorough search for the causative agent is made.

These examinations will rule out anal fissures, prolapsed hemorrhoids, proctitis, or inflamed mucous membranes that could be the causative agents. Proctoscopy is essential for diagnosing proctitis, parasitic infections, or diseases above the anal canal that might be causing itching.

Laboratory Data. Stool examination for ova, cysts, and parasites, and cultures for idiopathic organisms or fungus are also important in diagnosis, particularly in problem cases.

Barium enema examination, gastrointestinal series, and small bowel examination may be necessary to rule out other organic diseases that may be causing the symptoms.

Treatment. Supportive treatment with compresses, steroid ointments or creams, soft dressings for absorption of moisture, and rest generally provides some relief and will cure 50 per cent of the patients. Definitive management in the remaining 50 per cent of the patients will depend on a correct diagnosis followed by appropriate therapy directed toward the specific causative agents. The most common causes are organic anal disease, pinworms, and fungus infection.

HIDRADENITIS SUPPURATIVA

This is an infection of the skin and subcutaneous tissue of the perianal area. It also occurs in the inguinal region and the axillae, but all of these regions are not necessarily affected in the same patient. Once the physician has seen a previous case, the diagnosis is not difficult to make. It is most often mistaken for fistula-in-ano. Any patient who has recurrent, multiple abscesses on the buttocks or in the perianal region should be considered to have this disease until proved otherwise. The abscesses occur insidiously within the skin and subcutaneous tissue and, when drained, heal adequately. At first the abscesses are individual, but later they coalesce, form sinuses and indurated scar tissue, and become difficult to heal. The diagnosis is easily made when the patient has repeated abscesses, as the skin becomes more and more indurated and is characteristically packed. This is a rare disease, but when it occurs, it can be difficult to treat.

Treatment. Treatment consists of incision and drainage of the abscesses when they occur and prophylactic use of hexachlorophene detergent (pHisoHex or Dial soap) to decrease the bacterial content on the skin in this area. Occasionally, when the condition is recurrent and severe, excision of this area with skin grafting may be necessary.

PILONIDAL DISEASE

Any inflammation, draining sinus, or abscess of the sacrum or coccyx that is not drained into the anal canal is a pilonidal cyst, abscess, or sinus. Formerly, these were thought to be congenital, but proof is now available that they are acquired in most patients. Today, there is available clinical and pathologic evidence that hair is forced intradermally and subdermally to produce pilonidal disease.

Treatment. All patients with pilonidal disease must be treated surgically. There are three predominant methods of treatment: excision with primary closure, incision or excision with open packing, and incision with marsupialization or exteriorization—the latter method being preferred by us. Small sinuses can be treated by using office procedures under local anesthesia. The sinuses are simply incised and drained. However, they must be followed up at weekly intervals to prevent premature closure until wound healing is complete. Larger abscesses, complicated sinuses, or both, are treated in the operating room under general anesthesia. Each one is exteriorized and not excised. Exteriorization consists of determining the extent of the cyst cavity, and of all of its ramifications and of opening them. The wounds are then marsupialized with a continuous locking chromic 00 suture. It is a method that provides adequate drainage, conserves tissue, and requires only simple postoperative care. This more conservative approach has a much lower morbidity and allows the patient to return to full activity at an earlier date.

VENEREAL DISEASES OF THE ANORECTUM

When dealing with problems of the anorectal area, one should be ever alert to the possibility of venereal diseases. If a hard, painless, indolent ulcer with a firm, raised border is found, one should suspect the presence of a luetic chancre. Multiple small ulcers coalescing in the perianal area with accompanying inguinal lymphadenopathy should alert one to the possibility of anal chancroid. Extensive scarring and stricture formation in the anus and rectum in the female may be evidence of lymphogranuloma venereum. The Frei test should be used for confirmation. Mild-to-severe proctitis in the sexually active male or female may be caused by *Neisseria gonorrhoeae*. In the office, the use of Thayer-Martin media for culture is an important adjunct in the diagnosis of this condition. Once the diagnosis is confirmed, appropriate antibiotic therapy should be instituted.

Condyloma Acuminatum

Condyloma acuminatum, also called anal or venereal warts, is becoming more and more common. These papillomatous growths occur in the perianal skin and also on the mucous membrane, as high as 1 to 2 cm. above the dentate line. From 75 to 80 per cent of these growths are caused and spread by anal intercourse. The only symptoms may be warty growths, severe itching, frequent bleeding, and soreness. The lesions are characteristically reddish-pink, soft protuberances that are cauliflower-shaped and may be friable and moist. They can be difficult to cure.

Diagnostic studies should always include a test for syphilis. Condyloma acuminatum and the anogenital papule caused by secondary syphilis can be difficult to differentiate clinically. Treatment of condyloma acuminatum consists of podophyllum in mineral oil applied by the physician directly on the lesions, with the normal skin protected. After each individual application, the solution is left on the lesions for 3 hours and then is thoroughly washed off. It may be applied at weekly intervals and will be sufficient to eradicate the small, localized warts. To prevent recurrences, the area must be kept dry and if anal intercourse causes recurrence, this practice must be discontinued. Patients with condyloma acuminatum must be thoroughly examined, and the area above the dentate line must be carefully inspected. If the lesions on the mucous membrane within the anal canal are not treated also, the condition will recur. If the lesions are multiple and extend above the dentate line, electrosurgical coagulation with use of a general or a local anesthetic may be the only treatment advised. In many patients, even those undergoing electrosurgical cauterization, recurrences are frequent.

The patient must be informed that the lesions, although not malignant, are difficult to treat and require constant observation for many months with continuous therapy.

Other measures, such as bichloracetic acid applications, freezing techniques, and autogenous vaccines, have all been used. Topical treatments are successful if the physician and the patient both persist in the treatment.

CARCINOID OF THE RECTUM

Carcinoid of the rectum, although unusual, is an easily recognizable but significant finding. It can appear in any area of the rectum and is a submucosal deposit of argentaffin cells that have a characteristic yellow color. They might be mistaken for polyps, but because of the distinctive color and because they are firmer than polyps and are submucosal, they should be distinguishable. They are usually small, varying from 0.5 to 1 mm. in size, but can become large. When they are larger than 1.5 cm. in diameter, they are generally considered to be malignant. Ulcerations in the center are also a characteristic sign of malignancy. It is sufficient for the examining physician to recognize these lesions and to refer the patient immediately to a colon and rectal surgeon for appropriate treatment.

DIAGNOSIS AND TREATMENT OF CHILDREN WITH ANORECTAL DISEASE

The symptoms that bring infants and children to your office are usually limited to constipation, rectal bleeding, and anal pain. In a study performed by Levin on 250 private patients under the age of 12 years, the presenting symptom in 85 per cent of these patients was constipation. To most of the mothers, the constipation meant no bowel movement for at least 3 to 5 days, and when the patient had a bowel movement, it was painful. Careful histories often reveal that these patients are not as much disturbed by this symptom as are the parents. The other major symptom in conjunction with inability to have bowel movements is the constant soiling of underclothes. This sign may occur about the time the child has begun to be toilet-trained. Careful examination to rule out organic disease is necessary in such children. Once the problem is identified, it is important to encourage the child to try to have a bowel movement daily, at a time when the mother is not too busy. Stool softeners such as mineral oil may be helpful. Stimulant laxatives such as senna concentrate (Senokot) granules may also be of benefit.

The second most common symptom in children is that of pain during a bowel movement. During an episode of constipation or diarrhea, the child tears the anal canal, and this becomes tender. Then a vicious cycle begins. The child has pain and does not want to have a bowel movement, which results in a hard stool that eventually reinjures the anal canal. Many times the child will come to the office, the anal fissure will be healed, and yet the same symptoms persist. This is a postfissure syndrome. The child remembers the pain he had and delays having a bowel movement, which again results in hard stools and reinjury of the anal canal. Thus, the cycle starts over again. The judicious use of stool softeners and analgesic ointments is usually sufficient to remedy the situation.

The third symptom is bleeding. Usually bright red and not of an alarming amount, the blood occurs on the diaper or, in an older child, on the toilet tissue or in the toilet bowl. It occurs with bowel movements and may happen at any age. The most common cause in these patients is anal fissure.

Another cause in the differential diagnosis of rectal bleeding in children, besides anal fissure, is a juvenile polyp. These are benign and easily removed. The treatment of juvenile polyps should include use of an anesthetic and examination by proctoscopy or colonoscopy with snaring of the polyps. Removal of these polyps by either method is an acceptable procedure and will make laparotomy for polypectomy a thing of the past.

In older children with rectal bleeding, such as those between the ages of 8 and 12 years, it is important to consider a diagnosis of ulcerative colitis.

Children with any of these symptoms should be examined carefully; in the great majority of them, proctoscopic examination for a distance of about 10 to 12 cm. is relatively easily done. Only in rare instances should proctoscopy with use of anesthesia be necessary, as when the child is uncooperative or unmanageable and a

diagnosis is difficult. The diagnosis is usually easy to make without proctoscopy, and with the incidence of malignancy being practically zero in this age group, it is not necessary to subject the child to the dangers of a general anesthetic in most instances. Should the bleeding persist, a barium enema study may be necessary.

Hirschsprung's Megacolon (Disease). All patients with chronic constipation should be thoroughly evaluated, and those patients for whom the diagnosis is doubtful should be referred to a pediatric surgeon or a general surgeon for evaluation. The characteristic patient with this disease is an emaciated, pot-bellied child who complains of constipation although his rectum is found to be empty. It is unusual for a child to have encopresis and to have megacolon.

Anal Stenosis in the Newborn. Although rare, true incomplete anal stenosis in the newborn will usually respond to two or three digital dilatations by the physician. The presence of a true imperforate anus should be diagnosed during the initial examination of the newborn, and the patient should immediately be referred to a surgeon for appropriate treatment.

REFERENCES

1. `Behringer, G. E.: Changing concepts in histopathologic diagnosis of polypoid lesions of the colon. Dis. Colon Rectum, 13:116, 1970.
2. Bockus, H. L. (ed.): Gastroenterology. 3d Ed., Vol. 3. Philadelphia, W. B. Saunders Co., 1974.
2a. Burkitt, D. P.: Epidemiology of cancer of the colon and rectum. Cancer, 28:3, 1973.
3. Fansler, W. A.: Causes of error in proctologic diagnosis and therapy. J. Lancet, 68:278, 1948.
4. Kellogg, C. S.: Diseases of the anus, rectum, and colon. In Conn, H. F., Rakel, R. E., and Johnson, T. W. (eds.): Family Practice. 1st Ed., Philadelphia, W. B. Saunders Co., 1973.
5. Nesselrod, J. P.: Clinical Proctology. Philadelphia, W. B. Saunders Co., 1964.
6. Rubin, P.: Current Concepts in Cancer, Introduction. In Cancer of the Gastrointestinal Tract. Amer. Cancer Soc., Inc., 1975.
7. Spratt, J. S. Jr., Ackerman, L. V., and Moyer, C. A.: Relationship of polyps of colon to colonic cancer. Ann. Surg., 148:682, 1958.
8. Sterns, W.: Prophylaxis of bowel. Cancer. J. Med. Soc. NJ, 51:415, 1954.

Chapter 44

PEDIATRICS

by JOHN E. ALLEN,
VYMUTT J. GURURAJ,
and RAYMOND M. RUSSO

A thorough knowledge of the principles of growth and development is the foundation upon which the health care of children is based. Growth is defined as an increase in the physical size of the child's body or any of its components and can be observed and measured in terms of inches or centimeters, pounds or kilograms. Development is a functional process, increasing in complexity and dexterity until the full potential of an individual's abilities is reached. The normal processes resulting in normal growth and development are powerful forces, yet genetic aberrations, malnutrition, a wide range of acute and chronic infections, endocrine abnormalities, psychologic problems, or a noxious environment may result in significant deviations. Interpretation of charts, tables, and schedules depicting "normal" rates of growth and development must be carefully individualized for each child. The family physician, by utilizing his knowledge of growth and development, should join with parents, teachers, and other professionals to see that each child has the opportunity to reach his full potential.

The examination of the child differs from that of the adult, and techniques must be adapted to the degree of cooperation of the child. The variation between normal and abnormal may be subtle, particularly in the infant. A thorough physical examination should be done with the child completely undressed, regardless of the presenting complaint. The physician should examine those body areas last to which the patient will object most often, in order to avoid excessive concern and resistance.

THE NEWBORN

THE EVALUATION OF THE NEWBORN

A quick and reliable assessment of the status of the newborn can be made by using a numerical scoring system described by Virginia Apgar. The score has a significant correlation with morbidity and mortality during the newborn period. The Apgar score is the sum total of five individual scores, on a scale of 0 to 2, assigned to five objective signs (Table 44–1). The score is documented at 1 minute and at 5 minutes after the birth by an observer other than the physician who delivered the baby. The closer the score is to 10, the better the general status of the child and the prognosis. Generally a score between 8 and 10 signifies a normal, healthy infant.

The next step in the evaluation of the newborn is an assessment of the gestational age of the infant. This assessment is important, as it enables one to determine if the body measurements, such as the height and weight, are consistent with the postconceptual age of the infant. An inconsistency signifies a deviation from normal intrauterine growth. Although an approximate estimation of gestational age can be made by the obstetric history, the more accurate method is by noting certain physical and neurologic signs in the newborn (Fig. 44–1). By correlating these findings with the birth weight, one can classify newborns into three categories: normal for gestational age, small for gestational age, and large for gestational age. The gestational age also defines three other important categories

TABLE 44–1. APGAR SCORE

Sign	0	1	2
Heart rate	Absent	Slow	Over 100
Respiratory effort	Absent	Slow, irregular	Good, crying
Muscle tone	Limp	Some flexion of extremities	Active motion
Reflex irritability	No response	Grimace	Cry
Color	Blue, pale	Body pink, extremities blue	Completely pink

into which infants are placed. Those infants with a gestational age less than 37 weeks are classified as premature, those with a gestational age greater than 41 weeks as postmature, and those in between as term infants. Unlike former classification, weight is not considered.

Because the old classification termed all infants weighing less than 2500 grams premature, it must be stressed that a clear distinction should be drawn between a true premature infant (born before 37 weeks of gestation) and a term infant, both of whom weigh less than 2500 grams. The latter infant is the typical small-for-gestational-age newborn. This distinction is important because the immediate neonatal and perhaps long-term prognosis differs for these two categories of infants.

Small-for-Gestational-Age Infants

These infants are defined as newborns whose weight at birth is less than that

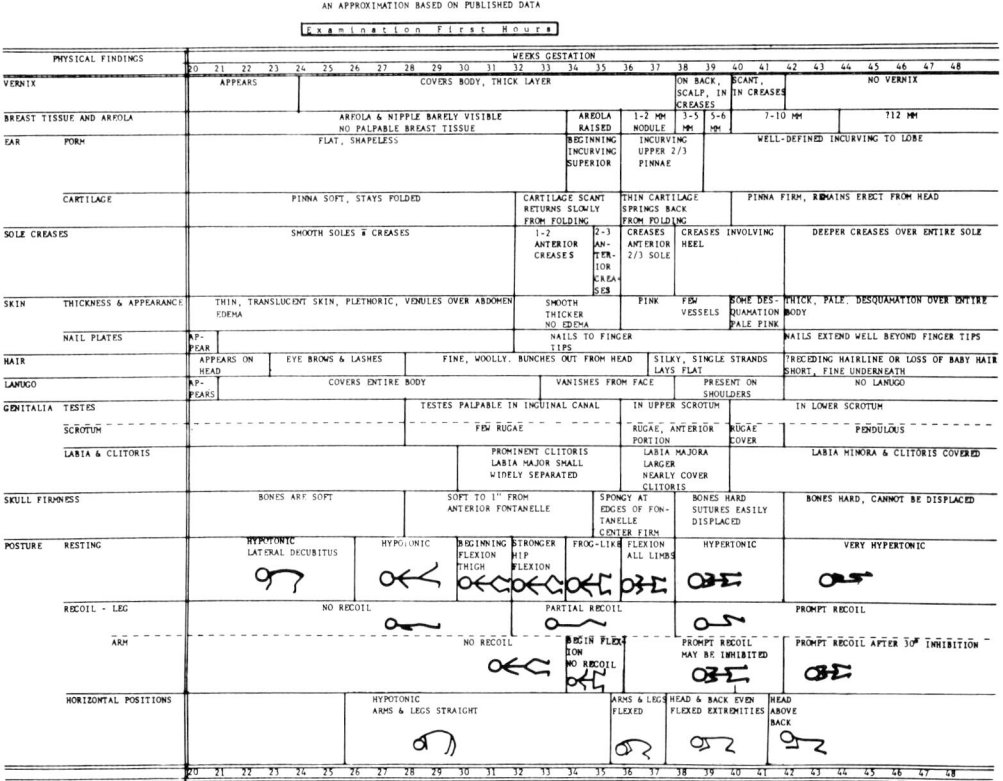

Figure 44–1. *A guide to the estimate of gestational age on the basis of physical and neurologic findings.* *(From Lubchenco, L. O.: Assessment of gestational age and development at birth. Pediatr. Clin. North Am., Vol. 17, No. 1, Feb., 1970.)*

predicted for the gestational age. The weight lag is attributed to an intrauterine growth retardation. This could be on the basis of an impaired uteroplacental support to the growing fetus or an intrinsic disorder of the fetus itself. Although fetal malnutrition exemplifies the former situation, newborns exposed to viral infection in utero or those having chromosomal aberrations are examples of the latter category. One should therefore obtain a careful prenatal history and also look for any congenital problems when examining these newborns. Hypoglycemia is noted in many of these infants, and early feedings are therefore recommended. If there are no associated congenital problems, the long-term prognosis seems to be generally good.

Large-for-Gestational-Age Infants

Babies born to diabetic mothers are often large for their age. However, with this exception, not much else is known about this category of infants. Prognosis is poor for those large babies who are born prematurely, particularly at 24 to 28 weeks of gestation.

Prematurity

As mentioned before, infants with a gestational age of less than 37 weeks are termed premature. Many factors are associated with prematurity. Among the maternal factors thought to cause premature birth are toxemias of pregnancy, age less than 16 or more than 35 years, repeated pregnancies, cigarette smoking, narcotic addiction, and a number of chronic illnesses. Premature births are particularly common among lower socioeconomic populations.

Physical and neurologic examinations of a premature infant reveal findings consistent with the gestational age. A crown-heel length of less than 47 cm. and a crown-rump length of less than 32 cm. are usually characteristic. The head and chest circumferences are less than 33 and 30 cm., respectively.

The management of premature infants includes maintenance of normal body temperature, administration of adequate oxygen in hypoxic infants, and maintenance of adequate nutrition.

Because these infants have difficulty in conserving their body heat, supplemental incubator heat is necessary to maintain a normal body temperature. The goal is to maintain a skin temperature of 36° C. An incubator air temperature between 33 and 36° C. at a relative humidity between 40 and 46 per cent will usually accomplish this. Oxygen need not be administered routinely. When supplemental oxygen is given, careful monitoring of arterial oxygen tension is necessary, as increased oxygen tension (60 to 100 mm. Hg) is associated with retrolental fibroplasia. Unless specially indicated, it is best not to exceed an oxygen concentration of greater than 40 per cent in the ordinary management of a premature infant.

Early feeding (4 to 8 hours after birth) is generally recommended, not only to provide the needed calories but also to reduce the dangers of hyperbilirubinemia and hypoglycemia. The amount of fluid per feeding depends on the general condition of the child and on his ability to take and retain feedings. Usually, small amounts (4 to 6 ml.) of glucose water are given for one to two feedings, then feeding is switched to a regular formula. The amount is increased by 1 to 2 ml. per feeding until a total of 140 to 160 ml. per kg. per day is reached, providing between 120 and 150 calories per kg. per day. Very small infants may have to be tube fed and sometimes may require intravenous fluids. Supplementation with iron (10 to 15 mg. of elemental iron per day) and with vitamins A, C, and D is generally recommended.

Postmaturity

Placental dysfunction is often associated with postmaturity. Clinical features include an absence of vernix caseosa and long nails and dry skin. Unless the postmaturity exceeds 3 weeks, the prognosis is generally excellent.

JAUNDICE IN THE NEWBORN

Most infants develop physiologic jaundice during the first week of life. The jaundice is due to an accumulation of unconjugated bilirubin that fails to become conjugated and is not excreted rapidly enough by the liver. The jaundice does not usually appear before the infant is 24 hours

TABLE 44–2. SOME COMMON CAUSES OF JAUNDICE DURING THE FIRST WEEK OF LIFE

Diagnosis	Clinical and Laboratory Data
Physiologic Jaundice	Observed 2 to 4 days after birth. Elevated indirect serum bilirubin. Peak 12 to 14 mg.
Hemolytic Diseases Rh incompatibility	Onset usually within 24 hours. Hepatosplenomegaly. Petechiae. Rh negative mother. Rh positive infant. Anemia with reticulocytosis. Positive Coombs' test. Elevated indirect serum bilirubin. Nucleated red cells in peripheral blood smear.
ABO incompatibility	Jaundice appears within 24 hours. Mild anemia and hepatosplenomegaly. Mother—0 blood group, and infant—either A or B group. Anemia with reticulocytosis. Peripheral blood smear reveals microcytosis and nucleated red cells. Elevated indirect serum bilirubin.
Congenital spherocytosis	Anemia and splenomegaly. Spherocytes on peripheral blood smear. Elevated indirect serum bilirubin. Coombs' test negative.
Infections Bacterial sepsis	Symptoms of sepsis, e.g., fever, vomiting, irritability, hepatosplenomegaly, indirect serum bilirubin elevated, positive cultures, and so forth.
Viral infection, e.g., rubella, cytomegalovirus infections	Low birth weight infants. Petechiae, hepatosplenomegaly. Both direct and indirect serum bilirubin elevated. Diminished platelets, congenital anomalies (rubella). Chorioretinitis (cytomegalovirus infections).
Neonatal hepatitis	Jaundice may be present at birth. Males outnumber females. Hepatomegaly. Both direct and indirect serum bilirubin elevated. Elevated SGOT and SGPT levels.
Biliary atresia	Jaundice usually appears late. Females outnumber males. Laboratory findings same as in hepatitis.

Other causes of jaundice in the first week: hemolytic disease due to red cell enzyme deficiency, e.g., glucose 6-phosphate dehydrogenase deficiency; infantile pyknocytosis; enclosed hemorrhage (cephalohematoma); drug-related jaundice.

old. The bilirubin levels may reach as high as 10 to 12 mg. per 100 ml., and icterus may last as long as 10 to 14 days. A greater accumulation may occur in premature infants. Physiologic jaundice should be distinguished from other causes of jaundice in the newborn (Table 44–2). Blood group incompatibilities (Rh and ABO) are the most common causes of nonphysiologic jaundice (see page 881).

Most of the unconjugated bilirubin remains in the blood bound to albumin. When albumin-binding sites become saturated, the unbound bilirubin diffuses into the body tissues. Diffusion into the central nervous system causes the clinical syndrome termed kernicterus in some infants. The syndrome is characterized by convulsions, rigidity, and opisthotonos. Infants who survive often show either frank or subtle signs of brain damage. Factors that predispose an infant to develop kernicterus include low levels of serum albumin (in premature infants); the presence of substances in the blood that compete with bilirubin for albumin-binding sites (e. g., sulfonamides, unesterified fatty acids, and so forth), hypoxia, and acidosis.

The work-up of an infant with jaundice includes:

1. An estimation of serum bilirubin levels, both direct and indirect. Repeated estimations must be made to assess the rate of accumulation.

2. Rh and blood grouping of both the infant and the mother.

3. An estimation of hemoglobin levels and a thorough examination of the peripheral blood smear.

4. Direct and indirect Coombs' testing.

5. If sepsis is suspected, appropriate cultures of blood, urine, and cerebrospinal fluid (CSF) should be obtained. If viral infection is a consideration, viral studies should be done.

6. If excessive hemolysis is causing the jaundice, without any evidence of obvious blood group incompatibilities, red cell enzyme studies should be done.

Irrespective of the cause, the central consideration in the management of neonatal jaundice is the prevention of kernicterus. This is accomplished by keeping the serum bilirubin from reaching critically high levels (20 mg. per 100 ml.), by the use of phototherapy, exchange transfusions, or both.

INFECTIONS IN THE NEWBORN

Generalized bacterial infection of the newborn is a frequent consideration in the hospital nursery. The incidence of sepsis is approximately 1 per 1000 full-term infants and 1 per 250 premature infants. Sex, prematurity, perinatal factors, and functional immaturity of some of the bodily defense mechanisms are some of the predisposing factors. Because a high degree of morbidity and mortality is associated with sepsis, prompt diagnosis and treatment are essential. Diagnosis, however, may present difficulties because most of the clinical features are rather nonspecific.

Infants may manifest signs of sepsis either shortly after birth or a few days later. In the early-onset type, presumably the infection is acquired in utero, either by way of the placenta or by ingestion of infected amniotic fluid or vaginal secretions during birth. Some of the circumstances often associated with early sepsis are premature rupture of the membranes, extended difficult deliveries, and systemic or local (vaginal) maternal infections. Although gram-negative organisms such as *Escherichia coli*, *Klebsiella*, or enterococci are the usual pathogens, infections caused by streptococci are on the increase.

The organisms causing late sepsis include staphylococci, *Klebsiella*, and *Pseudomonas*. These organisms commonly contaminate nursery equipment, particularly in intensive care units. Some of these organisms, such as *Klebsiella*, not only are frequently cultured from this equipment but also have developed resistance to the commonly used antibiotics.

The presenting manifestations in most newborns with sepsis are nonspecific. Thus, prompt diagnosis often becomes difficult. It is good practice, therefore, to assume the presence of sepsis in any "not-doing-well" infant, particularly when there are other predisposing factors that could be associated with that infant. The manifestations include feeding difficulties, lethargy, irritability, vomiting, diarrhea, cyanosis, jaundice, respiratory distress, convulsions, abdominal distention, hepatosplenomegaly, and mild temperature elevations. In advanced cases, pallor, hypothermia, and mottling of the skin can also be observed.

Because the manifestations are nonspecific, the differential diagnosis includes a number of conditions commonly encountered in the newborn nursery. Thus, for an infant with sepsis who is convulsing, other diagnostic considerations include intracranial hemorrhage, metabolic disturbances (hypoglycemia or hypocalcemia), and electrolyte imbalances (hyponatremia, hypernatremia, hypomagnesemia, and so on). Pneumonia and pneumothorax should be ruled out in an infant whose septic manifestations include respiratory distress and cyanosis.

Infection with group B streptococcal organisms requires special mention. Two clinical syndromes have been described: the early septicemic form and the delayed meningitic form. In the septicemic form, the symptoms appear early. Pneumonia is a constant finding. The course is usually fulminant, and the mortality is approximately 50 per cent. Aspiration of infected amniotic fluid or vaginal secretions is thought to be the cause. In the meningitic form, manifestations of sepsis and meningitis usually appear about 2 to 12 weeks after birth. The infection is probably acquired postnatally, and the prognosis is generally better.

The diagnostic work-up for neonatal sepsis includes obtaining blood, urine, spinal fluid, and nasopharyngeal cultures. Blood cultures may be negative in a large percentage of these infants, but this does not necessarily rule out sepsis. When the cultures are positive, the diagnosis is established. The spinal fluid culture may be positive in about one-third of these infants. An examination of the gastric aspirate for the presence of bacteria and neutrophil leukocytes is also carried out. These are not confirmatory findings but, when present, substantiate a suspicion of sepsis. The peripheral blood smear is examined for evidence of leukopenia, leukocytosis, thrombocytopenia, and occasionally for hemolysis.

Antibiotic treatment should be started immediately once the diagnosis of sepsis is suspected, even before confirmatory laboratory results are available. Ampicillin, 100 to 150 mg. per kg. per day (intravenously or intramuscularly) and kanamycin, 15 to 20 mg. per kg. per day (intramuscularly) in two divided 12 hour doses (this dose is higher than that listed in the manufacturer's official directive) constitute the treatment of choice for sepsis of unknown cause. Kanamycin may be replaced by gentamicin, 5 to 7.5 mg. per kg. per day in two divided doses (this dose of gentamicin may be higher than that listed in the manufacturer's official directive), in nurseries where organisms have developed resistance to kanamycin. Methicillin should replace ampicillin in a dose of 200 mg. per kg. per day (intramuscularly or intravenously) given in four 6 hour doses when staphylococcal sepsis is suspected. Similarly, if a serious *Pseudomonas* infection is suspected, carbenicillin should replace ampicillin. The dose of carbenicillin is 225 to 300 mg. per kg. per day (intramuscularly or intravenously) given in three to four divided doses. Gentamicin and carbenicillin should *not* be mixed in the same solution and given intravenously.

Once a definitive organism is isolated and its antibiotic sensitivities are known, the most appropriate drug or drugs should be selected. Treatment should continue for a period of 5 to 7 days after the clinical symptoms have subsided.

Infants with meningitis should be treated for a period of 2 to 3 weeks. Also, they should receive additional intrathecal gentamicin in a daily dose of 0.5 to 1.0 mg. for 3 to 5 days. (The intrathecal use of gentamicin is not listed in the manufacturer's official directive.)

Congenital Rubella

Infections caused by the rubella virus have received much attention because of the teratogenic effects of the virus on the fetus. The effect on the fetus is most pronounced if the infection is acquired by the mother during the first 6 to 8 weeks of pregnancy. Many abnormalities related to the intrauterine infection are seen in newborns. Among the more common ones are low birth weight, hepatosplenomegaly, congenital heart lesions, deafness, cataracts, microphthalmia, thrombocytopenia, purpura, bone lesions, and retinopathy. The diagnosis is established by isolating the virus from nasopharyngeal secretions. With the advent of rubella vaccine and its routine administration during childhood, a significant drop in the incidence of this infection is expected.

Herpes Simplex Infection

Clinical manifestations in the newborn affected by herpes virus infection (usually by Type II strains) consist of fever, jaundice, hepatosplenomegaly, encephalitic symptoms, and bleeding tendencies with anemia and thrombocytopenia. The infection is transmitted either transplacentally or during birth from the vaginal lesions of the mother. The mortality in disseminated infection is about 75 to 80 per cent.

The most rapid serologic means of establishing the infection is by demonstrating type specific IgM antibodies, using an indirect fluorescent antibody technique.

Antiviral agents such as 5-iodo-2–deoxyuridine (IDU), cytosine arabinoside (Ara-C), and adenine arabinoside (Ara-A) are currently being evaluated.

Cytomegalovirus Infection

Although the incidence of maternal cytomegalovirus infection, as assessed by virologic studies, is very high, infection in the newborn is relatively infrequent. The usual mode of transmission is via the placenta and, less frequently, by exposure to infected cervical secretions at the time of delivery. Encephalitis, microcephaly, intracranial calcifications, thrombocytopenia with petechiae, jaundice with hepatitis, and chorioretinitis are some of the clinical findings seen in infants with symptomatic congenital cytomegalovirus infection.

The diagnosis is best confirmed by the isolation of the virus from the urine and from nasopharyngeal secretions. A serologic confirmation is obtained by demonstrating the presence of specific IgM antibodies in the infant's blood, using a fluorescent antibody technique. The three antiviral agents just described for use in herpes simplex infection are currently being evaluated for use in this infection also.

Toxoplasmosis

The protozoan responsible for this infection is *Toxoplasma gondii*. The overall rate of transmission from the mother to the fetus is approximately 40 per cent and is related to the time of gestation. The later the transmission occurs during this period, the greater is the frequency of fetal infection. Fever, jaundice, hepatosplenomegaly, lymphadenopathy, chorioretinitis, seizures, abnormal CSF and anemia are some of the more frequent manifestations seen in infants with congenital toxoplasmosis. A demonstration of the specific IgM antibodies for toxoplasmosis establishes the diagnosis. Treatment with sulfadiazine and pyrimethamine is recommended for all infected infants.

Congenital Syphilis

Fetal infection caused by *Treponema pallidum* occurs by way of transplacental passage consequent to maternal spirochetemia. The gestational age influences the fetal infection. A maternal spirochetemia occurring before 16 to 20 weeks of pregnancy does not usually result in the transmission of the disease to the fetus.

Clinical findings of early congenital syphilis include polymorphic rashes, hepatosplenomegaly, adenopathy, mucocutaneous lesions, hemolytic and other anemias, and jaundice with hepatitis. X-ray examinations of the bones reveal osteochondritis and periostitis.

The presence of *T. pallidum*-specific IgM antibody as determined by the fluorescent treponemal antibody-absorbed (FTA-ABS) IgM assay confirms the diagnosis.

Prevention of congenital infection is successfully achieved by prompt identification and treatment of the maternal infection. Penicillin G procaine, 10,000 units per kg. per day, given for 10 days is the recommended treatment regimen for infected infants.

THE INFANT OF THE DIABETIC MOTHER

Most infants born to a diabetic mother are large for their gestational age. Typically, these infants are plethoric with abundant fat and hair, and their resemblance to one another is striking. Certain metabolic derangements produce some special problems shortly after birth. Hypoglycemia (blood glucose determination less than 20 mg. per 100 ml. in premature infants and less than 30 mg. per 100 ml. in full-term infants) is the most frequent of these problems, occurring in more than 50 per cent of the infants during the first few hours of life. Despite hypoglycemia, the majority of the infants are asymptomatic. Symptoms, when present, include jitteriness, tremors, convulsions, sweating, cyanosis, and feeding difficulties. These may appear at any time during the first 24 hours after birth. A smaller percentage of infants develop hypocalcemia. Also, increased bilirubin levels 2 to 3 days after birth are noted more often in these infants than in others of similar gestational age and weight. Hyaline membrane disease occurring in some infants accounts for a significant degree of perinatal mortality. Renal vein thrombosis is an occasional finding. The incidence of congenital anomalies is greater than in normal newborns.

Careful monitoring and supervision of the diabetic mother go a long way in preventing problems in the neonate. An early interruption of pregnancy by initiating labor at 35 to 37 weeks may be considered in some instances to assure the highest infant survival rates. Glucagon (300 mg. per kg.) is recommended for infants with asymptomatic hypoglycemia. In symptomatic babies, hypertonic glucose solutions (10 to 15 per cent glucose, 60 to 70 ml. per kg.), given intravenously, are usually sufficient to maintain normoglycemia. If hypoglycemia persists, hydrocortisone, 5 mg. per kg. per day, or adrenocorticotropic hormone (ACTH), 4 units per kg. per day, both in divided doses, may be given.

FEEDING OF INFANTS AND CHILDREN

Understanding the fundamentals of nutrition is necessary for professionals responsible for counseling parents about the proper feeding of their infants and children. Proper feeding habits result in normal physical growth and also strongly influence the psychologic and emotional well-being of the infant or child. Mealtime should be a pleasurable and satisfying experience for both mother and child. The counseling of the mother must impart a practical interpretation of nutritional needs, as well as emphasize the wide range of variation in the appetite and the feeding behavior of growing babies and children. For the majority of parents of normal babies, a self-regulatory feeding schedule is found to be most effective during the first month or so of life. For most babies, an acceptable schedule will be adopted by 4 to 6 weeks of age. For parents who have a special need for order, a more formal schedule should be provided.

Despite the relative lack of popularity of breast-feeding and despite the availability of excellent prepared formulas, breast-feeding continues to be a practical and psychologically sound method of feeding young infants. Breast-feeding should be offered as an alternative to all mothers when no contraindications exist, either on her part or on the part of the infant. Breast milk is readily available, preparation is not needed, and bacterial contamination does not exist. Feeding difficulties such as colic, "spitting up," and allergic reactions are fewer in breast-fed babies. Breast milk is the natural food for infants during the first few months of life, as all nutritional requirements except vitamin D, fluoride, and iron are supplied.

There are contraindications to breast-feeding. Fissures or cracking of the nipples requires temporary cessation, if breast shields are not useful. Mastitis generally necessitates permanent discontinuation. Serious maternal illnesses such as septicemia, active tuberculosis, or nephritis, and chronic or debilitating conditions such as poor nutrition, convulsive disorders, severe neurosis, and postpartum psychosis are also contraindications for breast-feeding. Premature infants whose weight is less than 2000 grams generally do better on modified cow's milk formulas than on breast milk. The resumption of menstruation is never a contraindication to continuing breast-feeding. A working mother who must return to her employment within 6 weeks of her delivery is not a good candidate for breast-feeding.

Nursing mothers should be advised that complete emptying of the breast is the most effective method of stimulating the secretion of milk. Emptying should be accomplished by the vigorous sucking of the infant, but artificial suction should be used if necessary. Breast-feeding should be begun as soon as practicable after birth, preferably within 6 to 12 hours. The infant should be fed at both breasts until the milk supply is adequate for a complete feeding. The first 2 weeks are crucial for establishing successful breast-feeding. When early supplemental bottle feedings are given, breast-feeding is usually doomed. The baby finds it far easier to get milk from a bottle than from the breast. If a normal infant is satisfied at the completion of a nursing period and sleeps 3 to 4 hours, it can be assumed that the milk supply is sufficient.

There are many forms of cow's milk formulas and milk substitutes available. If fed in proper amounts, using proper technique, infants will thrive on most of them, provided that additional requirements such as vitamins and iron are included in the formula or are given as a supplement. The required daily intake of vitamins C and D, and possibly of vitamin A, must be supplied by fortified formulas or by water-miscible preparations of these essential nutrients. Vitamin D, 400 IU; vitamin C, supplied as 25 to 50 mg. of ascorbic acid; and vitamin A, 3000 to 5000 IU, should be given from early in the neonatal period through 12 to 18 months of life. The physician must be familiar with the vitamin content of commercial formulas and must supplement the amount of formula taken by the infant with an appropriate vitamin preparation if the daily requirements are not met.

A supplemental source of iron, other than from solid foods, should be given in the amount of 12 mg. per day from age 6 weeks through age 18 months. The iron, in ferrous form, may be provided by iron-fortified formulas or by oral iron preparations. A convenient method is to utilize an oral vitamin preparation containing the necessary amount of vitamins and iron. If fluoride is not present in adequate amounts in the drinking water, it should be supplied in oral drops, 0.5 to 1.0 mg. per day.

Solid foods should be first offered in 1 to 2

TABLE 44–3. GUIDE FOR FEEDING
SOLID FOODS

Food	Age to Begin
Precooked infant cereals	3 weeks to 2 months
Strained or puréed fruits	4 weeks to 3 months
Vegetables	6 weeks to 4 months
Eggs – hard-boiled yolk only	4 to 6 months
Strained meat	4 to 6 months
Starchy foods – potatoes, rice, spaghetti, bread, and so forth	Second 6 months of life, after above foods are well tolerated
Desserts – puddings, junket, and custards	Same as above

teaspoonful amounts (Table 44–3). Infants
often push food out of their mouth with
their tongue, rather than pushing it back,
until they learn to swallow efficiently. This
must be explained to the mother, as she
often feels that the baby is "spitting up" and
therefore discontinues the food. One food
should be given until it is accepted and
tolerated before another is added. The
infant's appetite will determine how much
solid food he will take. There is no point in
forcing any particular food when an infant
definitely dislikes it.

Colic is characterized by excessive crying
and apparent abdominal pain in infants less
than 3 months of age. The baby's legs are
pulled up to his abdomen, his hands are
tightly clenched, and his feet are often cold.
Numerous explanations have been given as
to the cause. These include underfeeding,
overfeeding, failure to "burp," allergy,
excessive carbohydrate fermentation, and
emotional problems in the mother or other
family members. Intestinal obstruction and
infection may mimic colic and should be
ruled out. Management is often unsatisfactory. Holding the baby upright or permitting him to lie prone on a hot water bottle or
heating pad or causing the passage of flatus
or rectal contents with the aid of a supposi-
tory may help. Reviewing feeding techniques and formula preparation may also
relieve the discomfort. During prolonged
attacks, sedation for the infant may be indicated.

By the end of the first year of life, the
infant is usually on a three-meal-a-day
schedule and is eating vigorously. As he
enters the second year, he begins a deceleration in his rate of growth and, hence, a
gradual reduction in his caloric need. He
often has temporary periods when he is not
interested in eating food in general, or
rejects only certain types of food. If the
parents are unprepared for this, they may
attempt to force-feed the child. His reaction
is rebellion, and feeding and psychologic
problems may ensue. Mothers, fathers, siblings, and relatives should all be educated
to the normal reduction in caloric needs for
the toddler.

IMMUNIZATION

Routine immunizations should not be
given during the course of febrile illnesses.
Mild, convalescent, or healing infections
are not absolute contraindications. The
preferred site of injection in infants is
intramuscularly into the lateral thigh. In
older children, the deltoid or triceps muscle
is utilized. Each injection should be given
at a different site. Deep injection followed
by massage reduces the incidence of antigenic cysts.

Administration of aspirin or acetaminophen in age-appropriate dosages will often
prevent febrile reactions. When a convulsion follows a DPT injection, further pertussis immunization is *contraindicated*.

Anergy to tuberculin may develop and
persist for a month or longer after administration of live, attenuated measles vaccine.
A tuberculin test should, therefore, be done
prior to giving the measles vaccine. Use of
live measles vaccine is not recommended
for children with debilitating diseases such
as leukemia or for those receiving immunosuppressive drugs. When measles prophylaxis is indicated in this group, immune
serum globulin (human) in a dose of 0.25
ml. per kg. should be given as soon as possible after exposure.

A personal immunization record, such as
the one designed by the American Academy
of Pediatrics, should be provided for each
child. Pregnant women should not be given
live rubella virus vaccine. Routine immunization of adolescent girls and adult women
should not be undertaken because of the
danger of inadvertently administering the
vaccine before pregnancy becomes evident.
Table 44–4 provides recommendations
for routine immunizations.

TABLE 44–4. SCHEDULE FOR ACTIVE IMMUNIZATION AND TUBERCULIN TESTING OF NORMAL INFANTS AND CHILDREN IN THE UNITED STATES*

2 months	DTP[1]	TOPV[2]
4 months	DTP	TOPV
6 months	DTP	TOPV
1 year	Measles[3], Rubella[3]	Tuberculin test[4]
1½ years	DTP	Mumps[3]
4–6 years	DTP	TOPV
14–16 years	Td[5]	TO V and thereafter every 10 years

*This table was prepared by the Committee on Infectious Diseases of the American Academy of Pediatrics in 1974. Reproduced with permission of the American Academy of Pediatrics.

[1]DTP—diphtheria and tetanus toxoids combined with pertussis vaccine.

[2]TOPV—trivalent oral poliovirus vaccine. This recommendation suitable for breast-fed as well as bottle-fed infants.

[3]May be given at 1 year as measles-rubella or measles-mumps-rubella combined vaccines.

[4]Frequency of repeated tuberculin tests depends on risk of exposure of the child and on the prevalence of tuberculosis in the population group. The initial test should be at the time of, or preceding, the measles immunization.

[5]Td—combined tetanus and diphtheria toxoids (adult type) for those more than 6 years of age in contrast to diphtheria and tetanus (DT), which contains a larger amount of diphtheria antigen. Tetanus toxoid at time of injury: For clean, minor wounds, no booster dose is needed by a fully immunized child, unless more than 10 years have elapsed since the last dose. For contaminated wounds: A booster dose should be given if more than 5 years have elapsed since the last dose. Routine smallpox vaccination is no longer recommended.

INFECTIONS IN CHILDREN

The Common Cold

No single illness affects more children than the common cold. The average child can expect to experience about 30 such infections after the first year of life (when passively acquired maternal antibodies decline) through adolescence. Many viruses, as well as a few kinds of bacteria, have been shown to cause upper respiratory infection (URI). Symptoms include coryza, sneezing, and sore throat. Fever is seldom very high, and children do not usually appear to be very ill. As sinusitis from infection is uncommon in children, allergic rhinitis is the most prevalent condition likely to be confused with the common cold. Table 44–5 outlines the salient differentiating points.

TABLE 44–5. DIFFERENTIAL POINTS BETWEEN THE COMMON COLD AND ALLERGIC RHINITIS

Common Cold	Allergic Rhinitis
Lasts 1 week	Intermittent and persistent
Communicable to others	Noncommunicable
Injected nasal mucosa	Pale, boggy nasal mucosa
Mucopurulent discharge by day 3 or 4	Clear, watery discharge
Lymphocytes or neutrophils on nasal smear	Eosinophils on nasal smear

No specific therapy is effective, but antibiotics are useful for bacterial complications such as otitis media or sinusitis (Table 44–6). Children with chronic, debilitating illnesses, e.g., cystic fibrosis, should be protected from contact with patients suffering from a common cold. Infants will require measures to keep the nasal passages patent, as they are obligate nose breathers. Saline nose drops and gentle suctioning with a bulb syringe are suggested.

Otitis Media

See Chapter 39, Otorhinolaryngology, page 638.

Conjunctivitis

See Chapter 40, Ophthalmology, page 706.

Cervical Adenitis

Cervical lymph node infection generally follows an upper respiratory tract infection or represents spread from local infections involving the face, scalp, or neck. It is most often caused by the group A beta hemolytic streptococcus or by *Staphylococcus aureus.* Less commonly, pneumococcal or tuberculous organisms may be found. Clinically, the nodes are tender, discrete, indurated, and mobile and may be red. Later, they may soften and, finally, drain. Fever and anorexia are also common findings. There is generally a rise in polymorphonuclear leukocytes, and the throat culture or aspiration

TABLE 44-6. RECOMMENDED ANTIBIOTICS FOR COMMON BACTERIAL INFECTIONS

Condition	Preferred Antibiotic	Alternate	Condition	Preferred Antibiotic	Alternate
Group A streptococcal pharyngotonsillitis	Penicillin	Erythromycin	Endocarditis		
			Unknown cause	Penicillin and streptomycin	
Otitis media	Ampicillin or penicillin and sulfisoxazole	Erythromycin and sulfisoxazole	*Streptococcus viridans*	Penicillin and streptomycin	
			Enterococcus	Penicillin and streptomycin	
Cervical adenitis					
Beta streptococcus	Penicillin	Erythromycin	*Staphylococcus aureus*		
Staphylococcus aureus	Penicillin	Methicillin	Penicillin-sensitive	Penicillin	
Pneumonia			Penicillin-resistant	Methicillin	
Unknown cause	Penicillin	Erythromycin	Pericarditis		
Pneumococcus	Penicillin	Erythromycin	Unknown cause	Methicillin	
Mycoplasma	Erythromycin	Tetracycline	*Hemophilus influenzae*	Ampicillin	Chloramphenicol
Staphylococcus			Pneumococcus	Penicillin	
Penicillin-resistant	Methicillin	Cephalosporin	Impetigo	Penicillin or benzathine penicillin	Erythromycin or cephalexin
Penicillin-sensitive	Penicillin	Cephalosporin			
Meningitis					
Hemophilus influenzae	Ampicillin (if sensitive) Chloramphenicol (if resistant)	Chloramphenicol	Cellulitis	Penicillin or ampicillin	Erythromycin or cephalexin
Pneumococcus	Penicillin	Chloramphenicol	Septic arthritis		
Meningococcus	Penicillin	Chloramphenicol	Unknown	Methicillin	
Neonatal meningitis			*Staphylococcus*		
Unknown cause	Ampicillin and kanamycin	Penicillin and gentamicin	Penicillin-resistant	Methicillin	
			Penicillin-sensitive	Penicillin	
Neonatal sepsis			*Hemophilus influenzae*	Ampicillin	
Unknown cause	Ampicillin and kanamycin	Penicillin and gentamicin	*Streptococcus*	Penicillin	
			Gonococcus	Penicillin	
Gastroenteritis			Meningococcus	Penicillin	
Escherichia coli (pathogenic)	Neomycin	Polymyxin B or colistin	Pneumococcus	Penicillin	
Shigellosis	Ampicillin	Trimethroprim-sulfamethoxazole (TMP-SMX)	Osteomyelitis		
			Unknown cause	Methicillin	
			Staphylococcus		
			Penicillin-resistant	Methicillin	
Salmonellosis			Penicillin-sensitive	Penicillin	
Uncomplicated	No antibiotic		*Salmonella*	Ampicillin	
Septicemia (salmonellosis) and typhoid	Chloramphenicol	Ampicillin or TMP-SMX	Gonorrhea	Penicillin and probenecid	Tetracycline
Urinary tract infection			Syphilis		
			Congenital		
Initial attack	Sulfisoxazole or ampicillin	Cephalexin	Without CNS involvement	Benzathine penicillin	
Recurrent episodes	Gentamicin, kanamycin or carbenicillin		With CNS involvement	Penicillin (procaine)	
			Primary, secondary	Benzathine penicillin	Tetracycline

culture of an affected lymph node may demonstrate the causative organism.

The differential diagnosis includes various systemic viral illnesses such as rubella, infectious mononucleosis, or mumps, or neoplastic processes such as leukemia or Hodgkin's disease. The lack of characteristic symptoms of the various viral syndromes serves to rule out these disorders. In addition, neoplastic nodes are usually not tender or red and evolve in a different manner than the nodes in bacterial adenitis. A tuberculin test should be performed.

Antibiotic therapy is outlined in Table 44-6. Incision and drainage are indicated if the node softens and points.

Croup

Two types of croup exist: spasmodic or allergic croup and laryngotracheobronchitis or infectious croup. Allergic croup tends to recur in the absence of other symptoms of upper or middle respiratory tract infection, but laryngotracheobronchitis tends to occur as a single episode, with signs of infection such as coryza, fever, and cough. Infectious croup is usually a benign disease, but an occasional child (usually of preschool age) will require a tracheostomy when conservative therapy fails and breathing is seriously compromised. However, this occurs more often with measles and *H. influenzae* infections.

Symptoms consist of hoarseness, inspiratory stridor, a brassy cough, and suprasternal retractions that become more severe at night. The presence of tachypnea, tachycardia, restlessness, and cyanosis should cause the physician to consider hospitalization and preparation for tracheostomy.

Mild croup can usually be helped by the use of a vaporizer. In the event that fluid intake is decreased to the point of dehydration, intravenous fluid replacement should be undertaken. Antibiotics such as ampicillin are useful when *H. influenzae* is the causative agent. Antihistamines, which inspissate secretions, should not be used, and steroids do not appear to be helpful.

Laryngeal diphtheria, foreign bodies, tumors, congenital laryngeal malformations and epiglottitis should be considered in the differential diagnosis.

Epiglottitis

This life-threatening emergency presents as pain in the pharyngeal area with inspiratory stridor, dysphonia, and fever. Swallowing is painful, and drooling may be observed. If the diagnosis of epiglottitis is suspected based on these findings, examination of the larynx or pharynx is deferred until one is prepared to perform either an immediate tracheostomy or a laryngeal intubation. The finding of a swollen, injected epiglottis confirms the diagnosis, and intubation or tracheostomy should not be further delayed. Ampicillin is useful for combating *H. influenzae*, which is the most common bacterial cause of epiglottitis.

Bronchiolitis

Bronchiolitis is chiefly a viral illness that affects children between 3 months and 3 years of age and involves the small and terminal bronchioles. Symptoms of cough and increasing respiratory distress, retractions, and either low-grade or normal body temperature characterize the clinical picture. On auscultation, crepitant rales and wheezing are heard. The differential diagnosis is chiefly between asthma and pneumonia (Table 44–7). The chest x-ray may show overinflated lungs and patchy atelectasis.

Therapy is supportive. Fluids are given intravenously if the degree of respiratory distress prevents an adequate oral intake. Bronchodilators are not very helpful. Anti-

TABLE 44–7. DIFFERENTIAL DIAGNOSIS OF BRONCHIOLITIS, ASTHMA, AND PNEUMONIA

Bronchiolitis	Asthma	Pneumonia
Onset – 3 months to 3 years	Onset – infancy to adulthood	Onset – all ages
Previous history negative	Previous history often positive	Previous history often negative
Frequent in winter	Frequent all seasons	Frequent in winter
Afebrile or mildly febrile	Usually afebrile	Febrile
Prolonged expiration	Prolonged expiration	No prolonged expiration
Inspiratory and expiratory obstruction	Expiratory obstruction	Obstructive respiratory pattern usually lacking
Respiratory distress marked	Respiratory distress mild to marked	Respiratory distress mild to marked
Usually hyperresonant	Usually hyperresonant	Usually hyperresonant
Wheezing, rales, or ronchi	Wheezing	Rales
Chest findings bilateral	Chest findings bilateral	Chest findings either unilateral or bilateral
Lymphocytosis	Eosinophilia	Lymphocytosis or "viral" or "bacterial" white count and differential, polymorphonuclear leukocytosis
Hyperaeration	Hyperaeration	Pneumonic infiltrate or consolidation

biotics (ampicillin) are indicated for the occasional child with *H. influenzae* bronchiolitis.

Pneumonia

Pneumonia is most commonly caused by a great variety of viral agents and a few types of bacteria. The bacteria that most commonly cause pneumonia in small children are the pneumococcus, *H. influenzae, Mycoplasma pneumoniae*, group A streptococcus, and *Staphylococcus aureus.* Symptoms and signs are similar, but children with bacterial pneumonia tend to "look sicker," incur complications such as pleural effusion and pneumothorax more often, and have a rise in polymorphonuclear leukocyte counts. Cough, fever, a variable degree of tachypnea, dyspnea, and fine rales heard over one or both lung fields are characteristic findings (see Table 44–7).

The best single examination is by chest x-ray (anterior and lateral views), which may demonstrate pulmonic infiltrates, consolidation, atelectasis, effusion, or a combination of these. The presence of pneumatoceles in a baby whose illness is rapidly worsening suggests staphylococcal pneumonia. Sputum smears and cultures of both sputum and blood are occasionally helpful in determining a cause, and the tuberculin test should be done to rule out tuberculosis. Other serologic and viral studies are usually not as helpful because results are not quickly forthcoming and therapy cannot be delayed.

Treatment for viral pneumonia is supportive. A mist tent and oxygen are useful for the child who is dyspneic, or cyanotic, or both. An appropriate antibiotic is added for treatment of bacterial pneumonia (see Table 44–6). The course of therapy should last from 7 to 10 days in the uncomplicated case and longer (from 2 to 4 weeks or upon complete resolution) when pleural effusion or extensive involvement is present or when the illness is caused by a staphylococcus. Therapy by the intravenous route is preferred for the sicker child. Surgical therapy (closed water seal drainage via a chest tube) may be required for large effusions or for a pneumothorax.

Measles (Rubeola)

Measles is caused by a specific virus that is found in the respiratory tract secretions,

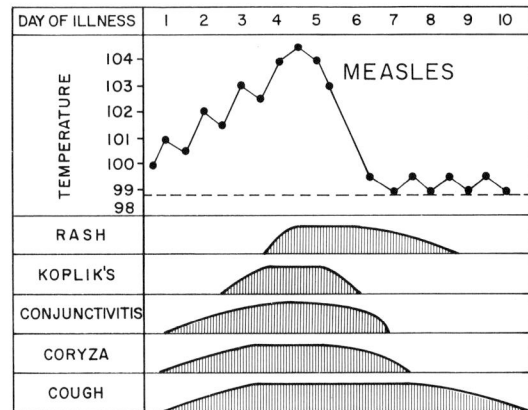

Figure 44–2. *Schematic diagram illustrating clinical course of typical case of measles. The rash appears 3 to 4 days after the onset of fever, conjunctivitis, coryza, and cough. Koplik's spots usually develop 2 days before the rash appears. (From Krugman, S., and Ward, R.: Infectious Diseases of Children and Adults. 5th ed. St. Louis. The C. V. Mosby Co. Reproduced with permission.)*

blood, and urine of infected patients. Measles is transmitted by direct contact with droplets, which may be airborne, from an infected person or by indirect contact with freshly contaminated articles. The incubation period is 10 to 12 days. The clinical course of measles is illustrated in Figure 44–2.

The development of a maculopapular rash preceded by a 3 to 4 day period (occasionally as long as 7 days) of fever, conjunctivitis, coryza, and cough associated with pathognomonic Koplik's spots is diagnostic of measles. No confirmatory laboratory tests are needed. Diagnostic tests such as virus isolation or neutralization, complement fixation, or hemagglutination inhibition techniques demonstrate rising antibody titers and may be utilized in the difficult diagnostic case.

The rash of measles must be differentiated from the rashes of rubella, roseola, enteroviral infections, toxoplasmosis, infectious mononucleosis, erythema infectiosum, scarlet fever, endemic typhus, and eruptions caused by drugs. Hemorrhagic measles may resemble meningococcemia or Rocky Mountain spotted fever.

Pulmonary complications are the primary cause of death resulting from measles. Otitis media is also one of the more common complications. Obstructive laryngitis may require tracheostomy. Acute encephalitis is a potentially crippling or fatal complication.

Less common complications include thrombocytopenic and nonthrombocytopenic purpura, appendicitis (lymphoid hyperplasia in the appendix), and subacute sclerosing panencephalitis (Dawson's encephalitis). No specific therapy is available. Antibacterial agents should be used only for the treatment of secondary bacterial complications.

The schedule for active immunization against measles is included in Table 44–4.

Care of exposed, susceptible children or adults: If previously unimmunized, give Edmonston B live measles vaccine together with 0 04 ml. per kg. of immune serum globulin (ISG) at separate sites. An alternative method is to give a preventive dose of 0.25 ml. per kg. of ISG. ISG should be given as soon after exposure as possible and is to be followed in 8 weeks by immunization with live measles vaccine. If the exposed, susceptible child is known to have leukemia, disseminated malignancy, chronic immunosuppression, or the "Swiss" type of agammaglobulinemia, (lymphopenia with thymic agenesis), give 20 to 30 ml. of ISG intramuscularly immediately.

Rubella (German Measles, Three Day Measles)

Rubella is caused by a specific virus that can be isolated and cultivated in tissue cultures. Rubella is rare in infants and uncommon in preschool children. There is an increased incidence of the disease in older children, adolescents, and young adults. Since 1941, great attention has been given to this disease because of the association between it and the presence of congenital malformations in the newborn infant when the disease occurs in pregnant women during the first trimester (see page 835). The incubation period is usually 16 to 18 days, with a range of 14 to 21 days. In the child, the usual initial symptom is the characteristic rash. In adolescents and young adults, the rash often is preceded by a 1 to 5 day prodromal period characterized by low-grade fever, headache, malaise, anorexia, mild conjunctivitis, sore throat, cough, and lymphadenopathy, particularly of the postauricular type.

A diagnosis of rubella is considered when the clinical features just described are present. Confirmation is by virus isolation or by serologic testing. The hemagglutination inhibition antibody test is the most useful and most rapid method, yielding results within 24 hours. Both an acute and a convalescent serum must be obtained for serologic diagnosis. The acute serum should be obtained as soon as possible after the onset of the rash and the convalescent serum 2 to 4 weeks later. A rise in rubella antibody titer is indicative of a recent infection. Although complications are unusual in rubella, arthritis does occur in adolescents and young adults, especially in females. The arthritis usually manifests itself as the rash is fading, with a return of fever, transient joint pain, or massive effusion in one or more joints. One or more larger or smaller joints may be involved. (For active immunization see Table 44–4.)

Roseola Infantum (Exanthem Subitum)

Although final confirmation is not available, all evidence points to a virus as the infecting agent in cases of roseola infantum. More than 95 per cent of the cases occur in patients between 6 months and 3 years of age. The disease occurs throughout the year, with some concentration of cases in the spring and autumn months. It has been estimated that 30 per cent of children less than 3 years of age develop the clinical picture of this disease. The remaining 70 per cent probably have either inapparent infection or fever without the rash. The duration of the incubation period is difficult to determine because contact is rarely known. However, the information that is available indicates a range of 9 to 15 days. The typical course of roseola infantum is illustrated in Figure 44–3.

Fever is high and continuous, often lasting from 3 to 4 days. Typically, the fever drops abruptly to normal levels after this period. Generally, the rash develops at the time the fever subsides. However, it may appear just prior to the drop in body temperature or up to 24 hours after the temperature reaches normal. The rash is composed of rose-pink maculopapular lesions that tend to remain discrete. The rash appears on the trunk and may be limited to that area of the body, or it may spread to the extremities, neck, and face. The lesions may be evanescent, disappearing in a few hours, or they may persist for 2 or 3 days.

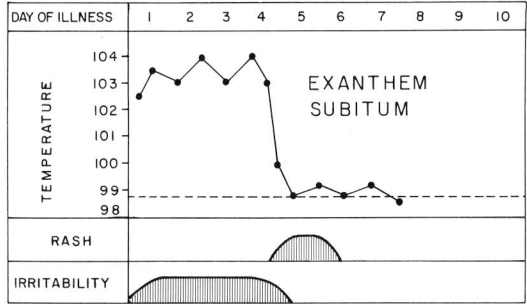

Figure 44–3. Schematic diagram illustrating typical clinical course of exanthem subitum. Between the third and fourth days, the temperature drops to normal and a maculopapular eruption appears. (From Krugman, S., and Ward, R.: Infectious Diseases of Children and Adults. 5th ed. St. Louis, The C. V. Mosby Co., 1973. Reproduced with permission.)

The child may not appear ill and often is quite playful, despite the marked elevation of temperature, or he may be quite irritable. Puffiness of the upper eyelids provides a clinical hint that one may be dealing with roseola. Lymphadenopathy of the subocci-pital, cervical, and postauricular nodes is frequently present. A string of BB shot-sized nodes along the inferior aspect of the occipital bulge in a child with markedly elevated temperature and a paucity of other physical findings is very suggestive of roseola. The onset of roseola may be ushered in by a generalized seizure. A bulging fontanelle with normal cerebro-spinal fluid findings may be noted. A marked leukopenia often develops toward the end of the febrile period, with an increase in the percentage of lymphocytes and monocytes. During the febrile stage, when the rash is not present, all acute infectious processes must be considered in the differential diagnosis, especially men-ingococcemia and sepsis. During the rash stage, all conditions mentioned in the sec-tion on the differential diagnosis of measles must be considered.

Seizures are the most common complica-tion, and their incidence appears to parallel the incidence of other forms of febrile convulsions. Sequelae are very rare. Treat-ment is symptomatic. Aspirin, or acetamin-ophen is indicated for its antipyretic effect, and administration may be repeated at 4 hour intervals. Elixir of phenobarbital, 15 mg. three times daily, is indicated for children who have had a febrile convulsion either during this illness or previously.

Chickenpox (Varicella)

Chickenpox and herpes zoster are both caused by the varicella-zoster (V-Z) virus. Chickenpox is predominantly a disease of childhood, with the highest incidence oc-curring in children between 2 and 8 years of age, but it may occur in early infancy, despite maternal immunity. Intrauterine infection may be followed by clinical chickenpox in the newborn infant. The majority of infants whose mothers had chickenpox during labor develop the dis-ease after an appropriate incubation period. The incubation period is from 14 to 16 days, with a range of from 10 to 21 days.

The disease usually beings with low-grade fever, malaise, and the appearance of the characteristic rash. The lesions pass rapidly through the stages of macules, papules, vesicles, and crusts, often in 6 to 8 hours. As the typical vesicle begins to dry, an umbilicated appearance (pseudoumbili-cation) may be apparent. The scabs fall off without scarring in 5 to 20 days. The number of lesions varies from one or two in some patients to thousands in others. Le-sions appear on the palms, soles, and mucous membrane surfaces. The complica-tion of varicella pneumonia is rarely seen in otherwise healthy children.

The typical case of chickenpox can be clinically identified without laboratory con-firmation. In typical cases, the virus may be readily isolated from the vesicular fluid within the first 3 or 4 days following the appearance of the rash. Complement-fixing antibody can be detected in serum obtained as early as 7 days after the onset of the rash. Chickenpox must be differentiated from impetigo, insect bites, papular urticaria, herpetic dermatitis, scabies, rickettsialpox, eczema herpeticum and vaccinatum, and herpes zoster. A severe case of chickenpox, particularly in an adult, must be differen-tiated from smallpox.

Secondary bacterial infection is the most common complication. Encephalitis occurs in less than 1 of every 1000 patients and generally is milder than postmeasles en-cephalitis. However, chickenpox encepha-litis may be overwhelming, even fatal. Varicella pneumonia is common in adults and has been found at autopsy in infants who died as a result of varicella neonato-rum. Fulminating, often fatal chickenpox may occur in children who have received corticosteroids just prior to contracting the disease.

Routine care includes keeping the child cool by dressing him lightly and by controlling the environmental temperature. Fingernails should be trimmed very short to prevent scratching and excoriation. Daily, gentle bathing and the use of calamine lotion, with or without antihistamines, are helpful in relieving itching.

Scarlet Fever

Group A beta hemolytic streptococci are the causative agents for a wide spectrum of clinical infections in children, including scarlet fever, tonsillitis or pharyngitis, and erysipelas. Scarlet fever occurs in children who have not developed immunity against the erythrogenic toxin that is common to the 40 or more types of group A beta hemolytic streptococci. Antibacterial immunity, on the other hand, is type-specific, so that a patient may have repeated streptococcal infections, each caused only by a type to which the patient is not immune. The punctate, papular rash of scarlet fever is a "red flag" that denotes the presence of a group A beta hemolytic streptococcal infection. This is the only streptococcal infection that can be correctly diagnosed clinically and is an absolute indication for adequate antibiotic therapy to eradicate the causative organism.

Pertussis (Whooping Cough)

The causative agent of pertussis is *Bordetella pertussis (Hemophilus pertussis)*, a small, gram-negative, nonmotile rod. *B. pertussis* is best isolated from the nasopharynx by means of a nasopharyngeal swab rather than by a cough plate. The Bordet-Gengou medium (glycerin-potato-blood agar) is preferred for the greatest yield. The bacillus is isolated with greatest frequency during the prodromal stage (first 1 to 2 weeks of illness).

Pertussis is worldwide in distribution and continues to be a serious health problem in all countries of the world. In many developing countries, the disease is a major problem, with high morbidity and mortality rates. Females have a higher morbidity and mortality than males, reversing the usual pattern of common childhood infectious diseases. The period of communicability can be considered to extend from 7 days after exposure to 3 weeks after the onset of the paroxysmal cough. The disease is more often spread by the patient before the characteristic whoops have occurred and thus before the disease is generally diagnosed. The incubation period is 7 to 10 days.

The prodromal stage manifests itself by nonspecific upper respiratory symptoms associated with a hacking cough, which gradually becomes more severe. A history of exposure to someone with pertussis is the only reliable evidence that the patient may have whooping cough during this stage. The paroxysmal stage usually lasts from 4 to 6 weeks but may be prolonged to 10 to 12 weeks. It is recognized by the characteristic series of expiratory coughs climaxed in many children by an inspiratory whoop and often by vomiting. Infants less than 6 months of age and patients with modified disease may not have this whoop. During the convalescent stage, there is a gradual cessation of whooping and vomiting. However, with subsequent respiratory infections, the coughing and vomiting may recur. These episodes may occur over a period of 1 to 2 years.

Although during the paroxysmal stage the clinical picture and the history of exposure point toward the diagnosis, the laboratory culture is most useful when pertussis is suspected in the prodromal stage. The application of the fluorescent antibody technique offers a rapid method of identifying organisms. The results of the white blood count often aid in establishing a diagnosis, and elevated counts (20,000 to 100,000 per cu. mm.) with a predominance of lymphocytes are characteristic. Young infants, however, may respond to a variety of viral and bacterial infections with lymphocytosis. Differential diagnoses include bronchiolitis, bronchopneumonia, fibrocystic disease, tuberculosis, tracheobronchial lymphadenopathy, foreign body in a bronchus, and parapertussis *(Bordetella parapertussis)*.

The most common, and generally the most serious, complication is bronchopneumonia, especially in children less than 3 years of age. The pneumonia is usually caused by secondary invaders, but may be primary *(B. pertussis)*. Atelectasis followed by bronchiectasis may occur. Convulsions may occur secondary to gastric tetany, hypoxia, or hemorrhage. Often, all these factors contribute to a diffuse encephalopathy with cerebral edema and subsequent cortical atrophy. Hemorrhage may occur in the conjunctiva or may be manifested by epistaxis, skin petechiae, or ecchymoses. Other complications include prolapsed rectum, nutritional disturbances, and hernias.

Specific treatment of the infant includes the use of pertussis immune globulin, 1.25 ml. by injection, repeated every other day for three or four doses, and the use of an antibiotic such as erythromycin or ampicillin for at least 10 days. Questions remain concerning the effectiveness of these agents, but the balance of evidence would indicate their continued use in most children less than 2 years of age.

Passive immunization of exposed, susceptible infants may be attempted, using pertussis hyperimmune gamma globulin in two doses of 1.25 ml. given at 3 to 5 day intervals. Active immunization can be accomplished with plain or alum-precipitated vaccine, preferably given during infancy in combination with diphtheria and tetanus toxids (see Table 44–4).

Mumps (Epidemic Parotitis)

Mumps is caused by the virus Myxovirus parotiditis, which has predilection for glandular and central nervous system tissue. Mumps is generally an endemic disease, but epidemics occur under conditions favorable to virus dissemination, such as those in children's institutions or in military establishments. Although the majority of cases of mumps occur in children between 5 and 10 years of age, the average age of those affected with mumps is older than of those affected with measles, chickenpox, and pertussis.

The incubation period is 16 to 18 days. In 30 to 40 per cent of patients, mumps infection is clinically nonapparent. In clinically apparent cases, there are a wide variety of clinical symptoms, depending upon the site or sites of the infection. In the majority of patients, mumps is characterized by involvement of one or both parotid glands. Involvement of the submaxillary and sublingual glands is next in frequency. Orchitis and meningoencephalitis are not uncommon. Pancreatitis, oophoritis, thyroiditis, and other disorders of glandular involvement are relatively rare.

Epididymo-orchitis is a relatively common manifestation of mumps in postpubertal males, as it occurs in 20 to 30 per cent of these patients. Although parotitis is generally present, orchitis may occur as the only manifestation of the disease. Only 2 per cent of patients with orchitis have bilateral involvement. The adult male's frequent concern is that sexual impotence and sterility will follow his testicular infection. There is little factual basis for these fears, even with the rare instances of bilateral involvement, as complete atrophy probably does not occur. Meningoencephalitis is another common manifestation of mumps, as it occurs in at least 10 per cent of the patients. It may precede, follow, or occur without the clinical picture of parotid mumps. The infection is characterized by a marked predominance of lymphocytes in the spinal fluid and by a generally favorable outcome. Pancreatitis, thyroiditis, mastitis, dacryoadenitis, and bartholinitis are rare manifestations of mumps.

Diagnosis by clinical findings is very inaccurate. A history of exposure, typical parotitis, or aseptic meningitis points to mumps as a likely diagnostic possibility, but confirmatory tests are frequently indicated to establish a definite diagnosis. The mumps complement fixation test, utilizing acute and convalescent serum, is the most practical method. The serum amylase level is elevated in 70 per cent of patients with mumps parotitis and thus can be a helpful tool in ruling in or out the presence of mumps. As mumps may be confused with other disorders involving the parotid glands or regional lymph nodes, other conditions to be considered are anterior or preauricular adenitis, suppurative parotitis, and calculi that obstruct Stensen's duct. Recurrent parotitis, usually of unknown cause, can best be differentiated by use of the complement fixation test. Meningoencephalitis without parotitis can be distinguished from other viral central nervous system (CNS) infections only by viral or complement fixation tests.

Treatment is symptomatic and supportive. Antibiotics are not useful. Treatment of moderate or severe orchitis includes the use of corticosteroids, which characteristically alleviate pain and may reduce swelling. For prevention of mumps, the live attenuated mumps virus vaccine is recommended (combined with measles and rubella vaccines) for all children and should be given at 12 months of age (see Table 44–4). If the mumps vaccine is not given as part of a child's basic immunization program, it should be given to boys who are approaching puberty, adolescent and adult males, and children living in institutions, camps, and so forth.

Urinary Tract Infection

Two types of urinary tract infection may be encountered: cystitis, or lower urinary tract infection, and pyelonephritis, or upper urinary tract infection. Symptomatology differs significantly between the two types. Dysuria, frequency, tenesmus, enuresis, and lower abdominal pain are frequent findings in patients with cystitis. Fever and other constitutional symptoms are usually absent. In patients with pyelonephritis, constitutional symptoms tend to predominate, particularly in younger children. Fever, chills, malaise, vomiting, and costovertebral tenderness are more characteristic. An occasional infant will have signs of sepsis with jaundice. It must be remembered, however, that the urinary tract is a single unit and infectious processes tend to involve the entire tract to some degree. Females are more likely to have a urinary tract infection than males.

Escherichia coli is the chief cause of infection. *Klebsiella pneumoniae, Enterobacter (Aerobacter) aerogenes, Pseudo-monas,* or *Proteus* are also frequently isolated. Other bacterial pathogens are found less often.

Making the diagnosis is helped considerably by finding white blood cells (>10 per high power field) and bacteria in a properly collected, clean-catch urine specimen. Clumps or casts of white blood cells are highly significant. The definitive test, however, is the urine culture. Colony counts in excess of 100,000 per ml. are considered diagnostic in untreated patients. Sensitivity testing should be done to help in choosing an effective antibiotic. Most patients, if not all, will require an intravenous pyelogram and a voiding cystourethrogram to rule out anomalies of the genitourinary tract that may have predisposed the patient to infection. As a rule, all males should have these studies done, and females definitely should if more than one attack of urinary tract infection is noted or if resolution of the initial attack is slow. Cystoscopy can also be done when the infection is difficult to control or is recurrent.

Prognosis is excellent if proper management is provided. Since the recurrence rate after an initial episode is high (10 per cent within the first year), frequent follow-up visits and urine cultures are necessary. Cultures should be performed for at least 1 year following an effective course of therapy if chronic pyelonephritis, with its high morbidity and mortality in later life, is to be avoided. Therapy is outlined in Table 44–8.

TABLE 44–8. MANAGEMENT OF ACUTE URINARY TRACT INFECTIONS°

Initial Urinary Tract Infection (Pyelonephritis and/or Cystitis)	Persistent and/or Recurrent Urinary Tract Infection (Pyelonephritis and/or Cystitis)
Sulfisoxazole — 150 mg./kg./24 hours orally for 2 weeks or Ampicillin — 100 mg./kg./24 hours orally for 2 weeks or Cephalexin — 25 mg./kg./24 hours orally for 2 weeks	Antibiotics — chosen by sensitivity testing and given for 2 months or more Followed by — one of the medications listed below for 1 year: Nitrofurantoin — 5 to 7 mg./kg./24 hours orally Nalidixic acid — 40 to 80 mg./kg./24 hours orally Methenamine mandelate — 4 mg./kg./24 hours orally
Pyridium (if analgesic is required) as long as needed for relief of symptoms	Surgical correction of anomalies — including persistent reflux and dilation of small urethral meatus

°Note: If symptoms do not improve and bacteriuria persists following 48 to 72 hours of therapy, consider changing antibiotics. See manufacturers' official directives before using these agents in young infants.

Gastroenteritis

The most important pathogens causing gastroenteritis are viral agents (ECHO, adenoviruses, Coxsackie) and enteric bacteria (especially *Escherichia coli, Shigella,* and *Salmonella).*

Symptoms include anorexia, diarrhea, and weakness. Fever and vomiting are encountered less often. High fever and prostration may be seen with *Salmonella* (salmonellosis) and *Shigella* (shigellosis).

If fluid loss exceeds fluid intake, dehydration results. This occurs more often in children less than 2 years old. Skin turgor is decreased, the mucous membranes dry, and the eyes are sunken (as is the fontanelle in younger children) whenever fluid loss amounts to 3 to 5 per cent of total body weight.

Treatment consists of eliminating known bacterial pathogens isolated by stool culture by giving a course of antibiotic therapy for 1 to 2 weeks or until stool cultures are repeatedly negative (see Table 44–6). In addition, fluid and electrolytes must be replaced in deficit states or must be maintained if no loss has occurred (see section on Fluid and Electrolytes).

Meningitis

Meningitis is an inflammatory process of diverse causes that is best considered by grouping patients by age. In the neonatal period, the gram-negative organisms (*Escherichia coli* in particular) and the group B streptococci are the chief bacterial agents. After 2 to 3 months and until 4 years of age, *Hemophilus influenzae* type B is the major causative organism. Beyond the age of 4 years, the pneumococcus is predominant. The meningococcus does not have a particular age predilection.

Often preceded by an upper respiratory tract infection, meningitis tends to have an insidious, deceptively mild onset. The classic findings of headache, vomiting, fever, and signs of meningeal irritation may not be observed until the second or third day of illness, and in infants and children less than 2 years of age, meningeal signs may never be observed. In this latter age group, fever, vomiting, and behavioral manifestations such as irritability or lethargy are common findings. Occasionally, a bulging fontanelle may signal the diagnosis. Even in the presence of frank meningeal signs, lumbar punctures are negative in slightly more than half the youngsters (meningismus). Thus, a high index of suspicion and a ready disposition to perform a lumbar puncture are the best guarantees that the diagnosis of meningitis will not be overlooked.

Pyelonephritis, salmonellosis, shigellosis, and exanthem subitum are some of the illnesses whose presenting signs are most likely to be confused with meningitis. The lumbar puncture findings serve to rule out meningitis, although some caution is urged because, rarely, spinal fluid without significant numbers of white cells will be found that will return a positive bacterial culture.

Positive cell counts consist of 10 or more mononuclear cells and more than one polymorphonuclear cell per cu. mm. Other characteristics of the spinal fluid of patients with meningitis are an elevated protein determination (greater than 40 mg. per 100 ml.), a low glucose content (less than 50 per cent of the glucose content of a simultaneously-taken blood specimen), and a positive Gram's stain. The quellung reaction, or capsular swelling test, and the fluorescent antibody test may provide rapid identification of the causative agent. In the event that antibiotics have previously been administered and the causative organisms may therefore be inhibited from growing in culture media, the counter immunoelectrophoresis test is advised. This test depends on the reaction between an antigen (the organism) and an antibody. The presence of dead organisms does not affect the outcome, as these organisms are still antigenically active.

Viral meningitis is usually characterized by a predominance of mononuclear cells in the spinal fluid, while bacterial meningitis will cause a rise in polymorphonuclear cells. This is not a foolproof finding, however, particularly during the early phases of infection or after antibiotics have been given for bacterial meningitis.

Meningitis is a medical emergency. No delay in therapy should be allowed to occur. The patient may need supportive measures (fluid and electrolyte therapy and anticonvulsants such as phenobarbital); specific antibiotic therapy for a bacterial or suspected bacterial-induced meningitis; and close monitoring, preferably in an intensive care unit initially. Isolation is needed during the first 48 hours. Table 44–6 outlines the use of antibiotics.

Until a specific cause is determined,

ampicillin should be given for suspected bacterial meningitis in doses of 200 to 300 mg. per kg. per day by intravenous push every 4 hours rather than by continuous drip (degradation occurs in the intravenous bottle). It should be accompanied by chloramphenicol, 100 mg. per kg. per day, intravenously, particularly in areas in which ampicillin-resistant strains of *H. influenzae* are encountered. Pencillin is administered, similarly, in doses of 250,000 units per kg. per day intravenously, in place of ampicillin when the cause is determined to be a pneumococcal or a meningococcal organism. For neonates, these doses will vary, as will the choice of antibiotics (see section on Infection in the Newborn).

Treatment is continued for at least 5 days after the patient's temperature returns to normal. A second lumbar puncture should be done within 1 to 2 days after the start of therapy to gauge the efficiency of the antibiotic, or antibiotics, chosen. The culture should be negative at this point, and the cerebrospinal fluid glucose should be returning to normal. The clinician must be alert for complications such as septic shock (Waterhouse-Friderichsen syndrome), disseminated intravascular coagulopathy, or electrolyte disturbances (hyponatremia) during the acute phase of illness. The physician should also be alert to the possibility of problems developing later on, e.g., subdural effusions, hydrocephaly, and behavioral sequelae.

Prophylactic therapy is unnecessary for contacts, unless the meningococcus organism is isolated. Current therapy, although debated, is sulfisoxazole or sulfadiazine, 2 grams per day for 4 days. A high percentage of meningococci are now resistant to the sulfonamides. In areas in which such strains are operative, rifampin, 10 mg. per kg. every 12 hours for four doses, is recommended.

Childhood Viral Hepatitis

There are two known varieties of acute hepatitis, type A and type B. As a rule, type A has a shorter incubation period (15 to 40 days) and runs a more acute course. It is spread by the fecal-oral route. Type B may incubate from 50 to 180 days and is usually spread by inoculation. Other important differentiating features are: Type A affects children and young adults and displays transient rises in serum glutamic oxaloacetic transaminase (SGOT) levels and decided increases in thymol turbidity and IgM levels. Type B affects all ages and displays a prolonged elevation in the SGOT level but generally shows no rise in thymol turbidity or IgM levels. In addition, hepatitis-B antigen (Australia antigen) may be isolated in the blood, particularly during the incubation period and the acute phase.

Clinically, type A hepatitis has a sudden onset, with fever, fatigue, gastrointestinal symptoms, tenderness over the liver, and, in two-thirds of the patients, apparent jaundice. Type B hepatitis is insidious, with a protracted but otherwise similar course. There is generally little or no fever associated with it. Occasionally, arthralgia, arthritis, or urticaria is observed. Other helpful laboratory test results include a rise in the total and direct bilirubin levels, urobilirubin in the urine, elevated alkaline phosphatase levels, and increased alpha and beta globulins.

It should be realized that children will appear to be far less ill than adults, and rarely is it necessary to confine them to bed or to provide elaborate diets. Often they are out of bed and eating normally after the first week or two of illness. B complex vitamins and analgesics (not aspirin) may be useful. Steroids are recommended for a protracted or chronic course (more than 12 months). Prednisone, 10 to 40 mg. per day, slowly decreased over many weeks, is recommended. Recent reports have indicated that interferons may be of value in therapy.

Prevention of type A hepatitis consists of administering immune serum globulin (ISG), 0.02 ml. per pound of body weight, which can modify the illness (Table 44–9). Infected patients should be isolated during the first 2 weeks of illness. A hepatitis vaccine is still being perfected. High titer ISG is also promising in helping to modify type B hepatitis. It is tentatively being recommended in known cases of accidental inoculation with infected material.

Childhood Tuberculosis

Many of the features of childhood tuberculosis are similar to those of adult tuberculosis and will not be elaborated here. The chief differences center on presenting signs and symptoms, degree of communicability, and prevention. There are four common modes of presentation: adenitis, pneumonia, meningitis, and the inapparent infection.

TABLE 44–9.   TYPE A HEPATITIS – INDICATIONS FOR PROPHYLAXIS WITH
IMMUNE SERUM (GAMMA) GLOBULIN*

Type of Exposure	Cases Given Gamma Globulin	Dose, Ml./Lb. Body Weight	Comments
Household contact	All	0.01 to 0.02	
School contacts	Usually none		Immune serum globulin is given if the infection tends to spread
Work contacts	Usually none		Immune serum globulin is given if the infection tends to spread
Institutions, orphanages, playing schools	All exposed	0.01 to 0.02	Immune serum globulin given if type of contact is similar to that of household contacts or if poor hygiene is prevalent
Common source outbreaks	All exposed	0.01 to 0.02	As restricted as possible to individuals known to have been exposed
Medical personnel	Usually none		Immune serum globulin given if cases occur among the personnel
Travelers to countries with a high incidence of hepatitis			
short-term travel (1 to 2 months)		0.01 to 0.02	
Extended travel (more than 2 months)		0.01 to 0.04	Repeated every 5 to 6 months

*From Ringertz, O.: Am. J. Dis. Child., *123*:427, April, 1972. Copyright 1972, American Medical Association.

In tuberculous adenitis, most often the cervical lymph nodes enlarge, display few signs of pyogenic infection, and, finally, coalesce and become adherent to nearby structures. If untreated, fistula formation commonly occurs. The atypical or Battey strains of bacilli are the most likely causative organisms. Skin testing with atypical mycobacteria, as well as with ordinary tuberculin, is indicated. Early therapy is often effective in preventing fistula formation and spread to other sites.

In the pneumonia form, onset is insidious and respiratory symptoms do not predominate. Usual findings consist of anorexia, weight loss, and fever. Chest findings are generally minimal: occasional rhonchi or rales and sometimes a pleural friction rub. Cough, night sweats, hemoptysis, and cavity formation are all infrequent in the childhood form. The chest x-ray will often show more extensive involvement than the clinical findings suggest. The tuberculin test is almost always positive. Cultures of sputum, if an adequate specimen can be obtained, and of gastric washings should be undertaken.

Tuberculous meningitis is usually clearly discernible from ordinary bacterial menin- gitis by its very slow, gradual onset over a period of several days or weeks. Headache, increasing lethargy, behavioral changes, anorexia, and fever are the usual manifestations. Cranial nerve signs (eyelid ptosis) help localize the process to the base of the brain. Spinal fluid will usually show an increase in mononuclear cells and a low glucose content (less than 50 per cent of the blood glucose). It should be realized that the tuberculin reaction is frequently negative (as often as 50 per cent of the time). A chest x-ray study may demonstrate pulmonic lesions. A Ziehl-Neelsen stain may reveal acid-fast bacteria in the cerebrospinal fluid (CSF), and cultures may be positive in 4 to 8 weeks. Therapy should not be delayed; otherwise both subsequent morbidity and mortality are great.

The patient with inapparent tuberculosis infection presents with intermittent fever and anorexia. The physical examination usually reveals nothing more than a somewhat "run-down" child. Chest x-rays are negative. The diagnosis is suggested by a positive tuberculin test.

In none of these forms is communicability usually a real problem nor is isolation necessary. But if an infected lymph node drains or if cavitary disease of the lung should develop, isolation will be necessary. These are unusual occurrences, however.

Prevention and Therapy. Bacille Calmette-Guérin (BCG) vaccine should be given to infants who are in continuous and intimate contact with an actively infected adult.

Surgical excision is indicated in tuberculosis adenitis if the nodes are few in number and discrete. Needle aspiration may help when nodes that cannot be removed are softening. Isoniazid (INH) and para-amino-salicylic acid (PAS) should be given for 1 year.

Patients with tuberculous pneumonia are given INH and PAS for at least 1 year. Streptomycin and other antituberculous agents may be useful if resolution does not occur. Prednisone is indicated for endobronchial involvement, particularly when accompanied by atelectasis.

INH and PAS are given for at least 1 year to children with tuberculous meningitis. Streptomycin is continued for 1 month after a good clinical response is noted. Prednisone, 1 mg. per kg. per 24 hours, is continued for 6 to 12 weeks. For inapparent infections, INH should be used for 1 year in a child of any age from infancy through adolescence.

In the event of a poor response in any of these forms of tuberculosis, other chemotherapeutic agents can be substituted, e.g., cycloserine, ethionamide, ethambutol, and rifampin (before using these agents, see manufacturers' official directives for recommendations and precautions for use in children).

Septic Arthritis

Septic arthritis is usually caused by group A streptococci, *Staphylococcus aureus*, pneumococci, and *H. influenzae,* but one may also encounter gonococci and, in infants, gram-negative organisms as causative agents.

Symptoms consist of pain, swelling, redness, warmth, and limitation of movement. Most often, systemic signs of fever, an ill appearance, and anorexia coexist. Occasionally, the child will look remarkably well, and the presence of persistent joint symptoms, with no adequate explanation for them, will lead to the diagnosis. The white

blood cell count usually shows a polymorphonuclear response. Cultures of joint fluid and blood cultures may allow precise identification of the causative organisms. Synovial fluid will show 25,000 to 250,000 lymphocytes with a decrease in glucose content. X-ray studies may demonstrate widening of the joint space and, later, destruction of joint cartilage.

Treatment consists of antibiotic therapy administered without delay (see Table 44–6). Splinting the joint may provide relief from pain, but when local signs abate, the joint should be increasingly mobilized. Incision and drainage or repeated aspirations are indicated for treating large collections of pus, particularly if 48 to 72 hours of antibiotic medication have not led to any improvement. Antibiotic therapy should be continued for 4 to 6 weeks, until all signs of acute infection are gone.

Osteomyelitis

Osteomyelitis generally involves the long bones, most often of the lower extremities. The bacterial causes are similar to the causes of septic arthritis, which can coexist when osteomyelitis involves bone tissue adjacent to a joint space. *Salmonella* osteomyelitis may be seen in children with sickle cell disease.

Symptoms include joint tenderness over the infected area with a variable degree of swelling, redness, and warmth; fever; anorexia; and a toxic appearance of the patient. The white blood cell count is elevated. Blood cultures and aspirates from the bone may allow identification of the organisms. Early x-ray examinations may show evidence of a deep-seated myositis, but these findings are not diagnostic. Later (>1 week or more), destruction of bony tissue and periosteal elevation with new bone formation may be observed.

Therapy consists of the administration of antibiotics (see Table 44–6) and analgesics. The duration of antibiotic treatment is from 4 to 6 weeks, depending on response. Intravenous administration of drugs is used during the first 2 to 5 days at the very least. If response is rapid, the intramuscular or oral route can be used. Surgery is needed for removal of large collections of pus and dead bone.

Parasite Infestation

The most common human parasites found in the United States are pinworms, roundworms, whipworms *(Trichuris)*, tapeworms, and hookworms.

Pinworm infestation is the most prevalent. It causes rectal pruritus and emotional irritability, but nutrition does not suffer. Communicability by the hand-to-mouth route is most common. The diagnosis is made by recovering ova on Scotch tape applied overnight to the rectum. Entire families may be affected and should be screened when a target case is discovered.

Roundworms *(Ascaris)* cause colicky abdominal pain, poor nutrition, fatigue, and irritability. Eosinophil counts may be elevated, but three or more stool examinations are more valuable in establishing the diagnosis. A chest x-ray study to detect possible pulmonary involvement should be obtained. The parasite passes through the lungs (Loeffler's syndrome).

Whipworms *(Trichuris)* are small and threadlike. Symptoms are mild, generally consisting only of slight pain in the abdomen. Nutrition is unaffected. The stool examination establishes the diagnosis, and eosinophilia is common.

The tapeworm infests the intestinal tract, causing nutritional compromise, abdominal pain, and hunger. Stool examinations or worm recovery confirms the diagnosis.

The hookworm is usually found in the southern regions of the United States. It enters the host by penetrating the skin. Initial symptoms may be of respiratory origin but later consist of abdominal pain, diarrhea, weight loss, and anemia. The ova can be identified in the stool.

Table 44–10 outlines the treatment of parasitic infestations.

EMERGENCIES

Cardiac Arrest

Abrupt or unexpected cardiac arrest can occur for a variety of reasons—anaphylaxis, anesthesia, myocarditis, suffocation, and so forth. The endpoint, however, is basically the same, that is, insufficient perfusion and oxygen transport to body tissues. As a result, organic acids rapidly increase, potassium ions are displaced from the intracellular to the extracellular compartment, and hyperkalemia develops. For these reasons, the PaO_2 level, base excess, and blood pH decrease while the $PaCO_2$ and serum K^+

TABLE 44–10.   TREATMENT OF PARASITE INFESTATION*

Parasite	Drug	Dose
Pinworm	Antiminth (pyrantel pamoate)	11 mg./kg. dose, not to exceed 1 gram; to 3 doses at 2 to 3 week intervals
	Povan (pyrvinium pamoate)	5 mg. per kg. per dose; to 3 doses at 2 to 3 week intervals
Roundworm	Antiminth	As for pinworms
	Antepar (piperazine citrate)	75 mg. per kg. per dose, not to exceed 3 grams; give 2 consecutive days
Whipworm	Vermox (mebendazole)	100 mg. twice daily for 3 days
Tapeworm	Yomesan (niclosamide)†	<20 lb.—0.5 gram, <60 lb.—1 gram, >60 lb.—2 grams for 5 days; repeat after 10 days
Hookworm	Antiminth‡	As for pinworms

*Modified from Rajkumar, S. V., and Laude, T. A., Pediatric Ambulatory Service Manual, Brooklyn, N.Y., Downstate Medical Center, Kings County Hospital, 1976.
†May be obtained from Parasitic Disease Drug Service, Center for Disease Control, Atlanta, Georgia 30333.
§The use of Antiminth in the treatment of hookworm infestations is not listed in the manufacturer's official directive.

levels increase. One of the devastating effects of these changes is a refractory heart, difficult to resuscitate; another, of course, is damage to the central nervous system.

Successful therapy demands rapid institution of the following measures: artificial ventilation by the mouth-to-mouth or self-inflating bag technique, after clearing the airway; cardiac massage; the administration of alkaline solutions to combat acidosis; and the administration of calcium, 100 mg. per kg. per dose, or of glucose and insulin to counter hyperkalemia. Coordinated massage and ventilation with a 4 to 1 ratio respectively at three-fourths the normal heart rate is recommended. An intravenous infusion of isoproterenol (Isuprel), 0.5 to 1.0 microgram per kg. per minute, as well as of sodium bicarbonate, 3 mEq. per kg. per dose, repeated every 8 minutes until a response is obtained or the effort is abandoned, is necessary.

If a total of 15 mEq. per kg. of sodium bicarbonate is reached, tromethamine with electrolytes (THAM) is substituted to avoid hypernatremia. Aqueous epinephrine may be used in place of isoproterenol (1.0 microgram per kg. per minute), but isoproterenol has the advantage of improving perfusion because it causes peripheral vasodilation. If ventricular fibrillation occurs, defibrillation should be used. Success rates depend on the cause of the fibrillation, the promptness with which therapy is initiated, and the skill of the resuscitators.

Shock

Shock leads to physiologic changes similar to those that occur in cardiac arrest, i.e., poor tissue perfusion, acidosis, and loss of precapillary sphincter tone with splanchnic pooling and hypotension. The causes of shock are many: hemorrhage, sepsis, hemolytic-uremic syndrome, and so forth. For this reason, clinical manifestations may vary; however, pallor, cyanosis, cold or clammy skin, tachycardia, oliguria, and hypotension are common to all patients in shock. The central venous pressure is decreased, and blood gases demonstrate a decreased pH, base excess, and PO_2 level. The PCO_2 level is variable.

Treatment, in addition to measures directed toward managing the primary disease, includes ensuring the maintenance of a good airway and adequate ventilation.

Intubation or tracheostomy, as well as oxygen, may be required. Acidosis will need to be corrected with either sodium bicarbonate or THAM. If pulmonary edema occurs, a phlebotomy and digitalization are necessary. Isoproterenol will improve cardiac output, as well as peripheral vasodilation and perfusion. When blood volume is low, whole blood or plasma expanders are useful. In instances of oliguria or renal shutdown without hypovolemia, or both, mannitol is administered. The use of steroids is controversial but has been recommended (dexamethasone, 5 mg. per kg. per 24 hours). Vasopressors are now used only temporarily, when the abrupt onset of hypotension may lead to cardiac arrest.

Anaphylaxis

Anaphylaxis is an immune reaction associated with the release of chemical mediators producing severe, life-threatening symptoms. It occurs most often after the parenteral administration of such medications as penicillin, treatment allergens, or antitoxins.

Nasal congestion, sneezing, and conjunctival tearing followed by dyspnea, vomiting, stridor, and cardiovascular collapse are some of the symptoms that may occur. Delay in initiating immediate therapy could prove fatal. The following steps should be instituted: A tourniquet is placed above the injection site (if any), 0.5 ml. of aqueous epinephrine (1 to 1000) is injected in the opposite arm, and 0.2 ml. of epinephrine is administered in the injection site as well. Then diphenhydramine (Benadryl), 1 mg. per kg., is given intramuscularly. After these initial steps, if further treatment is necessary, an intravenous infusion should be started, oxygen administered, and an adequate airway provided. In the event of severe hypotension and shock, vasopressors can be used. Aminophylline may be helpful for bronchospasm. Hydrocortisone sodium succinate (Solu-Cortef), 100 mg. intramuscularly is useful in controlling recurrent symptoms, although the onset of action of this drug is from 2 to 6 hours.

Accidental Poisoning

Every year more than 300 children die in the United States from self-poisoning, despite the increasing emphasis on both prevention and therapy. The risk is highest in preschool aged children and adolescents, with the risk in boys exceeding that in girls by 3 to 2 in preschoolers. However, the reverse is true in adolescents. The agents most likely to be ingested are medications, household preparations, cosmetics, and insecticides.

Diagnosis can be difficult in the absence of a specific history of poisoning. Unusual signs and symptoms, characteristic odors, and analysis of body fluids (particularly vomitus, urine, and blood) may indicate the offending agent.

Management consists of identifying the poison, estimating the quantity ingested, removing or neutralizing it, and providing support for life functions. Identification depends on obtaining an accurate history, having access to the material ingested, and, if necessary, consulting poison control centers or reference books for advice.

Several methods exist for removing or neutralizing the poison. The most effective is inducing vomiting by using an emetic agent. The most practical agent is syrup of ipecac because it can be obtained without a prescription, can be stored for long periods at home, can be given by mouth, and is an effective emetic. The child is given 15 ml. of ipecac followed by 6 to 8 oz. (180 to 240 ml.) of water. The dose may be repeated once if vomiting fails to occur after 20 minutes; otherwise, gastric lavage may be required. Lavage results in less efficient gastric emptying and is usually reserved for unconscious patients. However, if large, potentially lethal amounts of hydrocarbons are ingested, careful lavage is indicated and the induction of emesis is avoided. In this manner, the risk of aspiration pneumonia is reduced. If a cuffed endotracheal tube is used, the risk of aspiration is virtually eliminated.

Purgatives and enemas are useful in causing rapid elimination of the poison. More specialized methods such as alkalinizing or acidifying the urine, peritoneal dialysis and hemodialysis, and exchange transfusion may also be helpful.

A few poisons may be neutralized with specific antidotes (Table 44–11). Activated charcoal, if given within 2 hours of ingestion, is effective for aspirin, barbiturate, chlorpromazine, propoxyphene, and acetaminophen poisoning. It is given in a dose of

TABLE 44–11. SPECIFIC ANTIDOTES FOR ACCIDENTAL POISONING

Compound	Antidote
Arsenic	British anti-lewisite
Mercury	(BAL)
Bismuth	Penicillamine
Antimony	
Gold	
Lead	Ethylenediaminetetra-acetic acid (EDTA) and BAL Penicillamine
Caustic alkali	Weak acids (vinegar, fruit juices)
Strong acids	Weak bases that do not produce CO_2 (magnesium oxide, aluminum hydroxide [Amphojel], milk of magnesia)
Iodine	Sodium thiosulfate
Methemoglobin	Methylene blue
Formaldehyde	Ammonium hydroxide
Iron	Deferoxamine
Cyanide	Sodium nitrite Sodium thiosulfate
Phosphorus	Copper sulfate
Anticoagulants	Vitamin K
Morphine	Naloxone
Meperidine (Demerol)	
Methadone, etc.	
Parathion and other organic phosphate esters	Atropine
Parasympathomimetics (pilocarpine, muscarine)	

5 to 10 times the amount of the injested poison.

Salicylate Poisoning. Of all medications, aspirin is the most frequently involved in self-poisoning. The diagnosis and management require special mention for this reason, as well as for the difficulties they present.

Symptoms, when significant ingestion has occurred, tend to be insidious and to resemble other illnesses, e.g., pneumonia. In the first few hours after ingestion, anorexia, vomiting, fever, and sweating occur, but the most characteristic sign is hyperventilation. It is this latter sign that causes confusion with the signs of respiratory illnesses. However, on auscultation, the chest is clear. Later on, dehydration and sensorium changes leading to convulsions and coma dominate the clinical picture. In the initial or respiratory phase, there is a tendency for respiratory alkalosis to develop, although this is generally observed only in adults. After a short time, metabolic acidosis becomes the predominant process, and laboratory findings reflect this change. The PCO_2 level is decreased, as is base excess and plasma bicarbonate, while the blood pH remains normal in the compensated state but falls in the uncompensated state.

Reducing substances and ketones appear in the urine. An occasional child will have hypernatremia or hyperglycemia, or both. The most helpful test for both diagnosing and gauging the severity of salicylate poisoning is the determination of the serum salicylate level. The level itself is most valuable when it is compared with the known excretion rates of salicylate over the several hours following a single ingestion (Fig. 44–4). It should be understood that this nomogram loses its predictive value in instances of chronic ingestion. As a rule, toxic levels of salicylate are likely to be reached when 50 mg. per pound (110 mg. per kg.) of body weight is ingested.

Management of acute salicylate poisoning depends on the amount ingested, the elapsed time after ingestion, and the state of the patient. If the child is alert and ingestion has occurred within 2 hours, give 15 ml. of ipecac, 200 ml. of isotonic saline, and 10 mg. of activated charcoal for each mg. of salicylate ingested. Obtain a blood salicylate level to determine further therapy.

For asymptomatic patients with a salicylate level in the asymptomatic-to-mild range, force fluids by mouth, observe the child for 12 to 24 hours, and counsel the parents on prevention. For symptomatic patients with a salicylate level in the mild-to-moderate range, obtain blood gas and serum electrolyte determinations, monitor the vital signs, record intake and output, start intravenous fluids, and correct dehydration. The following solution may be used: 3000 ml. per square meter of body surface of a 1/3 isotonic, balanced electrolyte solution containing 5 per cent glucose to help replace liver glycogen. After urine flow is established, add potassium chloride, 40 mEq. per square meter, to correct hypokalemia and add sufficient sodium bicarbonate or sodium lactate to correct the negative base excess. Acetazolamide (Diamox), 5 mg. per kg., given subcutaneously to alkalinize the urine is effective in increasing salicylate excretion via the kidneys but results in an obligate loss of base, which may make the acidosis worse. Extreme caution is advised in using this medication, and frequent blood gas and urine pH determinations ought to be done. For acetazolamide to be effective, the urine pH should equal or exceed 7.5. Twentyfold more salicylate will be excreted at this pH than at a pH of 6.5.

Severely symptomatic patients with salicylate levels in the severe range or with hyperpyrexia, poor renal function, coma, and pulmonary edema, should be considered for either exchange transfusions or peritoneal dialysis or hemodialysis. Bleeding tendencies may be corrected with vitamin K.

POISONING

A. SALICYLATE POISONING

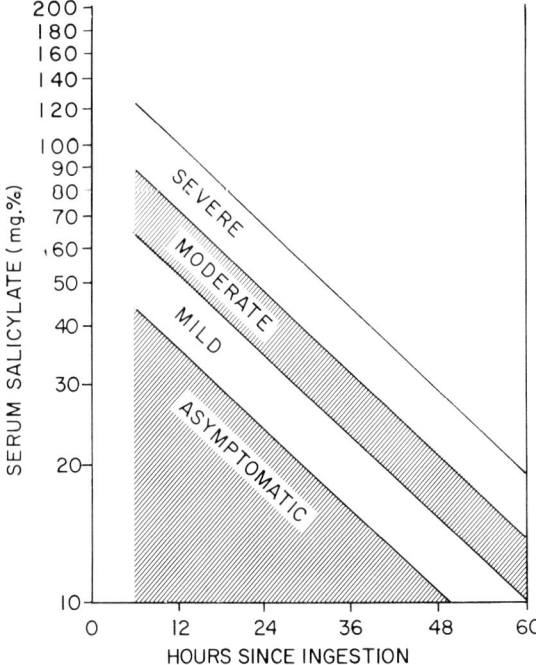

Figure 44–4. A nomogram comparing the serum salicylate level and the severity of intoxication following single dose ingestions of salicylate. (From Done, A. K.: Pediatrics, 26:800, 1969. Courtesy of the American Academy of Pediatrics, Inc., Publisher.)

CONVULSIVE DISORDERS IN CHILDREN

A wide variety of disorders of the central nervous system cause convulsions in children. Convulsions can be either acute and nonrecurring or chronic and recurring. The term epilepsy is used to describe the latter category.

The following are some of the frequent disorders of infancy and childhood that result in acute convulsions:

1. Febrile conditions—febrile seizures.
2. Intracranial infections—bacterial, viral, parasitic infections.
3. Intracranial injuries—birth trauma, anoxic damage, hemorrhages.
4. Metabolic and nutritional disorders—pyridoxine deficiency, hypernatremia, hypoglycemia, hypomagnesemia, hypocalcemia.
5. Encephalopathies—lead poisoning, shigellosis, immunization reactions.

Other less frequent causes of acute convulsions include congenital defects of the brain, cerebral degenerative diseases, and brain tumors.

Epilepsy can be either idiopathic (cause unknown) or organic (cause known). The residual damage following an acute insult to the brain from many of the causes just listed may contribute to the organicity of epilepsy.

Febrile Convulsions

Seizures occurring with fever that are unattributable to any specific illness within the nervous system are termed febrile seizures. This is one of the most frequent causes of convulsions in pediatric patients. Febrile seizures generally occur in children between the ages of 6 months and 6 years, being very infrequent after the age of 3 years. A familial pattern is frequently noted.

Two types of febrile seizures are defined: simple febrile convulsions and fever-precipitated epileptic seizures. In simple febrile seizures, fever produces convulsions in a child who is otherwise normal. Convulsions are generalized and brief, and the prognosis is uniformly good. In fever-precipitated epileptic seizures, fever precipitates convulsions in a youngster who is potentially an epileptic child. Convulsions may be prolonged, recurring, and either generalized or focal. A majority of children in this category go on to develop epilepsy.

A diagnosis of febrile convulsions must be made only after carefully ruling out other causes of convulsions also associated with fever, e.g., meningitis.

Seizure Patterns

Most seizures fall into a few identifiable patterns. A definition of the seizure pattern is essential, as it forms the basis for the selection of an appropriate anticonvulsant medication.

Grand Mal Seizures. These are generalized convulsions, usually with tonic and clonic muscular spasms, that are generally preceded by an aura. The aura most frequently consists of spasms or muscle twitching, vague abdominal sensations, dizziness, and headache. The convulsion that follows the aura starts with the tonic phase, consisting of a generalized contracture of the musculature, and simultaneous loss of consciousness. This is followed by the clonic phase, characterized by rhythmic muscular contractions. During the tonic-clonic phases, the child may bite his tongue, develop cyanosis, urinate, and defecate. The clonic phase may last for variable periods of time. The postconvulsive state is marked by fatigue, drowsiness, and generalized headache.

Focal Seizures. Focal seizures may be either sensory or motor (jacksonian epilepsy). Sensory seizures are rare in children. In jacksonian epilepsy, the seizures are generally clonic in nature. The seizures beginning in one group of muscles spread to the other groups, according to a pattern based on the representation of the muscle groups in the precentral gyrus (fingers to wrist to arm to face, and so forth). If the seizure remains confined to one area, a loss of consciousness may not occur. However, if the convulsion becomes widespread and generalized, the patient usually loses consciousness. The diagnosis of a focal seizure implies the presence of a localized organic lesion in the brain, although a discrete lesion may not always be demonstrable.

Petit Mal Seizures. Petit mal attacks are usually described by parents as "staring spells" or "dizzy spells." There is a very brief loss of consciousness, usually lasting for not more than 30 seconds. This is often accompanied by manifestations such as nodding movements of the head and rolling of the eyes. During the spell, the child will momentarily stop whatever he is doing at the time, such as writing or reading, and will resume normal activity once the attack is over, without being aware of having had a convulsion. The frequency of attacks varies from two to three a month to as many as several hundred a day. Petit mal seizures rarely occur in children under the age of 3 years.

Psychomotor Seizures. Clinically, this seizure pattern is difficult to recognize, as seizure manifestations are varied. An aura, similar to the one occurring with a grand mal seizure, usually precedes an attack. The attack itself may include psychic, sensory, and motor phenomena. These may occur in combination or singly. When motor symptoms mark an attack, one can see the affected child performing purposeful but inappropriate motor acts, e.g., masticatory and swallowing movements. Psychic symptoms include anger, fear, hallucinations, and feelings of depression. Numbness or paresthesia may be experienced by some children. Postictal phenomena such as headache, drowsiness, and fatigue usually follow an attack.

Myoclonic Seizures. The infantile myoclonic seizures (also called infantile spasm, lightning seizures, or jackknife seizures are characterized by sudden forceful contractions of the musculature of the trunk, neck, and extremities. In the flexor type of seizure, the child doubles up on himself and the neck is flexed. In the extensor type, the neck is extended and the arms are spread out. There is no apparent loss of consciousness. The attacks may be over in a matter of seconds. Repeated attacks may occur in a single day. The electroencephalogram (EEG) in 90 per cent of the patients is characterized by a pattern known as hypsarrhythmia. In many children, seizures spontaneously disappear before the age of 4 years. The prognosis is generally poor, with more than 90 per cent of the affected children showing significant mental retardation.

Akinetic Seizures. These are also known as "drop fits." Such seizures usually occur in conjunction with organic brain disease. The history in many patients strongly suggests a diffuse encephalopathy following a central nervous system infection. The attack is characterized by a sudden loss of muscle tone, resulting either in an abrupt nodding motion of the head if the child is sitting or in

his dropping to the floor if he is standing. Several attacks may occur in a single day.

Autonomic Seizures (Seizure Equivalents). These are paroxysmal attacks of autonomic disturbances that result in a variety of symptoms commonly encountered in pediatric practice. Such symptoms include headache, abdominal pain, cyclic vomiting, and enuresis. Behavioral disturbances such as fits of rage and uncontrollable laughter have also been observed.

Work-up of a Child with Seizures

A good history is an essential part of the total work-up. Particular attention should be given to the prenatal, neonatal, and family history. The age of onset and the association of fever are important considerations. The seizure pattern should be carefully determined. Physical examination should include complete neurologic and funduscopic examinations.

A spinal tap must be performed whenever meningitis is considered in the differential diagnosis. Although it is desirable to routinely tap all children being evaluated for a first convulsion to rule out meningitis, it is worthwhile to note that only rarely is such a diagnosis established. An urinalysis and complete blood tests should be done routinely. Blood glucose, calcium, and electrolyte values should be determined, and radiologic examination of the skull may occasionally provide valuable information.

Electroencephalography is a useful procedure, often helping not only to identify a seizure pattern but also to differentiate diffuse encephalopathies from localized lesions.

More specific investigations such as air studies and cerebral angiography may be considered if vascular or neoplastic lesions are suspected. Other studies such as urine tests for the presence of porphyria, aminoaciduria, cytomegaloinclusion bodies, and so forth, and blood tests for lead levels and sickle cell anemia should be done, if warranted on the basis of the history and physical examination. Computerized tomography should also be performed when intracranial lesions are suspected.

Management of a Child with Acute Convulsions

The child should be protected from injuries by placing him on his side on a firm mattress. All tight clothing should be loosened. Tongue-biting can be prevented by placing a padded tongue blade between the teeth. Prompt suctioning of nasopharyngeal secretions should be done. Oxygen, if necessary, should be administered. The drug of choice in the treatment of acute convulsions is diazepam (Valium) (see manufacturer's official directive about safety in neonates). This is given intravenously in a dose not exceeding 10 mg. (0.3 mg. per kg.) at a rate of 1 mg. per minute. The dose of diazepam can be repeated in 20 to 30 minutes if necessary.

Alternatively, phenobarbital sodium, 30 to 60 mg. per year of age up to a maximum of 240 mg., may be given intravenously. Half the initial dose may be repeated in 20 minutes if necessary.

Management of a Child with Chronic, Recurrent Convulsions (Epilepsy)

Success in the management of an epileptic child depends on the correct selection and dosage of the anticonvulsant medications, based on the seizure pattern; early and prompt institution of treatment, and strict patient compliance in taking the

medications, which is greatly influenced by the type of rapport a physician develops with the child.

The overall goal should be to enable a child with epilepsy to lead as nearly normal a life as possible. Patient and parent education concerning the nature of the illness and the duration of therapy is an essential part of the management.

The specific medications and their doses are shown in Table 44–12. It should be remembered that a second drug should not be added unless an adequate trial with a maximum-tolerated dose of the first medication has failed to control the convulsions. Medications should be taken in divided doses on a schedule that least interferes with the patient's routine activities. Periodic laboratory tests should be done during the course of the therapy with certain drugs.

FLUID AND ELECTROLYTES

Dehydration

A loss of body water and electrolytes without a loss of supporting tissues is

TABLE 44–12. RECOMMENDED MEDICATIONS FOR CHRONIC, RECURRENT CONVULSIONS (EPILEPSY)

Type	Medication	Dose
Grand mal seizures	Phenobarbital	3 to 5 mg./kg./day
	Phenytoin (diphenylhydantoin)	5 to 10 mg./kg./day
	Primidone	12 to 25 mg./kg./day
Petit mal seizures	Ethosuximide	15 to 30 mg./kg./day
	Trimethadione	20 to 30 mg./kg./day
Psychomotor seizures	Carbamazepine (Tegretol)°	12 to 24 mg./kg./day
	Primidone	12 to 25 mg./kg./day
	Phenytoin (diphenylhydantoin)	5 to 10 mg./kg./day
Myoclonic seizures	Diazepam°	0.1 to 0.8 mg./kg./day
	ACTH	5 to 10 units/day; up to 50 units/day
Akinetic seizures	Diazepam°	0.1 to 0.8 mg./kg./24 hrs.
Autonomic seizures	Phenobarbital	3 to 5 mg./kg./day
	Phenytoin (diphenylhydantoin)	5 to 10 mg./kg./day

°Consult package insert for pediatric restrictions.

TABLE 44–13.   CHARACTERISTICS OF THE THREE TYPES OF DEHYDRATION

	Isotonic	Hypotonic	Hypertonic
History	Acute onset of diarrhea Vomiting or refusal to feed	Severe diarrhea with excessive water ingestion, or chronic diarrhea with inadequate salt replacement	Acute diarrhea with intake of high–solute-load fluids (newborns with renal immaturity particularly susceptible)
Physical Examination	Apathetic, inactive Skin cold, with poor turgor Dry mucous membrane Sunken eyeballs and fontanelle Rapid pulse	Apathetic, inactive Skin cold and clammy, with poor turgor Dry mucous membrane Sunken eyeballs and fontanelle Rapid pulse	Hyperirritable Skin usually warm, with doughy feeling Turgor fairly well maintained Sunken fontanelle Moderately rapid pulse
Serum Sodium Values	Normal	Less than 130 mEq./L.	More than 150 mEq./L.

termed dehydration. Clinical signs of dehydration in infants usually do not become apparent until a loss of more than 60 ml. of fluid per kg. of body weight has occurred. A loss of more than 160 ml. of fluid per kg. of body weight represents the maximum dehydration tolerable. A loss greater than this amount leads to shock and death. In older children with relatively less body water, a loss of smaller amounts (about 75 per cent of the figures just cited) would produce similar degrees of dehydration.

The most common clinical entity causing dehydration in pediatric patients is diarrheal disease. Here, the abnormal losses of water and electrolytes in the stool occur in conjunction with a curtailed fluid intake, either because of vomiting or because of an unwillingness of the child to ingest adequate amounts of fluid. Metabolic acidosis is often an accompanying feature.

Dehydration occurs in three forms: isotonic, in which the loss of water and solute from the body is proportionately equal; hypertonic, in which the loss of water is proportionately greater than that of the solute; and hypotonic, in which the loss of solute is proportionately greater than that of water.

Clinically, it is important to distinguish the three types of dehydration, as therapy is different for each type. The differentiating factors of dehydration are summarized in Table 44–13.

When planning therapy for patients with dehydration, three basic questions should be answered. How much fluid? What kind of fluid? How should the fluid be administered?

How Much Fluid?

In order to calculate the amount of fluid a child requires in a given clinical situation, three factors should be taken into account: (1) the deficit that has already occurred when the child is first examined, (2) the normal losses that occur irrespective of the illness, and (3) the abnormal losses that continue to occur throughout the duration of the illness.

The Deficit that Has Already Occurred. The deficit is related to the body mass and is reflected in the weight change before and after the start of illness. The deficit in body weight equals the deficit in body fluid, as only fluid loss accounts for weight change in acute dehydration. Thus, if a child weighed 10 kg. before the onset of illness and weighs 9.5 kg. at the time of evaluation, the deficit is 0.5 kg., or 500 ml. of fluid. In many instances, however, the preillness weight is usually not available, so that an educated guess of the existing deficit has to be made on the basis of the degree of dehydration observed clinically. Mild dehydration usually represents a loss of about 3 to 5 per cent of body weight, moderate dehydration 6 to 9 per cent, and severe dehydration 10 to 15 per cent.

Normal Losses that Occur Irrespective of the Illness. Replacement of the normal fluid loss constitutes maintenance therapy. The following can be used in the assessment of maintenance fluid requirements: caloric expenditure, surface area, and body weight in kilograms.

MAINTENANCE NEEDS BY CALORIC EXPENDITURE. The normal loss is a reflection of body metabolism and therefore of caloric expenditure. Thus, in the strictest sense, the maintenance requirement is calculated on the basis of calories expended. Roughly, 150 ml. of water and 2 to 3 mEq. of sodium and potassium, the principal electrolytes, are expended by the body per 100 calories metabolized.

Calories expended per 24 hours by children with different body weights during parenteral therapy are given in Table 44–14. Thus, according to the table, a child weighing 10 kg. is expected to expend 450 calories per 24 hours and therefore his maintenance requirement of water is 675 ml. (150 ml. per 100 calories) and that of sodium and potassium is 9 mEq. (2 mEq. per 100 calories).

TABLE 44–14.   CALORIES EXPENDED PER 24 HOURS DURING FASTING*

Subject	Calories/Kg.
Newborn	45–50
3–10 kg.	60–80
10–15 kg.	45–65
15–25 kg.	40–50
25–35 kg.	35–40
35–60 kg.	30–35
Over 60 kg.	25–30

*From Darrow, D. C.: Pediatr. Clin. North Am., *11*:823, 1964.

MAINTENANCE NEEDS BY SURFACE AREA. With certain exceptions, caloric expenditure and therefore fluid requirement correlate well with the surface area of the body. Therefore, the latter can also be used as a convenient factor in the estimation of maintenance requirements of fluid and electrolytes. For a quick calculation, one needs to remember that 1500 to 2000 ml. of water and 40 mEq. of sodium and potassium are required for maintenance needs in a child per 1 square meter (m^2) of body surface area. These figures do not apply to newborns during the first few days of life, when the requirements are about two-fifths of these amounts.

To calculate the surface area, one needs to consult standard nomograms, but for a quick reference the following figures can be useful: a 10 kg. child has approximately 0.5 m^2 of surface area, a 30 kg. child has approximately 1 m^2 of surface area, and a 60 kg. child has approximately 1.5 m^2 of surface area. According to this method of calculation, a 10 kg. child needs the following amounts of water and electrolytes for maintenance: water—750 ml. (1500 × 0.5) and sodium and potassium—20 mEq. (40 × 0.5).

MAINTENANCE NEEDS BY BODY WEIGHT. This is yet another way to estimate the maintenance requirement of water and electrolytes. Calculating fluid requirements by body weight is popular because in the pediatric age group, the body weight, expressed generally in kilograms, is a constant consideration in an overall evaluation of the child. A reasonably satisfactory estimate of fluid requirements can be arrived at by using the guidelines in Table 44–15. According to this method, a 10 kg. child

TABLE 44–15. ESTIMATING FLUID REQUIREMENTS BY BODY WEIGHT

	Age of Patient	Fluid Requirements (Per Kg. of Body Weight)
Water	0–10 days	65–150 ml.
	10 days–1 year	150 ± 30 ml.
	1–5 years	120 ± 30 ml.
	Over 5 years	90 ± 30 ml.
Sodium and Potassium	(All ages)	3–5 mEq.

approximately 1 year of age would require 1500 ml. of water (150 × 10) and 30 mEq. of sodium and potassium (10 × 3).

The figures for the amount of maintenance fluids required for a 10 kg. child, as calculated by the three different methods just described, vary sometimes by as much as 50 per cent, but they nevertheless fall within the range of body tolerance provided by homeostatic mechanisms and therefore are equally well tolerated by the body. This simple truth cannot be stressed too much and should indicate to a clinician that he has, indeed, a good deal of flexibility in the management of fluid therapy. It must be remembered, however, that this liberal range of tolerance can become considerably narrower if body homeostatic mechanisms are not functioning optimally (e.g., renal disease).

Abnormal Losses. The abnormal losses that continue to occur throughout the duration of illness are the final consideration. The amount lost depends on the nature of illness. Losses should be replaced volume for volume by appropriate solutions. In a child with diarrheal disease, once the child is on parenteral therapy, the losses usually do not exceed 10 to 25 ml. per kg. per day. Approximately this same amount may be added to the total requirement calculated.

In summary, to arrive at an answer to the question "how much fluid?" calculate the amounts needed to cover the existing deficit, the ongoing, normal (maintenance) requirements, and the abnormal (supplemental) losses, and add these up.

What Kind of Fluid?

Except during the initial phase of the therapy for children with severe dehydration, most types of dehydration can ordinarily be corrected with hypotonic solutions containing the principal ions, sodium, potassium, bicarbonate or lactate, and chloride. In severe dehydration in which there is a significant contraction of the extracellular fluid compartment, it is necessary to expand the compartment as quickly as possible by using isotonic solutions such as isotonic saline, plasma, blood, and so forth, in order to prevent shock. A portion of the total amount calculated to correct the deficit can be used for this purpose. Usually, about 20 to 30 ml. of isotonic fluid per kg. of body weight given over a period of 30 to 60 minutes will be sufficient for this purpose.

Once this emergency phase is over, it is not physiologic to use isotonic saline to correct fluid and electrolyte imbalance. This is simply because the dehydrated body needs free water (water that is unaccounted for by the electrolytes in a given solution) to attain a normal fluid and electrolyte status. Isotonic saline (15 mEq. of sodium per 100 ml. of fluid) does not provide this free water, as the water content of this solution has been "accounted for by its electrolytes," either for its retention or excretion. The body needs free water because it generally loses more water than it does electrolytes under both normal and abnormal conditions. Given this fact, one would expect to find hypertonic dehydration in most clinical situations. However, this is not the case; isotonic dehydration is the most common type found. This occurs because the renal mechanism maintains isotonicity by producing concentrated urine and thus conserving body water. It must be remembered that simply because an isotonic dehydration is present, isotonic solutions are not necessarily justified to correct it, as the state of isotonicity is being maintained by a renal mechanism that is working extra hard. One must recreate the isotonicity of body fluids without demanding this extra work by the renal mechanism. This is done by providing the extra free water afforded by the hypotonic solution in the repair fluids referred to before.

Most hypotonic solutions that are commercially available for fluid repair are usually one-third to one-half the tonicity of an isotonic solution. One can prepare a satisfactory hypotonic solution by mixing 7 parts of 5 per cent glucose in water, 2 parts of isotonic saline, and 1 part of one-sixth molar sodium bicarbonate and by adding potassium chloride to provide 20 mEq. of potassium per liter (7:2:1 solution with potassium). To prevent hyperkalemia, potassium must be administered only after making sure that the child is voiding. In general, fluids used for intravenous therapy should not contain more than 40 mEq. of potassium per liter. If the dehydration is accompanied by significant metabolic acidosis (carbon dioxide is less than 10 mEq. per liter and the blood pH is less than 7.1), the fluid for correction may be prepared by replacing the chloride part of the 7:2:1 solution just

described with bicarbonate ions. Thus, a solution may be prepared by mixing 7 parts of 5 per cent glucose in water and 3 parts of one-sixth molar sodium bicarbonate with added potassium to give 20 mEq. of potassium per liter (7:3 solution with potassium).

How to Administer the Fluid

1. If the child is severely dehydrated, administer 20 to 30 ml. per kg. of isotonic saline intravenously slowly over a period of about 30 to 60 minutes. Subtract this amount from the total amount calculated for deficit therapy.

2. Compute the total amount of fluid requirement for 24 hours less any amount used in step one.

3. Divide the amount into four bottles given at 6 hour intervals and administer the solution on time, adjusting the number of drops per minute as needed. Continue intravenous therapy for 24 hours.

4. Periodically, evaluate the clinical condition of the patient by observing the child's activity, alertness, status of hydration, urine output and specific gravity, and, finally, weight gain. The urine specific gravity, which can be easily and quickly estimated, is a particularly good indicator of the adequacy of fluid therapy. Normally, the specific gravity of the urine is approximately 1.010. The kidneys can, however, produce an extremely dilute urine, with a specific gravity of approximately 1.001, when excess body water has to be excreted or a highly concentrated urine, with a specific gravity of approximately 1.030, when body water has to be conserved. The latter situation occurs in a dehydrated child. One must question the adequacy of fluid therapy if the urine specific gravity is repeatedly close to either of these two extremes. A gradual return of specific gravity to normal from previously high values should be observed in a dehydrated child who is receiving appropriate amounts of fluids and electrolytes.

Flexibility is a key word that should be constantly remembered. One must be prepared to revise the initial estimate downward if the patient shows improvement more rapidly than expected or upward if the reverse is true and signs of dehydration persist.

5. After the first 24 hours, reassess the

fluid requirement. Fluid for deficit therapy need no longer be computed at this stage. Continue intravenous therapy only if necessary. If the hydration is good and the patient is able to accept adequate amounts of fluids by mouth, gradually put the child on oral fluids.

Examples of Fluid Therapy

Patient A.   A 10 kg. child with moderate dehydration without significant metabolic acidosis: percentage of dehydration = 8 per cent and body surface area = 0.5 m².

TOTAL FIRST 24 HOUR AMOUNT:

Amount for deficit therapy = 800 ml. (8 per cent of 10 kg.).

Amount for maintenance therapy = 1000 ml. (2000 ml. per m²).

Amount for abnormal losses = 50 ml. (5 ml. per kg. per 24 hours).

Total = 1850 ml. per 24 hours.

COMPOSITION:

7:2:1 solution with potassium 20 mEq. per liter (7 parts of 5 per cent glucose in water = 1295 ml.; 2 parts of isotonic saline = 370 ml.; 1 part of 1/6 molar sodium bicarbonate = 185 ml.)

Add if patient is voiding or as soon as he voids – potassium chloride solution (2 mEq. per ml.) = 18 ml. (36 mEq. of potassium for 185 ml. of fluid at 20 mEq. per liter).

Corrected total = 1868 ml.

ADMINISTRATION:

Divide 1868 ml. into four bottles, give one bottle every 6 hours, and run intravenously on time.

Patient B.   A 10 kg. child with severe dehydration and with significant metabolic acidosis: percentage of dehydration = 10 per cent and body surface area = 0.5 m².

TOTAL FIRST 24 HOUR AMOUNT:

Amount for deficit therapy = 1000 ml. (10 per cent of 10 kg.).

Amount for maintenance therapy = 1000 ml. (2000 ml. per m²).

Amount for abnormal losses = 50 ml. (5 ml. per kg. per 24 hours).

Total = 2050 ml. per 24 hours.

Isotonic saline for intravenous push = 300 ml. (30 ml. per kg.).

Balance of fluid for 24 hours = 1750 ml.

COMPOSITION:

7:3 solution with 20 mEq. per liter of potassium (7 parts of 5 per cent glucose in water = 1225 ml. and 3 parts of 1/6 molar sodium bicarbonate = 525 ml.).

Add if patient is voiding or as soon as he voids – potassium chloride solution (2 mEq. per ml.) = 18 ml. (36 mEq. for 1750 ml. at 20 mEq. per liter).

Corrected Total = 1768 ml.

ADMINISTRATION:

Administer isotonic saline 300 ml. in 30 to 60 minutes intravenously.

Divide 1768 ml. into four bottles, give 1 bottle every 6 hours, and run on time.

CHRONIC AND COMPLEX DISEASES

Recurrent Headaches

The clinician can expect to encounter the problem of recurring headaches in school-aged children frequently. A knowledge of the variety of causes will be of great value in pinpointing the exact cause. Among the more common inciting conditions are allergy, with or without secondary sinusitis; eye disease (poor visual acuity, glaucoma); local infections (ear, scalp, tooth); migraine; and psychogenic headache. Less commonly found are hypertensive states, cranial nerve disease (trigeminal neuralgia), head trauma (concussion), chronic poisoning (lead, mercury), and central nervous system disease (tumor, abscess).

A thorough history and physical examination, including a blood pressure determination, a complete neurologic examination, and visual testing are essential in making an accurate determination of cause. Other helpful tests are a nasal smear for eosinophils, dental examination with x-ray studies, sinus and skull x-rays, and urinalysis. If a central nervous system disorder appears to be the likely cause, electroencephalogram (EEG) and a brain scan should be ordered. Therapy will depend on the cause of the headache.

Migraine Headaches

The patient with typical migraine (less than 50 per cent of cases) presents with a one-sided headache of unusual severity associated with transitory neurologic or sensory phenomena (vertigo, visual aura, dysarthria, and so forth) that tends to last several hours to 1 day and often clears following vomiting. A family history is frequently positive for recurrent headaches.

These bouts recur from once yearly to several times a day. The child will usually display a degree of somnolence after the headache abates.

Nonspecific EEG abnormalities are occasionally seen. It should be recalled that there is a higher incidence of migraine among patients with seizure disorders.

Therapy is directed toward eradicating existing conditions, i.e., stress, allergens, and so forth, if they can be discovered. Symptomatic relief is often achieved in younger children by the use of common analgesics. When this fails, one has resort to ergotamines. Ergotamine tartrate and caffeine (Cafergot) administered during the first few minutes of onset is usually successful. Occasionally, when headaches recur frequently, or are refractory to therapy, a prophylactic agent, methysergide maleate, may help (see warning in manufacturer's official directive before considering use in children). Two tablets daily for small children and three tablets for children over 10 years of age for a period not to exceed 6 months are recommended. Complications such as pulmonary and retroperitoneal fibrosis can develop if therapy is protracted.

Enuresis

Enuresis is the involuntary passage of urine beyond the age when normal bladder control is attained. Most children gain bladder control by about 3 years of age and are able to keep themselves dry during the day and through most of the night. Nocturnal bladder control is attained at about 4 years of age in most children. Some children continue to have intermittent nocturnal enuresis until about 5 or 6 years of age. Males are at least twice as commonly afflicted as females. In a small percentage of children, bedwetting recurs after a variable period of complete bladder control.

Enuresis may reflect normal variations in growth and development. Psychologic trauma during the early formative years; parental indifference to the toilet-training of a child who is physiologically ready; or, conversely, too early attempts at toilet-training and a small bladder capacity are all postulated as possible factors that cause enuresis in children. Although its significance and pattern are unclear, there is frequently a positive familial incidence.

Enuresis is also considered by some as a seizure equivalent. Occasionally, urinary tract infection is associated with enuresis, and, very rarely, enuresis may be a manifestation of lesions of the genitourinary tract. Diabetes mellitus or diabetes insipidus may cause bedwetting in an occasional child.

Diagnostic procedures include routine urinalysis and urine culture; careful neurologic evaluation, including x-ray examination of the spine (defects of the lower part of the spine may or may not be associated with neurologic defects) to rule out abnormalities of the sphincter mechanism; and careful urologic investigation, including intravenous pyelogram and voiding cystourethrogram studies when abnormalities of the urinary tract are suspected.

Management includes parental education about the nature of the problem, which will help allay anxiety and will prevent the development of undesirable attitudes. Punishing and shaming the child only tend to aggravate the situation. Pointing out that the child is suffering too and that he is not wetting to annoy the parents can be helpful. Bladder exercises to increase the bladder capacity have been advocated by some, particularly for those patients with diurnal enuresis. Bladder-stretching exercises consist of increasing fluid intake during the day and supressing the urge to void to the point of discomfort. The most popular medication is the use of imipramine for a varying period of time, usually 8 weeks, in doses between 25 and 75 mg. per day (the manufacturer's official directive does not recommend use of imipramine for children under 6 years of age). Recurrence of the problem after a course of therapy is not uncommon. The use of a conditioning alarm that awakens the child as soon as he begins to void has had reasonably good success.

Failure to Thrive

This term implies a condition of multiple causes in which a failure to attain or maintain a normal rate of growth and a normal course of development is a dominant feature. Since a child's growth is affected by any ongoing chronic disease state, it can be readily appreciated that the causes are numerous.

The approach to such a patient must be

systematic. It is absolutely essential to take a detailed history of all genetically-related persons. Prenatal and perinatal events as well as a dietary and a sociopsychoeconomic profile may be extremely important. Finally, a detailed review of organ systems is warranted to focus on possible causes.

The physical examination should emphasize precise measurements of height and weight and cranial, chest, and limb size as well as body proportions (sitting-to-total-height ratio). These same measurements should be obtained in parents and siblings. Any previous, reliable measurements should be compared with the current findings, and future measurements should be planned.

About 75 per cent of cases will be found to be caused by nutritional failure resulting from psychosocial or economic factors. Whenever nutrition is unquestionably normal, genetic causes must be suspected. Other frequent causes are chronic infections (tuberculosis, pyelonephritis), infestations (hookworm, tapeworm), and chronic intoxication (mercury, lead). Metabolic disorders (diabetes mellitus), malabsorptive states, central nervous system (CNS) damage, respiratory diseases such as severe asthma, and cystic fibrosis are encountered occasionally. Endocrine diseases such as hypopituitarism or hypothyroidism are discovered infrequently. An important clue to hypopituitarism is tooth eruption, which rarely proceeds normally in this disorder. Also, disproportionate body measurements tend to indicate an endocrinopathy.

Laboratory tests should be selected according to the clinical leads uncovered by the history and physical examination. The tuberculin test (PPD), urinalysis and urine culture, bone age determination, and stool examination for unabsorbed nutrients are usually indicated when the cause is obscure.

Management and long-term prognosis are directly related to the cause. In the majority of instances, normal growth patterns can be re-established.

CONGENITAL CARDIAC DISEASE

The problem of identifying the child with a congenital heart disorder sits squarely in the lap of the primary care physician. He must detect the first signs of illness if the whole process culminating in a referral to a pediatric cardiologist or surgeon is to be initiated. Frequently, the obstetrician is the first physician aware of the problem, but more often it is the physician providing well-baby care.

Some of the common presenting signs and symptoms that will arouse the examiner's suspicions include a history of congenital heart problems in the family; prenatal infections, particularly rubella, in the mother; and poor feeding, profuse sweating, grunting, and fatigue in the child. The physical examination is of very great importance, since it may reveal some of the cardinal signs of cardiac defects such as cyanosis, lagging growth, tachypnea, tachycardia, and a heart murmur. It is important that a complete physical examination be done, including a blood pressure determination and careful palpation of pulses in both the upper and lower extremities, since aortic coarctation may be discovered this way. Palpation of the liver, auscultation of the chest, and attention to the extremities and eyes (to detect edema) may give important clues to the presence of cardiac failure. An inspection of the mucous membranes and the skin may help to establish the presence of cyanosis.

The examination of the heart should center on the position of the point of maximal impulse (PMI). This is usually found in the fourth left intercostal space just left (lateral) of the midclavicular line in children less than 7 years old and at the fifth intercostal space just right (medial) of the midclavicular line in older patients. If the PMI is displaced downward and laterally, it is indicative of left ventricular enlargement, whereas downward displacement alone is more likely to result from right ventricular enlargement.

In addition, the heart sounds (often three, rather than the two in normal children) and their components will need to be carefully auscultated. A decreased or absent second sound over the pulmonic area indicates pulmonic stenosis, and an absent second sound over the aortic area signifies aortic stenosis. Increased sounds may indicate increased pressure, and a fixed splitting of the second sound is commonly found in an atrial septal defect. Muffled sounds are likely to mean a myocardiopathy, such as myocarditis.

The precise nature of any murmur must

be appreciated—its pitch, intensity, and time of appearance or disappearance during the cardiac cycle and whether it is crescendo-decrescendo or blowing or machinery-like. Of great importance, also, is the ability to distinguish venous hums and innocent murmurs from organic heart lesions.

The venous hum is a continuous, low-pitched sound heard over the neck and upper sternum. It is easily distinguished from an organic murmur, as it is completely abolished when pressure is applied over the internal jugular veins, which give rise to the sound.

Innocent murmurs tend to be short in duration; to occur only in systole and not in diastole; to be soft, musical, or blowing in quality; and to be located over the pulmonary area and base of the heart. In addition, they do not transmit well or radiate, and they change characteristics with change of position and from one visit to the next. Over a period of time, they tend to disappear, particularly as the chest wall increases in thickness. In the absence of other signs or symptoms of organic heart disease, the only management that need be undertaken is expectant, with reassurance given to the parents.

A summary of the x-ray findings in the common congenital heart diseases is listed in Table 44–16.

Congenital Cardiac Lesions

The following 12 disorders represent the more common congenital heart lesions for which either a surgical cure is available or a medical management program can materially affect long-range outcome. In most instances, the primary physician will want the consultative services of a competent pediatric cardiologist for both the diagnostic and the therapeutic phases of management. Therefore, those details that enable a presumptive clinical diagnosis to be reached are stressed.

Aortic Stenosis. Aortic stenosis occurs most often at the valvular or subvalvular level and only occasionally is supravalvular. Symptoms vary from the asymptomatic child to the child with dyspnea, easy tiring, and chest pain to, in serious cases, the child with syncope. This latter symptom may be the forerunner of left-sided heart failure and sudden death. Arrhythmias are also known to occur, as well as endocarditis

On auscultation, a loud systolic ejection murmur is heard, and which is loudest at the right base. It tends to transmit to the neck along the left sternal border. The second aortic sound is decreased, and occasionally the murmur of aortic insufficiency is heard. An ejection click is present with aortic dilatation. The pulse pressure is narrowed.

TABLE 44–16. SUMMARY OF X-RAY FINDINGS IN COMMON CONGENITAL HEART DISEASE

	X-ray Signs	Disease
No Clinical Cyanosis	Heart size normal Normal pulmonary vascular markings	Coarctation of the aorta Aortic stenosis Pulmonic stenosis

	Heart enlarged
	Prominent pulmonary vascular
	    markings
		Left ventricular hypertrophy:
		    Patent ductus arteriosus
		    Ventricular septal defect
		    Atrioventricular communis
		    Endocardial sclerosis
		Right ventricular hypertrophy:
		    Atrial septal defect

Clinical Cyanosis	Heart size normal Decreased pulmonary vascular markings	Tetralogy of Fallot

	Heart enlarged
	Prominent pulmonary vascular
	    markings
		Complete transposition of the great
		    vessels
		Total anomalous pulmonary drainage

X-ray studies in mild disease are normal, but in moderate or severe cases, left ventricular enlargement is observed. A dilated ascending aorta may be visualized, and angiography should be undertaken. The electrocardiogram (ECG) is also nonrevealing in mild cases but will show evidence of left ventricular hypertrophy in the more severe cases.

Surgery, with reasonably good results, may be performed for the valvular, supravalvular, and subaortic varieties of aortic stenosis, using cardiopulmonary bypass techniques.

Pulmonic Stenosis. This entity is infundibular and usually occurs with septal defects. Symptoms are similar to aortic stenosis, ranging from the asymptomatic child to the child with dyspnea, easy tiring, cyanosis, and heart failure.

A loud ejection systolic murmur heard best at the upper left sternal border and transmitted to the back and neck is characteristic. The second pulmonic sound is decreased. The ECG and x-ray films are normal in mild cases. In severe cases, the ECG will show a strain pattern, a wide QRS-T angle, and "P" pulmonale. The x-ray study will demonstrate a dilated pulmonary artery and right ventricular and right atrial hypertrophy. Pulmonary flow is usually decreased. Angiography is indicated to demonstrate the defect.

The Brock procedure or valvulotomy may be corrective. Operative risk is low, particularly in children. In mild, nonprogressing cases, no surgery need be done. On the other hand, an enlarging heart and a strain pattern noted on the ECG argue for early intervention.

Aortic Coarctation. Aortic coarctation may be pre- or postductal, and findings will vary between these. Symptoms tend to occur after early childhood, with leg pains and headache being the most common ones. In adult life, dissecting aortic aneurysm, hypertension, left-sided heart failure, endocarditis, or cerebrovascular accidents are final outcomes. On physical examination, the blood pressure is increased in the arms but is decreased in the legs. Femoral pulses are not palpable. A systolic murmur, heard best over the back on the left side, is typical. The ECG varies from a normal tracing to one displaying left ventricular hypertrophy. X-ray films show a normal heart size in most

instances, but occasionally left ventricular hypertrophy is observed. The left anterior oblique and posteroanterior views may reveal the coarcted aorta. In older patients, rib notching is frequently found.

Surgery is best performed when the patient is between 4 and 12 years of age. Surgery is recommended for even asymptomatic patients to avoid complications in later life. End-to-end anastomosis is suitable for short coarcted segments. Longer segments will require a graft to bridge the gap.

Patent Ductus Arteriosus. This is a fetal vascular remnant that allows communication between the aorta and the pulmonary artery. Although frequently asymptomatic and diagnosed on physical examination only, a patent ductus can give rise to exertional dyspnea, fatigability, delayed growth, and frequent bouts of lower respiratory tract infection. When pulmonary blood flow is markedly increased, obstructive pulmonary vascular disease may develop, giving rise to cyanosis. A wide pulse pressure with bounding pulses and a crescendo-decrescendo, machinery-like murmur may be best heard at the left heart base. The characteristic continuous murmur is not generally heard in infants and younger children.

X-rays vary, ranging from normal (small ductus) to showing left atrial, left ventricular, and aortic enlargement. When obstructive pulmonary vascular disease occurs, right atrial and right ventricular hypertrophy may also be observed. Pulmonary blood flow decreases in these instances. Angiography is not indicated in clear-cut cases but is necessary in atypical ones. The ECG may reflect the left ventricular hypertrophy or show the right ventricular hypertrophy resulting from obstructive pulmonary vascular disease.

Surgical correction is optimally done when the patient is between 3 and 10 years of age, and the mortality rate is under 2 per cent. It is most convenient to operate before the child reaches school age. Ligature or division of the ductus are the procedures done.

Atrial Septal Defect—Secundum Type. In this condition, unlike the more severe ostium primum type, the septal defect is usually high and is above the mitral or tricuspid valves. Early in the course of this disorder, symptoms are usually lacking; however, easy tiring, dyspnea, and eventual heart failure accompany large defects. The murmur is systolic and heard best over the upper left sternal border. Often there is a concomitant mid-diastolic murmur at the lower left sternal border. The second sound tends to be widely split and fixed. The ECG shows right axis deviation and right bundle branch block. Larger defects may give rise to right ventricular hypertrophy.

X-rays will show an enlarged right atrium and ventricle with increased pulmonary blood flow. Angiography, although not absolutely necessary, may reveal abnormal pulmonary veins on occasion.

Surgical correction can accomplish a closure of the defect by suturing. The operative risk is below 5 per cent, and childhood is the optimum time for repair.

Ventricular Septal Defect. Children with more than a small defect may exhibit the dyspnea, easy fatigability, and frequent respiratory infections commonly observed in many of the patients with congenital cardiac lesions. In addition, heart failure and obstructive pulmonary vascular disease can also occur from the left-to-right shunt of blood under systemic pressure.

The murmur tends to be loud and harsh. It is pansystolic and best appreciated over the lower left sternal border. It transmits over the precordium and is sometimes accompanied by an apical diastolic rumble. The second pulmonic heart sound may be increased.

X-rays may not reveal abnormalities (small defects) or may show left atrial and ventricular enlargement with increased pulmonary blood flow. With obstructive pulmonary vascular disease, pulmonic blood flow is decreased. Angiography is often not necessary, but aortography is done when obstructive pulmonary vascular disease is present to rule out the presence of a patent ductus or an aortic abnormality.

Surgery is undertaken when a patient becomes increasingly symptomatic and particularly whenever pulmonary hypertension is observed. When obstructive pulmonary vascular disease develops and a bidirectional shunt has occurred, the operative mortality rate is excessive, and medical management alone is relied upon. In asymptomatic patients with small or even moderate defects, surgery is delayed in the

hope that spontaneous closure will take place. The ideal time for repairing the defect is about the fourth year of life or whenever the child attains a weight no less than 25 pounds (11 kg.) and preferably closer to 40 pounds (20 kg.) or more. Pulmonary artery banding is a useful, temporary measure in infants too small to be operated on definitively. It stalls the development of pulmonary vascular obstructive disease and is indicated in the face of intractable cardiac failure or pulmonary hypertension.

Endocardial Cushion Defect. Failure of the endocardial cushion to fuse properly may allow communication between any or all of the four heart chambers.

Again, symptomatology includes dyspnea and easy tiring with frequent pulmonary infections. In the complete form, obstructive pulmonary vascular disease and early death can occur. Cyanosis is absent or mild. A harsh, holosystolic murmur is found at the apex, and the second heart sound is loud and split. Splitting will disappear in the presence of obstructive pulmonary vascular disease.

The ECG shows a superior electrical axis. A counterclockwise vector loop in the frontal plane and combined ventricular hypertrophy are characteristic findings. X-rays show right ventricular, left atrial, and left ventricular enlargement and increased pulmonary blood flow. Angiography should be done.

Surgical correction for the incomplete form of endocardial cushion defect is associated with a reasonably low mortality rate (2 to 5 per cent), but in the complete form the mortality rate is high (15 to 50 per cent). Pulmonary artery banding can be done when the shunt is primarily at the ventricular level, but it is less effective than banding for ventricular septal defects. It should not be done for predominantly atrial shunts.

Total Anomalous Pulmonary Drainage (Transposition of the Pulmonary Veins). Two varieties of this defect exist: supra-diaphragmatic and infradiaphragmatic. Mild-to-moderate bouts of cyanosis are typical, with heart failure occurring in infancy. Dyspnea, easy fatigability, and respiratory infections are also part of the picture. Early death, frequently associated with obstructive pulmonary vascular disease, is also common.

The murmur is systolic and is frequently located along the left sternal border. The second heart sound is split, and a third or even fourth heart sound may be present. Occasionally, a presystolic murmur and a continuous murmur are heard. The ECG shows right axis deviation and right atrial and right ventricular enlargement.

In the supracardiac variety, the x-ray shows a striking figure-of-eight configuration. The right atrial and ventricular enlargement is evident, and pulmonary blood flow is increased. In the infradiaphragmatic type, the heart appears small. Angiography should be performed, as well as pulmonary artery injection.

During catheterization, atrial balloon septostomy is often a helpful procedure. However, corrective surgery will usually be needed, using cardiopulmonary bypass or hypothermic techniques, to provide definitive repair. The mortality rate in the best medical centers has been reduced in recent years but is still considerable.

Tetralogy of Fallot. The principal defect is pulmonic stenosis. The ventricular septal defect overriding the aorta and the right ventricular hypertrophy tend to be secondary.

Early cyanosis, polycythemia, clubbing, paroxysmal dyspnea, squatting, poor growth, and intermittent cyanosis are typical. Because of the presence of mural thrombi and the existing shunt, cerebral emboli and brain abscesses may occur. A loud systolic murmur heard along the left sternal border and a decreased second sound heard over the pulmonic area are consistent with the diagnosis.

In the cyanotic form, right axis deviation and right ventricular hypertrophy are observed on the ECG. In the acyanotic form, a combined ventricular hypertrophy is found. The x-ray shows a normal-sized, boot-shaped heart. There may be a right-sided aortic arch, and the pulmonary vasculature is decreased. Angiography should be done.

Several surgical procedures exist. The Blalock procedure (subclavian to pulmonary artery anastomosis) and the Potts procedure (aorta to pulmonary artery anastomosis) are two that are frequently used. Infants and young children who are severely compromised or have syncopal episodes should have this type of shunt procedure. The risk is fairly low compared with

definitive correction in which cardiopulmonary bypass is needed.

Transposition of the Great Vessels. In this condition, the aorta arises from the right ventricle while the pulmonary artery springs from the left ventricle. Life is possible only if a second defect permits communication between the two circulations. Cyanosis, dyspnea, and progressive cardiac failure with death during the first 6 months are common. A systolic murmur is frequently (but not always) heard. The ECG shows right ventricular or combined ventricular hypertrophy. Occasionally, though, isolated left ventricular hypertrophy may be seen. X-rays will demonstrate a large, egg-shaped heart with a narrow, supracardiac stalk. Pulmonary blood flow may be either increased or decreased, but the former is more common. Angiography should be done.

Palliative surgery, permitting blood to flow between the arterial and venous systems, has a high risk but has been successful for some patients. Total correction using bypass procedures has also been performed, but with a high mortality rate.

Tricuspid Atresia. Not only is the valve atretic in this condition, but the right ventricle is as well. Hypoxic spells, early cyanosis, and dyspnea with death during the first year of life are characteristic of tricuspid atresia. Cerebrovascular accidents may also be encountered. A systolic murmur is often present at the left sternal border. A normal-sized, boot-shaped heart will be seen on x-ray, with decreased pulmonary blood flow. The left axis deviation and left ventricular hypertrophy on ECG help distinguish this entity from tetralogy of Fallot. A "P" pulmonale may also be seen.

The Blalock, Potts, or Glenn (superior vena cava to right pulmonary artery anastomosis) procedures may be helpful (if only palliative) surgery for patients with severe cyanosis and decreased pulmonary blood flow. A new, corrective procedure consisting of connecting the right atrium to the pulmonary artery is being evaluated.

Truncus Arteriosus. A single vessel arising from the ventricular area and branching into pulmonary and aortic arteries is known as truncus arteriosus. Other associated defects are ventricular septal defect, common pulmonary artery anomalies, and right aortic arch. Symptoms include dyspnea, lagging growth, pulmonary infections, and a variable amount of cyanosis. Death usually occurs during the first 6 months. The continuous murmur is harsh and best heard during systole along the left sternal border. The second sound is increased with no splitting.

X-rays will tend to show cardiac enlargement and increased pulmonary blood flow. The ECG shows right ventricular or combined ventricular hypertrophy. Angiography is indicated.

Palliative surgery consists of pulmonary artery banding. Recently, corrective surgery consisting of separating the pulmonary arteries from the truncus and closing the ventricular septal defect has been developed. The mortality rate appears to be high but must be considered in light of the grave prognosis.

PHYSICAL ACTIVITY. Reduction of physical activity is not necessary for most children with congenital heart lesions. Impending cardiac failure and hypoxia lead to self-restriction. Patients with aortic or pulmonic stenosis will have to be taught to avoid strenuous activity if they are symptomatic.

Referral

Ultimately, the primary care physician will need the services of a qualified pediatric cardiologist to establish a definitive diagnosis and help advise on management.

There are certain indications that will suggest the need for an early referral. The presence of cyanosis or cardiac failure is a rather obvious one. However, growth failure, syncopal attacks, progressive deterioration, squatting, and repeated respiratory tract infections should also constitute sufficient cause to seek further help. A newborn with a cardiac murmur or other signs of heart disease should also receive the benefit of early consultation.

Chest Pain

Chest pain, when it is of cardiac origin, is an alarming symptom. When it is associated with aortic stenosis, it can be an early warning sign of sudden cardiac decompensation. It should be realized, however, that chest pain in a pediatric population is rarely of cardiac origin. Once aortic stenosis or pericarditis can be ruled out, the cause will almost always be found elsewhere.

Bacterial Endocarditis

Bacterial endocarditis is a major complication of any of the congenital heart diseases. Unexplained fever and any acute infection should alert the physician to this possibility. Prevention includes antibiotic therapy during the course of suspected bacterial infections and whenever transient bacteremia may occur (for example, following tooth extraction).

TABLE 44–17.   DIGOXIN (LANOXIN)*

How Supplied	Age	Estimated Total Digitalizing Dose (Oral or Intramuscular)†	Maintenance Portion of Total Digitalizing Dose
Elixir: 0.05 mg./ml. Tablets: (scored) 0.25 and 0.5 mg.; (unscored) 0.125 mg.	Premature infant (< 2500 grams)	0.04 mg./kg.	¼ to ⅓ in two divided doses per 24 hours
	Newborn infant (1 to 14 days)	0.05 mg./kg.	¼ to ⅓ in two divided doses per 24 hours
Ampules: 0.1 and 0.25 mg./ml.	Infant (14 days to 2 years)	0.06 to 0.075 mg./kg.	¼ to ⅓ in two divided doses per 24 hours
	Child (> 2 years)	0.03 to 0.05 mg./kg. (maximal total dose of 1.5 mg.)	¼ to ⅓ in two divided doses per 24 hours

*From Fink, B. W., and Moss, A. J.: Congestive heart failure. *In* Gellis, S. S., and Kagan, B. M. (eds.): Current Pediatric Therapy 7. Philadelphia, W. B. Saunders Co., 1976, p. 133.

†For intravenous administration, use 75 per cent of the dose shown.

Cardiac Failure

Cardiac failure in children differs from that of adults by being predominantly a failure of the right rather than the left ventricle. It usually develops slowly. Early symptoms include poor feeding, exertional sweating, and weak cry in infants and tachycardia, tachypnea, excessive weight gain, and edema in both infants and older children. Cardiomegaly and hepatomegaly are observed on physical examination or on x-ray and electrocardiography. Unlike the findings in left ventricular failure, pulmonary rales are not generally present.

The hallmark of therapy is administration of digitalis. Digoxin is well suited for this purpose because of its rapid peak effect (8 hours), quick onset of action (1 hour), and rapid excretion (3 days). It can be given by oral, intramuscular, or intravenous routes. See Table 44–17 for dosage schedules for the various age groups. With each dose of digoxin the patient should be monitored electrocardiographically for signs of arrhythmia, extrasystoles, and heart block. Symptoms of toxicity include vomiting and diarrhea. Toxicity may be countered by administering potassium chloride, 1 gram orally every 8 hours, or 40 mEq. per 500 ml. of 5 per cent glucose in water (not to exceed 0.5 mEq. per kg. per 24 hours) given intravenously and carefully monitored by ECG.

Diuretics such as chlorothiazide or ethacrynic acid are used to decrease the accumulated burden of body fluids. Bed rest should be strictly enforced and oxygen administered.

Myocarditis

Myocarditis or inflammation of the myocardium can occur as a specific entity or can accompany an inflammatory process of other areas of the heart (pancarditis) or tissues of the body (rheumatic fever). It can be a primary disease process or can represent a secondary one (collagen disease). The most common causes are infectious (bacterial, viral, or rickettsial) followed by connective tissue disorders. Diphtheria, typhoid fever, and hepatitis are frequently associated disease states. Metabolic, hematologic, and parasitic diseases can also lead to development of myocarditis.

Clinical findings consist of dyspnea, fever, chest pain or discomfort, muffled heart sounds, and a tachycardia out of proportion to the rise in body temperature. Occasionally, an arrhythmia (tic-tac rhythm in which both diastole and systole are of equal duration) is observed. Congestive heart failure may result.

The x-ray shows cardiac dilatation, and the ECG may reveal nonspecific ST segment and T wave abnormalities or AV conduction defects. Blood cultures and serologic tests are done to help isolate a pathogen.

The prognosis is reasonably good, even though dangerous arrhythmias may develop and lead to an unexpectedly sudden death. Therapy consists of treating the underlying cause. Certain general measures may also be helpful. Bed rest and avoidance of strenuous activity well into the convalescent period are advisable. Cardiac arrhythmias may require procaine amide or quinidine for control. If this fails, the administration of oxygen, a diuretic, and digitalis will be necessary. Steroids have also been recommended, particularly with connective tissue disorders. However, they are not curative but only suppressive.

RHEUMATIC FEVER

Rheumatic fever is an inflammatory, systemic disease bearing an etiologic relationship to certain rheumatogenic strains of group A streptococci. It occurs most frequently in children between 5 and 15 years of age, with a peak incidence of first attacks in children between 6 and 8 years of age. It is extremely uncommon in children who are less than 3 years old. The clinical picture usually begins to appear 1 to 5 weeks after an upper respiratory tract illness. In about half of the patients, the history of this preceding illness can be elicited.

Diagnostic Criteria. Arthritis is one of the important features of the disease. The large joints of the extremities are the ones most frequently affected. The arthritis migrates from one joint to another, gradually involving multiple joints over a period of several days. Swelling, redness, tenderness, and limitation of normal movements characterize the arthritis.

Symptomatology referable to carditis may be absent in many children with cardiac involvement. Occasionally, affected children may be seen with cardiac failure or pericarditis, with or without friction rub. More often, the diagnosis of carditis is based on the presence of tachycardia that persists during sleep and afebrile periods; prolongation of the PR interval on ECG; cardiomegaly, with or without congestive cardiac failure; and significant cardiac murmurs. Both the appearance of characteristic new murmurs or a change in the quality of a murmur that was previously present are significant. The characteristic murmur is an apical, pansystolic murmur occasionally accompanied by an apical, mid-diastolic murmur, suggesting mitral regurgitation, and by an early, diastolic murmur heard best along the left sternal border at the base of the heart, suggesting aortic regurgitation. The presystolic murmur of mitral stenosis and the systolic murmur of aortic stenosis are later manifestations. Pericardial rub or effusion may be present.

Subcutaneous nodules are pea-sized nodules usually found along the extensor surfaces of the hands, feet, and knees. Association of these nodules with the presence of carditis is frequently noted. Subcutaneous nodules may also be present in other disorders, such as rheumatoid arthritis and systemic lupus erythematosus.

Erythema marginatum is characterized by an erythematous rash with a serpiginous border and a clear center, usually distributed over the covered part of the body, such as the trunk and proximal part of the extremities. Such rashes may appear intermittently throughout the course of the active disease.

Chorea consists of awkward, purposeless, involuntary movements, principally of the extremities and face, often bilateral and usually associated with muscle weakness.

Chorea occasionally may be the only manifestation of rheumatic fever or may appear when other manifestations have disappeared. The onset of awkward movements is usually gradual, and the intensity varies from child to child. Emotional disturbances in the affected child are common.

Laboratory findings include an elevated erythrocyte sedimentation rate (ESR), a positive C-reactive protein (CRP) test, leukocytosis, and anemia. Group A streptococci may be isolated on repeated throat cultures in a small number of patients. Antistreptolysin-O (ASO) titers equal to or greater than 500 Todd units are clearly significant. Titers between 250 and 320 Todd units are highly suspicious. ASO titers may not be elevated in children showing late manifestations of the disease, such as chorea and occasionally carditis. Elevation of other antibodies that inhibit streptococci, such as antistreptokinase (ASK), antihyaluronidase (AH), antideoxyribonucleotidase B (anti-DNase B), and antinicotinamide adenine dinucleotidase (anti-NADase) may occur. These are useful determinations in children in whom the ASO titer is borderline. Roentgenographic examination of the chest may demonstrate cardiac enlargement, and ECG tracings may reveal prolongation of the PR interval and other findings consistent with carditis and pericarditis.

The presence of two major or of one major and two minor criteria supported by evidence of recent streptococcal infection indicates a high probability of acute rheumatic fever (Table 44–18). Absence of this supporting evidence should raise doubts concerning a diagnosis of rheumatic fever. Strict adherence to these guidelines should enable the physician to avoid overdiagnosis of the disease, with its long-term implica-

TABLE 44–18. JONES CRITERIA (MODIFIED) FOR DIAGNOSIS OF RHEUMATIC FEVER*

Major Manifestations	Minor Manifestations	Supporting Evidence of Streptococcal Infection

1. Carditis
2. Polyarthritis
3. Chorea
4. Erythema marginatum
5. Subcutaneous nodules
	1. Arthralgia
	2. Fever
	3. Rheumatic fever or rheumatic heart disease in the past
	4. Increased ESR
	   Positive CRP
	   Leukocytosis
	   Prolonged PR interval
		1. Recent scarlet fever
		2. Positive throat culture for group A streptococci
		3. Increased ASO or other streptococcus-inhibiting antibodies

*Adapted from recommendations of the Committe of the American Heart Association.

TABLE 44–19. DIFFERENTIAL DIAGNOSIS OF RHEUMATIC FEVER, RHEUMATOID ARTHRITIS, AND SYSTEMIC LUPUS ERYTHEMATOSUS*

	Rheumatic Fever	Rheumatoid Arthritis	Systemic Lupus Erythematosus
Age trend	5 years	5 years	5 years
Sex ratio	Equal	Girls 1.5:1	Girls 5:1
Joint findings:			
Pain	Severe	Moderate	—
Swelling	Nonspecific	Nonspecific	Nonspecific
Tenderness	Severe	Moderate	—
Bony x-ray	None	Frequent	Occasional
Morning stiffness	Yes	Yes	Yes
Rash	Erythema marginatum	Rheumatoid arthritis rash	Malar flush
Chorea	Yes	No	Rarely
Clinical carditis	+	Rare	Late
Laboratory tests:			
WBC	Normal to high	Normal to high	Decreased to normal
Latex	—	+ (10%)	+ occasionally
Sheep cell agglut.	—	+ (10%)	—
L.E. cell prep.	—	+ (5%)	+
Biopsy:			
Skin rash	Nonspecific	Nonspecific	Diagnostic
Nodules	Nonspecific	Nonspecific	Nonspecific
Response to salicylates	Rapid	Slow, usually	Slow or none

*From Brewer, E. J., Jr.: Juvenile Rheumatoid Arthritis. Philadelphia, W. B. Saunders Co., 1970, p. 91.

tions. Differential diagnosis includes suppurative arthritis; osteomyelitis; rheumatoid arthritis; systemic lupus erythematosus (SLE); sickle cell anemia; Henoch-Schönlein purpura; drug sensitivity reactions associated with polyarthritis, fever, and skin rash; and myocarditis and pericarditis of viral origin (Table 44–19).

Management. Strict bed rest, in the absence of carditis or acute pain of arthritis or disabling movements of chorea, is of no recognized medical value. Even though no evidence of active streptococcal infection exists at the time of the diagnosis of rheumatic fever, it is desirable to administer a therapeutic course of penicillin to assure complete eradication of the organisms. Salicylates and steroids are the anti-inflammatory drugs used in the symptomatic management of the illness. Except in patients with rheumatic carditis, the drug of choice is a salicylate. Even in children with carditis, the superiority of steroids is not clearly established in terms of reducing the subsequent damage to the heart. Post-therapeutic rebounds are more frequent after steroid therapy than after salicylate therapy.

The starting dose of salicylate (aspirin) is 100 mg. per kg. per day in four divided doses. The dose may be gradually increased up to 200 mg. per kg. per day (maximum not to exceed 10 grams per day) and monitored by repeated serum salicylate levels until therapeutic results are achieved. For steroid therapy, prednisone, 50 to 75 mg. per day in divided doses, is recommended. Higher doses of up to 120 to 160 mg. per day may be given to children showing no response to the lower dose.

The duration of therapy depends on the severity of the disease. Abatement or disappearance of symptoms indicates the adequacy of the dosage, while the erythrocyte sedimentation rate (ESR) and C-reactive protein test are good indices of anti-inflammatory therapeutic progress. Salicylate therapy can be discontinued in children with arthritis but without carditis as soon as the ESR shows a significant fall. This period may vary from 2 to 6 weeks. Steroid therapy in children with carditis may have to be maintained up to 4 to 6 weeks or even longer, depending on the severity of carditis. The steroid therapy should be tapered gradually, with the substitution of salicylate as the dosage of steroid is gradually cut, to avoid rebound phenomena. The salicylate therapy is then continued for an additional 2 to 3 weeks. Phenobarbital and tranquilizers such as chlorpromazine may be used to control the movements of children with chorea. In addition, adequate reassurance to the patient and his family as to the nature of the problem must be given.

The disease usually subsides spontaneously after a period of 1 or 2 months. No restriction of physical activity is indicated after complete recovery from an attack unless the child has cardiac enlargement. Children with cardiac enlargement who are asymptomatic can usually tolerate moderate exercise and should be encouraged to do so, but should be cautioned to avoid strenuous, competitive sports.

Continuous prophylaxis against recurrent streptococcal infection with an antimicrobial agent constitutes the most effective method of preventing recurrences of rheumatic fever. Monthly benzathine penicillin, 1.2 million units given intramuscularly, is the most effective method. Oral penicillin, 200,000 to 250,000 units once or twice daily, or sulfadiazine, 1 gram daily, has also been used with satisfactory results. Prophylaxis should be continued for at least several years after the diagnosis has been made and at least through the child's school years.

ACUTE GLOMERULONEPHRITIS

Acute glomerulonephritis appears to be an antigen-antibody reaction that follows an infection, most often caused by group A beta hemolytic streptococci. The nephritogenic strains of streptococci are types 4 and 12 and, less frequently, types 25 and 45. The peak incidence occurs in children between 6 and 7 years of age and is extremely rare in those under 1 year of age. Boys are affected more often than girls.

Diagnostic Criteria. Clinical manifestations often include an episode of upper respiratory tract infection, such as pharyngitis or tonsillitis, preceding the onset of symptoms by about 1 to 3 weeks. Less commonly, streptococcal infection of the skin may precede the onset of symptoms. In most instances, the manifestations are mild, and only very occasionally is the onset abrupt and severe. Urinary abnormalities, edema, and hypertension are the classic findings. Hematuria is the most common presenting complaint. The urine is smokey in appearance. Further examination of urine

reveals proteinuria and cylindruria. Red blood cell casts and increased numbers of white blood cells are usually present. Rarely, children may have acute glomerulonephritis without any of these urinary abnormalities.

Edema is usually mild and mainly manifested as puffiness around the eyelids. Posture determines the site of edema elsewhere in the body.

Hypertension is present in about 60 to 70 per cent of all affected children. The elevated systolic pressure may range from 160 to 200 mm. Hg and the diastolic pressure from 100 to 120 mm. Hg. Hypertension is attributed to expanded plasma volume and generalized vasospasm. Symptoms of hypertensive encephalopathy (drowsiness, headache, convulsions, vomiting, visual disturbances, and restlessness) may occur. The symptoms usually disappear within 1 or 2 days after the fall in blood pressure.

Cardiovascular disturbances often associated with congestive failure may occur. The roentgenogram of the chest in these instances will show increased pulmonary markings and cardiac enlargement. Laboratory findings include elevated ASO titers, hypocomplementemia, hypoalbuminemia, mild hypercholesterolemia, mild degrees of anemia, and an elevated ESR. ECG findings show flattening or inversion of T waves and prolongation of the PR interval. Abnormal renal function values are present.

The condition most frequently confused with acute glomerulonephritis is acute urinary tract infection. The presence in the urine of a larger number of leukocytes in comparison with erythrocytes, bacteria, and significantly elevated bacterial colony counts ($\geq$ 100,000 per cu. mm.) should differentiate this condition from acute nephritis. Other conditions associated with hematuria such as blood dyscrasias, renal tumors, and tuberculosis of the urinary tract should also be considered. Nephritic findings associated with conditions such as the Henoch-Schönlein syndrome and systemic lupus erythematosus can be differentiated on the basis of the other clinical manifestations present in these conditions. Severe renal function impairment and a past history of chronic nephritis usually help to identify children in whom acute exacerbation of their chronic nephritis mimics acute glomerulonephritis. The nephrotic syndrome with gross hematuria as well as other conditions associated with proteinuria (orthostatic proteinuria and other benign proteinurias) are additional disorders considered in the differential diagnosis.

Management. Prompt diagnosis and treatment of streptococcal infection may help prevent acute glomerulonephritis. Once nephritis is established, the treatment is symptomatic. The child should have bed rest until the major manifestations of the disease—edema, hematuria, and hypertension—subside. This period usually lasts for 3 to 4 weeks. Dietary management in terms of protein restriction is necessary only in children who develop excessive edema and hypertension. Appropriate antibiotic therapy (penicillin for 10 days) is indicated when nasopharyngeal cultures are positive for streptococci. Prophylactic penicillin therapy following recovery is not necessary.

When administering fluids during the oliguric or anuric phase of the disease, care must be taken to avoid overhydration. An average amount that allows for insensible water loss of about 300 to 400 ml. per square meter of body surface per day plus the amount equal to urine output should be administered. The use of potassium-containing solutions is strictly contraindicated. Salt restriction and administration of diuretics (ethacrynic acid, chlorothiazide) and digitalis are some of the measures that should be instituted in children who develop severe edema or congestive cardiac failure or both (read manufacturer's official directive before considering use of ethacrynic acid in infants). It should be remembered that diuretics are usually ineffective in clearing the edema and that the beneficial value of digitalis is not clearly established. Antihypertensive medications are indicated in children who develop a diastolic blood pressure of 90 mm. Hg or more. The following regimen may be used:

1. Children with very mild hypertension: bed rest; salt restriction; and phenobarbital, 2 to 3 mg. per kg. per day orally. A single dose of phenobarbital may be all that is necessary.

2. Children with moderate to severe hypertension: combination of reserpine, 0.07 mg. per kg., and hydralazine hydrochloride (Apresoline), 0.1 mg. per kg., administered intramuscularly. Often a single dose is sufficient. The combined therapy may be repeated in 12 hours, if necessary.

Management of children who develop hyperkalemia (serum potassium level of 6.5 mEq. per liter or higher) and renal insufficiency consists of:

1. Avoidance of all potassium-containing dietary foods or fluids.

2. Administration of sodium polystyrene sulfonate (Kayexalate), 1000 mg. per kg., either orally or rectally as a 20 to 30 per cent solution. The dose may be repeated after 6 to 12 hours, if necessary. Periodically, serum calcium concentration must be checked while the child is being treated. An alternative to Kayexalate therapy consists of the administration of insulin and glucose (1 unit of insulin to 3 grams of glucose).

3. Use of peritoneal dialysis or hemodialysis for persistent hyperkalemia.

The administration of steroids or immunosuppressive agents is justified only when used as investigational drugs in established pediatric renal centers at the present time.

THE NEPHROTIC SYNDROME

The nephrotic syndrome is characterized by proteinuria resulting in hypoproteinemia, edema, hypovolemia, ascites, and hyperlipemia. Hypertension, hematuria, azotemia, and hypocomplementemia may also be seen. The syndrome can be grouped into three categories: congenital, secondary, and idiopathic. The cause of the nephrotic syndrome is unknown, although it is generally considered a hypersensitivity disease.

The congenital nephrotic syndrome is inherited as an autosomal recessive trait. The affected children do not respond to treatment and die within the first 1 or 2 years of life. The secondary nephrotic syndrome occurs in association with a specific disease such as a collagen disorder (systemic lupus erythematosus, anaphylactoid purpura), parasitic infection, and other conditions (amyloidosis, renal vein thrombosis, sickle cell disease, syphilis, chronic glomerulonephritis, diabetes mellitus, and so on). The nephrotic syndrome may also result following administration of drugs (trimethadione, paramethadione) and heavy metal preparations (gold salts, mercury). Bee stings and poison oak dermatitis are associated findings in some cases. The idiopathic nephrotic syndrome constitutes the vast majority of cases. The peak incidence is in children 2 to 3 years of age, with onset relatively rare after 8 years of age.

Diagnostic Criteria. Edema is the hallmark of the nephrotic syndrome and is insidious in onset. The early periorbital edema gradually becomes generalized, producing ascites, scrotal edema, and occasionally pleural effusion. In some untreated children, the initial edema may disappear, only to come back again after 1 or 2 weeks. Increased susceptibility to infection, peritonitis in particular, has been noted in edematous children. Diarrheal episodes, seen frequently during the acute stage, are presumably due to edema of the gastrointestinal mucosa. Anorexia and excessive loss of protein in the urine may result in malnutrition. Respiratory embarrassment due to marked ascites may be present. Laboratory findings include proteinuria, hypoproteinemia and hypoalbuminemia, hyperlipemia, hypocalcemia, elevated erythrocyte sedimentation rate (ESR), occasionally reduced beta 1c component of serum complement, and variable renal function values.

Management. This includes a high protein (3 to 4 grams per kg. per day) and low salt (40 to 80 mEq. of sodium per day) diet. Prompt therapy with antimicrobial agents for coexisting infections is indicated. Diuretic agents are usually not required, since diuresis occurs in most children after the start of steroid therapy. In patients in whom there are contraindications to using steroids, a diuretic such as hydrochlorothiazide (2 to 4 mg. per kg. per day) may be used. Corticosteroid therapy is the mainstay in the management of the nephrotic syndrome. The International Cooperative Study of Kidney Disease recommends the following schedule:

1. Prednisone, 60 mg. per square meter of body surface per day (maximum 80 mg. per day), for 4 weeks. Follow with 40 mg. per square meter of body surface per day (maximum 60 mg. per day) for 3 consecutive days in a week for 4 more weeks. If the patient responds during the last 4 weeks, continue intermittent (3 days a week) therapy for 4 more weeks and then discontinue the drug.

2. Children showing relapse, after responding to the steroid therapy, are again treated with steroids; first, continuously for 4 weeks and then intermittently for 4 more weeks, as just outlined.

Cytotoxic therapy is considered for steroid-nonresponsive children, as well as for children who show frequent relapses while on steroids. A number of drugs such as 6-mercaptopurine, azathioprine, chlorambucil, and cyclophosphamide are being clinically evaluated at present. Recent data seem to indicate that azathioprine is ineffective in the treatment of steroid-resistant children.

DIABETES MELLITUS

Diabetes mellitus is an inheritable, complex metabolic disorder affecting carbohydrate as well as fat and protein metabolism. The incidence of childhood diabetes varies between 1 in 2000 to 1 in 3000 children. Three types can be recognized among children with the disease: overt diabetes (growth onset juvenile diabetes), latent diabetes ("maturity onset" diabetes mellitus), and transient diabetes in the newborn.

Overt Diabetes. In overt diabetes, insufficient insulin activity is the primary factor. The average age at onset is 10 to 11 years. In one-fourth of the children, the onset is before 5 years of age. The remaining three-fourths of children will have the onset of overt diabetes between 5 and 15 years of age. Usually the onset of symptoms is sudden, although the precipitous development of symptoms is not always characteristic. The signs and symptoms that should alert the physician to the diagnosis are polyuria, polydipsia, polyphagia, weight loss, enuresis, pruritus vulvae, irritability, lassitude, and visual difficulties. A state of ketoacidosis may exist when the diagnosis is first established.

The diagnosis is based upon a characteristic history and the presence of glycosuria and ketonuria, with a random blood glucose level above 180 mg. per 100 ml. Glucose tolerance tests are rarely necessary.

Hospitalization is mandatory when the diagnosis is first established, in order to closely monitor and evaluate the child's response to initial treatment. Also, the period of hospital stay can be used to educate the child and his family about the nature of the disease and its implications for the child's new way of life. The primary thrust of therapy is to enable the child and his family to lead a normal or near normal life with minimal psychosocial and physical problems to contend with.

INITIAL MANAGEMENT. Initial management includes insulin therapy utilizing regular insulin, in a dosage of 0.5 to 2.0 units per kg., depending on the severity of initial manifestations (0.5 unit per kg. for glucosuria and 2.0 units per kg. for severe ketoacidosis). The insulin is to be administered subcutaneously. In case of vascular collapse, half the calculated dose given intravenously is indicated. Regular insulin may be repeated at 2 to 4 hour intervals. A dose of 0.5 to 1.0 unit per kg. is utilized, depending on the response to the previous therapy (fall in serum acetone levels, lowering of glucose and ketone concentrations in urine). During the second 24 hours, approximately four injections of regular insulin before meals are administered. The daily insulin requirement is determined by the previous day's dosage and by urinary glucose and ketone concentrations (5 units for the presence of 1+ urinary glucose, 10 units for 2+ glucose, and so on, and an additional 5 to 10 units for the presence of acetone).

Except in very mild cases (children with glucosuria only), intravenous fluids are necessary. Usually after the first 24 hours on intravenous therapy, clear fluids of high carbohydrate content can be given orally in sufficient amount. Regular meals can also be given during this period. Two or 3 days after the initial therapy, administer one injection of NPH or Lente insulin about 30 minutes before breakfast. The exact requirement varies from individual to individual. Such factors as the duration of the disease and the age of the patient influence the need. Usually a dose of 0.5 to 2.0 units per kg. of body weight will be required per day. If the child develops nocturnal hyperglycemia, divide the daily dose and give approximately 1/3 to 1/4 of the daily requirement before supper or at bedtime.

Caution: Following the initial control of the new diabetic, the insulin requirement drops precipitously during the remission phase. A regular diet as eaten by the child at home may be allowed, restricting only concentrated carbohydrate items. Between-meal snacks may be helpful in preventing mild hypoglycemic symptoms. Several factors such as exercise, infection, growth, and so forth influence the caloric and insulin needs. Hunger should be a useful guide in determining the caloric needs in these situations.

LONG-TERM MANAGEMENT. Effective long-term management depends on the degree of emotional acceptance and adjustments that the child and his family can make. Discussions concerning the nature of the disease, the feasibility of leading a normal life, and the genetic aspects of the problem help the family to cope with the disease. The parents or the child, or all three, should be taught to give injections at home. Steps to be taken in case the child develops either intercurrent infections or hypoglycemia should be explained. These include the use of crystalline insulin in addition to routinely administered insulin and the administration of antibiotics for infections. Participation in regular school activities should be encouraged. Additional food intake prior to any vigorous activities may be needed to prevent hypoglycemic symptoms.

Latent Diabetes. Children with latent diabetes have intermittent symptoms (polyuria, polydipsia, and polyphagia) and distinctive laboratory findings (abnormal glucose tolerance tests) but ordinarily do not require insulin or become ketotic. Under conditions of strain, such as surgery or during an acute illness, they may become acidotic and require insulin. The insulin levels of plasma during a glucose tolerance test are normal and, in some cases, above normal in these children, a finding that differentiates them from children with insulin-dependent, overt diabetes mellitus. Approximately 20 per cent of these children eventually develop overt diabetes. Oral hypoglycemic agents are of no value in children.

Transient Diabetes in the Newborn. Transient diabetes appears shortly after birth and is more common in "small-for-gestational-age" babies. The cause is unknown. The characteristic features of the syndrome are weight loss, dehydration with acidosis, failure to thrive, and polyuria. Laboratory findings include marked glucosuria and hyperglycemia. Management consists of administration of fluids parenterally to correct dehydration and insulin for the duration of the diabetic state. Newborns are very sensitive to insulin, and frequent estimations of blood glucose levels are necessary to avoid hypoglycemia. Approximately 1 to 3 units of regular insulin per kg. per day in divided doses may be required to control hyperglycemia.

MUSCLE AND NEUROMUSCULAR DISEASES

Hypotonia is most often caused (50 per cent of the time) by spinal cord disease, i.e., trauma, tumor, viral infections, and so forth. About 20 per cent of the cases are due to central nervous system processes (mental retardation, congenital cerebral defects) and the remaining hypotonias are due to muscle disorders, connective tissue problems, peripheral nerve disease, diseases of the neuromuscular junction, and skeletal disorders. Approximately 10 per cent are not diagnosed. The following are some of the more common hypotonias:

Werdnig-Hoffmann Disease (Infantile Spinal Muscular Atrophy). The onset of this autosomal recessive condition begins in the first $1\frac{1}{2}$ years of life. The earlier the onset, the more severe and rapidly progressive is the course. Proximal muscles are more extensively afflicted (limb girdle and trunk). No sensory or sphincter changes are noted. The electromyogram (EMG) shows scattered peaked waves and fibrillation potentials, indicative of anterior horn cell damage. Muscle biopsy will demonstrate muscular atrophy. The course is relentlessly progressive, with death caused by paralysis of respiratory muscles or intercurrent pulmonary infection. No therapy exists currently.

A more benign variant is amyotonia congenita. This illness presents similar findings but progresses far less rapidly, with death occurring only toward middle age.

Congenital Hypotonia. The onset of weakness dates from birth and is nonprogressive. The family history displays no familial incidence. Remission occurs before puberty in some, while others will have residual muscle weakness, particularly of the smaller muscles, beyond puberty. Electromyography shows polyphasic, short duration potentials but serum enzyme levels, nerve conduction, and muscle biopsies are normal.

Muscular Dystrophy of the Landouzy-Déjerine or Facioscapulohumeral Variety. This is a slowly progressive condition that begins anywhere from early childhood to adult life. Difficulty in closing the eyes, an expressionless face, drooping of the shoulders, and inability to raise the arms are early signs. Deep tendon reflexes are decreased or absent. In later stages lower limb weakness develops and contractures may form. A full life span is frequently attained.

The Erb's or limb-girdle variety also begins between early childhood and early adult life. It is more rapidly progressive than Landouzy-Déjerine dystrophy but not as fast as the Duchenne variant. Shoulder girdle muscles are primarily affected, and the patient has difficulty in moving the upper extremities. If pelvic girdle muscles are involved, the condition is termed Leyden-Moebius dystrophy. The course is similar, although more rapid, than Landouzy-Déjerine dystrophy, with death occurring in the third to fifth decades. The electromyogram shows short duration, low amplitude waves, and the muscle biopsy reveals fiber atrophy. Nerve conduction is normal, but enzyme levels are elevated (creatine phosphokinase, serum glutamic-oxaloacetic transaminase, and aldolase).

There is no specific therapy that reverses or halts the disease process, although much good can be accomplished by supportive therapy, i.e., counseling, physiotherapy and occupational therapy, good general care, and so forth.

THE ANEMIAS

Although a diagnosis of anemia is generally made on the basis of hemoglobin and hematocrit values, the most useful red cell index is the mean corpuscular hemoglobin concentration (MCHC). The normal MCHC in children is 32 to 34 per cent and in neonates is 34 to 36 per cent.

Anemias in children fall into two major groups:

1. Anemias due to an inadequate production of red cells or hemoglobin. Physiologic anemia of the newborn and iron deficiency

anemia are two of the most frequently encountered clinical entities in this category.

2. Hemolytic anemias due to a premature destruction of red blood cells. This could be on the basis of either an intrinsic or corpuscular abnormality of the red cells (e.g., hemoglobinopathies such as sickle cell disease, thalassemia, and so forth) or extrinsic or extracorpuscular abnormalities (e.g., Rh and ABO incompatibilities).

Physiologic Anemia

Anemia due to a physiologic depression of erythropoiesis and hemoglobin synthesis occurs in all newborn infants at about 2 to 3 months of age. The anemia is normochromic and normocytic and occurs with reticulocytosis. It may be especially severe in premature infants. No treatment is usually necessary, but in some premature infants packed red blood cell transfusion may be indicated if the hemoglobin falls to very low levels (below 6 to 7 grams per 100 ml.).

Iron Deficiency Anemia

This is the most common form of anemia encountered in pediatric practice. The incidence in children between 6 and 36 months of age varies from 17 to 44 per cent. The peak incidence is noted in the 10 to 15 month age group.

Causes of iron deficiency anemia fall into four major categories: (1) deficient intake, (2) increased demand, (3) blood loss, and (4) impaired absorption.

1. Deficient intake—Normally an iron intake of 1.0 mg. per kg. per day to a maximum intake of 15 mg. (2.0 mg. per kg. per day in low birth weight infants) is required to maintain normal hemoglobin levels in children. Milk is poor in iron, containing only 1 mg. of iron per liter. Milk alone, therefore, cannot provide an adequate iron supply for a growing infant unless it is fortified with iron or unless other iron-rich dietary items are introduced early in an infant's life. A diet deficient in iron is perhaps the chief cause of iron deficiency anemia in the United States.

2. Increased demand—The frequent occurrence of iron deficiency anemia in low birth weight infants is a result of an increased demand for iron. Low birth weight infants are born with low iron stores and have a greater need for iron than normal birth weight babies because of their more rapid growth. A combination of these two factors almost invariably produces anemia unless supplemental iron is provided in the diet.

3. Blood loss—Prenatal factors such as blood loss across the placenta or into a twin fetus, placental bleeding, and so forth result in inadequate body stores of iron at birth, leading to a deficiency during the infant's rapid growth period. Also in areas where hookworms are prevalent an iron deficiency anemia is frequently seen in children in whom chronic blood loss occurs as a result of the hookworm infestation. Another factor is the blood loss resulting in further aggravation of anemia that occurs in children who are already suffering from iron deficiency anemia. The loss of blood in these children is from the gastrointestinal tract, supposedly on the basis of mucosal changes brought about by an iron deficiency state. Hypersensitivity to cow's milk has also been known to cause blood loss from the gastrointestinal tract.

4. Impaired absorption—Anemia can result when iron absorption is impaired, e.g., in many of the malabsorption syndromes and in chronic diarrheal states.

Pallor, listlessness, irritability, and loss of appetite are some of the symptoms generally seen in children with moderate to severe degrees of iron deficiency anemia. Splenomegaly and a blowing apical systolic murmur are other findings one may notice on physical examination. Pica, an abnormal urge to ingest nonfood items, has been observed occasionally.

The peripheral blood smear examination reveals microcytic and hypochromic red blood cells. Target cells, stippled red cells, and normoblasts can also be seen on the blood smear in severe anemia. The total red blood cell count may be normal. The hematocrit and mean corpuscular hemoglobin concentration (MCHC) levels are lower than normal. The serum iron level is usually less than 50 micrograms per 100 ml. (normal level is 120 micrograms per 100 ml.) and the iron binding capacity is approximately 450 micrograms per 100 ml. (normal 250 micrograms per 100 ml.).

Prevention of iron deficiency anemia, particularly in susceptible infants (low birth weight infants), can be achieved by the use of an iron fortified formula until the child is 12 months of age.

Oral therapy with any form of ferrous iron is effective. Ferrous sulfate, which contains 20 per cent of elemental iron, is the drug of choice. The usual dosage is 5 to 6 mg. of elemental iron per kg. per day. Therapy is continued for about a month after normal hemoglobin values are achieved. Parenteral iron (iron-dextran) can be used if the patient's compliance in taking the medication is a problem, if the patient is unable to tolerate oral iron, or if the intestinal absorption of iron is defective.

Transfusion of packed red blood cells may be indicated in an occasional child with severe anemia complicated by infection. Correction of anemia should be done gradually in these children.

Finally, attention must be given to the basic causative factor of the anemia. Dietary alterations should be made and counseling should be done when necessary.

Sickle Cell Disease

This is one of the most common genetic diseases and is characterized by the presence of an abnormal red blood cell hemoglobin. The frequency of the gene for sickle hemoglobin (HbS) varies in different populations of the world. In the United States it is seen primarily in the black population, with approximately 10 per cent of the population carrying the trait and 1 per cent being affected by the disease.

The presence of abnormal hemoglobin causes sickling of red blood cells, which then become prone to early destruction by reticuloendothelial cells and hemolysis. The disease occurs in two forms: the heterozygous (sickle cell trait, or SA) in which the percentage of abnormal hemoglobin (HbS) varies between 24 and 45 per cent and the homozygous (sickle cell disease, or SS) in which the percentage of HbS varies between 80 and 100 per cent.

Children with sickle cell trait are usually symptom-free and maintain normal hemoglobin, hematocrit, and reticulocyte values. Identification of children who have the trait is usually made by examining a sickle cell preparation and, if positive, by performing hemoglobin electrophoresis.

Symptoms in children with sickle cell disease (SS) apart from those attributable to chronic hemolysis (anemia, jaundice, and so forth) result mainly from sequestration of sickled cells in the vasculature of different organs of the body, producing obstruction of blood flow and infarction. This results in a sickle crisis. The presenting symptom in a child with "crisis" depends on the site of infarction. Thus, abdominal pain may be the presenting symptom in a child with infarctions occurring in the omentum, mesentery, liver, and spleen. Medullary and cortical infarcts of the long bones result in local tenderness, swelling, and, if the lesion is close to a joint, limitation of movement and joint pain. Painful swelling of the hands and feet is noticed in those who suffer a circulatory impairment to the metacarpal and metatarsal bones. An obstruction of blood flow to the vital portions of the central nervous system may result in monoplegia or hemiplegia. The involvement of the kidneys results in polyuria and defective concentration of urine. An acute sequestration of blood in the spleen may produce a sudden drop in the blood volume, leading to shock. The spleen may become greatly enlarged in the first few years of life. By contrast, in later years, because of chronic sequestration of blood, the spleen becomes fibrotic and reduced in size.

These changes in the spleen result in splenic reticuloendothelial dysfunction and may account for the unusual susceptibility of these patients to pneumococcal infections. Pneumococcal pneumonia, septicemia, and meningitis are all repeatedly observed in these children. An unusual susceptiblity to infection caused by *Salmonella* organisms has also been well documented. The involvement of the liver produces symptoms often indistinguishable from hepatitis. The presence of gallstones is frequently demonstrated.

Other manifestations include "aplastic crisis," during which, because of erythroid hypoplasia, the child's anemia may suddenly worsen and "hyperhemolytic crisis" marked by an accentuated rate of hemolysis that results in a precipitous fall in the hematocrit value and a rise in the reticulocyte count. Hyperhemolytic crisis probably occurs only in those patients with associated glucose 6-phosphate dehydrogenase deficiency.

The hematologic picture in affected children consists of hemoglobin values of 6 to 9 grams per 100 ml., increased reticulocyte and white blood counts, and the presence of sickled cells on a routine blood smear. The diagnosis is established by hemoglobin electrophoresis.

Specific therapy to reverse or inhibit sickling is not presently available. Symptomatic treatment for children with painful crises includes administration of fluids and analgesics. If an infection is suspected, it must be promptly treated with appropriate antibiotics. Because infections caused by pneumococcal organisms are frequent and can often be fulminant, it is best to treat all children with a high unexplained fever with either penicillin or ampicillin. Blood transfusions may be indicated for patients with aplastic and hyperhemolytic crises.

Beta-Thalassemia

Beta-thalassemia is one of the more common hereditary hemolytic anemias in which there is suppression of normal hemoglobin (HgA) production because of a defective synthesis of the beta chain of the hemoglobin molecule. In the heterozygous form it is called thalassemia minor and in the homozygous form thalassemia major. There is also an intermediate form, beta thalassemia intermedia.

Thalassemia Minor.   In thalassemia minor, the patient is asymptomatic and exhibits no abnormal findings except perhaps splenomegaly. Blood smears, however, are abnormal (showing hypochromia, anisocytosis, and target cells). Elevated A_2 levels are noted on hemoglobin electrophoresis.

Thalassemia Major.   A profound hemolytic anemia occurring in children usually when they are about 4 months of age is the presenting manifestation. The chronic hemolytic process results in hyperplasia of the reticuloendothelial system. Hepatosplenomegaly, lymphadenopathy, and enlarged tonsils and adenoids are manifestations of this hypertrophy. Significant expansion of the marrow of the facial and skull bones produces a characteristic facies (enlarged head with bossing and maxillary prominence with protruding and maloccluded teeth).

The cardiac dilatation and hypertrophy seen in affected children are directly related to the degree of anemia. Pigmentation of the skin results from an excessive deposition of melanin and hemosiderin consequent to the repeated transfusions required by children with thalassemia major. Multiple endocrinologic abnormalities—diabetes mellitus, hypothyroidism, hyperparathyroidism, and so forth have been noted in some thalassemic children.

The hematologic picture consists of a blood smear showing hypochromia, microcytosis, anisocytosis, basophilic stippling of the red blood cells, target cells, and normoblasts, hemoglobin levels of 6 to 8 grams per 100 ml., elevated white blood cell count, increased levels of hemoglobin, and a decreased osmotic fragility of the red blood cells.

Repeated transfusions to maintain normal (10 grams or more per 100 ml.) or safe (6 grams per 100 ml.) levels of hemoglobin constitute the principal treatment modality. Prevention and prompt management of infection are essential. Splenectomy is indicated in the presence of hypersplenism. Secondary hemochromatosis resulting from repeated transfusions may improve with the use of chelating agents. Folic acid administration may be necessary in some patients.

Thalassemia Intermedia.   In thalassemia intermedia the patient may exhibit symptoms similar to those observed in thalassemia major but to a far lesser degree. The prognosis is generally good for these children.

Rh and ABO Incompatibilities

Hemolysis resulting from a passive transplacental transfer of maternal antibodies active against the red blood cells of the fetus occurs in Rh and ABO incompatibilities.

In Rh incompatibility, the mother is Rh negative and the fetus is Rh positive. The antibodies formed by the mother against the fetal red blood cells (usually from a previous pregnancy) cross the placenta to the fetus, and a hemolytic process is set in motion. In a small percentage of patients, the disease is mild. However, a greater number of affected infants present with varying manifestations at birth. In very severe incompatibility, a profound anemia, leading to cardiac decompensation and a generalized anasarca (hydrops fetalis), results in death in utero or shortly after birth. In less severe disease, significant hyperbilirubinemia, developing shortly after birth, is the invariable manifestation.

The direct Coombs' test is positive. Anemia is present. The peripheral blood smear shows macrocytosis and many nucleated red cells. Reticulocytes are also increased in number. The cord bilirubin level is usually greater than 3 mg. per 100 ml., and the level of bilirubin rises rapidly postnatally. The billirubin is of the indirect type.

The management is directed toward the detection and treatment of the severe form of the disease in utero and of the hyperbilirubinemia to prevent kernicterus (see page 833). Prevention of Rh sensitization can be achieved by parenteral administration of human anti-D gamma globulin to appropriate mothers.

In ABO incompatibility, the mother is type O and the infant is type A or B. The affected infant usually has only mild symptoms. Jaundice appears within the first 24 hours of life and may become progressively worse. The bilirubin in the blood is of the indirect type.

Although the infant's hemoblobin level is usually normal, the peripheral blood smear shows increased numbers of nucleated red cells and an unusual number of spherocytes. Reticulocytes are increased. The direct Coombs' test result is generally negative, but the indirect Coombs' test result is almost always positive. The indirect serum bilirubin may reach a critically dangerous level.

The prevention of a significant accumulation of bilirubin is achieved by phototherapy or exchange transfusion, or both.

BIBLIOGRAPHY

1. Allen, J. E., Gururaj, V. J., and Russo, R. M.: Practical Points in Pediatrics. 2nd ed. New York, Medical Examination Publishing Co., Inc., 1976.
2. Avery, G. B.: Neonatology: Pathophysiology and Management of the Newborn. Philadelphia, J. B. Lippincott Co., 1975.
3. Barness, L. A. (ed.): Symposium on fluid and electrolyte problems. Pediatr. Clin. North Am., 11:789, 1964.
4. Barnett, H. L., and Einhorn, A.: Pediatrics. 15th ed. New York, Appleton-Century-Crofts, 1972.
5. Gellis, S. S., and Kagan, B. M.: Current Pediatric Therapy. 8th ed. Philadelphia, W. B. Saunders Co., 1978.
6. Krugman, S., and Ward, R.: Infectious Diseases of Children and Adults. 5th ed. St. Louis, C. V. Mosby Co., 1973.
7. Nadas, A. S., and Fyler, D. C.: Pediatric Cardiology. 3rd ed. Philadelphia, W. B. Saunders Co., 1972.
8. Vaughan, V. C., III, McKay, R. J., and Nelson, W. E.: Nelson Textbook of Pediatrics. 10th ed. Philadelphia, W. B. Saunders Co., 1975.

Chapter 45

PULMONARY MEDICINE

by THOMAS J. GODAR,
ALEXANDER BERGER,
and JOHN E. DONNELLY

DEFINITIONS

Anatomic

Acinus (primary lobule, or terminal respiratory unit). Those structures distal to the end of a terminal bronchiole, usually consisting of three divisions of respiratory bronchioles, their alveolar ducts, and alveoli.

Dead space. The air in the respiratory tract that does not take part in gas exchange. It includes the "anatomic dead space" or the volume of gas in the conducting airways including the mouth, nose, pharynx, and tracheobronchial tree and the "alveolar dead space" or the volume of alveoli that are ventilated without perfusion (i.e., pulmonary embolism).

Lobule (secondary lobule). The smallest division of lung parenchyma bounded by connective tissue septa. It arises from a terminal bronchiole with variable numbers of terminal respiratory units.

Small airway. Terminal bronchi or bronchioles of less than 2 mm. internal diameter.

Physiologic

Dyspnea. A subjective symptom of shortness of breath or awareness of increased respiratory effort.

Hypercapnia. A term used to describe an elevated carbon dioxide tension in arterial blood, usually with a PCO_2 of 45 mm. Hg or greater.

Hyperpnea. An increase in minute ventilation, usually in response to pulmonary or metabolic needs (diabetic acidosis, renal failure), that is characterized by an increased volume of air exchanged, usually with an increased tidal volume and an increased rate.

Hyperventilation. An increase in ventilation in excess of metabolic needs or carbon dioxide production that leads to hypocapnia and can be identified by a low arterial PCO_2.

Hypocapnia. A carbon dioxide tension below normal (less than 35 mm. Hg.)

Hypoxemia. An arterial oxygen tension below normal (less than 85 to 90 mm. Hg during ambient air breathing).

Respiratory failure. A condition in which there is failure of the lungs to carry out adequate gas exchange either at rest or on exertion. A PaO_2 of less than 60 mm. Hg or a $PaCO_2$ of more than 50 mm. Hg, or both, are generally accepted as values that define respiratory failure.

Respiratory insufficiency. A condition in which there is abnormal respiratory physiology producing dyspnea either with exertion or at rest, but not denoting respiratory failure, which is established physiologically.

Shunt (venous admixture). This term describes a reduced ventilation/perfusion ratio leading to inadequate or incomplete oxygenation of blood during its passage through the lungs that is associated with and produces hypoxemia.

Stridor. A high-pitched inspiratory sound, as heard in croup, that is caused by obstruction of the upper airways, including the major bronchi, larynx, trachea, or hypopharynx. This is to be differentiated from the predominantly expiratory wheeze characteristic of distal airway obstruction.

Tachypnea. Rapid breathing, the respiratory frequency exceeding the normal 16 to 18 breaths per minute at rest.

Wheeze. Expiratory sibilant rhonchus (musical sound) caused by turbulent air flow in the large airways.

Disease Entities

Bronchial asthma. Recurrent, generalized expiratory airway obstruction associated with musical rhonchi. This is paroxysmal and reversible in the early stages.

Bronchiectasis. The condition characterized by chronically dilated bronchi with destroyed mucociliary clearance and a chronic bronchial infection.

Chronic bronchitis. A clinical continuum ranging from a slight morning cough or throat clearing to severe obstructive airway disease associated with cough and sputum production. A minimum definition is daily productive cough for at least 3 consecutive months for more than 2 years in the absence of a specific cause such as tuberculosis, bronchiectasis, or tumor.

Emphysema. A condition of the lung characterized by an abnormal increase in the size of air spaces distal to the terminal bronchioles and accompanied by destruction of lung tissue.

Empyema. A purulent pleural effusion.

Honeycomb lung. The presence on a chest radiograph of multiple, relatively thick-walled cavities, measuring 0.5 to 2 cm. in diameter. This is usually the end-stage of a diffuse pulmonary fibrosis and is nonspecific.

Interstitial fibrosis (Fibrosing alveolitis, or usual interstitial pneumonia [UIP]). A bilateral diffuse process with lung scarring that produces a nodular or reticular pattern in the lung fields. This is often referred to as interstitial, though in the early stages it is intra-alveolar followed later by an interstitial element resulting in thick, fibrotic alveolar walls and septa. The term pneumonia is a misnomer.

Lung abscess. A suppurative, cavitated lesion caused by infection by pyogenic organisms, but excluding cavities due to tuberculosis or necrotic tumors.

Pneumoconiosis. Both the accumulation of dust (as an aerosol composed of solid inorganic particles) in the lung and the tissue reaction resulting from its presence.

Pneumonia (pneumonitis). An inflammation of the parenchyma of the lungs involving alveolar ducts, alveolar sacs, and alveoli.

Sarcoidosis. A systemic granulomatous disease of unknown cause and pathogenesis, involving mediastinal and peripheral lymph nodes, lungs, liver, spleen, skin, eyes, and phalangeal bones. Histologic composition consists of epithelioid tubercles without necrosis in the absence of tuberculosis, fungus infection, and berylliosis.

Solitary pulmonary nodule. A sharply demarcated oval or round lesion appearing as a solitary density on the chest x-ray, usually 0.5 to 4 cm. in diameter and occurring with or without calcification.

COMMON PROBLEMS IN PULMONARY MEDICINE

Recently, an article in the *Journal of the Family Practice* logged problems encountered in multiple practices and ranked them by order of frequency.[6a] Table 45–1 lists these problems, broken down into two categories: acute, usually time-limited problems and chronic, usually current or progressive problems. The number beside each indicates the rank order of frequency

TABLE 45–1.   ORDER OF FREQUENCY OF PULMONARY MEDICINE PROBLEMS IN FAMILY PRACTICE*

Acute Problems	Order	Chronic Problems	Order
Upper respiratory infection	1	Allergic rhinitis	5
Acute bronchitis	2	Emphysema	7
Pneumonitis	3	Chronic bronchitis	9
Asthma	4	Neoplasm of the lung	10
Laryngitis and tracheitis	6	Excessive smoking	12
Pleuritis and pleurisy	8	Pulmonary tuberculosis	13
Pulmonary emboli	11	Cor pulmonale	14
Atelectasis	16	Bronchiectasis	15

*From Marsland, D. W., Wood, M. B., and Mayo, F.: J. Fam. Prac., 3:37, 1976.

in terms of problems of the respiratory tract. A few, such as allergic rhinitis and laryngitis, will be dealt with in other, more appropriate chapters in this book.

UPPER RESPIRATORY TRACT INFECTIONS

Although they are among the most common illnesses to beset man, upper respiratory tract infections remain a challenge to the diagnostic and therapeutic skills of the physician. Almost all (95 per cent) are viral in cause, running their natural course with significant morbidity and little mortality. School and work absenteeism is a significant complication and perhaps reflects one mode of transmission. Healthy adults suffer one to three "colds" per year, and young children suffer twice as many. Mortality does occur, usually during sporadic epidemics, such as influenza, and usually in a patient with a compromised host-response mechanism. These same patients are the target of massive vaccination programs when spread of viral infections to epidemic proportions is predictable.

Current methods of identification of viruses causing infections are expensive and slow. In addition, effective antiviral agents have not been developed, so that the physician must still rely on a clinical diagnosis and symptomatic therapy for most of these infections. The clinical classifications listed in Table 45–2 are helpful in quickly identifying those infections that have a specific treatment regimen.

TABLE 45–2. PRINCIPAL VIRUSES ASSOCIATED WITH UPPER RESPIRATORY SYNDROMES

Disorder	Virus
Common cold	Rhinovirus Parainfluenza I and II ECHO 28 Coxsackie A21 Respiratory syncytial virus
Influenza	Influenza A and B
Pharyngeal syndrome	Adenovirus Influenza Coxsackie ECHO Parainfluenza
Herpangina	Coxsackie A

The Common Cold

Truly known to all are the annoying common cold symptoms of nasal discharge (first watery, then purulent), obstruction, conjunctival irritation and discharge, sneezing, sore throat, malaise, headache, myalgia, and lassitude. Calls to the physician's office usually mirror the seasonal variation in incidence, starting in the fall, peaking in the winter, and slowly subsiding each spring. With an incubation period of 2 to 4 days and a variable duration and severity (3 days to 3 weeks), the usual family must face a total of a month of distracting illness. The pattern is more predictable in overcrowded homes and in homes with young children, especially those in the age groups between 2 and 7 years.

Faced with an index case, there is little that the family can do to prevent spread, but most do attempt to partially isolate the patient, especially for airborne droplet spread. Significant data indicate that these measures are not helpful, but why this is is not known. Preclinical spread may be the reason.

Therapeutic measures for the uncomplicated cold include the standard regimen of increased rest, fluid nourishment, and symptomatic therapy. Analgesics, antihistamines, and vasoconstrictors are commonly recommended for treatment, but all carry some hazards of adverse effects and little or no proof of efficacy. Use of ascorbic acid remains controversial as both a preventative and a therapeutic regimen, with insufficient data currently available to recommend its use for the general population.

Antibiotics enjoy the unenviable reputation of being unfashionable and are considered a reverse index of the professional skill of the physician; this despite early data, largely from British literature, that their use does shorten the duration of the illness and is beneficial to "high risk" patients (those with an already compromised host-response system).

There is little argument, however, concerning the benefit of antibiotics in the treatment of the complications of the cold, as most complications are superimposed bacterial infections. These commonly include sinusitis, otitis media, bronchitis, and pneumonia. It therefore becomes necessary for each physician to develop a mechanism for identification of patients with complications of the common cold and to initiate a program for both isolation and early intervention in "high risk" patients.

The Pharyngeal Syndrome

Patients afflicted with pharyngeal infections complain of a sore throat and swollen glands and occasionally of conjunctivitis. In other respects, the symptoms mirror the common cold. It is not uncommon to discover a bacterial causative agent, including the group A beta hemolytic streptococcus and the gonococcus. Infectious mononucleosis also frequently presents this way, and examination of the abdomen for hepatosplenomegaly can be rewarding in leading to an accurate diagnosis of that ailment.

As mentioned previously, culture techniques for viral identification are costly and tedious. However, culture techniques for bacteria are readily accessible to a small office and permit rapid, accurate diagnosis of a group A beta hemolytic streptococcal infection. More sophisticated equipment and culture media are required to accurately diagnose a gonococcal pharyngitis. Thus, most physicians still rely on a high index of suspicion; a history of oral sex, especially with multiple partners; and a fully equipped outside microbiologic laboratory for accurate diagnosis.

Screening tests for infectious mononucleosis are inexpensive and readily useful in an office setting. It is wise to wait 7 to 10 days before running the test and to run controls with each test, so as to maximize the cost benefit to the patient.

The specific treatment regimens include penicillin for streptococcal infections and penicillin plus probenecid for gonococcal disorders. Frequent changes in the treatment regimens are logged for the practicing physician by the Communicable Disease Center in Atlanta, Georgia, and their weekly newsletter is a valuable, free asset when determining therapy.

Steroids are mentioned in the literature as being useful to control the symptoms of infectious mononucleosis but are not recommended for general use.

Complications are essentially the same as for the common cold and are treated similarly when encountered.

A healthy concern for well members of an index family will occasionally permit identification of a subclinical infection caused by a streptococcus, and of course all contacts with an index case of gonococcal pharyngitis should be sought for specific cultures.

Last, but not least, a peritonsillar or retropharyngeal abscess may present as a "sore throat" syndrome. The toxicity of the patient and the inability to swallow saliva point quickly to the correct diagnosis and permit emergency treatment.

Influenza

This illness, named after the "influence of the stars," has been noted to occur in epidemics caused by a new strain of organism every 10 to 30 years. Sporadic illness within any community does occur every year, however. Characterized by a short incubation period and a propensity to infect young children, this infection masquerades as other viral respiratory infections that occur during the colder months, until it spreads to the older populations. The severe toxicity, myalgias, and involvement of the respiratory tract then become more obvious, permitting an accurate clinical diagnosis. Young children continue to shed the virus for 4 to 7 days, and this probably facilitates spread.

The usual course is completed in 7 to 10 days, and the denuded ciliated epithelium of the respiratory tract has healed by 14 days. Postinfectious asthenia and depression, however, are commonly found to last 2 to 4 weeks longer.

Treatment for the uncomplicated disease in a healthy host remains symptomatic. Common complications include bacterial pneumonias, usually caused by streptococcal or pneumococcal organisms. This usually appears as a "relapse" of the disease and requires appropriate therapy with a penicillinase-resistant penicillin. Less common complications include carditis, encephalitis, and myelopathy, all obviously serious and potentially morbid complications. In a family, anyone stricken with influenza who does not run the "usual" course deserves to be re-evaluated in light of these possible complications.

Prevention of influenza has become possible through worldwide tracking of the existing strains of virus and rapid production of a safe vaccine for new strains. Patients with heart disease and chronic lung disease and women in the third trimester of pregnancy are at highest risk, and anyone with a chronic illness is also considered at risk. The introduction of a new strain or the reintroduction of one that has not cycled frequently (e.g., the New Jersey swine strain) broadens the "at risk" population to include everyone. The older swine influenza strains carried a significant mortality among healthy adults aged 20 to 40 years. These two facts were focal in the national immunization effort of 1976.

Herpangina

Infection with the Coxsackie A virus, especially in young children, at first exposure can produce a toxic illness with a severe sore throat. The classic vesicles found in the mucous membrane usually permit an accurate clinical diagnosis. Of the many different methods of treatment that have been tried, none seem to be specific or superior to simple supportive measures,

and complications in previously healthy children are rare.

Other Upper Respiratory Tract Infections

Prior to massive vaccination, both measles and rubella presented with upper respiratory tract symptoms and challenged the diagnostic skills of the physician. Other common viral diseases (of children) such as varicella usually present in obvious fashion and require no specific therapy.

PNEUMONITIS

Pneumonitis is an inflammatory reaction of the parenchyma of the lung. The many diverse causes of this common disorder are outlined in Table 45–3. Those asterisked are the more common and will be discussed

TABLE 45–3.   CAUSES OF PNEUMONITIS

1. Bacterial pneumonias:
   °*Streptococcus pneumoniae:* pneumococcus
   °*Staphylococcus pyogenes*
   °*Mycobacterium tuberculosis*
   Klebsiella pneumoniae: Friedländer's bacillus
   Hemophilus influenzae
   Escherichia coli
   Pseudomonas aeruginosa or *pyocyanea*
   Bacteroides
   Streptococcus pyogenes
   Streptococcus viridans
   Bacillus cereus
   Loefflerella whitmori
   Malleomyces mallei

2. Bacterial pneumonias as a manifestation of a specific bacterial disease:
   Pertussis
   Typhoid-paratyphoid
   Brucellosis

3. °Viral pneumonias:
   Pneumonia commonly complicating infection:
   Psittacosis-ornithosis group
   Respiratory syncytial virus
   Influenza: pneumonia usually bacterial
   Measles: pneumonia usually bacterial
   Cytomegalovirus
   Pneumonia occasionally complicating infection:
   Adenoviruses
   Parainfluenza viruses
   Rhinoviruses
   Varicella: chickenpox
   Herpes zoster
   Smallpox
   Lymphocytic choriomeningitis
   Infectious mononucleosis

4. Rickettsial pneumonias

5. °Mycoplasmal pneumonias

6. Pneumonias due to yeasts, fungi, and protozoa

7. Allergic pneumonias and pneumonias complicating collagen diseases

8. Chemical pneumonias

9. Radiation pneumonias

°Commonly encountered causes.

in more detail. For less common pneumonias, the reader is referred to appropriate sections of standard medical texts that provide an organized list of causative agents.

Pneumococcal Pneumonia

Of the 80 types of pneumococci, seven are responsible for causing most lung infections, with type 3 being the most virulent. It is believed that all pneumococcal lung infections originate in the upper respiratory tract and are aspirated distally. Why some patients develop lobular involvement while others have segmental or lobar involvement is not entirely clear. Probably a combination of the virulence of the invader, the status of the lung parenchyma, and the state of the patient's host-response mechanisms all play an important role. We do know that epidemics of colds and influenza, air pollution, exposure to cold and wetness, smoking, ingestion of alcohol, anesthetics, chronic pulmonary disease, achalasia, chronic sinusitis, carcinoma of the bronchus, steroid therapy, and immune defects are all associated with increased incidence and risks of pneumococcal pneumonia.

The typical presentation of sudden high fever, chills, pleuritis, pain, cough, tachypnea, and cyanosis is common. Cough productive of a rusty sputum is also common. Physical examination usually reveals the location of the infection, and a leukocytosis with a shift to the left, elevated sedimentation rate, and positive chest radiographs are also common. Obtaining blood cultures and sputum for cultures and for Gram's stain will help to identify the pneumococcus.

Almost all physicians agree that penicillin remains the drug of choice, as 60,000 units per day for 7 days will be curative. Most would recommend at least 1 million units per day, with oral administration reserved for the less toxic patient. Cephalothin and erythromycin are alternative choices for those patients allergic to penicillin. Oxygen, fluid replacement, and analgesics are usually required as supportive measures.

Interestingly enough, use of this regimen has caused a shift in mortality from the pediatric to the geriatric population, but the total mortality rates remain unaffected. In this regard, a polyvalent polysaccharide vaccine is being tested for use in the high risk older population in an attempt to reduce the overall mortality rate.

Common complications of this form of pneumonia include pleural effusion and thrombophlebitis. Less common but more serious complications are empyema, pericarditis, meningitis, and glomerulonephritis.

Staphylococcal Pneumonia

Although staphylococcal pneumonia is less common than pneumococcal pneumonia, it still carries a significant mortality, which can be lowered by prompt and aggressive therapy.

Infection probably occurs through aspiration or by hematogenous spread and is most common in the very young and the very old. Patients who have significant cutaneous injuries (burns); or chronic diseases such as diabetes, emphysema, or carcinomatosis; or who have undergone recent treatment with steroids or broad-spectrum antibiotics are all at risk for this type of pneumonia.

As there are a variety of presentations and radiographic findings may mimic the findings of pneumococcal pneumonia, heavy reliance should be placed on staining and culture of sputum, blood, and pleural fluid, especially in the population at risk. A recent history of influenza followed by septic fever and pulmonary infiltrate should alert one to the possibility of staphylococcal pneumonia. Even with early diagnosis and appropriate treatment, patients recover slowly. Most therapists recommend the use of parenteral antibiotics for 2 to 4 weeks to adequately treat the bacterial endocarditis that accompanies this type of pneumonia in 20 per cent of the patients. Empyema may occur, complicating the clinical course, and bronchiectasis may follow, especially if the clinical course was protracted.

The antibiotic of choice is the penicillinase-resistant penicillin or cephalosporin drug that is most successful in eradicating the staphylococcus organisms peculiar to a geographic area. Pleural effusions require aggressive drainage. Although lower than in the preantibiotic era (when the mortality was 75 to 80 per cent), the mortality is still high (15 to 50 per cent) and is highest in the very old and the very young.

Viral Pneumonia

Many of the viral infections associated with the upper respiratory syndrome may cause pneumonitis—influenza, measles, and varicella commonly do. Their clinical importance differs very little from that described in the discussion of upper airway disorders. Patients have a cough and are usually mildly ill, but rarely are toxic. Chest x-ray films show patchy infiltrates that clear with time, irrespective of treatment regimens. Coughing may continue for several weeks, but the patients usually feel well and ignore the cough.

Perhaps the greatest error of all is to forget to correlate the patient's symptoms with the radiographic picture. An infiltrate that fails to clear within 2 weeks may represent an obstructing lesion rather than viral pneumonia, while one that clears within several days may well have been a pulmonary infarction.

Mycoplasma Pneumoniae Infection

Mycoplasma pneumoniae is a small organism that lacks a cell wall, grows in (rather than on) blood agar, and belongs to the pleuropneumonia-like organism (PPLO) species.

Although their favorite site of infection is the respiratory tract, mycoplasma organisms may also infect the middle ear, the central nervous system, and the blood, skin, and myocardium. There have been reports of a Stevens-Johnson-like syndrome in patients with skin infection and of a Guillain-Barré syndrome in those with a central nervous system mycoplasmal infection. Other complications are septicemia with thrombocytopenia and hemolysis and myocarditis with joint symptoms that mimic acute rheumatic fever.

By far the most common site of infection is the respiratory tract, and it is estimated that mycoplasmal infections are responsible for as much as 10 per cent of all pneumonias. The target population seems to be children and young adults, with infection being uncommon in those over the age of 40. The spread of infection is postulated to occur by airborne droplets, and there is relatively high infectivity. This may explain why the infections are more common during the school year. Classroom spread probably occurs first, followed by child-to-family spread at home. Most infections probably invade the upper respiratory tract only, and pneumonia occurs in only a few of those with this infection.

The incubation period is long, from 8 to 35 days (average 14 days), and the illness begins as a "cold." The disease slowly progresses down the respiratory tract, and substantial pain with coughing is common. The associated malaise, fever, headache, and joint aches mimic influenza, but the patients are less toxic in general than those with influenza.

Physical findings are usually limited to the pharynx, ears, and chest. Auscultation of the chest commonly reveals fine rales, usually at both bases, or less frequently at one base. Upper lobe involvement is uncommon. Frequently, physical findings are present but a routine chest x-ray may be normal, or an infiltrate may be found but physical findings are absent. With this constellation of presentations, accurate diagnosis is often difficult, if not impossible.

Sputum culture requires special media and considerable time and is therefore not helpful. The various antibody agglutination and complement fixation tests are specific but also require weeks, not hours, to perform and cannot be considered helpful to the family physician except in a retrospective sense or as confirmatory evidence of a previous diagnosis. Influenzal, pneumococcal, and adenoviral pneumonias may all cause a similar clinical picture. Less frequently seen, but also similar in presentation, are psittacosis, Q fever, tularemia, and even streptococcal or staphylococcal pneumonia. Acute pulmonary tuberculosis may also mimic the clinical picture of mycoplasmal pneumonia.

In establishing the differential diagnosis, the physician should suspect mycoplasmal infection, when faced with a patient who is ill but not toxic, who is 5 to 40 years old, and who has a history of an upper respiratory infection that migrated distally to produce a clinically evident pneumonia in the lower lobes.

Treatment with tetracycline or erythromycin results in an excellent clinical response in 50 per cent of patients, with a rapid clearing of the chest as shown by radiography. However, abundant evidence indicates that the actual protracted course of infection is unaltered, and infectivity by droplet spread continues for 4 to 6 weeks.

Fortunately, the infection afflicts a population that is usually healthy, and morbidity and mortality are low. It does behoove the family physician to isolate the patient with mycoplasmal pneumonia from the critically ill adult who might not tolerate a serious lower respiratory tract infection.

Neonatal Pneumonia

Neonatal pneumonia accounts for over 15 per cent of stillbirths near the time of delivery and for about 10 per cent of infant deaths during the first 48 hours of life.

Intrauterine infections resulting in pneumonia are more likely following (1) prolonged rupture of the membranes, (2) prolonged labor, and (3) excessive obstetric intervention. Infection caused by vaginal micro-organisms following the ascending route is most common, but hematogenous transplacental infection plays a role when specific organisms such as *Listeria* and cytomegalovirus are associated with pneumonia.

The symptoms of neonatal pneumonia depend on the maturity of the infant and on whether the infection was acquired in the antepartum or the postpartum period. It is important to stress that these symptoms are nonspecific and differ from the symptoms associated with pneumonia in older children and adults.

The onset of respirations may be delayed, labored, and inadequate. Hypothermia is prevalent, especially in premature infants. Cyanosis and irregular respirations with periods of apnea are frequently observed. Low-grade fever may develop hours or days after birth, usually in full-term infants.

Leukocytosis may or may not be present; either leukopenia (<5000 leukocytes per cu. mm.) or leukocytosis (>15,000 leukocytes per cu. mm.) is suggestive of infection. The infective organisms are most frequently coliform, gram-negative bacteria, streptococci, and staphylococci.

The pneumonia is almost always a diffuse process that appears in chest x-ray films as a bilateral, ill-defined, streaky density, with peribronchial thickening resulting in "ring signs" in the perilobar region.

ACUTE BRONCHITIS

Acute bronchitis is a common infection of the tracheobronchial tree that primarily involves the larger bronchi and most commonly is produced by viral infections. The onset is acute and is characterized by cough, at times paroxysmal, and by variable sputum production, with sputum varying from white to yellow in color. Patients may experience dyspnea, although usually only with a paroxysmal cough. However, there is an increased frequency of dyspnea in the very young because of the small size of the airways and the potential for airway obstruction caused by increased secretions. In a debilitated patient and in the elderly, a nonproductive cough may contribute to stasis of secretions with secondary atelectasis and superinfection. The most common causative agents are a variety of viruses, followed in frequency by the pneumococcus, *Hemophilus influenzae*, and *Mycoplasma pneumoniae*. Symptoms ordinarily subside in 3 to 7 days, with an occasional residual nonproductive cough remaining for the ensuing week.

Adequate oral hydration and the use of expectorants such as a saturated solution of potassium iodide (SSKI) or glyceryl guaiacolate that does not contain cough suppressants may help increase the water content of secretions and the mobilization of these secretions by inducing a bronchorrhea. Such therapy also probably helps prevent secondary superinfection.

In the absence of a specific and predominant bacterial organism in the sputum smear and culture, the majority of patients improve without antibiotic therapy. A change in the quality of the sputum, especially an increase in volume and a change to green sputum, suggests a more purulent bronchitis and the need for antibiotic therapy, which should rarely be given for less than 7 days. The early use of antibiotics is indicated more in patients with underlying chronic airway disease, cardiovascular disease, or other debilitating diseases and also in those patients who have undergone immunosuppression. If the cough persists and if there are focal rales or musical rhonchi (wheeze), either atelectasis associated with a foreign body or an intrinsic obstructing lesion such as an adenoma should be ruled out. A chest x-ray film might be helpful at this stage, but this study cannot be relied upon to exclude these diagnoses. The occasional patient with minimal secretions but with a continuing disabling paroxysmal cough may be treated cautiously with daily oral steroids to accelerate the clearing of the inflammatory changes that are causing the increased cough reflex. A failure to respond indicates need for further evaluation.

BRONCHIAL ASTHMA

Definition

Bronchial asthma is a state characterized by a hyper-reactivity of the bronchial tree with paroxysmal and reversible broncho-constriction that produces expiratory airway obstruction associated with dyspnea and cough, increased mucus production, and wheeze (sibilant rhonchi). Lung function is normal or near normal between episodes. The severity of the bronchospasm and expiratory airway obstruction may vary widely, as will the reversibility of this disorder with treatment, the frequency of episodes, and the etiologic mechanisms. Most patients have an allergic basis for their asthma, although they may subsequently respond with an asthmatic attack to a variety of environmental stimuli. The potential reversibility with treatment and the normal lung function between episodes differentiate asthma from chronic bronchitis and emphysema when bronchoconstriction is a part of the presenting picture. The incidence of bronchial asthma is estimated to be 5 per cent of the general population.

Etiology and Pathogenesis

A bronchial hyper-reactivity exists in asthmatic patients, which leads to an exaggerated bronchoconstriction following the inhalation of the mediator histamine. The same reactivity occurs with exposures to allergens, irritants, pollutants, and cold air; following infection of the bronchial tree; or after exercise. There is an unpredictable and variable pattern among patients and in the same patient from one time to another.

Asthma begins before 10 years of age in 50 per cent of patients and is more frequent in boys. It begins by age 30 in 85 per cent of patients, at which time the sex incidence is equal. Because of better recognition of asthma and of its differentiation from bronchitis and emphysema, its incidence in the middle-aged or elderly patient is apparently increasing. In this age group, the process usually has an onset associated with a respiratory infection and persists thereafter. Most of these patients will recall some wheezing in childhood and a third will have a family history of allergy.

Asthmatics are characterized by having a blockade of the beta-2 receptors of the sympathetic nervous system, which prevents activation of the beta-2 adrenergic system responsible for intracellular transformation of adenosine triphosphate (ATP) to adenosine 3',5'-monophosphate (cyclic AMP). Deficient cellular cyclic AMP levels are responsible for bronchoconstriction in response to many stimuli, including allergens.

Asthmatics are often classified as having "extrinsic" or "intrinsic" asthma. Extrinsic (atopic) asthma is the form that begins in childhood or young adulthood, often in conjunction with other allergic syndromes such as hay fever or eczema and with a positive family history of allergy. It is usually mediated by the IgE immunoglobulin (reagin) and is associated with positive skin tests to common allergens. These allergens include antigens from grass and tree pollens, mold, animal dander, and house dust (including the house dust mite). There is an immediate Type I reaction between the antigen and the reaginic antibody (IgE) present on the surface of the bronchial mast cells. This reaction causes mast cell degranulation and release of bronchoconstrictors, primarily histamine and slow-reacting-substance of anaphylaxis (SRS-A). Also serving as mediators of bronchoconstriction are kinins, serotonin, and prostaglandins. High levels of cyclic AMP inhibit the release of bronchoconstrictor mediators, resulting in bronchodilatation.

In some patients the levels of IgE are normal and the reaginic antibody is IgG. In contrast to patients with the Type I reaction who have almost immediate symptoms after exposure to the allergen, these patients have Type III reactions that are mediated by precipitating antibodies with airway obstruction and symptoms developing 6 to 12 hours after exposure. This variety is commonly seen in industrial exposures (e.g., polymer fume fever, reaction to toluene diisocyanate [TDI] in the plastics industry, and reaction to substances in the manufacture and use of detergents) in which the late onset of symptoms may hamper recognition of the causative agent, as symptoms often occur at night.

Intrinsic asthma is the term often applied to late onset asthma, usually precipitated by a respiratory infection with an associated

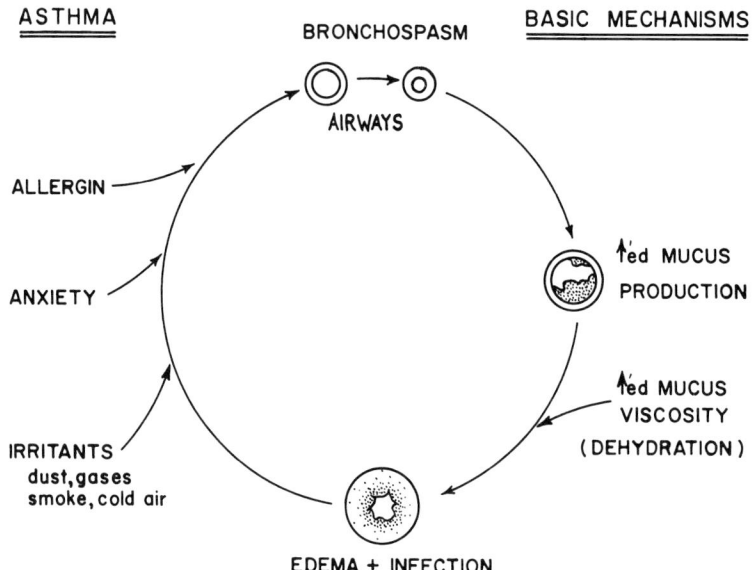

Figure 45-1. *Cascading effect of causative factors in asthma attacks.*

history of nasal polyposis, a common finding of aspirin sensitivity, negative skin tests to common allergens, and normal IgE levels. However, these patients often have a history of allergy in the past or of allergy in other family members, and they do have an increase in peripheral blood eosinophils.

The changes in the airways during an asthmatic attack include widespread bronchoconstriction, increased bronchial capillary permeability with edema of the mucous membranes, and marked hypertrophy with hypersecretion of bronchial mucous glands. This leads to tenacious mucous plugs that obstruct many bronchi and result in areas of lung that have blood supply but little ventilation. Such areas lead to hypoxemia because of inadequate oxygen transfer to perfusing blood. Obstructing mucous plugs are often colonized by bacteria, leading to further local inflammatory changes. Infection aggravates asthma further, both by producing and by intensifying the hyper-reactivity of airways, and is recognized as a common precipitating factor, as well as a cause for intractable asthma. The response of such patients to antibiotic treatment is further evidence of the key role infection may play in both intrinsic and extrinsic asthma.

Figure 45-1 illustrates the cascading effect of various causative factors in promoting and prolonging asthmatic attacks, regardless of the starting point or primary initiating mechanism. Special aggravating factors are the common urban pollutants (sulfur dioxide, nitrogen dioxide, and ozone), high levels of ambient air humidity, emotional stress, or vagal stimulation.

Clinical Manifestions

The patient first experiences a sense of chest tightness or congestion. Coughing and gradual onset of audible expiratory musical rhonchi (wheezes) begin. The patient has dyspnea and notes difficulty in the expiratory phase of respiration. Sputum is white but may be copious and is often tenacious. Anxiety generally exists and further aggravates the asthma. The onset may be related to recent contact with a known allergen or with cold air or may follow exercise or exposure to a nonspecific irritant such as smoke. Onset in conjunction with an upper respiratory tract infection is common, and attacks may be limited to periods of concurrent infection with prolonged symptom-free intervals. Most episodes are self-limited and respond readily to removal of the allergen and the use of bronchodilators.

Examination reveals tachypnea, a prolonged expiratory phase (greater than 3 seconds), expiratory wheeze, cough with secretions, anxiety, tachycardia, and a distended chest with low diaphragms and reduced excursion of both diaphragms and the chest cage. The subject tends to sit leaning forward with arms resting on a support and often uses accessory respiratory muscles. Intercostal retraction and flaring of the alae nasi are seen mostly in severe attacks. With more severe obstruction, the wheeze is audible in both expiratory and inspiratory phases, with respirations becoming more shallow and rapid and the patient becoming more restless. It should be noted that a reduction in audible wheeze may be associated with poor air motion and deterioration in ventilation rather than with improvement of the patient.

Laboratory Studies

Chest x-ray usually reveals distention and streaky densities that represent mucous plugs with local atelectasis. Definite pneumonic patches associated with a high peripheral blood eosinophilia (15 to 40 per cent of white blood cells) suggest the syndrome pulmonary infiltrates with eosinophilia (PIE). This syndrome is associated with asthma and responds dramatically to corticosteroids, which serve as a diagnostic and therapeutic test. Segmental and lobar collapse due to inspissated mucous plugs is seen in asthmatic patients, especially in children. Peribronchial cuffing by infection with cellular infiltrate may be seen in intrinsic asthmatics.

Pulmonary function tests reveal a reduction in forced vital capacity (FVC), moderate to severe reduction in FEV_1 (often less than 50 per cent of the FVC), and a large residual volume caused by dynamic and reversible air trapping. Expiratory flows improve 15 per cent or more in patients following the use of an aerosol bronchodilator, indicating that bronchoconstriction is a significant factor in the airway obstruction. The reduction in caliber of bronchi in the expiratory phase is usually greater than 40 per cent of the inspiratory caliber. Gas distribution is abnormal only during attacks because of mucous plugging during airway constriction. The diffusion capacity in patients with asthma is normal.

The key to evaluating the asthmatic is staging the patient by arterial blood gas and pH analysis. As noted in Figure 45–2 and Table 45–4, four stages are generally recognized. In the early stages, there is chest congestion with expiratory obstruction, but hyperventilation leads to normal oxygen tension, hypocapnia, and alkalosis (Stage I). In Stage II, there is more widespread mucous plugging and air trapping (See Fig. 45–2) with definite hypoxemia, although hypocapnia and alkalosis persist.

Status Asthmaticus. In more severe episodes, especially when there is failure to respond to treatment after 18 to 24 hours, the term status asthmaticus or intractable asthma is applied. In Stage III, hyperventilation is no longer possible despite progressive hypoxemia generated by ventilation/perfusion imbalance, and the chest is very distended. Therefore, the arterial pH and PCO_2 approach normal levels, but this

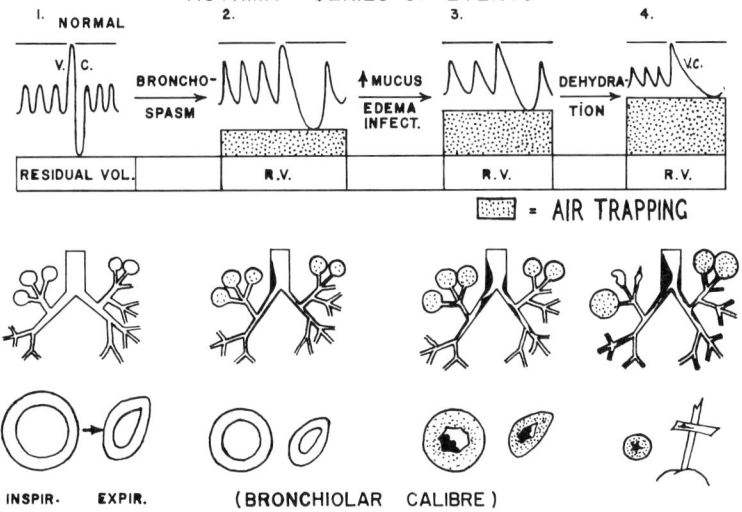

Figure 45–2. Four stages of asthma attack.

TABLE 45–4. STAGES OF ASTHMA

Stage	Expiratory Airway Obstruction	Arterial Oxygen Tension (mm. Hg)	Arterial Carbon Dioxide Tension (mm. Hg)	pH
I	Minimal	Normal: 80–95	Hypocapnia: 30–36	Alkalosis: 7.45–7.55
II	Mild	Mild hypoxemia: 70–80	Hypocapnia: 30–36	Alkalosis: 7.45–7.55
III	Moderate	Moderate hypoxemia: 50–70	Normal: 37–45	Normal: 7.35–7.45
IV	Severe	Severe hypoxemia: 30–50	Hypercapnia: 50–90	Acidosis: 7.15–7.35

must not be considered a good sign. The asthmatic who does not have hypocapnia and alkalosis is decompensating. Stage IV represents advanced respiratory failure with profound and often dangerous hypoxemia, underventilation manifested by a P_{CO_2} greater than 45 mm. Hg, and acidosis. Hypoxemia can be controlled with oxygen supplementation, but a significant elevation of Pa_{CO_2} indicates the need for intubation and mechanical ventilator support before respiratory arrest supervenes. Intubation is best carried out before the Pa_{CO_2} exceeds 55 mm. Hg, as this value will occur only in the intractable patient. There are still approximately 4000 deaths from asthma each year caused by both the excessive use of sympathomimetic drugs and the profound hypoxemia of status asthmaticus.

Treatment

In atopic asthma, environmental control is crucial, including avoidance of known allergens; a dust-free house with a minimum of carpets, drapes, and overstuffed furniture; and the elimination of fur-bearing animals. Skin testing of children may identify potential allergens but is usually of no help in those with adult-onset asthma. The patient should avoid vagal stimulation associated with cold air and cold food or drink.

Hydration. Good oral hydration helps control the viscosity of mucus in conjunction with use of expectorants. Alcohol, coffee, and soft drinks are generally dehydrating and should be avoided or moderated. A daily fluid intake of 3000 to 4000 ml. may be needed in warm climates.

Expectorants. The best expectorant is saturated solution of potassium iodide (SSKI), 10 to 15 drops three times daily after meals, although it often causes rhinorrhea and prolonged use may lead to hypothyroidism or simple goiter. About 15 per cent of

patients experience "iodism," with tender, swollen salivary glands, necessitating discontinuation of the iodide. Intravenous sodium iodide in doses of 1.5 grams per day is helpful in status asthmaticus and rarely causes iodism, although patients complain of a metallic taste in the mouth.

Antibiotics. Patients having asthma for several days with the onset associated with an upper respiratory tract infection or with purulent sputum should receive a broad-spectrum antibiotic such as ampicillin or tetracycline in doses of 1 to 2 grams per day for 7 to 10 days. For prophylaxis, cromolyn sodium powder, which inhibits release of bronchoconstrictors from mast cells, may be inhaled in 20 mg. doses four times a day to control allergic asthma. This drug may reduce the required dose of bronchodilators and is useful if taken before exercise in controlling exercise-induced asthma. Though worthy of a 2 week trial, the majority of patients taking cromolyn sodium do not respond dramatically, and some have increased wheeze with inhalation of the powder. It has no use in patients with status asthmaticus.

Sympathomimetic Amines. These drugs are beta-2 receptor stimulators and increase conversion of ATP to cyclic AMP, thus producing bronchodilatation. Epinephrine is given in acute attacks, especially in children. The adult dosage is 0.2 to 0.3 ml. of an aqueous solution of 1:1000 epinephrine given subcutaneously and repeated every 15 to 20 minutes, if needed, until there is a response or a total dose of 1.0 to 1.5 ml. has been given, with correspondingly smaller doses in children. Acidosis (pH less than 7.30) may render the airways unresponsive to epinephrine but will not block the side effects. Common side effects are hypertension and tachycardia, so that epinephrine is avoided in cardiac or hypertensive patients.

Ephedrine is useful orally in doses of 25 to 30 mg. every 4 to 6 hours in children and young adults, but the effect is brief (4 hours). In addition, it causes tachycardia, tremulousness, and central nervous system stimulation. Evening doses may cause insomnia. In elderly males, ephedrine aggravates symptoms of prostatism, at times leading to acute urinary retention, which renders it a drug to avoid in the elderly male. Terbutaline (not recommended for children under the age of 12 years) is also prone to cause effects similar to ephedrine, but this oral medication, in doses of 2.5 to 5 mg. every 6 to 8 hours, is effective and has a longer action than does ephedrine.

Theophylline is the mainstay of oral maintenance therapy, generally used in doses of 6 to 7 mg. per kg. in acute therapy and 3 to 4 mg. per kg. every 6 to 8 hours is routine treatment. It causes gastric irritation, which may improve when the theophylline is administered orally after meals. Theophylline is a central nervous stimulant and may cause insomnia as well as dizziness, postural hypotension, and tachycardia. In status asthmaticus, it is given in an intravenous dose of 250 to 500 mg., administered slowly at rates below 25 mg. per minute, and then at a level of 1.5 grams per 24 hours (5 mg. per kg. every 6 hours), preferably as a continuous intravenous drip. Theophylline can be administered as a rectal enema in patients with moderate asthma. Suppositories are slower in their onset of action but are less expensive. Theophylline acts to inhibit phosphodiesterase breakdown of cyclic AMP, so it is complementary to the sympathomimetic amines.

Isoproterenol. An aerosol solution of 1:200 isoproterenol may be given by intermittent positive pressure breathing (IPPB) or by powered nebulizer every 2 to 4 hours, using 0.3 to 0.5 ml. diluted with 1 to 2 ml. of isotonic saline for rapid effect. The rapid bronchodilating effect helps the mobilization of sputum and provides reassurance to the acutely ill patient. Freon powered nebulizers are useful but require careful control to avoid patient overuse that may delay proper treatment and result in serious arrhythmias. As the drug effects dissipate in 15 to 20 minutes, this often encourages excessive use. Metaproterenol aerosols may have a prolonged effect of 3 to 4 hours. These agents are useful when given

before postural drainage to assist in mobilization of bronchial secretions.

Corticosteroids. As corticosteroids stimulate beta-2 receptors, inhibit the breakdown of cyclic AMP by phosphodiesterase, restore beta-2 receptor responsiveness to sympathomimetic amines, and enhance bronchodilatation by their anti-inflammatory effects, they are very effective in treating patients with status asthmaticus and recalcitrant, chronic asthma. When administered intravenously, the response is delayed 4 to 6 hours, so steroids should be given early and in conjunction with other drugs in the treatment of status asthmaticus. A dose of 100 to 250 mg. of hydrocortisone is given intravenously initially and then 100 mg. is administered every 6 to 8 hours. Doses as high as 8 mg. per kg. every 6 hours may be needed. Less ill patients can be given prednisone in doses of 5 to 10 mg. orally every 6 to 8 hours. Many patients' attacks are controlled only when 5 to 7.5 mg. per day is used for long-term therapy, and at times patients respond satisfactorily to alternate-day therapy, which diminishes the adrenal suppression.

Side effects are salt and water retention, hypertension, and aggravation of diabetes mellitus, and in long-term therapy, muscle wasting and osteoporosis also occur. Osteoporosis is a special problem in the elderly. Poor response to oral prednisone often occurs when the concomitant ingestion of antacids prevents adequate absorption. Therefore, antacid and prednisone doses should be given at least 2 hours apart.

Beclomethasone. This newly available aerosol steroid has little systemic absorption and few side effects when used in doses of 100 micrograms per dose four times a day (two puffs from a dispenser equal 100 micrograms). Its use commonly reduces reliance on oral steroids, thereby controlling steroid side effects. It is never given only when needed (PRN), as no acute response will be noted, and most patients require four doses a day. Significant absorption begins only at doses of 1000 micrograms per day. Beclomethasone must not be substituted for another steroid without an appropriate period of oral steroid tapering in order to avoid the possibility of adrenal insufficiency.

Significant side effects consist of bronchospasm caused by the irritation of inhaling an aerosol and a 20 to 30 per cent incidence of thrush with prolonged use, usually associated with a pharyngeal exudate and a history of persistent hoarseness. This may be obviated by the use of a commercial mouthwash used as a gargle after inhalation, since concentrated drug in the posterior pharynx seems to be a mechanism for causing secondary monilial infection.

Oxygen. Patients in Stages II and III usually need oxygen supplementation that is best administered in a 28 per cent Venturi mask mixture or by nasal cannula at 2 liters per minute flow to approximate a 28 per cent oxygen mixture. Arterial blood gas analysis is essential to establish an adequate response, with the PaO_2 being kept above 60 mm. Hg.

Sedatives and Tranquilizers. Sedatives and tranquilizers are helpful in modest doses in the earlier stages of asthma, but patients should not be overly sedated because anxiety is often associated with physiologic abnormalities and accompanied by severe hypoxemia rather than being purely psychogenic in origin.

Supportive Care. Patients experiencing status asthmaticus require intravenous therapy, including fluids and drugs; cardiac monitoring; careful observation of arterial blood gas values and pH; and early, vigorous treatment with aerosol bronchodilators and theophylline. Hospitalized patients often experience progressive benefit from vigorous postural drainage and good control of bronchospasm, which repeatedly reinforces the impression that most treatment of asthma is less than adequate, leading to prolonged bouts of asthmatic bronchitis in which lung function remains poor for extended periods. The most common error in treatment is undertreatment with drugs, which results from the well-intended but unwise effort to reduce total drug therapy to a minimum of pills and a minimal cost to the patient. Patients are guilty of fragmented use of drugs and develop a tolerance for poor symptomatic relief, permitting persistence of bronchial hyper-reactivity that prevents long remissions.

Prognosis

The prognosis for childhood atopic asthma is good, with many patients having marked improvement during adolescence and the majority having few significant attacks after the second decade. Many of these patients will present years later with what appears to be adult-onset asthma of the extrinsic variety that follows a respiratory infection. At that point, prompt treatment may prevent a prolonged symptomatic course in adult life. Those smoking cigarettes should unequivocally be encouraged to discontinue smoking entirely. Special forms of asthma attributed to ambient air pollutants have been described and are increasing in frequency. Attacks associated with industrial exposure require a careful medical history and high index of suspicion on the part of the family physician. Often a trial away from the work environment has immediate salutary effects, corroborating the impression of occupational asthma.

HYPERVENTILATION SYNDROME

The hyperventilation syndrome describes a constellation of symptoms that are a frequent cause of visits to the family physician or the emergency room, followed by a search for organic disease. Hyperventilation is a common undiagnosed cause of dyspnea in young adults, despite their having undergone extensive medical evaluation, mainly resulting from failure to recognize the syndrome.

The respiratory centers control breathing primarily to maintain the pH and PCO_2 in a normal range. Oxygen tension represents no significant controlling mechanism except in the patient with severe hypoxemia, in whom it becomes a significant respiratory driving mechanism. Any person can override respiratory control mechanisms and hyperventilate either at will or in response to stimulants, including both pharmacologic agents and external stress. Chronic anxiety is a very common cause of intermittent, symptomatic hyperventilation in young persons who have no demonstrable respiratory disease, being especially prevalent among young women between the ages of 20 and 40.

Although ordinary exercise induces hyperventilation, this is associated with a compensated pH and a normal PCO_2, and the increased ventilation precisely matches the carbon dioxide liberation with steady-state exercise. However, when increased ventilation occurs at rest, as when a person is driven by chronic anxiety, it may become symptomatic because there is no increased carbon dioxide production. Furthermore, the episodes are evanescent and are associated with frightening symptoms related to hypocapnia and secondary alkalosis. Not only does alkalosis induce a reduction in ionized calcium, but it has been shown to cause cerebrovascular constriction, leading to widespread neurologic complaints that masquerade as a variety of acute cardiorespiratory problems.

Diagnosis

The diagnosis is readily made when there is a high index of suspicion arising from the pattern of respiratory symptoms. The episodes are intermittent, lasting from minutes to hours. Also, they generally occur with the subject at rest rather than during exercise, which immediately distinguishes these episodes from dyspnea due to cardiopulmonary disease. Episodes frequently occur in the evening, and there is no pattern of progression to suggest organic disease. When present in young people, especially in young women, in whom there is no evidence of organic disease and when a history of increased anxiety or stress is obtained, the diagnosis is not difficult to make. The following is a list of commonly observed symptoms, not all of which will be present in every case:

1. Shortness of breath. This is described as a desire for a deep breath or an inability to inhale deeply enough rather than as true air hunger or tachypnea. Patients generally describe the frequent sighing respiratory pattern quite well.

2. Lightheadedness, dizziness, blurred vision, or feeling faint. Occasionally, patients describe a sensation of floating in space.

3. Palpitations. Patients may describe tachycardia or irregular rhythm that follows the onset of respiratory symptoms rather than initiating such episodes.

4. Substernal pain or pain over the precordium that is dull rather than pleuritic and occurs without radiation.

5. Paresthesias. Patients describe a "pins and needles sensation," numbness, "a woody feeling," or other altered sensations noted commonly in the mouth, tongue, or face or in all extremities, which are bilateral and usually symmetrical.

6. Sweats, nausea or vomiting, and pain radiation are notably absent.

Physical Examination

The patient characteristically is young, appears quite tense, and demonstrates frequent sighing breaths during the history and physical examination, coupled with normal pulmonary and cardiovascular systems. The physician will do well to take a great deal of time examining the chest and having the patient carry out deep breathing during auscultation, while watching the facial expression and observing the onset of symptoms secondary to the acute hyperventilation induced by the procedure. The patients are then asked if any of the symptoms have been reproduced, because this maneuver reassures them that you understand the problem and that they have some control over symptoms.

Laboratory Studies

Patients may show acute hyperventilation with alkalosis and hypocapnia when arterial blood samples are taken, although this may be induced by pain during the procedure because of poor technique. One may observe chronic hyperventilation evidenced by hypocapnia associated with a normal pH, indicating compensation. Spirometry may be helpful in documenting frequent deep sighing breaths during recording of the spontaneous respiratory pattern. Such breaths often occur with a frequency of 2 to 3 per minute, which is sufficient to cause hypocapnia and symptomatic alkalosis.

Treatment

Treatment consists of an evaluation of the mechanism causing anxiety and of a careful description of the symptom mechanism. The physician should appreciate the fact that the symptoms are not imagined, although they have been generated by hyperventilation rather than by organic disease. Deliberate relaxation and breath-holding will often control symptoms, although such procedures will not prevent their recurrence until the anxiety is controlled. Drugs such as tranquilizers may be helpful on a short-term basis. Symptoms severe enough to induce carpopedal spasm and syncope have often been treated by the rebreathing of carbon dioxide, which is carried out by having the patient breathe into a paper bag. Administration of carbon dioxide and oxygen mixtures has been used but has no rationale.

The prognosis is excellent, although recurrence is common. Prompt diagnosis will prevent extensive, unnecessary evaluations for nonexistent cardiac or pulmonary disease.

ACUTE UPPER AIRWAY OBSTRUCTION

The upper airways are defined as those above the lobar bronchi, including the main stem bronchi, the trachea, and both the nasal and oral passages. Upper airway obstruction can be differentiated readily from lower airway disease. It often presents as a life-threatening disorder requiring prompt diagnosis and treatment to maintain a patent airway and prevent asphyxia.

Etiology

1. Anatomic
   a. Unconsciousness with hypopharyngeal obstruction because of flaccid tongue falling posteriorly.
   b. Paralysis involving neck muscles.
   c. Tracheomalacia and other congenital defects.
   d. Substernal thyroid (rare).
2. Local disease states
   a. Severe tonsillitis with peritonsillar abscess.
   b. Angioneurotic edema due to drugs or insect stings or bites.
   c. Neck trauma—tracheal fractures, hematoma, and so forth.
   d. Neoplasms—extrinsic (lymphoma, carcinoma) or intrinsic (adenoma, bronchogenic carcinoma).
   e. Epiglottitis, acute.
   f. Croup (laryngotracheitis).
   g. Acute laryngospasm.
   h. Flash burns, chemical burns.

3. Obstruction due to foreign bodies
   a. Teeth, dentures.
   b. Candy, peanuts, gum, fruit pits, toys.
   c. Food aspiration—"café coronary."

Diagnosis

Acute upper airway obstruction is characterized by an acute onset of frantic inspiratory efforts with no evident ventilation. Inspiratory stridor (crowing) is common, associated with anxiety, pallor followed by cyanosis, and intercostal and subclavicular retractions, followed shortly by collapse. Usually the cause will be evident from the associated history and physical findings, although in the case of food aspiration the onset is very sudden, occurring while the subject is eating and in the absence of associated disease. Food aspiration is most often caused by a poorly chewed bolus of meat, and the acute events are generally confused with a myocardial infarction. The bolus of food is generally in either the hypopharynx or the trachea. Food aspiration is the sixth leading cause of accidental death in the United States.

Treatment

When possible, the level of obstruction should be identified to determine the likely diagnosis and the appropriate method of establishing an airway. In the case of angioneurotic edema, epinephrine is administered immediately. Oxygen may be administered if some airway persists. Obstruction due to posture and neck flexion should be ruled out immediately. In the unconscious patient, the head is extended with the chin and tongue elevated to prevent posterior pharyngeal obstruction. Foreign bodies are identified and extracted to clear the airway.

If a foreign body cannot be seen or reached and acute, complete airway obstruction has occurred while the subject was eating, the Heimlich maneuver should be performed. This consists of standing behind the victim, wrapping the arms around the waist, placing a fist in the epigastrium, grasping it with the other hand, and pressing the fist into the abdomen with a quick upward thrust. This will suddenly elevate the diaphragm, generate a high tracheal pressure, and eject the foreign body. Several upward thrusts may be required, and one must be alert to the need for extricating the bolus of food to avoid reaspiration. On occasion, victims have self-administered the maneuver by falling against a table or sink. The foreign body is usually beef, chicken, bread, fruit, or candy. The food bolus can be felt by the fingertip but is not readily removed in many instances unless extraction instruments are available. Improper use of the Heimlich maneuver may cause fractured ribs, injury to the liver, or a hollow viscus. The maneuver has been safely used in infants and children.

Patients with burns and tumors and many of those with massive edema of the hypopharynx may require a tracheostomy rather than endotracheal intubation. Mouth-to-mouth or mouth-to-nose breathing should be attempted when complete obstruction by a foreign body has been ruled out and cyanosis is present. If the obstruction is at or above the pharynx and no immediate corrective treatment is possible, a tracheostomy is indicated. For lesions in the hypopharynx, a puncture can be made using a 16 gauge or larger needle via the cricothyroid membrane immediately below the thyroid notch. This will establish an avenue for oxygen supplementation while a definitive diagnosis is being made. Every effort should be made to ensure that an orderly tracheostomy can be carried out when it is needed, obviating the morbidity associated with emergency tracheostomies. Airway edema may respond within hours to intravenous administration of corticosteroids, but establishment of an adequate airway has first priority.

PLEURISY AND PLEURAL EFFUSION

Pleurisy implies a sharp chest pain associated with respirations and aggravated by deep inspiration. It is usually well localized and unilateral and represents either a pleural inflammation with an associated pleural effusion or fibrinous (dry) pleurisy without effusion. The appearance of an effusion often causes rapid relief of pleuritic pain secondary to the separation of parietal and visceral pleural surfaces. Pain is generally better localized and more common in the lower lung fields, owing to the increased excursion at the lung bases, and is definitely increased with deep inspiration. The pain commonly causes involuntary splinting of the involved area. Involvement of the diaphragmatic pleura may cause radiation of pain to the neck, and because of the frequent lower chest involvement, confusion with abdominal disease is common.

Auscultation may reveal a grating sound that is usually well localized in the respiratory cycle. This sound occurs in both inspiration and expiration but is noted most commonly at a reproducible point during deep inspiration. Deep breathing and cough fail to clear the sound, although it may disappear spontaneously within hours. Pleuritic pain with a rub is common in patients with bacterial pneumonia and pulmonary infarction, as well as in those with viral infections, including Coxsackie and adenovirus infections. Immobilization of the chest to control pain is not desirable, as it leads to underventilation and atelectasis. Oral analgesics are preferred for control of pain. Treatment is dependent on the associated clinical picture and the likely diagnosis. When of viral cause, pleurisy is benign and requires little treatment.

Pleural effusion is a common finding when the chest radiograph is included in the diagnostic evaluation, as effusions as small as 300 ml. are evidenced by blunting of the costophrenic angle. A lateral film may reveal a small quantity of fluid in the posterior gutter, and a lateral decubitus film often demonstrates a thin rim of free fluid. Fissure lines are often outlined by a thin film of pleural fluid.

Etiology

The most common causes of pleural effusion are infections, including tuberculosis and a variety of bacterial pneumonias; tumors of both bronchogenic and metastatic origin; and the frequent right pleural effusion associated with congestive heart failure. Other common mechanisms are pulmonary infarction, cirrhosis of the liver, and trauma (the effusion is generally hemorrhagic). Less common causes of pleural effusion are atelectasis, subdiaphragmatic abscess in postoperative patients, pneumothorax with an effusion produced by lung collapse, mycotic and viral infections, myxedema, Meigs' syndrome, nephrotic syndrome, rheumatoid arthritis, systemic lupus erythematosus, and pancreatitis.

There are four mechanisms commonly responsible for pleural effusion, either alone or in combination. The first is increased pressure in subpleural capillaries that leads to a transudate fluid with low specific gravity (less than 1.016), as in patients with congestive heart failure and superior vena caval obstruction. Another cause is decreased oncotic pressure with fluid leak resulting from hypoalbuminemia, as seen in patients with nephrosis and cirrhosis of the liver. Anatomic disease of the pleura associated with infection, neoplasms, and vasculitis is the third mechanism. The fourth mechanism is an increased intrapleural negative pressure, as noted in patients with moderate atelectasis resulting from bronchial obstruction. Pleural effusion results from an imbalance between production and normal drainage mechanisms. With the main channels of lymphatic drainage in the parietal and mediastinal pleura, most of the lymphatic fluid drains to the right lymphatic duct and the remainder to the thoracic duct. Respiratory excursions and venous pressure are important mechanisms in promoting lymphatic drainage.

Protein content analysis is more helpful than specific gravity determination in distinguishing transudate from exudate when the transudate contains less than 3 grams of protein per 100 ml. An exudate is a fluid, generally associated with infections, tumor, or pulmonary infarction, that has a protein content greater than 3 grams per 100 ml. and often clots on withdrawal. Effusions may be grossly hemorrhagic or blood-tinged (serosanguinous). Milky-appearing fluid with a specific gravity greater than 1.020, a protein content of 3 to 4 grams per 100 ml., and a fat content of more than 1 gram per 100 ml. may be due to obstruction of major lymphatic channels and is called chylous effusion. When pleural fluid is grossly purulent, empyema is present.

Transudates are most often caused by congestive heart failure, ascites, nephrotic syndrome, or other conditions with low serum albumin and water retention. Exudates are generally caused by infection or tumor. Hemorrhagic effusions are associated with tumor or pulmonary infarction. Traumatic effusions are also hemorrhagic. Tuberculous effusions may be hemorrhagic, but the vast majority are serous. Pancreatitis also causes hemorrhagic effusion, most often either on the left or bilateral. Bilateral serous pleural effusion is usually due to congestive heart failure, ascites, or nephrotic syndrome and is uncommon in patients with tumor or tuberculosis.

Diagnosis

Transudates have less than 3 grams of protein per 100 ml., but occasionally reabsorption of water leads to an increase in protein content when the effusion has been present for many days. A transudate will appear yellow and translucent, while an exudate may appear cloudy and opalescent.

The presence of more than 5000 leukocytes per cu. mm. with predominant polymorphonuclear leukocytes suggests a bacterial infection. However, this does not rule out tuberculosis, although lymphocyte predominance is more characteristic of tuberculous effusion.

When serial thoracentesis reveals a daily increase in leukocytes and the appearance of cloudy effusion fluid, empyema is likely and thoracotomy tube drainage is indicated before the effusion becomes grossly purulent. The appearance of eosinophils in the effusion is nonspecific and not suggestive of tuberculosis. In pancreatitis, pleural fluid amylase levels may be very high, often several thousand units. An elevated lactic dehydrogenase (LDH) may be found in patients with effusion from metastatic neoplasm. The presence of basophilic mesothelial cells rules out tuberculosis.

The pleural fluid glucose value, when measured simultaneously with blood glucose, is slightly lower than the blood glucose when the cause is an active bacterial infection. Extremely low pleural fluid glucose levels of 5 to 10 mg. per 100 ml. are typical of rheumatoid arthritis. Cholesterol effusions suggest the presence of an old hemorrhagic effusion with a breakdown of blood. Lupus erythematosus (L.E.) preps may be done on pleural fluid when pleural disease is evident in patients with systemic lupus erythematosus.

Thoracentesis is performed with the patient in the sitting position after the fluid has been localized by percussion and chest x-ray. The skin of the puncture area is thoroughly cleansed and infiltrated with lidocaine (Xylocaine). The aspiration needle is advanced over the superior margin of a rib to avoid the intercostal vessels and nerves. The fluid is collected in sterile containers and cultured for common bacteria, tuberculosis organisms, and fungi. Cytologic studies may be done when malignancy is suspected.

A pleural biopsy using the Abrams' needle has a significant yield (70 to 80 per cent) in diagnosing patients with suspected malignancy or tuberculosis and should be performed in conjunction with the pleural fluid aspiration. The withdrawal of more than 1500 ml. of pleural fluid should be avoided to prevent complications such as vascular collapse and pulmonary edema following the thoracentesis.

Follow-up studies of asymptomatic patients under the age of 40 who have serofibrinous effusions and who have a positive intermediate tuberculin skin test reveal active tuberculosis in up to 70 per cent. Twenty-five per cent have typical pleuritic pain. Since these effusions clear spontaneously in 2 to 4 months, spontaneous clearing does not rule out tuberculosis. Culture of pleural fluid is diagnostic for tuberculosis in only 5 per cent of patients.

Failure to adequately remove empyemic fluid or hemorrhagic effusion may lead to a thick, permanently scarred pleura, restricting the lung by entrapment and impairing lung function. An organized empyema requires surgical resection, which should be carried out as early as 1 to 2 months after its formation to avoid restrictive disease.

PULMONARY THROMBOEMBOLISM

Pulmonary thromboembolism is caused by the passage of a fresh or organized thrombus from the systemic venous system, usually from the leg or pelvic veins through the right heart, impacting and occluding one or more pulmonary arteries. In about 5 per cent or less of these patients, infarction of distal lung tissue will result. Pulmonary infarction is more common with underlying pulmonary or cardiovascular disease and with larger emboli. Pulmonary embolism is a leading cause of sudden death and the leading cause of death and disability in the hospitalized patient. The vast majority of embolic episodes are minor, are undiagnosed, and may even occur commonly in the general population (being cleared rapidly by normal lytic mechanisms). It is estimated that 500,000 nonfatal episodes occur each year in the United States and that more than 100,000 deaths annually are due to pulmonary embolism. Evidence of pulmonary thromboembolism is found in 24 per cent of general hospital autopsies and 60 per cent of autopsies on patients with heart failure. Embolic episodes are common after surgery, trauma, or prolonged immobilization and in the elderly.

Pathogenesis

The factors predisposing to thromboembolism are (1) hypercoagulability of blood, (2) venous stasis, and (3) vascular endothelial damage. Hypercoagulable states may be caused by platelet disorders, increased thrombin or fibrinogen, polycythemia or dehydration that increases blood viscosity, sickle cell disease, stress, endotoxic shock, and dysproteinemias. Venous stasis is often caused by varicose veins; immobilization by bed rest; surgical anesthesia using muscle relaxants, which eliminate muscle tone that supports the venous flow; myocardial infarction associated with poor cardiac output and prolonged bed rest; casting of leg fractures; mitral stenosis; congestive heart failure from any cause, especially in conjunction with atrial fibrillation; pregnancy; hypotension; and cramped posture during long trips by automobile, bus, or plane. Vascular damage is a cause of turbulent blood flow and exposure of platelets to adenosine diphosphate (ADP), which promotes platelet aggregation that initiates thrombus formation. Other conditions associated with thromboembolism are obesity, diabetes mellitus, the postpartum state, burns and contusions, pelvic inflammatory disease, carcinoma, and the use of tight leg bands and birth control pills.

Clinical Manifestations and Diagnosis

Massive pulmonary embolism with occlusion of more than 60 per cent of the pulmonary arterial tree is associated with sudden death or with shock, cyanosis, and tachypnea leading to rapid death, apparently caused by a critical reduction in venous return to the left heart and inadequate cardiac output. More often, the embolism occludes segmental arterial branches; emboli are multiple and often bilateral and cause the sudden onset of lateralized pleuritic pain (usually basilar) and dyspnea. Hours later, hemoptysis, cough, and low-grade fever appear, and a transient wheeze may be noted. Symptoms may recur hours or days apart because of recurring emboli. In 95 per cent of the patients, infarction will not occur, as the clots are lysed and cleared. In these patients, symptoms clear in hours to days, with the result that many episodes go undiagnosed.

Dyspnea occurs in more than 90 per cent of the patients, cough in 75 per cent, pleuritic pain in greater than 50 per cent, and hemoptysis in from 30 to 60 per cent in different series. Fever occurs in most patients and infarctions are visible by x-ray. Patients manifest hyperpnea, anxiety, diaphoresis, cyanosis, and chest splinting because of the pain. Less than half have evidence of phlebitis initially. A friction rub may by heard along with tachycardia and wheezing because of the widespread release of bronchoconstrictors by platelets. Focal rales that are usually at the lung bases and a loud pulmonic component of S_2 with frequent wide splitting of the second sound may be present. There may be a right ventricular heave and an S_3 gallop rhythm.

Arterial blood gas analysis reveals hypoxemia, often severe, with an oxygen tension (PO_2) below 70 mm. Hg in the majority of patients, which responds poorly to supplemental oxygen administration. There is usually hyperventilation with hypocapnia and alkalosis. Acidosis as a terminal event or lactic acidosis induced by hypoxemia may occur. The release of vasoactive amines causes marked shunting of blood with resultant hypoxemia, and vascular occlusion leads to a large dead space and broad arterial-alveolar carbon dioxide tension difference characteristic of pulmonary embolism and other vascular lung disorders. The triad of increased serum lactic dehydrogenase (LDH), increased serum bilirubin, and normal serum glutamic-oxaloacetic transaminase (SGOT) levels has proved of little diagnostic value.

The electrocardiogram helps establish a diagnosis in only 15 per cent of the patients, revealing sinus tachycardia, atrial arrhythmias, right heart strain, acute right axis shift, clockwise rotation of the QRS axis, and occasionally a very helpful (for diagnosis) sudden onset of right bundle branch block, which is generally seen only with severe embolism. Small emboli rarely produce infarction and cause few clinical or laboratory findings.

The chest film is very helpful, often because the findings are so minimal in even a very ill patient. Common findings are an elevated hemidiaphragm, pleural effusion (usually small), a peripheral density along the pleural border, and platelike atelectasis. These findings are usually seen at the lung bases, more often on the right, with involvement of the upper lobes in a minority of patients. There may be local ischemic lung fields and large main pulmonary arteries, but these are difficult to appreciate.

A lung scan using ^{131}I albumin macroaggregates is helpful in revealing focal perfusion defects if pneumonia, bullae, or asthma can be ruled out. The scan is most helpful when the clinical picture is compatible with pulmonary thromboembolism and the chest film appears normal.

A more definitive but technically demanding study is pulmonary angiography with selective dye injection. Such a study may reveal complete occlusion of vessels at segmental and subsegmental levels, a "pruned tree" appearance to the general arterial tree, retention of dye locally in the venous phase, webs (partial filling defects in arteries representing partly lysed thrombi), or focal ischemic areas. Both scans and angiography are best done within hours of onset and become less diagnostic with each passing day.

Treatment

The treatment of pulmonary thromboembolism consists of intravenous heparin, 10,000 units immediately and 5000 to 10,000 units every 4 to 6 hours intravenously in a bolus or by continuous infusion after obtaining a baseline coagulation time or partial thromboplastin time (PTT). The dose is modified as needed to maintain these clotting times at prolonged levels of 2 to 3 times normal, and levels are obtained prior to administering a dose of heparin and periodically thereafter to monitor the response. Heparin is continued for 7 to 10 days, and then anticoagulation is maintained in patients with severe illness by using sodium warfarin orally, which is regulated by the prothrombin time values. Recurrence of thromboembolism is prevented by continued anticoagulation, but not beyond 2 months after the acute event. However, if the patient has a continuing, highly predisposing disease process, long-term anticoagulation may be indicated.

Prophylaxis is rational in high risk patients, and its use in surgical patients has proven value. Heparin in doses of 5000 units is given every 8 hours, beginning several hours before surgery and continuing in the postoperative period until mobilization is initiated. Vena caval plication can be lifesaving in patients with recurrent large emboli in whom the risk is high that further embolization may be lethal. Thrombolytic therapy is experimental and useful mainly in patients with massive emboli, as it accelerates clot lysis but is accompanied by a high incidence of bleeding. Thromboembolectomy is rarely useful and probably of no value once a patient has survived the first hour after onset. Virtually all patients surviving the first hour will recover, as 75 per cent of deaths occur during this time period. Probably 20 to 30 per cent of patients are left with residual symptomatic pulmonary function loss, especially those with pre-existing pulmonary or vascular disease.

PNEUMOTHORAX

Pneumothorax is the presence of free air in the pleural space with lung collapse caused by an air leak through the visceral pleura. It may be spontaneous, associated with established lung disease, or secondary to acute trauma. Pneumothorax may occur at any age, including the newborn period. Eighty-five per cent occur in males and 75 per cent occur in persons less than 40 years of age, with the highest frequency being in the 15 to 40 age group. Most patients are physically inactive at onset, and the onset is acute, with dyspnea and chest pain localized to the side of the pneumothorax.

The most common type is called *spontaneous pneumothorax* and is caused by rupture of an intrapleural bleb that results from a defect in the subpleural alveoli. These blebs are almost always at the lung apices and are frequently bilateral, although not visualized by x-ray. Some patients experience the acute symptoms while stretching or bathing or engaging in some other activity with the arms elevated above the head. However, it is also common for symptoms to begin during sleep. The majority of patients have a benign course, and both pain and dyspnea have improved by the time the patient is first seen. There may be transient cyanosis and respiratory distress, which gradually improves over a period of minutes to hours.

Many patients have a *closed pneumothorax*, which implies that the leak through the ruptured subpleural bleb has sealed and that the air will be slowly absorbed with re-expansion of the lung, often with no more treatment indicated than rest and serial x-ray examinations to document re-expansion. A pneumothorax with less than 30 per cent lung collapse, as estimated by x-ray, may commonly be treated expectantly.

Pneumothorax associated with a disease is most commonly seen in both children and adults with acute bronchial asthma. It is also seen in association with vigorous positive pressure resuscitation efforts, as administered to infants with respiratory distress syndrome. Pneumothorax also occurs in patients with bronchiectasis, emphysema, and diffuse pulmonary fibrosis, especially with honeycomb lung and especially during intercurrent infections. Coughing is probably not the causative mechanism, as a cough normally generates pressures greater than 160 cm. of water without inducing a pleural leak. Air leak likely occurs during repeated deep inspiration, causing a stretch of pleural structures at the apex or in diseased segments. Distended alveoli may rupture, with air escaping along the perivascular sheath toward the peripheral pleural surface or medially toward the mediastinum. In these instances, the pleural leak may occur at either site. Additional causes are subpleural abscess, as seen in staphylococcal infections; esophageal trauma during endoscopy; or pneumothorax occurring in association with malignancy.

Traumatic pneumothorax commonly occurs with open chest wounds, such as gunshot or stab wounds, as well as secondary to fractured ribs lacerating the visceral pleura, and often is associated with a hemothorax.

A closed pneumothorax is usually treated expectantly. There is gradual reabsorption of air and re-expansion of the lung, generally over a 1 to 4 week period, depending upon the volume of air and extent of collapse. The term *open pneumothorax* is used when patients develop a bronchopleural fistula with a persistent communication between the pleural space and airways characterized by failure of the lung to re-expand and generally when there is a more extensive collapse (exceeding 20 per cent). This type is seen in patients with pulmonary tuberculosis, tumors of the lung, pulmonary infarction with or without secondary infection, chronic pulmonary fibrosis in which large tears may occur and the lung is slow to re-expand, emphysema, or after thoracic surgery. The open pneumothorax not only is persistent but also tends to be associated with greater collapse and more respiratory distress. It therefore warrants the use of a thoracotomy tube with immediate removal of the pleural space air either by underwater seal or by the application of negative pressure.

The presence of a large pleural tear and the development of a ball-valve phenomenon, with air entering the pleural space on inspiration and failing to escape on expiration, will rapidly lead to a true medical emergency. This is because the development of a tension pneumothorax, associated with generation of pressures in the diseased pleural space that are greater than atmospheric pressure; the concomitant collapse of the affected lung; and a shift of the mediastinum with vascular structures to the opposite side result in venous obstruction and a compromised cardiovascular system. These patients rapidly develop tachypnea with tachycardia, respiratory distress, cyanosis, and vascular collapse. Shock may occur as the result of impaired venous return and inadequate cardiac output.

The immediate withdrawal of air is life-saving, causing a dramatic return of cardiac output and improvement in the patient's clinical status. As a tension pneumothorax most commonly occurs within minutes to hours of the initial pneumothorax, but has also been observed even days after onset, all patients with pneumothorax should be evaluated and observed carefully for the development of this potentially lethal complication.

Diagnosis

The diagnosis is suggested by unilateral or substernal chest pain associated with transient respiratory distress and at times by pallor with diaphoresis and a gradual improvement over a period of minutes to hours. The examination may reveal hyperresonance, with a decrease in excursion, an increased volume of the involved hemothorax, and diminished breath sounds. Findings may be altered by the associated presence of blood or fluid on the collapsed side with dullness at the lung base. Patients experience hypoxemia initially, but often oxygen tensions improve rapidly, as there is an adjustment in ventilation and perfusion matching.

The chest x-ray is crucial in localizing and quantitating the collapse. Demonstration of a small pneumothorax is improved by obtaining full inspiration and full expiration films. The pleural line is more evident in the latter because of the increased contrast between the air and the more dense collapsed lung. The lung may be seen to be locally adherent to the pleural surface because of superficial adhesions or may collapse freely away from the chest wall.

Treatment

As 85 per cent of pneumothoraces are spontaneous and tend to close early, and half reveal less than 30 per cent collapse, many patients are treated expectantly, as long as there is no evidence of cardiovascular impairment or respiratory distress. It is important to observe such patients carefully during the initial 48 hours, but those with few symptoms at rest ordinarily do not develop tension pneumothorax. In a patient with a larger collapse or in someone with symptoms and in any patient with underlying lung disease, it is essential that a thoracotomy tube be used to remove free air and re-expand the involved lung as soon as possible, thereby improving lung function and probably improving the rate at which the pleural leak seals. Large thoracotomy tubes are indicated, and when the lung is scarred, stiff, or grossly abnormal, negative pressure application may improve re-expansion and recovery by irritating the pleura and promoting pleural adhesions.

The first episode of pneumothorax may be treated either by simple tube drainage or expectantly. The recurrence rate is approximately 25 per cent with conservative therapy and 15 per cent with tube thoracotomy treatment. More aggressive management further reduces the recurrence rate but should only be applied when recurrence has occurred. Once a second pneumothorax has occurred, especially if on the same side, further recurrences are very likely and pleurodesis by the instillation of an irritant solution to induce scarring of the pleura is indicated. Open pleurodesis is a relatively benign and probably more successful treatment. It is occasionally combined with a wedge resection of the abnormal lung tissue considered to be the source for the air leak, the latter procedure being almost universally successful. Aggressive management of recurrent pneumothorax is indicated, as acute bilateral pneumothorax may occur and threaten the patient's life. Bilateral pneumothorax is uncommon, but not rare.

ATELECTASIS

The term *atelectasis* implies incomplete expansion of the lung tissue, with alveoli in the affected area either partly collapsed or airless. *Microatelectasis* describes reduction in lung volume from incompletely expanded alveoli, commonly due to diffuse lung injury or prolonged underventilation. This disorder is not visible as a density on x-ray but is associated with ventilation/perfusion abnormalities and hypoxemia.

Atelectasis usually occurs at lung bases at which impairment of diaphragmatic motion by ascites, abdominal distention, abdominal binders, or splinting secondary to chest pain may lead to the progressive collapse of alveolar units, as they may become unstable at low volumes and may close entirely. Focal atelectasis, visible by x-ray, is a characteristic of pulmonary infarction. The release of bronchoconstrictors and alterations in circulation cause subsegmental collapse sufficient to be visualized as a platelike or discoid density on the chest x-ray. Obstruction of a bronchus will cause absorption of alveolar gas if pulmonary capillary perfusion continues, and there will be slow reduction in alveolar volume with variable collapse of lung units that produces clinical atelectasis. Atelectasis is more likely to occur in the young infant who lacks collateral ventilation, but in adults bronchiolar obstruction may not lead to collapse of distal units because of collateral ventilation from adjacent alveoli and bronchioles via alveolar pores.

As atelectasis is usually associated with airway secretions or with an obstructing lesion, re-expansion of an atelectatic lung depends on clearing the airways and re-establishing ventilation. Even then, complete re-expansion may require hours to days because of alterations in surface tension and the need to clear alveolar secretions.

Diagnosis

Symptomatic atelectasis is often a postoperative phenomenon, especially after general anesthesia and abdominal surgery, and is associated with low-grade fever and paroxysmal cough and with notable dyspnea in some patients. Physical examination reveals local dullness and diminished breath sounds when the atelectasis is more than segmental. There may be signs of a pleural effusion that results from the negative pleural pressure created by atelectasis involving multiple segments or a lobe. The chest film reveals a wedge-shaped density with its apex toward the hilum or simply shows platelike densities that are commonly horizontal and just above the diaphragms. There will be shifting of the minor fissure, the mediastinum, or the cardiac border toward the atelectatic area when the volume is sufficient, but in the vast majority of patients this is absent. The distribution of atelectasis from all causes is illustrated in Figure 45–3.

The sputum reveals no specific abnormalities except when the atelectasis is caused by an acute bronchitis with purulent secretions plugging larger bronchi. Arterial blood gas analysis generally reveals hypoxemia and a low or normal arterial carbon dioxide tension. In cigarette smokers, especially over the age of 40, bronchogenic carcinoma should be ruled out as a cause of obstruction with atelectasis, and bronchoscopy is indicated.

Treatment

Treatment consists of the use of bronchodilators, both systemically and in aerosol form, with adequate hydration and repeated hyperinflation of the lung by coughing. Postural drainage may be effective, and the patient should be positioned to drain the specific anatomic site of atelectasis. If re-expansion does not occur or if recurring atelectasis is noted in one area, an obstructing bronchial foreign body or an adenoma should be suspected. These are generally associated with focal rales and coarse musical rhonchi best described as "squeaks." Preoperative bronchial toilet in the patient with chronic bronchitis or bronchial asthma will help prevent postoperative atelectasis. It is likely that persistent atelectasis does lead to focal bronchopneumonia.

LUNG ABSCESS

A lung abscess is a collection of pus within a dense wall in the lung parenchyma that is produced by a suppurative (necrotizing)

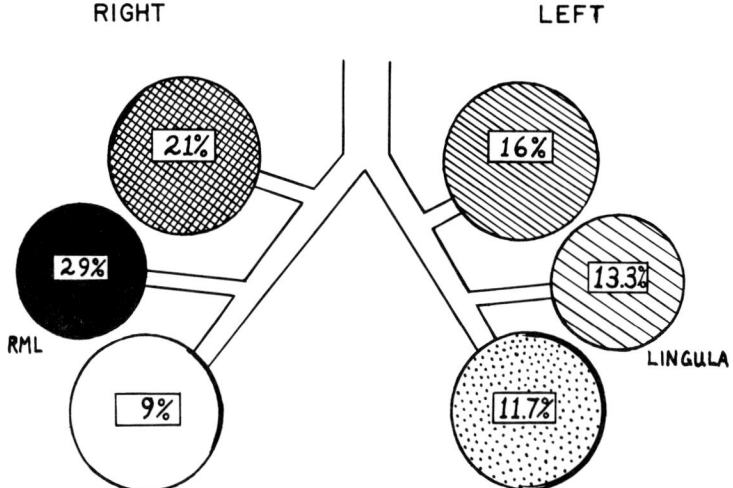

Figure 45–3.   *Diagram illustrating distribution of atelectasis from all causes.*

bacterial or fungal infection. The tuberculosis cavity may be considered an indolent abscess. The abscess arises from a local necrotizing bacterial pneumonia. It eventually communicates with a bronchus to drain a putrid, often blood-tinged material containing lung tissue and pus, leaving a cavity with an air-fluid level and a dense cavity wall. The cavity is usually round to oval in shape, and is surrounded by a rim of pneumonic infiltrate.

A single lung abscess commonly is associated with aspiration of foreign material or with bronchial obstruction, or both. It is seen in patients in the postanesthetic state or in those with alcoholic stupor, cerebrovascular accidents with coma, depressed gag reflex, or impaired deglutition; in patients with oversedation (especially in the elderly and the debilitated); and following oral or sinus surgery or dental procedures from extraction to simple fillings. Lung abscess is strongly associated with patients who have seizures. As aspiration is a common causative mechanism, the abscess is often in dependent segments of the lung. Therefore, it commonly occurs in the superior segment of a lower lobe in the supine patient, in the upper lobes in patients lying flat but not supine during aspiration, and in dependent zones if aspiration occurs while sitting. An anterior location suggests an associated primary lung tumor.

When lung abscesses are caused by bronchogenic tumors with bronchial obstruc-

tion, their location varies, and they must be differentiated from tumors undergoing avascular central necrosis. Tumors have a more lobulated inner border, thick walls, and sharply demarcated outer margins. Evidence of suppuration is absent, and cavitation most frequently occurs in a squamous cell (epidermoid) carcinoma. An infected pulmonary infarction may lead to abscess formation and is commonly located in the posterior lung bases. An abscess may result from bacterial pneumonia, especially in the debilitated or immunosuppressed patient. In these patients, it usually follows pneumonia caused by a staphylococcal infection, *Klebsiella pneumonia* (Friedländer's bacillus), *Pseudomonas aeruginosa, Escherichia coli,* hemolytic streptococcus, or virulent strains of pneumococcus. The majority of putrid lung abscesses are associated with gingival infection or dental caries with a mixed infection caused by saprophytic mouth flora, usually anaerobic streptococci, *Bacteroides,* fusospirochetes, and *Actinomyces.* They are virtually all penicillin-sensitive.

Multiple lung abscesses are characteristically nonputrid and may result from hematogenous dissemination of staphylococcal or gram-negative bacterial infection elsewhere in the body or from septic emboli commonly seen in patients who have septic pelvic thrombophlebitis. Septic emboli may lead to subpleural abscesses that may rupture and produce a pneumothorax.

Clinical Manifestations and Diagnosis

The onset may be characterized by fever and chills, pleuritic pain, cough, and sweats and days later by purulent sputum with hemoptysis. Fully 30 per cent of patients present with an indolent course and uncertain onset, even in the absence of a history of seizures or alcoholism. When first seen on x-ray films, the abscess may be sharply demarcated, with surrounding pneumonic infiltrate having partly cleared and a sharp air-fluid level in the abscess demonstrating open drainage (Fig. 45–4).

Putrid sputum suggests a mixed infection caused by anaerobes and fusospirochetes. Hemoptysis is present at some time in 70 per cent of the patients, and the leukocytosis is usually greater than 15,000 per cu. mm., with a preponderance of immature forms. The course may be modified by partial antibiotic treatment. A peripheral abscess may rupture into the pleural space, producing empyema or a bronchopleural fistula. The insidious type of onset is associated with malaise, weight loss, and sweats, and the patient may not appear acutely ill. Finger clubbing occasionally is seen and improves with treatment.

Pneumonitis with infected pre-existing bullae has a benign prognosis and must be differentiated from a lung abscess. A history of coma, seizures, aspiration, alcoholism, and oral or dental surgery is very suggestive of lung abscess. The chest film is usually typical, confirming the diagnosis, helping to locate the lesion, and thereby guiding proper postural drainage treatment. The rupture of an abscess into a bronchus with the sudden appearance of purulent sputum is associated with slow defervescence and improvement in constitutional symptoms.

Treatment

In the absence of a single known causative organism, such as following staphylococcal or *Klebsiella* pneumonia, a mixed infection should be suspected, and sputum

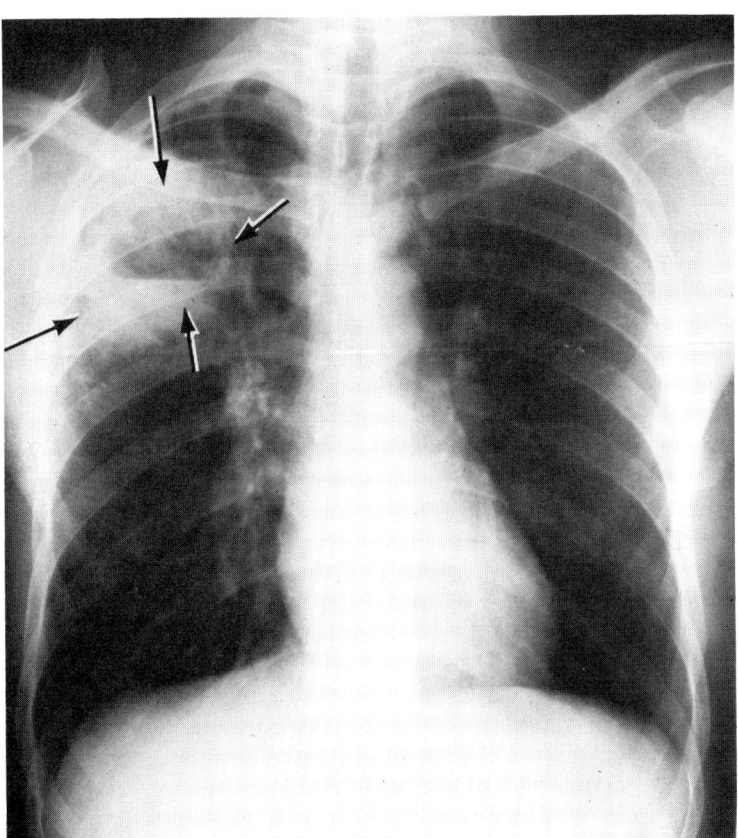

Figure 45–4. *This young alcoholic male has a right upper lobe abscess caused by mixed organisms, probably secondary to aspiration. Note the round outline, the air–fluid level, and the surrounding pneumonic infiltrate. The calcified right hilar nodes are caused by tuberculosis.*

or transtracheal aspirate should be cultured for aerobic and anaerobic organisms. Initial treatment is 10 to 12 million units of penicillin G intravenously, given daily in divided doses, usually every 6 hours, with reduced doses and oral therapy reserved for the period following a good clinical response. Therapy should continue for a minimum of 6 weeks to prevent relapse, and during this period, there should be good clearing of the infiltrate and fading of the abscess wall shadow. Often treatment has to be extended, with the administration of oral penicillin in smaller doses, such as 250 to 500 mg. every 6 hours for additional weeks, because improvement is delayed, although radiographic improvement may be seen to continue for 6 weeks or more. Treatment should not be aborted because the patients feel well. They commonly do not feel ill by the second or third week of treatment, and treatment acceptance may be a problem. In patients allergic to penicillin, cephalothin, 8 to 12 grams intravenously daily, may be used or erythromycin, 2 to 4 grams daily, may be given to less toxic patients.

A failure of the abscess to drain or a refilling of the abscess cavity with disappearance of the air-fluid level, especially when associated with fever spikes and increased toxicity, should be treated by aggressive drainage efforts, such as by bronchial brushing under fluoroscopic guidance or preferably by bronchoscopy, using the flexible fiberoptic technique to provide re-establishment of bronchial drainage. Early bronchoscopy can rule out an obstructing foreign body or tumor and should be considered if drainage is not clearly established early in the course of the illness.

The use of aerosol bronchodilators and inhaled mist followed by postural drainage with percussion or vibration of the chest in appropriate segmental drainage positions, carried out two to four times a day, can be invaluable in improving drainage and accelerating recovery. The management of an abscess caused by a single organism differs only in the need to select an appropriate antibiotic and evaluate sensitivities.

Complications

Surgical resection is rarely needed. If the abscess fails to clear after 6 weeks of treatment, it is considered a chronic abscess. However, medical management may be continued for up to 3 months to obtain cure, as long as radiographic improvement continues. The mortality is less than 10 per cent, and generally deaths are limited to the immunosuppressed patient, the patient with chronic debilitating disease, alcoholics, and patients with chronic obstructive pulmonary disease or cerebrovascular accidents. Attention should be given to improving oral and dental hygiene in order to prevent recurrent episodes. Recurrence is seen primarily in alcoholics.

CHRONIC BRONCHITIS

Chronic bronchitis is one of the most underdiagnosed respiratory conditions despite its marked prevalence, especially in urban areas and especially in males. It may occur in 15 to 20 per cent of adults and represents a leading cause of disability in patients with respiratory diseases. This disorder can be defined as a chronic cough with sputum production that occurs daily for at least 3 successive months in 2 successive years. This is the minimum requirement for diagnosis when bronchiectasis, tuberculosis, or lung tumor has been ruled out as a possible cause. In the absence of these diseases, chronic bronchitis can be suspected from the history alone. Significant cough and sputum often masquerade as throat clearing, and it is common for the patient to deny both cough and sputum production, despite their presence while the patient is being examined.

Chronic bronchitis is associated with hypertrophy of both the epithelial goblet cells and the bronchial mucous glands, the latter contributing 80 to 90 per cent of the secretions. Mucociliary drainage is ordinarily impaired, requiring the patient to pool secretions, thereby stimulating cough and expectoration when these secretions irritate major bronchi. The majority of patients are responding to irritants, of which the most significant is cigarette smoke. This is undoubtedly the most important determinant, followed by the common but less significant ambient air pollution and industrial exposure to dusts and fumes.

The significance of ambient air pollution is demonstrated by the finding of increased symptoms in both nonsmokers and heavy smokers in communities with dirty air as compared with fewer symptoms in comparable persons living in communities with clean air. This suggests that the effects of ambient air pollution have been underestimated. In general, the severity of symptoms correlates roughly with the amount of smoking by those who inhale cigarette smoke, and the severity increases steadily with the years of exposure. It is likely that patients who develop emphysema as a consequence of cigarette smoke exposure will have symptoms only of chronic bronchitis for many years, during which time the characteristic lung parenchymal damage of emphysema progresses insidiously. Although the mechanisms are not clear, it does appear that some patients have an increased sensitivity to cigarette smoke or pollutants and develop chronic bronchitis at lower exposure levels. Repeated cigarette smoke exposure may lead to bronchoconstriction that probably originates in the upper bronchial tree, with smoke serving as an irritant as well as a toxin to ciliary function.

Sulfur dioxide in high-humidity air is capable of inducing a low-grade chronic bronchitis. It is likely that other pollutants share this potential, and chronic bronchitis may occur in city dwellers who do not smoke cigarettes or have direct exposure to industrial pollutants.

The role of infection in the development of chronic bronchitis is controversial, although in patients with chronic bronchitis, the distal airways are usually colonized by organisms capable of producing active infection. These organisms are not found in the airways of normal persons. The predominant organisms are *Hemophilus influenzae* and *Diplococcus pneumoniae*. It is also established that cigarette smoke impairs lung macrophage function and the clearance of micro-organisms from the lung. Cyclic broad-spectrum antibiotic therapy with tetracycline or ampicillin during the winter months significantly reduces the infectious complications in these patients. Further, unlike the normal person with an acute respiratory infection, these patients often require the addition of broad-spectrum antibiotics to their regimen to guarantee prompt recovery because of their predisposition to significant superinfection with *H. influenzae* and *D. pneumoniae*.

Clinical Manifestations and Diagnosis

The disease ordinarily begins after many years of cigarette smoking in patients who have had a periodic cigarette cough with minimum sputum production occurring most often in the morning. With continued smoking, symptoms may increase following upper respiratory infections, and the patient presents for treatment. Early during the course of the disease, the patient denies dyspnea but may note periodic blood streaking of sputum associated with paroxysmal cough, especially during periods of intercurrent infections. Some experience wheezing, especially during acute infections. As the disease progresses, prolonged productive cough paroxysms in the morning are characteristic. The patient may begin to note dyspnea with moderate exertion, as well as increasing fatigue, but may show no respiratory distress at rest despite the prevalence of hypoxemia. The heavier smokers may demonstrate plethora because of an increase in red cell mass and bouts of cyanosis of the mucous membranes and nailbeds that occur primarily with intercurrent infections.

Examination of the chest reveals some increase in the anteroposterior diameter, and the diaphragm motion may be 1 inch or less, as measured by percussion during full inspiration and expiration. Medium rhonchi at the lung bases with an occasional wheeze are frequently heard. There may be an increase in chest resonance, depending partly on the degree to which it is associated with developing emphysema (a common accompaniment). Cor pulmonale often occurs in patients in the fifth or sixth decade, especially in the heavier smokers, and is characterized by jugular venous distention with enlargement or tenderness of the liver. Usually, peripheral edema is a first manifestation of cor pulmonale, occurring in the evening and clearing by morning. Patients commonly continue to deny dyspnea even at this stage, although the history reveals a marked reduction in their general activity.

The electrocardiogram often reveals a vertical P-axis consistent with chronic obstructive pulmonary disease and evidence of right ventricular hypertrophy. The chest radiograph usually shows some distention, with hyperinflation of lung fields and low diaphragms with diminished excursion. There may be an increase in perivascular and peribronchial markings, commonly referred to as "dirty lung," and one should look for fibrotic cuffing of the bronchial wall, as shown by prominent ring shadows in the hilar area.

Pulmonary function tests commonly reveal a decreased forced vital capacity associated with an increased residual volume. Flow studies, including measurement of the FEV_1, reveal significant expiratory airway obstruction, usually with a 5 to 10 per cent improvement after administration of an aerosol bronchodilator. Intrapulmonary gas distribution is ordinarily normal unless there is associated emphysema with parenchymal damage. Arterial blood gas analysis reveals hypoxemia, with a PaO_2 commonly in the range of 45 to 65 mm. Hg. Carbon dioxide retention occurs early in the disease, often while the patient is still actively employed and ambulating.

Hypercapnia in the absence of visible respiratory distress is a characteristic of advanced chronic bronchitis. Because of the plethora associated with cyanosis and the lack of cachexia that is characteristic of emphysema, patients have been called "blue-bloaters." The chronic bronchitis syndrome is clearly associated with concomitant degrees of pulmonary emphysema in the majority of patients, leading to the adoption of the term "chronic obstructive pulmonary disease."

Treatment

Treatment consists of the discontinuation of smoking and pollutant exposures and the use of hydration and expectorants, with antibiotics added in the presence of purulent sputum. Both systemic and aerosol bronchodilators are helpful prior to physiotherapy, which includes postural drainage to improve mobilization of secretions. Bronchodilators are used without regard for the presence or absence of clinical wheezing. Early stages of bronchitis are probably entirely reversible with the discontinuation of smoking and pollutant exposure, but the prognosis changes with the appearance of cor pulmonale. Episodes of acute right heart failure associated with intercurrent infections often respond well to oxygen supplementation, the oxygen supplementation being given to prevent reflex pulmonary hypertension, which will occur if the arterial PO_2 is less than 50 mm. Hg. Digitalis, diuretics, and vigorous bronchial toilet are also indicated. Some reversibility remains even in the late stages of disease, thus warranting vigorous efforts at treatment.

PULMONARY EMPHYSEMA

Emphysema, derived from the Greek word meaning overinflation, is defined by the American Thoracic Society as "an anatomical alteration of the lung characterized by an abnormal enlargement of the air spaces distal to the terminal, non-respiratory bronchiole, accompanied by destructive changes of the alveolar walls." The airway obstruction that is invariably present and the vascular bed loss accompanying the destruction of alveolar walls are not included in the definition. Emphysema develops insidiously, usually accompanied by chronic bronchitis, and is probably the result of parenchymal destruction produced by constituents of cigarette smoke on which are superimposed air pollutants such as ozone, nitrogen dioxide, sulfur dioxide, and particulates and at times by industrial fumes and chemicals. The poor airway clearance produced by chronic bronchitis may impair removal of toxic substances, with resultant slow destruction of alveoli and small airways in a nonhomogeneous manner. Serum alpha$_1$-antitrypsin deficiency is associated with a familial form of emphysema that occurs at an early age, often without cigarette exposure; has an equal sex incidence; and is limited to the white population.

The terms "compensatory emphysema," following lung resection, and "senile emphysema," represented by a less elastic and more inflated but functional lung that occurs with age, are misnomers with no clinical significance. A focal emphysema occurs in patients with tuberculosis, coal workers' pneumoconiosis, and bronchiectasis.

Pathologic classifications are of little clinical use. Emphysema may be associated with bullae representing focal areas of destroyed lung that are bounded by fibrous strands but that lack an epithelial lining. They are visible on the chest radiograph as holes in the lung resembling cysts. Such bullae represent focal emphysematous destruction, may enlarge slowly because of retraction of surrounding healthy tissue, and are often multiple. Basilar bullae are characteristic of the familial emphysema seen in young nonsmokers. In general, early emphysema is not diagnosed by x-ray studies or clinical evaluations, although sophisticated pulmonary function tests may detect changes in small airways.

The important functional and structural alterations in patients having chronic obstructive pulmonary disease (COPD) with predominant emphysema are as follows:

1. Parenchymal damage predominates, in contrast to chronic bronchitis in which large airway involvement is primary.

2. Disruption of alveolar architecture takes place, with loss of alveoli and membrane surface for gas diffusion.

3. Destruction of capillary beds and precapillary vessels and even obliteration of small arteries occur.

4. Loss of elastic recoil impairs passive exhalation.

5. Bronchioles collapse on expiration because of loss of adjacent supportive structures, including alveoli and septa.

6. Large airway collapse occurs in the expiration phase, involving the bronchi and even the trachea.

7. Distention occurs, and the depressed diaphragms are rendered functionless, leading to poor ventilation of the basilar zones.

8. Prominent ventilation of upper lung zones takes place, using accessory respiratory muscles with their inefficient mechanics.

9. Distention of the lungs and chest cage produces an increased respiratory drive and induces dyspnea out of proportion to hypoxemia and other physiologic derangement.

10. High energy costs of breathing are due to both upper zone breathing and use of energy in the ordinarily passive expiratory phase.

11. Uneven gas distribution occurs in lung units, with ventilation-perfusion mismatch leading to shunting and a large dead space.

Clinical Manifestations and Diagnosis

The clinical diagnosis may be difficult to make. In the mild form, slight distention of the chest with low position of the diaphragms but fair diaphragmatic motion (more than 1 inch excursion), increased resonance, slightly distant breath sounds, and a prolonged expiratory phase with an inspiration/expiration time ratio greater than 1:2 may be the early clues. In the moderate to severe form, the diagnosis can frequently be made by clinical evaluation. The following findings are suggestive of

pulmonary emphysema: (1) a prolonged expiratory phase with pursed lips and a forced exhalation time of longer than 4 seconds; (2) the use of accessory respiratory muscles, causing the patient to lean forward with the shoulders elevated; (3) flat diaphragms with less than 1 inch of excursion between peak inspiration and expiration; (4) en bloc movement of the chest cage, with little anteroposterior or lateral expansion and increased anteroposterior diameter; (5) hyper-resonant lung fields; (6) distant breath sounds, especially at bases, but louder in the upper zones, and diminished heart sounds best heard at the xiphoid; (7) loss of subcutaneous fat and muscle mass; and (8) chronic anxiety.

Dyspnea occurs only with exertion in the early form, but this progresses to dyspnea during functions of daily living such as shaving, dressing, and bathing, and finally to dyspnea at rest. The frequency of the advanced form of pulmonary emphysema increases with age and is most prevalent in the sixth to eighth decade, with bronchitis generally peaking 10 years earlier. The incidence is highest in males, probably reaching 10 to 15 per cent in elderly males, with rates in females rising in relation to cigarette smoking. Cough and sputum are minimal in those with little accompanying bronchitis. Cyanosis and clubbing do not occur in the absence of complications. These patients have an increased incidence of peptic ulcer disease, recurrent pulmonary embolism, and peripheral neuropathy caused by stress, sedentary existence, and respiratory posturing respectively.

Pulmonary Function Tests. With moderate to advanced disease, there is a reduced vital capacity, usually caused by airway collapse when carrying out a forced vital capacity (FVC) maneuver with a large residual volume encroaching on the FVC. The functional residual capacity (resting respiratory position at end expiration) is enlarged because of the increased residual volume, and the residual volume/total lung capacity (RV/TLC) ratio is increased to 40 to 60 per cent from a normal of 25 to 35 per cent. The TLC is also enlarged, reflecting the hyperinflated chest cage and flat diaphragms. Associated pulmonary fibrosis may reduce the observed volumes. The FEV_1 is below 70 per cent of the FVC, and often below 50 per cent, because of severe expiratory obstruction with no improvement following use of

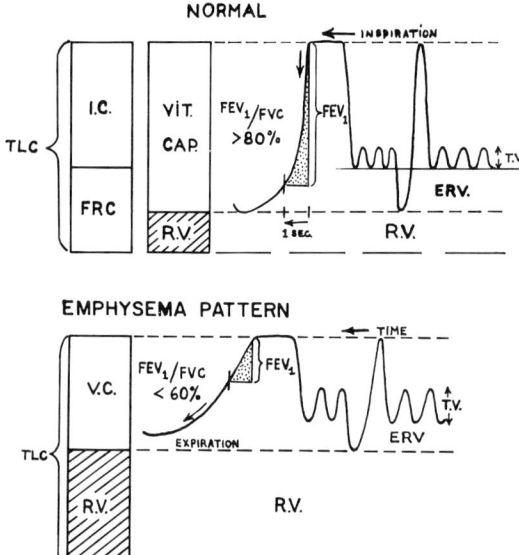

Figure 45–5. *Spirometric tracing and lung volume diagram of normal person (top) and a patient with emphysema (bottom). Note the expiratory obstruction and distention evidenced by a large residual volume.*

an isoproterenol (Isuprel) aerosol. This suggests a mechanism of airway collapse rather than of bronchoconstriction or blocking by secretions. The resting minute ventilation is increased to 10 to 12 liters or more per minute, and the tidal volume increases from a normal of 450 to 500 ml. to 700 to 1000 ml. per breath. This allows airways to remain patent and permits the patient to exchange air despite the severe obstruction that forces slow respiratory rates and a prolonged expiratory time of 3 to 6 seconds at rest. Large tidal volumes compensate for an increased dead space produced by the ventilated but underperfused or nonperfused lung (Fig. 45–5).

The maximum voluntary ventilation (MVV) is below 50 liters per minute, and gas distribution in the lung is abnormal because of disrupted alveolar architecture. Abnormal gas mixing is measured by demonstrating delayed nitrogen washout from the lung while the patient breathes pure oxygen. There is mild to moderate hypoxemia, with the arterial PO_2 usually ranging from 60 to 75 mm. Hg and the PCO_2 being 40 mm. Hg. Hypercapnia is a late event precipitated by infections or by other complications. The diffusion capacity is moderately to severely reduced because of alveolar-capillary surface loss. Lung compliance is increased, but elastic recoil is decreased, so passive emptying of the lung is impaired.

Because of inefficient muscle use, loss of diaphragm function, and the distended chest cage, the work of breathing is very high, resulting in fatigue and subjective dyspnea.

Respiratory failure is associated with a sudden increase in hypoxemia and the appearance of hypercapnia and cor pulmonale. It is usually caused by acute respiratory infections such as bronchitis or pneumonia. Other causes are inspissated secretions caused by dehydration or sedation, atelectasis, left heart failure, or pneumothorax. The administration of high concentrations of oxygen may reduce the hypoxic respiratory drive, leading to further underventilation and hypercapnia.

Radiologic Manifestations. Moderate or severe disease is associated with hyperradiolucent, overinflated lungs; flat, low diaphragms; lucency below the cardiac apex with a small vertical heart; and an increased retrosternal air space. An increased anteroposterior diameter is common but can be due to kyphosis or familial habitus rather than to emphysema. The most valid findings are loss of pulmonary vascular markings and an angle between the body of the sternum and the anterior half of the diaphragm of 90° or greater when viewed on the lateral chest film. The presence of bullae helps confirm the diagnosis, but these may also be seen in otherwise normal lungs. Obesity may obscure the hyperlucency, and congestive heart failure may obscure the loss of vascular markings. Diagnosis should never be made on the basis of a chest x-ray alone (Fig. 45–6).

Electrocardiogram. The electrocardiogram reveals a vertical P-axis "P" pulmonale is present if P waves in leads II, III, and AVF exceed 2.5 mm. in height. There is low QRS voltage and a vertical electrical axis. Right ventricular hypertrophy (RVH) is seen primarily in complicated cases and in terminal stages.

Treatment

Patients must stop further lung destruction by discontinuing smoking and avoiding air pollutants. They are told that lung regeneration does not occur. Patients are treated with hydration and expectorants and when bronchospasm or bronchitis is present, with oral and aerosol bronchodilators delivered by a compressor and nebulizer or

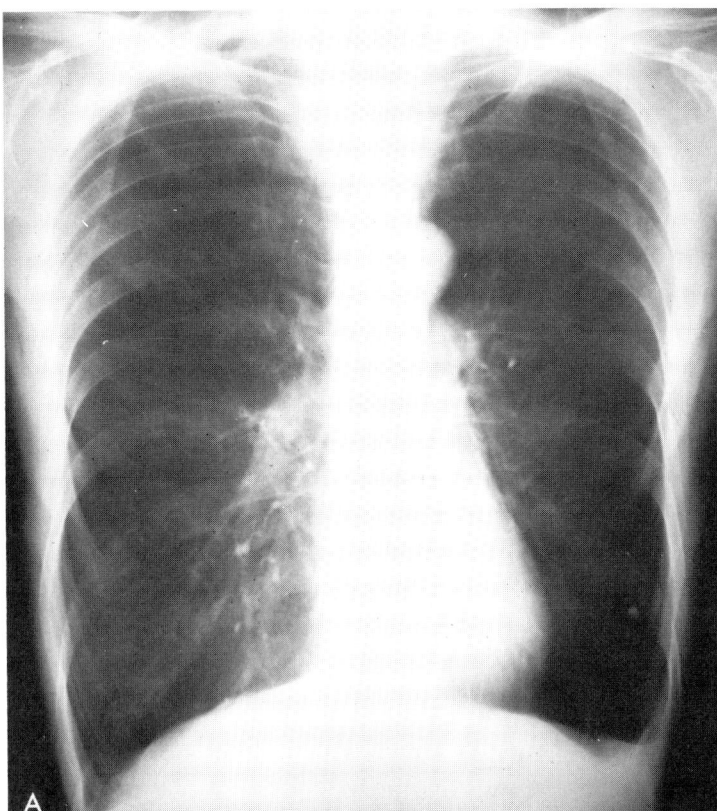

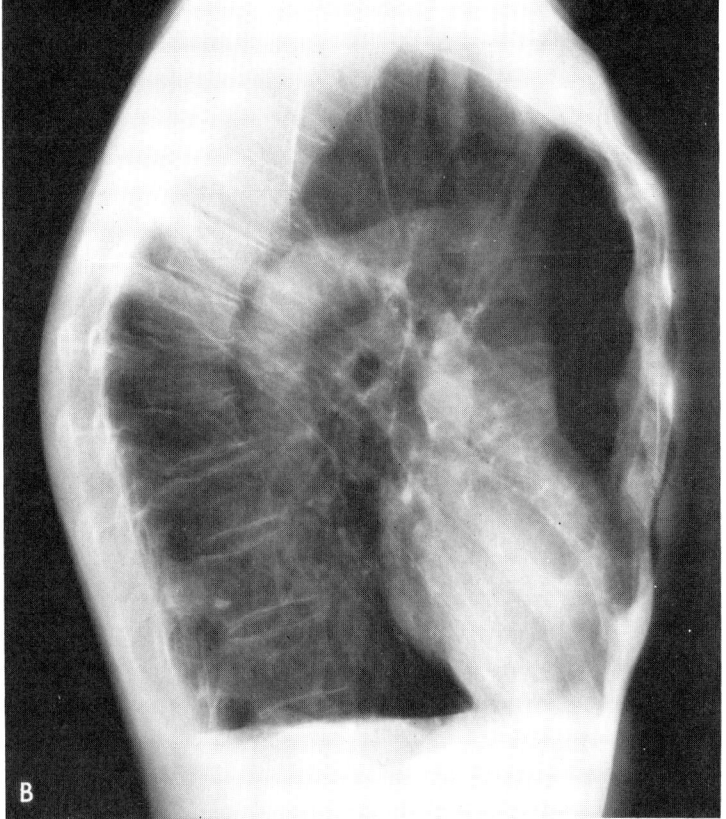

Figure 45-6. *Radiologic manifestations of emphysema.*

A.   This PA chest film with hyperlucent lung fields; low, flat diaphragms; separation of heart shadow and left hemidiaphragm; and loss of normal lung vascular markings is characteristic of emphysema.

B.   This lateral view of the chest in COPD reveals the findings of emphysema, with an increased AP diameter, a large retrosternal air space, a prominent right ventricle approaching the sternum, and an anterior diaphragm–sternal angle over 90 degrees.

by intermittent positive pressure breathing (IPPB). Intractable bronchospasm is a cause of respiratory failure and often responds to administration of a daily or alternate day low-dose steroid, such as prednisone, 5 to 10 mg. daily. Steroid therapy is often withheld too long from those patients with bronchospasm; its use may prolong life by years and reduce periods of hospitalization and episodes of acute respiratory failure.

Low flow oxygen (1 to 2 liters per minute) is used for patients with chronic cor pulmonale and acute exacerbations, which ordinarily occur when the arterial PO_2 falls below 50 mm. Hg. Breathing exercises with diaphragm retraining, when possible, and training in relaxation techniques as well as in efficient muscular use may improve functional status and quality of survival. Many patients benefit from vigorous and early treatment of respiratory infections with broad-spectrum antibiotics. Ampicillin or tetracycline is utilized early, as secretions are often colonized by *Hemophilus influenzae* and pneumococcus.

The risk of pulmonary embolism and lung cancer is increased in patients with emphysema. Death is usually due to respiratory failure and is precipitated by a respiratory infection leading to cor pulmonale and right heart failure. Cor pulmonale is manifested by cardiomegaly, an enlarged right ventricle, peripheral edema, a tender and enlarged liver, and jugular venous distention. Temporary respiratory support by intubation and mechanical ventilation may permit survival from the episode and prolong life. Permanent tracheostomies are rarely indicated.

CARCINOMA OF THE LUNG

Carcinoma of the lung is now the most common lethal malignancy afflicting males, with an increased incidence that parallels the incidence of cigarette smoking. In 1930, it was a rare tumor. In 1973, approximately 72,000 people died of bronchogenic carcinoma in the United States. The ratio of males to females with carcinoma of the lung is 7:1, but the rate in females is accelerating, matching their increasing total cigarette consumption. Lung cancer is ten times more common in cigarette smokers than in nonsmokers, and the rate parallels the amount of cigarette consumption. At high risk are males with chronic obstructive

pulmonary disease (COPD), with the peak incidence being between the ages of 50 and 60 years. The median age is now down to 59 years. More than 3 per cent of the patients are under the age of 40, and occurrence is not rare in the fourth decade.

The correlation between cigarette smoking and bronchogenic carcinoma is strongest with squamous cell carcinoma, as well as with both small cell and large cell undifferentiated types, but is minimal with adenocarcinoma and nonexistent with alveolar-bronchiolar carcinoma. Pipe smoking and cigar smoking are not implicated, probably because the smoke is rarely inhaled in a large volume. Cigarette smoke contains many volatile compounds, including 3,4-benzpyrene, a potent carcinogen that has been demonstrated to produce airway tumors. Ambient air pollutants may be one cause of increased cancer rates in urban centers. Exposure to several industrial agents increases the risk of lung cancer. Asbestos is the cocarcinogen best studied, with data revealing that bronchogenic carcinoma is eight times more frequent in smokers exposed to asbestos in contrast to smokers with no asbestos exposure and is 50 times more frequent in smokers with asbestos exposure than in the nonsmoking general population without such exposure. Cigarette smoking is crucial to this relationship, as bronchogenic carcinoma is rare in asbestos workers who do not smoke. Tumors originating in scars are usually associated with tuberculosis or a honeycomb lung.

Classification

Hilar tumors involving the main stem bronchus are most common, with 25 per cent originating in segmental bronchi and 10 per cent more peripherally. The hilar node extension often is larger than the primary tumor and is mistaken for the primary site.

The histologic classification and frequency of bronchogenic carcinoma are outlined in Table 45–5.

Squamous cell carcinoma reveals intercellular bridging, keratinization, and pearl formation when well differentiated, but may be classified as epidermoid carcinoma by pathologists when these findings are less evident. The tumors are central in location, spread to regional nodes, and 14 per cent cavitate to resemble an abscess. Hypercal-

TABLE 45-5. HISTOLOGIC CLASSIFICATION AND FREQUENCY OF BRONCHOGENIC CARCINOMA

Histologic Type	Frequency
Squamous cell carcinoma (epidermoid)	30%
Adenocarcinoma	26%
Small cell undifferentiated (oat cell)	23%
Large cell undifferentiated	16%
Mixed cell types	5%

location and metastasizes early with 75 to 90 per cent spread to bone marrow by the time of diagnosis (Fig. 45–8). Surgical procedures are not indicated except in extremely rare instances. The mean survival of patients is 6 to 9 months. About 50 per cent of small cell carcinomas produce endocrinopathies, such as Cushing's syndrome or inappropriate secretion of antidiuretic hormone.

Large cell undifferentiated tumors manifest early spread by lymphatic and hematogenous routes. There is evidence that the better differentiated tumors may be present for years before diagnosis. Growth appears to be slower in the very elderly patient.

Clinical Manifestations

About 10 per cent of patients are asymptomatic when neoplasm is first diagnosed. Symptoms relate to cell type, stage, and location of tumor. Unilateral pain occurs in 20 per cent of patients initially and up to 60

cemia occurs in 25 per cent of the patients, and significant bleeding is common. This type has the best prognosis for 5 year survival.

Adenocarcinoma is only slightly more common in men than in women. It is not related to smoking and is usually a peripheral lesion with silent, early hematogenous metastases. The primary tumor often is very large before being diagnosed because the metastases are silent (Fig. 45–7).

Small cell (oat cell) cancer is central in

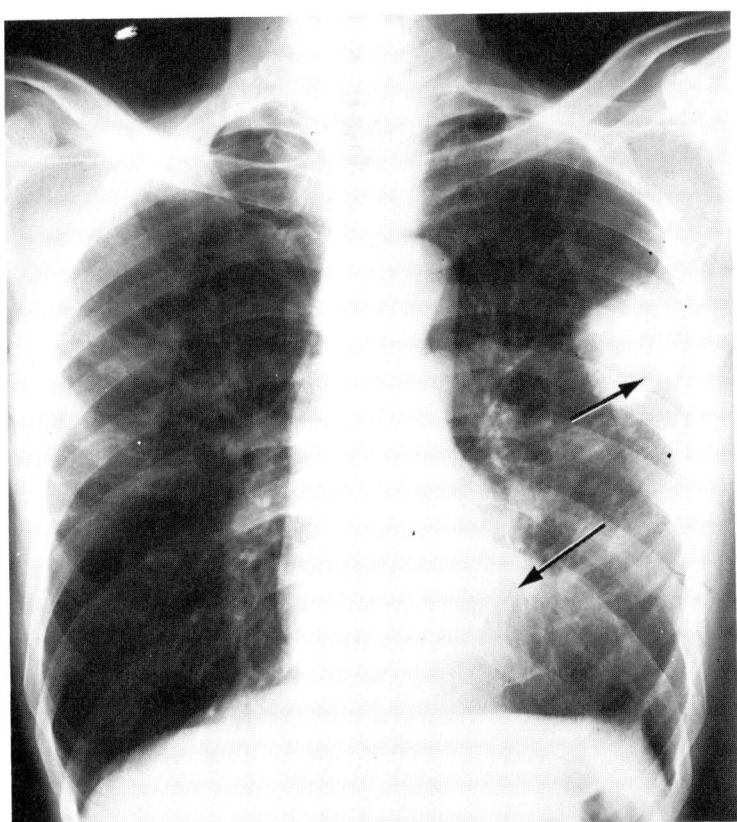

Figure 45–7. The well-circumscribed, dense, lobulated lesion in the left upper lung field is typical of a lung tumor, and the large, peripheral mass is a common presentation for adenocarcinoma. Note that the left heart border is obscured by a contiguous infiltrate in the lingular segments of the left upper lobe.

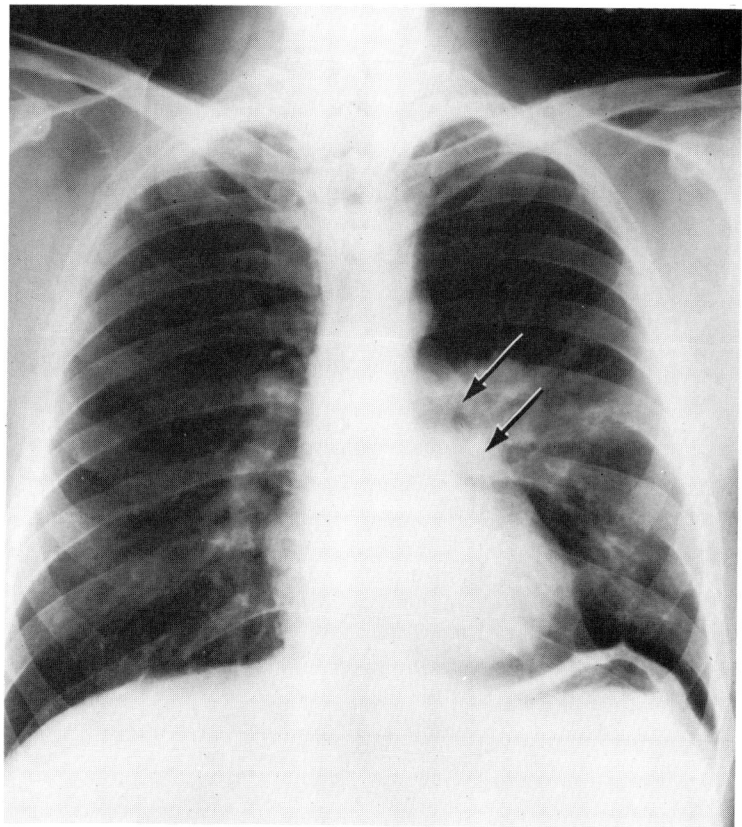

Figure 45-8. *This chest film reveals a central mass with contiguous node involvement at the left hilum. Biopsy revealed oat cell carcinoma, and the bone marrow was positive by both aspiration and biopsy. The patient was 31 years of age and had smoked three packages of cigarettes a day for 19 years.*

per cent at later stages. Cough is present in 75 per cent of patients and dyspnea in 15 per cent initially, the true nature of which may be obscured by coexistent airway disease. Asthenia or weight loss occurs in 33 per cent of patients initially and 25 per cent have hemoptysis in the early course, if intermittent blood streaking of sputum is noted. Massive hemoptysis is not common. A smoldering, postobstructive pneumonia is present in 5 per cent of patients. Other symptoms are wheeze, hoarseness, night sweats, and anorexia. Finger clubbing occurs in 12 per cent of the patients, and if of recent onset in an adult, is usually a sign of lung cancer. Hypertrophic osteoarthropathy may occur and may even precede the radiographic findings of tumor. Neuromuscular symptoms may occur in up to 15 per cent of patients, with over half presenting as a myasthenia. Migratory thrombophlebitis is associated with 1 to 2 per cent of lung cancers and also may precede the radiographic appearance of the tumor.

Staging

The staging of lung cancer involves many diagnostic studies and usually requires biopsy via bronchoscopy or mediastinoscopy or by scalene node biopsy. Cytologic examination of pleural fluid and pleural needle biopsy are also performed. Stage 0 refers to a persistently positive sputum cytology with negative x-ray and is associated with a 60 per cent 5 year survival, and Stage I to a local tumor without symptoms with a 34 per cent 5 year survival. Survival decreases with regional node involvement (Stage II) and with more malignant cell types. Diagnostic studies are directed toward proving the presence of bronchogenic carcinoma, demonstrating the histologic type, and delineating involvement of regional and mediastinal nodes, as well as ruling out distant metastases that will affect the therapeutic approach. The following data regarding frequency of occurrence of distant metastases have been obtained from postmortem examinations: regional nodes (90 to 96 per cent), brain (45 per cent), distant nodes (45 per cent—epidermoid [30 per cent], small cell type [60 per cent]), liver (45 per cent), adrenal (34 per cent), and bone (30 per cent, especially vertebrae). New staging techniques should improve selection of patients for surgery.

Diagnosis

Diagnostic techniques include cytologic examination of spontaneous sputum or sputum induced by aerosol inhalation, bronchoscopy with biopsy or bronchial brush exfoliation of tumor cells, pleural biopsy when effusion is present, and mediastinoscopy to evaluate the pattern of hilar and mediastinal node involvement and to assist in staging, while providing tissue diagnosis in some patients. Peripheral tumors may be accessible to aspiration needle biopsy. Laminography may reveal multiple tumors that suggest secondary tumor rather than primary bronchogenic carcinoma or may demonstrate hilar and mediastinal metastases in primary lung tumor.

Treatment

The single most productive treatment is surgery without preoperative radiation and occasional selective postoperative radiation. Lobectomy is adequate in 50 per cent of the patients, and pneumonectomy is needed for more extensive or central tumors that compromise the main stem bronchi. Stage I carcinoma with local disease has a 5 year survival of 16 per cent, Stage II with regional spread has a 4 per cent 5 year survival, and Stage III with distant spread has a 1 per cent 5 year survival. The tumor is inoperable when there are metastases to the brain, bone, liver, or the contralateral lung. Other signs of inoperability are vocal cord paralysis, positive scalene node biopsy, involvement within 2 cm. of the carina, and pleural effusion with positive cytologic findings. All small cell carcinomas are also inoperable. Relative contraindications to surgical resection are chest wall involvement, simple pleural effusion with negative cytologic findings, phrenic nerve paralysis, poor pulmonary function, or associated cardiovascular disease. After clinical study, only 25 per cent of tumors are found to be resectable and after mediastinoscopy, only 15 per cent.

Radiation therapy and chemotherapy are primarily palliative in unresectable tumors. Radiation of painful bone metastases is often beneficial in relieving pain.

Prognosis

Oat cell cancer is rapidly fatal. The overall 5 year survival for bronchogenic carcinoma is 5 to 10 per cent and is best for those with squamous cell carcinoma. For the latter group, the 5 year survival is 18 per cent in asymptomatic patients, 12 per cent in those with only primary tumor symptoms, and 6 per cent in patients with systemic symptoms when first seen. None survive 5 years who have demonstrated metastatic symptoms. An annual chest x-ray in a predisposed population has not improved prognosis, but cytologic examination of sputum in the high risk group may increase the early recognition of tumors that are surgically resectable. Discontinuing exposure to cigarettes and other carcinogens has demonstrated benefits in the prevention of bronchogenic carcinoma. The ex-smoker has a reduced risk of this form of cancer that improves from the time of initial withdrawal and is maximum after 5 to 7 years following the discontinuation of cigarette smoking.

METASTATIC LUNG TUMORS

The lung is a common site of metastatic tumor, most commonly by lymphangitic spread from breast cancer or from multiple tumor masses from the colon, kidney, prostate, bone, and thyroid. The tumors are usually multiple with a distribution consistent with hematogenous spread. They do not produce clubbing of the fingers, are often silent, and require a search for the primary site. When a hemorrhagic pleural effusion is present, concurrent liver metastases are common.

PULMONARY TUBERCULOSIS

Pulmonary tuberculosis still has a high rate of occurrence in lower socioeconomic groups, in urban centers, and in blacks, American Indians, and Spanish-speaking populations, with a higher rate among alcoholics. It is two to three times more frequent in males than in females, with the greatest difference in the high prevalence groups. The annual death rate from tuberculosis was greater than 500 deaths per 100,000 population in the year 1800, or 20 per cent of all deaths, thus establishing it as the leading killer at that time. Death rates fell as a result of improved public health measures, housing, and nutrition, even before the chemotherapy era. Further reductions occurred with the availability of chemotherapy, leading to current death rates of less than 5 per 100,000 population annually.

The new active case rate is now 15 cases per 100,000 population annually, with lower rates in rural areas. Primary infection rates in high school students have fallen from 50 per cent in 1930 to less than 1 per cent in suburban and rural areas presently. Large cities have case rates of 30 to 40 per 100,000 population annually, and small cities with less than 100,000 population have rates of 10 per 100,000. Alcoholics have rates 55 times the national average and tend to reactivate their disease. Treatment failures occur almost exclusively in alcoholic males.

Pathogenesis

Mycobacterium tuberculosis organisms are spread by coughs and sneezes. These droplets are inhaled and deposited in the susceptible recipient's lung, and numerous organisms are probably needed to establish a local infection in most persons. The organisms are killed by macrophages in a previously infected person, but in a susceptible host, they multiply locally and enter the lymphatics to reach regional nodes. They disseminate via the blood stream to the liver, spleen, other nodes, kidney, bones, and serosal surfaces. However, in the majority of persons, these foci are benign and heal with scar formation.

The primary lung infection leads to the formation of a granuloma that may undergo central caseation necrosis, usually followed by healing with fibrous encapsulation. There is commonly calcification of the primary lung and regional node focus occurring within 2 or more years after the initial infection. The primary lung focus is usually in the mid or lower lung fields. It is ordinarily small and difficult to visualize until there is calcification of both the primary focus and the regional node that produces the "primary complex" or Ghon complex visible on the chest film. Throughout this period of early primary infection, the patient is generally asymptomatic but develops a positive skin test and will have a persistent tuberculin-positive status and a stable healed primary complex throughout life.

The primary infection may follow several courses. *Progressive primary tuberculosis* represents a slowly progressing tuberculous pneumonia with fever, sweats, cough, weight loss, and malaise that are present without remission for weeks. Another course is that of *disseminated tuberculosis*, which is a lymphohematogenous dissemination of tuberculosis with the formation of caseous granulomas in multiple organ systems, including the central nervous system, bone, kidney, liver, and spleen. These patients are severely ill, having fever and weight loss and often the symptoms of tuberculous meningitis. The chest film may reveal diffuse 1 to 2 mm. densities representing local tubercles, a pattern termed *miliary tuberculosis*.

In a third course, there is a tuberculous effusion caused by rupture of a subpleural or pleural caseous tubercle into the pleural space, generally occurring within 1 year following primary infection. This form of tuberculosis is a self-limited disease characterized by unilateral serofibrinous effusion, mild pleuritic symptoms, or low-grade fever, but with no impressive parenchymal lesion. It clears spontaneously. Despite this deceptive spontaneous remission, this form is followed by overt pulmonary tuberculosis in 60 to 70 per cent of the patients in whom the majority of overt disorders will occur within 2 years of the pleuritis. Culture of the pleural fluid will be positive in up to 30 per cent of these patients and pleural biopsy will be positive in 80 per cent.

About 90 per cent of clinical pulmonary tuberculosis is *reactivation disease*, presenting as an indolent tuberculous parenchymal infiltrate that occurs within several years of the primary infection and is often confused with the much less common reinfection. Reactivation disease is increasing in the elderly and the debilitated. It now occurs 40 to 60 years after the primary infection, with an increasing frequency.

Delayed Hypersensitivity and the Tuberculin Skin Test

After the primary infection, a cell-mediated immunity develops, and antibodies denoting an infection by *Mycobacterium tuberculosis* can be demonstrated in the patient's skin within 2 to 8 weeks after the primary infection. A specific purified protein derivative (PPD) is extracted from tubercle bacilli by heat and precipitation, and the antigen material is currently being rendered stable by the addition of Tween-80. There are three strengths of PPD antigen, the most useful being equivalent to 5 tuberculin units (TU) of old tuberculin antigen and called 5-TU PPD or the "intermediate" skin test. First and second strength antigens contain 1-TU and 250-TU respectively. The first strength is used when strong reactions are anticipated, as in suspected active disease.

The standard skin test is performed by injecting 0.1 ml. of PPD intermediate antigen (5-TU) intradermally via a 26 gauge needle on the volar surface of the forearm and reading the induration that results at 48 to 72 hours. Induration is measured as the maximum dimension transversely across the forearm. The surrounding erythema has no diagnostic value and should be ignored. The induration is carefully palpated, measured with a millimeter ruler, and recorded in millimeters of induration. An indication of the interpretation as positive or negative is also entered in the patient's permanent record. The United States Public Health Service guidelines for interpreting the tuberculin skin test are: less than 5 mm. induration—negative, 5 to 9 mm. induration—doubtful, and 10 mm. or more induration—positive.

In practice, many regard induration over 7 mm. as a likely positive and treat their patients accordingly. Patients generally "convert" skin tests to positive within 3 to 8 weeks of primary infection. False-negative skin tests may occur in elderly, cachectic patients; patients with active sarcoid; those on immunosuppressive drugs, including moderate doses of steroids; and those with febrile illness during skin testing. A common cause of false-negative reactions is poor skin test technique that results from too little solution being injected or using a solution that has lost potency. Repeating the PPD intermediate skin test and obtaining two definitive negatives in the average individual rules out active tuberculosis with 98 per cent confidence. Knowing that a general population is largely negative by skin test makes the skin test very valuable in detecting new infections.

Clinical Reactivation Tuberculosis

This is the ordinary tuberculosis seen in the majority of patients who present with minimal symptoms, usually a low-grade fever, especially occurring in afternoons and evenings, with associated night sweats, malaise, some weakness, and easy fatigability, followed by weight loss in the later stages. It must be realized that in the early stages there may be no symptoms, and the disease is only detected by observation of abnormalities in a routine chest x-ray. Cough is usually, but not invariably, present, along with modest sputum volume. In later stages, local chest pain with hemoptysis occurs. The physical examination generally reveals only focal rales, most often in the upper lung zones, especially the right upper lobe, and routinely induced by coughing.

The chest radiograph is vital in the diagnosis and usually reveals a necrotizing pneumonia with cavitation, pleuritis, linear fibrosis, and nodular densities coupled with old calcified lesions. This is the telescoped picture of an indolent necrotizing pneumonia. There are multiple tuberculous granulomas with caseation necrosis in the centers. The caseous material extrudes and spreads organisms to the adjacent lung as well as to other segments and lobes by bronchogenic spread. The tuberculous organisms grow best in areas of high oxygen tension; therefore, areas of predilection are the upper lobes, especially the right upper lobe, and most often the apical and posterior segments (Fig. 45–9). Involvement of the anterior segment alone is unusual in tuberculosis. A second common site is the superior segment of the lower lobes, again more common on the right. Bilateral disease is not unusual, and large cavities may form, although they may be visible only on a laminogram of the chest.

Diagnosis

The diagnosis of tuberculosis is usually made by the physician's having a high index of suspicion, by evidence of a positive skin test in 95 per cent of patients with active tuberculosis, by detecting acid-fast organisms on a Ziehl-Neelsen or Kinyoun stain of sputum, or by culture of sputum. At least three sputum specimens should be smeared and cultured for tuberculosis, preferably using the early morning sputum. Twenty-

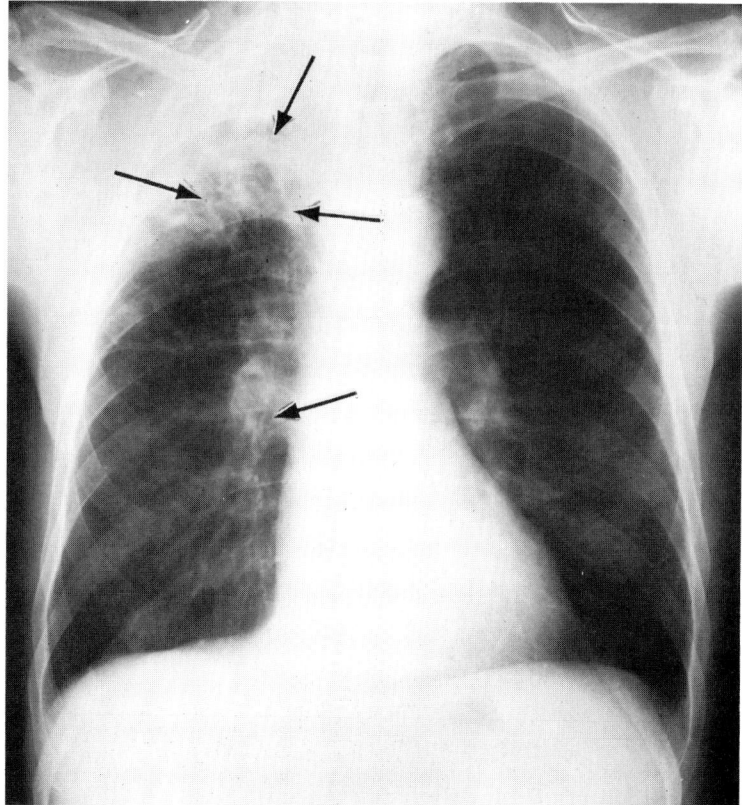

Figure 45-9. *This chest x-ray reveals the right upper lobe apical and posterior segment disease typical of adult, reactivation tuberculosis. Note the lucent areas characteristic of a necrotizing infection, suggesting early cavity formation.*

four hour collection of sputum is not necessary with the present bacteriologic techniques. Sputum can be induced by aerosol inhalation when there is little cough or sputum production. Bronchoscopy can aid in obtaining good specimens, and the bronchoscopic washings or the sputum obtained in the postbronchoscopic period is often positive. In miliary tuberculosis, the recovery of organisms is very difficult, and failure to demonstrate them does not rule out the diagnosis.

Treatment

Treatment of moderate or advanced disease should begin in the hospital. Criteria for treatment are symptoms of activity; a change in the chest x-ray that indicates increasing disease, even in the absence of symptoms; and a positive sputum smear or culture. Activity should be suspected in a patient with old established but untreated disease in whom a change is seen by x-ray. Medication can be given before all cultures

are obtained, and in the case of early or moderate disease, sputum can usually be rendered noninfectious after 2 to 3 weeks from the beginning of treatment. This thus allows patients to return to their homes without risk to household members. Alcoholic patients and those with large cavities (greater than 4 cm.) or those with many organisms in the sputum smear should receive several months of hospital treatment to ensure control before discharge.

The average patient requires treatment with two drugs, the usual treatment regimen being isoniazid (INH) for 2 years and ethambutol or rifampin for the first 12 to 18 months. Isoniazid is bactericidal and is given in a dose of 300 mg. per day for adults either in divided doses or in one morning dose. In children the dose is 10 to 14 mg. per kg. per day, but should not exceed a total dose of 300 mg. daily. Peripheral neuropathy may occur, especially in the alcoholic patient, and responds to 25 to 50 mg. of pyridoxine daily with continuation of INH. Hepatitis may occur in patients receiving INH, usually in the early weeks of therapy, but unless the serum glutamic oxaloacetic transaminase (SGOT) rises above three times the baseline level or symptoms of hepatitis occur, the drug may be continued while monitoring enzyme levels. The incidence of INH hepatitis is 1 per cent in young patients and increases to 4 per cent in patients over the age of 35.

Ethambutol is the best second drug administered in combination with isoniazid. It is given orally in a single morning dose of 15 mg. per kg. per day and is supplied in 400 mg. and 100 mg. tablets (ethambutol is not recommended for children under 13 years of age, as its safety has not been established). Larger doses have caused optic nerve toxicity. Therefore, monthly visual acuity and color discrimination examinations are done in some clinics, but almost all toxicity reported was in patients who received the 25 mg. per kg. doses used in earlier years. The optic nerve toxicity reverses on discontinuation of the drug.

Rifampin is a new and very effective drug, although it should never be used alone because of the rapid development of resistance by tuberculosis organisms. This drug may cause liver toxicity and may augment the hepatotoxicity of INH. It is given orally in a single daily dose of 600 mg. per day in adults and 15 mg. per kg. per day in children. Rifampin is very useful in retreatment regimens and in patients with resistant disease.

At least 95 per cent of patients can and should be managed by the family physician. The very ill patient who needs multiple drugs requires more specialized knowledge and techniques, as well as drug sensitivity studies, and is best treated in the hospital. Surgery is limited to the management of patients having cavitary disease with drug resistance and tuberculous empyema, both now unusual. Most patients feel better after 1 to 3 weeks of chemotherapy, although fever may persist for 2 to 3 weeks while cough and systemic symptoms are clearing. A failure to respond suggests (1) failure to take the prescribed drugs, (2) the presence of resistant organisms (usually in an alcoholic), (3) and the possibility that the organisms are atypical mycobacteria, not *M. tuberculosis*. In the case of atypical mycobacterial infection, the chest film findings may resemble those of tuberculosis, but cultures will differentiate the organism from *M. tuberculosis*. Infections with atypical mycobacteria are not contagious.

After 2 years of adequate treatment and resolution of the disease, the patient may be considered cured rather than one in whom the process is simply arrested. Patients at special risk of reactivation tuberculosis include:

1. The recent tuberculin converter—3 per cent reactivate during the first year.

2. Household contacts, especially children.

3. Patients with pulmonary silicosis.

4. Patients with diabetes mellitus who are insulin-dependent and poorly controlled.

5. Postsubtotal gastrectomy patients.

6. Immunosuppressed patients with malignancy.

7. Patients on large doses of steroids for many months.

8. The debilitated and the elderly.

9. The alcoholic.

Patients with pulmonary silicosis, immunosuppressed patients, and patients on steroids who have a positive skin test are often maintained on INH permanently because of the risk of tuberculous reactivation.

Prophylactic treatment with INH, 300 mg. daily for 1 year, is recommended following the conversion of the skin test in a patient under 35 years of age and known to be PPD-negative previously. Treatment for 1 year has successfully reduced the incidence of reactivation tuberculosis in children and adults, as well as virtually eliminating lymphohematogenous tuberculosis in children. At special risk is the adolescent female, and INH treatment is strongly recommended on conversion of the skin test. The benefit must be weighed against the risk of treatment, as the incidence of INH hepatitis reaches 4 per cent by age 35. Therefore, prophylactic INH therapy after PPD conversion over the age of 35 is arbitrary and at the physician's discretion.

When a patient with tuberculosis is identified and treated, the physician must examine the skin test reactions of household contacts and obtain a chest film on those with a positive skin test. If active disease is found, a treatment regimen should be started, and the physician should work closely with local public health officials to maintain proper reporting and surveillance. Bacille Calmette Guérin (BCG) immunization is reserved for especially high risk groups, being used primarily in developing countries that have very high tuberculosis rates. It has been used in the United States in selected high risk groups, such as nurses and physicians. BCG immunization eliminates the PPD conversion as a diagnostic test. Tuberculosis is a medical disease and is the family physician's responsibility; it is not the responsibility of the Public Health Department, alone.

BRONCHIECTASIS

Bronchiectasis is a condition characterized by permanent dilatation with fusiform or saccular distortion of the bronchial tree, at times extending to the smaller bronchioles but usually involving predominantly the first eight subdivisions of the lobar bronchi. It is not related to chronic obstructive pulmonary disease, has been seen with decreasing frequency in recent decades, and involves both sexes equally. Many patients have the onset of symptoms in childhood, as bronchiectasis often follows pertussis or similar viral illness, although generally a prolonged bacterial infection is the cause. In some series there is a history of bronchitis or pneumonia in at least 40 per cent of the patients with childhood onset.

True congenital bronchiectasis is probably rare. The disease is almost entirely caused by necrotizing infection that is associated with irreversible bronchial damage and fibrosis with contraction of surrounding lung tissue. Airway obstruction from a foreign body or other mechanism may be a factor in some patients who have focal disease, as the obstruction intensifies the effects of the distal infection. Bronchi are irregularly dilated to a cystic or fusiform shape with the muscular small bronchi showing more dilatation, as they have less bronchial wall support. In general, the ciliated columnar epithelium is destroyed and is replaced by a squamous epithelium, and purulent secretions pool in these dilated blind sacs, implying complete destruction of peripheral lung units. Ordinarily, multiple bronchi are involved and are crowded together, with contracted, collapsed lung tissue intervening but with a marked reduction in the volume of the involved segment or lobes.

Although bronchiectasis in adults is never reversible, a condition termed *chronic bronchitis* or *cylindrical bronchiectasis* seen in children shortly after a bacterial infection may be reversible. It is characterized symptomatically by chronic cough and sputum production and anatomically by the loss of the normal tapering of the bronchial tree with segmental or lobar distribution. Reversibility of these lesions in adults has never been demonstrated, and the term cylindrical bronchiectasis is appropriate.

Bronchiectasis occurs more commonly in the lower lobes and lingula, with involvement of the right middle lobe being next in frequency. It may be multisegmental or lobar. Bilateral involvement is present in approximately 40 per cent of patients. The distribution of lesions generally corresponds well with the distribution of the necrotizing pneumonia responsible for this residual damage.

Postprimary tuberculosis in adults is an indolent necrotizing pneumonia that involves primarily the upper lobes, especially the apical and posterior segments. Consequently, bronchiectasis caused by tuberculosis is localized to the upper lobes. In this type, mucopurulent secretions may be minimal because of effective drainage when the patient is in the erect position. Bronchiectasis may be suspected only by noting the contracted lobar shadow on the chest x-ray film or upon bronchographic study.

Diagnosis

The clinical manifestations are predominantly those of cough and sputum production. The sputum has a purulent character, and the volume generally exceeds 50 ml. per day. The voluminous and malodorous purulent secretions noted in past decades are not as common now because of more effective treatment of the bacterial pneumonias. The extent of lung damage and the chronic infection are also better controlled by long-term treatment. Patients have daily cough and sputum production despite all measures, as the normal mucociliary mechanisms are permanently destroyed. It is therefore essential that the patients cough to raise the secretions, and although cough frequency and sputum volume may be markedly improved by treatment, it is unlikely that they will clear completely.

There is a high incidence of associated

sinusitis, and exacerbation of a sinus infection may aggravate symptoms of bronchiectasis. Patients may complain of dyspnea and easy fatigability. In addition, there may be weight loss and night sweats and an increase in cough and sputum volume associated with intercurrent infection. Acute superinfections commonly are heralded by the appearance of hemoptysis caused by the exuberant bronchopulmonary arterial collaterals that form in bronchiectasis. Patients may also complain of vague chest pain that is not always pleuritic and is commonly related to an increased local infection. Many patients develop secondary erythrocytosis with plethora, and finger clubbing is common.

Auscultation of the chest ordinarily reveals coarse, medium-pitched inspiratory rales in the areas overlying the bronchiectasis, and breath sounds have a bronchial or even a tubular quality. Variable rhonchi that change with deep breathing and coughing may be present.

The x-ray film reveals curvilinear lines with saccular lucencies in the segments or lobes involved and evident volume loss and extensive fibrosis. In the case of saccular bronchiectasis, it may be possible to visualize air-fluid levels if there are large, cystic, blind bronchial pouches. Peribronchial fibrotic streaks radiating from the hilum downward are common.

The localization of bronchiectasis should be carried out, although never during the immediate recovery phase of an acute infection, as the airways will temporarily be filled with secretions and the changes noted may be reversible. Bronchograms are best performed after a minimum of 6 weeks following an acute infection, and an iodine-containing radiopaque medium should be used to demonstrate the fusiform or saccular changes and localize them to appropriate segments or lobes. This is an important procedure because it establishes the diagnosis and additionally because focal, segmental, or lobar bronchiectasis may be associated with symptoms that can be cured by surgical resection.

Pulmonary function tests ordinarily demonstrate a reduced vital capacity reflecting volume loss and mild to moderate airway obstruction. Borderline abnormalities in gas distribution are considered by some to reflect associated local emphysema. Patients may maintain adequate oxygen levels for some time because of proper ventilation/perfusion matching, although those having acute infections may suffer from severe hypoxemia and may develop hypercapnia with acute cor pulmonale.

Treatment

Those patients without local disease who are not candidates for surgical resection benefit from an increased fluid intake, the use of expectorants such as a saturated solution of potassium iodide, (SSKI), and the daily use of bronchodilators. This is followed by postural drainage for the segments or lobes involved, in accordance with the distribution demonstrated by the bronchogram. This should diminish the severity of cough and the volume of secretions, lead to less purulent secretions, and greatly reduce the incidence of acute infections. Hemoptysis, pleuritic pain, and the progressive disability associated with chronic infection are also ameliorated. Occasionally, proper treatment leads to reduction or even disappearance of finger clubbing and to improvement in nutrition as well as in the sense of well-being. It is important to note that pulmonary toilet must be practiced on a permanent basis, as mucociliary drainage mechanisms are permanently damaged.

PNEUMOCONIOSES

Pneumoconiosis is a lung disease associated with fibrosis and secondary to inhaled dusts, which are commonly industrial in origin. The disease may involve all components of the lung from pleura to airways and is produced by the inhalation of small mineral particles (1 to 5 microns) in sufficient concentration that the lungs' defenses, including mucociliary clearance of airways, lung macrophages, and lymphatic channels, are overwhelmed. This results in retention of dust particles. Prolonged exposure to and retention of substances that are fibrogenic will induce several patterns of lung fibrosis and calcification, depending upon the deposition site and the type of mineral. Often, years of exposure are needed to produce dyspnea or positive findings by x-ray, and the family physician must obtain a careful and complete work history with details of specific substances used in the various jobs held by the patient.

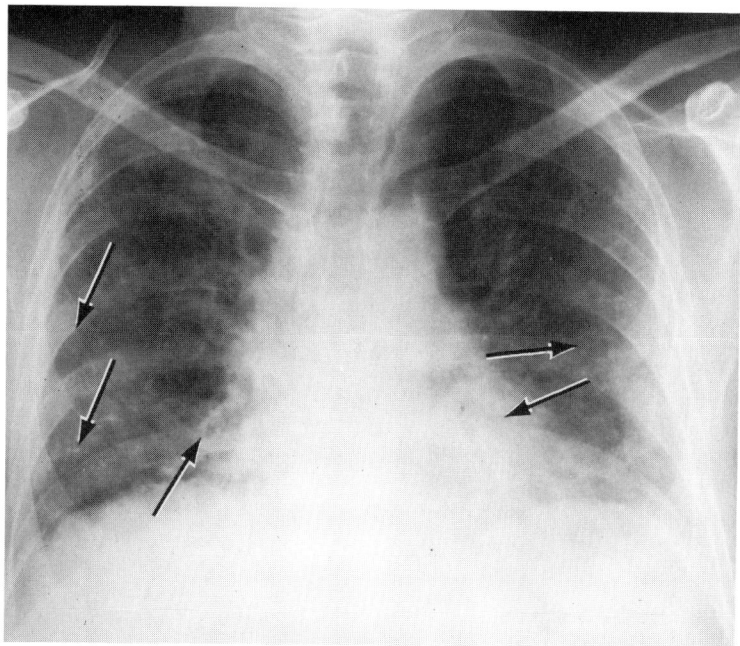

Figure 45-10. *This patient with asbestosis has a chest film revealing the typical fibrosis of the mid and lower lung fields and a shaggy heart border caused by intense pleural and subpleural fibrosis. Pleural plaques are evident along the lateral chest margin.*

Silicosis

Silicosis is caused by the inhalation of free crystalline silica or silicon dioxide particles that are engulfed by phagocytes and carried into lymphatics draining to regional and hilar nodes. Hydration of silica dioxide produces silicic acid, which induces fibrosis. Further, silica crystals cause the death of the macrophage and the liberation of its lysozymes, contributing to tissue damage. Fibrosis appears as discrete 2 to 5 mm. nodules, especially in the mid and upper lung zones, that reveal fibrous whorls and lamination. They are avascular and tend to calcify. In progressive massive fibrosis, the fibrotic nodules tend to coalesce and produce large conglomerate masses 2 or more cm. in diameter. Probably this is a combined silicotic and granulomatous process, which in most patients is either tuberculosis or histoplasmosis.

The x-ray appearance is that of conglomerate dense nodules with calcification of the hilar nodes resembling "eggshells," and frequently emphysematous changes are seen in the lower lung fields with evidence of retraction and scarring. Pulmonary function tests commonly reveal physiologic findings consistent with emphysema, probably because most silicotic patients are smokers, but silicosis occasionally occurs in nonsmokers.

Fibrosis is progressive, and conglomerate masses may cavitate with occasional liberation of tuberculosis organisms.

These patients have a history of exposure to silicotic rock dust (sandstone, granite, slate) from working in quarries or other similar operations or in the mining of gold, tin, silver, nickel, uranium, mica, and graphite. In addition, quartz and mica contain silicon dioxide. The most intense exposures occur in foundry workers dealing with casted metals when sand is used to line the mold, in polishers and chippers of casted metals, in anthracite coal miners when silica content is high in the coal ore, in tunnel workers, and in those producing or using abrasives, particularly sandblasters. The exposure during sandblasting may be so intense that a fulminant form of silicosis develops in a short period of time. Milder varieties are seen in pottery workers, stone cutters, and brickyard workers.

Asbestosis

Asbestos is a hydrated magnesium silicate that is mined and used by numerous industries and is commonly used in construction and insulation trades. The fibers are long and filamentous and tend to gravitate to the mid and lower lung fields, whereupon, after ingestion by a macrophage, the phagocytic cell dies and discharges the fiber and its enzyme content. The fiber is then re-engulfed and the process continues. Asbestos fibers vary in composition, but all produce intense fibrosis in the lower lung fields as well as marked fibrosis of the pleura leading to thickening that may entrap the lung. Fibrosis appears as a reticular network, often so dense that it obscures the heart and diaphragm border. The fibrosis often causes dense calcification of the pleura and fibrotic plaques along the pleural surface (Fig. 45–10).

Many years after an initial exposure that may be as brief as 3 months, there is a striking incidence of malignant pleural tumors (mesotheliomas) that are otherwise rare. Asbestos is a cocarcinogen that causes asbestos workers who smoke to have eight times the incidence of cancer as other smokers and 50 times that of the general nonsmoking population. Lung cancer is rare in asbestos workers who do not smoke.

Diagnosis

The diagnosis is suspected from the work history and the pattern of pulmonary fibrosis with pleural disease. Most patients work in construction or insulation industries, and asbestosis is common in shipyard workers, including steamfitters. Asbestos is used in filters, clutch facings, and brake linings, thus providing additional industrial and general exposure.

Pulmonary function is characterized by severe restriction of lung volumes caused by fibrosis and normal to high air flows produced by peribronchial fibrotic traction that prevents collapse of airways. Hypoxemia with impaired gas diffusion and respiratory insufficiency is common and generally occurs 20 to 30 years after initial exposure. There is no treatment, but limitation of exposure and improvement in industrial hygiene are essential.

Coal Workers' Pneumoconiosis

Coal workers' pneumoconiosis (black lung) is common and potentially disabling. It occurs in coal miners exposed to both soft (bituminous) and hard (anthracite) coal. Some miners have fibrosis because of the associated silica content in coal ore, and some have simple deposition of carbon, which is visible by x-ray but is not very fibrogenic. Carbon deposition occurs at respiratory bronchioles. This causes local bronchiolar dilatation (focal emphysema), but in many patients little physiologic abnormality occurs. For reasons that are not clear, but that may possibly be due to combined silica exposure, some patients go on to develop progressive massive fibrosis with pulmonary fibrosis and emphysema. The majority of patients have simple pneumoconiosis with multiple nodules made up largely of carbon, and despite the frequent expectoration of black sputum, their lung function remains good.

Exposure to Metals

Inert metals that may be seen on x-ray as lung densities but that induce no fibrosis are iron and iron oxide, tin, barium, pure talcum, and aluminum. As some talcum is contaminated with up to 20 per cent asbestos fibers, heavy exposure to talcum (e.g., in the rubber industry) can be associated with pulmonary fibrosis and pleural disease, as seen in asbestosis.

The family physician should be aware of the many types of occupational dust exposures that may produce pulmonary fibrosis. These are:

1. Silica and silicates—coal ore, sandstone, granite, quartz, mica, sands.
2. Diatomaceous earths (kaolin)—china, clay, pottery.
3. Asbestos—chrysotile, crocidolite, anthophyllite.
4. Beryllium oxides, phosphors—powders, heated alloys.
5. Nickel carbonyl.
6. Tungsten carbide.
7. Cadmium.
8. Bauxite—alumina, abrasives, corundum.
9. Graphite—electroplating.
10. Mercury vapors.
11. Zinc and magnesium oxide—welding, galvanizing.

Metal Fume Fever

This is a syndrome often occurring 4 to 8 hours after exposure to zinc or magnesium oxide that is liberated during welding or galvanizing. It has also been called "Monday morning fever" or "brass fever" and is seen in workers who are new to the industry following recurrent exposures. The syndrome consists of sweats, headache, cough, dyspnea, wheeze, malaise, and joint pains and in general is a syndrome suggestive of influenza. Symptoms may begin hours after exposure, therefore confusing the diagnosis. The syndrome is self-limited in that tolerance develops after repeated exposures. Other metal oxides known to cause symptoms are those of copper, cadmium, manganese, nickle, tin, and selenium.

SARCOIDOSIS

Definition

Sarcoidosis is a disease process characterized by noncaseating epithelioid granulomas involving the lymph nodes and lungs, as well as other structures. It generally has a benign and self-limited course, and an abnormal chest x-ray is often the only finding. Since sarcoidosis may be a complex of symptoms and findings rather than a specific disease and since it is often confused with tuberculosis, berylliosis, and other diffuse lung processes, an attempt at definition was made by the Second International Conference on Sarcoidosis:

Sarcoidosis is a systemic granulomatous disease of undetermined etiology and pathogenesis. Mediastinal and peripheral lymph nodes, lungs, liver, spleen, skin, eyes, phalangeal bones and parotid glands are most often involved, but other organs and tissues may be affected. The Kveim reaction is frequently positive, and tuberculin-type hypersensitivities are frequently depressed. Other important laboratory findings are hypercalciuria and increased serum globulins. The characteristic histologic appearance of epithelioid tubercles with little or no necrosis is not pathognomonic and tuberculosis, fungal infections, beryllium disease, and local sarcoid reactions must be excluded. The diagnosis should be regarded as established for clinical purposes in patients who have characteristic clinical features, together with biopsy evidence of epithelioid tubercles or a positive Kveim test.

Etiology

Numerous causative mechanisms have been implicated, including both *Mycobacterium tuberculosis* and the atypical mycobacteria, as well as pine pollen, various virus or fungus infections, and occupational exposures (e.g., with beryllium). It is likely that a number of causative agents exist, any of which may lead to a complex of tissue reactions and symptoms that are generally benign in course and appear so similar as to fulfill the criteria just noted.

Epidemiology

Sarcoidosis occurs in virtually a worldwide distribution, although it is apparently rare among Oriental and African races. Its low incidence in Orientals may be due to confusion of sarcoidosis with the more common tuberculosis. The incidence tends to rise with improved recognition of the entity and improved medical care, especially since it is often identified in routine chest x-rays. The highest incidence is in the third and fourth decades of life, with a slight female preponderance. Sarcoidosis is rare below the age of 14 and above the age of 60. There is an increased prevalence in blacks, with an overall incidence of 6 to 40 per 100,000 population in the United States. A familial incidence is reported.

Pathology

Involved organs, predominantly the lungs and lymph nodes, reveal studding with small granulomatous nodules of uniform size and distribution that usually lack necrosis and never show caseation. The nodule generally remains discrete, with palisading of histiocytes around a center with round cell infiltration and giant cells of the Langhans type. The epithelioid granuloma is characteristic, with rare necrosis and eventual hyalinization. The Kveim test is positive in active sarcoidosis. This test consists of the intradermal injection of 0.1 to 0.2 ml. of a saline suspension of sarcoid tissues, followed by biopsy and histologic examination of the injection site in 4 to 6 weeks. The presence of typical sarcoid granulomas is considered a positive test. The availability of Kveim reagent is a problem, but the test is 85 per cent positive in detecting active disease when a good reagent is used. Interpretation of the Kveim test requires an experienced pathologist.

Clinical Manifestations

Probably 75 per cent of patients are young adults who have few or no symptoms and a chest film revealing symmetrical hilar adenopathy and right paratracheal adenopathy. The disease is often diagnosed on a routine chest film in an asymptomatic person. There is a preceding history of erythema nodosum in 15 to 30 per cent of patients, often months before the initial diagnosis. Approximately 60 to 90 per cent will have disease that is limited to hilar and mediastinal lymphadenopathy with spontaneous resolution in a 1 to 3 year period.

The presence of hilar adenopathy without parenchymal densities is called Stage I. Ten to 30 per cent of patients have Stage II disease on initial diagnosis. Their chest films show parenchymal densities with symmetrical distribution, varying from streaky fibrotic shadows to fluffy nodules or miliary lesions and are characterized by extention to the lung periphery and concentration in the mid-lung zone. A number of patients will have clearing of the adenopathy but persistent pulmonary infiltrate. This is generally called Stage II-B and is considered a later stage in development. Lesions may remain stable and usually regress spontaneously within 3 years or as late as 11 years without treatment. A small number of patients progress to Stage III, which is represented by extensive pulmonary fibrosis with bullous formation and is associated with respiratory insufficiency and eventual cor pulmonale.

Although the hilar nodes and lungs are most commonly affected, other findings are those of endobronchial sarcoidosis leading to bronchostenosis and atelectasis, pleural involvement with only rare effusion, and perivascular involvement. Other manifestations of sarcoidosis include peripheral adenopathy in 42 to 88 per cent of patients, skin lesions with nodules or plaques in 15 to 37 per cent, and liver involvement in as many as 50 per cent, though hepatomegaly is uncommon. Eye involvement characterized by conjunctivitis and uveitis is generally associated with pain and altered vision. Splenic enlargement occurs in 15 to 33 per cent of patients. There is occasional involvement of the central nervous system, bone, kidney, and the myocardium. Myocardial involvement may cause conduction disorders. A commonly quoted but unusual presentation is termed *uveoparotid fever,* consisting of swelling of the parotid glands, uveitis, low-grade fever, and facial nerve palsy.

Symptoms are usually absent in Stage I disease, with an occasional history of erythema nodosum and a vague substernal soreness being the only complaints. Stage II-A or II-B may be associated with a bronchitic syndrome or with dyspnea on exertion that is accompanied by cough and findings consistent with multi-organ system involvement. These include fever, tender liver and spleen, joint pains in the absence of objective findings, and occasionally tachycardia or palpitations. About 25 per cent of patients will present with only cough and dyspnea, coupled with typical chest x-ray findings.

Laboratory Studies

A mild anemia is common, but leukocytosis is absent. There is hyperglobulinemia with either a diffuse elevation of gammaglobulins or, more specifically, elevation of IgA and IgG. Hypercalcemia occurs in 2 to 3 per cent of patients, usually those with severe sarcoidosis, and is apparently caused by increased sensitivity to vitamin D, with resultant increased calcium absorption from the gut. This hypercalcemia responds promptly to corticosteroid treatment. Hypercalciuria may result in nephrocalcinosis, with the symptoms secondary to the renal disorder. The electrocardiogram may reveal conduction defects, which include bundle branch block.

Cutaneous anergy is commonly present during active disease, although delayed hypersensitivity may return when the disease process remits. In addition, an associated active tuberculosis would probably result in the tuberculin skin test "breaking through" the anergy and giving a positive reaction. Anergy is commonly evaluated by the use of PPD, mumps antigen, trichophytin, and other common antigens. Patients exhibit the immunologic phenomenon of adequate to increased humoral immunity (B-lymphocyte mediated) and a deficiency of cell-mediated immunity (T-lymphocyte mediated). Patients with a previously reactive tuberculin test may be nonreactive after acquiring active sarcoidosis.

Pulmonary function tests reveal no significant abnormality in Stage I (adenopathy alone), but in Stage II, tests commonly reveal a restrictive disorder with variable levels of hypoxemia and a 'diffusion defect when parenchymal infiltrates are extensive. In general, there is a discrepancy between the alarming radiographic findings of multiple lesions and the relatively intact lung function, with the exception of reduced volumes. A characteristic of Stage II-A and II-B disease is a reduction in vital capacity coupled with a reduction in both total lung capacity and residual volume; however, these increase following effective treatment or spontaneous remission. Response to steroid therapy should be followed by the determination of lung volume measurements coupled with serial diffusion capacity measurements.

Generally, symptomatology and pulmonary function tests correlate better than do symptoms and chest x-ray findings. The Kveim test is not needed in a typical case in which the patient's age and the silent onset and characteristic x-ray findings, possibly preceded by erythema nodosum, would establish the diagnosis in conjunction with the various laboratory abnormalities noted.

Clinical Course

Over 80 per cent of patients have stable disease, the vast majority undergoing a remission without treatment. A great number of patients are never diagnosed simply because a chest film is not obtained. In addition, the subtle hilar adenopathy and right paratracheal adenopathy are often missed after casual examination of the chest film. Such films are useful later if the patient enters Stage II-A or II-B and becomes symptomatic. The diagnosis is easy because of the discrepancy brtween a markedly abnormal chest film and a relatively asymptomatic patient.

The patient should be observed clinically and by chest x-ray on a monthly basis for 3 to 6 months to establish that the disease is not progressing. Some will progress to Stage II-A or II-B during this

period, and their symptoms or the marked abnormality in pulmonary function tests may force intervention with corticosteroid therapy. The physician should be careful to note that sarcoidosis often improves during pregnancy but is followed by a prompt and alarming relapse of chest x-ray abnormalities and symptoms in the postpartum period. It is also pertinent that improvement in chest radiographic abnormalities may occur because of concurrent estrogen therapy.

Treatment

The majority of patients require no treatment because they are in Stage I. Further, the majority of those in Stage II-A or II-B require no treatment if they have only mild symptoms, especially when pulmonary function tests reveal fair preservation of function. Stage III disease with fibrosis and bullous formation does not respond to treatment and represents terminal and irreversible fibrosis. Treatment of Stage III patients had led physicians to the erroneous concept that sarcoidosis does not respond to steroid therapy. Treatment is initiated with prednisone, generally 30 mg. daily, with a gradual reduction to 10 to 15 mg. over a period of weeks to months. Stable symptomatic relief and x-ray improvement are the major guidelines in determining reduction of dosage. The value of following serum lysozyme levels in evaluating remission or control is not firmly established. Symptomatic relief and improvement in the x-ray picture are evidence of control. The diffusion capacity and lung volumes should improve, although the former is the last to be corrected, even with adequate treatment.

The principle is to treat for the 2 to 3 year period prior to the anticipated spontaneous remission that will occur in the majority of patients who are symptomatic and require treatment. The goal is the prevention of irreversible fibrosis. Steroids are tapered and discontinued when remission has occurred. The lowest effective dose of steroid medication is generally recommended for long-term treatment.

Treatment is considered mandatory for the following serious forms of sarcoidosis: (1) sarcoidosis with eye involvement—to prevent permanent visual loss, (2) progression of parenchymal disease with severe dyspnea and marked loss in pulmonary function, (3) persistent hypercalcemia or hypercalciuria—to prevent nephrocalcinosis and renal failure, (4) central nervous system symptoms attributed to sarcoidosis, (5) myocardial sarcoidosis with arrhythmias or congestive heart failure, (6) uveoparotid fever, (7) splenic enlargement with pain suggesting splenic infarction, and (8) sarcoidosis with a toxic onset characterized by high fever, severe hypoxemia, and tachycardia.

The prognosis for the vast majority of patients is quite benign, but only careful observation of the patient will determine that an individual patient will have a benign course. Intervention with steroids in the selected patient may prevent irreversible pulmonary fibrosis, cor pulmonale, and death.

RESPIRATORY FAILURE

The terms respiratory failure and respiratory insufficiency are often confused, so that some clarification is indicated before respiratory failure is discussed. When there is abnormality of the respiratory apparatus sufficient to produce an awareness of breathing difficulty or subjective dyspnea, the patient has respiratory insufficiency, although not necessarily respiratory failure. If respiratory insufficiency is characterized by dyspnea, the condition is based on a subjective complaint rather than an objective finding. Dyspnea may result from diverse mechanisms, such as increased work required for breathing, hypoxemia, distention of the chest as seen in emphysema or status asthmaticus, or hyperventilation related simply to anxiety in patients who do not have lung disease. It is useful to think of the causes of dyspnea in terms of the three major categories of patients experiencing this complaint. These groups are classified in Table 45-6.

To assist in quantitation of dyspnea, the American Thoracic Society in 1962 developed the following standards:

Grade I. Can keep pace walking on the level with a normal person of his (her) age and body build, but not on hills or stairs. Dyspnea on exertion.

Grade II. Can walk a mile at his (her) own pace without dyspnea,

TABLE 45-6. CATEGORIES OF DYSPNEA

Patient Types	Arterial Blood Gases	
A. No disease, *hyperventilation*	↑Po_2	↓Pco_2
B. Disease with *hyperventilation*—Primary defect is hypoxia, not corrected by hyperventilation	↓Po_2	↓Pco_2
C. Disease and *hypoventilation* (B) often progresses to (C)	↓Po_2	↑Pco_2

but cannot keep pace on the level with a normal person.

Grade III. Becomes breathless after walking about 100 yards or for a few minutes on the level.

Grade IV. Becomes breathless while dressing or talking.

Differentiation of Respiratory Failure

To differentiate the subjective dyspnea characterizing respiratory insufficiency from respiratory failure, one is forced to define the latter by physiologic terms, using objective laboratory data. A patient may be said to be in respiratory failure when the arterial Po_2 is below 60 mm. Hg or when the arterial Pco_2 is above 50 mm. Hg, or both. The blood gas levels indicated are arbitrary levels, but are used by most laboratories. This definition permits the diagnosis of respiratory failure in patients who have severe hypoxemia associated with diffuse lung disease and who, in the early stages, have hypocapnia rather than hypercapnia.

The blood gas tensions must be known to establish the state of respiratory failure. The majority of patients will have both hypoxemia and hypercapnia, representing alveolar hypoventilation. Those with severe hypoxemia as the primary abnormality usually have severe impairment in oxygen transfer to the pulmonary capillary blood (often called ventilation/perfusion imbalance, or shunting) and tend to be hyperventilators with low carbon dioxide tensions. The degree of resultant acidosis commonly seen in respiratory failure depends on the severity of failure (both tissue hypoxia and hypercapnia may contribute) and the acuteness of onset. Gradual onset allows the kidneys time to elevate bicarbonate levels to compensate for carbon dioxide retention, restoring the bicarbonate-carbonic acid ratio.

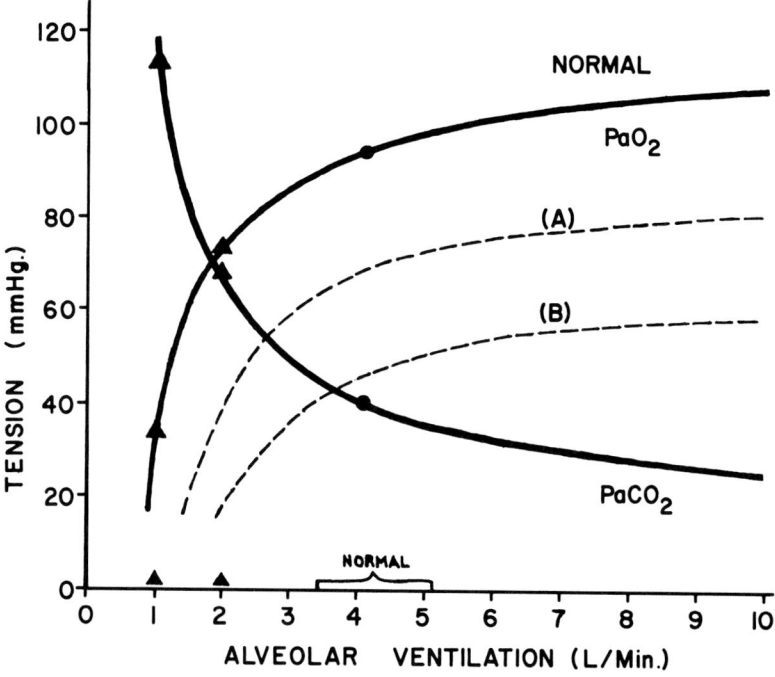

Figure 45–11. *Diagram illustrating two types of arterial hypoxemia.*

Hypoxia

An element of arterial hypoxemia is common to all patients with respiratory failure, but there are two types, A and B, as seen in Figure 45–11.

The Type B patient is hypoxic even at normal ventilation levels, indicating hypoxemia of the arterial blood. Type A patients develop hypoxemia only when ventilation of the lung is reduced. Note that Figure 45–11 reveals that as people with normal lungs underventilate progressively (as with drug overdose), the gas tensions move in opposite directions. Both hypercapnia and hypoxemia occur simultaneously, and changes in gas tensions that occur with each unit reduction in ventilation accelerate as we move to the left. Therefore, even slight further reductions in ventilation become important when alveolar ventilation is low. By the same token, at low ventilation levels, it is possible to sharply increase oxygen tensions and lower carbon dioxide tensions with less change in ventilation than at higher ventilation levels, since the expired air has a higher carbon dioxide tension and content and the inspired oxygen tension is much higher than the resident alveolar PO_2. This clarifies how underventilation

may lead to hypercapnia, but the carbon dioxide tension stabilizes at levels of 50 to 70 mm. Hg, as the reduced ventilation becomes adequate to control carbon dioxide elimination when higher tensions are being used in exchange.

The changes in both oxygen and carbon dioxide tension can be followed by observing the sequential triangular points in the ventilation graph, using the normal curve. It will be noted that blood gas tensions are stable in a wide range of ventilation levels when ventilation is normal or in the high range. For example, lowering the arterial PCO_2 from 40 to 30 mm. Hg ordinarily requires a doubling of the alveolar ventilation.

In Type A disease, characterized by only mild hypoxemia, considerable hypercapnia can occur before the hypoxemia becomes critical. Supplementation with oxygen allows even lower ventilation levels to exist by averting the catastrophe of sudden death secondary to hypoxemia. Therefore, if given oxygen, these patients become progressively underventilated until they develop levels of carbon dioxide tension greater than 100 mm. Hg, which lead to carbon dioxide narcosis and ultimately to death.

In Type B disease, characterized by

more severe hypoxemia at rest and seen in restrictive disorders associated with an oxygen diffusion abnormality, significant hypoxemia characterizes the patient, even at normal ventilation levels. This patient is likely to die of the consequences of tissue hypoxia before hypercapnia of any significance can develop via progressive hypoventilation, since critical oxygen tensions will be reached early, leading to cardiac arrest or arrhythmias. Therefore, in this group of patients, the hypercapnia tends to be only a transient and terminal event. Death is usually due to severe, untreated hypoxemia and characteristically occurs with little warning.

The Effects of Hypoxia. Hypoxemia is associated with tissue hypoxia and produces a number of symptoms and findings. Hypoxia leads to subjective dyspnea and stimulates ventilation to produce tachypnea and hyperpnea. Hypoxemia leads to tachycardia and to an increase in both cardiac output and renal blood flow. Hypoxemia characterized by a PO_2 below 50 mm. Hg causes reflex vasoconstriction of the pulmonary arterial and venous bed, leading to pulmonary hypertension, and is a prime reason for the treatment of oxygen tensions below 50 mm. Hg. Hypoxemia may result in tissue lactic acidosis, which then sensitizes the heart to epinephrine and other catecholamines. Hypoxemia can produce cerebral edema with an increased cerebrospinal fluid pressure, restlessness, confusion, euphoria, and seizures.

Although significant hypoxemia frequently produces cyanosis, it must be remembered that 5 grams per 100 ml. of reduced hemoglobin is required to produce cyanosis, so that anemic patients may die of hypoxemia without cyanosis appearing. In addition, cyanosis is subjective and can be due to poor peripheral circulation or to an increase in red cell mass (polycythemia), or a patient may appear cyanotic because of poor lighting. Cyanosis generally is not accurately quantitated even among trained observers. Since total body oxygen stores equal approximately 11 ml. per kg. of body weight, the average man has 840 to 900 ml., or enough for 4 to 5 minutes of survival if respirations cease and circulation continues. With severe anemia, the oxygen stores are further reduced. It is pertinent that raising the arterial oxygen tension from 25 to 40 mm. Hg will increase hemoglobin oxygen saturation from 40 to 70 per cent. With this change, oxygen delivery rises from 200 ml. per minute to 500 ml. per minute, a critical difference.

Hypercapnia

Hypercapnia is usually produced by alveolar hypoventilation in obstructive airway disease and less often occurs because of abnormal chest bellows or central nervous system depression. Furthermore, hypercapnia is the indicator of underventilation, as oxygen levels are quite variable in patients with a variety of lung diseases. It is unwise to use the arterial oxygen tension as a measure of ventilation.

The effects of hypercapnia are numerous. Mild elevations are stimulating to the respiratory center, inducing increased effort to correct the underventilation. However, arterial PCO_2 tensions greater than 80 mm. Hg may contribute to lethargy or coma, as carbon dioxide at high levels acts as a narcotic on the central nervous system. Hypercapnia dilates the cerebral arteries, which increases cerebrovascular flow and cerebrospinal fluid pressure and induces papilledema, an indicator of cerebral edema. After inducing increased PCO_2 levels from 35 mm. Hg to 75 mm. Hg in subjects in an experimental chamber for 5 days, investigators noted drowsiness, loss of concentration, irritability, insomnia, anorexia, headache, and mild hypertension, but *no dyspnea*. Hypercapnia causes a reduction in renal blood flow, which often produces oliguria; this effect depends on a reduction in pH. At higher levels, hypercapnia produces asterixis. Arterial PCO_2 tensions above 100 mm. Hg generally produce narcosis and hypotension.

Acidosis

Acidosis occurs when carbon dioxide retention is acute, depending on the rate and degree of hypercapnia. Often an additional metabolic component is superimposed because of lactic acidosis resulting from tissue hypoxia. Table 45–7 may be useful in predicting the levels of acidosis or alkalosis that might occur with acute changes in carbon dioxide tension. It assumes that the pH is initially normal and

TABLE 45–7. PREDICTING ARTERIAL pH
WITH ACUTE P_{CO_2} CHANGES

1. For each 10 mm. Hg rise in P_{CO_2}, the pH falls 0.07 unit.
2. A corresponding P_{CO_2} fall causes greater changes in pH than a rise in carbon dioxide.

P_{CO_2} mm. Hg.	pH	
20	7.65	HYPERVENTILATION
30	7.50	
40	7.40	
50	7.33	HYPOVENTILATION
60	7.26	
70	7.19	
80	7.12	

allows for the detection of combined metabolic and respiratory components when a given P_{CO_2} tension has not produced the anticipated arterial pH.

Acidosis has several serious effects, especially when the pH is below 7.25, by reducing responsiveness to beta-adrenergic-stimulating drugs and by reducing the saturation of hemoglobin at any existent oxygen tension. Acidosis contributes to pulmonary arterial vasoconstriction. It is then an important mechanism in producing cor pulmonale, right heart failure, and death.

Etiology

Table 45–8 provides an incomplete list of conditions that may be associated with alveolar hypoventilation. The list does not include the commonly encountered drug overdose as a cause for underventilation, as this is often seen in patients with no underlying pulmonary pathology.

Pathophysiology

The complex factors that may contribute to alveolar hypoventilation with resultant hypoxemia, hypercapnia, and acidosis are diagrammed in Figure 45–12 to permit inclusion of many contributing factors as well as of primary lung disease categories.

It should be noted that the most common disease producing respiratory failure is chronic obstructive pulmonary disease (COPD) with combined emphysema and chronic bronchitis as major factors.

Clinical Manifestations

The symptoms and appearance of the patient with respiratory failure may be those associated with a primary underlying disorder, and therefore will be variable.

TABLE 45–8. CAUSES OF RESPIRATORY FAILURE

General Alveolar Hypoventilation
I. Physiologic
   Sleep—significant in chronic obstructive pulmonary disease (COPD)
   Metabolic alkalosis
      Hypokalemic alkalosis
      Hypochloremic alkalosis
      Primary hydrogen ion depletion (vomiting)
   CO_2 retention (hypercapnia)

CO_2 elevation itself depresses the respiratory centers, but usually at high levels only. Respiratory centers may be "reset."

II. Anatomic
   Diseases of the respiratory centers—tumors, toxins, etc.
   Neuromuscular diseases
      Poliomyelitis
      Guillain-Barré syndrome (ascending myelitis)
      Myasthenia gravis
      Multiple sclerosis
      Toxic myopathy of carcinomatosis
      Neuromuscular blockage
      (curare, succinylcholine)
         Synergism with drugs—neomycin, etc.
         Pseudocholinesterase
         Electrolyte abnormalities
   Chest cage deformity—kyphoscoliosis, thoracoplasty, etc.
   Restrictive lung disease
      Granulomatous disease
      Pulmonary fibrosis
      Pleural disease
   Obesity—cardiopulmonary failure—"pickwickian syndrome"
   Myxedema

Hypoventilation Associated with Ventilation/Perfusion Abnormalities
I. Obstructive Pulmonary Diseases
   Bronchial asthma
   Chronic bronchitis
   Emphysema
   Cystic fibrosis
   Bronchiectasis

   Mechanisms
      Airway collapse
      Bronchial secretions
      Bronchial edema
      Inflammatory changes
      Bronchospasm

II. Vascular Disease
   Acute pulmonary embolism
   Chronic recurrent pulmonary embolism

PATHOPHYSIOLOGY

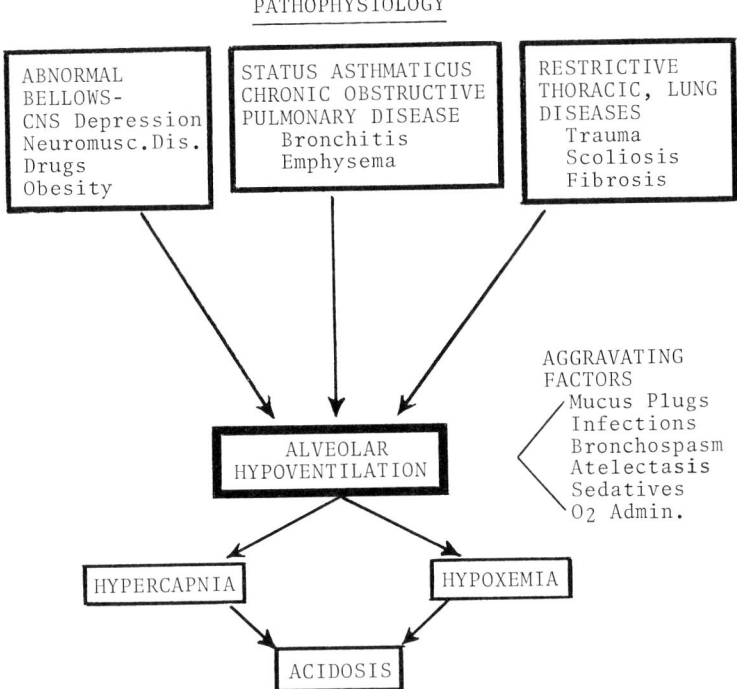

Figure 45-12. *Mechanisms of respiratory failure common to obstructive and restrictive pulmonary disease, as well as extrapulmonary disorders.*

Since there now exist more patients in the community with obstructive lung disease and other respiratory disorders who are in borderline respiratory failure and since treatment prolongs their survival, it becomes important that the family physician be aware of the clinical manifestations, even though many patients will require intensive care management for acute episodes.

Respiratory distress and overt anxiety will be noted in patients with chronic obstructive pulmonary disease, but patients with cardiorespiratory failure associated with massive obesity or hypothyroidism may appear lethargic despite cyanosis caused by intense hypoxemia. Somnolence is an early sign of hypercapnia, especially useful in patients with predominant chronic bronchitis. Agitation, restlessness, irritability, and euphoria may all be due to hypoxemia. Plethora is often not recognized as a sign of secondary erythrocytosis induced by prolonged hypoxemia. Cyanosis is often absent until the arterial PO_2 is well below 50 mm. Hg, so that its absence should not be considered reassuring.

Dehydration may be evident and may be associated with inspissated secretions precipitating acute failure in COPD. Evidence of twitching of the extremities or headaches related to hypercapnia should be noted. The signs of cor pulmonale with venous distention and peripheral edema require an early identification.

Treatment

The treatment is based on correction of the pathophysiologic mechanisms and will vary widely according to the underlying disease. The majority of patients will have chronic obstructive pulmonary disease (COPD), and it is important to keep airways clear by inducement of frequent coughing, hydration of secretions, and the use of expectorants and bronchodilators to improve mobilization of secretions. Postural drainage may improve airway management and obviate the need for intubation and mechanical ventilation. In the presence of hypoxemia associated with an arterial oxygen tension below 50 mm. Hg, it may be necessary to give controlled supplemental oxygen administered by Venturi mask in concentrations of 24, 28, or 35 per cent, or comparable concentrations delivered by nasal cannula at oxygen flows of 1, 2, or 4 liters per minute.

Patients with pre-existing hypercapnia should be given oxygen supplementation with caution, as because of long-term hypercapnia, their respiratory center has become less sensitive to carbon dioxide. Their ventilation is abnormally dependent on the presence of hypoxemia as a respiratory drive. Therefore, oxygen supplementation may destroy that hypoxic respiratory drive and result in progressive reduction in ventilation and further carbon dioxide elevation to the point of narcosis. Serial evaluation of arterial carbon dioxide tensions hourly will detect ventilatory depression secondary to oxygen therapy. Hypercapnic patients require ventilation in the most practical manner from use of intermittent positive pressure breathing (IPPB) to continuous ventilation if the hypercapnia is acute in onset (as evidenced by lack of pH compensation) and if a proper search is made for the precipitating event. The work of breathing may be so high that it leads to exhaustion (e.g., patients with status asthmaticus). Clinically this may require ventilator support, as was traditional even before arterial oxygen and carbon dioxide measurements became available to evaluate the patient's status.

Bronchospasm should be corrected whenever possible by intravenous bronchodilators. Theophylline is the primary drug used and is administered by continuous intravenous infusion in a dose of 1.0 to 1.5 grams in a 24 hour period. A slowly injected bolus of 250 mg. may be given to provide an immediate result. Theophylline is a respiratory stimulant and is useful in counteracting the depressing effects of supplemental oxygen. Hydrocortisone sodium succinate (Solu-Cortef), 100 to 150 mg. intravenously every 4 to 6 hours, may help control bronchospasm and reduce airway edema when it exists. When infection is a precipitating event, it should be treated after appropriate sputum smears and cultures have been obtained, but it is a secondary consideration in acute respiratory failure. Acidosis with a pH below 7.30 should be treated with alkali or increased ventilation if it is entirely caused by hy-

percapnia. Such treatment will improve hemoglobin oxygen saturation, render the patient more responsive to bronchodilating drugs, and control pulmonary hypertension.

A careful search should be made for the four most common causes of acute respiratory failure in the usual patient with chronic obstructive pulmonary disease. These are, in order of frequency: acute respiratory infections, inspissated secretions caused by dehydration or drugs, left heart failure, and pneumothorax. The prognosis for patients with acute respiratory failure is almost entirely based on the causative mechanisms and the reversibility of the underlying disease.

Acute Respiratory Distress Syndrome

In recent years, a special type of respiratory failure resembling that seen in the respiratory distress syndrome of the newborn has been observed in adults with increasing frequency. It is estimated that there may be 150,000 cases each year with a 50 per cent mortality. The acute respiratory distress syndrome (ARDS) in adults is characterized by wet, hemorrhagic lungs, which are noncompliant (stiff), and corresponding severe hypoxemia resistant to oxygen supplementation, associated with a very high work of breathing. The onset may occur several hours to a day after the acute events, and tachypnea and hypoxemia are the initial findings. Early recognition is needed, as patients require intubation with mechanical ventilation, use of very high concentrations of oxygen, and special techniques to improve oxygen transfer, such as positive end expiratory pressure (PEEP). The prognosis is dependent on early recognition, adequate oxygenation, and, in large measure, on the underlying causative mechanism.

This syndrome is seen in a very heterogeneous group of conditions, including gram-negative sepsis, prolonged shock, fat embolism, hemorrhagic pancreatitis, thoracic and extrathoracic trauma, or a chemical pneumonitis following aspiration or exposure to noxious fumes. In some patients, the acute respiratory distress syndrome results from prolonged exposure to high oxygen mixtures (usually greater than 80 per cent oxygen for longer than 10 days).

COR PULMONALE

The pulmonary circulation is a large volume-low pressure system capable of accommodating three to four times the usual cardiac output that occurs with vigorous exercise without causing an elevation of pulmonary artery pressure. Pulmonary hypertension (pulmonary artery pressure greater than 25/10 mm. Hg) caused by an increased pulmonary vascular resistance can be induced by several mechanisms. These include hypoxemia with a PO_2 less than 50 mm. Hg, moderate acidosis (pH below 7.25), vasoconstriction of the arterial or venous bed, or occlusion of the pulmonary arterial tree limiting the flow capacity. Cor pulmonale with pulmonary hypertension occurs with restrictive disorders, such as pulmonary fibrosis; with primary vascular occlusion, as in multiple pulmonary emboli; and with hypoventilation caused by neuromuscular or skeletal disease. However, the vast majority of patients have underlying chronic obstructive pulmonary disease (COPD) with coexisting bronchitis and emphysema. Pulmonary hypertension is initially present only with exercise or with other causes for increased cardiac output. Later, it occurs at rest and persists in association with the development of right ventricular hypertrophy. Right heart failure may not appear until later in the course, and its presence is not necessary for the diagnosis of cor pulmonale.

Diagnosis

The symptoms are dyspnea and easy fatigability, as well as a vague anterior chest pain that is often confused with angina pectoris. Some patients experience palpitations with exertion. The onset of right heart failure causes complaints of abdominal fullness and right upper quadrant tenderness, although invariably the first sign is evening peripheral edema, which is symmetrical and which initially clears during sleep.

Physical examination reveals the findings of the underlying pulmonary disease and commonly shows cyanosis and plethora associated with a secondary polycythemia involving the mucous membranes as well as the nailbeds.

Common physical findings of cor pulmonale without right heart failure are:

1. A loud pulmonic second sound with splitting of the second sound.
2. S_3 right ventricular gallop (heard over the sternum).
3. Right ventricular heave.
4. Early systolic pulmonary ejection click or murmur, or both.

Cor pulmonale with right heart failure reveals:

1. Peripheral edema, maximum at night.
2. Jugular venous distention that fails to clear on forced inspiration.
3. Hepatojugular reflux.
4. Enlarged and tender liver.
5. Ascites, when peripheral edema is marked.

The electrocardiogram reveals a vertical electrical axis, usually over 90°; indeterminate axis (S_I, S_{II}, S_{III} pattern); and QR or qR in lead aVR. Precordial leads reveal qR, RVH with large R waves and ST-T changes in leads V_{1-3}. There may be an incomplete or complete right bundle branch block (RBBB) pattern. Clockwise rotation is seen with prominent S waves in V_{5-6}.

The chest x-ray reveals the primary pulmonary disease and may demonstrate large main pulmonary arteries (Fig. 45–13). A right ventricular bulge approaching the sternum is seen on the lateral film. A prominent right ventricular outflow tract bulging out of the left heart border between the apex and aortic knob is common.

Treatment

Management begins with treatment of the underlying pulmonary disease, which may respond if reversible. Patients with hypoxemia with a PaO_2 below 50 mm. Hg should be treated with supplemental oxygen to elevate the oxygen tension above 60 mm. Hg, thereby preventing reflex pulmonary vasoconstriction. Acidosis should be corrected by the use of intravenous bicarbonate or a reduction in arterial PCO_2, when the latter is an important mechanism. Therapy should always be guided by sequential arterial pH and PCO_2 determinations. Bed rest, salt restriction, diuretics, and digitalis are useful. Antibiotics and bronchial toilet are important when chronic bronchitis is present, and the treatment of bronchospasm is mandatory when it plays a role in acute cor pulmonale. The patient often responds with massive diuresis within hours after the

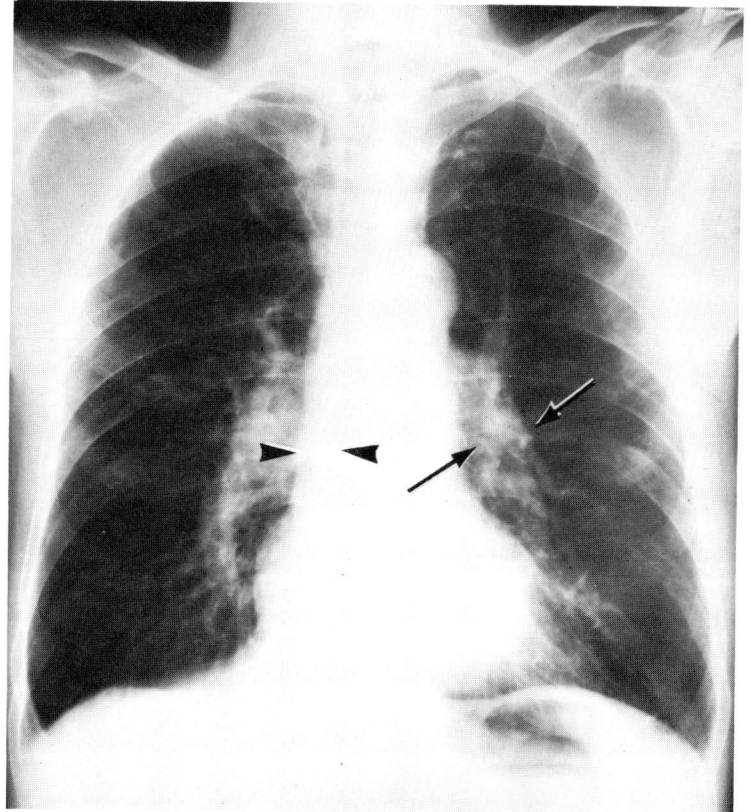

Figure 45–13.   *This 60 year old man had severe COPD with chronic bronchitis, severe hypoxemia, pulmonary hypertension and cor pulmonale. Note the very large right and left main pulmonary artery segments.*

correction of hypoxemia and acidosis. Digitalis should be used cautiously because of the sensitivity to this drug noted in patients with pulmonary disease. It has a secondary role in managing cor pulmonale.

Chronic treatment may require nasal oxygen by cannula at 1 to 2 liters per minute flow for 16 to 24 hours per day to control chronic cor pulmonale with right heart failure. Such treatment reduces mortality by 50 per cent in those patients with cor pulmonale who have experienced right heart failure. With the use of supplemental oxygen, digitalis, diuretics, salt restriction, and appropriate treatment of the primary pulmonary disease, the patient may survive for a period of years, even when in advanced COPD. Survival is dependent upon the correction of hypoxemia and the reversibility of the underlying pulmonary disease.

PULMONARY FUNGUS INFECTIONS

Mycotic infections can be divided into (1) primary infections with prominent lung involvement and (2) infections by "opportunistic fungi" specifically associated with other medical disorders. The most common primary pulmonary fungus infections are histoplasmosis, coccidioidomycosis, North American blastomycosis, and cryptococcosis (torulosis). The majority of other fungus infections represent superinfections preceded by colonization in some patients and associated in others with diseases that cause an altered immune system.

PRIMARY FUNGUS INFECTIONS

Histoplasmosis

This infectious disease is caused by *Histoplasma capsulatum,* a fungus found in the soil of chicken yards; in bird droppings, including those of pigeons and starlings; and in bat dung present in caves. The disease is endemic in the Ohio and Mississippi River basins. It is transmitted by inhalation of dust containing the *H. capsulatum* organism measuring 1 to 3 microns with its capsule. A bronchopneumonia then ensues and spreads to regional nodes. Most infections are benign and are detected as calcifications in the lung and hilar nodes, which represent healed lesions. Another form is a progressive, primary infection with significant fever and constitutional symptoms. Wandering pneumonic infiltrates have been noted, and spread to the mediastinum leads to mediastinitis with fibrosis. Benign hematogenous dissemination is common with primary histoplasmosis. A chronic reactivation or reinfection form also occurs. The majority of patients with primary histoplasmosis are asymptomatic, or their disease resembles a mild upper respiratory infection.

Healed and calcified granulomas with calcified hilar nodes, as found in tuberculosis, are seen in the chest films of patients living outside the endemic area. Patients with residual nodules (histoplasmoma) often present with calcification of hilar nodes in a stippled pattern. A skin test is available, and the organism grows well on Sabouraud's agar or cystine blood agar. The tissue reaction is the formation of a granuloma with occasional caseation. The histoplasmin skin test is positive in 80 per cent of proven cases and in 90 per cent of acute symptomatic forms. Complement fixation and precipitin tests become positive in both acute pulmonary and chronic active forms in 80 per cent of patients. The yeast-phase antigen may persist for years. Treatment is not needed in the vast majority of patients. Primary treatment for both progressive disease and severe disease is amphotericin B.

Coccidioidomycosis

This disease is often known as San Joaquin fever and is endemic in arid regions of the southwestern United States. The causative organism, *Coccidioides immitis,* is a spherule with endospores that when inhaled produces infections varying from bronchopneumonia with abscesses to granuloma. Infection occurs at the end of the wet season when the subsoil is damp and the surface soil has dried. Large numbers of arthrospores are aerosolized, and infection is almost exclusively via the respiratory tract. Infection, usually subclinical, is virtually universal in endemic areas. It occurs in many persons when they travel through such areas, as evidenced by development of a positive skin test. There is an incubation period of 1 to 4 weeks, and the illness resembles influenza. As many as 40 per cent of females and 20 per cent of males manifest erythema nodosum. Pregnant women and nonwhite races are predisposed to a disseminated form.

Diagnosis is made by identifying spherules in KOH preparations and by culture of sputum. The skin test is positive within 1 week of infection in 85 per cent of patients, with a positive precipitin test occurring early in the infection. The precipitin test becomes negative within weeks, but if a test remains persistently positive, it suggests dissemination. The complement fixation test becomes positive 2 to 3 months after infection and is a good indicator of active disease. The organism is highly infectious to laboratory personnel.

Prolonged active disease or dissemination requires treatment with amphotericin B, but the vast majority of patients require no treatment.

North American Blastomycosis

This disease is found in the central and southeastern United States and is caused by the fungus *Blastomyces dermatitidis*, a thick-walled sphere with characteristic single budding in the yeast-phase. It commonly produces indolent pulmonary and cutaneous infections. The pulmonary lesion is often a peripheral pneumonic infiltrate that has streaky infiltrates radiating from the hilum to the peripheral lesion. Skin test results are unreliable, as are serologic tests. Sputum examination and skin biopsy easily lead to the diagnosis. The tissue reaction varies from pneumonic to granulomatous. Progressive disease is treated with amphotericin B.

Cryptococcosis

Cryptococcosis (torulosis) is caused by *Cryptococcus neoformans*, a budding fungus frequently isolated from pigeon excreta. The pulmonary lesion is usually an asymptomatic solitary nodule, but pneumonic infiltrate with cavitation may occur. Pleural effusion is uncommon. The respiratory infection is usually benign, but when dissemination does occur, the neurotropic organism produces a serious meningoencephalitis. Central nervous system symptoms may be chronic and indolent but eventually are fatal. Diagnosis is made when a characteristic capsule or white halo is seen around organisms in India ink preparations obtained from sputum or from cerebrospinal fluid.

INFECTION WITH OPPORTUNISTIC FUNGI

Opportunistic fungi may invade the lungs of a patient who is compromised by an underlying disease. The disease states generally associated with opportunistic infections are diabetes mellitus, malignancies (lymphoma, leukemia), and alcoholism. Patients undergoing prolonged steroid treatment or prolonged treatment with irradiation or chemotherapeutic agents or those in the immunosuppressed states associated with organ transplants are also susceptible.

Actinomycosis

Actinomycosis is a widespread disease caused by *Actinomyces israelii*, an organism normally found in the mouth. Infection presents as the cervicofacial form (lumpy jaw) or the abdominal form; the pulmonary variety results from aspiration that is usually a complication of tooth extraction or other oral surgery. A pneumonic process results, causing a tendency to abscess formation, pleural effusion, and fistula formation. Treatment consists of penicillin in large doses for an extended period of weeks.

Candidiasis

Pulmonary candidiasis (moniliasis) is rare as an infiltrative lesion, but the organism causing this infection is commonly found as yeastlike bodies in the mucous membranes of the mouth and esophagus in patients who have received broad-spectrum antibiotic treatment for extended periods. Systemic infection with invasion of the lung and the blood stream occurs primarily in the immunosuppressed patient. Systemic infections require treatment with amphotericin B.

Aspergillosis

The organism has worldwide distribution caused by several species of *Aspergillus (A. fumigatus, A. versicolor, A. niger)*. The tissue reaction may be pneumonic or may produce a granuloma, and the host is generally a patient with underlying disease.

Four varieties of pulmonary aspergillosis occur: (1) the pneumonic form, (2) the fungus ball form, (3) the form with progressive pneumonia, and (4) the form with pulmonary eosinophilia. The pneumonic form is rarely seen in healthy persons except after overwhelming exposure to spores found on grain, but it may lead to abscess. A common variety is the fungus ball or aspergilloma, which is an indolent mass of organisms within a pre-existing cavity seen in tuberculosis, bronchiectasis, or end-stage sarcoid. The fungus ball is not associated with local or systemic invasion but rarely may cause a serious hemoptysis that necessitates surgical resection. A third form is aspergillosis with a progressive pneumonia. Another important form is aspergillosis associated with pulmonary eosinophilia (allergic bronchopulmonary aspergillosis). This is observed as a syndrome of fever, fleeting infiltrates, and eosinophilic mucous plugs in patients presenting with bronchitis or bronchial asthma. The syndrome responds to steroid therapy, and the infiltrates are often caused by masses of aspergillus organisms mixed with mucous that obstruct small airways.

Treatment is usually not needed for a fungus ball, and only progressive pulmonary infection with cavitation requires therapy. Amphotericin B is not very effective, but potassium iodide may be added to the regimen. The disseminated form usually causes death before sufficient drugs can be given.

CYSTIC FIBROSIS

Definition

Cystic fibrosis (mucoviscidosis) is an hereditary disease of children and young adults that is associated with chronic pulmonary disease, pancreatic insufficiency, and variable exocrine gland dysfunction involving the sweat, mucous, and salivary glands. A characteristic finding is an abnormally high level of sweat electrolytes. Cystic fibrosis was first recognized as a distinct disease entity in 1936. It was described as a disease of children, with the common occurrence of neonatal meconium ileus; intestinal obstruction; malabsorption,

especially of fat-soluble vitamins; and progressive pulmonary disease leading to death from respiratory complications.

Etiology and Pathogenesis

Cystic fibrosis is inherited as an autosomal recessive defect that causes no symptoms in heterozygotes who have only high-normal levels of sweat electrolytes. The parents are both heterozygotes, with one out of four children being homozygous. The carrier frequency is 1:25, and the disease incidence is 1:1600 to 2000 live births. It is rare in blacks, being unheard of in native African blacks, and is very rare in Orientals.

A serum factor that impairs ciliary activity has been identified that perhaps contributes to progressive obstructive pulmonary disease associated with mucus plugging, atelectasis, and secondary infection. Autonomic nervous system dysfunction is one possible mechanism that has been postulated to explain the bizarre pattern of multisystem disease. Abnormal membrane permeability and calcium flux have been suggested because of elevated salivary calcium and phosphorus levels, as well as elevated sodium and chloride levels in sweat and saliva. The mucus secreted in the bronchial tree has a high viscosity, leading to inspissation with atelectasis, secondary infection, and eventual bronchiectasis. Common features are pancreatic achylia, fat malabsorption, and steatorrhea associated with malnutrition and failure to thrive, often from infancy. No single hypothesis has as yet reconciled the diverse clinical manifestations of cystic fibrosis.

Clinical Manifestations

Approximately 10 to 18 per cent of the affected infants present with meconium ileus in the neonatal period. More than 80 per cent have pancreatic achylia and resultant malabsorption of fat with frequent, bulky, greasy, foul-smelling stools that float; steatorrhea; and deficiency of fat-soluble vitamins A, D, and K. About 10 per cent have normal pancreatic function, and another 10 per cent have isolated enzyme defects. Rectal prolapse or acute abdominal pains occur in 15 to 20 per cent, together with failure to thrive. Patients also have daily cough and tenacious bronchial mucus.

The initial lesion is a bronchiolar obstruction caused by impacted mucus that results from increased mucus viscosity and abnormal bronchial ciliary activity. Secondary infection with *Staphylococcus aureus* and *Pseudomonas aeruginosa* supervenes, and bronchial secretions are subsequently permanently colonized. Widespread atelectasis occurs that is associated with the slow loss of lung volumes, a subsequent obstructive airway disease with distention of the chest, the appearance of cystlike shadows in upper lung fields, and a chest configuration suggesting COPD combined with patchy pneumonia. Bronchiectasis occurs and emphysema develops, but only focally. In later years, the pulmonary complications of chronic infection, pneumothorax, atelectasis, and repeated bouts of hemoptysis are the predominant clinical features, and the majority of patients die of respiratory infection or respiratory failure with cor pulmonale.

All patients have hypoxemia, and finger clubbing is almost universal. A focal fibrosis of the liver is common, but only 2 to 3 per cent of patients develop portal hypertension. Males are virtually 100 per cent aspermic and have fibrosed or absent vas deferens, 50 per cent abnormal sperm, and low sperm counts. Sinusitis and nasal polyps are very common. Several women with cystic fibrosis have borne children.

Diagnosis is usually made by identifying the presence of steatorrhea and malabsorption combined with a persistent cough and sputum production and an abnormal sweat test. The sweat test is performed by iontophoresis with pilocarpine into the sweat glands, followed by sweat electrolyte analysis. The mean sweat chloride in normals is 20 mEq. per liter, with a range of 5 to 60 mEq. per liter. The mean sweat chloride in patients with cystic fibrosis is 95 to 100 mEq. per liter, with a range of 50 to 120 mEq. per liter. The sweat test thus provides results with virtually no overlap between normals and patients with cystic fibrosis.

Treatment

Bronchial toilet with bronchodilators, expectorants, and postural drainage for all lobes twice a day and the chronic use of antibiotics have improved the prognosis and diminished the rate of respiratory function loss. Severe infections are usually caused by *Pseudomonas* organisms and respond to 10 to 14 day courses of gentamicin and carbenicillin. Gastrointestinal symptoms and malabsorption respond well to pancreatic enzyme replacement, using doses sufficient to control stool frequency and volume. Multivitamins are usually administered.

Prognosis

Death is invariably caused by respiratory failure or infection associated with common complications of repeated hemoptysis, pneumothorax, or lobar collapse due to mucoid impaction. With current treatment regimens, mortality has been reduced to 2 to 4 per cent per year, and 50 per cent of the patients survive beyond age 18.

REFERENCES

1. American Lung Association: Chronic Obstructive Pulmonary Disease—A Manual for Physicians. 4th Ed. New York, American Lung Assoc., 1973.
2. American Lung Association: Diagnostic Standards and Classification of Tuberculosis. Revised Ed. New York, American Lung Assoc., 1973.
3. Baum, G. L.: Textbook of Pulmonary Diseases. 2nd Ed. Boston, Little, Brown & Co., 1974.
4. Cherniack, R. M., Cherniack, L., and Naimark, A.: Respiration in Health and Disease. 2nd Ed. Philadelphia, W. B. Saunders Co., 1972.
5. Crofton, J., and Douglas, A.: Respiratory Diseases. 2nd Ed. London, Blackwell Scientific Publications, 1975.
6. Illingworth, R. S.: Common Diseases in Children. London, Blackwell Scientific Publications, 1975.
6a. Marsland, D. W., Wood, M., and Mayo, F.: Content of family practice. J. Fam. Prac., 3:37, 1976.
7. Morgan, W. K., and Seaton, A.: Occupational Lung Disease. Philadelphia, W. B. Saunders Co., 1975.
8. West, J. B.: Respiratory Physiology—The Essentials. Baltimore, Williams & Wilkins Co., 1974.
9. Williams, H. E., and Phelan, P. D. Respiratory Illness in Children. London, Blackwell Scientific Publications, 1975.

Chapter 46

GASTROENTEROLOGY

by JOHN D. BARKER, JR.,
and LARRY LAWHORNE

This chapter is divided into sections discussing common gastrointestinal disorders frequently seen by the primary physician. No attempt has been made to turn this chapter into a synopsis of gastroenterology. Rather, we have selected for discussion those gastrointestinal complaints and diseases that we feel the family physician will encounter. Certain diseases have been omitted, either because of their rarity or because they are discussed elsewhere in this text. At the end of the chapter are selected references for the further understanding of gastroenterology. They are grouped by topic for easy reference.

THE APPROACH TO THE PATIENT WITH GASTROINTESTINAL DISEASE

Today, most physicians have at their disposal an impressive array of complex diagnostic gastrointestinal procedures that would have confused the practitioner of 30 years past. But with this technological advancement comes the danger of physicians' becoming too reliant on glamorous procedures and techniques in dealing with the gastroenterology patient. This must not occur. There is still no substitute for a thorough history and physical examination.

When obtaining the history, the physician must be sure that he and the patient are speaking the same language. As the level of patient sophistication changes, so do their definitions of words such as indigestion, heartburn, gas, or diarrhea. Indigestion, a common gastrointestinal complaint, can be a symptom of many disorders ranging from an acute myocardial infarction to a dietary indiscretion. The physician must be sure of

what the patient is telling him. He should gently guide the patient toward a precise description of his symptoms and then try to relate this description to the events that occur within the gastrointestinal tract. Emphasis should be placed on the timing of complaints as they relate to meals, the patient's activity, the ingestion of certain foods, the time of day, and defecation patterns.

The interaction of organic gastrointestinal disease and emotional factors contributes to the complexity of many patient histories in gastroenterology. The gastrointestinal tract is a prominent target organ for anxiety, depression, the daily stress of living, and even more severe forms of emotional disease. Sorting out the functional from the organic components of gastrointestinal complaints takes skill and a basic understanding of normal gastrointestinal physiology.

The examination of the abdomen is the most important part of the physical examination in gastroenterology patients. The examiner should adhere to a precise ritual, making full use of inspection, auscultation, palpation, and percussion, similar to the examination of the cardiovascular system. Armed with a proper understanding of the historical data and possessing a pathophysiologic approach to gastrointestinal disease, the physician will commit few errors if the abdominal examination is performed in a manner similar to that outlined in Table 46–1. Remember that the digital rectal examination, bimanual pelvic examination, testing of the stool for occult blood, and sigmoidoscopy are standard components of the abdominal examination.

In gastroenterology, numerous special

TABLE 46-1. OUTLINE OF THE ABDOMINAL EXAMINATION

1. Inspection: contour, scars, striae, masses, visible peristalsis, veins, body hair pattern, umbilicus, flanks, abdominal distention
2. Auscultation: bowel sounds, vascular bruits and hums, peritoneal and hepatic friction rubs
3. Palpation: light and deep palpation; tenderness; rebound tenderness; muscular spasm—voluntary and involuntary; rigidity; organ size, shape and consistency; masses; ascites; hernia; defects and tenderness of the abdominal wall; femoral pulses
4. Percussion: liver span, loops of bowel, shifting dullness, diaphragm location and mobility, fist percussion for hepatic tenderness
5. Special tests and maneuvers: iliopsoas test, obturator test, puddle sign, Murphy's sign
6. Bimanual pelvic examination: tenderness, cervix, uterus, adnexa, Douglas' pouch, masses
7. Digital rectal examination: prostate, masses, rectal shelf, mucosal texture, stool consistency
8. Test stool for occult blood
9. Sigmoidoscopy

tests and procedures are available to confirm objectively the lesion or the pathogenesis responsible for the patient's complaints and physical findings. First, try to utilize noninvasive tests such as plain x-ray views of the chest or abdomen and stool analysis. The majority of the more complicated invasive procedures seldom are helpful unless a specific lesion or diagnosis is suspected prior to the test. Although many patients with gastrointestinal disease will need a barium enema examination and an upper gastrointestinal radiographic series because of vague symptoms and a long differential diagnosis, specific reasons for doing these studies should be demanded. Avoid allowing the radiologist to make a diagnosis for you and altering your impressions to fit the radiologic findings. Many errors occur when one treats x-rays instead of patients.

Management of gastrointestinal disease must not be only symptomatic treatment. Too often a pill is given for nausea or paregoric is prescribed for diarrhea with no thought to the underlying mechanisms of that particular symptom. The average physician usually knows what to do. The outstanding physician understands why. Knowing why means understanding basic pathophysiology, the key to success in the diagnosis and management of patients with diseases of the gastrointestinal tract.

CHRONIC ABDOMINAL PAIN

The evaluation and management of patients with chronic abdominal pain is as challenging as and more frequently encountered than the management of an acute abdomen. The differential diagnosis of chronic abdominal pain is nearly endless. Pain sensed in the abdomen may not be of abdominal origin. Diseases of the thoracic cavity, abnormalities of the thoracic and lumbar spine, disease within the retroperitoneal space, irritation or defects of the muscular and cutaneous coats of the abdominal wall, disorders of the central and peripheral nervous system, abnormalities of the musculoskeletal system, and general metabolic or systemic diseases all can cause chronic abdominal pain.

Abdominal pain is purely subjective. There are no useful ways to objectively measure or quantify abdominal pain. The physician must rely totally on the patient's description of the pain. Therefore, during the initial evaluation, the physician must have the patient characterize the pain as precisely as possible. Table 46-2 lists components of abdominal pain that may help characterize the pain.

A careful description of the pain is necessary because the anatomic pathways and

TABLE 46-2. CHARACTERIZING ABDOMINAL PAIN

1. Quality: dull, boring, aching, gnawing, lightning-like, cutting, stabbing
2. Severity: takes breath away, doubles one over, annoying
3. Location: point with one finger to area of pain; if diffuse, from where does it originate
4. Referral: shoulder, back, scrotum, thigh, chest, neck
5. Timing: constant, intermittent, night pain, before breakfast, before or after meals, menstrual cycles, bowel movements, daily pattern
6. Duration: seconds, hours, days, comes in waves, steady
7. Special times of occurrence: how does pain relate to normal daily gastrointestinal functions—eating, swallowing, belching, flatus, defecation, physical activity, body position
8. Aggravating factors: position, meals, defecation, emotion, movement, lying still
9. Relieving factors: position, meals, defecation, emotion, movement, lying still
10. Associated symptoms: flatulence, distention, abdominal noises, nausea, vomiting, salivation, regurgitation, sweating, pallor, diarrhea, skin rashes, drugs, previous surgery, certain foods, weight loss

neurophysiology of pain fibers within the abdomen are complex and poorly understood. Pain patterns and associations must be used to construct differential diagnoses. Although differentiating visceral from parietal pain is helpful in the patient with an acute abdomen, the distinguishing features of these pains tend to become fused and clinically difficult to separate when the abdominal pain is chronic.

No matter how clinically astute the physician is, his history and physical examination alone cannot make a definite diagnosis of the cause of the chronic abdominal pain. A good guess from a well constructed differential diagnosis can be made, but must be confirmed objectively. For example, a patient may have classic symptoms of the irritable bowel syndrome, but in addition have a carcinoma of the colon as well. The irritable bowel complaints may completely mask any symptoms caused by the malignancy. On the other hand, to totally ignore the history and physical examination and rely exclusively on diagnostic tests also can lead to errors. Such practice can result in treating patients for a hiatal hernia or sigmoid diverticula, which were demonstrated radiographically, when in fact the abdominal pain has an entirely different cause.

What do you do with patients whose evaluation for chronic abdominal pain leads nowhere? Data from the history and physical examination fit no pathophysiologic pattern. The differential diagnosis is difficult to construct. An extensive radiographic and laboratory search has yielded no clues. At this point consider the differential diagnosis listed in Table 46-3.

Abdominal wall pain mimics the symptoms of many serious causes of chronic abdominal pain. It is more common than generally appreciated, and the pathogenesis is obscure. Surgical scars can heal with persistent tender areas. The intercostal nerve of a lower rib may become entrapped within the costal cartilage, spreading pain into the upper abdomen. Small muscular defects in the midline of the abdominal wall or along the lateral border of the rectus muscle may allow the formation of ventral hernias. Surgical scars may overlie small ventral hernias.

Most abdominal wall pain is constant, aching, and accentuated by sudden move-

TABLE 46–3. SUGGESTED DIFFERENTIAL DIAGNOSIS OF CHRONIC ABDOMINAL PAIN WHEN THOROUGH EVALUATION IS NEGATIVE

1. Abdominal wall pain
2. Occult neoplasms, particularly of pancreatic origin
3. Irritable bowel syndrome
4. Functional pain
5. A condition overlooked in the initial differential diagnosis or a disease in its early stages that is difficult to recognize

ments or by putting pressure on the painful area. On physical examination, the tenderness is more intense when the abdominal muscles are contracted. Ask the patient to hold his head or legs off the examining table while you palpate his abdomen. If intra-abdominal disease is present, this maneuver diminishes the tenderness, but it accentuates abdominal wall pain. A ventral hernia may be felt when the abdominal wall musculature is tensed or when the patient is standing.

Reassure the patient that no intra-abdominal pathology exists. Infiltration of the painful area with local anesthetic may give relief. A rib belt may ease the pain of an irritated intercostal nerve. Have a surgeon examine the patient if you suspect a ventral hernia. A patient with abdominal wall pain deserves close follow-up to be sure that the abdominal wall tenderness is not masking another condition.

Carcinoma of the pancreas occasionally causes vague chronic abdominal pain. It is a difficult malignancy to demonstrate because the pancreas is inaccessible to most standard diagnostic procedures. Chronic abdominal pain is frequently the only manifestation of the tumor. It is a dull, deep-seated, boring pain, usually located in the epigastrium or the left upper quadrant, with referred pain traveling straight through to the mid-back region or occasionally to the left shoulder. Some patients obtain relief by drawing their knees toward their chest. The pain tends to change in character when adjacent structures near or within the gland become involved with the malignancy. There is usually associated weight loss, which can be extreme. One reason the diagnosis can be overlooked is that the constant aggravating nature of the discomfort can provoke other functional-sounding complaints, depression, and despair, which cause the patient to appear neurotic.

The irritable bowel syndrome is responsible for more cases of unexplained chronic abdominal pain than any other cause, and its manifestations are protean. It will be discussed at length later in this chapter.

Could the abdominal pain be emotional or functional? Some people do over-react to normal daily gastrointestinal function, which they interpret as abdominal pain, and then expand it out of proportion because of their emotional make-up. The pain may be a shifting pain or an "all-over" pain that is either difficult for the patient to describe or described in a bizarre manner. It may be unbearable for several consecutive days. Serious organic causes of pain can elicit similar pathologic emotional responses. When a patient's abdominal pain is labeled as functional, careful observation should continue to be sure that this diagnosis is correct.

Finally, the physician must remember that the cause of the chronic abdominal pain may be a condition that he has not included in his differential diagnosis or some disease in an early stage that is difficult to recognize. He may not appreciate this until he has evaluated the patient on several different occasions. During these return visits, the physician must remain as objective and open-minded as possible and must not be inflexible about changing his impressions or the differential diagnosis. If after several visits the patient's pain remains unrelieved and unexplained, a consultation with another physician is in order for fresh ideas and a new approach to this patient. It probably is better to get another opinion prior to any extensive in-hospital evaluation.

ACUTE DIARRHEA

The sudden onset of diarrhea in a previously healthy individual usually is a mild, self-limited disease. Most of these acute diarrheal states are a result of nonspecific infections, presumably viral in origin. Only if the symptoms of acute diarrhea are particularly severe or persistent do patients seek medical assistance.

Some cases of acute diarrhea are not caused by viruses, are not self-limited, and

TABLE 46-4. EVALUATION OF ACUTE DIARRHEA

1. History and physical examination: ask about recent travel, medications, contact with people with diarrheal disease, recent food consumption, previous history of diarrhea
2. Routine blood studies: look for leukocytosis, eosinophilia, serum electrolyte abnormalities, anemia—all implying a more severe disease
3. Stool guaiac test: a positive test suggests inflammation, infection, or neoplasm
4. Stool leukocytes: if present—inflammatory bowel disease and bacterial infections that invade the mucosa are likely causes; if absent—viral disease, parasites, or the irritable bowel syndrome are the most likely causes
5. Sigmoidoscopy: do *without* prepping the bowel with cleansing enemas, take stool samples, scrape and biopsy abnormal mucosa
6. Stool examination for ova and parasites: several fresh stool specimens must be examined
7. Gram's stain of stool: staphylococcal and monilial overgrowth can be recognized

are potentially serious. These are the conditions that must be sought in the evaluation of the patient with acute diarrhea. Most serious conditions can be diagnosed by means of a complete history and physical examination and a few simple tests. One approach to the evaluation is shown in Figure 46-1. While attempting to find the cause of the acute diarrhea, give the patient good supportive care. If the patient is very young or elderly or if there are signs of toxicity, fever, or dehydration, hospitalization usually is necessary.

Every patient with acute diarrhea should undergo the diagnostic tests listed in Table 46-4. Although negative results are common, it is necessary to perform these tests in order to discover those potentially serious causes of the diarrhea. A differential diagnosis of acute diarrhea seen in patients living in the United States can be found in Table 46-5.

TABLE 46-5. ACUTE DIARRHEA— DIFFERENTIAL DIAGNOSIS

Infections: shigellosis, salmonellosis, amebiasis, giardiasis, viral and nonspecific gastroenteritis, traveler's diarrhea

Toxic: food poisoning—*Staphylococcus, Clostridium perfringens*

Drug-induced: antibiotics, especially lincomycin, clindamycin; some antacids, colchicine, antihypertensive agents, quinidine

Other causes: inflammatory bowel disease, pseudomembranous colitis

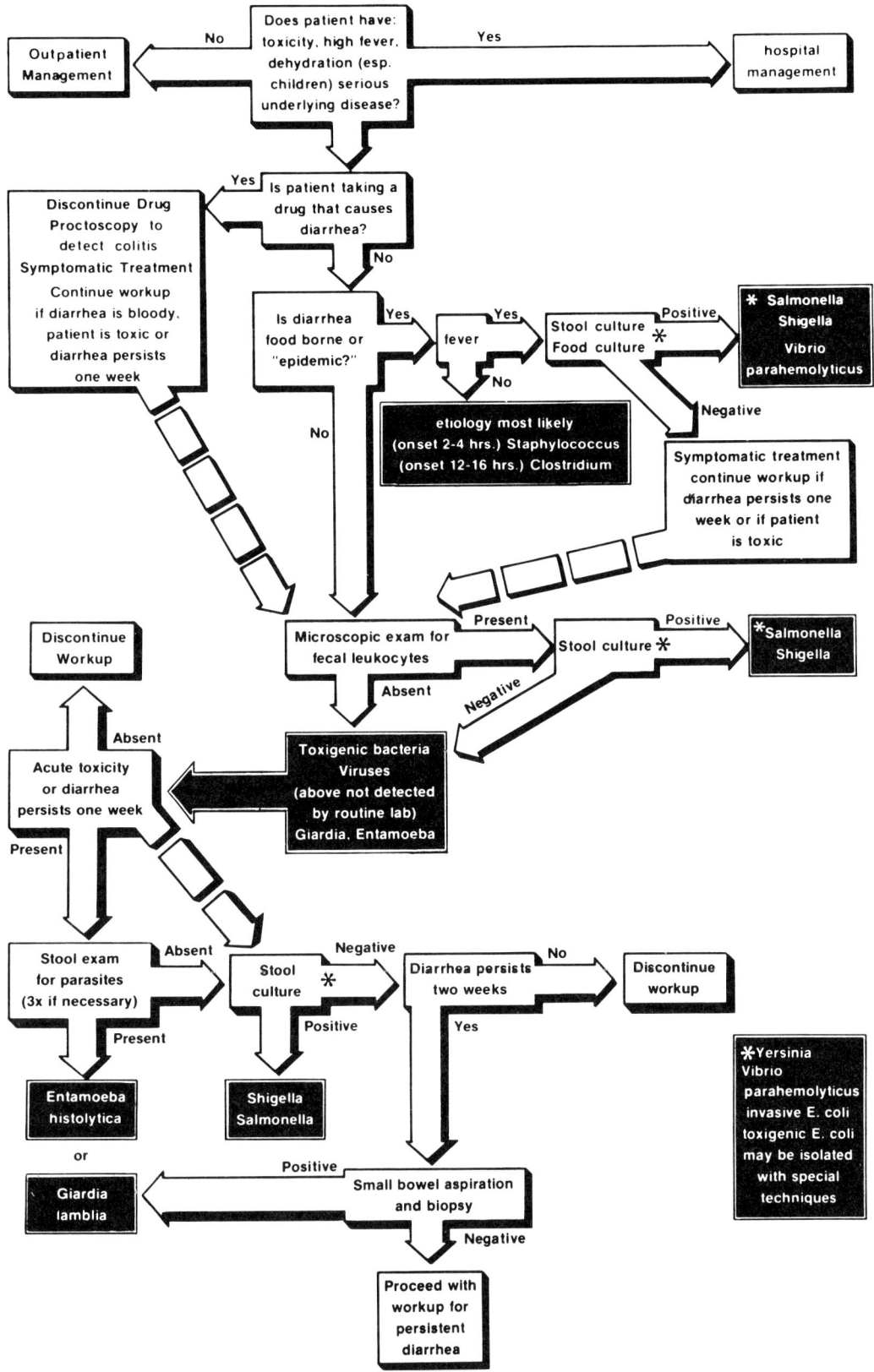

The patient with acute diarrhea.

Figure 46–1. An algorithm for diagnosing the patient with acute diarrhea. (From Satterwhite, T. K., and Du-Pont, H. L.: J.A.M.A., 236:2663, 1976. Copyright 1976 The American Medical Association.)

The sigmoidoscopic examination is a simple way to rule out generalized colonic mucosal disease as a cause for the acute diarrhea. A normal examination eliminates shigellosis, acute ulcerative colitis, salmonellosis, and amebiasis from the differential diagnosis. The mucosal inflammation caused by these diseases is recognized easily at sigmoidoscopy. Unfortunately, it usually is impossible to distinguish these diseases from one another by the sigmoidoscopic appearance. Further testing is necessary.

The stool leukocyte count is an excellent screening test for patients with acute diarrhea. Leukocytes appear in the stool in association with bacterial infections that invade the mucosa and with other inflammatory diseases of the colon, such as ulcerative colitis. Stool leukocytes are absent in viral or parasitic diseases.

Stool cultures can document a bacterial cause for the acute diarrhea. Stool for culture must be handled carefully and expediently. The *Shigella* organisms are very fragile. If the stool is not immediately plated onto culture media, pathogenic bacteria may not survive.

Have someone trained in stool parasitology examine fresh stool specimens for the presence of ova or parasites. Several stool samples collected at different times should be examined. Warm stage examination of stool for ameba is best done from material scraped off the mucosa at the time of sigmoidoscopy.

Since most causes of acute diarrhea are either infectious or toxic or are due to medication, an extensive history into these areas may help in making the diagnosis. Make sure that the diarrhea is not related to a food poisoning incident. Obtain a good travel history. Giardiasis is endemic in certain areas of Colorado and parts of the Soviet Union. Traveler's diarrhea may occur during any foreign travel. Antibiotic treatment can initiate diarrhea by altering the bacterial flora of the bowel, allowing a resistant organism to populate the bowel, or by some toxic effect on the colonic mucosa, as seen with the use of clindamycin or lincomycin.

The majority of evaluations for acute diarrhea have few positive findings. If the diarrhea is not self-limited and if the acute diarrhea evaluation is negative, approach the patient as someone with chronic diarrhea.

CHRONIC DIARRHEA

Diarrhea is the result of intestinal failure. It may be a failure of digestion, absorption, water and electrolyte transport, motility, or other intestinal functions. The localization and type of disease process in the intestinal tract enormously influence the pattern of diarrhea. Diarrhea is a nonspecific symptom caused by a variety of different diseases.

Steatorrhea

Failure of small bowel mucosal function causes malabsorption. Large amounts of residual small bowel contents escape in the stools. The stools contain unabsorbed dietary fat, giving them a bulky, frothy, greasy, malodorous quality. The diarrhea of malabsorption may be subtle. The patient may have only one or two bowel movements a day, but each movement is of considerable volume. The diarrhea does not cause the patient to seek medical help as much as do the secondary manifestations of malabsorption, such as weight loss, weakness, metabolic bone disease, and blood coagulation abnormalities.

The evaluation and management of malabsorption are complex. Documenting steatorrhea is the family physician's main goal prior to referring the patient to a general internist or a gastroenterologist. Only a quantitative 72 hour stool fat determination can document steatorrhea precisely. If screening tests for intestinal absorptive function (Table 46–6) are abnormal, proceed with this quantitative test (Table 46–7).

Steatorrhea and other signs and symptoms of small bowel diseases also are seen in maldigestive states in which the mucosal function remains normal. Maldigestion can occur from a deficiency of pancreatic secretions, as in chronic pancreatitis; from a lack of sufficient bile salts within the small bowel lumen; or from poor mixing of the chyme with digestive secretions as frequently occurs after partial gastrectomy with a Billroth II gastrojejunostomy. Although steatorrhea has many causes, documenting its presence is a big step toward finding the cause of the patient's diarrhea.

TABLE 46-6. SCREENING TESTS FOR INTESTINAL ABSORPTION AND DIGESTION

Serum Carotene:
  >70 micrograms per 100 ml.—normal
  30–70 micrograms per 100 ml.—may indicate malabsorption, maldigestion, generalized malnutrition,
    poor dietary intake, chronic disease
  <30 micrograms per 100 ml.—suggestive of maldigestion

Qualitative Stool Fat Analysis:
  Patient must have >60 grams of fat per day oral intake
  Stain stool suspension with Sudan III
    Increased fatty acids—malabsorption
    Increased neutral fats—maldigestion
    Presence of meat fibers—maldigestion

D-Xylose Absorption Test:
  Oral load—25 grams
  Measure urinary excretions for 5 hours or measure blood levels
    Normal >4.5 grams per 5 hours urinary excretion or >30 mg. % increase in blood level
    ↓—malabsorption; normal in maldigestion
    False ↓—incomplete urine collection, renal failure, ascites, blind loop syndrome

Gastrointestinal X-rays of Small Bowel:
  Structural mucosal abnormalities of small bowel
  Malabsorptive pattern
  Very nonspecific—many false negative examinations

Chronic Diarrhea of Colonic Origin

Diseases of the colon, particularly of the sigmoid colon and rectum, cause a type of diarrhea in which bowel movements may occur quite frequently, but each movement produces only small amounts of stool. The stool particles may be only small bits and pieces accompanied by liquid, mucus, pus, blood, or flatus. The bowel movements frequently relieve any lower abdominal cramping. The usual causes of this type of diarrheal pattern are motility disorders of the distal colon, such as diverticular disease and the irritable bowel syndrome, or inflammatory disorders involving the colon, such as ulcerative and granulomatous colitis and bacterial and parasitic infections The passage of blood with the stools implies an inflammatory, neoplastic, or infectious cause. Large amounts of mucus in the stools are present in motility disorders, particularly the irritable bowel syndrome. Transi-

TABLE 46-7. QUANTITATIVE 72 HOUR
STOOL FAT ANALYSIS

100 gram fat diet for 6 days
Collect all stools for last 3 days of diet period

Normal <5 grams of fat per 24 hours
More fecal fat excretion in maldigestion than in malabsorption, although both disorders cause gross abnormalities of fecal fat excretion

ent diarrheal states, such as viral gastroenteritis, can exacerbate a mild, underlying irritable bowel syndrome. Failure to fully recover from nonspecific gastroenteritis because it has exacerbated an underlying irritable bowel syndrome is a common cause of chronic, unexplained diarrhea.

Inflammatory Bowel Disease

The terminology of inflammatory bowel disease can be confusing. Table 46–8 lists a suggested classification. These are chronic diseases with protean manifestations encompassing a wide spectrum of complexity and severity. Many patients can be managed or at least coordinated by the family physician. He is in the best position to offer long-term supportive care.

Ulcerative Colitis. Ulcerative colitis is the most common chronic inflammatory disease of the colon in the United States. Its cause remains unknown. It afflicts patients of all ages but commonly has its onset in early adulthood. Diffuse inflammatory changes involve the rectum plus variable amounts of the colon proximal to the rectum, always in continuity. This inflammatory process makes that colonic mucosa congested, granular, friable, and highly vascular. (Only on microscopic examination does the colonic mucosa appear ulcerated.) Chronic involvement leaves the colon atrophic and scarred.

TABLE 46–8. CLASSIFICATION OF INFLAMMATORY BOWEL DISEASE

Ulcerative Colitis: predominantly mucosal disease confined to the colon, nearly always involves rectum, with involvement extending continuously to variable areas of remainder of the proximal colon

Pancolonic Ulcerative Colitis: entire colon involved with the inflammatory process

Backwash Ileitis: may be seen with pancolitis; disease extends a short distance into terminal ileum; terminal ileum appears dilated and featureless on retrograde filling during barium enema examination

Ulcerative Proctitis: mild form of the disease, inflammation limited to the rectum

Crohn's Disease: a transmural inflammatory disease of entire intestinal tract from mouth to anus; terminal ileum commonly involved with disease; skip areas of disease fairly frequent

Regional Enteritis: Crohn's disease limited to the small bowel

Granulomatous Colitis: Crohn's disease limited to large bowel

Crohn's Ileocolitis: Crohn's disease involving both large and small bowel

Bloody diarrhea is the predominant clinical symptom, abdominal cramps being of secondary importance to most patients with ulcerative colitis. The diarrhea results from the impairment of the normal colon function of water and electrolyte conservation; the rectal bleeding results from the vascular inflammation of the mucosa. The severity of the symptoms relates mainly to the amount of colon involvement. Those with total colonic involvement generally have a more severe course of the disease. With severe ulcerative colitis, systemic symptoms can predominate, particularly fever, hypoproteinemia, malnutrition, and anemia.

Sigmoidoscopy is diagnostic if bacterial and amebic infections can be ruled out. The rectal mucosa is always diffusely involved. The acute changes are congestion, diffuse granularity of the mucosa resembling a fine grade of sandpaper, purulent exudate, and friability. Friability is demonstrated by gently wiping the mucosa with a cotton swab and then watching for multiple pinpoint areas of bleeding. The more chronic changes are a blunting of the normally sharp rectal valves and a dullness to the mucosa through which the normal vascular pattern is not seen.

The barium enema examination is used to judge the extent of the disease. It need not be done initially to make the diagnosis. Frequently, early in the course of mild to moderate ulcerative colitis the barium enema study is normal.

The disease is one of exacerbations and remissions. The goal of medical management is to induce and sustain a remission. Corticosteroids help to induce a remission during a symptomatic phase. Once symptoms have abated and the changes in the rectal mucosa seen at sigmoidoscopy are no longer acute, gradually reduce the dose of the corticosteroids. They are not helpful during periods of remission. Sulfasalazine is effective in sustaining remissions. Two to 4 grams of sulfasalazine per day should be taken indefinitely by patients with ulcerative colitis.

COMPLICATIONS. The major complications of ulcerative colitis are toxic megacolon and carcinoma of the colon. The former is a complication of the severity of, the latter a complication of the duration of the disease.

Toxic megacolon frequently develops in acute fulminant cases of ulcerative colitis. The pathogenesis is poorly understood. The inflammatory process extends through the entire thickness of the wall of the colon, allowing dilatation to occur as the colon loses its muscular tone. This process usually affects the transverse colon. Toxic megacolon is a medical emergency, and many patients require immediate total colectomy. Mortality is high. Some cases of toxic megacolon probably are preventable. In patients with moderately severe symptoms of acute ulcerative colitis, a barium enema examination, a vigorous bowel preparation prior to the barium enema, or the use of opiates, including diphenoxylate with atropine (Lomotil), and all forms of anticholinergic medications may be instrumental in the development of a toxic megacolon. These medications are contraindicated in the management of ulcerative colitis. A barium enema study should not be performed during the acute stages of the disease.

The risk of cancer of the colon is much greater in patients with ulcerative colitis than in the general population. The risk is proportional to the duration of the disease and the extent of the colonic involvement. In patients whose entire colon has been diseased with ulcerative colitis for more than 10 years, the risk becomes significant enough to warrant prophylactic colectomy.

Ulcerative Proctitis. Ulcerative proctitis is a mild form of ulcerative colitis. Mucosal involvement rarely extends beyond the rectum. At sigmoidoscopy, one is able to pass the instrument beyond the proximal extent of involvement. Administration of corticosteroids per rectum helps to reduce inflammation and promote remissions in this form of ulcerative colitis. Patients with ulcerative proctitis have a brighter outlook. The disease does not progress to other areas of the colon, and no increased risk of carcinoma occurs.

Crohn's Disease. Crohn's disease can involve any part of the intestinal tract from the mouth to the anus. The presenting symptoms are more variable than those of ulcerative colitis. Diarrhea is usually of secondary importance compared with the abdominal pain and cramps caused by this disease. Patients can present with complaints of having many months of vague symptoms not necessarily related to the gastrointestinal tract. Fever, weight loss, arthritis, perirectal abscesses, or weakness may be the predominant symptoms.

Pathologically, a chronic inflammatory process involves the entire bowel wall and the surrounding mesentery and lymph nodes. The bowel wall is thickened and edematous, which narrows the lumen, causing stricture formation. The mucosa has a cobblestone appearance because of deep transverse and longitudinal fissure-ulcers. Abscesses and fistulas between the bowel and adjacent structures are common.

The diagnosis of Crohn's disease is more dependent on radiographic contrast studies of the bowel than is ulcerative colitis. The rectum frequently is free of disease. Proctoscopic abnormalities may be limited to the perianal region (fistulas, perianal abscesses, fissures), a common site of involvement with Crohn's disease. The barium enema study and small bowel series demonstrate a variety of changes. The thickened loops of bowel are separated from adjacent loops; the lumen is narrowed, the bowel

proximal to the narrowed segments is dilated; the mucosa may have a cobblestone appearance; mucosal folds are blunted, irregular, and ulcerated; and ulcers extend deep into the wall of the bowel. Skip areas of disease interposed with normal bowel are characteristic. The most common areas of the bowel involved with Crohn's disease are the terminal ileum, cecum, and ascending colon. If the disease is limited to the colon, the involvement is far more excessive in the right colon than further distally.

Management of Crohn's disease can be a true test of a physician's ability. The total patient must be looked after, using a combination of medical, surgical, and emotional support. Remissions and exacerbations are not as obvious as with ulcerative colitis. The course is more steadily chronic. The inflammation is controlled with corticosteroids and sulfasalazine. A multicenter cooperative study of the treatment of Crohn's disease has shown that there is some benefit from these drugs. Azathioprine is not helpful and should not be used. Surgical therapy is reserved for complications of the disease, such as intestinal obstruction and abscess formation, which are not uncommon. Removal of diseased bowel is not curative because of the high postsurgical recurrence rate. Close attention must be paid to keeping the patients' nutrition as adequate as possible. Routinely give folate and multiple vitamins. Patients with Crohn's disease involving the terminal ileum usually require parenteral vitamin B_{12}. Encourage reasonable dietary habits. A frequent problem is bile salt diarrhea due to ileal involvement with the disease. Cholestyramine therapy can improve the symptoms of bile salt diarrhea in many of these patients.

Although the course of the disease may be depressingly chronic, the long-term prognosis for Crohn's disease is not that grim. The risk of carcinoma is far less than with ulcerative colitis. With proper medical management of the chronic inflammation and with the judicious use of surgical therapy for complications of the disease, patients with Crohn's disease can lead long, productive lives.

Secretory Diarrhea

Abnormalities of intestinal secretion are rare but severe causes of diarrhea. Specialized secretory cells abound in the stomach, which is primarily a secretory organ. Although overshadowed by absorptive cells, specialized secretory cells also are present in the small and large bowel. What normal function they play is unknown. Secretory diarrhea occurs when the function of these cells accelerates at unchecked rates.

The Zollinger-Ellison syndrome can produce a secretory diarrhea in addition to an acid peptic disease diathesis. In this condition, the massive amount of fluid and acid secreted by the stomach overwhelms the absorptive capacity of the small and large bowel, resulting in a secretory diarrhea.

The enterotoxin elaborated by *Vibrio cholerae* stimulates adenyl cyclase of small bowel secretory cells, causing high intracellular levels of adenosine 3',5' monophosphate (cyclic AMP) and marked functional overactivity by these cells. The large amount of fluid that is secreted overwhelms the still intact absorptive capacity of the small bowel and a characteristic watery secretory diarrhea results. A similar syndrome can be caused by a pancreatic islet cell neoplasm producing a hormone, possibly vasoactive intestinal polypeptide (VIP), that also has the capacity to maximally stimulate small bowel secretory cells.

Large villous adenomas of the colon can secrete enough fluid to produce a similar secretory diarrheal picture.

Stool volumes are large in patients with secretory diarrhea; more than several liters of watery stool per day are not unusual. A secretory diarrhea will continue unaffected after having the patient fast for more than 24 hours.

Bile Salt Diarrhea

Bile salts play a major role in facilitating fat absorption. Above certain minimal intraluminal concentrations, bile salts aggregate into micelles, which aid in keeping fatty acids and monoglycerides in suspension within the lumen of the small bowel.

Bile salts are produced from cholesterol in the liver. Efficient active reabsorption of bile salts occurs in the ileum, so that only a small fraction are lost with the stools each day. The remainder recirculate via the enterohepatic circulation.

Surgical resection or disease of the terminal ileum compromises this efficient system. More bile salts are lost in the stools.

The liver compensates for this loss by manufacturing increased amounts of bile salts to reach a new steady state. Fat absorption remains normal. However, the nonabsorbed bile salts in the colon tend to impair water and electrolyte absorption and can cause a watery diarrhea. This complication is encountered frequently in Crohn's disease involving the terminal ileum. Cholestyramine, an ion-binding resin, is effective treatment for bile salt diarrhea. It binds the bile salts and prevents them from impairing colonic absorptive function.

If the ileal disease or resection is extensive, large amounts of bile salts are lost in the stools, exceeding the liver's capacity to produce an adequate amount. Fat malabsorption occurs. Cholestyramine is of no benefit in this condition.

Osmotic Diarrhea

The ingestion of some poorly absorbable substances creates osmotic diarrhea. These substances are osmotically active during their passage through the bowel, retarding normal water and electrolyte absorption. Diarrhea results. Osmotic diarrhea ceases with fasting.

Lactase deficiency is a common clinical example of osmotic diarrhea. Patients with this disorder have an isolated small bowel mucosal deficiency of lactase, the disaccharidase that splits lactose into the monosaccharides glucose and galactose prior to absorption. Lactose is nonabsorbable. Ingestion of milk and milk products, the primary dietary sources of lactose, causes abdominal distention, cramps, and diarrhea because of the osmotic effect of the nonabsorbed lactose within the intestinal lumen. The diagnosis can be made by obtaining a good dietary history. Patients totally lacking lactase can have symptoms merely from the milk they put in their coffee or on their breakfast cereal.

Primary lactase deficiency seems to be hereditary but is symptomatic only after adolescence. It is very common in blacks, Indians, and Spanish Americans.

An acquired lactase deficiency can occur with a variety of gastrointestinal disorders that injure the small bowel mucosa. This enzyme occupies a position near the tips of the microvilli and easily can be lost by inflammatory small bowel diseases such as Crohn's disease, celiac sprue, and nonspecific gastroenteritis. Lactase function rapidly recovers as the primary disease improves.

Measuring a rise in blood glucose levels after an oral lactose load (lactose tolerance test) or assaying a small bowel biopsy specimen for lactase activity are objective ways to confirm this diagnosis. Obviously, avoidance of milk products is effective therapy.

CONSTIPATION, IRRITABLE BOWEL SYNDROME, AND DIVERTICULAR DISEASE

Constipation

Patients have a variety of definitions for constipation. No matter if they suffer from hard stools, straining during bowel movements, infrequent stools, stools of small volume, or the sensation of incomplete evacuation, the complaint is constipation. Table 46–9 contains a partial list of the more common causes of constipation. In most patients, chronic constipation is the result of either the irritable bowel syndrome or habitual constipation.

Defective rectal emptying leads to the disorder of habitual constipation. These

TABLE 46–9. SOME CAUSES OF CONSTIPATION

Habitual constipation: defective defecation reflexes, poor bowel habits

Fecal impaction: complication of habitual constipation, more frequent in the aged, dehydration a contributing factor

Motility disorders of the large intestine: irritable bowel syndrome, diverticular disease, scleroderma, pregnancy, Hirschsprung's disease

Psychiatric illness

Laxative abuse

Constipating medications: opiates, ganglionic blocking agents, antidepressants, aluminum hydroxide antacids, sedatives, many others

Local rectal disease causing painful defecation: hemorrhoids, fissures, fistulas, rectal prolapse

Partially obstructing lesions of the colon: carcinoma, extrinsic lesions

Neurologic disorders: paraplegia, multiple sclerosis, parkinsonism

Endocrine and metabolic disorders: hypothyroidism, dehydration, hyperparathyroidism

TABLE 46–10. GENERAL MANAGEMENT OF CONSTIPATION

1. Rule out other causes of constipation in addition to the irritable bowel syndrome and habitual constipation by a thorough history and physical examination, an extensive medication history, routine blood studies, stool guaiac determination, sigmoidoscopy, barium enema examination, and upper gastrointestinal radiographic series
2. Discontinue all laxatives
3. Eliminate fecal impaction if present by digital disintegration and soapsuds enema
4. Treat any irritating local lesions of the anus and rectum
5. Increase fluid intake
6. Increase bulk in the diet and supplement with bulk-forming laxatives such as psyllium hydrophilic mucilloid (Metamucil, Konsyl)
7. Re-establish a regular time for bowel movements—have the patient sit at stool each day for 10 to 15 minutes after breakfast in a leisurely fashion to retrain his bowels
8. Reassure the patient of his benign condition and how this type of management takes many weeks before he will notice beneficial effects

patients let their life situations interfere with normal bowel function. After years of improper bowel habits and reliance on a variety of laxative preparations, their defecation reflexes become so atonic and their constipation so severe that they seek medical attention. These patients rarely have a normal bowel movement without the aid of a laxative. Being chronically constipated has become their way of life. Impactions can form from dehydrated stool being retained for days in the rectum or sigmoid colon.

Constipation due to the irritable bowel syndrome is caused by a colonic motility disorder that limits proper filling of the rectum with feces. The stool that reaches the rectum is of insufficient volume to provoke a proper defecation reflex. These patients may sit at the stool several times a day but never have a bowel movement of any considerable volume.

Other causes of constipation may occur in patients already suffering from the irritable bowel syndrome or habitual constipation and may magnify the symptoms. All possible causes of constipation, whether primarily causing the constipation or secondarily adding to the symptoms of the irritable bowel syndrome, must be sought before proper management can occur. Table 46–10 offers some suggestions for the management of constipation.

Irritable Bowel Syndrome

The irritable bowel syndrome accounts for 30 to 50 per cent of patients with gastrointestinal complaints seen by the family physician. Although it has a number of synonyms, of which several imply a psychiatric cause (nervous diarrhea, colonic neurosis, functional bowel), the irritable bowel syndrome is not an emotional disease. The colon is a frequent target for the physical effects of stress, anxiety, and neurosis. Because of some poorly defined motility disturbance of the large bowel, patients with the irritable bowel syndrome respond in an exaggerated manner to common life stresses, giving the impression that their bowel disease is caused by emotion. Anxiety, neurosis, and depression certainly magnify the symptoms of the irritable bowel syndrome but are not responsible for the basic motility disturbance underlying the disorder. Other older terms for the irritable bowel syndrome (mucous colitis, spastic colitis) imply an inflammatory process. This is not true. There is no inflammation. The word colitis should not be used when describing the syndrome of the irritable bowel.

Patients with the irritable bowel syndrome have abnormal intestinal motility. Their colonic motor activity is exaggerated and less coordinated in response to a variety of normal stimuli, such as eating, stress, certain drugs, and some hormones that influence intestinal motility. Intestinal transit is abnormal, and intraluminal pressures, particularly in the distal colon, are increased. These disturbances may in part be responsible for the frequent abdominal pain and altered bowel habits in patients with this disorder.

Diet may influence the irritable bowel syndrome. The diet of the developed Western countries of the world today lacks fiber and bulk. The addition of unprocessed bran or undigestable fiber to the diet of normal subjects causes a shortening of the intestinal transit time and an increase in stool weight and water content. Fiber may modify fecal flow patterns and reduce intraluminal pressures in the distal colon.

Diagnosis. The typical triad of symptoms of the irritable bowel syndrome is abdominal pain, alternating constipation and diarrhea, and a small caliber of the stools. The abdominal pain is steady rather than colicky and can be quite severe. The majority of the pain is in the left lower quadrant but can migrate to all areas of the abdomen. Defecation and flatus commonly relieve the pain. Nocturnal pain is unusual. Although the pain may be described as excruciating, there seems to be no physical deterioration of the patient in spite of a long history of suffering from the discomfort.

The bowel habits are abnormal. The patient may have constant diarrhea, intermittent diarrhea, or diarrhea alternating with constipation. The stools are pellet-shaped, usually quite hard, and are passed together with a variable amount of mucus and liquid stool. The patient usually describes his stools in a graphic manner. Diarrhea to these patients means frequency, urgency, and the passage of stools of little volume. Some bowel movements may be only mucus associated with tenesmus and flatus. The patient may complain of bloating, borborygmi, and explosive flatus, yet stool volume is small. Most stools occur in the morning, many before breakfast. As the day progresses, the symptoms tend to improve.

The physical examination is unremarkable. One commonly can palpate a tender sigmoid and a descending colon full of feces in the left lower quadrant. Sigmoidoscopy demonstrates normal mucosa, adherent to which are patches of mucus. The bowel contracts vigorously during the examination, and the patient is usually quite uncomfortable. The barium enema study is normal. Disturbances of colonic motility are difficult to demonstrate radiographically.

The diagnosis of the irritable bowel syndrome can be strongly suspected from the history alone. However, no specific tests exist to objectively prove the diagnosis. It must be one of exclusion. Carefully search for organic disease. The irritable bowel syndrome may coexist with other diseases, and the symptoms may mask those of other disorders. Suffering from the symptoms of the irritable bowel syndrome does not make the patient immune from acquiring other diseases. Fever, weight loss, rectal bleeding, steatorrhea, or progressively severe symptoms must not be ignored and blamed on the irritable bowel syndrome.

Management. Successful management of the irritable bowel syndrome begins with the patient's understanding the nature and pathophysiology of the disease. The physician must alleviate the patient's fears of cancer, colitis, colostomies, and surgery. Take a positive approach in discussing the natural history and prognosis of the disorder. Emphasize that the disease is not caused by a nervous condition and that the patient's colon responds abnormally to the stresses and anxieties of everyday life.

Be alert to discover additional disorders that may be contributing to the symptoms and altered motility pattern of the irritable bowel syndrome. All laxatives must be stopped. Symptoms of lactose intolerance should be looked for in the history and objectively documented by performing the lactose tolerance test if the symptoms warrant it. Be sure that there is no more than the normal amount of neurosis associated with the symptoms. Severe emotional disorders must be managed appropriately.

Do not prescribe a restrictive diet. Encourage adding fiber and bulk to the diet by the daily consumption of bran and other unprocessed grains. Each patient can discover on his own what foods tend to increase his symptoms. Beans, cabbage, and other foods containing undigestable disaccharides increase intestinal gas, which tends to worsen the symptoms of the irritable bowel syndrome.

Instead of a rigid bulk-filled diet, it is easier in Western societies to add a bulk-forming laxative to increase stool volume. Psyllium hydrophilic mucilloid (Metamucil, Konsyl) or other hydrophilic substances should be taken indefinitely by these patients two to three times a day.

Restrict the use of other medications. Antidiarrheal agents, antispasmodics, laxatives, tranquilizers, sedatives, and antidepressants generally are of little benefit and may aggravate the motility disturbance of the colon.

Symptoms of the irritable bowel syndrome never completely go away, but with proper management they will decrease in severity and frequency. The patient should be followed regularly to reinforce any improvement that slowly occurs and to re-emphasize the pathophysiology of the disease. Remember that this disorder does not give the patient protection from other diseases. If the symptoms change, a thorough re-evaluation is mandatory to look for organic disease.

Diverticular Disease

Diverticular disease is a collective term for diverticulosis and diverticulitis. Diverticulosis is the presence of colonic diverticula. Diverticulitis occurs when one or more of the diverticula become inflamed. The pathogeneses of the irritable bowel syndrome and diverticular disease are closely related. Both have similar chronic motility disturbances of the colon.

A colonic diverticulum is a herniation of the mucosa through the circular muscle at points at which the muscular wall is weak. These areas occur in places where nutrient blood vessels from the serosa penetrate the muscular layer to enter the submucosa. The motility disturbance in diverticular disease generates high intraluminal pressures within the colon, causing diverticula to form at these weak areas. Since higher intraluminal pressures occur in the sigmoid and descending colon, the majority of the diverticula form in these parts of the colon.

The incidence of diverticular disease increases with age. In some Western countries, more than 50 per cent of people past the age of 70 have colonic diverticula. The incidence of diverticular disease is very low in the underdeveloped areas of the world. Dietary habits may account for this difference. The diet of less developed countries includes large amounts of bulk and undigestable fiber, which tend to shorten intestinal transit time, increase the stool weight and volume, and perhaps reduce intraluminal colonic pressures by keeping the lumen of the bowel filled and normally distended. The diet of the developed countries of the Western world is rich in refined carbohydrate and deficient in bulk. This may be the answer to the cause of diverticular disease.

Diagnosis. Diverticulosis causes no clinical symptoms. The symptoms of patients with diverticulosis are the same as those with the irritable bowel syndrome. As previously mentioned, the formation of colonic diverticula and the irritable bowel syndrome probably have the same pathogenesis. Symptomatic diverticular disease results from one of the two major complications of this disorder—inflammation (diverticulitis) and hemorrhage.

Diverticulitis occurs when one or more of the diverticula perforate. With small perforations, an area of inflammation forms adjacent to the colon wall. It may be very localized or extensive enough to form large pericolic or pelvic abscesses. Partial or complete colonic obstruction can occur. The onset of symptoms may be abrupt, with fever, abdominal tenderness, and leukocytosis, and in the more severe cases evidence of peritonitis may be found on physical examination. A mass may be palpable in the left lower quadrant.

Management. Management should include plain films of the abdomen to detect free air within the peritoneum and radiographic signs of bowel obstruction or an associated ileus. Obtain blood cultures. Administer broad-spectrum antibiotics and maintenance intravenous fluids. Failure to improve in 48 hours makes the possibility of an extraluminal abscess likely, and surgical consultation should be obtained. A barium enema examination at this point may help localize the inflammatory process.

Many attacks of diverticulitis are mild. If the patient improves on medical management, be sure to perform a barium enema study at some time during the recovery period to be sure that you were dealing with diverticulitis and not a carcinoma of the colon. The differentiation can be difficult at times.

The anatomic relationship between diverticula and the nutrient perforating blood vessels may account for the increased risk of hemorrhage from diverticular disease. A large blood vessel frequently overlies the diverticulum. The vessel may be exposed to intraluminal abrasion, causing it to bleed. The onset of the bleeding is abrupt, with no preceding symptoms. The bleeding may originate as commonly from diverticula of the right colon as from the left. Bleeding can be massive and life-threatening. Angiography will locate the site of bleeding if the procedure is done during the time that the patient is actively bleeding.

BELCHING, FLATUS, AND INTESTINAL GAS

Origins of Intestinal Gas

Not all intestinal gas is due to aerophagia. Washout techniques that measure the total pool of intestinal gas find a mixture of nitrogen, oxygen, methane, hydrogen, and carbon dioxide. Bacterial metabolism within the colon produces the hydrogen, carbon dioxide, and methane. To produce gas, the bacteria must have substrate to metabolize. The substrate comes from food not absorbed in the small bowel. Gas production in the colon increases tremendously when the food consumed contains nonabsorbable substances such as the long chain polysaccharides of cellulose; stachyose and raffinose, the nondigestible oligosaccharides found in beans; and the lactose in patients deficient in the lactose-splitting enzyme, lactase. Bacterial fermentation of these compounds produces hydrogen and carbon dioxide. The same mechanism produces methane, but only in about one-third of the population. The tendency to harbor methane-producing colonic bacteria seems to be an inherited trait.

Flatus

Bothersome flatus is a frequent component of the irritable bowel syndrome. The symptoms of this disorder seem magnified when gas is expelled along with the stools and mucus. These patients have exaggerated colonic motility responses to a variety of stimuli, including the presence of excessive intraluminal gas that can cause abdominal pain, cramps, and flatus.

Analysis of flatus composition can determine the origin of the gas. Flatus composed mainly of nitrogen is caused by swallowed air. A predominance of carbon dioxide and hydrogen indicates flatus of colonic origin from the fermentation of nonabsorbed food.

Eliminating both sources of flatus can relieve many symptoms. Attempt to break the patient of his air-swallowing habit. He should avoid ingestion of the common nonabsorbable foodstuffs such as beans, cabbage, and other vegetables with a high cellulose content. Rule out mild malabsorptive states that may be contributing to the formation of intestinal gas. A mild lactase deficiency or fat maldigestion from chronic pancreatic disease can lead to marked excessive gas formation. Partially correcting these disorders may be a valuable therapeutic move.

Belching

The patient who complains of excessive belching represents an entirely different problem from those patients with colonic gas disorders. In nearly all cases, belching is due to swallowed air. The chronic repetitive belcher collects air in the esophagus by subtle swallowing maneuvers prior to the eructations. Many patients construe this nervous habit as a sign of gastrointestinal disease. However, not all belching is functional. It may be a conscious or unconscious habit to gain momentary relief from other unrelated symptoms. An underlying intestinal disease may increase the magnitude of the aerophagia and lead to symptoms overshadowing the primary disease.

Notice during the physical examination that these are the patients who try to belch. The patient may hyperventilate or sigh vigorously, facilitating the entrance of large amounts of gas into the stomach. Aggravating this habit are gum chewing, smoking, gulping food, poorly fitting dentures, carbonated drinks, using a straw to drink liquids, and the use of anticholinergic drugs. All must be eliminated in managing these patients.

Bloating, Abdominal Pain, and Distention

The air swallower does not trap all the air in his esophagus. Some travels into the stomach. If belching does not occur, the gas proceeds into the small bowel. Gas within the small bowel in some patients brings on complaints of abdominal distention, fullness, or feeling "gassy." A vicious circle may develop. Minimal intestinal distress causes more air swallowing, leading to more severe symptoms of distention, borborygmi, pain, and flatus.

Intestinal gas analysis of these "gassy" patients has failed to demonstrate any marked increase in the amount of gas contained within the intestine. Such patients seem to have painful responses to volumes of gas that are well tolerated by normal subjects. Attempts at reducing even this normal volume of gas, however, may diminish the symptoms.

Ingestion of fats and highly osmotic active substances such as refined sugars are strong inhibitors of gastric emptying. Any swallowed air accompanying a fatty or osmotically active meal is hindered from passing into the small bowel because of the delayed gastric emptying. This may explain the sensation of fullness and frequent eructations following a fatty meal.

Treatment is aimed at preventing gas formation within the intestine. A low fat diet may be useful. The patient should recognize his bad habit of air swallowing, although it is difficult to overcome. The use of anticholinergic drugs in these patients is a common mistake. There is no proof that they help relieve any gaseous symptoms. They also may worsen aerophagia by causing a dry mouth. Antacids theoretically can limit the carbon dioxide produced when gastric acid is neutralized by bicarbonate in the upper small bowel. The hydroxide groups of common antacids neutralize gastric acid without the generation of carbon dioxide.

Any nonabsorbable carbohydrate should be avoided. Lactose and beans are the main offenders. Even patients without a measurable deficiency of lactase may not totally hydrolyze a lactose load. A milk-free diet often is helpful. Feeding charcoal to "adsorb gas" or the use of antibiotics to lower intestinal bacterial counts is not effective therapy. Although advertised widely, simethicone-containing antacids have no more effect on gas symptoms than any other antacid.

ACID PEPTIC DISEASES

Acid peptic diseases are those conditions in which hydrochloric acid produced by the stomach has some influence on the pathogenesis. Reflux esophagitis, gastritis, gastric ulcer, duodenal ulcer, and duodenitis all fall within this broad category. Although a variety of different disease mechanisms underlie these disorders, they are linked by the common causative role played by gastric acid.

Duodenal Ulcer Disease

A duodenal ulcer is an inflammatory defect of the proximal duodenal mucosa extending into the submucosa. Edema, inflammation, and granulation tissue surround the necrotic debris of the ulcer crater. What leads to the formation of the ulcer is far more important to understand than the mere ulcer histology.

Duodenal ulcer disease is a chronic condition. Recurring remissions and exacerbations mark the usual course. The actual ulcer is but the end stage of a period of exacerbation. Duodenal ulcers may come and go, but the disease remains.

The cause of duodenal ulcer disease is closely related to gastric acid production, although the exact cause remains unclear. As a group, duodenal ulcer disease patients differ from the general population in the production of gastric acid (Table 46–11). Duodenal ulcer disease patients produce more acid in response to any stimulus for gastric acid secretion. Many other variables, such as emotional factors, genetic predisposition, and duodenal defense mechanisms against acid injury, may influence the determination of who suffers from duodenal ulcer disease and who does not.

Diagnosis. The diagnosis can be made from the history. If the abdominal pain in-

---

TABLE 46–11. COMPARISON OF DUODENAL ULCER DISEASE PATIENTS WITH THE NORMAL POPULATION

As a group, duodenal ulcer disease patients:

1. Have an increased capacity to secrete gastric acid because of their larger total gastric parietal cell mass
2. Produce more gastric acid when maximally stimulated with histamine or pentagastrin
3. Produce more gastric acid with submaximal stimuli such as eating a meal
4. Are more sensitive to the effects of gastrin on the parietal cell
5. Release more gastrin in response to physiologic stimuli
6. Cannot inhibit gastrin release as readily
7. Have more rapid gastric emptying times, so that gastric acid is delivered more quickly into the duodenum

---

TABLE 46–12. COMPONENTS OF DUODENAL ULCER DISEASE PAIN

1. Chronic, nonradiating epigastric pain, burning in character and perceived deep to the abdominal wall
2. A rhythmic cycle to the occurrence of the pain coinciding with periods of time when there are high concentrations of acid within the stomach. The pain generally occurs before meals, 1 to 3 hours after meals, and at night 1 to 2 hours after falling asleep
3. Temporary pain relief obtained from ingestion of food or antacids
4. Pain is not present upon awakening in the morning

---

cludes the four components listed in Table 46–12, it is very likely caused by duodenal ulcer disease. Directly looking at the duodenal mucosa by means of fiberoptic endoscopy or indirectly by radiographic barium contrast studies of the upper gastrointestinal tract helps to confirm this diagnosis. But remember that duodenal ulcer disease is a chronic condition. Both of these diagnostic tests look at the duodenal bulb only at one point in time. Inability to demonstrate an ulcer does not rule out the disease. The ulcer is but the end stage of an active period of the disease. Edematous duodenal mucosal folds, excessive secretions within the duodenum, or an erythematous appearance to the mucosa with multiple shallow erosions (a condition referred to as duodenitis) may indicate increased activity of the duodenal ulcer disease. A deformed duodenal bulb commonly seen in radiographic studies suggests that scarring has occurred from ulcer disease. This scarring could be current or could have formed years before. Interpret these tests with caution and with relevance to your patient's history.

Management. The goals of duodenal ulcer disease management are to relieve pain, hasten ulcer healing, prevent complications, and prevent recurrences. Whether any medical or surgical treatment actually is able to attain these goals is not certain with the present state of the art. Many treatment regimens for duodenal ulcer disease have not proved effective in controlled studies. Any treatment used should have sound pathophysiologic bases. Since duodenal ulcers do not form without the presence of acid, current treatment concentrates on reducing the amount of acid produced or on neutralizing that which is produced.

For years, antacids have been the cornerstone of duodenal ulcer disease therapy, yet they have never been shown to alter the natural history of the disease. Even the evidence that they relieve the pain of the disease is inconclusive, but we continue to prescribe them. Antacids are various combinations of inorganic compounds that buffer acid within the gastric lumen. Unlike food, which is also a good buffer, they cause no stimulation of acid secretion. This is not true of calcium-containing antacids. The calcium can stimulate parietal cells directly to produce acid. The use of food, milk, or antacids containing calcium as treatment for duodenal ulcer disease is unwise, as a hyperacidity state develops after the buffering capacity of these compounds has been exhausted.

In order for antacids to be effective, they must remain in the stomach to buffer the acid once it is produced. Therefore, antacids should be given when the gastric emptying time is not rapid. One hour after meals is the ideal time to take antacids, as this is when meal-stimulated acid secretion is reaching its peak, the buffering capacity of the food is nearly exhausted, and the gastric emptying time is delayed. Antacids taken 1 hour after meals will remain in the stomach for several hours.

Duodenal ulcer disease treatment also attempts to reduce the amount of acid produced by the gastric parietal cells. Anticholinergics will reduce acid secretion, but only with high doses. Bothersome side effects at these high doses limit their usefulness. When anticholinergics do not produce side effects, they do not effectively reduce acid secretion. There are no anticholinergics that act selectively on the parietal cell.

Controlled studies have shown that special ulcer diets, bland diets, milk and cream diets, or most other dietary adjustments have no effect on the course of duodenal ulcer disease. Patients should eat a regular diet, eliminating only those substances that may cause excessive acid production or break the gastric mucosal barrier. Alcohol, caffeine, smoking, and aspirin should be eliminated completely by the patient with duodenal ulcer disease, at least during exacerbations of the disease.

Cimetidine, an H_2-histamine receptor antagonist, blocks the effects of histamine on the gastric parietal cell. It markedly diminishes acid production, as all stimuli for increasing gastric acid secretion probably are mediated through histamine. Cimetidine also effectively decreases both basal and stimulated gastric acid secretion. The common antihistamines used for allergic rhinitis and other conditions have no effect on gastric acid production. They block only H_1-histamine receptors, none of which are present in the stomach. Controlled studies, some yet to be completed, suggest that cimetidine enhances the healing rate of duodenal ulcers when compared with a placebo. Long-term effects on recurrence rates are not known. The H_2-histamine receptor antagonist class of drugs offers great potential usefulness in the treatment of all the acid peptic diseases.

Surgical therapy for duodenal ulcer disease is reserved for the 10 to 20 per cent of patients who suffer a complication of the disease—hemorrhage, perforation, obstruction, or unrelenting symptoms refractory to medical management. The principle of surgical therapy is the same as medical management—reduce acid production. Sectioning the vagus nerve fibers innervating the stomach eliminates the vagal stimulation of the parietal cells and the cells in the antrum that release gastrin. Antrectomy removes the main source of gastrin. Combining the two, vagotomy and antrectomy, produces the operation for duodenal ulcer disease with the lowest recurrence rate, less than 1 per cent. A vagotomy and pyloroplasty operation results in higher recurrence rates but in less postoperative side effects, such as the dumping syndrome. A parietal cell vagotomy cuts only the vagal fibers innervating the body and fundus of the stomach, the areas containing the parietal cells. Innervation of the antrum, pylorus, and duodenum is preserved. No pyloroplasty need be done, as gastric motility is unaffected. Side effects of the operation are few. Hopefully, long-term follow-up evaluations of this operation will show the recurrence rate to be acceptably low.

Gastrin and the Zollinger-Ellison Syndrome

Gastrin is a true hormone that is released into the circulation by specialized cells of the gastric antrum. It acts primarily as a powerful stimulant for gastric acid secretion. A neoplastic collection of gastrin-producing cells, usually within the pancreas, causes the Zollinger-Ellison syndrome. This neoplasm continuously and autonomously produces large amounts of gastrin, causing constant maximal stimulation of the parietal cells. Enormous amounts of gastric acid are secreted. A serious ulcer diathesis occurs, with accompanying diarrhea and electrolyte abnormalities. The symptoms are refractory to standard ulcer therapy. Although rare, one should always suspect this diagnosis in patients with duodenal ulcer disease. Many patients present initially as having typical duodenal ulcer disease. Measuring the serum gastrin level and performing a standard basal and maximally stimulated gastric analysis will detect the patient with the Zollinger-Ellison syndrome.

Gastric Ulcer Disease

Peptic ulcer disease is not a single entity. The pathophysiology of gastric ulcer is distinctly different from duodenal ulcer, although the exact cause of either is unknown. A duodenal ulcer is associated with abnormal gastric acid secretion; a gastric ulcer is associated with abnormal responses of the gastric mucosa to the gastric acid secreted.

Normal gastric mucosa contains a built-in barrier, enabling the stomach to hold highly concentrated acid solutions without inflicting damage upon the mucosa. This gastric mucosal barrier protects the stomach from autodigestion. It seems to be a function of the gastric epithelial cell outer membranes. Certain chemicals, when placed within the stomach, alter this barrier and cause it to work less efficiently. These substances (aspirin, bile salts, ethanol) are said to "break" the gastric mucosal barrier. With the barrier broken, hydrogen ions are free to back-diffuse into the gastric mucosa, where they stimulate local release of histamine, cause injury to tissue within the mucosa, and further augment acid secretion. The end result is a gastritis that can lead to mucosal erosions and gastric ulcers.

Gastric ulcer patients seem to have some motility disturbance of the antrum, pyloris, and duodenum that allows duodenal contents containing bile salts to flow back into the stomach. The bile salts break the gastric mucosal barrier, allowing any acid normally produced to back-diffuse into the gastric mucosa and cause gastritis. Chronically, this disturbance may lead to gastric ulcer formation. Gastric acid secretion in patients with gastric ulcers is low when compared with normal subjects. Gastric ulcer formation is not due to the amount of acid produced but possibly to the amount of damage that the gastric mucosal barrier sustains, allowing the acid that is present to back-diffuse and cause mucosal damage.

When compared with duodenal ulcer patients, patients with gastric ulcers are older, have more associated chronic diseases, have a higher incidence of aspirin or alcohol abuse, and suffer higher recurrence rates. The symptoms of gastric ulcer are not as typical as those of duodenal ulcer. Patients may complain of many nonspecific symptoms, such as nausea, bloating, anorexia, and weight loss. Food may increase the pain. It is difficult to make a diagnosis from the history alone. Gastric x-rays and endoscopic inspection of the stomach are necessary for proper diagnosis.

The management of gastric ulcer disease is very nonspecific. Since the amount of gastric acid produced may be of secondary importance compared with the failure of the gastric mucosal barrier, treatment aimed at buffering the acid or reducing its secretion may not be beneficial. Antacids still are used, although many studies show that they do not relieve pain any better than a placebo. Bed rest in a hospital and cessation of cigarette smoking hasten gastric ulcer healing. Carbenoxolone, a drug that may strengthen the gastric mucosal barrier, does help gastric ulcers to heal but has many side effects and is not approved for use in the United States. H_2-receptor histamine antagonists may be useful therapy. Gastric mucosal damage will not occur with a broken gastric mucosal barrier unless acid is present in the stomach. Clinical trials with cimetidine in gastric ulcer patients are needed. No matter how they are managed, the vast majority of gastric ulcers heal within several months. Unfortunately, the recurrence rate is very high.

The major clinical problem in the management of gastric ulcer is the fear of malignancy. About 3 to 4 per cent of gastric ulcers are malignant. Although some gastric ulcers obviously are malignant at endoscopy or on x-ray examination, one can never be certain that an ulcer is benign—no matter what its appearance, where it is located in the stomach, or how big it may be. Fiberoptic endoscopy should be done on all patients with a gastric ulcer. With careful endoscopic inspection, directed biopsies, and brushings for cytology, a diagnostic accuracy of more than 95 per cent can be obtained. To be certain that the gastric ulcer is benign, the patient must have close follow-up to ensure that the ulcer heals and does not recur.

Surgical therapy is needed for the complications of gastric ulcer, which are the same as for duodenal ulcer disease—hemorrhage, perforation, obstruction, and ulcers refractory to medical therapy. The surgical procedure usually is a vagotomy, antrectomy, and excision of the ulcer. The postoperative recurrence rate is low.

Gastritis

The classification of gastritis is a confused area. Terminology varies, and little is known about the pathophysiology. One classification of gastritis is listed in Table 46–13.

Acute gastritis is a collective term for many descriptive clinical syndromes. Underlying all these conditions is acute generalized damage to the gastric mucosal barrier that allows gastritis to form suddenly. Excessive aspirin and alcohol use, sepsis, severe burns, central nervous system trauma, and uremia can cause acute gastritis. All these varied conditions break the gastric mucosal barrier, either locally by the compound's presence in the gastric lumen or systemically by somehow altering the blood flow to the stomach. Gastric acid then can back-diffuse massively and create acute gastritis, which commonly presents as acute, massive upper gastrointestinal bleeding. Treatment is supportive. If possible, remove the offending agent that broke the gastric mucosal barrier. H_2-histamine receptor antagonists may be helpful if they can eliminate acid production for a short period of time.

Chronic gastritis is altogether different. It

TABLE 46–13. CLASSIFICATION OF GASTRITIS

---

1. *Acute Gastritis:*
    Also called acute hemorrhagic gastritis, stress ulcers, erosive gastritis, and many other names
    Caused by a variety of conditions:
        Ingestion of drugs that break the gastric mucosal barrier, such as aspirin and alcohol
        Following severe burns
        Following severe trauma
        Associated with many severe illnesses
        Associated with acute central nervous system disease
    Can cause massive gastrointestinal bleeding

2. *Chronic Gastritis:*
    A degenerative process of the gastric mucosa of unknown cause; it may be a normal aging process or a destructive immunologic disease
    Usually causes few, if any, symptoms
    Subclassification based on increasing severity

    a. *Chronic Superficial Gastritis:*
        Mild form of chronic gastritis
        These patients have begun to gradually lose the secretory function of the stomach

    b. *Atrophic Gastritis:*
        More severe form
        Nearly all gastric secretory function is destroyed

    c. *Gastric Atrophy:*
        Completely achlorhydric
        Unable to secrete intrinsic factor
        Gastric mucosa resembles small intestine histologically
        10 per cent risk of developing gastric carcinoma

---

is a degenerative process of the gastric mucosa that causes few symptoms. The classification of chronic gastritis is based on histologic severity, as shown in Table 46–13. Chronic gastritis develops by the gradual loss of parietal and chief cells.. The gastric mucosa slowly changes from a secretory to an absorptive mucosa. In the later stages, it resembles intestinal mucosa. Achlorhydria, lack of intrinsic factor secretion leading to pernicious anemia, and an increased risk of gastric carcinoma are the end results of the most severe form of chronic gastritis—gastric atrophy. Symptoms are mild. Anorexia, nausea, and vague abdominal pain are the most frequent symptoms. There is no adequate treatment.

HEARTBURN, REFLUX ESOPHAGITIS

Heartburn is a burning retrosternal discomfort caused by the reflux of gastric contents into the esophagus. The acidic gastric contents stimulate sensory nerve endings within the esophageal mucosa and provoke spasms of the esophageal musculature. Both mechanisms produce the sensation of heartburn.

The Causes of Reflux Esophagitis

The pathogenesis of reflux esophagitis is confusing and controversial, and the subject is hotly debated. In the center of this controversy is the role of the lower esophageal sphincter (LES) in the prevention of reflux esophagitis. The LES is a 2 to 4 cm. segment of functionally specialized esophageal circular muscle located in the terminal portion of the esophagus. It is not a separate anatomic structure and can be demonstrated only by intraluminal esophageal pressure recording devices. By this method, the LES is considered a zone of intraluminal high resting pressure. It maintains a pressure gradient between the stomach and the esophagus, presumably to prevent reflux of gastric contents into the esophagus. The LES relaxes with swallowing but regains its high resting pressure once the peristaltic wave of swallowing has passed.

Patients with symptomatic reflux esophagitis have low resting pressures in their LES. However, the difference between them and normals is slight. In most cases, a single measurement of the LES resting pressure cannot determine if that patient has reflux esophagitis or not.

The presence of a sliding hiatal hernia does not alter the function of the LES. As many patients without a sliding hiatal hernia suffer reflux esophagitis as do those with a hernia. The sliding hiatal hernia is a radiologic curiosity with no clinical significance.

Evaluation of Heartburn Symptoms

A thorough investigation of heartburn symptoms should provide answers to the following questions:

1. Is reflux present? Obtaining a typical history may be all that is necessary to answer this question. The usual patient has burning substernal discomfort that is relieved temporarily by antacids, exacerbated in the recumbent position, and associated with nocturnal symptoms of pain, regurgitation, and coughing. But many patients do not behave so typically. To objectively demonstrate the presence of reflux is difficult. The barium swallow is an insensitive determinant of reflux. Only the spontaneous reflux of barium during this examination correlates well with the presence of reflux esophagitis. Fiberoptic esophagoscopy only detects gross mucosal changes of severe esophagitis. Probably the most sensitive method of demonstrating reflux is the intraluminal recording of pH in the distal esophagus. A normal endoscopy, barium swallow, and esophageal motility study or normal histologic findings on esophageal mucosal biopsy do not rule out the presence of reflux esophagitis.

2. Are the patient's symptoms due to reflux esophagitis? This question is answered best by performing the acid infusion test (Bernstein test), in which 0.1N hydrochloric acid and isotonic saline solutions are infused alternately through a tube placed in the upper third of the esophagus. If the acid infusion, but not the saline, reproduces the patient's symptoms, the symptoms are due to an acid-sensitive esophagus. It does not prove that reflux is occurring.

3. What has the reflux done to the esophageal mucosa? Changes in the esophageal mucosa from reflux esophagitis are a reflection of the severity of the disease. Histologic changes on biopsy are a more sensitive indicator than the appearance of the mucosa as seen through the endoscope. Answering this question helps grade the severity of the disease and recognize complications such as stricture formation, ulcerations, or friability.

Management of Reflux Esophagitis

About two-thirds of patients with reflux esophagitis will respond favorably to proper medical management. Any factors that may aggravate reflux esophagitis must be corrected. Table 46–14 outlines a physiologic approach to the medical management of reflux esophagitis.

The natural effects of gravity on the reflux of gastric contents must be minimized. The

TABLE 46–14. REFLUX ESOPHAGITIS—PATHOGENESIS AND MANAGEMENT

Factors Involved in Development	Pathophysiology	Therapy	
		Avoid	*Suggest*
Incompetent anti-reflux mechanisms	Incompetent LES allows reflux of gastric contents into the esophagus	Agents that decrease LES resting pressure (caffeine, fat, chocolate, cigarettes, anticholinergics); constricting garments; large meals; Recumbency after eating	Agents that increase LES resting pressure (bethanechol); elevate head of bed; weight loss
Concentration of acid-peptic mixture that is refluxed	The acidity and digestive enzyme content of refluxed material coupled with diminished esophageal clearance mechanisms allow caustic material to stay in the distal esophagus longer and increase chances of damaging the mucosa	Anticholinergics—decrease gastric emptying time	Antacids; H_2 blockers (cimetidine)
Susceptibility of esophageal tissue to injury	The wear-and-tear effect of the refluxed material diminishes the protective keratin layer of esophageal mucosa, exposing the neurovascular papillae and eliciting pain. Further damage progresses to gross esophagitis.	Anticholinergics—decrease gastric emptying time	Antacids; H_2 blockers (cimetidine)

patient should sleep on a bed that has its head elevated on 6 to 8 inch (15 to 20 cm.) blocks so that the thorax is higher than the stomach. Stooping and bending are discouraged. Try to diminish factors that will cause an increase in intragastric pressure. Avoid large meals; the overweight patient should lose weight. No tight clothing should be worn. The patient should not recline when the stomach is full. He should not eat for 1 to 2 hours before retiring for the night.

Antacids theoretically will reduce the acidity of the reflux material and may help strengthen the LES. Antacids containing alginate, a viscous substance that allegedly floats to the gastroesophageal junction, may create a physical barrier to prevent reflux. However, there is little clinical data showing additional benefit from these antacids compared with regular antacids. Cholinergic agents such as bethanechol raise LES resting pressure and help relieve symptoms of reflux esophagitis in many patients. Anticholinergics should be avoided. They delay gastric emptying, lower the LES pressure, and intensify the symptoms. Alcohol, smoking, fatty foods, and chocolate may adversely affect the LES resting pressure. They also should be avoided.

Patients with severe symptoms of reflux esophagitis who do not respond to medical management may be candidates for the various surgical procedures performed for this condition. Most of these procedures (Hill repair, Belsey anterior fundoplication, Nissen fundoplication) improve basal LES pressures by wrapping part of the gastric fundic musculature around the lower esophagus. The results generally have been good.

DYSPHAGIA

Dysphagia is the subjective sensation that food being swallowed is not traveling to the stomach in the usual manner. It is a reliable symptom of organic disease. Rarely is it a functional complaint. Every patient with dysphagia must be investigated and not labeled as suffering from globus hystericus or another functional diagnosis.

The family physician must be alert for complaints of dysphagia from his patients. Such complaints can be very subtle and not appreciated by the patient as symptoms of an abnormal esophagus. The patient casually may say that food hesitates on its way down or tends to pause at times. Just the awareness of food passing down the esophagus is abnormal. The patient may not think he has swallowing trouble. He may say he has no trouble swallowing but will admit that food does stick in his chest on its way down to his stomach.

Once dysphagia has been recognized, the family physician should expand his questioning. The cause of the dysphagia usually can be unraveled by a careful history. Try to obtain answers to the questions listed in Table 46–15. They can help to classify the type of dysphagia that the patient has (Table 46–16).

Oropharyngeal dysphagia is characterized by difficulty in initiating a swallow. Swallowing begins with the voluntary contraction of the various oropharyngeal muscles. Simultaneously, the upper esophageal sphincter relaxes, allowing the bolus to pass into the esophagus. Improper relaxation of the upper esophageal sphincter or weakness of the pharyngeal muscular contraction creates difficulties in initiating the swallow. Fluid may escape through the nose or fall into the trachea during swallowing. Coughing and episodes of aspiration pneumonitis commonly accompany this type of dysphagia.

Dysphagia from an obstructive lesion within the esophageal lumen generally occurs only with solid food, particularly large pieces of meat. Liquids are handled easily; in fact, drinking additional liquids may be a way for these patients to push the food bolus into the stomach to relieve their symptoms. The dysphagia may be intermittent. Vague intermittent dysphagia for only certain types of food may be the only early symptom of esophageal carcinoma.

The dysphagia of motility disorders of the esophagus occurs with ingestion of both liquids and solids. There may be severe pain associated with the dysphagia. The pain of diffuse esophageal spasm can mimic that produced by ischemic heart disease. Symptoms may be exacerbated by drinking liquids of extreme cold or hot temperatures. If regurgitation occurs, the material consists of undigested food. Symptoms tend to be worse at times of emotional stress, which commonly leads to these disorders being misdiagnosed as functional complaints.

TABLE 46–15. QUESTIONS TO ASK THE PATIENT TO HELP CHARACTERIZE DYSPHAGIA

1. Where does the food stick?
2. Is there any pain associated with the dysphagia?
3. Is there any difficulty in initiating the swallow?
4. How long has the swallowing disorder been symptomatic?
5. Is the dysphagia constant or intermittent?
6. Have the symptoms changed or progressed?
7. Does this sensation of "dysphagia" also occur when not swallowing?
8. What types of food or liquids tend to precipitate the dysphagia?
9. Is there any trouble swallowing very cold or hot liquids?
10. Once the dysphagia occurs, what can be done to relieve the symptoms?
11. Are there any problems with chewing, dentures, teeth?
12. Does coughing, aspiration, or wheezing occur at night?
13. Does regurgitation occur at night?
14. Are there food stains on the pillow in the morning?
15. Is undigested food that was eaten days before ever regurgitated?

ACUTE GASTROINTESTINAL BLEEDING

Symptomatic acute gastrointestinal bleeding occurs when approximately 1000 ml. of blood is lost over a period of a few minutes to several hours. It is a potentially fatal medical emergency. Mortality rates average nearly 10 per cent. The management can be organized into three sequential steps: (1) prevent hemorrhagic shock by correcting the hypovolemia, (2) determine the source of the bleeding, and (3) stop the bleeding by surgical or medical means.

Correcting the hypovolemia is the single most important step. The patient first must be stabilized. Preventing exsanguination has priority over making a diagnosis. Table 46–17 contains a brief outline of measures used initially to assess and stabilize the patient with acute gastrointestinal bleeding.

TABLE 46–16. A CLASSIFICATION OF THE COMMON TYPES OF DYSPHAGIA

I. Oropharyngeal Dysphagia:
   Painful dysphagia from intrinsic lesions of the oropharynx
      Carcinoma of tongue, piriform sinus
      Acute infections of oral cavity and pharynx
   Neuromuscular disease involving the mouth, tongue, pharynx, and hypopharynx
      Cerebrovascular disease
      Pseudobulbar palsy
      Poliomyelitis
      Myasthenia gravis
      Heavy metal poisoning
      Multiple sclerosis
   Incoordinated swallowing—cricopharyngeal dysfunction with or without an associated Zenker's
      diverticulum

II. Dysphagia Due to Partial Obstruction of the Esophageal Lumen:
   Benign esophageal stricture
      History of previous symptoms of reflux esophagitis
      Dysphagia is slowly progressive, mimics symptoms of esophageal carcinoma
   Esophageal carcinoma
      Progressive dysphagia, first solids, later liquids, occasional painful swallowing
   Lower esophageal mucosal ring (Schatzki's ring)
      Thin mucosal structure near gastroesophageal junction
      Intermittent lower esophageal dysphagia, especially for large pieces of meat
   Cervical esophageal webs (Plummer-Vinson syndrome)
      Iron deficiency anemia, intermittent sensation of dysphagia located high in chest or neck
      Thin mucosal membrane partially occluding lumen of upper esophagus

III. Dysphagia Due to Motor Disorders of the Esophagus:
   Achalasia
      Lower esophageal sphincter maintains a high resting pressure and fails to relax with swallowing
      Absence of normal peristaltic activity
      Esophagus empties only by gravity and hydrostatic pressure
      Esophagus behaves as a denervated organ
   Diffuse esophageal spasm
      Disordered peristalsis
      Intermittent severe chest pain
      Intermittent dysphagia
      Idiopathic motor disorder or secondary to reflux esophagitis
   Scleroderma
      Replacement of esophageal smooth muscle with fibrous tissue
      Involves lower two-thirds of esophagus
      Nonfunctioning lower esophageal sphincter
      Prone to reflux esophagitis
      Lower two-thirds of esophagus lacks peristaltic activity

While the resuscitative measures are under way, try to clinically determine the severity and possible source of the bleeding. The patient's impression of how much blood he vomited or passed per rectum is notoriously unreliable and tainted with emotion or hysteria. The resting pulse and blood pressure are not helpful for clinical assessment because of protective vasoconstriction and other compensatory reflexes to sudden blood loss. Examining the patient only in the supine position will mask the cardiovascular effects of acute blood loss. Blood pressure and pulse changes in response to rapidly assuming the upright posture must be sought. Compensatory reflexes do not mask these changes. A 20 per cent loss of total blood volume (about 1000 ml.) is a severe bleeding episode. Clinical signs of this amount of blood loss are listed in Table 46–18. Many patients, particularly previously healthy, younger individuals, may be completely asymptomatic despite significant blood loss and may demonstrate few physical signs.

Brisk bleeding proximal to the ligament of Treitz generally produces bright red hematemesis. Blood that remains in the stomach for longer periods of time has a coffee-ground appearance that results from gastric acid converting the hemoglobin to brown acid hematin, which precipitates. Blood from sources beyond the ligament of Treitz rarely gets back to the stomach. Melena can

TABLE 46–17. INITIAL MANAGEMENT OF THE PATIENT WITH ACUTE GASTROINTESTINAL BLEEDING

1. Insert one or two large bore intravenous lines, one of which is a central venous pressure monitoring catheter
2. Type and crossmatch for at least 6 units of blood
3. Monitor clotting factors—prothrombin time, partial thromboplastin time, platelet count
4. Accurate fluid intake and output records
5. Check serum electrolyte, blood urea nitrogen, and creatinine levels
6. Restore intravascular volume with isotonic solutions and plasma expanders until whole blood is available to administer
7. Gauge fluid and whole blood replacement by changes in the vital signs, urine output, and central venous pressure
   Keep central venous pressure > 5 cm. H_2O
   Keep vital signs normal, with no postural changes

occur from blood loss of more than 50 ml. from any location in the gastrointestinal tract. Bright red or mahogany stools imply massive bleeding from anywhere in the bowel or slower bleeding from a more distal colonic lesion.

Always insert a nasogastric tube. Blood aspirated from the stomach is good evidence that the bleeding source is proximal to the ligament of Treitz. Leave the tube in place to monitor further bleeding. Iced saline lavage helps clear the stomach prior to endoscopy and shows the presence of continuing bleeding. However, it never has been shown to control upper gastrointestinal bleeding.

The patient's response to the resuscitative efforts must be closely followed. Use a flow sheet to graphically assess the patient's course. Initially, entries should be made at hourly intervals. Most clinical assessment must be based on the postural changes of vital signs and on urinary output, central venous pressure, and the amount of fluid and blood replacement required. After 8 to 12 hours of hospitalization, most hemodilution has occurred, making serial hematocrit or hemoglobin determinations more valid as an index of further blood loss.

The family physician should seek consultation for the second and third sequential steps of acute gastrointestinal bleeding management previously referred to. With the advent of fiberoptic endoscopy and selective abdominal angiography, an aggressive approach is now advocated for obtaining an early diagnosis of the bleeding patient. These newer techniques should not detract from the importance of the early resuscitative measures. Prompt stabilization of the patient enables these diagnostic procedures to be carried out early in the course of the bleeding episode.

Perform endoscopy first. The three most common causes of acute gastrointestinal bleeding (peptic ulcer disease, especially a bleeding duodenal ulcer; acute gastritis; and esophageal varices) are recognized easily at endoscopy. With endoscopy, one not only sees the lesion but can tell if it is bleeding or not. Twenty per cent of patients with gastrointestinal bleeding have multiple lesions. Endoscopy can show which specific lesion is bleeding. If endoscopy can be done within several hours after hospital admission, a source for upper gastrointestinal tract bleeding can be found in more than 90 per cent of the patients. If the endoscopy is delayed for 48 hours, the accuracy falls to 50 per cent. Management and therapeutic decisions become more rational when knowing the exact site and cause of the bleeding.

Selective abdominal angiography or conventional barium contrast studies of the upper and lower gastrointestinal tract are useful if endoscopy fails to find the bleeding site. In the presence of continuing bleeding, angiography is the next step. It can be most helpful in the patient with massive rectal bleeding. Seventy per cent of these patients are bleeding from colonic diverticula. Angiography can tell the loca-

TABLE 46–18. MANIFESTATIONS OF 20 PER CENT BLOOD VOLUME LOSS

1. Syncope, lightheadedness, restlessness, anxiety, diaphoresis, thirst
2. Loss of pink coloration to creases of outstretched hands (caused by vasoconstriction)
3. Rapidly changing from a supine to a sitting or standing position causes the systolic pressure to fall > 20 mm. Hg and/or the pulse to rise > 20 beats per minute
4. Supine systolic blood pressure < 100 mm. Hg in a previously normotensive individual
5. Supine pulse rate > 100 beats per minute (sometimes unreliable)
6. Hemoglobin < 11.0 grams per dl. prior to any hemodilution
7. Blood urea nitrogen > 40 mg. per dl. from increased nitrogen load of the gut bacteria metabolizing protein of blood within bowel lumen; assumes normal renal function present

tion of the particular diverticulum that is bleeding.

Sigmoidoscopy is an important procedure in the initial evaluation of rectal bleeding. It allows the physician to be certain that there is no mucosal disease involving the rectum and that the bleeding is originating from above the area seen on sigmoidoscopy.

Specific therapy and management for gastrointestinal bleeding depend on the underlying lesion. These difficult therapeutic decisions are much easier to make if the patient initially has been well managed. The family physician plays a key role by vigorously correcting the hypovolemia and by then seeking assistance to quickly demonstrate the bleeding site and plan the appropriate therapy.

THE FAMILY PHYSICIAN'S ROLE IN THE MANAGEMENT OF CANCER OF THE GASTROINTESTINAL TRACT

Most cancer of the gastrointestinal tract has a poor prognosis. Chemotherapy or radiotherapy has had little influence on improving the prognosis for these malignancies. However, early detection of cancer of the gastrointestinal tract can prolong survival of patients with these malignancies. This important task is the responsibility of the primary physician. He can improve the prognosis for gastrointestinal cancer as much as can surgeons, oncologists, or radiotherapists. Those malignancies of the gastrointestinal tract that potentially can be detected in their early stages of development are discussed in this section.

Cancer of the Esophagus

The outlook for patients with cancer of the esophagus is grim. Since the esophagus has no protective serosa to contain tumor growth, the malignancy usually has spread beyond the local confines of the esophagus and is far advanced by the time it is discovered. Early symptoms are few. Management in most patients is palliative. Long-term survival is less than 2 per cent.

Earlier diagnosis of esophageal carcinoma could improve the eventual outcome. Any complaint of dysphagia, no matter how mild, must be investigated and explained. Dysphagia is the earliest symptom of carcinoma of the esophagus in more than 75 per

cent of patients. The dysphagia tends to occur only with solid food. The patient may not consider this mild annoyance serious and may only casually mention it during the history. Unfortunately, even dysphagia can be a late symptom. Swallowing difficulties may not be manifested until the tumor encases the entire circumference of the esophagus.

The initial investigation of dysphagia should include radiographic barium contrast studies and flexible fiberoptic endoscopy of the esophagus and stomach. Endoscopy permits the collection of tissue specimens with forceps biopsy and brush cytology of any esophageal mucosal irregularities. These procedures can produce a diagnostic accuracy of nearly 97 per cent. Do not confine your search to the esophagus. Many tumors of the lower esophagus are adenocarcinomas that originate in the proximal stomach and extend past the gastroesophageal junction into the distal esophagus.

There are certain patients who have an increased risk of developing esophageal carcinoma (Table 46–19). The diagnostic tests just mentioned are useful for periodic screening of these patients to detect the malignancy early in its development. Although there is no statistical evidence that screening at regular intervals will improve overall survival, it is known that if the carcinoma can be detected and removed prior to its spread beyond the local confines

TABLE 46–19. CONDITIONS ASSOCIATED WITH AN INCREASED RISK OF GASTROINTESTINAL MALIGNANCY

Esophageal Cancer:
    Chronic reflux esophagitis
    Barrett's esophagus
    Achalasia
    Lye stricture
    Plummer-Vinson syndrome

Gastric Cancer:
    Atrophic gastritis
    Pernicious anemia
    Gastric polyps
    Postgastrectomy stomach
    Positive family history of gastric cancer

Colon Cancer:
    Adenomatous polyps
    Villous adenoma
    Multiple polyposis syndromes
    Chronic ulcerative colitis
    Positive family history of colon cancer
    Crohn's disease of colon

of the esophagus, the patient has a much better prognosis.

Gastric Cancer

Ninety per cent of gastric malignancies are adenocarcinomas. In the United States, the overall 5 year survival for adenocarcinoma of the stomach is 10 to 15 per cent. Considerable growth and spread of the malignancy usually have occurred prior to its detection. The earliest symptoms of gastric carcinoma are weight loss, early satiety, anemia, intolerance to eating meat, and generalized weakness—all symptoms of extensive disease. The diagnosis at this point is easy; the treatment results are dismal. Again, the key for improving survival is early diagnosis and treatment of the malignancy before it has spread beyond the gastric mucosa. This is possible. In Japan, where the incidence of gastric cancer is very high, mass population screening by fiberoptic gastroscopy has detected early asymptomatic gastric cancer. Surgical resection of those lesions that have not spread beyond the gastric mucosa results in a 90 per cent 5 year survival.

The low incidence of gastric carcinoma does not make mass screening of Americans practical. Rather, screening should be directed toward those people known to have a greater risk of developing gastric carcinoma (see Table 46–19). Such patients should undergo periodic radiographic and endoscopic investigations, at which time any mucosal abnormality should be biopsied. These examinations are probably the best procedures for the screening of gastric cancer. Biochemical tests, determinations of enzyme levels in gastric juice, and serologic markers for cancer have not proved to be helpful in finding early gastric malignancies.

The approach to detecting malignancy in gastric ulcers has already been discussed. It should be emphasized again that fiberoptic endoscopy with multiple mucosal biopsies must be performed on all patients with gastric ulcers and should be repeated at regular intervals to document ulcer healing and rule out the possibility of cancer.

Cancer of the Large Intestine

Adenocarcinoma of the large intestine ranks as the second most common form of cancer encountered today. Although the prognosis for patients with this malignancy is better than for those with adenocarcinomas originating elsewhere in the gastrointestinal tract, the 50 per cent overall 5 year survival for patients with adenocarcinoma of the large intestine has been altered little by use of newer adjuvant forms of chemotherapy or radiotherapy. Early detection and surgical resection of adenocarcinoma of the colon will improve the patient's chances for survival. Seventy-five to eighty per cent of patients can be expected to survive 5 years or more following surgical resection of tumors that are free of any local extension or distal spread beyond the colon.

Unexplained symptoms must be investigated; simple periodic screening procedures must be performed. These tumors are usually slow-growing, and early detection is possible. Anyone past the age of 35 is a potential candidate for this malignancy.

The cardinal symptoms of colon carcinoma are a change in bowel habits, vague abdominal pain, rectal bleeding, and unexplained anemia. The change in bowel habits may be very subtle. It may be only the sensation that bowel movements seem incomplete or that stool caliber has changed. Any vague abdominal pain must be investigated and explained. *Rectal bleeding must not be ignored or blamed on hemorrhoids without an evaluation.* The cause of any anemia must be found. Profound iron-deficiency anemia can occur with carcinoma of the cecum or transverse colon prior to the tumor's causing any symptoms.

Diagnosis. Carcinoma of the large intestine can and should be detected even prior to the tumor's becoming symptomatic. Every physical examination must include testing of the stool for occult blood. The use of the impregnated guaiac slide (Hemoccult test) has improved this simple test. It has reduced the number of false positive and negative results. There are no longer graded reactions, as the test is either positive or negative. Any positive test should initiate an evaluation for carcinoma of the colon.

Sixty per cent of all cancers of the large intestine occur within the rectum or sigmoid colon, areas reached by the sigmoidoscope. Some rectosigmoid tumors are too high to be felt on the rectal examination, yet too low to be seen easily by barium enema. Hence, sigmoidoscopy is an indispensable tool for the evaluation of cancer of the large intestine. Any patient with rectal bleeding, occult blood in the stools, lower abdominal complaints, or questionable findings on rectal or abdominal examination must undergo sigmoidoscopy. Routine periodic sigmoidoscopic examinations of the general population over 35 years of age have not proved effective in detecting early rectosigmoid carcinoma. Only about 1.5 tumors will be found per 1000 examinations. But besides detecting malignancies, sigmoidoscopy also may detect asymptomatic adenomatous polyps, a premalignant lesion.

The barium enema examination, using good technique, can detect lesions as small as 5 mm. in diameter. However, some areas of the colon often are seen inadequately on barium enema study because of poor preparation of the colon prior to the study, technical problems, or spasm of the bowel. The cecum is probably the most difficult area of the colon to see well on barium enema examination. In the presence of rectal bleeding, unexplained occult blood in the stool, or symptoms suspicious of large bowel pathology, colonoscopy should be performed if the barium enema study is negative or equivocal or even if the barium enema shows a lesion. By colonoscopy, the physician can make a tissue diagnosis or remove the lesion with snare cautery if it appears to be benign, polypoid, and on a stalk.

Serologic means of screening for cancer of the large intestine have not proved helpful. When first discovered, the carcinoembryonic antigen seemed to be the answer to easily screening for early colon carcinoma. However, subsequent investigations have disclosed that it is less specific than originally thought and that its role in the evaluation of colon cancer is questionable. It may be useful in monitoring for recurrence of the disease once the initial surgical resection has been performed.

High-Risk Groups. There are three main groups of people at increased risk for developing carcinoma of the large intestine: patients with chronic ulcerative colitis, patients with one of the rare multiple polyposis syndromes, and patients with adenomatous polyps of the colon (see Table 46–19). Close relatives of patients with colon cancer also seem to be at a slightly higher risk of developing the same disease.

The problem of cancer in patients with ulcerative colitis has been discussed. Multiple polyposis syndromes are rare and are listed in Table 46–20. Remember that most are familial. All family members of patients with one of these syndromes must be carefully evaluated.

It is now generally accepted that there is a definite relationship between adenomatous polyps of the colon and the development of carcinoma. The exact relationship is debated. Do all polyps eventually become malignant? Do all malignancies originate in polyps? No matter what the answers to these questions are, patients with adenomatous polyps have an increased risk for developing cancer of the colon and should be screened periodically for early lesions.

A polyp is any circumscribed tumor that is raised above surrounding normal mucosa. Some have a stalk; some are sessile. Adenomatous polyps are but one of several different histologic types of polyps that can be present in the colon. Most of the other types are not true neoplasms and have no malignant potential (Table 46–21). The polyps that are related to cancer are the adenomatous polyp and the villous adenoma. The larger the polyp, the more likely the chance of its being malignant. Unfortunately, there is no way to tell the type of polyp or whether it contains a malignancy by looking at it radiographically or endoscopically. Small biopsies are not helpful. The polyp must be totally excised in order for the pathologist to make the histologic diagnosis. Once discovered, it should be removed. Because of the routine availability of fiberoptic colonoscopy, most colon polyps can be removed by snare electrocautery through the colonoscope.

Most polyps are discovered during routine sigmoidoscopy, during a barium enema study done for other reasons, or during the evaluation of rectal bleeding. Most will be benign. If the rest of the colon is normal, no further therapy is necessary once the polyp is removed.

However, once a patient has had a polyp, he is at an increased risk of developing recurrent polyps and later, cancer. These patients require periodic screening for any new polyps or tumors. A long latent period exists between the time an adenomatous polyp is formed and the time the malignancy occurs. After removing a polyp in a patient whose colon is otherwise free of

TABLE 46–20.   MULTIPLE POLYPOSIS SYNDROMES

Pathologic Type	Name	Clinical Points	Malignant Potential	Management
Adenomatous	Familial polyposis coli	Autosomal dominant; onset 4 months to 74 years; usually $> 10 < 40$ years; mucus, diarrhea, bleeding, anemia, abdominal pain	Ay least 95%, if symptoms — 50%; in propositus — 67%; family call up — 10%	Total colectomy vs. subtotal colectomy with ileorectal anastomosis and follow-up fulguration with 5% chance of malignancy, follow-up family
	Gardner's syndrome	Autosomal dominant, cutaneous cysts, desmoids, odontomas, lipomas, retroperitoneal fibrosis, sarcomas, and other cancers	Same as above and peri-ampullary carcinoma; other upper gastrointestinal adenomas, fibromas, desmoids	Colectomy late 20's
	Generalized familial polyposis	Bleeding, cramps, obstruction	High	Colectomy plus surgery for complications
	Turcot-Deprés-St. Pierre syndrome	? autosomal recessive, colon adenomas, nevi and central nervous system glial tumors, rare	? premalignant	Usually die of central nervous system tumor
Juvenile	Familial juvenile polyposis coli	Most autosomal dominant; bleeding, prolapse, autoamputation; associated congenital anomalies; cardiac, malrotation, hydrocephalus, etc.	Families that have cancer	Local excision and surgery for intussusception or obstruction
	Generalized juvenile	Symptoms develop at very young age (<1 yr), gastrointestinal blood loss, recurrent abdominal pain, obstruction, cachexia		Surgery for bleeding, obstruction
	Canada-Cronkhite syndrome	Alopecia, nail dystrophy, hyperpigmentation, protein-losing enteropathy, malnutrition vs. ectodermal defect	None reported	Treat complication — vitamins, iron, transfusions, etc.
Hamartomas	Peutz-Jeghers syndrome (small intestine — 100%, colon and rectum — 30%, stomach — 25%)	Autosomal dominant; muscularis mucosal overgrowth plus pigmentation of lips, buccal mucosa, digits; colicky abdominal pain, intussusception, obstruction, gastrointestinal bleeding	1 to 2%; ovarian 5%	Surgery for complications — obstruction, intussusception, or excessive bleeding
Inflammatory	Pseudopolyposis	Associated with ulcerative colitis, wormlike	Only that of longstanding ulcerative colitis	Colectomy if indicated for primary disease

TABLE 46–21. SOLITARY COLON POLYPS

Name	Gross Appearance	Microscopic Appearance	Clinical Points	Malignant Potential	Therapy
Villous adenoma (papilloma)	Velvety or shaggy, large, soft, flat, 20% pedunculated, especially right colon	Branching fronds reach base, no glands, loose vascular stroma	Bleeding—60%, watery diarrhea—30%, few—dehydration and hypokalemia	30% (approximate)	Local resection; radical surgery if malignant
Adenomatous polyp (Tubular adenoma)	Smooth or lobulated, oval, pedunculated, red color	Complex branching, glandular epithelium	No symptoms in 15%, bleeding in 50%	<1 cm.—0.5%, >2 cm.—10% (controversial)	Local resection
Metaplastic polyp (hyperplastic polyp)	Small, 1 to 5 mm., sessile, pale	Hypochromic, serrated epithelium	Harmless	0	None
Juvenile polyp (retention polyp)	Round, beefy red, short stalk, often ulcerated.	Dilated cystic glands, abundant stroma with inflammation and fibrosis	Often in children, 90% bleed, sometimes prolapse	0	Local resection
Polypoid carcinoma	Large, >2 cm., ulcerated, sessile, hard	Cellular atypia, invasion	Bleeding	100%	Radical resection

polyps, periodic evaluations with repeat barium enema examination and colonoscopy need be done only at about 3 year intervals. However, these patients must not be lost to follow-up.

Adenomatous polyps of the colon are not uncommon. If the family physician recognizes the importance of these polyps in the development of cancer and closely follows his patients with polyps, most of the malignancies that he detects will be small, localized, and easily resected. His patients then will enjoy a much better prognosis.

JAUNDICE AND THE INTERPRETATION OF LIVER FUNCTION TESTS

Jaundice is a sign of liver disease in the majority of patients. Many misconceptions still exist about jaundice. Its presence does not mean that an operation is imminent. Rarely is jaundice an emergency. The differential diagnosis includes the whole spectrum of liver disease. Grouping the common causes of jaundice into three broad disease categories eases the search for the specific cause (Table 46–22). A comprehensive clinical assessment plus the use of a small number of readily available liver function tests usually can place a jaundiced patient into one of these categories. Determining the precise cause of the jaundice within these broad categories requires more sophisticated procedures.

Unconjugated Hyperbilirubinemia

Unconjugated bilirubin is one of the breakdown products of hemoglobin. Prior to being excreted in the bile, it must be conjugated with glucuronide within the hepatocyte. Unconjugated bilirubin is water-insoluble, bound tightly to serum albumin, and not excreted in the urine. In the laboratory tests of serum bilirubin concentration, unconjugated bilirubin represents the indirect fraction.

Most diseases that cause predominantly unconjugated hyperbilirubinemia lead only to mild elevations of the total serum bilirubin level. The jaundice may not be clinically evident and may be discovered only during routine laboratory screening. To confirm that the serum bilirubin elevation is due to unconjugated hyperbilirubinemia,

TABLE 46–22.   THE COMMON CAUSES OF JAUNDICE*

Unconjugated Hyperbilirubinemia:
　Hemolysis
　Gilbert's syndrome

Hepatocellular Disease:
　Viral hepatitis
　Alcoholic liver disease
　Drug-induced hepatocellular damage
　Chronic active hepatitis
　Postnecrotic cirrhosis

Obstructive Jaundice:
　Choledocholithiasis
　Cancer of the region of the head of the
　　pancreas
　Drug-induced cholestasis

*These few diseases cause more than 90% of the cases of jaundice seen in adults.

fractionate the total serum bilirubin. Conjugated bilirubin (the direct fraction) normally is less than 20 per cent of the total. This is one of the few clinical settings in which fractionation of the bilirubin aids in the diagnosis.

What are the common causes of jaundice when the majority of the elevated bilirubin is the unconjugated fraction? The answer is far more difficult during the neonatal period when the numerous congenital causes of jaundice are included in the differential diagnosis. In an adult or older child who was not jaundiced during early life, the cause usually is hemolysis or Gilbert's syndrome.

Hemolysis increases unconjugated bilirubin production beyond the capacity of the normal liver to conjugate and excrete it effectively. Obtaining normal results from standard hematologic tests makes hemolysis an unlikely cause of the jaundice.

Gilbert's syndrome is a common cause of mild, asymptomatic cases of unconjugated hyperbilirubinemia. The exact pathophysiology of this syndrome remains unclear. Several abnormalities (impaired uptake of unconjugated bilirubin by the hepatocytes, diminished activity or concentration of glucuronyl transferase, occult hemolysis) have been demonstrated in patients with Gilbert's syndrome. The level of unconjugated bilirubin tends to fluctuate, rising with fasting, acute infections, and physical exertion. Intermittent scleral icterus may be noted by the patient. The liver biopsy in those with Gilbert's syndrome is normal, although it need not be done in most patients to make the diagnosis. If hemolysis can be ruled out as the cause of mild unconjugated hyperbilirubinemia and if other liver function tests are normal, Gilbert's syndrome is the likely cause.

While a mild, unexpected bilirubin elevation is detected, look at the results of the other liver function tests. Normal serum aspartate aminotransferase (serum glutamic oxaloacetic transaminase—SGOT) and serum alkaline phosphatase values indicate that hepatocellular destruction, extrahepatic biliary obstruction, and intrahepatic cholestasis are unlikely explanations. Check the urine for the presence of bilirubin. Unconjugated bilirubin is not filtered by the glomerulus, and the test should be negative. In other types of jaundice, bilirubin is present in the urine. But bilirubin is unstable in urine, and false negative values occur if the urine tested is not fresh.

Hepatocellular Jaundice

Viral hepatitis, alcoholic liver disease, drug-induced hepatocellular disease, chronic active hepatitis, and postnecrotic cirrhosis are the common diseases producing hepatocellular jaundice. Jaundice is not the only sign of hepatocellular disease, as these diseases directly involve the hepatocyte, producing many other liver function abnormalities. Both the serum aspartate aminotransferase (SGOT) and the serum alkaline phosphatase levels are abnormal. In acute cases of hepatocellular jaundice (viral hepatitis, drug-induced hepatitis), the predominant abnormality is the marked elevation of the hepatocellular enzyme levels, such as the SGOT and the serum glutamic pyruvic transaminase (SGPT). Bilirubin elevations in patients with cirrhosis occur as a late manifestation of the disease. Jaundice in cirrhotic patients indicates that little hepatic reserve remains. It occurs along with other signs of liver failure—ascites, encephalopathy, or portal hypertension.

All phases of bilirubin metabolism and excretion are disrupted by hepatocellular disease, but clinically the major dysfunction is the excretion of conjugated bilirubin. Hence, the jaundice is due to predominantly conjugated bilirubin. Bilirubin will be present in the urine.

Obstructive Jaundice

Obstructive or cholestatic jaundice is the most difficult type to evaluate. The main task is differentiating extrahepatic obstruction from intrahepatic cholestasis (Table 46–23).

The most common causes of extrahepatic obstruction are choledocholithiasis and carcinoma of the head of the pancreas, a rather loose term that includes carcinoma of the ampulla of Vater, the lower end of the bile duct, and the acini of the pancreas. Intrahepatic cholestasis is usually drug-induced, occurring most commonly with the use of phenothiazines, oral contraceptives, estrogens, and anabolic steroids.

The conjugated fraction constitutes most of the elevated bilirubin. Bilirubinuria is present. Less conjugated bilirubin reaches the intestine. Thus, intestinal bacterial breakdown products of bilirubin are reduced. Stools are pale or clay-colored from the lack of pigments ordinarily formed from these bilirubin breakdown products.

The serum alkaline phosphatase level in obstructive or cholestatic jaundice is elevated to a far greater extent than the level of hepatocellular enzymes (SGOT, SGPT), which may be normal or only raised slightly. But laboratory tests do not differentiate obstructive jaundice from intrahepatic cholestasis.

Choledocholithiasis should be a strong consideration in the differential diagnosis, as it occurs commonly and is a potentially curable lesion. Typical signs and symptoms

TABLE 46–23. DIFFERENTIATING EXTRAHEPATIC OBSTRUCTION FROM INTRAHEPATIC CHOLESTASIS

Factors that do not differentiate the two conditions:
  Elevated serum bilirubin, alkaline phosphatase
  Bilirubinuria
  Minimal elevations of hepatocellular enzymes
  Pruritus
  Light-colored stools

Factors favoring extrahepatic obstruction:
  History of biliary tract disease or surgery
  Signs of infection (fever, chills, leukocytosis)
  Tenderness in right upper quadrant
  History of pancreatic disease
  Occult blood in stools

Factors favoring intrahepatic cholestasis:
  Positive drug history (phenothiazines, oral contraceptives, anabolic steroids, etc.)
  Eosinophilia
  Presence of or recent history of skin rash

of gallbladder disease frequently are absent. The diagnosis depends on demonstrating a stone in the common bile duct. Any disorder of impaired bile excretion also affects the excretion of orally or intravenously administered contrast agents used to visualize the gallbladder or common bile duct. An intravenous cholangiogram generally will not visualize if the total serum bilirubin is greater than 3.0 mg. per 100 ml. However, radiologic visualization of both intra- and extrahepatic bile ducts can be accomplished with the newer techniques of endoscopic retrograde cholangiography or transhepatic cholangiography using a thin gauge needle. Consultation should be sought for radiographic bile duct visualization. Demonstrating normal bile ducts followed by performing a liver biopsy that shows intrahepatic cholestasis can avoid many surgical explorations for suspected obstructive jaundice.

Drug-induced cholestasis usually is reversible upon discontinuing the offending medication. The jaundice, however, may not disappear for many months. An extensive drug history is mandatory in the evaluation of jaundice.

Liver Function Tests

The large number of liver function tests available to today's clinician is exceeded only by the number of functions performed by the liver. A single liver function test neither supplies all the needed information nor effectively measures the total function of the liver.

The clinician should understand the functions of each liver function test—its specificity for hepatic disease, its ability to judge severity of disease, and its ability to discriminate between hepatocellular and extrahepatic disorders. The proper selection and interpretation of liver function tests occur when they are based on a thorough clinical appraisal of the patient.

Hepatocellular Enzymes. The SGOT and SGPT are the commonly used hepatocellular enzyme liver function tests. They are sensitive indicators of hepatocellular injury. Even minor hepatocyte injury will cause these enzymes to leak into the circulation. Quantitatively, they are not specific enough to judge the severity of hepatic disease, except in gross terms.

The SGPT is more specific for liver disease than is the SGOT, which also is present in skeletal muscle, cardiac muscle, and kidney tissue. The SGPT is also more sensitive to acute hepatocyte injury than the SGOT. For individuals at risk of developing liver injury, such as certain industrial workers exposed to potential hepatotoxins or hospital workers at risk from hepatitis B infections, the SGPT is a sensitive screening test.

Values of SGOT and SGPT exceeding 400 IU suggest acute, ongoing hepatic parenchymal cell damage. Obstructive or cholestatic processes only rarely elevate these values above 400 IU.

Alkaline Phosphatase. Elevated serum levels of the enzyme alkaline phosphatase can occur with liver disease, normal or abnormal osteoblastic activity, and during the third trimester of pregnancy from placental production. Several tests help confirm that an elevated alkaline phosphatase is of hepatic origin. The easiest way takes advantage of the heat lability of the osseous component ("bone burns"). Both serum 5'-nucleotidase and serum leucine aminopeptidase generally measure the same hepatic functions as alkaline phosphatase but are specific for the liver. The glutamyl transpeptidase (gamma GT) rises considerably with cholestasis and obstructive liver disease but also is elevated in hepatocellular liver disease. In the absence of elevations of the SGOT and SGPT, an abnormal gamma GT confirms that an alkaline phosphatase elevation is of hepatic origin.

In the absence of bone disease and pregnancy, an elevated alkaline phosphatase level generally reflects impaired hepatic excretory function. A normal alkaline phosphatase value in the presence of liver disease argues against obstructive jaundice or cholestasis. It is also a sensitive indicator of infiltrative liver disease. High levels are seen with granulomatous hepatitis, metastatic liver disease, and hepatic abscesses.

Lactic Dehydrogenase (LDH). The LDH is not a liver function test. The enzyme is distributed ubiquitously throughout tissues of the body. Fractionation into its five isoenzymes can enhance its specificity. High levels are seen in metastatic liver disease, reflecting extensive carcinomatosis. It has little utility in evaluating liver disease.

Serum Proteins. Older liver function tests based on quantitative changes of serum proteins (thymol turbidity, cephalin-cholesterol flocculation) are of historical interest only and no longer used. Even the quantitative measurements of albumin and total globulins and their components are liver function tests of limited value.

Albumin synthesis is a major hepatic function. However, the influence on serum albumin levels by nonhepatic factors makes its determination difficult to interpret. Hyperglobulinemia suggests chronic inflammatory liver disease, such as chronic active hepatitis and cirrhosis. Like serum albumin, serum globulin elevation is very nonspecific. The level of serum globulin plus the degree of hepatocellular enzyme abnormalities aids in following the disease activity of a chronic active hepatitis process.

Prothrombin Time. Although not a true liver function test, the prothrombin time is useful in judging the severity and prognosis of liver disease. In acute viral hepatitis, a prothrombin time less than 40 per cent of control and unresponsive to parenteral vitamin K administration suggests the presence of severe liver disease and the possibility of developing fulminant hepatic necrosis. The same degree of prothrombin time abnormality in patients with chronic liver disease carries poor prognostic implications. One always should try to correct the prothrombin time with vitamin K. Successful correction suggests that the liver disease may be due to extrahepatic obstruction.

Percutaneous Liver Biopsy. Histologic study of hepatic tissue is an indispensable tool for the proper evaluation of liver disease. Percutaneous liver biopsy is a safe, simple procedure that can produce a definitive diagnosis. A liver biopsy should be considered in any patient with suspected liver disease. Diffuse hepatocellular disease best lends itself to specific diagnosis on liver biopsy. Focal liver disease, such as metastatic lesions, can be diagnosed by biopsy under direct vision, with use of laparoscopy to direct the needle biopsy. Although it does not measure any function, liver biopsy is the best means today for making a specific diagnosis in hepatic disease.

ALCOHOL AND LIVER DISEASE

The Development of Laennec's Cirrhosis

The natural history of alcoholic liver disease is a slow process spanning many years. Only 10 to 20 per cent of chronic alcoholics develop liver disease. The reasons are poorly understood. In this group of alcoholics, regular consumption of alcohol for 5 to 15 years may produce only subcellular changes within the hepatocyte that are clinically silent and are detectable only with electron microscopy. However, these subcellular changes are the beginnings of alcoholic liver disease.

The fatty liver is the first clinically recognizable result of alcohol-induced liver disease. The accumulation of fat within hepatocytes is a morphologic response of the liver to chronic metabolism of alcohol. The liver becomes enlarged and slightly tender. Liver function tests are mildly abnormal. The patient usually is asymptomatic.

The fatty liver is a reversible lesion, as cirrhosis does not result from fat within hepatocytes. Improvement occurs when alcohol consumption ceases. The fatty liver, however, is a warning that chronic abuse of alcohol is causing structural hepatic damage. This is the stage of alcoholic liver disease that potentially is reversible if the patient stops his alcohol consumption.

The effects of alcohol are not the only cause of the fatty liver. Obesity, diabetes mellitus, kwashiorkor, and parenteral tetracycline therapy may cause similar hepatic histologic changes.

Alcoholic hepatitis is the key morphologic lesion in alcoholic liver disease. It lays the groundwork for cirrhosis. Eighty per cent of patients with alcoholic hepatitis will develop cirrhosis if they continue to consume alcohol. Why alcohol can cause fatty liver in some patients and alcoholic hepatitis in others is not known. It is not simply a reflection of the volume of alcohol ingested, although more severe cases of alcoholic hepatitis generally occur after a protracted period of binge drinking.

Liver biopsy specimens in patients with alcoholic hepatitis show diffusely scattered areas of hepatocellular necrosis with polymorphonuclear infiltration and varying degrees of fat accumulation. Degenerating hepatocytes may contain perinuclear clumps of eosinophilic material representing swollen, damaged cellular organelles called Mallory bodies. The active hepatic necrosis diffusely destroys hepatocytes, allows fibrosis to form as a healing process, distorts the hepatic vascular bed, and causes nodular regeneration of the remaining viable hepatocytes. Collectively, these changes lead to the formation of Laennec's cirrhosis.

Alcoholic hepatitis encompasses a broad clinical spectrum. The disease may cause no symptoms, or it can be a severe, acute, sometimes fatal febrile illness with jaundice, leukocytosis, abdominal pain, an exquisitely tender liver, and marked abnormalities of liver function tests. It can mimic acute cholecystitis, obstructive jaundice, or an acute abdomen.

Management of alcoholic hepatitis requires vigorous supportive care. Recovery from a clinically severe bout of the disease usually requires several weeks of hospitalization. Be sure that the patient receives adequate nutrition to aid recovery of hepatic function. Corticosteroids do not seem beneficial in the treatment of alcoholic hepatitis, although the data are conflicting.

Laennec's cirrhosis probably develops slowly from repeated episodes of alcoholic hepatitis, many of which may go undetected. The development of Laennec's cirrhosis is not a homogeneous process within the liver. At one point in time, a chronic alcoholic who is developing cirrhosis may have hepatic histologic findings that show various degrees of fatty infiltration, alcoholic hepatitis, fibrosis, scarring, and regenerative nodules. Some of these are reversible lesions, others are not.

Many patients with alcoholic liver disease have far advanced Laennec's cirrhosis prior to seeking medical assistance. Presumably, their previous episodes of alcoholic hepatitis that led to the cirrhosis were subclinical. Generally, one of four major complications of Laennec's cirrhosis will bring the patient to his physician. Table 46-24 lists these complications.

Hepatocellular Failure. Chronic hepatocellular failure develops when destruction of hepatocytes and distortion of the hepatic architecture by fibrosis and regenerative nodules are extensive enough to compromise many functions of the liver. Virtually every organ system may be indirectly affected. The patient is chronically ill. He may complain of weakness, fatigue, anorexia, and weight loss and suffer from many other clinical manifestations of chronic hepatocellular failure listed in Table 46-25.

In general, management consists of stopping the patient's ingestion of alcohol, feeding him a nutritious high calorie diet, and supplementing this diet with essential dietary factors of which he may be deficient because of his prolonged consumption of calories mainly from alcoholic beverages. He may require supplemental iron, folate, thiamine, vitamin B_{12}, or fat-soluble vitamins. Hospitalization for the initial evaluation and treatment is desirable. It will aid the patient in stopping his alcohol consumption and help to assess the patient's response to the initial management of his liver disease. Since cirrhosis develops at varying rates throughout the liver, even patients with severe hepatocellular failure may have some reversible components to their liver disease that proper symptomatic management can improve.

Portal Hypertension. Portal hypertension is a frequent complication of cirrhosis. Fibrosis and collapse of the normal hepatic architecture disrupt the intricate pathways for blood flow through the liver. High pressures develop within the normally low pressure portal venous system in an effort to overcome the increased resistance to flow within the diseased liver.

Portal hypertension causes no symptoms of its own. However, the increased resistance to portal blood flow through the liver allows collateral venous channels to open between the portal and systemic venous systems, bypassing the liver. The collateral veins produce hemorrhoids, distended abdominal wall veins, and esophageal varices.

Bleeding esophageal varices is a severe, life-threatening complication of portal hypertension. The mortality rate is about 30 per cent. The onset of variceal bleeding usually is spontaneous, without an obvious precipitating event other than the chronic portal hypertension. However, it is only one of several possible causes of acute upper gastrointestinal bleeding in patients with cirrhosis and portal hypertension. Early recognition of the source of bleeding is essential for proper management. Radiographic barium examination of the esoph-

TABLE 46-24. COMPLICATIONS OF LAENNEC'S CIRRHOSIS

1. Chronic hepatocellular failure
2. Portal hypertension
3. Hepatic encephalopathy
4. Ascites and fluid retention

TABLE 46–25. CLINICAL MANIFESTATIONS OF CHRONIC HEPATOCELLULAR FAILURE

Organ System	Manifestations
General	Weakness, fatigue, anorexia, weight loss, malaise, muscle wasting
Hepatic	Jaundice, hypoalbuminemia, splenomegaly, hepatomegaly
Renal	Edema, ascites, hepatorenal syndrome
Dermatologic	Spider angiomas, palmar erythema, loss of body hair, clubbing of fingers
Endocrinologic	Gynecomastia, testicular atrophy, diabetes mellitus, hypoglycemia
Hematologic	Blood clotting abnormalities; purpura; hypersplenism causing leukopenia, anemia, and thrombocytopenia; anemia from many causes—gastrointestinal blood loss, folic acid deficiency, hemolysis

agus, stomach, and duodenum is not very helpful, as it can only indicate the presence of varices. Fiberoptic endoscopy helps to properly diagnose and manage these patients by determining if the varices are indeed bleeding. Early consultation should be sought.

Hepatic Encephalopathy. Although alterations in ammonia metabolism continue to best explain the pathogenesis of hepatic encephalopathy, this theory remains to be proved. However, no matter if the offending substance is ammonia or some other compound, it has the following characteristics:

1. The substance is shunted around the liver, where it normally is detoxified.

2. The substance arises from the gastrointestinal tract.

3. It is of nitrogenous origin.

4. The bacterial flora of the gastrointestinal tract play an important role in producing the substance within the gut.

5. By avoiding detoxification in the liver, the substance is able to adversely affect function of the central nervous system, producing the signs and symptoms of hepatic encephalopathy.

Heptatic encephalopathy arbitrarily is divided into four stages of increasing severity (Table 46–26). Coma occurs only in Stage IV, the most severe stage. In Stage I, the level of consciousness and intellectual function are abnormal only to a slight degree. Euphoria, apathy, depression, restlessness, or an altered sleep pattern may be the only symptoms. Recognition of hepatic encephalopathy must occur in this early stage, prior to the patient's developing coma. The symptoms can be very subtle. The five main clinical features of hepatic encephalopathy are listed in Table 46–27. In the early stages of hepatic encephalopathy, only one or two of these characteristics may be evident. If the symptoms go unrecognized or are treated with sedatives or tranquilizers, deeper stages of encephalopathy can result.

The treatment of hepatic encephalopathy attempts to limit the amount of toxin produced in the gut. Since it is of nitrogenous origin, dietary protein is restricted to about 20 to 30 grams per day. Nonabsorbable antibiotics, such as neomycin, decrease the bacterial flora of the gastrointestinal tract, diminishing toxin production. Lactulose, a nonabsorbable disaccharide, acidifies the colonic contents, which diminishes absorption of the toxin.

Try to determine why hepatic encephalopathy has occurred (Table 46–28). There

TABLE 46–26. THE STAGES OF HEPATIC ENCEPHALOPATHY

STAGE I: Depressed or euphoric, mild confusion, apathy, disordered sleep pattern, slowed thinking, inappropriate behavior, and restlessness; a few patients have asterixis

STAGE II: Drowsiness; marked mental confusion to time, place and person; slowed responses to everyday stimuli, apathy, depression, long periods of sleep, marked asterixis, abnormal electroencephalogram (EEG), elevated serum ammonia level

STAGE III: Stupor, rousable sleep, incoherent speech, confusion, abnormal EEG, asterixis, gross neuromuscular changes

STAGE IV: Deep coma, absent tremor and asterixis, abnormal EEG, no limb rigidity, absent deep tendon reflexes

TABLE 46–27. THE CLINICAL FEATURES OF HEPATIC ENCEPHALOPATHY

Disturbance of consciousness: malaise, incoherent speech, stupor, deep coma

Impaired intellectual function: confusion, inappropriate behavior, slovenly dress, forgetfulness, illegible handwriting

Neuromuscular abnormalities: asterixis (flapping tremor) incoordination, muscle twitching, rigidity, hyper-reflexia, positive toe signs, seizures

Electroencephalogram changes: symmetrical slow triphasic waves, 2 to 5 per second

Elevated serum ammonia levels

usually is one event that has led to the development of encephalopathy in addition to the chronic liver disease. Gastrointestinal bleeding, which increases the protein load to the gut, is a common example. Correcting the precipitating cause may reverse the encephalopathy completely.

Ascites and Fluid Retention. Why ascites forms in patients with chronic liver disease remains poorly understood. Fluid escapes from the hepatic sinusoids because of the increased hydrostatic pressure of portal hypertension and the decreased oncotic pressure from the hypoalbuminemia of the chronic liver disease. Increased hepatic lymph flow attempts to handle the fluid that is leaving the sinusoids. Fluid not incorporated into the hepatic lymph weeps off the surface of the liver to become free fluid within the peritoneal cavity. A defective intravascular volume and a large extravascular fluid space result, to which the kidneys respond by clearing less free water and avidly retaining sodium.

Ascites is a complication of cirrhosis and not a disease on its own. Treatment should focus on the liver disease rather than on mechanically trying to remove the ascitic fluid. Rigid salt and fluid restriction and careful use of diuretics, particularly aldosterone antagonists, can be of some bene-

TABLE 46–28. EVENTS THAT MAY PRECIPITATE HEPATIC ENCEPHALOPATHY

Gastrointestinal bleeding
High protein diet
Use of diuretics
Use of sedatives, tranquilizers
Postoperative portacaval shunt
Uremia
Constipation
Hypokalemic alkalosis
Infections

fit if the patient stops drinking alcohol and eats a proper diet. Minimal ascites and edema usually disappear with bed rest and abstinence from alcohol alone. Any measures used to lessen ascites must be done in a slow, deliberate way. Rapid removal of ascites can precipitate hepatic encephalopathy and cause severe electrolyte disturbances.

The clinician's chief duty when dealing with alcoholic liver disease is to stop the patient's alcohol intake early in the course of the disease when some of the liver function is retainable and some damage is reversible. Most other forms of therapy merely try to compensate for a failing liver.

VIRAL HEPATITIS

Viral hepatitis is a diffuse inflammatory disease of hepatic parenchymal cells caused by several different viral agents. Since the discovery of the Australia antigen in 1965, the concepts of viral hepatitis have been altered extensively and the terminology has become complex. Some of the current nomenclature used in connection with viral hepatitis is listed in Table 46–29.

Diagnosis. Infections caused by both type A and type B hepatitis viruses begin with an asymptomatic incubation period after the patient is infected with the virus. The incubation period varies in length, averaging about 30 days with type A hepatitis and about 90 days with type B hepatitis, although with the latter type, it may last as long as 6 months. A prodromal period of nonspecific influenza-like complaints follows the incubation period and precedes by several days to weeks the appearance of bilirubinuria and clinical jaundice. Recovery begins soon after the jaundice appears, with the generalized symptoms subsiding more rapidly than the jaundice.

The history of the initial contact with the virus may be obscure. A history of close contact with sufferers of viral hepatitis can be obtained only about 20 to 30 per cent of the time. Infections with both type A and type B hepatitis viruses can be anicteric and subclinical. Many cases go undetected. This may explain the high incidence of circulating antibody to hepatitis A virus in urban adults and the many presumably sporadic cases of viral hepatitis.

TABLE 46-29. THE NOMENCLATURE OF VIRAL HEPATITIS

Term	Definition
Type A hepatitis	Viral hepatitis caused by the hepatitis A virus (HAV).
Type B hepatitis	Viral hepatitis caused by the hepatitis B virus (HBV).
Non-A, non-B viral hepatitis	Viral hepatitis following transfusions that does not seem to be caused by either hepatitis A or B viruses or by any other known virus that can give a hepatitis-like picture. A high percentage of post-transfusion hepatitis cases are due to this as yet unidentified agent, which is sometimes referred to as type C hepatitis.
Subacute hepatic necrosis	A severe form of viral hepatitis. Hepatocellular necrosis is extensive and occurs in broad bands, linking portal tracts and central veins (bridging necrosis). A high percentage of patients rapidly develop postnecrotic cirrhosis.
Acute fulminant viral hepatitis	An extremely severe, often fatal viral hepatitis infection.
HB_sAg	Hepatitis B surface antigen. The same as Australia antigen—now an outdated term. Represents the outer or surface coat of the hepatitis B virus. It is produced within the cytoplasm of hepatocytes and released into the circulation.
HB_cAg	Hepatitis B core antigen. Found in the nuclei of hepatocytes and the sera of patients infected with type B hepatitis.
Dane particle	A large particle consisting of an inner core containing HB_cAg (viral core) and a HB_sAg-containing outer coat. Represents the complete hepatitis B virus particle. Found in the sera and hepatocyte cytoplasm of type B hepatitis patients.
Anti-HB_s	Antibody to HB_sAg. Its presence indicates previous exposure to hepatitis B virus and that recovery has occurred. Patients with anti-HB_s are immune to future HBV exposures.
Anti-HB_c	Antibody to HB_cAg. Detectable in chronic carriers of HB_sAg. May indicate HBV replication.
DNA polymerase activity	A virus-specific enzyme whose activity indicates HBV replication.
e antigen	Found only in HB_sAg positive sera. Associated with Dane particles and clinical infectivity. Associated with HB_sAg carriers who have liver disease.
Anti-e	Antibody to e antigen. Found in asymptomatic HB_sAg carriers without liver disease.

The recognition of type B hepatitis occurs easily now because of the availability of serologic tests as markers of the hepatitis B virus, such as the hepatitis B surface antigen (HB_sAg). The use of these markers has shown that type B hepatitis (formerly called "serum hepatitis") can be transmitted not only parenterally but also by a variety of nonparenteral routes. Many of these transmissions go undetected. About 50 per cent of sporadic viral hepatitis cases in the United States are type B. These patients have no history to suggest parenteral exposure to blood or blood products. It is now well accepted that both type A and type B viral hepatitis may be transmitted by either parenteral or nonparenteral routes; hence, the terms "infectious" and "serum hepatitis" are outdated.

In most respects, the usual clinical picture of types A and B hepatitis are similar, except for the presence of HB_sAg in the sera of patients with type B hepatitis. The patient becomes ill in the prodromal stage, prior to becoming jaundiced, with nonspecific constitutional symptoms of nausea, vomiting, anorexia, fever, arthralgias, myalgias, and transient skin rashes. This stage lasts several days to a few weeks. Dark urine (bilirubinuria) is noted, and a few days later the patient becomes icteric. Once the jaundice is obvious, many of the constitutional symptoms begin to subside. Hepatocellular enzyme levels (SGOT, SGPT) tend to peak before the maximal increase in bilirubin. They may even be improving at the time the jaundice is recognized. In type B hepatitis, the HB_sAg, which is detectable even before the prodromal stage, usually vanishes when recovery begins. Later anti-HB_s appears. The jaundice slowly subsides over several weeks. Full biochemical recovery may take several months.

Management. There is no specific treatment for viral hepatitis. The physician should closely follow the patient through the stages of the disease and should frequently monitor the results of liver function tests. Hospitalization is necessary if there is any question about the diagnosis, if the disease is particularly severe, or if the patient is quite symptomatic, with vomiting and inability to eat. The prothrombin time is a useful guide in judging the severity of the disease. Prolongation more than 2 seconds over the control that fails to correct with administration of parenteral vitamin K denotes a patient with moderately severe viral hepatitis who deserves hospitalization. Other clinical features of severe viral hepatitis are a serum bilirubin level in excess of 25 mg. per dl., deepening jaundice occurring when hepatocellular enzyme levels are falling, a rapid decrease in liver size, ascites, and early signs of hepatic encephalopathy. These patients should be hospitalized immediately and followed closely. They could be suffering from fulminant viral hepatitis with acute hepatic failure or subacute hepatic necrosis—both fortunately rare complications of viral hepatitis that require specialized management.

When treating the usual patient with viral hepatitis, it is best to restrict physical activity until the clinical recovery phase begins, as judged by both the liver function tests and the generalized symptoms. Encourage consumption of a balanced high-calorie diet. Do not use any medications unless absolutely necessary for fear of side effects from delayed metabolism by the diseased liver. Corticosteroids are not useful, except perhaps in the rare patient with subacute hepatic necrosis. There is no evidence that corticosteroids shorten the course of the disease or change the ultimate outcome of viral hepatitis. Proper hygiene rather than strict isolation is a sounder way of handling the patient's infectivity of others. Proper hand-washing technique, a private bathroom, and careful handling of the patient's secretions, particularly blood samples, should be strictly enforced.

Use of Immune Serum Globulin. Conventional immune serum globulin (gamma globulin) has proved effective in attenuating infections following exposures to type A viral hepatitis. All intimate contacts of patients with type A hepatitis should receive 2 ml. of standard immune serum globulin. This includes the spouse and other household members having very close contact with the infected person. Classmates, neighbors, or visitors to the household need not receive the immune serum globulin. The immune serum globulin does not prevent the disease but rather attenuates the infection to a subclinical anicteric process. Active immunity still is obtained. Thus, both passive and active immunity occur in those exposed to type A viral hepatitis who receive immune serum globulin.

Because blood banks screen donors for circulating HB_sAg, the concentration of anti-HB_s in standard pooled immune serum globulin has increased in recent years. It now may be effective in attenuating type B viral hepatitis infections following certain exposures to small amounts of HB_sAg. Hospital workers pricked inadvertently by HB_sAg-contaminated needles and household contacts of patients with type B hepatitis may benefit from standard immune serum globulin administration. Because the titer of anti-HB_s is low in the standard immune serum globulin, the suggested dose is 5 ml. A specific hepatitis B immune globulin has been manufactured, but the limited supply restricts its use for investigational work only.

The food handler who develops hepatitis is a special case. Food-borne epidemics of viral hepatitis have occurred, but are unusual. Widespread use of immune serum globulin is not recommended in this situation unless cases of hepatitis can be traced to this source. The food handler should not return to his usual employment until his jaundice has disappeared.

Chronic Hepatitis. The vast majority of patients with viral hepatitis will recover completely with no residual liver disease. A few patients, however, will not. These patients must be detected. They may feel fit, not be jaundiced, and have a normal-sized, nontender liver, but biochemical evidence of complete recovery does not occur. Hepatocellular enzyme levels remain elevated. Total serum globulin levels may be elevated, and in patients with type B hepatitis, the HB_sAg persists in the serum. The patient should be evaluated thoroughly if the liver function tests remain abnormal for longer than 6 months after the onset of the acute disease. These patients have a form of chronic hepatitis—either chronic persistent hepatitis, a benign disease that requires no therapy, or chronic active hepatitis, a potentially serious disease that without corticosteroid and azathioprine therapy can lead to postnecrotic cirrhosis.

Although as a rule liver function test abnormalities are more severe in patients with chronic active hepatitis, the only definitive way to distinguish chronic active hepatitis from chronic persistent hepatitis is by the study of liver biopsy specimens. It is the responsibility of every physician who deals with patients having acute viral hepatitis to follow the patient closely to complete recovery and to evaluate properly those who develop manifestations of chronic hepatitis.

HB_sAg Carriers. A frequent problem facing physicians today is how to handle the patient with a positive test for HB_sAg. Because of the routine screening of blood donors for HB_sAg, this is not an uncommon situation. Approximately 0.1 to 0.2 per cent of the American population are asymptomatic carriers of HB_sAg. All carriers of HB_sAg should be screened for evidence of liver disease with a standard battery of liver function tests. Any abnormalities must be explained. This usually requires study of a liver biopsy specimen. Some of these carriers may have occult liver disease.

Whether they have liver disease or not, HB_sAg carriers represent a public health problem that has yet to be solved. Some may be infectious. At the present time, the blood of these carriers must be presumed to be infectious. They should not donate blood or share razors, toothbrushes, or needles. If the carrier has an occupation that brings him in close contact with other people, for example, physicians, dentists, barbers, food handlers, or health professional workers, proper hygiene must be stressed. There is not enough evidence at the present time to consider a change in occupation for this group of HB_sAg carriers.

DRUGS AND THE LIVER

The list of medications that may adversely affect the liver is extensive. Drug-induced hepatitis is an increasingly common cause of acute hepatic failure. *A detailed medication history is a must when evaluating patients with liver disease.*

The vast majority of drug-induced liver diseases occur as an idiosyncratic reaction in a small percentage of the recipients of any drug. Previous or chronic liver disease does not seem to predispose patients to an increased risk of developing drug-induced liver disease. The mechanisms responsible for individual susceptibility to various drugs are only partially understood. Some reactions may be due to aberrances in the metabolism of the drug. The hepatotoxic agent may not be the drug itself, but rather one of its metabolites. Other reactions possibly are due to an allergic susceptibility of the patient, in whom the drug somehow plays a sensitizing role. Commonly, extrahepatic manifestations of hypersensitivity are seen concurrently with the liver damage. Liver disease of recent onset is likely to be drug-induced in patients taking medication who also have fever, eosinophilia, a skin rash, arthralgias, or hemolytic anemia.

The clinical pattern of drug-induced liver disease varies. It may be cholestatic, which resembles obstructive jaundice, or hepatocellular, which mimics viral hepatitis. Frequently, features of both cholestasis and hepatocellular disease are seen. Fatty liver, chronic active hepatitis, and cirrhosis are less common histologic changes that result from drug-induced disease.

Drug-induced Cholestasis

Drug-induced intrahepatic cholestasis closely resembles the clinical picture of extrahepatic biliary obstruction. Jaundice, pruritus, and striking elevations of the serum cholesterol and alkaline phosphatase levels are the main clinical manifestations. Initially, the serum transaminase levels may be high. The onset of the jaundice usually is insidious.

Chlorpromazine is a frequent cause of cholestasis. Jaundice occurs in 1 to 2 per cent of chlorpromazine recipients. The reaction is not dose-related. Other phenothiazines also can cause cholestasis but do so less often, probably because of their less frequent clinical use.

The jaundice usually appears within the first month of therapy. Associated fever, rash, and eosinophilia are common. This reaction can sometimes be distinguished from extrahepatic obstructive jaundice by examination of liver biopsy specimens. Stopping the drug improves the cholestasis. Most cases resolve over several months. Other drugs that can cause a similar cholestatic picture are listed in Table 46–30.

The C-17-alpha-alkylated anabolic steroids (methyltestosterone, norethandrolone) adversely affect bile secretory function. The reaction is dose-dependent. Jaundice appears only after several months of treatment and is reversible in most cases by stopping the drug. No hepatocellular damage occurs.

Drug-induced Hepatitis

Hepatitis can be caused by a long list of drugs (see Table 46–30). The jaundice produced by drug-induced hepatocellular damage results from extensive hepatic necrosis rather than from cholestasis. The clinical picture closely resembles that of viral hepatitis. The onset of the disease may be quite abrupt, and the hepatocellular enzymes may be markedly elevated. The potential exists for serious liver disease, acute hepatic failure, and death, as may occur in viral hepatitis. Drug-induced hepatitis can be a far more serious reaction than cholestasis.

Halothane hepatitis has an extremely low incidence, but the disease is not rare because of the wide use of this anesthetic agent. An allergic or immune mechanism may be responsible for halothane hepati-

TABLE 46–30.   TYPES OF DRUG-INDUCED HEPATIC INJURY

Durg-induced cholestasis	Chlorpromazine and other phenothiazines Erythromycin estolate Tolbutamide Chlorpropamide Thiabendazole Methyltestosterone Norethandrolone Certain cholecystography agents

Drug-induced hepatitis	Anesthetic agents
	  Halothane
	  Methoxyflurane
	Analgesic agents
	  Aspirin (high doses)
	  Acetaminophen
	  Phenacetin
	Anticonvulsants
	  Phenytoin
	Other drugs
	  Methyldopa
	  Imipramine
	  Isoniazid
	  Phenylbutazone
	  Rifampin
	  Para-aminosalicylic acid
	  Papaverine
	  Sulfonamides

Drug-induced fatty liver	Tetracycline (parenterally administered) Methotrexate
Chronic active hepatitis	Oxyphenisatin Methyldopa
Cirrhosis	Methotrexate (prolonged use)
Hepatic adenoma Primary hepatocellular carcinoma	Oral contraceptives
Hepatic angiosarcoma	Industrial vinyl chloride exposure

tis. It usually occurs after several exposures to halothane and is associated with fever and eosinophilia. Halothane hepatitis is included in the differential diagnosis of postoperative fever, as the onset occurs within the first 2 weeks following anesthesia. Severe hepatitis is common, with very high transaminase levels and deep jaundice. Mortality is high. Acute hepatic failure is the usual cause of death.

Acetaminophen causes hepatic damage when large doses of the drug are ingested, usually in suicide attempts. Such doses shift the hepatic metabolism of acetaminophen to favor formation of a toxic metabolite that causes the hepatic damage, rather than being caused by the drug itself. A similar mechanism probably causes the hepatitis associated with the use of isoniazid.

Many drug-induced hepatocellular reactions are mild. Only minimal elevations of hepatocellular enzyme levels may occur. Always be suspicious of drug-induced liver disease in clinical settings in which abnormal liver function tests cannot be readily explained. Many drug reactions that produce hepatitis can cause a characteristic histologic appearance on liver biopsy.

Treatment of course includes stopping the use of the offending drug. Once this is done, the management is similar to that of viral hepatitis. No specific treatment exists once the liver disease has occurred. One gives supportive therapy and watches closely for complications of acute hepatic failure.

Oral Contraceptives and Liver Tumors

Prolonged use of oral contraceptives may cause hepatic adenomas, focal nodular hyperplasia of the liver, and primary liver cell carcinoma. Although the number of reported cases has been small, the high association of these rare tumors with the use of oral contraceptives for several years or more makes the association very suspicious, although not definitely proved.

Rather than presenting with liver function test abnormalities or jaundice, these women may complain of right upper quadrant pain, have a palpable mass in the right upper quadrant, or present with acute intraperitoneal hemorrhage from the tumor's rupturing and bleeding into the peritoneal cavity. Hepatic angiography best demonstrates these highly vascular lesions. A tumor more than 2 cm. in diameter will show up as a filling defect on liver scanning. Liver biopsy is contraindicated because of the risk of hemorrhage. Surgical excision, if possible, is the proper management. These rare tumors should be included in the differential diagnosis of any abdominal emergency developing in a woman of childbearing age. Rupture of the lesion and the subsequent hemorrhage can be fatal.

Industrial Toxins

Only recently have physicians begun to appreciate the potential of liver disease as an occupational hazard. Chronic industrial vinyl chloride exposure causes hepatic fibrosis and angiosarcoma of the liver. This may be only one example of the risk of hepatotoxins in industry, as more American workers become chronically exposed to synthetic chemicals. Not only should the physician be suspicious of drugs causing liver disease, but also of chronic industrial toxin exposures.

GALLBLADDER DISEASE

Cholelithiasis

Nearly all disease of the gallbladder is a consequence of cholelithiasis. The cholesterol gallstone, the most common gallstone found in Western countries, is responsible for most gallbladder disease. The fundamental defect causing cholesterol gallstone formation is not gallbladder malfunction but rather the hepatic secretion of bile supersaturated with cholesterol. Cholelithiasis is a hepatic disorder, the symptoms of which occur in the gallbladder.

Cholesterol gallstones form in the gallbladder by the precipitation of cholesterol microcrystals. These microcrystals represent that portion of cholesterol that is insoluble in bile. The liver actively secretes cholesterol, bile salts, and lecithin into the bile. The bile salts and lecithin together form small aggregates called mixed micelles, which greatly enhance the solubility of cholesterol. The relative proportions of the bile salts, lecithin, and cholesterol in the bile determine if the cholesterol will be soluble. If the bile salt concentration is low or the cholesterol concentration high, the bile becomes supersaturated with cholesterol. Supersaturated bile is lithogenic, as the cholesterol is able to precipitate and form microcrystals, leading to the formation of cholesterol gallstones. The liver produces a lithogenic bile in patients with cholesterol gallstones.

Many questions regarding the pathogenesis of cholelithiasis remain unanswered. Not everyone with lithogenic bile develops gallstones. The liver produces lithogenic bile in most people during the fasting state. It is uncertain what the primary biochemical defect in the liver is that causes the secretion of lithogenic bile. Not all gallstones are composed primarily of cholesterol. Many are calcium bilirubinate stones. The pathogenesis of these stones is poorly understood.

The incidence of gallstones is high. At least 5 to 10 per cent of persons past the age of 50 have cholelithiasis. Many of these persons are asymptomatic. Others develop acute cholecystitis or suffer the symptoms of chronic cholecystitis.

Cholecystitis

Acute cholecystitis is caused by the sudden obstruction of the cystic duct by a gallstone. The gallbladder distends, bacteria proliferate within the lumen, and signs of an acute illness ensue. Acute cholecystitis can present clinically with a wide spectrum of severity. Right upper quadrant abdominal pain, nausea, vomiting, fever, leukocytosis, and mild icterus are the common features. The pain may radiate to the shoulder or subscapular region. If the stone migrates into the common bile duct, severe pain of biliary colic and marked jaundice occur. Tenderness, guarding, and occasionally a tender, palpable gallbladder are felt in the right upper quadrant of the abdomen.

The liver function tests are only mildly abnormal. The oral cholecystogram is of no diagnostic help. It will not visualize the gallbladder. The intravenous cholangiogram will outline a normal biliary tree but will fail to opacify the gallbladder. However, this pattern frequently occurs in normal persons. If the gallbladder visualizes on intravenous cholangiography, acute cholecystitis is not the cause of the patient's symptoms.

Most episodes of acute cholecystitis subside within several days with supportive care. A few do not and require urgent surgical intervention. Seek early surgical consultation in patients with acute cholecystitis. Many surgeons now operate during the early course of the disease instead of waiting several weeks for the inflammation to subside. If a cholecystectomy is not done, repeated episodes of acute cholecystitis can be expected to occur.

Repeated attacks of mild to moderately severe episodes of acute cholecystitis define the clinical condition of chronic cholecystitis. The symptoms are not as well defined as in acute cholecystitis and may be difficult to recognize as those of gallbladder disease. Right upper quadrant abdominal pain, dyspepsia, flatulence, eructations, and intolerance to fatty foods are nonspecific symptoms. Only a small percentage of patients with these symptoms are suffering from gallbladder disease. A cholecystectomy commonly fails to relieve these symptoms. A nonvisualizing gallbladder or one containing stones on oral cholecystography does not tell you if the gallbladder disease is symptomatic.

Management of Gallbladder Disease

At least 30 per cent of patients with cholelithiasis are asymptomatic. Of these about one-third will develop symptoms within 5 years. Elective cholecystectomy removes this risk plus the risk of developing serious complications from acute cholecystitis. The decision for elective cholecystectomy is not easy in patients who have an increased surgical risk because of other diseases or their age. Cholecystectomy is not recommended for patients past the age of 60, as the risks of the surgery outweigh the risks of developing complications from the gallstones.

Symptoms similar to those of chronic cholecystitis that occur after cholecystectomy tend to be lumped into the vague condition called the postcholecystectomy syndrome. The majority of these symptoms are similar to those suffered prior to the cholecystectomy. Many are the symptoms of an irritable bowel, abdominal wall pain, or diseases of other organ systems. Stenosis of the sphincter of Oddi, a postoperative stricture of the common bile duct, a retained common bile duct stone, or a cystic duct remnant are uncommon causes of continued pain following cholecystectomy. Thorough preoperative evaluation of the patient can eliminate many of these symptoms from being blamed on the surgery.

Medical therapy for gallstones continues to be investigated. Oral administration of chenodeoxycholic acid (one of the primary bile acids) can convert lithogenic bile to normal and in functioning gallbladders can slowly dissolve noncalcified cholesterol gallstones that previously had formed. The feeding of this bile acid increases the concentration of bile salts within the bile, thus increasing the ability of the bile to keep cholesterol in solution. The feasibility of this treatment awaits the results of multicenter clinical trials currently in progress.

REFERENCES

General

1. Beck, E. R., Francis, J. L., and Souhami, R. L.: Tutorials in Differential Diagnosis. New York, Pitman Publishing Corp., 1974.
2. Bockus, H. L. (ed.): Gastroenterology. 3rd Ed. 4 Vol. Philadelphia, W. B. Saunders Co., 1974–1976.
3. Brooks, F. P. (ed.): Gastrointestinal Pathophysiology. New York, Oxford University Press, Inc., 1974.
4. DeGowin, E. L., and DeGowin, R. L.: Bedside Diagnostic Examination. 3rd Ed. New York, Macmillan Publishing Co., Inc., 1976.
5. Greenberger, N. J., and Winship, D. H.: Gastrointestinal Disorders: A Pathophysiologic Approach. Chicago, Year Book Medical Publishers, Inc., 1976.
6. Harvey, A. M., and Bordley, J., III: Differential Diagnosis. 2nd Ed. Philadelphia, W. B. Saunders Co., 1970.
7. Schiff, L. (ed.): Diseases of the Liver. 4th Ed. Philadelphia, J. B. Lippincott Co., 1975.
8. Sherlock, S.: Diseases of the Liver and Biliary System. 5th Ed. Oxford, Blackwell Scientific Publications, 1975.
9. Sleisenger, M. H., and Fordtran, J. S. (eds.): Gastrointestinal Disease. 2nd Ed. Philadelphia, W. B. Saunders Co., 1978.
10. Spiro, H. M.: Clinical Gastroenterology. 2nd Ed. London, The MacMillan Company, 1977.
11. Thorn, G. W., Adams, R. D., Braunwald, E., et al. (eds.): Harrison's Principles of Internal Medicine. 8th Ed. New York, McGraw-Hill Book Co., 1977.

Chronic Abdominal Pain

1. Cope, Z.: The Early Diagnosis of the Acute Abdomen. 12th Ed. New York, Oxford University Press, 1963.
2. Heffernon, E. W., and Reaves, L. E., III.: Considerations in the diagnosis of abdominal pain. Med. Clin. North Am., 50:439, 1966.
3. Spiro, H. M.: Visceral viewpoints: Pain and perfectionism—the physician and the "pain patient." N. Engl. J. Med., 294:829, 1976.

Acute Diarrhea

1. Harris, J. C., DuPont, H. L., and Hornick, R. B.: Fecal leukocytes in diarrheal illness. Ann. Intern. Med., 76:697, 1972.
2. NIH Conference. Acute Infectious Nonbacterial Gastroenteritis: Etiology and Pathogenesis. Moderator: Blacklow, N. R., Discussants: Dolin, R., Fedson, D. S., DuPont, H., et al.: Ann. Intern. Med., 76:993, 1972.
3. Satterwhite, T. K., and DuPont, H. L.: The patient with acute diarrhea. An algorithm for diagnosis. J.A.M.A., 236:2662, 1976.

Chronic Diarrhea, Inflammatory Bowel Disease

1. Beeken, W. L.: Remediable defects in Crohn's disease. Arch. Intern. Med., 135:686, 1975.
2. Kirsner, J. B., and Shorter, R. G.: Inflammatory Bowel Disease. Philadelphia, Lea and Febiger, 1975.
3. Phillips, S. F.: Diarrhea: Pathogenesis and diagnostic techniques. Postgrad. Med., 57:65, 1975.
4. Phillips, S. F.: Diarrhea—A broad perspective. Viewpoints Dig. Dis., 7:No. 5, 1975.
5. Schachter, H., and Kirsner, J. B.: Definitions of inflammatory bowel disease of unknown etiology. Gastroenterology, 68:591, 1975.
6. Schedl, H. P.: Water and electrolyte transport: Clinical aspects. Med. Clin. North Am., 58:1429, 1974.
7. Shorter, R. G., and Shephard, D. A. E.: Frontiers in inflammatory bowel disease. Am. J. Dig. Dis., 20:540, 639, 1975.

Irritable Bowel, Diverticular Disease

1. Connell, A. M.: Clinical aspects of motility. Med. Clin. North Am., 58:1201, 1974.
2. Findlay, J. M., Smith, A. N., Mitchell, W. D., et al.: Effects of unprocessed bran on colon function in normal subjects and in diverticular disease. Lancet, 1:146, 1974.
3. Harvey, R. F., Pomare, E. W., and Heaton, K. W.: Effects of increased dietary fibre on intestinal transit. Lancet, 1:1278, 1973.
4. Irritable bowel syndrome (Editorial): Brit. Med. J., 1:197, 1972.
5. Reilly, R. W., and Kirsner, J. B. (eds.): Fiber Deficiency and Colonic Disorders. New York, Plenum Medical Book Co., 1975.
6. Waye, J. D.: Diverticular disease. Prim. Care, 3:91, 1976.

Intestinal Gas

1. Bayless, T. M.: Lactase deficiency and intolerance to milk. Viewpoints Dig. Dis., 3:No. 2, 1971.
2. Bond, J. H., and Levitt, M. D.: A rational approach to intestinal gas problems. Viewpoints Dig. Dis., 9:No. 2, 1977.
3. Lasser, R. B., Bond, J. H. and Levitt, M. D.: The role of intestinal gas in functional abdominal pain. N. Engl. J. Med., 293:524, 1975.

4. Welsh, J. D.: Isolated lactase deficiency in humans: Report on 100 patients. Medicine, *49*: 257, 1970.

Acid Peptic Disease

1. Isenberg, J. I.: H_2-receptor antagonists in the treatment of peptic ulcer. Ann. Intern. Med., *84*:212, 1976.
2. Spiro, H. M.: Moynihan's disease? The diagnosis of duodenal ulcer. N. Engl. J. Med., *291*:567, 1974.
3. ULCA Conference. A New Look at Peptic Ulcer. Moderator: Grossman, M. I. Discussants: Guth, P H., Isenberg, J. I., Passaro, E. P., Jr., et al.: Ann. Intern. Med., *84*:57, 1976.
4. When is gastric ulcer really a cancer? (Editorial): Lancet, *1*:233, 1976.

Heartburn, Reflux Esophagitis

1. Behar, J., Biancani, P., and Sheahan, D. G.: Evaluation of esophageal tests in the diagnosis of reflux esophagitis. Gastroenterology, *71*:9, 1976.
2. Bennett, J. R.: Medical management of gastro-oesophageal reflux. Clin. Gastroenterol., 5:175, 1976.
3. Clearfield, H. R.: Heartburn. Am. Fam. Phys., *15*:158, 1977.
4. Dodds, W. J., Hogan, W. J., and Miller, W. N.: Reflux esophagitis. Am. J. Dig. Dis., *21*:49, 1976.
5. Farrell, R. L., Roling, G. T., and Castell, D. O.: Cholinergic therapy of chronic heartburn. Ann. Intern. Med., *80*:573, 1974.
6. Goyal, R. K.,: The lower esophageal sphincter. Viewpoints Dig. Dis., 8:No. 3, 1976.
7. Pope, C. E., II: Pathophysiology and diagnosis of reflux esophagitis. Gastroenterology, *70*:445, 1976.

Dysphagia

1. Bennett, J. R., and Hendrix, T. R.: Diffuse esophageal spasm: A disorder with more than one cause. Gastroenterology, 59:273, 1970.
2. Edwards, D. A. W.: Discriminatory value of symptoms in the differential diagnosis of dysphagia. Clin. Gastroenterol. 5:49, 1976.
3. Schroder, J. S., and Hatcher, C. R., Jr.: Achalasia of the esophagus. Diagnosis and treatment. J.A.M.A., *202*:168, 1967.

Gastrointestinal Bleeding

1. Katon, R. M., and Smith, F. W.: Panendoscopy in the early diagnosis of acute upper gastrointestinal bleeding. Gastroenterology, 65:728, 1973.
2. Katz, D., Pitchumoni, C. S., Thomas, E., et al.: The endoscopic diagnosis of upper-gastrointestinal hemorrhage: Changing concepts of etiology and management. Am. J. Dig. Dis., *21*:182, 1976.
3. Malt, R. A.: Control of massive upper gastrointestinal hemorrhage. N. Engl. J. Med., *296*:1043, 1972.
4. Moody, F. G.: Rectal bleeding. N. Engl. J. Med., *290*:839, 1974.

Cancer of the Gastrointestinal Tract, Polyps of the Colon

1. Dilemma of esophageal carcinoma (Editorial): J.A.M.A., *235*:1044, 1976.
2. Erbe, R. W.: Inherited gastrointestinal polyposis syndromes. N. Engl. J. Med., *294*:1101, 1976.
3. Levin, B., Riddell, R. H., and Kirsner, J. B.: Management of precancerous lesions of the gastrointestinal tract. Clin. Gastroenterol., 5:827, 1976.
4. Machado, G., Davis, J. D., Tudway, A. J. C., et al.: Superficial carcinoma of the stomach. Brit. Med. J., *iii*:77, 1976.
5. Malt, R. A., and Ottinger, L. W.: Carcinoma of the colon and rectum. N. Engl. J. Med., *288*:772, 1973.
6. McIllmurray, M. B., and Langman, M. J. S.: Large bowel cancer: Causation and management. Gut, *17*:815, 1975.
7. Morson, B. C.: Genesis of colorectal cancer. Clin. Gastroenterol., 5:505, 1976.
8. Welch, C. E., and Hedberg, S. E.: Polypoid Lesions of the Gastrointestinal Tract. 2nd Ed. Philadelphia, W. B. Saunders Co., 1975.
9. Winawer, S. J., Sherlock, P., Schottenfeld, D., et al.: Screening for colon cancer. Gastroenterology, 70:783, 1976.
10. Wolff, W. I., and Shinya, H.: Definitive treatment of "malignant" polyps of the colon. Ann. Surg., *182*:516, 1975.

Jaundice, Interpretation of Liver Function Tests

1. Berk, R. D., Wolkoff, A. W., and Berlin, N. I.: Inborn errors of bilirubin metabolism. Med. Clin. North Am., 59:803, 1975.
2. Bissell, D. M.: Formation and elimination of bilirubin. Gastroenterology, 69:519, 1975.
3. Kaplan, M. H.: Current concepts: alkaline phosphatase. N. Engl. J. Med., *286*:200, 1972.
4. NIH Conference. Unconjugated Hyperbilirubinemia: Physiologic Evaluation and Experimental Approaches to Therapy. Moderator: Berk, P. D. Discussants: Martin, J. F., Blaschke, T. F., Scharschmidt, B. F., et al.: Ann Intern. Med. 82:552, 1975.
5. Ostrow, J. D.: Jaundice in older children and adults: Algorithms for diagnosis. J.A.M.A., *234*: 522, 1975.

Alcohol and Liver Disease

1. Gabuzda, G. J.: Cirrhosis, ascites, and edema; clinical course related to management. Gastroenterology, 58:546, 1970.
2. Gabuzda, G J.: Nutrition and liver disease, practical considerations. Med. Clin. North Am., *54*: 1455, 1970.
3. Leevy, C. M., Tamburro, C. H., and Zetterman, R.: Liver disease of the alcoholic. Med. Clin. North Am., 59:909, 1975.
4. Maddrey, W. C., and Weber, F. L., Jr.: Chronic hepatic encephalopathy. Med. Clin. North Am., 59:937, 1975.
5. Resnick, R. H.: Portal hypertension. Med. Clin. North Am., 59:945, 1975.
6. Schenker, S., Brien, K. J., and Hoyumpa, A. M.: Hepatic encephalopathy — Current status. Gastroenterology, 66:121, 1974.
7. Webster, M. W.: Current management of esophageal varices. Surg. Clin. North Am., 55:461, 1975.
8. Zieve, L., and Nicoloff, D. M.: Pathogenesis of hepatic coma. Ann. Rev. Med., 26:143, 1975.

Viral Hepatitis

1. Aach, R. D.: Viral hepatitis — Update 1976. Viewpoints Dig. Dis., 8:No. 1, 1976.

2. After Type B Hepatitis (Editorial): Brit. Med. J., *iv*:311, 1975.
3. Barker, J. D., Jr., Anuras, S., and Summers, R.: Gamma globulin prophylaxis of viral hepatitis—An update. Postgrad. Med., *60*:90, 1976.
4. Boyer, J.: Chronic hepatitis—A perspective on classification and determinants of prognosis. Gastroenterology, *70*:1161, 1976.
5. Holland, P. V., and Alter, H. J.: The clinical significance of hepatitis B virus antigens and antibodies. Med. Clin. North Am., 59:849, 1975.
6. Mosley, J. W.: Type A hepatitis. Med. Clin. North Am., 59:831, 1975.
7. Sherlock, S.: Progress report: Chronic hepatitis. Gut, *15*:581, 1974.
8. Summerskill, W. H. J.: Chronic active liver disease re-examined: Prognosis hopeful. Gastroenterology, 66:450, 1974.
9. UCLA Conference. The Liver and the Antigens of Hepatitis B. Moderator: Gitnick, G. L. Discussants: Goldberg, L. S., Koretz, R., and Walsh, J. H.: Am. Int. Med., 85:488, 1976.

Drugs and the Liver

1. Mitchell, J. R.: Drugs and the liver. Viewpoints Dig Dis., 5:No. 5, 1974.
2. Mitchell, J. R., and Jollows, D. J.: Metabolic activation of drugs to toxic substances. Gastroenterology, *68*:392, 1975.

3. NIH Conference. Vinyl Chloride-associated Liver Disease. Moderator: Berk, P. D. Discussants: Martin, J. F., Young, R. S., Creech, J., et al.: Ann. Int. Med., *84*:717, 1976.
4. Sherlock, S.: Progress report: Hepatic adenomas and oral contraceptives. Gut, *16*:753, 1975.
5. Stauffer, J. Q., Lapinski, M. W., Honold, D. J., et al.: Focal nodular hyperplasia of the liver and intrahepatic hemorrhage in young women on oral contraceptives. Ann Intern. Med., *83*:301, 1975.
6. Zimmerman, H. J.: Liver disease caused by medicinal agents. Med. Clin. North Am., 59:897, 1975.

Gallbladder Disease

1. Dawson, J. L.: Cholecystitis and cholecystectomy. Clin. Gastroenterol., 2:85, 1973.
2. Hermann, R. E.: Acute cholecystitis. J.A.M.A., *234*:1261, 1975.
3. Hofmann, A. F., and Thistle, J. L.: Chenodeoxycholic acid: The Mayo Clinic experience. Hosp. Prac., Aug. 1974, pp. 41–48
4. Rosenbaum, H. D.: An Evaluation of oral cholecystography. J.A.M.A., *229*:76, 1974.
5. Schoenfield, L. J., and Coyne, M. J.: Cholesterol gallstones, 1975. Viewpoints Dig. Dis., 7:No. 1, 1975.

Chapter 47

CARDIOLOGY

by ROBERT H. SELLER

This chapter on cardiology covers the common cardiac illnesses and problems that the family physician is called upon to deal with in an ambulatory setting. Each of the following topics is covered in a separate section: (1) hypertension, (2) congestive heart failure and heart failure in the elderly, (3) cardiac murmurs, (4) chest pain, (5) cardiac arrhythmias, and (6) hyperlipidemias. A short review of helpful clinical suggestions for dealing with patients and families of patients with these illnesses concludes each section.

Myocardial infarctions are not discussed because the subject has been extensively covered in many monographs, textbooks, and articles. Likewise, for the interpretation of electrocardiograms, the reader is referred to the many excellent textbooks that are available.

HYPERTENSION

Introduction

Innumerable studies have shown that hypertension is one of the most common illnesses seen by the practicing family physician. This disorder afflicts 15 to 20 per cent of the adult population, a figure that places hypertension alongside obesity and coronary artery disease in prevalence in the United States. It is important to note that studies have shown that only 50 per cent of the entire hypertensive population is recognized. Of these, only half are under the care of a physician; and, finally, of those who are under the care of a physician, only half have achieved adequate control of their blood pressure. This means that in only one-eighth of all the hypertensive patients in the United States is the blood pressure

adequately controlled. In view of the prevalence and seriousness of this disease, plus the fact that the most patients with hypertension are cared for by family physicians, it behooves the family physician to be particularly expert in the diagnosis and management of hypertensive cardiovascular disease.

Definition

For the purposes of this discussion, hypertension will be defined only as a diastolic blood pressure greater than 90 mm. Hg. If increased, the pressure reading should be recorded on at least two visits before therapy is initiated. In instances of severe diastolic hypertension or if there is significant diastolic hypertension despite antihypertensive therapy, the requirement that the diastolic hypertension be found on two successive visits can be waived.

Etiology

Although approximately 90 per cent of hypertensive patients have essential hypertension, a precise physical examination and history may give clues to a specific cause of the hypertension. Lower blood pressure in the legs than in the arms suggests the presence of *coarctation of the aorta.*

Bruits in the flanks or in the costovertebral region suggest a *renovascular* cause. The following historical clues also suggest a renovascular cause for hypertension: (1) onset of diastolic hypertension in patients under the age of 35, (2) documented onset of diastolic hypertension after the age of 60, (3) all cases of malignant or rapidly progressive hypertension, (4) sudden, severe exacerbation of pre-existing mild-to-moderate hypertension, and (5) onset of diastolic hypertension associated with renal trauma or a history compatible with renal infarction, such as flank pain associated with hematuria.

Other patients may present with some of the clinical characteristics of *Cushing's disease*, including pigmentation, hirsutism, or abnormal fat distribution.

A history of episodic weakness (particularly after the administration of diuretics), polyuria, nocturia, hypokalemia, and hypernatremia suggests the possibility of *primary aldosteronism*. Glucosuria and tachycardia associated with sustained or episodic hypertension suggest a *pheochromocytoma*, as does episodic orthostatic hypotension. Albuminuria or a history of renal disease, including *glomerulonephritis* or *pyelonephritis*, should suggest a renal cause. One unusual clue that suggests a *congenital abnormality* of the kidneys is the finding of deformed or malplaced ears. This correlation is found because the ears and the genitourinary system develop during the same fetal time period. Occasionally, congenital abnormalities of the kidney are associated with congenital malformations of the ear on the same side.

Pathophysiology

Although the precise cause of essential hypertension is not well understood, several contributing causes are well established. In addition to renal and adrenal factors, these include increased vascular reactivity, increased sensitivity to catecholamines, abnormal sodium metabolism, and hereditary and psychogenic factors. Decreased glomerular filtration rate, increased reabsorption of sodium, and increased levels of renin and aldosterone all contribute to the fundamental abnormality of essential hypertension, i.e., increased peripheral vascular resistance.

Signs and Symptoms

It must be emphasized that hypertension is a silent disease. The patient has no symptoms of hypertension until it results in end-organ disease. Although many patients think that various complaints are related to elevated diastolic blood pressure, this is rarely, if ever, the case. Patients often think that headaches are related to their high blood pressure. To the contrary, most patients with headaches do not have high blood pressure; most patients with high blood pressure do not have headaches. When patients with hypertension do have headaches, it is rare to find a causal relationship. Occasionally, some patients with hypertension have typical hypertensive headaches, i.e., throbbing, which is worse in the morning after prolonged recumbency and is relieved when hypertension is treated.

Hypertensive retinopathy, including retinal hemorrhage, usually occurs only after several years of sustained hypertension. On the other hand, papilledema may develop soon after the onset of severe hypertension. Cardiac symptoms usually develop after several years of sustained hypertension, although a sudden onset of severe hypertension may rapidly precipitate cardiac symptoms. These cardiac symptoms include congestive heart failure, as well as angina pectoris. Signs or symptoms of progressive renal function impairment are protean and again occur only after sustained hypertension. A patient may present with epistaxis or a subarachnoid hemorrhage when diastolic hypertension is severe. Although the precise mechanism is not clear, atherosclerotic processes are accelerated in patients with hypertension. Some investigators feel that this is particularly true in patients with the so-called hyper-reninemic hypertension. Accelerated atherogenesis may manifest itself by cerebrovascular symptoms, cardiac symptoms, and renal symptoms, as well as by peripheral vascular insufficiency.

Diagnostic Work-up

Once the physician has determined that sustained diastolic pressure (greater than 90 mm. Hg on two or more successive visits) is present and after performing a precise history and physical examination, he should proceed with a diagnostic work-up (Table 47–1) aimed at ruling out a specific cause of the hypertension. The physician should recognize that in most instances essential hypertension will be found. All hypertensive patients should have a complete urinalysis, determination of blood urea nitrogen (BUN), or preferably of serum creatinine, and a serum potassium determination. The urinalysis and serum creatinine determination help to assess renal function and screen for a renal cause of the hyper-

TABLE 47-1. WORK-UP OF HYPERTENSIVE PATIENTS

Urinalysis
Blood urea nitrogen and/or creatinine determination
Serum potassium determination

Electrocardiogram
Chest x-ray
Blood glucose determination
Uric acid determination
Cholesterol determination

Hypertensive intravenous pyelogram

tension. The serum potassium level is determined as a screen for primary aldosteronism, although the serum potassium level may be normal, rather than low, in some patents with primary aldosteronism. As mentioned previously, the presence of episodic weakness, polyuria, nocturia, hypokalemia, and hypernatremia are all clues to the presence of primary aldosteronism. If this is suspected, appropriate tests are performed to confirm the diagnosis. These tests must include the finding of low-to-absent renin levels under conditions of maximal stimulation of renin production, as well as high serum and urinary aldosterone levels under conditions of maximal suppression. These tests have been described in detail elsewhere in the literature. They must be performed under close monitoring in a hospital.

In addition, a hypertensive (rapid sequence) intravenous pyelogram also should be performed. It should be noted that some physicians do not do a hypertensive intravenous pyelogram initially, but reserve it for patients with more severe hypertension or for those in whom hypertension is not adequately controlled with diuretic therapy alone. I feel that, whenever possible, a hypertensive intravenous pyelogram should be done in all patients in order to assess renal function, rule out gross structural abnormalities, and screen for unilateral renal disease.

Since oral contraceptives contribute to hypertension, they should be discontinued for at least 3 months before the work-up, so that the possible hypertensive effect of these drugs will be dissipated.

To estimate prognosis and evaluate cardiovascular risk factors the following studies are performed: determinations of blood glucose, uric acid, cholesterol and triglycerides, electrocardiogram (ECG), and chest x-ray. When indicated, more specific tests are performed; these may include serum aldosterone and renin levels; urine levels of steroids, aldosterone, vanillylmandelic acid, metanephrine, and catecholamines; and renal arteriography.

Management

Once the indicated diagnostic work-up has ruled out the uncommon but specific causes of hypertension, the physician next can direct his attention to therapy. The most important components of a successful therapeutic regimen include initiating the rational use of antihypertensive drugs, enlisting the patient's participation in the management of this chronic illness, and facilitating compliance by educating the patient about therapeutic regimens and low salt diets. Patient education and compliance are reviewed at the end of this section.

In most instances, the choice of therapy depends on the severity of the hypertension and the altered pathophysiologic mechanisms (i.e., decreased renal function, levels of renin and/or aldosterone).

In order to select the most appropriate drugs, the physician must understand the altered pathophysiology of essential hypertension (Fig. 47-1) as well as the clinical pharmacology of the various agents (Figs. 47-2 and 47-3). All patients with essential hypertension have increased peripheral vascular resistance and may have decreased renal blood flow, decreased glomerular filtration rate, and increased renal vascular resistance. The ideal antihypertensive agent therefore should decrease peripheral vascular resistance while maintaining cardiac output, renal blood flow, glomerular filtration rate, and cerebral blood flow at constant levels. Likewise, the ideal antihypertensive agent would be effective in both the supine and erect positions, have minimal or no side effects, and have a sustained antihypertensive effect despite prolonged administration.

The diuretic agents, despite having only moderate antihypertensive effectiveness, come close to representing the ideal antihypertensive agent in that they are effective in both the supine and erect positions, have a relatively low incidence of side effects, have a sustained antihypertensive

HEMODYNAMIC ALTERATIONS IN ESSENTIAL HYPERTENSION

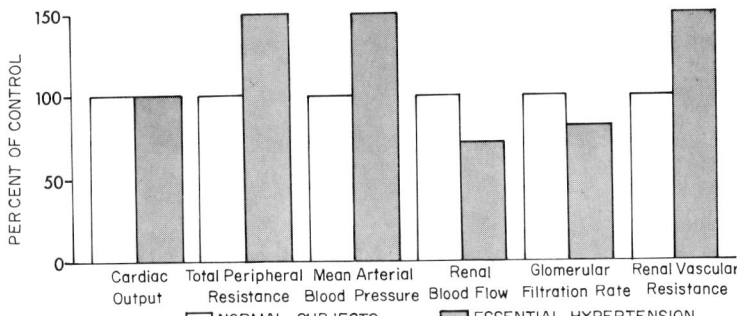

Figure 47-1. Hemodynamic alterations in essential hypertension.

The basic hemodynamic defect is increased peripheral vascular resistance with normal cardiac output.

Progressive renal function impairment is an inevitable consequence of chronic diastolic hypertension.

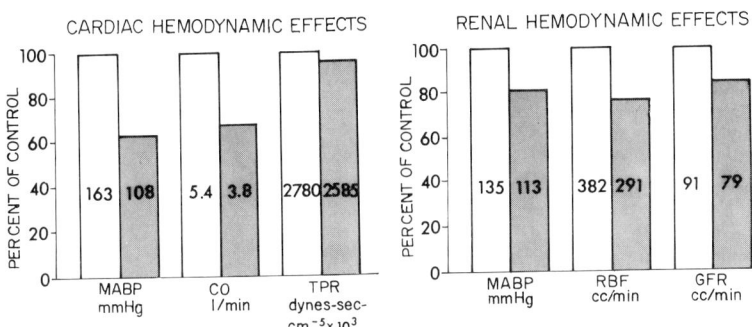

Figure 47-2. Hemodynamic effects of guanethidine on mean arterial blood pressure, cardiac output, total peripheral resistance, renal blood flow, and glomerular filtration rate.

Pharmacodynamic Effects

1 Lowers blood pressure by reducing cardiac output.

2 Renal hemodynamics are reduced to a moderate extent.

3 Marked antihypertensive potency. 4 Predominant orthostatic effect.

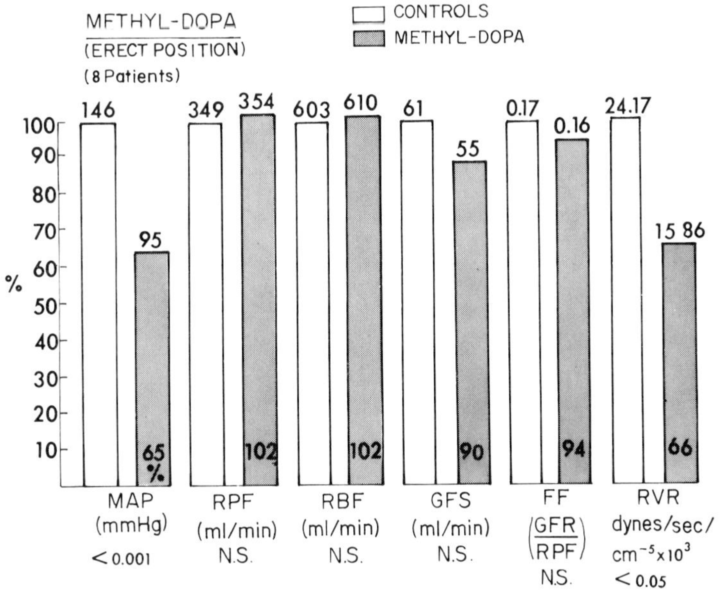

Figure 47-3. Hemodynamic effects of methyldopa on mean arterial blood pressure, renal plasma flow, renal blood flow, glomerular filtration rate, filtration fraction, and renal vascular resistance.

effect despite prolonged administration, and—most important—potentiate the antihypertensive effect of more potent agents. Because they can potentiate other antihypertensive agents, diuretics should be given initially to almost all hypertensive patients (Table 47-2).

If normotension is not achieved, a "second-line" drug can be added. In most instances, the second- and third-line antihypertensive agents have more frequent and serious side effects than do the oral diuretics (Table 47-2). Because diuretics potentiate the more potent agents, it is possible to reduce the doses of these

second- and third-line drugs and thus decrease their side effects (Fig. 47-4 and Table 47-3). Generally, the oral diuretics, whether benzothiadiazines, chlorthalidone, or a "loop diuretic," such as furosemide or ethacrynic acid, represent good initial therapy for all hypertensives. Most patients with minimal hypertension (diastolic pressure 90 to 110 mm. Hg) become normotensive on appropriate diuretic therapy and modest salt restriction.

The presence of hyperuricemia and hyperglycemia are relative but not absolute contraindications to oral diuretic therapy. In a few instances, therapy with spironolac-

TABLE 47-2.   ANTIHYPERTENSIVE DRUGS

Drug	Dosage° Initial	Usual	Maximum	Side Effects	Comments
INITIAL THERAPY					
Thiazide Diuretics:					
Hydrochlorothiazide (Hydrodiuril, etc.)	50 mg. o.d.	50 mg. b.i.d.	100 mg. b.i.d.	Hypokalemia, hypomagnesemia, hyperuricemia, hyperglycemia, alkalosis, pancreatitis, dermatitis, leukopenia, hypercalcemia, dry mouth, gastrointestinal disturbance	All thiazides equipotent in equivalent doses
Chlorothiazide (Diuril)	500 mg. o.d.	500 mg. b.i.d.	1000 mg. b.i.d.		
Trichlormethiazide (Naqua)	2 mg. o.d.	4 mg. o.d.	4 mg. b.i.d.		
Bendroflumethiazide (Naturetin)	2.5 mg. o.d.	5 mg. b.i.d.	5 mg. t.i.d.		
Chlorthalidone: (Hygroton)	50 mg. o.d.	100 mg. o.d.	200 mg. o.d.		Long-acting
Metolazone: (Zaroxolyn)	5 mg. o.d.	5 mg. b.i.d.	10 mg. b.i.d.		Useful in renal insufficiency
Loop Diuretics:				As above and in addition: severe hypokalemia, dehydration, ototoxicity	
Ethacrynic acid (Edecrin)	50 mg. o.d.	50 mg. b.i.d.	100 mg. b.i.d.		Useful in renal insufficiency
Furosemide (Lasix)	40 mg. b.i.d.	40 mg. b.i.d.	200 mg. t.i.d.	Liver disease, gastrointestinal disturbance, pruritus	Useful in renal insufficiency
Potassium-sparing Diuretics:					
Spironolactone (Aldactone)	25 mg. b.i.d.	50 mg. b.i.d.	50 mg. q.i.d.	Hyperkalemia, gastrointestinal disturbance, gynecomastia, rash, metabolic acidosis	Contraindicated in renal insufficiency, useful in low renin hypertension
Triamterene (Dyrenium)	50 mg. b.i.d.	100 mg. b.i.d.	100 mg. t.i.d.	Hyperkalemia, gastrointestinal disturbance, photosensitivity, azotemia, metabolic acidosis	Contraindicated in renal insufficiency
"SECOND LINE" THERAPY					
Methyldopa (Aldomet)	250 mg. b.i.d.	500 mg. q8h	2 to 3 grams o.d.	Bradycardia, sedation, fever, abnormal liver function tests, positive Coombs' test, postural hypotension	Additive effect to propranolol, inhibits effect of levodopa
Prazosin (Minipress)	1 mg. t.i.d.	2 to 5 mg. t.i.d.	20 mg. o.d.	Orthostatic hypotension, headache, sedation	A vasodilator

TABLE 47–2. ANTIHYPERTENSIVE DRUGS *(Continued)*

Drug	Dosage° Initial	Dosage° Usual	Dosage° Maximum	Side Effects	Comments
"THIRD LINE" THERAPY					
Hydralazine (Apresoline)	25 mg. q8h	50 mg. q6h	100 mg. q8h	Tachycardia, headache, gastrointestinal disturbance, exacerbation of angina and heart failure, lupus-like syndrome	A vasodilator
Reserpine derivatives (Serpasil, etc.)	0.1 mg. o.d.	0.2 mg. o.d.	0.5 mg. o.d.	Bradycardia, depression, drowsiness, nightmares, impotence, gastrointestinal disturbance	Not commonly used anymore, central nervous system excitability with MAO inhibitors, additive effect to propranolol, facilitates peptic ulcer disease
Clonidine (Catapres)	0.1 mg. t.i.d.	0.2 mg. t.i.d.	2.4 mg. o.d.	Bradycardia, dry mouth, rash, postural hypotension, gastrointestinal disturbance, severe drowsiness	Must be tapered when stopping, additive to propranolol
Guanethidine (Ismelin)	10 mg. o.d.	25 mg. t.i.d.	150 mg. o.d.	Bradycardia, postural hypotension, impotence, diarrhea, may aggravate asthma, loss of ejaculation	Pressor effect of phenylephrine enhanced; effects antagonized by ephedrine, amphetamines, MAO inhibitors; alcohol may aggravate hypertension, may aggravate asthma
Propranolol (Inderal)	10 mg. q.i.d.	50 mg. t.i.d.	320 mg. o.d.	Bradycardia; may precipitate congestive heart failure, gastrointestinal disturbance; may precipitate bronchial asthma attacks, diarrhea	Usually used in conjunction with hydralazine and a diuretic, blocks sympathetic response to hypoglycemia, useful in high renin hypertension
Pargyline (Eutonyl)	25 mg. o.d.		100 mg. o.d.	Potent MAO inhibitor	Rarely used, rise in blood pressure on eating tyramine-rich food (contraindicated with other drugs), used in depressed patients

°Abbreviations: o.d.—once daily; b.i.d.—twice daily; t.i.d.—three times daily; q8h—every 8 hours.

tone alone, in doses of up to 50 mg. four times daily, may result in normotension. Combining spironolactone or triamterene with an oral diuretic permits a 50 per cent reduction in the usual dose of the oral diuretic and thus decreases hyperglycemia or hyperuricemia. Triamterene (50 mg.) in combination with 25 mg. of hydrochlorothiazide (Dyazide) administered as 1 capsule twice daily produces approximately the same natriuresis, diuresis, and antihypertensive effect as does hydrochlorothiazide, 50 mg. twice daily.

In recent years, more specific therapy has been indicated when high or low renin levels are recognized.

Therapy for Low Renin Hypertension. Hypertensive patients who have low renin essential hypertension often respond well to large doses of spironolactone (200 to 400 mg. daily).

High doses of spironolactone also have been reported to be effective antihypertensive therapy in some patients with primary aldosteronism. Although surgical removal of the adenoma causing the aldosteronism is

Therapeutic Regimen	No. of Patients	Supine				Erect			
		Normotensive[1] No.	%	Responsive[2] No.	%	Normotensive[1] No.	%	Responsive[2] No.	%
Guanethidine	30	5	17	12	40	13	43	27	90
Guanethidine + Hydrochlorothiazide	25	6	24	13	52	14	56	22	88
Pargyline	33	5	15	7	21	19	57	27	82
Pargyline + Hydrochlorothiazide	11	1	9	4	36	5	45	9	82
Methyldopa	38	6	16	13	34	9	24	16	42
Methyldopa + Hydrochlorothiazide	19	8	42	12	63	10	53	17	89
Clonidine (Catapres)	16	1	6	3	19	0	0	6	37
Clonidine (Catapres) + Chlorthalidone	20	1	5	16	80	2	10	16	80

Normotensive[1] = blood pressure reduced >140/90 mmg. Hg
Responsive[2] = mean blood pressure reduced >20 mm. Hg or normotensive

Figure 47–4. *Comparative antihypertensive effects of guanethidine, pargyline, methyldopa, and clonidine (Catapres), alone and in combination with oral diuretics.*

generally recommended, this pharmacologic therapy has been used when patients have been considered a poor operative risk.

Therapy for High Renin Hypertension. Other antihypertensive agents should be selected in the presence of high renin essential hypertension. Several antihypertensive drugs suppress the production of renin, i.e., the beta-blocking agents, such as propranolol, hydralazine, and methyldopa. The combination of propranolol, hydralazine, and furosemide is particularly effective in hyper-reninemic hypertension. Propranolol lowers blood pressure by suppressing renin formation, minimally reducing cardiac output and blocking the effect of catecholamines on the arterioles. Hydralazine reduces peripheral vascular resistance by having a direct effect on vascular muscle. The tachycardiac effect of hydralazine is neutralized or reduced by the bradycardiac effect of the propranolol. The diuretic agent reduces both the peripheral vascular resistance and the increased salt and fluid retention caused by the propranolol.

Therapy for Hypertension with Renal Insufficiency. It is important to recognize that the blood urea nitrogen level does not rise above the upper limits of normal until there is at least a 50 per cent loss of renal function. Patients more than 65 years old, without any renal disease, have a 40 to 60 per cent decrease in renal blood flow and glomerular filtration rate. Furosemide or ethacrynic acid is preferred in patients with even minimal azotemia because the benzothiadiazines do not usually have as great an antihypertensive effect in patients with renal insufficiency as do the "loop" diuretics. Hydralazine and methyldopa are the preferred second-line antihypertensive drugs, as these more potent agents are able to decrease blood pressure without causing a corresponding decrease in renal blood

TABLE 47–3. ANTIHYPERTENSIVE DRUG SELECTION BASED ON DIASTOLIC BLOOD PRESSURE

Severity of Diastolic Pressure (mm. Hg)	Initial Therapy	If Necessary, Add
90–110	Hydrochlorothiazide or other diuretic	Methyldopa or prazosin
110–130	Diuretic plus methyldopa	Hydralazine
	Diuretic plus prazosin	Methyldopa or clonidine
>130	Diuretic plus guanethidine	Methyldopa and/or hydralazine or prazosin
	Diuretic plus clonidine	Hydralazine or prazosin and/or methyldopa

flow and glomerular filtration rate (Fig. 47–3). They somewhat selectively decrease renal vascular resistance. This effect is desirable in patients who already have impaired renal function and increased renal vascular resistance. A combination of furosemide (40 to 160 mg.), methyldopa (1 to 2 grams), and hydralazine (100 to 300 mg.) in divided doses is often a particularly effective antihypertensive regimen in patients with renal insufficiency.

Selection of Drugs Based on Severity of Hypertension. If no special instances of high or low renin levels, renal impairment, mineralocorticoid excess, diabetes, hyperuricemia, or hypersensitivity are present, hypotensive drugs can be selected according to the severity of the hypertension (Table 47–3). In these instances, it is best to start with an oral diuretic agent such as hydrochlorothiazide, 50 mg. twice daily. Some studies suggest that the benzothiadiazines are more effective hypotensive agents than are equivalent natriuretic doses of the loop diuretics. Omitting the diuretic drug on Saturdays and Sundays significantly reduces the incidence of hypokalemia. It is particularly advisable to omit diuretic therapy on the weekends if the patient is receiving a digitalis glycoside, as in these instances it is especially desirable to avoid hypokalemia. The use of the optimum diuretic dosage and appropriate salt restriction results in the achievement of normotension in approximately 40 per cent of patients with minimal hypertension (diastolic pressure 90 to 110 mm. Hg).

Most often, if the diastolic level exceeds 110 mm. Hg, or if the response to diuretic therapy alone is inadequate, a second-line drug is usually required. The most frequently used second-line drug is methyldopa in doses of up to 2 grams. Side effects of methyldopa include drowsiness, loss of libido, and orthostatic hypotension. The soporific effects can be reduced by administering the drug in a single night-time dosage. Patients should be advised that they may temporarily experience more drowsiness on institution of methyldopa therapy or when increasing the dose. It is important to recognize that although patients may not complain about the soporific or libido-suppressing properties of the drug, these side effects invariably will impair compliance. If these side effects are present, it is advisable for the physician to prescribe other drugs.

The decreased libido effect is as likely to occur in females as it is in males.

Prazosin is a potent, newly introduced drug that may be added to the diuretics as a "second-line" drug. Its action is similar to hydralazine, in that it is a direct vasodilator. Prazosin does not cause a tachycardia and therefore can be used without the concomitant administration of a bradycrotic agent. If an inadequate antihypertensive response is obtained with double drug therapy or if undesirable side effects occur, a third drug should be added.

At this point, I would like to emphasize the fact that all antihypertensive drugs should be administered so that each individual drug is pushed to (1) the maximum therapeutic dosage, (2) the establishment of normotension, or (3) the production of undesirable side effects. The same thing should be done with the addition of a second, third, or fourth drug. It is not appropriate to have a patient on hydrochlorothiazide, 50 mg. daily, which is not optimum dosage, and then add methyldopa, 250 mg. twice daily, and then add a third drug. Each drug should be pushed to optimum dosage: hydrochlorothiazide to 50 mg. twice daily, or furosemide to 80 mg. twice daily, and then a second drug should be added. This second drug then should be administered in increasing dosage until normotension is achieved or undesirable side effects are produced. If side effects are produced, the dosage of that drug should be reduced to a level at which these effects are not present, and a third drug should be added. Here, again, the third drug is pushed to maximum therapeutic dose, achievements of normotension, or production of undesirable side effects.

Third-line drugs include hydralazine, guanethidine, and clonidine. When a patient is receiving a diuretic and methyldopa, hydralazine can be administered in divided doses (every 8 hours) up to 300 mg. daily. Hydralazine should always be administered in conjunction with another agent that causes bradycardia (propranolol, methyldopa, guanethidine, or clonidine). Guanethidine can be added to a diuretic or to methyldopa. Clonidine can be added to a diuretic and hydralazine. Clonidine and methyldopa probably should not be used together, as their individual soporific effects may be additive and result in marked drowsiness. Rarely do patients require a combination of four antihypertensive drugs, i.e., a diuretic, methyldopa, hydralazine, and guanethidine.

Practical Suggestions for Dealing with Hypertensive Patients and Their Families

The majority of hypertensive patients cannot be cured. As they require long-term management, it is important that both the patients and their families be well-informed concerning the goals of therapy. They must understand and participate in the treatment plan. Hypertensive patients must understand that this disease is rarely cured and that their treatment in almost all instances must continue for the remainder of their life. The patients and their families should be told that the presence of well-controlled hypertension should in no way interfere with the patients' life style. They must, however, avoid excessive salt intake and adhere to a reasonable low salt diet. The importance of the low salt diet must be explained to the other members of the family to enlist their cooperation with a dietary management plan. Positive aspects of dietary management should be stressed, e.g., the replacement of salt with other spices, such as garlic, onion, pepper, or vinegar, as well as with salt substitutes.

Techniques of simplifying the administration of medications and the development of constructive means for family members to remind the patient to take medications may be useful, particularly when the patient is forgetful. Other members of the family should be interviewed to make sure that the patient is informing the physician of undesirable side effects, such as orthostatic hypotension, drowsiness, and decreased libido. Very often, a spouse will inform the physician of the patient's increased fatigability and decreased libido more readily than the patient will.

CONGESTIVE HEART FAILURE

Diagnosis and Differential Diagnosis

The classic symptoms of heart failure include dyspnea, dyspnea on exertion, orthopnea, paroxysmal nocturnal dyspnea, cough, occasional hemoptysis, and peripheral edema. Physical signs that are commonly present include cardiac enlargement; tachycardia; gallop rhythm; distended neck veins; enlarged, tender liver; pulmonary edema with rales, particularly at the bases; pleural effusions; and pulsus alternans. When several of these symptoms or signs are present in a patient with cardiovascular disease (e.g., hypertension, acquired valvular disease, or severe coronary artery disease), the diagnosis is easily and accurately made.

The picture may be confusing, however, when one or more of these cardinal signs and symptoms are present but are due to another disease entity. *Dyspnea* can be caused by obesity, acidosis, anemia, or pulmonary disease. *Rales* at the bases can be caused by pulmonary fibrosis, bronchitis, asthma, pneumonia, or bronchiectasis or just by basilar atelectasis. The causes of *tachycardia* are legion. It is particularly important to note that most patients (60 per cent) with *edema* of the legs do not have congestive heart failure. Most commonly, peripheral edema is caused by venous disease. Renal disease, hypoalbuminemia, liver disease, and lymphatic obstruction also lead to edema. The classic physical finding of *distended neck veins* is seen in patients with constrictive pericarditis, tricuspid insufficiency, and superior vena caval obstruction. An *enlarged, tender liver* can be seen in patients with hepatitis, hepatic vein obstruction, and tricuspid disease.

Obese patients with deep vein insufficiency often complain of exertional dyspnea and pedal edema. The former symptom may be due to their obesity and possibly to associated pulmonary disease. The latter is due to deep vein insufficiency without dilatation of the superficial leg veins. It must be recognized that these patients do *not* have congestive heart failure, as they do not demonstrate enlarged liver, distended neck veins, tachycardia, gallop rhythm, or cardiac enlargement.

The symptoms of congestive heart failure must be differentiated from those primarily due to pulmonary disease, as both conditions cause cough, dyspnea, dyspnea on exertion, hemoptysis, and occasionally wheezing. A chest x-ray that does not show cardiac enlargement or pulmonary congestion suggests that chronic heart failure is not present. Furosemide, 40 to 80 mg. twice daily orally for 3 or 4 days, is a useful tool in establishing the diagnosis of congestive heart failure. Although edema resulting from mostly all causes will respond to diuretics, the alleviation of dyspnea, orthopnea, and rales at the bases after the induction of significant diuresis is fairly substantial evidence that congestive heart failure was present. Marked right-sided failure without significant left ventricular failure may result from severe chronic obstructive pulmonary disease and may cause dyspnea, cough, venous engorgement, enlarged, tender liver, and marked peripheral edema. Although there are rare instances in which only left ventricular or right ventricular failure is present, in most instances combined left and right ventricular failure occurs; the symptoms usually attributed to one or the other may predominate, however.

Precipitating or Aggravating Factors

Before the physician begins therapy, he must direct his attention to the precipitating or aggravating factors. Myocardial infarctions may be typical or, particularly in the aged, silent or atypical. Arrhythmias, including supraventricular tachycardias, atrial fibrillation, and heart block, may contribute to the development of heart failure. Infections, particularly pulmonary and renal infections, may contribute to the development of congestive heart failure. The fever that complicates infection processes put an additional strain on diminished myocardial reserve and can precipitate or aggravate heart failure.

Electrolyte imbalance, most commonly observed in patients receiving diuretic therapy, not only can lead to digitoxic arrhythmias but also may contribute to diuretic refractoriness. Hyperthyroidism, whether overt or "masked," also places additional demands on the myocardium. Renal insufficiency, including obstructive uropathies, contributes to the development of congestive heart failure. Pulmonary emboli, particularly small recurrent ones, as well as pleural effusions, may either precipitate or aggravate congestive heart failure.

Sex hormones and anti-inflammatory agents, such as steroids, indomethacin, and phenylbutazone, all cause salt and water retention. Drugs that interfere with myocardial contractility, such as propranolol and other beta-blocking agents, may pre-cipitate profound heart failure. Although beta-blockers are relatively contraindicated in patients with heart failure, such drugs may be given cautiously to these patients as long as they also receive a digitalis glycoside simultaneously. In these instances, the patient must be examined carefully at frequent intervals.

Remediable Cardiac and Extracardiac Conditions

In addition to the axiom "first do no harm," the physician also must bear in mind another, which is "treat the untreatable." To accomplish the latter, the clinician must search for remediable cardiac and extracardiac conditions. The treatable cardiac conditions that contribute to the development of heart failure include active myocardial processes, constrictive pericarditis, congenital and acquired valvular lesions, subacute bacterial endocarditis, arrhythmias, and coronary artery disease. Rarely are myocardial tumors and congenital heart defects present in adult patients with congestive heart failure. The two most common congenital heart defects found in adults are atrial septal defects and patent ductus arteriosus. In adulthood, these conditions do not give rise to typical murmurs. The patient with an atrial septal defect may present with a grade 3 to 4 apical systolic murmur, which can be confused with mitral insufficiency. Likewise, the murmur of patent ductus arteriosus in an adult is not usually continuous but is more often just systolic. When the latter condition is present in adulthood, it is not uncommonly associated with cyanosis, most evident in the lower extremities and left hand. This is due to a shunting of unoxygenated blood to these areas through the ductus.

It is particularly important to identify and correct remediable extracardiac factors in refractory cases. These include inadequate restriction of activity; excessive salt intake; inappropriate dosage of digitalis or diuretics, or both; electrolyte imbalance; and pulmonary infections or effusions, or both. Special attention should be paid to the detection of the previously enumerated conditions that contribute to high-output heart failure. Finally, diastolic hypertension (pressure greater than 95 mm. Hg) is one of the most common remediable conditions in patients with heart failure.

Pathophysiology

A thorough understanding of the major pathogenic mechanisms underlying congestive heart failure is essential if one is to treat patients with this disease effectively. Figure 47–5 elucidates most of the major factors in the development of edema in patients with congestive heart failure. Although abnormal cardiac function initiates the process of congestive heart failure, many of the associated signs and symptoms are due to abnormalities in the renal and adrenal function induced by the abnormal cardiac function. Patients with left ventricular failure (or so-called forward failure) invariably demonstrate an elevated end-diastolic pressure in the left ventricle. Although minimal dilatation of the left ventricular chamber and stretch of the myocardial fibers initially lead to an increased force of contraction of the left ventricular musculature, progressive dilatation and increasing preload gradually lead to a reduction in cardiac output.

It is notable that although anemia, hyperthyroidism, beriberi, arteriovenous fistula, and Paget's disease can cause so-called high-output failure, most patients with heart failure have a decreased cardiac output. This reduced cardiac output leads to a decreased renal blood flow and an increased reabsorption of salt and water. In addition, the decreased renal blood flow is sensed by the juxtaglomerular apparatus, and the subsequent release of renin leads to increased production of aldosterone-stimulating hormone and secondary aldosteronism. The increased aldosterone effect on the distal renal tubule also contributes to the increased reabsorption of salt and water. As shown in Figure 47–1, these factors facilitate excessive fluid retention and the production of edema.

Right ventricular failure, to even a slight degree, results in elevated venous pressure and increased transudation of fluids from the intravascular bed into the interstitial spaces, which causes edema. This elevated venous pressure also leads to hepatic congestion and the transudation of fluids into the peritoneal cavity. Likewise, patients with hepatic congestion demonstrate an impaired degradation of aldosterone, which also contributes to excessive salt and water retention.

For additional discussion of the pathophysiology of congestive heart failure, the reader is referred to the many recent articles on the subject. However, it should be apparent from this brief discussion that the use of appropriate pharmacologic agents is directed primarily toward (1) improving cardiac function, (2) diminishing the excessive renal reabsorption of salt and water, and (3) blocking the effect of aldosterone on

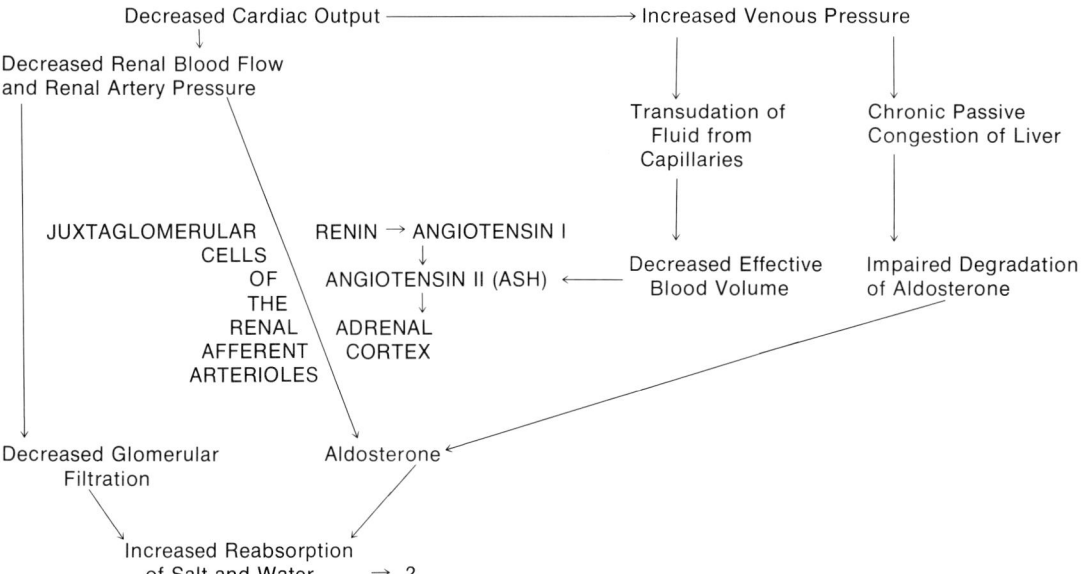

Figure 47–5. Pathophysiologic mechanisms in congestive heart failure.

the distal renal tubule, thus facilitating diuretic responsiveness.

Management

Digitalis. After the precipitating and aggravating factors have been corrected and remediable cardiac and extracardiac conditions treated, the physician can direct his attention to appropriate therapy. This generally includes restricted physical activity, a low salt diet, digitalis, and diuretics.

Digitalis is most effective in patients whose heart failure is due to hypertension, valvular disease, or ischemic heart disease. It is particularly useful when heart failure is associated with atrial fibrillation or flutter, especially when these are associated with rapid ventricular rates.

Digitalis is less effective but occasionally useful in patients with cardiomyopathy and right ventricular failure. One must be particularly careful in the use of digitalis in patients with right ventricular failure and cor pulmonale when hypoxia is present. These patients are particularly prone to the development of digitalis toxicity. Therefore, the presence of cor pulmonale and hypoxia is a relative, but not an absolute, contraindication to the use of digitalis. In these patients, it is best to treat the pulmonary insufficiency with antibiotics, bronchodilators, tracheal toilet, and oxygen and to correct the congestive symptoms with diuretic therapy.

Currently, digoxin is the most commonly used glycoside in the initial and maintenance treatment of patients with congestive heart failure. The usual oral digitalizing dose is 2 to 3 mg. given in divided doses over a 24 to 48 hour period. The usual maintenance dose is 0.25 mg. orally per day. These doses should be reduced in older patients and in those with renal insufficiency. The dosage can be increased or decreased according to the needs of the individual patient, but it should be remembered that the therapeutic dose is close to that dose at which toxic side effects and arrhythmias may be seen. In addition, patients with electrolyte imbalance (hypokalemia, hypomagnesemia, and hypercalcemia), hypoxia, hypothyroidism, and other disorders may develop digitalis toxicity even though serum levels are in the therapeutic rather than the toxic range. Digitalis is relatively contraindicated in the presence of atrioventricular block.

Not uncommonly, patients receiving maintenance doses of digoxin complain of anorexia and nausea, especially after eating. This is often due to a direct gastric effect of the digoxin rather than being a manifestation of toxic dosage. In these instances, serum digoxin levels are not abnormally high, and there are no electrocardiographic manifestations of digitalis toxicity. When this occurs, the patients can be switched to digitoxin, which rarely causes gastrointestinal side effects. Paradoxically, the absence of these side effects is considered one of the disadvantages of digitoxin, as patients often manifest cardiac toxicity before any other manifestations of excessive dosage. Unfortunately, when digitoxin arrhythmias appear, they may persist for 2 to 4 weeks after the drug is stopped.

Recent studies have shown that vasodilator drugs such as the long-acting nitrites and prazosin are helpful in the treatment of severe heart failure.

Diuretics. Hydrochlorothiazide, 50 mg. twice daily, usually is adequate diuretic therapy. Many clinicians have found that if the patient skips the diuretic on Saturdays and Sundays, the likelihood of developing electrolyte imbalance is reduced. Hypokalemia and hypomagnesemia, which facilitate digitalis toxicity, are most commonly caused by diuretic therapy. Triamterene, 100 mg. twice daily, or spironolactone, 25 mg. three times daily to 50 mg. four times daily, can be added to potentiate the diuretic and natriuretic effectiveness of diuretic therapy and also to reduce kaliuresis and the subsequent development of hypokalemia. Needless to say, potassium-sparing agents should be avoided in azotemic patients, and these drugs should not be given concomitantly with supplemental potassium except in extraordinary cases of severe hypokalemia. The latter combination should be used only under close monitoring of hospitalized patients by daily serum potassium determinations.

Spironolactone is a specific aldosterone antagonist and is particularly effective in instances of secondary aldosteronism, which usually is present in patients with refractory congestive heart failure. Therefore, spironolactone should be added to the more potent "loop" diuretics in the treatment of all patients with refractory heart failure. For these patients or for those with renal insufficiency, furosemide or ethacrynic acid generally are more effective than the benzothiadiazine derivatives. Furosemide can be given in doses of 40 to 80 mg. twice daily. This dose need rarely be exceeded except in patients with severe renal insufficiency. In addition to their potent diuretic and natriuretic effects, furosemide and ethacrynic acid elicit significant kaliuresis. Serum potassium levels must be monitored at regular intervals, particularly when high doses are administered. Potent diuretics should be given cautiously to elderly patients, as these patients are more susceptible to true depletional hyponatremia and dehydration.

Acute pulmonary edema is best managed by parenteral furosemide (80 mg. intravenously), nasal oxygen, morphine sulfate (8 mg. intravenously and 8 mg. subcutaneously), rotating tourniquets, and appropriate digitalization. Dramatic relief of the symptoms of pulmonary edema can be obtained with the use of parenteral furosemide (Table 47–4). After intravenous administration of furosemide, diuresis begins within 5 minutes, peaks at 30 minutes, and has a total duration of action of approximately 4 hours. It is not at all uncommon to see a patient diurese 2 liters within 2 hours after administration of furosemide, 80 mg. intravenously. In elderly patients with chronic lung disease and possible hypoxia or hypercapnia, or both, use of diuretics offers a prompter and safer treatment for acute pulmonary edema than does the use of morphine sulfate. Morphine sulfate should be given most carefully in patients who are hypoxic, as it can, on occasion, cause significant respiratory depression. Finally, once the patient has been stabilized, pleural effusions should be removed by paracentesis.

Heart Failure in the Elderly

Thorough knowledge of heart failure in the elderly is essential for the family physician because it is the most common cause of death in geriatric patients. These patients are difficult to treat and prone to develop complications of therapy. Essentially, the pathophysiology of congestive heart failure in elderly patients is similar to that in middle-aged patients, except that the former demonstrate significantly reduced renal function and often have multiple diseases. Mostly all elderly patients with congestive heart failure demonstrate a decreased cardiac output. This leads to a decrease in renal blood flow and glomerular filtration rate and an enhanced reabsorption of sodium in the proximal and distal renal tubule. It is particularly important to realize that elderly patients, because of aging alone, have a decrease in renal function of 50 per cent or more. In elderly patients, the blood urea nitrogen (BUN) level may be within normal limits despite a marked and significant reduction in renal blood flow and glomerular filtration rate. Because of their decreased renal function, elderly patients may require the use of potent "loop" diuretic agents.

Diagnosis and Differential Diagnosis. Older patients frequently have multiple diseases of aging, such as chronic obstructive pulmonary disease, cerebrovascular disease, arthritis, and diabetes. These multiple diseases, plus impaired mental function, may impede the establishment of a precise diagnosis. For instance, a patient with congestive heart failure and severe arthritis may not complain of dyspnea on exertion because the arthritis precludes significant exertion. Likewise, a patient with chronic obstructive pulmonary disease may constantly complain of shortness of breath and dyspnea on exertion—yet congestive heart failure may not be present.

Since impaired mental function and the presence of multiple diseases may confuse the diagnosis, the physician often must employ more precise physical examination techniques and objective measurements than are necessary in the usual examination. For example, patients with congestive heart failure usually have a tachycardia, yet disease of the sinus node or conduction system (recognition of which can require special

TABLE 47–4. ETHACRYNIC ACID AND FUROSEMIDE

Route	Onset of Action	Peak Action	Duration
I.V.	Within 5 minutes	Within 30 minutes	2 to 4 hours
Oral	20 to 60 minutes	2 hours	6 to 8 hours

diagnostic tests) may preclude the development of a significant tachycardia. Other confirmatory signs of congestive heart failure include gallop rhythm, distended neck veins, enlarged liver, and positive hepatojugular reflux. In some instances, chest x-rays and venous pressure determinations are helpful in establishing the diagnosis.

When dealing with elderly patients, physicians often incorrectly assume that congestive heart failure is due to arteriosclerotic coronary artery disease. Since coronary artery disease does not lend itself to simple correction, it is essential that the physician not assume this diagnosis: he must search specifically for precipitating, aggravating, and remediable factors, as mentioned previously. Silent or atypical infarctions, arrhythmias, hypertension, "masked" hyperthyroidism, pulmonary disease, and obstructive uropathy are not uncommonly found in elderly patients with congestive heart failure.

When congestive heart failure develops in the elderly, it is important to rule out "masked" hyperthyroidism, as the usual symptoms may be absent and the heart rate may be normal or only minimally elevated.

Management. Since elderly patients already have a 50 to 60 per cent decrease in renal function, any further decrement, whether it be due to obstructive uropathy, renal infection, or nephrotoxic drugs, can lead to impaired salt and water excretion and the subsequent development of congestive heart failure. Inadequate salt restriction and inadequate or inappropriate dosage of digitalis and diuretics can also contribute to refractoriness of the disease process in elderly patients, as discussed previously. Although the physician should not restrict physical activity excessively, there are some instances in which inadequate restriction of physical activity in geriatric patients does, in fact, contribute to cardiac decompensation.

Elderly patients, because of presbycardia (aging of the myocardium) and hypoxia, often are particularly sensitive to digitalis toxicity. In addition, because of decreased renal function, there is impaired excretion of digoxin. For the aforementioned reasons, in elderly patients it is most appropriate to use less than the usual dose of digoxin. Instead of a maintenance dose of 0.25 mg. daily of digoxin, these patients should re-

ceive digoxin, 0.25 mg. five times a week. If the creatinine level is minimally elevated, digoxin, 0.125 mg. daily, is usually adequate therapy. When more severe renal insufficiency is present, the appropriate dose of digoxin must be calculated or digitoxin substituted. When congestive heart failure is resistant to usual treatment, it is preferable to "push" diuretics rather than to give additional digitalis. "Pushing" digitalis may be lethal because of the development of fatal arrhythmias; therefore, it is much safer to administer extra diuretics.

Although it is important to understand the clinical pharmacology of diuretic agents in all patients, it is particularly important when dealing with elderly patients. For instance, in older patients who do not sleep well, it is probably best to prescribe a short-acting diuretic, such as furosemide, earlier in the day. Generally, furosemide, 40 to 80 mg., is prescribed in the morning, and the second dose is administered at 1:00 or 2:00 P.M. As this drug has a duration of action of approximately 6 to 8 hours, the diuretic response is over by bedtime. This is preferable to prescribing hydrochlorothiazide, 50 mg. in the morning and 50 mg. in the middle of the afternoon, as its 12 hour duration of action may contribute to nocturia and thus to wakefulness. Although many elderly patients require the administration of "loop" diuretics, *most* elderly patients respond adequately to one of the thiazide diuretics in optimal doses, such as hydrochlorothiazide, 50 mg. twice daily.

Patients should be instructed not to take their diuretic on Saturdays and Sundays in order to reduce the induction of hypokalemia. If the response to hydrochlorothiazide is inadequate, furosemide, 40 mg. twice daily, increasing to 80 mg. twice daily, is prescribed instead of the benzothiadiazine derivative. If there is an inadequate diuretic response to furosemide, spironolactone is added in doses of up to 50 mg. four times daily. If the dose of furosemide, 80 mg. twice daily, is exceeded, it is essential to monitor patients carefully for dehydration, prerenal azotemia, and electrolyte imbalance.

When patients require larger than usual doses of diuretics, e.g., furosemide, 80 mg. twice daily, it is important for the physician to maintain them on that dose of diuretics that keeps them at their "dry" weight.

Often, patients who have responded in-adequately to furosemide, 40 mg. twice daily, will diurese significantly on double that dose. If that dose is inappropriately reduced, congestive symptoms and findings may recur.

The prognosis for heart failure in the elderly is poorest when hypertension, atrial fibrillation, or severe pulmonary disease is an associated finding. Prompt and vigorous therapy, therefore, should be directed toward patients with these conditions.

Practical Suggestions for Dealing with Patients with Congestive Heart Failure and Their Families

The physician must recognize that symptoms of fatigue, shortness of breath, and sleeplessness may be caused by minimal-to-mild congestive heart failure but that they may also be caused by anxiety related to the disease entity. It is important, then, that changes in the level of symptomatology be correlated with objective measurement of the patient's cardiovascular status. For instance, if a patient's sleeplessness or fatigue increases as his weight increases, these nonspecific symptoms may be related to progressive cardiac decompensation.

I generally encourage all my patients to weigh themselves daily in the morning—before having breakfast and after having emptied their bladder. When a patient begins to complain of symptoms of increasing fatigability, insomnia, or breathlessness, I determine if there has been a concomitant weight gain, which generally is synchronous with excessive fluid retention. If the patient has developed mild weight gain, larger doses of diuretics are administered.

Some patients complain of increased fatigability, which may be related to sleeplessness; yet they may not voluntarily state that they are having trouble sleeping. Often this symptom must be elicited by close questioning. The physician should inquire: "When do you retire? When do you fall asleep? Do you awaken during the night? Do you awaken feeling reasonably rested?" Symptoms of fatigability often may be improved by adjusting the therapeutic regimen to provide better and sounder sleep. This can be accomplished by use of increased diuretic therapy administered early in the day, raising the head of the bed, administration of aminophylline supposito-ries, use of nitroglycerin ointment if nocturnal angina is present, and administration of hypnotic drugs, such as flurazepam hydrochloride (Dalmane).

Here again, family members should be educated as to the patient's problems. I find it most useful, after having examined the patient in private, to bring family members into the consultation room as I discuss the patient's condition, therapeutic regimen, and prognosis. Upon completion of the conference, I then can ask both the patient and his family whether they have any questions. When family members do not generally accompany the patient, I encourage the patient to set up an appointment at a time when appropriate family members can be present.

Summary

When treating patients with congestive heart failure, the physician first must establish a complete and accurate diagnosis. Next, all remediable cardiac and extracardiac conditions, such as anemia, electrolyte imbalance, and arrhythmias must be corrected. The physician must diligently search for and treat all precipitating and aggravating factors, such as arrhythmias, renal insufficiency, hypertension, and use of salt-retaining drugs. Next, optimal conditions for diuresis must be established; these include bed rest and full digitalization. Then, potent diuretic regimens can be instituted, including the utilization of benzothiadiazines or "loop" diuretics (furosemide, ethacrynic acid) in combination with either spironolactone or triamterene.

CARDIAC MURMURS

The etiology of cardiac murmurs has been widely debated, but the exact cause remains unknown. The most widely accepted theory is that turbulence in the cardiac chambers and great vessels is audible, whereas laminar flow is silent. Turbulence can be caused by rapidly moving streams of blood striking the cardiac wall, a relatively large volume of blood being forced through an opening, blood being forced through a narrowed or deformed opening, or some abnormal structural components, such as ruptured chordae tendineae.

Although the description and classification of murmurs have progressed immensely since the advent of phonocardiography, this section will stress the use of the stethoscope and the evaluation of other clinical findings in diagnosis. The need for patient education and appropriate consultations will be reviewed. The reader is referred to cardiology texts and articles for review of pathologic heart sounds.

In most articles about cardiac murmurs, the organic murmurs are reviewed in detail, but there is little discussion of functional or innocent murmurs. Family physicians must realize that more harm is apt to result from misinterpretation of an innocent murmur than from missing an insignificant organic lesion. There are too many instances in which children have been unnecessarily labeled as having organic disease and restricted from play, candidates for the armed services have been turned down, or applicants for life insurance coverage have been either rated as extremely high risks or rejected, as well as incalculable amounts of mental anguish caused by an unjustified diagnosis of organic heart disease. Certainly, the identification of an innocent murmur is as important as the recognition of a murmur signifying disease. Classification of the functional or innocent murmur needs definite criteria to facilitate the diagnosis and make it more certain. Generally, functional murmurs have the following characteristics: systolic, not pansystolic; loudest along the left sternal border; occasionally harsh; not transmitted; and modified by change in position or respiration. It should be noted that *just about all diastolic murmurs are pathologic* but that systolic murmurs may be of no clinical significance.

In order for the family physician to discharge a person as having an innocent murmur without requesting consultation or referral, there should be (1) a negative clinical history, (2) typical characteristics of an innocent systolic murmur (just noted), (3) normal cardiac size and contour by x-ray, and (4) a normal electrocardiogram.

Incidence of "Innocent" Murmurs

Many children and young adults demonstrate functional murmurs. A basal systolic murmur has been described in many older adults with no evidence of organic heart disease. Although the terms "innocent" and "functional" have frequently been used interchangeably by many authors, it is more appropriate to state that an "innocent" murmur is found in normal subjects with healthy hearts; a "functional" murmur is found when the heart is structurally normal but the cardiac blood flow is markedly increased (e.g., due to exercise or excitement). One of the simplest methods of classification divides innocent systolic murmurs into three categories: (1) short, early parasternal systolic murmur, or Still's murmur (most commonly found in children between 3 and 7 years of age and decreasing in frequency with adolescence); (2) basal (pulmonic) ejection murmurs (commonly found in adolescents, thin people, and pregnant women); and (3) late systolic murmurs. Of these murmurs, Still's murmur and the basal ejection murmur have been reported to account for as much as 98.6 per cent of all innocent murmurs.

These murmurs, as well as the organic murmurs, can be characterized by several criteria: (1) location, (2) transmission, (3) intensity, (4) quality and pitch, (5) timing, (6) effect of respiration, (7) effect of posture, and (8) effect of pharmacologic agents. The three major innocent murmurs are described according to these criteria in Table 47–5.

The venous hum is another common murmur (found in 50 per cent of children under 12 years of age). It is not systolic in timing but often is a high-pitched, continuous murmuring sound that frequently has a louder diastolic component. The venous hum usually is heard best (i.e., loudest) in the supraclavicular area but also may be heard parasternally. Its most unique characteristic is that it decreases markedly or disappears with recumbency, rotation of the head, or pressure on the neck veins.

When the family physician finds an organic murmur, it is important to determine whether it is hemodynamically significant. Often patients will have a grade 1 to 2 apical pansystolic murmur that may reflect hemodynamically insignificant mitral insufficiency. If there is any doubt about the significance of the murmur, the patient should be referred for consultation with a cardiologist. Although cardiac catheterization may be required, noninvasive techniques such as phonocardiography and echocardiography often can determine whether the murmur is hemodynamically significant and whether more invasive diagnostic tests are necessary.

TABLE 47–5. COMMON INNOCENT MURMURS

Characteristics	Early Systolic (Still's)	Basal Ejection	Late Systolic
Location	Left lower sternal border at third or fourth intercostal space	Pulmonic area	Apex (occasionally confused with murmur of mitral insufficiency)
Transmission	Usually not transmitted, may be minimally transmitted toward axilla	Usually not transmitted, may be minimally transmitted along the sternum	Usually not transmitted
Quality and Pitch	Low-pitched; like a "twanging string"	Low-pitched "blowing"	Low-pitched
	Pitch is determined by frequency of vibrations; if vibrations are regular, the murmurs have a musical quality.		
Intensity	It must be noted that the hemodynamic significance of murmurs should not be graded by their loudness. Although loud murmurs are often organic, soft murmurs may represent organic pathology also. In most instances the innocent murmurs are no louder than a grade 2 to 3. A thrill, which is tactile evidence of vigorous vibrations, is unlikely to be found with innocent murmurs.		
Timing	First 1/2 or 2/3 of systole	Early systole, during rapid flow of blood through right ventricular outflow tract	Late systole, may begin with systolic click
Effect of Respiration	Intensity is often increased with inspiration, during which venous return to right side of heart is increased.		
Effect of Posture	Often is influenced by change in position, while organic murmurs are but slightly influenced.		
Effect of Pharma-cologic Agents		Increased after amyl nitrate	

Practical Suggestions for Dealing with Patients with Heart Murmurs and Their Families

Generally, all patients with benign but unusual heart sounds or murmurs, or both, should be informed that these findings are present. The physician can best built rapport with his patients by informing them of these findings. The patient's immediate concern can be alleviated by the reassurance that this finding (systolic ejection murmur, late apical systolic murmur, systolic clicks) is entirely within normal limits. If, at a later date, another physician detects this auscultatory finding, the patient not only will know that it was present but also will know that the family physician was aware of this finding. Certainly, patients with murmurs of questionable hemodynamic significance should be referred to a cardiologist and followed periodically by both the family physician and the cardiologist.

Occasionally, a family physician is told by a patient or relative that an innocent murmur had been found by another physician. With this statement, the patient or the family may be implying that you missed the murmur or that you found it but did not inform them of the finding. The former situation may strain the doctor-patient relationship a good deal. This is an opportunity for candor as well as for patient education. The patient and family should be told about heart murmurs, what they mean, and why they may vary in their manifestations. In the latter instance, it is important that you underscore your philosophy of patient care, i.e., that in certain instances you prefer not to burden patients unnecessarily with what are insignificant findings.

Finally, it must be remembered that consultations also can be ùsed constructively to allay a patient's anxiety. Even if the family physician is quite confident that the murmur is innocent, functional, or of no hemodynamic significance, a consultation with a cardiologist may do a great deal to reassure both the patient and his family. When suggesting consultations for cardiac patients, it is considerate to assist them in arranging the consultation without undue delay, as they may experience unnecessary concern if they must wait a protracted length of time before seeing the cardiologist.

CHEST PAIN

Differential Diagnosis of Angina Pectoris and Noncardiac Chest Pain

Chest pain is one of the most common complaints of patients presenting at a physician's office. Needless to say, most patients—whether they admit it or not—are concerned that this pain reflects some type of cardiac disease. Therefore, it is incumbent upon the physician to know well the differential diagnosis of chest pain. The distinctive clinical characteristic of angina pectoris is paroxysmal, brief, dull, pressing substernal pain, occasionally radiating to the precordium or upper extremities, or to both areas. The pain is usually related to exercise, relieved by rest or nitroglycerin, or both, and rarely, if ever, is described as knifelike, sharp, or sticking. An accurate diagnosis usually can be made by a precise history. The diagnosis of angina is questionable if there is no history of precipitation by effort and relief by rest or nitroglycerin, or both. Although there are many causes of chest pain, the following are detailed because they often mimic the pain

of angina pectoris, except that they usually are not precipitated by exertion (Table 47–6).

1. Often patients with *psychoneurosis* are younger and demonstrate marked concern about their chest pain, as well as other bodily concerns. There is no consistent relationship to exercise, and the pain often is described as constant or lasting several hours, and is characterized as sharp, sticking, or knifelike.

2. *Costochondritis* usually causes localized pain that can be replicated by pressure on the affected costochondral junction. The pain may be associated with exercise, which causes movement of the affected costochondral joint. This pain also may be brought on by specific movements of the arm or chest or may be associated with deep breathing. Directing the patient to move arm or chest muscles may elicit the pain.

3. *Nonspecific myositis* may cause chest pain, but in this instance the pain is often sharp and sticking. The astute clinician, by having the patient move certain muscles, can often bring on the pain. For example, one can have the patient push his arms together, pull them forward or backward, and push against resistance, thus exercising different muscles in the chest in an attempt to bring on the chest pain of which the patient complains. If the chest pain is related to a particular musculoskeletal action or position, it is very important to reassure the patient that the pain is not of cardiac origin—that cardiac pain occurs only after exertion and not with a particular muscular movement or change in posture.

TABLE 47–6. NONCARDIAC CAUSES OF CHEST PAIN

Resembles Angina Slightly	Not Typical of Angina
Psychoneurosis°	Psychoneurosis°
Pulmonary hypertension (mitral stenosis)°	Costochondritis
Esophagitis and esophagospasm°	Nonspecific myositis
	Radiculitis
	Cervicodorsal arthritis
	Bursitis
	Shoulder disease
	Pericarditis
	Pneumonia
	Aneurysm
	Gastrointestinal distention with gaseous entrapment°
	Peptic ulcer
	Gallbladder disease°
	Diaphragmatic or paraesophageal hernia°

°Relieved by nitroglycerin

4. *Pain associated with peptic esophagitis or spasm of the esophagus* is often indistinguishable from the pain of angina pectoris, except that it usually is not related to exertion. This pain frequently is described as dull, pressing, and substernal and occasionally as burning. When it occurs in the recumbent posture or at night, the diagnosis is more readily made. Esophagitis with reflux may be the cause of chest pain, despite negative x-ray findings. The diagnosis can definitely be established by acid perfusion studies (Bernstein test) or by intraluminal manometric esophageal recording, or both. Symptoms of chest pain may be reproduced in these patients by the instillation of dilute acid or the distention of a balloon in the distal esophagus. Often the pain of peptic esophagitis is referred to one or both arms or shoulders, while in the same patient the angina pain may be more typical—limited to the substernal or precordial region, associated with exertion, and relieved by nitroglycerin.

The pain of esophagitis or esophageal spasm may be relieved by nitroglycerin (which relaxes the smooth muscle of the esophagus) and by antacids. It should be treated with liquid antacids, antacid tablets (to be dissolved slowly, not chewed or swallowed), bland diets, smaller and more frequent meals, and sleeping with the head of the bed elevated. Long-acting nitrites are also useful in the treatment of esophageal spasm.

5. *Gaseous distention* of the stomach, esophagus, or splenic flexure (splenic flexure syndrome) may cause dull chest pain. These pains are not related to exercise and are often relieved by belching or passing flatus. The chest pain of gas entrapment can be made worse by bending over to tie shoes or by putting on a girdle. Occasionally, this pain can be replicated by applying pressure over the colon or by flexing the left thigh over the abdomen. This discomfort frequently is relieved by nitroglycerin.

6. The pain of *cholelithiasis* /or *cholecystitis*, or both, may manifest itself by pain in the chest. Again, this pain may be relieved by nitroglycerin, which gives the physician an erroneous clue to the diagnosis of angina pectoris. Patients with gallbladder disease may *also* have angina pectoris.

7. The pain of diaphragmatic or paraesophageal *hiatal hernia* may be a dull, pressing substernal pain. It is important to note that despite x-ray evidence of hiatal hernia, most patients with hiatal hernias do *not* have chest pain. All too often, cardiac pain has been attributed erroneously to hiatal hernia, particularly because the latter also may be relieved by nitroglycerin.

8. As patients with *peptic ulcer* disease rarely present with pain in the chest, this diagnosis should not be confused with angina pectoris.

9. The pain of *pleurisy* is related to a specific phase of respiration.

10. *Cervical or dorsal arthritis* is one of the most common causes of chest pain, particularly when C4–C5 and T1–T4 are involved. It is relatively simple to differentiate this arthritis from angina pectoris because the pain is often described as being sharp, generally not being related to exercise, coming on any time of the day or night while the patient is either sitting or moving, and often lasting 30 minutes or more. This pain is not relieved promptly by nitroglycerin. In all instances in which the pain has no relation to exercise, time of day, or position and particularly if it is described as sharp or sticking, an x-ray of the cervical and dorsal spine is in order. On the other hand, it is important to note that most patients with cervicodorsal arthritis do not have chest pain. Therefore, its presence should *not* necessarily be assumed to be the cause of chest pain.

11. The chest pain that patients with *mitral stenosis* occasionally develop on exertion is thought to be related to *pulmonary hypertension*. It is said that this pain more often radiates down the right arm than the left. This chest pain is *particularly difficult* to differentiate from that of coronary artery disease, as it is precipitated by exertion and is relieved by nitroglycerin or rest. Occasionally, bronchial asthma is associated with chest pain.

It is particularly important to note that *six* common causes of chest pain other than angina pectoris are often relieved by nitroglycerin. They include: (1) cholelithiasis; (2) esophagospasm and esophagitis; (3) diaphragmatic or paraesophageal hernias; (4) gas entrapment syndromes, including the splenic flexure or hepatic flexure syndromes; (5) pulmonary hypertension, particularly in patients with mitral stenosis; and (6) psychoneurosis. As these noncardiac causes of chest pain are relieved by nitroglycerin, many physicians have the erroneous idea that the pain is due to coronary heart disease. Please note that the several causes of chest pain generally can be established by a precise history and physical examination with but minimal laboratory testing. As stated previously, any of them can be present in patients who also have coronary artery disease, and the physician therefore must be particularly certain that coronary artery disease is not present also. A well-performed negative exercise electrocardiogram (ECG) coupled with a normal resting electrocardiogram usually, but not always, means that there is no significant coronary artery disease present. In rare instances, typical angina pectoris that is relieved by nitroglycerin and that occurs with or without an abnormal ECG may be present even in patients with normal coronary arteriography.

Management of Noncardiac Chest Pain. It is absolutely essential that patients with noncardiac causes of chest pain be reassured that the pain is not caused by heart disease. They should *not* be restricted in physical activity, and it is particularly important for the physician to stress that there is no need for them to restrict such activity. Too often, physicians give a double message by telling patients that their pain is not cardiac but also that they should avoid strenuous physical acivity "just to be on the safe side." This mixed message not only confuses patients and reduces their confidence in their physician, but also tends unnecessarily to make invalids out of them.

Angina Pectoris

As mentioned previously, this pain is usually paroxysmal; brief in duration; brought on by exertion, especially after a heavy meal or in cold weather; and is relieved by rest or nitroglycerin, or both. It often is precipitated by emotional stress, tachycardia, or hypoglycemia. The pain usually is described as dull, squeezing, pressing, viselike, or burning; rarely, if ever, is it characterized as sharp, sticking, or knifelike. If, after close questioning, the patient still describes it as sharp, sticking, or knifelike, the physician should be particularly wary of making the diagnosis of angina pectoris. The pain of angina pectoris is usually located substernally but may pres-

ent precordially or radiate to the precordium. It can also radiate to the neck and jaw or to the upper extremities. Rarely will patients have only anginal equivalents, i.e., pain in the shoulder, arm, hand, or jaw with no pain in the chest. This occurs more frequently after thoracic or cardiac surgery, when for unexplained reasons, some patients who had previously complained of typical angina pectoris no longer develop chest pain but present with pain in their jaw, shoulder, arm, or hand.

Premonitory angina, unstable angina, coronary insufficiency, and the intermediate coronary syndrome all connote a progression in the severity, duration, or frequency of angina that is thought to herald an actual myocardial infarction on occasion. It is particularly important for the physician to keep accurate records of the severity, duration, and frequency of anginal attacks, including the number of nitroglycerin tablets consumed per day or per week. Any significant change in the usual pattern should alert the physician to the possibility of an impending myocardial infarction.

Angina decubitus is the term for angina that occurs while the patient is in the recumbent posture. In these patients, the physician should pay particular attention to the possibility that the chest pain is due to peptic esophagitis or hiatal hernia. If it appears that the pain is due to coronary artery disease, one should consider the possibility of associated minimal congestive heart failure. If the latter is present, the angina decubitus often can be prevented by appropriate management of the congestive heart failure with diuretics or digitalis, or both.

Nocturnal angina comes on while the patient is sleeping and is without apparent cause. It occasionally is related to disturbing dreams of which the patient may or may not be aware. In addition, the possibility of nocturnal hypoglycemia as a precipitating cause of nocturnal angina should be considered in all patients who are taking insulin.

The Electrocardiogram in Angina Pectoris. Although angina pectoris is a diagnosis made by history, at times certain diagnostic studies may be useful. Although the ECG often is normal, abnormalities of the electrocardiogram such as transient T wave inversion or ST segment depression that occurs coincidentally with the chest pain suggest that coronary artery disease probably underlies the chest pain. When the ECG is within normal limits between episodes of chest pain, an accurately performed exercise electrocardiogram, which can include a Master's two-step test or preferably a treadmill or bicycle ergometer test may suggest the presence of coronary artery disease. An abnormal exercise ECG, although confirmatory of coronary artery disease, is not necessarily diagnostic of the fact that the chest pain is due to angina pectoris. For instance, a patient could have asymptomatic coronary artery disease, and the chest pain could be due to peptic esophagitis or cervical arthritis, or both.

Management of Angina Pectoris

Physical Activity. Moderate physical activity to tolerance should be a major management principle of patients with coronary artery disease. Strenuous exertion and specific activities that consistently result in pain (such as walking uphill in cold weather, lifting garage doors, or carrying food parcels) should be avoided. In some instances, patients may be instructed to take sublingual nitroglycerin tablets prophylactically to avoid pain, e.g., a nitroglycerin tablet before walking to the store or before sexual intercourse. The most important principle in the management of patients with angina pectoris is to avoid making them cardiac invalids. I encourage patients to participate in any regular physical activity that they can tolerate, whether it be swimming, bicycling, or jogging. When necessary, I advise patients to slow their pace by reducing their total number of working hours by resting in midmorning or midafternoon or by returning home early. This is preferable to severe, often unnecessary, restriction of occupational activity.

Life Style. Vacation time should be increased, if possible, and scheduled to avoid extremes of both hot and cold weather. Large meals should be avoided. Patients should stop smoking, but if they cannot, they should at least reduce their number of cigarettes, stop inhaling, or switch to a pipe, cigar, or denicotinized cigarettes.

Weight and Diet. Patients should be vigorously encouraged to achieve their ideal weight. Although low fat diets are generally recommended, it may be that this is closing the barn door after the horse has gotten away. Lipid profiles should be done in all patients, and appropriate therapeutic regimens (caloric restriction, fat restriction, sucrose restriction, or lipid-lowering agents) should be utilized when there are *marked* abnormalities in the lipid levels.

Antianginal Drugs. I generally prescribe sublingual nitroglycerin (0.3 to 0.6 mg.), which acts within 1 minute. It is useful for the patient to record the number of nitroglycerin tablets taken daily before long-acting nitrites and beta-blockers are added to the therapy. If the patient is taking more than three or four nitroglycerin tablets per day, a long-acting drug such as isosorbide dinitrate (Isordil), usually in the long-acting form (Isordil Tembids, 40 mg.), is prescribed. The dose of Isordil may be increased gradually from 40 mg. twice daily up to 80 mg. twice daily, or rarely to 80 mg. three times daily. (These doses are higher than those given in the manufacturer's official directive.) If anginal episodes persist and if there is no contraindication, propranolol (Inderal) is then added in doses of 20 to 40 mg. three or four times daily. The use of nitrites and beta-blockers is complementary. The nitrites exert their antianginal effect primarily by decreasing venous return and thus decreasing cardiac work. The beta-blockers also decrease cardiac work and oxygen consumption, as well as reduce the myocardial response to catecholamines. These two types of drugs also antagonize each other's undesirable side effects, particularly their effect on heart rate. Nitroglycerin ointment (2 per cent Nitrol) applied to the chest or forearm is particularly useful in the treatment of nocturnal angina. When angina appears to be related to emotional stress, the addition of a minor tranquilizer, such as chlordiazepoxide (Librium) or diazepam (Valium) or phenobarbital, 15 to 30 mg. three times daily, is often helpful.

Practical Suggestions for Dealing with Patients with Coronary Artery Disease and Their Families

Dealing with patients and families of patients with coronary artery disease can be quite trying but also very gratifying. Unfortunately, the unnecessary development of cardiac "cripples" is an all too common iatrogenic disease. In my experience, physicians tend to err on the side of being overly conservative in restricting the physical activity of patients with coronary artery disease. This results in both fearful patients and fearful and guilt-ridden family members. When a patient is encouraged to participate in certain moderate physical activities, including sexual intercourse, there may be tremendous feelings of guilt on the part of a family member if chest pain is subsequently induced in the patient. I believe it is particularly important to tell patients and their families that the patients should be encouraged to do as much as possible—up to the point at which chest pain is elicited.

Once it is determined that a particular activity usually results in angina pectoris, the strenuousness of this activity should be reduced or the patient should be instructed to take nitroglycerin prophylactically, or both. For instance, a patient who often experiences chest pain while walking to the train station in cold weather should be instructed to dress warmly, possibly walk somewhat more slowly, and take nitroglycerin before setting out. Likewise, nitroglycerin can be taken before sexual intercourse to avoid angina. As mentioned previously, if more than three or four nitroglycerin tablets are consumed per day, the patient may benefit from long-acting nitrites, often given in combination with propranolol.

Often the tolerance for exercise in patients who have sustained a myocardial infarction can be increased by regularly prescribed physical activity. Physical activity can be measured and increased gradually over several months, while observing the patient's clinical tolerance, pulse rate, and electrocardiographic changes. Recognition that they can increase their physical activity without resultant chest pain often provides a great psychologic lift to cardiac patients. Appropriate weight reduction and treatment of hypertension, if present, can provide an additional extension of these patients' exercise tolerance.

If at all possible, patients should resume work on a part-time basis for a few weeks before resuming their full-time occupation. Although persistent complaints of weakness and shortness of breath may be related to minimal cardiac decompensation or residual muscle weakness from prolonged inactivity, these symptoms not uncommonly represent a depressive reaction. The patient's ability to resume regular activity without undue discomfort often suggests that the prognosis is a good one. The

physician should seize every opportunity to provide enthusiastic encouragement to cardiac patients, pointing out to them that their ability to resume usual activities without discomfort is a particularly good prognostic sign.

ARRHYTHMIAS

It is essential that the family physician evaluate all arrhythmias comprehensively; this includes making a specific diagnosis of the type of the arrhythmia as well as recognizing the arrhythmia in the context of the patient's total clinical condition. An electrocardiogram should be performed on all patients with arrhythmias or symptoms compatible with arrhythmias. It is particularly important for the physician to be able to differentiate supraventricular arrhythmias, which may be disabling, from ventricular arrhythmias, which are potentially lethal. Arrhythmias result from one or more of the following factors: abnormal rate of impulse formation (too fast or too slow), abnormal site of impulse formation, and abnormal conduction.

From the clinical standpoint, arrhythmias may be divided into (1) those with regular rhythm (bradycardia or tachycardia) and (2) those with irregular rhythm.

Arrhythmias with a Regular Rhythm

Sinus bradycardia (less than 60 beats per minute) is one of the most common arrhythmias. It generally is due to either decreased sympathetic tone or increased vagal tone. This arrhythmia frequently is seen in athletes or former athletes and most particularly in people who in earlier years had participated in regular, vigorous exercise, such as long-distance running. Characteristically, this type of bradycardia disappears with minimal to mild exercise. Running in place or the performance of several "situps" may result in an increase of rate to within normal limits. When a patient has a regular bradycardia of 30 to 50 beats per minute that does not increase with exercise, complete heart block with an idioventricular rhythm should be suspected. It should be noted that when premature ventricular contractions (PVC's) are present in patients with sinus bradycardia, the disappearance of PVC's after exercise strongly suggests that the premature contractions are of negligible clinical significance.

Sinus bradycardia can also be seen in patients with hypothyroidism, jaundice, and coronary artery disease. In addition, conditions that lead to increased vagal tone, such as carotid sensitivity, glaucoma, and distended viscera (gastric dilatation, esophageal dilatation, hydroureter, and distended urinary bladder) may all contribute to the development of bradycardia. Digitalis and propranolol, as well as certain antihypertensive drugs (alpha-methyldopa, reserpine derivatives, guanethidine, and clonidine) all tend to produce bradycardia.

Although digitalis can cause a sinus bradycardia, it also can produce a high degree of or even complete atrioventricular (A-V) block manifested as bradycardia. Bradycardia due to digitalis excess is often a slow (50 to 60 beats per minute) nodal "escape" rhythm. A nodal rhythm of approximately 80 to 100 beats per minute, "nodal tachycardia," also may be caused by excess digitalis. Most often, complete A-V block is due to heart disease (either congenital or coronary artery) or some other disease of the conduction system that results in complete A-V block.

Sinus bradycardia rarely requires therapy. Propantheline bromide (Pro-Banthine), 15 mg. three times daily, may be useful on occasion. Isoproterenol (Isuprel), sublingual, can be used to increase the sinus rate as long as there is no ventricular irritability, which may be exaggerated by the administration of the Isuprel. In most instances, patients with chronic symptomatic sinus bradycardia and those with the so-called "sick sinus" (bradytachycardia) should be treated by the use of a pacemaker.

Sinus tachycardia (greater than 100 beats per minute) is probably the most common arrhythmia. When it is present, the physician must search for its cause, which can include fever, anxiety, exercise, hyperventilation, hypoglycemia, or emotional stress. It also is seen in patients with minimal to severe congestive heart failure, hyperthyroidism, pheochromocytoma, anemia, hypoxia, chronic lung disease, and coronary insufficiency. Excessive stimulants such as caffeine, alcohol, tobacco, and drugs (amphetamines, hydralazine, thyroid drugs, and several psychotropic drugs) also cause sinus tachycardia. When evaluating a

patient with sinus tachycardia, the patient should be allowed to rest quietly for a few minutes to determine if the tachycardia abates. If the tachycardia persists, the aforementioned clinical conditions should be considered.

Paroxysmal tachycardia can be supraventricular or ventricular in origin. Paroxysmal supraventricular tachycardias, although sometimes seen in patients with no organic heart disease, are due most often to rheumatic heart disease, ischemic heart disease, or hyperthyroidism. Reactive hypoglycemia should always be considered a possible cause for paroxysmal supraventricular tachycardia. A history that the tachycardia occurs in the mid- to late morning, mid- to late afternoon, or mid-evening or appears after fasting should make the physician suspect reactive hypoglycemia. It is thought that epinephrine release subsequent to hypoglycemia serves as a stimulus to the production of the paroxysmal tachycardia. In most patients, the cause of paroxysmal supraventricular tachycardia is metabolic. On the other hand, most patients with *sustained supraventricular tachycardia* (other than sinus tachycardia) have either heart disease or chronic obstructive pulmonary disease. As mentioned previously, digitalis toxicity may cause a nonparoxysmal supraventricular tachycardia.

The pre-excitation (Wolff-Parkinson-White) syndrome should be considered particularly in patients with paroxysmal tachycardia. It may be detected by a delta wave (initial slurring of the R wave) in the QRS complex, which may be of prolonged duration, although it is usually of normal duration.

Increasing vagal tone by either carotid sinus massage or gag reflex may result in the abrupt cessation of a paroxysmal supraventricular tachycardia, although these same measures cause but minimal transient slowing in patients with nonparoxysmal tachycardia. In applying carotid sinus pressure, it is important that the pressure be applied from cephalad to the carotid sinus down to the carotid sinus. This is most effectively accomplished with the patient recumbent and the neck in mild hyperextension, achieved by elevating the shoulders on a pillow or blanket. Pressure on the eyeballs is dangerous and not particularly effective. Paroxysmal supraventricular tachycardia can also be terminated by use of parenteral digitialis or intravenous propranolol. When resistant, the tachycardia can be converted by overdriving with a transvenous atrial pacer. Once-converted patients who have recurrent bouts of tachycardia should be placed on quinidine, propranolol, or digoxin, or combinations thereof. Paroxysmal supraventricular tachycardia with block must be considered digitalis toxicity until proved otherwise.

Atrial flutter with block is another form of regular supraventricular tachycardia. Whenever the heart rate is approximately 150 beats per minute and regular, atrial flutter with 2:1 block should be suspected. Another bedside clue to its presence is the halving of the rate with carotid sinus pressure (decreasing from 150 beats per minute to 75 beats per minute, i.e., from 2:1 to 4:1 block). Atrial flutter with 2:1 conduction is best treated by rapid digitalization or DC cardioversion. Recurrence is best prevented by long-term administration of digoxin in combination with quinidine.

Sustained ventricular tachycardia usually results in cardiopulmonary collapse. On the other hand, patients may have short bouts of a regular ventricular tachycardia on clinical examination. If an electrocardiogram reveals this to be runs of three or more consecutive premature ventricular contractions, this should be considered paroxysmal ventricular tachycardia, a potentially lethal condition. It should be treated as a medical emergency. These patients should be treated promptly with parenteral lidocaine or procainamide and hospitalized immediately. DC cardioversion is useful in resistant cases. Paroxysmal ventricular tachycardia is frequently due to digitalis excess or electrolyte imbalance (low potassium or magnesium), or both. In these instances, treatment should include termination of digitalis, correction of the electrolyte imbalance, and the parenteral administration of lidocaine, propranolol, or phenytoin.

Arrhythmias with Irregular Rhythms

The most common irregular rhythms, other than sinus arrhythmia, which is of no clinical consequence, are ventricular and atrial premature beats, atrial fibrillation, and second degree A-V block.

Ventricular premature beats often occur in healthy individuals and may be without clinical significance. They often become more frequent under conditions of fatigue, emotional upset, or excessive ingestion of stimulants such as caffeine or tobacco. If ventricular premature beats disappear with mild exercise and increased sinus rate, they probably do not represent clinically significant cardiac disease. On the other hand, if they become more frequent with exercise or if the electrocardiogram reveals multifocal ventricular premature beats (nonfixed coupling with a varying QRS configuration), some form of heart disease is probably present. Digitalis toxicity, with or without electrolyte imbalance (hypokalemia or hypomagnesemia, or both), is a frequent cause of ventricular premature beats.

If the ventricular premature beats are not due to heart disease, digitalis excess, or some other pathologic condition and if the patient is not troubled by these beats ("palpitations"), there is no need for treatment. On the other hand, if the patient is annoyed by these premature beats or if they occur near the vulnerable period (near the peak of the T wave), then therapy is indicated. Intravenous lidocaine is most effective in emergency situations. Oral quinidine, procainamide, or phenytoin is useful occasionally in the prevention of premature ventricular contractions.

Atrial premature beats, in contradistinction to premature ventricular contractions (PVC's), are usually pathologic and indicate cardiac or pulmonary disease. If they are frequent or multifocal, or both, they may be precursors of atrial fibrillation. When they are manifestations of chronic lung disease with hypoxia, treatment must first be directed toward correcting the underlying pulmonary insufficiency. Atrial premature beats can be treated with quinidine, 300 mg. every 4 to 6 hours.

Atrial fibrillation, with its irregular irregularity, may occur rarely in patients without heart disease but most often is a manifestation of rheumatic heart disease (particularly mitral stenosis), hyperthyroidism, or arteriosclerotic heart disease. It is best treated by rapid digitalization. If atrial fibrillation is not converted to sinus rhythm, quinidine can be added. DC cardioversion is particularly effective in instances of recent onset. Once converted to sinus rhythm, patients should receive digitalis and quinidine. In chronic atrial fibrillation, the ventricular rate is best controlled with digoxin. If signs of excess digitalization appear before the ventricular rate is adequately controlled, propranolol should be added.

In *patients with chronic atrial fibrillation, the regularization of ventricular response* should alert the physician to the possibility of digitalis excess. In other words, if a patient with chronic atrial fibrillation develops a relatively regular ventricular response (55 to 85 beats per minute), the physician should suspect excess digitalis as causing a relatively high degree of A-V block with a nodal escape rhythm. An electrocardiogram should be performed and digitalis withheld until the high degree of A-V block has abated.

It is particularly important to note that when atrial fibrillation or so-called chaotic rhythms occur in patients with chronic lung disease, therapy should be directed toward correction of the hypoxia rather than just the administration of digitalis. Patients with chronic lung disease and hypoxia are particularly sensitive to the toxic effects of digitalis, and therefore digitalis is relatively, but not absolutely, contraindicated.

Patients who have arrhythmias that result in cardiopulmonary collapse, evidence of cerebral insufficiency as manifested by episodic syncope, or falling or transient episodes of lightheadedness should be referred for investigation by a cardiologist. In addition, it should be noted that some patients with what may appear to be minor conduction disturbances are potential candidates for cardiac catastrophes. For example, transient episodes of cerebral insufficiency in patients with (1) second degree A-V block, (2) first degree A-V block and complete right bundle branch block, or (3) bifascicular block (right bundle branch block with left axis deviation [left anterior hemiblock]) may be due to the development of intermittent complete heart block. These patients are candidates for the prophylactic insertion of cardiac pacemakers *before* permanent complete heart block develops. Pacemakers also are indicated in patients with Adams-Stokes attacks, symptomatic heart block, and some cases of recurrent tachyarrhythmias, as well as the "sick sinus" syndrome.

The reader is referred to review articles on arrhythmias and textbooks on electrocardiography for illustrations of arrhythmias, reviews of conduction disturbances, indications for bundle of His recordings in the evaluation of patients with A-V block, and indications for pacemaker therapy, both permanent and temporary.

Practical Suggestions for Dealing with Patients with Arrhythmias and Their Families

What can the family physician do when the patient complains of palpitation but the clinical examination does not reveal an arrhythmia? In these instances, it is useful to get the patient to try to tap out the pulse beat that he thought he had felt. If the patient is unable to do this, I tap out a regular fast rhythm, an irregular fast rhythm, a slow irregular rhythm, and a regular rhythm with premature beats in order to get the patient to provide more precise identification of the nature of the palpitation that he experienced. This procedure is particularly useful when the arrhythmia cannot be documented on electrocardiogram.

In addition, it is important to teach patients how to take their pulse, either radially or at their temple, so they can report to the physician their rate and rhythm at the time of their "palpitation." Also, they are instructed to go the nearest physician's office or hospital when they experience a palpitation, in order that it can be documented electrocardiographically. The patient should be instructed to request a strip of this electrocardiogram, so the attending physician can make it a part of his records. If these procedures fail or if the patient experiences symptoms of lightheadedness or syncope with the arrhythmia, Holter tape monitoring should be instituted, as it is essential to know the type of the arrhythmia prior to instituting antiarrhythmic pharmacologic therapy.

HYPERLIPIDEMIA

It must be emphasized that the hyperlipidemias are most often asymptomatic. Only a fraction of patients with hyperlipidemia have cutaneous manifestations or a lactescent serum. Hyperlipidemias are best diagnosed, therefore, by routine laboratory determinations. This should include the determination of serum cholesterol and triglyceride levels after a 12 hour fast without alcohol consumption for the preceding 24 to 48 hours. Weight-reducing diets should be discontinued for 2 weeks prior to the determination of serum lipids, as they may reduce the serum lipid level. The turbidity of the serum should be noted after it has stood overnight at 4° C. All abnormal tests should be rechecked to make sure that there has not been a laboratory error.

If hyperlipidemia is detected, secondary causes of hyperlipidemia should be ruled out first. These include hypothyroidism, nephrotic syndrome, Cushing's syndrome, diabetes, alcoholic hyperlipidemia, stress hyperlipidemia, and biliary obstruction. Certain drugs, particularly thyroid hormones, adrenocorticoids, and the estrogenic component of contraceptive steroids, may alter serum lipid levels. Other drugs that interfere with the estimation of serum cholesterol levels include phenytoin, anabolic steroids, chlorpromazine, sulfonamides, testosterone, mestranol, allopurinol, tetracycline, monoamine oxidase (MAO) inhibitors, and phenformin.

Once hyperlipidemia is confirmed by a repeat laboratory determination and secondary causes have been ruled out, the physician should first type and then correct the hyperlipidemia, as premature atherosclerosis and coronary artery disease appear to be associated with the hyperlipidemias.

The cholesterol and triglyceride levels in the five types of primary hyperlipidemia are listed in Table 47–7. In this chapter only three of the more common types of hyperlipidemia will be discussed—Types IIA, IIB, and IV.

Type IIA, "pure" hypercholesterolemia, is due to increased beta lipoproteins; the serum is clear. In Type IIB (the "mixed" type), the serum is slightly turbid, and there is an elevation of the pre-beta lipoproteins as well as the beta-lipoproteins. In Type IIB, the cholesterol level is elevated, and the triglyceride levels are modestly elevated. A diagnosis of Type II hyperlipoproteinemia or hypercholesterolemia requires that the cholesterol exceed 400 mg. per 100 ml.; xanthomas are often present. Since Type II is inherited as a mendelian dominant trait, one parent also will have hypercholesterolemia, if this diagnosis is correct.

The treatment of pure hypercholesterolemia (Type IIA), although inadequate, should be instituted when the serum cholesterol level exceeds 300 to 400 mg. per 100 ml. Dietary fats, including cholesterol, should be restricted; saturated fat intake reduced; and polyunsaturated fat intake increased. Drugs such as cholestyramine 15 to 30 grams daily in divided doses with meals (see manufacturer's official directive for doses over 24 grams daily) or nicotinic acid 2 to 12 grams daily in divided doses are useful in lowering cholesterol levels in Type II disorders. Cholestyramine interferes with the reabsorption of bile acids and cholesterol from the gut; D-thyroxine is also occasionally effective. Clofibrate (Atromid-S) (approximately 2 grams per day) may be minimally effective, although it is usually more effective when both cholesterol and triglyceride levels are elevated, such as in the Type IIB and Type IV. Patients with Type IIB hyperlipidemia should be instructed to restrict carbohydrates and to lose weight. If these measures do not produce an adequate lowering of lipids, clofibrate therapy should be initiated.

Type IV is another of the common hyperlipidemias. Here the pre-beta lipoprotein level is elevated, and the serum is cloudy. Both cholesterol and triglyceride levels are elevated. Xanthomas are rare in Type IV hyperlipidemia. Clofibrate is particularly effective in lowering lipid levels, and nicotinic acid also may be effective. As mentioned previously, dietary management should include weight reduction, restriction of carbohydrates, and decreased cholesterol intake, as well as an increased ingestion of unsaturated fats. It should be mentioned that clofibrate potentiates the action of anticoagulants, and therefore doses of warfarin (Coumadin) probably should be reduced by 50 per cent.

TABLE 47–7. HYPERLIPIDEMIA

Type of Hyperlipidemia	Serum Cholesterol Level	Serum Triglyceride Level
Type I	Normal or elevated	Elevated
Type IIA	Elevated	Normal
Type IIB	Elevated	Elevated
Type III	Elevated	Elevated
Type IV	Normal or elevated	Elevated
Type V	Elevated	Elevated

Therapeutic regimens should be continued until the cholesterol levels are consistently reduced to below 300 mg. per 100 ml. and the triglyceride levels to below 200 mg. per 100 ml. Finally, it should be pointed out that there has been *no conclusive evidence that reduction of the lipid levels results in a decreased incidence of atherosclerosis or of coronary artery disease.*

Practical Suggestions for Dealing with Patients with Hyperlipidemia and Their Families

When implementing low-fat diets, as in all other types of dietary restriction, the physician should do *more* than just tell the patient what not to eat; rather, the patients should also be told what should be eaten (i.e., the positive aspects of dietary changes should be stressed). The patient should be encouraged to eat foods high in polyunsaturated fats as well as foods such as poultry, fish, and vegetables, which are low in fats. Encouraging the patient to keep a diet notebook that is reviewed with the physician during office visits reinforces and encourages the patient's active participation. The latter is preferable to a situation in which the patient is just a passive recipient of the doctor's orders.

Since familial hyperlipidemia is common, it is important to test families of patients with hyperlipidemia to detect asymptomatic afflicted relatives.

SUGGESTED ADDITIONAL READINGS

Hypertension

1. Laragh, J. H.: Modern system for treating high blood pressure based on renin profiling and vaso-constriction—Volume analysis. Am. J. Med., *61*:797, 1976.

Heart Failure

1. Braunwald, E.: Vasodilator therapy—a physiologic approach to the treatment of heart failure. N. Engl. J. Med., 297:331, 1978.
1a. Cohn, J. N.: Indications for digitalis therapy—A new look. J.A.M.A., 229:1911, 1974.
2. Seller, R. H., and Brest, A. N.: Heart failure in the elderly. Geriatrics, *22*:225, 1967.
3. Seller, R. H., Banach, S., Neff, S., et al.: Cardiac effect of diuretic drugs. Am. Heart J., 89:493, 1975.
4. Seller, R. H., Ramirez-Muxo, O., Brest, A. N., et al.: Refractory heart failure, differential diagnosis and management. Postgrad. Med., *40*:599, 1966.

Cardiac Murmurs

1. Evans, W.: Heart murmurs. Brit. Heart J., 9:1, 1947.
2. Leatham, A., Segal, B., and Shaffer, H.: Auscultatory and phonocardiographic findings in healthy children with systolic murmurs. Brit. Heart J., 25:451, 1963.
3. Shabetai, R., and Marsbald, W. J.: Systolic murmurs. Am. Heart J., 65:412, 1973.

Chest Pain

1. Brest, A. N., and Moyer, J. H.: Cardiovascular Disorders. Philadelphia, F. A. Davis Co., 1968.
2. Friedberg, C. K.: Diseases of the Heart. 3rd Ed. Philadelphia, W. B. Saunders Co., 1966.

Arrhythmias

1. Salerni, R., and Lion, D. F.: Current status of cardiac pacing. Disease a Month, October, 1972.
2. Seller, R. H.: The role of magnesium in digitalis toxicity. Am. Heart J., 82:551, 1971.
3. Surawicz, B.: Arrhythmias and anti-arrhythmic therapy in context. Hosp. Practice, *11*:59, 1976.
4. Wright, K. E., and McIntosh, H. D.: Artificial pacemakers—Indications and management. Circulation, 47:1108, 1973.

Hyperlipidemia

1. Fisher, W. R., and Truitt, D. H.: The common hyperlipoproteinemias. Ann. Intern. Med., 85:496, 1976.
2. Hazzard, W. R.: A pathophysiologic approach to managing hyperlipidemia. Am. Fam. Phys., *14*:78, 1976.

Chapter 48

NEUROLOGY

by JOHN GILROY,
and JOSEPH W. HESS

NEUROLOGIC HISTORY, PHYSICAL EXAMINATION, AND DIAGNOSTIC PROCEDURES

This section outlines the components of a complete neurologic examination that can be used in office practice by the family physician (Table 48–1). The object of this examination is to facilitate localization and diagnosis for the majority of patients with neurologic problems. In addition, the family physician will be able to recognize neurologic abnormalities in the remainder of his patients and proceed logically to further evaluation or consultation.

HISTORY

The *neurologic history* is a modification of the history taken in the evaluation of any medical problem. The physician obtains information from the patient but may have to add to this information by an interview with a close relative, particularly when the patient shows dementia, language problems, or episodic loss of consciousness. The interview begins by eliciting the chief complaint, followed by obtaining a history of the present illness in chronologic order. There is then a deviation from the usual order, and before moving on to the past history, the physician asks a series of questions that can be termed the neurologic review. It is important to interject the neurologic review, as it is an immediate supplement to the history obtained from the patient or relative, or both. The information obtained, added to that from the history, may give such a clear picture of the patient's condition that a diagnosis or differential

diagnosis can be made at that point. This occurs in about 80 per cent of patients, and the neurologic examination becomes a confirmatory act rather than a search for additional information toward establishing a diagnosis.

The neurologic review is a series of short questions covering the following symptoms: (1) headache, (2) visual abnormalities, (3) diplopia, (4) hearing deficit, (5) tinnitus, (6) vertigo, (7) ataxia, (8) focal weakness, (9) focal numbness, (10) sphincter problems, (11) speech problems, (12) writing problems, (13) difficulty swallowing, (14) memory and mentation patterns, and (15) syncopal episodes and seizures.

Simple terms are used when posing questions so that the patient will understand and respond more accurately. When a positive response is obtained, the physician must determine its significance in the history. If he decides that it is significant, a series of additional questions are asked in order to bring out as much information as possible concerning the symptoms. This procedure should be followed by the physician in each step throughout the neurologic review. The information thus derived will provide a good differential, if not the diagnosis, by the end of the neurologic review.

The neurologic review is followed by the history of previous illnesses. This should be documented chronologically, including the usual diseases of childhood.

Many neurologic problems are genetically determined, and the family history is important in patients who appear to have degenerative diseases, movement disorders, or seizures. Details of illnesses suffered by the parents and siblings should

TABLE 48–1.   THE NEUROLOGIC HISTORY AND EXAMINATION

History	Examination
Chief complaint	Mentation
History of present illness	Cranial nerves
Neurologic review	Motor system
Past history	Coordination
Family history	Gait
Social history	Station and Romberg test
Birth and developmental history	Sensation
	Reflexes
	Skull, spine, murmurs (bruits), nuchal rigidity

be documented and supplemented by information about close relatives such as uncles, aunts, and cousins when this seems to be appropriate.

A social history is often important in the evaluation of neurologic problems, particularly in our complex society. A patient should be asked about his occupation and should also be asked to give some description of that occupation. This has two purposes: it may reveal some association between the patient's activities or work and the neurologic problem, and at the same time it enhances physician-patient rapport. The number of children of the patient and whether the children are well should be recorded, as well as the history of smoking, alcohol consumption, and exposure to drugs. It is useful to make a list of the medications that the patient has been taking during the past year, including dosage and reasons for the prescription, if the patient is aware of this information. It is also useful to ask about exposure to any unusual chemicals or toxic substances in the past year or two.

The birth and developmental history may be of crucial importance when interviewing a child or an adolescent with a neurologic problem. This should include obtaining some history of the pregnancy from the mother, involving such information as whether this was a normal pregnancy, whether there were any unexplained fevers during pregnancy, whether the maternal weight gain was normal, and whether it was a full-term pregnancy. Duration of labor, complications, need for resuscitation of the baby, and birth weight should also be recorded. The physician will then want to know whether the child fed well and

whether there was prolonged jaundice following birth. A notation should be made about the common developmental milestones up to the age of 2 years.

The neurologic examination of every patient must include a complete general physical examination. Neurologic problems rarely exist in isolation, and many of them are complications of other systemic disease, the extent of which will be revealed only by a detailed general physical examination.

PHYSICAL EXAMINATION

Examination of Cerebral Function

The *neurologic examination* begins with assessment of cerebral function. A great deal of information about intellectual function will have already been obtained by the physician from observation of the patient up to this point. *Disorientation, impaired judgment, poor insight, memory deficits,* and *inappropriate emotional responses* may well have been detected during the period of history-taking and should be recorded. However, it is wise to spend some time in further evaluation of mental status when the physician suspects that there may be a cerebral lesion. In evaluating the mental status, the physician should assess the following:

1. *Dysphasia.* A difficulty in comprehension or production of language symbols caused by disease of the central nervous system. A patient's responses will obviously be modified in the presence of dysphasia, and this must be considered in an overall assessment of intellectual capacity.

2. *Dysarthria.* A difficulty in articulation, resulting from a disturbance of neuromuscular control of the muscles involved in articulation.

3. *Dysphonia.* A condition in which there is disturbance of sound, tone, or quality of speech.

4. *Awareness.* The patient's awareness of his environment, whether he is oriented to time, place, and person.

5. *Mood and affect.* Whether the patient is depressed, elated, anxious, and so forth, and whether he shows appropriate affect, that is, the appropriate emotional response to a given situation.

6. *Delusions and hallucinations.* These perceptual difficulties may be seen in pa-

tients with neurologic and psychiatric disorders and may be defined as follows:

    a. Delusions—a false belief.

    b. Illusions—a false interpretation of a sensory perception.

    c. Hallucination—a sensory perception that is not founded on objective reality.

7. *Memory.* Assessment of the patient's recent and remote memory may be obtained from the history.

8. *Frontal lobe function:*

    a. Judgment—the ability to respond appropriately to a situation that provides several alternative responses.

    b. Insight—the awareness of the significance of a situation. Does the patient know why he is undergoing a medical examination?

    c. Dyspraxia—the inability to perform a complex task requiring motor integration in the absence of paralysis of the muscles involved.

    d. Abstraction—the ability to abstract is usually tested by asking the patient to interpret proverbs.

9. *Temporal lobe function:*

    a. Retention and recall—the ability to retain information and recall that information within a period of a few minutes.

    b. Calculation—the ability to understand arithmetic symbols.

    c. Auditory agnosia—the inaccurate recognition of an auditory stimulus in the absence of impairment of hearing.

    d. Right-left confusion—the inability to identify right and left sides of the body.

    e. Agraphia—the inability to write in the absence of paralysis of the hand.

10. *Parietal Lobe Function:*

    a. Dyslexia—the inability to read in the absence of visual impairment.

    b. Tactile localization—two point discrimination, stereognosis—usually performed with sensory examination.

    c. Autotopagnosia—the inability to recognize a body part.

    d. Anosognosia—the denial of abnormality (usually paralysis) in a limb.

11. *Occipital lobe function:*

    a. Visual agnosia—the inability to accurately recognize objects visually in the absence of visual impairment.

    b. Aprosognosia—the nonrecognition of familiar faces.

    c. Visual-spatial agnosia—the nonrecognition of familiar objects or places, such as the home or its surrounding areas.

    d. Constructional dyspraxia—dyspraxia caused by malfunction of visual association areas. The patient cannot copy simple designs.

    e. Visual field defects with cortical pattern.

Examination of the Cranial Nerves

The cranial nerves are examined in numerical order, as outlined in Table 48–2.

Examination of the Motor System

When examining the motor system in the upper or lower limb girdles, the following sequence should be followed: (1) inspection, (2) tone, (3) power, (4) posture, and (5) development.

Inspection. The patient should be seated comfortably on an examining table facing the examiner. The examiner rapidly compares the muscle bulk in the shoulder girdle on both sides, then compares the upper arms, forearms and hands followed by the thighs and legs. If there is any suspicion of wasting in the muscles, the girth of the part in question should be measured and recorded. This will confirm (or exclude) wasting on one side and will provide a reference for subsequent measurement if the patient is experiencing progressive wasting of muscle. Inspection includes observation of any involuntary movement arising centrally (e.g., caused by chorea, athetosis, tremor, or myoclonus) or peripherally (e.g., caused by fasciculations).

Tone. Tone is assessed by moving the limb passively and using the other hand to palpate the muscle that is being stretched. The physician examines each muscle group, alternating between the two sides (e.g., right biceps to left biceps) so that a comparison of tone can be made between the two sides. The palpation of the muscle during passive movement assures that subtle changes in tone, such as minor degrees of cogwheeling, will be detected. When tone is examined in the calf, the foot should be suddenly dorsiflexed and held firmly. This

TABLE 48-2.   CRANIAL NERVE EXAMINATION

Cranial Nerve Number	Name	Method
1st	Olfactory	Not necessary
2nd	Optic	1. Examine optic disc with ophthalmoscope 2. Test visual fields by confrontation for binocular vision and for each eye independently 3. If optic nerve abnormal or visual fields abnormal, obtain perimetry and tangent screen examination
3rd	Oculomotor	1. Test pupillary reaction to light and accommodation
4th	Trochlear	2. Test extraocular movements internally, upward, downward;
6th	Abducens	note smoothness of movement, impersistence, nystagmus, deviation of ocular axis, diplopia, dysfunction of conjugate eye movements 3. Note presence or absence of ptosis, enophthalmos, exophthalmos.
5th	Trigeminal	1. Check corneal reflex 2. Test facial sensation to touch and pinprick 3. Test strength of masseter and temporal muscles 4. Test jaw jerk
7th	Facial	1. Note strength of facial muscles
8th (Auditory)	Acoustic division	1. Test hearing, comparing each side by whispering or by tick of a watch 2. Rinne test—If air conduction is better than bone conduction, Rinne test is positive 3. Weber test—Tuning fork lateralizes to affected side in patients with middle ear disease or to opposite (normal) side with cochlear or nerve impairment
9th	Glossopharyngeal	1. Palate elevates symmetrically and uvula remains in midline
10th	Vagus	on phonation 2. If voice has nasal quality, soft palate may be paralyzed 3. If there is dysphonia or aphonia, do indirect laryngoscopy to examine vocal cords
11th	Accessory	1. Test contraction of trapezius muscle bilaterally 2. Test contraction of sternocleidomastoid muscles bilaterally
12th	Hypoglossal	1. Tongue normally protrudes in midline; deviation indicates weakness on side of deviation 2. Examine tongue as it lies in mouth for fasciculations, wasting, or scarring.

will produce ankle clonus if the tone is sufficiently increased in the calf muscles.

Power.   The power of each muscle group is tested, alternating between the two sides in the upper and lower limbs.

Posture and Development.   The patient, eyes closed, is asked to hold his arms outstretched, hands supinated. The examiner notes any deviation that might indicate dystonia or drifting. Pronation of one limb, indicating a minor degree of weakness or a loss of proprioception, is also noted. Muscle bulk and bone development should be equal on the two sides of the body. There may be minor differences in development of the limbs, hands, or feet in patients with longstanding or congenital lesions of the central nervous system.

Coordination.   Rapid alternating movements of the outstretched arms, rhythmical hand patting, finger tapping on each side, and foot tapping are used to measure coordinated movement. Finger-nose-finger and heel-knee-shin testing measures more proximal coordination in the limbs.

Gait.   Much can be learned by observing the gait. The ambulatory patient should be closely observed while walking backward and forward across the examining room several times. This will disclose subtle changes in gait, such as the absence of associated movement of one arm as seen in patients with an early corticospinal or extrapyramidal tract lesion. The abnormalities of gait listed in Table 48-3 are commonly seen in patients with neurologic disease.

Station.   A great deal can be learned from observing the patient standing. The patient should be observed for abnormal posture, tremor, involuntary movements, and abnormal position of the limbs or head that may be seen in spasmodic torticollis or dystonia.

TABLE 48-3. ABNORMALITIES OF GAIT

Type	Description	Clinical Correlation
Hemiplegia	Arm does not swing, flexed at elbow and wrist, hand pronated, lower limb circumducted when walking, foot scrapes ground	Unilateral corticospinal tract lesion anywhere above C5 level
Spastic	Lower limbs affected more than upper, with increase in tone predominantly in adductor muscles, producing typical "scissor gait"	Bilateral involvement corticospinal tracts
Festinating gait	Generalized flexion of body, short shuffling steps with slowed movement (bradykinesis), no associated arm movement	Extrapyramidal disorders, particularly Parkinson's disease
Dystonic gait	Sudden flinging or writhing movements interfering with gait caused by choreoathetosis or ballism	Huntington's chorea, Wilson's disease, double athetosis, dystonia musculorum deformans, drug side effects (especially phenothiazines)
Cerebellar ataxia	Wide-based staggering gait with truncal and limb ataxia	Cerebellar disorders
Proprioceptive ataxia	Wide-based staggering gait, feet slapping the ground (locomotor ataxia of visual compensation essential)	Severe peripheral neuropathy or posterior column disease (e.g., tabes dorsalis, subacute combined degeneration, diabetic neuropathy)
Steppage gait	Bilateral foot drop, foot plantar flexes when limb elevated, limb raised excessively high to avoid foot catching on ground	Peripheral neuropathy
Apraxia of gait	Inability to initiate gait, feet stick to floor, walking begins after rapid shuffling movements	Cerebral degeneration from any cause
Waddling gait	Name describes gait, seen in patients with weakness of gluteal and iliopsoas muscles	Duchenne muscular dystrophy, polymyositis, other myopathies
Hysterical gait	Bizarre theatrical gait with body movements that can only be accomplished with an intact nervous system	Psychologic dysfunction

The generalized flexed posture of the patient with Parkinson's disease that is accompanied by the typical tremor involving the fingers of one or both hands is easily recognized.

Patients who can stand unaided are asked to place their feet together and their hands by their side, fixing their gaze on a distant object. If this posture can be maintained, the patients are then asked to close their eyes to perform the Romberg test. Any movement of the feet in order to maintain balance indicates a positive Romberg test due to lack of proprioceptive impulses passing from the lower limbs to the central nervous system or to disease involving the posterior columns of the spinal cord.

Testing Sensation

The sensations of touch, pinprick, and vibration should always be tested by comparing similar sites on the two sides of the body. Small areas of sensory loss or impairment should be carefully marked out and the affected dermatome or peripheral nerve should be identified, using a standard anatomic chart. Tests of vibration are usually carried out over the bony prominences, and, again, a comparison should be made with each side. Position sense is a well developed sensation, and the patient should be asked to indicate awareness of movement of digits with the eyes closed.

Cortical sensation should be tested only

when the examiner is certain that the primary sensations are normal. The most reliable tests of cortical sensation include:

1. Tactile localization, the ability to identify the site of stimulation, is tested by using a piece of cotton.

2. Two-point discrimination is easily performed with calipers or two pins and should be less than 0.5 cm. on the fingertips.

3. Double simultaneous stimulation is a test in which homotopic areas are stimulated simultaneously, using cotton or the fingertips. Appreciation of one stimulus may be lost when there is an early lesion involving the parietal lobe on the opposite side, a phenomenon that has been called "sensory extinction."

4. Graphism is identification of letters or numbers written on the fingertips with a sharp pencil, with comparison of correct results on the two sides.

5. Stereognosis is the ability to recognize and name simple objects placed in the hands with the eyes closed.

Testing Reflexes

A list of the commonly used tendon reflexes and their level of segmental innervation is given in Table 48–4. These reflexes should always be examined by comparing the two sides of the body, and the reflex response should be graded from 0 to 4, 0 being absent response and 4 being sustained clonus. Examination of tendon reflexes is followed by performance of the plantar reflex. This response is elicited by gently stroking the lateral aspect of the sole of the foot and extending the stimulus across the heads of the metatarsal bones. A normal response is one of flexion of the great toe (plantar flexor response). The

extensor plantar response (Babinski's sign) consists of extension of the great toe, with fanning of the other toes. The extensor plantar response is seen in patients with lesions involving the corticospinal tract.

A number of superficial reflexes are tested in the neurologic examination. These include:

1. *Abdominal reflexes*, which are elicited by stroking the skin of the abdominal wall toward the midline on the two sides above and below the umbilicus; there should be an immediate contraction of the muscles below the stimulus—the reflexes are lost in the presence of corticospinal tract lesions.

2. The *cremasteric reflex* is similar to the abdominal reflex and is elicited in the male by stroking the skin on the inside of the thigh, which produces a contraction of the cremasteric muscle with movement of the testis on the same side.

3. The *anal reflex* is elicited by stroking the skin on the buttock near the anus, which produces contraction of the sphincter. This response may be lost in patients with lesions of the sacral segments of the spinal cord.

A number of reflex responses are seen in degenerative diseases of the central nervous system. These responses are usually present in infants but disappear with maturation of the central nervous system. They include:

1. The *glabellar reflex*, which is elicited by tapping the glabella on the forehead between the orbits. Normally, this elicits blinking of the eyes, which ceases after tapping has proceeded for a short period of time. This reflex is increased and persists in patients with lesions involving the extrapyramidal system and is commonly seen in those with Parkinson's disease.

2. The *snout reflex*, which is elicited by gently tapping the skin immediately above the upper lip and below the nose. When positive, this produces a symmetrical grimacing movement of the mouth. This reflex is positive in patients with corticospinal tract lesions and those with degenerative conditions involving the frontal lobes.

3. The *sucking reflex*, which can be produced by stroking the upper lip with the finger. In degenerative conditions, the patient responds by making sucking movements of the lips.

4. The *chewing or biting reflex*, which is elicited by placing a tongue depressor in

TABLE 48–4. REFLEXES AND THEIR LEVEL OF INNERVATION

Reflex	Level
Jaw jerk	lower pons
Pectoralis major	C4–C5
Biceps	C5–C6
Brachioradialis	C5–C6
Triceps	C6–C7
Finger jerk	C7–C8
Knee jerk	C2–C3–C4
Ankle jerk	L5–S1

the mouth. In degenerative conditions involving the central nervous system, the patient chews or bites the tongue blade tightly between the teeth.

Examination of the Skull, Neck, and Spine

The neurologic examination is completed with the examination of the skull, neck, and spine. Any abnormalities in the shape of the skull should be noted, as well as in the position of the neck and spine. The position

of the ears should be noted; they are frequently seen in a low-set position in patients who have developmental abnormalities. The neck may be unduly short and the hairline low in patients who have congenital abnormalities involving the base of the skull or the cervical spine. The examiner should always listen to the major vessels in the neck for the presence of bruits, which may occur with a significant stenosis of the carotid arteries. Patients should always be tested for the presence of nuchal rigidity by flexing the head on the

TABLE 48–5. NEURODIAGNOSTIC PROCEDURES

Procedure	Indications	Contraindications
Lumbar puncture	Suspected meningitis, suspected encephalitis, brain tumor suspect, suspected subarachnoid hemorrhage, multiple sclerosis, postinfectious polyneuropathy (Guillain-Barré syndrome)	Marked increase in intracranial pressure with papilledema, infection in lumbar area
X-ray, skull and chest	Brain tumor suspect for metastatic disease or intracranial calcification	None
Electroencephalography	Epilepsy, brain tumor suspect, head trauma, any condition with altered consciousness	None
Echoencephalography	Good screening procedure in emergency room examination following head trauma; will show suspected subdural hematoma	None
Computerized tomography (CT)	Useful in confirming presence of intracranial lesions such as tumor, hematoma, hydrocephalus, cerebral atrophy	Allergy to iodine, if enhancement is used
Pneumoencephalography	Rarely performed now, superseded by CT scanning	
Myelography	Suspected spinal cord or spinal nerve root lesions; occasionally used for suspected posterior fossa lesions (clivogram)	Allergy to iodine
Arteriography	Any intracranial mass lesion; disease of extra- and intracranial blood vessels (carotid and vertebral-basilar systems)	Use arteriography as a logical sequence to other studies; check heart and kidney function first
Other studies	Radioactive cisternogram in suspected normal pressure hydrocephalus, auditory evoked potentials in suspected brain stem lesions, audiogram in suspected lesions of 8th cranial nerve, visual evoked potentials in suspected lesions of optic nerve, neuropsychologic testing in all children with seizures or behavior disorders and in all cases of dementia	
Electromyography	Suspected anterior horn cell diseases or diseases of peripheral nerves, myoneural junction, or muscle; of no value in diseases of central nervous system except when anterior horn cell involvement suspected	
Nerve conduction velocities	Peripheral neuropathy, entrapment syndromes	

neck. Early nuchal rigidity may indicate inflammation of the subarachnoid space, as seen in those with meningitis or encephalitis.

Scoliosis of the spine may indicate hereditary diseases, such as spinocerebellar degeneration or previously acquired disease affecting the spinal column. Midline tufts of hair may indicate the presence of a dermal cyst.

DIFFERENTIAL DIAGNOSIS AND MANAGEMENT OF NEUROLOGIC PROBLEMS

The material presented in this section is organized according to the following rationale:

1. The first step in diagnosis is to identify the general neuroanatomic location of the patient's problem ("where is it?").

2. The second step is to begin to identify the most likely sites and etiologic causes of the problem within the affected part of the system ("what is it?").

3. The third step is to systematically test the most likely possibilities by appropriate use of neurologic examination techniques, ancillary diagnostic studies, therapeutic trials, or a combination of these (Table 48–5).

HEADACHE

Headaches are among the most frequent types of pain experienced by man and consequently are one of the most common problems encountered in family practice. Knowledge of prodromal symptoms, onset, location, frequency, type of pain, and aggravating, alleviating, and associated factors are fundamental to a rational approach to assessment (differential diagnosis) of headache. A basic question that the physician must try to answer is: Are the headaches due to a disturbance in function (vascular tone, muscle tension, chemical factors, and so forth), or are they due to a condition involving pathologic changes in or near pain-sensitive structures of the head?

Table 48–6 lists and describes the clinical characteristics, recommended management, and caveats associated with the various forms and causes of headache under the two broad categories of disturbance of function

and pathologic abnormalities. The table is followed by supplementary information, including additional details concerning therapy.

MIGRAINE

Definition

Migraine is a condition of paroxysmal headaches accompanied by a wide range of other symptoms.

Epidemiology

Migraine is a common complaint, often occurring in families. However, the occurrence in families is probably due to no more than the chance of occurrence of any common condition, rather than to any hereditary factor. Migraine occurs in both sexes and can appear at any age, but it is unusual for the first attack of migraine to occur after 40 years of age.

Etiology

Migraine is the result of excessive vasodilatation in the craniocerebral circulation that produces local ischemia and malfunction. The vasoconstriction is followed by vasal dilatation that is associated with a release of fluid from the affected blood vessels, leading to local edema and pain. In classic migraine, the headaches are associated with marked increase in blood flow through the external carotid system, including the superficial temporal, middle meningeal, and occipital arteries. An injection of ergotamine or epinephrine reduces blood flow to these vessels and results in a prompt resolution of the headache. This suggests a close correlation between increased blood flow and headache.

It has been suggested that migraine is biochemically mediated and that one or more biochemical changes may produce the vasal constriction and vasal dilatation that are the hallmarks of this condition. It is also possible that there is a release of a pain-producing substance in the edema fluid during the stage of vasodilatation. Many biochemical abnormalities have been investigated and described, but the results of these investigations are not uniformly reproducible and must be considered inconclusive at this time.

Migraine may be associated with some known metabolic abnormalities, incuding hypoglycemia and water retention, and there is a close association between migraine headaches and an abnormal menstrual cycle in some women.

Clinical Features

Classic Migraine. Classic migraine has a well-developed aura or prodromal stage that precedes the headache. This usually consists of visual abnormalities that often occur in a homonymous field. The patient may experience flashing lights or various scotomata, including bright, jagged lines that have been called fortification spectra. In some patients, these prominent visual symptoms are accompanied by vertigo or lightheadedness, some degree of dysphasia, dyslexia, some impairment of judgment and ability to concentrate, impaired memory, and occasionally by micropsia.

The headache usually begins approximately 20 minutes after the aura. It may be unilateral or bilateral. It frequently begins as a dull ache or a painful pulsation but rapidly develops to a severe, constant pain. At that point, the patient becomes nauseated and frequently vomits. There is considerable prostration, and the patient frequently complains of photophobia and may prefer to lie quietly in a darkened room. The headache begins to subside after several hours but may last for as long as 2 or 3 days in some patients. There is often recovery after a night's sleep. Following recovery, the patient experiences a feeling of lassitude, and there may be a mild sensation of pain in the head for 2 or 3 days and some tenderness of the scalp.

Common Migraine. Symptoms of common migraine are exactly the same as those of classic migraine except that the aura is ill-defined or absent and the patient usually describes the attack as beginning with a headache. However, careful questioning may reveal a change in personality or activity for 2 or 3 days prior to the headache. Thus, a patient may complain of feeling depressed or irritable or occasionally of feeling elated with an unusual sense of well-being for 24 to 48 hours before the headache. Other patients complain of excessive drowsiness and yawning or of increased appetite with a desire for particular food. The headache is identical to the headache of classic migraine, as is the recovery phase.

Complicated Migraine. This is the most fascinating form of the disease to the neurologist, and the condition is often misdiagnosed because of the prominence of the accompanying symptoms

Complicated migraine may follow an aura or may begin without this feature. The following types have been recognized:

1. Ophthalmoplegic migraine. Migraine accompanied by paralysis of one or more of the ocular motor nerves with associated diplopia.

2. Facioplegic migraine. Migraine accompanied by temporary paralysis of one side of the face.

3. Basilar migraine, sometimes called cerebellar or vestibular migraine. Migraine accompanied by vertigo, ataxia, and signs of cerebellar dysfunction.

4. Dysphrenic migraine. Migraine accompanied by personality changes or sudden, unexplained changes in behavior.

5. Hemiplegic migraine. This type of migraine takes two forms:

    a. Familial hemiplegic migraine is a condition occurring in many family members. The hemiplegia accompanies the migraine and always resolves without neurologic complications.

    b. Nonfamilial hemiplegic migraine is a sporadic case of hemiplegic migraine. A number of patients with this disorder have developed permanent neurologic deficits following one of the attacks.

6. Sensory migraine. The patient with this form of migraine may present with numbness or paraesthesias in the perioral area or involving the hand and fingers on one side, or occasionally there may be a hemisensory loss. Recovery is usually complete.

7. Dysphasic or aphasic migraine. The migraine headache is accompanied by severe dysphasia or loss of language function, i.e., aphasia, with complete recovery after several hours.

Differential Diagnosis

Classic and common migraine do not usually present problems of differential diagnosis. The more complicated forms of

TABLE 48–6. CLASSIFICATION AND THERAPY OF HEADACHE

Type	Typical Characteristics	Usual Therapy (See Text for Dosage)	Comments
I. *Disturbances of Function:*			
Tension headache	Recurrent generalized band or pressure-like headaches. Symptoms described with wealth of embellishment. Patient does not look sick or appear to be in as much pain as described.	Taking the patient's complaint seriously, counseling, nonnarcotic analgesics, relaxation techniques, all have a role in management. Look for and treat other contributory factors.	Always be prepared to change diagnosis. This headache may mask a more serious underlying neurologic or psychiatric problem.
Common migraine	Throbbing unilateral or bilateral, recurrent or sporadic. Nausea, sometimes vomiting, photophobia. Relieved by pressure over painful area. Scalp may be tender during and after attack. Neurologic examination and other studies negative except for occasional electroencephalogram (EEG) changes.	*For all forms of migraine:* *Analgesia:* aspirin, propoxyphene, or codeine. To reduce vasodilatation: ergotamine tartrate or ergotamine tartrate with caffeine. *Sedatives:* barbiturates, etc. *Prophylaxis:* imipramine, propranolol, methysergide. (This use of imipramine and propranolol is not mentioned in the manufacturers' official directives.)	Do not use ergotamine during pregnancy or in presence of peripheral arterial disease or coronary artery disease. Use with caution in hypertensives. Be aware of complications of long-term methysergide therapy, such as retroperitoneal fibrosis, cardiopulmonary fibrosis, etc.
Classic migraine	Headache preceded by well-defined aura. This is usually visual, with dot scotomata, bright lights, fortification spectra (moving streaks of light around scotoma), photophobia, chromophobia. Family history often positive. Neurologic examination and ancillary diagnostic studies negative except for EEG changes in some patients.		
Unusual forms of migraine	This includes "complicated," ophthalmoplegic, facioplegic, dysphrenic, hemiplegic, sensory and dysphasic forms (defined in more detail in text).		
"Hypertensive" headaches	Headaches are a feature of hypertension only if it is extremely severe, i.e. hypertensive encephalopathy. Pain often worse in A.M. and associated with slowed mentation and drowsiness. Papilledema with or without retinal hemorrhages and exudates may be present. Blood pressure usually above 200/125.	Promptly lower blood pressure. Aspirin, acetaminophen, propoxyphene, codeine for pain.	
Cluster headaches (histamine headaches)	Episodic attacks occur in clusters, unilateral sudden onset, severe pain with lacrimation and nasal stuffiness.	Avoid alcohol. Prophylaxis: cyproheptadine, propranolol, imipramine. (This use of these agents is not listed in the manufacturers' official directives.)	Sphenopalatine ganglionectomy may be considered in intractable cases but relief may not be permanent.
Benign intracranial hypertension (pseudotumor cerebri)	Generalized headache with papilledema. No other abnormal neurologic signs. Often seen in the presence of obesity, menstrual irregularities, vitamin A intoxication, corticosteroid withdrawal, hypoparathyroidism (see Table 48–13 for complete list).	Treat underlying problem. Nonnarcotic analgesics for pain. Surgical shunt may be required if vision begins to deteriorate.	Midline brain tumor must be excluded. Monitor visual fields, especially size of physiologic blind spot, and peripheral field, in chronic cases.
Ocular refractory errors	Rare cause of headache, except in children who are hypermetropic. Frontal headache, usually worse after prolonged reading.	Prescription glasses.	Refer to ophthalmologist.

Table continued on opposite page

TABLE 48-6. CLASSIFICATION AND THERAPY OF HEADACHE—*Continued*

Type	Typical Characteristics	Usual Therapy (See Text for Dosage)	Comments
Miscellaneous conditions associated with headache	A number of conditions have headache as part of their symptom complex. These include posthead trauma, postlumbar puncture, severe anemia, acute infections, hangover syndrome, hypoglycemia, hypercapnia, anoxia, heat exhaustion, menopause, premenstrual syndrome, cervical arthritis.	Treatment is directed toward correction of underlying pathophysiology when possible, plus use of mild analgesics.	
II. *Headaches with Demonstrable Pathologic Abnormalities:*			
Meningitis/encephalitis—acute	Fever, severe generalized headache, often clouding of sensorium, neck stiffness, Kernig's sign positive. Cerebrospinal fluid (CSF) shows increased cells and protein. Culture usually positive in bacterial meningitis. CSF glucose usually low in bacterial infections and normal in viral encephalitis.	Antibiotics if bacterial (see treatment outline, Table 48–10).	Complications include subdural effusions in infants, brain abscess, hydrocephalus at any age, ventriculitis. Recovery usually complete.
Meningitis/encephalitis—chronic	Dull, generalized headache, personality changes, cranial nerve palsy. Subtle degree of neck stiffness. CSF protein increased, glucose markedly decreased in patients with tuberculosis. Cells increased. Positive acid-fast bacilli smear or India ink preparation for fungi helpful, but negative smear doesn't exclude diagnosis.	Tuberculosis: streptomycin, INH. Cryptococcosis: amphotericin B.	
Intracranial tumor	Unilateral headache, often without papilledema in early cases, but with abnormal neurologic signs, such as personality change or increased reflexes, loss of sensation, etc. on the opposite side. Headache worse on awakening in the morning. Signs/symptoms vary, depending on tumor size and location.	Should be recognized and neurologic consultation obtained promptly.	Usually preferable to let consultant obtain x-rays and other diagnostic studies.
Subarachnoid hemorrhage	Sudden onset, severe generalized headache, restless patient, neck stiffness, Kernig's sign positive. Diagnosis confirmed by grossly bloody CSF.	Analgesia, control blood pressure, support vital functions, correct blood clotting defects if present.	Cerebral arteriography should be done in most, if not all, cases. Convalescent phase is preferred time.
Subdural hematoma	Intermittent headache, particularly in elderly patients or alcoholics, or following head trauma at any age. Personality changes, waxing and waning level of consciousness. Focal neurologic signs usually present. Lumbar puncture shows xanthochromia in 70% of cases.	Prompt neurosurgical consultation should be obtained if diagnosis suspected.	Prompt evacuation of hematoma reduces likelihood of permanent neurologic deficit.
Hydrocephalus	Vomiting, loss of appetite, weight loss in infants and children. Bulging fontanelle in infants.	Prompt neurosurgical consultation for consideration of bypass for trapped CSF.	Prompt reduction of intraventricular pressure is essential in progressive cases.
Temporal arteritis	Unilateral pain, constant in character. Exquisite tenderness over affected temporal artery or branches. Elevated edimentation rate often present. Biopsy of tender artery with typical histology confirms diagnosis.	Treat promptly with steroids. Adult dosage methylprednisolone, 96 mg. orally, 4 times per day.	50% of patients lose vision because of involvement of ophthalmic artery.
Sinusitis	Steady pain over sinus usually accompanied by upper respiratory infection. Percussion tenderness over affected frontal or maxillary sinuses often present. Clouding of sinus air spaces on x-ray.	Nasal decongestants, antibiotics, analgesics	Infections of the frontal or sphenoidal sinuses can spread intracranially to produce phlebitis and cavernous sinus thrombosis.

migraine may present considerable difficulty in diagnosis, particuarly when episodes occur with little or no headache. However, a careful neurologic history will usually reveal that episodes are recurrent and are usually accompanied by severe migraine headache, nausea, and vomiting. The neurologic examination is normal between attacks.

Treatment

Management of a migraine attack includes:

1. Ergotamine tartrate (see manufacturer's official directive before using).
   a. Orally or sublingually, 2 to 4 mg. at onset, then 2 mg. every hour, maximum 10 mg.
   b. Rectally, 2 to 4 mg. at onset, then 2 mg. every hour, maximum 8 mg.
   c. Intramuscularly, 0.5 mg. at onset.
   d. An ergotamine-caffeine preparation (Cafergot) contains 1 mg. of ergotamine and 100 mg. of caffeine per tablet and is used in doses of two tablets every 30 minutes for no more than three doses.
2. Analgesics
   a. Aspirin, 640 to 960 mg. (10 to 15 grains) every 4 hours as needed. To this may be added:
      (1) Codeine, 32 to 64 mg. every 4 hours as needed, or
      (2) Propoxyphene, 32 to 65 mg. every 4 hours as needed.
3. Sedatives. Barbiturates such as amobarbital sodium (Amytal Sodium), phenobarbital, or newer hypnotics such as flurazepam hydrochloride (Dalmane) may be used to induce sleep, which may relieve an acute attack of migraine.

Prophylaxis includes:

1. Methysergide (Sansert). This was the first effective drug in the prophylaxis of migraine and comes in 2 mg. tablets. The initial dose is one tablet at night, increasing by one tablet every 3 to 5 days to a maximum of one tablet four times a day. Increments should be made only if the patient does not show side effects such as drowsiness or lightheadedness. Treatment should be continued for a maximum of 6 months only, in order to avoid the development of retroperitoneal, pleuropulmonary, and cardiac fibrosis.

2. Propranolol. This beta-sympathetic blocking agent is effective as a prophylactic medication in many cases of migraine. Many patients respond to small doses of 10 mg. three or four times a day. If partial control is obtained, the drug can be increased to a maximum of 120 mg. per day (this use of propranolol is not listed in the manufacturer's official directive).

3. Imipramine hydrochloride. This drug has also been reported to be effective as a prophylactic in migraine. The usual dosage is 25 mg. one to three times per day (this use of imipramine is not listed in the manufacturer's official directive).

4. Cyproheptadine. This serotonin and histamine antagonist has been reported to be effective in migraine prophylaxis in doses of 4 to 16 mg. per day.

5. Estrogen and progesterone, i.e., oral contraceptives, may provide relief for some women who have migraine headaches that occur during the menstrual cycle.

6. Diuretics are of questionable value in patients with migraine that is associated with premenstrual edema.

HYPERTENSIVE ENCEPHALOPATHY

The severe, prolonged elevation of blood pressure resulting in cerebral edema is an unusual finding in current practice. Hypertensive encephalopathy should be diagnosed only in the presence of severe hypertension and papilledema when other causes of papilledema have been eliminated. This is a medical emergency that requires immediate lowering of the blood pressure with intravenous trimethaphan or sodium nitroprusside or other rapidly acting antihypertensive drugs.

CLUSTER HEADACHES

It is possible that cluster headaches are a migraine variant, but they are distinctive and easily diagnosed by history. Patients experience severe unilateral headache of sudden onset, which often awakens them in the early hours of the morning. The severe pain is associated with nasal stuffiness and excess tearing of the eye on the same side. Attacks last for a few hours and then subside. They tend to occur in "clusters," with several attacks per week for several weeks followed by months of freedom. The neurologic examination is normal, but a Horner's syndrome may develop on the affected side after several years.

Treatment includes:

1. Avoidance of alcohol, if this seems to be a precipitating factor.

2. Use of prophylactic medication as for migraine, including imipramine, propranolol or methysergide, may help (this use of these agents is not listed in the manufacturers' official directives).

SEIZURE DISORDERS AND SYNCOPE

"Blacking out" or "passing out" are common symptoms and may be due to any one of a number of causes, ranging from epilepsy to the micturition syncope. The common and more well-defined causes are listed in Table 48–7. Epilepsy is the most complex disorder of the group and is discussed in detail.

EPILEPSY

Definition

Epilepsy may be defined as a sudden, uncontrolled, electrical discharge of neurons in the brain that may remain localized or spread to involve other parts of the entire central nervous system.

Etiology and Pathology

Epilepsy is a syndrome. There are many causes. However, the pathogenesis remains unknown in about 50 per cent of the patients.

Generalized Seizures (Grand Mal)

Definition. Seizure activity due to a generalized and simultaneous discharge of both cerebral hemispheres. Generalized seizures may be:

1. *Primary.* This type of seizure has been called centrencephalic, idiopathic, or cryptogenic and is believed to be due to seizure activity arising in a deep central site, producing simultaneous discharge of electrical activity in both hemispheres.

2. *Secondary.* These seizures may occur following any focal seizure activity. They

are not uncommon in patients with psychomotor seizures.

Clinical Features. In the primary type of generalized seizure, there is a sudden loss of consciousness without symptoms or signs of focal epileptic activity. In secondary generalized seizures, the patient may experience a partial seizure before development of a generalized seizure.

When a generalized seizure occurs, there is sudden loss of consciousness with tonic contraction of all muscles. A marked resemblance to sudden decerebration is apparent. This tonic phase rapidly gives way to symmetrical clonic movements, which may be associated with tongue-biting and bladder and bowel evacuation. The clonic movements gradually decrease in severity until the patient is left completely comatose in a flaccid state. At this point, respirations become regular, and there are bilateral extensor plantar responses. After several minutes to several hours, the patient may be roused, and confusion is apparent. The only complaint is that of severe headache. If left alone, the patient will sleep heavily for 2 or 3 hours. Recovery is associated with confusion or at least with some degree of mental dulling that may last for several days.

Differential Diagnosis. The differential diagnosis includes:

1. *Conversion reaction.* This is probably the most common condition encountered in practice that may mimic generalized seizures. However, generalized seizures are quite stereotyped. A conversion reaction can be distinguished by obtaining a careful history or by observing the bizarre movements, wild thrashing of limbs, and vocalization.

2. *Tetanus.* The painful spasms of tetanus may give rise to opisthotonos and may resemble a seizure; however, there is no loss of consciousness in this condition.

3. *Decerebrate rigidity.* This condition is commonly mistaken for a generalized seizure in an emergency room situation. The extension of the arms with rotation, associated with opisthotonos of the body, extension of the lower limbs, and plantar flexion of the feet, is characteristic of decerebrate rigidity and is not seen in generalized seizures.

Evaluation. Patients seen for the first time with generalized seizures should be immediately checked for hypoglycemia or exposure to toxic substances such as cam-

TABLE 48-7. SYNCOPE AND SEIZURES

Clinical Disorder	Clinical Manifestations	Comments
Epilepsy	Sudden loss of consciousness with tonic then clonic phase in generalized (grand mal) seizures. Psychomotor seizures are more difficult to identify and require good history. Absence (petit mal) is often over-diagnosed. Most cases of brief loss of consciousness are due to psychomotor seizures.	Subtle forms need good history from patient and observer to cover period immediately before, during, and after attack. May have normal EEG in intraictal period. Diagnosis depends on history, not EEG.
Fainting	Individual typically "feels faint" before loss of consciousness, accompanied by light-headedness, with or without tinnitus. Immediate recovery without mental confusion after event, although weakness may persist for short periods. During the attack, the pulse may be slow and blood pressure somewhat lower than usual (vasovagal reaction). In others, pulse may be rapid and weak.	May be precipitated by fright, emotional stress, acute infections, an overheated room, hunger, etc. Most episodes are transient and require no specific treatment. Anemia, hypotension, electrolyte imbalance, and endocrine dysfunction should be considered if attacks recur.
Tussive syncope	Sudden loss of consciousness in an adult immediately preceded by severe bout of coughing. Cerebrovascular disease, chronic bronchitis, and pulmonary emphysema are predisposing factors.	Symptoms produced by decreased cardiac output by mechanism similar to Valsalva maneuver.
Micturition syncope	Sudden loss of consciousness immediately after micturition with loss of muscle tone. Full, immediate recovery in supine position.	Occurs in presence of bladder outlet obstruction with straining and Valsalva maneuver, pooling of blood in abdominal vascular bed, and decreased venous return.
Carotid sinus hypersensitivity	Loss of consciousness after pressure on carotid sinus. May be from head turning or tight collar. May indicate arteriosclerotic plaques in carotid artery in older patient. Confirmed by inducing bradycardia or fall in blood pressure with light carotid sinus pressure.	May be ameliorated by ephedrine sulphate, 25 mg. three times a day; dextroamphetamine sulfate; or atropine.
Stokes-Adams attack	Sudden loss of consciousness in an older person with partial or complete heart block or paroxysmal ventricular arrhythmias.	Attacks may be fatal; therefore, appropriate and prompt cardiac therapy is essential. Permanent pacemaker often required.
Orthostatic hypotension	Loss of consciousness on standing after sitting or lying. Check blood pressure when patient supine, then standing.	May be due to antihypertensive drugs or associated with multiple sclerosis, amyotrophic lateral sclerosis, peripheral neuropathy, diabetic neuropathy, postsympathectomy primary autonomic insufficiency, or Parkinson's disease treated with levodopa or carbidopa. Sympathomimetic amines, high salt diet (5 to 10 grams Na per day), or 9-fluorohydrocortisone, 0.1 to 0.5 mg. per day, may be helpful.
Vertebral-basilar insufficiency	Loss of consciousness in a patient who has symptoms of brain stem insufficiency: dimness of vision, diplopia, dysarthria, ptosis, transient facial weakness, etc.	Control hypertension and diabetes if present. Consultation should be obtained from a neurologist/neurosurgeon in suspected cases to determine if there are correctable extracranial vascular lesions.
Breath-holding spells	Infants and children under age 4 years. Episodes of crying, sudden cessation of respiration and loss of consciousness with either pallor or cyanosis. May make a few clonic movements.	Do NOT diagnose or treat as epilepsy. Assessment of family dynamics and conditions under which attacks occur is of primary importance. Small doses of atropine may be helpful in pallid form.
Conversion reaction (hysteria)	Dramatic, theatrical event with loss of consciousness often preceded by bizarre behavior. Individual may respond verbally to voice even though "unconscious." Neurologic examination normal during episode. Careful history and observation will reveal characteristics of hysterical personality.	Assessment of the psychologic function of the attacks and helping the patient to develop a healthier response to stress should be attempted. Psychiatric consultation may be necessary with difficult cases.

phor. The electroencephalogram shows generalized slowing following seizure activity with gradual restoration of EEG activity to the normal preictal recording over a period of several days.

TONIC SEIZURES. Very occasionally, the generalized seizures stop with the tonic phase without a subsequent clonic phase. This is a rare event seen in infants and children.

CLONIC TYPE OF GENERALIZED SEIZURES. This type of generalized seizures is also more common in infants and children and is characterized by generalized clonic movements from the onset of the seizure. It is the usual manifestation of febrile convulsions in children. The EEG shows bifrontal spike wave activity recorded during the seizure. The interictal record is normal in children with febrile convulsions.

Petit Mal (Absence)

Definition. A seizure disorder characterized by brief lapses of consciousness and associated with 3 cycles per second generalized spike wave activity in the electroencephalogram.

Clinical Features. Petit mal is a condition seen only in children and does not occur before the age of 3 years or after maturity. The attacks tend to disappear as the child grows older, and there is a change in pattern to other seizure disorders in about 50 per cent of the patients.

Petit mal is characterized by an episode during which the child suddenly stops whatever action he is performing. The child stares, and occasionally it may be possible to see 3 cycles per second eye blinking or eye movement. The attack terminates within a few seconds, and the previous activity is resumed. The condition is very sensitive to the effects of hyperventilation, and attacks may be induced by having the child hyperventilate in the office.

Differential Diagnosis. The majority of children who have a brief loss of consciousness associated with seizure activity have psychomotor epilepsy, which should be differentiated from absence (petit mal). The characteristic electroencephalogram and accentuation by hyperventilation are diagnostic of petit mal.

Treatment. See Table 48–8.

Myoclonic Seizures

Definition. Seizures characterized by very brief myoclonic movements that may produce falling, followed by immediate recovery.

Clinical Features. These seizures occur in children. They are more common in the morning and characteristically occur after the child awakens, either during dressing or during breakfast. A brief, shocklike myoclonic movement affects the whole of the body but is often seen more prominently in the limbs. Objects may be flung from the hands, or the shock may be sufficient to throw the child to the floor. There is a brief loss of consciousness and no recollection of falling. Recovery is almost immediate.

The electroencephalogram frequently shows paroxysmal spike wave activity of very brief duration occurring symmetrically over both hemispheres. This activity is not always present, however.

Treatment. See Table 48–8.

Psychomotor Seizures (Temporal Lobe Epilepsy)

Definition. A complex form of epileptic activity that may be associated with clouding or loss of consciousness. The attack is associated with sensory or motor components, or both, of varying complexity.

Clinical Features. Psychomotor seizures can occur at any age and are not uncommon in children but are frequently mistaken for absence (petit mal). In fact, psychomotor seizures are the most common form of brief lapses of consciousness caused by epilepsy in children. Seizures consist of some clouding of consciousness and are very often associated with a sense of hallucination of the olfactory, visual, auditory, or alimentary type. Complex motor movements, including walking, fumbling with objects, rearranging objects, and fumbling with clothing, may be seen. These seizures have the potential to become generalized at any time, and psychomotor seizures with generalized seizures are not uncommon.

Differential Diagnosis. These seizures should be differentiated from petit mal in children, as the treatment is totally different. There may be some difficulty in differentiating psychomotor seizures from migraine or transient ischemic attacks in adults.

TABLE 48–8. DRUG THERAPY OF CONVULSIVE DISORDERS

Drug	Therapeutic Serum Level	Dose	Seizure Type	Side Effects	Preparations
Phenytoin (Dilantin)	20–25 μg./ml.	Adults: begin 200 mg. q. 12 h. and adjust to achieve therapeutic levels; children: 5 mg./kg./day, and adjust to therapeutic serum levels	1. All generalized convulsive seizures 2. Psychomotor seizures 3. All partial (focal) seizures	Gastrointestinal upset, hirsutism, megaloblastic anemia, skin rash, gingival hyperplasia, ataxia, drowsiness	Capsules, 100 mg.; tablets, 50 mg.; oral suspension, 125 mg./5 ml. and 30 mg./5 ml.
Phenobarbital	15–20 μg./ml.	Adults: 30 mg. q. 8. h., adjust to achieve therapeutic serum levels; children: 2–3 mg./kg./day, adjust to therapeutic serum levels	1. All generalized seizures 2. Psychomotor seizures 3. All partial (focal) seizures 4. May be useful in some children with absence (petit mal)	Drowsiness, nystagmus, ataxia, morbilliform rash, megaloblastic anemia	Tablets, 15 mg., 30 mg., 60 mg.
Primidone (Mysoline)	5–10 μg./ml.	Adults: begin 125 mg. at night, increase by 125 mg. every 3 days in divided doses to achieve therapeutic serum levels; children: under 8 yrs., start at half adult dose	1. Psychomotor seizures	Drowsiness, ataxia, nausea, skin rash, anemia	Tablets, 50 mg., 250 mg.; suspension 250 mg./5 ml.
Carbamazepine (Tegretol)	(Not established), probably 8–10 μg./ml.	Adults: begin 200 mg., h.s., increase to between 800–1200 mg./24 hrs.	1. Psychomotor seizures	Drowsiness, ataxia, skin rash, anemia, thrombocytopenia, hepatocellular damage	Tablets, 200 mg.
Ethosuximide (Zarontin)	50–100 μg./ml.	Adults: 250 mg. q. 12 h., increasing to seizure control or therapeutic serum levels; children: 250 mg. initially, increase by 250 mg. at weekly intervals	1. Absence (petit mal)	Nausea, vomiting, anorexia, skin rash, anemia, leukopenia	Capsules, 250 mg.; suspension, 250 mg./5 ml.
Diazepam (Valium)		Use in status epilepticus—adults: 5–10 mg. IV, repeat at 10–15 min. intervals to maximum of 30 mg.; children: under 5 yrs., 0.2–0.5 mg. q. 15 min. to maximum of 5 mg.; over 5 yrs., 1 mg. q. 5 min. to maximum of 10 mg.			

Evaluation. The electroencephalogram may show focal spike or sharp wave activity in one or both temporal lobes. This activity may be accentuated by drowsiness and light sleep.

Treatment. See Table 48–8.

Narcolepsy

Definition. A condition in which there are frequent episodes of irresistible desire to sleep.

Clinical Features. Narcolepsy can occur in either sex and usually affects young adults who experience "attacks" in which there is an overwhelming desire to sleep. Periods of sleep last a few minutes, and the person awakens refreshed until the next attack.

Narcolepsy may be accompanied by:

1. Cataplexy—sudden attacks of loss of muscle tone that are precipitated by emotion, such as fright, joy, amusement, or anger.

2. Hypnagogic hallucinations—auditory or visual hallucinations occurring just as the person is falling asleep.

3. Sleep paralysis—brief periods of inability to move the limbs immediately preceding sleep or on awakening.

Treatment. Methylphenidate (Ritalin) is effective in controlling narcolepsy. Cataplexy responds to imipramine, 50 to 75 mg. daily (this use of imipramine is not listed in the manufacturer's official directive).

Epilepsia Partialis Continua

Partial (focal) epileptic discharges that are confined to one area of the brain may occasionally occur over prolonged periods of time. The seizure discharges produce focal neurologic abnormalities such as clonic movements affecting the thumb, hand, arm, one side of the face, or foot. This may cease at any time, spread slowly (jacksonian seizure), or occur in explosive fashion, resulting in a secondarily generalized seizure. Epilepsia partialis continua is a seizure discharge, indicating focal irritation of neurones in the brain. This disorder is usually seen after trauma and anoxia or in the presence of infarction or tumor. The condition warrants full investigation and treatment. It is, however, not an emergency and does not require immediate intravenous therapy, as outlined under status epilepticus.

Status Epilepticus

Status epilepticus may be defined as a condition in which there are repeated generalized seizures without recovery of consciousness between episodes. Status epilepticus is a medical emergency, and patients should be treated promptly and adequately in order to control seizures as soon as possible. The repeated seizures are associated with episodic cerebral anoxia, and this may produce cerebral edema in some patients. In addition, the metabolic demands of intense seizure activity lead to dehydration and electrolyte imbalance that may compound the cerebral dysfunction.

Treatment. Therapy is as follows:

1. Establish the airway and keep the airway clear.

2. Correct any fluid or electrolyte imbalance.

3. Drug therapy—adults:
   a. Diazepam (Valium), 10 mg. intravenously, administered *slowly*. Repeat in 15 minutes if seizures continue. Can repeat at 15 minute intervals as long as seizures continue and *airway is secure*. Maximum dose is 30 mg.
   b. Amobarbital sodium (Amytal Sodium), 250 mg. intravenously at rate of 50 mg. every 30 seconds. May repeat after 30 minutes if *airway is secure.*
   c. Phenobarbital, 300 mg. intravenously, at the rate of 50 mg. every 30 seconds.
   d. Phenytoin sodium injection (Dilantin), 1000 mg. intravenously (if patient has not had phenytoin previously). Do not exceed 50 mg. per minute (see manufacturer's official directive).

4. Drug therapy—children:
   a. Diazepam (Valium), 0.3 mg. per kg. (not exceeding 10 mg.) intravenously, administered *slowly.*
   b. At the same time give phenobarbital, 5 mg. per kg. (not exceeding 300 mg.) intramuscularly.

5. Once the seizure activity is under control, investigate the patient for the cause

of the status epilepticus and treat accordingly.

DIZZINESS AND VERTIGO

One of the symptoms frequently encountered in office practice is that of "dizziness." Dizziness is an ambiguous word without precise medical meaning. It is the physician's responsibility to know how to question and examine the patient in a manner that will efficiently determine:

1. If the patient is experiencing a light-headed feeling or an unsteadiness of gait (ataxia) or has a definite sensation of rotation (true vertigo).

2. Whether ear symptoms (tinnitus, diminished hearing) are present and, if so, are they unilateral or bilateral?

3. If objective abnormalities such as nystagmus, ataxia, hearing loss, or other neurologic signs are present.

4. Whether special investigations such as audiometry, skull x-rays, electronystagmograph (ENG), and so forth are indicated.

Table 48–9 is a listing of causes of dizziness and some of the differentiating features.

CONDITIONS WITH DIFFUSE CENTRAL NERVOUS SYSTEM EFFECTS

There are a group of conditions that do not have a predictable localized effect or that are not easily classified or discussed on a neuroanatomic basis. In many instances, the nervous system is only one of several systems that are affected.

Diffuse Cerebral Sclerosis (Leukodystrophies)

There are a group of demyelinating (leukodystrophic) diseases of probable genetic origin that occur sporadically. Several eponyms familiar to neurologists are attached to specific syndromes within this group (Schilder, Krabbe, Greenfield, and so forth). Clinically, these disorders may produce spastic paralysis, peripheral neuropathy, progressive failure of vision, and mental deterioration. They are due to genetically determined biochemical defects in the metabolism of myelin.

The age of onset may be in infancy, childhood, or early adult life. Neurologic consultation should be obtained for patients suspected of having this condition to confirm the diagnosis. There is no definitive treatment.

Wilson's Disease

This condition is associated with an abnormality in copper metabolism. Patients with Wilson's disease show an increased absorption of copper, failure of conversion of copper to ceruloplasmin, and elevation of serum copper levels but decrease in total serum copper because of decreased ceruloplasmin levels and increased excretion of copper in the urine. The pathologic changes in this condition are caused by the deposition of copper in the liver cells; brain, particularly in the basal ganglia; and kidneys.

In long-standing or terminal cases of Wilson's disease, the brain is atrophic, and there is a generalized increase in copper content. However, the copper tends to be concentrated in the area of the globus pallidus and putamen. There is diffuse neuronal degeneration and increased gliosis.

Clinical Features. Wilson's disease usually appears in children and young adults, but the onset has been delayed as late as the fourth decade. In the dystonic form of the disease, the patient develops generalized rigidity, bradykinesis, dysarthria, and a picture somewhat resembling parkinsonism. In the choreoathetotic form of the disease, the patient develops dystonic movements affecting the limbs, trunk, and face. Facial grimacing produces a characteristic but changing open-mouthed appearance. Dystonic movements produce a dancing-like quality of gait. Very occasionally, Wilson's disease presents in a hepatic form, in which the neurologic manifestations are minor.

Patients with neurologic manifestations of Wilson's disease show progressive dementia, often followed by the development of epileptic seizures and progressive weakness, leading to a bedridden state and death in 4 to 5 years without treatment.

Examination shows the presence of Kayser-Fleischer rings, which are brownish, red, or brownish-green rings at the corneoscleral junction. This finding is

TABLE 48–9. CAUSES OF DIZZINESS AND VERTIGO

Disorder	Clinical Manifestations
A. *Nonvertiginous Dizziness* (i.e., lightheadedness):	A sensation of giddiness or "lightheadedness" without a definite rotatory component. Nystagmus and other objective signs of involvement of the labyrinthine apparatus and its central connections are absent.
1. *Decreased cerebral perfusion:* Transient hypotension with normal heart	Symptoms most pronounced in erect position, relieved by lying down. Associated with transient vasomotor instability induced by drugs, especially antihypertensives; emotional stress; acute infections; dehydration; hyponatremia, etc.
Narrowing of cerebral arteries	Focal neurologic symptoms or signs in the distribution of the affected portion of the brain may be present. A bruit may be heard over an affected extracranial artery. If the vestibular apparatus is involved, true vertigo and nystagmus may be present.
Cardiac dysfunction	Associated with persistent or intermittent cardiac arrhythmia, atrioventricular (A-V) block, carotid sinus hypersensitivity, myocardial infarction, valvular disease (especially aortic and subaortic stenosis).
2. *Changes in arterial blood gas concentration:* Hyperventilation	Hypocapnia typically occurs in anxious young adults who hyperventilate in response to emotional stress.
Hypoxia	Transient hypoxic episodes from any cause may induce a sensation of lightheadedness.
3. Drugs	A wide variety of drugs may induce lightheadedness. Review of medications and adjustments to test this hypothesis should be done in suspected cases.
B. *True Vertigo:*	
1. *With ear symptoms:* Acoustic neurilemona and other cerebellopontine angle (CPA) tumors	Asymmetric hearing loss, tinnitus, facial weakness, depressed corneal reflex, ataxia, asymmetric deep tendon reflexes. Signs and symptoms may be episodic at first. Obtain audiogram, tomograms of petrous ridge, electronystagmograph (ENG), and auditory evoked potentials.
Meniere's syndrome	Episodic and more common over age 40. Classic triad is tinnitus, vertigo, and deafness, although the latter may be absent. Pure tone audiometry and ENG should be obtained to demonstrate unilateral lesion. Petrous ridge tomograms should be done to exclude CPA tumor in chronic or progressive cases.
2. *Without ear symptoms:* Labyrinthine disease	Vertigo increased by turning the head in the direction of the quick phase of nystagmus. Caloric stimulation by cold water ear irrigation on the affected side produces increased nystagmus with irritative lesions and reduced or no response with destructive lesions. Acute labyrinthitis may be associated with nausea and vomiting.
Benign positional vertigo	Vertigo induced by turning in bed or other positional change. Thought to be due to degeneration of nerve endings in semicircular canals.
Cervical injury or disease	May produce vertigo and nystagmus caused by interference with proprioceptive impulses or by concussion to brain stem damaging the sensitive vestibular nuclei.
Drugs	Antihistamines, sedatives, tranquilizers, antihypertensives, and other drugs can produce vertigo in some patients.
Migraine	Changes in vascular perfusion of the brain stem in association with migraine attacks may induce vertigo.
Menopause	May be associated with hot flashes. Thought to be due to changes in microcirculation of the inner ear.

pathognomonic of Wilson's disease and is due to the deposition of copper in Descemet's membrane.

Evaluation. Diagnostic studies reveal the following:

1. Examination of the blood shows elevated free serum copper levels and reduced ceruloplasmin levels.

2. There is increased excretion of copper in the urine.

3. Kayser-Fleischer rings are often difficult to see or cannot be seen with the naked eye but can be readily confirmed by slit lamp examination.

4. Liver function tests show the presence of impairment of liver function and cirrhosis

Treatment. Management of the patient is as follows:

1. Dietary copper should be restricted, and intestinal copper absorption can be decreased by the use of potassium sulfide, 40 mg., given with each meal.

2. Copper can be removed by the use of chelating agents. The oral preparation penicillamine is probably the most effective agent, given in doses of 1 to 4 grams per day in divided doses.

Acute Bacterial Meningitis

Despite the widespread use of antibiotics, acute bacterial meningitis remains a serious illness with a high mortality under certain circumstances. There are many bacteria that can cause acute meningitis. The most common infections are listed in Table 48–10. It should be noted that with age there is distinct change in the bacterial type causing the meningitis.

Etiology and Pathology. Acute bacterial meningitis is the result of contamination of the subarachnoid space with bacteria. The infection may gain direct entry following compound fractures of the skull, particularly if these involve the petrous temporal bone or the paranasal sinuses. Infection may also spread from chronically infected sinuses or mastoidal cells into the subarachnoid space. Bacterial meningitis is frequently due to contamination of the subarachnoid space during septicemia, associated with a remote focus of infection. The infection may be direct or may result from the intermediate development of an extradural, subdural, or brain abscess.

The cerebrospinal fluid provides an ideal culture medium for bacteria that are rapidly disseminated throughout the subarachnoid space. There is an acute inflammatory response that also involves the bridging blood vessels, many of which will thrombose, producing small areas of infarction in the superficial layers of the brain and spinal cord. Bacterial meningitis, then, should be regarded as an acute meningoencephalitis.

Clinical Features

Infants. It is not unusual for bacterial meningitis to occur in infants with few localizing signs. There may be a history of premature delivery or of prolonged labor with a traumatic delivery. The infant is usually seriously ill, is febrile and dehydrated, and has convulsions, neck stiffness, and a bulging fontanelle.

Children and Adults. Bacterial meningitis may present as a fulminating infection with rapid onset of fever, headache, neck stiffness, clouding of consciousness, and seizures. In other patients, the onset is somewhat slower, with a prodromal period of fever and headache followed by the gradual development of nuchal rigidity and clouding of consciousness. Occasionally, the patient may present with fever followed by the rapid development of a shocklike state associated with hypotension. Under these circumstances, the meningitis is part of an overwhelming septicemia.

Examination of children and adults with meningitis shows the presence of clouding of consciousness and coma in some patients. Cranial nerve involvement is not unusual. There may be asymmetry of reflexes, and in some patients frank hemiparesis may be present. Both Kernig's and Brudzinski's signs are positive. A petechial rash is not unusual in meningococcal and *Hemophilus influenzae* infections.

Evaluation. When evaluating a patient with acute bacterial meningitis, the physician should:

1. Look for a focus of infection in the middle ear, mastoidal cells, or paranasal sinuses. An x-ray of the chest may detect a pneumonic process or lung abscess.

2. Lumbar puncture should be performed as soon as bacterial meningitis is suspected. The fluid is under increased pressure and is often cloudy or purulent. The cell count varies, but the white cells are overwhelmingly polymorphonuclear in type. The glucose content is markedly reduced. Staining of a centrifuged specimen with Gram's stain will reveal intracellular or extracellular

TABLE 48–10. BACTERIAL MENINGITIS

Type	Age Group Incidence (Infant, Child, Adolescent, Adult)	Treatment	Complications
Escherichia coli	Infant, child	Gentamicin—adults: 4 mg./kg./day IM divided doses q. 8 h., 5 mg. intrathecally° daily for 7 days, alternate days for 10 days; children: 5 mg./kg./day IM, 2 mg. intrathecally°	Subdural effusion, ventriculitis, seizures, hyperthermia, septicemia and shock, disseminated intravascular coagulation (DIC), cerebral edema
Hemophilus influenzae	Child, adolescent	Ampicillin and chloramphenicol—adults: ampicillin, 1 gram IV bolus, 1 gram q. 3 h. IM; children: 200 mg./kg./day q. 3 h. Chloramphenicol, 50 mg./kg./day given q. 6 h.†	Cerebral edema, septicemia and shock seizures, DIC, hyperthermia
Neisseria meningitidis	Adolescent, adult	Penicillin G—adults: 1 million units bolus IV, 2 million units q. 2 h. constant IV; children: 1 million units bolus IV, 500,000 units q. 2 h. constant IV drip	Septicemia and shock, DIC, cerebral edema, seizures, hyperthermia
Streptococcus pneumoniae	Adult	Same as for *N. meningitidis*	Septicemia and shock; severe fever; infection, particularly pneumonia; DIC; cerebral edema; hyperthermia
Unknown		Ampicillin and gentamicin	

°The intrathecal use of gentamicin is not mentioned in the manufacturer's official directive.
†When culture results are available, continue with ampicillin, if sensitive. If not sensitive to ampicillin, continue chloramphenicol and stop ampicillin.
Note: Rare meningitis—staphylococcal meningitis: use methicillin. *Pseudomonas* meningitis: use gentamicin.

organisms in many cases. All fluid should be cultured for organisms in many cases. All fluid should be cultured for organisms.

3. Since septicemia is a common concomitant of acute bacterial meningitis, serial blood specimens should be taken for culture.

Treatment. The antibiotic treatment is outlined in Table 48–10. Patients with acute bacterial meningitis are seriously ill and need expert nursing care. Fluid and electrolyte balance should be maintained. Stuporous or comatose patients should have indwelling bladder catheters. Patients should be turned frequently in bed. Secretions should be suctioned and drainage assisted. Artificial respiration should be administered to those who develop depression of respiratory function. If shock occurs, it should be corrected by adequate fluid replacement and the use of pressor agents. Disseminated intravascular coagulation should be suspected in patients who develop hypotension with bleeding from one or more sites.

Cerebral edema is not an unusual complication of acute meningitis and may be treated with dexamethasone, 12 mg. intravenously, followed by 6 mg. every 12 hours.

Complications. Infants and children who appear to respond to the antibiotic medication but continue to show depression of the level of consciousness should be investigated for the possibility of ventriculitis or subdural effusion. Serial electroencephalograms are useful in adults when marked focal slowing may indicate the presence of a cerebral abscess. Hydrocephalus is a late complication of acute meningitis and should be suspected in patients who appear to improve and then deteriorate. Diagnosis may be confirmed by computerized tomography (CT) scan, followed by radioactive cisternography. There is good response to ventriculoatrial or ventriculoperitoneal shunting.

Brucellosis

Brucellosis may also cause a chronic meningoencephalitis and should be consid-

ered in all cases of chronic meningitis or
chronic myelitis.

Protozoal Infections

Toxoplasma is a ubiquitous organism that
infects most of the population asymptomatically. Transplacental infection of the fetus
may result in death prematurely or in
encephalitis followed by brain damage and
mental retardation.

Localized toxoplasmosis may produce
pulmonary lesions, myocarditis, myositis,
and chorioretinitis in adults. It is occasionally complicated by meningoencephalitis or
the development of a granuloma in the
brain.

Treatment. Sulfadiazine and pyrimethamine are effective in the treatment of toxoplasmosis.

Tuberculous Meningitis

This formerly fatal disease is encountered
occasionally in Canada and the United
States but is seen more frequently in other
areas of the world, occurring particularly in
infants and children.

Tuberculous meningitis may occur during
any stage of tuberculosis. It is, however,
more common in primary tuberculosis and
is believed to be due to the entry of
tubercular bacilli into the subarachnoid
space through the choroid plexus. Other
causes, such as extension from an extradural
abscess or rupture of a tuberculoma, are
rare.

Clinical Features. The disease begins insidiously with headache, fever, and neck
stiffness. Infants and children often become
listless, lose appetite, and lose weight.
Patients may show bulging of the anterior
fontanelle. Meningeal irritation produces
neck stiffness in both children and adults.
There is early involvement of the cranial
nerves, particularly of the oculomotor system, with production of diplopia. The development of hydrocephalus leads to increasing headache and clouding of
consciousness.

Evaluation. The cerebrospinal fluid is
usually under increased pressure. It is often
clear, but when left standing, a small fibrin
coagulum may be seen in the bottom of the
test tube. There is a moderate lymphocytic
pleocytosis, the protein is elevated, and the
glucose content is markedly reduced.
Staining of the fibrin coagulum or of a
centrifuged specimen with Ziehl-Neelsen
stain may reveal the presence of *Mycobacterium tuberculosis* organisms. All cerebrospinal fluid specimens should be cultured when tuberculosis is suspected.

Treatment Therapy includes the following:

1. A combination of streptomycin and
isoniazid (INH) is still the most widely
used treatment. Streptomycin sulfate
should be given in doses of 20 to 30 mg. per
kg. per day by intramuscular injection to
infants and children. This dosage should be
changed to two or three times per week
after 2 weeks and should be continued for
approximately 2 years. In adults, streptomycin is given in doses of 1 gram daily by
intramuscular injection. INH should be
given in doses of 3 to 5 mg. per kg. daily to
infants and children and 400 mg. daily to
adults.

2. A number of other drugs have been
used in the treatment of tuberculous meningitis. These include para-amino-salicylic
acid, ethambutol, and ethionamide (see
manufacturers' directives before using ethambutol or ethionamide in children). Generally speaking, these should be reserved
for patients who show resistance or toxic
reaction to streptomycin.

3. Treatment should be continued in all
patients until the spinal fluid is free of
cellular response, glucose content is normal, and cultures are negative. When treatment is discontinued, usually after 2 years,
repeated lumbar punctures should be done
at 3 month intervals for the first year and at 6
month intervals for the next 2 years to detect
relapsing disease.

Diabetes Mellitus

The neurologic complications of diabetes
mellitus are frequently encountered in
family practice.

Coma occurs in both ketotic and nonketotic diabetic states associated with marked
elevation of blood glucose levels. Cerebrovascular disease is accelerated in the
diabetic, who is more prone to strokes,
spinal cord infarction, and heart disease,
particularly when the diabetes is associated
with hypertension. Diabetics may develop
isolated mononeuropathies or a symmetrical peripheral neuropathy. The latter may
lead to severe disability in a small number
of patients, with the development of lower
limb weakness, ataxia, bladder paralysis,

and Charcot's joints (so-called diabetic pseudotabes).

Hypoglycemia

Cerebral metabolism is almost entirely dependent on adequate levels of glucose and oxygen, and glucose depletion is followed by the prompt appearance of neurologic symptoms. Mild hypoglycemia produces reversible symptoms, but severe hypoglycemia may lead to neuronal degeneration or to the development of laminar infarcts in the cortical grey matter.

Symptoms include:
1. Confusion, sweating, and syncope.
2. Seizures. All new patients with epileptic seizures, whether children or adults, should be screened for hypoglycemia.
3. Cerebellar degeneration in patients with chronic intermittent hypoglycemia.
4. Coma, with either full recovery or variable permanent neurologic deficits, including dementia.

Treatment. The treatment of hypoglycemia depends upon identification of the cause. The high protein diet given to a patient with functional or alimentary hypoglycemia would be detrimental to a patient who has leucine-sensitive hypoglycemia.

Alcohol and the Nervous System

The neurologic complications of alcohol are, with the exception of acute intoxication, primarily the result of a chronic nutritional deficiency in the long-time alcoholic.

Acute Intoxication. Although acute intoxication is a common and reversible condition, it should not be regarded as invariably innocuous. Respiratory arrest and death have occurred during periods of acute alcoholic intoxication, particularly if the condition has been complicated by drug ingestion (barbiturates are especially lethal). Patients with severe alcoholic intoxication may require respiratory assistance as a life-saving measure.

Alcoholic Dementia. Considerable controversy has been raised about the occurrence of dementia in the chronic alcoholic. There is now no doubt that it can occur, and computerized tomography scanning has demonstrated ventricular dilatation in chronic alcoholics. The condition can be arrested by complete abstinence from alcohol.

Delirium Tremens. This is an acute psychosis that follows acute withdrawal after a bout of heavy drinking. It is often precipitated by infection or may follow an epileptic seizure. Treatment should be directed toward:
1. Maintaining fluid and electrolyte balance.
2. Providing adequate sedation, using a phenothiazine or chlordiazepoxide (Librium) or diazepam (Valium).
3. Controlling any concurrent infection with antibiotics.
4. Supplementing thiamine hydrochloride, 200 mg. intravenously or intramuscularly daily.

Wernicke's Encephalopathy. This condition is the classic example of acute thiamine deficiency. It is seen in the chronic alcoholic who has had a continuously poor diet. Wernicke's encephalopathy presents with the acute onset of strabismus, diplopia, and cerebellar ataxia. This may be followed by changes in mentation, often presenting as Korsakoff's psychosis. The latter is characterized by loss of both retention and recent memory and may be permanent, despite prompt treatment of the Wernicke's encephalopathy. Peripheral neuropathy is often demonstrable when the patient is able to cooperate.

TREATMENT. There is a dramatic resolution of the strabismus and ataxia following parenteral administration of 100 mg. of thiamine twice daily. Prompt treatment is essential, as the syndrome can be fatal.

Alcoholic Seizures. There are three causes of epilepsy in alcoholics:
1. Alcohol withdrawal in a chronic alcoholic associated with lowering of serum magnesium levels.
2. Precipitation of seizures in an epileptic who abuses alcohol.
3. Repeated head injury in the chronic alcoholic.

Alcoholic Hallucinations. The chronic alcoholic may experience severe auditory or visual hallucinations as the only symptom.

Pathologic Intoxication. An uncontrolled rage reaction may occur in some chronic alcoholics after taking relatively small amounts of alcohol.

Alcoholic Cerebellar Degeneration. This is a specific form of cerebellar degeneration that occurs in alcoholics, characterized by specific and severe degeneration of the anterior lobe of the cerebellum. This produces a severe lower limb ataxia with minor involvement of the upper limbs and absence of nystagmus. Recovery is possible after the first attack if the patient completely abstains from alcohol.

Alcoholic Myelopathy. Spastic paraplegia with ataxia caused by spinal column degeneration is a rare complication of alcoholism.

Hyperthyroidism

The clinical features of systemic hyperthyroidism are discussed elsewhere. Neurologic complications or concomitants of hyperthyroidism include optic neuritis thyroid myopathy, myasthenia gravis, and hypokalemic periodic paralysis.

Hypothyroidism

Classic myxedema is associated with headache and mental dullness. Hypothermia and coma may occur in patients with severe myxedema. The cerebellar degeneration of hypothyroidism shows an excellent response to replacement therapy with thyroid hormone. Other complications of hypothyroidism include myopathy, peripheral neuropathy, delayed relaxation of deep tendon reflexes, and the carpal tunnel syndrome.

Hyperparathyroidism

Neurologic symptoms are not infrequent in hyperparathyroidism. Patients experience chronic headache, and frank psychosis can occur if serum calcium levels are greater than 16 mg. per 100 ml.

TABLE 48–11.   CLINICAL MANIFESTATIONS OF ELECTROLYTE IMBALANCE

Sign or Symptom	Electrolyte Disturbance
Drowsiness, lethargy, stupor, coma	Hypo- or hypernatremia, acidosis, alkalosis, hypercalcemia
Muscular weakness	Hypo- or hyperkalemia, hyponatremia, hypercalcemia
Neuromuscular hyperirritability	Hypocalcemia, hypomagnesemia

Hypoparathyroidism

The lowered serum calcium levels that occur in hypoparathyroidism result in tetany, seizures, and increased intracranial pressure with papilledema. X-ray studies of the skull often show calcification of the basal ganglia, a somewhat paradoxical finding in the presence of chronic low serum calcium levels.

Electrolyte Imbalance

Extreme variations in electrolyte balance can lead to aberrations in function of nerve and muscle cells. The neuromuscular system ordinarily tolerates moderate deviations from normal quite well. The obvious reason for neuromuscular dysfunction is the key role that sodium, potassium, pH, calcium, and magnesium play in membrane threshold excitability and recovery of resting potential. The clinical manifestations are listed in Table 48–11.

Management should be directed toward

TABLE 48–12.   HEAVY METAL POISONING

Metal	Clinical Features	Diagnostic Findings	Treatment
Lead	Children: encephalopathy; adults: anemia, peripheral neuropathy, colic	CBC—anemic basophilic stippling; urine and stool—lead content elevated; coproporphyrin III in urine; lead line on bone x-ray	Reduce cerebral edema in encephalopathy; use chelating agent EDTA to remove lead
Arsenic	Dermatitis, anemia, peripheral neuropathy	Arsenic level in urine elevated; nerve conduction velocities prolonged	Dimercaprol, BAL
Mercury (organic compounds)	Encephalopathy, cerebellar degeneration, peripheral neuropathy	Presence of mercury in urine and hair	Eliminate source
Thallium	Encephalopathy, peripheral neuropathy, alopecia	Thallium in urine	Eliminate source
Manganese	Emotional lability, hallucinations, paranoia, parkinsonism	Elevated blood and urine levels of manganese	Eliminate source; levodopa for parkinsonism

correcting the specific aberrations present and searching for the underlying cause.

Heavy Metal Poisoning

The clinical features, diagnosis, and treatment of specific types of heavy metal poisoning are listed in Table 48–12.

Decompression Sickness (Caisson Disease)

Sudden decompression from increased pressure to normal pressure (lower) or from normal to decreased atmospheric pressure (aviation) can lead to the development of nitrogen bubbles in the blood or tissues. This may be followed by multiple cerebral infarctions or spinal cord infarction. Affected persons often develop paraplegia caused by spinal cord involvement, but seizures, altered consciousness, or hemiparesis may indicate cerebral involvement.

Treatment consists of rapid recompression followed by slow decompression to normal atmospheric pressure.

Multiple Sclerosis

Definition. Multiple sclerosis is (1) a condition in which there is loss of myelin with relative preservation of axons and (2) a disease due to destruction of the cytoplasmic process of the oligodendrocyte.

The myelin sheath is formed by the cytoplasm of the oligodendrocyte in the central nervous system and by the Schwann cell in the peripheral nervous system. The axon is surrounded by concentric layers of the cytoplasm, as though it were "wrapped" in insulating material. In multiple sclerosis, the oligodendrocyte is involved, but the Schwann cell is spared. Multiple sclerosis is a disease strictly confined to the central nervous system.

Etiology. There are two current hypotheses:

1. Multiple sclerosis is an autoimmune disease in which the body produces antibodies against myelin. This occurs periodically in response to some unidentified stimulus and produces the periodic scattered demyelination seen in multiple sclerosis.

2. Multiple sclerosis is a viral disease in which the virus, which is believed to belong to the papovavirus group, combines with the protein of the membrane of the oligodendroglial cell, resulting in alteration of cell metabolism, cell damage, or death.

It should be noted that these two hypotheses are not exclusive. A virus could produce focal damage to oligodendroglial cells in the central nervous system in conjunction with the liberation of an antigen that stimulates the production of antibodies locally, thus leading to the characteristic demyelination seen in this disease.

Pathology. Areas of demyelination, so-called "plaques," are scattered throughout the central nervous system. Demyelination tends to be concentrated in certain areas of the brain and spinal cord, particularly in the periventricular areas of the cerebral hemispheres and the periaqueductal area of the brain stem. The typical lesions show loss of myelin centrally, with degeneration of myelin at the periphery. There is relative preservation of axons. With the passage of time, gliosis occurs, and distortion and fragmentation of axons are later features of this disease.

Clinical Features. Attacks can occur almost anywhere in the central nervous system, and, therefore, the clinical features of this disease are of infinite variation. Many cases begin with optic neuritis, characterized by blurring of vision rapidly leading to loss of central vision and even complete blindness on one side. There is associated pain on movement of the eye, and examination shows papilledema if the plaque is near the surface of the optic disc. This may be the only symptom of multiple sclerosis in many patients, and resolution of the optic neuritis may be followed by a latent period extending from several weeks to several years before the periods of further symptoms. Onset characterized by motor weakness, sensory loss, or ataxia is not uncommon. Bladder involvement with urgency is also an early symptom in many patients.

It is possible to recognize three types of multiple sclerosis:

1. The relapsing, remitting form. This is a common form of the disease in which the patient has an attack of multiple sclerosis with some degree of recovery, leaving residual neurologic deficits. The patient does not show any further evidence of the disease for a period varying from several weeks to several years, at which time a second attack occurs. This second attack produces a further increase in neurologic

deficit. Relapses then recur at irregular intervals, each with some further neurologic damage. These patients become restricted in their activities after the second or third attack.

2. The benign group. These patients also show a relapsing and remitting course, but the recovery is good following each attack with little residual neurologic damage. Such patients continue to lead almost normal and productive lives and are never disabled by the disease.

3. The chronic, progressive form. This form, in which the patient appears to regress steadily following the onset of the disease, is the most pernicious. There are never good signs of remission, and there is a steady increment of neurologic deficit.

It is important to recognize the benign form of multiple sclerosis, and it is possible to do so if one follows the patient for many years. If a patient is able to ambulate independently and is fully employed 10 years after the diagnosis of multiple sclerosis, this patient can be considered to have the benign form of the disease.

Differential Diagnosis. The differential diagnosis includes:

1. Postinfectious leukoencephalopathy. This condition may be indistinguishable from multiple sclerosis because of patchy involvement of the central nervous system. It may be suspected if the onset of the condition occurred 2 to 3 weeks after inoculation or following a documented viral infection. However, the diagnosis of multiple sclerosis will be established if there is a second episode occurring weeks or months after the first episode, as postinfectious leukoencephalopathy does not recur.

2. Spinocerebellar degenerations. These conditions are multisystem diseases and therefore might be considered a form of multiple sclerosis, particularly if there is an absence of family history.

3. Brain or spinal cord tumor. When the first episode of multiple sclerosis produces predominantly unilateral cerebral or spinal cord involvement, the question of tumor must be considered.

4. Vasculitis. The artery diseases associated with collagen diseases such as systemic lupus erythematosus and polyarteritis nodosa causing patchy infarction of the central nervous system may resemble multiple sclerosis.

Evaluation. There is no specific test for multiple sclerosis at this time. Evaluation should include:

1. Visual fields testing should be performed to detect and document scotomata. Serial testing may reveal evidence of remission or exacerbation of the disease.

2. Lumbar puncture should be done. The cerebrospinal fluid is clear and of normal pressure. There may be a slight pleocytosis of mononuclear cells with normal glucose and slightly elevated protein content. The gamma globulin content is elevated in 80 per cent of the patients and exceeds 40 per cent of total protein content.

3. Appropriate studies should be carried out if a brain or spinal cord tumor is suspected.

4. Cystometrogram should be performed in patients with bladder involvement.

5. Neuropsychologic testing is useful, in that these tests give an actual score for purposes of comparison in suspected relapses.

6. Electroencephalography (EEG) may show impairment of background activity and focal slowing during acute exacerbations. Serial EEG's may be of value in assessing progress.

Treatment. To treat patients during the acute phase or an exacerbation:

1. Place the patient on bed rest during exacerbation.

2. Treat any associated respiratory or urinary tract infection promptly.

3. Give methylprednisolone, 128 mg. in a single dose on alternate days in the morning, gradually reducing the dose as improvement occurs.

4. As soon as improvement begins, place the patient in a physical therapy program.

5. Refer the patient to a vocational rehabilitation facility for job retraining in an attempt to keep the patient employable, whenever this is appropriate.

Sarcoidosis

Sarcoidosis may produce:

1. Polymononeuropathy.

2. Meningeal involvement with hydrocephalus.

3. Involvement of the optic chiasma and pituitary, with optic atrophy and pituitary insufficiency.

4. Granulomatous infiltration of cerebral blood vessels, producing cerebral infarction.

The diagnosis is usually established by lymph node biopsy or biopsy of a large nerve in patients with mononeuropathy.

Treatment. The condition usually shows some response to long-term corticosteroids, which should be given on an alternate day basis to minimize side effects. Pituitary insufficiency and diabetes insipidus can be treated with replacement therapy. Hydrocephalus should be treated by ventriculoatrial shunting procedures.

DISORDERS OF HIGHER BRAIN FUNCTION (CONSCIOUSNESS, COGNITION, MOTOR AND SENSORY CONTROL)

There are a number of pathologic or pathophysiologic processes of widely differing causes that produce acute or chronic abnormalities of higher brain function, i.e., cognition (mentation), and reduction or interruption of functions controlled by the various lobes of the cerebrum.

Anoxic Encephalopathy

This condition is becoming a greater problem in medical practice because of the increasing efficiency in the resuscitation of patients who have suffered from respiratory or cardiac arrest. As brain metabolism is almost entirely dependent upon adequate oxygen and glucose, brain damage can occur within a short period of oxygen deprivation from any cause.

Etiology. Anoxia may be caused by:

1. Obstruction of the airway from any cause.

2. Impairment of function of respiratory muscles from any cause.

3. Depression of the brain stem respiratory center.

4. Impairment of pulmonary function and absorption of oxygen from the lungs.

5. Anesthesia.

6. Exposure to low pressures of oxygen, such as high altitudes.

7. Cardiac arrest.

8. Blood loss.

9. Carbon monoxide poisoning.

Pathology. The pathologic changes in the brain depend upon the time of survival following the anoxic episode. If there is immediate death, the brain is congested. If death occurs in several hours, the brain becomes edematous, and there may be scattered necrotic changes, particularly in the area of the basal ganglia. Necrotic neurones are replaced by astroglial cells, and later changes include widespread gliosis and in some cases quite prominent demyelination.

Clinical Features. There may be:

1. Complete recovery.

2. Neurologic deficits that may improve over a period of several months or years.

3. A period of apparent recovery after the anoxic episode that is followed by the development of neurologic deficits after several weeks.

The neurologic deficits of anoxic encephalopathy may indicate involvement of any portion of the cerebral hemispheres, basal ganglia, brain stem, or cerebellum.

Differential Diagnosis. Hypoglycemia produces an almost identical clinical picture.

Evaluation. The following procedures should be carried out:

1. The airway is secured, and the patient is placed on oxygen as soon as possible.

2. Blood samples should be obtained for carboxyhemoglobin and serum barbiturate levels.

3. Serum electrolyte and arterial blood gas determinations should be obtained at frequent intervals, particularly if respiratory assistance is needed.

4. X-rays of the chest should be obtained to rule out pulmonary causes for the anoxic episode.

5. An electrocardiogram and serum enzyme levels should be obtained to rule out the possibility of cardiac arrest and myocardial infarction.

6. Serial electroencephalograms should be obtained, as these are of great value in assessing progress toward recovery in patients who survive.

Treatment. The patient should be admitted to an intensive care unit. Respiratory assistance should be given if necessary, and associated conditions such as myocardial infarction should be treated promptly. Transfusion may be required for patients suffering from carbon monoxide poisoning or from barbiturate intoxication.

Benign Intracranial Hypertension (Pseudotumor Cerebri)

Definition. A condition of high elevation of cerebrospinal fluid pressure appearing in children or adults.

TABLE 48-13. CAUSES OF BENIGN INTRACRANIAL HYPERTENSION

Infants and Children
1. Vitamin A deficiency or excess
2. Tetracycline therapy
3. Withdrawal of corticosteroids
4. Dural sinus thrombosis (so-called otitic hydrocephalus)

Adolescent and Young Adult Women
1. Onset at menarche
2. Obesity and menstrual irregularities
3. Pregnancy

Adults and Children
1. Hypoparathyroidism
2. Addison's disease
3. Vitamin A excess
4. Carbon dioxide retention

Etiology and Pathology. The causes are listed in Table 48-13. There does not seem to be any common causative factor. The occurrence in adolescents and adults suggests that there may be some unidentified hormonal imbalance in this group. In other patients, some evidence suggests that there is interference in absorption of cerebrospinal fluid into the dural sinuses.

Clinical Features. Infants present with irritability, lack of appetite, vomiting, and bulging fontanelles. Children and adults show changes in personality associated with headache, nausea, and vomiting.

Examination shows the presence of papilledema without other neurologic deficits except for the occasional presence of sixth nerve paresis.

Evaluation. The presence of a midline tumor must be excluded in all patients by adequate evaluation. (See evaluation of brain tumors.)

Treatment. Therapy includes:
1. Omission of all offending substances.
2. A short course of corticosteroids may be of benefit in adults suffering from this condition.
3. Adults failing to improve, in whom there is progressive visual failure, should have a ventriculoatrial shunt procedure to relieve intracranial pressure.

Hepatic Encephalopathy

Hepatic encephalopathy may be seen in patients with both acute and chronic liver failure. The cause is not clear, but it appears to be related to abnormalities in ammonia metabolism. However, it is clear that other factors, including deficiencies in carbohydrate metabolism and the tricarboxylic acid cycle, may be involved.

Clinical Features. Acute hepatic encephalopathy usually occurs in patients with severe liver damage who have gastrointestinal bleeding. This is followed by some impairment in the level of consciousness, often with somnolence, in which the patient's level of consciousness waxes and wanes. When aroused, the patient is disoriented and may hallucinate. Examination shows an irregular alternating extension and flexion of the hands when the arms are outstretched, the so-called flapping tremor or asterixis. These movements are often associated with some degree of choreoathetosis.

Evaluation. A number of metabolic abnormalities may be present, including elevated blood ammonia levels, hyponatremia, hypokalemia, elevated serum bilirubin levels, and alterations in blood pH. The electroencephalogram shows progressive and generalized slowing in both hemispheres with bilaterally synchronous triphasic waves that appear bifrontally.

Treatment. Therapy includes:
1. Correction of dehydration and electrolyte imbalance.
2. Exchange transfusion.
3. Levodopa, 3 to 5 grams daily, may produce dramatic improvement in some patients.

Cerebrovascular Disease

Cerebral Arteriosclerosis. Cerebral circulation is almost entirely dependent upon blood supplied through the carotid and vertebral arterial systems. There is an efficient collateral circulation between the two systems at the base of the brain through the circle of Willis, which permits compensation for vascular insufficiency in one of the systems. However, in practice, it is possible to accurately distinguish between symptoms of carotid artery insufficiency and vertebral basilar insufficiency.

CAROTID (MIDDLE CEREBRAL) ARTERIAL INSUFFICIENCY. Transient ischemic attacks (TIA) involving the carotid or middle cerebral artery produce episodic hemiparesis and hemisensory loss on the side opposite the ischemic hemisphere. Transient homonymous hemianopia may occur in some patients, and associated dysphasia, dyslexia, and dyscalculia occur when the dominant hemisphere is involved. In carotid artery insufficiency, there may be blindness in the eye on the same side because of an associated insufficiency of the circulation of the ophthalmic artery (amaurosis fugax).

VERTEBRAL BASILAR INSUFFICIENCY. Insufficiency is dependent upon the ·ischemic effect involving the occipital lobe or brain stem, or both. Patients might present with episodic dimness of vision or transient blindness when the occipital lobes are involved. Brain stem involvement produces diplopia, ptosis, facial weakness, tinnitus, vertigo, ataxia, dysphagia, dysarthria, nausea, and vomiting, singly or in any combination. There is occasional bilateral involvement of the medullary pyramids that results in sudden loss of tone and collapse, with or without loss of consciousness (drop attacks).

Prognosis of Transient Ischemic Attacks (TIA). Transient ischemic attacks indicate that the patient is in a high risk category for the development of a stroke. Twenty-five per cent of patients with transient ischemic attacks develop a stroke within the first year following the initial attack, with the majority developing cerebral infarction within the first month. The risk of cerebral infarction is high in patients with carotid artery insufficiency. Long-term follow-up has shown that about 33 per cent of patients with transient ischemic attacks develop cerebral infarction, while 33 per cent cease to have attacks, presumably because of the development of adequate collateral circulation. The remaining 33 per cent of patients continue to have attacks and, therefore, remain in a high risk category for a stroke.

Predisposition to Cerebral Arteriosclerosis and TIA. Factors that may contribute to the acceleration of cerebral arteriosclerosis and factors that may precipitate a stroke in patients with cerebral arteriosclerosis are listed in Table 48–14. All patients with transient ischemic attacks should be inves-

TABLE 48–14. MECHANISMS OF TRANSIENT ISCHEMIC ATTACKS

Mechanism	Investigations	Therapy
Stenosis in carotid and/or basilar-vertebral arteries	Listen for bruit; perform four vessel cerebral angiography	Surgical repair if lesion is accessible
Emboli from atherosclerotic plaques	Look for increased serum uric acid, cholesterol, triglyceride and beta-lipoprotein, and blood glucose levels	Lower uric acid and lipids by diet and appropriate drug therapy; aspirin, dipyridamole,° sulfin-pyrazone (Anturane) may reduce platelet aggregation; consider anticoagulants
Transient hypotensive episodes	Monitor blood pressure hourly for several hours; check blood pressure in supine and erect positions	Adjust antihypertensive drugs if being used; ephedrine sulfate, 25 mg. 3 times a day, if chronically hypotensive
Hypertension	Monitor blood pressure carefully	Reduce blood pressure gradually to normal or near normal levels; alpha-methyldopa is especially useful
Temporary compression of neck vessels	Determine whether specific head positions or brief compression of carotid produces symptoms; perform four vessel angiography with neck manipulation	Have patient wear loose collar; limit neck movement with special collar if necessary; consider surgery if stenotic lesion present
Transient reduction in cardiac output secondary to arrhythmia or heart block	ECG, frequent monitoring of heart rate and rhythm; consider 24 hour cardiac monitoring	Therapy directed toward correcting cardiac dysfunction
Small vessel occlusion in the brain, producing microinfarcts	May be difficult to confirm; angiography usually reveals plaques in larger vessels	Control of other factors such as hypertension, diabetes, hyperlipidemia, etc.; drugs that decrease platelet aggregation or anticoagulants may be tried
Transient hypoglycemia	Five hour glucose tolerance test; blood glucose during attack; consider pancreatic tumor	If diabetic, adjust medication; high protein, low carbohydrate diet, frequent feedings; insulin-producing tumors should be removed if possible

°This use of dipyridamole is not listed in the manufacturer's official directive.

tigated for the presence of any of these factors, as many of them are treatable, and treatment will immediately reduce the risk in the affected individual.

Investigation of a Patient with Transient Ischemic Attacks. Investigative procedures and therapy are outlined in Table 48–14. Any associated medical condition should be treated. It is particularly important to treat hypertension and to emphasize to the patient that treatment will be indefinite. This means that patients will have to be followed closely, as many will abandon treatment once attacks of ischemia cease. Patients with significant extracranial stenotic lesions should have vascular surgery, and, again, patients should be as healthy as possible at the time of the procedure, and every effort should be made to identify and treat those conditions associated with arteriosclerosis before the patient comes to surgery.

Cerebral Infarction

Thromboembolism of the Middle Cerebral Artery. Cerebral infarction in the distribution of the middle cerebral artery that is caused by thrombosis or embolism is usually of sudden onset and in many cases occurs during sleep. The patient develops a contralateral hemiparesis or hemiplegia and a sensory loss and homonymous hemianopia in most instances. Involvement of the dominant hemisphere produces dysphasia and, when the lesions are extensive, dyslexia, dysgraphia, dyscalculia, and right-left confusion. The combination of dyscalculia, right-left confusion, finger agnosia, and dysgraphia is well recognized as Gerstmann's syndrome. In lesions involving the nondominant hemisphere, it is not uncommon to find denial of symptoms (anosognosia) or denial and nonrecognition of an affected limb (autotopagnosia).

Brain Stem Infarction. Infarction of the brain stem is usually due to occlusion of the vertebral artery, posterior inferior cerebellar artery, or basilar artery. Occlusion of the vertebral artery or posterior inferior cerebellar artery produces the lateral medullary syndrome in which the onset is sudden with intense vertigo and vomiting and in which the patient presents with Horner's syndrome, loss of sensation over the face on the side of the lesion, nystagmus and ataxia maximal on the side of the lesion, dysarthria due to involvement of the dorsal pharyngeal

vagal complex, and a contralateral hypalgesia to pinprick involving the trunk and extremities.

Basilar artery occlusion carries a high mortality and is associated with disturbance of consciousness, coma in many instances, bilateral signs of brain stem involvement, and bilateral corticospinal tract involvement with quadriparesis or quadriplegia.

Patients with posterior cerebral artery occlusion are occasionally encountered. They may present with a sudden onset of contralateral homonymous hemianopia, or the so-called sensory stroke, in which there is little motor involvement but quite dense sensory loss on the opposite side of the body due to infarction involving the posterolateral ventral nucleus of the thalamus.

Diagnostic Procedures in Cerebral Infarction. Patients should be evaluated as outlined in the section on transient ischemic attacks.

Treatment. Therapy is as follows:

1. Correct electrolyte and fluid imbalance.

2. Maintain airway with frequent suctioning if necessary.

3. Reduce cerebral edema, using dexamethasone, 6 mg. every 12 hours, for 10 days.

4. Correct hypertension and treat any associated cardiac abnormalities.

5. Correct any metabolic abnormalities present.

6. Treat any associated infection; pneumonia is not uncommon.

7. Begin physical therapy on the first day with passive movements of the affected limbs.

8. Ambulate the patient as soon as possible.

9. Consider arteriography to demonstrate extracranial stenotic lesions when the patient is in a stable condition; this is usually in 2 weeks after the onset of the stroke.

10. Treat the patient on a long-term basis, as outlined under transient ischemic attacks.

Cerebral Hemorrhage

This condition is usually due to massive bleeding into the deeper structures of a cerebral hemisphere and carries a high mortality. Pontine hemorrhage and cerebellar hemorrhage are not uncommon.

Cerebral hemorrhage occurs against a

background of chronic hypertension, which produces accelerated arteriosclerotic changes in the penetrating vessels arising from the middle cerebral artery. Some of these vessels develop small aneurysms (Charcot-Bouchard aneurysms). These aneurysms rupture, and because the rupture occurs in the high pressure system, there is pouring of blood into the area of the internal capsule, thalamus, and basal ganglia. The pathologic background is similar in pontine and cerebellar hemorrhages.

In cerebral hemorrhage, the onset is sudden and is characterized by the development of severe headache, followed by clouding of consciousness, progressing rapidly to coma. There is contralateral hemiplegia and a rapid rise in intracranial pressure, producing brain stem compression and death in a high percentage of patients. The lumbar puncture shows the presence of a bloody spinal fluid in 80 per cent of the patients because the hemorrhage ruptures into the ventricular system.

In pontine hemorrhage, the onset is acute, with rapid progression to coma. The pupils are pinpoint, and there is quadriplegia.

In cerebellar hemorrhage, the onset is acute, and coma may develop in a short period of time. In some patients, however, consciousness is maintained, and there are signs of cerebellar ataxia predominantly occurring on one side, It is important to recognize this group of patients, as surgical treatment with evacuation of the clot produces good results.

The treatment of cerebral hemorrhage and pontine hemorrhage is largely supportive. Hypertension should be controlled, fluid electrolyte balance maintained, and cerebral edema reduced with the use of dexamethasone.

Subarachnoid Hemorrhage

The most common cause of subarachnoid hemorrhage is cerebral trauma. The most common cause of nontraumatic subarachnoid hemorrhage is rupture of a berry aneurysm. These aneurysms may occur in the majority of vessels in the circle of Willis or at the origin at the first branches of the major vessels arising from the circle of Willis.

Rupture of a berry aneurysm produces bleeding into the subarachnoid space and into the substance of the brain. The type of

symptoms is related to the relative severity of bleeding in these areas.

The onset is sudden and is associated with the development of severe headache. When the bleeding is predominantly in the subarachnoid space, the patient may retain consciousness and appear extremely restless and distressed, with severe headache and nuchal rigidity. On the other hand, when there is destruction of the brain parenchyma, the patient may show stupor, semicoma, or coma with focal neurologic deficits.

The development of coma in patients with subarachnoid hemorrhage indicates a poor prognosis and carries a high mortality.

There is still some difference of opinion regarding the surgical treatment of subarachnoid hemorrhage caused by ruptured berry aneurysms. However, the majority of neurosurgeons favor the performance of arteriography after about 7 days of medical treatment. Total surgery within the first few days carries a higher mortality than does interval surgery after a week. There is, of course, a considerable risk of a second subarachnoid hemorrhage occurring during the period of waiting, but the best results seem to be obtained when surgery is performed after the 7 day delay.

Patients with subarachnoid hemorrhage who are in the good risk category, that is, those who have few abnormal neurologic findings, should be treated with adequate analgesics to relieve the headache. This frequently requires intramuscular injections of meperidine, 100 to 150 mg., or equivalent amounts of morphine. The patient should be kept absolutely quiet at complete bed rest. Fluid electrolytes should be strictly maintained, and added sedation with the use of phenobarbital or chlorpromazine is helpful.

Subarachnoid Hemorrhage Due to Arteriovenous Aneurysms and Other Causes. Subarachnoid hemorrhage following the rupture of an arteriovenous aneurysm carries a better prognosis than does the rupture of a berry aneurysm, as an arteriovenous aneurysm tends to be in a low pressure system, and the rupture does not produce the devastating damage seen with rupture of a berry aneurysm. Nevertheless, patients with subarachnoid hemorrhage from the rupture of an arteriovenous aneurysm should be treated in a manner similar to those suffering rupture of a berry aneurysm. Some arteriovenous aneurysms can be excised surgically as an interval procedure.

There are a number of other rare causes of subarachnoid hemorrhage, including rupture of arteriosclerotic vessels or vessels affected with arteritis. Subarachnoid hemorrhage caused by bleeding from a tumor is rare but is occasionally seen in patients with hemangioblastomas of the cerebellum.

Cerebral Arteritis

Arteritis of the cerebral vessels is uncommon. Changes in cerebral vessels can occur in infectious conditions such as syphilis, tuberculosis, or brucellosis and in autoimmune conditions such as polyarteritis nodosa, systemic lupus erythematosus, and temporal arteritis. The symptoms are usually those of patchy infarction of the brain or spinal cord, and seizures are not uncommon. Most cerebral arteritides are treatable with steroids and other drugs, once correct identification has been made.

HEAD TRAUMA

There is a high risk of head injury in modern society because of the widespread use of the automobile. In addition, head injury is not unusual in industry and in contact sports.

Skull Fracture

It should be realized that severe intracranial damage can occur in the absence of skull fracture. Skull fracture may occur at the site of impact or in some cases may be remote. Examples of the latter are fractures of the cribriform plate that occur following a blow to the occipital area. Fractures of the skull may be as follows:

1. Incidental findings without neurologic deficit.
2. Associated with contusion or laceration of the brain immediately beneath the fracture site.
3. Linear fractures may produce laceration of meningeal blood vessels, resulting in extradural hemorrhage.
4. Fractures at the base of the skull may produce laceration of the internal carotid artery with subsequent development of aneurysm.
5. Fracture of the skull may be associated with acute subdural hematoma.

6. Fractures at the base of the skull may be associated with tearing or evulsion of cranial nerves.
7. Fractures involving the cribriform plate or temporal bone may be associated with cerebrospinal fluid rhinorrhea.
8. Fractures of the cribriform plate or temporal bone or fractures into the paranasal sinuses carry a risk of intracranial infection.

Treatment. The treatment is directed toward the underlying intracranial damage. When there is risk of intracranial infection, the patient should be placed on prophylactic antibiotics. All patients with new skull fractures seen in the emergency room should be kept under observation for at least 24 hours to detect any delayed intracranial complications of the fracture.

Concussion

Definition. Concussion may be defined as a completely reversible neurologic deficit that occurs following head injury.

Etiology and Pathology. Concussion follows a blow to the head that sets up a pressure wave passing through the intracranial contents. The pressure wave can only resolve by passing through the foramen magnum, and, in doing so, its effect is felt at the level of the brain stem. The passage of the pressure wave through the brain stem produces a cessation of activity in the neurones of the reticular activating system and loss of consciousness. This neuronal dysfunction resolves in a short period of time.

Clinical Features. There is sudden loss of consciousness subsequent to a blow to the head, followed by return of consciousness and amnesia for the traumatic event.

Evaluation. All patients who have had a head injury followed by loss of consciousness should have a skull x-ray. Further studies will depend upon the development of abnormal neurologic findings.

Treatment. The patient should be placed under observation for a period of 24 hours following the head injury, and vital signs should be recorded every 15 minutes.

Head Injury with Damage to the Intracranial Contents

Although extensive damage may occur to the cerebral hemispheres without loss of consciousness (e.g., to the frontal lobe of the brain), long periods of unconsciousness following head trauma are usually associated with severe contusion or laceration of the brain.

Clinical Features. There is immediate loss of consciousness and prolonged coma following the head injury. Examination of the patient may show signs of injury to the face or orbits, laceration of the scalp, bleeding from the nose or ears, or an obvious depressed skull fracture. If the patient is in shock, additional injuries to internal viscera should be considered.

The patient may be categorized as being in:

1. Coma. Patient shows lack of response to painful stimuli.

2. Semicoma. Patient makes affirmative withdrawal movements as a response to painful stimuli.

3. Stupor. Patient is restless and can be stimulated sufficiently to respond to simple commands.

4. Obtundity. Patient is restless and may show delirium. Response to the examiner is immediate, but replies to questions are inappropriate.

When the patient is comatose, an assessment should be made for signs of brain stem involvement.

Evaluation. X-rays of the skull and cervical spine should be performed as soon as possible after the patient has been examined in the emergency room and an adequate airway has been established. The frequent association of cervical spine fractures with head injuries requires the combined study of the skull and cervical spine in all patients.

Echoencephalography is a useful technique that should be available in all emergency rooms. If there is a shift in the midline of more than 2 mm., the possibility of an epidural or subdural hematoma should be considered.

Arteriography should be performed as an emergency procedure in all patients in whom there are neurologic signs that indicate a focal deficit following head injury or in whom the echoencephalogram is abnormal.

Serial electroencephalograms should be obtained on all patients who are being followed after head injury that is associated with prolonged periods of stupor or coma. These records are useful in assessing the progress of the patient. Deterioration in the EEG should lead to the consideration of a complication such as subdural hematoma.

Treatment. Patients should be treated as follows:

1. Establish an adequate airway.

2. Comatose and stuporous patients should be turned in bed every 2 hours to improve pulmonary exchange and to drain the dependent parts of the lung.

3. Airways should be suctioned frequently to remove accumulating secretions.

4. Serum electrolyte balance should be maintained initially by the use of intravenous fluids. In more prolonged instances of coma, use nasogastric feeding after the first few days.

5. The bladder should be catheterized with a Foley catheter, using aseptic technique.

6. Cerebral edema can be treated by intramuscular injections of dexamethasone, beginning with 12 mg. and followed by 6 mg. every 12 hours.

7. Prophylactic antibiotics should be given when there are demonstrable skull fractures entering the paranasal sinuses and nasal cavity or the middle ear.

8. Restlessness during recovery may be controlled by the use of phenothiazine drugs.

Epidural Hematoma

Definition. An accumulation of blood between the inner table of the skull and the dura.

Etiology. This condition usually occurs following head injury causing a linear fracture of the skull that severs the middle meningeal vessels. Occasionally, the complication of tearing of blood vessels at other sites occurs.

Pathology. There is tearing of the middle meningeal vessels or occasionally of the vessels at other sites, such as the superior sagittal sinus, as they traverse the linear fracture site. This produces bleeding into the epidural space with pressure on the brain that might accumulate in this space.

Clinical Features. The classic situation is that of head injury followed by immediate loss of consciousness due to concussion, recovery of consciousness, and a second period of drowsiness, stupor, and coma. This situation occurs only in about 33 per cent of patients who have an epidural hematoma. The majority of patients have an initial loss of consciousness that is not followed by return of consciousness, but there is increasing evidence of intracranial pressure as the hematoma accumulates.

Evaluation. Diagnostic studies will reveal the following:

1. X-rays of the skull may disclose a linear fracture, usually in the temporoparietal area, crossing the course of the middle meningeal vessels.

2. Echoencephalography shows displacement of midline structures.

3. A computerized tomography (CT) scan may reveal a laterally situated mass before the presence of the mass can be confirmed by arteriography, if this is necessary.

Treatment. Surgical exploration, drainage of the hematoma, and sealing of all bleeding points should be performed as soon as possible.

Acute Subdural Hematoma

Definition. The acute accumulation of blood in the subdural space following head injury.

Etiology. Differences in acceleration or deceleration of intracranial contents in the bony vault following head injury result in tearing of bridging veins. There is an accumulation of blood in the subdural space.

Pathology. In most cases of acute subdural hematoma, the accumulation of blood in the subdural space is associated with severe contusion or laceration of the underlying brain. The brain damage is, in fact, the major concomitant of acute subdural hematoma.

Clinical Features. In most patients, there has been a severe head injury with immediate loss of consciousness. This is followed by progressive deterioration, ranging through stupor to coma. Signs of brain stem compression caused by uncal herniation are an indication for immediate treatment.

Evaluation. Findings include:

1. X-ray of the skull may reveal a fracture or displacement of the calcified pineal.

2. Echoencephalography will demonstrate a shift of the midline structures unless there are bilateral subdural hematomas.

3. Computerized tomography will reveal a mass between the surface of the brain and the inner table of the skull.

4. The presence of a mass lesion can be confirmed by arteriography.

Treatment. Acute subdural hematoma should be treated as a surgical emergency and drained as soon as possible.

Chronic Subdural Hematoma

Definition. The slow accumulation of fluid in the subdural space usually following head injury.

Etiology. Chronic subdural hematomas usually follow minor head injury; however, they may occur spontaneously following the use of anticoagulants in patients with blood dyscrasias and following pneumoencephalography.

Pathology. The rupture of bridging veins leads to the accumulation of blood in the subdural space. Initial clotting is followed by hemolysis, and the fluid attracts cerebrospinal fluid by osmosis through the arachnoid membranes. As the subdural hematoma increases in size, there is tearing of small vessels at the periphery of the hematoma. This produces fresh bleeding into the subdural space and further osmotic attraction of the fluid into the space. In time, there is proliferation of fibroblasts in the dura and arachnoid, which gradually forms a "membrane" around the subdural hematoma.

Clinical Features. It is not always possible to obtain a history of head injury, which may have been relatively minor in the elderly or debilitated patient. The condition is also frequent in alcoholic patients, who have no recollection of their multiple head injuries. Patients usually exhibit alteration in personality with clouding of consciousness that may wax and wane. Focal neurologic signs occur according to the site of the hematoma. Eventually, there will be signs of brain stem compression and deepening of the level of coma, followed by death.

Differential Diagnosis. Subdural hematoma may be indistinguishable from subdural hygroma caused by tearing of the arachnoid following head injury and the accumulation of cerebrospinal fluid in the subarachnoid space.

Evaluation. Diagnostic procedures are as follows:

1. X-ray of the skull may show a calcified pineal gland.

2. Cerebrospinal fluid is characteristically xanthochromic in about 80 per cent of patients with subdural hematoma.

The electroencephalogram shows decreased voltage on the side of the subdural hematoma with focal slowing of activity in the theta and delta range on that side.

4. Echoencephalography may demonstrate a shift of the midline structures.

5. The CT scan demonstrates a biconvex area between the brain and the midtable of the skull.

6. The presence of the hematoma may be demonstrated by arteriography.

Treatment. In some patients, the subdural hematoma may be drained through burr holes. In others, it can only be removed through a bone flap because of the membranes around the hematoma.

Cerebral and Intracerebellar Hematoma

Definition. The presence of a hematoma within the parenchyma of the brain.

Etiology and Pathology. Tearing of blood vessels within the substance of the cerebral hemispheres or cerebellum may result in accumulation of blood and the formation of a hematoma.

Clinical Features. It may be possible to demonstrate focal neurologic signs in those patients who are not comatose following head injury. Thus, the patient with a hematoma in the cerebral hemisphere might show a contralateral hemiparesis on painful stimulation. A patient with a cerebellar hematoma may show progressive signs of pressure on the brain stem and unilateral-bilateral signs of cerebellar dysfunction on examination.

Evaluation. As for chronic subdural hematoma.

Treatment. The hematoma is evacuated either through burr holes or following the creation of a bone flap by a neurosurgeon.

The Dementias

There are a number of neurologic conditions in which dementia is the primary and most prominent symptom. The diagnosis in many cases is described in such meaningless terms as "presenile dementia," "senile dementia," or "chronic brain syndrome," which not only illustrates lack of knowledge but implies lack of treatment and often lack of interest. Many dementias are *treatable*; therefore, correct diagnosis is mandatory in good medical practice.

Etiology and Pathology. The cause is unknown in many, but not all, of the dementias. It is probable that Jakob-Creutzfeldt

disease is a neuronal degeneration caused by a slow viral infection, indicating the possibility of viral involvement in other neuronal degenerations. Normal pressure hydrocephalus is caused by an alteration in cerebrospinal fluid dynamics, and if this disorder is diagnosed, it is possible to obtain a most gratifying response to treatment.

Clinical Features. The essential symptom is dementia, which usually begins with a loss of operational judgment.

Evaluation. All patients with dementia should be evaluated for a treatable cause. If the evaluation covers the conditions listed in Table 48–15, the diagnosis is likely to be established in the great majority of patients.

Diagnostic studies include:

1. A complete history from the patient and family.

2. Neurologic examination. Spend time on mentation.

3. Neuropsychologic examination. Provides an accurate assessment of the patient's current status and is a reference for determination of later deterioration.

4. X-rays of skull and chest. Look for a shift of a calcified pineal or occasionally for a calcification in a tumor or a subdural hematoma.

5. Lumbar puncture. Pleocytosis suggests infarction; lowered glucose content suggests infection; elevated protein content suggests tumor; perform serologic test for syphilis.

6. Electroencephalography. Focal slowing is seen with focal lesions, such as tumor or subdural hematoma. Electroencephalography is useful as a serial indicator of deterioration, demonstrated by progressive slowing in serial EEG's.

7. Computerized tomography (CT) scan. The scan not only discloses the majority of focal lesions but also indicates the shape and size of ventricles and the presence or absence of cortical atrophy.

8. Arteriography. This study indicates the localization of tumors, the presence of arteritis, and the presence of treatable stenotic lesions in multi-infarct dementia.

9. Radioactive cysternography. This should be performed in all patients with generalized ventricular dilatation to exclude normal pressure hydrocephalus, i.e., delayed absorption of cerebrospinal fluid (CSF).

10. Complete blood count and measurement of serum folic acid. These studies are

TABLE 48–15. DEMENTIAS

	Alzheimer's Disease	Normal Pressure Hydrocephalus	Multi-Infarct Dementia
Etiology	Unknown	Intermittent increase in ventricular pressure	Arteriosclerosis
Pathology	Loss of neurones, neurofibrillary tangles in surviving neurones, excess senile plaques	Ventricular dilatation	Multiple scattered infarcts in both hemispheres and brain stem
Clinical Features	Slowly progressive dementia	Slowly progressive dementia, early incontinence, early spasticity of lower limbs	Stuttering, progressive focal neurologic abnormalities; hypertension, arteriosclerotic heart disease
Evaluation			
Spinal fluid	Normal	Normal	Normal
Chest x-ray	Normal	Normal	Enlarged heart
EEG	Symmetrical loss of alpha, appearance of excess theta activity	Symmetrical loss of alpha, appearance of excess theta activity	Asymmetrical focal theta activity, often episodic
Radioactive brain scan	Normal	Normal	May show excess uptake in areas of infarction
Computerized tomography	Ventricular enlargement, cortical atrophy	Ventricular enlargement, no cortical atrophy	Ventricular enlargement may be asymmetrical, infarcted areas may be seen
Neuropsychologic tests	Impaired abstraction, poor judgment, decreased insight, auditory and visual memory impairments, dysphasia	Spatial disorientation, any combination of signs of frontal lobe impairment such as decreased judgment, insight, abstraction, or decreased, fast, tapping speed	Lateralized motor-slowing dysphasia, visual-spatial disorientation, lateralizing signs depending on sites of infarction
Arteriography	No arteriosclerotic change, vessels patent, bowing of anterior cerebral vessels due to ventricular enlargement	No arteriosclerotic change, vessels patent, bowing of anterior cerebral vessels due to ventricular enlargement	Extracranial and/or intracranial arteriosclerotic vessel occlusion, major and minor
Radioactive cysternography	Normal	Abnormal, delay in passage over hemispheres and abnormally long assimilation in lateral ventricles	Normal
Treatment	Supportive: adequate diet, prompt treatment of infections, phenothiazines for agitation or combative behavior; social service involvement when patient cannot be supported in home	Ventriculoatrial shunt	As for cerebrovascular insufficiency

required to exclude pernicious anemia and vitamin B_{12} deficiency.

11. Sedimentation rate. The sedimentation rate is elevated in cerebral arteritis.

12. Serologic test for syphilis. Central nervous system syphilis is a potent and treatable cause of dementia.

13. Thyroid profiles. These are necessary to exclude hypothyroidism.

14. Serum calcium and phosphorus determinations. Such tests exclude hypo- or hypercalcemia.

15. Fasting blood glucose determination. Required to exclude hypoglycemia.

16. Biopsy of muscle, skin, or temporal artery. Biopsies are necessary to exclude arteritis.

17. Other tests as appropriate. These include sickle cell preparation, urine testing for porphobilinogen.

Treatment. Treat the cause in treatable cases. In nontreatable progressive dementia:

1. Counsel the family and give frank opinion about the patient's ability to manage his affairs.

2. The patient should be managed at home as long as possible.

3. Involve social service facilities when home conditions are deteriorating.

4. Use sedation cautiously, but do not hesitate to use when necessary. When using phenothiazines to reduce agitation, anxiety, and combative behavior, use a mild preparation; begin with low dose and increase slowly to effect.

5. Treat infections immediately. Patients with dementia have reduced resistance to all infections.

DISORDERS AFFECTING THE CEREBELLUM AND EXTRAPYRAMIDAL SYSTEM (MOTOR COORDINATION, MOVEMENT DISORDERS)

These are neurologic disorders that produce prominent effects on the coordination of motor activity, either by involvement of the cerebellum and its connections or by disrupting the function of the extrapyramidal system. Determining whether the patient's disease affects other parts of the nervous system is a key step in the differential diagnosis. Table 48–16 summarizes the usual pattern of involvement of the disorders listed. Additional detail is given for some of these disorders in the paragraphs that follow.

Ballism

This is the most violent of all involuntary movements, consisting of flinging movements of the limbs that are irregular in time and amplitude and often affect only one side of the body (hemiballismus). The condition usually begins with an acute episode, following a discrete infarction in the area of the subthalamic nucleus. Other causes, including primary and metastatic tumors or abscess, are uncommon.

Treatment. The condition is extremely exhausting and may be so violent that the patient is flung out of bed. There is prompt but temporary improvement following a slow intravenous injection of diazepam (Valium). Response to oral diazepam is unpredictable, and oral haloperidol is probably more effective. The movements tend to decrease spontaneously over a period of several weeks.

The Choreas

Sydenham's Chorea. This condition is seen almost exclusively in children and adolescents.

Etiology and Pathology. There is a definite association between Sydenham's chorea and rheumatic fever, with the eventual development of signs of rheumatic fever in a considerable number of patients who have Sydenham's chorea. This disorder is believed to represent a vasculitis with predominant involvement of the basal ganglia.

Clinical Features. Sydenham's chorea appears in children and young adolescents and is often preceded by a period in which the individual is regarded as being "clumsy." This is followed by the development of definite choreiform movements, which are essentially rapid and nonrepetitive movements affecting the limbs and later the trunk, head, and neck. When the symptoms are fully developed, the child is dysarthric, and there is an explosive quality to the speech. Facial grimacing is present, and there is inability to protrude the tongue, which is retracted during involuntary movements.

TABLE 48–16. DISORDERS OF COORDINATION AND MOVEMENT

Clinical Disorder	Major Clinical Manifestations	Other Possible Nervous System Involvement
Cerebellar Disorders:		
Cerebellar ischemia, infarction	Sudden onset of ataxia and intention tremor	Occipital cortex; cranial nerves III, IV, VI, VII, IX, XII; corticospinal tracts
Cerebellar tumors	Nausea, vomiting, headache, ataxic gait, papilledema ± unsteady when seated ± nystagmus ± hypotonia, dysmetria, adiadochokinesia	Brain stem, cranial nerves
Cerebellopontine angle tumors	Hearing loss and tinnitus, loss of balance, unsteady gait, facial numbness and weakness, dysarthria, dysphagia, nystagmus, positive Romberg's sign, papilledema a late feature	Corticospinal tracts, cranial nerves V, VII, IX, X, XI, XII
Cerebellar degeneration with cancer	Progressive limb and truncal ataxia, loss of ability to walk an early feature	Other signs of degeneration may be present in spinal cord, peripheral nerve, or muscle
Phenytoin intoxication	Drowsiness and ataxia occurring in a patient receiving this anticonvulsant	
Myxedematous cerebellar degeneration	Increasing ataxia of gait in a myxedematous patient, with prompt response to thyroid replacement	
Alcoholic cerebellar degeneration	Ataxia of gait, acute and transient, or chronic; lower limbs most affected; usually no nystagmus or dysarthria	Cerebrum, spinal cord, peripheral nerve, muscle
Familial spinocerebellar degenerations of infancy and childhood	Ataxia is the common feature in this group; the other manifestations provide the distinguishing characteristics	Telangiectasia, optic atrophy, retinal degeneration, congenital cataracts, mental retardation
Familial spinocerebellar degenerations of adult life	Progressive ataxia, dysarthria	Occasional optic atrophy, retinitis pigmentosa, myoclonus

Predominantly cerebellar group	Ataxia, tremor, other cerebellar signs	Cerebral cortex, autonomic nervous system, brain stem
Predominantly spinal (Friedreich's, Roussy-Lévy, Marie's, Charcot-Marie-Tooth disease)	Wide-based gait, ataxia, dysarthria, Romberg's sign positive, intention tremor, dysdiadochokinesia, dysmetria, change in muscle tone	Optic nerve, brain stem, posterior columns, corticospinal tracts

Extrapyramidal System Disorders:

Ballism	Sudden onset of severe flinging movements of limbs, usually due to infarction near subthalamic nucleus	
The choreas	Rapid flexion, extreme movements of fingers, hands, tongue, lips	
The dystonias	Comprises a diverse group of disorders of muscle tone and movement, ranging from athetosis to prolonged, inappropriate muscular tone; individual disorders are discussed in the text	
Drug-induced movement disorders	May be parkinsonian tremor or choreoathetosis (tardive dyskinesia)	
Parkinson's disease	Rhythmical rest tremor of extremities, beginning with fingers; so-called pill-rolling tremor, often associated with rigidity, bradykinesia, and hypokinesia	Gradual deterioration of mental function may be seen in some forms
Benign familial tremor	Bilaterally symmetrical tremor (4 to 10 cps), typically beginning in the fingers, later spreading to the hands and head; the voice may be affected and symptoms are exaggerated by fear, anger, anxiety; begins in youth or middle age and progresses slowly; partial response to propranolol or diazepam (this use of these agents is not listed in the manufacturers' official directives)	Typically lacks the rigidity, bradykinesia, and hypokinesia of parkinsonism; mild cerebellar signs may be present

TREATMENT. In the acute phase, the patient should be treated with bed rest and sedation. The most effective drug appears to be haloperidol, beginning with small doses of 0.5 mg. and gradually increasing to effect (see manufacturer's official directive before using haloperidol in children). If, however, haloperidol is not effective, phenobarbital may help in some patients.

In the convalescent stage, the child should be observed frequently for the development of signs of rheumatic fever, and penicillin therapy should be considered as a prophylactic measure.

Chorea Gravidarum. The appearance of choreiform movements in young women during pregnancy is believed to represent a recrudescence of Sydenham's chorea. The condition usually resolves promptly after delivery.

Familial Benign Chorea. This form of chorea seems to be transmitted as an autosomal dominant trait and appears in two or more members of the affected families. The condition is essentially nonprogressive but persists throughout life. The symptoms may respond to use of haloperidol or reserpine.

Secondary Chorea. Choreiform movements may occur in a number of other degenerative conditions or toxic conditions affecting the central nervous system. Such conditions include viral encephalitis, in which choreiform movements may appear during the acute stage or as a sequel to this condition. Choreiform movements also occur in demyelinating diseases such as the leukodystrophies and postinfectious leukoencephalopathy. They have been seen in anoxic encephalopathy and in other toxic conditions affecting the brain, including carbon monoxide poisoning. Such movements are not unusual as a complication of long-term use of phenothiazine drugs. Patients with multiple small infarcts in the brain (multi-infarct dementia) occasionally display choreiform movements. It should be recognized that these choreiform movements are occurring against a background of diffuse cerebral arteriosclerosis and multiple infarction. Such cases should not be termed "senile chorea."

The Dystonias

Spasmodic Torticollis. Both familial and sporadic cases of spasmodic torticollis have been described, and there is little doubt that the condition is a form of dystonia and not a psychiatric disorder.

The pathologic changes are unknown. The spasm producing the dystonic posture occurs in the sternocleidomastoid muscle or the posterior cervical muscles, or both. Spasmodic torticollis can occur in both children and adults. The head is turned forcibly to one side, often with a series of jerks, before it shows a forced dystonic posture. The chin is often elevated and the occiput depressed toward the shoulder.

TREATMENT. Haloperidol, trihexyphenidyl and amantadine may be effective, singly or in combination (see manufacturers' official directives before using these agents in children). Electromyographic biofeedback has been successful in treating some patients.

Dystonia Musculorum Deformans. Autosomal dominant, autosomal recessive, and sporadic cases of dystonia musculorum deformans occur. The condition is caused by a bilateral disorder of the basal ganglia with neuronal degeneration within these structures.

Symptoms usually appear in childhood and are characterized by intermittent dystonia of the axial musculature. The dystonia increases in severity with later involvement of the limbs, and the body is contorted into a severely dystonic posture in the fully developed case.

TREATMENT. There may be some response to haloperidol in the early stages of the disease (see manufacturer's official directive before using haloperidol in children). Surgical treatment by thalamotomy has produced temporary improvement, which may be dramatic in some patients.

Athetosis

Athetotic movements may occur in:
1. Double athetosis (athetotic cerebral palsy).
2. Huntington's disease.
3. Hepatolenticular degeneration (Wilson's disease).
4. Patients on phenothiazine therapy.
5. Paroxysmal choreoathetosis.
6. Miscellaneous conditions:
   a. Anoxic encephalopathy.
   b. Alzheimer's disease.
   c. Postinfectious leukoencephalopathy.
   d. Viral encephalitis.
   e. Hepatic encephalopathy.

Double Athetosis. This condition is one of the forms of cerebral palsy, although the choreoathetotic movements do not appear until after the first year of life. The majority of cases are caused by anoxia at birth. Kernicterus, formerly the other major cause of double athetosis, is now an unusual factor in this condition, as kernicterus can be treated adequately by exchange transfusion.

Double athetosis, or athetotic cerebral palsy, is a result of damage to the basal ganglia, particularly to the putamen and globus pallidus. It results in loss of neurones and increased gliosis with a haphazard myelination of the area. There is usually a history of anoxia at birth, with the need for resuscitative measures, or a clear history of kernicterus can be obtained. These infants are usually hypotonic and fail to show the usual milestones in motor development during their first year, or occasionally later. This stage is eventually superseded by the development of involuntary movements which include alternating flexion and extension of limbs, facial grimacing, head turning, and truncal dystonia. The speech is affected and shows a characteristic slurred dysarthria. Intelligence is usually normal.

Huntington's Disease (Huntington's Chorea). Huntington's disease is a condition that is inherited as an autosomal dominant trait and is apparently caused by a deficiency of the neurotransmitter gamma-aminobutyric acid (GABA). There is early, diffuse neuronal loss that is most marked in the basal ganglia and particularly in the caudate nucleus and putamen.

These patients develop athetotic movements that first appear in the fourth decade; however, the movements may occasionally be manifested in childhood or adolescence. The athetotic movements affect the face, causing facial grimacing, and the extremities. Gait is ataxic, and speech is expressive and dysarthric. There is a progressive dementia in Huntington's disease that usually begins after the appearance of the choreoathetotic movements. The course is progressive, and death from intercurrent infection occurs between 10 and 15 years after onset.

The involuntary movements may respond to reserpine in gradually increasing doses, to haloperidol or deanol, or occasionally to phenothiazines. There is a high risk of suicide in patients with Huntington's dis-

ease, and the depression seen in this condition may be treated with imipramine or amitriptyline.

Paroxysmal Choreoathetosis. Paroxysmal choreoathetosis is a condition of paroxysmal episodes of sudden, intermittent choreoathetosis of the extremities, trunk, and face in children. Attacks usually occur when the child makes sudden movements, such as abruptly getting to his feet to run. There is immediate falling to the floor and distortion of the limbs and trunk with choreoathetotic movements. The attacks usually last about 30 seconds and are followed by complete recovery. The electroencephalogram is reported to be normal in this condition; nevertheless, the good response to phenytoin supports the view that paroxysmal choreoathetosis is a form of epilepsy.

Neurologic Complications of Phenothiazines

1. *Coma.* Phenothiazines may be used in a suicide attempt and produce a coma that is accompanied by respiratory arrest, hypotension, and, in some cases, hypothermia. Patients need treatment in an intensive care unit and require respiratory assistance and management of hypotension.

2. *Acute dystonia.* This is an idiosyncratic reaction that occurs after exposure to small doses of a phenothiazine. Acute dystonia involves the facial muscles, platysma, and neck. Opisthotonos may occur. The dystonia occurs episodically and has a superficial resemblance to tetanus. The condition is self-limiting. Patients with mild episodes need only be observed. When the dystonia causes distress, attacks can be terminated by an intravenous injection of diazepam, 10 mg., benztropine mesylate, 2 mg., or diphenhydramine, 25 mg.

3. *Parkinsonism.* This is a not unfrequent complication of chronic phenothiazine therapy. As phenothiazines block the release of dopamine, the condition will not respond to L-dopa. It does respond to anticholinergics such as benztropine mesylate.

4. *Tardive dyskinesia.* Choreoathetotic movements producing a marked restlessness of arms and lower limbs with constant, irregular, and repetitive movements of the lips and jaws (akathisia) may occur after prolonged use of phenothiazines. This condition also occurs in elderly patients with cerebral arteriosclerosis. Treatment consists

of withdrawal of the phenothiazine and giving reserpine. There is usually a good response to the reserpine, beginning with 0.25 mg. daily and slowly increasing to effect. Haloperidol and deanol have also been used in this condition.

Parkinson's Disease

Parkinsonism is really syndromic, and the condition is better named the parkinsonian syndrome.

Etiology and Pathology. The biochemical disturbance in parkinsonism is probably located in the dopaminergic pathway that connects the substantia nigra and the putamen. In theory, failure of synthesis, failure of storage, failure of release of dopamine, or a block at the dopamine receptor site in the putamen could result in the imbalance in the nigrostriatal thalamic pathway that is believed to produce the rigidity and tremor of parkinsonism. One theoretical scheme postulates that the dopaminergic nigrostriatal system acts as an inhibitor of a cholinergic putamen-pallidal pathway. Failure of the dopaminergic system removes the inhibition of the cholinergic pathway, and this release of activity results in the symptoms of parkinsonism.

Clinical Features. Parkinsonism is characterized by:

1. *Rigidity.* There is an increase in tone in both antagonist and protagonist muscle groups, and the rigidity is observed by the examiner as a "lead pipe" or cogwheel phenomenon when passively moving the limbs of the affected individual.

2. *Tremor.* Arrhythmical discharges giving rise to tremor probably originate in the thalamus, but the exact mechanisms of tremor are still a matter of conjecture. The tremor of parkinsonism is seen in the periphery. It usually begins on one side before the other and affects the index finger and thumb. When fully developed, it produces the characteristic "pill-rolling tremor" of Parkinson's disease. In the later stages, the tremor may be seen in the tongue and the more proximal muscle groups of the affected limbs. It is not unusual for one side of the body to be affected by tremor and rigidity for several years before symptoms are noted on the other side.

3. *Bradykinesis.* The combination of rigidity and tremor produces the characteristic bradykinesis seen in the patient with parkinsonism who shows a stooped posture associated with flexion of the head on the chest, flexion of the trunk, and a typical lack of facial expression. When walking, the arms do not show associated movements, and the steps are small and shuffling. The rigidity prevents rapid correction of balance by contraction of antagonists and protagonists, so that the patient tends to lose balance easily. This may give rise to a phenomenon known as propulsion, in which the patient moves forward at a progressively increasing rate in an attempt to maintain balance. He will eventually fall unless he comes up against some restraining object.

Patients with parkinsonism show a number of other features, including easy fatigue, muscle weakness, marked slowness of finger movements, impaired handwriting that becomes small and cramped (micrographia), and slow, monotonous speech of poor volume. There is a variable deterioration in intellect. In many patients, this loss is hardly noticeable and can be documented only by detailed neuropsychologic testing. In some patients, however, the dementia is progressive and adds a further complication to this disabling disease.

A number of the conditions associated with the parkinsonian syndrome have additional characteristic features. Postencephalitic parkinsonism is rarely seen nowadays, as the majority of cases resulted from the pandemic of encephalitis lethargica that occurred from 1918 to 1928. Patients with postencephalitis parkinsonism tend to show more intellectual deterioration and emotional disturbance. There is increased drooling and periods of forced deviation of the eyes, usually in an upward direction, which may last up to 20 minutes (oculogyric crises).

Arteriosclerotic parkinsonism should be diagnosed only in patients with documented cerebral arteriosclerosis who have shown the intermittent progression of symptoms in conjunction with a series of small strokes. The majority of these patients have additional pseudobulbar features with laughing and crying on minimal emotional stimulus and with marked dysarthria.

Evaluation. In order to assess the progression of the disease or therapeutic response in patients with parkinsonism, a series of tests that can be easily repeated should be given at each visit to the office. The patient should be asked to draw a square, write his name, bisect a straight line, and draw concentric circles with each hand at each visit. Comparison of these records will indicate progression or amelioration of the condition under therapy.

Treatment. Adequate treatment of Parkinson's disease will produce alleviation of symptoms in the majority of patients, and improvement may be maintained for many years. It should be realized, however, that Parkinson's disease is a slowly progressing, deteriorating condition and that this deterioration continues despite treatment. Nevertheless, patients may remain comfortable for many years when given adequate drug therapy plus periodic adjustment of medication.

One form of treatment of Parkinson's disease is based upon the partial restoration of activity in the inhibitory dopaminergic pathway from the substantia nigra to the putamen.

In theory, the imbalance in the dopaminergic-cholinergic system can be countered by (1) increasing dopaminergic activity in the putamen or (2) inhibiting cholinergic activity in the putamen and globus pallidus.

Drugs available for enhancement of dopaminergic activity include: (1) L-dopa (levodopa), (2) carbidopa-levodopa (Sinemet), and (3) amantadine (Symmetrel). Dopamine does not cross the blood-brain barrier; however, its precursor, dopa, does cross the blood-brain barrier in small amounts when given orally. This fact has led to the use of L-dopa in the treatment of Parkinson's disease.

DOSAGE. Begin with a small dose of L-dopa, such as 250 mg. with the evening meal. Add increments of 250 mg. every 3 to 5 days, giving the medication with meals. Increase dosage until the symptoms are alleviated or until the amount is limited by side effects.

SIDE EFFECTS. The most common side effects are nausea and vomiting. These can be minimized by giving L-dopa with meals. Postural hypotension is often a problem and may limit the dosage of levodopa; therefore, take the blood pressure frequently with the patient both lying and standing. Other side effects include dystonias of the head, trunk, and limbs; hallucinations; and agitation.

DISORDERS OF THE CRANIAL NERVE, MIDBRAIN, BRAIN STEM, AND SPINAL CORD

DISORDERS OF THE CRANIAL NERVES AND CONTIGUOUS STRUCTURES

The cranial nerves are extensions of the brain in the cranial area. As such, they are valuable indicators of dysfunction or disease of those portions of the brain that contain the cranial nerve nuclei and the central connections of the cranial nerves. Table 48–17 gives a listing of the various conditions that affect the central and peripheral portions of each cranial nerve and adjacent neural structures in the midbrain and brain stem.

Papilledema

Definition. Papilledema is edema of the optic disc. The condition may be inflammatory or noninflammatory. It is not possible to differentiate between these two basic causes by the appearance of the disc. However, when the papilledema is known to be inflammatory, it is called "optic neuritis."

Noninflammatory papilledema can be caused by:
1. Raised intracranial pressure.
    a. Obstruction to flow of cerebrospinal fluid
    b. Brain swelling from any cause.
    c. Intracranial mass.
       (1) Extradural.
       (2) Subdural.
       (3) Intracerebral.
    d. Impairment of venous drainage.
       (1) Thrombosis of central retinal vein.
       (2) Orbital venous obstruction due to cellulitis, abscess, or tumor.
       (3) Cavernous sinus thrombosis.
       (4) Carotid cavernous fistula.
       (5) Mediastinal obstruction.
       (6) Intrathoracic obstruction due to emphysema or heart failure.
2. Nutritional—vitamin B_1 or B_{12} deficiency.
3. Metabolic—diabetes mellitus, gout.
4. Neoplastic—tumors of optic nerve or chiasm.
5. Blood dyscrasias—anemia, leukemia, polycythemia.

TABLE 48–17.   CONDITIONS AFFECTING CRANIAL NERVES AND RELATED STRUCTURES

Cranial Nerve	Clinical Manifestations	Diseases of Central Tracts and Contiguous Structures	Diseases of Peripheral Tracts and Contiguous Structures
I (Olfactory)	Anosmia	Tumor, infarction of frontal lobe	Fracture of cribriform plate, colds, sinusitis, heavy smoking, chemical injury
II (Optic)	Retina and optic disc—hemorrhage, exudates, vascular disease	Subarachnoid hemorrhage	Hypertension, diabetes mellitus, toxemia of pregnancy, eclampsia, arteriosclerosis, blood dyscrasias, arteritis, arterial emboli, retinitis pigmentosa, chorioretinitis, cherry red spot, angiomatous malformations
	Papilledema	Increased intracranial pressure, central nervous system (CNS) infections, hypertensive encephalopathy, toxemia	Optic neuritis; infectious and idiopathic; retrobulbar neuritis
	Optic atrophy *Visual field defects:*	See text for listing	See text for listing
	Enlarged physiologic blind spot, constriction of peripheral fields	Increased intracranial pressure with chronic papilledema	Optic neuritis
	Nonquadrantal scotomata		
	Blindness with loss of light reflex		Retinal disease, i.e. detachment hemorrhage, etc.
	Bitemporal partial or complete hemi- or quadrantal anopia	Pressure on or injury to optic chiasm (pituitary tumor, suprasellar tumor, trauma, etc.)	Complete destruction of optic nerve
	Homonymous hemianopia	Optic tract, optic radiation, calcarine cortex	
	Upper homonymous quadrantanopia	Temporal lobe lesion of Meyer's loop	
	Lower homonymous quadrantanopia	Optic radiation, parietal lobe	
	Blindness with preservation of light reflex	Destruction of occipital cortex	
III (Oculomotor)	Unilateral, dilation of pupil	Compression of 3rd nerve	Benign dysfunction of pupil (Holmes-Adie syndrome)
	Argyll Robertson pupil (myotic pupil that reacts to accommodation but not to light)	Tertiary syphilis, encephalitis, diabetic vascular disease, multiple sclerosis, midbrain tumors	
	Horner's syndrome (ptosis, miosis, enophthalmos, anhidrosis)	Syringobulbia	Interruption of cervical sympathetic nerves due to surgery, tumor, aneurysm, etc.

Nerve	Sign/Symptom	Lesion	Associated Conditions
III (Oculomotor) IV (Trochlear) VI (Abducens)	Diplopia, ptosis, paralysis of extraocular movements	Brain stem lesions causing pressure or injury, diabetic vascular disease, inflammatory CNS disease, multiple sclerosis, syphilis, syringobulbia	Ophthalmoplegic migraine, cavernous aneurysm, superior orbital tumor, orbital abscess, myasthenia gravis, exophthalmic ophthalmoplegia, cyclic oculomotor paralysis
V (Trigeminal)	Trigeminal neuralgia (tic douloureux)	Multiple sclerosis, tumor, aneurysm near foramen ovale	Degeneration of gasserian ganglion or peripheral fibers, tumors of root
	Loss of corneal reflex, facial sensation	Midbrain or sensory tract lesions	Cavernous sinus lesions
VII (Facial)	Paralysis of forehead, periorbital, and lower facial muscles	Nuclear or supranuclear infarct, tumor, syringobulbia, etc.	Bell's palsy, Guillain-Barré syndrome, tumors of facial canal, trauma, herpes zoster
	Paralysis of periorbital and lower facial movement only		Sequel to Bell's palsy or idiopathic
	Hemifacial spasm		
VIII (Auditory)	Facial myokymia	Idiopathic or multiple sclerosis	
	Decreased auditory acuity	Tumors of cerebellopontine angle or pons, neurilemoma	Aminoglycoside antibiotics, nerve degeneration, chronic noise exposure
	Tinnitus		Cochlear inflammation, degeneration
	Vertigo	Vascular, neoplastic, or degenerative involvement of vestibular nuclei and/or tracts	Disorders of vestibular apparatus, Meniere's syndrome, benign paroxysmal vertigo
IX (Glossopharyngeal)	Nasal voice, weakness of palate, dysphonia	Tumors, infarcts of pons and adjacent areas	Glomus jugular tumor
X (Vagus)	Hoarseness, unilateral vocal cord paralysis		Interruption of recurrent laryngeal nerve due to tumor, thyroid surgery, aortic aneurysm, etc.
XI (Spinal Accessory)	Weakness of sternocleidomastoid and trapezius muscles	Vascular, degenerative, and neoplastic lesions of lower pons and medulla and supranuclear motor tracts	Polyneuropathy, amyotrophic lateral sclerosis, post-traumatic
XII (Hypoglossal)	Deviation of protruded tongue toward affected side	Vascular, degenerative, and neoplastic lesions of medulla and supranuclear motor tracts, syringobulbia	Same as XI
	Hemiatrophy of tongue		

6. Toxic—due to methyl alcohol, lead, arsenic, uremia.

7. Vascular—due to severe hypertensive encephalopathy.

8. Degenerative—due to multiple sclerosis.

Inflammatory papilledema can be caused by:

1. Infections of the optic nerve.
    a. Bacterial—due to orbital cellulitis, acute meningitis.
    b. Syphilis.
    c. Tuberculosis.
    d. Viral encephalitides.
    e. Fungal—cryptococcosis.
    f. Protozoal—malaria and toxoplasmosis.

2. Idiopathic optic neuritis

Clinical Features. Patients with early papilledema usually present with blurring of vision and some scintillation in any part of the visual field. As papilledema progresses, perimetry and tangent screening will show peripheral constriction of the visual fields with enlargement of the blind spot.

In the inflammatory form of papilledema, i.e., optic neuritis, the onset may be abrupt, with sudden diminution of visual acuity or even complete blindness in one eye. There is pain on eye movement, and when some vision is retained, the patient shows a central, paracentral, or cecocentral scotoma.

Differential Diagnosis. The history and physical examination of the patient will usually reveal the cause of the papilledema and dictate the appropriate investigative procedures.

Treatment. A primary disease process, if present, should be treated promptly. The consultative assistance of a competent ophthalmologist is recommended.

Disorders Affecting Cranial Nerves III, IV, and VI

Paralysis of one or more of these nerves is commonly encountered in neurologic practice. When considering the cause of the paralysis, it is well to begin at the level of the brain stem and proceed in an orderly fashion toward the periphery.

Causes of paralysis of the third, fourth, and sixth cranial nerves need to be considered as follows:

1. *Brain stem.* Involvement at this level is likely to produce a neurologic abnormality that indicates tract signs and involvement of the cerebellar connections. Common causes are encephalitis, syphilis, multiple sclerosis, Wernicke's encephalopathy, tumors of the brain stem, and infarction.

2. *Intracranial.* There may well be signs of involvement of the cranial nerves apart from the third, fourth, and sixth cranial nerves. Common causes include acute or chronic basal meningitis; polyneuritis, particularly acute infectious polyneuropathy (Guillain-Barré syndrome); diabetes mellitus; tumors; and raised intracranial pressure.

3. *Intracavernous.* Isolated third nerve lesions are more common when the fault lies at this level. Consider the presence of ophthalmoplegic migraine or an aneurysm of the terminal carotid or posterior communicating artery.

At the level of the superior orbital fissure, lesions of the third, fourth, and sixth cranial nerves occur exclusively. The causes include tumor, Paget's disease, and the superior orbital fissure syndrome. At the level of the orbit, again the third, fourth, and sixth cranial nerves are usually involved alone. Common causes include tumors, abscesses, and exophthalmic ophthalmoplegia. At the level of the extraocular muscles, lesions do not involve all muscles supplied by the third, fourth, and sixth cranial nerves but may mimic such lesions. Botulism and myasthenia gravis should be considered.

Miscellaneous Causes. Paralysis of one or more ocular motor nerves may occur in cyclic fashion. This is known as cyclic oculomotor paralysis and is an episodic condition in children.

Tic Douloureux

Definition. Tic douloureux is a spasmodically painful condition occurring in the distribution of the trigeminal nerve.

Etiology. The cause is unknown, although there are many theories, such as pressure on the gasserian ganglion by an arteriosclerotic carotid artery, stretching of the preganglionic nerve root or irritation of the spinal tract trigeminal nerve. The condition is rarely symptomatic in posterior fossa tumor, basilar artery aneurysm, or multiple sclerosis.

Pathology. Demyelination of fibers in gasserian ganglion has been described.

Clinical Features. Tic douloureux is a

disease of late onset with lightning-like pain occurring in second or third divisions, or both, of the trigeminal nerve. Pain, associated with involuntary exclamations and tic-like grimacing of face, lasts for only a few seconds. The condition is rare in the ophthalmic divisions of the nerve. There are long remissions between attacks initially, which gradually get shorter. Pain may be triggered by light pressure on trigger zones in the face, usually near the upper lip and nostril. Pain is also triggered by facial movements, chewing, and exposure to drafts of cold air. The neurologic examination is normal.

Differential Diagnosis. Conditions to be excluded are:

1. Dental pain. The lightning-like pain of tic douloureux shooting across the face is not associated with dental disease.

2. Sinusitis. The pressure pain of sinusitis does not resemble tic douloureux.

3. "Atypical facial pain." This pain is characterized by a dull ache of long duration in trigeminal distribution.

4. Cluster headaches. The pain in the temple and orbit is of longer duration than the pain of tic douloureux.

5. Temporomandibular joint disease. A dull ache exacerbated by chewing occurs in this form of joint disease.

Treatment. Treatment is as follows:

1. Phenytoin (diphenylhydantoin) is effective in some early cases. Increase the dose until serum phenytoin is in the therapeutic range of 15 to 25 micrograms per ml. (This use of phenytoin is not listed in the manufacturer's official directive).

2. Carbamazepine (Tegretol) is the drug of choice. Begin with 200 mg. at night and increase slowly to avoid side effects, prescribing up to 1200 mg. per day in divided doses.

3. Surgical. Electrocoagulation of the trigeminal ganglion is the procedure of choice when carbamazepine is not effective.

Bell's Palsy

Definition. Bell's palsy is a condition of unknown cause in which there is an isolated paresis of the facial muscles of peripheral type.

Etiology. It has been postulated that Bell's palsy is caused by a virus infection of the peripheral nerve in the facial canal. A similar condition occurs following infection by herpes zoster virus, in which the virus produces inflammation of the geniculate ganglion. This is associated with herpetic vesicles in the external auditory meatus and is known as the Ramsay Hunt syndrome.

Pathology. It is believed that the paralysis of facial nerve function follows acute edema of the nerve, which then undergoes strangulation in the facial canal. The increased pressure on the nerve produces paralysis of function followed by degeneration of the nerve fibers. As the edema subsides, the surviving fibers begin to function, and there is a gradual regeneration of degenerated fibers that produces the recovery seen in most patients.

Clinical Features. A prodromal stage of pain in the region of the sternomastoid area is not uncommon in the 24 hours preceding the onset of facial paralysis. The onset of the paralysis is usually acute, with sagging of the face and inability to close the eye. There may be excess watering of the eye because of inability to move secretions across the cornea by lid closure. Drooling may also occur from the paralyzed side of the mouth. It is not uncommon for food to accumulate in the side of the mouth because of paralysis of the buccinator. Some 10 per cent of patients show loss of taste on the affected side because of involvement of the chorda tympani, as the edema extends up the facial canal. More than 90 per cent of patients show recovery in a period of several weeks. The majority of the remainder show incomplete recovery, and a few develop contractures of the face, facial spasms, and ectopia.

Differential Diagnosis. Bell's palsy is an isolated paralysis of facial nerve function. If the neurologic examination shows involvement of other cranial nerves or of the central nervous system, other conditions should be considered.

Evaluation. Some idea of the prognosis may be obtained by measurement of the amplitude of evoked response on stimulation of the facial nerve at the sternomastoid foramen. If the response is good 7 days after the onset of facial weakness, the prognosis is excellent.

Treatment. The patient is given:

1. ACTH, 40 to 60 units, injected intramuscularly daily for 2 weeks.

2. Methylprednisolone, 90 to 120 mg. once every 48 hours for 10 days.

Both ACTH and methylprednisolone are

believed to contribute to a significantly high rate of improvement in Bell's palsy.

Hemifacial Spasm

Repetitive contractions of the facial muscles in random fashion may occur following partial recovery from Bell's palsy. Some episodes appear spontaneously in older individuals. The condition is often mild and is exacerbated by stress. If the condition is troublesome, some improvement may be obtained with the use of phenytoin or carbamazepine in some patients.

Cerebellopontine Angle Tumor

Of the tumors that occur in the cerebellopontine angle, the neurilemoma is by far the most frequently encountered. Meningiomas, dermoid cysts, cholesteatomas, and metastatic tumors may also occur at this site.

Clinical Features. These are as follows:
1. Pressure on the eighth nerve produces progressive loss of hearing and intermittent vertigo.
2. Pressure on the fifth nerve produces loss of corneal reflex.
3. Pressure on the seventh nerve produces facial weakness.
4. Pressure on the brain stem produces contralateral increase in tendon reflexes.
5. Pressure on the cerebellum produces ipsilateral limb ataxia.

Treatment. The tumor can be removed completely in the early stages, followed by resolution of symptoms.

Glomus Jugular Tumors

These are rare tumors arising in the jugular foramen and invading the petrous temporal bone. They produce paralysis of the ninth and tenth cranial nerves and may present as a bleeding mass in the external auditory meatus.

Other Neuralgias

Glossopharyngeal neuralgia is a rare condition in which the patient experiences paroxysmal, lightning-like pains in the throat, often precipitated by swallowing, chewing, or talking. The pain frequently radiates into the ear and into the upper cervical area. Patients with this condition

should be investigated for the possibility of a cerebellopontine angle tumor or infiltration at the base of the skull, as this has occasionally been reported in association with glossopharyngeal neuralgia. Most cases are idiopathic and respond to carbamazepine.

Geniculate neuralgia is somewhat similar to glossopharyngeal neuralgia and consists of paroxysmal, lightning-like pains in the area of the external auditory meatus, sometimes radiating into the throat. It also responds to carbamazepine.

Superior laryngeal nerve neuralgia is an unusual condition in which there is paroxysmal pain recurring over the anterior portion of the neck. This pain may radiate backward toward the angle of the mandible or downward into the anterior chest. An attack of pain can be precipitated by stroking the skin of the neck just above the thyroid cartilage and can be alleviated by injection of local anesthesia into trigger areas in the neck. This form of neuralgia also responds to carbamazepine.

Occipital neuralgia is more frequently encountered in medical practice and consists of paroxysmal attacks of pain occurring in the distribution of the greater occipital nerve situated just to the left or right of the midline in the occipital and posterior parietal areas of the scalp. Paroxysmal pain usually occurs in the background, along with a dull ache in the same area, and the condition is probably due to irritation of the roots of the second or third cervical nerve by arthritic changes in the upper cervical spine. It frequently responds to heat, rest, and analgesics. Patients with more persistent pain should be treated by injection of the nerve with a local anesthetic and methylprednisolone. If this treatment fails, surgical section of the nerve should be considered.

DISORDERS OF THE SPINAL CORD

The function of the spinal cord may be impaired by a variety of mechanisms ranging from mechanical injury and compression to inflammation; interference with metabolism or nutrition, or both; toxic injury; or degeneration due to genetic or other causes. Table 48–18 provides a summary of the majority of known disorders of the spinal cord, with supplementary information included in the text.

TABLE 48–18. CONDITIONS THAT MAY AFFECT THE SPINAL CORD

Condition	Areas Usually Affected	Comments
Degenerative/Genetic		
Amyotrophic lateral sclerosis	Anterior horn cell degeneration of brain stem and spinal cord; cervical cord often affected early	Onset after age 35 (see text)
Progressive spinal muscular atrophy	Degeneration of anterior horn cells with weakness and muscular wasting, especially of limb girdle musculature in juvenile and adult forms	Werdnig-Hoffmann syndrome in infants, diffuse disease involving brain stem and cord; Kugelberg-Welander syndrome in juveniles and adults, more slowly progressive than infant form
Spinocerebellar degeneration	Usually diffuse involvement, beginning in cervical or lumbar cord	
Syringomyelia	Usually cervical and dorsal, occasionally lumbar cord. Loss of anterior horn cells, sensory fibers, corticospinal tracts	Loss of pain, sensation in hands, muscle wasting with fasciculations, spastic paraparesis below lesion if corticospinal tracts involved; light touch, vibration, and position sense intact
Carcinomatous degeneration	Diffuse	Nonmetastatic effect of certain cancers, especially lung cancer
Nutritional		
Vitamin B_{12} deficiency	Patchy demyelination of posterior and sometimes lateral columns of cord, usually maximal in thoracic cord	Associated with megaloblastic anemia and defective absorption of vitamin B_{12}; peripheral neuropathy may be present
Infections		
Syphilis	Posterior columns, vasculitis, epidural	A manifestation of tertiary lues
Epidural abscess	Usually thoracic area	Often associated with diabetes
Intramedullary abscess	Any area	Rare condition, usually a secondary site of infection
Tuberculous abscess	Mid- or upper thoracic cord	Typically a complication of Pott's disease
Neoplastic		
Chordoma	Sacral, clival, mid-cranial fossa	Presacral extension is common, benign tumor
Intramedullary tumors, epidural cysts, and other extramedullary tumors	Most common in thoracic area but can occur anywhere	Many types occur (see text for more detail), this group is difficult to distinguish prior to surgery
Physical Injury		
Trauma, contusion, compression laceration	Any level	Manifestations depend on level of injury and portions of cord affected
Vertebral collapse with cord and/or root compression	Usually thoracic or lumbar	May be caused by osteoporosis, myeloma, bone metastases, metabolic bone disease
X-irradiation	Level of irradiation injury	May produce vascular injury and ischemia, transverse myelitis
Hematomyelia	Usually cervical cord, primarily involving grey matter	Post-traumatic fracture of whiplash of cervical spine. Produces sensory and/or motor loss below level of lesion
Vascular Disease		
Cord infarction	May occur anywhere in cord	Associated with arteriosclerosis, myocardial infarction, cord irradiation, heroin abuse, thrombosis or aneurysm of aorta
Arteriovenous malformations	Usually thoracic, occasionally cervical or lumbar	Leaks may produce back pain, subarachnoid hemorrhage, paraparesis

Amyotrophic Lateral Sclerosis

Definition. Amyotrophic lateral sclerosis (motor neurone disease) is a degenerative disease involving the anterior horn cells of the spinal cord, the motor neurones of the cranial nerve nuclei, and, to a lesser extent, the motor neurones of the frontal lobes of the brain.

Etiology. The cause is unknown. It may be due to:

1. Abiotrophy—a premature dying of neurones.

2. Slow viral infection of the motor neurones.

3. Autoimmune disease in which anterior horn cells are destroyed by circulating antibodies.

Pathology. There is marked loss of motor neurones in the spinal cord and brain stem, with some loss of motor neurones in the frontal lobes of the brain. The cortical spinal tract shows marked degeneration in the brain stem and spinal cord. The anterior nerve roots contain motor fibers, and the muscles supplied by defective neurones show atrophy of muscle fibers in a fascicular fashion.

Clinical Features. The disease usually occurs after 35 years of age, with the maximum incidence in the fourth and fifth decades. Three types are recognized.

1. *Progressive muscular atrophy.* The patient presents with atrophy of one or more muscle groups, often atrophy of the small muscles of the hands in which there is wasting of interossei, thenar, and hypothenar muscles. Other sites, such as the lower limbs and shoulders, may be involved first in some patients. The atrophy gradually spreads and eventually becomes generalized. Respiratory insufficiency occurs, with involvement of the intercostal muscles and diaphragm. In the terminal stages, this form usually shows signs of bulbar palsy and lateral sclerosis.

2. *Progressive bulbar palsy.* This form of amyotrophic lateral sclerosis usually runs a more rapid course, with wasting of the bulbar muscles. The patient presents with dysarthria, dysphagia, regurgitation of food through the nose, and inability to handle secretions.

3. *Primary lateral sclerosis.* In this form of the disease, there is progressive spasticity in all four extremities, which is slowly progressive but not necessarily symmetrical. Wasting and fasciculations are not present in the early stages of the disease, but do appear later.

Differential Diagnosis. The possibility of nerve root compression due to cervical spondylosis might well be considered in the early stages, in which the wasting and fasciculations are confined to the hands or upper limbs. Spinal cord compression caused by Arnold-Chiari malformation, odontoid compression, or basilar invagination should be excluded in patients with early primary lateral sclerosis. The generalized form of amyotrophic lateral sclerosis has been described as a remote effect of carcinoma. The successful removal of a malignant tumor has been followed by remission of the amyotrophic lateral sclerosis in some patients.

Evaluation. Diagnostic procedures are as follows:

1. Search for a neoplasm.

2. Electromyography will show the presence of fibrillations and fasciculations in affected muscles; nerve conduction velocities will be normal.

3. Myelography should be performed to exclude spinal cord compression when this is suspected or nerve root compression caused by cervical spondylosis.

4. Muscle biopsy will show typical neurogenic atrophy.

5. Serum creatine phosphokinase levels are usually elevated.

6. Barium swallow may be helpful when there is pharyngeal weakness.

7. Pulmonary function tests should be performed in serial fashion when there is impairment of pulmonary function.

Treatment. There is no specific treatment for this condition. Patients should be kept as active as possible for as long as possible. When dysphagia occurs, attention should be paid to diet so that nutrition is maintained. The patient and relatives should be taught suctioning to remove secretions in the pharynx. Small doses of atropine may reduce secretions if these become troublesome. A tracheotomy may be required in some patients in the late stages of the disease to aid in removal of secretions and prevent aspiration pneumonia. A gastrostomy may be necessary to maintain nutrition when swallowing is impaired.

Progressive Spinal Muscular Atrophy

There are a spectrum of conditions that are associated with loss of anterior horn cells and muscle wasting. Infantile spinal muscular atrophy (Werdnig-Hoffmann syndrome) is inherited as an autosomal recessive trait and produces a rapidly fatal generalized muscle wasting in infants with early death due to respiratory insufficiency. More chronic cases of spinal muscle atrophy are occasionally encountered in children, adolescents, and adults. These conditions are often slowly progressive but in some patients may apparently cease to progress. Some patients have predominantly proximal limb girdle wasting, and this may be misdiagnosed as polymyositis or muscular dystrophy. The diagnosis of spinal muscular atrophy can be established by electromyography and muscle biopsy.

Syringomyelia

This is a disease of the spinal cord, and the process extends into the brain stem (syringobulbia). Syringomyelia is a condition in which there is a cavity in the substance of the spinal cord. The cavity that usually occurs in the cervical area may be the result of degeneration occurring in embryonic cell rests that have been enclosed in the cauda during the development of degeneration in a chronic low-grade glioma. The condition is extremely chronic, and the cavity gradually increases in size, sometimes expanding into the brain stem (syringobulbia).

The disease usually appears in adult life. As the cavity occurs in the center of the cord and extends longitudinally as well as laterally, it produces characteristic symptoms:

1. Involvement of the decussating pain fibers in the cervical cord produces a loss of pain sensation, usually beginning in the hands. Patients develop painless cuts and infections of the hands or may burn their hands without experiencing any discomfort.

2. Extension of the cavity in a lateral direction involving the corticospinal tract produces spasticity and increased reflexes below the level of the lesion and extensor plantar responses.

3. Extension anterolaterally will involve the anterior horn cells, with resultant wasting of the muscles supplied by these cells that often begins with wasting of the small muscles of the hands. This wasting is associated with fasciculations.

4. Lateral extension involves the cortical relay to the sacral nerves subserving bladder function, producing a small spastic bladder with urgency and eventually causing incontinence.

The typical patient presents with wasting of the small muscles of the hand, extending into the forearm muscles and later to muscles of the shoulder girdles accompanied by a dissociated sensory loss in the upper quadrant, spastic paraparesis with increased reflexes and extensor plantar responses, and a small spastic bladder. Loss of sensation in the joints of the upper limb may produce an arthropathy that resembles that of the Charcot joints of tabes dorsalis.

Extension into the brain stem with syringobulbia produces cranial nerve involvement, Horner's syndrome, nystagmus, and eventual loss of touch, vibration, and position sense caused by involvement of the decussating fibers of the medial lemniscus.

All patients with syringomyelia should undergo myelography for detection of a possible intramedullary tumor. Development of abnormalities of the cervical spine are not unusual in patients with syringomyelia.

The disease is extremely chronic and usually advances slowly. It is possible that irradiation of the cervical cord produces some slowing of the process. The usual dose is 5000 roentgen units. When the myelogram shows considerable widening of the cord, the syrinx may be drained surgically and drainage maintained by the use of intramedullary polyethylene tubing. In some patients, the decompression is also said to be of benefit.

Infarction of the Spinal Cord

Infarction of the spinal cord is relatively unusual but may occur with vascular occlusion in patients with syphilitic vasculitis or in diabetics with severe arteriosclerosis. The onset is usually acute and is associated with loss of function below the level of the cord infarction. Acute and chronic vascular lesions of the cord may occur as a complication of x-ray therapy.

Hematomyelia

Acute flexion or extension injuries to the cervical cord occasionally rupture blood vessels within the substance of the cord, causing the formation of a linear or cylindrical blood clot stretching over several segments.

Chordoma

Remnants of the notochord may develop into tumors that occur at the level of the clivus or in the sacral area. The former produces symptoms of compression of cranial nerves and the brain stem. The sacral chordoma produces progressive involvement of sacral nerves.

Epidural Cysts and Tumors

Tumors (neurilemomas, meningiomas, fibromas, lipomas, and metastases) and cysts (dermoid, echinococcal) are not uncommon in the spinal epidural space. They usually grow slowly and produce:
1. Nerve root or girdle pains, with pressure on emerging spinal nerves.
2. Progressive neurologic signs of cord compression, including paraparesis and bladder dysfunction.

Diagnosis is established by myelography. Surgical decompression is imperative in all patients with cord compression. Prognosis for return of function is excellent if decompression is carried out before paraplegia occurs.

Extramedullary Tumors

Extramedullary tumors of the cord are clinically indistinguishable from epidural tumors.

Intramedullary Tumors

Astrocytomas are the most frequently encountered intramedullary tumors of the spinal cord, but ependymomas are not uncommon, particularly in the lowest portion of the cord and the cauda equina. Intramedullary tumors affect:
1. The corticospinal tracts, usually producing asymmetrical progressive spastic paraparesis.
2. The anterior horn cells, producing weakness, wasting, and fasciculation of muscle supplied by the cells at the level of the tumor.
3. The cortical control of bladder function, resulting in increasing urgency and later in incontinence of micturition.
4. The decussating sensory fibers sub-serving the mechanisms of pain and temperature, with loss of these modalities in the dermatomes corresponding to the level of the tumor.

Diagnosis and treatment are the same as for extradural tumor. Gliomas cannot usually be removed surgically and should be treated by irradiation.

SPINAL ROOTS, PLEXUSES, AND PERIPHERAL NERVES

DEGENERATIVE ARTHRITIS OF THE SPINE

Cervical Spondylosis

Cervical spondylosis is a chronic, progressive, degenerative process of the cervical spine manifested by degenerative changes in the intervertebral discs, thickening of the anulus fibrosis, and osteoarthritic changes in the vertebrae, the adjacent vertebral joints, and interpeduncular surfaces. Symptoms of pain, paresthesias, or weakness in the neck or arm are usually produced when osteophytes project into the spinal canal or the intervertebral foramina and compress adjacent spinal arteries or nerve roots. Many patients have radiologic changes without neurologic signs or symptoms. To confirm the diagnosis of root disease caused by cervical spondylosis, characteristic changes on cervical spine films should be demonstrated. These include narrowed disc spaces, vertebral deformities, and projection of osteophytes into the neural foramina on oblique views. In addition, there is often straightening of the cervical lordotic curve.

Treatment. Treatment, particularly of acute exacerbations, includes cervical traction, analgesics, and muscle relaxants. Equipment is available for home application of regular cervical traction. A physical therapist or properly trained nurse can be very helpful in establishing a home treatment program. A properly adjusted cervical collar also may be helpful. Skilled application of these measures can produce substantial symptomatic improvement in many patients.

Lumbar Osteoarthritis

Osteoarthritis of the lumbar spine is very common, especially in older age groups, and usually is asymptomatic. Caution must be exercised in attributing neurologic symptoms to this disorder. When present, neurologic signs are produced by generation and herniation of an intervertebral disc or by compression of vessels and nerve roots by large osteophytes. X-ray films show an advanced degree of degenerative change. Electromyography may be used to demonstrate denervation potentials in affected muscles.

Treatment. Therapy consists of administering analgesics and muscle relaxants and advising the patient to sleep on a firm mattress. Lumbosacral traction and a back brace may be of value in some patients. Bed rest with pelvic traction may be necessary during severe exacerbations. If significant motor or sensory deficits are progressive, the possibility of more serious disease, such as disc or cord tumor, should be considered.

DISORDERS OF THE VERTEBRAL COLUMN

Herniated Intervertebral Discs

The majority of disc herniations occur in the lower lumbar and lower cervical areas.

Pathology. The intervertebral disc consists of an inner gelatinous nucleus pulposus surrounded by a fibrous anulus fibrosis. There is a progressive loss of water content in the nucleus fibrosis with increasing age, and as the disc decreases in width, there is a bulging of the anulus fibrosis. Sudden rupture may occur spontaneously or after trauma, which may be relatively minor, and the protruded contents of the nucleus may impinge on adjacent spinal nerves or on the spinal cord when rupture occurs in the cervical area.

Clinical Features. Cervical disc herniation produces pain in the dermatomal distribution of the affected cervical nerve, weakness and later wasting of the appropriate muscles, and loss of tendon reflexes (e.g., C5, C6—brachioradialis and biceps reflexes; C6, C7—triceps reflex). Pressure on the cervical cord produces spastic paraparesis and increasing urgency of micturition in response to the development of a small spastic bladder.

Herniated lumbar discs usually occur at the L4–L5 or L5–S1 levels. This results in pain in the sciatic nerve that radiates into the appropriate dermatome, weakness of muscles supplied by the involved nerve, and loss of the ankle jerk. Movements of the lumbar spine are restricted, and there is spasm of the erector spinae with scoliosis. Straight leg raising is limited on the affected side.

Treatment. Patients with early disc disease should be treated with strict bed rest, heat, analgesics, and corticosteroids to reduce edema in the compressed nerve root (e.g., dexamethasone in an initial dose of 40 mg. and decreasing by 5 mg. each day). Recurrence of symptoms or failure of medical treatment is an indication for myelography to localize the site of herniation and for possible surgical treatment.

PLEXUS SYNDROMES

Brachial Plexus Birth Injury

Injury to the upper brachial plexus (Erb's paralysis), lower plexus (Klumpke's paralysis), or the entire plexus (Erb-Klumpke paralysis) has been described. Erb's paralysis produces a characteristic posture of the affected limb, which is adducted and internally rotated at the shoulder. There is paralysis of the deltoid, supraspinatus, infraspinatus, biceps, brachialis, and brachioradialis muscles. Klumpe's paralysis produces weakness and atrophy of the forearm flexors and the small muscles of the hand.

Brachial Plexus Neuropathies

The brachial plexus is vulnerable to injury by stabbing or gunshot wounds and from contact sports injury in which there is sudden widening of the angle between the head and the point of the shoulder. Dislocation of the head of the humerus may also damage the brachial plexus on the axilla.

Infiltration of the lower plexus by neoplasm, particularly by a bronchial carcinoma arising in the apical area of the lung, results in Pancoast's syndrome. This is characterized by pain down the medial aspect of the arm (C8, T1), wasting of the small muscles of the hand, and a Horner's syndrome. The nerve roots of the brachial plexus are occasionally involved by viral infections. Brachial neuritis is characterized by the sudden onset of pain in the affected dermatome, muscle weakness and wasting, and the appearance of typical vesicles if the virus is that of herpes zoster.

Treatment. Traumatic injury to the brachial plexus demands prompt attention by a qualified surgeon. Other conditions are treated medically. Analgesics for pain and physical therapy are important for treating the reversible form.

Lumbosacral Plexus

The signs and symptoms are pain, paresthesias, and weakness of the pelvic girdle or lower extremities in the distribution of the affected nerve roots. The problem may be produced by trauma, inflammation, neoplastic infiltration, or ischemia. Therapy depends on the nature and location of the lesion. Plexus lesions may be difficult to differentiate from cord or root lesions.

PERIPHERAL NEUROPATHIES

Hereditary Neuropathies

Hereditary neuropathies are all uncommon neurologic diseases. The most common is chronic interstitial hypertrophic polyneuropathy, which is a slowly progressive disease involving the limbs and associated with marked hypertrophy of the peripheral nerves. A similar hypertrophy is seen in the even rarer condition of heredopathia atactica polyneuritiformis, or Refsum's disease, in which the enlargement of the peripheral nerves is associated with progressive deterioration hearing, retinitis pigmentosa, development of polar cataract, and mild cerebellar ataxia. Refsum's disease is a metabolic abnormality in which there is an excess of 3,7,11,15 tetramethylhexadecanoic acid (phytanic acid) in the serum of affected persons.

Mild peripheral neuropathies have been described in families with alpha-lipoprotein deficiency and in those with hypobetalipoproteinemia. Familial forms of amyloid neuropathy are also described.

It is also believed that familial hyperlipidemias may be associated with a mild peripheral neuropathy. Many of these patients are also mildly diabetic, and it is difficult to determine whether or not the peripheral neuropathy is diabetic peripheral neuropathy or is caused by the hyperlipidemia.

Infectious Neuropathies

Bacterial Neuropathy. Diphtheria may cause neurotoxic peripheral nerve damage. Usually the cranial nerves are also involved. Leprosy is associated with focal-sensorimotor neuropathy caused by bacterial invasion of the nerves.

Viral Neuropathy. Causes include herpetic infections, infectious mononucleosis, measles, mumps, infectious hepatitis, Coxsackie infections, and so forth. Herpes zoster produces a characteristic pattern of pain and vesicular skin lesions along the distribution of a cranial or spinal nerve that is typically unilateral. Neuropathies may occur in association with other viral diseases, as just above.

ACTH or steroids may be useful in the treatment of herpetic facial nerve palsy. If there is involvement of the eye, ophthalmologic consultation should be obtained. With supportive care, most viral neuropathies resolve in a few days or weeks.

Acute Postinfectious Polyradiculoneuropathy (Landry-Guillain-Barré Syndrome)

DEFINITION. An acute, symmetrical, predominantly motor polyradiculoneuropathy, usually occurring after an infectious process.

ETIOLOGY. A history of an antecedent viral infection may be obtained in approximately half of the patients. It is postulated that this is a secondary immunologic condition arising after a viral infection because of an immunologic cross-reaction involving the protein in the virus membrane and protein in the peripheral myelin sheath.

PATHOLOGY. An autoimmune reaction that affects the Schwann cells is responsible for the maintenance of peripheral nerve myelin. This results in the destruction of myelin around ventral nerve roots, causing impaired axial conduction at that site. The demyelination is followed by a severe inflammatory response around the ventral nerve root and the removal of damaged myelin by macrophages. Recovery occurs following regrowth of myelin from surviving Schwann cells. If there is delay in recovery, there may be some destruction of the underlying axons, and chromatolysis and later destruction of the anterior horn cells in the spinal cord may occur.

CLINICAL FEATURES. The onset of the peripheral neuropathy is usually acute and is associated with some paresthesias in the lower extremities. In a few hours this is followed by lower limb weakness that ascends symmetrically to involve the trunk and the arms. In about 25 per cent of patients, the weakness will remain in the lower extremities. In others, it becomes more generalized, and cranial nerve involvement may occur. Bilateral involvement of the seventh cranial nerve is the most common sign when cranial nerve involvement is present.

Sensory symptoms are usually subjective. In many patients, some patchy sensory change may be found on examination. Respiratory involvement occurs in severely affected patients, and there is an added risk of aspiration pneumonia because of bulbar paralysis. Recovery occurs in the majority of patients over a period of several weeks to several months. About 10 per cent make an incomplete recovery and show chronic symmetrical peripheral neuropathy with muscle wasting and fasciculations.

DIFFERENTIAL DIAGNOSIS. Other conditions to be considered are:

1. Acute anterior poliomyelitis. Paralysis usually occurs with fever. The paralysis is asymmetrical, and there is an early pleocytosis in the cerebrospinal fluid.

2. Botulism. This condition begins with cranial nerve and pupillary involvement occurring before the onset of respiratory and limb paralysis.

3. Diphtheritic polyneuropathy. This condition also begins with cranial nerve involvement. It does not present with *symmetrical* polyneuropathy.

4. Acute transverse myelitis. There is usually marked sensory loss below the level of the lesion with an abrupt change to normal above the lesion.

EVALUATION. Cerebrospinal fluid is usually normal and shows minimal pleocytosis, usually less than 10 cells per ml., all of which are mononuclear cells. There is a characteristic elevation of protein content during the third week, when the protein may gradually increase to several hundred mg. per 100 ml.

Tests of respiratory function should be carried out for all patients in serial fashion when the disease appears to be active, in an attempt to anticipate respiratory insufficiency.

TREATMENT. All patients should be observed closely and moved to an intensive care unit at the first signs of respiratory insufficiency. Respiratory assistance should be carried out using the pressure ventilator

as soon as respiratory insufficiency develops, and assistance may have to be maintained for several weeks in some patients. The potential value of corticosteroids is currently under critical review.

Metabolic-Toxic Neuropathies

Alcoholic Neuropathy. Alcohol produces a distal symmetrical neuropathy that usually begins in the lower extremities and later involves the upper limbs. It appears first as a sensory neuropathy, but when severe, there may be motor involvement as well. Therapy includes abstinence from alcohol, a nutritious diet, supplementary thiamine (50 to 100 mg. per day), and other B-complex vitamins in therapeutic doses.

Carcinomatous Neuropathy. Carcinomatous neuropathy is a toxic rather than a metastatic effect of carcinoma. Typically, it presents as a symmetrical peripheral neuropathy. The neuropathy usually improves if the cancer is responsive to therapy.

Chemical Neuropathy. Industrial, agricultural, and household chemicals such as methylbromide, organophosphates, orthocresyl phosphate, and many others may damage peripheral nerves. In most instances of acute or chronic poisoning, peripheral neuropathy is only one part of a complex of neurologic manifestations. Careful investigation of work and leisure time exposure to chemicals is essential in pinpointing the specific agent. Guidance about specific therapy should be obtained from a poison control center or from an appropriate medical text.

Diabetic Neuropathy. This rather frequent complication of diabetes mellitus may produce either a distal symmetrical or an asymmetrical single or multiple mononeuropathy. The symmetrical type is usually mild and may be asymptomatic until detected by the examiner, or it may be associated with paresthesias, including a burning sensation of the feet. Symptoms may be worse at night. Vibratory and position sense may be reduced, and ankle jerks are reduced or absent. The mononeuropathic variety may involve the sciatic or lateral femoral cutaneous nerve and the peroneal, median, or other nerve trunks. It produces pain, paresthesias, and often weakness in the affected area. Therapy includes close control of the diabetes, analgesics for pain, and physical therapy if motor involvement is present. Supplementary B-complex vitamins may be given but may do little to alter the course.

Diabetic amyotrophy is less common than diabetic neuropathy and is a combination of nerve and muscle involvement. The manifestations include weakness and wasting of the muscles in the lower extremities, especially the thighs, sometimes accompanied by pain and paresthesias. Treatment is similar to that of diabetic neuropathy.

Heavy Metal Neuropathies. Lead and other heavy metals may produce peripheral neuropathy. This variety of neuropathy should be suspected in persons with occupational exposure to such metals. The primary therapeutic approach is to remove the heavy metal from the body by the use of chelating agents or other measures.

Hyperuricemia. Hyperuricemia is a rare cause of neuropathy. Therapy consists of analgesia and maintaining a normal uric acid level over an extended period of time by the use of uricosuric agents.

Nutritional Neuropathy. Inadequate intake or absorption, or both, of vitamins B_1, B_2, B_6, and B_{12} or of pantothenic acid may contribute to the development of peripheral neuropathy. The basis for the nutritional neuropathy may be cancer, hyperemesis gravidarum, severe starvation, chronic alcoholism, impaired intestinal absorption, or bizarre dietary patterns. The typical picture is that of symmetrical distal sensory deficit, with motor manifestations in more severe forms. Distal deep tendon reflexes are diminished or absent, and calf tenderness may occur along with numbness, paresthesias, and weakness. Pyridoxine, B_{12}, and pantothenic acid deficiencies often involve the central nervous system as well as the peripheral nerves. Panthothenic acid may be associated with unpleasant paresthesias and burning of the feet. Pyridoxine deficiency may cause seizures in the neonatal infant. B_{12} deficiency can lead to subacute combined degeneration.

Therapy is directed toward oral or parenteral replacement therapy with B-complex vitamins. Except for addisonian pernicious anemia, B-complex deficiencies usually occur as multiple rather than single deficiencies. The oral replacement route is appropriate except in situations in which an absorptive defect has been demonstrated. During the initial phase, the therapeutic dose should be several times the recommended daily dietary allowance. The recommended daily allowance is listed in Table 48–19.

Uremic Neuropathy. Uremia may occasionally be associated with peripheral neuropathy. The neuropathy is usually distal and may begin by distressing burning of the feet, progressing to numbness, paresthesias, and weakness. In adddition to control of the uremia, high doses of B-complex vitamins and an analgesic combined with a phenothiazine if pain is present are usually effective.

Vascular Neuropathies

The vasa nervorum may be involved by arteritis in connective tissue disorders such as polyarteritis nodosa or systemic lupus erythematosus or following x-irradiation. The pattern is usually that of single or multiple peripheral nerve involvement. Irradiation neuropathy may appear as long as 20 years after receiving x-ray therapy. The treatment is directed toward the primary disease plus use of analgesics and other supportive measures.

Amyloidosis and Neuropathy

Both primary and secondary amyloidosis may be associated with chronic peripheral neuropathy caused by deposition of amyloid in nerve trunks. The distribution is symmetrical, and there may be palpable enlargement of some nerves. Cranial neuropathy may also be present. Nerve involvement is more common if other organs such as the heart, tongue, and skin are also sites of amyloid deposition. There

TABLE 48–19. RECOMMENDED DAILY DIETARY ALLOWANCE OF B-COMPLEX VITAMINS

	Thiamine	Nicotinic Acid	Vitamin B_6	Vitamin B_{12}
Children	1.1 mg.	15 mg.	1 mg.	2 mcg.
Adults	2 mg.	20 mg.	2 mg.	2 mcg.

is no specific therapy other than control of the primary disease in secondary forms of amyloidosis.

Entrapment Neuropathies

Carpal Tunnel Syndrome. Compression of the median nerve as it passes beneath the flexor retinaculum at the wrist is a common cause of pain and weakness in the hands. The condition is frequently encountered in industrial workers and is not infrequent in patients with hypothyroidism, diabetes mellitus, and rheumatoid arthritis.

CLINICAL FEATURES. The early symptoms of pain and paresthesias in the thumb and index and middle fingers are followed by pain in the forearm and upper arm. Discomfort is worse at night. Muscle atrophy of the thenar eminence is a late complication. The diagnosis is established by demonstration of prolonged distal latency on median nerve stimulation.

TREATMENT. Patients with early impairment are frequently relieved by injecting 40 mg. of methylprednisolone in 1 per cent lidocaine beneath the flexor retinaculum around the nerve. When injection fails, the pressure on the nerve should be relieved by surgical incision of the flexor retinaculum.

Entrapment neuropathy may be seen in other sites, such as the tarsal tunnel and the ulnar notch. In the latter instance, fibrous thickening may be palpated in the ulnar notch. Management is similar to that described for carpal tunnel syndrome.

PERIPHERAL PAIN SYNDROMES

Causalgia

This condition occurs when there is incomplete severance of a peripheral nerve, particularly the median nerve. Injury results in cross-stimulation between sensory and autonomic fibers and in intermittent pain and excessive sweating in the distribution of the affected nerve. Causalgia responds to sympathectomy or excision of false neurones at the site of nerve injury.

Meralgia Paresthetica

This condition is characterized by pain or paresthesias, or both, in the distribution of the lateral cutaneous nerve of the thigh. It usually occurs in persons who have sudden loss of weight or in diabetics, but it can also occur in young and otherwise healthy people, especially following prolonged exercise. Examination shows hypalgesia to pinprick over the affected area on the lateral aspect of the thigh and tenderness on palpation of the nerve as it enters the thigh just medial to the anterosuperior iliac spine below the inguinal ligament. There is usually prompt and permanent relief when the nerve is injected at that point with 40 mg. of methylprednisolone in 2 ml. of a local anesthetic.

DISEASES OF THE MYONEURAL JUNCTION AND SKELETAL MUSCLE

Polymyositis

Definition. Polymyositis is an acute, subacute, or chronic inflammatory disorder of skeletal muscle that occurs in childhood or throughout adult life. It is characterized clinically by weakness, especially of proximal limb and girdle muscles, and in some patients is accompanied by skin rash (dermatomyositis).

Etiology. The cause of polymyositis is unknown, but multiple hypotheses have been proposed. Virus-like particles have been found in association with affected muscle, although their relationship to the disease remains to be established. Lymphocytes from the blood of polymyositic patients are toxic for cultured muscle cells, suggesting a cell-mediated immune process. Infection with toxoplasmosis has also been suggested.

Clinical Features. The most characteristic feature of polymyositis is weakness in the hips, thighs, shoulders, and upper arms. The onset may be sudden (i.e., within a few days) or gradual. Patients complain of difficulty arising from a sitting position, getting out of the bathtub, combing their hair, or climbing stairs. In the acute form, there may be muscle tenderness and even myoglobinuria. In the chronic form, pain is typically absent. Muscle wasting becomes apparent as the disease progresses but is not an early feature.

Skin rash, when present, may vary in appearance but typically is erythematous to bluish in appearance and is seen on the eyelids, cheeks, or pretibial surfaces. Erythema of the dorsal surfaces of the interphalangeal joints and fingers, the periungual areas, and the extensor surfaces of the elbows and knees also occurs and is a useful diagnostic sign.

Diagnostic Procedures. Elevation of serum concentrations of enzymes found in muscles, i.e., creatine phosphokinase (CPK), aldolase, glutamic oxaloacetic transaminase (GOT), and lactic dehydrogenase (LDH), is typically present. The level of enzyme elevation correlates roughly with disease activity and is a useful method to help monitor clinical progress and response to therapy.

Muscle biopsy is usually positive and shows patches of interstitial inflammatory infiltrate along with abnormalities of size and configuration of muscle fibers.

Electromyography (EMG), which is usually abnormal, reveals a myopathic pattern with increased insertion potentials, decreased amplitude of action potentials, increased numbers of polyphasics, and spontaneous discharge at rest.

X-ray studies are helpful, in that pulmonary infiltrates may coexist. Calcification of subcutaneous tissue and muscle may be demonstrable, particularly in children.

Treatment. Corticosteroids (nonfluorinated) are the mainstay of drug therapy. For the acute and subacute forms of the disease, 60 to 80 mg. per day of prednisolone is recommended for at least a month. If clinical improvement has been observed, the dose can then be gradually decreased every 2 to 4 weeks by 5 mg. per day until a dose of 20 mg. per day has been reached.

Serum creatine phosphokinase (CPK) levels and reproducible measures of muscle strength should be used to monitor progress. Clinical regression after dosage reductions have begun may require maintaining or increasing the prednisolone dose temporarily. Alternate-day double-dose steroid therapy may be instituted when the daily dose has been reduced to 20 to 25 mg.

Immunosuppressive drugs (methotrexate, cyclophosphamide and 6-mercaptopurine) have been used for patients unresponsive to steroids. These drugs (investigational) should be instituted by a neurologist or rheumatologist experienced in the treatment of polymyositis.

Physical therapy is fully as important as drug therapy. In the acute phase, emphasis is on passive range of motion exercises and measures to prevent shortening of muscles and contractures. In the subacute and chronic stages, and especially as clinical improvement begins, the emphasis should shift to more active exercises designed to promote the gradual return of muscle strength.

Myoglobinuria

Myoglobinuria occurs when a large number of muscle cells break down and release their intracellular contents into the extracellular fluid. Muscle enzymes such as CPK, aldolase, LDH, and SGOT are released along with myoglobin and other intracellular components. Serum proteins bind myoglobin to a limited degree, and myoglobin is quickly filtered by the kidney and appears in the urine as a burgundy to brown pigment. Hemoglobin, by contrast, is bound to haptoglobin and is cleared from the serum more slowly. Table 48–20 lists criteria for making a presumptive differentiation between hemoglobinuria and myoglobinuria. Definitive confirmation is by

TABLE 48–20. DIFFERENTIATING BETWEEN HEMOGLOBINURIA AND MYOGLOBINURIA

Determination	Hemoglobinuria	Myoglobinuria
Color of urine	Red to brown	Red to brown
Urine test for occult blood	Positive	Positive
Urine microscopic exam	RBC's if urinary tract bleeding; no RBC's if intravascular hemolysis	No RBC's
Color of centrifuged serum	Pink if intravascular hemolysis	Clear
Serum CPK	Normal	Marked elevation

spectrophotometric examination of the urine. The maximum absorption band for myoglobin is 58 nanometers.

The immediate clinical concern in the presence of myoglobinuria is acute renal failure with hyperkalemia. Urine output needs to be monitored carefully for 3 to 4 days after the episode of myoglobinuria. Dialysis may be necessary for patients with severe disease, although most do well on careful control of fluid and electrolyte balance.

The variety of causes of myoglobinuria are listed in Table 48–21.

Muscular Dystrophy and Related Inherited Disorders

Definition. These are inherited diseases of muscle that are believed to be due to as yet unidentified metabolic abnormalities affecting the muscle cell. Muscular dystrophies may be divided into two subgroups, conditions without myotonia and conditions with myotonia (Table 48–22)

Treatment. There is no specific treatment for any of the muscular dystrophies. Patients should be kept in the best functioning state by long-term physical therapy. In later stages, respiratory infections may be fatal and should be treated promptly.

Myotonic atrophy sometimes responds to quinine, procaine amide, or phenytoin.

Muscle Diseases Due to Known Metabolic Abnormalities

Myopathies have been described in patients with hyperthyroidism, hypothyroidism, hyperparathyroidism, hypoglycemia, and Cushing's disease. Exophthalmic ophthalmoplegia is a condition of exophthalmos with paralysis of extraocular muscles that occurs as a rare complication of primary hyperthyroidism. It may also occur in patients with myasthenia gravis associated with hyperthyroidism. The presence of myasthenia gravis should be suspected if the edrophonium (Tensilon) test is positive.

Phosphorylase Deficiency. The myopathy of myophosphorylase deficiency (McArdle's disease) is associated with an abnormality of glycogen metabolism and accumulation of glycogen in muscle fibers. The patient presents with muscle cramping that occurs after exercise. The condition begins in childhood and persists throughout life. Myoglobinuria has been reported after prolonged exertion. The diagnosis is established by demonstrating lack of increase in lactic acid in an exercised limb. Muscle biopsy shows the presence of excess glycogen in muscle fibers and the absence of muscle phosphorylase. A similar myopathy has been described in phosphofructokinase deficiency.

OTHER DISEASES OF THE MYONEURAL JUNCTION

Botulism

This condition, which carries a high mortality, is the result of blocking of neurotransmission by the exotoxin or *Clostridium botulinum*. The organism multiplies under anaerobic conditions in contaminated canned foods that are usually home prepared. After ingestion, the exotoxin pre-

TABLE 48–21.   CAUSES OF MYOGLOBINURIA

Exertional myoglobinuria:
  Anterior tibial syndrome
  Prolonged exercise
  Prolonged or recurrent seizures
Idiopathic acute rhabdomyolysis
Hyperthermia (heat stroke, anesthesia)
Ischemia with acute necrosis of muscle
Polymyositis, acute phase
Trauma (crush injuries)
	Metabolic/toxic:
	  Alcoholic myopathy
	  Amphotericin B therapy
	  Barbiturate overdose
	  Carbon monoxide poisoning
	  Diabetic acidosis
	  Drug withdrawal in chronic abusers:
	    Alcohol
	    Barbiturates
	    Heroin
	  Hypokalemia
	  Hypothermia
	  McArdle's syndrome (phosphorylase deficiency)
	  Prolonged coma
	  Succinylcholine therapy

TABLE 48–22.   MUSCULAR DYSTROPHIES

Condition	Inheritance	Age of Onset	Clinical Features	Remarks
WITHOUT MYOTONIA				
Pseudohypertrophic (Duchenne)	Sex linked, recessive	0–4 years	Waddling gait, wheelchair often by age 10 years, generalized involvement including heart muscle; death may occur by age 15–20 years but some live longer	CPK elevated, ECG often abnormal
Benign X-linked (Becker)	Sex linked, recessive	6–16 years	As above, wheelchair 18–22 years, death 25–35 years	CPK elevated, ECG often abnormal
Facioscapulohumeral (Landouzy-Déjerine)	Autosomal dominant	Children, teens	Progressive wasting of facial muscles and shoulder girdle muscles, does not usually affect span of life	A few later develop lower limb-girdle weakness
Limb-girdle dystrophy (Erb)	Autosomal recessive	Children, teens	Lower limb girdle, upper limb girdle weakness	Some may be indistinguishable from progressive muscular atrophy
Distal type (Gowers)	Autosomal recessive	Children, teens	Slow wasting distal muscles	Rare, some probably myotonic dystrophy without myotonia
Ocular	—	—	—	Probably does not exist
WITH MYOTONIA				
Myotonic dystrophy (atrophy)	Autosomal recessive	Children, teens, adults	Proximal or distal wasting, myotonia, frontal balding, cataracts, testicular atrophy, cardiac involvement	Probably combined neurogenic and dystrophic condition, biopsy shows both neuropathic and myopathic changes, ECG often abnormal
Myotonic congenita (Thomsen)	Autosomal recessive	Childhood	Hypertrophy may be present, myotonia worse in cold temperatures, no wasting of muscle	Myotonia tends to lessen with age, biopsy normal.
Paramyotonia	Autosomal	Childhood	Stiffness, weakness or paralysis often after exposure to cold, no atrophy	Biopsy normal, is a form of periodic paralysis

vents the release of acetylcholine at the presynaptic membrane.

Symptoms occur within a few hours of ingesting food. The initial diplopia is followed by paralysis of bulbar muscles that may proceed to a fatal respiratory paralysis.

Treatment consists of respiratory assistance, using a mechanical respirator. Polyvalent botulinum antitoxin should be given after testing for serum sensitivity. Guanidine given through a nasogastric tube may be effective.

Myasthenia Gravis

Myasthenia gravis is a condition in which there is progressive weakness, paresis, or paralysis of voluntary muscle after exercise, followed by recovery of strength at rest.

Etiology and Pathology. Myasthenia gravis is believed to be caused by a defect in neuromuscular junction transmission, probably due to the blocking of acetylcholine receptors at the postsynaptic membrane. There is some evidence that these receptors are blocked by circulating antibodies to receptive protein that may be forming in the thymus gland. If this theory is correct, myasthenia gravis should be classified as an autoimmune disease.

Clinical Features. Myasthenia gravis is a relatively rare condition and is often misdiagnosed as anxiety neurosis or depression in patients with mild symptoms. It is a sporadic disease with a somewhat higher incidence in families and is more common in women. The late onset myasthenia is more common in the male. Myasthenia gravis may be classified into four grades, as follows:

1. *Ocular myasthenia.* This condition is confined to one or more extraocular muscles. It is associated with the production of diplopia and in some cases with ptosis, which becomes increasingly severe in the afternoon and evening.

2. *Mild generalized myasthenia.* This condition often begins with ocular myasthenia and progresses to mild and generalized involvement of muscle. Patients in this category are able to function relatively normally.

3. *Severe generalized myasthenia.* This is a more rapidly progressive form of myasthenia gravis with severe generalized involvement of muscle. The patient is unable to function normally and leads a severely restricted existence. There is an ever present danger of crisis.

4. *Myasthenic crisis.* This may be defined as severe generalized myasthenia with respiratory insufficiency.

Deterioration in the myasthenic patient tends to occur within the first year or 18 months after developing the disease. After that time, patients tend to remain stabilized in the same category of myasthenia gravis.

Differential Diagnosis. A number of conditions may be present with a myasthenic-like picture. These include thyrotoxic myopathy, histochemical hemiplegia, lupus erythematosus, and polymyositis.

Evaluation. Edrophonium (Tensilon) is an extremely rapidly acting anticholinesterase drug when given intravenously. When testing patients, a weak muscle group should be selected for observation and the degree of weakness determined in the pretest state (e.g., the degree of ptosis, the degree of diplopia, or the ability of the patient to bite the tongue blade). The Tensilon test is performed by injecting 2 mg. of Tensilon intravenously. The patient is observed for 30 seconds for any side effects, such as excessive salivation, sweating, or tachycardia. If these do not occur, a further 8 mg. of Tensilon is given. Patients with myasthenia gravis show a dramatic increase in strength of the affected muscles within 20 to 30 seconds. The increase in strength lasts for only a few minutes.

Electromyography in Myasthenia Gravis. There is a characteristic line of amplitude of the muscle action potential on repetitive stimulation of the nerve at the rate of 2 per second. This defect can be corrected by rest or by injection of edrophonium (Tensilon).

All patients with myasthenia gravis should have x-rays of the chest to exclude the possibility of thymic tumor or thymic hyperplasia. They should also receive full investigation for concomitant thyrotoxicosis or lupus erythematosus.

Patients with respiratory involvement should have daily respiratory function tests to detect an early increase in respiratory muscle involvement.

Treatment. Therapy is as follows:

1. Patients with thymic tumor should have the tumor removed surgically because of the potential neoplastic properties.

2. Any concomitant metabolic abnormality or autoimmune disease should be treated.

3. Patients with mild myasthenia gravis can be treated in an outpatient setting by use of anticholinesterase drugs. The patient should be given 15 mg. of neostigmine or 60 mg. of pyridostigmine every 4 hours during the day. At the next office visit, the patient should be given a Tensilon test immediately before the next dose of anticholinesterase drug is scheduled. If the Tensilon test is positive, the patient can take more of the oral preparation; if it is negative, there is no point in increasing the dosage of the oral anticholinesterase. The frequent use of the intravenous Tensilon test prior to the oral dose of anticholinesterase preparation allows the physician to prescribe the optimum dose of preparation for the patient.

Some 50 per cent of patients show good response to oral anticholinesterase drugs.

Those patients who show some improvement may experience further improvement with the addition of ephedrine, 25 mg. three times daily, and potassium chloride, 0.5 mg. three times daily, to their therapy. The muscarine-like side effect of anticholinesterase drugs, including colic and diarrhea, are very troublesome in some patients and may be reduced by the use of small doses of atropine (1 mg. three times daily).

Patients with severe myasthenia gravis should be admitted to the hospital for initial treatment, and the amount of the anticholinesterase drug should be governed by the results of the Tensilon tests.

Corticosteroids may be used in patients with severe generalized myasthenia. However, it is recommended that the administration of these drugs should be considered after consultation with a physician who is familiar with the use of corticosteroids in the treatment of myasthenia gravis.

The place of thymectomy in treating patients with myasthenia gravis remains controversial. There is a tendency to perform thymectomy in the early stage of the disease in patients who have obtained maximum benefit from the use of anticholinesterase drugs and corticosteroids but whose symptoms are not well controlled.

Myasthenic crisis is a medical emergency that should be treated in an intensive care unit. It is imperative to treat the respiratory insufficiency or failure as the first priority, and patients should be intubated and placed on a mechanical respirator. Myasthenic crisis should be treated by a team consisting of a specialist in respiratory diseases, an anesthesiologist, and a physician who is familiar with the handling of medications used in this condition.

Myasthenia Syndrome with Cancer (Lambert-Eaton Syndrome)

Failure of release of acetylcholine may occur as a nonmetastatic complication of neoplasia. Most cases occur in patients with bronchial carcinoma, but other neoplasms may cause this condition. Patients present with easy fatigability and symmetrical weakness of limb girdle muscles. The diagnosis is established by electromyography, which shows a poor response to supramaximal stimulation. Repetitive stimulation at 20 Hz. shows a gradual facilitation of evoked responses.

Treatment consists of removal of the neoplasm when resection is possible. There is improvement in strength following use of guanidine, 125 mg. daily, increasing to a maximum of 900 mg. daily.

Tick Paralysis

Both wood ticks and dog ticks may attach themselves to human skin. The adult female tick liberates a toxic substance that is believed to block release of acetylcholine at the myoneural junction. The condition presents as a rapid generalized paralysis, and respiratory muscles may be involved. There is rapid recovery when the tick is removed.

Hypokalemic Periodic Paralysis

This disorder is inherited as an autosomal dominant trait. The attacks usually begin between the ages of 10 and 25 years, often following trauma, exercise, exposure to cold, or a high carbohydrate meal. The weakness often occurs on awakening. The paralysis is generalized, but the respiratory muscles are spared. The duration of the attack is from 6 to 24 hours. Frequency varies from one attack per week to one per lifetime. Abortive attacks producing weakness in one limb or muscle group may occur and are usually of brief duration. The clinical phenomena are due to passage of potassium ions into the muscle fibers with hyperpolarization. Some cases are associated with a defect in carbohydrate metabolism, and sporadic cases have been observed in hyperthyroid patients. Attacks can be precipitated by thiazides and intravenous glucose.

Evaluation. Laboratory studies show an elevated white blood cell count (polymorphonuclears) during an attack, low serum potassium levels, electrocardiographic changes compatible with hypokalemia, and decreased amplitude of action potentials with increased numbers of polyphasics on electromyography.

Treatment. Treatment consists of administration of 5 to 15 grams of potassium chloride during the attack. Prophylaxis includes avoidance of high carbohydrate meals, use of a low sodium diet, and, for patients with recurrent attacks, administration of spironolactone, 100 to 200 mg. per day.

AUTONOMIC DYSFUNCTION

Raynaud's Disease and Raynaud's Phenomenon

Raynaud's disease is characterized by sympathetic vasomotor hyper-reactivity to cold, and emotional stimuli that occurs in the upper extremities. It is seen primarily in women and usually begins in the teens or twenties. Patients experience pain and paresthesias in the fingers and observe that color in the fingers changes from white to blue to red. Ulcers on the fingers are rare.

Raynaud's phenomenon is a similar physiologic manifestation but occurs at any age and is a manifestation of another disease process that has already appeared or is still clinically unrecognized, such as progressive systemic sclerosis, systemic lupus erythematosus, or dysproteinemia. It also occurs in pneumatic drill operators, in patients who have suffered other kinds of trauma, and in patients with thromboangiitis obliterans.

Treatment should focus on minimizing factors that trigger the vasospastic response, such as protection from cold, dealing with emotional factors, and avoiding trauma. Cervical sympathectomy is usually not very effective. Drugs such as reserpine and methyldopa may afford some benefit.

Disturbance of Bowel and Bladder Control

Trauma, tumors, multiple sclerosis, irradiation, congenital malformations, or other noxious processes that damage neural tissue may also involve autonomic fibers. Disturbances of bladder and bowel function are the usual clinical manifestations.

Therapy is directed toward maximizing partial function, when present, i.e., bethanechol chloride (Urecholine) for a partially denervated bladder. When function is destroyed, substitute methods of control, such as surgical diversion, ileal conduit, and so forth, have to be employed.

SUPPLEMENTARY REFERENCES

1. Chusid, J. G.: Correlative Neuroanatomy and Functional Neurology. 16th Ed. Los Altos, Cal., Lange Medical Publications, 1976 (contains a collection of useful neurologic illustrations and diagrams to assist in the localization of neurologic lesions).
2. Gardner, E.: Fundamentals of Neurology. A Psychophysiological Approach. 6th Ed. Philadelphia, W.B. Saunders Co., 1975 (a summary of basic anatomy, physiology, and chemistry of the nervous system written for clinicians).
3. Gilroy, J., and Meyer, J. S.: Medical Neurology. 2nd Ed. New York, The Macmillan Co., 1975 (a comprehensive textbook on neurology).
4. Mayo Clinic and Mayo Foundation: Clinical Examinations in Neurology. 4th Ed. Philadelphia, W.B. Saunders Co., 1976 (describes in detail the neurologic history, physical examination, and various neurodiagnostic procedures).

Chapter 49

NUTRITION

by KATHARINE A. MUNNING,
and L. J. FILER, JR.

Nutritional problems in the United States are primarily those of overconsumption and undereducation in proper eating habits. Malnutrition (faulty nutrition) is prevalent in American society, and improper diet has been connected with six of the leading causes of death in the United States: heart disease, stroke and hypertension, cancer, diabetes, arteriosclerosis, and cirrhosis of the liver. Of these, arteriosclerotic heart disease, diabetes, hypertension, and cancer account for approximately two-thirds of all deaths in the United States today.

Nutrition has been cited as one of the most important components of preventive health care. Breslow[7d] indicates that seven health-related behaviors have more impact on our health than all of the medical innovations that have been developed since the turn of the century. Four of these seven behaviors are related to nutrition: (1) limiting alcohol consumption to one to two drinks per day, (2) eating three meals daily without eating between meals, (3) eating breakfast, and (4) keeping weight within normal range. The other three health behaviors are: (1) participating in regular physical exercise, (2) getting seven or eight hours of sleep, and (3) not smoking cigarettes. A white male who follows all of these behaviors will live 11 years longer than a person who follows three or less of them. Since 1900, all developments in medical care have added less than 4 years to the life expectancy of men 45 years of age.

Hegsted[7d] has asserted that everything that is known about the killer diseases indicates that it would be wise for Americans to modify their diets. Americans should eat less food in general and specifically should consume less meat, fat (especially saturated

fats and cholesterol), salt, and sugar. They should also increase their intake of unsaturated fats, dietary fiber, fruits, vegetables, and whole grain cereals. Health risks are high with our present diet, and there are no identifiable nutritional risks associated with changing the American diet to meet the recommendations of Hegsted.

The family physician possesses a unique opportunity to ensure proper dietary patterns in his patient population. The nature of his practice—continuing, comprehensive family care with an emphasis on prevention and early intervention—allows the family physician to educate patients concerning individualized nutritional recommendations to promote health and, when necessary, to manage illness. To determine the nutritional needs of his patients, the physician must gather a baseline of data about the dietary habits and physical condition of the patient (Table 49–1). These data can then be reviewed for risk factors and other signs of "malnutrition."

THE LIFE CYCLE AND NUTRITION

Food consumption (eating) usually occurs in conjunction with social groups. It is associated with a wide variety of learned attitudes and responses toward the preparation, selection, and consumption of both individual food items and combinations of items. Behavior modification directed toward changing these learned dietary habits requires sensitivity, not only to existing behaviors but also to the priority that these behaviors have in the patient's life and that of the family unit. Because the majority of eating patterns are learned within the fam-

TABLE 49–1. DATA FOR THE DETERMINATION OF NUTRITIONAL STATUS

Historical Data

A. Food intake pattern:
1. Number of meals and snacks
2. Weekdays versus weekends
3. Ethnic, religious influences
4. Location of meals (home, restaurant, etc.)
5. Social/psychologic importance of food to the patient and family unit
6. Recent changes in intake pattern
7. Use of supplements (vitamin/mineral preparations or special food products)
B. Resources:
1. Facilities available for preparation and storage of foodstuffs
2. Source of foodstuffs (grocery store, garden, etc.)
3. Use of community nutrition programs:
   a. Food stamps
   b. Supplemental food programs
   c. Meal programs (i.e., Meals on Wheels)
4. Approximate weekly expense for foodstuffs
C. Alterations in nutritional habits:
1. Physician-prescribed diets – date, type, compliance
2. Self-prescribed diets – date, type, compliance
3. Involvement in "diet groups"
D. Approximate daily dietary intake:
1. Methods of data collection:
   a. 24 hour recall of food intake
   b. Daily food diary – written record for specified length of time
2. Evaluation for healthy eating habits:
   a. Moderate intake of sodium (8 grams of salt per day)
   b. Moderate intake of cholesterol, saturated fats (300 mg. per day of cholesterol)
   c. Moderate intake of energy (calories) – avoidance of foods that contain *only* calories
   d. Adequate intake of dietary fiber
   e. Moderate use of alcohol, caffeine

Biochemical Data

A. Hemoglobin/hematocrit (especially children and elderly)
B. Serum cholesterol
C. Triglycerides and electrophoresis for type of hyperlipoproteinemia (if history warrants – 14 hour fasting)
D. Blood glucose (fasting)
E. Uric acid
F. Serum albumin (especially elderly and hospitalized patients)

Clinical Signs

A. Blood pressure
B. Adiposity
C. Specific signs of nutritional deficiencies

Anthropometric Data

A. Height
B. Weight
C. Skin fold thickness
D. Head circumference (infant and child)

ily system, the family physician is in a unique position to guide the families under his care, especially those with infants and children, toward the formation of healthful nutritional habits. The family physician has the opportunity to provide a higher quality adulthood and old age for his patient population by continuing guidance concerning sensible nutritional habits and by health/illness care. The following sections will describe important nutritional considerations that the family physician can utilize at specific intervention points throughout the life cycle.

MATERNAL NUTRITION

Concepts about maternal nutrition have ranged from "semi-starvation is a blessing in disguise" to "the pregnant woman is eating for two, so requirements are doubled." Neither extreme presents a realistic format for optimal nutritional care of the pregnant patient. The alterations in nutritional requirements from the normal nonpregnant state are simple and logical.

Energy (caloric) requirements are increased by approximately 300 kcal. per day. Therefore, if your patient is consuming the recommended level of 2000 kcal. per day in the nonpregnant state, she would be advised to consume approximately 2300 kcal. daily during her entire pregnancy (the requirement does not change during the various trimesters). These requirements are based on moderate activity expenditure that in some instances may not be the patient's norm of behavior. Modification in energy intake will need to be made for the extremely active or the sedentary individual. Energy requirements should be met through the consumption of foods of high nutritional quality.

Protein intake must be adequate during pregnancy to meet the demands for (1) the rapid growth of the fetus, (2) the enlargement of maternal tissue (uterus, mammary glands, and placenta), (3) the increase in maternal circulating blood volume with the concurrent need for increased synthesis of hemoglobin and plasma proteins, and (4) the formation of amniotic fluid and energy storage (fat) for labor, delivery, and lactation.

Because of the risk to the mother and fetus from an inadequate intake of protein, a generous allowance is recommended—an increase of 30 grams daily. In other words, the recommended allowance for a nonpregnant 25 year old woman is 46 grams of protein daily; while pregnant, the same person would require 76 grams of protein per day.

Because of their integral roles in metabolism and tissue growth, the requirements for calcium, iron, vitamin A, the B-complex vitamins, and vitamin C are increased during pregnancy. Vitamin D is the only nutrient whose requirements remain unchanged.

To provide optimal nutrient intake during pregnancy, a recommended daily food pattern would be:

Milk or milk substitute (cheese, ice cream, yogurt, and so forth). Three to 4 servings, 8 ounces (240 grams) each, as a good source of protein, calcium, and phosphorus. One ounce (30 grams) of cheese is equivalent to one 8 ounce (240 ml.) serving of milk.

Meat, fish, eggs (other high biologic value protein sources). At least 4 ounces (120 grams) per day as a source of essential amino acids and minerals.

Vegetables. Cooked or raw, at least 3 servings (1/2 cup each) per day. The frequent use of dark green leafy and yellow vegetables, sources of vitamin A and folacin, is recommended.

Fruits. At least 2 servings, with 1 serving being a citrus fruit, strawberries, or tomatoes as a good source of vitamin C.

Breads, cereals, starches. Three to 4 servings of whole grain or enriched bread, cereals, or starch items as a source of B-complex vitamins.

Butter or fortified margarine. As desired to meet energy requirements and as a source of essential fatty acids.

Fluids. Eight to 10 glasses of water or other non-fattening fluids.

Consideration must be given to antenatal factors that might affect the nutritional status of the nonpregnant woman and consequently both maternal health and the development of the fetus. For instance, the woman who had previously taken oral contraceptives may enter pregnancy with lowered plasma levels of folacin and vitamins B_6 and B_{12} because of drug-nutrient interactions. Neither the mechanism of these interactions nor the subsequent effects upon the mother and fetus have been defined. Therefore, these altered laboratory findings need to be handled conservatively.

Other factors of nutritional concern during pregnancy are those involving the overweight or underweight woman, the adolescent, the mother with a past history of unfavorable obstetric outcome, and the person with pre-existing medical conditions. These women warrant careful dietary instruction to assure optimal maternal health, fetal development, and obstetric outcome.

Supplementation

The prescription of multivitamin supplements for pregnant women has almost become a routine practice. Clinical studies, however, have failed to indicate that the use of such supplements in themselves has influenced the outcome of pregnancy. Vitamin supplements should not be considered innocuous medications, especially to be taken ad libitum. Because of the possible serious side effects of high doses of vitamin A (central nervous system anomalies in experimental animals) and vitamin D (hypercalcemia with craniofacial abnormalities and supravalvular aortic and pulmonic stenosis in human infants), careful consideration should be given to the type of supplement to be prescribed for the patient. The recommended daily intake of vitamin A is 6000 I.U. (a 20 per cent increase over the nonpregnant state). An adequate intake of these vitamins can be obtained by daily consumption of 1 serving (1/2 cup) of a dark green or yellow vegetable and 1 quart (1 liter) of vitamin D enriched milk. The physician should ascertain whether the patient uses over-the-counter vitamin/mineral supplements and should educate the patient concerning the potential hazards of indiscriminate use of supplements, especially during pregnancy.

Because of the stress that pregnancy places on the maternal hematologic system and because the normal American diet provides inadequate intake of iron and folacin, both of these nutrients need to be supplemented to prevent iron deficiency anemia and megaloblastic anemia. Recommendations for supplementation of iron and folacin are:

1. All pregnant women should receive ferrous iron in doses of 30 to 60 mg. daily during the last two trimesters of pregnancy

and the period of lactation. For the mother who does not breast-feed her infant, supplementation should be continued for 2 or 3 months after delivery to replenish maternal iron stores.

2. Folacin should be supplemented in doses of 200 to 400 micrograms daily as prophylaxis against folacin deficiency. A physician's prescription will be required to comply with the Food and Drug Administration (FDA) regulations for preparations containing more than 100 micrograms of folacin.

The use of these supplements can give the physician or patient, or both, a false sense of security regarding the adequacy of nutrient intake, as an adequate intake of protein and energy cannot be assured by the use of vitamin/mineral supplements.

Weight Gain

The definition of optimal or ideal weight gain during pregnancy has been subject to much debate. Current authorities consider that total weight gain during pregnancy should range from 10 to 12 kg. (22 to 27 pounds). The normal curve of weight gain during pregnancy is sigmoid in shape, with little gain during the first trimester (approximately 1 kg., or 2.2 pounds), then rapid increase during the second trimester, followed by a slight reduction in rate during the third trimester (0.3 to 0.4 kg., or 0.8 pound, per week).

During pregnancy, it is important to obtain accurate periodic maternal weights. Insufficient weight gain may jeopardize both maternal health and fetal development. Excessive weight gain needs to be evaluated for differentiation between fluid retention and tissue accumulation. Weight gain due to excessive tissue accumulation has not been convincingly correlated with toxemia or other complications. Obviously, the possible relationship to obesity must be considered.

Overweight women sometimes view pregnancy as an opportunity to lose their excess weight. If energy intake is reduced to the extent that maternal fat deposits are broken down to meet energy requirements, ketosis and acetonuria occur. A recent study has suggested that maternal acetonuria from any cause may be correlated with decreased intellectual ability of the offspring. The energy intake of healthy women should not be reduced below 36 kcal. per kg. of pregnant weight in order to ensure adequate utilization of protein. Therefore, weight reduction regimens should *not* be instituted until pregnancy has been terminated.

Sodium

Sodium metabolism during pregnancy has been studied extensively, and it has been shown that sodium retention for both maternal and fetal needs seems to be a normal physiologic happening. Therefore, the use of routine sodium restriction during pregnancy is of unknown value. Moderate sodium restriction (no added salt), although not an effective factor in the prevention of toxemia is probably harmless because of the renin-angiotensin-aldosterone mechanism for conserving body sodium. However, severe sodium restriction could lead to electrolyte imbalance and compromise the intake of other essential nutrients because of unpalatability or limited food choices. Sodium restriction and the concurrent prescription of diuretics is a potentially dangerous practice and has no place in the management of normal pregnant patients.

Morning Sickness

Although gastric hypomotility during pregnancy may allow for more complete digestion, it probably contributes significantly to the common complaint of nausea. Certain foods have been identified as frequently aggravating nausea and vomiting. These include fatty foods, fried foods, and large amounts of fluids, especially with meals. Relief is achieved by withholding fluids for 1 to 2 hours before and following meals and by consuming a dry diet. This diet includes dry breads, such as Melba toast or Saltines; baked potatoes; and dry toast served at 2 hour intervals, in addition to meals containing foods of low fat content.

Constipation

Constipation can become a significant problem as the pressure of the enlarging uterus in the lower intestine makes elimination more difficult. Increased fluid intake, physical exercise, and the use of laxative bulk foods (whole grain or bran breads and cereals, dried fruits, other fruits, and juices) will help to establish regularity. Laxatives such as mineral oil should be avoided because of their effect on the absorption and utilization of fat-soluble vitamins.

LACTATION

Breast-feeding is the most natural way of providing adequate nutrition for the human infant. The desire of the mother to breast- or bottle-feed will be affected by many factors—one important factor being the advice and attitude of her family physician. Advice concerning the desirability of breast-feeding should start early during prenatal care, and not just before delivery.

From a nutritional point of view, breast-feeding is the preferable method of infant feeding. The advantages of breast-feeding are:

1. The composition of human milk is specifically designed for the human infant and cannot be exactly duplicated in commercial formulas.

2. Due to the presence of various antibodies in human milk, breast-feeding has an immunologic effect against certain infections (poliomyelitis, Coxsackie virus, and enteropathogenic strains of *Escherichia coli*, *Salmonella*, *Shigella*, and other enteric organisms).

3. The most efficient method for reduction of the maternal fat stores of pregnancy is lactation, which utilizes an additional 500 kcal. daily for milk production.

4. Breast-feeding is more economical than bottle-feeding.

5. Overfeeding of the infant is less likely to occur in the breast-fed infant because the mother correctly assumes that her infant is satiated when he stops sucking and swallowing. However, the formula-fed infant is sometimes forced to finish the entire contents of the bottle, as determination of satiation is based upon an empty bottle rather than upon the infant's internal feelings of satiation.

Obviously, not all women can or want to breast-feed, and they should be reassured that formula-fed infants can also maintain an adequate nutritional intake.

Nutritional Requirements

Besides utilizing an additional 500 kcal. per day, lactation also requires an increase in protein intake of 20 grams daily. Intake of proteins of high biologic value (meat, fish, eggs, milk, and so forth) should be stressed. Vitamin and mineral needs are also increased, as both the mother and infant are being nourished from the mother's daily intake of nutrients.

As the composition of human milk is largely water, the secretion of milk requires sufficient maternal fluid intake. The recommended intake of fluids should total 2 to 3 quarts (2 to 3 liters) per day of water or other beverages such as juice, tea, or milk.

If the mother's diet is deficient in quantity and quality, the volume of the milk will be reduced, but the quality (composition) of the milk will remain the same by drawing on the nutritional reserves of the mother. For example, if the calcium intake of the mother is inadequate, calcium will be drawn from her bones, the organic matrix of the bones will be broken down, and, if the condition persists, permanent consequences to the maternal skeletal system can result. Therefore, the physician needs to communicate at periodic intervals with the lactating mother to ascertain her continued intake of an adequate diet.

Contaminants of Human Milk

Human milk can become less than the perfect infant food when contaminated with toxicants ingested by the mother. These toxicants can be medicinal, such as antibiotics, phenytoin, thiazides, and so forth; social, such as alcohol; and ecologic, such as the chemicals DDT, the PCB's and the PBB's. These substances may cause a variety of responses in the lactating mother and in the infant. For example, oral contraceptives not only decrease milk production but the circulating metabolites may have a long-term effect on the developing endocrine system of the suckling infant.

Differing opinions exist as to when the maternal use of medications may contraindicate breast-feeding. Arena[2] advises against the use of the following types of drugs while breast-feeding: any drug or chemical in excessive amounts, diuretics, oral contraceptives, atropine, reserpine, steroids, radioactive preparations, morphine and its derivatives, hallucinogens, anticoagulants, bromides, antithyroid drugs, anthraquinones, dihydrotachysterol, and antimetabolites. Most experts agree that breast-feeding is contraindicated in mothers with illnesses requiring large doses of any drug or in those taking new and unusual drugs. However, the vast majority of mothers requiring medications should be encouraged to breast-feed.

INFANT NUTRITION

The human infant is a dependent organism who must rely upon parents, family, or surrogates for survival. Adequate nutrition is an essential component for normal growth and development, both physically and psychologically. Furthermore, early nutritional experiences contribute to the development of food choices and eating practices that will extend into the adult years. The family physician has the opportunity to temper the cultural habits and societal pressures toward undesirable dietary patterns by giving the mother healthful advice, so that she can guide her infant into an adulthood uncomplicated by obesity, hypercholesterolemia, or other nutritionally related conditions.

Growth and Development

Growth and development of the infant progress rapidly after birth. Normal growth and development are significantly dependent upon the nutritional status of the infant. Nutritional status is related to numerous factors, including the dietary intake of essential nutrients. The infant born with a poor nutritional rating needs special dietary attention to achieve normal growth and central nervous system development.

In the human infant, approximately two-thirds of the brain cells are present at birth and the remaining one-third develop during the first year of life. Almost 80 per cent of total brain weight is gained by 1 year of age. Malnutrition during this critical period results in suboptimal growth and development of the brain and central nervous system.

Energy intake is an important consideration for normal growth and development. The Food and Nutrition Board of the National Research Council, National Academy of Sciences, advises an energy intake of approximately 120 kcal. per kg. of body weight at birth, reducing this to 100 kcal. per kg. by the end of the first year. Determination of the adequacy of energy intake is relatively simple. After gathering data from the parents or caretaker about the 24 hour dietary intake of the infant, utilize Table 49-2 and calculate the average daily energy intake; then divide by weight (kg.) of the infant. An example of this calculation is shown in Table 49-3.

The other essential nutrients are of equal importance during this rapid growth period. Because of the formation of new tissue, protein intake is especially important. The Food and Nutrition Board of the National Research Council advises providing 2.4 grams of protein per kg. per day during the first month, with a gradual decline to 1.5 grams per kg. per day by the sixth month. The calculation for adequacy of protein intake can be accomplished in the same manner as that described for energy intake.

Breast-Feeding Versus Formula-Feeding

Human milk is specifically designed for the human infant. Any substitute feeding (commercial formula, cow milk, and so forth) should be similar in composition (protein, fat, and carbohydrate content) to human milk. The percentages of energy from protein, fat, and carbohydrate present in human milk, whole milk, skim milk, and commercial formula are shown in Table 49-4. To approximate human milk, skim milk would have to be extensively altered because of its excessive protein content and inadequate energy and fat content. Skim milk should not be used in an infant's diet until the second year of life. A simple formula that is acceptable to the infant is 13 ounces (390 ml.) of evaporated milk, 19 ounces (570 ml.) of water, and 1 ounce (30 ml.) of corn syrup.

Of the various milks available, the following are not recommended for infant feeding: (1) raw milk (not pasteurized), (2) filled milk (combination of skim milk and vegetable oil), (3) imitation milk (often inferior to milk and very low protein content), (4) condensed milk (added sugar), and (5) skim milk before 2 years of age (inappropriate ratio of protein, fat, and carbohydrate).

There are a wide variety of commercial formulas available for use by the normal infant or the child with specific problems that benefit from changes in composition of the formula. Information about these formulas can be obtained from the manufac-

TABLE 49-2.   AVERAGE ENERGY AND PROTEIN CONTENT OF FOODS
COMMONLY CONSUMED BY INFANTS

Milk/Formula°	Energy— kcal./100 ml. (3 oz.)	Protein— gm./100 ml. (3 oz.)
Human milk	75	1.1
Whole milk	66	3.5
Skim milk	36	3.6
2% milk	59	4.2
Commercial formula	67	1.5–1.6

Food†	kcal./100 gm. (7 tbsp.)	gm./100 gm. (7 tbsp.)
Baby foods (strained):		
Cereal:		
Dry, mixed with milk	109	5.2
(one part cereal with six parts milk)		
Wet, packed with fruit	78	1.0
Egg yolk	195	9.7
Fruit juice	57	0.04
Fruit	67	0.4
Dinners:		
High meat	82	6.2
Meat and vegetables	55	2.1
Desserts	85	1.1
Meats	104	13.7
Vegetables	42	1.7

° Data from Fomon, S. J.: Infant Nutrition. 2nd Ed. Philadelphia, W. B. Saunders Co., 1974.
† Data from Gerber Products Co., 1976.

turing firms. These formulas have been designed to closely approximate the composition of human milk.

Because of the necessity for proper distribution of carbohydrate, protein, and fat, there is adequate reason to delay the change in the infant's diet from human milk or formula (commercial or evaporated milk) to whole milk until the child is receiving approximately two jars of commercially strained food or the equivalent of mashed table foods.

Introduction of Solid Foods

It seems relatively unimportant whether an infant's entire energy intake is derived from formula or partly from other sources as long as he consumes adequate energy (calories), all the essential nutrients, and a reasonable distribution of energy from protein, carbohydrate, and fat. There has been no substantiation of the opinion that if the infant isn't offered a variety of strained foods during the first months of life, he will be reluctant to accept new foods later on. Rather, supplementary foods are added according to the age, level of development, and growth demands. The Committee on Nutrition of the American Academy of Pediatrics states that a normal infant can thrive on human milk or formula accompanied by necessary vitamin supplementation for 2½ to 3 months.

At 10 to 12 weeks, the oral musculature plus salivary and intestinal enzymes are

TABLE 49-3.   ENERGY INTAKE OF 6 MONTH OLD INFANT WEIGHING 8 KG.

	Amount Consumed	Energy (kcal.)
Milk, whole	840 ml. (28 oz.)	560
Strained fruit	133 gm. (1 jar)	89
Strained dinner	133 gm. (1 jar)	73
Cereal with milk	100 gm.	108
		830
		104 kcal./kg.

TABLE 49–4. PERCENTAGE OF ENERGY FROM PROTEIN, FAT, AND CARBOHYDRATE °

	Desirable Range	Type of Milk			Commercial Formula
		Human	Whole	Skim	
Protein	7–16	7	20	40	9
Fat	30–55	55	50	3	48–50
Carbohydrate	35–65	38	30	57	41–43

° Data from Fomon, S. J.: Infant Nutrition. 2nd Ed. Philadelphia, W. B. Saunders Co., 1974.

usually adapted to the utilization of solid foods. Biting movements begin at about 3 months of age. Chewing movements begin at about 7 to 9 months of age, and foods such as zwieback and chopped meat can then be added. A general guideline to follow regarding the introduction of supplementary foods is if the infant is hungry after the daily consumption of 1 quart (1 liter) of formula, semisolid foods are needed to satisfy hunger.

An adequate intake of all essential nutrients can be provided by human milk or commercial formulas without use of solid foods; thus, there appears to be no advantage to introducing solid foods during the first 6 months of life. If solid foods are introduced, intelligent choices must be made to combine these with other energy sources (formula, human milk) so that the proper distribution of carbohydrate, protein, and fat can be maintained. For example, most infants on whole milk require the inclusion of solid food with low protein content. Because the protein content of human milk is significantly less than that of whole milk, the breast-fed infant may have a marginal intake of protein if the food choices are low in protein and are substituted for a significant quantity of human milk. Detailed lists of the nutrient composition are available upon request from the manufacturers of infant food.

Other considerations to remember when advising mothers about the introduction of solid foods into the infant's diet are (1) homemade strained foods prepared with care can be as nutritious and economical as commercial items; (2) proper dilution of cereals includes mixing with milk or formula, not water; and (3) the early introduction of solid foods is not a sign of achievement or advancement of the child. The primary consideration is the digestive capabilities of the developing intestine of the infant.

Supplementation

Recommendations for supplements for the normal full-sized infant are summarized in Table 49–5. It is wise to caution parents about the use of vitamin supplements. They should be carefully instructed concerning the proper dosage, as hypervitaminosis A and D can and have occurred in infants because of the overutilization of supplements.

Iron

Because of its integral role in the hemoglobin molecule and iron-containing oxidative enzyme systems, iron is an essential element. Iron stores present at birth are often depleted by 6 months of age, thus potentiating the development of iron deficiency anemia if adequate iron intake is not attained.

The recommendations for iron increase from 10 mg. daily at 0 to 6 months to 15 mg. daily at 6 months to 1 year. This allowance is related to rate of growth and not to body size. The increase in the recommended intake relates to increased need caused by the decrease in body stores of iron.

Attention must be directed to the infant's intake of food items that are sources of iron. Table 49–6 outlines the iron content of various foods commonly fed to infants in the United States. Note that both human and cow milk are poor sources of iron, while commercial formulas fortified with iron provide a substantial amount of this element. Studies of consumption patterns have shown that relatively few infants receive iron-fortified formulas after 5 months of age, yet this age represents the potentially vulnerable period for the infant, who is rapidly utilizing his iron stores. The family physician can intervene either by prescribing iron supplements or by strongly advising

TABLE 49–5. SUPPLEMENTATION FOR THE NORMAL, FULL-SIZED INFANT°

Energy Source	Vitamin A	Vitamin D	Vitamin C	Iron
Human milk		400 I.U.		10–15 mg.
Cow milk:				
Whole, fresh fluid		400 I.U.†	20 mg.	10–15 mg.
Whole, powdered		400 I.U.†	20 mg.	10–15 mg.
2%	500 I.U.†	400 I.U.†	20 mg.	10–15 mg.
Skim, fresh fluid	500 I.U.†	400 I.U.†	20 mg.	
Skim, powdered			20 mg.	
Evaporated			20 mg.	10–15 mg.
Goat milk, fresh fluid‡		400 I.U.†	20 mg.	10–15 mg.
Commercially prepared formula				10–15 mg.†

Fully breast-fed infants should receive supplements of fluoride (0.25 mg. per day).

°Modified from Fomon, S. J.: Infant Nutrition. 2nd Ed. Philadelphia, W. B. Saunders Co., 1974.
†Supplement only if product is unfortified.
‡Folacin, 50 micrograms, daily should be given.

the continuation of iron-fortified formula or iron-fortified cereal until the child is 1 year of age.

Most commercially prepared strained foods, except for iron-fortified cereals, contain only a small amount of iron. As research continues, the future food market may supply the consumer with products con-

TABLE 49–6. AVERAGE IRON CONTENT OF FOODS FED TO INFANTS IN THE UNITED STATES

Milk/Formula°	Mg. of Iron/100 ml. (3 oz.)
Human	0.05
Cow milk	0.05
Iron-fortified formula	0.9–1.3
Formula unfortified with iron	0.05

Food	Mg. of Iron/100 gm. (7 tbsp.)
Infant cereals:†	
Iron-fortified (dry) mixed with milk (one part cereal with six parts milk)	7.0
Wet, packed with fruit	5.0
Strained and junior foods:†	
Meats:	
Liver	3.9
Other meats	1.3–1.5
Egg yolks	2.8
Dinners:	
High meat	0.7
Vegetables and meat	0.5–0.7
Vegetables	0.4
Fruits	0.2–0.3
Desserts	0.3

°Data from Fomon, S. J.: Infant Nutrition. 2nd Ed. Philadelphia, W. B. Saunders Co., 1974.
†Data from Gerber Products Co.

taining absorbable forms and adequate amounts of iron. At present, the infant who consumes several jars of strained foods daily is not necessarily receiving an adequate intake of iron, as these foods average 1.5 mg. of iron per jar (7 tbsp.).

Certain factors concerning the absorption and excretion of iron must be considered. Age, iron status of the individual, condition of the gastrointestinal tract, amount and form of iron consumed, and other components of the diet all affect the absorption of iron. Iron from food is usually less bioavailable than iron from inorganic salts. Iron from vegetable sources tends to be absorbed less well than iron from animal sources. The iron present in egg yolk seems to not only be poorly absorbed but may also interfere with the absorption of iron from other food sources. Ferrous sulfate is absorbed better than other compounds, such as sodium iron pyrophosphate.

Normal infants lose iron from the gastrointestinal tract in the form of occult blood loss and desquamated intestinal epithelial cells, as well as from the skin and in the urine. An important consideration is the effect that chronic steatorrhea during infancy may have on gastrointestinal loss of iron. Infants receiving a high percentage of energy from whole milk often develop steatorrhea because of the butterfat content. The possibility exists that steatorrhea can be accompanied by increased desquamation of gastrointestinal mucosal cells and thus contributes significantly to the anemia seen in children consuming whole milk as a major energy source.

Infant Nutrition — Long-Term Effects

Numerous viewpoints exist concerning the effects of the early eating patterns of the infant upon the future health status of the adult. Three major areas for concern have been the development of obesity, arteriosclerosis, and hypertension.

It is impossible to say if there are specific infant feeding practices that cause the development of obesity in childhood or adult life. The increased potential for force-feeding the infant who is being bottle-fed may be a factor. If parents are intolerant and insensitive to the appropriate meaning of the crying infant (crying does not always indicate hunger), they often succumb to the temptation to feed the infant to stop his crying. As a result, the infant's sensitivity to his internal physiologic cues of satiation may be altered. The formation of healthful eating habits in the infant should undoubtedly begin early and should be reinforced throughout childhood, adolescence, and adulthood.

The influence of early nutrition on the subsequent development of coronary artery disease has been suggested, but the data are not conclusive. The Committee on Nutrition of the American Academy of Pediatrics recommends that dietary restriction of cholesterol content is *not* applicable for all children. However, those children with Type II hypercholesterolemia, with diabetes mellitus, or with a significant family history of Type II hypercholesterolemia, early heart disease, or diabetes mellitus can benefit from appropriate dietary intervention.

Hypertension and sodium intake are of equal concern to the health of the American public. The Committee on Nutrition of the American Academy of Pediatrics points out that 20 per cent of the children in the United States run the risk of developing hypertension as adults. Genetic factors help identify the population of children at risk. The genetic factors that predispose the infant to this disease cannot be modified; however, the environmental factors that affect blood pressure, such as dietary intake of sodium, can be modified. Infants with a family history of hypertension, myocardial infarction, stroke, or renal disease may benefit from a lowered sodium intake, even though conclusive evidence of the effectiveness of this restriction is not present.

The committee recommends that more information regarding the sodium content of foods be presented to the consumer via nutrition labeling of food products by the manufacturers and increased education programs by qualified health professionals.

CHILDHOOD AND ADOLESCENT NUTRITION

Growth and Development

Both heredity and environment affect the potential of the developing child. Environmental factors such as nutrition are susceptible to change through the use of educational programs initiated at critical periods during the growth process.

Development is an orderly progression that leads to maturity. However, the rate at which an individual proceeds through developmental phases is varied. Therefore, rigid compliance to any standard measurements of growth and development is unwise. The variables that affect the standard nutritional requirements during growth and development are the chronologic age of the child, rate of growth, level of physical exercise, maturational stage, and ability to absorb and utilize nutrients.

Four basic stages of growth in height and weight have been delineated:

Phase I: Rapid growth during infancy.
Phase II: Slow but uniform gain throughout early and middle childhood.

TABLE 49–7. ESTIMATIONS OF NUTRIENT ALLOWANCES DURING LIFE CYCLE°

Age	Energy (kcal./kg./day)	Protein (gm./kg./day)
Birth–1 year	120–100	2.4–1.5
1–3 years	100–95	1.8
3–6 years	95–80	1.8
6–9 years	80–75	1.5
10–13 years	75–60	1.3
Girls:		
14–15	50–45	1.3
16–17	45–40	1.3
18–19	40–35	1.3
Boys:		
14–17	60–65	1.3
18–19	55–50	1.3
Adults	35–40	0.8
Pregnancy	+300	+30 gm.
Lactation	+500	+20 gm.

° Kg. of body weight determined from desirable weights of height-weight charts.

TABLE 49–8. ADEQUATE DIET DURING CHILDHOOD AND ADOLESCENCE

Food	Amount per Day
Milk, milk products	Children – 1 pint to 1 quart (500 to 1000 ml.) Adolescents – 1 quart (1000 ml.) or more
Protein foods – meat, fish, poultry, eggs, or equivalent	1 or 2 servings of 2 to 3 oz. (60 to 90 ml.)
Cereals and breads, whole grain, enriched	4 or more servings
Vegetables	2 servings besides potato
Dark green or yellow	1 serving
Fruits	2 servings
Citrus fruit	1 serving
Butter, margarine	4 teaspoons
Snacks – use foods mentioned above	As required by child

Phase III: Marked acceleration during adolescence.

Phase IV: Gradual decline and cessation of growth.

The recommended nutritional allowances reflect these four phases. Table 49–7 presents an estimation of energy and protein needs throughout the life cycle. Vitamins and minerals are required for normal growth and development, so careful consideration must be given to dietary intake to determine if nutrient requirements are being met or if supplements should be taken. The basic outline of an adequate diet during childhood and adolescence is given in Table 49–8.

The Preschool Child (1 to 6 Years)

At this time the child has entered the period of slower, somewhat erratic growth and has left behind the accelerated growth of infancy. Because of this, the appetite decreases, growth is slow, and sometimes weight may even decrease. The child possibly becomes a little more selective and independent about food; actually, the "won't eat" phase is normal. The normality of these eating patterns needs to be communicated to the parents, along with the warning that overanxious bribing or urging may foster the establishment of improper eating habits. Parents should be reassured that as the child reaches school age, his appetite will improve.

Because they like to identify foods, toddlers seem to prefer simple foods that can be eaten easily with their fingers. The 4 to 5 year old often goes on food jags, and the 5 to 6 year olds are imitators. As eating habits are primarily learned behavior patterns, parents should be counseled concerning the importance of not utilizing foods or mealtimes as scolding, praising, or conflict mechanisms. Rather, food selection and consumption should be exhibited by parents as unemotional, enjoyable, healthful experiences, so that favorable, self-controlling attitudes toward food consumption will be fostered in the child.

The School-Aged Child (6 to 12 Years)

Growth (height and weight) during the school years is slow but steady. Additional height of 10 to 12 inches (25 to 30 cm.) and weight of 30 to 35 pounds (14 to 16 kg.) may be accumulated. Food intake increases in a constant manner. Exposure to the school environment adds some stresses to the nutritional habits of the child. The mealtimes are determined by the school schedule rather than by the individual needs of the child. The child is exposed to numerous alternatives of food choices (cafeteria, vending machines, or food brought from home), which represent varying degrees of nutritional quality. Peer pressure becomes an important factor in food selection and in the establishment of eating patterns. Nutrition education programs by both health professionals and teachers are a necessary component for the acquisition and retention of healthy eating habits.

The Adolescent (12 to 19 Years)

The teenage years represent the second period of rapid growth. The rate of growth varies among individuals. These are often the years of the highest level of physical activity. Teenagers may have either tremendous appetites or rather finicky consumption patterns. The experimentation with independence that is characteristic of adolescence may be reflected in eating patterns and food choices. Preoccupation with body size and form may affect the dieting behaviors of both the weight conscious female and the athletic contender. The family physician must be knowledgeable about the current trends in dieting and should express his professional judgments about these trends through individual or group education programs. Three problem areas in adolescent nutrition will be discussed: the pregnant adolescent, the underweight or overweight adolescent, and nutrition and athletics.

The Pregnant Adolescent. The number of adolescent pregnancies in the United States has risen to the point that more adolescents become pregnant in this country than in any other Western or developed nation. The inherent risks (biologic and psychologic) of adolescent pregnancy are numerous. The greatest biologic risk occurs among those girls who become pregnant before the cessation of growth. Growth and gynecologic maturity are achieved usually at 17 years of age. Before this age, a biologic risk exists and is demonstrated by the higher rates of neonatal, postneonatal, and infant mortality for the offspring of these young mothers. The rates are even higher among adolescents with repeated pregnancies. The incidence of low birth weight babies is also appreciably higher in the adolescent mother, especially in those under 15 years of age. After 17 years of age, pregnancy does not seem to represent any special hazard, as growth has ceased and physical and gynecologic maturity have been reached.

Gynecologic maturation proceeds in an orderly sequence. Similar to linear growth, the rate and nature of this maturation in individual females vary widely. In girls who mature early, menarche occurs during the peak of the prepubertal growth spurt when the skeletal maturation is less advanced than in those girls whose physical development is slower. The early maturer may be able to conceive at an earlier age, even though her skeletal development, specifically her pelvic capacity, is incomplete. If these early maturers become pregnant during the active anabolic stage of linear growth, the additional demands may affect the final adult stature.

The nutritional considerations for the pregnant adolescent center around the need for adequate nutrient intake to promote both optimal maternal linear growth and normal fetal development. Energy needs during this period will parallel the individual growth curve of the adolescent. An additional 300 kcal. per day is recommended for the pregnant teenager. Caloric reduction in the pregnant adolescent would be unwise and potentially harmful to both maternal and fetal growth. Weight reduc-

tion is *not* a component in the prenatal care of an adolescent. The physician needs to stress the importance of *adequate* energy intake for the teenaged mother, who is at an extremely weight conscious age.

Protein intake should be increased by 30 grams per day. Foods containing protein of high biologic value (meat, fish, eggs, poultry, milk) need to be stressed. Protein requirements will vary according to the stage of maturational process—more protein is required during the prepubertal growth acceleration than during the slowed growth rate of puberty. Therefore, the physician needs to make periodic assessments of the pregnant adolescent's diet for adequacy of protein and energy intake.

Surveys have suggested that the dietary intakes of adolescent girls are often erratic and affected by food faddism. Inadequate intakes of calcium, iron, ascorbic acid, and vitamin A have been documented. Therefore, special attention must be given to the adequate intake of all essential nutrients. If appropriate intake of nutrients cannot be achieved, supplements must be given. Iron and folacin supplements should be administered in dosages similar to those given to a nonadolescent pregnant woman.

The psychologic stress of pregnancy to the adolescent may affect her eating habits and food choices. The physician needs to support and counsel the pregnant teenager so that compliance with all aspects of prenatal care, including nutritional recommendations, will be attained.

The Underweight or Overweight Adolescent. A teenager is defined as being underweight when his or her weight is 10 per cent or more below the ideal standard of weight for height and age. Underweight can be due to the inadequate intake of energy and possibly of other essential nutrients over a period of time. Data must be gathered to determine the cause of the inadequate intake, and appropriate intervention methods must be initiated. An uncommon form of undernutrition in the adolescent female is anorexia nervosa, a neurosis reflected as severe malnutrition. These adolescents need to be referred to a mental health agency for treatment.

Approximately 20 per cent of the adolescents in the United States are overweight (obese). Studies have indicated that the obese child and the obese adolescent (after the prepubertal growth spurt) will become obese adults. The incidence of obese parents having obese children is high—80 per cent if both parents are obese, 40 per cent if one parent is obese, and only 8 or 9 per cent if neither parent is obese.

The cause of obesity in the adolescent is varied and has to be approached in an individualized manner. Before management can be determined, historical data need to be gathered about birth weight, age of onset of obesity, rates of growth and maturation, family occurrence of obesity, physical activity level, and the role food plays in the functioning of the family unit. Other data concerning dysfunction within the family; the emotional status of the adolescent; personality characteristics, such as passivity; and body image concepts will also be helpful in determining the appropriate therapy and the probable response of the adolescent to the therapy.

The weight reduction program for the moderately obese adolescent should center around a daily rigorous physical exercise plan and improved eating habits without caloric restriction, in order to assure adequate energy intake for growth. Both the patient and the family unit need to be involved in the definition and implementation of the program. The school physical fitness program or summer camp experiences can be beneficial. An extremely important component for successful weight reduction in the adolescent is the attitude of parents (and other family members), who should not display anxious or punitive overconcern for the teenager's obesity. Studies have suggested that parental preoccupation with weight control in their teenager produces negative effects rather than successful weight reduction and behavior change in eating habits.

The extremely obese adolescent can probably be placed on a weight reduction diet without any resultant impairment in growth. A daily exercise program plus nutrition education concerning proper food choices, serving sizes, and eating behaviors should be stressed. Because of the peer alienation that most obese adolescents feel, family members should be counseled to provide adequate, nonjudgmental support for the teenager. In some communities, self-help groups for obese adolescents are available and should be considered as adjunct therapy.

Nutrition and Athletics

Proper nutrition is an important factor in athletic performance. Surveys have indicated that coaches recommend a wide variety of dietary programs for their young athletes. The fundamentals for a nutritionally sound diet remain relatively simple and straightforward. Special foods and high doses of supplements are unnecessary and expensive and in the case of fat-soluble vitamins are potentially harmful to the athlete.

The essentials for an adequate diet of approximately 2500 calories are outlined in Table 49–9.

The amount of energy necessary to maintain ideal weight can be determined by utilizing standard height-weight charts to determine ideal weight and then multiplying by the energy needed per kg. per day, as depicted in Table 49–7. These figures are based on moderate activity level, so that alterations must be made for increased energy output. Consideration must also be given to the underweight or overweight athlete. Additional servings of a variety of nutritional foods should be utilized to meet the requirements of increased energy expenditure.

Athletic performance does require energy, and the harder and longer muscular work is performed, the more energy is utilized. Sports that are single effort events, such as diving or ski jumping, or are of short duration, such as skiing, hurdle racing, or sprinting, require a very small increase in energy needs, especially if practiced less than an hour a day. Sports that require

TABLE 49–9.   2500 CALORIE DIET FOR ATHLETES

Food	Amount per Day
Milk	4 cups
Protein foods (meat, fish, poultry, cheese, eggs)	5 ounces (150 gram)
Dark green or dark yellow vegetable	1/2 cup serving
Citrus fruit	1/2 cup serving
Other fruits and vegetables	2 servings—1/2 cup each
Bread (enriched or whole grain bread, cereal, potato, starches such as spaghetti, plain desserts)	13 servings
Fats (butter, margarine, salad dressings	10 teaspoons

energy expenditure over an extended period of time, such as middle or long distance swimming, running, and so forth, may increase the need for total caloric intake to 4000 to 5000 kcal. per day, depending on body size and weight.

Protein is a necessary nutrient for increasing muscle mass but does not have to be supplied in the form of supplements or in a particular food item, such as steak. The important point is that proteins of high biologic value (containing all essential amino acids) should be utilized; therefore, milk, meat, fish, poultry, and eggs are good sources of protein.

Water is required by the body for the digestion and utilization of foods, as a transportation medium for nutrients, and to control body temperature through insensible water loss. Dehydration limits the capacity for physical exercise, primarily because of impaired cardiovascular function. Water loss exceeding 10 to 20 per cent of body water can lead to death. Also, heat exhaustion can develop if fluid loss from sweating is not replaced at frequent intervals during physical activity. Replace fluid at a rate of 2 cups of water for every pound (0.5 kg.) of weight lost. This should be replaced on an hour to hour basis. Frequent fluid intake must be emphasized to those on the practice field.

Various methods have been utilized by athletes to "make weight," ranging from crash diets to sweat baths to self-induced vomiting. The hazards of methods that quickly and substantially reduce body water are obvious. Studies show that weight losses up to 5 per cent of body weight that occur in less than 24 hours are apt to not only decrease performance but also to place stress on the cardiovascular system. Any dieting effort should be accomplished over a period of several weeks to several months, depending on the amount of weight to be gained or lost.

Preseason conditioning for the athlete requires an increased energy intake because of the frequent practice sessions and in contact sports for the development of the necessary fat pads as protective layers around internal organs, such as the kidneys. An additional 500 kcal. per day may be needed during preseason training. This requirement will probably decrease when the regular season begins.

The pre-event meal should be eaten about 3 hours before competition, as this will allow for digestion and absorption of nutrients but will maintain satiation because gastric emptying is completed by 3 to 4½ hours. Excessive fat and foods that form gas should be restricted to avoid problems of cramping. Reduction of protein and bulk foods in the pre-event meal will help avoid the necessity for urinary or bowel excretion, especially during a prolonged event. Fluids should be given up until 1½ hours of competition and as needed thereafter to compensate for sweat loss and prevention of dehydration.

Sugar has often been utilized as a quick energy source during athletic events. Although quick energy foods do not seem to affect performance in short-term events, supplements may aid in endurance events. A hypertonic solution of sugar may distend the stomach and cause nausea, cramps, and distention of the small intestine. Also, large amounts of carbohydrate may increase fermentive activity of intestinal flora and result in gas and diarrhea. No more than 50 grams of sugar (3 rounded tablespoons) in solution should be taken each hour. This should be given in diluted form, as water is necessary for the absorption of glucose.

GERIATRIC NUTRITION

Research has generated numerous theoretical explanations for the aging process. Any explanation will need to allow for the individual pathophysiologic, social, environmental, and economic variables in each elderly person's life. Obviously, the nutritional recommendations for the elderly also need to be approached in an individualized manner with focus on specific needs. The assurance of optimal nutritional status during the aging process begins with healthy eating patterns during the prenatal and infancy periods. Nutrition, as an environmental factor, is a health variable over which people have extensive control to alleviate some of the disease present in the elderly.

Determining Nutritional Status

The physical and metabolic changes during old age have not been unequivocally attributed to an unchangeable aging process. For example, as persons age, they usually experience an increase in body fat, a decrease in musculature, and an increase in bone demineralization. These components of aging require consideration of different guidelines for nutritional requirements and drug dosage in the elderly patient. Initially, a nutrition history, including an approximation of the adequacy of intake over a period of time, should be obtained to aid in determination of nutritional status. Elderly persons oftentimes have erratic eating patterns, so analysis of a single 24 hour period would not be representative for determination of adequacy of intake. Dietary studies such as the Ten State Nutrition Survey and biochemical studies have demonstrated that the diets of seemingly normal elderly persons were deficient in protein plus one or more B-complex vitamins, vitamins A and C, iron, and calcium. Therefore, special attention should be given to the *quality* of the diet, as well as to the adequacy of energy intake.

Evaluation of body weight should be made in relation to the standard height-weight tables and to the patient's body composition or ratio of body fat to muscle mass. Instruments such as skin fold calipers are available for the determination of fat thickness. Simple visual observation plus pinching between thumb and forefinger the area over the triceps, subscapular region, and lateral abdominal wall will also supply data about the fat deposition of the person. The accumulation of fat in comparison to muscle provides information about both the nutritional and exercise patterns of the older person.

Laboratory data that are extremely useful in the estimation of the nutritional status of the geriatric patient are the values of hemoglobin, hematocrit, and serum albumin. These values are indicators of possible dietary iron or protein deficiencies. Evidence indicates that well nourished older patients have hemoglobin values in the same normal range as younger adults. Hematocrit values below 40 (in males) and 38 (in females) should be considered abnormal for the elderly person, and dietary deficiency should be considered as a possible cause. The serum albumin level tends to decrease with a marginal protein intake. Levels below 3.5 grams per 100 ml. are considered below normal and indicate decreased intake or utilization of protein or protein losses. Deficient dietary intake should be considered as a possible cause for abnormal laboratory findings, especially for the institutionalized (hospital, nursing home) elderly patient.

Impaired Nutritional Status

The inadequacy of the dietary intake of elderly persons is a consequence of many factors in the United States. These factors include social isolation from a food supply; frequent ingestion of cheap convenience foods (such as bakery and snack items) that are poor sources of protein; loss of teeth, which makes chewing of protein and bulk foods difficult; and the rejection of food by the elderly person as a response to a variety of social stigmata and physical conditions associated with old age in this country. The geriatric patient is also susceptible to the promises of the food faddist and is seduced into senseless expenditures for supplements and youth-restoring foods.

Elderly patients should be instructed about the importance of protein, along with the other essential nutrients. Foods such as milk, meat, eggs, fish, and cheese, which contain high quality protein, should be stressed. Fruits and vegetables are necessary as a source of vitamins and also for bulk to help avoid the problem of constipation. Whole grain or enriched bread should be utilized. Adequate water intake (6 to 8 glasses per day) also helps alleviate constipation and if consumed early in the day will not result in nocturia. The importance of a diet consisting of a wide variety of foods is necessary to stress but often difficult to attain because of the environmental circumstances. Community programs that offer nutritious meals to the elderly at a low cost are widely available.

Osteoporosis in the Geriatric Patient

A common affliction of the elderly is osteoporosis. Osteoporosis must be distinguished from osteomalacia. Osteomalacia is decreased bone density primarily caused by loss of calcium content from the bone matrix. This results from lack of vitamin D and occurs in persons who have poor dietary intake of vitamin D or who have limited exposure to sunshine, such as some institutionalized patients. On the other hand, osteoporosis is decreased bone density without change in the chemical composition (normal protein/calcium ratios). Approximately 6 million spontaneous fractures, resulting from osteoporosis are estimated to occur annually in the United States in persons 45 years of age or older. About 5 million of these fractures occur in women. In fact, osteoporosis is a major orthopedic disorder in 25 per cent of postmenopausal women. Nutritional surveys indicate that approximately 30 per cent of the American population have intakes of calcium below the recommended levels of 800 mg. per day.

The higher incidence of subnormal bone density in women may be due to several nutritional factors:

1. Weight-reducing diets may result in loss of skeletal mass as well as of soft tissue mass. Prevention of this deleterious side effect to weight reduction can be achieved by education concerning the proper intake of calcium or calcium supplementation.

2. Pregnancy may deplete the system of calcium. If this deficit is not adequately replenished by supplements or dietary intake, the depletion could intensify with each subsequent pregnancy.

3. Lactation also places an additional burden on total body calcium supplies. The physician should advise and periodically document adequate daily intake of calcium (1200 mg. daily during lactation).

Consideration must also be given to factors that affect the absorption and retention of calcium. One important factor is the changed calcium/phosphorus ratio of the American diet. This change is undoubtedly due to a variety of factors, one of which is the increased consumption of foods containing added phosphates, such as soft drinks and bakery products. The retention of calcium has been proved to be adversely affected by emotional stress, inactivity, and immobility.

The dietary intake of calcium should not be underestimated as a factor contributing to osteoporosis, as deficient dietary intake of calcium has been documented repeatedly in the elderly population. Effort should be made to assure the adequate intake of 800 mg. per day of calcium by elderly patients to help combat osteoporosis and alveolar bone loss. The role of sodium fluoride in the treatment of osteoporosis is still controversial.

NUTRITIONAL MANAGEMENT IN COMMON DISEASES

The family physician cares for patients presenting with a broad spectrum of disease conditions, some of which may benefit from nutritional management. Obviously not all such regimens or their detailed description can be outlined in this chapter. A wide variety of high quality diet manuals from public health agencies or hospitals are available for this purpose. The remainder of this chapter will describe the important components of the dietary management of diseases most common in family practice.

Patients rarely require care for a single problem. Therefore, treatment priorities must be established for the unique combination of therapies necessary to control the patient's unique combination of problems. The task of coordinating various medications, dietary management, and exercise programs is difficult for both physician and patient. However, the continuity and comprehensiveness of the care in every family practice office allow these treatments to be approached in an empathetic, individual, and family-oriented manner. As with all therapies that require significant behavior change, nutritional treatments will take both time and sharing of information on the part of the patient and the physician. Table

TABLE 49–10 COMPONENTS OF NUTRITIONAL COUNSELING

1. Obtain appropriate diagnostic data to verify the use of nutritional therapy.
2. Explain the pathophysiology of the disease condition and the relationship of the proposed diet to this condition to the patient and to other persons who routinely participate in his nutritional environment.
3. Obtain a data base of information about the patient's current eating patterns. The use of a daily food diary for 1 to 3 weeks is helpful.
4. Establish realistic alterations in eating patterns in conjunction with other required therapies and with the patient's and physician's expectations for outcome. If possible, appropriate family members should be present.
5. If diet therapy is complicated or requires outside assistance, refer to appropriate health professional (registered dietitian or nutritionist, social worker, visiting nurse).
6. Check with the patient at frequent, regular intervals to support and reinforce efforts toward compliance.

Remember that eating habits have become ingrained with time, so that changing these habits will take time and encouragement.

49–10 lists some of the important components for successful nutritional counseling. The interest and attitudes projected verbally and nonverbally by the physician toward the patient and his efforts toward compliance are most important.

Cancer

Cancer is the second biggest killer in the United States. Cigarette smoking is related to 30 per cent of the cases of cancer, and there is now strong preliminary evidence that nutritional imbalances in the diet contribute to at least another 30 per cent of cancers in men and 50 per cent in women. For example, a positive correlation has been found between high fat consumption and cancer of the breast and colon and between a lack of dietary fiber and cancer of the lower intestinal tract. It must be emphasized that correlation does not mean causation; however, proof of definitive causation should not be required before thorough consideration and preventive measures are instituted.

Diabetes Mellitus

Newer concepts in the dietary management of diabetes mellitus stress both the need for individualization of therapy and a concern for preventive measures against commonly occurring disease in the diabetic.

Although some differentiation needs to be made between the dietary management of the insulin-dependent, growth-onset diabetic patient and the maturity-onset, ketosis-resistant diabetic patient, diet is essential in the treatment of both of these types of diabetes. Some principles of nutritional care are common to both types. The diet pattern needs to be adapted to the specific needs of the diabetic patient. These needs may result from the presence of other chronic conditions such as hyperlipoproteinemia or hypertension, which may require additional dietary recommendations. The patient also possesses individual needs concerning the use of certain foods or the frequency of meals because of ethnic, familial, or religious reasons; economic reasons; or reasons relative to food supply available in his environment. All of these needs can carry a high priority with the patient and

have to be considered when establishing the dietary management.

Occlusive atherosclerotic heart disease is a most important cause of morbidity and mortality in the diabetic patient. Therefore, lowering the proportion of dietary fat and cholesterol in the diet may help reduce the predisposition to coronary artery disease, as lowering the fat content of the diet of the diabetic patient increases the percentage of total energy consumed as carbohydrates. The increased carbohydrate content of the diet does not affect diabetic control. This increase in carbohydrate content can lead to a greater degree of diversity of food choices in the diet and thus possibly can improve compliance behavior.

After having identified and discussed the medical, social, and psychologic needs of the patient, the diet (meal patterns, food choices, and so forth) can be determined by the physician, patient, and consultant registered dietitian (if necessary). The exchange list diet pattern has been the traditional tool utilized to instruct the patient with diabetes. This diet plan is only an instructional tool, readily modified to meet the individual needs of the patient rather than requiring that the patient conform to a standardized written format and eating pattern. Above all, the diet should conform to the eating habits of the family and to the patient's own life style (including occupation, recreational habits, and so forth), provided, of course, that these habits are healthful and not contraindicated by the disease. Simplicity of diet prescription is most desirable.

Foods do not have to be weighed, as common serving size measurements (1/2 cup, 4 ounces, 2 tbsp.) are adequate. Concentrated sweets should be avoided as a rule, as they may result in hyperglycemic peaks. However, a piece of birthday cake or consumption of similar foods on special occasions can be included in the diet of diabetic patients. Also, alcoholic beverages in moderation are allowable and can be calculated into food choice lists. Special food products, often labeled diabetic or dietetic, are not required and in the majority of cases are unwise items to include in the diet. These foods are expensive and most are *not* calorie-free, as is assumed. Foods utilized by the rest of the family can usually be consumed by the diabetic patient.

Energy requirements for the patient with

diabetes are based on the same factors as in other persons — age, sex, height, weight, and exercise level. In the insulin-dependent young diabetic patient who is usually underweight, the first priority is to provide adequate energy to promote desirable weight gain and normal growth and development. However, in the patient with maturity-onset diabetes who is usually overweight, the most important consideration is a nutritionally adequate diet restricted in energy to promote weight loss and to protect and improve beta cell function.

The frequency of meals and snacks varies with the person and the type of medication. Patients on insulin or oral hypoglycemic agents require regular spacing of meals to avoid intermittent hypoglycemia. Meal spacing needs to be coordinated with the type of insulin used and its peak action time. The patient being treated by dietary management alone does not have to adhere as closely to an established pattern of meal consumption. Snacks, especially at bedtime, are often essential in the care of diabetic patients, especially children, adolescents, or adults with high energy requirements. The bedtime snack should preferably consist of foods containing protein and fat, such as milk or a sandwich, rather than food items containing primarily carbohydrate, such as fruit juice or crackers. Protein and fat are absorbed and utilized at a slower rate and thus control hypoglycemia in the early morning hours.

During periods of illness, the diabetic patient, especially the insulin-dependent patient, should be advised to consume an equivalent of the carbohydrate content of his usual meals as sweetened beverages such as ginger ale, 7 Up, or fruit juice. This will help combat insulin reaction.

Diverticular Disease

In the early 1970's Burkitt[5] hypothesized that the reduction in dietary fiber of peoples living in developed countries contributed to the increased incidence of diverticular disease, cancer of the colon, appendicitis, gallbladder disease, obesity, diabetes mellitus, and ischemic heart disease. Epidemiologic data indicate that these diseases are almost nonexistent in communities and cultures in which high fiber diets are consumed.

Burkitt demonstrated that an inverse relationship exists between the intake of fiber and intestinal transit time. In contrast to the formed stools passed by persons eating a diet low in fiber content, the persons consuming a high fiber diet tend to pass large, soft, often unformed stools. The effect of dietary fiber in altering stool volume and shortening transit time may be attributed to (1) the water-absorbing properties of fiber, especially of cellulose, (2) the production of volatile fatty acids by bacterial metabolism of fiber, and (3) the sequestering of substances such as bile salts and fatty acids by fiber in the small intestine and their subsequent release and possible cathartic effect in the colon.

As symptoms of diverticular disease are usually relieved by a high fiber diet, patients should be advised to consume raw fruits and raw vegetables in addition to or in lieu of canned or cooked items. Bran cereals and 100 per cent whole wheat bread and cereal products should also be included in the diet. Labels need to be read carefully to ensure that the product is a 100 per cent whole wheat product. Vegetarians tend to consume more dietary fiber than the average American, who may find it difficult to increase consumption of such fiber. Persons who consume extremely high levels of dietary fiber may adversely affect the absorption of nutrients, as various minerals are bound by compounds present in the vegetable and cereal products and consequently decrease absorption.

Hyperlipoproteinemias

Controversy has surrounded the role of cholesterol in the development of atherosclerosis. Ever since an elevated serum cholesterol level was determined to be a risk factor for coronary artery disease, researchers have attempted to describe the mechanism of involvement and the subsequent importance of dietary intervention. Various dietary components and their relationship to serum cholesterol levels have been studied extensively; these include dietary cholesterol, total dietary fat, levels of saturation of dietary fat, and dietary carbohydrate. Several studies have indicated that serum cholesterol levels can be lowered effectively by 8 to 18 per cent by dietary means. To date, one of these studies has conclusively proved that a lowered serum cholesterol level will prevent or delay coronary heart disease. The other risk factors, i.e., hypertension, diabetes mellitus, obesity, positive family history of heart disease, electrocardiographic abnormalities, cigarette smoking, decreased physical activity, and social stress, undoubtedly require control.

Hyperlipoproteinemias occur on a genetic basis, as a seondary component to certain disease states, and from environmental factors such as dietary intake. As such, they will respond to the appropriate dietary management. However, if the condition is secondary to another disease state, the primary disease should be treated before such a diet is prescribed for a patient with hyperlipoproteinemia. Only about 5 per cent of the American public has severe, genetically determined hyperlipoproteinemia. The vast majority of Americans who develop atherosclerosis have mild hyperlipoproteinemias that are primarily diet-induced. These persons usually have cholesterol levels of 220 to 280 mg. per 100 ml. and triglyceride concentrations of 150 to 300 mg. per 100 ml. Although this is a mild form of hyperlipoproteinemia, these persons still run an increased risk of developing coronary artery disease as compared with a person with a serum cholesterol *below 220 mg. per 100 ml.* This mild form is extremely susceptible to dietary treatment.

Types I, III, and V of the hyperlipoproteinemias are rare entities and will not be seen in the average family practice office. Types II and IV are common abnormalities and may be seen frequently in a primary care setting (Table 49–11).

In Type II hyperlipoproteinemia, the beta lipoprotein fraction is increased, resulting in an elevated serum cholesterol level. Type II has also been further subdivided into Type IIa (serum triglyceride levels normal) and Type IIb (serum triglyceride levels elevated). Patients with Types IIa and IIb hyperlipoproteinemia are placed on diets low in cholesterol (100 to 200 mg. per day) and fat (20 per cent total energy). Such a diet differs markedly from that consumed by the average American, i.e., 800 mg. of cholesterol per day with 40 per cent of total energy from fat. Maintenance of ideal weight is a very important constituent of dietary management.

Type IV hyperlipoproteinemia is characterized by increased amounts of normal pre-beta lipoprotein with a high triglyceride content. These patients usually have elevated serum triglyceride levels and elevated serum cholesterol levels and are frequently overweight, have overt diabetes mellitus, or have an abnormal glucose tolerance test. Weight reduction is the most decisive therapeutic approach to Type IV hyperlipoproteinemia. The serum lipid response to weight loss is prompt (within a few days) and provides motivation for continued compliance by the patient. As long as weight loss continues at a reasonable rate of 1 to 2 pounds (0.5 to 1.0 kg.) per week, triglyceride levels will stay reduced. When ideal weight is reached, the diabetes or the abnormal glucose tolerance test will become normalized.

The dietary management of Type IV hyperlipoproteinemia includes:

1. Weight reduction and maintenance of normal weight.

2. If serum cholesterol level remains elevated after normal weight is achieved, a low cholesterol (100 to 200 mg.) diet with 20 per cent of total energy from fat should be used.

3. Sucrose need not be restricted except for its contribution to total energy intake.

4. Alcohol need not be restricted except for its contribution to total energy intake. After normal weight has been achieved, most patients can tolerate small amounts (3 ounces [90 ml.]) of alcohol.

Detailed copies of the dietary treatments to be utilized for patients with the hyperlipoproteinemias can be obtained from the American Heart Association.

Hypertension

Approximately 20 per cent of the adult population (18 to 74 years) suffer from hypertension or hypertensive heart disease. Various dietary treatments have been utilized over the decades, beginning in the 1940's with the Kempner rice-fruit diet that restricted sodium to 200 mg. daily. This extreme salt restriction was found to substantially decrease blood pressure. Obviously, this diet was not only too restrictive to be palatable but was also too restrictive to contain all essential nutrients.

After confirmation of the effect of sodium

TABLE 49-11. CLASSIFICATION OF HYPERLIPOPROTEINEMIAS

Type	Secondary Causes	Clinical Findings	Genetics	Dietary Management	Drug Therapy
Type I: Cholesterol normal or mildly elevated, triglycerides markedly elevated—very rare	None	Fat tolerance abnormal; abdominal pain, may in fact be pancreatitis on some occasions; hepatosplenomegaly; lipemia retinalis	Autosomal recessive: expression in childhood	Caloric restriction to achieve normal weight; then extremely low fat diet (12% of calories from fat)	Drugs neither necessary or effective
Type IIa: Cholesterol elevated, triglycerides normal—common	May be secondary to dietary excess, myxedema, hypothyroidism, myeloma, porphyria, dysglobulinemia, nephrotic syndrome, glycogen storage disease, biliary obstruction	Corneal arcus (25%), tendon xanthoma (5%), xanthelasma (5%), premature coronary atherosclerosis	Autosomal dominant: form appears in childhood; polygenic form appears later in life	Low cholesterol (100–200 mg. per day) with 20–25% of calories from fat	Cholestyramine (note: not established that drug treatment beneficial)
Type IIb: Cholesterol elevated, triglycerides elevated—common	Same as IIa plus obesity, alcohol	Glucose intolerance may be present, tendon xanthomas rare, premature coronary atherosclerosis	Autosomal dominant: onset usually early adulthood; polygenic factors also	Caloric restriction to achieve normal weight, low cholesterol (100–200 mg. per day) with 20–25% of calories from fat	Clofibrate° (note: not established that drug treatment beneficial)
Type III: Cholesterol elevated, triglycerides usually elevated—relatively uncommon	May be secondary to diabetes mellitus, hypothyroidism, myxedema, liver disease	Glucose tolerance often abnormal, fat tolerance often abnormal, xanthomatosis—planar tuberoeruptive, corneal arcus, xanthelasma, peripheral artery disease	Autosomal dominant: and recessive possible	Caloric restriction to achieve normal weight, low cholesterol (100–200 mg. per day) with 20% of calories from fat	Clofibrate°
Type IV: Cholesterol normal or elevated, triglycerides elevated—very common	May be secondary to obesity, alcohol, diabetes mellitus liver disease, nephrosis. oral contraceptives	Glucose tolerance usually abnormal, uric acid often abnormal, hepatosplenomegaly, eruptive xanthomas rare	Autosomal dominant: expression in early adulthood; sporadic forms also	Caloric restriction to achieve normal weight, low cholesterol (100–200 mg. per day) with 20–25% calories as fat	Clofibrate°
Type V: Cholesterol elevated, triglycerides elevated—rare	May be secondary to alcohol, uncontrolled diabetes mellitus, myxedema, pancreatitis, nephrotic syndrome, glycogen storage disease, obesity	Fat tolerance abnormal, glucose tolerance abnormal, pancreatitis, hepatosplenomegaly, lipemia retinalis, xanthomas—eruptive	Autosomal dominant: sporadic forms also	Caloric restriction to achieve normal weight, extremely low fat diet (12% of calories as fat)	Clofibrate,° nicotinic acid (note: drug therapy not usually effective except after weight loss)

° May need to discontinue oral contraceptives (estrogens).

TABLE 49–12. FOOD CATEGORIES CONTRIBUTING TO DAILY SODIUM INTAKE OF THE AVERAGE AMERICAN*

Food Category	Grams of Sodium/Day
Processed meats	1.9
Baked goods	1.8
Processed vegetables	0.6
Processed fruits	0.6
Soups	0.4
Condiments	0.3
Cereals	0.2
Milk products	0.2
Poultry	0.1

*Data from a comprehensive survey of industry on the use of food chemicals generally recognized as safe (GRAS): Table 13: Part A possible daily intakes of NAS Appendix A substances (Group I and II), per food category and total dietary intake, based on food consumption by total sample. National Research Council, 1973.

on blood pressure, the pendulum of treatment swung toward prevention. Researchers then faced the issue of whether or not the high salt content of the American diet was predisposing the population to hypertension. Evidence now seems to indicate that unless a person has a family history of hypertension, there is probably no indication for restriction of salt intake. Salt intake is probably only one of many factors that contribute to the manifestations of hypertension in a person who is genetically predisposed to the disease.

Because of the severe level of sodium restriction necessary to facilitate a significant, stable lowering of blood pressure, dietary management is not the primary choice of treatment of moderate or severe hypertension. However, sodium restriction may be an extremely useful adjunct therapy. Moderate salt restriction to 5 grams per day (the average American intake reaches 6 to 18 grams of salt per day) stabilizes the patient's intake of sodium so that the appropriate antihypertensive medication dosage can be determined more efficiently.

When counseling a patient about sodium restriction, moderation is the primary precept. The sodium in processed and convenience foods constitutes a large portion of the daily sodium intake of the average American (Table 49–12). Certain popular items such as cured meats, sausages and luncheon meats, TV dinners, pizza, canned soups, and

so forth have extremely high sodium contents (Table 49–13). Therefore, complete abstinence from high sodium foods is unrealistic — but *controlled* indulgence can be attained.

The sodium ion is present in other components of our environment in addition to food. Drinking water may contain appreciable amounts of sodium, owing to natural composition or to chemical additives as part of the water softening process. Each state public health department has access to data about the sodium content of public water supplies. Individual wells or water supplies can be analyzed for sodium content.

Medications, either physician-recommended or self-prescribed, may contain significant amounts of sodium. Numerous prescribed drugs or over-the-counter preparations (e.g., Alka Seltzer) as well as home remedies (e.g., sodium bicarbonate) have extremely high sodium concentrations. Information about the sodium content of these preparations can be obtained from the local pharmacist or from the pharmaceutical manufacturer. Other less common sources of high sodium intake are chewing tobacco and cough medicines.

Iodized salt is an important source of iodine in the United States. If salt intake has been decreased or eliminated, the diet needs to be analyzed for iodine content, especially in geographic areas with iodine-deficient soil.

A side effect of the treatment of hypertension with certain agents is hypokalemia. Although potassium supplements are often used, there are natural foods available as alternatives. Bananas, oranges and orange juice, apricots, tomatoes, prunes, dates, dried fruits, dried beans, white and sweet potatoes (especially baked), and spinach are all excellent sources of potassium. Salt substitutes frequently contain potassium chloride compounds.

Patients with hypertension may also have additional problems, such as diabetes mellitus, obesity, or hypercholesterolemia. A moderate reduction of sodium intake is not contraindicated in the treatment of any of these disease states.

The American appetite for salt is a learned behavior and does *not* reflect salt needs, which have been estimated to be only 500 mg. per day. The average American intake of 6 to 18 grams of salt per day is dependent on many factors, including eth-

TABLE 49–13. APPROXIMATE SODIUM CONTENT OF COMMONLY CONSUMED FOODS *

Food Item	Serving Size	Mg. of Sodium
Cheese (except cottage)	1 ounce	200
Condiments:		
Catsup	1 tbsp.	180
Mustard, prepared	1 tbsp.	195
Olives	2 medium	240
Pickle, dill	1 large	1400
Salad dressings	1 tbsp.	80–200
Convenience foods:		
Chili, canned	2/3 cup	730
Macaroni and cheese	1 cup	1220
Pot pie	1 pie	800–1000
TV dinner	1 dinner	700–1300
Fish, canned in oil	1/2 cup	500–800
Meats:		
Bacon	1 slice	75
Luncheon meat, sausage	1 ounce	390–450
Canadian bacon	1 ounce	440
Canned meats	1 ounce	295–400
Corned beef	1 ounce	270
Frankfurter	1	540
Ham, cured	1 ounce	390
Sauerkraut	1/2 cup	750
Soups:		
Bouillon cube	1 cube	425
Canned	1/3 of can	570–1000
Frozen	1 serving	750–950

* Data from Church, C. F., and Church, H. N.: Bowes and Church's Food Values of Portions Commonly Used. 11th Ed. Philadelphia, J. B. Lippincott Co., 1970.

nic and geographic customs. Moderation of sodium intake would be a healthful behavior change for the American population.

Obesity

The cause of obesity is complex, and many hypotheses exist concerning the possible physiologic (metabolic and regulatory) or psychologic mechanisms that can effect the excess accumulation of adipose tissue. Current discussion centers around the concept that obesity is related to the number and size of adipose cells, which has brought about the classification of obesity as either hyperplastic or hypertrophic. Whatever mechanisms exist, environmental factors such as familial eating habits, quantity and quality of food supply, lack of exercise, and so forth also contribute significantly to the development of obesity.

A few of the disease entities that have been correlated with obesity are hyperten-sion, diabetes mellitus, hyperlipoprotein-emias, cerebrovascular disease, mechanical burden on the body frame, and accelerated deterioration of the joint surfaces. Mann[17] has suggested five general mechanisms by which obesity might be detrimental to health:

1. The additional weight of the stored fat might, through its burden on the frame and circulatory system, overwork some systems and lead to poor health.

2. The greater food intake of obese persons might damage health by increasing the intake of some unspecified noxious agents in the food.

3. The excessive intake of food energy necessarily promotes glyceride synthesis and transport.

4. Physical inactivity, regarded by some as the most convincing indictment for the cause of obesity, has been considered the prime cause of several chronic diseases.

5. There is a possibility that a genetic

linkage exists between a tendency to obesity and metabolic disease.

Differentiation between overweight and obesity needs to be established. Height-weight charts indicate if a person is overweight in comparison with the population from which the chart was determined. Adiposity versus muscle mass can be estimated by physical examination, utilization of skin fold calipers, or a "pinch test" of the triceps muscle area.

The diagnosis and management of obesity are important medically and should be approached by a rational, non–value-laden evaluation of the patient. The physician needs to establish a weight history, with emphasis on the *chronologic record* of body weight at specific milestones such as birth, completion of elementary school, graduation from high school and college, marriage, and retirement. Also record weight changes following specific life events such as death of a parent, change in marital status, pregnancy, trauma, and job change and following *earlier attempts at weight reduction* (diets, medications, exercise programs—document successful regimens). A dietary history

should be elicited, with special attention being given to eating patterns and quantification of intake of specific foods. The physician should also seek out any psychologic problems that may be leading the patient to view food as a compensatory mechanism. A form, as shown in Table 49–14, can be helpful in gathering information about both dietary and social/psychologic data. Information regarding potential support from concerned family members or friends will be an important factor in estimating the success of the treatment plan.

The traditional aspects of family history, review of systems, laboratory tests, and physical examination have to be completed to rule out any medical causes for obesity, with special attention being given to obesity-related findings.

To determine the daily energy allowance to be recommended to the patient, the physician's first task is to establish the daily energy requirement to maintain weight. The food nomogram (Fig. 49–1) can be utilized to determine the maintenance energy level. Once this maintenance level has been determined, the calculation of the

TABLE 49–14.   BASELINE EATING MONITORING FORM*

Food Eaten		Time	Social		Where Eaten	Mood When Eaten
Quantity	Type of Food	Circle Time If Food Was Part of Meal	Alone?	With Whom?	Home Work Restaurant Recreation	A–Anxious B–Bored C–Tired D–Depressed E–Angry

*From Stuart, R. B., and Davis, B.: Slim Chance in a Fat World: Behavioral Control of Obesity. Champaign, Ill., Research Press Co., 1972, p. 78.

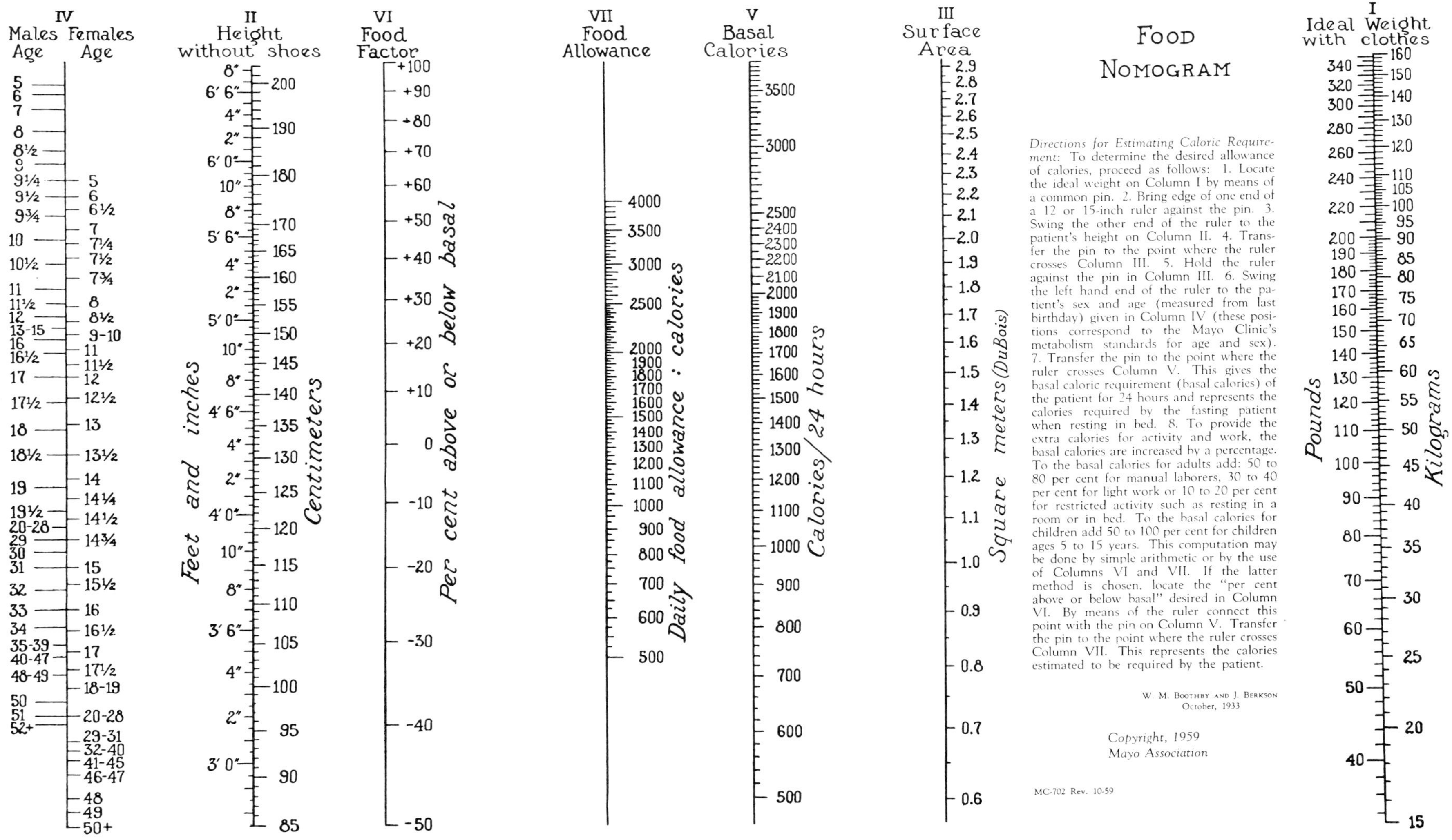

FOOD NOMOGRAM

I
Ideal Weight with clothes

Kilograms

340 320 300 280 260 240 220 200 190 180 170 160 150 140 130 120 110 100 90 80 70 60 50 40

Pounds

Directions for Estimating Caloric Requirement: To determine the desired allowance of calories, proceed as follows: 1. Locate the ideal weight on Column I by means of a common pin. 2. Bring edge of one end of a 12 or 15-inch ruler against the pin. 3. Swing the other end of the ruler to the patient's height on Column II. 4. Transfer the pin to the point where the ruler crosses Column III. 5. Hold the ruler against the pin in Column III. 6. Swing the left hand end of the ruler to the patient's sex and age (measured from last birthday) given in Column IV (these positions correspond to the Mayo Clinic's metabolism standards for age and sex). 7. Transfer the pin to the point where the ruler crosses Column V. This gives the basal caloric requirement (basal calories) of the patient for 24 hours and represents the calories required by the fasting patient when resting in bed. 8. To provide the extra calories for activity and work, the basal calories are increased by a percentage. To the basal calories for adults add: 50 to 80 per cent for manual laborers, 30 to 40 per cent for light work or 10 to 20 per cent for restricted activity such as resting in a room or in bed. To the basal calories for children add 50 to 100 per cent for children ages 5 to 15 years. This computation may be done by simple arithmetic or by the use of Columns VI and VII. If the latter method is chosen, locate the "per cent above or below basal" desired in Column VI. By means of the ruler connect this point with the pin on Column V. Transfer the pin to the point where the ruler crosses Column VII. This represents the calories estimated to be required by the patient.

W. M. Boothby and J. Berkson
October, 1933

Copyright, 1959
Mayo Association

MC-702 Rev. 10-59

III
Surface Area

Square meters (DuBois)

2.9 2.8 2.7 2.6 2.5 2.4 2.3 2.2 2.1 2.0 1.9 1.8 1.7 1.6 1.5 1.4 1.3 1.2 1.1 1.0 0.9 0.8 0.7 0.6

V
Basal Calories

Calories/24 hours

3500 3000 2500 2400 2300 2200 2100 2000 1900 1800 1700 1600 1500 1400 1300 1200 1100 1000 900 800 700 600 500

VII
Food Allowance

Daily food allowance : calories

4000 3500 3000 2500 2000 1900 1800 1700 1600 1500 1400 1300 1200 1100 1000 900 800 700 600 500

VI
Food Factor

Per cent above or below basal

+100 +90 +80 +70 +60 +50 +40 +30 +20 +10 0 -10 -20 -30 -40 -50

II
Height without shoes

Centimeters

8' 200 6'6" 4" 2" 6'0" 10" 180 8" 170 5'6" 165 4" 160 2" 155 5'0" 150 10" 145 8" 140 4'6" 135 4" 130 2" 125 4'0" 120 10" 115 8" 110 3'6" 105 4" 100 2" 95 3'0" 90 85

Feet and inches

IV
Males Females Age
Age

5 6 7 8 8½ 9 9¼ 9½ 9¾ 5
6 10 6½
10½ 7
11 7¼ 7½ 7¾
11½ 8 12 8½ 13-15 9-10 16 16½ 11 17 11½ 12 17½ 12½ 18 13 18½ 13½ 19 14 19¼ 14¼ 20-28 14½ 29 14¾ 30 15 31 15½ 32 16 33 16½ 34 17 35-39 17½ 40-47 17¾ 40-49 18-19 50 20-28 51 23-31 52+ 32-40 41-45 46-47 48 49 50+

Figure 49-1. Food nomogram. (Copyright 1959, The Mayo Association.)

energy intake to recommend for weight loss is straightforward.

Sample Calculation for Recommending Energy Intake

Fact: A deficit of 3500 calories is required to lose 1 pound of body weight.

Example: Weekly goal for weight loss — 2 pounds.

2 pounds × 3500 calories = 7000 calories per week (deficit).

7000 calories per 7 days = 1000 calories per day (deficit).

Maintenance requirement minus 1000 calories = calories to lose 2 pounds per week.

Precaution: 1200 calories is recommended as the minimum daily caloric allowance. Lower levels may be deficient in essential nutrients.

Numerous dietary plans and caloric counting lists are available to aid the patient in controlling energy intake, but consideration must be given to adjunct therapy, such as an exercise program and behavior modification techniques. Behavior modification, as it applies to the treatment of obesity, involves several basic concepts.

First, patients must provide a description of the eating behavior to be controlled. To facilitate this, patients should be asked to keep daily food records, which lead them to a keen awareness of the quantity and quality of foods consumed in connection with the wide variety of environmental and psychologic situations associated with eating. Second, a method for modification and control of the discriminative stimuli governing eating habits has to be designed. For example, eating is to be restricted to one area in the house, and mealtime is to be a singular experience, not accompanied by reading, television, or arguing with the family. Third, techniques to control eating are developed. The patient is encouraged to become aware of the components of eating and to control those components, e.g., counting each mouthful eaten during a meal or placing utensils on the plate after every second mouthful until food is chewed and swallowed. Fourth, prompt reinforcement (positive reward) of behavior that controls or delays eating must be instituted. A point system can be devised to serve as instant rewards for positive behaviors. These points can be accumulated and converted into more tangible rewards, such as money. Strong support by family members is essential for successful behavior modification.

There is some evidence to indicate that group therapy is more effective in the treatment of obesity than individual management. In addition to medically oriented group therapy, there are several nonmedical groups in most communities — TOPS (Take Off Pounds Sensibly), Weight Watchers, and Overeaters Anonymous.

The best treatment for obesity is prevention. The family physician can effectively monitor weight and eating patterns during critical periods in the life cycle, especially during pregnancy and during the periods of formation of eating habits in the infant and young child. Unwise eating patterns are health hazards that can be changed by consistent, concerned nutrition education. Weight gains should be noticed and corrected before weight reduction becomes an insurmountable task. Every effort should be made to help patients stop overfeeding themselves and their families, as their health does depend upon it.

REFERENCES

1. American Association for Health, Physical Education and Recreation: Nutrition for Athletes, A Handbook for Coaches. Washington, D.C., Am. Assoc. for Health, Physical Education and Recreation, 1971.
2. Arena, J. M.: Contamination of the ideal food. Nutr. Today, 5:2, 1970.
3. Bruch, H.: Eating Disorders: Obesity, Anorexia Nervosa and the Person Within. New York, Basic Books, Inc., 1973.
4. Brunzell, J. D., Lerner, F. L., Hazzard, W. R., et al.: Improved glucose tolerance with high carbohydrate feeding in mild diabetes. New Engl. J. Med., 284:521, 1971.
5. Burkitt, D. P., Walker, A. R. P., and Painter, N. S.: Dietary fiber and disease. J.A.M.A., 229:1068, 1974.
6. Cheek, D. B.: Fetal and Postnatal Cellular Growth. New York, John Wiley & Sons, Inc., 1975.
7. Committee on Maternal Nutrition: Maternal Nutrition and the Course of Pregnancy. Food and Nutrition Board. National Academy of Sciences, Washington D.C., 1970.
7a. Committee on Nutrition: Iron balance and requirements in infancy. Pediatrics, 43:134, 1969.
7b. Committee on Nutrition: Childhood diet and coronary heart disease. Pediatrics, 49:305, 1972.
7c. Committee on Nutrition: Salt intake and eating patterns of infants and children in relation to blood pressure. Pediatrics, 53:115, 1974.
7d. Congressional Record: Proceedings and Debates on the 94th Congress. Second Session. Vol. 122, No. 131, Sept. 1, 1976.

8. Dahl, L. K.: Salt intake and salt need. New Engl. J. Med., *258*:1152,1205, 1958.

9. Fomon, S. J.: Infant Nutrition. 2nd Ed. Philadelphia, W. B. Saunders Co., 1974.

10. Freis, E. D.: Salt, volume, and the prevention of hypertension. Circulation, *53*:589, 1976.

11. Givin, W. H., Ejarque, P. M., Hines, C., et al.: Diet vs drugs in hyperlipidemia. Patient Care, August 1, 1976.

12. Goodhart, R. S., and Shils, M. E. (eds.): Modern Nutrition in Health and Disease. 5th Ed. Philadelphia, Lea & Febiger, 1973.

13. Kiell, H. (ed.): The Psychology of Obesity: Dynamics and Treatment. Springfield, Ill., Charles C Thomas Co., 1973.

14. Krause, M. V., and Hunscher, M. A.: Food, Nutrition and Diet Therapy. 5th Ed. Philadelphia, W. B. Saunders Co., 1972.

15. Lechtig, A., Habicht, J. P., Delgado, H., et al.: Effect of food supplementation during pregnancy on birthweight. J. Pediatr., *56*:508, 1975.

16. Lees, R. S., and Wilson, D. E.: The treatment of hyperlipidemia. New Engl. J. Med., *284*:186, 1971.

17. Mann, G. V.: The influence of obesity on health. New Engl. J. Med., *291*:178, 226, 1974.

18. Mayer, J.: Overweight: Causes, Cost and Control. New York, Prentice-Hall, Inc., 1968.

19. Mendeloff, A. I.: Dietary fiber. Nutr. Rev., *33*:321, 1975.

20. Meneely, G. R., and Battarbee, H. D.: Sodium and potassium. Nutr. Rev., *34*:225, 1976.

21. Pitkin, R. M., Kaminetsky, H. A., Newton, M., et al.: Maternal Nutrition, a selected review of clinical topics. Obstet. Gynecol., *40*:773, 1972.

22. Recommended Dietary Allowances. Washington, D.C., National Academy of Sciences, National Research Council, 1974.

23. Report: A Maximal approach to the dietary treatment of the hyperlipidemias. Subcommittee on Diet and Hyperlipidemia Council on Arteriosclerosis. New York, 1973. American Heart Association, 1973.

24. Report: Drugs in breast milk. Med. Lett. Drugs Ther., *16*:25,1974.

25. Report: Nutrition in pregnancy. Med. Lett. Drugs Ther., *16*:67, 1974.

26. Review: Water deprivation and performance of athletes. Nutr. Rev., *132*:9, 1974.

27. Stuart, R. R., and Davis, B.: Slim Chance in a Fat World: Behavioral Control of Obesity. Champaign, Ill., Research Press Co., 1972.

28. Symposium: Nutrition in the causation of cancer. Cancer Res. 35(No. 11), 1975.

29. Trowell, H.: Definition of dietary fiber and hypothesis that it is a protective factor in certain diseases. Am. J. Clin. Nutr., *29*:417, 1976.

30. Weisier, R. L., Seeman, A., Herrera, M.G., et al.: High and low carbohydrate diets in diabetes mellitus: a study of effects on diabetic control, insulin secretion and blood lipids. Ann. Intern. Med., *80*:332, 1974.

31. Winick, M.: Malnutrition and Brain Development. New York, Oxford University Press, 1975.

32. Wood, F. C., and Bierman, E. L.: New concepts in diabetic dietetics. Nutr. Today, 7:4, 1972.

Chapter 50

DERMATOLOGY AND SYPHILOLOGY

by WILLIAM WELTON

It would be helpful to have a complete compendium of the diagnosis and therapy of skin diseases. A patient walks in with a rash, and you slip out to the book and find the answer. Although this chapter does not pretend to be a complete compendium of dermatology, it is hoped that it will aid the family physician in the diagnosis of these diseases by the grouping of entities that have some common characteristics. Because of the scope of dermatology, the discussions must of necessity be brief.

THE INFLAMMATORY (PAPULOSQUAMOUS) GROUP

The inflammatory skin diseases are the most difficult to diagnose. However, if we start with three diseases of this group that can be recognized by their morphology and distribution, the common pool can be reduced. Psoriasis, lichen planus, and pityriasis rosea are examples of this papulosquamous group.

Psoriasis (Figures 50–1 to 50–7)

Location. Elbows, knees, intergluteal area, scalp, nails, but may be anywhere, localized or generalized, and often symmetrical.

Duration. Chronic, life-long, onset at any age, remissions and exacerbations.

Etiology. Unknown.

Pathology. Epidermis grows too rapidly. Other members of the family may be affected. A new lesion induced at the site of skin injury is called the Koebner phenomenon (also occurs in lichen planus).

Symptoms. Itching in some occasional patients.

Appearance. Small, round papules to large plaques. Scale is thick and silvery and may be diminished or absent in new, treated, or rubbed lesions. There is a small bleeding point at the site of scale removal.

Color. Deep red.

Differential Diagnosis. Bowen's disease, basal cell carcinoma, lichen simplex chronicus, lupus erythematosus, mycosis fungoides, lichen planus, fungus, nummular eczema, parapsoriasis, and seborrheic dermatitis.

It is particularly difficult to differentiate psoriasis from seborrheic dermatitis. Instead of psoriasis being in its usual distribution pattern, it may be in the pattern of seborrhea: i.e., on the scalp, in the center of the chest, under the breasts, and in the groin. This unusual pattern may be explained by the Koebner phenomenon: First

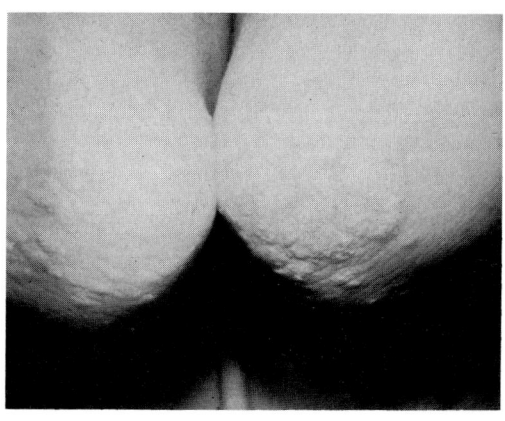

Figure 50–1. Psoriasis. Typical elbow location.

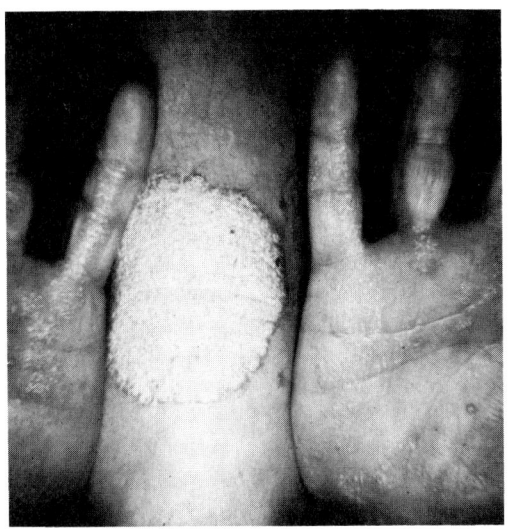

Figure 50-2. Psoriasis. White scale and palm lesions.

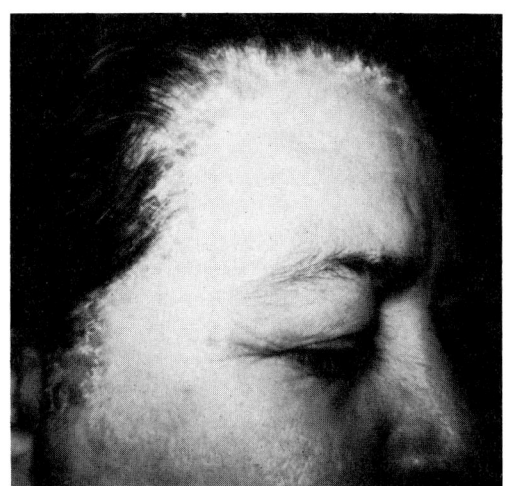

Figure 50-4. Psoriasis resembling seborrheic dermatitis.

the patient has seborrheic dermatitis, and then psoriasis develops in this area as a result of skin trauma. In a dandruff of the scalp that is particularly resistant to treatment, psoriasis should be considered the cause.

Superficial basal cell carcinoma and Bowen's disease are in the differential diagnosis. Bowen's disease (Fig. 50-55) is a squamous cell carcinoma in situ. These lesions can be excluded by biopsy. A biopsy should be performed on any persistent solitary lesion not responding to therapy. Under the microscope, psoriasis itself can be diagnosed, but is not always diagnostic.

Treatment. Tars, anthralin, local steroids, sunlight, or ultraviolet light. The exposure to sun should be gradual. Sunburn can bring on new lesions; also, some psoriatics may be made worse by sun. In the acute spreading phase, exposure to sunlight is not indicated.

The best therapy for the localized plaques is a topical steroid covered with an occlusive dressing (Saran Wrap) or steroid-impregnated tape (Cordran Tape). This may be left on for 12 to 48 hours. In warmer weather, a shorter wearing time and periods of open exposure are recommended. At any sign of irritation or heat rash, the wrap

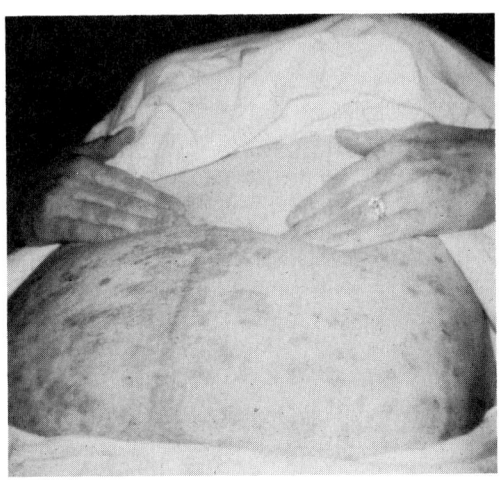

Figure 50-3. Psoriasis occurring in postoperative scar (Koebner phenomenon).

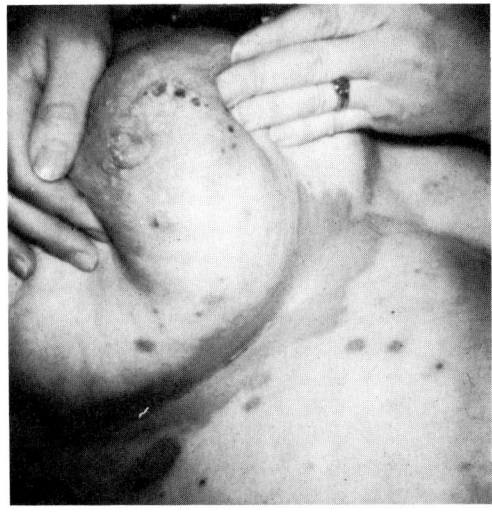

Figure 50-5. Psoriasis resembling intertrigo, fungus, and Paget's disease of the nipple.

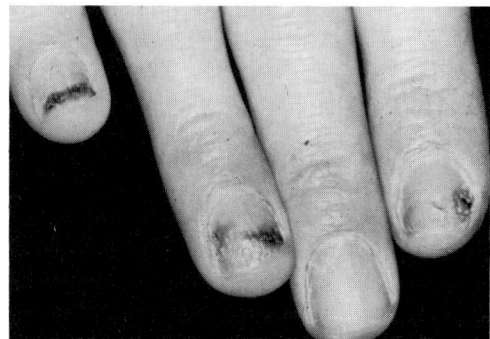

Figure 50-6. Psoriasis of the nails with the characteristic pitting.

should be discontinued. The wrap should be held in place with nonirritating tape or an elastic bandage. Lesions of the trunk and of other large areas are more difficult to manage this way. Plastic suits are available to be worn over the topical steroid, or plastic dry-cleaning bags can be used. The high price of the steroid creams is a drawback.

For severe psoriasis, dermatologists have been using methotrexate (investigational for this use). This antimetabolite is effective,

but side effects such as cirrhosis of the liver make its future uncertain. The use of internal steroids is not recommended.

Oral psoralen followed by long-wavelength ultraviolet is undergoing clinical trials at a few centers with good results.

Lichen Planus (Figure 50--8 and Plate 2F, p. 1115)

Location. Wrists, lower legs, mouth, and areas of clothing pressure. (The Koebner phenomenon as described in psoriasis is applicable here.) Lesions may be generalized and located anywhere, including on the nails.

Duration. Months or sometimes a few years. It occurs more often in the middle years of life.

Etiology. Unknown. Drugs, particularly antimalarials, may sometimes be the cause. Emotional stress may be a precipitating factor.

Symptoms. Pruritus is usual and may be severe.

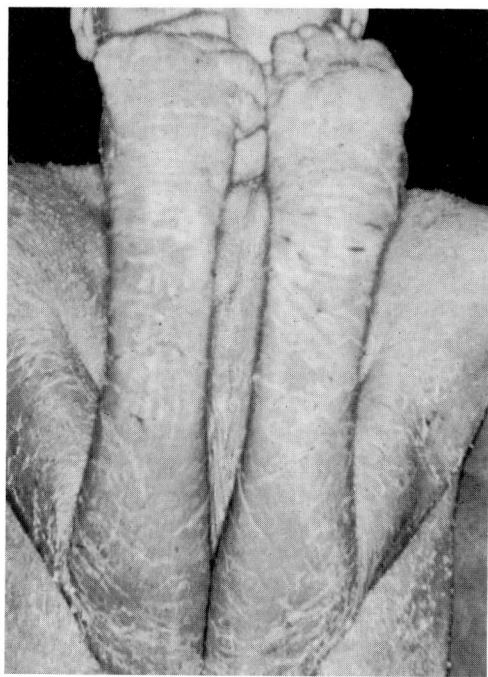

Figure 50-7. Generalized exfoliative psoriasis.

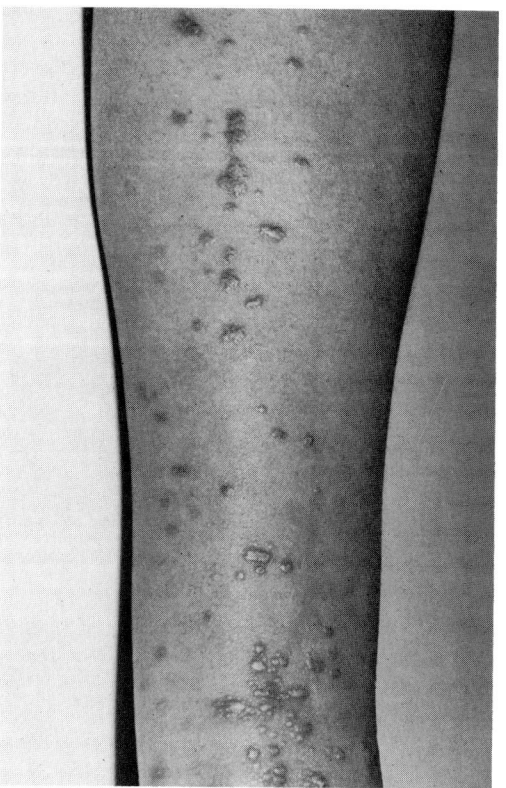

Figure 50-8. Lichen planus. (From Domonkos, A.: Andrews' Diseases of the Skin. 6th Ed. Philadelphia, W. B. Saunders Co., 1971, p. 240.)

Appearance. Flat-topped polygonal, shiny to scaling violaceous papules. The angularity of the circumscribed margin helps differentiate lichen planus from the others in this papulosquamous group. The papules may be small and occur in linear groups, or they may coalesce to form large hypertrophic plaques resembling psoriasis or lichen simplex chronicus. The mucosal lesions, usually located on the buccal mucosa and tongue, form a diffuse white reticulated network with thicker nodes at the points of intersection. The epithelium may separate, leaving an eroded surface. As the skin lesions heal, they leave hyperpigmentation as a result of melanin dropping into the dermis.

Differential Diagnosis. Flat warts, psoriasis, lichen simplex chronicus, pityriasis rosea, other rarer lichens, melanin pigmentations, drug eruptions, and other white mucosal lesions of *Candida albicans* (thrush), leukoplakia, and syphilis. Mouth lesions may be present without skin lesions. If the diagnosis is in doubt, the biopsy is quite helpful and is the most specific in this group. It should show basal layer degeneration and a band of lymphocytes.

Treatment. Local steroids with or without occlusive bandage (described under psoriasis). Internal steroids (prednisone) may be needed for the acute generalized form (prednisone, 5 mg. tablets, 6 tablets each A.M. for 2 weeks; then, every other day, 6 tablets for 2 weeks; then reduce to 3 tablets and then 2 tablets over the next month). Hopefully, local therapy will then be sufficient treatment.

Other therapy is aimed at controlling the itching: tranquilizers, aspirin, antihistamines, cool compresses, and lotions (Keri Lotion, Lubriderm). Stop previous drugs and solve emotional problems. For symptomatic mouth lesions, local application of Orabase Emollient, promethazine hydrochloride (Phenergan Elixir), or a couple of 5 mg. prednisone tablets dissolved in the mouth daily may be used.

Pityriasis Rosea (Figures 50–9 and 50–10; Plate 2A, p. 1114)

Location. Trunk. Characteristic distribution in lines of skin cleavage. Quite unusual on face, palms, and soles.

Duration. Four to ten weeks. Rare to have a second attack.

Etiology. Unknown. Usually several cases seen at a time. Spring and fall occurrence, but no apparent contagion.

Symptoms. Pruritus occasionally.

Appearance. Oval lesions with long axis in lines of cleavage. A collarette of fine scale may start centrally and move peripherally (Fig. 50–10 and Plate 2A). The severity is variable.

The first lesion or herald patch is larger and usually precedes the generalized eruption by 2 weeks. At this stage the diagnosis is often missed. Fungus infection is the

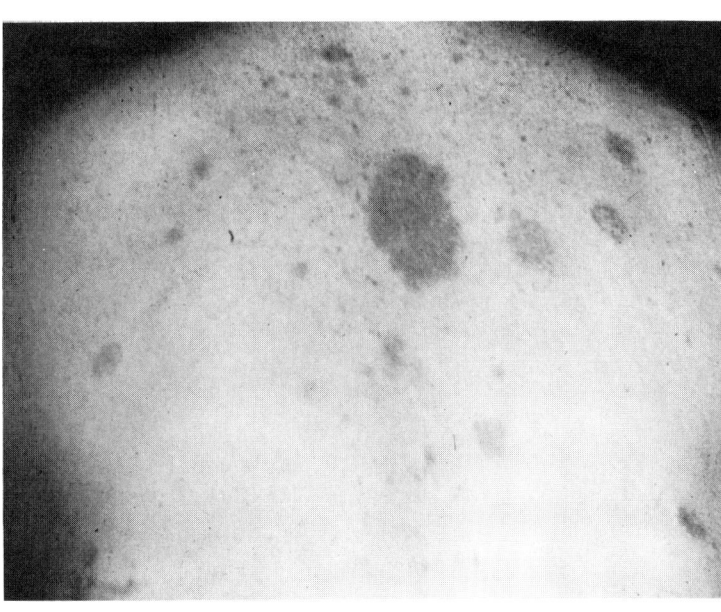

Figure 50–9. Pityriasis rosea with herald patch.

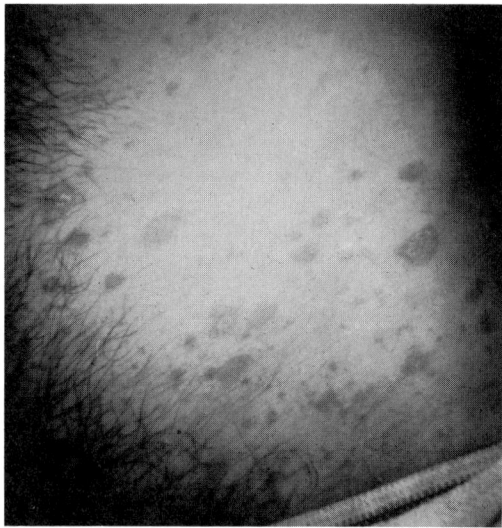

Figure 50-10. *Pityriasis rosea. Oval lesions in lines of skin cleavage.*

usual diagnosis, griseofulvin is given, and when the rest of the rosea erupts, the natural conclusion is drug eruption.

Differential Diagnosis. Psoriasis, lichen planus, drug eruption, fungus, nummular eczema, and, particularly, secondary syphilis. A blood test for syphilis is recommended if there is any atypicality: e.g., peripheral lesions (palms, face), mucosal lesions, adenopathy, sore throat, and lack of the herald patch.

Treatment. None, Treat pruritus if it occurs. Ultraviolet therapy helps some patients. The eruption is often disturbing to the patient. Diagnosis and subsequent reassurance are the most important factors.

THE BULLOUS DERMATOSES GROUP

Early diagnosis by biopsy is important in this group because of the life-threatening nature of pemphigus and severe erythema multiforme.

Pemphigus (Plate 2C, p. 1114)

Location. Generalized. May start in the mouth.

Duration. Rare to start in childhood; more likely to begin in middle years. It may be acute, with early death resulting either from the disease or from the necessarily high prednisone dosage (septicemia, bleed-

ing ulcer), or it may be chronic and controlled by a low dosage of prednisone.

Etiology. Unknown. The epidermal cells separate from each other (acantholysis). An immune mechanism is demonstrated by fluorescent antibodies to the epidermal cell membrane.

Symptoms. Usually not too pruritic.

Appearance. The vulgaris form shows large, flaccid bullae on a noninflamed base. The blisters rupture easily and spread when pressed; firm stroking may bring on a new lesion (Nikolsky's sign). This makes biopsy difficult because the epidermis tends to rub off when one tries to excise around the bulla. Intertriginous lesions may be vegetative.

The foliaceous type is more difficult to recognize because the bullae are so superficial that they rupture before they are seen by the physician. Thus, the lesion looks like exfoliating skin. When the dermatosis is on exposed areas, it resembles lupus erythematosus. To add to the confusion, the two diseases may be seen together.

Differential Diagnosis. Bullous pemphigoid, erythema multiforme, dermatitis herpetiformis, contact dermatitis, burn and comatose patient from drug overdose. There is a benign familial form of pemphigus seen in intertriginous areas.

Treatment. Therapy is best started in the hospital under specialist care with about 100 mg. of prednisone a day. If there is no response in a couple of days, increase the dose to 200 mg. a day. Even higher doses may be needed. After control is achieved, the dose can be lowered, rapidly at first and then more slowly to maintenance level. Epidermal cell membrane antibodies in the patient's serum can be measured; titer change indicates the effectiveness of therapy. Immunosuppressive drugs are now being added to the therapy. If there is evidence of infection, internal antibiotics can be used.

Bullous Pemphigoid (Figure 50-11)

Location. Generalized, but not in mouth. Some tendency to grouping and to occurring on sides of trunk, toward axillae.

Duration. Occurs most often in the older age group. May have acute onset and then become chronic with remissions and exacerbations.

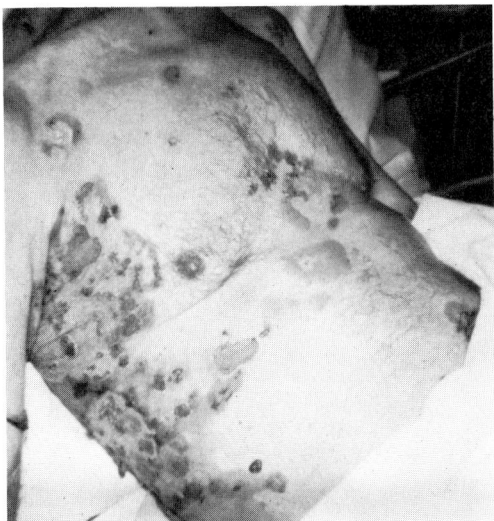

Figure 50-11.   Pemphigoid.

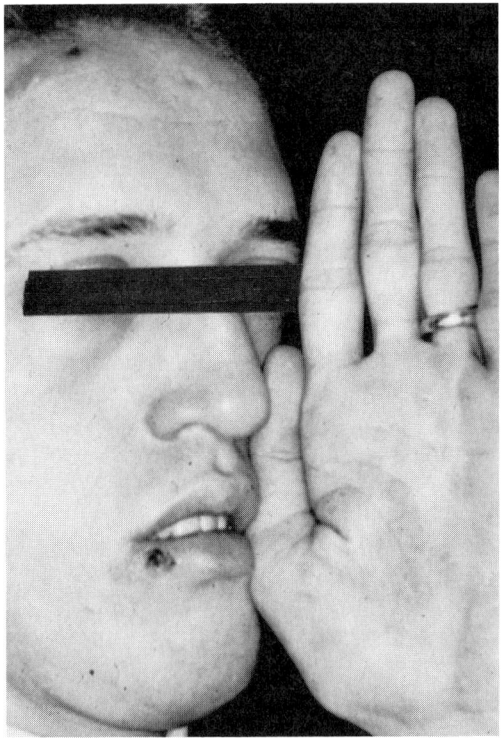

Figure 50-12.   Erythema multiforme on the palm and herpes simplex on the lip.

Etiology.   Unknown. An antibody to the epidermal basement membrane is found in the serum and by direct examination of the blister.

Symptoms.   Some burning and itching.

Appearance.   May resemble pemphigus, with large bullae on noninflamed base. These are easily ruptured and hemorrhagic and spread when pressure is applied. There may also be some erythema and grouping, resembling dermatitis herpetiformis.

Differential Diagnosis.   Pemphigus, erythema multiforme, and dermatitis herpetiformis.

Pemphigus can be ruled out by finding the subepidermal location of the blister.

Erythema multiforme and dermatitis herpetiformis may be excluded, respectively, by finding the basement membrane antibody and by the lack of clinical responses to sulfapyridine (p. 1109).

Treatment.   Prednisone, 40 mg. a day each morning after breakfast, reduce to 20 mg. a day, then to 20 mg. every other day.

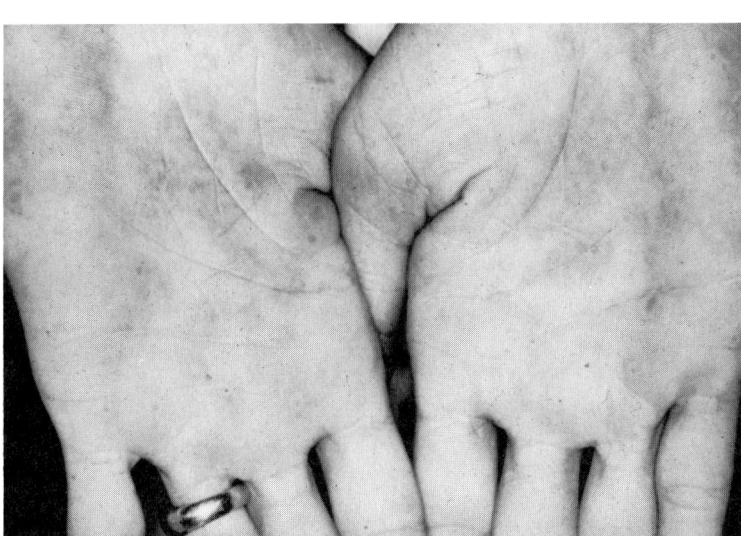

Figure 50-13.   Erythema multiforme with iris lesions of the palms.

Higher maintenance doses may be needed. Recently, immunosuppressive drugs have been added to the therapy with some benefit. Even though pemphigoid is not as severe as pemphigus, it may be life-threatening because of extensive lesions or therapy complications, particularly because the patient is older and may have other diseases.

Erythema Multiforme (Figures 50–12 to 50–14)

Location. Palms, soles, dorsum, mucous membranes, or generalized.

Duration. Acute and self-limited, but recurrent following inciting cause, such as herpes simplex.

Etiology. Drugs or infection (herpes simplex, streptococcal). The usual history is that the patient had fever, was given drug therapy, and the eruption followed.

Appearance. The characteristic lesion is the target or iris (Figs. 50–13 and 50–14), a round ring with redder periphery and edematous center. There may be various-sized

bullae on an erythematous base, and these may be hemorrhagic or necrotic. The mouth, eyes, and genitalia may be involved (Stevens-Johnson syndrome). There may be a diffuse, dusky, or hemorrhagic erythema. The blood vessels are the main site of damage here, with a secondary lifting away of the epidermis.

Differential Diagnosis. Pemphigoid and dermatitis herpetiformis. These two are chronic as compared with the acute erythema multiforme. Syphilis, Rocky Mountain spotted fever, and smallpox are included in the differential diagnosis because they also involve the skin of the palms.

Treatment. The main problem is to find the cause. The picture is usually complicated by signs of infection and prior antibiotic therapy. Hospital management is indicated for the sick patient, who should receive throat culture, antistreptolysin titer, blood culture, urine culture, and x-rays. Change the antibiotic and start prednisone. The eruptions that recur with every herpes simplex infection are usually mild and can be treated with prednisone, 20 mg. a day, for about a week.

Dermatitis Herpetiformis (Figures 50–15 and 50–16)

Location. Grouped lesions over scapula, sacrum, and extensors of arms and legs. Not mucosal.

Duration. Chronic and recurrent, occurring at almost any age.

Etiology. Unknown.

Symptoms. Severe burning and itching. Dermatitis herpetiformis should be considered and ruled out in any patient with these severe symptoms.

Appearance. The main lesion is a vesicle on a red base. Biopsy of an intact lesion is difficult because lesions are scratched off. Excoriations, crusts, and pigmented scars are seen (Fig. 50–16). Occasionally there are large bullae, some with peripheral extension. These may resemble bullous impetigo in children. Urticarial lesions may be present.

Differential Diagnosis. Scabies and neurotic excoriations. Also consider the other bullous lesions and impetigo. The biopsy shows subepidermal lesions, and they may be confused with those of erythema multiforme and pemphigoid. Peripheral eosin-

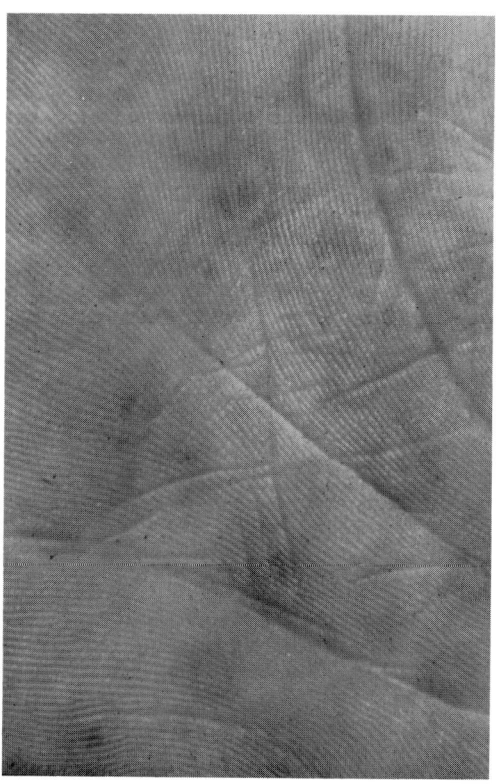

Figure 50–14. Close-up of Figure 50–13.

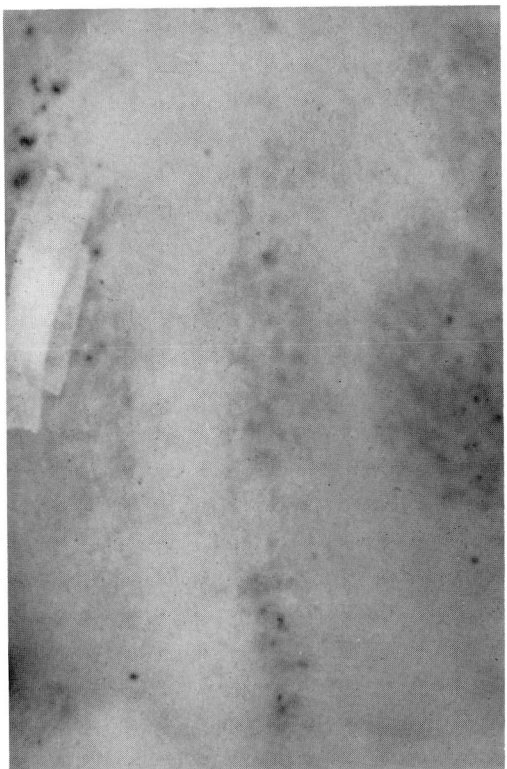

Figure 50–15. *Dermatitis herpetiformis. Grouped lesions below scapula and above sacrum.*

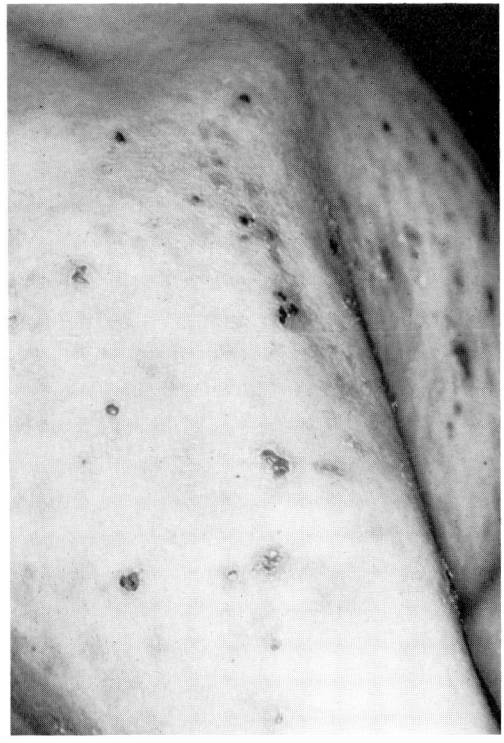

Figure 50–16. *Dermatitis herpetiformis. Excoriated lesions.*

ophilia and small bowel malabsorption with gluten sensitivity may be associated.

Treatment. The diagnosis is often made by a therapeutic trial of sulfapyridine, 1 gram three times daily, with dramatic relief of itching. Because the diagnosis of dermatitis herpetiformis is often missed, this trial is worthwhile in an excoriated pruritic dermatitis. After control of the disease, the dosage can be reduced to maintenance levels. With exacerbations, increase the dose. Most patients learn to regulate the dose themselves. Urine examination and blood count should be performed about every 4 months. Some patients do not tolerate the sulfapyridine, and headache, gastrointestinal upset, or allergic skin reaction may subsequently occur. They may tolerate a lower dosage of the drug.

Dapsone, 100 mg. one to three times daily, can be used. A blood count is indicated when dapsone therapy is initiated and on follow-up visits. Some hemolysis may occur. Other sulfas and antibiotics are not effective.

Bullae may be seen also in porphyria cutanea tarda, diabetes, congenital ichthy-osis and epidermolysis bullosa, congenital syphilis, toxic epidermal necrolysis, and mast cell disease.

THE SUPERFICIAL FUNGUS GROUP

Tinea Versicolor (Figures 50–17 to 50–19)

Location. Trunk and upper arms. May be more generalized.

Duration. Chronic and recurrent, usually starting in young adults.

Etiology. *Malassezia furfur.*

Symptoms. Not contagious. Occasional itching, which is worse in warm weather.

Appearance. Round, scaling macules that tend to become confluent. They may vary in color from brown to red to white. It is too often misdiagnosed as vitiligo (Fig. 50–18). The diagnosis is easily confirmed by finding many organisms on a skin scraping put on a slide with 10 per cent KOH and cover slipped (see description of KOH slide technique at end of chapter). Short hyphae and spore clusters are seen.

Differential Diagnosis. Other fungi, viti-

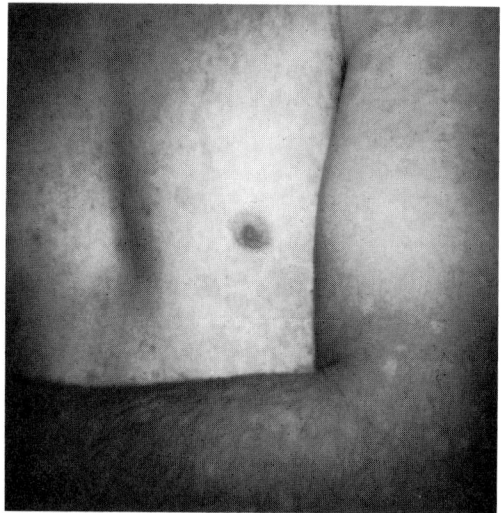

Figure 50–17. *Tinea versicolor in varying stages of pigmentation and depigmentation.*

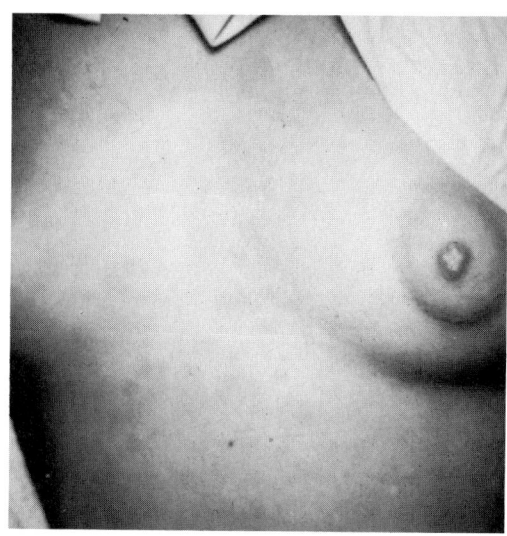

Figure 50–19. *Tinea versicolor. Pigmented areas.*

ligo, other pigmentary changes, leprosy, Addison's disease, pinta, and pityriasis rosea.

Treatment. Local therapy is effective but not curative. Griseofulvin is not helpful. Sodium hyposulfite, 20 per cent, applied to the skin for 3 or more weeks, is the traditional treatment. Selsun shampoo, a total of three washings, is helpful but can be too irritating. Repeated courses of therapy are usually necessary.

Candida Albicans (Candidiasis, Moniliasis) (Figure 50–20)

Location. Intertriginous, groin, under breasts, interphalangeal, periungual, and mucosa of the mouth and genitalia. Can be generalized or systemic.

Duration. May be chronic and occur at any age.

Etiology. The yeast *Candida albicans.* Usually there is some other factor causing low resistance, such as diabetes, antibiotic

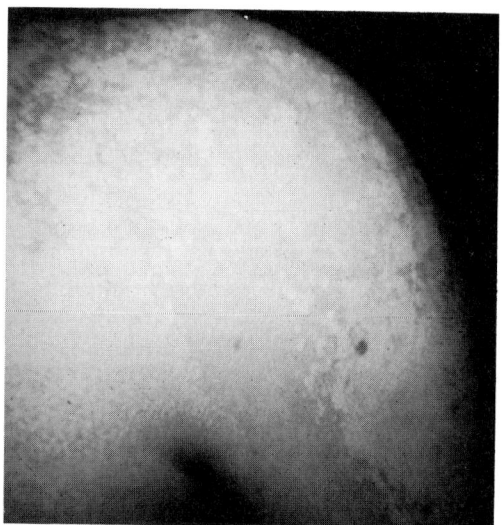

Figure 50–18. *Tinea versicolor, the depigmented area resembling vitiligo.*

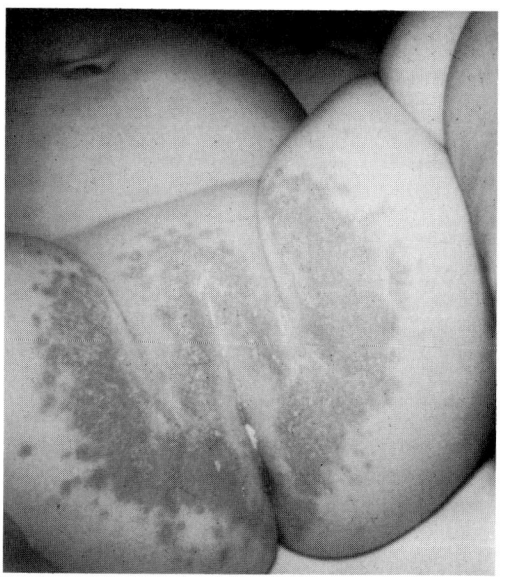

Figure 50–20. *Candidiasis.*

or steroid therapy, overhydration of the skin with maceration, exposure to water, sweat, or wet diapers.

Appearance. The skin lesion is red, macerated, and confluent, with white pustules and small satellite lesions (Fig. 50–20). In the mouth and genitalia the patches are white. The chronic paronychias are often thought to be bacterial, and treatment with soaks and antibiotics makes them worse.

Differential Diagnosis. Other fungi, intertrigo, and contact dermatitis. On the mucosa, lichen planus and leukoplakia. The skin scraping on KOH slide shows yeasts and sometimes, on the heavy white lesions, long pseudohyphae. Cultures are also helpful. (See discussion on KOH slide and culture technique, p. 1134). There are two problems: many artifacts look like yeasts, or yeasts may be seen incidentally in eczemas.

Treatment. Local iodochlorhydroxyquin (Vioform), or nystatin (Mycostatin) creams. In caring for the skin, avoid maceration and water. The diaper area is a problem. Keep it as dry as possible and leave uncovered. Castellani's paint is strong but may be needed in more resistant skin areas, such as in the therapy of paronychia.

THE DERMATOPHYTES— GRISEOFULVIN-SENSITIVE

Tinea Pedis (Figures 50–21 and 50–22)

Location. Feet.
Duration. Chronic or acute.
Etiology. *Trichophyton mentagrophytes* or *Trichophyton rubrum.*
Symptoms. Itching and burning.
Appearance. Two types (there are other rare ones):

1. *T. mentagrophytes:* This is the common dermatophyte occurring between the toes, causing scaling maceration, fissures, and in some patients, acute blisters over the soles of the feet.

2. *T. rubrum:* More subtle and chronic. Diffuse red scaling over the bottom and up the sides of the foot. Nails and other areas involved also.

Differential Diagnosis. Psoriasis and eczema. Under eczema, one might consider intertrigo or nonspecific irritation. Hyperhidrosis, maceration of keratin, and lividity of the soles may be mistaken for fungus

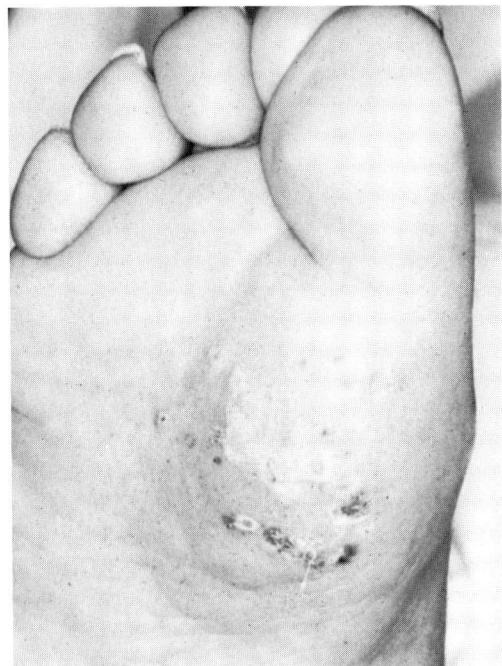

Figure 50–21. *Tinea pedis. Macerated acute type.*

infection and may often be overtreated. Confirm the diagnosis by skin scrapings on KOH slide and by culture (p. 1134).

Treatment. The more acute type (*T. mentagrophytes*) will often cure itself by the more intense skin reaction and blistering. The feet are kept dry and exposed to air. In

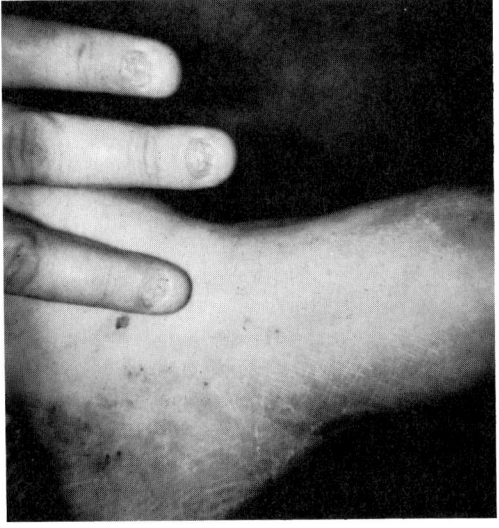

Figure 50–22. *Tinea pedis. Chronic rubrum type. Nails also involved.*

more resistant cases, 2 per cent iodine or 10 per cent undecylenic solution (Desenex) can be used. Secondary bacterial infection is common and internal antibiotics such as erythromycin are recommended.

In *T. rubrum* infection, the skin of the feet does not reject the fungus, and griseofulvin is given internally for about 4 weeks. Recurrence is common.

Tinea of the Nails

Location. Nails.

Duration. Chronic.

Etiology. *T. rubrum* in most cases.

Appearance. Yellow spots and streaks are the most helpful finding, along with some red scaling of the feet or hands. The nail becomes thick and friable. Some nails may be spared.

Differential Diagnosis. *Candida albicans* more frequently involves the paronychia, with swelling and some secondary undermining and ridging of the nails. Psoriasis may show a similar thickening but is associated with pitting. Peripheral vascular disease may cause the nails to thicken.

Treatment. Toenails respond poorly even to removal and long-term (6 months) griseofulvin therapy.

The fingernails are more responsive and noticeable. A 4 month course is suggested. Confirm the diagnosis first by direct KOH slide technique or by culture examination from friable material under the nails (p. 1134).

Tinea Cruris (Figure 50–23 and Plate 2 B, p. 1114)

Location. Groin.

Duration. Chronic.

Etiology. Several *Trichophyton* organisms and *Epidermophyton*.

Appearance. The progressive circumscribed active margin with some central clearing differentiates tinea cruris from *Candida* and intertrigo. It may extend more diffusely over the buttocks, thighs, and further, and may be mistaken for an eczema. This type may go unrecognized for years. It may be erroneously treated with steroid creams as an eczema, with little result.

Differential Diagnosis. Eczema, *C. albicans*, intertrigo, seborrheic dermatitis, and psoriasis.

Treatment. Local fungicides may help,

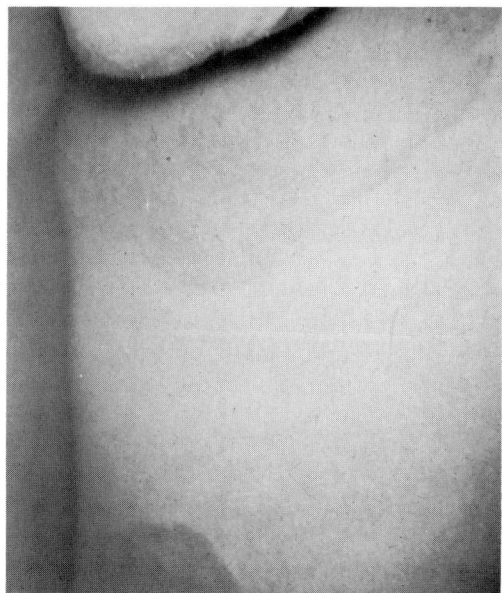

Figure 50–23. Tinea cruris.

but in this tender area internal griseofulvin is more practical.

Tinea Capitis (Figure 50–24)

Location. Scalp.

Duration. More often seen in children and may be self-limited. Rare and endemic in adults.

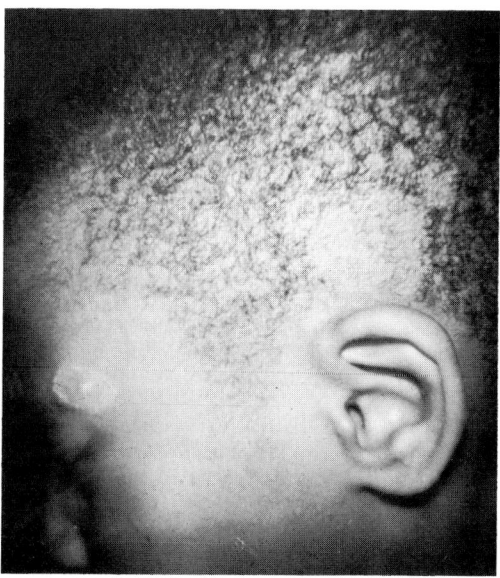

Figure 50–24. Tinea capitis. Round areas of broken hairs, and some scale.

Etiology. *Microsporum* organisms mostly. Occasionally a *Trichophyton*. May be contracted from children or animals.

Appearance. Round areas of broken hairs and scaling in the human form. When caused by *M. canis* (animal form), more inflammatory reaction is seen. Here the Wood's light is helpful in demonstrating the fluorescence around the involved hairs. Some experience in interpretation is necessary. The direct KOH slide examination of a hair and culture on Sabouraud's medium are indicated (p. 1134). This identification will be of epidemiologic help in finding the source of the infection. Try the Wood's light on family pets, particularly the young ones (puppies, kittens). As the hormones of puberty become active, the infection may clear spontaneously.

Differential Diagnosis. Seborrheic dermatitis and psoriasis. Often alopecia areata is misdiagnosed as fungus of the scalp (Fig. 50–33), but in alopecia there are round patches of complete hair loss with no scale. Trichotillomania is included in the differential diagnosis. This occurs particularly in children, who twist the hair and break it off or pull it out. The area is less well defined than in tinea infection.

Treatment. Griseofulvin.

Tinea of the Hands

Location. Hands.
Duration. Chronic.
Etiology. *T. rubrum*, mostly.
Appearance. The striking thing about tinea of the hands is that just one palm is involved and not the other. There is redness, diffuse scaling, and an occasional pustule. The fingernails and feet may be involved too. Confirm by culture and KOH slide technique (p. 1134).

Differential Diagnosis. Round eczema on the hands is usually misdiagnosed as fungus infection. The chronic recurrent vesicular eruptions could be ids (allergic reaction to fungus on the feet), but they are usually just a form of eczema.

Treatment. Griseofulvin.

Tinea Corporis

Location. Trunk.
Duration. Variable.
Etiology. Several *Trichophyton* organisms and *Microsporum* organisms.

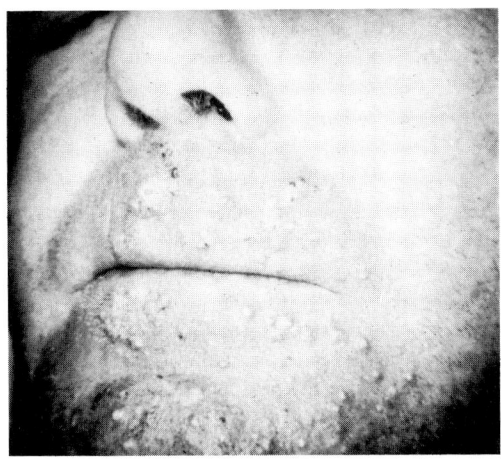

Figure 50–25. *Tinea barbae resembling a bacterial folliculitis.*

Appearance. Round rings with central clearing. Some may look more like bacterial folliculitis. Some may be chronic, irregular eczematous-looking extensions of *T. rubrum* of feet or groin. Others may be the result of animal contact.

Differential Diagnosis. Again, the round or nummular eczema is often misdiagnosed as a fungus infection.

Treatment. Usually internal griseofulvin.

Tinea Barbae (Figure 50–25)

Location. Beard.
Appearance. May have false appearance of a bacterial infection. KOH and culture techniques should give correct diagnosis.

Treatment. Griseofulvin.

All the preceding superficial fungus infections, including candidiasis and tinea versicolor, will respond somewhat to three new topicals: haloprogin (Halotex), clotrimazole (Lotrimin), and miconazole nitrate (MicaTin).

THE DEEP FUNGUS GROUP

Sporotrichosis (Figure 50–26)

This is usually easy to diagnose clinically because of the chain of nodules extending up the arm or leg from the initial ulcer inoculation site. There is usually a history of skin puncture, such as from a rose thorn, or

A

B

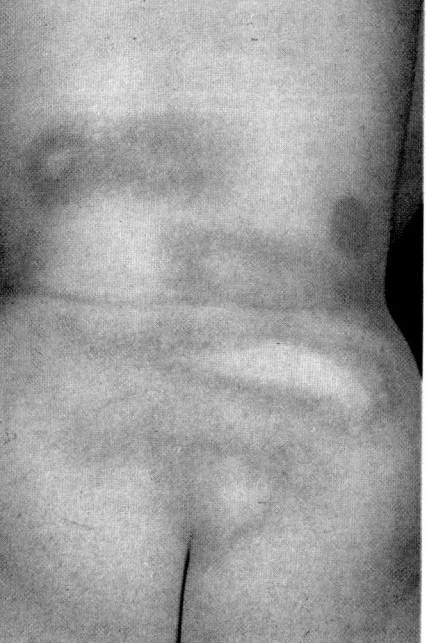

Plate 2. A, *Pityriasis rosea, primary plaque and secondary lesions. Typical marginal scaling (collarette); B, tinea cruris et inguinalis, sharply defined, raised erythematovesicular border; C, pemphigus vulgaris, large, tense bullae containing clear fluid and surrounded by clinically normal skin; D, localized scleroderma, older plaques show peripheral hyperpigmentation; active lesions are characterized by violaceous border. (From Kimming, J., and Jänner, M.: Frieboes/Schönfeld Colar Atlas of Dermatology. Philadelphia, W. B. Saunders Co., 1966.)*

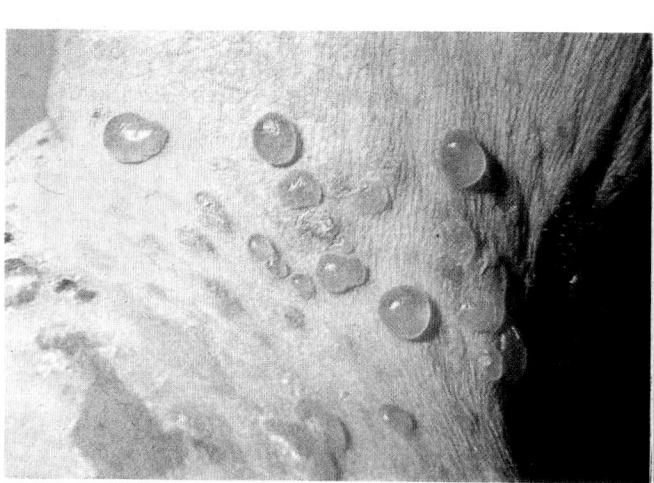

C

D

E

F

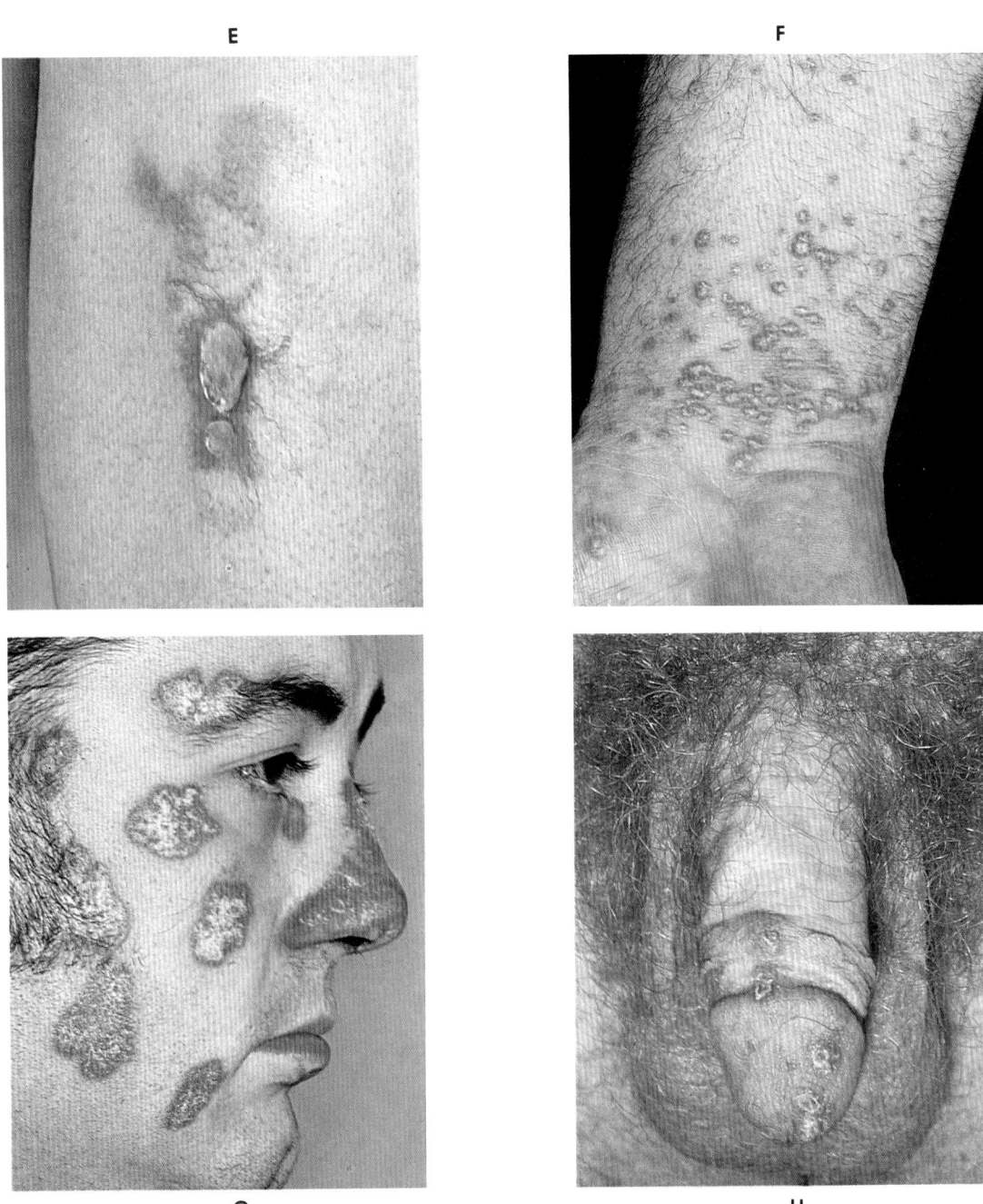

G

H

***Plate 2* (continued).** E, *Necrobiosis lipoidica with ulcerations; F, lichen planus, typical localization on the wrist; G, chronic discoid lupus erythematosus of the face; erythematosus with central atrophy; H, scabies, eroded papules on the penis. (From Korting, G. W., and Denk, R.: Differential Diagnosis in Dermatology. Philadelphia, W. B. Saunders Co., 1976.)*

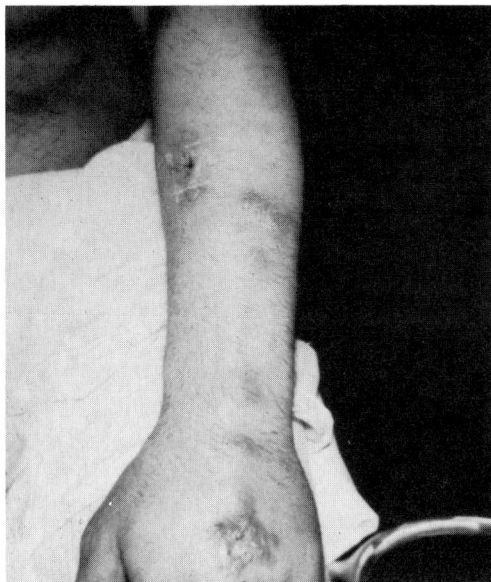

Figure 50-26.   Sporotrichosis.

of exposure to gardening, floral work, or clearing ground. Sporotrichosis is usually unilateral and rarely systemic or in lymph nodes. The fungus is easily cultured on Sabouraud's agar.

Treatment. Saturated solution of potassium iodide. Start with 3 drops twice a day, add a drop a day up to 30 drops, and then reduce dosage at same rate. If generalized pustules of iodide eruption develop, the drug may have to be reduced or stopped.

Blastomycosis (Figure 50-27)

The first thought in the diagnosis of this representative deep fungus is tumor. When tumor is considered, deep fungus should be kept in mind. The diagnosis is often made by biopsy of the suspected lesion. The organism can easily be missed if fungus infection is not mentioned as a possibility when the specimen is given to the pathologist.

Treatment. Amphotericin B or hydroxystilbamidine intravenously.

THE ECZEMAS

Atopic Dermatitis (Figure 50-28)

Location. Antecubital and popliteal areas, cheeks, neck, scalp, or generalized.

Duration. Chronic. May start in infancy and recur throughout life, or clear without recurrence.

Etiology. Unknown. Probably not allergic directly, although it is associated with asthma and hay fever in the patient or in other members of the family. Inherent dry itching skin that tends to thicken (lichenify) on scratching is a factor. In occasional patients, contact with a food, dust, mold, inhalant, or wool may cause a flare. Emotional stress aggravates it. The child may

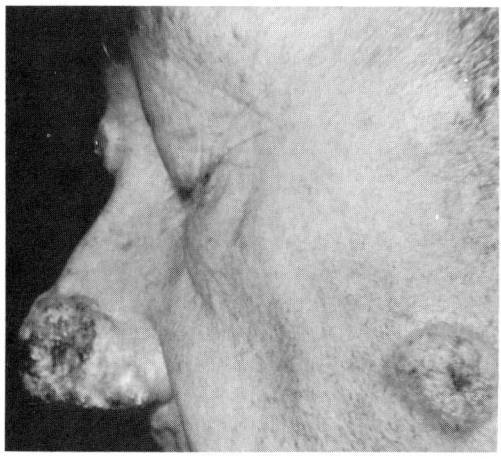

Figure 50-27.   Blastomycosis.

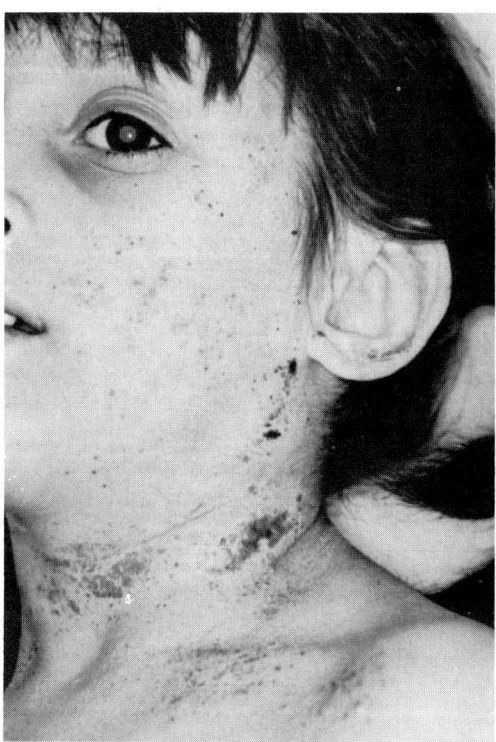

Figure 50-28.   Atopic dermatitis.

get attention by scratching himself into a bloody mess.

Symptoms. Pruritus.

Appearance. The most helpful features are the location and the lichenification (thick skin with accentuation of skin lines). The lesions are ill-defined in various stages of dryness, scaling, oozing, crusting, and excoriation.

Differential Diagnosis. Contact dermatitis, seborrheic dermatitis, fungus, ichthyosis, psoriasis, and drug eruptions. Rarer syndromes occur in infancy, such as Leiner's disease, Letterer-Siwe disease, or Wiskott-Aldrich syndrome.

Treatment. These patients are miserable because of the chronic itching. Both doctor and patient become frustrated. The basis of treatment is to relieve the itching and combat the dryness of the skin. Avoid soap and water and use a lotion such as Cetaphil to clean and lubricate the skin. Keep down the dust. In cool climates increase the humidity in the house in winter. The disease may clear in summer. In some areas high summer humidity may cause occlusion of the sweat pores and exacerbation of the disease. A salve that is too greasy may occlude the skin and make it itch more.

Local steroid cream is the primary treatment. Because of long-term use often over large areas, the expense may be prohibitive. Weaker solutions and larger quantities are helpful. They can be used in conjunction with the less expensive lotions such as Cetaphil and Keri. Oral antihistamines, such as diphenhydramine hydrochloride (Elixir of Benadryl for children and the capsules for adults), given in high enough dosage help sedate and relieve itching. Tranquilizers are also helpful.

Internal steroids are not recommended. The condition is chronic and tends to flare when corticosteroid therapy is discontinued. It will be difficult to get the patient off steroids once they are started. Secondary infection should be treated with an internal antibiotic, such as erythromycin.

Smallpox vaccination should not be done. The patient should be isolated from anyone in the family who has been vaccinated. Eczema vaccinatum may be fatal. Herpes simplex is milder but the patient is better off away from those with fever blister. The parents and patient are helped by some psychotherapy and understanding

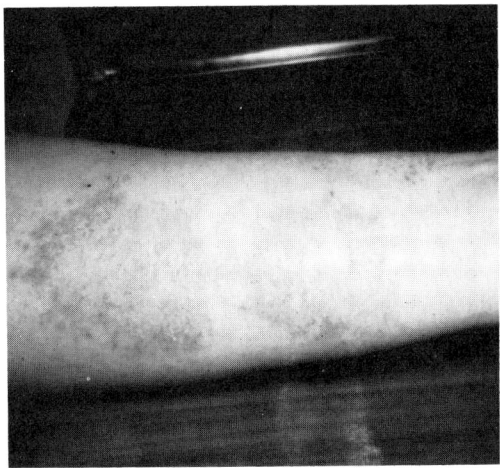

Figure 50-29. Nummular eczema.

of the disease. Allergic reaction to medications may develop and confuse the picture.

Nummular Eczema (Figure 50-29)

Location. Hands and extremities. May be anywhere.

Duration. Some patients have chronic, localized, and recurrent episodes. Some have acute generalized flares.

Etiology. Unknown. There may be some relation to atopic dermatitis. Dry skin is a factor, as well as soaps, cold weather, irritants, and venous stasis of the legs.

Symptoms. Pruritus.

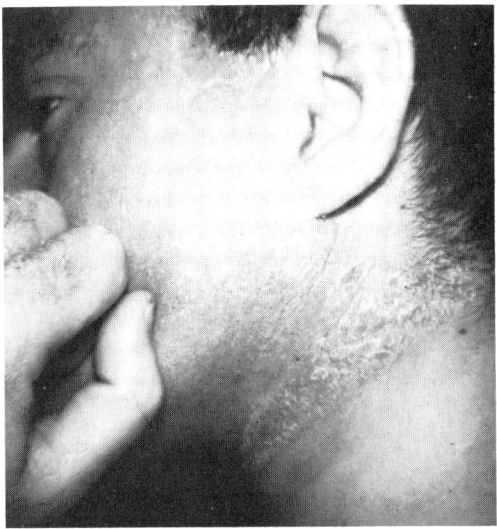

Figure 50-30. Contact dermatitis. Photoallergic. Note sparing of area behind ear and under chin as well as that covered by the shirt.

Appearance. The lesions are round (coin-shaped, as the name implies), oozing, vesicular, cracking, and scaling. Some may become confluent. The dermatitis may start as a chronic area on the leg, then flare as a generalized eruption of small lesions over the whole body.

Differential Diagnosis. Fungus (ringworm; see the discussion on pp. 1111 to 1113), contact dermatitis, mycosis fungoides, psoriasis, and pityriasis rosea.

Treatment. See the treatment for atopic dermatitis. Local steroid creams help the itching and dryness. Avoid soap, water, and so forth. The only difference from atopic dermatitis therapy is that internal steroids may be used during the acute generalized flares, in which case the dose is gradually reduced over a 6 week period.

Contact Dermatitis (Allergic) (Figures 50–30 to 50–32)

Location. Anywhere the allergen touches. The location of the eruption is helpful in making the diagnosis and in finding the cause (e.g., if on the ear lobes and anterior and posterior thighs, the cause may be nickel in earrings and garters). Exposed areas suggest photocontact allergy (Fig. 50–30).

Duration. Acute to chronic.

Etiology. Delayed type of cellular reac-

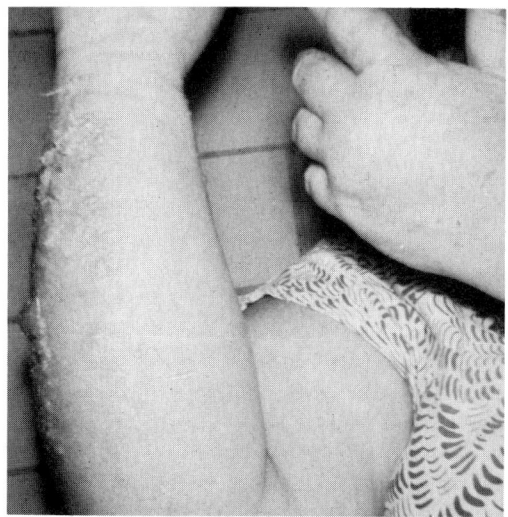

Figure 50–32. Poison ivy aggravated by allergic contact dermatitis to local antihistamine.

tion to many chemical antigens that form by combining with skin protein. A first exposure and then a refractory period of several weeks' duration is necessary for the sensitized lymphocyte to form. Then, after subsequent exposures it takes 24 to 48 hours for the contact reaction of vesicles to start. The oil of the poison ivy leaf is a common example. It is not the spread of vesicle fluid by scratching that causes the linear lesions (Fig. 50–31), but just the way the leaf went across the skin. Local medication and cosmetics are common causes, particularly benzocaine and diphenhydramine. These are usual ingredients of over-the-counter poison ivy and sunburn remedies. Other causes of contact dermatitis are neomycin, thimerosal, nitrofurazone, mercury, and paraben preservatives in cream bases. Nail polish sensitivity usually manifests itself on the eyelids. Consult dermatology texts or Fisher's *Contact Dermatitis*[5] for complete lists of allergens.

Symptoms. Itching, often severe.

Appearance. The vesicle is the main lesion, then edema and larger fluid-filled bullae. Secondary changes follow, such as crusts, oozing, and infection.

Differential Diagnosis. Other eczemas, primary irritant contact to soap, and so forth. Patch tests can be used to find the allergens. Put some of the suspected material on a 2 inch square Band-Aid and apply to the skin for 48 hours. There may be surrounding tape irritation. A positive

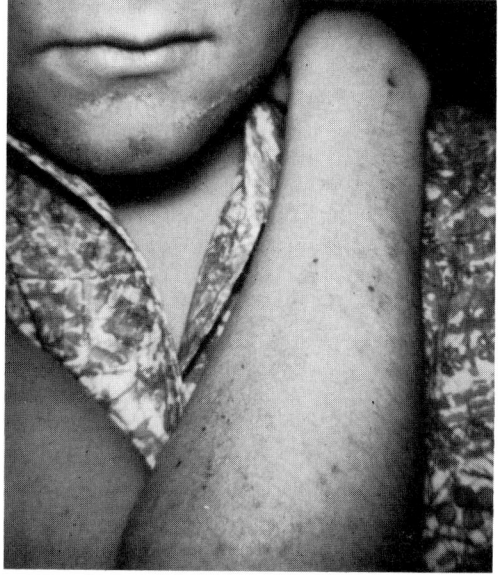

Figure 50–31. Contact dermatitis due to poison ivy.

reaction shows as a red, edematous, or vesiculobullous area under the center of the patch. Local medicines and cosmetics may be tested without dilution. For trays of routine testing and dilutions of irritants, consult Fisher.[5] With a severe eruption, a positive patch test may make all the lesions worse.

Treatment. For acute poison ivy, as for other extensive lesions, early internal steroids should be used for about a week (e.g., prednisone, 5 mg. tablets, 8 tablets immediately and 6 each morning after breakfast for a week, and then 4 tablets every other morning for 2 doses and stop). Locally, cool water compresses can be used at the oozing stage, then a steroid cream.

The chronic recurrent lesions are the difficult ones to prevent and treat. The cycle of itching and scratching may keep the lesions going. Secondary allergic reactions to local therapy can also perpetuate them. Part of the therapy is to find out what the patient is doing to the lesions. Some scrub them, soak them in Clorox, or use hot water and many substances from the drugstore that make the lesions worse. Find out what the patient does at work and what his hobbies are at home. This takes some time, but it is often more fruitful than handing over the latest pharmaceutical sample, which usually does not contain enough ointment to cover the lesions adequately. Instruct the patient to protect the area and avoid the use of irritants.

An allergic contactant may start the eruption, and soap perpetuates it. The hands are a particular problem. If housewives must wash dishes, cotton gloves covered by rubber gloves should be used. The rubber, heat, and sweating may aggravate the lesions. The cotton gloves can be used alone over the ointment, particularly at night. This helps protect the hands from scratching while the patient is asleep and keeps the ointment in contact with the skin. Internal steroids are not recommended as treatment for prolonged periods in chronic contact dermatitis. Sedatives or tranquilizers may be beneficial.

Contact Dermatitis (Primary Irritant)

Location. Hands, most commonly.
Duration. Acute, but often chronic.

Etiology. Soap and solvents, cleaning solutions, acids, and alkalis. This group is responsible for a high incidence of occupational skin disease.

Symptoms. Itching.

Appearance. Diffuse crusting, scaling, and oozing. Sometimes there are vesicles.

Differential Diagnosis. Allergic contact dermatitis, atopic dermatitis, nummular eczema, psoriasis, and fungus. The patch test is not indicated. These substances (primary irritants) will cause a reaction even in most normal people if occluded under a Band-Aid. The chronic hand or housewives' eczema is most often caused by primary irritants.

Treatment. In general, treatment is the same as for allergic contact dermatitis, particularly the protective measures and care of chronic cases. Internal prednisone is not recommended except in occasional cases of widespread dermatitis.

OTHER SKIN ALLERGIES

Urticaria

Location. Generalized.
Duration. Acute and chronic.

Etiology. In the acute form, a food or drug allergy is often obvious from the history. The chronic form presents the difficulty. The cause is not often found and emotions are therefore assumed to be causative. Factors to be considered are sun, heat, cold, inhalants, lymphomas, collagen disease, infections, dermatitis herpetiformis, and mast cell disease.

Appearance. A raised red wheal is the primary lesion. Swelling of the lips and eyelids is more representative of the angioedema form. Swelling of the hands and joints is characteristic of the serum sickness form, often due to penicillin.

Differential Diagnosis. Insect bites and erythema multiforme.

Treatment. Some reactions may be very acute with laryngeal edema and require immediate subcutaneous injection of epinephrine (0.5 ml. of 1:1000) or intravenous corticosteroids. The usual reaction can be controlled by oral antihistamines—e.g., chlorpheniramine (Chlor-Trimeton) 4 mg. four times daily—while attempts are made to find and eliminate the cause. Consider current medication.

If the reaction becomes chronic, continue the chlorpheniramine (Chlor-Trimeton) 4 to 8 mg. four times daily, investigate any symptoms, and do a routine blood count, urinalysis, and chest x-ray. Experiment with the diet by eliminating and adding back items. If the urticaria recurs on reducing the antihistamine, the administration of a tranquilizer is suggested.

Drug Eruptions

Location. Generalized, fixed localized, or on exposed areas.

Duration. Usually acute. The fixed type is chronic and recurrent.

Etiology. May be caused by almost any drug: penicillin, tranquilizers, and so forth. The fixed drug eruption is often caused by phenolphthalein in laxatives.

The eruptions on exposed areas are caused by exposure to the sun plus the drug: e.g., demeclocycline (Declomycin), oral hypoglycemics, chlorpromazines, diuretics, and others.

Appearance. A variety of lesions (hives, vesicles, bullae, purpura, erythema), not specific for a particular drug, are seen.

Differential Diagnosis. Many skin diseases, measles, other viral exanthemas, and lupus erythematosus.

Treatment. Stopping the drug may be sufficient. If there are no contraindications, give internal prednisone, 20 mg. daily for 1 week. Penicillin eruptions may be delayed in starting (2 months) and then persist for several months.

Alopecia Areata (Figure 50–33)

Location. Localized to any hairy area (e.g., scalp, eyebrow, eyelash, or beard) or total loss of all hair.

Duration. Some patients recover in a few months, but there is a tendency for the alopecia to recur. In others, there is total hair loss with a poor prognosis.

Etiology. Unknown. Emotions are a factor.

Symptoms. None.

Appearance. Round areas of complete hair loss, smooth without scale or scar; there may be some erythema. Gray hairs may not fall out, leaving a relative appearance of the hair turning gray.

Differential Diagnosis. Tinea capitis is most often suspected. The tinea shows broken hairs and scaling. The endocrine

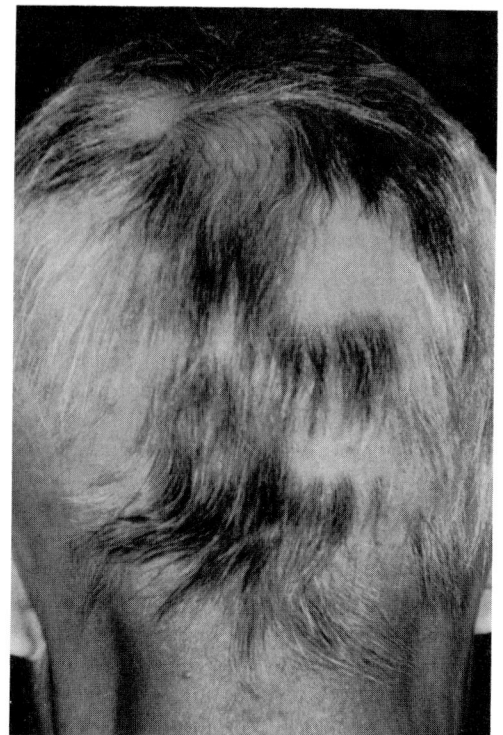

Figure 50–33. Alopecia areata.

disorders and drugs cause a more diffuse alopecia.

Treatment. Attempt to solve the emotional problem; give tranquilizers. The local patches can be injected with steroid suspension—e.g., triamcinolone acetonide (Kenalog) diluted to 3 mg. per ml. Steroid lotions or solutions can be rubbed into the scalp. For women, a wig will cover the bald areas and minimize their concern over scalp hair loss.

THE ACNE-SEBORRHEA GROUP

Acne

Location. Face, mostly. Also chest and back.

Duration. Starts at puberty and may persist for many years.

Etiology. Plugging and continued sebum production of sebaceous glands with rupture of the gland and tissue reaction. The increase in hormone production at puberty starts the process.

Appearance. Black points of plugged follicles, comedones, papules, pustules, abscesses, and scars.

Differential Diagnosis. Boils and rosacea.

Treatment. Treatment can be simplified by a regimen of soap, alcohol, lotion, and tetracycline, 250 mg. twice daily. At present, long-term tetracycline seems to be safe. Occasional *Candida* vaginitis and, even rarer, diarrhea may necessitate cessation of the drug. The psychologic benefits outweigh the small long-term risk. Milder, smaller, and less scarring lesions can be handled by local therapy only. The scalp should be kept clean. It takes 4 to 6 weeks to see results with tetracycline. The patient should be encouraged· to continue the therapy and not just told that he will outgrow the acne.

Diet therapy is not believed to be as important as it was thought to be in the past. Some patients may notice a flare with chocolate or excess milk. Summer sun or sun lamp therapy is helpful.

Seborrheic Dermatitis

Location. Scalp, center of chest and back, groin, axillae, ears, eyebrows, nasal crease.

Duration. Starts at puberty, sometimes during infancy, or in later life.

Etiology. The hormones of puberty stimulate the sebaceous glands. Patients with Parkinson's disease have an increased incidence.

Symptoms. Pruritus.

Appearance. The lesions are red, diffuse, and scaling. The disorder may be associated with acne and dandruff.

Differential Diagnosis. Psoriasis may begin in the scalp. Psoriasis should be considered when any seborrheic dermatitis does not respond well to therapy. Fungus infection, eczema, contact dermatitis, lupus erythematosus, and dermatomyositis are considered in the differential diagnosis.

Treatment. Prescribe the use of a shampoo containing a keratolytic. The red areas on the face may be irritated by soap. A hydrocortisone cream, 1/2 per cent, is most helpful here as well as on other generalized areas of seborrhea. The other more potent steroid creams should not be used on the face because they can induce an acneiform eruption. A mild dermatitis with just some scaling of the scalp may be controlled by using regular soap or shampoo and brushing away the scales.

Rosacea

Location. Face.

Duration. Begins later in life than acne.

Etiology. Unknown. Thought to be precipitated by too much cleansing cream, stimulants, alcohol, hot coffee, or spices.

Appearance. Presence of papules, pustules, and telangiectasia. The oil and comedones of acne are absent. The end result may be a rhinophyma or "rum nose."

Differential Diagnosis. Acne, seborrheic dermatitis, and lupus erythematosus.

Treatment. Avoid cleansing creams. The stronger lotions and soaps used in acne may be too drying. An acne lotion may be used in conjunction with iodochlorhydroxyquin (Vioform) cream. Oral tetracycline, 250 mg. twice daily, is helpful. In resistant cases a short course of internal prednisone may start a remission. Avoid internal stimulants and alcohol.

Hidradenitis Suppurativa

Location. Axillae and groin.

Duration. Chronic.

Etiology. Hidradenitis is placed in this group because of its association with acne. The apocrine gland is involved.

Symptoms. Pain.

Appearance. Hidradenitis starts as deep abscesses, with subsequent rupture and sinus and scar formation.

Differential Diagnosis. Boils and adenopathy.

Treatment. If the diagnosis is in doubt, try a regular course of antibiotic first (erythromycin, 250 mg. four times daily). The patients with chronic disease can be treated with long-term tetracycline administration, 250 mg. twice daily, and the use of antibacterial soaps for washing. Surgical drainage or removal of affected glands may be necessary.

THE PYODERMAS

Impetigo (Figure 50–34)

Location. Face, mostly. Sometimes other areas. Entity is called ecthyma when deeper in other areas.

Duration. More acute than other infections of the skin.

Etiology. Pathogenic *Staphylococcus aureus* is the most common cause. Beta strepto-

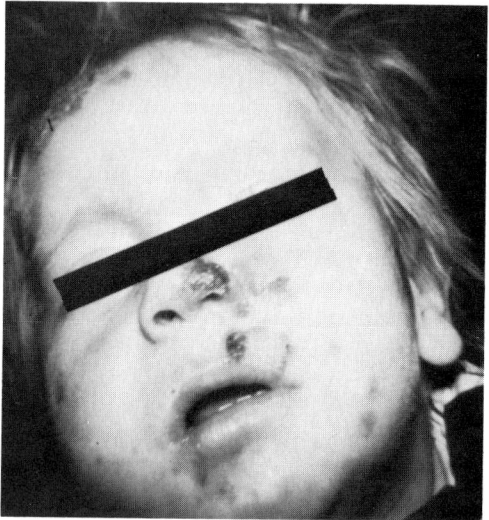

Figure 50–34. Impetigo.

coccus is the second most frequent cause.

Appearance. The lesions are crusted, round, and oozing. They are sometimes bullous, particularly in the infant, at the advancing edge of the lesion (Fig. 50–34).

Differential Diagnosis. Ringworm (fungus), nummular eczema, erythema multiforme, and dermatitis herpetiformis.

Treatment. Immediate internal antibiotic therapy shortens the course and complications. To kill the streptococcus and staphylococcus, give an antibiotic such as erythromycin, 250 mg. four times daily or less, according to the child's weight. Try to prevent spread of the infection by isolation of the patient, and do not allow others to use his washcloth or towel.

Boils

Location. Anywhere.
Duration. Acute but recurrent.
Etiology. Usually staphylococcus.
Appearance. Red, swollen, raised areas that later "point" as a pustule, become fluctuant, rupture, and drain.
Differential Diagnosis. Acne and folliculitis.
Treatment. The chronic cases are the problems. Antiseptic soap and internal antibiotics are prescribed. Culture and sensitivity tests are suggested.

Folliculitis

Location. More often found on extensors of arms and legs and on the buttocks.

Duration. Chronic, recurrent.
Etiology. Some lesions may be caused by bacterial invasion of the follicle. Others may be related to dry skin, atopic dermatitis, and plugged follicles. Oral iodide can also cause folliculitis.
Symptoms. Few.
Appearance. Small pustules about hair follicles, plugged follicles, little surrounding redness or swelling.
Differential Diagnosis. Acne, boils, and atopic dermatitis.
Treatment. Bacitracin ointment. If more severe, internal antibiotic. Use antiseptic soap but avoid drying out the skin.

VIRAL INFECTIONS

Herpes Simplex

Location. The lip is the usual location, but herpes may occur in several other areas, such as the fingertips, buttocks, and genitalia.
Duration. Recurrent vesicles at the same site is the most common form. Infants or debilitated persons may have more widespread infection.
Etiology. Virus.
Symptoms. Burning and pain.
Appearance. There are grouped vesicles, which go on to crusting.
Differential Diagnosis. Impetigo.
Treatment. None. Internal antibiotics should be given if secondary infections develop.

Herpes Zoster (Figure 50–35)

Location. On one-half of the body, over certain nerve distributions. Zoster of the ophthalmic branch may involve the conjunctiva or cornea. Occasionally, herpes zoster may become generalized in debilitated patients.
Duration. Rarer in childhood. Lasts about 2 weeks.
Etiology. Chickenpox virus. The patient has previously had chickenpox; the virus is then reactivated along a particular nerve distribution.
Symptoms. Pain may precede the eruption by a couple of days, mimicking the pain of appendicitis or of coronary heart disease, depending on the location. The pain may persist for months or years afterwards.

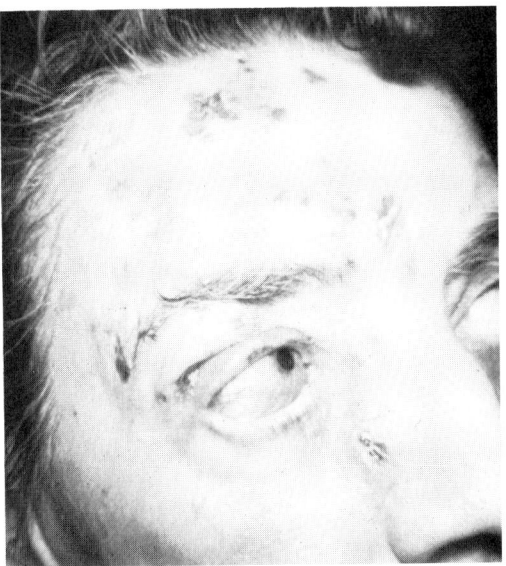

Figure 50-35. *Herpes zoster with eye involvement.*

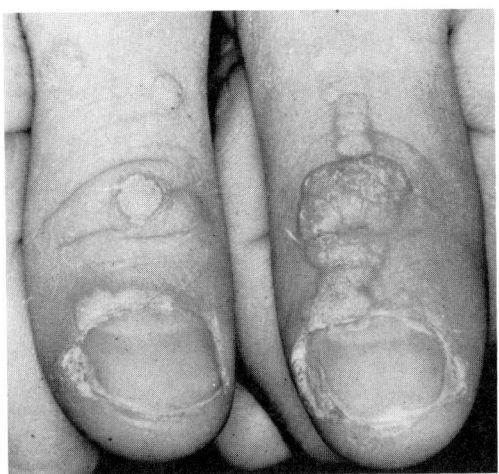

Figure 50-36. Warts. Some of the periungual warts resemble fungus.

Appearance. Grouped vesicles and pustules, sometimes hemorrhagic or necrotic; different sizes in a neural distribution.

Treatment. For patients under 50 years of age, analgesics for pain are suggested. When the patient is 50 years of age or older, analgesics plus internal prednisone are suggested: 40 mg. of prednisone for 2 days, then 30 mg. a day for 4 days, then 30 mg. every other day for four doses, then 15 mg. every other day for two doses and stop. This hopefully will prevent the posttherpetic neuralgia that occurs in older people.

Warts (Figures 50-36 to 50-38)

Location. Anywhere.
Duration. Chronic. More often seen in children. They may disappear spontaneously.
Etiology. Virus.
Appearance. Raised, verrucous, scaly, round lesions that may be linear in the scratch of inoculation. The flat, small warts are more difficult to diagnose, as are the periungual ones that mimic fungus (Fig. 50-36). Plantar lesions are often misdiagnosed and may in reality be corns. The wart has regular small blood vessels perpendicular to the plantar surface. By paring off some of the keratin layer, these vessels can be seen. The warts in the

genital area (condylomata acuminata) are more pedunculated and proliferative.

Differential Diagnosis.
1. Flat warts resemble lichen planus, sarcoid, and acne.
2. Plantar warts resemble corns.
3. Periungual warts resemble fungus.
4. Genital warts resemble secondary syphilis (condylomata lata) or carcinoma.

Treatment. The success of many remedies in the past may be attributed to spontaneous remission, antibodies to the virus, or suggestion. In therapy the main thing is to avoid scarring. Curettage and cautery is most definitive and can be used in areas where scarring will not be a problem. For multiple warts, freezing with liquid ni-

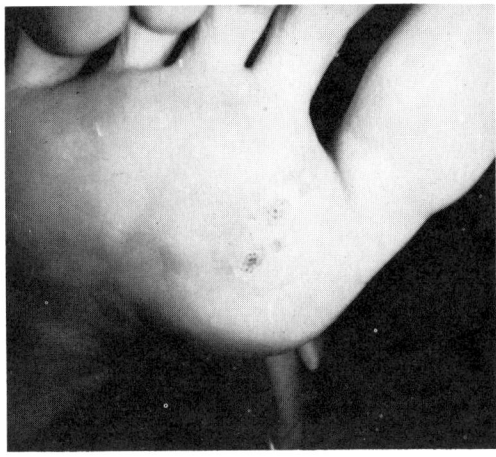

Figure 50-37. Plantar wart with dark blood vessels.

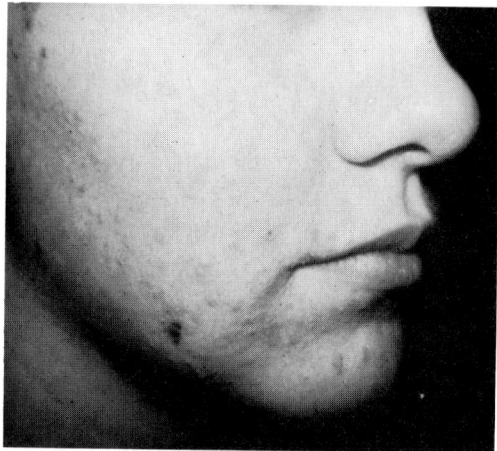

Figure 50–38. *Flat warts, many over the face, some forming in rings following recurrence after liquid nitrogen therapy.*

trogen is most effective. The flat warts disappear most readily. Application of a dye such as gentian violet may help by suggestion alone. The plantar warts are best treated by paring, followed by application of 90 per cent trichloroacetic acid and covering with a 40 per cent salicylic plaster. Leave plaster on for a week and have the patient return for new paring and plastering. Because this often takes months, the patient may use the plaster at home and make less frequent visits to the physician. This therapy may be used on warts in other areas or on plantar corns. Excision is contraindicated.

Molluscum Contagiosum (Figure 50–39)

Location. Anywhere. Genital area in adults.

Duration. Chronic. More often seen in younger patients.

Etiology. Virus.

Appearance. The main lesion is a round, shiny papule with a dimple in the center. This dimple can be accentuated by spraying with dichlorotetrafluoroethane (Frigiderm) (Fig. 50–39), or ethyl chloride spray. The lesions may be solitary (mimicking tumors) or multiple.

Differential Diagnosis. Warts, tumors, and basal cell carcinoma. The biopsy is specific.

Treatment. The papules are easily scraped off the skin with a curet. They may also clear spontaneously. Excision is not recommended.

THE SYSTEMIC DISEASE GROUP

Lupus Erythematosus (Figures 50–40 to 50–42 and Plate 2G, p. 1115)

Location. Face, hands, and exposed areas. Distribution may be extensive.

Duration. Acute to chronic.

Etiology. Autoimmune mechanism.

Appearance. The chronic discoid type presents as chronic, red, irregular plaques with some scale and follicular plugs that heal with scars. The plaques may occur in

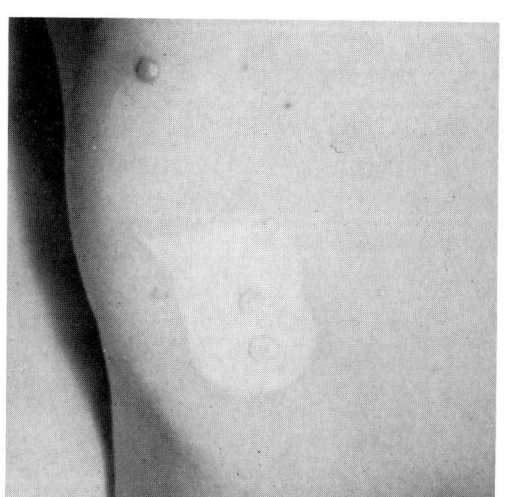

Figure 50–39. *Molluscum contagiosum.*

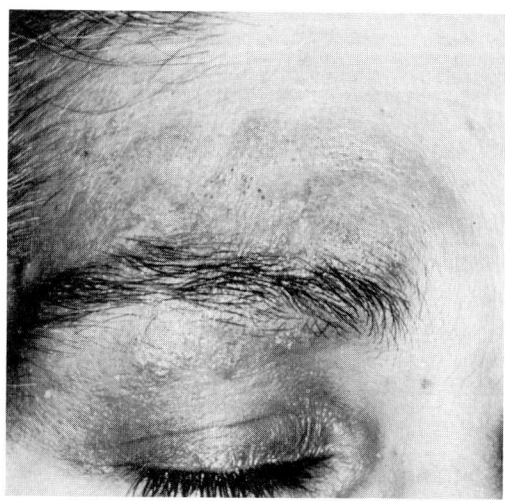

Figure 50–40. *Lupus erythematosus. Chronic discoid.*

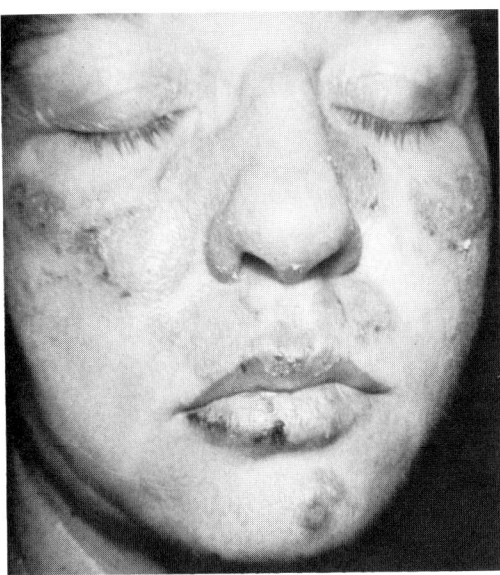

Figure 50–41. *Lupus erythematosus. Acute.*

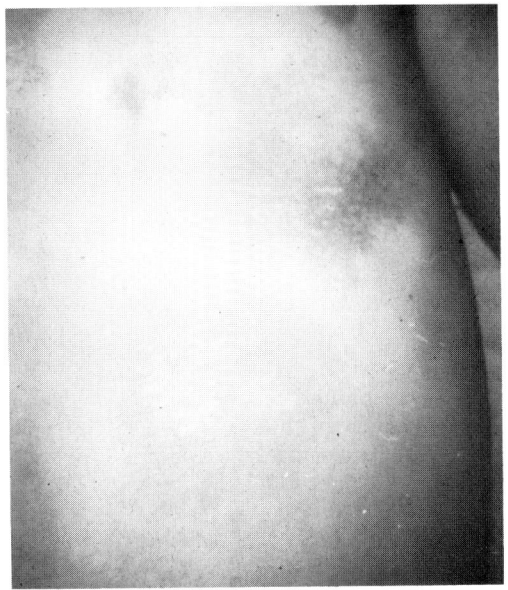

Figure 50–43. *Scleroderma. Localized with hyper- and hypopigmentation on the chest.*

the scalp and cause alopecia. The acute type may be less well defined and involve the palms, the periungual region, or larger areas. Systemic lupus erythematosus is confirmed by laboratory tests. The biopsy is helpful. The discoid type remains in the chronic benign form in many patients. The start of the acute type may follow exposure to the sun; thus, all of these patients should stay out of sunlight.

Differential Diagnosis. Psoriasis, rosacea, and photoallergy.

Treatment. Cordran Tape and intralesional triamcinolone acetonide (Kenalog).

10 mg. per ml. (dilute to 3 mg. per ml.; too much may cause atrophy), are used for the discoid form. If there are systemic symptoms and positive laboratory tests, internal drugs are used: chloroquine, prednisone, and immunosuppressives.

Scleroderma (Figure 50–43 and Plate 2D, p. 1114)

Location. Hands and face. May be more extensive. The local form is often linear, down an arm or leg.

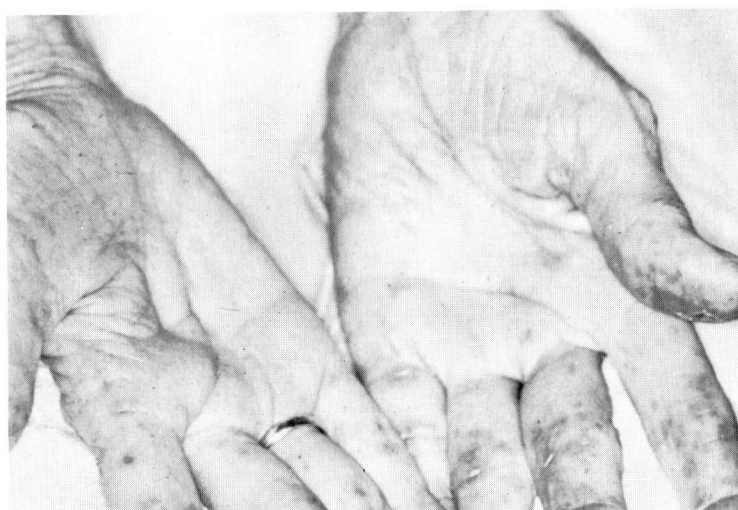

Figure 50–42. *Acute vascular lesions of the hands in lupus erythematosus.*

Duration. Chronic. Localized in the young.

Appearance. The skin is tight, shiny, and indurated, with areas of increased and decreased pigmentation. The hands become stiff, the face masklike. This systemic form may go on to involve the esophagus, kidneys, and lungs.

Patients with a localized plaque on the trunk or linear lesions down the leg have a good prognosis, and the disease does not become systemic.

Treatment. Unsatisfactory. Intralesional triamcinolone acetonide (Kenalog) can be used in the local form.

Dermatomyositis (Figure 50–44)

Location. Eyelids, extensors of joints, and periungual area.

Duration. Acute onset.

Symptoms. Muscle pain and weakness, particularly in the shoulder and hip girdle, and difficulty getting out of a deep chair. May progress to affect the muscles used in eating and breathing. There is a high incidence of internal malignancy.

Appearance. Redness and swelling of eyelids, face, and around scalp. There are redness and dilated vessels over joints.

Differential Diagnosis. Seborrheic dermatitis, angioedema, contact dermatitis, and lupus erythematosus. Muscle biopsy and elevated enzymes confirm the diagnosis.

Treatment. Early diagnosis and treatment with prednisone are important.

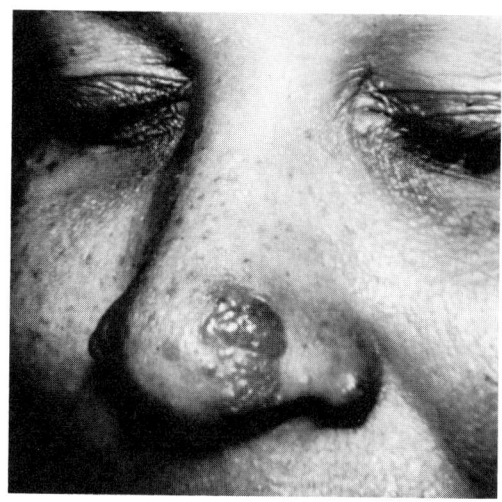

Figure 50–45. Sarcoid.

Sarcoid (Figure 50–45)

Recognition and biopsy of the papules about the face may help confirm the diagnosis of sarcoidosis.

Necrobiosis Lipoidica Diabeticorum (Figure 50–46 and Plate 2E, p. 1115)

Location. The lesions occur most often on the lower leg.

Duration. Chronic.

Etiology. Diabetes and vascular disease in some patients.

Appearance. Circumscribed, atrophic

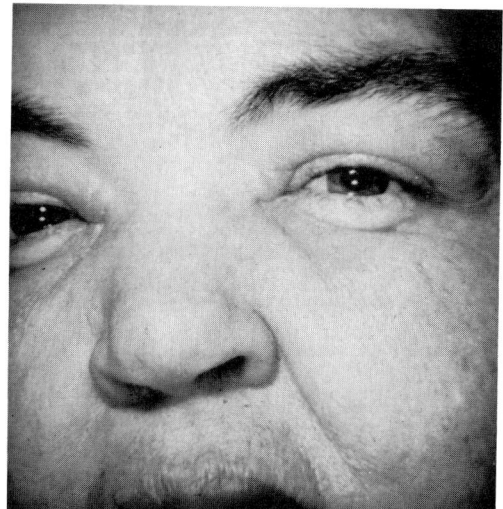

Figure 50–44. Dermatomyositis, with swollen face and eyelids.

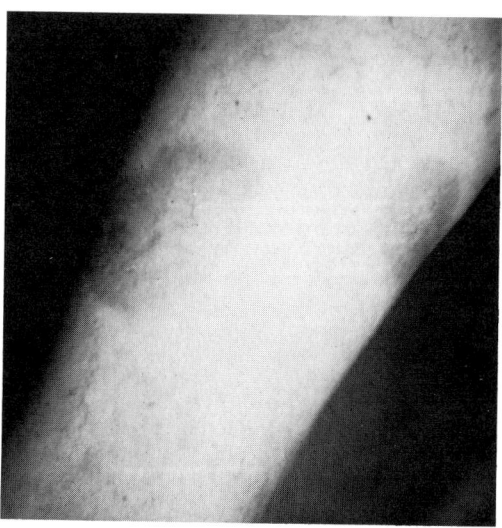

Figure 50–46. Necrobiosis lipoidica diabeticorum.

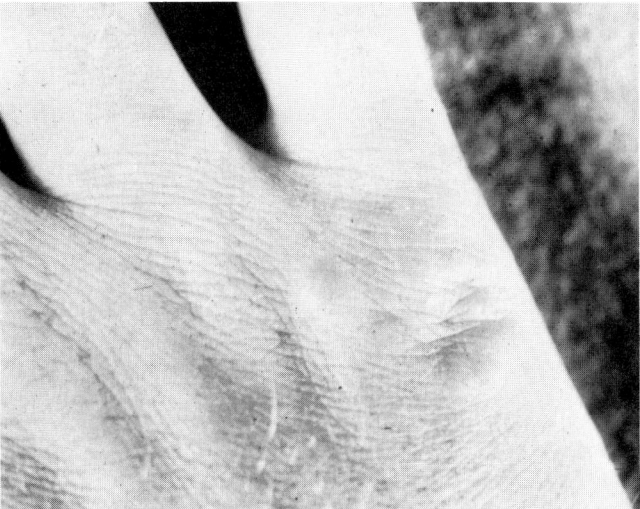

Figure 50–47. Granuloma annulare.

plaque, yellow to red, with the vessels showing through. There may be multiple plaques.

Differential Diagnosis. Localized scleroderma and scars. Diabetic patients may also have pigmented atrophic shin spots.

Treatment. None is satisfactory. Avoid trauma. If ulcer occurs, treat as other leg ulcers (soaks and internal antibiotics).

Granuloma Annulare (Figure 50–47)

Location. About the joints, fingers, and ankles, but may be anywhere.

Duration. Chronic with spontaneous resolution and some recurrence. More often seen in children.

Etiology. Unknown. Some tendency to occur in adult diabetics.

Appearance. Papules to nodules forming raised peripheral rings and central clearing. Flesh-colored or slightly pigmented. The lack of scale distinguishes it from tinea.

Differential Diagnosis. Granuloma annulare may be misdiagnosed as tinea or ringworm, particularly when it occurs on the feet. It also resembles fixed drug eruption, erythema multiforme or marginatum, and nummular eczema. The deeper nodules may be mistaken for erythema nodosum or for rheumatoid nodules. Some lesions have been unnecessarily excised because the raised shiny margin resembled basal cell carcinoma. The biopsy will usually confirm the diagnosis. Microscopically, the granuloma resembles a rheumatoid nodule.

Treatment. The lesions are usually only a cosmetic problem and will eventually resolve spontaneously. The newer local steroids applied under a plastic sheet (Saran Wrap) can be used.

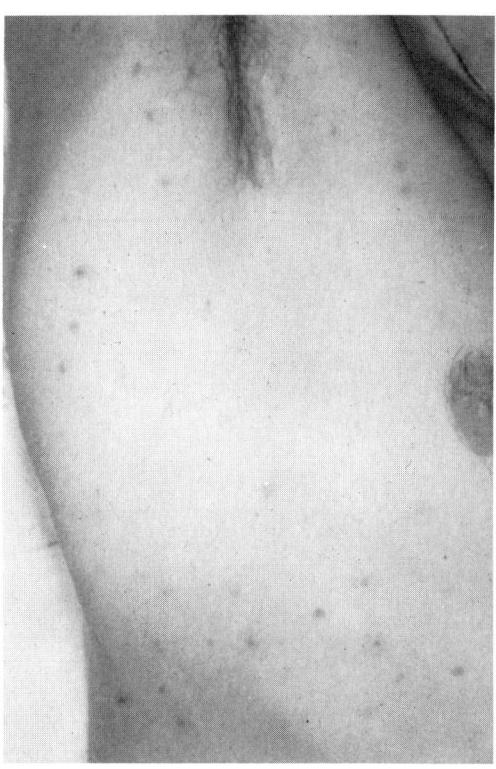

Figure 50–48. Syphilis. Secondary, generalized.

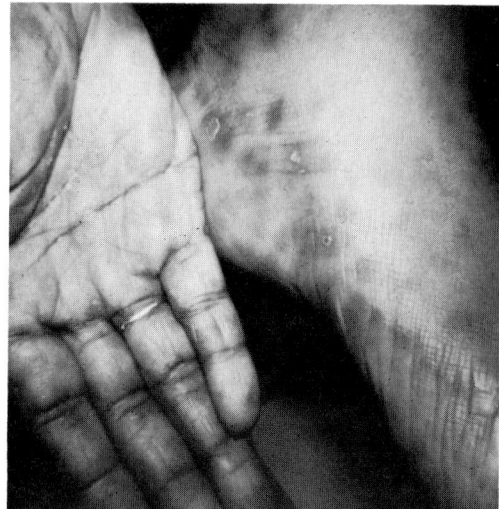

Figure 50–49. *Syphilis. Characteristic palmar and plantar location.*

Syphilis (Figures 50–48 and 50–49)

Location. The primary lesion (chancre) usually occurs in the anogenital region but may occur anywhere. The early signs of secondary syphilis tend to appear first on the lateral aspects of the chest and abdomen and on the flexor surfaces of the arms, palms, and soles.

Duration. The chancre appears approximately 21 days after infection, with a range of 10 to 90 days. Untreated, the lesion disappears in 9 to 12 weeks; the chancre in a treated patient should disappear in about a week.

Secondary lesions usually begin to appear after 2 months from the date of the original infection, but this time period may vary greatly. Occasionally the chancre may still be present when the signs of secondary syphilis appear.

Etiology. Infection with *Treponema pallidum.*

Appearance. Typically, the chancre appears as a hard, eroded papule with a clean base. A serosanguineous discharge may cover the eroded area or may be expressed by applying gentle pressure. Secondary lesions show extreme variation, from early macular (roseola) lesions to papular syphilids.

Excellent detailed descriptions and illustrations of the skin lesions of syphilis can be found in older textbooks of dermatology and syphilology. *Diseases of the Skin* by Sutton and Sutton[9] and *Modern Dermatology and Syphilology* by Becker and Obermayer[2] are excellent references and contain numerous illustrations of the various forms of syphilitic skin lesions before the advent of more effective therapy.

Differential Diagnosis. Syphilitic lesions may be confused with those of rubella, pityriasis rosea, acute psoriasis, fungus infections, drug eruptions, and viral exanthemas. The white mucous patches in the mouth mimic lichen planus, erythema multiforme, drug eruption, viral and bacterial infections, and infectious mononucleosis.

Maintain a high index of suspicion and

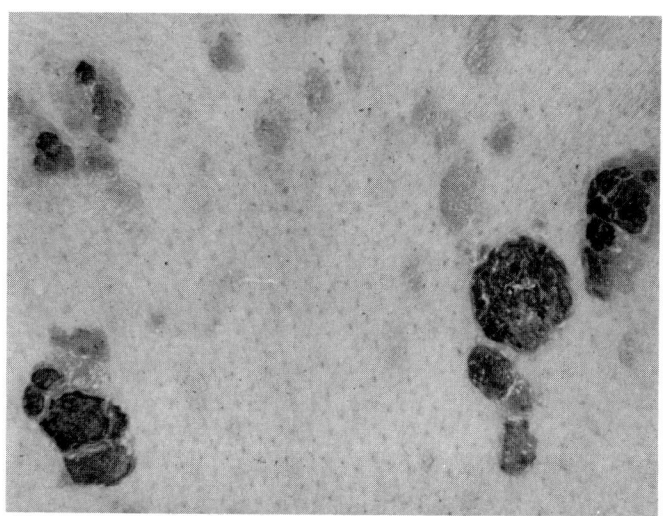

Figure 50–50. *Seborrheic keratoses.*

obtain a darkfield examination of any lesion if even the slightest doubt exists. Serologic tests for syphilis may not be reactive in the early infection but should be obtained for follow-up and therapy. For more detailed discussion of darkfield examinations and serologic tests, see Norins and Olansky.[7] Consult your local public health office for case finding and treatment.

TUMORS

Seborrheic Keratosis (Figure 50-50)

Location. Anywhere.
Duration. Slow-growing. Appears with age.
Etiology. Unknown.
Appearance. Circumscribed, stuck on the skin, verrucous, and scaly. Varying shades of pigment. Often multiple.
Differential Diagnosis. Warts, nevus, melanoma, and actinic keratoses.
Treatment. Shave off the lesion at the skin surface, then scrape away any rough base with a curet. A smooth firm base indicates complete removal. Light coagulation with Monsel's solution (ferric subsulfate solution) or trichloroacetic acid can be used to stop bleeding. Gelfoam or just a pressure dressing may give a better cosmetic result. Have the specimen submitted for histologic examination. If there is some doubt as to the clinical nature of the lesion, excision biopsy is recommended.

Skin Tags (Figure 50-51)

Location. Neck and axillae.
Duration. Slow appearance.
Appearance. Pedunculated, narrow base. Pigmented to flesh-colored. Usually multiple.
Differential Diagnosis. Nevus and neurofibroma.
Treatment. The small ones with a very narrow base may be cut quickly with a small scissors without anesthesia. A dressing usually stops any bleeding. The larger lesions with more pigmentation and without a narrow base should be submitted for histologic examination. Local anesthesia is desirable for excision of larger lesions.

Nevi (Figures 50-52 and 50-53)

Location. Anywhere.
Duration. Little change.
Appearance. Lesions variable in form from flat, dark to raised, nonpigmented.
Treatment. The raised, nonpigmented lesions about the face may be shaved at the base and lightly coagulated and the specimen submitted for examination. If the lesion turns out to be something other than a nevus, further excision can be done.

The flatter, more pigmented, irregular, growing, or ulcerated lesions should be excised.

Actinic (Senile) Keratosis (Figure 50-54)

Location. Exposed areas, hand, arms, face.

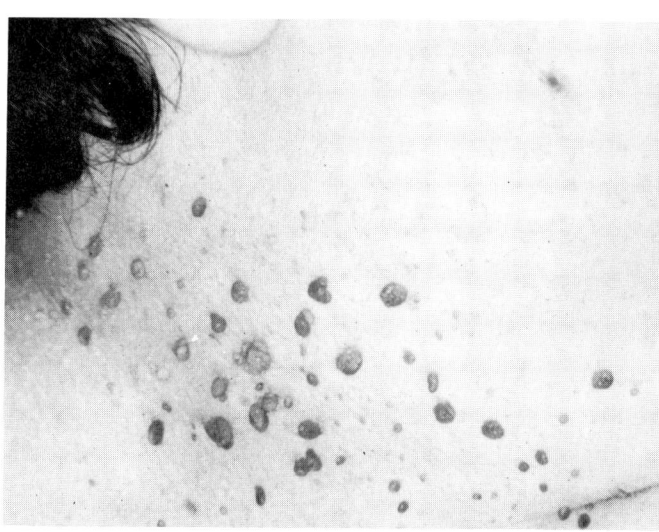

Figure 50–51. *Skin tags.*

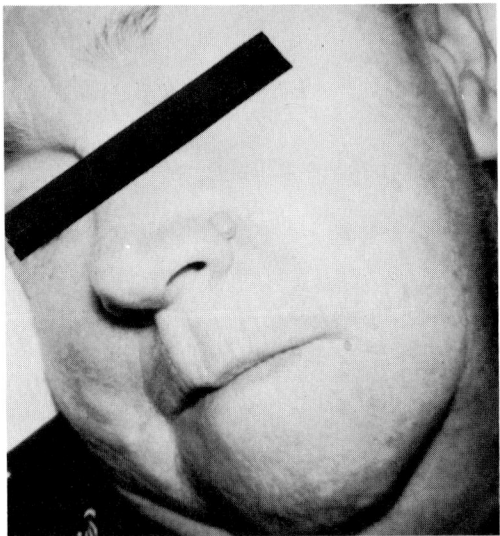

Figure 50–52. Nevus. Raised, nonpigmented.

Duration. Increase with age and fair skin.

Etiology. Sun exposure.

Appearance. Red, flat, scaling, and ill-defined lesions, sometimes with thick crust or horn.

Differential Diagnosis. Seborrheic keratosis, eczema, lupus erythematosus, early squamous cell carcinoma, and Bowen's disease.

Treatment. Local solution or cream of 5–fluorouracil (5–FU) 1 to 5 per cent works well (Fluoroplex, Efudex). It may

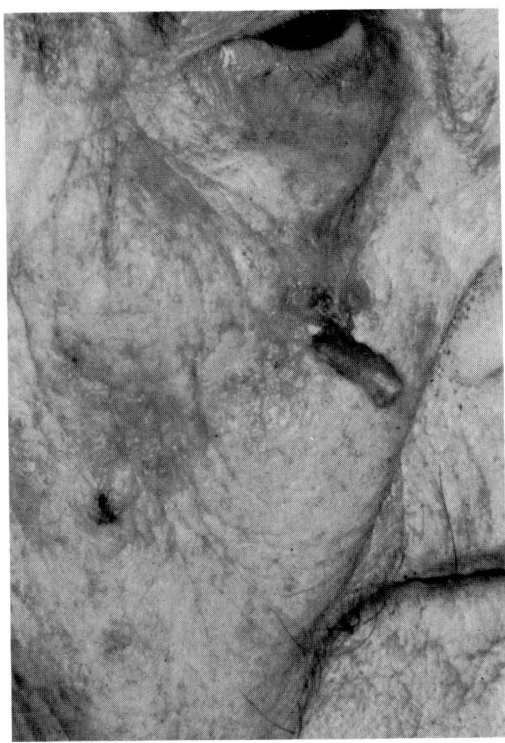

Figure 50–54. Actinic keratosis. Note horn, scaling, and age of individual.

be applied over large areas. Only the sun-damaged skin is affected. In a few days the areas become irritated, and the application should be continued for a total of 10–14 days. After healing, more persistent areas can be re-treated. A biopsy should be performed on any raised, doubtful, persistent areas. The 5-FU on the more keratotic lesions on the hands can be covered with a Band-Aid to produce more reaction. These lesions are precancerous and can develop into squamous cell carcinoma.

Bowen's Disease (Figure 50–55)

Location. Anywhere.

Duration. Chronic and slow growing.

Etiology. This is a form of squamous cell carcinoma in situ and may rarely become invasive or metastic. Arsenic is a cause, such as in Fowler's solution, tonics, and insect sprays, but not the arsenic used formerly in syphilis therapy.

Appearance. Round, scaling, circumscribed plaques, single or multiple. They are slow growing and often mistaken for eczema, fungi, or psoriasis. A biopsy

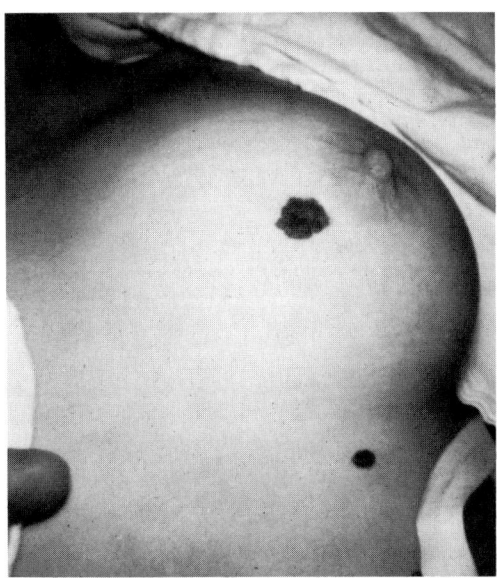

Figure 50–53. Nevus. Flatter, darker.

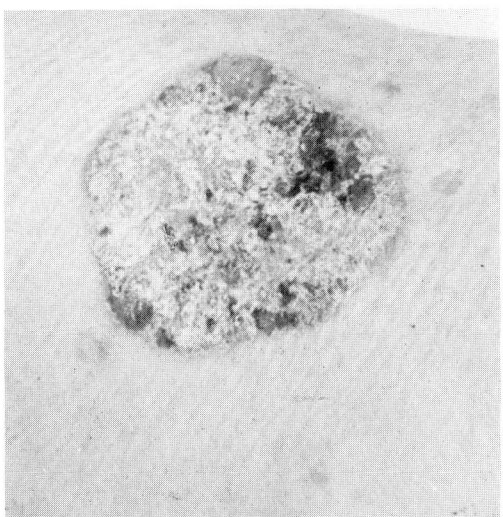

Figure 50–55. Bowen's disease. Plaque on wrist.

should be taken of any long-standing localized dermatitis not responding to local steroids. The palms and soles may show the discrete, punctate, arsenical keratoses. There is a high incidence of other internal primary carcinoma in association with Bowen's disease.

Differential Diagnosis. In addition to the inflammatory lesions mentioned at the beginning of this chapter, superficial basal cell carcinoma should be considered.

Treatment. After confirmation by biopsy, smaller lesions may be primarily excised. Larger lesions can be treated with local 5–fluorouracil, using two or three courses as described under *Actinic Keratosis.* Those lesions not responding should be excised, and, if needed, the area covered with skin grafts.

Basal Cell Carcinoma (Figures 50–56 to 50–58)

Location. Mostly seen on the face, but may be found anywhere on the skin.

Duration. Slow growing.

Etiology. The main cause is exposure of fair skin to sun plus some congenital factor to account for the frequency in more shaded areas (e.g., the nasal crease and the inner canthus of the eye). Chronic use of arsenic may cause the superficial lesions on covered areas. Previous x-ray therapy is also a cause.

Appearance. Round, raised, pearly edge, depressed or crusted ulcerated center, and telangiectasia. The superficial lesions are often missed. They grow slowly on the trunk or scalp and are usually thought to be a dermatitis or fungus (as mentioned under *Bowen's Disease*). They have a small pearly margin (Fig. 50–58).

Differential Diagnosis. Besides those entities just mentioned for the superficial lesions, nonpigmented nevi, sebaceous hyperplasia, molluscum contagiosum, keratoses, and squamous cell carcinoma should be included in the differential diagnosis.

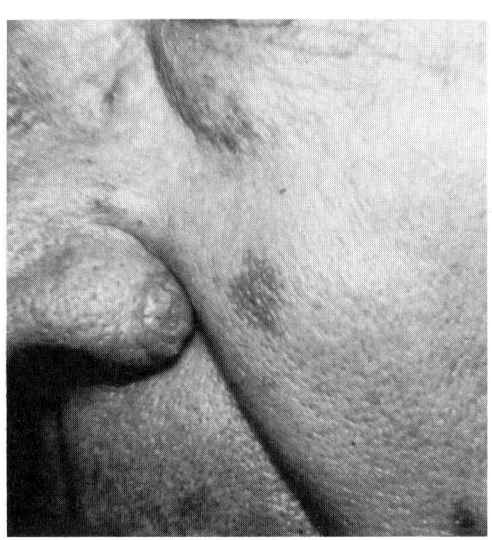

Figure 50–56. Basal cell carcinoma.

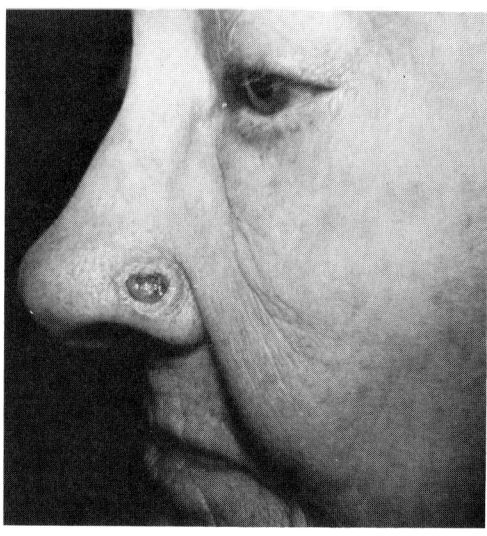

Figure 50–57. Nodular basal cell carcinoma on nose.

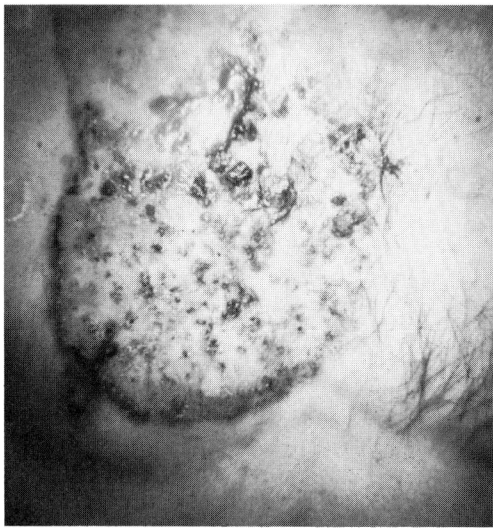

Figure 50–58. *Basal cell carcinoma. Superficial.*

Treatment. They respond equally well to curettage, x-ray, or excision. The size and location influence the type of treatment. The details are not within the scope of this book.

Squamous Cell Carcinoma of Skin

Location. More on exposed areas, hands, face, and ears.

Duration. Slow to arise in the actinic keratoses. Some may grow more rapidly.

Etiology. Sun, x-ray, and burns.

Appearance. This section is mainly concerned with the low-grade lesions that arise in actinic keratosis (see previous section). The lesions become raised and keratotic and proceed to ulcerations and friable vegetation.

Differential Diagnosis. Deep fungus (see section on *Blastomycosis*), keratoacanthoma, gumma, lymphoma, metastatic carcinoma, amelanotic melanoma, wart, and keratosis.

Treatment. Adequate prior biopsy is recommended. The smaller lesions that do not respond to the local 5–fluorouracil (see treatment for *Actinic Keratosis*) can be treated by curettage or excision. Larger lesions may be treated with excision and grafting or by x-ray.

Keratoacanthoma (Figures 50–59 and 50–60)

Location. Exposed areas.

Duration. Rapid growth in 3 months. Squamous carcinoma is slower.

Etiology. Unknown.

Appearance. Raised, with keratotic center.

Differential Diagnosis. Same as that for squamous carcinoma. It is important to note that although keratoacanthoma clinically and histologically resembles a squamous cell carcinoma, it does not require radical treatment.

Treatment. The lesion may disappear spontaneously after biopsy (see Figs. 50–59 and 50–60, before and after). Only an adequate biopsy is done, removing a wedge from the center along with some deep and lateral margin. For those lesions that do not regress, further consultation and diagnostic measures are suggested.

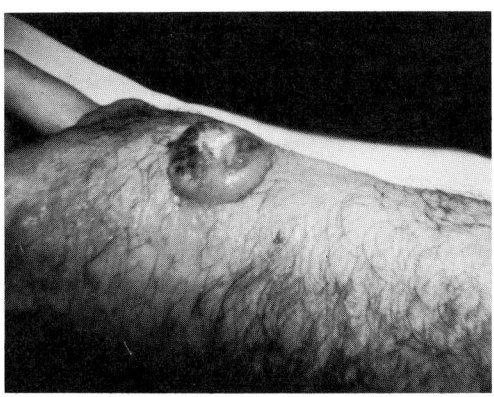

Figure 50–59. *Keratoacanthoma.*

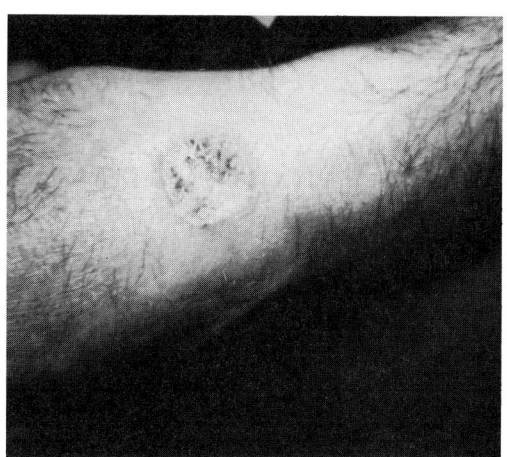

Figure 50–60. *Keratoacanthoma following a wedge biopsy.*

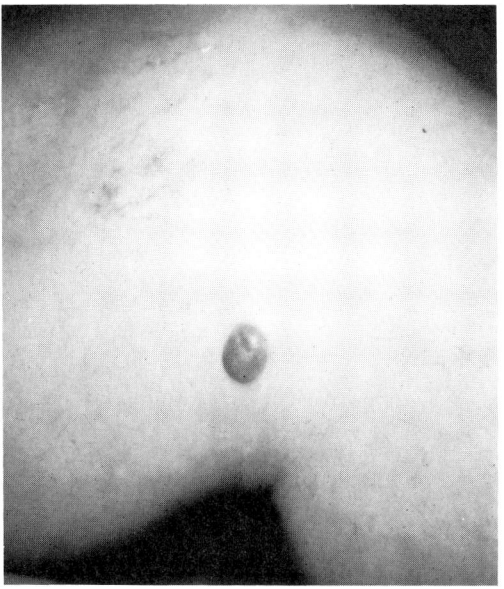

Figure 50–61. *Dermatofibroma.*

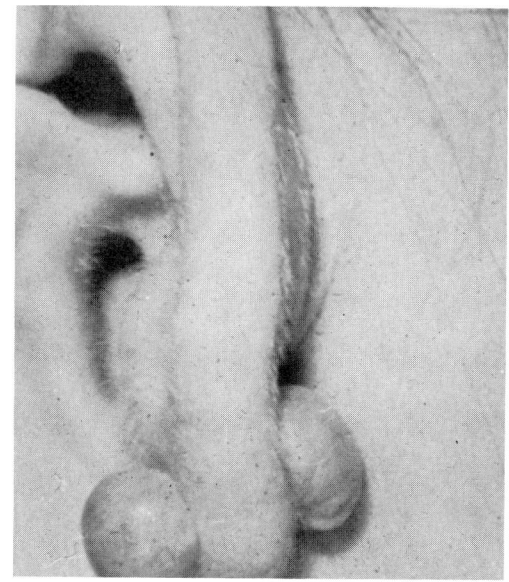

Figure 50–62. *Keloid from pierced ears. (Courtesy Harold Saferstein, M.D.)*

Dermatofibroma (Figure 50–61)

Location. Occurs on lower legs most often, but may be anywhere.

Duration. Chronic. Little change.

Etiology. May follow trauma.

Appearance. Firm, raised nodule. Reddish-brown. Some are more palpable than raised.

Treatment. Excise with narrow margin, and suture. The lesions are not premalignant but could be mistaken for early dermatofibrosarcoma.

Keloid (Figure 50–62)

Location. More often located on ear lobes, chin, neck, shoulders, upper trunk, and lower legs.

Duration. Chronic but may regress spontaneously. Less often seen in infants and aged patients.

Etiology. Hereditary predisposition. Trauma, even very minor trauma, such as vaccination or piercing ears.

Symptoms. Some patients complain of itching or burning.

Appearance. Firm, raised, brownish, red-purple, smooth areas. May be in dumbbell-shaped bands on chest.

Differential Diagnosis. Dermatofibroma and hypertrophic scar.

Treatment. Try to prevent by avoiding procedures in those persons with a tendency to form keloids. Avoid tension on sutures and consider some x-ray therapy as the excision site is healing. Excision of the keloid often results in a larger one, plus keloids at the suture marks. Intralesional injection of steroids—e.g., triamcinolone acetonide (Kenalog) 10 mg. per ml.—is recommended.

Mycosis Fungoides (Figures 50–63 and 50–64)

Location. Generalized and multicentric.

Duration. Chronic.

Etiology. Lymphoma of skin.

Symptoms. Itching.

Appearance. Starts as a scaling dermatitis, becomes indurated plaques, and finally develops into tumors.

Differential Diagnosis. Psoriasis, nummular eczema, fungus, and atopic dermatitis. This lymphoma is important because it may progress for years diagnosed as an eczema. Early therapy does seem to alter the course. The reverse may happen, also: an eczema may be diagnosed histologically as mycosis fungoides.

Treatment. For the early stage, local nitrogen mustard works well. Later, x-ray and cytotoxic drugs are used.

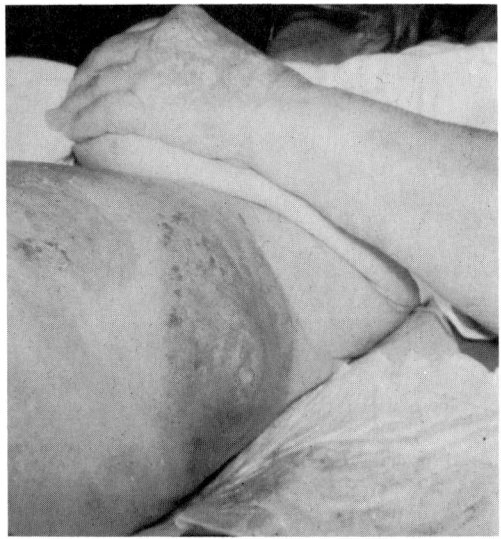

Figure 50-63. Mycosis fungoides.

Scabies (Plate 2H, p. 1115)

Location. The hands, feet, and genitalia are more favored than the arms, legs, and trunk.

Etiology. Mite.

Symptoms. Severe itching, especially at

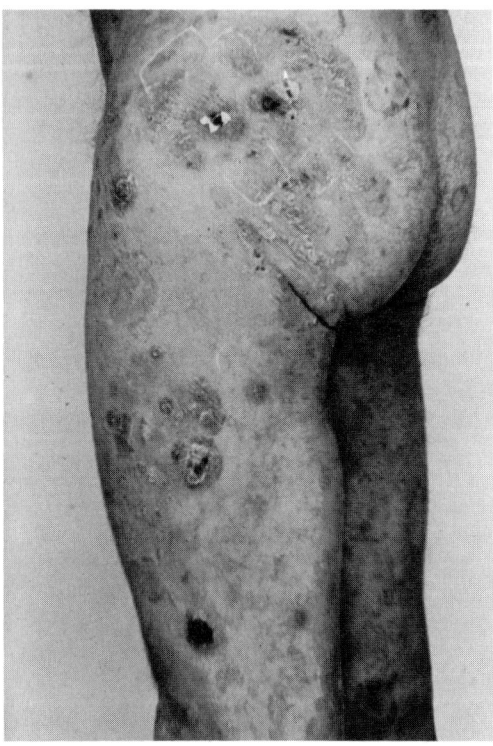

Figure 50-64. Mycosis fungoides.

night. Other people in the family may have the same thing.

Appearance. Excoriations, crusts, oozing, secondary infection, eczematization. Edematous papules or nodules, especially on the penis and scrotum. The linear burrows are not often seen.

Diagnosis. The mite and eggs are easy to identify under the microscope, but it may be difficult to get a positive scraping. Scrape several areas with a curet, put on a slide with 10 per cent KOH or oil, and cover slip.

Treatment. Use 1 per cent gamma benzene hexachloride cream or lotion applied from the neck down one time and washed off in 24 hours and change clothes. It may be repeated in a week. Until we know more about gamma benzene hexachloride absorption and toxicity, sulfur 6 per cent ointment is recommended for small infants and pregnant women. Apply once a day for 3 days.

Pediculosis Pubis

Location. Hairy areas except scalp.

Etiology. Louse *(Phthirus pubis)*. This louse can be seen on the skin or hair. Also the dewdrop egg attached to the hair.

Symptoms. Itching.

Treatment. Same as for scabies.

KOH SLIDE TECHNIQUE

Wet the skin lightly with alcohol gauze (not cotton), so that the scales will stick to the No. 15 blade. It is best to take the scales from the active margin.

Smear the scales on a slide, add a drop of 10 per cent KOH, and warm gently, or let it sit for 20 minutes to make the epidermal cell margins less distinct. Then look for the long, branching septate hyphae. They may be hard to find. Some practice is needed. Perhaps a nurse or physician's assistant could be trained to do this.

CULTURE TECHNIQUE

For culture, try the dermatophyte test medium (DTM) available from Chester A. Barker Laboratories, Miami, Florida. DTM comes with an orange color and turns red owing to pH change as a pathogen grows. Contaminants do not change the color. If the growth is a pathogen, it will in most cases respond to griseofulvin. If further identification is desired, the culture could be sent to a laboratory for identification. Read the culture after 2 weeks' incubation at room temperature.[1]

With DTM, false positives and false negatives occur. For best results use Sabouraud's agar with antibiotics.

Yeasts such as *Candida albicans* will grow on both media and do not respond to griseofulvin. There should be no trouble telling the small, shiny yeast colonies from other fungi.

The Sabouraud's agar implanted with lesion scales is also kept at room temperature and observed after 2 weeks. If there is growth, ask someone to identify it. Check with a dermatologist or teaching center in your area for the best place to obtain media and accurate identification of cultures. Contaminants do grow on Sabouraud's agar.

BIOPSY TECHNIQUE

The punch biopsy is a helpful diagnostic technique requiring little equipment. The 4 to 5 mm. punch is most often used. Dome Labs., West Haven, Connecticut, has a disposable punch, but it is not quite as sharp as the conventional ones.

A small amount of alcohol is applied to the skin, and a wheal raised with lidocaine (Xylocaine) and epinephrine. The punch is applied perpendicular to the skin and rotated between the thumb and index finger. Go through the dermis to the fat. Usually you can feel penetration. The plug of tissue will usually pop up a little, and a blade or sterile scissors is used to cut loose the underlying fat. Handle the tissue carefully with the forceps. Avoid crushing, particularly the surface. Put the tissue in 10 per cent formalin.

Choosing the biopsy site is difficult. A typical well-formed lesion is usually best; e.g., those in lupus erythematosus or lichen planus. For bullous lesions a new, small lesion is best. Try to get a whole, intact blister. A large punch or an elliptical excision may be needed.

A biopsy of two different areas may be helpful. Some people prefer to put a suture in the punch site, but this is unnecessary and requires additional equipment and sterilization.

REFERENCES

1. Allen, A. M., Drewry, R. A., and Weaver, R. E.: Evaluation of two new color indicator media for diagnosis of dermatophytosis. Arch. Derm., *102*:68, 1970.
2. Becker, S. W., and Obermayer, M. E.: Modern Dermatology and Syphilology. Philadelphia, J. B. Lippincott Co., 1943.
3. Conn, H. F.: Current Therapy 1978. Philadelphia, W. B. Saunders Co., 1978.
4. Conn, H. F., and Conn, R. B.: Current Diagnosis 5. Philadelphia, W. B. Saunders Co., 1977.
5. Fisher, A. A.: Contact Dermatitis 2nd Ed. Philadelphia, Lea & Febiger, 1975.
6. Korting, G. W.: Diseases of the Skin in Children and Adolescents. A Color Atlas. (Translated by Drs. William and Helen Curth.) Philadelphia, W. B. Saunders Company, 1970. [This is a good collection of color plates of the diseases discussed in this chapter.]
7. Norins, L. C., and Olansky, S.: Syphilis. *In* Conn, H. F., and Conn, R. B.: Current Diagnosis. Philadelphia, W. B. Saunders Co., 1971, p. 223.
8. Rook, A., Wilkinson, D. S., and Ebling, F. J. G.: Textbook of Dermatology. 2nd Ed. Oxford, Blackwell Scientific Publications Ltd., 1972.
9. Sutton, R. L., and Sutton, R. L., Jr.: Diseases of the Skin. St. Louis, The C. V. Mosby Co., 1939.
10. Syphilis. Modern Diagnosis and Management. Washington, D.C., U.S. Government Printing Office, 1961.

Chapter 51

ALLERGY AND IMMUNOLOGY

by ALAN A. WANDERER,
and CARL FLAXER

EVALUATION OF SUSPECT IMMUNODEFICIENCY DISORDERS

General

Immune responses can be classified into four major categories, as proposed by Gell and Coombs[3]:

1. Type I—Anaphylactic reactions. This class refers to the interaction between reaginic antibodies and antigen. The reaginic antibodies primarily belong to the IgE immunoglobulin class. The interaction between IgE reaginic antibodies and antigen results in the release of pharmacologic mediators such as histamine. Examples of Type I reactions include extrinsic asthma, allergic rhinitis, and some urticarial responses.

2. Type II—Cytotoxic reactions. This class of immune responses refers to the interaction of circulating antibodies with cell-bound antigen. Examples are transfusion reactions.

3. Type III—Immune complex reactions (Arthus's reactions). These reactions are due to the deposition of antigen-antibody complexes, which results in complement activation and tissue damage. Examples include serum sickness and hypersensitivity pneumonitis.

4. Type IV—Delayed hypersensitivity. This refers to the interaction between antigen and sensitized lymphoid cells. Examples include the classic tuberculin skin test response and contact dermatitis reactions.

Immunologic and allergic manifestations may involve more than one of these immune mechanisms.

Type I through Type III responses involve humoral antibodies that belong to one of five different classes of immunoglobulins. These antibodies are produced by plasma cells, which in turn are derived from B lymphocytes originating in the bone marrow and lymphoid patches, such as Peyer's patches. Each class of immunoglobulins differs chemically and functionally, and each is part of the globulin moiety in serum protein electrophoretic patterns. IgG is the immunoglobulin with the largest blood concentration and the only one that passes the placenta and accounts for most neonatal antibody. It is the principal antigen-binding immunoglobulin in the circulation of adults and children. IgA antibody is detected in the serum and in the respiratory and gastrointestinal tracts as secretory antibody. IgM is the first antibody produced after antigen stimulation. If detected in neonatal serum, it implies the existence of intrauterine infection, as the antibody does not cross the placental barrier. IgD is present in small quantities, and its function is still not understood. IgE is the immunoglobulin present in the smallest quantities and appears to be identified as the reaginic factor that is responsible for immediate hypersensitivity reactions. It is elevated in atopic persons with extrinsic asthma, atopic eczema, and parasitic infestations.

Type IV reactions involve so-called cell-mediated immunity. The cell-mediated immune response, also referred to as delayed-type hypersensitivity, is responsible for the major host defense against pathogens that are capable of intracellular survival, such as viral, fungal, and protozoal agents. Cell-mediated immunity is also responsible for graft rejection and contact dermatitis reactions. The lymphocytes responsible for this immune response are referred to as T lymphocytes, as they are under thymic influence. The T cells secrete various lymphokines that are responsible for delayed hypersensitivity responses and host defenses against intracellular proliferating organisms. Some of the important lymphokines that have been identified include interferon, migration-inhibition factor, macrophage-activating factor, and chemotactic factors.

Evaluation of host defense systems has led to the recognition of various immunodeficiency disorders. Approximately 60 per cent result from defects of the humoral antibody system, 20 per cent are caused by combined failure of the humoral antibody and cell-mediated systems, and 10 per cent are related to deficiencies of cellular immunity alone. Disorders of the phagocytic and complement systems account for less than 1 per cent of immunodeficiency problems.

Clinical Features

Table 51–1 refers to various known immunodeficiency disorders.

The most characteristic symptom of immunodeficiency is an increased susceptibility to infections. This includes not only increased frequency of infection but also prolonged duration of infection and unusual manifestations and complications. In general, respiratory infections are the most common, but disorders of other organ systems may be involved, such as osteomyelitis, meningitis, and sepsis.

There are four classes of infections that suggest immunodeficiency: (1) infections by bacteria of high virulence, such as *Staphylococcus aureus* and *Hemophilus influenzae*; (2) infections by bacteria of low virulence, such as *Streptococcus viridans*; (3) fungal infections, such as *Candida albicans*; and (4) reactions to live attenuated vaccines, such as smallpox vaccine.

Diagnosis

The diagnosis of an immunodeficiency can be ascertained only by laboratory tests. Table 51–2 lists an outline for evaluation of suspect immunodeficiency diseases.

A complete blood count (CBC) is requested along with a total lymphocyte count. The latter is often depressed in disorders of cell-mediated immunity. Examination or x-ray, or both, of the lateral

---

TABLE 51–1. IMMUNODEFICIENCY DISORDERS

Disorders of the Immunoglobulin System (Humoral Antibody)
1. Transient disorders in infancy (4 to 6 months)
2. X-linked agammaglobulinemia (Bruton's disease)
3. Functional antibody deficiency despite normal Ig levels
4. Acquired hypogammaglobulinemia
5. Dysgammaglobulinemias
6. IgA deficiency
7. IgM deficiency

Cell-mediated Immunodeficiency
1. Thymic hypoplasia (DiGeorge's syndrome)
2. Chronic candidiasis

Combined Immunodeficiency (Humoral Antibody and Cell-mediated Deficiencies)
1. Swiss type
2. Autosomal recessive type (Nezelof's syndrome)
3. Ataxia telangiectasia
4. Reticular dysgenesis
5. Wiskott-Aldrich syndrome
6. Acquired deficiency
7. Thymomas

TABLE 51–2. DIAGNOSTIC EVALUATION FOR SUSPECT IMMUNODEFICIENCY DISORDERS

History

Physical Examination

Assessment of Humoral Antibody Deficiency
1. Screening tests:
   a. Complete blood count and differential with total lymphocyte count
   b. Lateral x-ray of pharynx and chest x-ray if indicated
   c. Quantitative determination of serum immunoglobulins
   d. Specific tests for antibody function, such as Schick test (IgG) and serum isohemagglutinin titers (IgM)
2. Specialized tests for humoral antibody:
   a. Quantitation of B cell rosettes
   b. Lymph node biopsy
   c. B cell immunofluorescence

Assessment of Cell-mediated Immunity
1. Screening tests:
   a. Total peripheral lymphocyte count
   b. Chest x-ray for thymus shadow in neonates
   c. Skin tests for delayed hypersensitivity (SK-SD, *Candida, Trichophyton*, PPD, mumps)
2. Specialized tests for cell-mediated function:
   a. DNFB sensitization (dinitrofluorobenzene)
   b. T cell determination by sheep red cell rosette assay
   c. Phytohemagglutinin lymphocyte stimulation
   d. Lymph node biopsy

pharynx may reveal decreased tonsillar and adenoid tissue, indicative of decreased lymphoid development. Humoral immunity can be assessed by radial immunodiffusion quantitation of serum immunoglobulins to include IgG, IgA, and IgM. This method is more specific and accurate than other techniques such as serum electrophoresis and immunoelectrophoresis. These determinations vary with the age of the patient, and therefore interpretation of these tests must be made by comparing age-dependent norms. Assessment of humoral antibody must also include determination of functional antibody production. A Schick test can be utilized to assess IgG function in a person previously immunized with diphtheria toxoid. Erythema and induration at the skin test site (a positive Schick test) suggest deficient IgG diphtheria antitoxin. A negative test shows that the patient has circulating antitoxin to neutralize the injected toxin, which signifies the presence of specific and effective antibody of the IgG type. IgM functioning antibody can be assessed by measuring serum isohemagglutinin titers. Antibody function can also be determined by measuring antibody levels in response to vaccines such as diphtheria-tetanus antigens.

The evaluation of cell-mediated immunity includes a total lymphocyte count. Normally, peripheral blood contains 1000 to 2000 lymphocytes per cu. mm. A total lymphocyte count lower than 1000 per cu. mm. is compatible with a deficiency of cell-mediated immunity. Lymphopenia may also occur secondary to viral infection. A normal total lymphocyte count does not exclude cell-mediated immune deficiency. A neonatal chest x-ray for thymus shadow is worth obtaining, as many immunodeficiency syndromes are associated with the absence of a thymus gland. Intradermal skin tests with certain antigens provoke delayed-type hypersensitivity reactions at 24 to 72 hours. A panel of antigens is used to detect the presence of delayed-type hypersensitivity in order to increase the likelihood of a positive reaction. These antigens include: (1) streptokinase-streptodornase (SK-SD, 10 units and 2.5 units respectively) injected intradermally; if negative, a higher concentration may be used (40 units and 10 units respectively), (2) *Candida albicans,* diluted 1:1000 and injected intradermally and then diluted 1:100 if the first dilution is negative, (3) *Trichophyton,* same as *Candida albicans,* (4) intradermal tuberculin skin tests, and (5) mumps antigen skin test. Approximately 9 out of 10 adults should have a positive reaction to one of these delayed-type hypersensitivity skin tests. If the skin tests are negative, further tests for cellular-immune function can be performed by specialized immunology laboratories (see Table 51–2).

Treatment

The major emphasis in treating immunodeficiency disorders should be in the prevention and early treatment of infectious illnesses. Antibiotic therapy is encouraged after appropriate cultures are obtained If the infection does not respond to antibiotics, the physician should consider that the infection may be caused by opportunistic infectious agents, for example, *Candida albicans,* or *Pneumocystis carinii.* Continuous prophylactic use of antibiotics is often beneficial in treating immunodeficiency disorders. Penicillin or ampicillin, adult oral doses of 0.5 to 1.0 gram per 24 hours, is recommended. This approach is particularly useful in treating patients with recurrent pulmonary infections, for example, bronchiectasis.

Gamma globulin is the mainstay for treatment of humoral antibody deficiency disorders. However, it should be reserved for severe deficiency of serum IgG. Exogenous gamma globulin injection cannot raise serum IgG levels above 300 to 400 mg. per 100 ml. Deficiencies of IgA or IgM will not benefit from injections of gamma globulin, as 95 per cent of commercially prepared gamma globulin is IgG. The recommended intramuscular dose of gamma globulin is 0.7 ml. per kg. in divided doses per month.

Patients with cellular-immune deficiency should not receive:

1. Fresh whole blood transfusions, because of the possibility of a graft vs. host reaction from the transfused lymphocytes. In the graft vs. host response, deficient cellular immunity in the host prevents elimination of the transfused foreign lymphocytes. As a result, the transplanted lymphocytes induce a host response characterized by rash, hepatic dysfunction, bone marrow aplasia, and death.

2. Live attenuated viral vaccines (smallpox, poliomyelitis, measles, mumps, ru-

bella), because of the risk of vaccine-induced infection.

Therapy for cellular-immune deficiency currently includes: (1) bone marrow replacement, (2) thymus gland transplantation, and (3) transfer factor injections. Transfer factor is a low molecular weight extract of sensitized lymphocytes that impart cellular immunity to nonsensitized lymphocytes. These procedures are experimental and require expert supervision.

URTICARIA AND ANGIOEDEMA

Urticaria may be defined as an eruption of transient circumscribed edema of the skin that is usually, but not always, pruritic. Angioedema, sometimes referred to as giant urticaria or angioneurotic edema, is a similar process involving the subcutaneous tissues. This symptom complex is not associated with a neurotic predilection, and the term angioneurotic edema has therefore been replaced by the more appropriate term, angioedema.

It is customary to differentiate between acute and chronic urticaria based on duration of symptoms. In general, symptoms that persist more than 2 months are classified as chronic. Urticaria is a very common disorder, and it is estimated that 20 per cent of the general population experience at least one episode of urticaria during their lifetime. It occurs more frequently in young women, regardless of the cause. The mean duration of chronic undifferentiated urticaria that occurs alone is 6 months, chronic angioedema lasts an average of one year, and chronic urticaria associated with angioedema persists an average of 5 years.

There is an unfortunate tendency of clinicians to view urticaria or angioedema, or both, as benign, self-limiting processes that are not worthy of significant attention. This attitude should be dispelled, as these symptoms may be the harbinger of other features of anaphylactic shock and laryngeal edema. In addition, urticaria and angioedema may be a manifestation of more serious underlying illnesses.

Histopathology and Pathogenesis

The histopathology of urticaria is a mixture of dilation of small cutaneous blood vessels and edema of the upper corium. The blood vessel dilation causes the erythema associated with this eruption, while the increased capillary permeability and transudation of fluid induce a characteristic pale swelling, i.e., a wheal. Similar changes in subcutaneous tissues produce more diffuse swelling, and the term angioedema refers to this dermal process. An intracutaneous injection of histamine can mimic the aforementioned histologic changes, which supports the hypothesis that urticaria is a result of histamine release. Other chemical mediators can increase capillary permeability, and there is considerable investigative interest in whether urticaria can be induced by mediators such as slow-reacting substance of anaphylaxis (SRS-A), kinins, and prostaglandins. Histamine release typically occurs as a result of allergic mechanisms (Type I reagin antibody mediation); however, immunologic mechanisms other than immediate hypersensitivity may also evoke urticarial responses. For instance, hives may accompany transfusion reactions in which IgG or IgM antibodies react with antigens on red cells (Type II cytotoxic mechanism). Similarly, antigen-antibody immune complexes (Type III Arthus's reactions) are associated with urticaria induction, as observed in serum sickness and following injections of aggregated gamma globulin.

Nonimmune release of histamine and other mediators can also result in urticarial induction. For example, a wide variety of chemical compounds such as dextran, opiates, and polymyxin, can release histamine by nonimmunologic processes. There are many additional factors that may induce urticaria. These include endocrine influences (increased thyroid activity), viral infections (infectious hepatitis virus) exercise (cholinergic urticaria), physical factors (cold-induced urticaria, solar urticaria), and genetic influences (hereditary angioedema). Obviously, the mechanisms of urticaria and angioedema are multiple, which underscores the clinical difficulty in establishing the etiologic basis of this symptom complex.

Diagnosis

Table 51–3 lists some of the etiologic considerations when diagnosing urticaria and angioedema. In view of the multiple diseases with which urticaria can be asso-

TABLE 51–3. DIFFERENTIAL DIAGNOSIS OF URTICARIA AND ANGIOEDEMA

1. Drugs:
   a. Immunologic mechanism—example: penicillin (IgE mediation)
   b. Nonimmunologic mechanism—example: opiates, dextran, polymyxin, and aspirin
2. Food antigens
3. Infectious agents:
   a. Viral infection—examples: infectious hepatitis, infectious mononucleosis
   b. Parasitic infestations
   c. Bacterial agents (considered very rare)
4. Inhalant allergens—example: seasonal pollens, animal danders
5. Physical factors:
   a. Pressure—example: dermographism, deep pressure urticaria
   b. Cold urticaria—example: acquired idiopathic variety, familial inherited variety
   c. Heat urticaria—example: cholinergic variety
   d. Solar urticaria
6. Insect allergy—example: Hymenoptera sensitivity
7. Connective tissue disorders—example: rheumatoid arthritis, systemic lupus erythematosus
8. Neoplasms—example: Hodgkin's disorder, large carcinomas
9. Genetic disorders—example: hereditary angioedema
10. Endocrinopathies—example: hyperthyroidism
11. Immune complex disorders—example: serum sickness secondary to penicillin

ciated, it is obvious that patients merit a complete history and physical examination. The evaluation might also include: (1) routine skin stroking for dermographia; (2) routine blood count, urinalysis and panel of blood screening tests, such as liver function tests, thyroid function tests, and antinuclear antibody determinations to rule out serious underlying diseases; (3) appropriate allergen skin tests for suspect inhalant or food allergies; (4) food elimination and challenges; and (5) evaluation for parasitic infestations.

One of the most intriguing causes of chronic urticaria is due to acquired idiopathic cold sensitivity. This can be easily diagnosed in most patients by direct application of a cold stimulus (plastic bag filled with ice cubes) to a skin site such as the forearm for 5 minutes. A wheal will develop after skin temperature rewarming. Idiopathic cold sensitivity is an important diagnosis to establish, as some patients may develop anaphylactic reactions to cold temperatures and are susceptible to drowning while swimming. Furthermore, the sensitivity can be reversed by prophylactic therapy with cyproheptadine (Periactin).

Treatment

The successful therapy for urticaria and angioedema depends on the identification and elimination of the cause. This is feasible when the causative agent is known, such as a food, drug, or insect sensitivity or hypersensitivity to physical factors such as cold temperatures.

Various pharmacologic agents are helpful in controlling urticaria. Epinephrine injections are useful for the acute phase but are impractical to repeat for relief of continuous symptoms Antihistamines are useful adjuncts for long-term suppressive therapy. Hydroxyzine (Atarax, Vistaril) has been demonstrated to have a superior suppressive effect in the therapy of chronic undifferentiated urticaria. Corticosteroids should be reserved for severely afflicted persons with chronic urticaria who cannot be controlled with antihistamines, singly or in combination. Immunotherapy has no apparent benefits in the therapy of chronic urticaria except for treatment of Hymenoptera sensitivity.

ALLERGIC RHINITIS

Allergic rhinitis is one of the most common forms of atopic disorders and is estimated to afflict 10 per cent of the general population. Its symptoms can be mild in degree, but in some patients more generalized symptoms, such as fatigue, malaise, and disorders of collateral organ involvement (i.e., conjunctivitis, serous otitis, and sinusitis), may accompany the local nasal discomfort. Seasonal allergic rhinitis signifies recurrent nasal disease that occurs during seasonal exposure to sensitizing aeroallergens such as tree, grass, and weed pollens. Perennial allergic rhinitis is induced by continuous exposure to indoor inhalants such as housedust, mold spores, and epidermals (animal danders).

Mechanism

Allergic rhinitis both seasonal and perennial, must be viewed as a hypersensitivity state to inhaled aeroallergens. Significant evidence exists to implicate the Type I Gell and Coombs' immunologic reaction in this disease state. Over a period of time, the genetically predisposed allergic patient becomes sensitized to inhaled antigens. This primary sensitization results in the development of reaginic antibody. This peculiar antibody has been characterized as a separate physicochemical class of immunoglobulins, namely IgE. The IgE antibodies are low in concentration in the serum and normally measure 0.1 to 0.4 microgram per ml. They are produced by plasma cells and have an unusual tissue affinity, lasting in the skin for over 2 weeks. The IgE antibody adheres to target cells, tissue mast cells, and blood basophils. Small amounts of antigen are absorbed through the nasal mucosa and react with the IgE antibody fixed to the mast cells that reside in the nasal tissue. This results in the liberation of vasoactive mediators. Histamine is considered the primary chemical mediator, although the slow-reacting substance of anaphylaxis prostaglandins, and the eosinophilic chemotactic factor may all have potential import in the pathogenesis of this disorder. These substances alter vascular permeability, causing the classic features of mucosal edema and hypersecretion. Understanding the immunopathology of allergic rhinitis is further complicated by other proposed mechanisms such as the role of IgG reaginic antibody and delayed hypersensitivity reactions. For the sake of simplicity in this discussion, we will refer to the basic immunologic mechanism as being IgE mediated.

The pathophysiology of allergic rhinitis has been studied by various investigators who have suggested the presence of a priming effect. Repeated challenges of nasal membranes with a single pollen cause classic mucosal edema associated with an objective increase in nasal airway resistance. After repeated challenges of the nasal mucosa with the same antigen over several weeks' duration, the reactivity of the nasal membranes can be reproduced with as little as 1/40 of the initial antigen dose required to significantly increase nasal airway resistance. When this priming effect occurs, the patient may then develop similar nasal reactivity to antigens to which he is minimally sensitive.

The allergens that are etiologically important in the induction of allergic rhinitis are mostly airborne. Most pollen antigens that induce allergic rhinitis are light and windborne. The warmer air currents of midday presumably keep these pollens aloft, while the cooler air currents of early morning and late evening allow them to descend. This phenomenon may explain why some patients note increased symptoms during the cooler hours Pollen from plants that are insect pollinated is heavy and not buoyant enough to be carried by air currents. Consequently, such pollens are not thought to be a significant cause of allergic rhinitis. It is beyond the scope of this discussion to describe the specific pollens capable of inducing allergic rhinitis. The pollen types and concentrations vary markedly in each geographic region.

Mold spores are perennial aeroallergens that are capable of inducing allergic rhinitis. They are derived from saprophytic fungi and thrive especially in moist climates. The mold spore count is generally highest during the peak rainfall months of the spring and early autumn. Indoors, mold growth is noted wherever there is a dormant collection of water, such as in humidifiers, air conditioning units, vaporizers, potted plants, bathrooms, and basements. Delineation of mold sensitivity by history is more difficult, as there is no well-defined season, as with pollens. Nevertheless, clues as to etiologic role of mold can be established by asking appropriate questions, such as whether the patient has increased symptoms after turning on an air conditioning unit or humidifier.

Housedust allergy is another antigen considered to be a major inducer of perennial allergic rhinitis. Until recently, little experimental assay had been undertaken to define the major allergenic component of housedust. Studies now indicate that insect antigens are major allergens in housedust antigen, particularly mite allergen. Housedust is obviously heterogeneous antigenically and has been shown to include epidermal proteins and insect antigens. Symptoms from housedust sensitivity are considered perennial, but often the housedust-sensitive patient has increased symptoms during the colder months of the year when central heating systems are operative.

Animal dander (i.e., epidermals) are significant sensitizers in the nasal mucosa. It is thought that the true sensitizing protein antigen is not derived from insoluble hair matrix but rather from decomposing epidermal cells and salivary secretions. These antigens are easily dispersed and become part of the household environment.

Food allergens have occasionally been implicated in the induction of allergic rhinitis. This association is generally very low in frequency. The observant physician will occasionally elicit a history of increased rhinorrhea in a patient after ingestion of certain foods. Often the patient exhibits other manifestations of anaphylaxis, such as bronchospasm or urticaria, which establish a clearer clinical diagnosis of food allergy. Foods such as legumes, melons, whole milk, and seafoods may induce rhinorrhea in markedly sensitive persons.

Symptoms

The most prominent symptoms include intermittent or persistent rhinorrhea; paroxysmal sneezing; nasal obstruction; nasal or ocular pruritus, or both; and excessive lacrimation. Symptoms may fluctuate in intensity daily during the season of maximal exposure to the sensitizing pollens, but often the symptoms seem more severe during the cooler time of the day, i.e., early morning or late evening. Other symptoms include habitual nasal rubbing (allergic salute), palatal pruritus epistaxis, bruxism, sinus pattern of cephalalgia, and fatigue. If the allergic process involves the lower respiratory tract, the patient may exhibit features of bronchospasm, coughing, paroxysms, and dyspnea. There is an increased association of serous otitis media with chronic allergic rhinitis. Eustachian tube dysfunction secondary to swelling of the nasopharyngeal mucosa is thought to be of primary importance in the pathogenesis of serous otitis media. Fluctuating impairment of hearing is often observed in younger children.

Physical Features

The nasal mucosa is typically edematous and often appears pale and gray in color. Occasionally the inferior turbinates appear markedly swollen. The nasal discharge is characteristically clear and watery. Marked edematous swelling of the nasal mucosa may result in polypoid formations. More widespread membranous edema may extend into the paranasal sinuses, producing mucosal thickening and even polypoid tumors on sinus x-ray. Purulent nasal discharge may be observed if the sinus mucosa becomes secondarily infected. Impairment of hearing may be observed in patients with eustachian tube dysfunction secondary to swelling of nasopharyngeal mucosa. Audio-metric studies may reveal significant air conduction loss, and the presence of fluid behind the tympanic membrane may be further documented by pneumatic otoscopic examination and tympanogram studies. The hearing loss of allergy-induced serous otitis may not be fully appreciated in younger children. As a result, serious learning disability and behavior problems may result from an overlooked hearing problem.

Diagnosis

The diagnosis of allergic rhinitis is based primarily on historical features, physical findings and certain laboratory aids. Examination of nasal mucus from patients with allergic rhinitis commonly reveals eosinophilia. The nasal mucus is best obtained by having the patient blow his nose into wax paper. It is worth noting that inadequate sampling of mucus may lead to false negative results. The mucus is smeared on a glass slide and stained with Hansel or Wright's stain and then examined for eosinophils. A positive nasal smear is noted if the eosinophil count is greater than 10 per cent. Infants 3 months of age or younger may normally have nasal eosinophilia. Peripheral blood eosinophilia may also be observed in allergic patients.

Skin testing is very useful in establishing the existence of reaginic (IgE) antibodies to suspect antigens. The immediate skin test reaction is caused by the interaction between the test antigen and specific reaginic antibody bound to tissue mast cells. The resultant reaction leads to a wheal and flare response. The basic scratch technique involves the application of a drop of glycerinated aqueous antigen on the epidermis, preferably the posterior thoracic surace. A scratch through the droplet allows the antigen to pass the epidermal barrier. Within minutes a flare and whealing response can be observed. Whenever these tests are performed, proper controls should be included, namely a saline control to rule out false positive reactions, as in dermographic patients, and histamine controls to rule out false negative reactions caused by poor scratch technique or drug suppression. Intradermal skin testing may be indicated in situations in which a scratch test is negative for a suspect antigen. The customary concentration of antigen for intradermal testing is 1:1000 weight by volume of nonglycerinated aqueous extract. Skin testing should be carefully supervised by the physician. Signs of anaphylaxis may result from the testing, and this should be treated as a medical emergency. Improper interpretation of test results may relegate a patient to unnecessary immunotherapy.

The serum radioallergosorbent (RAST) test has become available for detection of IgE antibody to specific antigens. The test is costly and requires large volumes of serum, thus obviating its use as a standard method for detecting reaginic antibodies.

A variety of poorly defined diagnostic techniques exist, such as provocative skin challenges, leukopenic index, and the leukocyte cytotoxic test. Reviews indicate that these techniques have no scientific basis for their use in clinical allergy testing.

Differential Diagnosis

The diagnosis of allergic rhinitis is generally not difficult to establish. Other entities that require exclusion are (1) vasomotor rhinitis, a condition clinically similar to allergic rhinitis, but in which there is no evidence of reaginic antibody mediation; (2) rhinitis medicamentosa secondary to abuse of topical alpha-adrenergic agents (nosedrops); (3) reserpine-induced rhinitis; (4) nasal tumors; (5) foreign bodies; (6) nasal polyps secondary to aspirin sensitivity, cystic fibrosis, or chronic bacterial infection; (7) hypothyroidism; and (8) sarcoidosis (lupus pernio).

Treatment

Symptomatic therapy for allergic rhinitis is relatively effective in controlling mild to moderate degrees of nasal discomfort. Antihistamines, of which there are four chemical classes, constitute the major drugs used for symptomatic control of rhinitis They act as competitive inhibitors of histamine at receptor sites. Maximal therapeutic effects of these drugs are often achieved only if patients maintain high dose around-the-clock prophylaxis. Side effects, such as somnolence and behavior alteration, or poor therapeutic results may be indications to choose other antihistamines from a different chemical class. The addition of sympathomimetics, such as pseudoephedrine or phenylpropanolamine, may be indicated to obtain vasoconstriction and reduction of nasal mucosal edema. Topical alpha-adrenergics, i.e., nosedrops, should be used only for short periods of time in order to prevent rebound congestion and ultimately rhinitis medicamentosa. Steroid therapy is rarely indicated systemically, although topical corticosteroids such as aerosolized dexamethasone, have significant suppressive effects. Close surveillance is required if steroids are administered by this route, as the cortisone analog may be systemically absorbed if used over extended periods In addition, nasal mucosal atrophy and sinusitis may occasionally develop after prolonged use of steroid therapy.

Specific therapy for allergic rhinitis can be achieved by (1) avoidance of causal antigens, such as animal dander, dust, and suspect foods and (2) parenteral injections of antigens (termed immunotherapy). In vivo and in vitro studies have demonstrated that injection therapy of certain pollens, such as ragweed and grass antigens, is clinically effective. Immunotherapy with these antigens has been shown to be especially effective in patients receiving high dose therapy over a prolonged period of time (weight by volume concentrations between 1:10 and 1:20). By use of objective measurements of in vitro immunologic indices these same studies have shown that significant changes occur in patients receiving high dose therapy of antigens. The specific changes in immunologic indices that occur include (1) increased titers of blocking antibodies of the IgG type; (2) decline in reaginic antibody titers, namely IgE antibodies; and (3) diminution of cellular sensitivity to the administered antigens, i.e., histamine-releasing capacity of basophilic leukocytes. Although these studies provide supportive evidence of the benefits of immunotherapy, it is important to realize that this form of therapy rarely leads to complete resolution of the disease process; however, in most patients amelioration of symptoms occurs. Studies with other antigens have not been as conclusive. Supportive evidence for efficacy of mold and housedust antigens is not convincing. Nevertheless their use continues and is primarily based on anecdotal evidence. Bacterial vaccine antigens are also used empirically, but there is a substantial body of evidence that is not supportive of their benefits.

Formulation of allergenic extracts requires an intelligent and reasonable approach. One should include those antigens in the formulation that are implicated in causing the patient's symptoms and should exclude those antigens that can be avoided. The addition of unnecessary antigens will only serve to dilute the immunogenicity of the allergenic extract. Certain commercial laboratories offer the service of formulating allergenic extracts based only on skin test results. Although this approach is tempting for the busy physician, it often leads to poor standards of allergy care. Physicians who are truly interested in providing excellence in allergy care should seek the advice of competent allergists. The specific methodology of allergenic extract formulation and the administration of immunotherapy are unfortunately beyond the scope of this discussion.

BRONCHIAL ASTHMA

Bronchial asthma has been defined as a reversible obstructive disease of the bronchial airways. Its hallmark for differentiation from other chronic obstructive lung disorders, such as emphysema and chronic bronchitis, is the significant reversibility of the airway obstruction. The definitive diagnosis of bronchial asthma requires demonstration of a significant bronchodilatory response to certain pharmacologic agents such as epinephrine, steroids, theophylline or combinations of these.

Pathophysiology

Heterogeneous factors have been implicated as causes of bronchospasmodic episodes. Such variable triggering mechanisms as exercise, respiratory infection, emotional outbursts, weather changes, inhaled allergens, and aspirin ingestion exemplify the multitude of factors that may induce bronchospasm. Involvement of Type I immune reactions (immediate hypersensitivity reactions mediated by IgE reaginic antibodies) has been thoroughly described and physiologically reproduced by the induction of bronchospasm with bronchial inhalation challenges of suspect allergens. Nevertheless, asthma is erroneously thought of as being primarily an immunologically induced disorder. The underlying basis of this

disorder is probably nonallergic and is thought to be an autonomic functional imbalance, described as the beta-adrenergic blockade theory. The basis of this concept is the observation that the asthmatic bronchial airway is hyper-responsive to various chemical mediators, such as histamine or acetylcholine, released by allergic or nonallergic factors. Immune reactions of Type I, which may cause the release of chemical mediators, may, therefore, act as important but not exclusive triggers of the bronchospasmodic response.

Clinical Classification

Asthma can be classified into certain types, depending on the various mechanisms of induction. A common approach to classification includes:

1. Extrinsic bronchial asthma, in which clearly defined external inducers of bronchospasm, such as pollen antigens, are established. This group has been described as reagin-mediated asthma.

2. Intrinsic bronchial asthma, in which there is no known definitive cause of the disorder. These patients characteristically are nonatopic, do not demonstrate reaginic mediation, and seem to flare with viral respiratory infections. In young children, the most important infectious agents are respiratory syncytial virus and parainfluenza virus, while in older children and adults rhinovirus and influenza virus are more commonly associated with the induction of bronchospasm.

3. Aspirin-induced asthma, in which the asthma is associated with aspirin ingestion, is considered to be a special class. These patients often exhibit associated chronic rhinitis, sinusitis, and nasal polyposis. The asthma associated with this syndrome is often severe and is occasionally fatal in extremely sensitive persons. Certain other chemically dissimilar compounds such as indomethacin and coloring dyes (tartrazine yellow) may cause similar reactions. The basic mechanism of this syndrome is not understood, but current evidence excludes reaginic mediation.

4. Exercise-induced asthma is another common form of wheezing that is more frequently seen in younger adults and children. Generally, the bronchoconstriction occurs after termination of exercise. The mechanism for the exercise induction

of bronchospasm is not understood, but it can be modified and prevented with pharmacologic agents such as theophylline and cromolyn.

It is common to see patients exhibiting mixed forms of these types of asthma. In addition, patients are seen whose asthma seems to be triggered by irritant factors such as fumes, smoke, cold air, emotional outbursts, and so forth. These patients presumably have a hyper-responsiveness of their bronchial airway and might be considered prime examples of those persons with presumed underlying autonomic imbalance.

Clinical Features

The manifestations of bronchial asthma are protean and depend, for the most part, on the degree and persistence of increased airway resistance. Mild forms may be sporadic, with episodic bronchospasm resulting from exposure to seasonal allergens such as pollens. Occasionally, increased airway resistance may exhibit as coughing spasms only. Asthma in early life is frequently associated with viral respiratory infections, and, in infancy, recurrent bronchiolitis may eventually be transformed into conventional asthma. Similarly, the older child or adult may exhibit intermittent bronchospasm secondary to viral infections, and often this entity is termed asthmatic bronchitis.

As the episodes of bronchospasm become more frequent and severe, the patient may exhibit stationary signs of increased airway resistance. Prolongation of the expiratory phase of respiration may be noted, along with expiratory wheezing and eventually hyperinflation of the thoracic cavity. The latter disorder has been termed the barrel chest deformity of asthma, and frequently this is confused with and diagnosed as emphysema. The term emphysema is rarely used appropriately in this condition, as it signifies chronic irreversible obstructive lung disease with histologic evidence of damaged lung parenchyma.

Eventually, long-standing bronchial asthma will lead to significant dyspnea. Progression to respiratory failure may result, with evidence of hypercapnia, hypoxemia, respiratory acidosis and cyanosis. The clinician may underestimate the developing respiratory failure, as some patients may not exhibit pronounced bronchospasm as a result of inadequate air exchange. The sudden development of a "silent chest" during a severe episode of bronchospasm may be a harbinger of rapidly increased airway resistance and marked clinical deterioration. It is worth noting that the patient with chronic asthma rarely demonstrates clubbing, a sign more often seen in other chronic pulmonary disorders, such as cystic fibrosis and emphysema.

The most frequent complications of long-standing asthma are:

1. Status asthmaticus, which may be defined as a state of bronchospasm that is unresponsive to conventional drugs, such as epinephrine and theophylline. These patients require close medical attention and treatment to prevent respiratory failure.

2. Pneumomediastinum and pneumothorax. Rupture of alveoli caused by hyperdistention leads to this complication. Crepitation over the supraclavicular space is often the most significant clinical sign of this complication, which may be verified by chest x-ray. If the pneumothorax is considerable, treatment with a water-sealed intercostal tube may be indicated. However, the air is usually absorbed rapidly, especially after the patient is treated with high nasal oxygen tension.

3. Atelectasis is a common feature of long-standing asthma and may occur asymptomatically. It may be observed in some patients after a routine chest x-ray without any clinical correlation to indicate its existence. More often, it is associated with a sudden clinical exacerbation of asthma, and in children the most common location involves the right middle lobe. Atelectasis in the asthmatic patient will often resolve rapidly, and it is best to avoid bronchoscopy in this situation.

Laboratory Evaluation and Diagnosis

There are no specific laboratory data that are diagnostic of bronchial asthma except for pulmonary function findings that demonstrate evidence of reversible obstructive lung disease. The most common pulmonary function evaluation includes volumetric measurement of lung compartments. Several of these studies can be performed as an office procedure, such as spirometric determination of vital capacity, 1 second forced expiratory volume (FEV_1), maximal mid-expiratory flow rate, or maximum breathing capacity. A Jones Pulmonor or the more sophisticated Monaghan Pulmonary Function Analyzer is a useful instrument that permits rapid determination of these indices. The Wright Peak Flow Meter is useful as a rapid detector of increased airway obstruction. Other lung compartment measurements, such as functional residual capacity (FRC), residual volume (RV), and total lung capacity (TLC) require access to a pulmonary function laboratory for their determination. In general, spirometric analysis of resting and forced breathing patterns provides sufficient data for the diagnosis of bronchial asthma. These studies are usually coupled with repeat measurements following inhalation of a bronchodilator in order to demonstrate the reversibility of the airway obstruction.

Even in the mild asymptomatic asthmatic patient, the spirometric indices may be abnormal. As a patient becomes more symptomatic, the degree of airway obstruction will become more pronounced with obvious reduction of forced vital capacity, FEV_1/VC ratio, maximum breathing capacity (MBC), and maximum mid-expiratory flow rate (MMEF). The RV, FRC, and TLC will increase because of increased air trapping, but these measurements are not essential to establishing the diagnosis of this disorder. Arterial blood gas measurements should be obtained as part of the pulmonary evaluation. Often there is hypoxemia even in the mildly asthmatic patient, which suggests the presence of ventilation-perfusion abnormalities. As the degree of airway obstruction increases, the blood gas determination will reveal more pronounced hypoxemia, hypercapnia, and respiratory acidosis.

Roentgenograms of the chest may reveal evidence of hyperinflation and depression of the diaphragm. Increased bronchial markings or segmental atelectasis may also be observed. Forced expiration and inspiration films are helpful in order to appreciate the degree of airway obstruction and also to rule out an unsuspected foreign body that may induce wheezing. Sinus x-rays may reveal a concomitant pansinusitis.

Determination of quantitative serum immunoglobulins is recommended to rule out IgG or IgA deficiency. Deficiency of secretory IgA, which most often occurs with absence of serum IgA, may increase a patient's susceptibility to respiratory infection. Serum IgE levels are often elevated in patients with extrinsic reagin-mediated asthma. The routine laboratory evaluation should include appropriate skin testing and RAST tests, as described in the section on allergic rhinitis The differential diagnosis of asthma may sometimes be confusing and, therefore, other laboratory tests may be required in the evaluation. These include:

1. Alpha$_1$-antitrypsin determination to rule out deficiency of this enzyme, which is associated with familial emphysema.

2. Sweat test to rule out cystic fibrosis.

3. Serum precipitin test to demonstrate the presence of precipitating antibodies to antigens capable of inducing immune complex reactions of the lung. Examples of antigens include thermophilic fungi, avian proteins, and wood dust.

4. Sputum analysis for eosinophils.

5. Antigen inhalation challenges to establish that the lung is indeed a target organ for a specific antigen identified by positive skin test. These tests are hazardous as an office procedure.

6. Aspirin and other ingested challenges of suspect foods or food additives (tartrazine). The patient may be extremely sensitive to these challenges, especially to aspirin, and it is recommended that these tests be performed in a hospital setting with close supervision.

Differential Diagnosis

In general, the diagnosis of bronchial asthma can be suspected by the previously described historical and physical features. The definitive diagnosis should be based on pulmonary physiology data that are demonstrative of reversible airway obstruction. The mere presence of wheezing that improves clinically with use of a bronchodilator is not diagnostic of bronchial asthma, as reversible wheezing may occur with acute bronchitis, tracheobronchitis, and aspirated foreign bodies. As some patients are denied insurance coverage because of the loosely used diagnosis of bronchial asthma, it is important to have supportive physiologic data before suggesting the diagnosis.

Asthma should be differentiated from other causes of airway obstruction. Upper airway obstruction may present with stridor and may be mistaken for wheezing. Nasal and laryngeal tumors and congenital anomalies may also present in this manner. Lower airway obstruction with expiratory wheezing may occur with aspirated foreign bodies, congenital anomalies, bronchial compression from tumors, and vascular anomalies. Wheezing may accompany transient infectious processes, such as viral diseases, and it is also noted occasionally with cystic fibrosis. Other pulmonary disorders with obstructive lung features should be considered in the differential diagnosis, such as alpha$_1$-antitrypsin deficiency, immune complex diseases of the lung, chronic bronchitis, emphysema, and immunodeficiency disorders.

Treatment

The therapy for bronchial asthma may be divided into three basic approaches: (1) preventive measures, (2) specific therapy (immunotherapy), and (3) pharmacologic management.

Treatment of asthma consists of reducing exposure to suspect allergens or irritants. Identification of causal factors in the home environment such as animal danders and tobacco smoke may be important. In addition, the patient should note any relationship of symptoms to high air pollution index, change in air temperature (especially cooler temperatures), physical activities, and stress. Once a relationship is established, the patient may subsequently notice a significant improvement if he can control exposure to the causal factor.

When environmental control is impossible or insufficient to control symptoms, specific therapy, such as immunotherapy, should be considered. The details of immunotherapy have been described in the section on allergic rhinitis It is worth stressing that this therapy should be reserved for patients with extrinsic asthma, especially those with a significant pollen sensitivity. Patients who receive high antigen doses seem to respond more successfully to this mode of therapy. Treatment of intrinsic asthma with bacterial vaccine is, at best, controversial and inconclusive.

The customary pharmacologic agents used in the therapy of asthma are described in Table 51–4.

The patient with frequent, mild episodes of asthma can be successfully treated using bronchodilators orally or by inhalation.

TABLE 51–4. AGENTS USED IN THE THERAPY OF ASTHMA

Methylxanthines: theophylline compounds
Adrenergic compounds:
  A. Catecholamines:
    1. Epinephrine
    2. Isoproterenol
    3. Isoetharine
  B. Noncatecholamines:
    1. Ephedrine
    2. Metaproterenol
    3. Terbutaline
Cromolyn sodium
Corticosteroids

Around-the-clock therapy is very often indicated for some of these patients in order to prevent the frequent recurrence of these symptoms. As patients frequently resist taking medications, it is important to prescribe a drug program that is therapeutic in dosage but has minimal side effects. For this reason, we prefer single drug prescriptions. Control studies have revealed that combination drugs such as theophylline-ephedrine compounds do not cause more bronchodilation than theophylline itself. Thus, ephedrine can often be eliminated and, therefore, the side effects associated with it can be reduced. For around-the-clock regimens, theophylline is the drug of choice, with a recommended dose of 3 to 5 mg. per kg. of body weight of anhydrous equivalent every 6 hours. Theophylline is available in various formulations, and physicians should become aware of the anhydrous equivalent of the drug they choose. For example, aminophylline is 85 per cent anhydrous theophylline, while oxtriphylline is only 60 per cent the equivalent of anhydrous theophylline. The physician prescribing theophylline products should refer to the *Physician's Desk Reference* *(PDR)* for anhydrous theophylline equivalents.

If a patient does not respond to anticipated oral anhydrous theophylline dosages a blood theophylline value should be obtained. A safe therapeutic blood level of theophylline is 10 to 20 micrograms per ml. If the blood level is low, the physician may be inclined to increase the oral anhydrous dosage. Theophylline toxicity, which may manifest as convulsions, often occurs if the blood theophylline level is higher than 20 micrograms per ml.

Catecholamines are also used on an as needed (PRN) basis both orally and by inhalation, to control mild episodes of asthma. Newer beta-2 adrenergic agonists, such as terbutaline, apparently cause less tachycardia than previous adrenergic analogs. The side effects of ephedrine, such as hyperactivity and tachycardia, make it a difficult choice as an around-the-clock bronchodilator. In addition, it seems to be less effective as a bronchodilator, as well as having a tendency to cause tachyphylaxis. Inhalation of adrenergic agents such as isoproterenol or isoetharine by aerosol is a useful adjunct to oral therapy, but excessive use may cause paradoxical bronchospasm.

Patients unresponsive to oral bronchodilators may be candidates for cromolyn sodium administration. Cromolyn sodium is a bischromone powder administered by inhalation four times a day. It is a prophylactic capable of preventing both allergen-induced and nonallergen-induced release of chemical mediators. Therapy with cromolyn sodium may be sufficient to control perennial asthma, with or without use of added bronchodilators. In addition, corticosteroid-dependent asthmatic patients may require less steroids when they receive this drug. There are no absolute criteria to ascertain which patient will respond to this drug; hence, a 6 to 8 week trial of cromolyn sodium is worthwhile in any patient with chronic asthma. It seems to be particularly successful in reducing exercise-induced bronchospasm, particularly in adolescents. Side effects are minimal and include hypersensitivity manifestations (rash, eosinophilic pneumonia). The drug should be discontinued during acute exacerbations of asthma, as it is not a bronchodilator and the powder may become an irritant and worsen the asthmatic symptoms

The chronic asthmatic patient may ultimately require corticosteroids in order to adequately control symptoms. The steroids prescribed should be short-acting, e.g., prednisone, prednisolone, or methylprednisolone. Triamcinolone, betamethasone, and dexamethasone are long-acting steroids that cause long-term adrenal suppression and do not lend themselves to alternate-day schedules. In addition, some of the long-acting steroids have been associated with the induction of myopathies in children. Starting doses of prednisone depend on the age and weight of the patient. The suppressive dose of prednisone in children is 2 mg. per kg. per 24 hours, given in two divided doses daily, and in adults the dose is 40 to 80 mg. per 24 hours, given also in two divided doses. For patients requiring maintenance therapy, the lowest possible dose compatible with adequate control of symptoms should be used. Reduction of long-term steroid side effects can be achieved by conversion to every-other-day (q.o.d.) administration. This conversion can best be achieved by tripling the minimal daily effective dose of prednisone. The prednisone q.o.d. dose then should be reduced by 5 to 10 mg. every 2 weeks.

Recently, aerosolized forms of nonpolar, insoluble steroids (beclomethasone) have become available for the management of asthma. These steroids seem to have minimal systemic effects, such as adrenal suppression, except when given in high doses. The main side effect associated with their use is the development of oral moniliasis. The chief indication for the use of inhaled beclomethasone is for the steroid-dependent asthmatic patient. Often the systemic steroid requirement may be reduced in these patients. Blood cortisol levels should be obtained during the process of steroid withdrawal in order to monitor early signs of adrenal insufficiency.

Management of Status Asthmaticus

Acute asthma management deserves special attention. Most acute episodes can be managed with aqueous epinephrine 1:1000 given subcutaneously in a dose of 0.05 to 0.2 ml. for children and 0.2 to 0.4 ml. for adults. Smaller doses may be repeated at 30 minute intervals two or three times. Alternatively, acute asthma may be treated with aerosolized adrenergic bronchodilators such as isoetharine or isoproterenol. Inadequate response to adrenergic agents is an indication for use of aminophylline (theophylline ethylenediamine) in a dose of 250 to 500 mg. every 6 hours intravenously for adults or 4 to 5 mg. per kg. intravenously every 6 hours for children. Status asthmaticus is a severe, life-threatening form of asthma that, by

TABLE 51–5. PROGRAM FOR TREATMENT OF STATUS ASTHMATICUS

1. Hospitalization, preferably in intensive care unit.
2. Laboratory studies: complete blood count, chest x-ray, arterial blood gas determinations.
3. Discontinue respiratory depressants such as sedatives and tranquilizers.
4. Proper hydration up to 1½ times normal maintenance.
5. Oxygen therapy using humidified oxygen in concentration of 2 to 3 liters per minute, as guided by arterial blood gas determinations.
6. Aminophylline intravenously. For children, 4 to 5 mg. per kg. of body weight diluted 1:1 with intravenous fluids administered over 20 minutes by piggyback method using Volutrol device. Repeat every 6 hours. For adults, 250 to 500 mg. intravenously administered over 20 minutes every 6 hours.
7. Corticosteroid therapy. For children and adults, hydrocortisone (Solu-Cortef) in the dose of 2 to 4 mg. per kg. every 4 hours intravenously. Alternatively, methylprednisolone (Solu-Medrol) may be used.
8. Aerosolized bronchodilators. For adults, isoproterenol, 5 drops of 1:200, or isoetharine, 10 drops in 2 ml. saline, every 2 to 4 hours as tolerated. For children, the dose is lowered, depending on age.
9. Sodium bicarbonate for metabolic acidosis. For children 2 mEq. per kg. intravenously every hour, as needed. For adults, 44 to 88 mEq. intravenously every hour as needed.
10. Consider ventilatory assistance with a volume respirator if respiratory failure develops. Criteria for blood gases is PO_2 less than 50 mm. Hg and PCO_2 greater than 50 mm. Hg.

definition, exists when the patient is unresponsive to adrenergic drugs and aminophylline. If improperly treated, its sequela is respiratory failure. Table 51–5 lists the recommended program for treatment of status asthmaticus.

REFERENCES

1. Connell, J. T.: Quantitative intranasal pollen challenges. The priming effect in allergic rhinitis. J. Allergy, 43:33, 1969.
2. Ellis, E. F.: Symposium on pediatric allergy. Pediatr. Clin. North Am., 22:(1), 1975.
3. Gell, P. G. H., and Coombs, R. R. A.: Clinical Aspects of Immunology. 2nd Ed. Philadelphia, F. A. Davis Co., 1968.
4. Golbert, T.: A review of controversial diagnostic and therapeutic techniques employed in allergy. J. Allergy Clin. Immunol., 56:170, 1975.
5. Henley, W. L.: Immunology in infancy and childhood. Pediatr. Ann., 5:(6), 1976.
6. Patterson, R.: Allergic Diseases. Philadelphia, J. B. Lippincott Co., 1972.
7. Samter, M.: Immunological Diseases. 2nd Ed. Boston, Little, Brown & Co., 1971.
8. Samter, M.: Symposium on Allergy in Adults. Med. Clin. North Am., 58:(1), 1974.
9. Stiehm, R. E., and Fulginiti, V. A.: Immunological Disorders in Infants and Children. Philadelphia, W. B. Saunders Co., 1973.
10. Wanderer, A. A., and Ellis, E. F.: Treatment of cold urticaria with cyproheptadine. J. Allergy Clin. Immunol., 48:366, 1971.
11. Warin, R., and Champion, R.: Urticaria. Major Probl. Dermatol., Vol. I, 1974.

INDEX

Note: Page numbers in *italics* indicate illustrations; those followed by (t) indicate tables.

Abdomen, acute. See *Abdomen, surgical.*
distension of, chest pain in, 1003(t), 1004
from air swallowing, 955
examination of, 941–942, 942(t)
injuries of, 529–531
surgical, diagnosis of, 486(t), 487–488
Abdominal pain, chronic, 942–944, 942(t), 943(t)
from intestinal gas, 955
in duodenal ulcer disease, 956(t)
in pancreatic carcinoma, 944
in pregnancy, 487
Abdominal reflexes, testing of, 1018
Abducens nerve, paralysis of, 726, 1057(t), 1058
ABO incompatibility, 881–882
Abortion, recurrent, spontaneous, genetic counseling for, 473
threatened, vaginal bleeding in, 744–745
Abrasions, corneal, 709
Abscess, anorectal, 804–806, *805*
and fistula-in-ano, 806–808, *807*
in hidradenitis suppurativa, 827
vs. anal fissure, 804
cervical, 679
parapharyngeal, 663
peritonsillar, 662–663
pulmonary, 905–908, *907*
defined, 884
retropharyngeal, 663
scrotal, 782
Absence attack, 1027, 1028(t)
Acetaminophen, and hepatic injury, 980(t), 981
Accidents, treatment in, 521–538
Achalasia, 683
Achilles tendon, pain in, 547
Achondroplasia, 672
genetic counseling for, 474
Acid peptic disease, 955–959
Acidosis, in respiratory failure, 931–932, 932(t)
Acinus, defined, 883
Acne, 1120–1121
and oral contraceptives, 459
Acromioclavicular joint, lesions of, 595–596, *595,
596*
Actinic keratosis, 1129–1130, *1130*
Actinomycosis, pulmonary, 938
Adenitis, cervical, in children, 839–840
tuberculous, in children, 850
Adenocarcinoma, of endometrium, 748-749
of kidney, 784
of lung, 915, 915(t)
Adenoid, hyperplasia of, 667
Adenoidectomy, indications for, 667
Adenoma, of kidney, 783
Adenomyosarcoma, of kidney, 784

Adenomyosis, 748
Adenosis, vaginal, 753
Adnexa, tumors of, 750–753
Adolescence, and family life cycle, 41–42
Adolescent(s). See also *Children.*
gynecologic examination in, 733
nutritional requirements of, 1085(t), 1086–1088,
1086(t)
overweight, nutritional requirements of, 1087–
1088
pregnant, nutritional requirements of, 1087
sexuality of, 437–438
underweight, nutritional requirements of,
1087–1088
Agenesis, pulmonary, 684
renal, 772
urinary bladder, 773
Aging, biological aspects of, 222–225, *224, 225*
Aglossodactyly, 660
Agnathia, 661
Air pollution, and chronic bronchitis, 908–909
Air swallowing, 955
Airway, injury to, in burn patients, 536–537
small, defined, 883
Airway obstruction, acute, 898–899
from foreign body, 522–525, 684–685, 898–899
emergency treatment of, 522–524
differential diagnosis of, 1146–1147
in chronic bronchitis, 909
in pulmonary emphysema, 910
Akinetic seizures, 857
Alcohol, and liver disease, 973–976
neurologic effects of, 1035–1036
Alcohol intoxication, acute, 1035
pathologic, 1035
Alcohol withdrawal syndrome, 333–334
Alcoholic cerebellar degeneration, 1035–1036,
1050(t)
Alcoholic dementia, 1035
Alcoholic hallucinations, 1035
Alcoholic hepatitis, 332, 973–974
Alcoholic myelopathy, 1036
Alcoholic neuropathy, 1067
Alcoholic psychosis, 1035
Alcoholic seizures, 1035
Alcoholism, 330–340
drug therapy for, 382(t)–388(t)
neurologic complications of, 1035–1036
physical complications of, 330–333
stages in, 335–339, 337(t)
treatment of, motivation for, 339–340
of alcoholic process, 334–340
of physical complications, 330–334
referral for, 334
withdrawal in, 333–334

Aldosteronism, primary, and hypertension, 987
Alkaline phosphatase, tests of, 972
Allergens, airborne, and allergic rhinitis, 1140–1142
Allergic dermatitis, *1117*, 1118–1119, *1118*
Allergic rhinitis, 650–651, 1140–1144
  allergens causing, 1140–1142
  diagnosis of, 1142–1143
  differential diagnosis of, 1143
  mechanism of, 1140–1142
  physical features of, 1142
  skin testing in, 1142
  symptoms of, 1142
  treatment of, 1143–1144
  vs. common cold, 839(t)
Allergy, 1137–1149
  animal dander, 1141
  dermatologic, *1117*, 1118–1120, *1118*
  drug, dermatologic, manifestations of, 1120
  food, and allergic rhinitis, 1141–1142
  housedust, 1141
  mold spore, 1141
  pollen, 1141
  respiratory, 650–651
Allied health professionals, 189–198
  and physician preceptors, 194
  consultation with, 206
  evolution of, 189–192
  role of, 192–194
  training of, 197
  utilization of, 194–197
Alopecia, and oral contraceptives, 459
Alopecia areata, 1120, *1120*
Alveolitis, fibrosing, 884
Alzheimer's disease, 229, 1048(t)
Amblyopia, 703–704
Amenorrhea, 753–754
  after use of oral contraceptives, 457–458, *458*
American Academy of Family Physicians, 4
American Academy of General Practice, 176
American Association of Marriage and Family Counselors, 423–424
American Board of Family Practice, 4
Aminoglycoside antibiotics, ototoxicity of, 645
Amitriptyline, dose, use and side effects of, 382(t)–383(t)
  for depression, 309(t)
Amyloidosis, and neuropathy, 1068–1069
Amyotrophic lateral sclerosis, 1061(t), 1062
Anal reflex, testing of, 1018
Anaphylaxis, 1136
  in children, 853
Anemia, hemolytic, in children, 880–882
  in children, 878–882
    periodic screening for, 126(t), 127(t), 128
  iron deficiency, in children, 879–880
  ocular manifestations of, 728
  physiologic, in children, 879
Anencephaly, genetic counseling for, 477
Aneuploidy, 466
Aneurysm, aortic, 508–509
  arteriovenous, rupture of, and subarachnoid hemorrhage, 1043–1044
  berry, rupture of, and subarachnoid hemorrhage, 1043
  intracranial, ocular nerve paralysis in, 726
Angina, Ludwig's, 662
  Vincent's, 661
Angina decubitus, 1005

Angina pectoris, 1005–1006
  drugs for, 1006
  electrocardiogram in, 1005–1006
  management of, 1006
  vs. noncardiac chest pain, 1003–1005, 1003(t)
Angina, nocturnal, 1005
Angioedema, 1139–1140
  vs. urticaria, 1140(t)
Angiofibroma, juvenile, 668
Angiography, selective visceral, 797
Angioid streaks, 729
Angiomyolipoma, renal, 783
Angioneurotic edema, 1139–1140
Animal dander, allergy to, 1141
Ankle, aspiration of, *622*
  sprain of, 554–555
  tenosynovitis in, 546–547
  weak, 555
Ankyloglossia, 660
Anorectal surgery, anal contracture after, 814
  by family physician, 787
  complications of, 811–814
  dysuria after, 812–813
  excess pain after, 811–812
  fecal impaction after, 814
  hemorrhage after, 812, 813
  postoperative care for, 808–811
  tissue sloughing after, 814
Anorectum. See also *Anus* and *Rectum.*
  abscess of, 804–806, *805*
    and fistula-in-ano, 806–808, *807*
  anatomy of, 787–790, *788, 789, 790*
  bleeding from, in children, 829
  blood supply of, 788–789, *789*
  carcinoma of, 181–820
  disorders of, diagnostic procedures for, 791–797
    history taking in, 790–791
    in children, 828
  examination of, 792–797
    anoscopic, 792–794
    carcinoembryonic antigen test in, 797
    digital, 792, *793*
    fiberoptic colonoscopy in, 797
    proctoscopic, 794–797, *795*
    selective visceral angiography in, 797
    sigmoidoscopic, 794–797, *795*
  innervation of, 789
  integumentary system of, 788
  lymphatic supply of, 789
  pectinate line of, 788, *788*
  surgery of. See *Anorectal surgery.*
  surgical spaces of, 790
  venereal disease of, 827–828
Anoscopy, 792–794
Anosmia, hereditary, 650
Anoxia, causes of, 1039
Anoxic encephalopathy, 1039
Antacids, in duodenal ulcer disease, 957
  in reflux esophagitis, 961, 961(t)
Anterior uveitis, 714–715, *714*
Antibiotics. See *Drugs, antibiotic.*
Anticoagulants. See *Drugs, anticoagulant.*
Anticonvulsants. See *Drugs, anticonvulsant.*
Antidepressants. See *Drugs, antidepressant.*
Antidotes, poison, 854(t)
Antisocial personality, 278
Anuria, 767
Anus. See also *Anorectum.*
  abscesses of, 804–806, *805*
    and fistula-in-ano, 806–808, *807*

Anus (*Continued*)
in hidradenitis suppurativa, 827
cancer of, 818–820
contracture of, postoperative, 814
diseases of, 797–808
fissure of, 808
vs. anal abscess, 804
fistula of, 806–808, *807*
hematoma of, 798
hemorrhoidal disease of, 797–803. See also *Hemorrhoids.*
imperforate, 829
infections of, 803, *804*
in hidradenitis suppurativa, 827
sequelae of, 804–808
pruritus of, 826–827
stenosis of, in newborn, 828
postoperative, 814
tissue sloughing in, postoperative, 814
venereal warts of, 828
Anxiety, and familial stress, 418
and phobias, 300–302
as symptom vs. syndrome, 290–291
behavior modification for, 300–302
chronic, hyperventilation syndrome in, 896
treatment of, 294
differential diagnosis of, 288–290
drugs for, 379, 382(t)–388(t)
in children, 292
in organic brain syndrome, 359
neurologic conditions causing, 290
organic diseases causing, 289–290
physiologic and personality traits in, 291
predisposition to, 291
psychiatric referral for, 295
psychologic causes of, 291–293
symptoms of, 288, 289(t)
transient situational, 290
treatment of, 293–295
community resources for, 295
vs. fear, 379(t)
Anxiety neurosis, defined, 291
Aortic aneurysm, 508–509
Aortic arch syndrome, ocular manifestations of, 729–730
Aortic coarctation, 867
and hypertension, 986
Aortic stenosis, 866–867
Apgar score, 830, 831(t)
Aphakia, 713
Appendicitis, 487–490
diagnosis of, 486(t), 488
in pregnancy, 487
treatment of, 489–490
vs. perforated peptic ulcer, 490
Appendix, perforation of, 489
Apraxia, 213–214
Arcus juvenilis, 728
Arcus senilis, 708, *709*
in systemic disease, 728
Arm, pain in, in children, 596–598
pseudoparalysis of, 597–598
Arrhythmias, cardiac, 1007–1010
Arsenic poisoning, 1036(t)
Arterial disease, chronic peripheral occlusive, 506–508
obliterative, of lower limb, 506–508
Arterial disorders, 504–511

Arterial embolism, 504–505
Arterial injuries, 504
Arterial occlusion, acute, 504–506
Arterial thrombosis, 505–506
Arteriolar sclerosis, ocular manifestations of, 728
ophthalmologic grading of, 716–718, *717*
vs. intimal atherosclerosis, 716–718
Arteriosclerosis. See also *Arteriolar sclerosis.*
and retinal degeneration, 715–718, *717*
cerebral, 1040–1042, 1041(t)
Arteriosclerotic dementia, 229
Arteriosclerotic heart disease, as surgical risk factor, 485
Arteriovenous aneurysm, rupture of, and subarachnoid hemorrhage, 1043–1044
Arteritis, cerebral, 1044
temporal, headache from, 1023(t)
ocular manifestations of, 726
Arthritis. See also *Osteoarthritis.*
cervical, chest pain in, 1003(t), 1004
degenerative. See *Osteoarthritis.*
dorsal, chest pain in, 1003(t), 1004
in rheumatic fever, 871–874
rheumatoid. See *Rheumatoid arthritis.*
septic, in children, 851
synovianalysis in, 622(t)
synovianalysis in, 621–622, 622(t)
traumatic, synovianalysis in, 622(t)
Arthrofibrosis, of shoulder, 591–595
Asbestosis, 924–925, *924*
Ascher's syndrome, 660
Ascites, in Laennec's cirrhosis, 976
Aspergillosis, pulmonary, 938–939
Aspiration, of joints, 621–622, *622*, 622(t), *623, 624, 625*
Aspirin, and bronchial asthma, 1144
for rheumatoid arthritis, 626
intoxication by, in children, 855–856, *855*
ototoxicity of, 645
Assertiveness training, 404
Asthenopia, 691
Asthma. See *Bronchial asthma.*
Astigmatism, 700
Atelectasis, 905, *906*
in bronchial asthma, 1145
Atherosclerosis, intimal, vs. arteriolar sclerosis, 716–718
Athetosis, 1052–1053
double, 1053
Athletic pseudonephritis, 778
Athletics, and nutrition, 1088–1089, 1088(t)
Atopic dermatitis, 1116–1117, *1116*
Atresia, choanal, posterior congenital, 649
laryngeal, congenital, 670
tricuspid, 869
Atrial fibrillation, 1009–1010
Atrial flutter with block, 1009
Atrial premature beats, 1009
Atrial septal defect (secundum type), 867–868
Atrophic rhinitis, 656
Atropinism, 346–347
Audiometry, 635, *636*
Auditory nerve, disorders of, 1057(t)
Autism, infantile, 320–321
Autonomic nerve dysfunction, 1075
Autonomic seizures, 857
Autosomes, defined, 465

Back. See also *Spine* and under the specific divisions of the spinal column.
disorders of, 574–584
examination of, 574–578, 574(t), 575, 577
exercises for, 216–217, 216, 217, 580, 583, 584
low-back syndrome in, 579–584
lumbosacral degeneration in, 582–584, 582(t), 583, 584
lumbosacral instability in, 580–581, 581(t)
muscle spasm in, 575–576, 576
osteoarthritis of, 582–584, 583, 584, 1064–1065
pain in, 579–584
physical therapy for, 215–218, 216, 217, 218
sprain of, 579–580, 579(t), 580
"sprung," 581
Backwash ileitis, 948(t)
Bacteriuria. See *Urinary tract infections*.
Balance, mechanics of, 632
Balanoposthitis, 781
Ballism, 1049, 1051(t)
Barbiturates, dose, use and side effects of, 388(t)
Basal body temperature, 756, 756
Basal cell carcinoma, 518–519
of ear, 644
of skin, 1131–1132, 1131, 1132
Baseball finger, 617–618, 617, 618
Beard, fungal infection of, 1113, 1113
Becker's dystrophy, 1072(t)
Beclomethasone, for asthma, 895–896
Behavior disorders, episodic, 280. See also *Learning disorders; Personality disorders*.
etiology of, 281–283
hospitalization in, 284–286
incidence of, 281–283
pathogenesis of, 281–283
psychotherapy for, 283
Behavior modification, 390–403
for phobias, 300–302
Behavior therapy, 395
Behaviorism, and preventive medicine, 115–120
Belching, 955
Bell's palsy, 643–644, 1059–1060
hemifacial spasm after, 1060
Belladonna derivatives, intoxication by, 346–347
Benzodiazepines, dose, use, and side effects of, 382(t)
Berry aneurysm, rupture of, and subarachnoid hemorrhage, 1043
Beta-thalassemia, in children, 881
Biceps, rupture of, 602–603, 602
strain of, 602
Bile duct, calculi in, and jaundice, 971–972
Bile salt diarrhea, 950
Biliary tract, extrahepatic obstruction of, vs. intrahepatic cholestasis, 971–972, 971(t)
Biopsy, breast, indications for, 515(t)
cervical, 734, 749–750
endometrial, 734–735
in infertility, 755–756
for dermatologic disorders, 1135
of pigmented nevi, 519–520, 520(t)
percutaneous hepatic, 973
Birth control, 450–464. See also *Contraceptives* and *Contraceptive counseling*.
Birth defects, and hydramnios, 764
and oral contraceptives, 455(t), 458, 736
Biting reflex, 1018–1019
Black eye, 705–706
Black hairy tongue, 665

Bladder. See *Urinary bladder*.
Blastomycosis, 1116, 1116
North American, 938
Bleeding. See also *Hemorrhage*.
anorectal, in children, 829
breakthrough, and oral contraceptives, 458, 735–736
control of, in trauma patients, 526
from nose, 655–656, 655
gastrointestinal, 497–499
acute, 963–965, 964(t)
in alcoholism, 332(t)
intermenstrual, 742–743
menstrual, excessive, 743
postcoital, 743
postmenopausal, 744
rectal, in children, 829
in diverticulosis, 815
uterine, dysfunctional, 744
vaginal. See *Vagina, bleeding from*.
Blepharitis, 704, 705
Blindness, from retinal artery occlusion, 718
in diabetic retinopathy, 719
in glaucoma, 712
Bloating, 955
Blood clotting, and oral contraceptives, 457
Blowout fractures, 680, 680, 682(t), 710
Blue phlebitis, 509
Boils, 1122
Botulism, 1071–1073
Bowel. See also *Colon* and *Small intestine*.
irritable. See *Irritable bowel syndrome*.
neurogenic, 211
Bowel disease, inflammatory, 947–949, 948(t)
Bowel function, disorders of, 821–823
neurologic disturbance of, 211, 1075
Bowel training, after spinal cord injury, 211
Bowen's disease, 781, 1130–1131, 1131
Boxer's fracture, 618–619, 618, 619, 620
Brachial plexus, birth injury of, 1065
disorders of, 1065–1066
neuropathies of, 1065–1066
Bradycardia, sinus, 1007–1008
Brain. See also names of specific anatomic parts.
decreased perfusion of, dizziness in, 1031(t)
injury of, in head injuries, 1045
organic syndromes of, in elderly, 228–231
vascular disease of, ocular manifestations of, 726
Brain concussion, 1044
anxiety following, 290
Brain function, examination of, 1014–1015
impairment of, in organic brain syndrome. See *Organic brain syndrome*.
higher, disorders of, 1039-1049
Brain stem, infarction of, 1042
Brain syndrome, acute, 228
Brass fever, 925–926
Breakthrough bleeding, and oral contraceptives, 458, 735–736
Breast, biopsy of, indications for, 515(t)
cancer of, 514–517, 515(t), 516(t), 517(t)
chemotherapy for, 515–516, 517(t)
diagnosis of, 514–515, 515(t)
periodic screening for, 133–134
recurrent, treatment of, 517
staging of, 514
treatment of, 515–517
cysts of, 512–513, 513

Breast (*Continued*)
    diseases of, 511–517, *513*, 513(t), 515(t), 516(t), 517(t)
    enlargement of, in males, 514
    examination of, 511–512, 514, 731
    fibroadenoma of, 513
    fibrocystic disease of, 512–513, *513*
    nipple discharge from, 513–514, 513(t)
    tenderness of, and oral contraceptives, 738
Breast feeding, 838
    advantages of, 1080
    nutritional requirements in, 1080–1081
    vs. formula feeding, 1081–1082
Breast milk, contamination of, 1080–1081
    nutritional content of, 1082(t), 1083(t), 1084(t)
Breath-holding, 1026(t)
Briquet's disorder, 277–278
Bronchi, carcinoma of, 685
    cysts of, 683–684
    foreign bodies in, 684–685
Bronchial asthma, 891–896, 1144–1149
    aspirin-induced, 1144
    attacks of, stages of, 893–894, *893*, 894(t)
        causes of, *892*
    clinical classification of, 1144–1145
    clinical manifestations of, 892–893, 1145
    defined, 891, 894
    diagnosis of, 1145–1146
    differential diagnosis of, 1146–1147
    drug therapy for, 894–895
    etiology and pathogenesis of, 891–892, *892*
    exercise-induced, 1144–1145
    extrinsic, 891, 1144
    intrinsic, 891–892, 1144
    laboratory studies for, 893–894, 1145–1146
    management of, 1148–1149, 1149(t)
    pathophysiology of, 1144
    prognosis in, 896
    status asthmaticus in, 893–894, 894(t), 1145
        management of, 1148–1149, 1149(t)
    treatment of, 894–896, 1147–1148, 1147(t)
    vs. bronchiolitis, 841(t)
    vs. pneumonia, 841(t)
Bronchiectasis, 922–923
    cylindrical, in children, 922
    defined, 884
Bronchiolitis, 841–482, 841(t)
Bronchitis, acute, 890
    chronic, 908–910
        and pulmonary emphysema, 909, 910
        defined, 884
        in children, 922
Bronchogenic carcinoma, 685, 914–917, 915(t), *916*
Bronchoscopy, 682
Bronchospasm, in bronchial asthma, 1145
    treatment of, 934
Brooke formula, for fluid therapy for burn patients, 537(t)
Brucellosis, 1033
Buccal mucosa, carcinoma of, 664
Bullous pemphigoid, 1106–1108, *1107*
Burns, corrosive esophageal, 685
    thermal, 536–538
        rule of nines for, 537(t)
Bursa, Tornwaldt's, 666
Bursitis, of elbow, 603–604, *603*
Butyrophenones, dose, use, and side effects of, 386(t)

Café coronary, 523–524
Caisson disease, 1037
Cake kidney, 773
Calcium deficiency, and osteoporosis, 1091(t)
Calculi, bile duct, and jaundice, 971–972
    salivary, 677
        detection of, 676
    urinary, 770–772, 772(t)
Cancer. See also *Carcinoma* and names of specific malignancies and sites.
    and nutrition, 1092
    and oral contraceptives, 455–456
    cerebellar degeneration in, 1050(t)
Candidiasis, 1110–1111, *1110*
    oral, 665
    pulmonary, 938
Canes, use of, 218–219, *219*
Cannulation, of external jugular vein, *522*
    of subclavian vein, *523*
Carbohydrate metabolism, and oral contraceptives, 456–457
Carcinoid, rectal, 828
Carcinoma, and ulcerative colitis, 816
    basal cell, 518–519
        of ear, 644
        of skin, 1131–1132, *1131, 1132*
    bronchogenic, 685, 914–917, 915(t), *916*
    gastrointestinal, diseases predisposing to, 965(t), 967–970, 968(t)–969(t)
        management of, 965–970
    of anorectum, 818–820
    of bladder, 784–786
    of breast. See *Breast, cancer of.*
    of cervix, 749–750
        screening for, 132–133
    of colon, 818–820, 966–970
        and colonic polyps, 967–970, 968(t)–969(t)
        and familial adenomatous polyposis, 818
        and ulcerative colitis, 816, 949
        diseases predisposing to, 965(t), 967–970, 968(t)–969(t)
        screening for, 134–136
    of endometrium, 748–749
    of esophagus, 685, 965–966
        diseases predisposing to, 965(t)
    of kidney, 783–784
    of larynx, 674–675
    of lung, 685, 914–917, 915(t), *916*
    of nasopharynx, 668
    of neck, 679
    of oral cavity, 664–665
    of pancreas, chronic abdominal pain in, 943–944
    of penis, 781
    of prostate, 783
    of rectum, 818–820
        screening for, 134–136
    of salivary gland, 678
    of stomach, 966
        diseases predisposing to, 965(t)
    of testis, 782
    of tongue, 664
    of ureter, 784
    of urethra, 781–782, 786
    of vagina, 753
    squamous cell. See *Squamous cell carcinoma.*
Carcinomatous neuropathy, 1067
Carcinoembryonic antigen test, 797
Cardiac arrhythmias, 1007–1010
Cardiac tamponade, 528–529, *529*

Cardiology, 986–1012
Cardiopulmonary resuscitation, 525–526
Cardiovascular system, and oral contraceptives, 455–456
  in alcoholism, 331
Carotid arterial insufficiency, 1040–1041, 1041(t)
Carotid artery, occlusive disease of, ocular manifestations of, 729
Carotid sinus hypersensitivity, 1026(t)
Carpal tunnel, anatomy of, 606
Carpal tunnel syndrome, 606–607, 606, 1069
Cartilage, discoid, of knee, and locked knee, 562–563
  tears of, in knee, 559–562
    and locked knee, 555–557, 556
Caruncle, urethral, 782
Case finding, defined, 123
Case history method, epideiologic, 148–149
Cataract, 712–714, 712
  complicated, 713
  congenital, 712–713
    genetic counseling for, 473–474
  extraction of, 713–714
  senile, 713
  toxic, 713
  traumatic, 713
Catatonia, schizophrenic, 320
Catheterization, central venous, 522, 523
  urethral, complications of, 777
    in urinary tract infection, 776–777
Causalgia, 1069
Cell-mediated immunity, 1136–1137
  evaluation of, 1137(t), 1138
Cerebellar degeneration, alcoholic, 1035–1036, 1050(t)
  carcinomatous, 1050(t)
  familial, 1050(t)
  myxedematous, 1050(t)
Cerebellar disorders, affecting movement and coordination, 1050(t)–1051(t)
Cerebellar hemorrhage, 1043
Cerebellar infarction, 1050(t)
Cerebellar ischemia, 1050(t)
Cerebellar tumors, 1050(t)
Cerebellopontine angle tumors, 1050(t), 1060
  vertigo in, 1031(t)
Cerebellum, disorders affecting, 1049–1055
Cerebral arteriosclerosis, 1040–1042, 1042(t)
Cerebral arteritis, 1044
Cerebral artery, middle, thromboembolism of, 1042
Cerebral concussion, 1044
  anxiety following, 290
Cerebral function, evaluation of, 1014–1015
Cerebral hematoma, 1047
Cerebral hemorrhage, 1042–1043
Cerebral infarction, 1042
Cerebral perfusion, decreased, dizziness in, 1031(t)
Cerebral sclerosis, diffuse, 1030
Cerebrospinal fluid rhinorrhea, 651–652
Cerebrovascular accident. See Stroke.
Cerebrovascular disease, 1040–1042
Ceruminoma, 644
Cervical adenitis, in children, 839–840
Cervical collar, 587, 587
Cervical disc, rupture of, 590, 590
Cervical spondylosis, 1064

Cervix, biopsy of, 734, 749–750
  carcinoma of, 749–750
    screening for, 132–133
  dysplasia of, 749
  examination of, 732
    examination of, in infertility, 756
  polyps of, 749
  tumors of, 749–750
Chalazion, 704, 705
Charcot knee, 565
Chemical neuropathy, 1067
Chemodectoma, of ear, 644–645
Chemosis, conjunctival, 727
Chest, flail, 528
  injuries of, 526–529, 527, 528
Chest pain, anginal. See Angina pectoris.
  cardiac, vs. noncardiac, 1003–1005, 1003(t)
  differential diagnosis of, 1003–1007, 1003(t)
  in congenital heart disease, 870
  noncardiac, vs. cardiac, 1003–1005, 1003(t)
  psychoneurotic, 1003, 1003(t)
Chest tubes, insertion of, 527, 528
Chewing reflex, 1018–1019
Chickenpox, 844–845
Child(ren). See also Adolescents, Infants, and under specific disorders.
  abdominal pain in, 488
  anxiety in, 292
  as rape victim, counseling for, 366
  birth of, and family life cycle, 37–39
  departure of from home, 42
  diet for, 837–838
  early and middle school years of, 40–41
  emergency treatment for, 852–855
  emerging sexuality of, 40
  epileptic, management of, 858
  failure to thrive in, 864–865
  fluid and electrolyte balance in, 858–863
  growth retardation in, 864–865
  gynecologic examination in, 733
  hyperactive, 269
  immunization for, 838–839, 839(t)
  individuation of, 39–40
  infections in, 839–852. See also names of specific infections.
  learning diabilities in, 267–275. See also Learning disabilities.
  nutrition for, 837–838, 838(t), 1085–1087, 1085(t), 1086(t)
  periodic health screening in, 126–128, 126(t), 127(t)
  poisoning in, 853–855, 854, 854(t), 855
  preventive medicine for, 108(t)–109(t)
  sexuality of, 40, 436–437
Chlorazepate, dose, use, and side effects of, 382(t)
Chlordiazepoxide, dose, use, and side effects of, 382(t)
  for anxiety, 293
Chlorpromazine, and cholestasis, 979–980, 980(t)
  dose, use, and side effects of, 385(t)–386(t)
  for schizophrenia, 325
Chlorprothixene, dose, use, and side effects of, 387(t)
Choanal atresia, posterior congenital, 649
Chochlea, anatomy of, 630–632, 631
Chocolate cysts, 752
Cholasma, and oral contraceptives, 459
Cholecystectomy, 495, 500

Cholecystitis, 982
    acute, 486(t), 494–495
    chest pain in, 1003(t), 1004
Cholecystography, 499–500, *499, 500*
Cholecystostomy, 495
Choledocholithiasis, and jaundice, 971–972
Cholelithiasis, 499–501, *499, 500,* 981–982
    chest pain in, 1003(t), 1004
Cholestasis, drug-induced, 979–980, 980(t)
    intrahepatic, vs. extrahepatic biliary obstruc-
        tion, 971–972, 971(t)
Cholesteatoma, 640–641
Cholesterol, and hyperlipoproteinemias, 1093–
    1094
Chondromalacia, of patella, 564–565, *566*
Chordoma, 1061(t), 1064
Chorea(s), 1049–1052, 1051(t)
    famililial benign, 1052
    Huntington's, 1053
    secondary, 1052
    Sydenham's, 1049–1052, 1051(t)
Chorea gravidarum, 1051(t), 1052
Choreoathetosis, paroxysmal, 1053
Chorioretinitis, 714
Choroid, malignant melanoma of, 721
Choroiditis, 714
Choristoma, nasopharyngeal, 666
Chromosome(s), aberrations in, 466–467
    deletions of, 466–467
    duplications of, 466–467
    errors in numbers of, 466
    karyotyping of, 465–466, *466*
        indications for, 467
    normal, 465–466, *466*
    rearrangements of, 467
Cigarette smoking. See *Smoking.*
Cirrhosis, Laennec's, complications of, 974–976,
    974(t)
    development of, 973–976
Claudication, intermittent, 506
Clavicle, fracture of, 597–598, *597, 598*
Cleft lip, 649–650, 660
Cleft palate, 649–650, 660–661
Cleft tongue, 660
Cleft uvula, 661
Client-centered psychotherapy, 399
Clitoris, hypertrophy of, 774
Cluster headache, 1022(t), 1024
Coal workers' pneumoconiosis, 925
Coarctation, aortic, 867
    and hypertension, 986
Coccidioidomycosis, 937–938
Cohabitation, and sexual counseling, 438-439
Cohort method, epidemiologic, 149
Coitus interruptus, 451(t), 452
Cold, common, 885–886, 885(t)
    in children, 839
    vs. allergic rhinitis, 839(t)
Cold urticaria, 1140
Colic, 838
Colitis, ulcerative, 815–816, 947–949, 948(t)
Colon, carcinoma of, 818–820, 966–970
    and colonic polyps, 967–970, 968(t)–969(t)
    and familial adenomatous polyposis, 818
    and ulcerative colitis, 816, 949
    diseases predisposing to, 965(t), 967–970,
        968(t)–969(t)
    screening for, 134–136

Crohn's disease of, 816–817, 949
    vs. fistula-in-ano, 807
disorders of, chronic diarrhea in, 947
diverticular disease of, 953–954
obstruction of, 491–494, 491(t)
perforation of, in diverticulosis, 815
    in ulcerative colitis, 816
polyps of, 817–818
    and colonic carcinoma, 967–970, 968(t)–969(t)
ulceration of, in colitis, 815–816, 947–949
Colonoscopy, fiberoptic, 797
Colostomy, care of, 820–821
Colposcopy, 734, 797
Coma, in head injuries, 1045
    in phenothiazine intoxication, 1053
Concussion, cerebral, 1044
    anxiety following, 290
Condom, 451(t), 463, 737
Condylomata acuminata, 741
Confusional reaction, acute, 228
Congenital anomalies, and hydramnios, 764
    and oral contraceptives, 458
Coniotomy, 524, *524*
Conjunctiva, chemosis of, 727
    congestion of, 727
    disorders of, 706–707
    hemorrhage under, 707
    in systemic disease, 727–728
Conjunctivitis, 706–707
    allergic, 707
    bacterial, 706
    drug-induced, 707
    vernal, 707
    viral, 706
Connective tissue disorders, ocular manifestations
    of, 727
Consciousness-raising groups, 404
Constipation, 823–824
    after anorectal surgery, 814
    causes of, 951, 951(t)
    in children, 828
    in irritable bowel syndrome, 951, 952
    in pregnancy, 1079–1080
    management of, 951(t)
Consultation. See also *Referral.*
    in marriage and family counseling, 431
    indirect, 202
    mechanisms for, 202
    medicolegal aspects of, 202–204
    organization of, 206–208
    timing of, 204–205
    types of, 205–206
    vs. referral, 200–202
    with allied health workers, 206
    with diagnostic specialists, 205
Contact dermatitis, allergic, *1117,* 1118–1119,
    1118
    primary, 1119
Contact lenses, 700–701
    for cataract, 713
Contraception, 735–737
    counseling for, 450–464
    history-taking in, 450
Contraceptive(s), efficacy of, 451(t)
    mechanical, 459–460, 463
    oral. See *Oral contraceptives.*
    post-coital, 460
    spermicidal, 463
Contraceptive foam, 737

Contrast baths, in rheumatoid arthritis, 214–215
Conversion hysteria, 297–298
    and syncope, 1026(t)
    vs. grand mal epilepsy, 1025
Convulsive disorders, 1025–1030. See also
        Epilepsy.
    drug therapy in, 858(t), 1028(t)
    in children, 855–858
    types of, 1026(t)
Convulsive seizures. See *Seizures.*
Coordination, motor, disorders of, 1049–1055,
        1050(t)–1051(t)
    neurologic examination of, 1016
Cor pulmonale, 935–937, *936*
Cornea, abrasions of, 709
    disorders of, 708–709
    foreign body in, 709
    herpetic infection of, 708
    inflammation of, 708
    injuries of, 709
    lacerations of, 709
    metabolic changes in, 708–709
    ulcers of, 708, *708*
Coronary artery disease. See also *Angina pectoris.*
    and infant nutrition, 1085
    family counseling in, 1006–1007
Coronary heart disease, and oral contraceptives,
        456
    early, genetic counseling for, 476
Cortical sensation, testing of, 1017–1018
Corticosteroids, for asthma, 895
    for rheumatoid arthritis, 626
Coryza, 652
Costochondritis, chest pain in, 1003, 1003(t)
Cough, in bronchiectasis, 922
    in chronic bronchitis, 908, 909
Counseling, contraceptive, 450–464
    for depression, 313–314
    for rape victims, 365–366
    genetic. See *Genetic counseling.*
    nutritional, 1091(t)
    psychiatric. See *Psychotherapy.*
    sexual. See *Sexual counseling.*
Cover testing, visual, 695–696, *695*
Cranial nerves, disorders of, 1055–1060, 1065(t)–
        1067(t)
    examination of, 1016(t)
Creatinine clearance, by age, *225*
Cremasteric reflex, testing of, 1018
Crohn's disease, 816–817, 949
    vs. fistula-in-ano, 807
Crossed eyes, 701–702, *703*
Croup, 672–673, 840–841
Crutches, use of, 219–220, *218, 219, 220*
Cryptococcosis, 938
Cryptorchidism, 774
Cue, in problem-solving, 140–141
Culture technique, for dermatoses, 1134–1135
Cupulolithiasis, 643
Cushing's disease, anxiety in, 289
    hypertension in, 987
Cyclitis, 714
Cyclothymic personality, 277
Cylindrical bronchiectasis, in children, 922
Cyst(s), breast, 512–513, *513*
    bronchogenic, 683–684
    cervical, 678
    chocolate, 752
    epidural, 1061(t), 1064

Cyst(s) *(Continued)*
    Gartner's duct, 753
    laryngeal, 670–671
    nasopharyngeal, 666
    ovarian, 750, 751(t)
    pilonidal, 827
        excision of, 521
    preauricular, 637
    renal, 773
    sebaceous, excision of, 521
    thyroglossal duct, 678
    vaginal, 753
Cystic fibrosis, pancreatic, genetic counseling for,
        474
    pulmonary, 939–940
Cystic hygroma, 678
Cystinuria, urinary calculi in, 770
Cystitis, in children, 847, 847(t)
    vs. vaginitis, 738–739
Cystocele, 755
Cytogenetic examination, indications for, 467
Cytomegalovirus, neonatal infection with, 835–
        836

Dacryocystitis, 706
Dander, animal, allergy to, 1141
Day care programs, for elderly, 235
Dead space, respiratory, defined, 883
Deafness, congenital, genetic counseling for,
        474–475
    drug-induced, 645–646
    from acoustic neuromas, 645
    from otosclerosis, 637–638
    iatrogenic causes of, 641
    in allergic rhinitis, 1142
    in Meniere's disease, 642
    in normal aging process, 642
    measurement of. See *Hearing, tests of.*
    noise-induced, 642
    sensorineural, 638
Death. See *Illness, terminal.*
Debridement, wound, 532, *533*
Decerebrate rigidity, vs. grand mal epilepsy, 1025
Decompression sickness, 1037
Defecation, disorders of, 821–825. See also
        Constipation; Diarrhea.
    in irritable bowel syndrome, 952
    painful, in children, 829
Dehydration, in children, 858–860, 859(t)
    fluid therapy for, 860–863, 860(t), 861(t)
    hypertonic, 859(t)
    hypotonic, 859(t)
    isotonic, 859(t)
    management of, 860–863
Delirium, and organic brain syndrome, 354, 354(t)
Delirium tremens, 1035
Delusions, neurologic evaluation of, 1014
Dementia(s), 1047–1049, 1048(t)
    alcoholic, 1035
    and organic brain syndrome, 354, 354(t)
    anxiety in, 290
    arteriosclerotic, 229
    clinical features of, 1047
    drug therapy for, 382(t)–388(t)
    etiology of, 1047
    evaluation of, 1047–1049
    management of, 230

Dementia(s) *(Continued)*
multi-infarct, 1048(t)
organic, 228–230
pathology of, 1047
presenile, 229
senile, 229
treatment of, 1049
Dental care, in pregnancy, 758
Delusion, in schizophrenia, 318–319
Depressants, central nervous system, 388(t)
intoxication by, 345–347
Depression, 303–316, 376–379
and family stress, 418
and oral contraceptives, 458
and suicide, 309–310
bipolar, 304, 304(t)
classification of, 304–305, 304(t)
complications of, 306
correlation of with life events, 306
course of, 305–306
diagnosis of, 303–304
differential diagnosis of, 306–308, 377(t)
drug-induced, 307
drug therapy for, 309–313, 309(t), 310(t), 311(t),
378(t), 382(t)–388(t)
side effects of, 312–313
electroshock therapy for, 315
family history in, 305–306
functional, differential diagnosis of, 377(t)–
378(t)
hospitalization for, 308–309
in elderly, 307
in systemic disease, 306–307
incidence of, by age and sex, 305–306
neurotic, differential diagnosis of, 377(t)–378(t)
physical causes of, 306–307
primary, 304, 304(t)
unipolar, vs. bipolar, 307–308
psychotic, differential diagnosis of, 377(t)–
378(t)
psychiatric referral in, 315
secondary, 304, 304(t)
success, 376
symptoms of, 305
treatment of, 308–315
medical, 378(t), 382(t)–388(t)
outpatient, 308
psychologic, 313–315
unipolar, 304, 304(t)
Dermatitis, allergic, *1117*, 1118–1119, *1118*
atopic, 1116–1117, *1116*
contact, *1117*, 1118–1119, *1118*
seborrheic, 1121
Dermatitis herpetiformis, 1108–1109, *1109*
ocular manifestations of, 727
Dermatofibroma, 1133, *1133*
Dermatology, 1102–1135
Dermatomes, of leg, 578
Dermatomyositis, 1126, *1126*
Dermatophytes, griseofulvin-sensitive, 1111–
1113
Dermatoses, bullous, 1106–1109
diagnostic techniques for, 1134–1135
inflammatory, 1102–1106
ocular manifestations of, 726–727
papulosquamous, 1102–1106
superficial fungal, 1109–1111
DES. See *Diethylstilbestrol.*

Desensitization, behavioral, 395
for anxiety, 300–301
for phobias, 300–301
Diabetes mellitus, and oral contraceptives, 456–
457
as surgical risk factor, 484
diet in, 1092
genetic counseling for, 476–477
in children, 876–878
latent, 878
maturity-onset, 877
overt, 876-877
transient, 878
in pregnancy, 761–762, 762(t)
and neonatal complications, 836
juvenile, 876–877
neurologic complications of, 1034–1035
ocular manifestations of, 728
ocular nerve paralysis in, 726
retinal pathology in, 719–720, *719*
skin lesions in, 1126–1127, *1126*
transient, in newborn, 877–878
White's classification of, 762(t)
Diabetic neuropathy, 1067–1068
Diabetic retinopathy, 719–720, *719*
Diagnosis, early, of undifferentiated problems,
138–146
epidemiologic principles for, 151–152
importance of, in family practice, 11–13
pay-off of, defined, 139
probability of, defined, 138–139
Diaphragm, contraceptive, 463, 737
Diarrhea, 824–825
differential diagnosis in, acute, 944–946, 944(t),
945
bile salt, 950
chronic, causes of, 946–951
in Crohn's disease, 949
in colonic disorders, 947
in inflammatory bowel disease, 947–949,
948(t)
in irritable bowel syndrome, 952
in malabsorption, 946, 947(t)
in regional ileitis, 816–817
in ulcerative colitis, 815–816, 947 949, 948(t)
in ulcerative proctitis, 949
osmotic, 950
secretory, 949–950
Diazepam, dose, use, and side effects of, 382(t)
for alcohol withdrawal, 333–334
for anxiety, 293
Dibenzoxazepines, dose, use, and side effects of,
388(t)
Diet. See also *Nutrition.*
for children, 837–838
for infants, 837–838, 838(t)
high-fiber, in diverticular disease, 1093
in diabetes mellitus, 1092
in disease, 1091–1101
in duodenal ulcer disease, 957
in hyperlipoproteinemias, 1093–1094
in pregnancy, 758, 1078
reducing, 1098–1100, 1098(t), *1099*
sodium-restricted, in hypertension, 1093–1096,
1096(t), 1097(t)
Diethylstilbestrol, as "morning after" pill, 460
Digitalis, for congestive heart failure, 997
in elderly, 999
in children, 870(t)

Digoxin, for congestive heart failure, 997
    in elderly, 999–1000
    in children, 870(t)
Dihydroindolones, dose, use, and side effects of,
    387(t)–388(t)
Diphtheria, immunization for, 839(t)
    laryngeal, 673
    tonsillar, 662
Disc, intervertebral. See *Intervertebral disc.*
Disc kidney, 773
Discoid lupus erythematosus, *1124*, 1124–1125
Disease. See also *Illness.*
    biological gradient of, defined, 148
    determinants of, study of, 148. See also
        Epidemiology.
    diet in, 1091–1101
    distribution of, study of, 148. See also
        Epidemiology.
    natural history of, 161, *161*
    prevention of. See also *Preventive medicine.*
        choice of strategies for, 150–151
        primary, 150
        secondary, 150
        tertiary, 150
    social and cultural determinants of, 58–60
    terminal. See *Illness, terminal.*
Dislocation, of acromioclavicular joint, 595–596,
    595, 596
    of elbow, 604
    of finger, 611–614, *612, 613*
    of hip, congenital, 573, *573*
    of patella, recurrent, 563, *564*
    of shoulder, 598, 599, *599*
    of thumb, 611–614, *612, 613*
    vascular injury in, 504
Dissociative hysteria, 298–299
Disulfiram, in alcoholism, 334
Diuretics, in congestive heart failure, 997–998,
    998(t)
    in elderly, 999–1000
Diverticulitis, 815, 953–954
Diverticulosis, 815, 953–954
    diet in, 1093
    urethral, 782
Divorce, and family life cycle, 42–43
Dizziness, causes of, 1030, 1031(t)
Double simultaneous stimulation test, 1018
Douching, in pregnancy, 758
Doughnut kidney, 773
Down syndrome, genetic counseling for, 473
Doxepin, dose, use, and side effects of, 382(t)–
    383(t)
    for depression, 309(t)
Drug(s). See also generic names of specific drugs.
    abuse of. See *Drug abuse.*
    addiction to. See *Drug addiction.*
    allergy to, dermatologic manifestations of, 1120
    antacid, in duodenal ulcer disease, 957
        in reflux esophagitis, 961, 961(t)
    antianginal, 1006
    antianxiety, 379, 382(t)–388(t)
    antiarthritic, 625–626
    antiasthmatic, 894–895, 1147–1148, 1147(t)
    antibiotic, for asthma, 894
        for bacterial infections, 840(t)
        for neonatal sepsis, 835
        for urinary tract infections in children, 847(t)
        for wound infection prophylaxis, 534–535
        oropharyngeal disorders from, 665
        ototoxicity of, 645

Drug(s) *(Continued)*
    anticoagulant, for arterial embolism, 505
        for deep venous thrombosis, 510
        for postphlebotic syndrome, 511
    anticonvulsant, 858(t), 1028(t)
        in alcohol withdrawal, 334
    antidepressant, 309–312, 309(t), 378(t)
        combinations of, 312
        tricyclic, 309–311, 309(t)
            dose, use, and side effects of, 382(t)–383(t)
    antihypertensive, 988–994, 991(t)–992(t)
    antischizophrenic, 325–326, 381
    anxiety from, 289
    breast milk contamination by, 1080–1081
    caractogenic, 713
    diuretic, in congestive heart failure, 997–998,
        998(t)
        in elderly, 999–1000
    depressant, 388(t)
        intoxication by, 345–347
    for behavior disorders, 283–284
    for congestive heart failure, 997–998, 998(t)
        in elderly, 999–1000
    for elderly, 232–234
    for psychiatric disorders. See *Psycho-
        pharmacologic drugs.*
    hepatotoxic, 979–981, 980(t)
    hypnotic, for depression, 312
    in pregnancy, 758
    intoxication by. See *Drug intoxication.*
    laryngeal disorders from, 675
    nasopharyngeal disorders from, 668
    oral disorders from, 665
    ototoxic, 645–646
    poisoning by. See *Drug intoxication.*
    psychopharmacologic, 374–389, 382(t)–389(t)
        diagnosis for, 374
        dose, use, and side effects of, 382(t)–389(t)
        precautions for, 375
        selection of, 374
    psychosis from vs. schizophrenia, 323
    rhinitis from, 657
    toxicity of, in elderly, 226, 232–233
    tranquilizing, and tardive dyskinesia, 326
        for alcohol withdrawal, 333–334
        for anxiety, 293
        for asthma, 896
        for behavior disorders, 284
        for depression, 312
        for schizophrenia, 325–326
Drug abuse, 341–352. See also *Alcoholism.*
    agents used in, 344(t)–345(t)
    behavioral components of, 342
    diagnosis of, 347
    incidence of, 341–342
    prevention of, 348–349
    rehabilitation and detoxification programs for,
        349–352
    social implications of, 342–343
    treatment of, 347–348
    types of, 341–342
    vocabulary of, 343–344, 344(t)–345(t)
Drug addiction, drug therapy for, 382(t)–388(t)
Drug intoxication, and organic brain syndrome,
    355
    antidotes for, 854(t)
    clinical monitoring in, 346
    drug therapy for, 346
    history-taking in, 346

Drug (*Continued*)
  treatment of, 345–347
    with belladonna derivatives, 346–347
    with depressants, 345–346
    with hallucinogens, 347
    with heroin, 348
Drusen, 722, *722*
Duchenne's dystrophy, 1072(t)
Duodenal ulcer disease, 956–957, 956(t)
  pain in, 956(t)
  patient characteristics in, 956(t)
Dupuytren's contracture, 608–609, *608*
Dust, allergy to, 1141
Dying patient, care of, 249–257. See also *Illness, terminal.*
Dysarthria, 213
  evaluation of, 1014
Dyskinesia, tardive, from phenothiazine, 1053–1054
  from tranquilizers, 326
Dyslexia, defined, 267
Dysmenorrhea, 745–746
  defined, 742
Dyspareunia, 448, 746
Dysphagia, 213
  causes of, 961–962, 962(t)
  classification of, 963(t)
  in esophageal carcinoma, 965
Dysphasia, evaluation of, 1014
Dysphonia, evaluation of, 1014
Dyspnea, categories of, 929(t)
  defined, 883
  in bronchial asthma, 1145
  in congestive heart failure, 994
Dystonia, 1051(t), 1052
  acute, from phenothiazine, 1053
Dystonia musculorum deformans, 1052
Dystrophy, Becker's, 1072(t)
  Duchenne's, 1072(t)
  Erb's, 878, 1072(t)
  facioscapulohumeral, 1072(t)
  Gower, 1072(t)
  Landouzy-Déjerine, 878, 1072
  Leyden-Moebius, 878
  limb-girdle, 1072(t)
  myotonic, 1072(t)
  pseudohypertrophic, 1072(t)
  X-linked, benign, 1072(t)
Dysuria, 767
  after anorectal surgery, 812–813

Ear, anatomy of, 628–630, *629, 630, 631*
  basal cell carcinoma of, 644
  ceruminomas of, 644
  chemodectomas of, 644–645
  disorders of, congenital, 637
    hereditary, 637–638
    iatrogenic, 641
    idiopathic, 642–644
  embryology of, 628
  examination of, 632–635, *632*
  external, anatomy of, 628–629, *629*
    infections of, 638
    malformations of, 637
      and renal anomalies, 987
    physiology of, 630
  foreign body removal in, 635, *635*

Ear (*Continued*)
  infections of, 639–641
  injuries of, drug-induced, 645–646
  inner, auditory function of, 630–632
    infections of, 641
    physiology of, 630–632, *631*
    vestibular function of, 632
  lop, 637
  Meniere's disease of, 642
  middle, infections of, 638–641
    physiology of, 630
  neoplasms of, 644–645
  neuromas of, 645
  physiology of, 630–632
  polyps of, 641
  preauricular cysts of, 637
  preauricular sinuses of, 637
  swimmer's, 638
  tumors of, 644–645
Eardrum, anatomy of, 629–630, *630*
Eclampsia, 763–764
Ectopic pregnancy, vaginal bleeding in, 744
Ectropion, 705
Eczema, 1116–1119
  nummular, 1117–1118, *1117*
  of nipple, and Paget's disease, 513(t), 514
Edema, and oral contraceptives, 736
  angioneurotic, 1139–1140
Effective communication pattern, 424–426, 425(t), *426–427*
Ejaculation, premature, 443–444
  retarded, 444–445
  retrograde, 445
Elbow, anatomy of, *599*
  aspiration of, *624*
  bursitis of, 603–604, *603*
  contusion of, 601
  dislocation of, 604
  disorders of, 599–604
  fractures of, 604
  pain in, 600–601, *600, 601*
  sprain of, 603
  stiff, 601
  subluxation of, in children, 596–597
  swelling of, 603 604, *603*
  tendon disorders in, 602–603, *602*
Elderly, aging process in, 222–225, *224, 225*
  care of, 222–238
  creatinine clearance in, *225*
  day care programs for, 235
  depression in, 307
  disease in, diagnosis of, 225–226
    latency of, 225–226
    misleading signs and symptoms in, 225–226
    multiple, 226
  drugs for, increased effect of, 226
    prescription of, 232–234
    toxicity of, 232–233
  food services for, 236
  glucose tolerance in, *224*
  home care programs for, 235
  homemaking services for, 236
  housing for, 236
  loss of physiologic capacity in, 224–225, *224, 225*
  medical records of, 227–228
  neuropsychiatric disorders in, differential diagnosis of, 230–231
  noninstitutional care of, 235–236
  nursing homes for, 237–238

Elderly (*Continued*)
  nutrition in, 1089–1091
  organic brain syndrome in, 228–231. See also
    Organic brain syndrome.
  periodic health screening in, 130–132
  population of, 222
  preventive medicine for, 110(t)
  sexuality of, 439–440
Electrocardiogram, in angina pectoris, 1005–1006
  in health screening, 132
  in pulmonary emphysema, 912
  preoperative, 485
Electrocardiographer, consultation with, 205
Electroconvulsive therapy, 315
Electroencephalogram, in organic brain syndrome, 358, 358(t)
Electrolyte imbalance, neurologic complications of, 1036–1037
Electrolyte therapy, in children, 858–863
Electronystagmography, 635–636
Embolectomy, 505
Embolism, arterial, 504–505
  pulmonary, 901–903
    in elderly, 231–232
Embryoma, renal, 784
Emergency treatment, for trauma, 521–538
Emotional problems. See also *Personality disorders.*
  after spinal cord injury, 212
  and functional bowel disorders, 821–823
  drug therapy for, 374–389, 382(t)–389(t)
  of rape victims, 367–368
  psychotherapy for. See *Psychotherapy.*
Emphysema, defined, 884
  infantile lobar, 684
  pulmonary, 910–914, *913*
Empyema, defined, 884
Encephalitis, acute, headache in, 1023(t)
  chronic, headache in, 1023(t)
Encephalocele, nasopharyngeal, 666
Encephalopathy, hepatic. See *Hepatic encephalopathy.*
  hypertensive, 1024
  secondary metabolic, defined, 355. See also *Organic brain syndrome.*
  Wernicke's, 1035
Endocardial cushion defect, 868
Endocarditis, bacterial, in congenital heart disease, 870
Endocrine ophthalmopathy, 725–726, *725*
Endometrial adenocarcinoma, 748–749
Endometrial biopsy, 734–735
  in infertility, 755–756
Endometriosis, 753
  internal, 748
Endometritis, 739
Endoscopy, in gastrointestinal bleeding, 964
Endotracheal intubation, 522–524
  and subglottic stenosis, 673
Enema, for colostomy patients, 820–821
Enterocele, 755
Entrapment neuropathy, 1069
Entropion, 705, *706*
Enuresis, 767
  in children, 864
Environmental hazards, limiting effects of, 156–157
Enzymes, hepatocellular, tests of, 972
Epicondylitis, 600–601, *600, 601*

Epidemic, community, management of, 155–156
  family, management of, 153–155
Epidemiologic survey, defined, 123
Epidemiology, and health care evaluation, 157–158
  and preventive medicine, 103–110, 111–112
  case history method in, 148–149
  cohort method in, 149
  defined, 147
  in diagnosis, 151–152
  in management of chronic illness, 152–153
  in management of terminal illness, 153
  in treatment, 152
  uses of, 147
Epidermolysis, ocular, 727
Epididymis, examination of, 780
Epididymitis, 782
Epidural cysts, 1061(t), 1064
Epidural hematoma, 1045–1046
Epigastric hernia, in children, 502
Epiglottis, bifid, 671
Epiglottitis, acute, 672
  in children, 841
Epilepsia partialis continua, 1029
Epilepsy, 1025–1030
  alcoholic, 1035
  and oral contraceptives, 459
  and personality disorders, 280
  fever precipitating, 856
  grand mal, 856, 1025–1027, 1028(t)
  in children, drugs for, 857(t)
    management of, 858
    patterns of, 856–857
  jacksonian, 856
  petit mal, 856–857, 1027, 1028(t)
  seizure patterns in, 856–857
  status epilepticus in, 1029
  temporal lobe, 1027–1029, 1028(t)
    anxiety in, 289
Episodic behavior disorders, 280
Episodic dyscontrol syndrome, 280
Epispadias, 774
Epistaxis, 655–656, *655*
  in juvenile angiofibroma, 668
Equifinality, in family system theory, 24
Erb's dystrophy, 878, 1072(t)
Erb's paralysis, 1065
Erection, penile, disorders of, 442–443, 781
Erythema multiforme, *1107*, 1108, *1108*
  ocular manifestations of, 727
Erythroplasia of Queyrat, 781
Esophagitis, peptic, chest pain in, 1003(t), 1004
  reflux, 960–961, 961(t)
Esophagoscopy, 682
Esophagus, anatomy of, 681–682
  carcinoma of, 685, 965–966
    diseases predisposing to, 965(t)
  corrosive burns of, 685
  disorders of, 681–685
    causing dysphagia, 963(t)
    congenital, 683–684
  duplication of, 683
  dysfunction of, 685
  embryology of, 682
  examination of, 682–683
  fistula of, 683
  foreign bodies in, 684–685
  neoplasms of, 685
  perforation of, iatrogenic, 684

Esophagus *(Continued)*
  spasm of, chest pain in, 1003(t), 1004
  stenosis of, congenital, 683
  varices of, bleeding from, diagnosis of, 497–498
      treatment of, 498–499
    in portal hypertension, 974–975
Esophoria, 695–696
Esotropia, 701–702, *703*
Estrogen(s), synthetic, as contraceptives, 453–455,
    453, 454(t), 455(t). See also *Oral contraceptives.*
Estrogen therapy, postmenopausal, and vaginal
    bleeding, 744
Ethacrynic acid, ototoxicity of, 645–646
Ethics, as academic discipline, 244–246
  and patient life-style change, 121
  normative, 244–245
  of consultation and referral, 202–204
Exanthem subitum, 843–844, *844*
Exercise(s). See also *Physical therapy.*
  and asthma, 1144–1145
  for back pain, 216–217, *216, 217, 580, 583, 584*
  for frozen shoulder, *594, 595*
  for knee injuries, 220–221, 557–558
  for rheumatoid arthritis, 215
  for spondylosis, 590, *590*
  in congenital heart disease, 870
  in pregnancy, 758
Exercise pseudonephritis, 778
Exhibitionism, 370(t). See also *Sexual variations
    and deviations.*
Existential psychotherapy, 399–400
Exophoria, 695–696
Exophthalmos, in thyroid disease, 725, *725*
Exotropia, 701–702, *701*
Extended family, 33–34
  and social class, 50
Extramedullary tumors, of spinal cord, 1061(t),
    1064
Extrapyramidal system, disorders of, 1049–1055,
    1051(t)
Eye(s). See also names of specific anatomic parts.
  anatomy of, *698, 699*
  angioid streaks in, 729
  black, 705–706
  contusions of, 709–710, *710*
  crossed, 701–702, *703*
  dermatitis herpetiformis of, 727
  discharge from, 691
  disorders of, floaters in, 691
    light flashes in, 691
    nonvisual signs and symptoms of, 691
    rainbows and halos in, 691
    visual signs and symptoms of, 690–691
  epidermolysis of, 727
  examination of, 691–698
    auscultation in, 697
    cover testing in, 695–696, *695*
    equipment for, *692*
    motility testing in, 695–696, *695*
    observation in, 692–693
    ophthalmodynamometry in, 729
    ophthalmoscopy in, 693–695, *694*
    palpation in, 696
    tonometry in, 696–697, *697*
    visual acuity testing in, 692
    visual field survey in, 697–698
  foreign bodies in, 710
  hemorrhage in, 709–710, *710*
  in systemic disease, 725–730

Eye(s) *(Continued)*
  injuries of, 709–710
  inner, pathology of, 711–715
  masses in, 691
  motility of, examination of, 695–696, *695*
  outer, pathology of, 701–710
  pain in, 691
  paralysis of, 726
  phoria of, 695–696
  pink, 706
  redness of, 691
    differential diagnosis of, 715(t)
  refractive errors of, 699–700
    headache from, 1022(t)
  tumors of, 721
  wall, 701–702, *701*
Eyelid(s), disorders of, 704–706
  ecchymosis of, 705–706
  lacerations of, 709
  retraction of, in thyroid disease, 725–726

Facial bones, injuries of, 679–681, 682(t)
Facial nerve, *644*
  disorders of, 1057(t)
  paralysis of, in Bell's palsy, 643–644, 1059–1060
Facioscapulohumeral dystrophy, 1072(t)
Failure to thrive, 864–865
Fainting, causes of, 1026(t)
Fallopian tubes, ligation of, for sterilization,
    461–462, *461*
  tumors of, 752–753
Familial benign chorea, 1051(t), 1052
Familial polyposis, 968(t)
Family, as cultural transmitter, 47–50
  as system, 21–30
  autonomy in, 421–422
  childbearing practices of, 419–420
  cultural heritage of, 48–49
  definition of, in family practice, 20–21
  economic issues in, 422
  epidemic in, management of, 153–155
  extended, 33–34
    and social class, 50
  homeostasis in, 24
  life cycle of. See *Family life cycle.*
  medical records of. See *Medical records.*
  problem-solving capacity of, 419
  recreational practices of, 420
  religious practices of, 420–421
  roles in, 420
  size of, and social class, 50
  social class of, 48, 49
  structure and function of, 20–32
  subsystems of, 25–26
  transformations in, 26–29
Family counseling, 415–432. See also *Marriage
    and family counseling.*
Family dynamics, 32–46
  and organic medicine, 415–417, *416*
  scope of, 33
Family life cycle, 33–44
  and adolescence, 41–42
  and birth of first child, 37–39
  and child's early and middle school years,
    40–41
  and departure of child, 42
  and divorce, 42–43
  and early marriage, 35–37

Family life cycle *(Continued)*
  and emerging sexuality of first child, 40
  and illness, 43–44
  and individuation of first child, 39–40
  and pregnancy, 37–39
Family pedigree chart, 85, 87, 88
Family physician(s), 3–19. See also *Family practice; Physicians.*
  and dying patient, 249–257
  and medical ethics, 241–248
  as consultant, 53–54
  as health care coordinator, 13–14
  as nursing home medical director, 237–238
  as preceptor for allied health professionals, 194
  as psychotherapist, 391–392. See also *Psychotherapy.*
  attributes of, 6–13
  comprehensive care by, 9–10
  consultation by, vs. referral by, 200–202
  contraceptive counseling by, 450–464
  defined, 5
  diagnostic skills of, 11–13
  effective communication by, 55–57
  evolution of, in United Kingdom, 181–182
    in United States, 176–177
  genetic counseling by, 465–478. See also *Genetic counseling.*
  interpersonal skills of, 10–11
  interviewing techniques of, 258–266
  knowledge of specialties needed by, 9–10, *10*
  legal responsibility of, to use consultants, 202–204
  marriage and family counseling by, 415–418, *418.* See also *Marriage and family counseling.*
  numbers of, in United Kingdom, 180(t)
    in United States, 178(t)
  ongoing care by, 6–8
  outpatient audit programs of, 96–97, *97*
  personalized care by, 5–6
  problem-solving techniques of, 138–140, *139*
  psychologic counseling by, 391–392. See also *Psychotherapy.*
  rate of patient consultations with, 15, *15, 16,* 52
  record-keeping by. See *Medical records.*
  referral to social services by, 186–187
  relation to patient of, 53–58
  role of in patients' behavioral change, 115–120
  sexual counseling by, 433–449. See also *Sexual counseling.*
  sexual education of, 372
  types of problems seen by, 15–18, *16,* 16(t), 17(t)
  use of consultants by, 199–209
  utilization of social and cultural factors by, 60–62, *61*
  use of social services by, 183–187
Family practice. See also *Family physician.*
  as specialty, 3–4
  constituent disciplines of, *10*
  content of, 15–18, *15–17,* 18(t)
  defined, 3, 5
  evolution of, 176–177
  family dynamics in, 21–30
  systems theory in, 21–30
Family systems theory, 21–30
Family therapy, 402. See also *Marriage and family counseling.*
Farsightedness, 699–700, *700*
Fatigue, chronic, and familial stress, 418

Feces, impaction of, 824
  after anorectal surgery, 814
Feedback, in family system theory, 23–24
Female(s), genital herpes in, 741
  infertility in, 755–757
  middle-aged and aging, sexuality of, 439
  reproduction in, physiology of, 450–451
  sexual dysfunction in, 440–442, 445–448
    general, 446–447
    in rape victim, 368
    orgasmic, 447–448
  venereal disease in, 739–741
Femoral epiphysis, necrosis of, 572–573, *572*
  slipped capital, 570–571, *571*
Femoral hernia, 502–503
Fetishism, 370(t). See also *Sexual variations and deviations.*
Fetus, growth retardation in, 831–832
  malformations of, and hydramnios, 764
    and oral contraceptives, 458
  metal fume, 925–926
  Monday morning, 925–926
  postmaturity of, 764–765
  preventive medicine for, 107(t)–108(t)
Fever, and convulsions, in children, 856
  hay. See *Allergic rhinitis.*
  rheumatic, 871–874, 872(t), 873(t)
    and Sydenham's chorea, 1049
  scarlet, 845
Fibroadenoma, of breast, 513
Fibrocystic disease, of breast, 512–513, *513*
Fibroid tumor, uterine, 746–748
Fibroma, nasal, 657
  ovarian, 752
Fibrosing alveolitis, defined, 884
Fibrosis, interstitial, defined, 884
  pulmonary, in pneumoconiosis, 923–926
Finger(s), aspiration of, *625*
  baseball, 617–618, *617, 618*
  crush injuries of, 616–617, *616, 617*
  dislocation of, 611–614, *612, 613*
  disorders of, 607–621
  Dupuytren's contracture of, 608–609, *608*
  examination of, *609*
  extensor tendon injury of, 617–618, *617, 618*
  fixed flexion deformity of, 608–609, *608*
  fractures of, 614–619, *615, 616, 671, 618, 619, 620*
  lacerations of, 609
  mallet, 617–618, *617, 618*
  pain in, nocturnal, 606–607
  puncture wounds of, 609–610
  sprain of, 610–611, *612*
  snapping, 621, *621*
  subluxation of, 610–611
  tingling in, 606–607
  trigger, 621, *621*
Fingernail(s). infection of, 620–621, *621*
  fungal, 1112
  injuries of, 619–621, *620, 621*
First branchial cleft anomalies, 676
Fistula-in-ano, 806–808, *807*
  palatal, 661
  tracheoesophageal, 683
Fixed flexion deformity, of fingers, 608–609, *608*
Flail chest, 528
Flat feet, 545–546, *545*
Flatus, 954–955
Flexion deformity, of fingers, 608–609, *608*

Floaters, vitreous, 691
Fluid retention, and oral contraceptives, 736
  in Laennec's cirrhosis, 976
Fluid therapy, in burn patients, 537, 537(t)
  in children, 858–863, 860(t), 861(t)
Fluphenazine, dose, use, and side effects of,
  385(t)–386(t)
Foam, contraceptive, 737
Focal seizures, 856, 1029
Folic acid supplements, in pregnancy, 1079
Folliculitis, 1122
Food(s). See also *Diet; Nutrition.*
  allergy to, and allergic rhinitis, 1141–1142
  aspiration of, 898
  infant, energy and protein content of, 1082(t)
    iron content of, 1084(t)
    sodium content of, 1097(t)
Food services, for elderly, 236
Foot, broken down, 554, *554*
  disorders of, 544–555
  flat, 545–546, *545*
  fungal infection of, 1111–1112, *1111*
  osteochondritis of, 543, *544*, 548–549, *549*
  pain in, 546–554
    in forefoot, 549–551
    in mid foot, 548–549
    lateral, 551–552
  splayed, *550*
  sprain of, 554–555
  strain of, 545
  tenosynovitis in, 546–547
  weight distribution in, *544*
Forearm, injuries of, 604–605
Foreign body, in airway, management of, 522–
  525, 684–685, 898–899
  in cornea, 709
  in ear, 635, *635*
  in esophagus, 684–685
  in eye, 710
  in nasopharynx, 667–668
  in oropharynx, 664
  in tracheobronchial tree, 684–685
Fracture, blowout, 680, *680*, 682(t), 710
  boxer's, 618–619, *618, 619, 620*
  LeFort, 680, *681*, 682(t)
  of clavicle, 597–598, *597, 598*
  of elbow, 604
  of facial bones, 679–681, 682(t)
  of fingers, 614–619, *615, 616, 617, 618, 619, 620*
  of hand, 614–619, *615, 616, 617, 618, 619, 620*
  of larynx, 672
  of malar complex, 679–680, *679*, 682*(t)*
  of mandible, 680, *681*, 682(t)
  of maxilla, 680–681, *681*, 682(t)
  of metacarpal head, 618–619, *618, 619, 620*
  of nose, 651
    reduction of, 652
  of orbit, 680, *680*, 682(t), 710
  of penis, 780
  of skull, 1044
  of thumb, basilar, 618–619
  of wrist, 606
  of zygomatic arch, 679–680, *679*, 682(t)
  vascular injury in, 504
Frigidity, 445. See also *Sexual dysfunction,
  female.*
Frontal lobe function, examination of, 1015
Frozen shoulder, 591–595, *592, 593, 594*

Fungal infections, dermatologic, deep, 1113–1116
  griseofulvin-sensitive, 1111–1113
  superficial, 1109–1111
  pulmonary, 937–939
Furosemide, ototoxicity of, 645–646
Furuncles, nasal, 652

Gait, abnormalities of, 1016, 1017(t)
Gait patterns, for walking aids, 218–220, *218, 219,
  220*
Galactorrhea, and oral contraceptives, 459
Gallbladder, disease of, 981–983
Gallstones, 499–501, *499, 500*, 981–982
Game analysis, 397
Ganglion, of wrist, 607, *607*
Gartner's duct, cysts of, 753
Gastric acid secretion, in duodenal ulcer disease,
  956(t)
  in gastric ulcer disease, 958–959
Gastric ulcer. See *Peptic ulcer.*
Gastrin release, in duodenal ulcer disease, 956(t)
  in Zollinger-Ellison syndrome, 957–958
Gastritis, 959, 959(t)
Gastroenteritis, in children, 848
Gastroenterology, 941–985
Gastroesophageal reflux, 683
Gastrointestinal bleeding, 497–499
  acute, 963–965, 964(t)
  in alcoholism, 332(t)
Gastrointestinal carcinoma, diseases predisposing
  to, 965(t), 967–970, 968(t)–969(t)
  management of, 965–970
Gastrointestinal disease, abdominal examination
  in, 941–942, 942(t)
  diagnosis in, 941–942, 942(t)
  history-taking in, 941
  predisposing to cancer, 965(t), 967–970,
  968(t)–969(t)
Gastrointestinal system, in alcoholism, 331–332,
  332(t)
Geller-Gesner Tables, 163, 164(t)–166(t), 171(t)
Gene(s), mutant, diseases caused by. See *Genetic
  diseases.*
  normal, 467–468
General practitioner. See *Family physician.*
Genetic counseling, 465–478
  diagnosis in, 470
  establishing probability in, 470, *471*
  family physician's role in, 470
  follow-up in, 462
  history-taking in, *471*
  illustrative cases of, 473–478
  indications for cytogenetic counseling in, 467
  informative, 472
  supportive, 472
Genetic diseases, 467–469
  autosomal dominant, 468
  autosomal recessive, 468–469
  case histories of, 473–478
  multifactorial, 469
  x-linked, 469
    with negative family history, 475
Geniculate neuralgia, 1060
Genitalia, anomalies of, 774
  female, herpetic infection in, 741
  male, disorders of, 780–783
    injuries of, 779–780

Genitourinary tract, anomalies of, 772–774
Geographic tongue, 660
Geriatric patients. See *Elderly.*
German measles. See *Rubella.*
Gestalt psychotherapy, 398–399
Gilbert's syndrome, 970–971, 970(t)
Gingiva, carcinoma of, 664–665
Gingivitis, 661
Glabellar reflex, 1018
Gland. See *Parotid gland; salivary glands.*
Glaucoma, 710–712, *711*
  congenital, 710
  differential diagnosis of, 715(t)
  narrow angle, 712
  open angle, 710–712
  testing for, 696–697, *697*
Glomerulonephritis, acute, in children, 874–875
Glomus jugulare tumors, 1060
Glossitis, median rhomboid, 660
Glossopharyngeal nerve, disorders of, 1057(t),
  1060
Glucose, effect of alcohol on, 332–333
Glucose tolerance, by age, *224*
Gold salts, for rheumatoid arthritis, 626
Goldblatt kidney, 786
Gonorrhea, anorectal, 827–828
  in female, 739–740
    complications of, 740
Gout, synovianalysis in, 622(t)
Gower dystrophy, 1072(t)
Grand mal epilepsy, 856, 1025–1027, 1028(t)
Granuloma, lethal midline, 657
Granuloma annulare, *1115,* 1127, *1127*
Granulomatosis, Wegener's, 656–657
Granulomatous ileitis, 807
Granulomatous ileocolitis, 807
Graphism, 1018
Grat's tumor, 784
Great vessels, transposition of, 869
Groin, fungal infection of, 1112, *1112*
Group therapy, 402, 404–412
  curative factors in, 406–408
  indications for, 405–406
  leader's role in, 408–411
  members of, rights of, 405(t)
    role of, 405
    selection of, 405–406
  objectives of, 404
  patient preparation for, 411
  referral to, 405–406
  vs. assertiveness training, 404
  vs. consciousness-raising groups, 404
  vs. human potential movement, 404
  vs. self-help groups, 404
Growing pains, 541–544
Growth, retarded, in children, 864–865
Guillain-Barré syndrome, 1066–1067
Gynecologic examination, 731–733
  cervical biopsy in, 734, 749–750
  colposcopy in, 734, 797
  endometrial biopsy in, 734–735
  for infertility, 755
  in adolescents, 733
  in children, 733
  in obese patient, 732–733
  Pap test in, 733–734
  Schiller test in, 734
  screening tests in, 733–735

Gynecology, 731–765
Gynecomastia, 514

Hair loss. See *Alopecia.*
Hallucinations, alcoholic, 1035
  in schizophrenia, 319
  neurologic evaluation of, 1014
Hallucinogens, intoxication with, 347
Hallux valgus, 553, *553*
Halo, visual, 691
Haloperidol, dose, use, and side effects of, 386(t)
Halothane hepatitis, 980–981, 980(t)
Hamartomas, colonic, and colonic carcinoma,
  968(t)
  renal, 783
Hand, abrasions of, 610
  contusions of, 610
  disorders of, 605–621
  examination of, *609*
  fractures of, 614–619, *615, 616, 617, 618, 619,*
    620
  fungal infections of, 1113
  lacerations of, 609
  pain in, nocturnal, 606–607
  puncture wounds of, 609–610
  tingling in, 606–607
Hay fever. See *Allergic rhinitis.*
Head injuries, 1044–1047
  with cerebral hematoma, 1047
  with damage to intracranial contents, 1045
  with epidural hematoma, 1045–1046
  with intracerebellar hematoma, 1047
  with subdural hematoma, 1046–1047
Headache, 1020–1025
  classification of, 1022(t)–1023(t)
  cluster, 1022(t), 1024
  from hydrocephalus, 1023(t)
  from intracranial tumor, 1023(t)
  from meningitis, 1023(t)
  from ocular refractive errors, 691, 1022(t)
  from subarachnoid hemorrhage, 1023(t)
  from temporal arteritis, 1023(t)
  histamine, 1022(t), 1024
  hypertensive, 1022(t), 1024
  migraine. See *Migraine headache.*
  ocular, 691
  recurrent, in children, 863
  sinus, 1023(t)
  tension, 1022(t)
  treatment of, 1022(t)–1023(t)
Health care delivery, 175–182
  in United Kingdom, 179–182
    and evolution of general practice, 181–182
    future trends in, 182
    National Health Service for, 179–180
    referral system for, 180–181
  in United States, 175–178
    and evolution of family practice, 176–177
    changes in, 177–178
    future trends in, 178
    national programs for, 175
    referral system for, 175–176
    utilization of community resources for, 183–
      187
    use of consultants for, 199–209
Health hazard appraisal, 163–168, *163, 164–166,*
  169(t)

Hearing, mechanics of, 630–632
  tests of, 633–634, *634*, 635–637, *636*
    audiometric, 635, *636*
    electronystagmographic, 635–636
    tuning fork, 633–634, *634*
Hearing loss. See *Deafness.*
Heart, arrhythmias, of, 1007–1110
Heart disease, anxiety in, 288
  as surgical risk factor, 485–486
  congenital, 865–871
    bacterial endocarditis in, 870
    chest pain in, 870
    diagnosis of, 865–866, 866(t)
    heart failure in, 871
    in elderly, 231–232
    lesions in, 866–870
    myocarditis in, 871
    physical activity in, 870
    radiographic findings in, 866(t)
    referral in, 870
  coronary, and oral contraceptives, 456
    early, genetic counseling for, 476
  dizziness in, 1031(t)
  effect of, on family, 43–44
  in elderly, 231–232
  in pregnancy, 761
  rheumatic, in elderly, 231
Heart failure, congestive, 994–1000
    aggravating factors in, 995
    as surgical risk factor, 485
    causes of, 995
    diagnosis of, 994
    differential diagnosis of, 994–995
    drug therapy for, 997–998, 998(t)
    family counseling in, 1000
    in children, 871
    in elderly, 231–232, 998–1000
    management of, 997–998
    pathophysiology of, 996–997, *996*
    precipitating factors in, 995
  in children, 852–853, 871
  in congenital heart disease, 871
  resuscitation in, 525–526
Heart murmurs, 1000–1003
  diastolic vs. systolic, 1001
  family counseling in, 1002–1003
  in children, 865–866
  innocent, 1001–1002, 1002(t)
  systolic vs. diastolic, 1001
Heart sounds, in children, 865–866
Heartburn, 960–961, 961(t)
Heat treatments, for back pain, 216
  for rheumatoid arthritis, 214–215, *214*
Heavy metal poisoning, neurologic complications
  of, 1036(t), 1037, 1068
Heel, pain in, 547–548
  Thomas, for flat feet, 546
Heimlich maneuver, 523–524, 898
Hemangioma, congenital laryngeal, 671
  congenital salivary, 676
Hemangiopericytoma, renal, 783
Hematoma, cerebral, 1047
  epidural, 1045–1046
  intercerebellar, 1047
  perianal, 798
  subdural, acute, 1046
    chronic, 1046–1047
Hematomyelia, 1061(t), 1063–1064
Hematopoietic system, in alcoholism, 331

Hemifacial spasm, 1060
Hemoglobinuria, vs. myoglobinuria, 1070(t)
Hemolysis, and unconjugated hyperbilirubinemia, 970, 970(t)
Hemolytic anemia, in children, 880–882
Hemophilia, genetic counseling for, 475
Hemophilus vaginalis vaginitis, 738
Hemorrhage. See also *Bleeding.*
  cerebellar, 1043
  cerebral, 1042–1043
  control of, in trauma patients, 526
  ocular, 709–710, *710*
  pontine, 1043
  postoperative, in anorectal surgery, 812, 813
  subarachnoid, 1043–1044
    headache from, 1023(t)
  subconjunctival, 707
    in systemic disease, 727–728
  transplacental, Rh immune prophylaxis for, 760
Hemorrhoid(s), 797–803
  combined internal and external, 799
  etiology of, 798
  excision of, 799–802, *801*
  freezing of, 803
  nonoperative management of, 802–803
  rubber band ligation of, 803
  sclerotic injection of, 802
  thrombosed external, 798
    vs. anal abscess, 804
Hemorrhoidectomy, 799–802, *801*
Hemothorax, 528
Heparin, for arterial embolism, 505
  for deep venous thrombosis, 510
  for postphlebotic syndrome, 511
  for pulmonary thromboembolism, 902–903
Hepatic encephalopathy, 1040
  clinical features of, 976(t)
  in Laennec's cirrhosis, 975–976
  stages of, 975(t)
Hepatitis, alcoholic, 332, 973–974
  chronic, 978–979
  drug-induced, 980–981, 981(t)
  halothane, 980–981, 980(t)
  jaundice in, 970(t), 971
  viral, 977–979, 977(t)
    carriers of, 979
    diagnosis of, 976–978
    immune serum globulin for, 978
    in children, 849, 850(t)
    management of, 978
Hepatocellular enzymes, tests of, 972
Hepatocellular failure, clinical manifestations of,
  975(t)
  in Laennec's cirrhosis, 974, 974(t)
Hepatocellular jaundice, 970(t), 971
Hernia, 501–504, *501, 502, 503*
  in adults, 502–504
    femoral, 502–503
    hiatal, chest pain in, 1003(t), 1004
    incisional, 503, *503*
    inguinal, 502
    umbilical, 503
  in children, 501–502, *501*
    epigastric, 502
    inguinal, 501, *501*, 502
    umbilical, 501
  recurrence of, 504
  repair of, 503–504
Herniated intervertebral disc, 1065

Heroin detoxification, 348
Herpangina, 885(t), 887
Herpes genitalis, 741
Herpes simplex, 1122
  neonatal infection with, 835
Herpes zoster, 1122–1123, *1123*
Herpes zoster oticus, 641
Hiatal hernia, chest pain in, 1003(t), 1004
Hidradenitis suppurativa, 827, 1121
Hip, arthritis of, 567–570, *570*
  aspiration of, *623*
  congenital dislocation of, 573, *573*
  disorders of, 567–574
  examination of, 568–569, *568–569*
  osteochondrosis of, 572–573, *572*
  pain and limp in, in children, 567–573
    with knee pain, in children, 543, 570–571, *571*
    in elderly, 567–570
    in infants, 573
  pain in, in adults, 574
  transient synovitis of, 571–572
Hirschsprung's disease, 829
Hirsutism, facial, and oral contraceptives, 459
Histamine headache, 1022(t), 1024
Histoplasmosis, 937
  laryngeal, 673
Home care, for elderly, 235
Homemaking services, for elderly, 236
Homeostasis, family, 24
Homeostatic impasse, in family system theory, 25
Homosexuality, 370(t). See also *Sexual variations and deviations.*
  sexual counseling for, 438
Honeycomb lung, 884
Hookworm, 852, 852(t)
Hordeolum, 704, *704*
Horseshoe kidney, 773
Housedust, allergy to, 1141
Housing, for elderly, 236
Human potential movement, 404
Huntington's chorea, 1053
Hydramnios, 764
Hydrocele, 774, 782
Hydrocephalus, headache from, 1023(t)
  in elderly, 229
  normal pressure, 1048(t)
Hydroxyzine hydrochloride, dose, use, and side effects of, 382(t)
Hydroxyzine pamoate, dose, use, and side effects of, 382(t)
Hygroma, cystic, 678
Hyperactivity, in children, 269
Hyperbilirubinemia, unconjugated, 970–971, 970(t)
Hypercalciuria, urinary calculi in, 770
Hypercapnia, defined, 883
  in respiratory failure, 931
  treatment of, 934
Hypercholesterolemia, 1010–1012, 1011(t)
Hyperlipidemia, 1010–1012, 1011(t)
  in alcoholism, 321
  ocular manifestations of, 729
Hyperlipoproteinemias, classification of, 1093–1094
  diet in, 1093–1094
Hypernephroma, 784
Hyperopia, 699–700, *700*
  headache from, 1022(t)
Hyperoxaluria, urinary calculi in, 770

Hyperparathyroidism, neurologic complications of, 1036
Hyperpnea, defined, 883
Hypertension, 987–994
  and infant nutrition, 1085
  and oral contraceptives, 456
  and pheochromocytoma, 987
  and sodium intake, 1093–1094
  anxiety in, 290
  benign intracranial, 1022(t), 1039, 1040
    causes of, 1040(t)
  defined, 986
  diagnostic work-up for, 987–988, 988(t)
  diseases associated with, 986–987
  drugs for, 988–994, 991(t)–992(t)
    selection of, 993–994
  encephalopathy in, 1024
  etiology of, 986–987
  family counseling in, 994
  headache in, 1022(t), 1024
  high renin, drugs for, 992
  in elderly, 232
  incidence of, 986
  low renin, drugs for, 991–992
  low-salt diet for, 994
  management of, 988–994
  ocular manifestations of, 715–718, *717*, 728
  ophthalmologic grading of, 716–718, *717*
  pathophysiology of, 987, *989*
  periodic screening for, 126(t), 127–128, 127(t), 129(t)
  portal, 974–975, 974(t)
  renovascular, 786, 986
  retinal degeneration in, 715–718, *717*
  signs and symptoms of, 987
  with renal insufficiency, drugs for, 993
Hyperthyroidism, drug-induced, 675
  neurologic complications of, 1036
  ocular manifestations of, 725–726, *726*
Hyperuricemia, 1068
Hyperventilation, defined, 883
  dizziness from, 1031(t)
Hyperventilation syndrome, 896–898
Hypnotic drugs, for depression, 312
Hypocapnia, defined, 883
Hypoglossal nerve, disorders of, 1057(t)
Hypoglycemia, and anxiety, 288–289
  in newborns of diabetics, 836
  neurologic complications of, 1035
Hypokalemic periodic paralysis, 1074
Hypoparathyroidism, neurologic complications of, 1036
Hypopharynx, anatomy of, 668–669, *669*
  congenital disorders of, 670–671
  embryology of, 668–669
  examination of, 670, *670*
  infectious disorders of, 672–673
  injuries of, 672
  neoplasms of, 674–675
Hypospadias, 774
Hypotension, orthostatic, 1026(t)
  transient, dizziness in, 1031(t)
Hypotheses, in problem-solving, 141
Hypothyroidism, drug-induced, 675
  neurologic complications of, 1036
  ocular manifestations of, 726
Hypotonia, congenital, 878
Hypoventilation. See *Respiratory insufficiency.*
Hypovolemia. See *Shock.*

Hypoxemia, arterial, 930–931, *930*
  defined, 883
Hypoxia, dizziness from, 1031(t)
  effects of, 931
  in respiratory failure, 930–931
Hysteria, 277–278, 297–299
  conversion, 297–298
    vs. grand mal epilepsy, 1025
  dissociative, 298–299
  drugs for, 382(t)–383(t)
  syncope in, 1026(t)

ICD. See *International Classification of Disease*.
ICHPPC. See *International Classification of Health Problems in Primary Care*.
Ileitis, 816–817
  backwash, 948(t)
  granulomatous, 807
Ileocolitis, granulomatous, 807
Ileostomy, care of, 821
Illness. See also *Disease*.
  chronic, management of, epidemiology and, 152–153
  effect of on family, 43–44
  perceptions of, and social class, 50–52
  self-care in, 52–53
  sexual intercourse in, 440
  terminal, appropriate death in, 256–257
    diagnosis in, 249–250
    helping patient cope with, 254–256
    informing patient of, 250–252
    management of, 249–257
      epidemiology and, 153
    palliation in, 256
    patient vulnerability in, 252–253
      varieties of, 253–254
    preterminal stage of, 256
    safe conduct in, 250
    treatment in, 250
Imipramine, dose, use, and side effects of, 382(t)–383(t)
Immune responses, categories of, 1136
  for depression, 309(t)
Immune serum globulin, for viral hepatitis, 978
Immunity, cell-mediated, 1137–1138
    evaluation of, 1137(t), 1138
Immunization, for infants and children, 838–839, 839(t)
  in pregnancy, 757
Immunodeficiency disorders, classification of, 1137(t)
  clinical features of, 1137
  diagnosis of, 1137–1138, 1137(t)
  evaluation of, 1136–1139
  treatment of, 1138
Immunology, 1137–1145
Impetigo, 1121–1122, *1122*
Impotence, 442–443
  defined, 781
Incision, herniation through, 503, *503*
Indomethacin, for rheumatoid arthritis, 626
Infant(s), breast feeding of. See *Breast feeding*.
  diet for, 837–838, 838(t)
  energy intake of, 1082(t)
  failure to thrive in, 864–865
  feeding of, 837–838, 838(t). See also *Breast feeding*.
    solid foods, 1082–1083
  formula for, vs. breast milk, 1081–1082

Infant(s) *(Continued)*
  formula for, nutritional content of, 1082(t), 1083(t), 1084(t)
  growth and development of, 1081–1085
  immunization for, 838–839, 839(t)
  iron supplements for, 837, 1082–1083
  newborn. See *Newborns*.
  nutrition in, 837–838, 838(t), 1081–1085
    long-term effects of, 1085
  nutritional requirements of, 1085(t)
  nutritional supplements for, 837, 1083, 1084(t)
  preventive medicine for, 108(t)
  sexuality of, 40, 436–437
Infantile autism, 320–321
Infantile lobar emphysema, 684
Infantile paralysis, immunization for, 839(t)
Infantile polycystic disease of kidney, 773
Infantile spasm, 857
Infantile spinal muscular atrophy, 878
Infarction, brain stem, 1042
  cerebellar, 1050(t)
  cerebral, 1042, 1048(t)
  of spinal cord, 1061(t), 1063
Infection(s). See also under body parts affected.
  anxiety following, 290
  fungal, dermatologic, 1109–1116
    pulmonary, 937–939
  in children, 839–852
  neonatal, 834–836
  parasitic, in children, 852, 852(t)
  protozoal, neurologic complications of, 1034
  surgical, 534–536
  susceptibility to, in immunodeficiency disorders, 1137
  wound, prevention and treatment of, 534–536
Infertility, 755–757
  and leiomyoma, 747–748
  female, evaluation of, 755–757
  in alcoholism, 333
  male, evaluation of, 783
Inflammatory bowel disease, 947–949
  classification of, 948(t)
Influenza, 885(t), 886–887
Ingrown toenail, 553–554
Inguinal hernia, in adults, 502
  in children, 501, *501*, 502
Insulin, dosage of, for surgical patient, 484
Insulin therapy, for children, 877
Intercourse, sexual. See *Sexual intercourse*.
Intermittent claudication, 506
International Classification of Disease, 15–16
International Classification of Health Problems in Primary Care, 16
Interphalangeal joint, dislocation of, 613, *613*
  sprain of, 612
Interstitial fibrosis, defined, 884
Intervertebral disc, cervical, rupture of, 590, 590(t)
  degeneration of, 587–590, *588*, 588(t), *590*
  herniated, 1065
  ruptured, 578–579, 578(t)
Interviewing, patient, in psychotherapeutic counseling, 390–391, 392–394. See also *Psychotherapy*.
  techniques of, 258–266
Intestinal gas, causes of, 954
Intestinal obstruction, 491–494, 491(t), *493*
  diagnosis of, 486(t), 492
  treatment of, 494
Intestine, large. See *Colon*.
  small. See *Small intestine*.

Intoxication. See also *Poisoning.*
    alcohol, 1035
    drug. See *Drug intoxication.*
Intracerebellar hematoma, 1047
Intracranial hypertension, benign, 1022(t), 1039–
    1040
    causes of, 1040(t)
Intracranial tumor, headache from, 1023(t)
Intracranial vascular disease, ophthalmologic man-
    ifestations of, 726
Intramedullary tumors, of spinal cord, 1061(t),
    1064
Intrauterine device, 736
    and endometritis, 739
    effectiveness of, 451(t)
    intact, in pregnancy, 460
Intrauterine growth retardation, 831–832
Intubation, endotracheal, 522–524
        and subglottic stenosis, 673
    thoracic, 527, 528
Iritis, 714–715, *714*
    differential diagnosis of, 715(t)
Iron, in infant food, 1084(t)
Iron deficiency anemia, in children, 879–880
Iron supplements, for infants, 837, 1083–1084
    in pregnancy, 1078
Irritable bowel syndrome, 952–953
    chronic abdominal pain in, 944
    constipation in, 951
    flatus in, 954
Ischemia, cerebellar, 1050(t)
    in extremities, diagnosis of, 504
    transient, 1041–1042, 1041(t)
Ischemic rest pain, 506
Isocarboxazid, dose, use, and side effects of,
    386(t)–387(t)
Isoproterenol, for asthma, 895
IUD. See *Intrauterine device.*

Jackknife seizure, 857
Jacksonian epilepsy, 856, 1029
Jaundice, causes of, 970–973, 970(t)
    cholestatic vs. obstructive, 971–972, 971(t)
    drug-induced, 979–981
    hepatocellular, 970(t), 971
    in unconjugated hyperbilirubinemia, 970, 970(t)
    liver function tests for, 972–973
    neonatal, 832–834, 833(t)
    obstructive, 970(t), 971–972, 971(t)
Jaw, congenital disorders of, 661
    fractures of, 680–681, *681*, 682(t)
Joint(s), arthritis of. See *Arthritis.*
    aspiration of, 621–622, *622*, 622(t), *623, 624, 625*
Jones criteria, for rheumatic fever, 872(t)
Jugular vein, cannulation of, *522*
Juvenile angiofibroma, 668
Juvenile diabetes, 876–877
Juvenile papillomas, 673
Juxtaglomerular cell adenoma, renal, 783

Karyotyping, 465–466, *466*
    indications for, 467
Keloid, 1133, *1133*
Keratitis, 708, *708*
Keratoacanthoma, 1132, *1132*

Keratosis, actinic, 1129–1130, *1130*
    seborrheic, *1128*, 1129
        excision of, 520
    senile, 1129–1130, *1130*
Kidney(s). See also *Renal.*
    abnormal location of, 772–773
    adenocarcinoma of, 784
    agenesis of, 772
    angiomyolipoma of, 783
    anomalies of, 772–773
        and ear anomalies, 987
    cake, 773
    cancer of, 783–784
    cystic disease of, 773
    disc, 773
    doughnut, 773
    ectopic, 773
    fusion anomalies of, 773
    Goldblatt, 786
    horseshoe, 773
    hypoplastic, 772
    injuries of, 778
    medullary cystic disease of, 773
    multicystic, 773
    polycystic, 773
    ptosis of, 772–773
    sponge, 773
    supernumerary, 772
    tumors of, benign, 783
        malignant, 794
    vascular anomalies of, 773
Kidney disease, and hypertension, 987
    in children, 874–876
Klumpke's paralysis, 1065
Knee, anatomy of, *542*
    aspiration of, *623*
    cartilage of, discoid, and locked knee, 562–563
        tears in, 559–562
            and locked knee, 555–557, *556*
    Charcot, *565*
    disorders of, 555–566
    injuries of, 559–566
        in children, 563–566
    instability of, 558–559, *558, 559*
    ligaments of, injuries of, 559–562
        laxity of, 558–559, *559*
    locked, 555–557, *556*
        in children, 562–563
    osteochondritis dissecans of, 542, *543*
    pain in, in children, 564–566
        with hip limp, in children, 570–571
    rehabilitative exercises for, 220–221, 557–558
    rheumatoid arthritis, of, *565*
    swelling of, in children, 565–566, *565*
    trick, 557–558
        in children, 563
    villous synovitis of, *565*
Kneecap. See *Patella.*
KOH slide technique, for scabies, 1134

Labile personality, 277
Laboratory tests, effects of oral contraceptives on,
    457, 457(t)
Labyrinthine disease, vertigo in, 1031(t)
Labyrinthitis, purulent, 640

Lacerations, of cornea, 709
  of eyelid, 709
  of finger, 609
  of hand, 609
  of lip, 661
  of palate, 661
  of tongue, 661
  of tonsil, 661
  treatment of, 532, 533
Lacrimal glands, stenosis of, 706
Lacrimal tract, disorders of, 706
Lactase deficiency, osmotic diarrhea in, 950
Lactation. See also Breast feeding.
  nutrition in, 1080–1081
Lactic dehydrogenase, test of, 972
Laennec's cirrhosis, complications of, 974–976,
    974(t)
  development of, 973–976
Lambert-Eaton syndrome, 1074
Landouzy-Déjerine dystrophy, 878, 1072
Landry-Guillain-Barré syndrome, 1066–1067
Large intestine. See Colon.
Laryngeal diphtheria, 673
Laryngeal nerve, superior, neuralgia of, 1060
Laryngocele, 671
Laryngomalacia, 671
Laryngoscopy, 670
Laryngotracheobronchitis, 672–673
  in children, 840–841
Larynx, anatomy of, 668–669, 669
  carcinoma of, 674–675
  congenital atresia of, 670
  congenital hemangioma of, 671
  congenital webs of, 671
  cysts of, 670–671
  disorders of, congenital, 670–671
    drug-induced, 675
    hereditary, 672
    idiopathic, 673–674
    infectious, 672–673
  embryology of, 668–669
  examination of, 670, 670
  fracture of, 672
  histoplasmosis of, 673
  injuries of, 672
  juvenile papillomas of, 673
  neoplasms of, 674–675
  physiology of, 669–670
  syphilis of, 673
  tuberculosis of, 673
Laxative abuse, and constipation, 951
Lead poisoning, 1036(t)
Learning disabilities, 267–275
  and personality disorders, 282
  and visual exercises, 696
  attention span and activity level in, 269
  diagnosis of, 268–273
  emotional and social development in, 271–272
  family counseling in, 275–276
  history-taking in, 272
  language and thought development in, 270–271
  movement and perceptual development in,
    269–270
  physical examination in, 272–273
  types of, 267–268
LeFort fractures, 680, 681, 682(t)
Leg, dermatomes of, 578
  obliterative arterial disease of, 506
Leiomyoma, 746–748

Leiomyosarcoma, uterine, 749
Lens, contact, 700–701
    for cataract, 713
  crystalline, of eye, opacities of. See Cataract.
Lesbianism, 370(t). See also Sexual variations and
    deviations.
Leukodystrophies, 1030
Leukoplakia, 664
Leukorrhea, 737
Leyden-Moebius dystrophy, 878
Lichen planus, 1104–1105, 1104, 1115
Ligament(s), injuries of. See Sprain.
  of knee, injuries of, 559–562
    laxity of, 558–559, 559
Light flashes, in ophthalmologic disorders, 691
Lightning seizures, 857
Limb-girdle dystrophy, 1072(t)
Limp, hip, in children, 570–573
  in elderly, 567–570
Lip, carcinoma of, 664
  cleft, 649–650, 660
  double, 660
  lacerations of, 661
Lipid metabolism, and oral contraceptives, 456
Lithium carbonate, dose, use, and side effects of,
    387(t)
  for behavior disorders, 284
  for depression, 311–312
Liver. See also Hepatic.
  alcoholic, cirrhosis of, 332, 973–976, 974(t),
    975(t)
  Laennec's cirrhosis of, 973–976, 974(t), 975(t)
  percutaneous biopsy of, 973
  tumors of, and oral contraceptives, 980(t), 981
Liver disease, and alcohol, 332, 973–976
  drug-induced, 979–981, 980(t)
  encephalopathy in. See Hepatic encepha-
    lopathy.
  occupational, 981
Liver failure, clinical manifestations of, 975(t)
  in Laennec's cirrhosis, 974, 974(t)
Liver function, and oral contraceptives, 457
  tests of, 972–973
Lobule, pulmonary, defined, 883
Locked knee, 555–557, 556
  in children, 562–563
Lop ear, 637
Low-back syndrome, 579–584
Loxapine, dose, use, and side effects of, 388(t)
LSD. See Lysergic acid diethylamide.
Ludwig's angina, 662
Lumbar osteoarthritis, 1064–1065
Lumbosacral degeneration, 582–584, 582(t), 583,
    584
Lumbosacral instability, 580–581, 581(t)
Lumbosacral plexus, disorders of, 1066
Lumbosacral sprain, 579–580, 579(t), 580
Lung(s). See also Pulmonary.
  abscess of, 905–908, 907
    defined, 884
  agenesis of, 684
  carcinoma of, 685, 914–917, 915(t), 916
  fibrosis of, in pneumoconiosis, 923–926
  fungal infections of, 937–939
  honeycomb, 884
  miners', 925
  tuberculosis of. See Pulmonary tuberculosis.
Lung disease, as surgical risk factor, 485

Lupus erythematosus, *1115*, 1124–1125, *1124*, *1125*
  vs. rheumatic fever, 873(t)
Lysergic acid diethylamide, intoxication with, 347

McArdle's disease, 1071
Macroglossia, 660
Macula, senile degeneration of, 720, *720*
Magnesium, effect of alcohol on, 333
Malabsorption, diagnosis of, 946, 947(t)
Malar complex, fractures of, 679–680, *679*, 682(t)
Male(s), breast enlargement in, 514
  genital disorders in, 780–783
  genital injuries in, 779–780
  infertility in, 783
  middle-aged and aging, sexuality of, 439–440
  sexual dysfunction in, 440–445
Malignant melanoma, 519–520, 520(t)
  choroidal, 721
Malingering, defined, 298
Mallet finger, 617–618, *617*, *618*
Mallory-Weiss syndrome, in alcoholism, 332(t)
Malnutrition, as surgical risk factor, 483–484. See also *Nutrition*.
Mammography, 514–515
  indications for, 512
  value of, 134
Mandible, congenital disorders of, 661
  fractures of, 680, *681*, 682(t)
  prognathism of, 661
Manganese poisoning, 1036(t)
Manic-depressive states, 381, 389
  diagnostic signs of, 381(t)
  drugs for, 382(t)–388(t)
Marriage, early, and formation of family, 35–37
  sexual adjustment in, 439
Marriage and family counseling, 415–432
  appointment scheduling in, 431
  as profession, 423–424
  consultation in, 431
  defined, 415
  diagnostic considerations in, 419–423
  effective communication pattern in, 424–426, 425(t), *426–427*
  fees in, 431
  methods of, 424–430
  patient expectations in, 417–418
  positive stroking in, 425–429, 428(t)
  presenting complaints in, 418–419
  referral in, 422–423
  structuring in, 429–431, 430(t), 431(t)
Massage, for back pain, 216, *216*
Mastectomy, 515–516
Mastoiditis, acute, 639–640
Masturbation, therapeutic, for female orgasmic dysfunction, 447
Maxilla, congenital disorders of, 661
  fractures of, 680–681, *681*, 682(t)
Measles, 842, *842*
  German. See *Rubella*.
  immunization for, 839(t)
Medicaid, 175
Medical ethics, 241–248
Medical identification card, 69, *70*
Medical records, consultation information and, 208–209
  of elderly, 227–228

Medical records (*Continued*)
  problem indexing of, 97–100, *99*
  problem-oriented, 67–100
    advantages of, 68, 73–75, 76(t)–77(t)
    and assessment of care, 96–97, *97*
    and improved communication, 68–69
    and information retrieval, 69
    chart organization of, 77
    data base of, 84–88, *86*, *87*, *88*, *90*, *91*
    filing of, 73
    flow sheets of, 93–96, *94*, *95*
    legibility of, 70–71
    minimum information for, 71–73, *71*, 72(t), 73(t)
    problem list of, 77–84, *78*, *79*, *80*, *81*, *82*, *83*
    progress notes on, 89–93, *91*, *92*, *93*
    transfer of information to, 69–70
    transfer to, 69–73
    types of, *71*, *74*, *75*
    use of, 75–96
    vs. source-oriented records, 67–68, 73–75, 76(t)–77(t), *93*
  source-oriented, 67–68
    vs. problem-oriented, records, 67–68, 73–75, 76(t)–77(t), *93*
Medicare, 175
Medicine, preventive. See *Preventive medicine*.
  prospective. See *Prospective medicine*.
Medullary cystic disease, renal, 773
Megacolon, Hirschsprung's, 829
  toxic, 816
    in ulcerative colitis, 948
Megalocornea, 708
Megaureter, 769
Megavitamin therapy, 388(t)
Meigs' syndrome, 752
Melanoma, malignant, 519–520, 520(t)
  choroidal, 721
Melasma, and oral contraceptives, 459
Meniere's disease, 642
  vertigo in, 1031(t)
Meningitis, acute bacterial, 1032–1033, 1033(t)
  headache in, 1023(t)
  in infants and children, 1032
  chronic, headache in, 1023(t)
  in children, 848–850, 1032
  tuberculous, 1034
    in children, 850
Menometrorrhagia, 743
Menopause, bleeding after, 744
  vertigo in, 1031(t)
Menorrhagia, 743
Menses, absence of, 753–754
  excessive, 743
    and leiomyomas, 747
  normal, 742
  pain during, 745–746
  "silent," and oral contraceptives, 736
Mental illness. See also *Emotional problems; Personality disorders;* and names of specific disorders.
  drugs for. See *Drugs, psychopharmacologic*.
  in elderly, differential diagnosis of, 230–231
  therapy for. See *Psychotherapy*.
Mental retardation, drugs used in, 382(t)–388(t)
  genetic counseling for, 473, 477–478
Meprobamate, dose, use, and side effects of, 384(t)
Mercury poisoning, 1036(t)

Mesoridazine, dose, use, and side effects of, 385(t)–386(t)
Metabolic-toxic neuropathy, 1067–1068
Metacarpal head, fractures of, 618–619, *618, 619, 620*
Metaethics, 245
Metal(s), poisoning from, 1036(t), 1037, 1068
  pulmonary fibrosis from, 925
Metal fume fever, 925–926
Metaphysics of morals, 245–246
Metatarsal bar, 550, *550*
Metatarsalgia, 549–551
Methadone, for heroin withdrawal, 348
Methylprednisolone, for rheumatoid arthritis, 627
Metrorrhagia, 742–743
Microatelectasis, 905
Microcornea, 708
Micrognathia, 661
Micropenis, 774
Microtia, 637
Micturition syncope, 1026(t)
Migraine headache, 1020–1024, 1022(t)–1023(t)
  and oral contraceptives, 458–459
  in children, 863–864
  vertigo in, 1031(t)
Mikulicz's disease, 677
Miliary tuberculosis, 918
Miners' pneumoconiosis, 925
Minimal brain dysfunction, and personality disorders, 282
  defined, 267
Mini-pill, contraceptive, 453–455, *453*, 454(t), 455(t). See also *Oral contraceptives.*
Mitral stenosis, chest pain in, 1003(t), 1004
Mittelschmerz, 742
Mold spores, allergy to, 1141
Moles. See *Pigmented nevus.*
Molindone, dose, use, and side effects of, 387(t)–388(t)
  and oral contraceptives, 459
Molluscum contagiosum, 1124, *1124*
Monday morning fever, 925–926
Mongolism. See *Down syndrome.*
Monilial vaginitis, 737–738
Moniliasis, 1110–1111, *1110*
  oral, 665
  vaginal, 737–738
    and oral contraceptives, 459
Monoamine oxidase inhibitors, dietary restrictions for, 310(t), 311, 311(t)
  dose, use, and side effects of, 386(t)–387(t)
  for depression, 309(t), 311–312
Mononucleosis, infectious, 662
Morning sickness, 1079
Morphogenesis, defined, 23
Morphostasis, defined, 23
Motor coordination, disorders of, 1049–1055, 1050(t)–1051(t)
Motor function, examination of, 1015–1017, 1017(t)
Motor neurone disease, 1061(t), 1062
Mouth, anatomy of, 657–659, *658*
  carcinoma of, 664–665
  disorders of, 657–665
    congenital, 660–661
    drug-induced, 665
    iatrogenic, 663
    idiopathic, 664
    infectious, 661–663
  embryology of, 657–658

Mouth *(Continued)*
  examination of, 659–660, *659*
  injuries of, 661
  moniliasis of, 665
  neoplasms of, 664–665
  physiology of, 659
Mucocele, nasal, 654
Mucoviscidosis, 939–940
Multifinality, in family system theory, 24
Multiple birth, 762–763
Multiple sclerosis, 1037–1038
  and organic brain syndrome, 355
Mumps, 677, 846–847
  ear infection in, 641
  immunization for, 839(t)
Muscle(s), disorders of, 1069–1071
  neurologic examination of, 1015–1017
Muscle spasm, in back, 575–576, *576*
Muscular dystrophy, 1071, 1072(t)
  in children, 878
Musculoskeletal system, in alcoholism, 332
Myasthenia gravis, 1072–1074
Myasthenia syndrome, with carcinoma, 1074
Mycoplasma pneumoniae infection, 887(t), 889
Mycosis fungoides, 1133, *1134*
Myelopathy, alcoholic, 1036
Myocardial disease, in elderly, 232
Myocarditis, 871
Myoclonic seizures, 857, 1027, 1028(t)
Myoglobinuria, 1070–1071, 1070(t), 1071(t)
Myoneural junction, disorders of, 1069–1074
Myopathies, metabolic, 1071
Myophosphorylase deficiency, 1071
Myopia, 699, *699*
  headache from, 1022(t)
Myositis, chest pain in, 1003, 1003(t)
Myositis ossificans, 566–567
Myotonia congenita, 1072(t)
Myotonic dystrophy, 1072(t)

Naloxone, for diagnosis of drug intoxication, 345–346
Narcolepsy, 1029
Nasopharyngoscope, 665
Nasopharynx, anatomy of, 665
  choristoma of, 666
  cysts of, 666
  disorders of, 665–668
    congenital, 666
    drug-induced, 668
    infectious, 667
  embryology of, 665
  encephalocele of, 666
  examination of, 665
  foreign bodies in, 667–668
  injuries of, 666–667
  neoplasms of, 668
  physiology of, 665–666
  stenosis of, 666
  teratomas of, 666
  tumors of, malignant, 668
National Health Service, 179–180
Nausea, and oral contraceptives, 735
  in pregnancy, 1079
Neck. See also *Cervical.*
  abscess of, 679
  anatomy of, 678

Neck (*Continued*)
  arthritis of, chest pain in, 1003(t), 1004
  carcinoma of, 679
  chronic pain in, 587–590, 588(t)
  cysts of, 678
  disorders of, 584–590, 678–679
  embryology of, 678
  examination of, 584(t), 585, 678
    neurologic, 1019–1020
  neoplasms of, 679
  ragging injury of, 586, 586
  range of motion of, 585
  sprain of, 584–587, 585(t), 586, 587
  stiff, 584–587, 585(t)
  wry, 679
Necrobiosis lipoidica diabeticorum, 1115, 1126–1127, 1126
Negligence, and duty to consult or refer, 203
Neonates. See Newborns.
Neoplasm. See names of specific lesions and body parts affected.
Nephroblastoma, 784
Nephrotic syndrome, in children, 875–876
Nerves. See also names of specific nerves.
  autonomic, dysfunction of, 1075
  cranial. See Cranial nerves.
  entrapment of, 1069
Nervous system, in alcoholism, 330–331
Neuralgia(s), 1060
  geniculate, 1060
  glossopharyngeal, 1060
  occipital, 1060
  superior laryngeal nerve, 1060
  trigeminal, 1058–1059
Neuritis, retrobulbar, 723
Neurogenic bladder, 211, 769–770
Neurogenic bowel, 211
Neurologic disorders, affecting motor coordination, 1049–1055, 1050(t)–1051(t)
  diagnostic procedures for, 1019(t)
  differential diagnosis of, 1020
  history taking in, 1013–1014, 1014(t)
  physical examination in, 1014–1020, 1014(t), 1016(t), 1017(t), 1018(t), 1019(t)
Neurology, 1013–1075
Neuroma, acoustic, 645
  of foot, 551, 551
Neuronitis, vestibular, 643
  viral, 641
Neuropathy, alcoholic, 1067
  bacterial, 1066
  carcinomatous, 1067
  chemical, 1067
  diabetic, 1067–1068
  entrapment, 1069
  heavy metal, 1036(t), 1037, 1068
  hereditary, 1066
  infectious, 1066
  metabolic-toxic, 1067–1068
  nutritional, 1068
  peripheral, 1066–1067
    and amyloidosis, 1068–1069
  uremic, 1068
  vascular, 1068
  viral, 1066
Neuropsychiatric disorders, in elderly, differential diagnosis of, 230–231

Neurosis, anxiety, 291
  chest pain in, 1003, 1003(t)
  diagnosis of, 297
  drugs for, 382(t)–388(t). See also Drugs, psychopharmacologic.
  hysterical, 297–299
Nevus, 1129, 1130
  pigmented, excision and biopsy of, 519–520, 520(t)
Newborn, 831–836
  anal stenosis in, 829
  Apgar score for, 830, 831(t)
  bacterial infections in, 834–835
  congenital rubella in, 835
  congenital syphilis in, 836
  cytomegalovirus infection in, 835–836
  evaluation of, 830–832, 831, 831(t)
  gestational age of, assessment of, 830–831, 831
  herpes simplex infection in, 835
  hypoglycemia in, 836
  infections in, 834–836
  intestinal obstruction in, 491(t)
  jaundice in, 832–834, 833(t)
  large-for-gestational-age, 832
  meningitis, in 848–849
  of diabetic mothers, 836
  pneumonia in, 887(t), 890
  postmature, 832
    defined, 831
  premature, 832
    defined, 831
  respiratory distress syndrome in, 934
  small-for-gestational-age, 831–832
  toxoplasmosis in, 836
  transient diabetes in, 877–878
Nipple, discharge from, 513–514, 513(t)
  ulcerated, and Paget's disease, 513(t), 514
Nocturia, 766–767
Nocturnal angina, 1005
Noise, and hearing loss, 642
Normal pressure hydrocephalus, 1048(t)
Normative ethics, 244–245
North American blastomycosis, 938
Nortriptyline, dose, use, and side effects of, 382(t)–383(t)
Nose, 646–657
  anatomy of, 646–648, 646, 647
  bleeding from, 655–656, 655
    in juvenile angiofibroma, 668
  disorders of, congenital, 649–650
    hereditary, 650–651
    iatrogenic, 654–655
    infectious, 652–654
  embryology of, 646
  examination of, 647, 648, 648
  fibroma of, 657
  fracture of, 651
    reduction of, 652
  furuncle of, 652
  mucocele of, 654
  neoplasms of, 657
  packing of, 655
  papillomas of, 657
  physiology of, 648–649
  polyps of, 651
  squamous cell carcinoma of, 657
  tumors of, congenital, 650, 650
Nummular eczema, 1117–1118, 1117

Nurse practitioners. See *Allied health professionals.*
Nursing homes, role of medical director of, 237–238
Nutrition, 1077–1101
  and cancer, 1092
  and life cycle, 1076–1091
  counseling on, 1091(t)
  evaluation of, 1077(t)
    in elderly, 1089–1090
  for athletes, 1088–1089, 1088(t)
  for children, 837–838, 838(t), 1085–1087, 1085(t), 1086(t)
  for elderly, 1089–1091
  for infants, 837–838, 838(t), 1081–1085
    long-term effects of, 1085
  in disease, 1091–1101
  in lactation, 1080–1081
  in pregnancy, 757–758, 1077–1080
Nutritional neuropathy, 1068
Nutritional supplements, for infants, 837, 1083–1084, 1084(t)
  in pregnancy, 1078–1079
Nystagmus, 726
  positional, 643

Oat cell carcinoma, of lung, 915, 915(t)
Obesity, 1097–1100
  and infant nutrition, 1085
  and pelvic examination, 732–733
  as surgical risk factor, 482
  in adolescence, 1088
  reducing diet for, 1098–1100, 1098(t), *1099*
Obstetrics, 731–765
Obstructive jaundice, 970(t), 971–972
Occipital lobe function, examination of, 1015
Occipital neuralgia, 1060
Occlusive carotid arterial disease, ocular manifestations of, 729
Occupational diseases, hepatic, 981
  pulmonary, 923–926
Occupational therapy, after spinal cord injury, 212
  after stroke, 213
Ocular headache, 691
Ocular motor paralysis, 726, 1056(t)–1057(t), 1058
Ocular pemphigus, 726–727
Olfaction, hereditary absence of, 650
Olfactory nerve, disorders of, 1056(t)
Ophthalmodynamometry, 729
Ophthalmology, 690–730
Ophthalmoscopy, 693–695, *694*
Optic nerve, atrophy of, 723
  crescents of, 722
  disorders of, 722–725, 1056(t)
  drusen of, 722, *722*
  hyaline bodies of, 722, *722*
  neuritis of, 723
  papillitis of, 722–723, *723*
Oral contraceptives, 451(t), 452–458, *453*, 454(t), 455(t), 457(t), *458*, 735–736
  and birth defects, 455(t), 458, 736
  and blood clotting, 457
  and breakthrough bleeding, 458, 735–736
  and carbohydrate metabolism, 456–457
  and coronary heart disease, 456
  and depression, 458
  and diabetes, 456–457

Oral contraceptives *(Continued)*
  and edema, 736
  and epilepsy, 459
  and galactorrhea, 459
  and hair loss, 459
  and hepatic function, 457
  and hepatic tumors, 980(t), 981
  and hypertension, 456
  and lipid metabolism, 456
  and melasma, 459
  and migraine headache, 458–459
  and nausea, 735
  and post-pill amenorrhea, 457–458, *458*, 736
  and smoking, 456
  and thromboembolic disease, 456
  and vaginitis, 459
  and weight gain, 735–736
  choice of, 453–455
  combination, 453–455, *453*, 454(t), 455(t)
  contraindications to, 455(t), 735
  effect of on laboratory tests, 457, 457(t)
  mini-pill, 453–455, *453*, 454(t), 455(t)
  side effects of, 455–459, 455(t), 457(t), *458*, 735–736
    carcinogenic, 455–456
    cardiovascular, 456
  types of, 453–455, *453*, 454(t), 455(t)
Orbit, fractures of, 680, *680*, 682(t), 710
  pain in, 691
Orchitis, in mumps, 846
Organic brain syndrome, 353–361
  acute, case histories of, 354–355
    characteristics of, 354(t)
  brain function impairment in, 353(t)
  causes of, 355–356, 356(t), 358(t)
  chronic, case histories of, 354–355
    characteristics of, 354(t)
    treatable types of, 360(t)
  diagnostic evaluation in, 356–358
  drug therapy for, 381, 382(t)–388(t)
  family counseling in, 360
  in elderly, 228–231
  laboratory studies in, 358
  patient referral in, 360
  physical findings in, 357
  signs and symptoms of, 379–381
Organic dementia, 228–230
Orgasmic dysfunction, female, 447–448
Oropharynx, abscess of, 662–663
  anatomy of, 657–659, *658*
  carcinoma of, 664–665
  disorders of, 657–665
    congenital, 660–661
    drug-induced, 665
    iatrogenic, 663
    idiopathic, 664
    infectious, 661–663
  embryology of, 657–658
  examination of, 659–660, *659*
  foreign body in, 663
  injuries of, 661
  neoplasms of, 664–665
  physiology of, 659
  tumors of, benign, 664
Orthomolecular therapy, 388(t)
Osmotic diarrhea, 950
Orthopedics, 541–627
Orthostatic hypotension, 1026(t)

Osteoarthritis, of hip, 567–570, *570*
    of spine, 582–584, 582(t), *583, 584,* 1064–1065
        chest pain in, 1003(t), 1004
    of thumb, 607–608
    synovianalysis in, 622(t)
Osteochondritis, dissecans, of knee, 542, *543*
    of tarsal navicular, 543, *544,* 548–549, *549*
    of tibial prominence, 562, *562*
Osteochondrosis, of hip, 572–573, *572*
Osteomalcia, vs. osteoporosis, 1090–1091
Osteomyelitis, in children, 851
Osteoporosis, in elderly, 1090–1091, 1091(t)
Otitis externa, 638
Otitis media, 639–640
    acute, 639
    and adenoidectomy, 667
    chronic, 639
    serous, 639
    tuberculous, 641
Otorhinolaryngology, 628–689
Otosclerosis, 637–638
Ovary(ies), cysts of, 750, 751(t)
    examination of, 732
    fibroma of, 752
    tumors of, 750–752, 751(t)
Oxalosis, urinary calculi in, 770
Oxazepam, dose, use, and side effects of, 382(t)
Ozena, 656

Paget's disease, 513(t), 514
Pain(s), abdominal. See *Abdominal pain.*
    ankle, in tenosynovitis, 546–547
    back, 579–584
        physical therapy for, 215–218, *216, 217, 218*
    chest, 1003–1007, 1003(t). See also *Angina
        pectoris; Chest pain.*
    during intercourse, in female, 746
    elbow, 600–601, *600, 601*
    finger, at night, 606–607
    foot, 546–554
    growing, 541–544
    hand, at night, 606–607
    hip, in adults, 574
        in children, 567–573
    in peripheral nerve disorders, 1069
    in upper extremity, in children, 596–598
    in urologic disorders, 767
    ischemic rest, 506
    knee, in children, 564–566
    neck, chronic, 587–590, *588,* 588(t)
    ocular, 691
    orbital, 691
    orthopedic, in children, 541–544
    pelvic, 745–746
    postoperative, in anorectal surgery, 811–812
    reaction to, and social class, 51
    shoulder, 595–596
    wrist, 604–605
Palatal insufficiency, 667
Palate, cleft, 649–650, 660–661
    fistula of, 661
    lacerations of, 661
Pancreas, carcinoma of, chronic abdominal pain
    in, 943–944
Pancreatitis, acute, 486(t), 495–497
    vs. perforated peptic ulcer, 490
Papanicolaou test, 132–133, 733–734

Papilledema, 722–723, *723,* 1055–1058, 1056(t)
Papillitis, of optic nerve, 722–723, *723*
Papilloma, juvenile, 673
    nasal, 657
    squamous, excision of, 520
Paralysis, Erb's, 1065
    facial nerve, 643–644, 1059–1060
    hypokalemic periodic, 1074
    infantile, immunization for, 839(t)
    Klumpke's, 1065
    nerve, causes of, 1056(t)–1057(t)
    ocular motor, 726, 1056(t)–1057(t), 1058
    rehabilitation in, 211–212
    tick, 1074
    vocal cord, congenital, 671
Paramyotonia, 1072(t)
Paranasal sinus(es), 646–657
    anatomy of, 646–648, *647*
    infectious disorders of, 652–654
Paranoia, vs. schizophrenia, 324
Parapharyngeal abscess, 663
Paraphimosis, 781
Paraplegia, rehabilitation in, 211–212
Parasitic infections, in children, 852, 852(t)
Parent Effectiveness Training, 400–402, *400*
Parietal lobe function, examination of, 1015
Parkinson's disease, 1051(t), 1054–1055
    and phenothiazine, 1053
Paronychia, 620–621, *621*
Parotid gland. See also *Salivary glands.*
    infections of, 677
Parotitis, epidemic, 677, 846–847
    suppurative, 677
Paroxysmal choreoathetosis, 1053
Pars planitis, 715
Paroxysmal tachycardia, 1008
Passive-aggressive personality, 279
Patella, chondromalacia of, 564–565, *566*
    recurrent, dislocation of, 563, *564*
Patent ductus arteriosus, 867
Pathologist, consultation with, 205
Patient(s), behavioral modification in, 115–120
    dying, care of, 249–257. See also *Illness,
        terminal.*
    geriatric. See *Elderly.*
    implementation of physician's instructions by,
        57–58
    interviewing of, 258–266
    life-style risk factors of, 111–122
        techniques for changing, 115–120
    medical records of. See *Medical records.*
    physician consultation by, 52–53
    self-care by, 52–53
    social class of, and perception of illness, 50–51
        and perception of pain, 51
        and reaction to stress, 51
Pectinate line, anorectal, 788, *788*
Pediatrics, 830–882
Pediculosis pubis, 1134
Pedophilia, 370(t). See also *Sexual variations and
    deviations.*
Pelvic examination. See *Gynecologic examination.*
Pelvic infections, 737–739
Pelvic inflammatory disease, and gonorrhea, 740
Pelvis, anomalies of, 773
    duplication of, 773
    pain in, 745–746
    relaxation of supporting structures of, 754–755

Pemphigoid, bullous, 1106–1108, *1107*
Pemphigus, 664, 1106, *1114*
  ocular, 726–727
Penis, anomalies of, 774
  Bowen's disease of, 781
  carcinoma of, 781
  disorders of, 781
    erectile, 442–443, 781
  erythroplasia of, 781
  examination of, 780
  fractures of, 780
  infection of, 781
  injuries of, 780
  Peyronie's disease of, 781
  precancerous lesions of, 781
  skin lesions of, 781
Peptic esophagitis, chest pain in, 1003(t), 1004
Peptic ulcer, 958–959
  and chest pain, 1003(t), 1004
  bleeding from, diagnosis of, 497–498
    treatment of, 498–499
  perforated, 486(t), 490
Pericardial disease, in elderly, 232
Pericardiocentesis, 529
Periodic health screening. See *Screening*.
Peritoneal lavage, diagnostic, 530, *530*
Peripheral arterial occlusive disease, chronic, 506–508
Peripheral nerves, and pain syndromes, 1069
Peripheral neuropathies, 1066–1067
  and amyloidosis, 1068–1069
Peritonsillar abscess, 662–663
Perphenazine, dose, use, and side effects of, 385(t)–386(t)
Personality, labile, 277
  passive-aggressive, 279
Personality disorders, 276–287
  classification of, 276–280
  diagnostic tests for, 280–281
  drug therapy for, 283–284, 382(t)–388(t). See also *Drugs, psychopharmacologic*.
  inheritance and, 281–282
  physiologic causes of, 280–281
  treatment of, 283–285. See also *Psychotherapy*.
Perthe's disease, 572–573, *572*
Pertussis, 845–846
  immunization for, 839(t)
Petit mal seizures, 856–857, 1027, 1028(t)
Petrositis, 640
Peyronie's disease, 781
Phallus. See *Penis*.
Pharyngeal syndrome, 885(t), 886
Pharyngitis, acute, 662
Pharynx. See *Oropharynx*.
Phenothiazines, dose, use, and side effects of, 385(t)–386(t)
  neurologic complications of, 1053–1054
Phenylbutazone, for rheumatoid arthritis, 626
Phenytoin, for alcohol withdrawal, 334
  for seizure disorders, 1028(t)
  intoxication with, 1050(t)
Pheochromocytoma, and hypertension, 987
  anxiety in, 289
Phimosis, 781
Phlebitis, 509–511
  and postphlebitic syndrome, 511
Phobias, 300–302
  behavior modification for, 300–302
  in rape victims, 368
  psychiatric referral for, 295

Phoria, 695–696
Phosphorylase deficiency, and myopathy, 1071
Physical therapy, after spinal cord injury, 212
  after stroke, 212–213
  for back pain, 215–218, *216, 217, 218*
Physician(s). See also *Family physician*.
  and medical ethics, 241–248
  as moral agent, 246–247
  consultation with, vs. referral to, 200–202
  decision-making by, and medical ethics, 241–248
  distribution of, 178(t)
  primary, defined, 4–5. See also *Family physician*.
Physician assistant, and physician preceptor, 194
  evolution of, 189–192
  role of, 192–194
  training of, 197
  utilization of, 194–197
Pigmented nevus, excision and biopsy of, 519–520, 520(t)
Pill, contraceptive. See *Oral contraceptives*.
Pilonidal cysts, 827
  excision of, 521
Pilonidal sinus, 521, 827
Pinguecula, 707, *707*
Pink eye, 706
Pinna. See *Ear, external*.
Pinworms, 852, 852(t)
Pityriasis rosea, 1105–1106, *1105, 1106, 1114*
Placenta, disorders of, and vaginal bleeding, 745
Plantar wart, 1123, *1123*
  excision of, 520–521
Pleural effusion, 899–901
Pleurisy, 899–901
Plissit model, for sexual counseling, 434–435
Pneumoconiosis, 923–926
  coal workers', 925
  defined, 884
Pneumonia, defined, 884
  in children, 842
  mycoplasmal, 887(t), 889
  neonatal, 887(t), 890
  pneumococcal, 887(t), 888
  staphylococcal, 887(t), 888
  tubercular, in children, 850
  usual interstitial, defined, 884
  viral, 887(t), 888–889
  vs. asthma, 841(t)
  vs. bronchiolitis, 841(t)
Pneumonitis, causes of, 887–890, 890(t)
  defined, 884
Pneumothorax, 527, *527*, 903–905
  closed, 903
  open, 903–904
  spontaneous, 903
  traumatic, 903
Poison ivy, 1118–1119, *1118*
Poisoning, antidotes for, 854(t)
  arsenic, 1036(t)
  aspirin, 855–856, *855*
  belladonna, 346–347
  drug. See *Drug intoxication*.
  heavy metal, neurologic complications of, 1036(t), 1037, 1068
  in children, 853–855, *854, 855*
  lead, 1036(t)
  manganese, 1036(t)
  mercury, 1036(t)

Poisoning (*Continued*)
  salicylate, 855–856, *855*
  thallium, 1036(t)
Polio, immunization for, 839(t)
Pollen, allergy to, 1141. See also *Allergic rhinitis.*
Pollution, air, and chronic bronchitis, 908–909
Polymyositis, 1069–1070
Polyp(s), colonic, 817–818
    and colonic carcinoma, 967–970, 968(t)–
      969(t)
  ear, 641
  nasal, 651
  rectal, 817–818
  uterine cervix, 749
  vocal cord, 673–674
Polyposis, familial adenomatous, 818
  types of, 968(t)
Polyposis syndromes, and colonic carcinoma,
  967–970, 968(t)–969(t)
Polyradiculoneuropathy, acute postinfectious,
  1066–1067
Pontine hemorrhage, 1043
Portal hypertension, 974–975, 974(t)
Positional nystagmus, 643
Positional vertigo, 643, 1031(t)
Postconcussion syndrome, anxiety in, 290
Postinfectious polyradiculoneuropathy, 1066–
  1067
Postinfective syndrome, anxiety in, 290
Postmaturity, neonatal, 831, 832
Postmenopausal bleeding, and endometrial
  adenocarcinoma, 748
Postphlebitic syndrome, 511
Posture, and back pain, 217–218, *217*
  examination of, in neurologic examination, 1016
Pre-eclampsia, 763–764
Pregnancy, 757–765
  abdominal pain in, 487
  and family life cycle, 37–39
  bleeding in, 744
  chorea in, 1052
  constipation in, 1079–1080
  dental care in, 758
  diabetes in, 761–762, 762(t)
    and neonatal complications, 836
  diet in, 758, 1078
  douching in, 758
  drugs in, 758
  ectopic, vaginal bleeding in, 744
  exercise in, 758
  fetal postmaturity in, 764–765
  genetic counseling for, 465–478. See also
    Genetic counseling.
  heart disease in, 761
  high risk, 759–765
  hydramnios in, 764
  immunization in, 757
  in adolescents, nutritional requirements in,
    1078
  morning sickness in, 1079
  multiple gestation in, 762–763
  nausea in, 1079
  nutrition in, 757–758, 1077–1080
  nutritional supplements in, 1078–1079
  patient instruction in, 757–758
  pre-eclampsia in, 763–764
  preventive medicine for, 107(t)–108(t)
  rubella in, 757
  sexual intercourse in, 439, 758

Pregnancy (*Continued*)
  smoking in, 758
  sodium restriction in, 1079
  toxemia of, 763–764
  use of oral contraceptives in, 458, 736
  weight gain in, 757–758, 1079
  with intact IUD, 460
Premature ejaculation, 443–444
Prematurity, neonatal, 831, 832
Presbycusis, 642
Presbyopia, 700
Presenile dementia, 229
Preventive medicine, 103–122
  and epidemiology, 103–110, 111–112
  and life style factors, 111–112
  behavioral view of, 114–115
  epidemiological view of, 111–112
  major problems in, 105(t)
  political view of, 112–114
  prenatal, 107(t)–108(t)
  primary prevention in, 103–104
  problem analysis in, 106(t)
  procedures for, 107(t)–110(t)
  secondary prevention in, 104
  tertiary prevention in, 104
Priapism, 781
Primary care, defined, 4
Primary physician, defined, 4–5
Proctalgia fugax, 825
Proctitis, ulcerative, 948(t), 949
Proctology, 787–829
Proctoscopy, 794–797, *795*
Proctosigmoidoscopy, in periodic screening,
  135–136
Progestogens, synthetic, as contraceptives, 453–
  455, *453*, 454(t), 455(t). See also *Oral
  contraceptives.*
Prognathism, 661
Progressive resistance exercises, for knee, 220
Progressive spinal muscular atrophy, 1061(t),
  1062–1063
Propanediols, dose, use, and side effects of, 384(t)
Propranolol, dose, use, and side effects of, 382(t)
Proptosis, in thyroid disease, 725–726
Prospective medicine, 161–174
  credibility of, 172–173
  health hazard appraisal in, 163–168, *163,
    164–166,* 169(t), 171(t)
Prostate, carcinoma of, 783
  disorders of, 782–783
  examination of, 781
  hyperplasia of, benign, 783
  infections of, 782–783
Prothrombin time, test of, 973
Protozoal infections, neurologic complications of,
  1034
Protriptyline, dose, use, and side effects of,
  382(t)–383(t)
  for depression, 309(t)
Pruritus ani, 826–827
Pseudohypertrophic dystrophy, 1072(t)
Pseudomotor cerebri, 1022(t)
Pseudonephritis, athletic, 778
  exercise, 778
Pseudostrabismus, 702, *702*
Pseudotumor cerebri, 1039–1040
  causes of, 1040(t)
Psoriasis, 1102–1104, *1102, 1103, 1104*

Psychiatric disorders. See also *Emotional prob-
    lems; Personality disorders;* and names of
    specific disorders.
    drugs for. See *Drugs, psychopharmacologic.*
    in elderly, differential diagnosis of, 230–231
    therapy for. See *Psychotherapy.*
Psychologic problems. See *Emotional problems.*
Psychopharmacologic drugs. See *Drugs, psycho-
    pharmacologic.*
Psychomotor seizures, 857, 1027–1029, 1028(t)
Psychophysiologic reactions, 376
Psychoses, affective, vs. schizophrenia, 323–324
    alcoholic, 1035
    defined, 317. See also *Depression; Schizo-
        phrenia.*
    drug-induced, vs. schizophrenia, 323
    drug therapy for, 382(t)–388(t)
    organic, vs. schizophrenia, 324
    symbiotic, 321
    drugs for, 382(t)–388(t)
Psychosomatic disorders, 376
Psychotherapy, 390–403
    behavior therapy in, 395
    client-centered, 399
    counselor's approach to, 393–394
    existential, 399–400
    family physician's role in, 391–392
    family therapy in, 402. See also *Marriage and
        family counseling.*
    for anxiety, 294
    for behavior disorders, 283
    for depression, 313–314
    for schizophrenia, 326–327
    gestalt, 398–399
    group. See *Group therapy.*
    history taking in, 390–391
    indications for, 390–391
    Parent Effectiveness Training in, 400–402, *400*
    patient referral in, 392
    techniques in, 394–402
    transactional analysis in, 395–397, *396, 397*
Pterygium, 707, *707*
Pulmonary disease, as surgical risk factor, 485
    chronic obstructive, 932–933
        treatment of, 933–934
    incidence of, in family practice, 844(t)
Pulmonary drainage, total anomalous, 868–869
Pulmonary emboli, in elderly, 231–232
Pulmonary fibrosis, in pneumoconiosis, 923–926
Pulmonary function tests, in chronic bronchitis,
        909–910
    in emphysema, 911–912, *912*
Pulmonary medicine, 883–940
    incidence of problems in, 884(t)
    terminology in, 883–884
Pulmonary nodule, solitary, defined, 884
Pulmonary thromboembolism, 901–903
Pulmonary tuberculosis. See *Tuberculosis, pul-
    monary.*
Pulmonary veins, transposition of, 868–869
Pulmonic stenosis, 867
    in tetralogy of Fallot, 869
Pyelonephritis, in children, 847, 847(t)
Pyoderma, 1121–1122

Quadriplegia, rehabilitation in, 211–212

Quervain's disease, 604–605, *605*
Quinine, ototoxicity of, 645

Radiologist, consultation with, 205
Ragging injury, cervical, 586, *586*
Rainbow, visual, 691
Ramsey Hunt syndrome, 641
Range of motion exercises, for knee, 220
Rape, 362–369, 370(t)
    defined, 362–363
    history taking in, 365
    incidence of, 363
    legal considerations in, 367
Rape crisis centers, 363–364
Rape victims, characteristics of, 363
    counseling for, crisis-intervention, 365–366
        immediate, 365–367
        long-term, 367–369
        methods of, 366
    medical follow-up for, 366–367
    physical examination of, 365
    post-rape symptoms in, sexual, 368
        somatic, 367–368
    preservation of physical evidence by, 364
    stages in response of, 365–366
    treatment of, 364–369
        crisis centers for, 363–364
        immediate, 364–367
        long-term, 367–369
Raynaud's disease, 1075
Raynaud's phenomenon, 1075
Rectocele, 755
Rectum. See also *Anorectum; Colon.*
    bleeding from, in children, 829
        in diverticulosis, 815
    carcinoid of, 828
    carcinoma of, 818–820
        screening for, 134–136
    polyps of, 817–818
Referral. See also *Consultation.*
    in marriage and family counseling, 422–423
    in sexual counseling, 372
    mechanisms for, in United Kingdom, 180–181
        in United States, 175–176
    medicolegal aspects of, 202–204
    psychiatric, 392
        for anxiety, 295
        for depression, 315
        for group therapy, 405–406
        for phobias, 295
    vs. consultation, 200–202
Reflexes, testing of, 1018–1019, 1018(t)
    in newborn, 831(t)
Reflux esophagitis, 960–961, 961(t)
Refractive errors, 699–700
    headache from, 1022(t)
Regional ileitis, 816–817
Rehabilitation, 210–222
    after spinal cord injury, 211–212
    after stroke, 212–214, 213(t)
    in drug abuse, 349–352
    in rheumatoid arthritis, 214–215
    in schizophrenia, 327–328
    postsurgical, 220–221
    progress monitoring in, 221
Renal cell carcinoma, 784
Renal function tests, 767

Renal insufficiency, hypertension in, drugs for, 993
Renovascular hypertension, 786, 986
Reproduction, female, physiology of, 450–451
Reproductive tract, female. See names of specific anatomic parts.
  male, disorders of, 780–783
    injuries of, 778–780
    normal, 780
Respiratory allergies, 650–651
Respiratory distress. See also *Airway obstruction.*
  defined, 883
  in burn patients, 536–537
  in newborn, 934
  vs. respiratory failure, 929
Respiratory distress syndrome, 934
Respiratory failure, 929–934
  acidosis in, 931–932, 932(t)
  defined, 883
  diagnosis of, 929
  etiology of, 932, 932(t)
  hypercapnia in, 931
  hypoxia in, 930–931, *930*
  in bronchial asthma, 1145
  pathophysiology of, 932–933, *933*
  treatment of, 933–934
  vs. respiratory insufficiency, 929
Respiratory infections, 885–887
  causative viruses of, 885(t)
Respiratory system, in alcoholism, 331
Resuscitation, cardiopulmonary, 525–526
Retarded ejaculation, 444–445
Retina, arteriosclerotic changes in, 715–718, *717*
  detachment of, 720–721, *721*
  diabetic changes in, 719–720, *719*
  disorders of, 715–721
  hypertensive changes in, 715–718, *717*
  in sickle cell disease, 728
  tumors of, 721
  vascular disorders of, 715–719, *718*
Retinal artery, occlusion of, 718–719, *718*
Retinoblastoma, 721
  genetic counseling for, 476
Retrobulbar neuritis, 723
Retrograde ejaculation, 445
Retropharyngeal abscess, 663
Rh incompatibility, 759–761, 881–882
Rheumatic fever, 871–874, 872(t), 873(t)
  and Sydenham's chorea, 1049
Rheumatic heart disease, in elderly, 231
Rheumatoid arthritis, drug therapy for, 625–626
  management of, 622–627
  ocular manifestations of, 727
  of knee, *565*
  rehabilitation in, 214–215, *214*
  synovianalysis in, 622(t)
  vs. rheumatic fever, 873(t)
Rhinitis, acute, 652
  allergic. See *Allergic rhinitis.*
  atrophic, 656
  chronic, 652
  drug-induced, 657
  vasomotor, 656
Rhinitis medicamentosum, 654
Rhinorrhea, cerebrospinal fluid, 651–652
Rhythm method, 451–452, 451(t)
Rinne test, for hearing, 633–634
Risk factors, 111–122
  age average, 171

Risk factors (*Continued*)
  reduction of, 170–172, *170*
  appraisal of, 163–170, *163*, *164—166*, 169(t), 171(t)
    techniques for, 115–120
  surgical, 481–482, 482(t)
Rosacea, 1121
Roles, family, 420
  ocular manifestations of, 726
Roseola infantum, 843–844, *844*
Rotator cuff, calcification in, *593*
Roundworms, 852, 852(t)
Rubella, 843
  congenital, 835
  immunization for, 839(t)
  in pregnancy, 757
Rubeola, 842, *842*
Rule of nines, for burn estimation, 537(t)

Sadomasochism, 370(t). See also *Sexual variations and deviations.*
Salicylates, and bronchial asthma, 1144
  intoxication with, in children, 855–856, *856*
  ototoxicity of, 645
Salivary glands, anatomy of, 675
  calculi of, 677
    detection of, 676
  carcinoma of, 678
  congenital hemangiomas of, 676
  disorders of, 675–678
    congenital, 676
    drug-induced, 678
    iatrogenic, 677
    idiopathic, 677
    infectious, 677
  embryology of, 675
  examination of, 675–676, *676*
  first branchial cleft anomalies of, 676
  injuries of, 676–677
  neoplasms of, 678
  physiology of, 675
Salt. See *Sodium.*
Sarcoid, 1126, *1126*
Sarcoidosis, 926–929, 1038–1039
  defined, 884
Sarcoma, renal, 783
  uterine, 749
  vaginal, 753
Scabies, *1115*, 1134
  KOH slide technique for, 1134
Scalp, fungal infection of, 1112–1113, *1112*
Scarlet fever, 845
Schiller test, 734
Schizoid state, 279–280
Schizophrenia, 317–329
  and family background, 322
  and social class, 322
  behavioral disturbances in, 319
  biochemical factors in, 321
  catatonic, 320
  childhood, 320–321
  chronic, 327
    undifferentiated, 320
  cognitive disturbances in, 318–319
  course of, 318
  defined, 317
  delusions in, 318–319

Schizophrenia (Continued)
  diagnosis of, 322–323, 379(t)
  differential diagnosis of, 323–324
  drug therapy for, 325–326, 381
  environmental factors in, 322
  etiology of, 321–322
  hallucinations in, 319
  hebephrenic, 320
  inheritance in, 321
  latent, 320
    anxiety in, 290
  motor disturbances in, 319
  onset of, 318
  paranoid, 320
  perceptual disturbances in, 318–319
  psychotherapy for, 326–327
  rehabilitation in, 327–328
  residual, 320
  schizoaffective, 320
  simple, 320
  subtypes of, 319–320
  symptoms of, 318–319, 379(t)
  treatment of, 324–328
    trends in, 317–318
  violent behavior in, management of, 324
Scleroderma, 1114, 1125–1126
Sclerosis, cerebral, 1030
  multiple. See Multiple sclerosis.
  of ear, 637–638
Screening, 123–137
  flow sheet for, 131, 136
  for anemia, in children, 126(t), 127(t), 128
  for bacteriuria, in children, 126(t), 127
  for breast cancer, 133–134
  for cervical cancer, 132–133, 733–734
  for colonic cancer, 134–136
  for hypertension, 126(t), 127–128, 127(t), 129(t)
  for rectal cancer, 134–136
  gynecologic, 733–735
  in adults, 128–136, 129–130(t)
  in children, 126–128, 126(t), 127(t)
  in elderly, 130–132
Screening programs, criteria for, 125, 125(t)
  types of, 124–125
Screening tests, sensitivity of, 124, 124(t)
  specificity of, 124
Script analysis, 397
Scrotum, abscess of, 782
  disorders of, 782
  examination of, 780
  injuries of, 780
Sebaceous cysts, excision of, 521
Seborrheic dermatitis, 1121
Seborrheic keratosis, 1128, 1129
  excision of, 520
Secretory diarrhea, 949
Sedatives, for asthma, 896
Seizures, 1025–1030. See also Epilepsy.
  akinetic, 857
  alcoholic, 1035
  autonomic, 857
  causes of, 1026(t)
  drug therapy for, 858(t), 1028(t)
  febrile, 856
  focal, 856, 1029
  grand mal, 856, 1025–1027, 1028(t)
  in children, diagnostic work-up for, 857
    management of, 857–858
  in hypoglycemia, 1035

Seizures (Continued)
  in organic brain syndrome, 359
  jackknife, 856, 1024
  jacksonian, 1029
  lightning, 857
  myoclonic, 857, 1027, 1028(t)
  partial, 1029
  patterns of, 856
  petit mal, 856–857, 1027, 1028(t)
  psychomotor, 857, 1027–1029, 1028(t)
  therapeutic, induced, 315
Semen, analysis of, in infertility, 755
Seminal vesicles, disorders of, 783
  examination of, 781
Senile cataract, 713
Senile dementia, 229
  drugs for, 382(t)–388(t)
Senile keratosis, 1129–1130, 1130
Senile macular degeneration, 720, 720
Sensate focus, in sexual counseling, 441–442
Sensation, testing of, 1017–1018
Septic arthritis, in children, 851
  synovianalysis in, 622(t)
Serum amylase, in acute pancreatitis, 496
Serum cholesterol level, in hyperlipidemia, 1011(t)
Serum proteins, tests of, 972–973
Serum triglyceride level, in hyperlipedemia, 1011(t)
Sexual assault, 362–369. See also Rape.
Sexual counseling, 433–439. See also Marriage and family counseling.
  as profession, 423–424
  for female sexual dysfunction, 440–442, 445–448
  for male sexual dysfunction, 440–445
  for sexual variations and deviations, 371–373
  history taking in, 435–436
  Plissit model for, 434–435
  sensate focus in, 441–442
Sexual deviations. See Sexual variations and deviations.
Sexual dysfunction, 440–448
  marital problems, 418–419
  female, 440–442, 445–448
    general, 446–447
  in alcoholism, 333
  in rape victims, 368
    orgasmic, 447–448
  male, 440–445
Sexual intercourse, after spinal cord injury, 212
  during illness, 440
  during pregnancy, 439, 758
  dysfunctional. See Sexual dysfunction.
  painful, 448, 746
Sexual variations and deviations, 369–373, 370(t)
  diagnosis of, 369–370
  patient referral in, 372
  physician counseling in, 371–373
  specialized treatments for, 373
  therapeutic goals in, 370–371
Sexuality, in infancy and childhood, 40, 436–437
    and family life cycle, 40
  in puberty and adolescence, 437–438
  of middle-aged and aging female, 439
  of middle-aged and aging male, 439–440
  of young adults, 438–439
SGOT, test of, 972
SGPT, test of, 972

Shock, in children, 853
    in gastrointestinal bleeding, 962–963, 964(t)
    venous catheterization in, 522, 523
Shoulder, anatomy of, 591
    arthrofibrosis of, 591–595
    aspiration of, 624
    calcification in, 593
    dislocation of, 598, 599, 599
    disorders of, 591–599
    frozen, 591–595, 592, 593, 594
    pain and deformity in, 595–596
    range of motion of, 592
    sprain of, 598–599
    stiff, 591–595, 592, 593, 594
Shunt, venous admixture, defined, 883
Sialadenitis, chronic recurrent, 677
Sialadenopathy, benign lymphoepithelial, 677
Sialectasis, chronic, 677
Sialography, 676
Sickle cell disease, in children, 880–881
    ocular manifestations of, 728
Sigmoidoscopy, 794–797, 795
Silicosis, 924
Sims-Huhner test, 756
Sinus(es), paranasal. See Paranasal sinuses.
    pilonidal, 521, 827
    preauricular, 637
Sinus bradycardia, 1007–1008
Sinus tachycardia, 1008
Sinusitis, acute, 652–653
    chronic, 653–654
    headache from, 1023(t)
Situational anxiety, 290
Skin, basal cell carcinoma of, 1131–1132, 1131,
    1132
    Bowen's disease of, 1130–1131, 1131
    cancer of, 518–519, 1130–1132, 1131, 1132
    care of, after spinal cord injury, 211–212
    disorders of. See Dermatitis; Dermatoses; and
        names of specific disorders.
    fungal infections of, 1109–1116
    lesions of, minor office surgery for, 518–521,
        518
        squamous cell carcinoma of, 1130–1132, 1131,
        1132
    systemic diseases affecting, 1124–1129
    tumors of, 1129–1134
    viral infections of, 1122–1124
Skin tags, 1129, 1129
    excision of, 520
Skull, fracture of, 1044
    neurologic examination of, 1019–1020
Small intestine, obstruction of, 486(t), 491–494,
    491(t), 493
Smoking, and bronchogenic carcinoma, 914
    and chronic bronchitis, 908–909
    and oral contraceptives, 456
    and pulmonary emphysema, 910
    in pregnancy, 758
Snapping finger, 621, 621
Snout reflex, 1018
Sodium restriction, in hypertension, 1093–1096,
    1096(t), 1097(t)
    in pregnancy, 1079
Soft tissue injuries, 531–532
Sore throat, 885(t), 886
Spasmodic torticollis, 1052
Speech therapy, after stroke, 213–214

Spermatic cord, anomalies of, 774
    examination of, 780
    hydrocele of, 774
    infections of, 782
    torsion of, 774, 782
    variocele of, 774
Spermatocele, 774, 782
Spermicides, contraceptive, 463
Spina bifida, genetic counseling for, 477
Spinal accessory nerve, disorders of, 1057(t)
Spinal cord, disorders of, 1060–1064, 1061(t)
    infarction of, 1061(t), 1063
    injuries of, rehabilitation after, 211–212
    tumors of, 1061(t), 1064
Spinal flexion exercise, for back pain, 216–217,
    216, 217
Spinal muscular atrophy, infantile, 878
Spine, arthritis of, 582–584, 582(t), 583, 584,
        1064–1065
    chest pain in, 1003(t), 1004
    neurologic examination of, 1019–1020
Spinocerebellar degeneration, familial, 1050(t)
Splay foot, 550
Spleen, rupture of, 531
Spondylosis, 587–590, 588, 588(t), 589, 590
    cervical, 1064
Sponge kidney, 773
Sporotrichosis, 1113–1116, 1116
Sprain, ankle, 554–555
    cervical, 584–587, 585(t), 586, 587
    elbow, 603
    finger, 610–611, 612
    foot, 544–555
    lumbosacral, 579–580, 579(t), 580
    shoulder, 598–599
    thumb, 611, 612
    wrist, 605–606
Sprung back, 581
Squamous cell carcinoma, 519
    of ear, 644
    of lung, 914, 915(t)
    of nose, 657
    of oral cavity, 664–665
    of skin, 1130–1132, 1131, 1132
Squamous papillomas, excision of, 520
Station, examination of, in neurologic examina-
    tion, 1016–1017
Status asthmaticus, 893–894, 894(t), 1145. See also
        Bronchial asthma.
    management of, 1148–1149, 1149(t)
Status epilepticus, 1029. See also Epilepsy.
Steal syndromes, ocular manifestations of, 730
Steatorrhea, 946, 947(t)
Stenosis, anal, congenital, 828
        postoperative, 814
    aortic, 866–867
    esophageal, congenital, 683
    lacrimal, 706
    mitral, chest pain in, 1003(t), 1004
    nasopharyngeal, 666
    pulmonic, 867
        in tetralogy of Fallot, 869
    subglottic, iatrogenic, 684
    tracheal, 683
        iatrogenic, 684
    ureterovesical, 768
    urethral, 769, 781
Stereogenesis, 1018

Sterility. See *Infertility*.
Sterilization, 451(t), 460–463, *461*
Steroids, and cataract, 713
  and increased intraocular tension, 710
  contraceptive. See *Oral contraceptives*.
  for rheumatoid arthritis, 626–627
Stiff neck, 584–587, 585(t)
Stiff shoulder, 591–595, *592, 593, 594*
Still's murmur, 1001, 1002(t)
Stokes-Adams attack, 1026(t)
Stomach, carcinoma of, 966
    diseases predisposing to, 965(t)
Strabismus, 701–703, *701, 702, 703*
  test for, 696
Stress, reaction to, and social group, 51
Stridor, defined, 883
  neonatal, 671
Stroke, predisposing factors in, 1041–1042, 1041(t)
  rehabilitation after, 212–214, 213(t)
Stye, 704, *704*
Subarachnoid hemorrhage, 1043–1044
  headache from, 1023(t)
Subclavian vein, cannulation of, *523*
Subconjunctival hemorrhage, 707
  in systemic disease, 727–728
Subdural hematoma, acute, 1046
  chronic, 1046–1047
Subglottic stenosis, iatrogenic, 684
Sucking reflex, 1018
Suicide, and depression, 309–310
Supraventricular tachycardia, sustained, 1008–1009
Surgery, 481–539
  anorectal. See *Anorectal surgery*.
  for patients with nipple discharge, 513(t)
  in family practice, 481
    minor office procedures for, 517–521
  patient assessment for, 481–482, 482(t)
  patient preparation for, 482–486
  preoperative tests for , 482(t)
  risk assessment for, 481–482, 482(t)
Swallowing, difficulty in. See *Dysphagia*.
Sweat test, for cystic fibrosis, 940
Swimmer's ear, 638
Symbiotic psychosis, 321
Sympathomimetic amines, for asthma, 895–896
Syncope, causes of, 1026(t)
  micturition, 1026(t)
  tussive, 1026(t)
Sydenham's chorea, 1049–1052, 1051(t)
Synovianalysis, 621–622, *622*, 622(t), *623, 624, 625*
Synovitis, transient, of hip, 571–572
  villous, of knee, *565*
Syphilis, anorectal, 827–828
  congenital, 836
  laryngeal, 673
  primary, in female, 740–741
  skin lesions in, *1127*, 1128–1129, *1128*
Syringomyelia, 1061(t), 1063
System, defined, 22
  closed, 22
  closed-loop, 22
  open, 22–25
  open-looped, 23
System theory, in family practice, 21–30
Systemic lupus erythematosus, *1115*, 1124–1125, *1125*
  vs. rheumatic fever, 873(t)

Tachycardia, paroxysmal, 1008
  sinus, 1008
  sustained supraventricular, 1008–1009
  sustained ventricular, 1009
Tachypnea, defined, 883
Tactile localization test, 1018
Tapeworm, 852, 852(t)
Tardive dyskinesia, from phenothiazine, 1053–1054
  from tranquilizers, 326
Teenagers. See *Adolescents*.
Teeth, care of, in pregnancy, 758
Temporal arteritis, headache from, 1023(t)
  ocular manifestations of, 726
Temporal lobe epilepsy, 1027–1029, 1028(t)
  anxiety in, 289
Temporal lobe function, examination of, 1015
Tendon(s), biceps, strain of, 602
  extensor, of finger, injury of, 617–618, *617, 618*
  of forearm, injuries of, 604
  of lower extremity, inflammation of, 546–547
  triceps, strain of, 602
Tenosynovitis, of lower extremity, 546–547
  stenosing, 604–605, *605*
Tension headache, 1022(t)
Teratogen, oral contraceptives as, 458
Teratomas, nasopharyngeal, 666
Terminal illness. See *Illness, terminal*.
Test(s). See also names of specific tests.
  diagnostic, choice of, 141–143
  routines of, 143–144
  screening, sensitivity of, 124, 124(t)
    specificity of, 124
Testis(es), anomalies of, 774
  carcinoma of, 782
  disorders of, 782
  ectopic, 774
  examination of, 780
  infections of, 782
    in mumps, 846
  injuries of, 780
  retractile, 774
  torsion of, 782
  tumors of, 782
  undescended, 774
Tetanus, immunization for, 839(t)
  prevention of, 839(t), 532–534
  vs. grand mal epilepsy, 1025
Tetralogy of Fallot, 869
Thalassemia, in children, 881
Thallium poisoning, 1036(t)
Thermal burns, 536–538
  rule of nines for, 537(t)
Thiamine deficiency, in alcoholics, 1035
Thigh, injuries of, 566
  mass in, 566–567
Thioridazine, dose, use, and side effects of, 385(t)–386(t)
Thiothixene, dose, use, and side effects of, 387(t)
Thioxanthenes, dose, use, and side effects of, 387(t)
Thomas heels, for flat feet, 546
Thomsen's disease, 1072(t)
Thoracostomy, tube, *527, 528*
Thromboembolism, and oral contraceptives, 456
  of middle cerebral artery, 1042
  postoperative, in cardiac patients, 486
  pulmonary, 901–903

Thrombosis, arterial, 505–506
    deep venous, 509–511
        and postphlebitic syndrome, 511
Thumb, base of, fracture of, 618–619
        pain in, 607–608
    dislocation of, 611–614, *612*, *613*
    osteoarthritis of, 607–608
    sprain of, 611, *612*
    subluxation of, 611
Thyroglossal duct cyst, 678
Thyroid disease, anxiety in, 288
    ocular manifestations of, 725–726, *725*
Tibial prominence, osteochondritis of, 562, *562*
Tic douloureux, 1058–1059
Tick paralysis, 1074
Tinea, of hands, 1113
    of nails, 1112
Tinea barbae, 1113, *1113*
Tinea capitis, 1112–1113, *1112*
Tinea corporis, 1113
Tinea cruris, 1112, *1112*, *1114*
Tinea pedis, 1111–1112, *1111*
Tinea versicolor, 1109–1110, *1110*
Tinnitus, 634
Toe, pain in, 552–553
Toenail, ingrown, 553–554
Tongue, absence of, 660
    black hairy, 665
    carcinoma of, 664
    cleft, 660
    congenital disorders of, 660
    embryology of, *658*
    enlargement of, 660
    geographic, 660
    lacerations of, 661
    sensory innervation of, *659*
Tongue-tie, 660
Tonometry, 696–697, *697*
Tonsil(s), abscess of, 662–663
    foreign bodies in, 664
    lacerations of, 661
Tonsillectomy, velopharyngeal insufficiency after, 663
Tonsillitis, acute, 662
Tornwaldt's bursa, 666
Torticollis, 679
    spasmodic, 1052
Torulosis, 938
Torus palatinus, 661
Toxemia of pregnancy, 763–764
Toxic megacolon, 816
    in ulcerative colitis, 948
Toxoplasmosis, 1034
    neonatal infection with, 836
Trachea, anatomy of, 682
    disorders of, 681–685
        congenital, 683–684
        infectious, 684–685
    embryology of, 682
    examination of, 682–683
    fistula of, 683
    foreign bodies in, 684–685
    stenosis of, 683
        iatrogenic, disorders of, 684
Tracheobronchial tree, neoplasms of, 685
Tracheoesophageal fistula, 683
Tracheomalacia, 683
Tracheostomy, and subglottic stenosis, 673
    emergency, 524–525, *525*

Tranquilizers. See *Drugs, tranquilizing.*
Transactional analysis, 395–397, *396*, *397*
Transitional cell carcinoma, of bladder, 784–785
Transplacental hemorrhage, Rh immune
    prophylaxis for, 760
Transsexualism, 370(t). See also *Sexual variations
    and deviations.*
Transvestism, 370(t). See also *Sexual variations
    and deviations.*
Tranylcypromine, dose, use, and side effects of,
    386(t)–387(t)
Trauma, management of, 521–538
Triceps, strain of, 602
Trichomonas vaginalis vaginitis, 738
Trick knee, 557–558
    in children, 563
Tricuspid atresia, 869
Trifluoperazine, dose, use, and side effects of,
    385(t)–386(t)
Triflupromazine, dose, use, and side effects of,
    385(t)–386(t)
Trigeminal neuralgia, 1058–1059
Trigger finger, 621, *621*
Trochlear nerve, paralysis of, 726, 1057(t), *1058*
Tropias, 701–703
    test for, 696
Truncus arteriosus, 869–870
Tubal ligation, for sterilization, 461–462, *461*
Tube thoracostomy, 527, *528*
Tuberculin skin test, 918–919
    schedule for, 839(t)
Tuberculosis, disseminated, 918
    in children, 849–851
    laryngeal, 673
    meningitis in, 1034
    miliary, 918
    progressive primary, 918
    pulmonary, 917–922
        clinical reactivation, 919, *920*
        diagnosis of, 919–920
        incidence of, 917–918
        pathogenesis of, 918
        treatment of, 920–922
    reactivation, 919, *920*
    tuberculin skin test for, 918–919, 839(t)
Tuberculous meningitis, 1034
Tumors. See names of specific tumors and body
    parts affected.
Tuning fork tests, for hearing, 633–634, *634*
Tussive syncope, 1026(t)
Twins, pregnancy with, 762–763
Two point discrimination test, 1018
Tympanic membrane, anatomy of, 629–630, *630*

Ulcer(s), contact, of vocal cords, 674
    corneal, 708, *708*
    duodenal, chronic, 956–957, 956(t)
    gastric, chronic, 958–959. See also *Peptic ulcer.*
    of nipple, and Paget's disease, 513(t), 514
    peptic. See *Peptic ulcer.*
Ulcerative colitis, 815–816, 947–949, 948(t)
Ulcerative proctitis, 948(t), 949
Ulnar nerve, contusions of, 601–602
Umbilical hernia, in adult, 503
    in chidren, 501
Unconjugated hyperbilirubinemia, 970–971,
    970(t)

Upper airway obstruction. See *Airway obstruction.*
Upper respiratory infections, 885–887
  causative viruses of, 885(t)
Uremic neuropathy, 1068
Ureter, anomalies of, 773
  dilated, 769
  duplication of, 773
  ectopic, 769
  injuries of, 779
  tumors of, 784
Ureteral calculi, 770–772, 772(t)
Ureteral orifice, anomalies of, 773
Ureteropelvic strictures, 768
Ureterovescial stenosis, 768
Urethra, carcinoma of, 781–782, 786
  caruncle of, 782
  disorders of, 781–782
  examination of, 780
  infection of 781
  injuries of, 779
  prolapse of, 782
  stenosis of, 769, 781
  stricture of, 781
  tumors of, 781–782, 786
Urethral catheterization, complications of, 777
  in urinary tract infections, 776–777
Urethral diverticulosis, 782
Urethral sphincter, neurogenic dysfunction of, 769–770
Urethral valves, posterior, 769
Urethritis, vs. vaginitis, 738–739
Urethrocele, 754
Urethrogram, 779–780
Uric acid, effect of alcohol on, 333
Uricosuria, urinary calculi in, 770
Urinalysis, 767
Urinary bladder, agenesis of, 773
  anomalies of, 773–774
  atonic, 770
  carcinoma of, 784–786
  duplication of, 773
  exstrophy of, 773
  flaccid, 770
  function of, neurologic disturbance of, 211, 769–770, 1075
  hypertonic, 770
  infection of, after spinal cord injury, 211
  injuries of, 778
  neck of, contracture of, 768–769
  neurogenic, 211, 769–770
  sensory paralytic, 770
  training of, after spinal cord injury, 211
  tumors of, 784–786
Urinary calculi, 770–772, 772(t)
Urinary frequency, 766
Urinary incontinence, 767
Urinary reflux, 769
Urinary tract, infections, 774–778
  antimicrobial treatment for, 776
  clinical manifestations of, 775
  contributing factors in, 774–775
  defined, 774
  diagnosis of, 775–776
  epidemiology of, 776
  in children, 847, 847(t)
    screening for, 126(t), 127
  incidence of, 776
  pathogenesis of, 774–775

Urinary tract *(Continued)*
  persistent, treatment of, 776
  recurrent, treatment of, 776
  treatment of, 776–778
  urethral catheterization in, 776–777
  urologic survey in, 776
Urinary tract injuries, 778–780
Urinary transport system, 766–770
  diagnosis of, 767–768
    obstructive, 768–769
    symptoms of, 766–767
  evaluation of, 767–768
Urinary urgency, 767
Urine, collection and voiding of, normal, 766
  examination of, in urinary tract infections, 775–776
Urography, 767–768
Urolithiasis, 770–772
Urology, 766–785
Urticaria, 1119–1120, 1139–1140
  giant, 1139
  vs. angioedema, 1140(t)
Usual interstitial pneumonia, defined, 884
Uterus, bleeding from, dysfunctional, 744
  examination of, 732
  prolapse of, 754–755
  tumors of, 746–750
Uveitis, 714–715, *714*
  anterior, differential diagnosis of, 715(t)
  peripheral, 715
Uvula, cleft, 661

Vaccination. See *Immunization.*
VACTERL syndrome, and oral contraceptives, 455(t), 458
Vagina, adenosis of, 753
  bleeding from, abnormal, 741–745
    during pregnancy, 744
    excessive, and leiomyomas, 747
    postcoital, 743
    postmenopausal, 744
      and endometrial adenocarcinoma, 748
  carcinoma of, 753
  cysts of, 753
  discharge, from excessive, 737
  examination of, 732
  tumors of, 753
Vaginismus, 448
Vaginitis, 737–739
  diagnosis of, 738–739
  Hemophilus vaginalis, 738
  monilial, 737–738
    and oral contraceptives, 459
  Trichomonas vaginalis, 738
Vaginitis emphysematosa, 753
Vagus nerve, disorders of, 1057(t)
Varicella, 844–845
Varices, esophageal, bleeding from, diagnosis of, 497–498
    treatment of, 498–499
  in portal hypertension, 974–975
Varicocele, 774, 782
  retinal, 715–719, *718*
Vascular disease, intracranial, ocular manifestations of, 726
Vascular injuries, in dislocations, 504
  in fractures, 504
Vascular neuropathies, 1068

Vascular rings, 684
Vasectomy, 462–463
Vasomotor rhinitis, 656
Veins, pulmonary, transposition of, 868–869
Velopharyngeal insufficiency, 663
Venereal disease, anorectal, 827–828
   in female, 739–741
Venereal warts, 828
Venous shunt, defined, 883
Venous thrombosis, deep, 509–511
   and postphlebitic syndrome, 511
Ventilation, emergency, 524–525, *524, 525*
Ventricular premature beats, 1009
Ventricular septal defect, 868
   in tetralogy of Fallot, 869
Ventricular tachycardia, sustained, 1009
Vernal conjunctivitis, 707
Vertebral-basilar insufficiency, 1026(t), 1041,
   1041(t)
Vertigo, causes of, 1030, 1031(t)
   in vestibular neuronitis, 643
   positional, 643, 1031(t)
Vesicoureteral reflux, 769
Vestibular neuronitis, 643
Vestibulitis, 652
Villous synovitis, of knee, *565*
Vincent's angina, 661
Viral hepatitis. See *Hepatitis, viral.*
Viruses, causing upper respiratory infections,
   885(t)
Vision, disorders of, 699–700
   loss of, as disease symptom, 690–691
   painful, 691
   refractive errors of, 699–700
      headache from, 1022(t)
   testing of, 692
Visual field, changes in, 723–725, *724*
   examination of, 697–698
Visual field defect, 691
Visual phenomena, as symptom, 691
Vitamin B, recommended dietary allowances of,
   1068(t)
Vitamin B deficiency, and peripheral neuropathy,
   1068
   in alcoholics, 1035
Vitamin supplements, for infants, 1083, 1084(t)
   in pregnancy, 1078–1079
   in megavitamin therapy, 388(t)
Vitreous floaters, 691
Vocal cords, congenital paralysis of, 671
   contact ulcers of, 674
   nodules on, 674
   polyps of, 673–674

Vocalization, mechanics of, 669–670
Vocational rehabilitation, for schizophrenics, 328
Voyeurism, 370(t). See also *Sexual variations and
   deviations.*

Walkers, use of, 220
Wall eyes, 701–702, *701*
Wall test, for posture, 217–218, *217*
Warfarin, for deep venous thrombosis, 510
Wart(s), 1123–1124, *1123, 1124*
   excision of, 520–521
   plantar, 1123, *1123*
      excision of, 520–521
   venereal, 828
Weber test, for hearing, 633
Wegener's granulomatosis, 656–657
Weight gain, and oral contraceptives, 735–736
   in pregnancy, 757–758, 1079
Weight loss, diet for, 1098–1100, 1098(t), *1099*
Werdnig-Hoffmann disease, 878, 1063
Wernicke's encephalopathy, 1035
Wheelchairs, use of, 220
Whipworm, 852, 852(t)
Whooping cough, 845–846
   immunization for, 839(t)
Wilm's tumor, 784
Wilson's disease, 1030–1032
Wolff-Parkinson-White syndrome, 1008
Wound, burn, treatment of, 537
   debridement of, 532, *532*
   infection of, 534–536
      prevention of, 534–535
      treatment of, 535–536
   soft tissue, treatment of, 531–532
Wrist, aspiration of, *624*
   contusion of, 605
   disorders of, 605–607
   fracture of, 606
   ganglion of, 607, *607*
   pain in, 604–605
   Quervain's disease of, 604–605
   sprain of, 605–606
Wry neck, 679

X-linked dystrophy, benign, 1072(t)

Zollinger-Ellison syndrome, 957–958
   secretory diarrhea in, 950
Zygomatic arch, fracture of, 679–680, *679*, 682(t)